W9-AUT-299

Dr. Williamson,

to your continued success in practice for many years to come!

Thank you for your continued support of Ortho Tri-Cyclen Lo, Ortho Evra, + all of the Ortho product line. You da man!

Best Wishes + Thanks,

- Anthony Porter '06

Novak's Gynecology

Novak's

Gynecology

Thirteenth Edition

Editor

Jonathan S. Berek, MD, MMSc

Professor and Chair, College of Applied Anatomy
Executive Vice Chair, Department of Obstetrics and Gynecology
Chief, Division of Gynecologic Oncology
David Geffen School of Medicine at UCLA
Los Angeles, California

Editorial Assistant

Rebecca D. Rinehart

Assistant Editors

Paula J. Adams Hillard, MD

Professor, Departments of Pediatrics, and Obstetrics and Gynecology
Director of Women's Health
University of Cincinnati College of Medicine
Cincinnati, Ohio

Eli Y. Adashi, MD

Presidential Professor of Obstetrics and Gynecology
John A. Dixon Professor and Chair
University of Utah Health Sciences Center
Salt Lake City, Utah

Illustration and Graphic Design

Timothy C. Hengst, CMI, FAMI

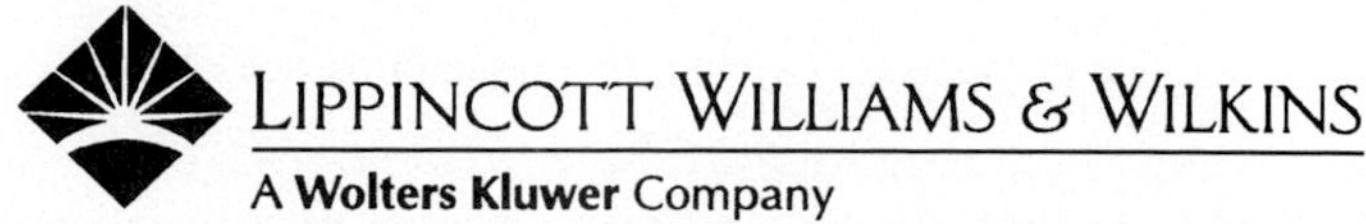

Philadelphia • Baltimore • New York • London
Buenos Aires • Hong Kong • Sydney • Tokyo

Acquisitions Editor: Lisa McAllister
Developmental Editor: Raymond Reter
Production Editor: Steven P. Martin
Manufacturing Manager: Benjamin Rivera
Cover Designer: Christine Jenny
Compositor: TechBooks
Printer: Quebecor-World/Dubuque

530 Walnut Street
Philadelphia, PA 19106 USA
LWW.com

Printed in the USA

Library of Congress Cataloging-in-Publication Data

Novak's gynecology.—13th ed. / editor, Jonathan S. Berek.
p. ; cm.
Includes bibliographical references and index.
ISBN 0-7817-3262-X
1. Gynecology. I. Title: Gynecology. II. Novak, Emil, 1883–1957.
III. Berek, Jonathan S.
[DNLM: 1.Genital Diseases, Female. 2. Gynecology—methods. 3. Pregnancy Complications. WP 100 N9351 2002]
RG101 .N69 2002
618.1—dc21 2002017858

Care has been taken to confirm the accuracy of the information presented and to describe generally accepted practices. However, the authors, editors, and publisher are not responsible for errors or omissions or for any consequences from application of the information in this book and make no warranty, expressed or implied, with respect to the currency, completeness, or accuracy of the contents of the publication. Application of this information in a particular situation remains the professional responsibility of the practitioner.

The authors, editors, and publisher have exerted every effort to ensure that drug selection and dosage set forth in this text are in accordance with current recommendations and practice at the time of publication. However, in view of ongoing research, changes in government regulations, and the constant flow of information relating to drug therapy and drug reactions, the reader is urged to check the package insert for each drug for any change in indications and dosage and for added warnings and precautions. This is particularly important when the recommended agent is a new or infrequently employed drug.

Some drugs and medical devices presented in this publication have Food and Drug Administration (FDA) clearance for limited use in restricted research settings. It is the responsibility of the health care provider to ascertain the FDA status of each drug or device planned for use in their clinical practice.

10 9 8 7 6 5 4 3 2 1

The publishers have made every effort to trace the copyright holders for borrowed material. If they have inadvertently overlooked any, they will be pleased to make the necessary arrangements at the first opportunity.

To my wife, Deborah, whose love, patience and understanding makes my work possible.

Foreword to the Twelfth Edition

In 1940, Emil Novak published the first edition of what has been known as "Novak's Textbook." Dr. Novak was a mentor and exemplar to so many of those of us who studied gynecology and gynecologic pathology. He clearly saw the importance of this study and this field of medicine, and he provided each of us who have followed in his footsteps with a wonderful example. To us, Emil Novak was the ultimate doctor, a man who saw the study of medicine as a way to provide aid to those who suffered illness. We are indebted to him for having begun this work, taught so many who have worked in this specialty, and provided the means by which his textbook could carry on his work.

It is a pleasure and a privilege to have been asked to pen this foreword, as it has been my pleasure and privilege to have worked on this textbook and to have as colleagues in this endeavor so many superb physicians. Dr. Novak would endorse and be thankful that the text is being updated for your use. He knew, as we do, that the pursuit of academic medicine is imperative to the development of medicine in general and our field in particular. In order to provide you with the same superb resource that Emil Novak began 55 years ago, Novak's ***Textbook of Gynecology*** must be updated, and a new generation of men and women must accept his challenge.

Medicine as a profession has changed and will continue to change, but the basic message that Emil Novak presented in the first textbook is the same: doctors must be concerned with the welfare of patients, and in order to accomplish this task, they must have access to the latest and best information and training. Jonathan Berek and his colleagues are well schooled in the legacy of Emil Novak and all of those who have worked on this book. It is with confidence in the quality of their work that I endorse this 12th edition of ***Novak's Gynecology.***

J. Donald Woodruff, MD
Richard W. TeLinde Professor Emeritus
Johns Hopkins University School of Medicine
Baltimore, Maryland

Dr. J. Donald Woodruff passed away in 1996. He was a particularly gifted teacher and clinician who helped guide the development of our specialty. I feel it is important to retain the thoughtful comments he contributed to our twelfth edition for this edition of ***Novak's Gynecology.***

Jonathan S. Berek

Preface to the Thirteenth Edition

Novak's Gynecology, 13th edition, has been thoroughly updated and revised to be certain that its contents and bibliography are current and accurate. Its essence is the same as the original—a comprehensive general textbook in gynecology. The substance reflects the wealth of information that has emerged and evolved during the 62 years since the inception of ***Novak's Textbook of Gynecology.*** It is an honor to have been asked to continue to shepherd this important book and I hope will retain its value to inform and assist our colleagues for many years.

The textbook, originated by the faculty of the Johns Hopkins University School of Medicine, continues to reflect the contributions of that great institution. The book was inaugurated by Dr. Emil Novak, a pioneer in gynecology and pathology. After the fifth edition and subsequent death of Dr. Novak in 1957, many physicians on the faculty of Johns Hopkins, and subsequently some members of the Vanderbilt faculty, have helped carry the torch—Dr. Edmund R. Novak through the ninth edition in 1979; Drs. Howard W. Jones, Jr. and Georgeanna Seegar Jones through the tenth edition in 1981; and Drs. Howard W. Jones, III, Lonnie S. Burnett, and Anne Colston Wentz through the 11th edition in 1988. These editors, assisted by many contributors who have been faculty at Johns Hopkins, especially Drs. J. Donald Woodruff and Conrad G. Julian, have helped define the specialty of gynecology over the latter half of the 20th century. These physicians and authors are responsible for the ideas that shaped the specialty of gynecology as we know it today—its surgical and medical therapies, reproductive endocrinology, assisted reproductive technologies, gynecologic oncology, urogynecology, and infectious diseases. As a graduate of Johns Hopkins University School of Medicine, I am proud to contribute to that rich tradition.

Starting with the twelfth edition, this textbook utilized a new format. The design of the book was established by Dr. Leon Speroff and his colleagues in the textbook ***Clinical Gynecologic Endocrinology and Infertility*** and was adapted for the book ***Practical Gynecologic Oncology.*** This presentation style should facilitate the study of gynecology for the student as well as the specialist.

Novak's Gynecology, 13th edition, is presented in six sections. The first, "Principles of Practice," includes the initial assessment of the gynecologic patient, the history and physical examination, and communication skills. This section addresses ethical principles of patient care, quality assessment and improvement, and the epidemiology of gynecologic conditions. The second section, "Basic Sciences," summarizes the scientific basis for the specialty—anatomy and embryology, molecular biology and genetics, and reproductive physiology. The third section, "Preventive and Primary Care," reflects the importance of primary health care for women, which has evolved to address preventive care, screening, family planning, sexuality, and common psychiatric problems. The fourth section, "General Gynecology," reviews benign diseases of the female reproductive tract, the evaluation of pelvic infections, pain, intraepithelial diseases, the management of early pregnancy loss and ectopic pregnancy, the evaluation of benign breast disease, and the operative management of benign gynecologic conditions. The fifth section, "Reproductive Endocrinology," summarizes the major disorders affecting the growth, development, and function of women from puberty through menopause. The sixth section, "Gynecologic Oncology," covers malignant diseases of the female reproductive tract and breast cancer.

I have purposely abbreviated the discussion of the historical development of the subjects in each chapter. Space limitations have required a shift in emphasis from the achievements of the past to the relevant issues of the present.

I am especially grateful to the many individuals who contributed to this book. Rebecca Rinehart provided superb editorial assistance, manuscript review, and revision. Drs. Paula Hillard and Eli Adashi served as excellent Assistant Editors. Tim Hengst, an outstanding medical illustrator, designed and created the original artwork. At the publishers, Lippincott Williams & Wilkins, Ms. Lisa McAllister supported the editorial process with great enthusiasm. Working with her, Ray Reter, Steven Martin and the rest of their team skillfully produced the manuscript. Expert secretarial support was provided by Kevin Wong and Sergio Huidor.

I acknowledge the efforts of my mentors and colleagues—Dean Sherman Mellinkoff, Drs. J. Donald Woodruff, Kenneth J. Ryan, Isaac Schiff, J. George Moore, William J. Dignam, Gautum Chaudhuri, and Neville F. Hacker. Each of these physicians and scholars provided me with guidance, wisdom, and encouragement during the years we shared at our respective university medical schools.

My thanks to Nicole Kidman, the chair of the advisory board for the UCLA Women's Reproductive Cancer Program—whose support and friendship has helped stimulate this project.

I hope that this book will be a useful resource for my colleagues and for students of the specialty of gynecology. I look forward to the continued impact of the specialty on the enhancement of health care for women throughout the world.

Jonathan S. Berek

Preface to the First Edition

Since the plan and scope of this book represent something of a departure from those followed in other textbooks of gynecology, the author feels impelled to state the ideas which furnished the incentive for the preparation of this work, and which dictated its character and scope.

First of all, no especial apology seems necessary for the combined title. While gynecology was formerly often spoken of as a branch of surgery, this is certainly not its present status. Only a small proportion of gynecological patients require surgical treatment. On the other hand, the biological aspects of gynecology have assumed vast importance, chiefly because of the amazing developments in the field of reproductive physiology and endocrinology. Many of these advances find daily application in the interpretation and management of functional disorders in women. In other words, female endocrinology is now an integral and important part of gynecology and it is so considered in this book.

Second, it has always seemed to me that the great majority of readers of textbooks on gynecology must be not at all interested in the details of operative technique, to the consideration of which most authors have devoted many pages. Certainly this applies to the general practitioner, while medical educators are now generally agreed that the medical student should not be burdened with such details in his undergraduate years. Since this book is designed for these two groups primarily, the indication seemed clear to omit the consideration of operative details. The plan followed is to carry the patient up to the point of operation, and to discuss the indications, scope and purpose of the latter, without going into descriptions of the technique itself.

Diagnosis and treatment have been accented throughout the book, as I believe most readers would wish. The traditional chapters on anatomy, history-taking, and methods of examination have been boiled down to the essentials. On the other hand, functional disorders, including especially the large group of gynecological endocrinopathies, have been treated rather elaborately, in keeping with the avowed plan of covering the combined fields of gynecology and female endocrinology. The list of references appended to each chapter makes no pretense of exhaustiveness, and preference has been given to publications most worth while, those most recent, and those written in English. The pathological aspects of gynecological disease, so fundamental to a proper understanding of the whole subject, have received adequate but not disproportionate consideration.

In the consideration of various endocrine disorders a disturbing problem presented itself. In the discussion of endocrine preparations which might be indicated in treatment, there is no doubt that the mention of various products by their commercial names would have had some advantages. On the other hand, these have appeared to be definitely outweighed by the disadvantages of such a plan, apart from its questionable delicacy. These proprietary preparations are constantly multiplying, and their commercial names are being changed from day to day. For example, there are now well over forty estrogenic preparations on the market. It would be almost impossible, in any enumeration of such therapeutic products, to avoid omission of some of them, and this might be very unfair to products perhaps just as effective as those which might be included. A complete list published today is quite likely to be very incomplete within a few months.

The sensible plan seemed to be to rely on the intelligence and initiative of the reader, who should have no difficulty in ascertaining good commercial preparations of estrogen, progesterone, chorionic hormone or any other hormone principle to which reference is made in the treatment of various disorders.

It will be noted that the work is devoted to "straight" gynecology and male endocrinology and that it does not include a consideration of disorders in allied fields which concededly obtrude themselves frequently into the practice of the gynecologist. For example, many gynecologists include female urology in their practices, while anorectal and abdominal surgical problems are often encountered, as may be problems in almost any field of medicine. For textbook purposes, however, the line must be drawn fairly sharply, and the reader will naturally expect to go to the proper sources for information in any of these allied fields.

In short, the purpose of this book is to present to the reader as much information as is possible in as practical a fashion as possible on the subjects of gynecology and female endocrinology. Whether right or wrong, the ideas behind the book represent the crystallization of many years of teaching and practice in gynecology. The author's goal has been to produce a book which would not only be suited to the needs of the medical student, but which could be carried with him into the practice of his profession.

It is a pleasant obligation to express my indebtedness to those who have been helpful to me in the preparation of this book. To a number of my friends, especially Dr. R.B. Greenblatt, of Augusta, Georgia, I am grateful for the loan of illustrations; to Dr. E.L. Krieg, for the excellent colored illustrations as well as for other photographic work; to Mr. Chester Reather, for most of the photomicrographs; to Miss Eva Hildebrandt, technician in the Laboratory of Gynecological Pathology at The Johns Hopkins Hospital and to Sister Mary Lucy, technician at Bon Secours Hospital for help in the preparation of sections for microscopic illustration; to my artist, Miss Frances Shultz, for many of the illustrations; and to my faithful secretary, Miss Helen L. Clayton, for much help throughout the project. For permission to use illustrations which have appeared in previously published articles of my own I am indebted to the publishers of the Journal of the American Medical Association; the American Journal of Obstetrics and Gynecology; Surgery, Gynecology and Obstetrics; and the Bulletin of The Johns Hopkins Hospital.

Certain illustrations which appeared in one of my previous books, Gynecological and Obstetrical Pathology, do not have a credit line in the caption. For permission to use these I wish to thank WB Saunders Company, the publishers.

Finally, it is a genuine pleasure to acknowledge the efficient and wholehearted cooperation of the publishers, Little, Brown and Co., throughout the preparation of this work.

Emil Novak
Baltimore

Contributors

Eli Y. Adashi, MD

Presidential Professor of Obstetrics and Gynecology
John A. Dixon Professor and Chair
Departments of Obstetrics and Gynecology
University of Utah Health Sciences Center
Salt Lake City, Utah

Angeles A. Alvarez, MD

Associate Professor
Department of Obstetrics and Gynecology
Duke University Medical Center
Durham, North Carolina

Lawrence S. Amesse, MD, PhD

Assistant Professor
Department of Obstetrics and Gynecology
Wright State University
Associate Program Director
Department of Obstetrics and Gynecology
Miami Valley Hospital
Dayton, Ohio

Jean R. Anderson, MD

Associate Professor
Department of Gynecology and Obstetrics
Johns Hopkins University School of Medicine
Baltimore, Maryland

Vicki V. Baker, MD

Professor
Wayne State University
Division of Gynecologic Oncology
Harper Hospital
Detroit, Michigan

David A. Baram, MD

Clinical Assistant Professor
Department of Obstetrics and Gynecology
University of Minnesota School of Medicine
Minneapolis, Minnesota
Attending Physician Regions Hospital
St. Paul, Minnesota

Jonathan S. Berek, MD, MMSc

Professor and Chair, College of Applied Anatomy
Executive Vice Chair, Department of Obstetrics and Gynecology
Chief, Division of Gynecologic Oncology
David Geffen School of Medicine at UCLA
Los Angeles, California

Ross S. Berkowitz, MD
William H. Baker Professor of Gynecology
Harvard Medical School
Director of Gynecologic and Gynecologic Oncology
Brigham and Women's Hospital
Dana Farber Cancer Institute
Boston, Massachusetts

Andrew I. Brill, MD
Professor
Obstetrics and Gyncology
University of Illionios at Chicago
Chief of General Obstetrics and Gynecology
Department of Obstetrics and Gynecology
University of Illinois
Chicago, Illinois

Joanna M. Cain, MD
University Professor and Chair
Department of Obstetrics and Gynecology
Oregon Health and Science University
Portland, Oregon

Daniel L. Clarke-Pearson, MD
James M. Ingram Professor and Director
Division of Gynecologic Oncology
Department of Obstetrics and Gynecology
Duke University Medical Center
Durham, North Carolina

Daniel W. Cramer, MD, ScD
Professor of Obstetrics, Gynecology and Reproductive Biology
Department of Obstetrics and Gynecology
Harvard Medical School
Gynecologist, Department of Obstetrics and Gynecology
Brigham and Women's Hospital
Boston, Massachusetts

Dayton W. Daberkow II
Associate Professor of Medicine
Internal Medicine Residency Program
Director, Louisiana State University Health Science Center
New Orleans, Louisiana

Thomas M. D'Hooghe, MD, PhD
Assistant Professor
Department of Obstetrics, Gynecology, and Reproductive Biology
Harvard Medical School
Brigham and Women's Hospital
Boston, Massachusetts

John Christopher Elkas, MD

Assistant Professor, Department of Obstetrics and Gynecology
Uniformed Services University of the Health Services
Bethesda, Maryland
Attending Physician, Department of Obstetrics and Gynecology
Walter Reed Army Medical Center
Washington, DC

Joseph C. Gambone, DO, MPH

Associate Professor
Department of Obstetrics and Gynecology
David Geffen School of Medicine at UCLA
Los Angeles, California

Rene Genadry, MD

Associate Professor
Department of Gynecology and Obstetrics
The Johns Hopkins Medical Institutions
Baltimore, Maryland

Armando E. Giuliano, MD

Chief of Surgical Oncology
John Wayne Cancer Institute
Santa Monica, California
Clinical Professor of Surgery
David Geffen School of Medicine at UCLA
Director, Joyce Eisenberg Keefer Breast Center
Saint John's Hospital and Health Center
Santa Monica, California

Paul A. Gluck, MD

Associate Clinical Professor
Department of Obstetrics and Gynecology
University of Miami School of Medicine
Attending Physician, Department of Obstetrics and Gynecology
Baptist Hospital of Miami
Miami, Florida

Donald P. Goldstein, MD

Associate Professor
Department of Obstetrics, Gynecology, and Reproductive Biology
Harvard Medical School
Department of Obstetrics and Gynecology
Brigham and Women's Hospital
Boston, Massachusetts

Baiba J. Grube, MD

Assistant Director
Joyce Eisenberg Keefer Breast Cancer
John Wayne Cancer Institute
Saint John's Health Center
Santa Monica, California

Kenneth D. Hatch, MD

Professor and Head
Department of Obstetrics and Gynecology
University Medical Center
Tucson, Arizona

Laura J. Havrilesky, MD

Fellow, Department of Obstetrics, Gynecology, and Gynecologic Oncology
Duke University Medical Center
Durham, North Carolina

Avner Hershlag, MD

Associate Professor of Obstetrics and Gynecology
Department of Obstetrics and Gynecology
New York University School of Medicine
New York, New York
Medical Director, Department of Obstetrics and Gynecology
North Shore University Hospital
Manhasset, New York

Joseph A. Hill, MD

Reproductive Endocrinologist
Fertility Center of New England
Reading, Massachusetts

Paula J. Adams Hillard, MD

Professor, Departments of Pediatrics, and Obstetrics and Gynecology
Director of Women's Health
University of Cincinnati College of Medicine
Cincinnati, Ohio

Christine H. Holschneider, MD

Assistant Professor
Department of Obstetrics and Gynecology
David Geffen School of Medicine at UCLA
Los Angeles, California

William W. Hurd, MD

Nicolas J. Thompson Professor and Chairman
Department of Obstetrics and Gynecology
Wright State University School of Medicine
Dayton, Ohio

Julie A. Jolin, MD

Resident, Johns Hopkins Hospital
Department of Obstetrics and Gynecology
Baltimore, Maryland

Thomas C. Krivak, MD

Fellow, Gynecologic Oncology
Walter Reed Army Medical Center
Washington, DC

Johnathan Lancaster, MD

Associate, Department of Obstetrics and Gynecology
Division of Gynecologic Oncology
Duke University Medical Center

John R. Lurain, MD

John and Ruth Brewer Professor of Gynecology and Cancer Research
Head, Section of Gynecologic Oncology
Northwestern University Medical School
Chief, Gynecologic Oncology
Department of Obstetrics and Gynecology
Northwestern Memorial Hospital/Prentice Women's Hospital
Chicago, Illinois

Otoniel Martínez-Maza, PhD

Associate Professor
Departments of Obstetrics and Gynecology, and Microbiology, Immunology, and Molecular Genetics
David Geffen School of Medicine at UCLA
Los Angeles, California

John W. McBroom, MD

Fellow, Gynecologic Oncology
Walter Reed Army Medical Center
Washington, DC

Howard D. McClamrock, MD

Associate Professor and Director
Department of Obstetrics, Gynecology, and Reproductive Sciences
Division of Reproductive Endocrinology and Infertility
University of Maryland School of Medicine
Baltimore, Maryland

Shawn A. Menefee, MD

Assistant Clinical Professor
Department of Reproductive Medicine
University of California, San Diego
Co-director, Section of Female Pelvic Floor Medicine and Reconstructive Surgery
Department of Obstetrics and Gynecology
Kaiser Permanente
San Diego, California

Malcolm Gordon Munro, MD

Professor of Clinical Obstetrics and Gynecology
Department of Obstetrics and Gynecology
David Geffen School of Medicine at UCLA
Los Angeles, California

Thomas E. Nolan, MD, MBA

Professor
Departments of Obstetrics, Gynecology, and Medicine
Louisiana State University
Hospital Center Director
Department of Women's and Newborn Services
Medical Center of Louisiana
New Orleans, Louisiana

Dean T. Nora, MD

Senior Surgical Oncology Fellow
John Wayne Cancer Institute
Santa Monica, California

David L. Olive, MD

Professor, Department of Obstetrics and Gynecology
Director, Department of Reproductive Endocrinology and Infertility
University of Wisconsin—Madison School of Medicine
Madison, Wisconsin

Steven F. Palter, MD

Medical and Scientific Director
Reproductive Medicine and Surgery Center
Plainview, New York
Clinical Assistant Professor
Division of Reproductive Endocrinology and Infertility
Yale University School of Medicine
New Haven, Connecticut

C. Matthew Peterson, MD

Associate Professor
Division of Reproductive Endocrinology
Department of Obstetrics and Gynecology
University of Utah Medical Center
Director of Reproductive Endocrinology
LDS Hospital
Salt Lake City, Utah

John F. Randolph, Jr., MD

Associate Professor
Department of Obstetrics and Gynecology
University of Michigan
Ann Arbor, Michigan

Andrea Rapkin, MD

Professor
Department of Obstetrics and Gynecology
David Geffen School of Medicine at UCLA
Los Angeles, California

Robert W. Rebar, MD

Associate Executive Director
American Society for Reproductive Medicine
Birmingham, Alabama

Robert C. Reiter, MD

Vice President for Quality Management
ProMedica Health Systems
Toledo Hospital
Toledo, Ohio

Wendy J. Schillings, MD

Clinical Associate Professor of Obstetrics and Gynecology
Pennsylvania State College of Medicine
Lehigh Valley Hospital
Allentown, Pennsylvania

Daniel J. Schust, MD

Clinical Fellow
Department of Obstetrics, Gynecology, and Reproductive Biology
Harvard Medical School
Brigham and Women's Hospital
Boston, Massachusetts

David E. Soper, MD

Professor and Vice Chairman
Departments of Obstetrics and Gynecology
Medical University of South Carolina
Charleston, South Carolina

Nada L. Stotland, MD, MPH

Professor
Department of Psychiatry and Obstetrics and Gynecology
Rush Medical College
Chicago, Illinois

Thomas G. Stovall, MD

Professor
Department of Obstetrics and Gynecology
University of Tennessee, Memphis
Memphis, Tennessee

Phillip G. Stubblefield, MD

Professor
Department of Obstetrics and Gynecology
Boston University School of Medicine
Boston Medical Center
Boston, Massachusetts

L. Lewis Wall, MD, DPhil

Associate Professor
Section of Female Pelvic Medicine and Reconstructive Surgery
Department of Obstetrics and Gynecology
Washington University School of Medicine
St. Louis, Missouri

Mylene W. M. Yao, MD

Assistant Professor
Department of Obstetrics and Gynecology
Columbia University College of Physicians and Surgeons
New York, New York

Contents

SECTION

I

PRINCIPLES OF PRACTICE

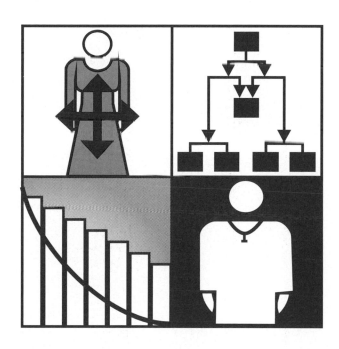

1 Initial Assessment and Communication

Jonathan S. Berek
Paula J. Adams Hillard

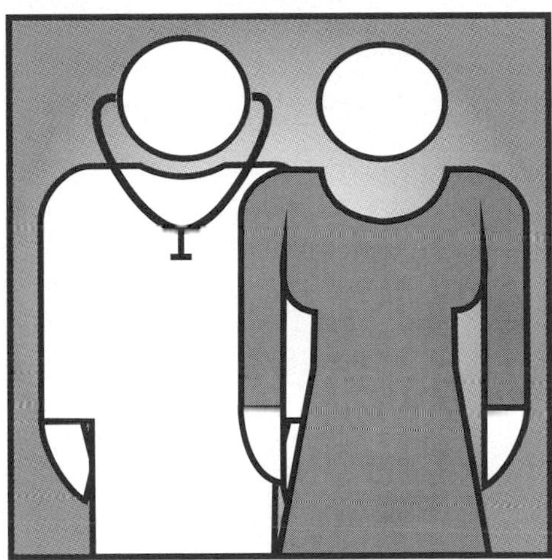

The practice of gynecology requires many skills. In addition to medical knowledge, the gynecologist should develop interpersonal and communication skills that promote patient–physician interaction and trust. The assessment must be of the "whole patient," not only of her general medical status. It should include any apparent medical condition as well as the psychological, social, and family aspects of her situation. Environmental and cultural issues that affect the patient must be taken into account to view her in the appropriate context. This approach is of value in routine assessments, providing opportunities for preventive care and counseling on a continuing basis, as well as in the assessment of medical conditions.

Communication

Good communication is essential to patient assessment and treatment. The patient–physician relationship is based on communication conducted in an open, honest, and careful manner so that the patient's situation and problems can be accurately understood and effective solutions determined. Good communication requires patience, dedication, and practice.

The foundation of communication is based on key skills: empathy, attentive listening, expert knowledge, and rapport. These skills can be learned and refined (1). After establishing the initial relationship with the patient, the physician must vigilantly pursue interviewing techniques that create opportunities to foster an understanding of the patient's concerns (2). Trust is the fundamental element that encourages the patient to communicate her feelings, concerns, and thoughts openly, without withholding information.

Although there are many styles of interacting with patients and each physician must determine the best way that he or she can relate to patients, physicians must convey that they are able and willing to listen and that they receive the information with utmost confidentiality (3).

Table 1.1. Variables that Influence the Status of the Patient
Patient
Age
History of illness
Attitudes and perceptions
Sexual preference
Habits (e.g., use of drugs, smoking)
Family
Patient's status (e.g., married, separated, divorced)
Siblings (e.g., number, ages)
History (e.g., disease)
Environment
Socioeconomic environment
Religion
Culture and ethnic background

The Hippocratic oath demands that physicians be circumspect with all patient-related information.

Variables that Affect Patient Status

Many external variables exert an influence on the patient and on the care she receives. Some of these factors include the patient's "significant others"—her family, friends, and personal relationships (Table 1.1). These external variables also include psychological, genetic, biologic, social, and economic issues. Factors that affect a patient's perception of disease and pain and the means by which she has been taught to cope with illness include her education, attitudes, understanding of human reproduction and sexuality, family history of disease, and, in some cases, need for attention (3–5). Cultural factors, socioeconomic status, religion, ethnicity, and sexual preference are important considerations in understanding the patient's response to her care in both illness and health.

We are all products of our environment, our background, and our culture. The importance of ascertaining the patient's general, social, and familial situation cannot be overemphasized (1). The context of the family can and should be ascertained directly. The family history, including a careful analysis of those who have had significant illnesses, such as cancer, must be obtained. The psychological and sexual practices of the patient should be understood, and her functional level of satisfaction in these areas should be determined. **The physician must avoid being judgmental, particularly with respect to questions about sexual practices and preferences** (see Chapters 11 and 12).

Communication Skills

It is essential for the physician to communicate with a patient in a manner that allows her to continue to seek appropriate medical attention. Not only the words used, but also the patterns of speech, the manner in which the words are delivered, even body language and eye contact, are important aspects of the patient–physician interaction. The traditional role of the physician has been rather paternalistic, with the physician being expected to deliver direct commands and specific guidance on all matters (1). Patients are now demanding more balanced communication with their physicians, and although they do not in most cases command an understanding of medicine, they do expect to be treated with appropriate deference, respect for their intellect, and a manner more equal in stature with the physician (6). There is some evidence that giving the patient more control in the relationship with her doctor can lead to better health outcomes (3, 7, 8).

Table 1.2. Important Components of Communication between the Patient and Physician: The Physician's Role

The physician is:
A good listener
Empathetic
Honest
Genuine
The physician uses:
Understandable language
Appropriate body language
A collaborative approach
Open dialogue
Appropriate emotional content
Humor and warmth
The physician is not:
Confrontational
Combative
Condescending
Overbearing
Judgmental

Physician–Patient Interaction

The pattern of the physician's speech can influence interactions with the patient. Some important components of effective communication between patients and physicians are presented in Table 1.2. For this communication to be effective, the patient must feel that she is able to discuss her problems fully. In addition, if the patient perceives that she participates in the decision and that she is given as much information as possible, she will react to the proposed treatment with lower levels of anxiety and depression. There is ample evidence that patient communication and understanding and treatment outcome are improved when discussions with physicians are more dialogue than lecture. In addition, when patients feel they have some room for negotiation, they tend to retain more information regarding health care plans (9).

The notion of collaborative planning between patients and physicians has developed (9). This means that the patient becomes more vested in the process of determining health care choices. For example, if the patient is informed about the risks and benefits of hormone replacement therapy and clearly understands them, she may be more likely to comply with the plan once it has been set jointly by she and her physician.

There is some evidence that when patients are heard, understood, more vocal, and more inquisitive, their health improves (2). **Good communication is essential for the maintenance of a relationship between the patient and physician that fosters ongoing care.** Health maintenance, therefore, can be linked directly to the influence of positive, genial interactions. Patients who are comfortable with their physician may be more likely to raise issues or concerns or convey information about potential health risks and may be more receptive to the physician's recommendations. This degree of rapport may promote the effectiveness of early interactions, including behavior modification. It also helps ensure that patients return for regular care because they feel the physician is genuinely interested in their welfare.

When patients are ill, they feel vulnerable, physically and psychologically exposed, and powerless. Because the physician has power by virtue of knowledge and status, this relationship can be intimidating. Therefore, it is essential that the physician be aware of this disparity so that the "balance of power" does not shift too far away from the patient. Shifting it back from the physician to the patient may help improve outcomes (3, 7, 8).

In assessing the effects of the patient–physician interaction on the outcome of chronic illness, three characteristics that are associated with better health care outcomes have been identified (8):

1. Empathetic physician and more patient control of the interview
2. Expression of emotion by both patient and physician
3. Provision of information by the physician in response to the patient's inquiries

These findings related to the control of diastolic blood pressure and the reduction of hemoglobin A_{1c} in patients with diabetes, who experienced improved function and subjective evaluation of health in the presence of these characteristics. The best responses were achieved when an empathetic physician provided as much information and clarification as possible, responded to the patients' questions openly and honestly, and expressed a full range of emotions, including humor, and when the relationship was not entirely dominated by the physician (8).

In studies of gender and language, men tend to talk more than women, successfully interrupt women, and control the topics of the conversation (10). As a result, male physicians may tend to take control and be more assertive than female physicians. Men's speech tends to be characterized by interruptions, command, and lectures, and women's speech is characterized by silence, questions, and proposals (11, 12). Some patients may simply feel more reticent in the presence of a male physician, whereas others may be more forthcoming with a male than a female physician (13). Although these generalizations clearly do not apply to all physicians, they can raise awareness about the various styles of communication. These patterns indicate the need for all physicians, regardless of their gender, to be attentive to their style of speech because it may affect their ability to elicit open and free responses from their patients (14, 15). Women tend to speak openly in order to express their feelings and to have them validated and shared in an attempt to gain understanding of their concerns (9–11).

With regard to communication relating to gynecologic issues, it is important to understand that different styles of communication may affect the physician's ability to perceive the patient's status and to achieve the ultimate goal of optimal assessment and compliance with medical and surgical therapies. The intimate and highly personal nature of many gynecologic conditions requires particular sensitivity to evoke an honest response.

Style

In general, the art of communication and persuasion is based on mutual respect and development of the patient's understanding of the circumstances of her health (2). Insight is best achieved when the patient is encouraged to query her physician and when she is not pressured to make decisions (3, 9). Patients who feel "backed into a corner" have the lowest compliance with recommended treatments (7).

Following are techniques to help achieve rapport with patients:

1. **Use positive language** (e.g., agreement, approval, and humor).
2. **Build a partnership** (e.g., acknowledgment of understanding, asking for opinions, paraphrasing, and interpreting the patient's words).

3. **Ask rephrased questions.**

4. **Give complete responses to the patient's questions.**

The manner in which a physician guides a discussion with a patient will determine the patient's level of understanding and her compliance. For example, in providing a prescription, if a command is given to take the medication without a discussion of the rationale for it, patients may not comply, particularly if they become confused about the instructions (9). It is obviously inappropriate to prescribe hormone replacement therapy with a statement of simply, "Just take one of these pills every night before you go to bed," without a discussion of the risks and benefits of taking estrogen and progesterone.

The style of the presentation of information is key to its effectiveness. The physician should avoid "speaking down" to patients, both figuratively and literally. The latter occurs when discussions take place with the patient in the supine or the lithotomy position. Such a position creates a vulnerable situation in which the patient does not feel she is an equal partner in the relationship. Serious discussions about diagnosis and management strategies should be conducted when the patient is fully clothed and face-to-face with a doctor in a private room, with or without an intervening desk.

Body language is also important in interactions with patients. The physician should avoid an overly casual stance, which can communicate a lack of caring or lack of compassion. The patient should be viewed directly and spoken to with eye contact so that the physician is not perceived as "looking off into the distance" (2).

Laughter and Humor

Humor is an essential component that promotes open communication. It can be either appropriate or inappropriate. Appropriate humor allows the patient to diffuse anxiety and understand that (even in difficult situations) laughter can be healthy (16). Inappropriate humor would horrify, disgust, or offend a patient or generally make her uncomfortable or seem disrespectful of her. Laughter can be used as an appropriate means of relaxing the patient and making her feel better.

Laughter is a "metaphor for the full range of the positive emotions" (16). It is the response of human beings to incongruities and one of the highest manifestations of the cerebral process. It helps to facilitate the full range of positive emotions—love, hope, faith, the will to live, festivity, purpose, and determination (16). Laughter is a physiologic response, a release that helps us all feel better and allows us to accommodate the collision of logic and absurdity. Illness, or the prospect of illness, heightens our awareness of the incongruity between our existence and our ability to control the events that shape our lives and our outcomes. We use laughter to combat stress, and stress reduction is an essential mechanism used to cope with illness.

Strategies for Improving Communication

All physicians should understand the art of communication during the medical interview. It is essential that interactions with patients are professional, honorable, and honest. Issues that are important to physicians regarding patient–physician interactions are presented in Table 1.3. Following are some general guidelines that can help to improve communication:

1. **Listen more and talk less.**

2. **Encourage the pursuit of topics introduced by and important to patients.**

3. **Minimize controlling speech habits such as interrupting, issuing commands, and lecturing.**

Table 1.3. Importance Attached to the Patient–Physician Relationship[a]

Rank	*Physicians' Support Services*	*Always or Often (%)*	*Rarely or Never (%)*
1	Answering the patient's questions about the disease and its treatment, side effects, and possible outcomes	99	1
2	Making sure that the patient clearly understands the explanation of the medical treatment procedures	99	1
3	Encouraging the patient to develop an attitude of hope and optimism concerning treatment outcome	95	5
4	Adjusting treatment plans to enhance compliance when the patient exhibits noncompliance	88	12
5	Directly counseling family members	87	13
6	Continuing to serve as primary physician when the patient receives supplementary treatment at another facility	85	15
7	Providing referral to social support groups	83	17
8	Providing the patient with educational materials	81	19
9	Helping the patient develop methods to improve the quality of his or her life	74	26
10	Assisting the patient in determining which of his or her coping mechanisms are most productive and helping to activate them	62	38
11	Providing referral to psychological counseling services	57	43

[a]Results of a physician survey of 649 oncologists in regard to patient–physician communication. Modified from **Cousins N.** *Head first: the biology of hope and the healing power of the human spirit.* New York: Penguin Books, 1989:220, with permission.

4. **Seek out questions and provide full and understandable answers.**
5. **Become aware of discomfort in an interview, recognize when it originates in an attempt by the physician to take control, and redirect that attempt.**
6. **Assure patients that they have the opportunity to discuss their problem fully.**
7. **Recognize when patients may be seeking empathy and validation of their feelings rather than a solution. Sometimes all that is necessary is to be there as a compassionate human being.**

In conducting interviews, it is important for the physician to understand the patient's concerns. In studies of interviewing techniques, it has been shown that although clinicians employ many divergent styles, the successful ones tend to look for "windows of opportunity" (i.e., careful, attentive listening with replies or questions at opportune times) (2). This skill of communication is particularly effective in exploring psychological and social issues during brief interviews. The chief skill essential to allowing the physician to perceive problems is the ability to listen attentively.

An interview that permits maximum transmission of information to the physician is best achieved by the following approach (2):

1. **Begin with an open-ended question.**
2. **As the patient begins to speak, pay attention not only to her answers but also to her emotions and general body language.**

3. **Extend a second question or comment, encouraging the patient to talk.**

4. **Allow the patient to respond without interrupting, perhaps by employing silence, nods, or small facilitative comments, encouraging the patient to talk while the physician is listening.**

5. **Summarize and express empathy and understanding at the completion of the interview.**

Attentiveness, rapport, and collaboration characterize good medical interviewing techniques. Open-ended questions are generally desirable, particularly coupled with good listening skills ("*How are you doing?*" "*How does that make you feel?*").

Premature closure of an interview and inability to get the complete information to the patient may occur for several reasons (2). It may arise from a lack of recognition of the patient's particular concern, from not providing appropriate opportunity for discussion, from the physician's becoming uncomfortable in sharing the patient's emotion, or perhaps from the physician's lack of confidence that he or she can deal with the patient's concern. One of the principal factors undermining the success of the interview is lack of time. However, skilled physicians can facilitate considerable interaction even in a short time by encouraging open communication (17).

Many patients lack accurate information about their illness. Lack of full understanding of an illness can produce dissatisfaction with medical care, increased anxiety, distress, coping difficulties, noncompliance with treatment, and poor treatment response (18–20). As patients increasingly request more information about their illnesses and more involvement in decisions about their treatment, and as physicians attempt to provide more open negotiation, communication problems become more significant. Poor patient understanding stems from poor communication techniques, lack of consultation time, patient anxiety, patient denial, and in some cases, the withholding of information considered detrimental to patient welfare (18).

If clinical findings or confirmatory testing strongly suggest a serious condition (e.g., malignancy), the gravity and urgency of this situation must be conveyed in a manner that does not unduly alarm or frighten the individual. Honest answers should be provided to any specific questions the patient may want to discuss (19, 20).

Allowing time for questions is important, and scheduling a follow-up visit to discuss treatment options after the patient has had an opportunity to consider the options and recommendations may be valuable (19, 20). The patient should be encouraged to bring a partner or family member with her to provide moral support and to assist with questions. The patient should also be encouraged to write down any concerns she may have and bring them with her because important issues may not come to mind easily during an office visit. If the patient desires a second opinion or if a second opinion is mandated by her insurance coverage, it should be facilitated.

Valuable information can be provided by interviews with ancillary support staff and by providing pamphlets and other materials produced for patient education. Some studies have demonstrated that the use of pamphlets is highly effective in promoting an understanding of the condition and treatment options. Others have shown that the use of audiotapes and videotapes has a positive impact on knowledge and can decrease anxiety (18).

There are numerous medicine websites on the Internet that can be accessed, although the accuracy of the information is variable and must be carefully reviewed by physicians before recommending to patients.

The relationship between the patient and her physician is subject to constant change, as is true of all features of social interchange. The state of our health is dynamic. Many of us are fortunate to be in a good state of health for much of our lives, but some are not so fortunate. The goal of open communication between patient and physician is to achieve maximum effectiveness in diagnosis, treatment, and compliance for all patients.

Talk to the heart, speak to the soul.

Look to the being and embrace the figure's form.
Reach deeply, with hands outstretched.
Talk intently, to the seat of wisdom,

as life resembles grace.
Achieve peace within a fragile countenance.
Seek the comfort of the placid hour.
Through joyous and free reflection
know the other side of the flesh's frame.

JSB

History and Physical Examination

After a dialogue has been established, the patient assessment proceeds with obtaining a complete history and performing a physical examination. Both of these aspects of the assessment rely on good patient–physician interchange and attention to details. During the history and physical examination, the identification of risk factors that may require special attention should be sought. These factors should be reviewed with the patient in developing a plan for her future care (see Chapter 8).

History

After the ascertainment of the chief complaint and characteristics of the present illness, the history of the patient should be obtained. It should include her complete medical and surgical history, her reproductive history (including menstrual history), and a thorough family and social history.

A technique for obtaining information about the present illness is presented in Table 1.4. The physician should determine what other consultations may be needed to complete the evaluation. In some cases, referral to a social worker, psychologist, psychiatrist, or sexual counselor would be helpful. These issues are covered in Section III, Primary and Preventative Care (see Chapters 8 through 12). Laboratory testing for routine care and high-risk factors are presented in Chapter 8.

Table 1.4. Technique of Taking the History of the Present Illness

1. **The technique used in taking the history of the present illness varies with the patient, the patient's problem, and the physician. Allow the patient to talk about her chief complaint.** Although this complaint may or may not represent the real problem (depending on subsequent evaluation), it is usually uppermost in the patient's mind and most often constitutes the basis for the visit to the physician.
   During the phase of the interview, establish the temporal relation of the chief complaint to the total duration of the illness. Questions such as, *"Then up to the time of this complaint, you felt perfectly well?"* may elicit other symptoms that may antedate the chief complaint by days, months, or years. In this manner, the patient may recall the date of the first appearance of illness.

Table 1.4.—*continued*

Encourage the patient to talk freely and spontaneously about her illness from the established date of onset. Do not interrupt the patient's account, except for minor promptings such as, *"When did it begin?"* and *"How did it begin?"* which will help in developing chronologic order in the patient's story.

After the patient has furnished her spontaneous account (and before the next phase of the interview), it is useful to employ questions such as, *"What other problems have you noticed since you became ill?"* The response to this question may reveal other symptoms not yet brought forth in the interview.

Thus, in the first phase of the interview, the physician obtains an account of the symptoms as the patient experiences them, without any bias being introduced by the examiner's direct questions. Information about the importance of the symptoms to the patient and the patient's emotional reaction to her symptoms are also revealed.

2. **Because all available data regarding the symptoms are usually not elicited by the aforementioned techniques, the initial phase of the interview should be followed by a series of direct and detailed questions concerning the symptoms described by the patient.** Place each symptom in its proper chronologic order and then evaluate each in accordance with the directions for analyzing a symptom.

   In asking direct questions about the details of a symptom, take care not to suggest the nature of the answer. This particularly refers to questions that may be answered *"yes"* or *"no."* If a leading question should be submitted to the patient, the answer must be assessed with great care. Subject the patient to repeated cross-examination until you are completely satisfied that the answer is not given just to oblige you.

   Finally, before dismissing the symptom under study, inquire about other symptoms that might reasonably be expected under the clinical circumstances of the case. Symptoms specifically sought but denied are known as negative symptoms. These negative symptoms may confirm or rule out diagnostic possibilities suggested by the positive symptoms.

3. **The data secured by the techniques described in the first two phases of the interview should now suggest several diagnostic possibilities.** Test these possibilities further by inquiring about other symptoms or events that may form part of the natural history of the suspected disease or group of diseases.

4. **These techniques may still fail to reveal all symptoms of importance to the present illness, especially if they are remote in time and seemingly unrelated to the present problem.** The review of systems may then be of considerable help in bringing forth these data. A positive response from the patient on any item in any of the systems should lead immediately to further detailed questioning.

5. **Throughout that part of the interview concerning the present illness, consider the following factors:**
   a. **The probable cause of each symptom or illness, such as emotional stress, infection, neoplasm.** Do not disregard the patient's statements of causative factors. Consider each statement carefully, and use it as a basis for further investigation. When the symptoms point to a specific infection, direct inquiry to water, milk, and foods eaten; exposure to communicable diseases, animals, or pets; sources of sexually transmitted disease; or residence or travel in the tropics or other regions where infections are known to exist. In each of the above instances, ascertain, if possible, the date of exposure, incubation period, and symptoms of invasion (prodromal symptoms).
   b. **The severity of the patient's illness, as judged either by the presence of systemic symptoms, such as weakness, fatigue, loss of weight, or by a change in personal habits.** The latter includes changes in sleep, eating, fluid intake, bowel movements, social activities, exercise, or work. Note the dates the patient discontinued her work or took to bed. Is she continuously confined to bed?
   c. **Determine the patient's psychological reaction to her illness (anxiety, depression, irritability, fear) by observing how she relates her story as well as her nonverbal behavior.** The response to a question such as, *"Have you any particular theories about or fear of what may be the matter with you?"* may yield important clues relative to the patient's understanding and feeling about her illness. The reply may help in the management of the patient's problem and allow the physician to give advice according to the patient's understanding of her ailment.

Modified from **Hochstein E, Rubin AL.** *Physical diagnosis.* New York: McGraw-Hill, 1964:9–11, with permission.

Physical Examination

A thorough general physical examination should be performed during each patient assessment (Table 1.5). In addition to evaluation of the vital signs, examination of the breast, abdomen, and pelvis is an essential part of the gynecologic examination.

Abdominal Examination

With the patient in the supine position, an attempt should be made to have the patient relax as much as possible. Her head should be leaned back and supported gently by a pillow so that she does not tense her abdominal muscles.

The abdomen should be inspected for signs of an intraabdominal mass, organomegaly, or distention that would, for example, suggest ascites or intestinal obstruction. Initial palpation of the abdomen is performed to evaluate the size and configuration of the liver, spleen, and other abdominal contents. Evidence of fullness or mass effect should be noted. This is particularly important in evaluating patients who may have a pelvic mass and in determining the extent of omental involvement, for example, with metastatic ovarian cancer. A fullness in the upper abdomen could be consistent with an "omental cake." All four quadrants should be carefully palpated for any evidence of mass, firmness, irregularity, or distention. A systematic approach should be used (e.g., clockwise, starting in the right upper quadrant). Percussion should be used to measure the dimensions of the liver. The patient should be asked to inhale and exhale during palpation of the edge of the liver.

Auscultation should be performed to ascertain the nature of the bowel sounds. The frequency of intestinal sounds and their quality should be noted. In a patient with intestinal obstruction, "rushes," as well as the occasional high-pitched sound, can be heard. Bowel sounds associated with an ileus may be less frequent but at the same pitch as normal bowel sounds.

Pelvic Examination

The pelvic examination is typically performed with the patient in the dorsal lithotomy position (Fig. 1.1). The patient's feet should rest comfortably in stirrups with the edge of the buttocks at the lower end of the table so that the vulva can be readily inspected and the speculum can be inserted in the vagina without obstruction from the table.

The vulva and perineal area should be carefully inspected. Evidence of any lesions, erythema, pigmentation, masses, or irregularity should be noted. The skin quality should be noted as well as any signs of trauma, such as excoriations or ecchymosis. The presence of any visible lesions should be quantitated and carefully described with regard to their full appearance and characteristics on palpation (i.e., mobility, tenderness, consistency). Ulcerative or purulent lesions of the vulva should be cultured as outlined in subsequent chapters, and biopsy should be performed on any lesions.

After thorough visualization and palpation of the external genitalia, including the mons pubis and the perianal area, a speculum is inserted in the vagina. In a normal adult who is sexually active, a Pederson or Graves speculum is used. The types of specula that are used in gynecology are presented in Fig. 1.2. In general, the smallest speculum necessary to produce adequate visualization should be used. The speculum should be warmed before it is inserted into the vagina, and warm water generally provides sufficient lubrication for this procedure. The patient should be alerted to the fact that the speculum will be inserted so that she is not surprised by its placement. After insertion, the cervix and all aspects of the vagina should be carefully inspected. Particular attention should also be paid to the vaginal fornices because lesions (e.g., warts) may be present in those areas and are not readily visualized unless care is taken to do so.

Table 1.5. Method of the Female Pelvic Examination

The patient is instructed to empty her bladder. She is placed in the lithotomy position (Fig. 1.1) and draped properly. The examiner's right or left hand is gloved, depending on his or her preference. The pelvic area is illuminated well, and the examiner faces the patient. The following order of procedure is suggested for the pelvic examination:

A. External genitalia

1. Inspect the mons pubis, labia majora, labia minora, perineal body, and anal region for characteristics of the skin, distribution of the hair, contour, and swelling. Palpate any abnormality.
2. Separate the labia majora with the index and middle fingers of the gloved hand and inspect the epidermal and mucosal characteristics and anatomic configuration of the following structures in the order indicated below:
   a. Labia minora
   b. Clitoris
   c. Urethral orifice
   d. Vaginal outlet (introitus)
   e. Hymen
   f. Perineal body
   g. Anus
3. If disease of the Skene glands is suspected, palpate the gland for abnormal excretions by milking the undersurface of the urethra through the anterior vaginal wall. Examine the expressed excretions by microscopy and cultures.
   If there is a history of labial swelling, palpate for a diseased Bartholin gland with the thumb on the posterior part of the labia majora and the index finger in the vaginal orifice. In addition, sebaceous cysts, if present, can be felt in the labia minora.

B. Introitus

With the labia still separated by the middle and index fingers, instruct the patient to bear down. Note the presence of the anterior wall of the vagina when a cystocele is present or bulging of the posterior wall when a rectocele or enterocele is present. Bulging of both may accompany a complete prolapse of the uterus.

The supporting structure of the pelvic outlet is evaluated further when the bimanual pelvic examination is done.

C. Vagina and cervix

Inspection of the vagina and cervix using a speculum should always precede palpation.

The instrument should be warmed with tap water—not lubricated—if vaginal or cervical smears are to be obtained for the test or if cultures are to be performed.

Select the proper size of speculum (Fig. 1.2), warmed and lubricated (unless contraindicated). Introduce the instrument into the vaginal orifice with the blades oblique, closed, and pressed against the perineum. Carry the speculum along the posterior vaginal wall, and after it is fully inserted, rotate the blades into a horizontal position and open them. Maneuver the speculum until the cervix is exposed between the blades. Gently rotate the speculum around its long axis until all surfaces of the vagina and cervix are visualized.

1. Inspect the vagina for the following:
   a. The presence of blood
   b. Discharge. This should be studied to detect trichomoniasis, monilia, and clue cells and to obtain cultures, primarily for gonococci, and chlamydiae.
   c. Mucosal characteristics (i.e., color, lesions, superficial vascularity, and edema)
      The lesion may be:
      1) Inflammatory—redness, swelling, exudates, ulcers, vesicles
      2) Neoplastic

Table 1.5.—*continued*

3) Vascular

4) Pigmented—bluish discoloration of pregnancy (Chadwick's sign)

5) Miscellaneous (e.g., endometriosis, traumatic lesions, and cysts)

d. Structural abnormalities (congenital and acquired)

2. Inspect the cervix for the same factors listed above for the vagina. Note the following comments relative to the inspection of the cervix:

a. Unusual bleeding from the cervical canal, except during menstruation, merits an evaluation for cervical or uterine neoplasia.

b. Inflammatory lesions are characterized by a mucopurulent discharge from the os and redness, swelling, and superficial ulcerations of the surface.

c. Polyps may arise either from the surface of the cervix projecting into the vagina or from the cervical canal. Polyps may be inflammatory or neoplastic.

d. Carcinoma of the cervix may not dramatically change the appearance of the cervix or may appear as lesions similar in appearance to an inflammation. Therefore, a biopsy should be performed if there is suspicion of neoplasia.

D. Bimanual palpation

The pelvic organs can be outlined by bimanual palpation; the examiner places one hand on the lower abdominal wall and the fingers (usually two) (Fig. 1.3) of the other hand in the vagina (or vagina and rectum in the rectovaginal examination) (Fig. 1.4). Either the right or left hand may be used for vaginal palpation.

1. Introduce the well-lubricated index and middle finger into the vagina at its posterior aspect near the perineum. Test the strength of the perineum by pressing downward on the perineum and asking the patient to bear down. This procedure may disclose a previously concealed cystocele or rectocele and descensus of the uterus.

Advance the fingers along the posterior wall until the cervix is encountered. Note any abnormalities of structure or tenderness in the vagina or cervix.

2. Press the abdominal hand, which is resting on the infraumbilical area, very gently downward, sweeping the pelvic structures toward the palpating vaginal fingers.

Coordinate the activity of the two hands to evaluate the body of the uterus for:

a. Position

b. Architecture, size, shape, symmetry, tumor

c. Consistency

d. Tenderness

e. Mobility

Tumors, if found, are evaluated for location, architecture, consistency, tenderness, mobility, and number.

3. Continue the bimanual palpation and evaluate the cervix for position, architecture, consistency, and tenderness, especially on mobility of the cervix. Rebound tenderness should be noted at this time. The intravaginal fingers should then explore the anterior, posterior, and lateral fornices.

4. Place the "vaginal" fingers in the right lateral fornix and the "abdominal" hand on the right lower quadrant. Manipulate the abdominal hand gently downward toward the vaginal fingers to outline the adnexa.

A normal tube is not palpable. A normal ovary (about $4 \times 2 \times 3$ cm in size, sensitive, firm, and freely movable) is often not palpable. If an adnexal mass is found, evaluate its location relative to the uterus and cervix, architecture, consistency, tenderness, and mobility.

5. Palpate the left adnexal region, repeating the technique described previously, but place the vaginal fingers in the left fornix and the abdominal hand on the left lower quadrant.

6. Follow the bimanual examination with a rectovaginal-abdominal examination.

Insert the index finger into the vagina and the middle finger into the rectum

Table 1.5.—*continued*

very gently. Place the other hand on the infraumbilical region. The use of this technique makes possible higher exploration of the pelvis because the cul-de-sac does not limit the depth of the examining finger.

7. In patients who have an intact hymen, examine the pelvic organs by the rectal-abdominal technique.

E. Rectal examination

1. Inspect the perianal and anal area, the pilonidal (sacrococcygeal) region, and the perineum for the following aspects:

a. Color of the region (note that the perianal skin is more pigmented than the surrounding skin of the buttocks and is frequently thrown into radiating folds)

b. Lesions

1) The perianal and perineal regions are common sites for itching. Pruritus ani is usually indicated by thickening, excoriations, and eczema of the perianal region and adjacent areas.

2) The anal opening often is the site of fissures, fistulae, and external hemorrhoids.

3) The pilonidal area may present a dimple, a sinus, or an inflamed pilonidal cyst.

2. Instruct the patient to "strain down" and note whether this technique brings into view previously concealed internal hemorrhoids, polyps, or a prolapsed rectal mucosa.

3. Palpate the pilonidal area, the ischiorectal fossa, the perineum, and the perianal region before inserting the gloved finger into the anal canal.
Note the presence of any concealed induration or tenderness in any of these areas.

4. Palpate the anal canal and rectum with a well-lubricated, gloved index finger. Lay the pulp of the index finger against the anal orifice and instruct the subject to strain downward. Concomitant with the patient's downward straining (which tends to relax the external sphincter muscle), exert upward pressure until the sphincter is felt to yield. Then, with a slight rotary movement, insinuate the finger past the anal canal into the rectum. Examine the anal canal systematically before exploring the rectum.

5. Evaluate the anal canal

a. Tonus of the external sphincter muscle and the anorectal ring at the anorectal junction

b. Tenderness (usually caused by a tight sphincter, anal fissure, or painful hemorrhoids)

c. Tumor or irregularities, especially at the pectinate line

d. Superior aspect: Reach as far as you can. Mild straining by the patient may cause some lesions, which are out of reach of the finger, to descend sufficiently low to be detected by palpation.

e. Test for occult blood: Examine the finger after it is withdrawn for evidence of gross blood, pus, or other alterations in color or consistency. Smear the stool to test for occult blood (guaiac).

6. Evaluate the rectum

a. Anterior wall

1) Cervix: size, shape, symmetry, consistency, and tenderness, especially on manipulation

2) Uterine or adnexal masses

3) Rectouterine fossa for tenderness or implants
In patients with an intact hymen, the examination of the anterior wall of the rectum is the usual method of examining the pelvic organs.

b. Right lateral wall, left lateral wall, posterior wall, superior aspect; test for occult blood

Modified from **Hochstein E, Rubin AL.** *Physical diagnosis.* New York: McGraw-Hill, 1964:342–353, with permission.

Figure 1.1 The lithotomy position for the pelvic examination.

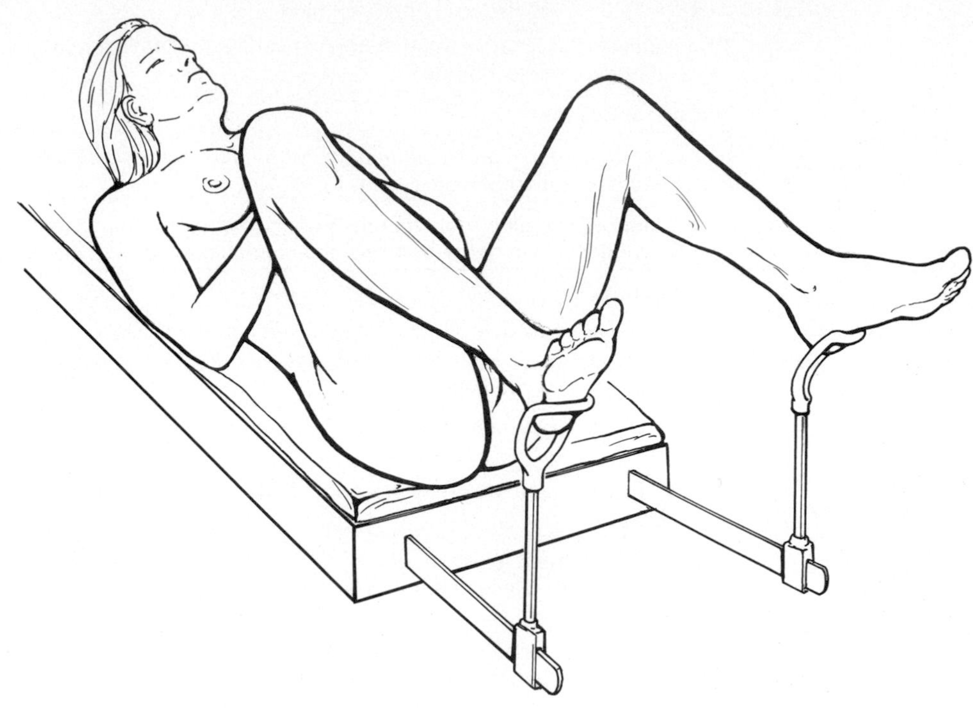

Figure 1.2 Vaginal specula: 1, Graves extra long; 2, Graves regular; 3, Pederson extra long; 4, Pederson regular; 5, Huffman "virginal"; 6, pediatric regular; and 7, pediatric narrow.

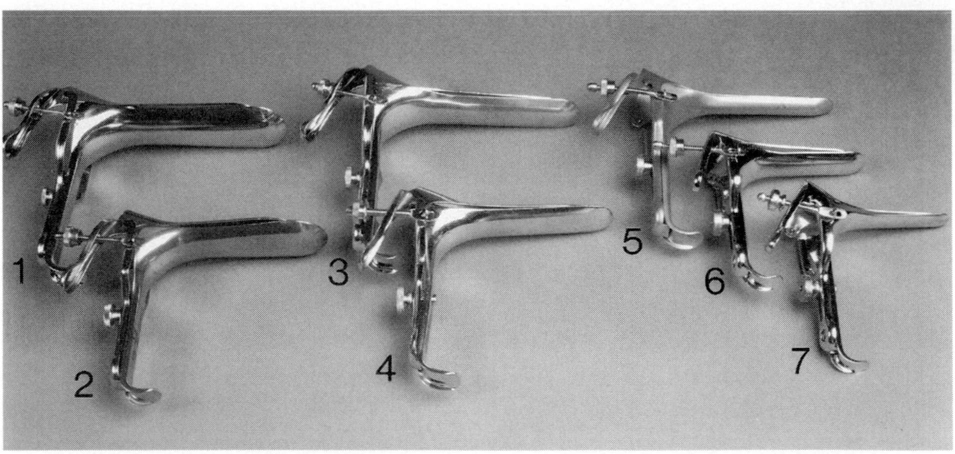

The appropriate technique for a Papanicolaou's (Pap) test is presented in Chapter 16. Any obvious lesions on the cervix or in the vagina should undergo biopsy. An endometrial biopsy is usually performed with a flexible cannula or a Novak curette (see Chapter 13). Any purulence in the vagina or cervix should be cultured (see Chapter 15).

After the speculum is removed and the pelvis palpated, the first and second fingers are inserted gently into the vagina after adequate lubrication has been applied to the examination glove. In general, in right-handed physicians, the right hand is inserted into the vagina and the left hand is used on the abdomen to provide counter pressure as the pelvic viscera are moved (Fig. 1.3). The vagina, its fornices, and the cervix are palpated carefully for any

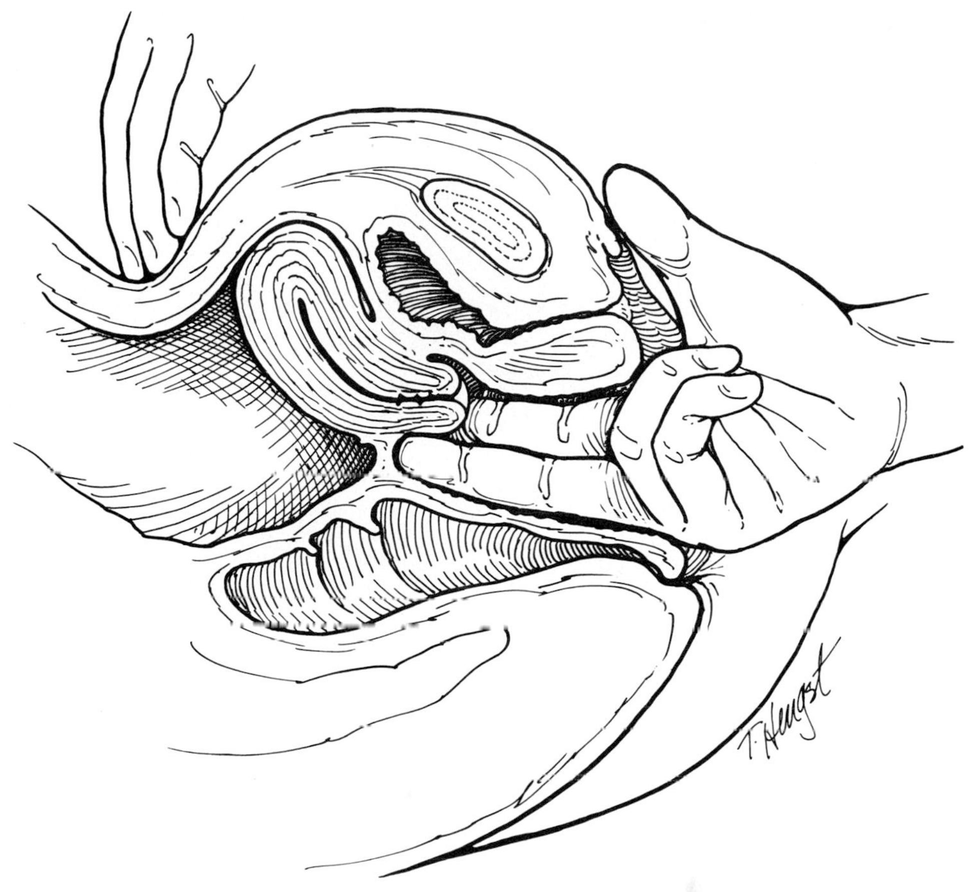

Figure 1.3 The bimanual examination.

masses or irregularities. The fingers are placed gently into the posterior fornix so that the uterus can be moved. With the abdominal hand in place, the uterus can usually be palpated just above the surface pubis. In this manner, the size, shape, mobility, contour, consistency, and position of the uterus are determined.

The adnexa are then palpated gently on both sides, paying particular attention to any enlargements. Again, the size, shape, mobility, and consistency of any adnexal structures should be carefully noted.

A rectal examination is suggested periodically in women 40 years of age and older (see American College of Obstetricians and Gynecologists guidelines, Chapter 8) and in all premenopausal women in whom there is any difficulty ascertaining the adnexal structures (Fig 1.4). Rectovaginal examination should also be performed in these women to exclude the possibility of concurrent rectal disease (21). In postmenopausal women who undergo rectal examination, a stool guaiac test can be performed. During rectal examination, the quality of the sphincter muscles, support of the pelvis, and evidence of masses such as hemorrhoids or lesions intrinsic to the rectum should be noted.

At the completion of the physical examination, the patient should be informed about the findings. When the results of the examination are normal, the patient can be reassured accordingly. When there is a possible abnormality, the patient should be informed immediately. A plan to evaluate the findings should be outlined briefly and in clear, understandable language. The implications of any proposed procedure (e.g., biopsy) should be discussed, and the patient should be informed when the results of any tests will be available.

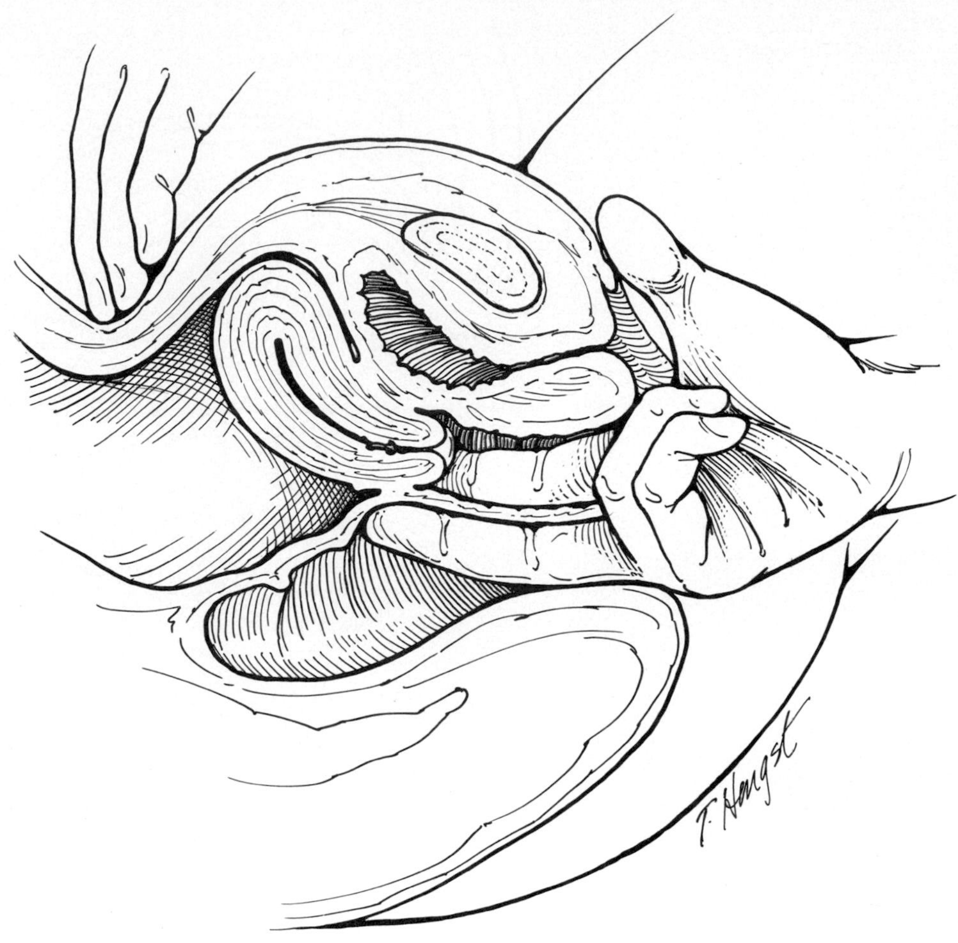

Figure 1.4 The rectovaginal examination.

Pediatric Patients

A careful examination is indicated when a child presents with genital complaints. The examiner should be familiar with the normal appearance of the prepubital genitalia. The normal unestrogenized hymenal ring and vestibule can appear mildly erythematous. The technique of examination is different from that used for examining an adult and may need to be tailored to the individual child based on her age, size, and comfort with the examiner. A young child can usually be examined best in a "frog-leg" position on the examining table. Some very young girls (toddlers or infants) do best when held in their mother's arms. Sometimes, the mother can be positioned, clothed, on the examination table (feet in stirrups, head of table elevated) with the child on her lap, the child's legs straddling her mother's. The knee-chest position may also be helpful for the examination (22). The child who is relaxed and warned about touching will usually tolerate the examination satisfactorily. Some children who have been abused, who have had particularly traumatic previous examinations, or who are unable to allow an examination may need to be examined with the use of anesthesia, although a gentle office examination should almost always be attempted first. If no obvious case of bleeding is visible externally or within the distal vagina, an examination under anesthesia may be indicated to visualize the vagina and cervix completely. A hysteroscope, cytoscope, or other endoscopic instrument can be used to provide magnification and light source.

Adolescent Patients

A pelvic examination may be less revealing in an adolescent than in an older woman, particularly if it is the patient's first examination or if it takes place on an emergency basis. Although other diagnostic techniques (such as pelvic ultrasound) can supplement an inadequate or poorly revealing examination, an examination should usually be attempted. The keys to a successful examination lie in earning the patient's trust, explaining the components of her examination, performing only the essential components, and using a very careful and gentle technique. It is important to ascertain whether the patient has had a previous pelvic examination.

An adolescent should have a pelvic examination if she has had intercourse, if the results of a pregnancy test are positive, if she has abdominal pain, if she is markedly anemic, or if she is bleeding heavily enough to compromise hemodynamic stability. The pelvic examination occasionally may be deferred in young teenagers who have a classic history of irregular cycles soon after menarche, who have normal hematocrit levels, who deny sexual activity, and who will reliably return for follow-up.

Before a first pelvic examination is performed, a brief explanation of the planned examination (which may or may not need to include a speculum), instruction in relaxation techniques, and the use of lidocaine jelly as a lubricant can be helpful. The patient should be encouraged to participate in the examination through voluntary relaxation of the introital muscles or by using a mirror if she wishes. If significant trauma is suspected or the patient finds the examination too painful and is truly unable to cooperate, an examination under anesthesia may occasionally be necessary. The risks of general anesthesia must be weighed against the value of information that would be obtained by the examination.

Confidentiality is an important issue in adolescent health care. A number of medical organizations, including the American Medical Association, the American Academy of Pediatrics, and the American College of Obstetrics and Gynecologists, have endorsed adolescents' rights to confidential medical care. Particularly with regard to issues as sensitive as sexual activity, it is critical that the adolescent be interviewed alone, without a parent in the room. The patient should be asked if she has engaged in sexual intercourse, if she used any method of contraception, and if she feels there is any possibility of pregnancy.

Follow-up

Arrangements should be made for the ongoing care of patients, regardless of their health status. Patients with no evidence of disease should be counseled regarding health behaviors and the need for routine care. For those with signs and symptoms of a medical disorder, further assessments and a treatment plan should be discussed. The physician must determine whether he or she is equipped to treat a particular problem or whether the patient should be directed to another health professional, either in obstetrics and gynecology or another specialty. If the physician believes it is necessary to refer the patient elsewhere for care, the patient should be reassured that this measure is being undertaken in her best interests and that continuity of care will be ensured.

Summary

The management of patients' gynecologic symptoms, as well as abnormal findings and signs detected during examination, requires the full use of a physician's skills and knowledge and poses challenges to practice the art of medicine in a manner that leads to effective alliances between physicians and their patients. Physicians must listen carefully to what patients are saying about the nature and severity of their symptoms. The art of medical history taking must not be minimized. Physicians also must listen carefully for what patients may not be saying: their fears, anxieties, and personal experiences that lead them to react in a certain manner when faced with what is often, to them, a crisis (the diagnosis of an abnormality on examination, laboratory testing, or pelvic imaging).

Physicians must use their knowledge of gynecology gained through formal education, personal experience, teachers and mentors, and textbooks, always striving to have the latest information about a given problem. Patients often present a unique set of circumstances, medical issues, or combination of diseases. Today, the use of a textbook chapter is only a beginning. Computers have made the world of information management accessible. Physicians must learn to practice evidence-based medicine—based on the very latest of what is known, not just impressions, recollections, or advice of colleagues. Physicians need to search the medical literature to help discover what they do not know. Patients are searching the medical literature, using computer online services to gain access to medical subject talk-groups, research reports, and the same literature read by physicians. Knowledge derived from an evidence base must be applied, using the art of medicine, to interact with patients to maintain health, alleviate suffering, and manage and cure disease.

References

1. **Lipkin M Jr.** The medical interview and related skills. In: **Branch WT,** ed. *Office practice of medicine.* Philadelphia: WB Saunders, 1987:1287–1306.
2. **Branch WT, Malik TK.** Using windows of opportunities in brief interviews to understand patients' concerns. *JAMA* 1993;269:1667–1668.
3. **Simpson M, Buckman R, Stewart M, et al.** Doctor-patient communication: the Toronto consensus statement. *BMJ* 1991;303:1385–1387.
4. **Ley P.** *Communicating with patients.* London: Croom Helm, 1988.
5. **Butt HR.** A method for better physician-patient communication. *Ann Intern Med* 1977;86:478–480.
6. **Mishler EG, Clark JA, Ingelfinger J, et al.** The language of attentive patient care: a comparison of two medical interviews. *J Gen Intern Med* 1989;4:325–335.
7. **The Headache Study Group of the University of Western Ontario.** Predictors of outcome on headache patients presenting to family physicians: a one year perspective study. *Headache* 1986;26:285–284.
8. **Kaplan SH, Greenfield S, Ware JE Jr.** Assessing the effects of physician-patient interactions on the outcomes of chronic disease. *Med Care* 1989;27:S110–S127.
9. **Fallowfield LJ, Hall A, Macguire GP, Baum M.** Psychological outcomes of different treatment policies in women with early breast cancer outside a clinical trial. *BMJ* 1990;301:575–580.
10. **Spender D.** *Man made language.* 2nd ed. New York: Routledge & Kegan Paul, 1985.
11. **Tannen D.** *You just don't understand: women and men in conversation.* New York: Ballentine, 1990.
12. **West C.** Reconceptualizing gender in physician-patient relationships. *Soc Sci Med* 1993;36:57–66.
13. **Todd AD, Fisher S.** *The social organization of doctor-patient communication.* 2nd ed. Norwood, NJ: Ablex Publishing, 1993:243–265.
14. **Roter D, Lipkin M Jr, Korsgaard A.** Sex differences in patients' and physicians' communication during primary medical care visits. *Med Care* 1991;29:1083–1093.
15. **Lurie N, Slater J, McGovern P, et al.** Preventive care for women: does the sex of the physician matter? *N Engl J Med* 1993;329:478–482.
16. **Cousins N.** The laughter connection. In: **Cousins N,** ed. *Head first: the biology of hope and the healing power of the human spirit.* New York: Penguin Books, 1989:125–153.
17. **Levinson W, Chaumetor N.** Communication between surgeons and patients in routine office visits. *Surgery* 1999;125:127–134.
18. **Dunn SM, Butow PN, Tattersall MHN, et al.** General information tapes inhibit recall of the cancer consultation. *J Clin Oncol* 1993;11:2279–2285.
19. **Baile WB, Kudelks AP, Beale EA, et al.** Communication skills training in oncology: description and preliminary outcomes of workshops on breaking bad news and managing patient reactions for illness. *Cancer* 1999;86:887–897.
20. **Maguire P, Faulkner A.** Improve the counselling skills of doctors and nurses in cancer case. *BMJ* 1999;297:847–849.
21. **Hochstein E, Rubin AL.** *Physical diagnosis.* New York: McGraw-Hill, 1964.
22. **Emans SJ, Goldstein P.** The gynecologic examination of the prepubital child with vulvovaginitis: use of the knee-chest position. *Pediatrics* 1980;65:758–760.

2 Principles of Patient Care

Joanna M. Cain

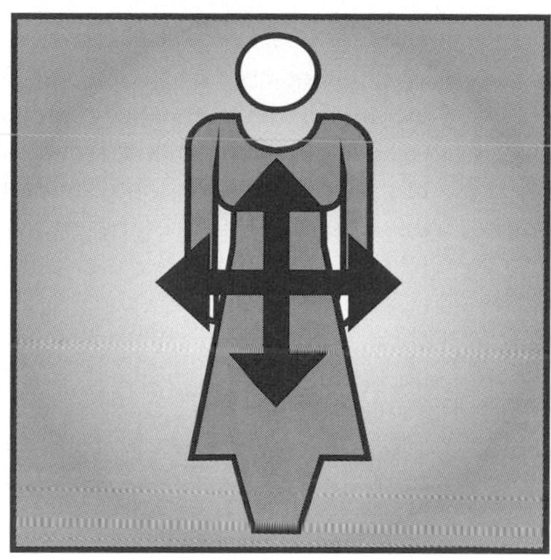

The practice of gynecology, as with all branches of medicine, is based on ethical principles that guide patient care. These principles and concepts create a framework for ethical decision making that applies to all aspects of practice:

- **Autonomy**: a person's right to self-rule, to establish personal norms of conduct, and to choose a course of action based on a set of personal values and principles derived from them
- **Beneficence**: the obligation to promote the well-being of others
- **Confidentiality**: a person's right to decide how and to whom personal medical information will be communicated
- **Covenant**: a binding agreement between two or more parties for the performance of some action
- **Fiduciary relationship**: a relationship founded on faith and trust
- **Informed consent**: the patient's acceptance of a medical intervention after adequate disclosure of the nature of the procedure, its risks and benefits, and alternatives
- **Justice**: the right of individuals to claim what is due them based on certain personal properties or characteristics
- **Maleficence**: the act of committing harm (*nonmaleficence* obliges one to avoid doing harm)

Patient and Physician

Health care providers fulfill a basic need—to preserve and advance the health of human beings. Despite the challenges imposed by the commercial aspects of the current medical environment, for most physicians, the practice of medicine remains very much a "calling," a giving of oneself to the greater good. Although much of medicine is contractual in nature, it cannot be understood in only those terms: "The kind of minimalism that a contractualist understanding of the professional relationship encourages produces a professional too grudging, too calculating, too lacking in spontaneity, too quickly exhausted to go the second mile with his patients along the road of their distress" (1). There is a relationship between physician and patient that extends beyond a contract and assumes the elements of a fiduciary relationship—a covenant between parties. **The physician, having knowledge about the elements of health care, assumes a trust relationship with the patient whereby her interests are held paramount. Both the patient and the physician have rights and responsibilities in this relationship, and both are rewarded when those rights and responsibilities are upheld. Confidentiality and informed consent are two expressions of that trust or covenantal relationship.**

Confidentiality

The patient seeking assistance from a health professional has the right to be assured that the information exchanged during that interaction is private. Privacy is essential to the trust relationship between doctor and patient. Discussions are privileged information. **The right to privacy prohibits a physician from revealing information regarding the patient unless the patient waives that privilege.** Privileged information belongs to the patient except when it impinges on the legal and ethical rights of institutions and society at large, regardless of the setting. In a court situation, for example, physicians cannot reveal information about their patients unless that privilege is waived by the patient. If privilege is waived, the physician may not withhold such testimony.

The privilege of privacy must be maintained even when it does not seem intrinsically obvious. A patient's family, friend, or spiritual guide, for example, has no right to medical information regarding the patient unless the patient specifically releases it. This may seem obvious but often can be overlooked, such as when a health care giver receives a call from a concerned parent, spouse, or relative inquiring about the status of a patient. The response may be a natural attempt to reassure and inform a caring individual about the patient's status. However, for her own reasons, the patient may not want certain individuals informed of her medical condition. Thus, confidentiality has been breached. It is wise to ask patients about who may be involved in decision making and who may be informed about their status. If a health care giver is unclear of the patient's wishes regarding the person requesting information, the reply should indicate that the patient's permission is necessary before discussing her status. Finally, when trying to contact individual patients for follow-up of medical findings, it is never appropriate to reveal the reason to an individual other than the patient.

Record Keeping

Health care professionals are part of a record-keeping organization. Those records are used for multiple purposes in medicine and are a valuable tool in patient care. Unfortunately, there is an increasing tendency for ancillary organizations to collect, maintain, and disclose information about individuals to whom they have no direct connection (2). Given the present lack of universal and nondiscriminatory access to health insurance in the United States, physicians must be aware of this practice and its ramifications. Patients sign a document, often without understanding its meaning, upon registering with a health care institution or insurance plan. That document waives the patient's privilege to suppress access and gives access to the medical record to insurers and often other health care providers who request it. The consequences of such disclosure for patients can be significant in terms of insurance coverage and potential job discrimination (3). This concern must be weighed against the need for all health care providers involved with an individual to be informed about past or present diseases or activities that may interfere with or complicate management. The use of illegal drugs, a positive human immunodeficiency virus (HIV) test result, and even a history of cancer or psychiatric illness are all exceptionally important to health care providers in evaluating individual patients. When revealed to outside institutions, however, these factors may affect the patient's ability to obtain and keep medical coverage, insurance, or even credit. It is axiomatic that everything that is written in a patient's record should be important to the medical care of that patient and that extrinsic information should be avoided. Furthermore, it is appropriate for physicians to discuss with patients the nature of medical records and their release to other parties so that patients can make an informed choice about such release. Additional guidelines from the Department of Health and Human Services (DHHS) to protect the security of patient records, known as the Healthcare Information

Privacy and Protection Act (HIPPA), will translate into additional requirements for access to these records for clinical research as well as guidelines for electronic medical records protections. The security of medical records, then, is a concern not just for individual patients and physicians but also for health systems and researchers.

Legal Issues

The privilege of patients to keep their records or medical information private can be superseded by the needs of society, but only in rare circumstances. The classic legal decision quoted for the needs of others superseding individual patient rights is that of Tarasoff v. Regents of the University of California (4). That decision establishes that the special relationship between a patient and doctor may support affirmative duties for the benefit of third persons. It requires disclosure if "necessary to avert danger to others" but still in a fashion "that would preserve the privacy of the patient to the fullest extent compatible with the prevention of the threatened danger." This principle also is compatible with the various codes of ethics that allow physicians to reveal information in order to protect the welfare of the individual or the community. In other words, "the protective privilege ends where the public peril begins" (4).

Legislation can also override individual privilege. The most frequent example is the recording of births and deaths, which is the responsibility of physicians. Various diseases are required to be reported depending on state law [e.g., HIV status may or may not be reportable in individual states, whereas acquired immunodeficiency syndrome (AIDS) is reportable in all states]. Reporting injuries caused by lethal weapons, rapes, and battering (e.g., elder and child abuse) is mandatory in some states and not others. The regulations for the reporting of these conditions are codified by law and can be obtained from the state health department. These laws are designed to protect the individual's privacy as much as possible while still serving the public interest. Particularly in the realm of abuse, physicians have a complex ethical role regardless of the law. Victims of abuse, for example, must feel supported and assured that the violent act they have survived will not make a difference in how they are treated as people. Their sense of vulnerability and their actual vulnerability may be so great that reporting an incident may increase their risk for medical harm. Despite the laws, physicians also have an ethical responsibility to see to the patient's best interest, and weighing that ethical responsibility can be difficult.

Informed Consent

Informed consent is a process that involves an exchange of information directed toward reaching mutual understanding and informed decision making. Ideally, informed consent should be the practical manifestation of respect for patient preferences (autonomy) (5,6). Unfortunately, an act of informed consent is often misunderstood as procurement of a signature on a document. Furthermore, the intent of the individual involved in the consent process often is the protection of the physicians from liability. Nothing could be further from either the legal or ethical meaning of this concept.

Informed consent is a conversation between physician and patient that teaches the patient about the medical condition, explores her values, and informs her about the reasonable medical alternatives. Informed consent is an interactive discussion in which one participant has greater knowledge about medical information and the other participant has greater knowledge about that individual's value system and circumstances affected by the information. This process does not require an arduous lecture on the medical condition or extensive examination of the patient's psyche. It does require adjustment of the information to the educational level of the patient and respectful elicitation of concerns and questions. It also requires acknowledgement of the various fears and concerns of both parties. Fear that the information may frighten patients, fear of hearing the information by the patient, lack of ability to decode technical information, and inability to express lack of comprehension are among the many barriers facing physicians and patients engaging in this conversation. Communication skills are part of the art of medicine, and observation of good role models, practice, and good intent can help to instill this ability in physicians (7).

Autonomy

Informed consent arises from the concept of autonomy. Pellegrino (8) defines an autonomous person as "one who, in his thoughts, work, and actions, is able to follow those norms he chooses as his own without external constraints or coercion by others." This definition contains the essence of what health care providers must consider as informed consent. The choice to receive or refuse medical care must be in concert with the patient's values and freely chosen, and the options must be considered in light of the patient's values.

Autonomy is not respect for a patient's wishes against good medical judgment. Consider the example of a patient with inoperable, advanced-stage cervical cancer who demands surgery and refuses radiation therapy. The physician's ethical obligation is to seek the best for the patient's survival (beneficence) and avoid the harm (maleficence) of surgery, even though that is what the patient wishes. Although physicians are not obligated to offer treatment that is of no benefit, the patient does have the right to refuse treatment if it does not fit into her values. Thus, this patient could refuse treatment for her cervical cancer, but she does not have the right to be given any treatment she wishes.

Surrogate Decision Makers

If the ability to make choices is diminished by extreme youth, mental processing difficulties, extreme medical illness, or loss of awareness, surrogate decision making may be required. In all circumstances, the surrogate must make every attempt to act as the patient would have acted (9). The hierarchy of surrogate decision makers is specified by statutory law in each state and differs slightly from state to state. For adults, the first surrogate decision maker is a court-appointed guardian if one exists and second is a durable power of attorney, followed by relatives by degree of presumed familiarity (e.g., spouse, adult children, parents).

For children, parents are the surrogate decision makers, except in circumstances in which the decision is life-threatening and might not be the choice a child would make later, when adult beliefs and values are formed. The classic example of this is the Jehovah's Witness parents who refuse life-saving transfusions for their child (10). Although this case is the extreme, it illustrates that the basic principle outlined for surrogate decision making should also apply to parents. Bias that influences decision making (in protection of parental social status, income, or systems of beliefs) needs to be considered by physicians because the potential conflict may lead parents to decisions that are not in the best interest of the child. If there is a conflicting bias that does not allow decisions to be made in the best interest of the child or that involves a medical threat to a child, legal action to establish guardianship (normally through a child protective agency) may be necessary. This action can destroy not only the patient (child)–physician relationship but also the parent–physician relationship and may affect the long-term health and well-being of the child, who must return to the care of the parents. Such decisions should be made only after all attempts to educate, clarify, and find alternatives have been tried.

The legal age at which adolescents may make their own decisions regarding their health care varies by state (11). However, there is a growing trend to increase the participation of adolescents who are capable of decision making in decisions about their health care. Because minors often have developed a value system and the capacity to make informed choices, their ability to be involved in decisions should be assessed individually rather than relying solely on the age criteria of the law and their parents' views.

A unique area for consideration of informed consent is in the international context, either conducting care or clinical research in foreign settings or caring for individuals from other countries with widely differing viewpoints regarding individual informed consent. For example, if the prevailing standard for decision making by a woman is that her closest male relative makes it for her, how is that standard accommodated within our present autonomy-based system? In international research, these issues have presented major concerns when women were assigned to placebo or treatment groups and consent was accepted from male relatives (12). Furthermore, the coercive effect of access to health care through clinical trials when no other access to health care is available creates real questions about the validity and freedom of choice for participants in these studies (13). Guidelines for limiting coercion and ensuring the ability to choose participation in research are being developed for international research. However, it is important to recognize that these same issues exist in a microcosm when caring for patients from certain cultures and foreign countries in daily practice. Ensuring that the patient can make the choice herself or freely chooses to have a relative make it for her remains an important element of informed consent between individual physicians and individual patients.

Beneficence and Nonmaleficence

The principles of beneficence and nonmaleficence are the basis of medical care—the "to do good and no harm" of Hippocrates. However, these issues are often clouded by other decision makers, consultants, family pressures, and sometimes financial constraints or conflicts of interests. Of all the principles of good medical care, benefit is the one that continually must be reassessed. Simple questions often have no answers. What is the medical indication? How does the proposed therapy address this issue? How much will this treatment benefit the patient? How much will it extend the patient's life? Furthermore, when confronted with multiple medical problems and consultants, physicians should ask how much treatment will be of benefit given all the patient's problems (e.g., failing kidneys, progressive cardiomyopathy, HIV-positive status, and respiratory failure) rather than necessarily attempting intubation and respiratory support to treat the immediate problem.

The benefit or futility of the treatment, along with quality-of-life considerations, should be considered in all aspects of patient care. It is best to weigh all of the relevant issues in a systematic fashion. Some systematic approaches depend on a sequential gathering of all the pertinent information in four domains: medical indications (benefit and harm), patient preferences (autonomy), quality of life, and contextual issues (justice) (5). Other approaches identify decision makers, followed by facts, and then ethical principles. It is important for physicians to select an ethical model of analysis with which to practice so that, when faced with troubling and complex decisions, a system is available to help clarify the issues.

Medical Futility

The essence of good medical care is to attempt to be as clear as possible about the outcomes of the proposed interventions. If the proposed intervention (e.g., continued respiratory support or initiating support) has a very low or highly unlikely chance of success, intervention might be considered futile. Physicians have no obligation to continue or initiate therapies of no benefit (14). The decision to withdraw or withhold care, however, is one that must be accompanied by an effort to ensure that the patient or her surrogate decision maker is educated about the decision and agrees with it. Other issues, such as family concerns, can and should modify decisions if the overall well-being of the patient and of the family is best served. For example, waiting (within reason) to withdraw life support may be appropriate to allow a family to reach consensus or a distant family member to see the patient for a last time.

Quality of Life

Quality of life is a much used, often unclear term. In the care of patients, quality of life is the effect of therapy on the patient's experience of living based on her perspective. It is perilous and wholly speculative to assume that physicians know what quality of life represents for a particular patient judging from a personal reaction. It is instructive, however, to attempt to guess what it means and then seek the patient's perspective. The results may be surprising. For example, when offered a new drug for ovarian cancer, a patient might prefer to decline the treatment because the side effects may not be acceptable even when there may be a reasonable chance that her life may be slightly prolonged. In some instances, the physician may not believe that further treatment is justified but the patient finds joy and fulfillment in preserving her existence as long as possible.

Controversy exists regarding whether currently available quality-of-life measurement systems will provide information to help patients make decisions (15). Information from quality-of-life studies might be judged by criteria that include whether the measured aspects of the patient's life were based on the patient's views or the physician's clinical experience (16). Informing patients of others' experiences with alternative treatments may help in their decision making, but it is never a substitute for the individual patient's decisions.

Professional Relations

Conflict of Interest

All professionals have multiple interests that affect their decisions. Contractual and covenantal relationships between physician and patient are intertwined and complicated by health care payers and colleagues, which creates considerable pressure. The conflict with financial considerations directly influences how patients' lives are affected, often without their consent. Rennie (17) described that pressure eloquently: "Instead of receiving more respect (for more responsibility), physicians feel they are being increasingly questioned, challenged, and sued. Looking after a patient seems less and less a compact between two people and more a match in which increasing numbers of spectators claim the right to interfere and referee." An honest response to this environment is for the physician to attempt to protect his or her efforts by assuming that the physician–patient relationship is contractual, and only contractual, in nature. This allocation of responsibility and authority for the contract precludes the need for the covenant between the physician and patient. For example, a contract, insurance, or managed care plan may discourage referral to a more knowledgeable specialist, removing the physician's responsibility. Thus, the contract establishes the extent of the physician–patient relationship. All health care providers must decide whether they will practice within a covenantal or contractual relationship and whether the relationship they develop remains true to this decision. In either setting, a reasonable perception of that relationship is "one that allows clients as much freedom as possible to determine how their lives are affected as is reasonably warranted on the basis of their ability to make decisions" (18).

Health Care Payers

An insurance coverage plan may demand that physicians assume the role of gatekeeper and administrator. Patients can be penalized for a lack of knowledge about their future desires or needs and the lack of alternatives to address the changes in those needs. Patients are equally penalized when they develop costly medical conditions that would not be covered if they moved from plan to plan. These situations often place the physician in the position of being the arbiter of patients' coverage rather than acting as an advocate and adviser. It is an untenable position for physicians because they often cannot change the conditions or structure of the plan but are made to be the administrators of it.

In an effort to improve physician compliance with and interest in decreasing costs, intense financial conflicts of interest can be brought to bear on physicians by health care plans. If a physician's profile on costs or referral is too high, he or she might be excluded from the plan, thus decreasing his or her ability to earn a living or to provide care to certain patients with whom a relationship has developed. Conversely, a physician may receive a greater salary or bonus if the plan makes more money. The ability to earn a living and to see patients in the future is dependent on maintaining relationships with various plans and other physicians. These are compelling loyalties and conflicts that cannot be ignored (19–21).

These conflicts are substantially different from those of older fee-for-service plans, although the ultimate effect on the patient can be the same. In fee-for-service plans, financial gain may result in failure to refer a patient, or referral is restricted to those cases in which the financial gain is derived by return referral of other patients (22). Patients may be unaware of these underlying conflicts, a situation that elevates conflict of interest to an ethical problem.

A patient has a right to know what her plan covers, to whom she is being referred and why, and the credentials of those to whom she is referred. The reality is that health care providers make many decisions under the pressure of multiple conflicts of interest. Physicians are potentially caught between self-interest and professional integrity. Whether it is the more blatant lying about indications for a procedure in order to receive reimbursement or a more subtle persuasion to sign up for a certain protocol because of points earned for a study group, the outcome for individual and society's relationship with health care providers is damaged by failure to recognize and specifically address conflicts of interest that impede decision making (23). Focusing clearly on the priority of the patient's best interest and responsibly rejecting choices that compromise the patient's needs are ethical requirements.

Institutions, third-party payers, and legislatures have avoided accountability for revealing conflicts of interest to those to whom they offer services. The restrictions of health care plans are never placed in as equally prominent a position as the coverage. The coverage choices can be quite arbitrary, and there is rarely an easily accessible and usable system for challenging them. The social and financial conflicts of interest of these payers can directly affect the setting and nature of the relationship between physician and patient. To deal with ambiguous and sometimes capricious decision making, revelation of the conflicts of interest and accountability for choices should be demanded by physician and patient (24).

Legal Problems

Abuses of the system (e.g., referral for financial gain) have led to proposals and legislation, often referred to as Stark I and II, affecting physicians' ability to send patients to local laboratories and facilities in which they have a potential for financial gain. Although there have been clearly documented abuses, the same legislation would affect rural clinics and laboratories in which the only capital available is obtained through the rural physicians. States vary on the statutory legislation regarding this issue. Regardless of the laws, however, it is ethically required that financial conflicts of interest be revealed to patients (25–28).

Another abuse of the physician–patient relationship caused by financial conflicts of interest is fraudulent Medicare and Medicaid billings. This activity resulted in the Fraud and Abuse Act of 1987 (42. U.S.C. at 1320a–7b), which prohibits any individual or entity making false claims or soliciting or receiving any remuneration in cash or any kind, directly or indirectly, overtly or covertly, to induce a referral. Indictments under these laws are felonies, with steep fines, jail sentences, and loss of the license to practice medicine. Physicians should be aware of the legal ramifications of their referral and billing practices (23,29).

Harassment

The goal of medicine is excellence in the care of patients and, often, research and education that will advance the practice of medicine. Thus, everyone involved in the process should be able to pursue the common goal on equal footing and without harassment that interferes with employees' or colleagues' ability to work or be equally promoted in that environment. Every office and institution must have written policies on discrimination and sexual harassment that detail inappropriate behavior and state specific steps to be taken to correct an inappropriate situation. The legal sanction for this right is encoded in both statutory law through the Civil Rights Act of 1964 [42 U.S.C.A. at 2000e–2000e–17 (West 1981 and Supp. 1988)] and reinforced with judicial action (case or precedential law) by state and U.S. Supreme Court decisions. In particular, charges of sexual harassment can be raised as a result of unwelcome sexual conduct or a hostile workplace (such as areas of medicine that have been known for antifeminist attitudes in the past). As stated in one legal case, "a female does not assume the risk of harassment by voluntarily entering an abusive, antifemale environment" (Barbetta v. Chemlawn Service Co., 669 F, Supp. 569, WDNY, 1989). The environment must change; it is not acceptable to expect the men or women to adapt because "they knew what it would be like." The tension in the legal debate regarding harassment (sexual, racial, disability) always hinges on the weight of protection of free speech and the right of the individual to equality and a nonhostile work environment.

Stress Management

There is little doubt that the day-to-day stress of practicing medicine is significant. Besides the acknowledged stress of the time pressures and responsibility of medicine, the current health care environment has had a detrimental effect on physicians' job security, with concurrent health risks (30). Stress takes a toll not only on cardiac function (31) but also on the practice of medicine and life outside of medicine (32).

Responding to stress through drug or alcohol abuse increases overall health and marital problems and decreases effectiveness in practice. In a long-term prospective study of medical students, individuals with high-risk (e.g., volatile, argumentative, aggressive) temperaments have been shown to have a high rate of premature death (particularly before 55 years of age) (33). Adequate sleep, reasonable working hours, exercise, and nutritional balance have been shown to be directly related to decreases in psychological distress (34). Simple relaxation training has been shown to decrease gastroesophageal reflux in response to stress (35).

The pace that physicians maintain has a seductive quality that can easily mask the need for stress reduction by means of good health practices, exercise, and relaxation training. The answer to increased stress is not to work harder and extract the time to work harder from the relaxing and enjoyable pursuits that exist outside medicine. The outcome (in terms of psychological and physical optimal functioning) of that strategy is in neither the physician's nor the patient's best interest. Both the welfare of the patient and the welfare of the physician are enhanced by a planned strategy of good health practices and relaxation. Furthermore, such a strategy is important to all members of the health care team. By providing such leadership, physicians can contribute to a better work and health care environment for everyone.

Society and Medicine

Justice

Some of the ethical and legal problems in the practice of gynecology relate to the fair and equitable distribution of burdens and benefits. How benefits are distributed is a matter of great debate. There are various methods of proposed distribution:

- Equal shares (everyone has the same number of health care dollars per year)
- Need (only those people who need health care get the dollars)
- Queuing (the first in line for a transplant gets it)
- Merit (those with more serious illnesses receive special benefits)
- Contribution (those who have paid more into their health care fund get more health care)

Each of these principles could be appropriate as a measure of just allocation of health care dollars, but each will affect individual patients in different ways. Only recently has just distribution become a major issue in health care. The principles of justice apply only when the resource is desired or beneficial and to some extent scarce (36).

The traditional approach to medicine has been for practitioners to accept the intense focus on the individual patient. However, the current changes in medicine will alter the focus from the patient to a population (37)—"in the emerging medicine, the presenting patient, more than ever before, will be a representative of a class, and the science that makes possible the care of the patient will refer prominently to the population from which that patient comes." Physicians are increasingly bound by accumulating outcomes data (population statistics) to modify the treatment of an individual in view of the larger population statistics. If, for example, the outcome of liver transplantation is only 20% successful in a patient with a certain set of medical problems, that transplant may instead be offered to someone who has an 85% chance of success. Theoretically, the former individual might have a successful transplant and the procedure might fail in the latter, but population statistics have been used to allocate this scarce resource. The benefit has been measured by statistics that predict success, not by other forms of justice allocation by need, queuing, merit, or contribution. This approach represents a major change in the traditional dedication of health care to the benefits of individual patients. With scarce resources, the overall benefits for all patients are considered in conjunction with the individual benefits for one patient.

There has always been an inequity in the distribution of health care access and resources. This inequity has not been seen by many health care providers who do not care for those patients who are unable to gain access, such as those who lack transportation or live in rural areas or where limits are imposed by lack of health care providers, time, and financial resources. Social discrimination sometimes leads to inequity of distribution of health care. Minorities are less likely to see private physicians or specialists, regardless of their income or source of health care funding (38–40). Thus, health care is rationed by default.

Health care providers must shift the paradigm from the absolute "do everything possible for this patient" to the proportionate "do everything reasonable for all patients" (5). To reform the health care system requires not just judicial, legislative, or business mandates but also attention to the other social components that can pose obstacles to efforts to expand health care beyond a focus on individual patients.

Health Care Reform

The tension between understanding health as an inherently individual matter (in which the receipt of health care is critical to individual well-being) and as a communal resource (in which distribution of well-being throughout society is the goal) underpins much of the political and social debate surrounding health care reform (41). The questions of health care reform are: What is the proper balance between individual and collective good? and Who will pay for basic health care? Because much of health care reform requires a balancing of competing goals, legislation should specifically address how this balance can be achieved. The role of government would be the following:

- Regulating access of individuals to health care
- Regulating potential harms to the public health (e.g., smoking, pollution, drug use)
- Promoting health practices of benefit to large populations (e.g., immunization, fluoridation of water)

Decisions regarding both the amount and distribution of resources are often made by health care payers, not individual providers. The health insurance industry determines what are "reasonable and customary" charges and what will be covered. The government decides (often with intense special-interest pressure) what will be covered by Medicare and Medicaid (42,43). These decisions directly affect patient care. For that reason, health care providers cannot ethically remain silent when the health and well-being of their individual patients and their communities are adversely affected by health care reform decisions. Health care providers should assess proposed reforms in light of their value to the community and to individual patients and then formulate their own criteria for judging proposals for health care reform (44–47). Furthermore, initiation and support of research focused on the outcomes of care delivered by gynecologists (financial aspects, quality-of-life measures, survival, morbidity, and mortality) will allow the discipline to have a real voice in determining what choices are made for health care for women.

References

1. **May WF.** Code and covenant or philanthropy and contract. *Hastings Cent Rep* 1975;5:29–38.
2. **Privacy Protection Study Commission.** *Personal privacy in an information society.* Washington, DC: U.S. Government Printing Office, 1977.
3. **Cain J.** Confidentiality. In: APGO Task Force on Medical Ethics. *Exploring medical-legal issues in obstetrics and gynecology.* Washington, DC: APGO, 1994:43–5.

4. **Tobriner MO.** Majority Opinion, California Supreme Court, 1 July 1976. *California Reporter* (West Publishing Company) 1976:14–33.

5. **Jonsen AR, Siegler M, Winslade WJ.** *Clinical ethics.* New York: McGraw-Hill, 1992:5–61.

6. **American College of Obstetricians and Gynecologists.** *Ethical dimensions of informed consent.* Committee Opinion, No. 108. Washington, DC: ACOG, 1992.

7. **Katz J.** Informed consent: must it remain a fairy tale? *J Contemp Health Law Policy* 1994;10:69–91.

8. **Pellegrino ED.** Patient and physician autonomy: conflicting rights and obligations in the physician-patient relationship. *J Contemp Health Law Policy* 1994;10:47–68.

9. **Buchanan AE, Brock DW.** *Deciding for others: the ethics of surrogate decision making.* New York: Cambridge University Press, 1989.

10. **Ackerman T.** The limits of beneficence: Jehovah's Witnesses and childhood cancer. *Hastings Cent Rep* 1980;10:13–16.

11. **Nocon JJ.** Selected minor consent laws for reproductive health care. In: APGO Task Force on Medical Ethics. *Exploring medical-legal issues in obstetrics and gynecology.* Washington, DC: APGO, 1994:129–136.

12. **Loue S, Okello D.** Research bioethics in the Ugandan context. II. Procedural and substantive reform. *J Law Med Ethics* 2000;28:165–173.

13. **Emanuel E, Wendler D, Grady C.** What makes clinical research ethical. *JAMA* 2000;283:2701–2711.

14. **Jecker NS, Schneiderman LJ.** Medical futility: the duty not to treat. *Camb Q Healthc Ethics* 1993;2: 151–159.

15. **Gill TM, Feinstein AR.** A critical appraisal of the quality of quality of life measurements. *JAMA* 1994;262:619–626.

16. **Guyatt GH, Cook DJ.** Health status, quality of life and the individual. *JAMA* 1994;272:630–631.

17. **Rennie D.** Let us focus your worries! Health care policy: a clinical approach. *JAMA* 1994;272:631–632.

18. **Bailees MD.** The professional-client relationship. In: *Professional ethics.* Belmont, CA: Wadsworth, 1981.

19. **Ellsbury K.** Can the family physician avoid conflict of interest in the gatekeeper role? An affirmative view. *J Fam Pract* 1989;28:698–701.

20. **Stephens GG.** Can the family physician avoid conflict of interest in the gatekeeper role? An opposing view. *J Fam Pract* 1989;28:701–704.

21. **Miles C.** Resource allocation in the National Health Service. In: **Byrne P,** ed. *Ethics and the law in health care and research.* New York: John Wiley and Sons, 1990.

22. **Cain JM, Jonsen AR.** Specialists and generalists in obstetrics and gynecology: conflicts of interest in referral and an ethical alternative. *Womens Health Issues* 1992;2:137–145.

23. **American College of Obstetricians and Gynecologists.** *Committee opinion: deception.* No. 87. Washington, DC: ACOG, 1990.

24. **Wrenn K.** No insurance, no admission. *N Engl J Med* 1985;392:373–374.

25. **Hyman D, Williamson JV.** Fraud and abuse: setting the limits on physicians' entrepreneurship. *N Engl J Med* 1989;320:1275.

26. **McDowell TN Jr.** Physician self referral arrangements: legitimate business or unethical entrepreneurialism. *Am J Law Med* 1989;15:61–109.

27. **Stark F.** Ethics in patient referrals. *Acad Med* 1989;64:146–147.

28. **Green RM.** Medical joint-venturing: an ethical perspective. *Hastings Cent Rep* 1990;20:22–26.

29. **Nocon JJ.** Fraud and abuse: employment kickbacks and physician recruitment. In: APGO Task Force on Medical Ethics. *Exploring medical-legal issues in obstetrics and gynecology.* Washington, DC: APGO, 1994:69–74.

30. **Heaney CA, Isreal BA, House JS.** Chronic job insecurity among automobile workers: effects on job satisfaction and health. *Soc Sci Med* 1994;38:1431–1437.

31. **Sloan RP, Shapiro PA, Bagiella E, et al.** Effect of mental stress throughout the day on cardiac autonomic control. *Biol Psychol* 1994;37:89–99.

32. **Serry N, Bloch S, Ball R, et al.** Drug and alcohol abuse by doctors. *Med J Aust* 1994;60:402–407.

33. **Graves PL, Mead LA, Wang NY, et al.** Temperament as a potential predictor of mortality: evidence from a 41 year prospective study. *J Behav Med* 1994;17:111–126.

34. **Ezoe S, Morimoto K.** Behavioral lifestyle and mental health status of Japanese workers. *Prev Med* 1994;23:98–105.

35. **McDonald HJ, Bradley LA, Bailey MA, et al.** Relaxation training reduces symptom reports and acid exposure in patients with gastroesophageal reflux disease. *Gastroenterology* 1994;107:61–69.

36. **Daniels N.** *Just health care.* Cambridge, UK: Cambridge University Press, 1985.

37. **Jonsen AR.** *The new medicine and the old ethics.* Boston: Harvard University Press, 1990.

38. **Watson SD.** Minority access and health reform: a civil right to health care. *J Law Med Ethics* 1994;22:127–137.

39. **Watson SD.** Health care in the inner city: asking the right question. *N C Law Rev* 1993;71:1661–1663.

40. **Freeman HE, Blendon RJ, Aiken LH, et al.** Americans report on their access to health care. *Health Aff (Millwood)* 1987;6:6–8.

41. **Burris S.** Thoughts on the law and the public's health. *J Law Med Ethics* 1994;22:141–146.

42. **Evans RW.** Health care technology and the inevitability of resource allocation and rationing decisions: part 2. *JAMA* 1983;249:2208–2210.

43. **President's Commission for the Study of Ethical Problems in Medicine and Biomedical and Behavioral Research.** *Securing access to health care: the ethical implications of differences in availability of health services.* Washington, DC: Government Printing Office, 1983:1–3.

44. **Eddy DM.** What care is essential? *JAMA* 1991;265:786–788.

45. **Sultz H.** Health policy: if you don't know where you're going, any road will take you. *Am J Public Health* 1991;81:418–420.

46. **Agich GJ.** Medicine as business and profession. *Theor Med Bioeth* 1990;2:311–324.

47. **Daniels N.** Is the Oregon rationing plan fair? *JAMA* 1991;265:2232–2235.

3 Quality Assessment, Performance Improvement, and Patient Safety

Joseph C. Gambone
Robert C. Reiter
Paul A. Gluck

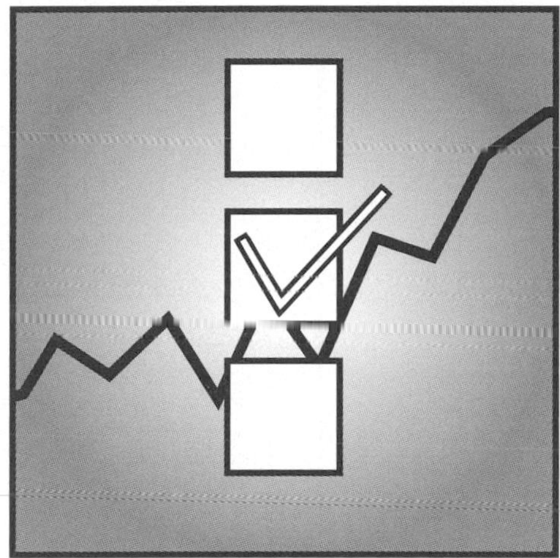

For more than 20 years, the need to maintain or increase the quality of health care while controlling its cost has stimulated a great deal of interest and activity in quality assessment and performance improvement. A report from the Institute of Medicine (IOM) on patient safety has generated intense public interest and concern about the high estimated number of preventable deaths caused by medical errors (1). Although the conclusions of this report are controversial, it raises fundamental and disturbing questions about health care quality and performance.

The annual United States per capita expenditure for health care (in constant dollars) had risen steadily from about $950 in 1970 to about $3,400 in 1992 (about 12% increase per year). Although efforts in the 1990s to "manage" care and its costs were reasonably successful in slowing annual health care cost increases, they have recently been returning to double digits. Currently, annual United States per capita expenditure is estimated to exceed $4,500 (about 3.2% increase per year since 1992). The "political" failure and public distrust of 1990s-style managed care has resulted in predictions of its demise despite well-documented economic success (2). Before the mid-1990s, much of the increase in health care costs had been shifted from individuals to state and federal governments and to employers (Fig. 3.1). More recently, employers have been setting limits on their contributions to health care benefits and shifting more of the increased costs to their employees. Currently, the United States spends more on health care (about 14% of gross domestic product) than on education and defense combined. Despite this enormous outlay of resources, there is concern about the overall quality of health care (3,4). The health status of U.S. residents (in terms of life expectancy, neonatal mortality, and rates of illness and disability) is poorer than that of people living in most European and Scandinavian countries, the United Kingdom, Japan, and Canada, although these countries spend far less per capita on health care. Quality improvement programs in other industries have shown that management methods can both increase quality and reduce costs. Because of concerns about quality, cost, and safety, patients, as well as private and public third-party payers, are demanding ongoing quality assessment and performance improvement programs in health care delivery systems.

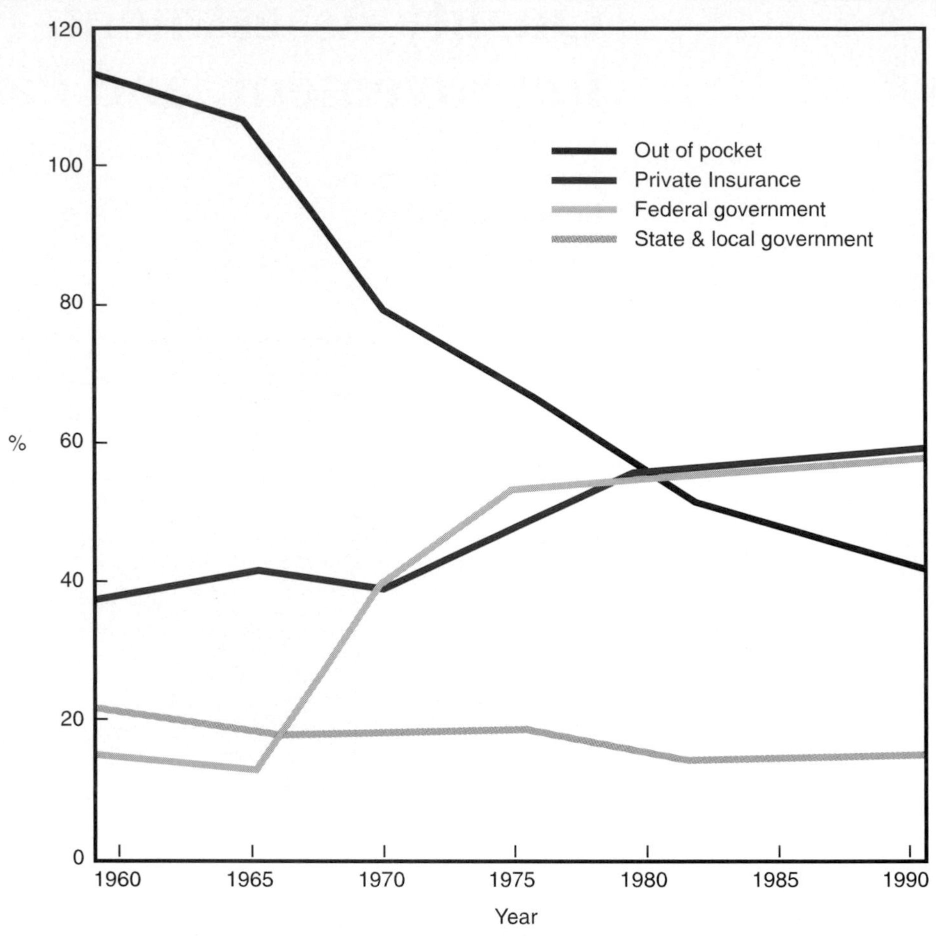

Figure 3.1 Sources of spending in U.S. health care, 1960–1990. Note that third-party payment steadily replaced direct payment during this interval. After a long decline, out of pocket spending is expected to rise. (Data from U.S. Congressional Budget Office, 1992).

Quality Assurance

The medical profession traditionally has focused its efforts on assessing and improving the quality of health services through internal, self-imposed, retrospective peer review. Examples of such mechanisms are morbidity and mortality (M&M) conferences, medical society–sponsored and state-legislated peer-review programs, surgical case reviews (tissue committees), and the specialty board certification processes. These programs review adverse occurrences retrospectively (e.g., assessment of medical and surgical complications and review of misdiagnoses). **Although useful as part of the peer-review process, these quality assurance (QA) programs are not aimed at prevention of errors and are not designed to assess and improve the effectiveness of health care services and procedures** (5).

The differences between traditional QA programs and newer performance improvement and quality management programs, such as continuous quality improvement (CQI) or total quality management (TQM), are presented in Fig. 3.2. QA programs are designed to identify and eliminate the small percentage of substandard care represented on the left side of the normal curve (the "bad apple" approach). Most "standard" care occurs in the middle of the curve, however, and is the focus of newer programs like CQI. Such programs are designed to study prospectively the processes of care based on need and to

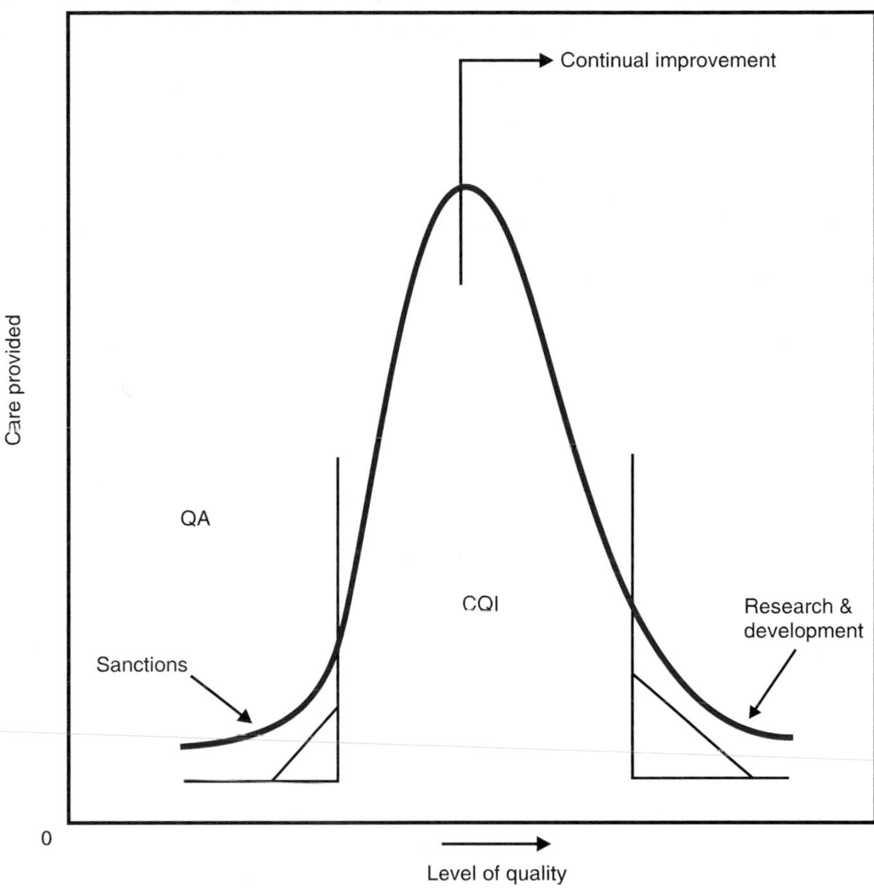

Figure 3.2 The hypothetical relationship between quality assurance (QA) and quality or performance improvement.

improve outcomes by the reduction of unintended variation (6). The right side of the curve represents state-of-the-art practice usually performed under protocols at universities and other large centers of excellence that are monitored by institutional review boards and national research groups such as the National Cancer Institute and the Gynecologic Oncology Group. As more emphasis is placed on quality management programs in health care, innovations should come from both traditional research and performance improvement efforts.

Quality management programs such as CQI, TQM, and performance improvement each have three essential elements (7):

1. To understand customers (patients, payers, and other clients) and to link that knowledge to the activities of the organization
2. To mold the culture (beliefs and performance characteristics) of the organization through the deeds of leaders; to foster pride, enjoyment, collaboration, and scientific thinking
3. To increase knowledge (of how to improve performance) continuously and to control variation (unintended and wasteful differences in performance) by scientific methods

Health care professionals often do not like to refer to health care services as products and patients as customers or consumers. The older, paternalistic attitude (i.e., patients passively agreeing to health care procedures that were determined largely by health care providers) is being replaced by a more egalitarian view of patients as intelligent and informed consumers who should participate in their care (8). The consumerism movement in health care is predicated on the belief that health care services should conform to acceptable standards of quality, efficiency, and safety (9). This newer attitude may lead to improved communication and shared decision making (between patient and provider) and should alter the wasteful practice of "defensive medicine," which has been shown to increase health care costs significantly (10,11).

Principles of Quality Assessment

Quality means different things in different situations. The concept of quality in products (e.g., consumer goods and state-of-the-art machinery) is different than that of complex services (e.g., health care delivery to people). However, many of the principles of quality assessment and improvement that have been shown to improve the quality of consumer goods and services can also be applied to the evaluation and improvement of health services. There are certain principles of quality assessment that should be considered when attempting to measure and improve health care quality.

Efficacy, Effectiveness, and Efficiency

***Efficacy* and *effectiveness* are similar terms that are often used interchangeably to describe evaluations of outcomes of health care services and procedures. As defined by the Institute of Medicine, *efficacy* refers to what an intervention or procedure can accomplish under ideal conditions and when applied to appropriate patients (12). *Effectiveness* refers to the actual performance in customary practice of an intervention or procedure.** An example of this difference is the theoretical success rate (*efficacy*) of oral contraception used for one year (99% successful at preventing pregnancy) versus the actual or *use-rate,* effectiveness, usually reported to be 93% to 97%. Most health care decisions have been based on efficacy rates obtained from controlled clinical trials rather than the actual effectiveness of such decisions. One of the major challenges for quality assessment and management programs is to develop and use measurements that reflect the actual, or real-life, success rates of treatment options so that *evidence-based* decision making can replace *authority-based* decision making. Also, strategies need to be developed to improve patient compliance rates in order to increase the likelihood that the actual effectiveness is as close as possible to theoretical efficacy (13).

***Efficiency* describes the relative "waste" or resource use (complications and costs) of alternative effective interventions.** To realize meaningful improvements in health services, health professionals and organizations must develop more efficient interventions (e.g., medical therapy or expectant management versus surgical treatment for abnormal bleeding) when appropriate. The goal of health care quality improvement is optimal value. ***Value* is defined as quality divided by the cost, or as the quotient of outcomes (benefits) divided by resources used:**

Value = outcomes/resource use

Optimal versus Maximal Care

The assessment of the quality of health care depends on whether the goal of the system is to provide maximally effective or optimally effective care (14). Figure 3.3 shows a theoretical representation of the difference between maximally effective health care *(Point B),* in which every conceivable intervention is offered regardless of cost to those who can afford it, and optimally effective health care *(Point A),* in which resources are used in a manner that will provide the most good for as many people as possible. Maximized health care emphasizes individual intervention, whereas optimized care emphasizes public health care and prevention. When optimal health care becomes the goal of a health care system, conflicting individual and societal needs must be resolved.

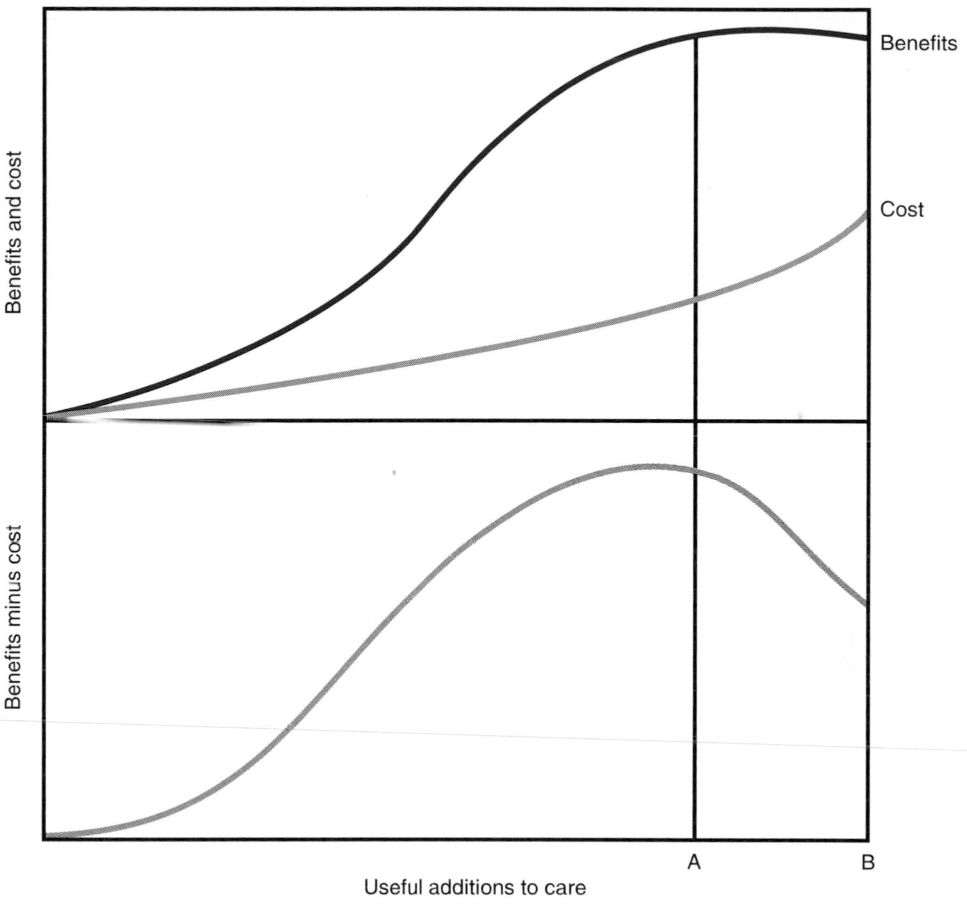

Figure 3.3 The "optimal" versus the "maximal" benefits and costs of medical treatments. On the *top panel,* the benefits to health and the costs of care are plotted. On the *bottom panel,* the cost is subtracted from the benefits, illustrating that after a certain point, additions of care may detract from the benefits. (From Donabedian A. The quality of care: How can it be assessed. *JAMA* 1988;260:1743–1748, with permission.)

Assessing Outcomes

A widely accepted system for assessing the quality of health care is based on the measurement of indicators of structure, process, and outcome (15). *Structure* includes the resources, equipment, and people who provide health care. *Process* is the method by which a procedure or course of action is executed. *Outcome* includes the complications, adverse events, and short-term results of interventions, as well as the patient's health status and health-related quality of life after treatment, which reflects the effectiveness of the intervention.

Evaluation of health care structure involves the assessment of the stable and tangible resources needed to provide care, such as safe and adequately sized operating rooms and properly functioning equipment. Other examples of structural elements include the aspects of the medical staff's qualifications, such as school accreditation, licensure, continuing medical education credits, and specialty board certification. Although these elements form the foundation of a health care organization or system, there is a weak correlation between structural assessment and other measures of the quality of care, such as clinical outcomes (16). Therefore, many health services researchers believe that organizations need to measure clinical outcomes directly (including not only death and short-term morbidity but also disability and health-related quality-of-life issues) if they hope to improve both the effectiveness and

Table 3.1. Clinical and Health Outcomes and Their Corresponding Intermediate or Surrogate Endpoints: Some Examples

Clinical or Health Outcomes	*Intermediate or Surrogate Endpoints*
Longevity	Dilated coronary arteries
Quality of life	Five-year survival rate
Take baby home	Pregnancy
Pain relief	Fewer adhesions
No transfusion	Less blood loss

efficiency of health care delivery. Their research also emphasizes measurement of clinical or health outcomes that are defined as those that patients can experience and value without the interpretation of a health care provider. Examples of clinical or health outcomes and their corresponding intermediate or surrogate end points are presented in Table 3.1. Ultimately, longevity and quality-of-life factors may be the only relevant outcomes of health care.

Quality-of-Life Measurement

In the past, traditional quality assessment programs have tended to focus on the assessment of short-term risks and the confirmation of pathologic diagnoses. This effort has usually been limited to quantification of mortality and major morbidity—such as infection, blood transfusion, and reoperation—occurring while the patient was hospitalized and verified by tissue diagnosis. Most standardized lists of clinical QA indicators are from the medical model of outcomes assessment. Although the importance of these kinds of indicators seems obvious, these indicators may have little or no relevance to the more fundamental question of actual effectiveness of a procedure in terms of preserving or enhancing quality of life. For example, if a patient with pelvic pain undergoes a hysterectomy for leiomyomas, experiences no short-term complications, and has a diagnosis that is confirmed histologically, the procedure may be considered successful from the standpoint of surgical risk management, short-term outcome, and histologic verification. However, if the patient continues to experience pain and has no improvement in the quality of her life, the surgery has been, in reality, unsuccessful. Short-term risk indicators often have little or no bearing on whether the procedure actually works.

Behavioral Model of Health Outcomes

Efforts to measure the success or the effectiveness of health care procedures in the United States are based on the traditional medical model in which a patient is evaluated for a symptom, diagnosed as having a condition, and treated for that diagnosis. A procedure is usually considered successful if the diagnosis is confirmed.

Medicine has traditionally relied on short-term risk indicators and histologic confirmation because these measurements seem more objective and quantifiable. Death and infection rates, blood loss, and rates of histologic verification can all be measured and expressed numerically. Crucial to the application of a more predictive behavioral model in clinical outcomes research are several statistically valid and reliable methods to measure health-related quality of life. Many measures have been developed and validated, but few are used in clinical practice (17).

Using the *behavioral model* of effectiveness, the concept of *quality-adjusted life-years* (QALY) has been proposed to measure the benefit, in both quantity and quality of life, of a health care procedure (18). The number of QALYs is determined by combining the extra years of life that a procedure offers with a validated measure of eight categories of disability and four measures of distress. The use of this methodology allows standardized comparison of the cost of entirely different health care procedures. Despite its inadequacies, the medical model has been the standard, but the behavioral model of outcomes is now becoming incorporated into health care evaluation and research (19). Scales of health-related quality-of-life issues, called the *SF-36* and the *SF-12* (short form 36 and short form 12, the health-status tool derived from the RAND Medical Outcomes Survey), have been developed (20).

Performance Improvement

Most methods for the assessment of the quality of health care and the delivery of health services have been based on the premise that quality is the sole responsibility of the health care practitioner. Because the practitioner's technical skills, knowledge, and interpersonal interactions are the basis for quality of patient care and its delivery, many regulatory agencies [e.g., the Joint Commission on the Accreditation of Health Care Organizations (JCAHO)] and hospitals have created traditional QA models that focus mostly on the practitioner. However, quality of care is determined by many interacting forces, and the practitioner clearly does not deliver care in isolation. The delivery of health care requires the integration and management of many processes. The practitioner's ability to deliver care is influenced by the environment, the ability and skill of support staff, policies and procedures, facilities, governing processes, methods of work, and equipment and materials available, as well as innumerable patient variables such as severity of illness, concurrent illness (comorbidity), and social support. Historically, QA efforts attempted to monitor these processes to document bad outcomes. However, this approach has not proved to be adequate in improving the quality of care (21). Regulatory agencies and hospitals are now focusing on the overall performance of health care organizations in terms of clinical or health outcomes.

Performance improvements in health care have been based on knowledge that physicians and other health care professionals acquired in medical and other professional schools. Improvements have been brought about by clinicians applying knowledge developed by discipline-specific experts (22). The recent national emphasis on health care reform is an indication that the past rate of improvements is not sufficient to meet the financial needs and expectations of society. Performance improvements in efficiency must be made at a faster pace because consumers are seeking greater value for and access to health care services. A theoretical basis for organizational change that promotes continuous improvement includes knowledge of a system, knowledge of variation, and the theory of knowledge (23,24).

Knowledge of a System

The first component of continuous performance improvement is knowledge of a system. A *system* is defined as a network of interdependent components that work together to accomplish its aim. A system does not exist without an aim and is only capable of improving if there is a connection between the aim, the means of production, and the means of improving. An *open system* is one that permits continued access from outside the system. Because health care organizations are accountable to patients and to the community as a whole, they are considered open systems. The aim of an organization involves the integration of the knowledge of the social needs and the needs of patients.

Knowledge of a system includes the following aspects:

Customer knowledge. This is the basis of an organization's aim. The aim is derived by identifying the organization's customers and by understanding the measures used to judge quality. Meeting patient expectations is one of the most accurate ways to define quality.

How the organization provides its services. This is the means of producing a service, which involves knowledge of what is delivered, the processes or steps taken to deliver the services, the information and materials used to provide services, and the suppliers.

How the organization improves what it delivers. This involves knowledge of the aim and identification of areas for improvement that are likely to have the greatest impact.

Understanding the interrelationships between the aim, the customers, the primary areas for improvement, and the specific processes that can be improved is known as *systems thinking.* When a health care organization is focused on providing as many services as possible without consideration for the needs of the community and their customers, it will eventually fail to deliver quality services. Proper perspective for customer needs and preferences gained through a process called *strategic planning* may even lead to a competitive advantage for a health care organization (25).

Knowledge of Variation

Another element of continuous improvement is knowledge of variation. Variation is present in every aspect of our lives. Variation is inherent to everyone's behavior, learning styles, and ways of performing a task. Although the presence of variation, or uniqueness, can be considered a kind of quality, most services are judged on the basis of predictability and a low level of variation. When a service is thought to be of high quality, we expect it to be exactly the same each time, and if there is to be any variation, it must be better.

To improve health products and services continually, it is necessary to know the customers, their needs, and how they judge the quality of health services. The processes by which health services are delivered must be understood and unintended variations reduced. If an organization is to improve and be innovative, it must plan changes that are based on knowledge of what can be better. Two types of variation found in production processes are those that occur by chance (common cause) and those due to assignable causes (special causes) (26). The ability to differentiate between these two types of variation is essential to making improvements in health care.

Clinicians regularly make decisions in their practices based on variation. For example, a physician making frequent rounds may note a change in a patient's temperature and may decide to treat or to observe the patient based on the temperature change and on experience (i.e., judgment). If the temperature variation is seen as special cause (i.e., infection), a decision may be made to add an antibiotic. However, if the change or variation is interpreted as common cause variation in temperature due to short-term, normal changes or chance, it may be ignored. If this happens often, the physician may alter the frequency of observation, thereby making an improvement to the monitoring process. Frequently, however, common cause variation is not recognized in health care, and the variation is acted on prematurely, resulting in the overuse of resources and a lower quality of care (7). If the approach is to measure and change, too many costly changes might be made.

Learning how to respond appropriately to variation in health care processes is a major challenge. Understanding and controlling variation in health care services should be the main emphasis of quality management. The notion of controlling variation, however, causes concern and skepticism in many health care professionals. Physicians who fear any effort to control variation are worried about the loss of options and about restrictions on their judgment. As Berwick points out (7), however, "The (problem) is not considered, intentional variation, but rather unintended or misinterpreted variation in the work of health care. Unintended variation is stealing health care blind today. In controlling it, the health care system could potentially recover a bounty in wasted resources that would dwarf the puny rewards of cost-containment to date."

Variation in Utilization

One of the earliest and most compelling influences on modern health care quality assessment in the United States was a series of investigations that demonstrated a wide variation in the use of health care procedures (27). Although previous investigations had documented a twofold to fourfold difference in the rates of selected procedures both within the United States and between the United States and other industrialized countries, these variations usually were disregarded as secondary to population differences. However, a small-area analysis documented similar or even greater magnitudes of variation within small (25 to 50 miles) geographic regions that could not be explained by differences in patient characteristics or appropriate differences in standards of care (28).

Variations in utilization have now been analyzed for virtually all major surgical procedures, including hysterectomy and cesarean delivery (29,30). Also, variation in the performance of medical procedures, such as those used in the management of acute myocardial infarction and sepsis, have been identified (31). On the basis of these analyses, significant variation has been documented in utilization and in important outcomes such as complications, cost, and derived benefit (32). This type of analysis does not usually allow accurate assessment of which rate of utilization or outcome is appropriate. However, it can help to focus attention on the quality of health services and the complexities of using statistically valid methods to measure health care quality.

Variation in utilization of health care services can be categorized as follows:

1. Necessary and intended variation because of well-recognized patient differences such as severity of illness, comorbidity, and legitimate patient preferences
2. Acceptable but reducible variation because of uncertainty and lack of accurate information about outcomes
3. Unacceptable variation because of nonclinical factors, such as habitual differences in practice style, which are not grounded in knowledge or reason

Most of the differences in utilization rates of many health care procedures result from the last two categories.

Variation in Women's Health Care

Overall, the rate of inpatient surgery for females aged 15 to 44 years is more than 3 times that of males, excluding vaginal deliveries. The most commonly performed major surgical procedure in the United States is cesarean delivery, with about 950,000 procedures performed annually in the United States. Rates of cesarean delivery vary by region, state, and small geographic areas. Overall, the rate of cesarean deliveries is 12% to 40%, and the national mean is about 23%. Comparative rates for the United Kingdom are 6% to 12%.

Hysterectomy is the second most frequent inpatient surgical procedure in the United States. The total annual occurrence of hysterectomy for all ages, all indications, and all institutions (federal and nonfederal) in the United States is about 550,000. Hysterectomy rates in the southern and western United States are 50% to 75% higher than those in the Midwest and New England. A twofold to fivefold variation in utilization rates has been documented within states and small geographic areas within the United States (29). National rates in the United States are twice those in the United Kingdom and more than 3 times the rates in Sweden and Norway (33).

Hysterectomy utilization in the United States varies by both provider and patient characteristics. Studies of utilization patterns have demonstrated that older physicians are more likely to recommend hysterectomy than are younger physicians and that (when controlled for age) gender does not appear to influence hysterectomy decision making (34). With respect to patient variables, although hysterectomy utilization is similar among African American women and white women (35,36), low income and low educational level are risk factors for hysterectomy (37). By 65 years of age, the prevalence of hysterectomy is 40% for women with a high school education and 20% for women with a college education.

Short-term outcomes of hysterectomy vary significantly by race. African American women have a substantially higher relative risk (RR) for morbidity and in-hospital mortality (RR = 3.1) compared with age- and condition-matched white women (38). The reasons for this variation are not known. Quality management techniques are being applied to research in an attempt to reduce these wasteful variations.

The Theory of Knowledge

The final component of knowledge for improvement is the theory of knowledge. The *theory of knowledge* refers to the need for the application of a scientific method for improving performance. One model for testing small-scale change is called the **P**lan, **D**o, **S**tudy, **A**ct (PDSA) method (24). Unlike the ideal scientific method recommended for clinical trials, the PDSA method does not include a control group. Although randomized controlled trials have been considered to be the best way to determine the value of health care interventions, they have two distinct disadvantages: they are expensive, and they tend to define the efficacy of an intervention such as a drug or a surgical procedure. Because efficacy is the way an intervention works under ideal conditions, compared with effectiveness, which is the way an intervention works in everyday practice, health services researchers now recognize that it may not be possible to generalize about an intervention's effectiveness based on its efficacy as measured in a randomized trial. Also, it is too expensive to perform randomized trials in all situations in which the effectiveness of health care services need to be improved.

The PDSA cycle has been modified as the **F**ind a process, **O**rganize a team, **C**larify the process, **U**nderstand the variation, and **S**elect an improvement (**FOCUS**). The PDCA cycle has tested FOCUS for application to health care improvements (24). In this model, the **P** represents the need to *plan* an improvement by first identifying a change that might lead to improvement and then testing the change on a small scale. During this phase, who will do what, when the change will occur, and how the change will be communicated to those who will be affected are detailed. The **D** stands for *doing* or implementing the plan (change to the process) and collecting the data. The **C** stands for *checking* the data to determine whether the change to the process represents an improvement, and the **A** stands for *acting* or incorporating the change into the process if it is found to be an improvement. A new cycle with another change is started if an improvement was not recognized.

Health care organizations are seeking efficient ways to optimize their delivery of and to improve health care services. The notion that high-quality health care automatically means high cost is no longer accepted without question. At a time when many businesses have transformed themselves by using newer methods of quality management, enabling them to deliver high-quality goods and services at reasonable costs, health care professionals and organizations are beginning to test these improvement methods in medical and surgical practice.

Newer Methods for Improving Performance

Health services researchers and clinicians are beginning to develop and validate newer methods for the measurement and improvement of health care quality. For example, there is a need to make valid comparisons of quality between divergent populations and to correlate clinical performance with measurable processes of care. The goal of a new branch of investigation called *clinical outcomes sciences* is to obtain valid measures of relevant outcomes that are correlated with measurable processes of care so that changes in process can be identified and initiated, thereby improving outcomes. This discipline incorporates methodologies from divergent areas, such as epidemiology, clinical research, management, engineering, economics, and behavioral sciences.

Statistical adjustments are used to allow clinically dissimilar populations, such as high-risk and low-risk patients and those with complicated and uncomplicated conditions, to be compared. This procedure is called *case-mix adjustment* and controls for severity of illness and comorbidity (39,40). Outcomes that are assessed include traditional (medical model) measures, such as complications and adverse occurrences, as well as newer, well-validated measures of satisfaction, health, and functional status.

Concurrently, the processes of care are assessed. This would include measurement of resources used during an episode of care (e.g., supplies, medications, specialized personnel) and practice parameters (e.g., physician orders and nursing practices).

Measurement of the processes and outcomes of health care can be prohibitively expensive if this measurement is not integrated into the daily clinical care. For this reason, another goal of clinical quality outcomes research is to develop and incorporate methods of quality assessment into routine practice. This mechanism could be accomplished, for example, by using the SF-36 as a standard nursing intake form at the time of admission.

Analytic methods in clinical outcomes science rely heavily on multivariate statistics and iterative outcomes databases to provide valid correlations between measurable (and changeable) processes and outcomes. However, the mere identification of process changes that would improve outcomes does not ensure that they will, in fact, be used. For this reason, process and outcomes data must be linked to methods that will allow this information to be incorporated into clinical and operational decision making if they are to change behavior and improve outcomes. These analyses must be readily available both geographically and temporally at the point of care (the place and time that the decision is made) if they are to improve outcomes.

One approach to QA, performance improvement, and medical decision making that has been recommended (the PREPARED system) uses a checklist to analyze the value of a health care procedure before it is performed (9,41). The purpose is to review sequentially the critical data categories of information, each represented by a letter in the word *PREPARED,* that should be used to determine the most appropriate course of action or choice (42):

Procedure:	the course of action being considered
Reason:	the indication or rationale
Expectation:	the chances of benefit and failure
Preferences:	patient-centered priorities (utilities) affecting choice
Alternatives:	other reasonable options
Risks:	the potential for harm from procedures
Expenses:	all direct and indirect costs
Decision:	fully informed collaborative choice

Standardized procedural analysis using this sequenced checklist has been shown to improve health care decision making by increasing patient satisfaction and self-efficacy, thereby facilitating patient choice. It has the potential to improve the assessment of the quality and appropriateness of both provider and patient decision making.

Outcomes Research and Outcome-derived Clinical Guidelines

In the past, clinical practice guidelines or parameters have been largely derived by expert opinion and consensus. A major goal of clinical outcomes science is to allow for the development of guidelines based on actual measured outcomes that could self-adjust based on performance and newer methods of diagnosis and treatment. One such process for incorporating outcomes data into clinical practice is the *critical pathway–case management* method (43). In this method, consensus practice parameters for a given condition (e.g., management of preterm labor) are initially developed by a multidisciplinary team consisting of all professional, allied, and support services involved in the care of the target population. This list of parameters is called a *critical path* or *clinical map.* The critical path details all laboratory, dietary, consultative, medical, teaching, and nursing activities that are thought to be necessary to obtain specific clinical outcomes. Outcomes of care, as well as variations from the "path," are monitored and collected continuously.

Positive and negative outcomes are then analyzed and correlated with variances from the critical pathway. These data are then returned to the multidisciplinary team, which recommends changes in the entire path based on the outcomes and variance analyses.

In one pilot study of a critical pathway method for cesarean delivery, length of stay and cost were reduced by 13% and 14%, respectively. Additionally, five of seven measurements of satisfaction, including quality of care, were improved, and health status was unchanged (43). A relatively new federal government agency, the Agency for Healthcare Research and Quality (AHRQ), formerly known as the Agency for Health Care Policy and Research (AHCPR), is responsible for funding developmental efforts, collecting information about clinical care guidelines, and disseminating information.

Managed Care

Measuring and improving health care quality and performance have received progressively greater support and validation. Health care reform activity and rapidly changing reimbursement patterns are moving away from traditional fee-for-service plans toward negotiated fee-for-service plans, prospective payment, and capitation-based contracting. This trend has led to a rapid application of modern quality management techniques and performance improvement activity aimed at reducing costs. Managed care contracts are being awarded on the basis of both clinical outcomes and cost.

Many states and federal agencies have enacted legislation that requires health care providers to collect and disseminate comparative outcomes data in their practices. The National Committee on Quality Assurance (NCQA), which is sponsored by managed care organizations, has mandated the collection of quality performance indicators, referred to as *HEDIS,* which stands for **H**ealthplan and **E**mployer **D**ata **I**nformation **S**et. If data are collected and analyzed appropriately, these initiatives could improve health care quality and reduce costs by facilitating rational decision making by consumers, providers, and third-party payers. If done hastily or inappropriately, efforts to use outcomes data, although well intended, could undermine these goals. For these reasons, standardized and validated methods for measuring the processes and outcomes of health care must be developed and integrated into daily clinical and operational practice (44).

Patient Safety

Patient safety has been identified by the IOM as one of the most important dimensions of health care QA and performance improvement. According to a recent report from the IOM, it is estimated that between 44,000 and 98,000 preventable deaths may be due to medical error (1). Although there continues to be controversy about the validity of methods used in these analyses, critics admit that even if the actual number of preventable deaths from error is much smaller than estimated, efforts should be made to eliminate as many as possible.

Patient safety has its roots in traditional risk management (RM) but there are important conceptual differences between the two (Fig. 3.4). RM is retrospective and is focused on individual outliers. It is also outcomes oriented and addresses significant adverse (sentinel) events. The goals of RM include sanctions for substandard providers with far less attention to finding systems-oriented improvements that could prevent recurrent medical errors. Patient safety initiatives are prospective, interdisciplinary, and focused on health care process in addition to outcomes. They are designed to be nonpunitive and to recognize that most adverse outcomes are because of systems deficiencies and not individual error. Therefore, system changes in the overall process of delivery of care are necessary to prevent future problems. For example, when the wrong extremity is removed during a therapeutic amputation, RM efforts usually focus on legal liability issues, holding surgeons and operating room personnel accountable. A patient safety initiative would ideally study the entire process of care using a root-cause analysis approach (Fig. 3.5). All of the members of the health care team, from admission to discharge, would be involved in order to identify and implement preventive measures. This "going beyond blame" approach was a significant

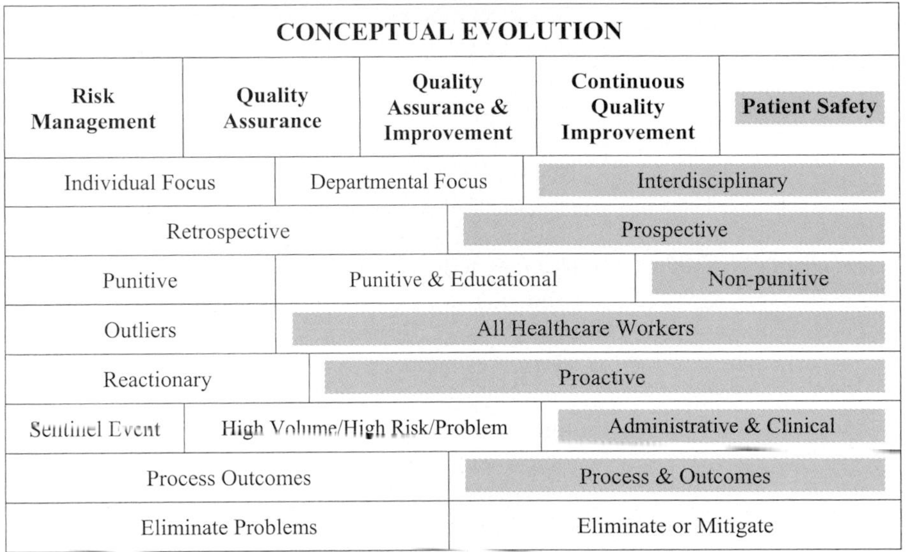

CONCEPTUAL EVOLUTION

Risk Management	Quality Assurance	Quality Assurance & Improvement	Continuous Quality Improvement	Patient Safety
Individual Focus	Departmental Focus		Interdisciplinary	
Retrospective			Prospective	
Punitive	Punitive & Educational			Non-punitive
Outliers	All Healthcare Workers			
Reactionary	Proactive			
Sentinel Event	High Volume/High Risk/Problem		Administrative & Clinical	
Process Outcomes			Process & Outcomes	
Eliminate Problems			Eliminate or Mitigate	

Figure 3.4 A conceptual evolution of the characteristics of risk management (RM), quality assurance (QA), continuous quality improvement (CQI), and patient safety.

recommendation in the IOM report, and it is the approach that is commonly used in other industries, such as aviation safety (1). Process changes and improvements, such as having the patient and surgeon sign the correct extremity using indelible ink at the time of admission and sharing the responsibility during the process so that several individuals (operating room personnel, anesthesia personnel, and members of the surgical team) would verify that the correct extremity is prepared and eventually removed. This team accountability approach is now being applied in all specialties, including obstetrics and gynecology.

The JCAHO has been very active and influential in the evolution of patient safety activities. Starting with an initial requirement that all significant (sentinel) events be reported, it now

Figure 3.5 Root-cause(s) analysis: getting to the single or multiple causes of adverse outcomes.

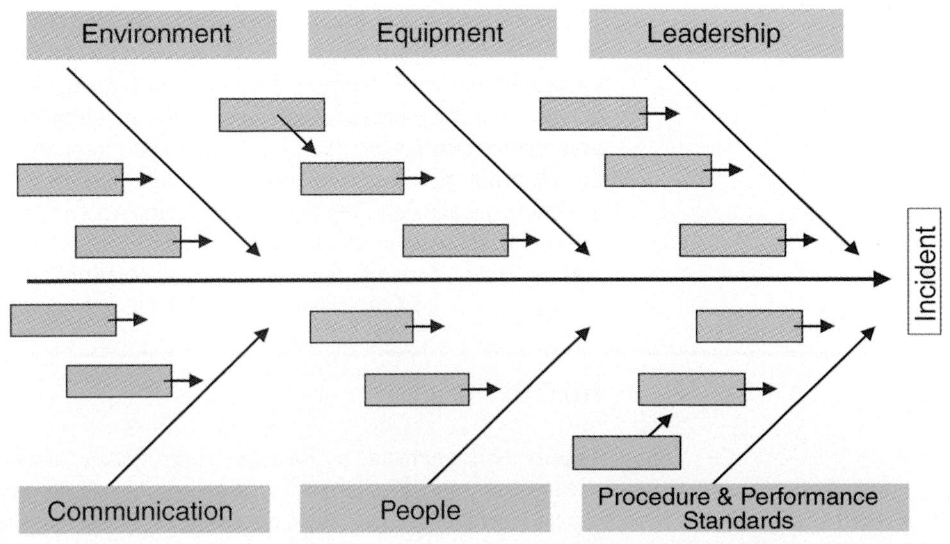

requires that root-cause(s) analysis be used to investigate the incident, identify contributing factors, and improve the process of care (45). Starting with all JCAHO surveys performed after June 2001, the Joint Commission requires documented evidence that a health care organization being reviewed has invested in a "top-down" commitment to patient safety improvement.

Business and government are also interested in promoting patient safety activities. A business committee called the Leapfrog Group representing the National Business Roundtable and corporations such as General Electric, General Motors, and Verizon have announced that they will give purchasing preference to health care organizations that have at least the following three patient safety programs that have been shown to improve performance: (a) 24-hour, 7 days per week in-house coverage by intensive care specialists; (b) computerized physician-order systems; and (c) high volume, optimal outcomes, and low complication rates for high-risk procedures such as cardiovascular and transplant surgeries. There are currently several legislative bills before the United States congress addressing patient safety issues, such as practice reform and confidentiality. In addition, government programs such as Medicare and Medicaid are putting into place financial and other incentives for patient safety initiatives.

Leaders in health care assessment and performance improvement have recommended five principles to help make health systems safer:

1. Leadership should commit to patient safety in the organization to provide the necessary personnel and financial resources.

2. System design should recognize human limitations. The noted health care improvement researcher, David Eddy, has stated that "the complexity of modern medicine exceeds the limitations of the unaided human mind." The one-person ("captain-of-the-ship") accountability of the past may actually lead to more errors in the current health care system.

3. Working and training in teams can help deliver safer care and more dependable accountability.

4. Training should anticipate the unexpected.

5. The organization should foster a learning environment for continual improvement of patient safety.

There is a growing consensus that there will need to be a nonpunitive reporting system to identify not only errors but also "near misses" and other hazards so that they may be corrected before the patient is harmed. The aviation industry is a prime example of how measures can be taken to improve safety. Operations are simplified and standardized. Crew resource management empowers the most appropriate individual to correct a problem, even if that person is not the pilot. Simulators and team training are widely employed. The industry has a system, the airline safety reporting system (ASRS), for reporting actual incidents and near misses. Furthermore, this system is confidential and separated from the Federal Aviation Agency (their main regulatory body) by the National Aviation and Space Agency (NASA).

Summary

Quality assessment and performance improvement activities are becoming increasingly important components of health care delivery. Although retrospective peer review and other QA efforts are still necessary, newer, prospectively focused methods to improve performance are being introduced. In the past, managing the cost of health care has been a major rationale for quality assessment and performance improvement programs. Recently, however, concerns about patient safety and deficiencies in quality have been prompted by several IOM reports (1,3). The complexity of modern health care delivery now requires a multidisciplinary team approach to quality management and error reduction. Health care professionals need to move away from an atmosphere of blame and individual accountability to a more effective *systems approach* to improve health care quality and safety significantly.

References

1. **Kohn L, Corrigan J, Donaldson M.** *To err is human: building a safer health system.* Washington, DC: National Academy Press, 2000.
2. **Robinson JC.** The end of managed care. *JAMA* 2001;285:2622–2628.
3. **Committee on Quality of Health Care in America.** *Crossing the quality chasm: a new health system for the 21st century.* Washington, DC: National Academy Press, 2001.
4. **Fuchs VR.** The best health care system in the world? *JAMA* 1992;268(7):916–917.
5. **Morris M, Gambone JC.** Making continual improvements to health care. *Clin Obstet Gynecol* 1994;37(1):137–148.
6. **Berwick DM.** Continuous improvement as an ideal in health care. *N Engl J Med* 1989;310:53–56.
7. **Berwick DM.** Controlling variation in health care: a consultation from Walter Shewhart. *Med Care* 1991;29(12):1212–1225.
8. **DiMatteo MR.** The physician-patient relationship: effects on the quality of health care. *Clin Obstet Gynecol* 1994;37(1):149–161.
9. **Reiter RC, Lench JB, Gambone JC.** Consumer advocacy, elective surgery, and the "golden era of medicine." *Obstet Gynecol* 1989;74:815–817.
10. **Hickson GB, Clayton EW, Entman SS, et al.** Obstetricians' prior malpractice experience and patients' satisfaction with care. *JAMA* 1994;272:1583–1587.
11. **Entman SS, Glass CA, Hickson GB, et al.** The relationship between malpractice claims history and subsequent obstetric care. *JAMA* 1994;272:1588–1591.
12. **DeFreise GH.** Measuring the effectiveness of medical interventions: new expectations of health services research. *Health Serv Res* 1990;25:691–695.
13. **DiMatteo RM, Reiter RC, Gambone JC.** Enhancing medication adherence through communication and informed collaborative choice. *Health Commun* 1994;6(4):253–265.
14. **Donabedian A.** The quality of care: how can it be assessed? *JAMA* 1988;260:1743–1748.
15. **Donabedian A.** *The methods and findings of quality assessment and monitoring.* Ann Arbor: Health Administration Press, 1985:3.
16. **Kaplan RM, Anderson JP.** The general health policy model: an integrated approach. In: Spilker B, ed. *Quality of life assessment in clinical trials.* New York: Raven Press, 1990:131–149.
17. **Deyo RA, Patrick DL.** Barriers to the use of health status measures in clinical investigation, patient care, and policy research. *Med Care* 1989;27:S254–268.
18. **Maynard A.** Developing the health care market. *Economic Journal* 1991;101:1277–1287.
19. **Kaplan RM.** An outcomes-based model for directing decisions in women's health care. *Clin Obstet Gynecol* 1994;37(1):192–206.
20. **Ware JE Jr, Kosinski M, Bayliss MS, et al.** Comparison of methods for the scoring and statistics of SF-36 health profile and summary measure: summary of outcomes study. *Med Care* 1995;33[Suppl 4]:AS264–79.
21. **Batalden PB, Buchanan DB.** Patient care process improvement. In: Batalden PB, Buchanan DB, eds. *A course, hospital wide quality: focus on continuous improvement.* Nashville: Hospital Corp. of America (QRG), 1990:12.
22. **Batalden PB, Nolen TW.** Knowledge for the leadership of continual improvement in healthcare. In: Taylor RJ, ed. *Manual of health services management.* Gaithersburg: Aspen, 1993:1–21.
23. **Deming WE.** *The new economics for industry, government and education.* Cambridge, MA: Massachusetts Institute of Technology, 1993.
24. **Bataldin PB, Stoltz PK.** A framework for the continual improvement of health care: building and applying professional and improvement knowledge to test changes in daily work. *Joint Comm J Qual Impr* 1993;19(10):424–452.
25. **Gambone JC, Chez RA.** Strategic planning: a modern tool for obstetricians and gynecologists in a competitive practice environment. *Prim Care Update Obstet Gynecol* 2000;7:177–180.

26. **Shewhart WA.** *Statistical method from the viewpoint of quality control.* Washington, DC: Department of Agriculture, 1993.

27. **Wennberg JE, Gittelsohn A.** Variations in medical care among small areas. *Sci Am* 1982;246:120–134.

28. **Wennberg JE, Freeman JL, Culp WJ.** Are hospital services rationed in New Haven or over-utilized in Boston? *Lancet* 1987;1:1185–1189.

29. **Roos NP.** Hysterectomy: variations in rates across small areas and across physicians' practices. *Am J Public Health* 1984;74(4):327–335.

30. **Centers for Disease Control and Prevention.** Rates of cesarean delivery—United States. *MMWR Morb Mortal Wkly Rep* 1993;42:285–289.

31. The Cardiology Working Group. Cardiology and the quality of medical practice. *JAMA* 1991;265:482–485.

32. **Bickell NA, Earp JA, Garrett JM, et al.** Gynecologists' sex, clinical beliefs, and hysterectomy rates. *Am J Public Health* 1994;84:1649–1652.

33. **Graves EJ.** *Summary: national hospital discharge survey.* Advance Data From Vital and Health Statistics: No. 199. Hyattsville: National Center for Health Statistics, 1989.

34. **Haas S, Acker D, Donahue C, Katz ME.** Variation in hysterectomy rates across small geographic areas of Massachusetts. *Am J Obstet Gynecol* 1993;169:150–154.

35. **Carlson KJ, Nichols DH, Schiff I.** Indications for hysterectomy. *N Engl J Med* 1993;328:856–860.

36. **Kjerulff K, Langenberg P, Guzinski G.** The socioeconomic correlates of hysterectomies in the United States. *Am J Public Health* 1993;83(5):106–108.

37. **Kjerulff KH, Guzinski GM, Langenberg PW, et al.** Hysterectomy and race. *Obstet Gynecol* 1993;82:757–764.

38. **Wilcox LS, Koonin LM, Pokras R, et al.** Hysterectomy in the United States, 1988–1990. *Obstet Gynecol* 1994;83(4):549–555.

39. **Boyle T.** Developing severity-adjusted critical paths using Medisgroups reporting. *Am J Med Qual* 1991;4:1–12.

40. **Zander K.** Nursing care management: strategic management of cost and quality outcomes. *J Nurs Adm* 1988;18:23–30.

41. **Gambone JC, Reiter RC.** Quality improvement in health care. *Curr Probl Obstet Gynecol Fertil* 1991;15(5): 170–175.

42. **Gambone JC, Reiter RC.** Promising innovation or needless intervention? *J Gynecol Techniques* 1995;1:59.

43. **Blegen MA, Reiter RC, Goode C, et al.** Outcomes of hospital based managed care: a multivariate analysis of cost and quality. *Obstet Gynecol* 1995;86:809–814.

44. **Loegering L, Reiter RC, Gambone JC.** Measuring the quality of health care. *Clin Obstet Gynecol* 1994;37(1):122–136.

45. **Gluck PA.** Patient safety: a new imperative. *ACOG Clin Rev* 2001, July/August.

Novak's Gynecology, 13th Edition. Edited by J.S. Berek. Lippincott Williams & Wilkins, Philadelphia © 2002

4 Epidemiology for the Gynecologist

Daniel W. Cramer

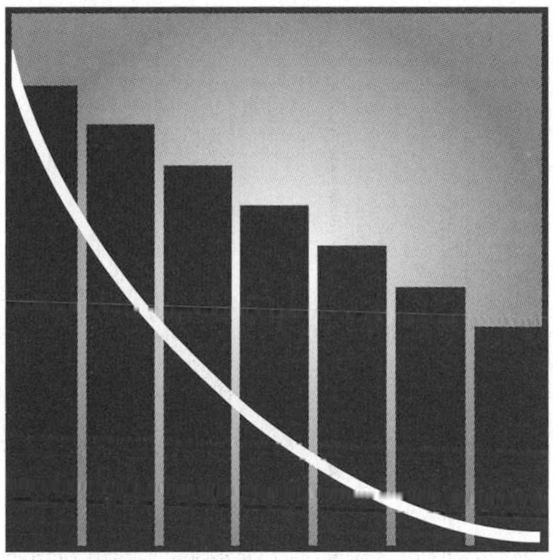

Epidemiology is the study of the occurrence of health events in human populations. Epidemiologic studies may encompass broad topics, such as how birth or death rates vary among people of different nationalities, or more narrow topics, such as how risk for a specific disease changes after a specific exposure. A common theme of most epidemiologic studies is the relationship between disease and exposure, but the design, strengths, weaknesses, and validity of epidemiologic studies vary considerably (1–6).

Some definitions that are commonly used in epidemiology are as follows:

- **Age-specific incidence:** the number of new events occurring in 5- or 10-year age groups per year
- **Attributable risk:** the difference between the occurrence measure in the exposed and the unexposed cohort
- **Bias:** a systematic error in the design, conduct, or analysis of a study
- **Clinical trial:** a prospective cohort study to evaluate treatments for disease in humans
- **Cohort:** a group of people who have some factor in common
- **Confidence interval (CI):** a component of statistical inference in which an interval is provided to give the reader some idea of the range in which the "true" statistical measure calculated (e.g., mean, proportion, and relative risk) is expected to occur
- **Confounder:** an extraneous variable that accounts for the apparent effect of the study variable or masks the true association
- **Incidence:** the rate of occurrence of new cases of a disease or condition over a specific time interval
- **Predictive value of a negative test:** the number of true negative results out of all those screened with negative results
- **Predictive value of a positive test:** the number of true positive results out of all those screened with positive results
- **Prevalence:** the existing number of cases at a specific point in time
- **Recall bias:** a type of information bias that may occur if cases are more likely than controls to remember or to reveal past exposures
- **Relative risk:** the occurrence in the exposed cohort divided by occurrence in the nonexposed cohort

- **Sensitivity:** the proportion of persons with a true positive screening result out of all those who have the disease
- **Specificity:** the proportion of persons with a true negative screening result out of all those who do not have the disease
- **Statistical significance:** the application of a statistical method to test the null hypothesis (i.e., the hypothesis that two or more factors are not associated)
- **Yield:** the exposure odds ratio (or simply *odds ratio*) in a case-control study (i.e., the ratio of exposed cases to unexposed cases divided by the ratio of exposed to unexposed controls)

Study Designs

Epidemiologic studies are primarily descriptive or analytic (i.e., designed to test a hypothesis about an association). This distinction is important in evaluating a medical study.

Descriptive Studies

Studies in which the characteristics of a disease are described are among the most common type of study. **The two principal types of descriptive studies are *case series* and *cross-sectional studies.***

Case Reports or Series

A simple type of study is the case report or case series in which the characteristics of individuals who have a particular disease are described. Hypotheses about the cause of the disease or its treatment are frequently developed from case series and then explored in analytic studies. For example, a link between oral contraceptives and thromboembolism was first suggested by case reports (7) and later confirmed in a case-control study (8). Occasionally, when case series describe the co-occurrence of rare exposures and rare diseases, they are compelling enough on their own to suggest a cause-and-effect relationship. Links between thalidomide and fetal limb reduction (9), the Dalkon shield intrauterine device and septic abortion (10), and sequential oral contraceptives and premenopausal endometrial cancer (11) emerged through case series that were persuasive enough to initiate public health action without the performance of formal epidemiologic studies. In general, however, just because a high number of members of a case series share a particular characteristic, one cannot assume that there is a cause-and-effect relationship. A number of selection factors could have contributed to the observation.

Because of their potential importance, attention should be paid to details of the case selection in case reports or series (e.g., incident or prevalent cases, record-based or personal contact with patients). Investigators should strive to be sure that clear criteria exist for the definition of disease or study variables and that identification of cases was complete. Case series that extend over a long period may suffer from changes in the diagnosis or treatment of the condition that may confuse objectives. Interobserver or reviewer reliability may need to be assessed. Careful assembly of a case series is the first step in performing a case-control study as the logical extension of a case series.

A case series does not usually yield any formal epidemiologic measures other than estimates of the frequency of a particular characteristic among members of the case series. This is often referred to as the *incidence* of a particular characteristic among cases, but *prevalence* is usually the more appropriate term.

Cross-sectional Studies

Design

Cross-sectional studies are larger in scope than case series and generally do not focus on a particular disease. Individuals are surveyed to provide a "snapshot" of health events in the population at a particular time. The U.S. Census Bureau counts the population by categories of age, sex, and ethnicity. The U.S. National Center for Health Statistics compiles a wide variety of data on the health of the population, such as occurrence of hospitalization for various conditions. State health departments are required to count the number of births and deaths annually in their population, and some maintain registries to count the number of individuals who have cancer.

Yield

***Incidence* is the rate of occurrence of new cases of diseases or conditions over a specific time.** Cross-sectional studies often yield incidence rates in which births, new disease cases, or deaths are counted annually for a specified census region and divided by the population size to yield events per population per year. The rate is usually multiplied by a base (1,000, 10,000, or 100,000) to give numbers that can more easily be tabulated. Incidence is an important concept in epidemiology and is often used to calculate other measures of disease frequency, such as prevalence and lifetime risk.

***Age-specific incidence* refers to the number of new events occurring in 5- or 10-year age groups per year.** Because of marked differences by age for most illnesses, age-specific incidence rates are the best way to describe event occurrence in a population. If the incidence rate is not specified with regard to age, it is described as "crude."

***Prevalence* is the existing number of cases at a specific point in time.** Prevalence is another measure frequently developed from cross-sectional studies. For example, in 1988, the Family Growth Survey Branch of the National Center for Health Statistics interviewed a sample of married couples and found the prevalence of infertility among married women younger than 45 years of age in the United States to be about 8.0% (12). Because prevalence measures disease status in a population rather than events occurring over time, prevalence is a proportion.

Although cross-sectional studies are primarily descriptive, they may contribute information on the cause of a disease by showing how that disease varies by age, sex, race, or geography. In *ecologic studies,* disease rates in various populations are correlated with other population characteristics (e.g., endometrial cancer rates worldwide are positively correlated with per capita fat consumption and negatively correlated with cereal and grain consumption) (13). Such observations are valuable in suggesting topics for analytic studies or supporting the consistency of an association.

Analytic Studies

The purpose of an analytic epidemiologic study is to test a hypothesis about and to measure an association between exposure (or treatment) and disease occurrence (or prevention) (Fig. 4.1). Analytic studies may be subdivided into *nonexperimental* and *experimental studies.*

Nonexperimental analytic studies include cohort and case-control studies and take advantage of "natural experiments" in which individuals do or do not have a particular disease and have or have not had an exposure of potential interest. *Experimental studies,* such as clinical trials, should meet more rigid criteria than nonexperimental studies. Features they should include are randomization (in which participants are randomly assigned to exposures) and measures to ensure unbiased assessment of outcome.

Nonexperimental Studies

Cohort Studies

Design **A cohort is a group of people who have some factor in common. In the context of a survival analysis, the cohort begins with a population that is 100% well at a particular time and is followed over time to calculate the percentage of the cohort**

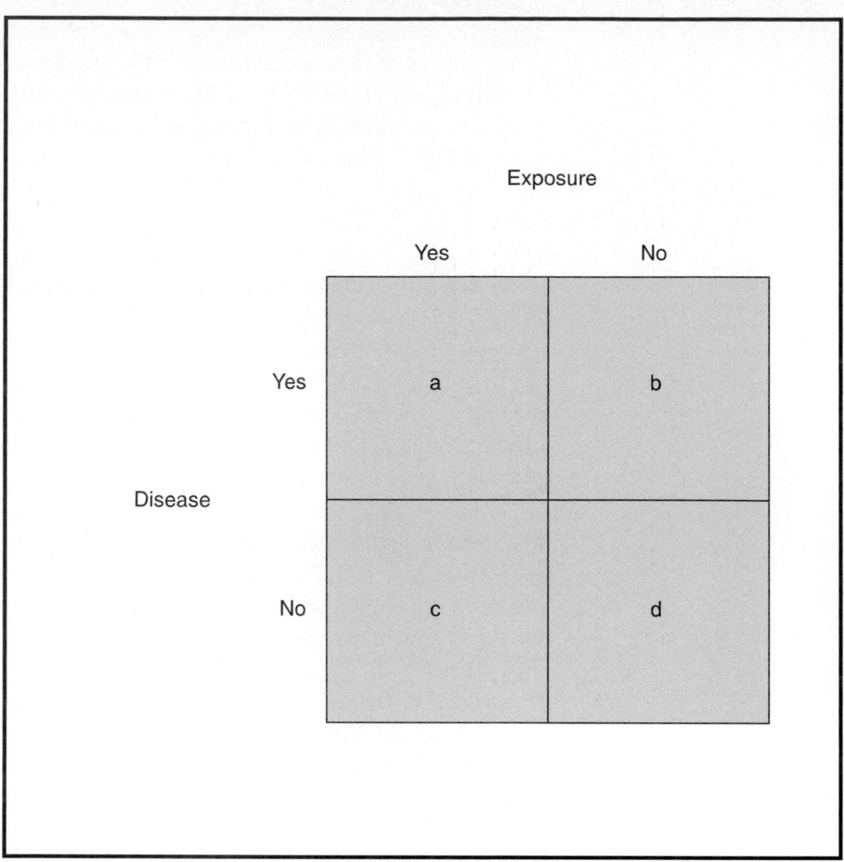

Figure 4.1 The essential design of an epidemiologic study showing the relationship between exposure (or treatment) and disease.

still well at later times. Survival analysis describes mortality after disease (i.e., cancer patients who died within 5 years) but can be adapted to other events (e.g., the percentage of women who continue to menstruate after 50 years of age or the percentage of infertile women who conceive after therapy).

A cohort is defined by subsets of a population who are, have been, or may in the future be exposed to factors hypothesized to influence the occurrence of a given disease (Fig. 4.2). The exposed and nonexposed subjects are observed long enough to generate *person-years* as the denominator for incidence or mortality rates in exposed and nonexposed subsets.

Cohort studies are also called *follow-up, longitudinal,* or *prospective studies.* Although these terms suggest that the exposure is identified before outcome, a retrospective cohort study may also be performed in which the exposure and outcome have already occurred when the study is begun. For example, studies of radiation and subsequent cancer are often based on records of patients who received radiation therapy many years previously. Medical records and death certificates are used to determine whether a second cancer occurred after the radiation therapy.

Yield Cohort studies may yield two measures of an association between exposure and illness. These measures are an *attributable risk* and a *relative risk.*

***Attributable risk* is the difference between the occurrence measure in the exposed and the unexposed cohort.** The null value is zero—a positive number indicates how many cases of disease may be caused by the exposure, and a negative number indicates how many cases of disease may be prevented by the exposure.

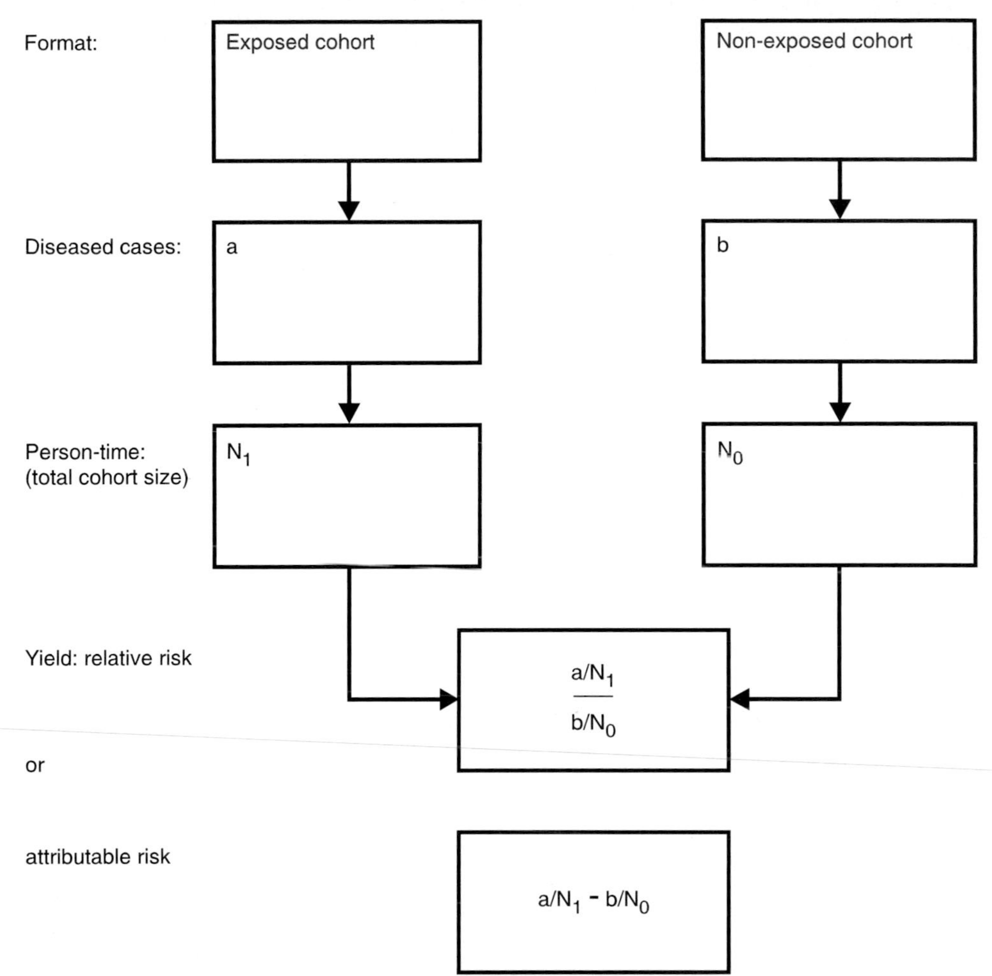

Figure 4.2 The format and calculations for a cohort study design.

Relative risk **divides occurrence in the exposed cohort by occurrence in the nonexposed cohort.** The null value for the relative risk is 1. A value greater than 1 indicates that exposure may increase risk for the disease (i.e., a relative risk of 1.5 indicates that exposed individuals had 1.5 times, or 50% greater, the risk for disease as unexposed individuals). A value less than 1 indicates that exposure may decrease risk for disease (i.e., a relative risk of 0.5 indicates that the rate in exposed individuals was half that of the rate in the nonexposed individuals).

Strengths and Weaknesses **The ability to obtain both attributable and relative risks is a strength of cohort studies. In addition, cohort studies are less susceptible to selection and recall bias.** Misclassification of exposure and confounding variables can occur, however. Disadvantages of a cohort study generally include higher cost and longer time for completion. Cohort studies are most useful for examining the occurrence of common diseases after a rare exposure. For rare exposures, an investigator may use the general population as the unexposed group. In this type of study, the observed number of cases in the exposed cohort is divided by the number of cases expected if general population rates had prevailed in the exposed cohort. This comparison is called the standardized morbidity or mortality ratio (SMR) and is equivalent to relative risk.

Case-control Studies

Design **A case-control study starts with the identification of individuals with a disease or outcome of interest and a suitable control population without the disease or outcome**

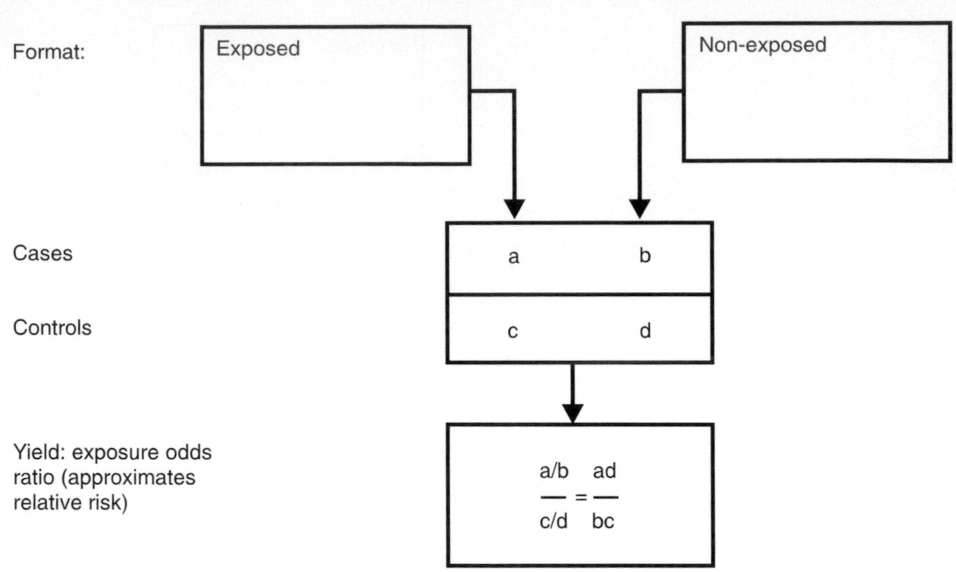

Figure 4.3 The case-control study design.

of interest. The relationship of a particular attribute or exposure to the disease is studied by comparing how the cases and controls differed in that exposure. An alternate term frequently used to describe a case-control study is *retrospective* because the exposures are assessed after the disease has occurred.

Yield **The yield of a case-control study is the exposure odds ratio.** It is the ratio of exposed cases to unexposed cases divided by the ratio of exposed to unexposed controls. If an entire population could be characterized by its exposure and disease status, the exposure odds ratio would be identical to the relative risk obtainable from a cohort study of the same population. Although it is not feasible to survey the entire population, so long as the sampling of cases or controls from the population was not influenced by their exposure status, the exposure odds ratio will approximate the relative risk. Attributable risk is not directly obtainable in a case-control study (Fig. 4.3).

Strengths and Weaknesses **The advantages of case-control studies are that they are generally lower in cost and easier to conduct than other analytic studies.** Case-control studies are most feasible for examining the association between a relatively common exposure and a relatively rare disease. Disadvantages include greater potential for selection bias, information bias, and confounding variables.

Because an investigator must assign exposures according to a strict protocol, human experimental studies are limited to the study of measures that will prevent disease or the consequences of disease. Examples of experimental studies are clinical trials and field and community intervention trials.

Experimental Studies

Clinical Trials

The clinical trial is a prospective cohort study to evaluate treatments for disease in humans. Randomization of the treatment assignment is the cornerstone of a good clinical trial because it minimizes bias, which can result from confounding variables or preferential assignment of treatment based on patient characteristics. Evidence must be provided that factors that might influence outcome, such as stage of disease, were similar in patients assigned to the study protocol compared with patients assigned to placebo or traditional treatment. Criteria for successful treatment must be clearly defined. Blinding

Table 4.1. Measures of Validity for a Screening Procedure

Status Determined by Screening	*True Disease Status*		
	Positive	*Negative*	*Total*
Positive	a (true positives)	b (false-positives)	a + b (all screened positives)
Negative	c (false-negatives)	d (true negatives)	c + d (all screened negatives)
Total	a + c (all diseased)	b + d (all nondiseased)	N (all subjects)
Measure	*Definition*	*Formula*	
Sensitivity	True positives / All diseased	$\frac{a}{a+c}$	
Specificity	True negatives / All nondiseased	$\frac{d}{b+d}$	
Predictive value of a positive screen	True positives / All screened positives	$\frac{a}{a+b}$	

From **Cramer DW.** Epidemiology and biostatistics. In: **Berek JS, Hacker NF,** eds. *Gynecologic oncology.* 3rd ed. Baltimore: Williams & Wilkins, 2000:263, with permission.

the subject and clinician to the treatment modality may help ensure unbiased assessment of the outcome. A properly designed clinical trial will have a sufficient number of subjects enrolled to ensure that a "negative" study is powerful enough to rule out a treatment effect.

Field and Community Intervention Trials

Field and community intervention trials evaluate measures that may prevent disease, such as vaccines, dietary interventions, or screening procedures. In a field trial, the intervention is applied to individuals. In a community intervention trial, the intervention (e.g., water fluoridation) is applied on a community-wide basis rather than to individuals. Both types of studies include subjects who do not yet have disease and may require large numbers of participants, especially for studies of screening procedures to prevent cancer. In the latter context, issues related to the validity of screening tests (i.e., *sensitivity, specificity,* and *predictive value*) are quite important (Table 4.1).

Features

Features of an analytic study that are considered in judging its scientific validity include statistical significance, biases, dose response, consistency, and biologic credibility.

***Statistical significance* is determined by application of a statistical method to test the null hypothesis (i.e., the hypothesis that two or more factors are not associated).**

The degree of conflict between the test result and the result predicted by the null hypothesis is indicated by the *p value.* Typically, $p \leq 0.05$ is used to determine statistical significance and indicates a 5% chance of incorrectly rejecting the null hypothesis.

Confidence Interval

The *confidence interval* (CI) is a component of statistical inference in which an interval is provided to give the reader some idea of the range in which the true statistical measure calculated (e.g., mean, proportion, and relative risk) is expected to occur. A 95% CI implies that, if a study were to be repeated many times within the same population, the measures assessed would be expected to fall in this interval 95% of the time. Confidence intervals of 95% for an odds ratio that includes the null value of 1 would not be statistically significant.

Bias

***Bias* is a systematic error in the design, conduct, or analysis of a study.** Such errors result in a mistaken conclusion and can take various forms.

Information Bias ***Information bias* occurs when subjects are classified incorrectly with respect to exposure or disease.** This may occur if records are incomplete or if the criteria for exposure or outcome were poorly defined, leading to misclassification.

***Recall bias* is another type of information bias that may occur if cases are more likely than controls to remember or to reveal past exposures.** In addition to adequate criteria and complete records, information bias may be reduced by making interviewers unaware of the status of the subjects or the purpose of the study.

Selection Bias ***Selection bias* may occur when correlates of the exposure or outcome influence sampling from the larger population of potentially eligible subjects.** An example of selection bias that may arise in a hospital-based case-control study occurs when the combination of the disease under study and a particular exposure is more likely to lead to hospital admission (14). Using incident cases from more than one hospital, obtaining high participation rates, and attempting to describe nonparticipants are several ways to reduce or at least evaluate the potential for selection bias.

Confounding

A third source of potential error is *confounding.* A *confounder* is an extraneous variable that accounts for the apparent effect of the study variable or masks the true association. When a factor differs between cases and controls or cohort members and is associated with both the study exposure and the study outcome, a distortion of the true association between the exposure and the disease may be produced. Age, race, and socioeconomic status are likely confounders; results must be adjusted for these variables by using statistical techniques such as stratification or multivariate analysis. Stratification involves examining the association of interest only within groups that are similar with respect to a potential confounder. Multivariate analysis is a statistical technique commonly used in epidemiologic studies that controls a number of confounders simultaneously. After an analysis to control for confounding variables, the investigator presents the adjusted risk ratio that presumably reflects an association free of confounding.

Dose Response

***Dose response* means that a change in the amount, intensity, or duration of an exposure is associated with either a consistent increase or decrease in risk for a specified disease or outcome.** Trend tests are used to determine whether a dose response exists.

Consistency and Metaanalysis

***Consistency* between findings in different populations, at different times, and by different methods or investigators is an important criterion used to judge whether there is likely to be a causal relationship.** A formal method for studying consistency and pooling results from different studies is metaanalysis. ***Metaanalysis* is the process of combining results from several independent studies examining the same exposure (or treatment) and same outcome in order to conduct a more powerful test of the null hypothesis.** A metaanalysis is conducted by assembling measures of the association from different studies, such as relative risks, weighting them by the variance of the measure, and taking an overall average. In the weighting process, the studies with the largest sample size contribute the greatest information. A properly performed metaanalysis also has a qualitative component that establishes criteria for acceptance of a study (e.g., only randomized studies might be chosen for a metaanalysis of the effect of a particular treatment on a particular disease).

Biologic Credibility

Biologic credibility **means that an association is plausible, taking into consideration all aspects of what is known about the natural history or demographics of a disease or what has been observed in relevant experimental models.** Whereas an imaginative epidemiologist can find an explanation for any single association, a key issue is whether a model can be proposed accounting for a variety of exposures as well as experimental data and cross-sectional observations.

Gynecologic Considerations

In epidemiologic terms, *exposure* refers to events that could be linked to an increased risk of disease. Exposures that are important to women's health are either gynecologic exposures that affect common diseases or common exposures that affect gynecologic diseases.

Reproductive Events

Age at menarche, characteristics of menstrual cycles, number of pregnancies, contraceptives or hormones used, and age at menopause are important events that may have broad impact on many diseases, including endometriosis (15), fibroids (16), heart disease (17), osteoporosis (18), and cancers of the breast, endometrium, or ovary (19–21). Gynecologists should maintain careful records of reproductive landmarks, both for their potential usefulness in advising patients and for their relevance to clinical research.

Contraception and Sterilization

Barrier Contraception

A protective effect of barrier contraception against pelvic inflammatory disease (PID) (22), tubal infertility (23), ectopic pregnancy (24), and cervical cancer (25) has been consistently observed.

Intrauterine Devices

Current or past use of an intrauterine device (IUD) has been linked with risk for PID (26), ectopic pregnancy (27), and tubal infertility (28). It is likely that these risks could be reduced by restricting IUD use to women at low risk for genital infections (e.g., parous women in a monogamous relationship).

Oral Contraceptives

Early epidemiologic literature on oral contraceptives (OCs) focused on adverse events, including thromboembolism (particularly with high-dose formulations) (29), hypertension (30), myocardial infarction (especially in women older than 40 years of age who also smoked) (31), and liver adenomas (32). Protective effects of OCs have more recently been appreciated, including lower risk for benign breast disease (33), ovarian cysts (34), ovarian cancer (35), and PID (36). Controversy exists concerning the relationship between OC use and cervical and breast cancer. Progression of intraepithelial cervical lesions may be more rapid among OC users (37). A large case-control study of breast cancer in England suggested use of preparations containing 50 μg or more of estrogen may increase the risk for breast cancer (38). However, the possible increased risk associated with past OC use for developing breast cancer at an early age may be more than offset by a decreased risk for developing breast cancer at an older age (39).

Sterilization

Concerns that sterilization might induce early menopause (40) have not been proved. An unexpected protective effect of female sterilization has been suggested for ovarian cancer (41). This protection may derive from the reduction of uterine growth factors that reach the ovary as a result of the interruption of the uteroovarian circulation or from closure of the female tract, which would prevent substances in the vagina or uterus from reaching the ovaries (42).

Hormone Replacement Therapy

Similar to early studies of OCs, studies of menopausal hormones focused on adverse events, including endometrial cancer, associated with unopposed estrogen use (43). This association has likely been obviated by the use of combined estrogen-progesterone regimens (44). More recent studies suggest protective effects on heart disease (45), osteoporosis (46), and even Alzheimer's disease (47). The association between menopausal hormones and breast cancer continues to be debated. However, a recent metaanalysis of studies of menopausal hormone use and breast cancer provided reassurance that the effect of such agents on breast cancer risk is modest (48).

Sexually Transmitted Disease

Worldwide, sexually transmitted diseases are possibly the most important preventable cause of morbidity in women. This morbidity includes not only PID from gonorrhea and chlamydia but also chronic disease from syphilis and genitally transmitted viruses, including hepatitis, human papillomavirus, and human immunodeficiency virus (HIV). The importance of public health measures to prevent the spread of sexually transmitted diseases, especially the use of barrier contraception, cannot be overemphasized because the morbidity from these infections may carry over to the offspring of those infected.

Lifestyle

Factors relating to an individual's lifestyle can increase the risk for potential problems. Often, the risk can be minimized by identifying these factors and altering behavior.

Smoking

Adverse effects of smoking on the lungs and heart are well known; however, it is less widely appreciated that smoking may be linked to tubal infertility (49), ectopic pregnancy (50), cervical cancer (51), and early menopause (52).

Alcohol

In moderation, alcohol use is associated with decreased risk for cardiovascular disease (53), which may come at the expense of an increased risk for breast cancer (54). It is possible that both of these effects are mediated by the ability of alcohol to retard the metabolism of estrogen, thereby leading to higher circulating levels of estrogen (55).

Exercise and Nutrition

Although aspects of exercise and nutrition cannot be fairly summarized in a single paragraph, it can be stated that gynecologic problems can occur at either extreme. The lean athlete in training who becomes amenorrheic may lose bone mass because of a lack of estrogen, as might the patient with anorexia (18). In obese women, menstrual difficulties may occur that are related to higher estrogen levels, which may, in the longer term, be associated with a higher risk for endometrial cancer (56).

Talc

Use of talc in genital hygiene is an exposure emphasized as a potential risk factor for ovarian cancer (57). Because there are no benefits of genital talc use, other than aesthetic, this practice should be discouraged.

Table 4.2. Reported Deaths for the 10 Leading Causes of Death by Age, United States, 1998

	All Ages	*1–19 Yr*	*20–39 Yr*	*40–59 Yr*	*60–79 Yr*	*80 + Yr*
	All causes: 1,179,996	All causes: 9,311	All causes: 30,538	All causes: 113,027	All causes: 411,516	All causes: 602,932
1	Heart diseases: 370,962	Accidents: 3,971	Accidents: 6,351	Cancer: 45,892	Cancer: 131,017	Heart diseases: 233,478
2	Cancer: 259,467	Cancer: 885	Cancer: 6,107	Heart diseases: 20,006	Heart diseases: 113,981	Cancer: 75,526
3	Cerebro-vascular diseases: 97,303	Homicide: 719	Heart diseases: 2,804	Accidents: 6,174	Chronic obstructive pulmonary diseases: 28,423	Cerebro-vascular diseases: 63,641
4	Chronic obstructive pulmonary diseases: 55,566	Congenital anomalies: 543	Suicide: 2,066	Cerebro vascular diseases: 5,197	Cerebro-vascular diseases: 27,366	Pneumonia and influenza: 37,147
5	Pneumonia and influenza: 50,892	Heart diseases: 377	Homicide: 1,930	Diabetes mellitus: 4,024	Diabetes mellitus: 16,506	Chronic obstructive pulmonary diseases: 23,217
6	Diabetes mellitus: 35,167	Suicide: 357	HIV infection: 1,626	Chronic obstructive pulmonary diseases: 3,421	Pneumonia and influenza: 11,010	Diabetes mellitus: 13,980
7	Accidents: 34,793	Pneumonia and influenza: 174	Cerebro-vascular diseases: 886	Cirrhosis of liver: 2,829	Accidents: 7,561	Alzheimer's disease: 12,551
8	Alzheimer's disease: 15,671	Cerebral palsy: 166	Diabetes mellitus: 620	Suicide: 2,389	Nephritis: 4,780	Accidents: 10,407
9	Nephritis: 13,621	Chronic obstructive pulmonary diseases: 122	Cirrhosis of liver: 576	Pneumonia and influenza: 1,835	Septicemia: 4,622	Nephritis: 7,820
10	Septicemia: 13,506	Cerebro-vascular diseases: 86	Pneumonia and influenza: 523	HIV infection: 1,299	Cirrhosis of liver: 4,184	Athero-sclerosis: 7,680

HIV, human immunodeficiency virus.
Data Source: US Mortality Public Use Data Tape 1998, National Cancer for Health Statistics, Centers for Disease Control and Prevention, 2000. From **Greenlee RT, Hill-Harmon MB, Murray T, et al.** Cancer statistics, 2001. *CA Cancer J Clin* 2001;51:15–36, with permission.

Illnesses

Many gynecologists are primary care providers for women, and they may increasingly assume this role in the future. It is important, therefore, for gynecologists to have an overview of the major causes of mortality in women. Reliable incidence data for gynecologic cancers and benign gynecologic problems are sometimes difficult to find, but statistics are available to guide clinical interventions.

Table 4.2 shows the 10 leading causes of death in 1998 for females in the United States by age from the National Center for Health Statistics data (58). Heart disease remains the major cause of death in women overall, but there is considerable age variation. Accidents, homicides, and suicides are most important at ages younger than 40 years, and cancer is most important at ages 40 to 79 years.

Table 4.3 shows the five leading causes of cancer mortality in women by various ages. In women, lung cancer now accounts for more deaths than breast cancer. Colon and rectal cancers are second overall, highlighting the importance of colon cancer screening in women older than 50 years of age. Pancreatic and ovarian cancers occur with about equal frequency, and both remain elusive to screening.

Figure 4.4 illustrates the age-specific incidence of genital malignancies in all females in the United States around 1991 (59). The incidence of invasive cervical cancer remains steady across all ages, whereas ovarian and endometrial cancer increase markedly during the perimenopausal years and predominate after 50 years of age. The sharp increase in endometrial and ovarian cancer rates around the time of menopause may reflect anovulatory cycles associated with unopposed estrogen and increased levels of gonadotropins. Although ovarian cancer appears to rank second to endometrial cancer in terms of incidence, mortality from ovarian cancer currently exceeds the combined mortality of endometrial and cervical cancer (58).

Table 4.3. Reported Deaths for the Five Leading Cancer Sites for Females by Age, United States, 1998

All Ages	*<20 Yr*	*20–39 Yr*	*40–59 Yr*	*60–79 Yr*	*≥80 Yr*
All sites: 259,467	All sites: 920	All sites: 6,107	All sites: 45,892	All sites: 131,017	All sites: 75,526
Lung and bronchus: 63,075	Leukemia: 280	Breast: 1,604	Breast: 11,889	Lung and bronchus: 39,077	Lung and bronchus: 13,392
Breast: 41,737	Brain and ONS: 233	Uterine cervix: 634	Lung and bronchus: 10,155	Breast: 18,292	Colon and rectum: 12,174
Colon and rectum: 28,950	Soft tissue: 73	Leukemia: 456	Colon and rectum: 3,472	Colon and rectum: 12,950	Breast: 9,949
Pancreas: 14,529	Endocrine system: 68	Lung and bronchus: 442	Ovary: 2,841	Pancreas: 7,454	Pancreas: 5,193
Ovary: 13,391	Bones and joints: 62	Brain and ONS: 401	Pancreas: 1,775	Ovary: 7,038	Non-Hodgkin's lymphoma: 3,881

Note: "All Sites" excludes *in situ* carcinomas except urinary bladder.
ONS, other nervous system.
Data Source: US Mortality Public Use Data Tape 1998, National Center for Health Statistics, Center for Disease Control and Prevention, 2000.
From **Greenlee RT, Hill-Harmon MB, Murray T, et al.** Cancer statistics, 2001. *CA Cancer J Clin* 2001;51: 15–36, with permission.

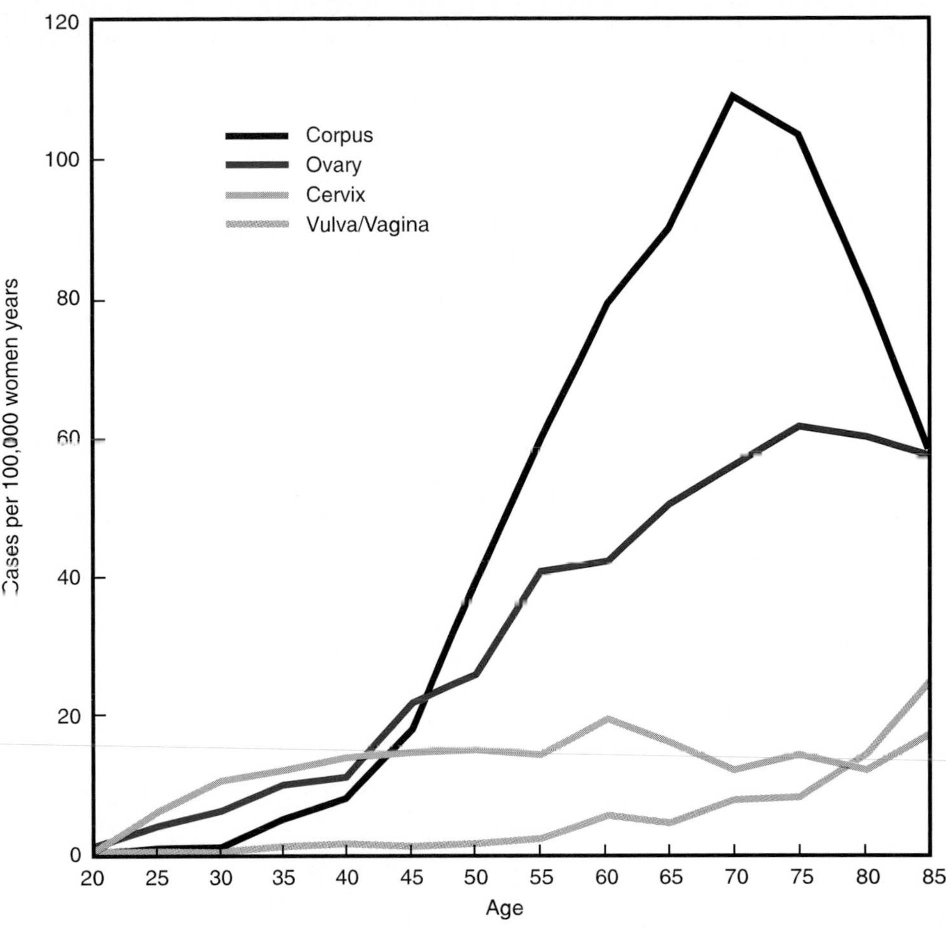

Figure 4.4 Age-specific incidence of gynecologic cancers, all U.S. females (1991). (From Ries LAG, Miller BA, Hankey BF, et al. *SEER cancer statistics review, 1973–1991, tables and graphs.* Bethesda, MD: Surveillance Program, Division of Cancer Prevention and Control, National Cancer Institute, NIH Pub No. 94–2789, 1994, with permission.)

The estimated number of hospital admissions listing various benign gynecologic conditions as a discharge diagnosis, shown in Table 4.4, is based on data collected by the National Hospital Discharge Survey for 1988 to 1990 and by the Division of Reproductive Health of the Centers for Disease Control and Prevention (60). These data pertain to women 15 to 45 years of age and are based on discharges from nonmilitary hospitals. PID is the most frequent discharge diagnosis, with nearly 300,000 women hospitalized annually. Of almost equal frequency are hospitalizations for benign ovarian cysts, endometriosis, and fibroids, each of which accounts for the hospitalization of almost 200,000 women annually.

The estimated age-specific incidence of PID, ovarian cysts, fibroids, and endometriosis is shown in Fig. 4.5. Notable are the higher incidence of PID in women in their 20s and the increasing incidence of endometriosis and fibroids into the 40s. The high frequency of the latter two conditions, combined with a lack of information on their cause, suggests that these conditions should be targets for more epidemiologic research.

In 1989, there were about 88,400 ectopic pregnancies in the United States, with a rate of about 16.0 per 1,000 reported pregnancies, compared with 4.5 per 1,000 in 1970 (61). In 1970, however, the case-fatality rate was 35.5 per 10,000 ectopic pregnancies, compared with 3.8 per 10,000 ectopic pregnancies in 1989, which accounted for about 13% of all

Table 4.4. Estimated Number of Annual Hospitalizations among Women of Reproductive Age in the United States

Group of Diagnosis	***Hospitalizations***[a]
Pelvic inflammatory disease	287,343
Benign cysts of the ovary	190,548
Endometriosis	188,805
Menstrual disorders	182,988
Uterine leiomyomas	177,082
Prolapse/stress incontinence	101,907
Cervical intraepithelial neoplasia	60,320

[a]Based on discharge diagnoses for women 15 through 45 years of age in nonmilitary hospitals averaged for the period 1988–1990.
From **Velebil P, Wingo PA, Xia A, et al.** Rate of hospitalization for gynecologic disorders among reproductive-age women in the United States. *Obstet Gynecol* 1995;86:764–769, with permission.

Figure 4.5 Age-specific incidence of hospitalization for various benign gynecologic conditions around 1990. (From Velebil P, Wingo PA, Xia A, et al. Rate of hospitalization for gynecologic disorders among reproductive-age women in the United States. *Obstet Gynecol* 1995;86:764–769, with permission.)

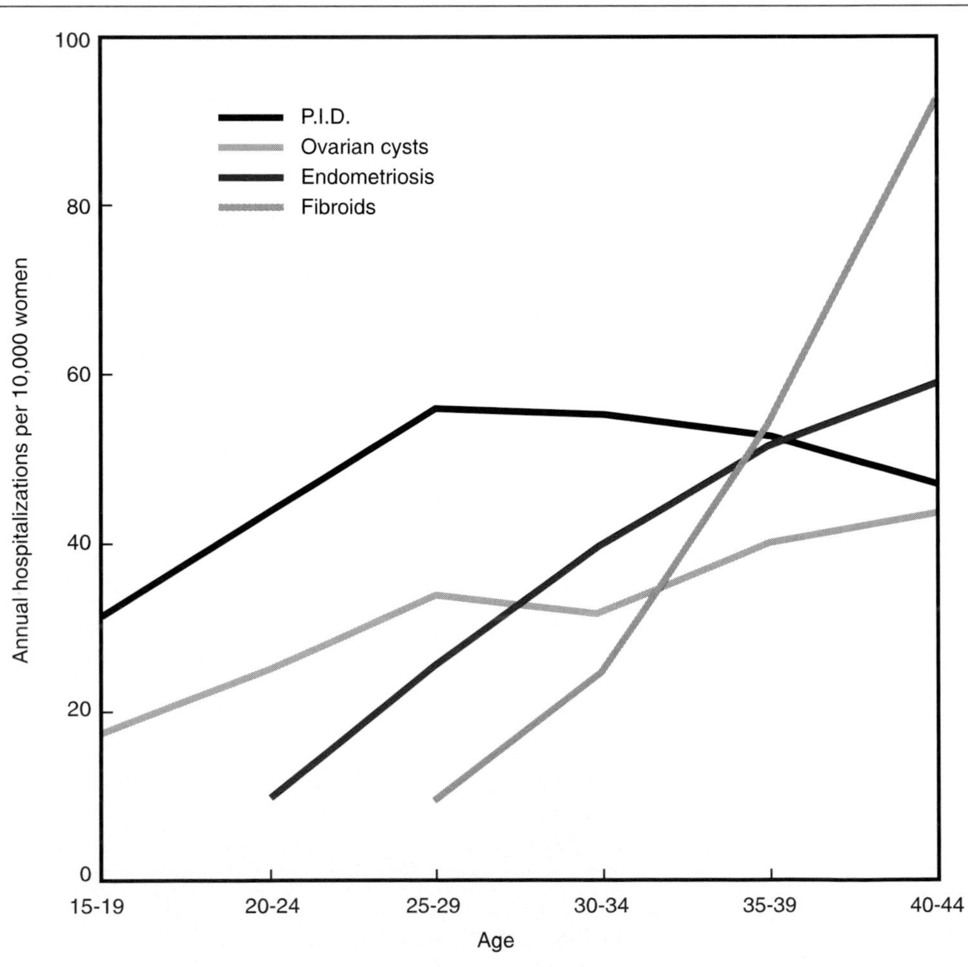

maternal deaths that year. Ectopic pregnancy continues to contribute to maternal mortality, particularly among nonwhite populations.

Gynecologic exposures and gynecologic diseases have always been major focuses for epidemiologic research. However, gynecologists have infrequently been involved in the design and interpretation of such studies, and therefore, the physiologic and clinical relevance of various associations often have been inadequately discussed. Even if the gynecologist does not actually perform epidemiologic research, an understanding of epidemiologic principles allows for a more critical reading of the medical literature and sharpens the practice of preventive medicine in gynecology.

References

1. **Dawson-Saunders B, Trapp RG.** *Basic and clinical biostatistics*. Norwalk, CT: Appleton & Lange, 1990.
2. **Last JM.** *A dictionary of epidemiology*. 2nd ed. New York: Oxford University Press, 1988.
3. **Peterson HB, Kleinbaum DG.** Interpreting the literature in obstetrics and gynecology. I. Key concepts in epidemiology and biostatistics. *Obstet Gynecol* 1991;78:710–717.
4. **Peterson HG, Kleinbaum DG.** Interpreting the literature in obstetrics and gynecology. II. Logistic regression and related issues. *Obstet Gynecol* 1991;78:717–720.
5. **Rothman KJ.** *Modern epidemiology*. Boston: Little, Brown, 1986.
6. **Schlesselman JJ.** *Case-control studies: design, conduct, analysis*. New York: Oxford University Press, 1982.
7. **Tyler FT.** Oral contraceptives and thromboembolism. *JAMA* 1963;185:131–132.
8. **Research Advisory Service of the Royal College of General Practitioners.** Oral contraception and thromboembolic disease. *J R Coll Gen Pract* 1967;13:267–279.
9. **McBride WG.** Thalidomide and congenital abnormalities. *Lancet* 1961;2:1358.
10. **Christian CD.** Maternal deaths associated with an intrauterine device. *Am J Obstet Gynecol* 1974;119:441–444.
11. **Silverberg SG, Makowski EL.** Endometrial carcinoma in young women taking oral contraceptive agents. *Obstet Gynecol* 1975;46:503–506.
12. **Chandra A, Mosher WD.** The demography of infertility and use of medical care for infertility in study designs and statistics for infertility research. In: **Cramer DW, Goldman MB,** eds. *Infertility and reproductive medicine clinics of North America.* Vol. 5. Philadelphia: WB Saunders, 1994:283–296.
13. **Armstrong B, Doll R.** Environmental factors and cancer incidence and mortality in different countries with special reference to dietary practices. *Int J Cancer* 1975;15:617–631.
14. **Berkson J.** Limitations of the application of fourfold table analysis to hospital data. *Biometrics Bull* 1946;2:47–53.
15. **Cramer DW, Wilson E, Stillman RJ, et al.** The relation of endometriosis to menstrual characteristics, smoking, and exercise. *JAMA* 1986;255:1904–1908.
16. **Ross RK, Pike MC, Vessey MP, et al.** Risk factors for uterine fibroids: reduced risk associated with oral contraceptives. *BMJ* 1986;293:359–362.
17. **Matthews KA, Meilahn E, Kuller L, et al.** Menopause and risk factors for coronary artery disease. *N Engl J Med* 1989;321:641–646.
18. **Jones KP, Ravnikar VA, Tulchinsky D, et al.** Comparison of bone density in amenorrheic women due to athletics, weight loss, and premature menopause. *Obstet Gynecol* 1985;66:5–8.
19. **MacMahon B, Cole P.** Etiology of human breast cancer: a review. *J Natl Cancer Inst* 1973;50:21–42.
20. **MacMahon B.** Risk factors for endometrial cancer. *Gynecol Oncol* 1974;2:122–129.
21. **Cramer DW, Hutchinson GB, Welch WR, et al.** Determinants of ovarian cancer risk I. Reproductive experiences and family history. *J Natl Cancer Inst* 1983;72:711–716.
22. **Kelaghan J, Rubin GL, Ory HW, et al.** Barrier-method contraceptives and pelvic inflammatory disease. *JAMA* 1982;248:184–187.
23. **Cramer DW, Goldman MB, Schiff I, et al.** The relationship of tubal infertility to barrier method and oral contraceptive use. *JAMA* 1987;257:2446–2450.
24. **Kalandidi A, Doulgerakis M, Tzonou A, et al.** Induced abortions, contraceptive practices, and tobacco smoking as risk factors for ectopic pregnancy in Athens, Greece. *Br J Obstet Gynaecol* 1991;98:207–213.
25. **Aitken-Swan J, Baird D.** Cancer of the uterine cervix in Aberdeenshire: aetiologic aspects. *Br J Cancer* 1966;20:642–659.

26. **Faulkner WL, Ory HW.** Intrauterine devices and acute pelvic inflammatory disease. *JAMA* 1976;235:1851–1853.

27. **Chow WH, Daling JR, Cates W Jr, et al.** Epidemiology of ectopic pregnancy. *Epidemiol Rev* 1987;9:70–94.

28. **Cramer DW, Schiff I, Schoenbaum SC, et al.** Tubal infertility and the intrauterine device. *N Engl J Med* 1985;312:941–947.

29. **Inman WHW, Vessey MP, Westerholm B, et al.** Thromboembolic disease and the steroidal content of oral contraceptives. *BMJ* 1970;2:203–209.

30. **Fisch IR, Frank J.** Oral contraceptives and blood pressure. *JAMA* 1977;237:2499–2503.

31. **Incidence of arterial disease among oral contraceptive users. Royal College of General Practitioners' Oral Contraceptive Study.** *J R Coll Gen Pract* 1983;33:75–82.

32. **Rooks JB, Ory HW, Ishak KG, et al.** Epidemiology of hepatocellular adenoma and the role of oral contraceptive use. *JAMA* 1977;237:2499–2503.

33. **Ory H, Cole P, MacMahon B, Hoover R.** Oral contraceptives and reduced risk of benign breast diseases. *N Engl J Med* 1976;294:419–422.

34. **Ory HW.** Functional ovarian cysts and oral contraceptives. *JAMA* 1974;228:68–69.

35. **Gross TP, Schlesselman JJ.** The estimated effect of oral contraceptive use on the cumulative risk of epithelial ovarian cancer. *Obstet Gynecol* 1994;83:419–424.

36. **Rubin GL, Ory HW, Layde PM.** Oral contraceptives and pelvic inflammatory disease. *Am J Obstet Gynecol* 1980;144:630–635.

37. **Swan SH, Brown WL.** Oral contraceptive use, sexual activity, and cervical carcinoma. *Am J Obstet Gynecol* 1981;139:52–57.

38. **UK National Case Control Study Group.** Oral contraceptive use and breast cancer risk in young women. *Lancet* 1989;1:973–982.

39. **Stadel BV, Schlesselman JJ, Murray PA.** Oral contraceptives and breast cancer. *Lancet* 1989;1:1257–1259.

40. **Cattanach J.** Oestrogen deficiency after tubal ligation. *Lancet* 1985;1:847–849.

41. **Hankinson SE, Hunter DJ, Colditz GA, et al.** Tubal ligation, hysterectomy, and risk of ovarian cancer. *JAMA* 1993;270:2813–2818.

42. **Cramer DW, Xu H.** Epidemiologic evidence for uterine growth factors in the pathogenesis of ovarian cancer. *Ann Epidemiol* 1995;5:310–314.

43. **Shapiro S, Kaufman DW, Slone D, et al.** Recent and past use of conjugated estrogens in relation to adenocarcinoma of the endometrium. *N Engl J Med* 1980;303:485–489.

44. **Key TJ, Pike MC.** The dose-relationship between "unopposed" oestrogens and endometrial mitotic rate: its central role in explaining the predicting endometrial cancer risk. *Br J Cancer* 1988;57:205–212.

45. **Stampfer MJ, Colditz GA, Willett WC, et al.** Postmenopausal estrogen therapy and cardiovascular disease. Ten-year follow-up from the nurses' health study. *N Engl J Med* 1991;325:756–762.

46. **Lindsay R, Aitken JM, Anderson JD, et al.** Long-term prevention of postmenopausal osteoporosis by oestrogen. *Lancet* 1976;i:1038–1041.

47. **Henderson VW, Paganini-Hill A, Emanuel CK, et al.** Estrogen replacement therapy in older women: comparisons between Alzheimer's disease cases and nondemented control subjects. *Arch Neurol* 1994;51:896–900.

48. **Dupont WD, Page DL.** Menopause estrogen replacement therapy and breast cancer. *Arch Intern Med* 1991;151:67–72.

49. **Phipps WR, Cramer DW, Schiff I, et al.** The association between smoking and female infertility as influenced by cause of the infertility. *Fertil Steril* 1987;48:377–382.

50. **Handler A, Davis F, Ferre C, et al.** The relationship of smoking and ectopic pregnancy. *Am J Public Health* 1989;79:1239–1242.

51. **Brinton LA, Schairer C, Haenszel W, et al.** Cigarette smoking and invasive cervical cancer. *JAMA* 1986;255:3265–3269.

52. **McKinlay SM, Bifano NL, McKinlay JB.** Smoking and age at menopause in women. *Ann Intern Med* 1985;103:350–356.

53. **Klatsky AL, Armstrong MA, Friedman GD.** Risk of cardiovascular mortality in alcohol drinkers, ex-drinkers and nondrinkers. *Am J Cardiol* 1990;66:1237–1242.

54. **Willett WC, Stampfer MJ, Colditz GA, et al.** Moderate alcohol consumption and the risk of breast cancer. *N Engl J Med* 1987;316:1174–1180.

55. **Cronholm T, Rudquist V.** Effects of ethanol metabolism on oxidoreduction at C-17 in vivo in the rat. *Biochem Biophys Acta* 1982;711:159–165.

56. **Elwood JM, Cole PH, Rothman KJ, et al.** Epidemiology of endometrial cancer. *J Natl Cancer Inst* 1977;59:1055–1060.

57. **Harlow BL, Cramer DW, Bell DA, et al.** Perineal exposure to talc and ovarian cancer risk. *Obstet Gynecol* 1992;80:19–26.

58. **Greenlee RT, Hill-Harmon MB, Murray T, et al.** Cancer statistics 2001. *CA Cancer J Clin* 2001;51:15–36.

59. **Ries LAG, Eisner MP, Kosary CL, et al.** *SEER cancer statistics review, 1973–1997, tables and graphs.* Bethesda, MD: Surveillance Program, Division of Cancer Prevention and Control, National Cancer Institute, NIH Pub. No. 94-2789, 2000.

60. **Velebil P, Wingo PA, Xia A, et al.** Rate of hospitalization for gynecologic disorders among reproductive-age women in the United States. *Obstet Gynecol* 1995;86:764–769.

61. **Goldner TE, Lawson HW, Xia Z, et al.** Surveillance for ectopic pregnancy-United States 1970-1989. *MMWR Morb Mortal Wkly Rep* 1993;42:73–85.

Novak's Gynecology, 13th Edition. Edited by J.S. Berek. Lippincott Williams & Wilkins, Philadelphia © 2002

SECTION

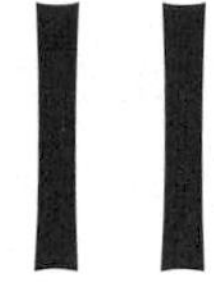

BASIC SCIENCE

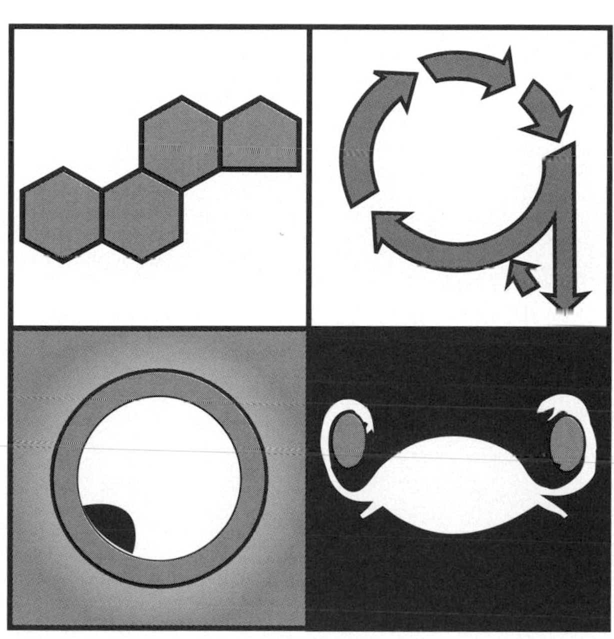

5 Anatomy and Embryology

Jean R. Anderson
Rene Genadry

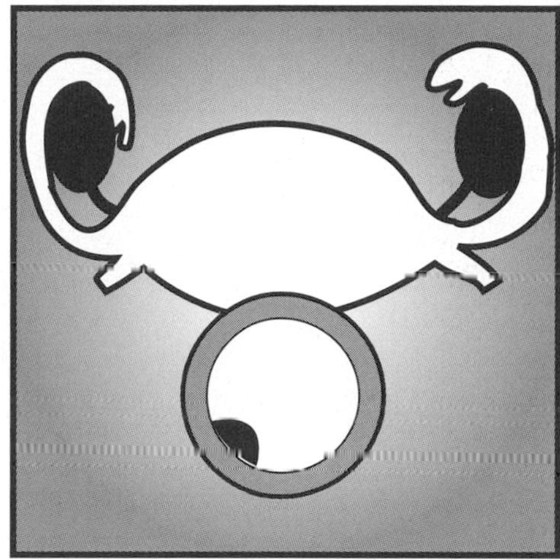

Nothing is more fundamental to the knowledge base of the practicing gynecologist than an understanding of the anatomy of the female pelvis. Although the basic facts of anatomy and their relevance to gynecologic practice do not change with time, our understanding of specific anatomic relationships and the development of new clinical and surgical correlations continue to evolve.

The anatomy of the fundamental supporting structures of the pelvis and the genital, urinary, and gastrointestinal viscera are presented in this chapter. Because significant variation has developed in the names of many common anatomic structures, the terms used here reflect current standard nomenclature according to the *Nomina Anatomica* (1); however, other commonly accepted terms are included in parentheses.

Pelvic Structure

Bony Pelvis

The skeleton of the pelvis is formed by the sacrum and coccyx and the paired hipbones (coxal, innominate), which fuse anteriorly to form the symphysis pubis. Figure 5.1 illustrates the bony pelvis as well as its ligaments and foramina.

Sacrum and Coccyx

The sacrum and coccyx are an extension of the vertebral column resulting from the five fused sacral vertebrae and the four fused coccygeal vertebrae. They are joined by a symphyseal articulation (sacrococcygeal joint), which allows some movement.

The essential features of the sacrum and coccyx are as follows:

1. **Sacral promontory**—the most prominent and anterior projection of the sacrum, this is an important landmark for insertion of a laparoscope. It is located at the level of bifurcation of the common iliac arteries.

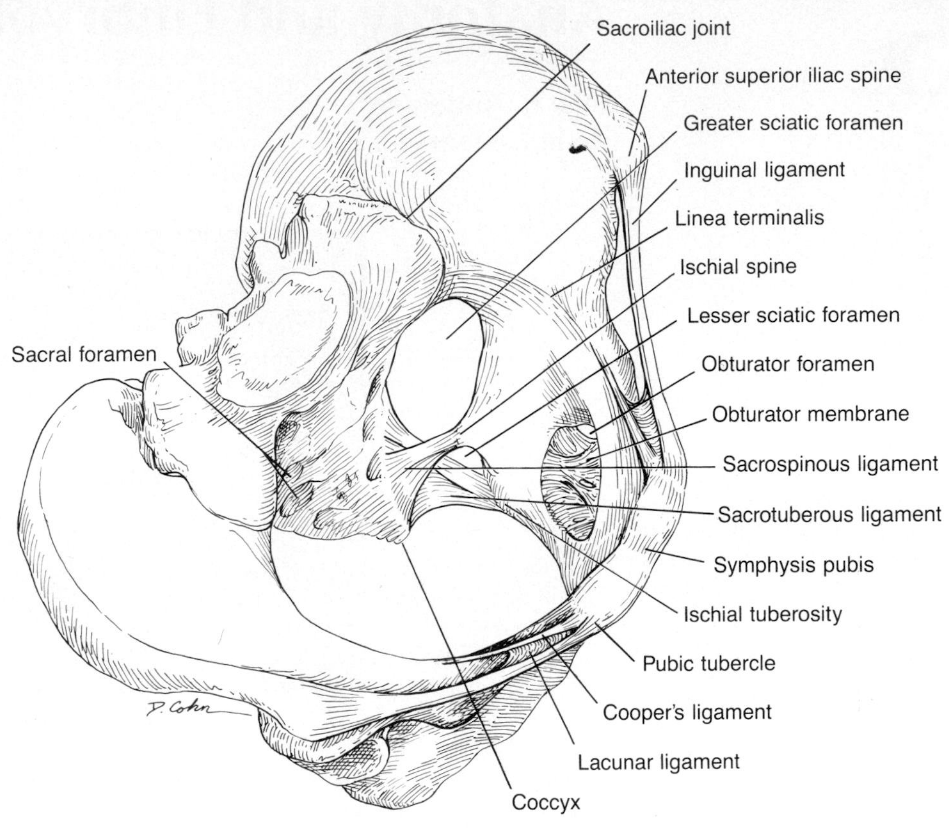

Figure 5.1 The female pelvis. The pelvic bones (the innominate bone, sacrum, and coccyx) and their joints, ligaments, and foramina.

2. **Four paired anterior and posterior sacral foramina**—exit sites for the anterior and posterior rami of the corresponding sacral nerves; anterior foramina are also traversed by the lateral sacral vessels.

3. **Sacral hiatus**—results from incomplete fusion of the posterior lamina of the fifth sacral vertebra, offering access to the sacral canal, which is clinically important for caudal anesthesia.

Laterally, the alae ("wings") of the sacrum offer auricular surfaces that articulate with the hipbones to form synovial sacroiliac joints.

Os Coxae

The paired os coxae, or hipbones, have three components: the ilium, the ischium, and the pubis. These components meet to form the acetabulum, a cup-shaped cavity that accommodates the femoral head.

Ilium

1. **Iliac crest**—provides attachments to the iliac fascia, abdominal muscles, and fascia lata.

2. **Anterior superior and inferior spine**—superior spine provides the point of fixation of the inguinal ligament.

3. **Posterior superior and inferior spine**—superior spine is the point of attachment for the sacrotuberous ligament and the posterior sacral iliac ligament.

4. **Arcuate line**—marks the pelvic brim and lies between the first two segments of the sacrum.

5. **Iliopectineal eminence (linea terminalis)**—the line of junction of the ilium and the pubis.

6. **Iliac fossa**—the smooth anterior concavity of the ilium, covered by the iliacus muscle.

Ischium

1. **Ischial spine**—delineates the greater and lesser sciatic notch above and below it. It is the point of fixation for the sacrospinous ligament; the ischial spine represents an important landmark in the performance of pudendal nerve block and sacrospinous ligament vaginal suspension; vaginal palpation during labor allows detection of progressive fetal descent.

2. **Ischial ramus**—joins that of the pubic rami to encircle the obturator foramen; provides the attachment for the inferior fascia of the urogenital diaphragm and the perineal musculofascial attachments.

3. **Ischial tuberosity**—the rounded bony prominence upon which the body rests in the sitting position.

Pubis

1. **Body**—formed by the midline fusion of the superior and inferior pubic rami.

2. **Symphysis pubis**—a fibrocartilaginous symphyseal joint where the bodies of the pubis meet in the midline; allows for some resilience and flexibility, which is critical during parturition.

3. **Superior and inferior pubic rami**—join the ischial rami to encircle the obturator foramen; provide the origin for the muscles of the thigh and leg; provide the attachment for the inferior layer of the urogenital diaphragm.

4. **Pubic tubercle**—a lateral projection from the superior pubic ramus, to which the inguinal ligament, rectus abdominis, and pyramidalis attach.

Pelvic Bone Articulations

The pelvic bones are joined by four articulations:

1. **Two cartilaginous symphyseal joints—the sacrococcygeal joint and the symphysis pubis**—these joints are surrounded by strong ligaments anteriorly and posteriorly, which are responsive to the effect of relaxin and facilitate parturition.

2. **Two synovial joints—sacroiliac joints**—these are stabilized by the sacroiliac ligaments, the iliolumbar ligament, the lateral lumbosacral ligament, the sacro-tuberous ligament, and the sacrospinous ligament.

The pelvis is divided into the *greater* and *lesser pelvis* by an oblique plane passing through the sacral promontory, the *linea terminalis (arcuate line of the ilium),* the pectineal line of the pubis, the pubic crest, and the upper margin of the symphysis pubis. This plane lies at the level of the superior pelvic aperture (*pelvic inlet*) or pelvic brim. The inferior pelvic aperture or *pelvic outlet* is irregularly bound by the tip of the coccyx, the symphysis pubis, and the ischial tuberosities. The dimensions of the superior and inferior pelvic apertures have important obstetric implications.

Ligaments and Foramina

Four ligaments of the bony pelvis are of special importance to the gynecologic surgeon.

Inguinal Ligament

The inguinal ligament is important surgically in the repair of inguinal hernia. The inguinal ligament:

1. Is formed by the lower border of the aponeurosis of the external oblique muscle folded back upon itself.
2. Is fused laterally to the iliacus fascia and inferiorly to the fascia lata.
3. Flattens medially into the lacunar ligament, which forms the medial border of the femoral ring.

Cooper's Ligament

Cooper's ligament is used frequently in bladder suspension procedures. Cooper's ligament:

1. Is a strong ridge of fibrous tissue extending along the pectineal line—also known as the pectineal ligament.
2. Merges laterally with the iliopectineal ligament and medially with the lacunar ligament.

Sacrospinous Ligament

The sacrospinous ligament is often used for vaginal suspension. This ligament offers the advantage of a vaginal surgical route. The sacrospinous ligament:

1. Extends from the ischial spine to the lateral aspect of the sacrum.
2. Is separated from the rectovaginal space by the rectal pillars.
3. Lies anterior to the pudendal nerve and the internal pudendal vessels at its attachment to the ischial spine.
4. The inferior gluteal artery, with extensive collateral circulation, is found between the sacrospinous and sacrotuberous ligaments and may be injured during sacrospinous suspension (2).

Sacrotuberous Ligament

The sacrotuberous ligament is sometimes used as a point of fixation for vaginal vault suspension. The sacrotuberous ligament:

1. Extends from the ischial tuberosity to the lateral aspect of the sacrum.
2. Merges medially with the sacrospinous ligament.
3. Lies posterior to the pudendal nerve and the internal pudendal vessels.

The bony pelvis and its ligaments delineate three important foramina that allow the passage of the various muscles, nerves, and vessels to the lower extremity.

Greater Sciatic Foramen

The greater sciatic foramen transmits the following structures: the piriformis muscle, the superior gluteal nerves and vessels, the sciatic nerve along with the nerves of the quadratus femoris, the inferior gluteal nerves and vessels, the posterior cutaneous nerve of the thigh, the nerves of the obturator internus, and the internal pudendal nerves and vessels.

Lesser Sciatic Foramen

The lesser sciatic foramen transmits the tendon of the obturator internus to its insertion on the greater trochanter of the femur. The nerve of the obturator internus and the pudendal vessels and nerves reenter the pelvis through it.

Obturator Foramen

The obturator foramen transmits the obturator nerves and vessels.

Muscles

The muscles of the pelvis include those of the lateral wall and those of the pelvic floor (Fig. 5.2; Table 5.1).

Lateral Wall

The muscles of the lateral pelvic wall pass into the gluteal region to assist in thigh rotation and adduction. They include the pyriformis, the obturator internus, and the iliopsoas.

Pelvic Floor

Pelvic Diaphragm

The pelvic diaphragm is a funnel-shaped fibromuscular partition that forms the primary supporting structure for the pelvic contents (Fig. 5.3). It is composed of the levator ani and the coccygeus muscles, along with their superior and inferior fasciae (Table 5.1). It forms the ceiling of the ischiorectal fossa.

Levator Ani

The levatores ani are composed of the pubococcygeus (including the pubovaginalis, pubourethralis, puborectalis, and the iliococcygeus). It is a broad, curved sheet of muscle stretching from the pubis anteriorly and the coccyx posteriorly and from one side of the pelvis to the other. It is perforated by the urethra, vagina, and anal canal. Its origin is from the tendinous arch extending from the body of the pubis to the ischial spine. It is inserted into the central tendon of the perineum, the wall of the anal canal, the anococcygeal ligament, the coccyx, and the vaginal wall.

The levator ani assists the anterior abdominal wall muscles in containing the abdominal and pelvic contents. It supports the vagina, facilitates defecation, and aids in maintaining fecal continence. During parturition, the levator ani supports the fetal head while the cervix dilates. The levator ani is innervated by S3 to S4, the inferior rectal nerve.

Urogenital Diaphragm

The muscles of the urogenital diaphragm reinforce the pelvic diaphragm anteriorly and are intimately related to the vagina and the urethra. They are enclosed between the inferior

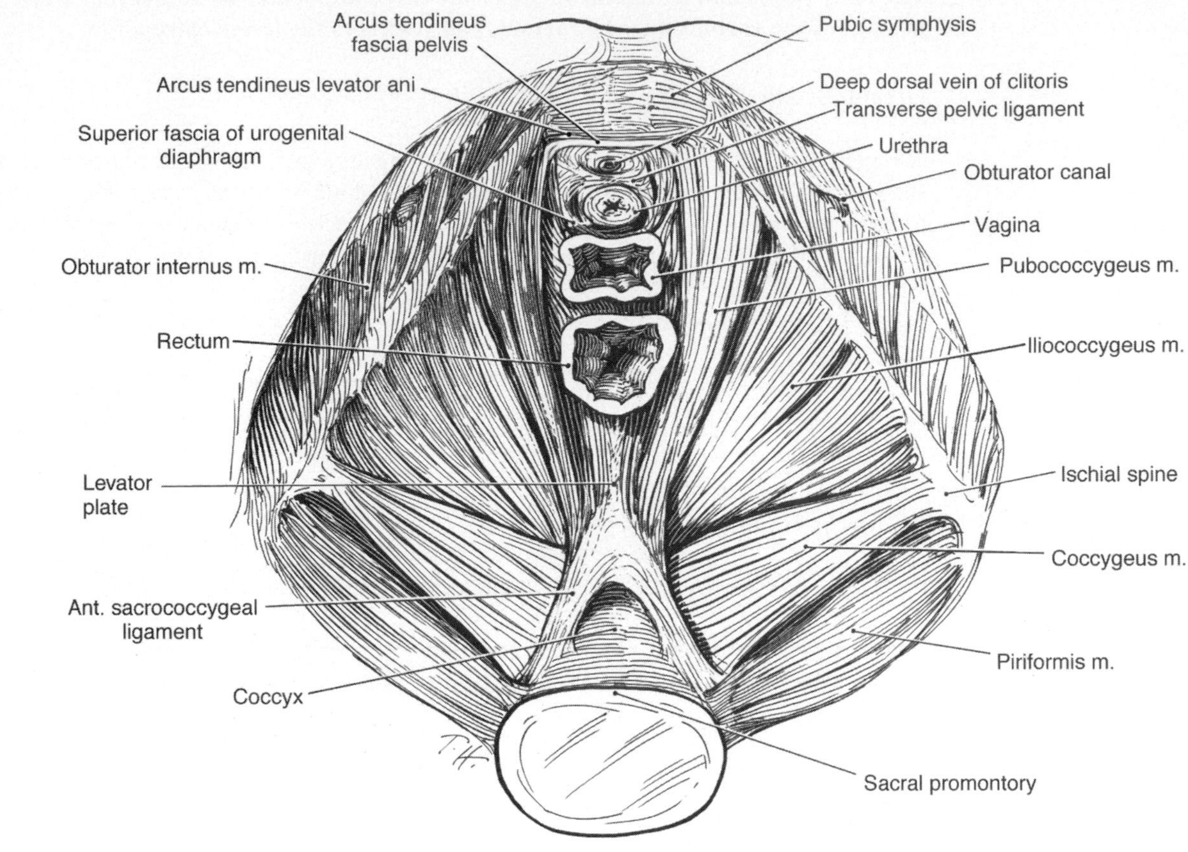

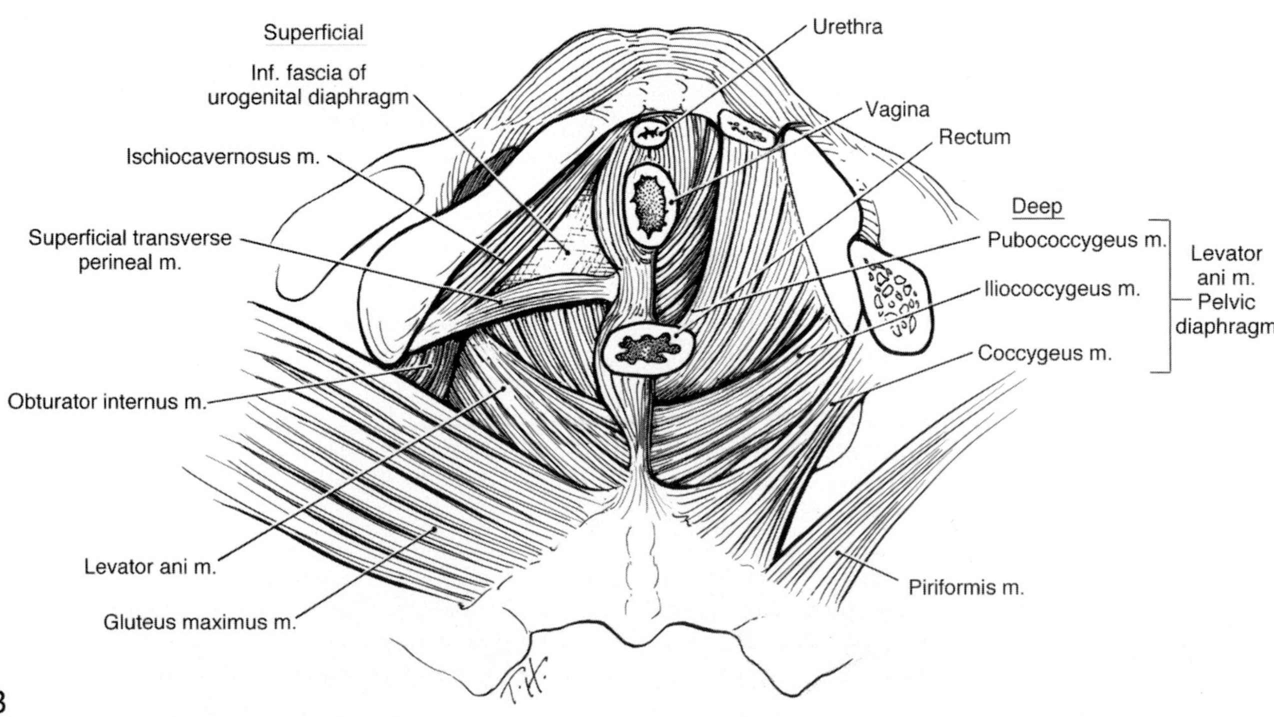

Figure 5.2 The pelvic diaphragm. A: A view into the pelvic floor that illustrates the muscles of the pelvic diaphragm and their attachments to the bony pelvis. **B:** A view from outside the pelvic diaphragm illustrating the divisions of the levator ani muscles (superficial plane removed on the right). **C:** A lateral, sagittal view of the pelvic diaphragm.

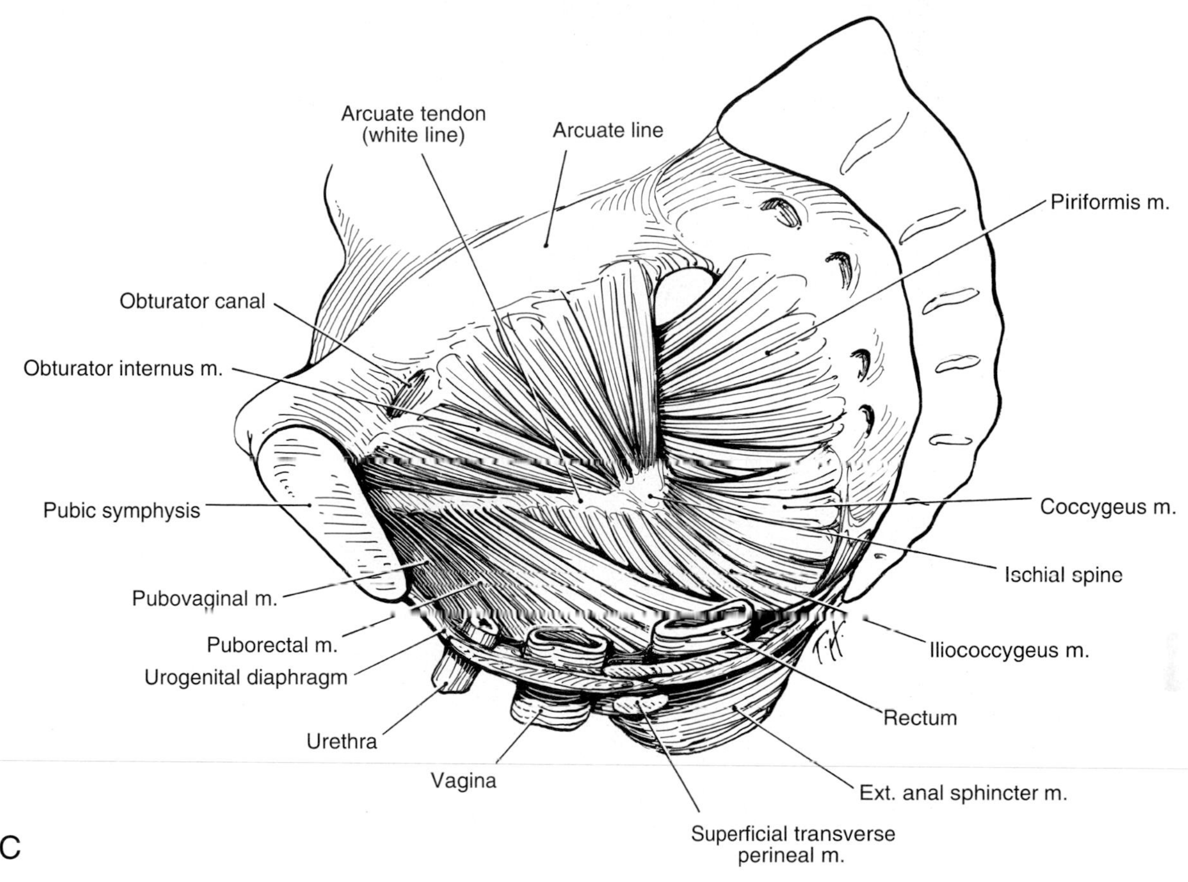

Figure 5.2—*continued*

and superior fascia of the urogenital diaphragm. The muscles include the deep transverse perineal and sphincter urethrae (Table 5.1).

Blood Vessels

The pelvic blood vessels supply genital structures as well as the following:

- Urinary and gastrointestinal tracts.
- Muscles of the abdominal wall, pelvic floor and perineum, buttocks, and upper thighs.
- Fasciae, other connective tissue, and bones.
- Skin and other superficial structures.

Classically, vessels supplying organs are known as *visceral vessels* and those supplying supporting structures are called *parietal vessels*.

Major Blood Vessels

The course of the major vessels supplying the pelvis is illustrated in Fig. 5.4; their origin, course, branches, and venous drainage are presented in Table 5.2. In general, the venous system draining the pelvis closely follows the arterial supply and is named accordingly. Not infrequently, a vein draining a particular area may form a plexus with multiple channels. Venous systems, which are paired, mirror each other in their drainage patterns, with the notable exception of the ovarian veins. Unusual features of venous drainage are also listed in Table 5.2.

Table 5.1. Muscles of the Pelvic Floor

	Origin	*Insertion*	*Action*	*Innervation*
Lateral Pelvic Wall				
Piriformis	Anterior aspect of S2–S4 and sacrotuberous ligament	Greater trochanter of the femur	Lateral rotation, abduction of thigh in flexion; holds head of femur in acetabulum	S1–S2; forms a muscular bed for the sacral plexus
Obturator internus	Superior and inferior pubic rami	Greater trochanter of the femur	Lateral rotation of thigh in flexion; assists in holding head of femur in acetabulum	(L5, S1) Obturator internus nerve
Iliopsoas	Psoas from the lateral margin of the lumbar vertebrae; iliacus from the iliac fossa	Lesser trochanter of the femur	Flexes thigh and stabilizes trunk on thigh; flexes vertebral column or bends it unilaterally	(L1–L3) Psoas-ventral rami of lumbar nerve (L2–L3) Iliacus-femoral nerve contains the lumbar plexus within its muscle body
Pelvic Floor				
Pelvic Diaphragm				
Levator Ani Pubococcygeus Pubovaginalis Puborectalis	From the tendinous arch, extending from the body of the pubis to the ischial spine	Central tendon of the perineum; wall of the anal canal; anococcygeal ligament; coccyx; vaginal wall	Assists the anterior abdominal wall muscles in containing the abdominal and pelvic contents; supports the posterior wall of the vagina; facilitates defecation; aids in fecal continence; during parturition, supports the fetal head during cervical dilation	S3–S4; the inferior rectal nerve
Coccygeus	Ischial spine and sacrospinous ligament	Lateral margin of the fifth sacral vertebra and coccyx	Supports the coccyx and pulls it anteriorly	S4–S5
Urogenital Diaphragm				
Deep transverse perineal	Medial aspect of the ischiopubic rami	Lower part of the vaginal wall; anterior fibers blend with those of the sphincter urethrae	Steadies the central perineal tendon	S2–S4; perineal nerve
Sphincter urethrae	Medial aspect of the ischiopubic rami	Urethra and vagina	Compresses the urethra	S2–S4; perineal nerve

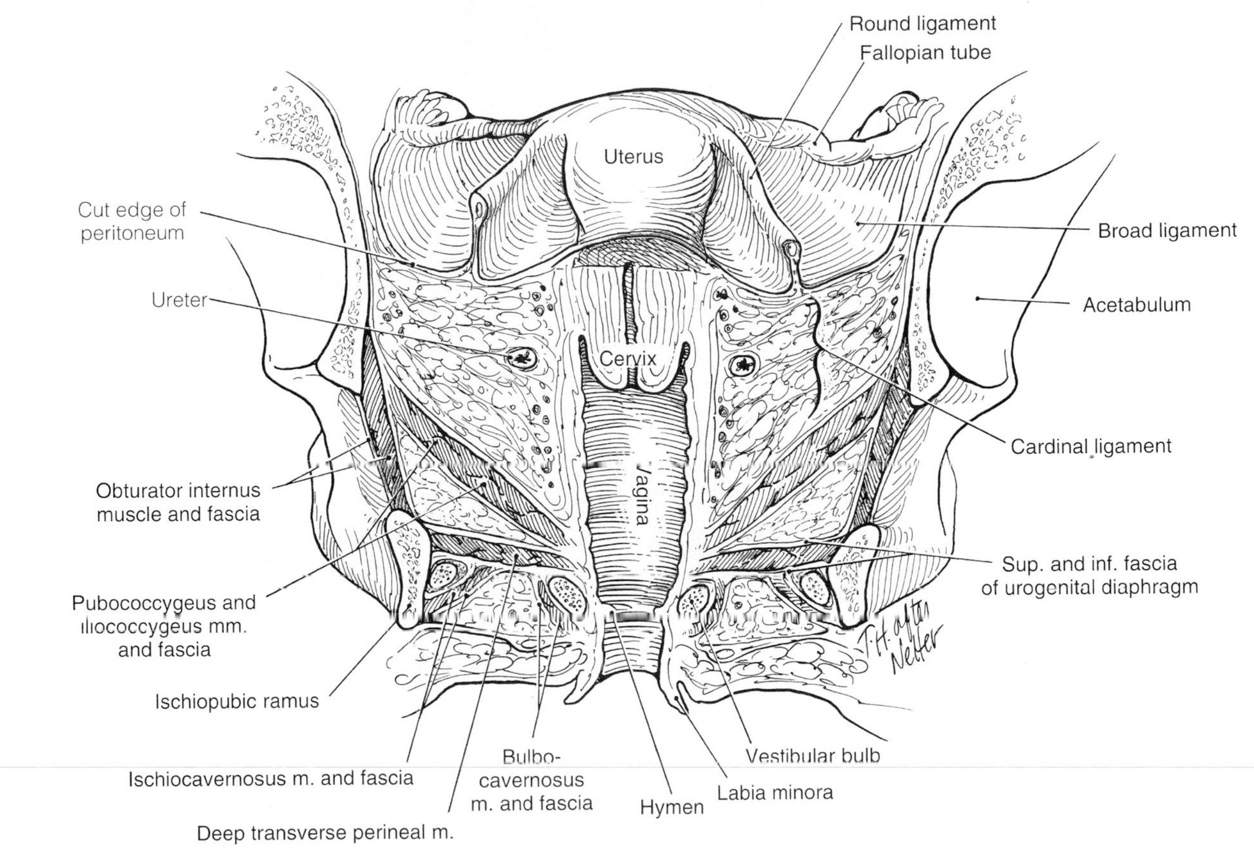

Figure 5.3 The ligaments and fascial support of the pelvic viscera.

General Principles

"Control blood supply" and "maintain meticulous hemostasis" are two of the most common exhortations to young surgeons. In developing familiarity with the pattern of blood flow in the pelvis, several unique characteristics of this vasculature should be understood and may have implications for surgical practice:

1. **The pelvic vessels play an important role in pelvic support.** They provide condensations of endopelvic fascia that act to reinforce the normal position of pelvic organs (3).

2. **There is significant anatomic variation between individuals in the branching pattern of the internal iliac vessels.** There is no constant order in which branches divide from the parent vessel; some branches may arise as common trunks or may spring from other branches rather than from the internal iliac. Occasionally, a branch may arise from another vessel entirely (e.g., the obturator artery may arise from the external iliac or inferior epigastric artery). This variation may also be found in the branches of other major vessels; the ovarian arteries have been reported to arise from the renal arteries or as a common trunk from the front of the aorta on occasion. The inferior gluteal artery may originate from the posterior or the anterior branch of the internal iliac (hypogastric) artery (2). Patterns of blood flow may be asymmetric from side to side, and structures supplied by anastomoses of different vessels may show variation from person to person in proportion of vascular support provided by the vessels involved. The pelvic surgeon must be prepared for deviations from "textbook" vascular patterns.

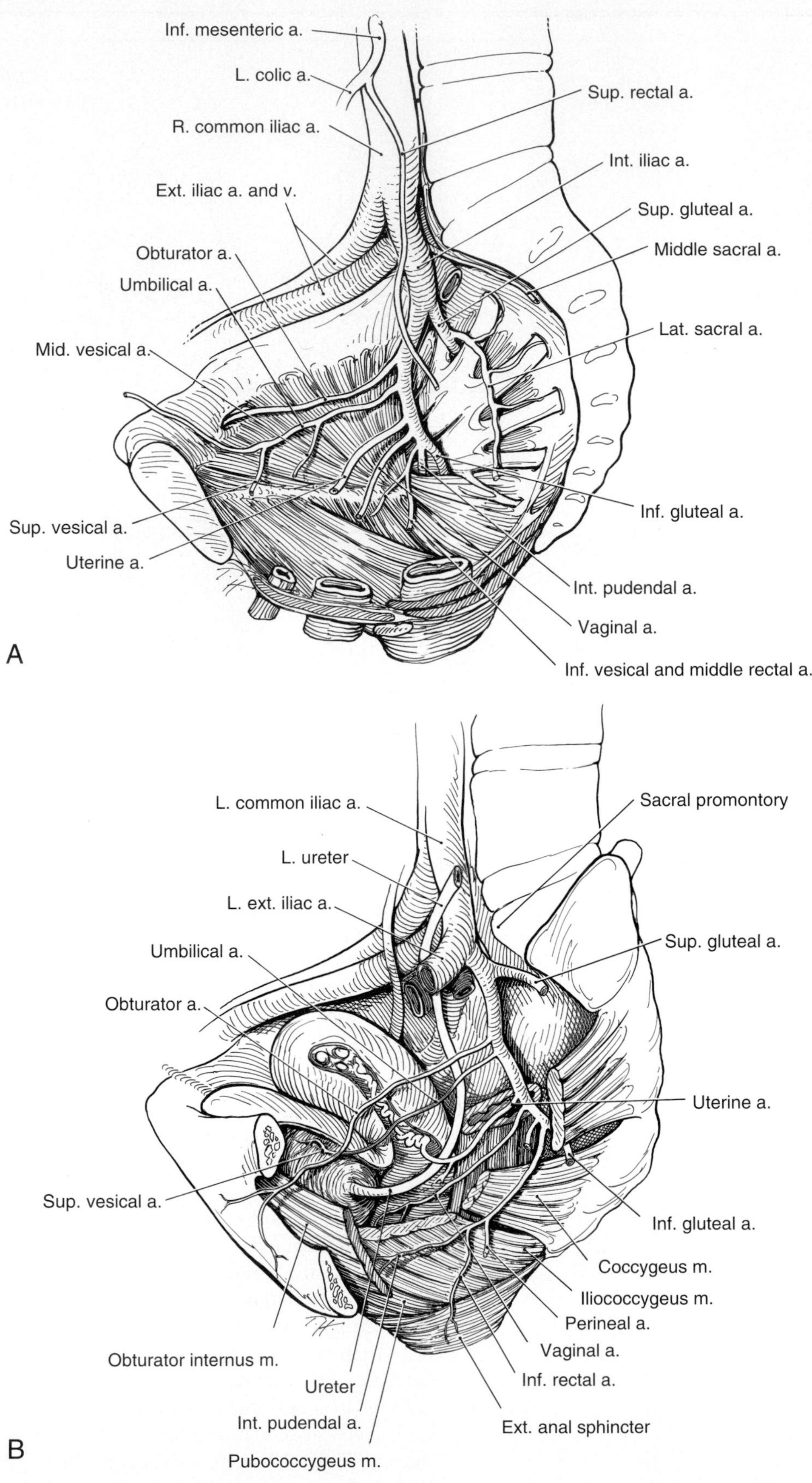

Figure 5.4 The blood supply to the pelvis. A: The sagittal view of the pelvis without the viscera. **B:** The blood supply to one pelvic viscera.

Table 5.2. The Major Blood Vessels of the Pelvis

Artery	*Origin*	*Course*	*Branches*	*Venous Drainage*
Ovarian	Arises from ventral surface of aorta just below the origin of the renal vessels	Crosses over common iliac vessels; in proximity to ureter over much of its course, crosses over ureter while superficial to the psoas muscle and runs just lateral to the ureter when entering the pelvis as part of the infundibulopelvic ligament	To ovaries, fallopian tubes, broad ligament; often small branches to ureter	Right side drains into the inferior vena cava; left drains into the left renal vein
Inferior mesenteric artery (IMA)	Unpaired left-sided retroperitoneal artery arising from the aorta 2–5 cm proximal to its bifurcation	IMA and its branches pass over the left psoas muscle and common iliac vessels; IMA courses anterior to the ureter and ovarian vessels above the pelvic brim	1. *Left colic*—originates above pelvic brim; supplies left transverse colon, splenic flexure, descending colon 2. *Sigmoid*—several branches; supply sigmoid colon 3. *Superior rectal (hemorrhoidal)*—divides into two terminal branches to supply rectum	Inferior mesenteric vein empties into the splenic vein
Common iliac artery	Terminal division of the aorta at fourth lumbar vertebra	Oblique and lateral course, about 5 cm in length	1. *External iliac* 2. *Internal iliac*	Lie posterior and slightly medial to arteries; drain into inferior vena cava
External iliac femoral artery	Lateral bifurcation of common iliac, begins opposite the lumbosacral joint	Along the medial border of the psoas muscle and lateral pelvic side wall; becomes femoral artery after passing under the inguinal ligament to supply lower extremity	1. *Superficial epigastric*—supplies skin and subcutaneous tissue of lower anterior abdominal wall 2. *External pudendal*—supplies skin and subcutanious tissue of mons pubis and anterior vulva 3. *Superficial circumflex iliac*—supplies skin/subcutaneous tissues of the flank 4. *Inferior epigastric*—supplies musculofascial layer of lower anterior abdominal wall 5. *Deep circumflex iliac*—supplies musculofascial layer of lower abdominal wall	Lie posterior and then medial to the artery as it enters the anterior thigh; drain into common iliac veins

Table 5.2.—*continued*

Artery	*Origin*	*Course*	*Branches*	*Venous Drainage*
Internal iliac (hypogastric) artery	Medial bifurcation of common iliac artery, begins opposite the lumbosacral joint; is major blood supply to the pelvis	Descends sharply into the pelvis; divides into an anterior and posterior division 3–4 cm after origin	*Posterior division:* 1. *Iliolumbar*—anastomoses with lumbar and deep circumflex iliac arteries; helps supply lower abdominal wall, iliac fossa 2. *Lateral sacral*—supplies contents of sacral canal, piriformis muscle 3. *Superior gluteal*—supplies gluteal muscles *Anterior division:* 1. *Obturator*—supplies iliac fossa, posterior pubis, obturator internus muscle 2. *Internal pudendal* 3. *Umbilical*—remnant of fetal umbilical artery; after giving off branches, as the medial umbilical ligament 4. *Superior, middle, inferior vesical*—supply bladder and one or more branches to the ureter 5. *Middle rectal (hemorrhoidal)*—supplies rectum, branches to mid vagina 6. *Uterine*—supplies uterine corpus and cervix, with branches to upper vagina, tube, round ligament, and ovary 7. *Vaginal*—supplies vagina 8. *Inferior gluteal*—supplies gluteal muscles, muscles of posterior thigh	Deep to arteries, from complex plexus; drain into common iliac veins

Table 5.2.—*continued*

Artery	*Origin*	*Course*	*Branches*	*Venous Drainage*
Internal pudendal artery	Internal iliac artery; provides the major blood supply to the perineum	Leaves the pelvis through the greater sciatic foramen, courses around the ischial spine, and enters the ischiorectal fossa through the lesser sciatic foramen. In its path to the perineum, lies with the pudendal nerve within Alcock's canal, a fascial tunnel over the obturator internus muscle	1. *Inferior rectal (hemorrhoids)*—supplies anal canal, external anal sphincter, perianal skin, with branches to levator ani 2. *Perineal*—supplies perineal skin, muscles of superficial perineal compartment (bulbocavernosus, ischiocavernosus, superficial transverse perineal) 3. *Clitoral*—supplies clitoris, vestibular bulb, Bartholin gland, and urethra	Drain into internal iliac veins
Middle sacral artery	Midline unpaired vessel arising from posterior terminal aorta Courses over lower lumbar vertebrae, sacrum, and coccyx Supplies bony and muscular structures of posterior pelvic wall Paired middle sacral veins usually drain into left common iliac vein			
Lumbar arteries	Segmental branches arising at each lumbar level from posterior aorta Supplies abdominal wall musculature (external/internal oblique, transversus abdominis) veins into inferior vena cava			

3. **The pelvic vasculature is a high-volume, high-flow system with enormous expansive capabilities throughout reproductive life.** Blood flow through the uterine arteries increases to about 500 mL/min in late pregnancy. In nonpregnant women, certain conditions, such as uterine fibroids or malignant neoplasms, may be associated with neovascularization and hypertrophy of existing vessels and a corresponding increase in pelvic blood flow. Understanding of the volume and flow characteristics of the pelvic vasculature in different clinical situations will enable the surgeon to anticipate problems and take appropriate preoperative and intraoperative measures (including blood and blood product availability) to prevent or manage hemorrhage.

4. **The pelvic vasculature is supplied with an extensive network of collateral connections (Fig. 5.5) that provides a rich anastomotic communication between different major vessel systems.** This degree of redundancy is important to ensure adequate supply of oxygen and nutrients in the event of major trauma or other vascular compromise. *Hypogastric artery ligation continues to be used as a strategy for management of massive pelvic hemorrhage when other measures have failed. Bilateral hypogastric artery ligation, particularly when combined with ovarian artery ligation, dramatically reduces pulse pressure in the pelvis, converting flow characteristics from that of an arterial system to a venous system and allowing use of collateral channels of circulation to continue blood supply to pelvic structures. The significance of collateral blood flow is demonstrated by reports of successful pregnancies occurring after bilateral ligation of both hypogastric and ovarian arteries* (4). Table 5.3 lists the collateral channels of circulation in the pelvis.

Special Vascular Considerations

When inserting a laparoscopic trocar into the anterior abdominal wall, the gynecologic surgeon must keep in mind certain anatomic relationships in order to avoid injury to vascular structures and resultant hemorrhage. The inferior epigastric artery is a branch of the external iliac artery, arising from the parent vessel at the medial border of the inguinal ligament and coursing cephalad lateral to and posterior to the rectus sheath at the level of the arcuate line. It lies about 1.5 cm lateral to the medial umbilical fold, which marks the site of the obliterated umbilical artery. The aortic bifurcation occurs at the level of L4 to L5, just above the sacral promontory. Palpation of the sacral promontory to guide trocar insertion allows the surgeon to avoid the major vascular structures in this area (see Fig. 21.4 in Chapter 21).

Lymphatics

The pelvic lymph nodes are generally arranged in groups or chains and follow the course of the larger pelvic vessels, for which they are usually named. Smaller nodes that lie close to the visceral structures are usually named for those organs. Lymph nodes in the pelvis receive afferent lymphatic vessels from pelvic and perineal visceral and parietal structures and send efferent lymphatics to more proximal nodal groups. The number of lymph nodes and their exact location is variable; however, certain nodes tend to be relatively constant:

1. Obturator node in the obturator foramen, close to the obturator vessels and nerve.

2. Nodes at the junction of the internal and external iliac veins.

3. Ureteral node in the broad ligament near the cervix, where the uterine artery crosses over the ureter.

4. The *Cloquet* or *Rosenmüller* node—the highest of the deep inguinal nodes that lies within the opening of the femoral canal.

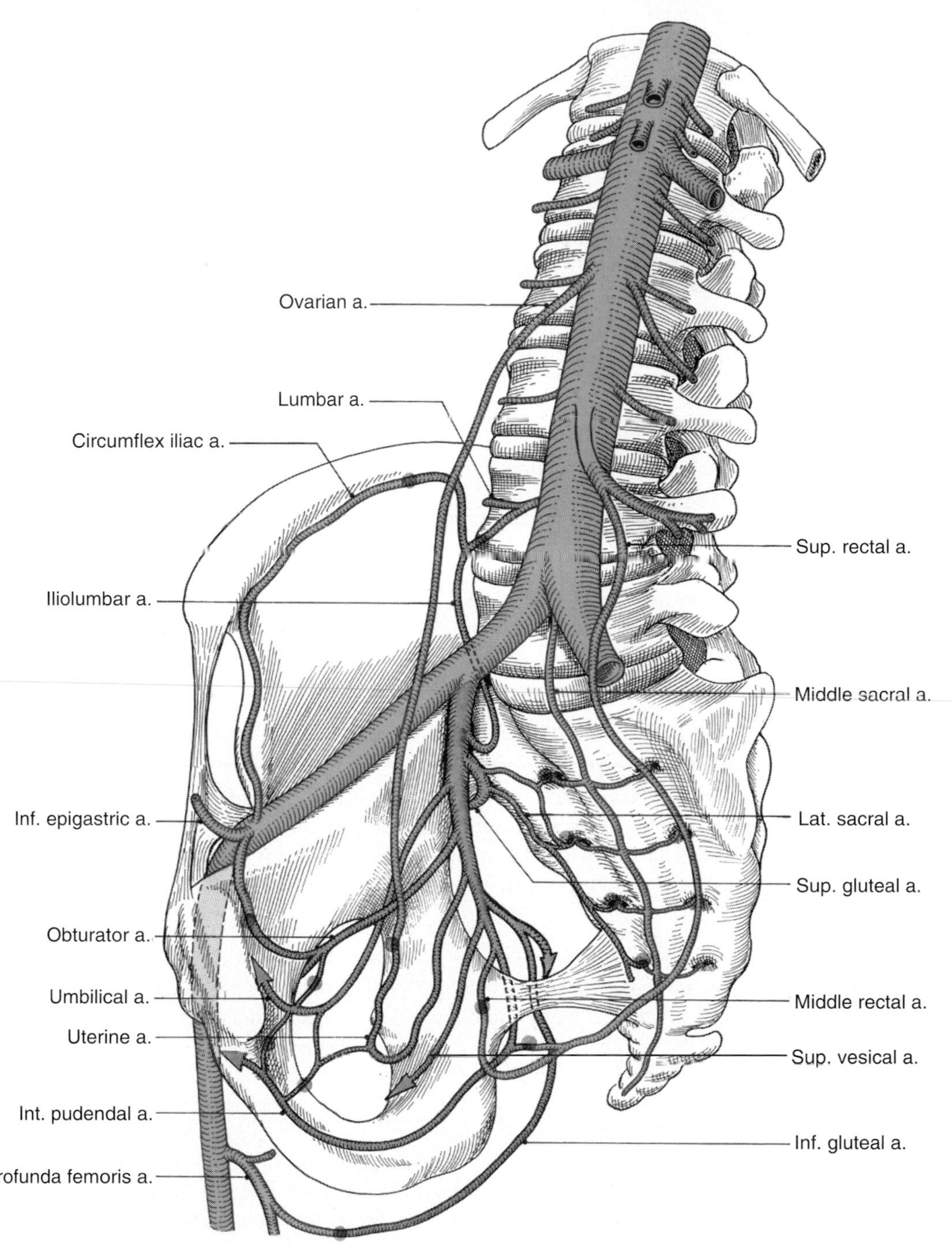

Figure 5.5 The collateral blood vessels of the pelvis. (Modified from **Kamina P.** *Anatomie gynécologique et obstétricale.* Paris: Maloine Sa Éditeur, 1984:125, with permission.)

Figure 5.6 illustrates the pelvic lymphatic system. Table 5.4 outlines the major lymphatic chains of relevance to the pelvis and their primary afferent connections from major pelvic and perineal structures. There are extensive interconnections between lymph vessels and nodes; more than one lymphatic pathway is usually available for drainage of each pelvic site. Bilateral and crossed extension of lymphatic flow may occur, and entire groups of nodes may be bypassed to reach more proximal chains.

The natural history of most genital tract malignancies directly reflects the lymphatic drainage of those structures, although the various interconnections, different lymphatic

Table 5.3. Collateral Arterial Circulation of the Pelvis

Primary Artery	*Collateral Arteries*
Aorta	
Ovarian artery	Uterine artery
Superior rectal artery (inferior mesenteric artery)	Middle rectal artery
	Inferior rectal artery (internal pudendal)
Lumbar arteries	Iliolumbar artery
Vertebral arteries	Iliolumbar artery
Middle sacral artery	Lateral sacral artery
External Iliac	
Deep iliac circumflex artery	Iliolumbar artery
	Superior gluteal artery
Inferior epigastric artery	Obturator artery
Femoral	
Medial femoral circumflex artery	Obturator artery
	Inferior gluteal artery
Lateral femoral circumflex artery	Superior gluteal artery
	Iliolumbar artery

paths, and individual variability make the spread of malignancy somewhat unpredictable. Regional lymph node metastasis is one of the most important factors in formulation of treatment plans for gynecologic malignancies and prediction of eventual outcome.

Nerves

The pelvis is innervated by both the autonomic and somatic nervous systems. The autonomic nerves include both *sympathetic* (adrenergic) and *parasympathetic* (cholinergic) fibers and provide the primary innervation for genital, urinary, and gastrointestinal visceral structures and blood vessels.

Somatic Innervation

The *lumbosacral plexus* (Fig. 5.7) and its branches provide motor and sensory somatic innervation to the lower abdominal wall, the pelvic and urogenital diaphragms, the perineum, and the hip and lower extremity. The nerves originating from the muscles, the lumbosacral trunk, the anterior divisions of the upper four sacral nerves (*sacral plexus*), and the anterior division of the coccygeal nerve and fibers from the fourth and fifth sacral nerves (*coccygeal plexus*) are found on the anterior surface of the piriformis muscle and lateral to the coccyx, respectively, deep in the posterior pelvis. Table 5.5 lists each major branch by spinal segment and structures innervated. In addition to these branches, the lumbosacral plexus includes nerves that innervate muscles of the lateral pelvic wall (obturator internus, piriformis), posterior hip muscles, and the pelvic diaphragm. A visceral component, the pelvic splanchnic nerve, is also included.

Nerves supplying the cutaneous aspects of the anterior, medial, and lateral lower extremities, as well as the deep muscles of the anterior thigh, primarily leave the pelvis by passing beneath the inguinal ligament. Nerves supporting the posterior cutaneous and deep structures of the hip, thigh, and leg lie deep in the pelvis and should not be vulnerable to injury during pelvic surgery. *The obturator nerve travels along the lateral pelvic wall to pass through the obturator foramen into the upper thigh, and it may be encountered in more radical dissections involving the lateral pelvic wall and in paravaginal repairs.*

The pudendal nerve crosses over the piriformis to travel with the internal pudendal vessels into the ischiorectal fossa, where it divides into its three terminal branches to provide the primary innervation to the perineum. Other nerves contribute to the cutaneous innervation

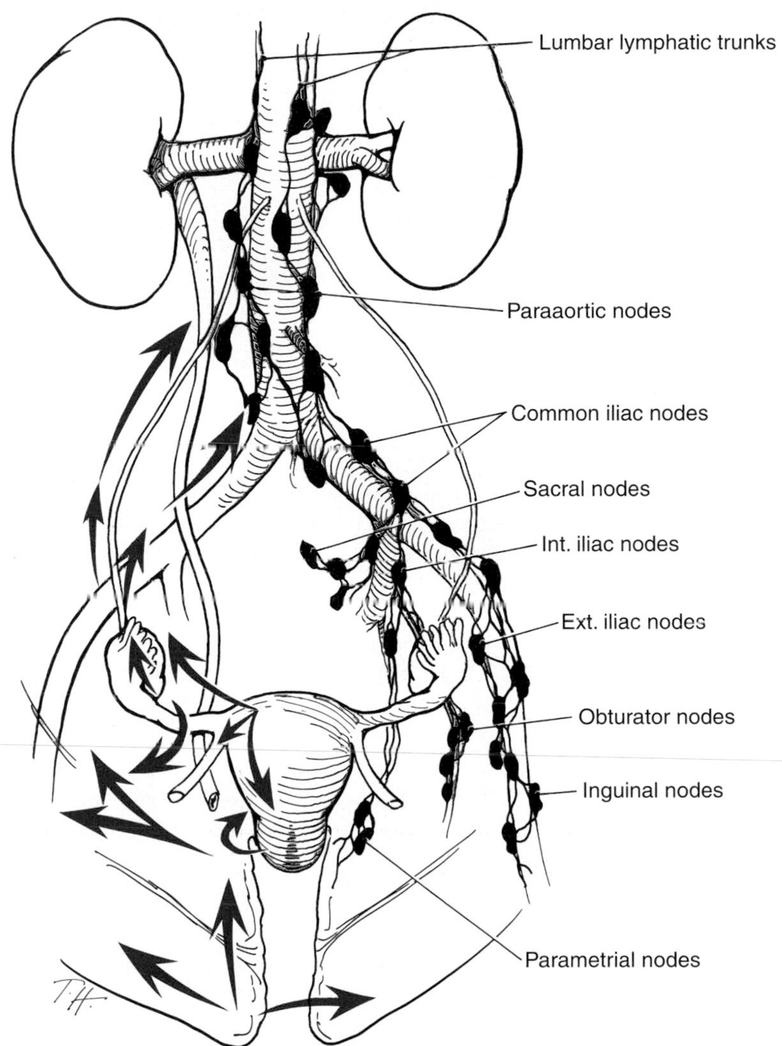

Figure 5.6 The lymphatic drainage of the female pelvis. The vulva and lower vagina drain to the superficial and deep inguinal nodes, sometimes directly to the iliac nodes (along the dorsal vein of the clitoris) and to the other side. The cervix and upper vagina drain laterally to the parametrial, obturator, and external iliac nodes and posteriorly along the uterosacral ligaments to the sacral nodes. Drainage from these primary lymph node groups is upward along the infundibulopelvic ligament, similar to drainage of the ovary and fallopian tubes to the paraaortic nodes. The lower uterine body drains in the same manner as the cervix. Rarely, drainage occurs along the round ligament to the inguinal nodes.

of the perineum:

1. **The anterior labial nerve branches of the ilioinguinal nerve**—these nerves emerge from within the inguinal canal and through the superficial inguinal ring to the mons and upper labia majora.

2. **The genital branch of the genitofemoral nerve**—this branch enters the inguinal canal with the round ligament and passes through the superficial inguinal ring to the anterior vulva.

3. **The perineal branches of the posterior femoral cutaneous nerve**—after leaving the pelvis through the greater sciatic foramen, these branches run in front of the ischial tuberosity to the lateral perineum and labia majora.

Table 5.4. Primary Lymph Node Groups Providing Drainage to Genital Structures

Nodes	*Primary Afferent Connections*
Aortic/paraaortic	Ovary, fallopian tube, uterine corpus (upper); drainage from common iliac nodes
Common iliac	Drainage from external and internal iliac nodes
External iliac	Upper vagina, cervix, uterine corpus (upper); drainage from inguinal nodes
Internal iliac Lateral sacral Superior gluteal Inferior gluteal Obturator Vesical Rectal Parauterine	Upper vagina, cervix, uterine corpus (lower)
Inguinal Superficial Deep	Vulva, lower vagina; (rare: uterus, tube, ovary)

4. **Perforating cutaneous branches of the second and third sacral nerves**—these branches perforate the sacrotuberous ligament to supply the buttocks and contiguous perineum.

5. **The anococcygeal nerves**—these nerves arise from S4 to S5 and also perforate the sacrotuberous ligament to supply the skin overlying the coccyx.

Figure 5.7 The sacral plexus. (Modified from **Kamina P.** *Anatomie gynécologique et obstétricale.* Paris: Maloine Sa Éditeur, 1984:90, with permission.)

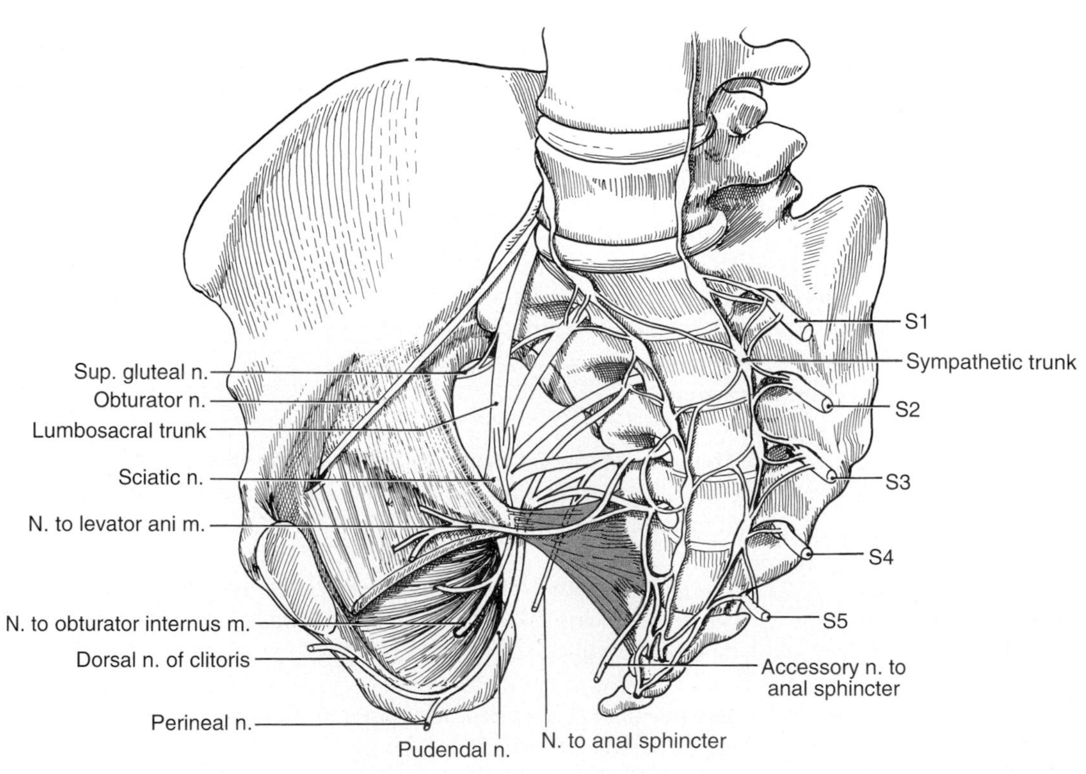

Table 5.5. Lumbosacral Plexus

Nerve	*Spinal Segment*	*Innervation*
Iliohypogastric	T12, L1	Sensory—skin near iliac crest, just above symphysis pubis
Ilioinguinal	L1	Sensory—upper medial thigh, mons, labia majora
Lateral femoral cutaneous	L2, L3	Sensory—lateral thigh to level of knee
Femoral	L2, L3, L4	Sensory—anterior and medial thigh, medial leg and foot, hip and knee joints Motor—iliacus, anterior thigh muscles
Genitofemoral	L1, L2	Sensory—anterior vulva (genital branch) middle/upper anterior thigh (femoral branch)
Obturator	L2, L3, L4	Sensory—medial thigh and leg, hip and knee joints Motor—adductor muscles of thigh
Superior gluteal	L4, L5, S1	Motor—gluteal muscles
Inferior gluteal	L4, L5, S1, S2	Motor—gluteal muscles
Posterior femoral cutaneous	S2, 3	Sensory—vulva, perineum
Sciatic	L4, L5, S1, S2, S3	Sensory—much of leg, foot, lower-extremity joints Motor—posterior thigh muscle, leg and foot muscles
Pudendal	S2, S3, S4	Sensory—perianal skin, vulva and perineum, clitoris, urethra, vaginal vestibule Motor—external anal sphincter, perineal muscles, urogenital diaphragm

Autonomic Innervation

Functionally, the innervation of the pelvic viscera may be divided into an *efferent* component and an *afferent,* or sensory, component. In reality, however, afferent and efferent fibers are closely associated in a complex interlacing network and cannot be separated anatomically.

Efferent Innervation

Efferent fibers of the autonomic nervous system, unlike motor fibers in the somatic system, involve one synapse outside the central nervous system, with two neurons required to carry each impulse. In the *sympathetic (thoracolumbar) division,* this synapse is generally at some distance from the organ being innervated; conversely, the synapse is on or near the organ of innervation in the *parasympathetic (craniosacral) division.*

Axons from preganglionic neurons emerge from the spinal cord to make contact with peripheral neurons arranged in aggregates known as *autonomic ganglia.* Some of these ganglia, along with interconnecting nerve fibers, form a pair of longitudinal cords called the *sympathetic trunks.* Located lateral to the spinal column from the base of the cranium to the coccyx, the sympathetic trunks lie along the medial border of the psoas muscle from T12 to the sacral prominence and then pass behind the common iliac vessels to continue into the pelvis on the anterior surface of the sacrum. On the anterolateral surface of the aorta, the *aortic plexus* forms a lacy network of nerve fibers with interspersed ganglia. Rami arising from or traversing the sympathetic trunks join this plexus and its subsidiaries.

The ovaries and part of the fallopian tubes and broad ligament are innervated by the *ovarian plexus,* a network of nerve fibers accompanying the ovarian vessels and derived from the aortic and renal plexuses. The *inferior mesenteric plexus* is a subsidiary of the *celiac plexus* and *aortic plexus* and is located along the inferior mesenteric artery and its branches, providing innervation to the left colon, sigmoid, and rectum.

The *superior hypogastric plexus (presacral nerve)* (Fig. 5.8) is the continuation of the aortic plexus beneath the peritoneum in front of the terminal aorta, the fifth lumbar vertebra, and the sacral promontory, medial to the ureters. Embedded in loose areolar tissue, the plexus overlies the middle sacral vessels and is usually composed of two or three incompletely fused trunks. It contains preganglionic fibers from lumbar nerves, postganglionic fibers from higher sympathetic ganglia and from the sacral sympathetic trunks, and visceral afferent fibers.

Just below the sacral promontory, the superior hypogastric plexus divides into two loosely arranged nerve trunks, the *hypogastric nerves.* These nerves course inferiorly and laterally to connect with the inferior *hypogastric plexuses (pelvic plexuses)* (Fig. 5.8), which are a dense network of nerves and ganglia that lie along the lateral pelvic sidewall overlying branches of the internal iliac vessels.

Figure 5.8 The presacral nerves.

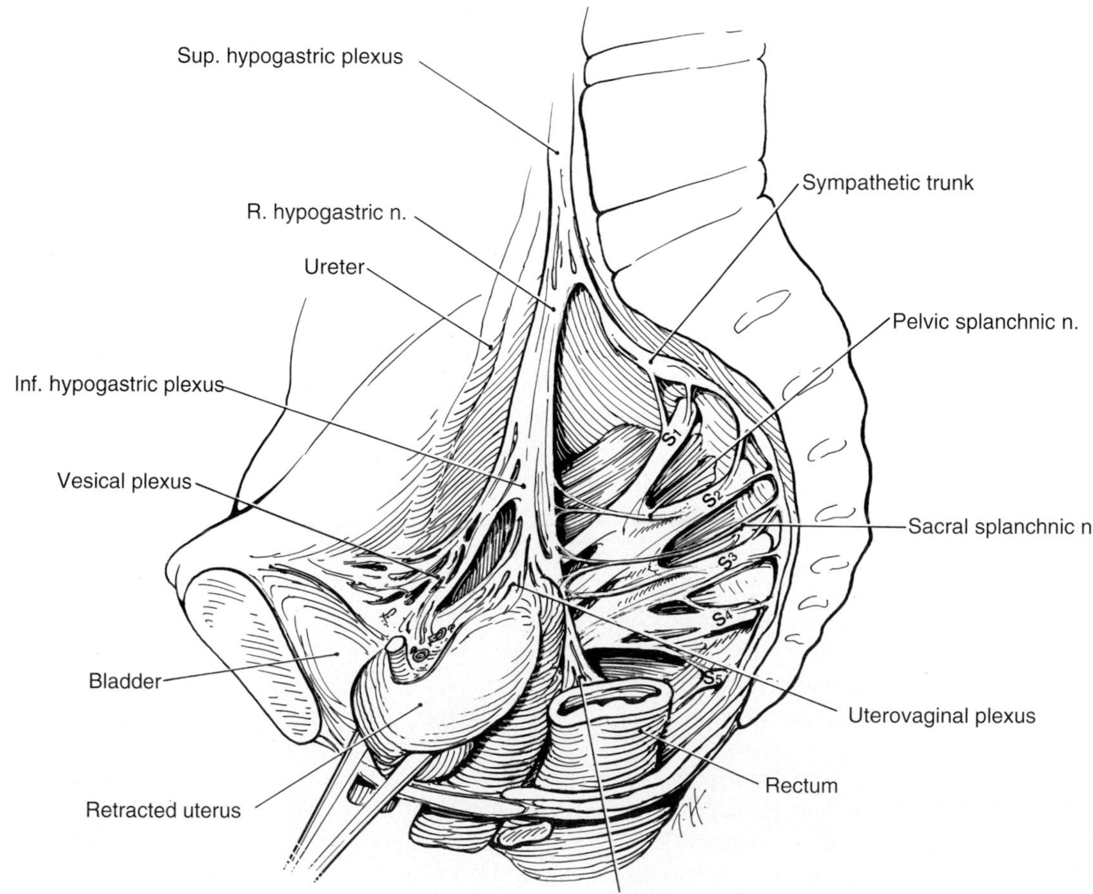

The inferior hypogastric plexus includes efferent sympathetic fibers, afferent (sensory) fibers, and parasympathetic fibers arising from the pelvic splanchnic nerves (S2 to S4, nervi erigentes).

This paired plexus is the final common pathway of the pelvic visceral nervous system and is divided into three portions, representing distribution of innervation to the viscera:

1. **Vesical plexus**
   - Innervation: bladder and urethra
   - Course: along vesical vessels

2. **Middle rectal plexus (hemorrhoidal)**
   - Innervation: rectum
   - Course: along middle rectal vessels

3. **Uterovaginal plexus (Frankenhäuser ganglion)**
   - Innervation: uterus, vagina, clitoris, vestibular bulbs
   - Course: along uterine vessels and through cardinal and uterosacral ligaments; sympathetic and sensory fibers derive from T10, L1; parasympathetic fibers derive from S2 to S4.

Afferent Innervation

Afferent **fibers from the pelvic viscera and blood vessels traverse the same pathways to provide sensory input to the central nervous system.** They are also involved in reflex arcs needed for bladder, bowel, and genital tract function. The afferent fibers reach the central nervous system to have their first synapse within posterior spinal nerve ganglia.

Presacral neurectomy, in which a segment of the superior hypogastric plexus is divided and resected in order to interrupt sensory fibers from the uterus and cervix, has been associated with relief of dysmenorrhea secondary to endometriosis in about 50% to 75% of cases in which it has been employed (5,6). Because efferent fibers from the adnexa travel with the ovarian plexus, pain originating from the ovary or tube is not relieved by resection of the presacral nerve. Because this plexus also contains efferent sympathetic and parasympathetic nerve fibers intermixed with afferent fibers, disturbance in bowel or bladder function may result. An alternative surgical procedure advocated in recent years is resection of a portion of the uterosacral ligaments; because they contain numerous nerve fibers with more specific innervation to the uterus, it is postulated that bladder and rectal function is less vulnerable to compromise.

An anesthetic block of the pudendal nerve is performed most often for pain relief with uncomplicated vaginal deliveries but may also provide useful anesthesia for minor perineal surgical procedures. This nerve block may be accomplished transvaginally or through the perineum. A needle is inserted toward the ischial spine with the tip directed slightly posteriorly and through the sacrospinous ligament. As anesthetic agent is injected, frequent aspiration is required to avoid injection into the pudendal vessels, which travel with the nerve.

Pelvic Viscera

Embryonic Development

The female urinary and genital tracts are closely related, not only anatomically but also embryologically. Both are derived largely from primitive mesoderm and endoderm, and there is evidence that the embryologic urinary system has an important inductive influence on the developing genital system. **About 10% of infants are born with some abnormality of**

Table 5.6. Development of Genital and Urinary Tracts by Embryologic Age

Weeks of Gestation	Genital Development	Urinary Development
4–6	Urorectal septum	Pronephros
	Formation of cloacal folds, genital tubercle	Mesonephros/mesonephric duct
		Ureteric buds, metanephros
	Genital ridges	Exstrophy of mesonephric ducts and ureters into bladder wall
6–7	End of indifferent phase of genital development	Major, minor calyces form
	Development of primitive sex cords	Kidneys begin to ascend
	Formation of paramesonephric ducts	
	Labioscrotal swellings	
8–11	Distal paramesonephric ducts begin to fuse	Kidney becomes functional
	Formation of sinuvaginal bulbs	
12	Development of clitoris and vaginal vestibule	
20	Canalization of vaginal plate	
32		Renal collecting duct system complete

the genitourinary system, and anomalies in one system are often mirrored by anomalies in another system (7).

Developmental defects may play a significant role in the differential diagnosis of certain clinical signs and symptoms and have special implications in pelvic surgery (7–11). This is important for the practicing gynecologist to have a basic understanding of embryology.

Following is a presentation of the urinary system, internal reproductive organs, and external genitalia in order of their initial appearance, although much of their development proceeds concurrently. The development of each of these three regions proceeds synchronously at an early embryologic age (Table 5.6).

Urinary System

Kidneys, Renal Collecting System, Ureters

The kidneys, renal collecting system, and ureters derive from the longitudinal mass of mesoderm (known as the *nephrogenic cord*) found on each side of the primitive aorta. This process gives rise to three successive sets of increasingly advanced urinary structures, each developing more caudal to its predecessor.

The *pronephros,* or "first kidney," is rudimentary and nonfunctional; it is succeeded by the "middle kidney," or *mesonephros*, which is believed to function briefly before regressing. Although the *mesonephros* is transitory as an excretory organ, its duct, the *mesonephric (wolffian) duct*, is of singular importance for the following reasons:

1. It grows caudally in the developing embryo to open, for the first time, an excretory channel into the primitive cloaca and the "outside world."

2. It serves as the starting point for development of the metanephros, which becomes the definitive kidney.

3. It ultimately differentiates into the sexual duct system in the male.

4. Although regressing in female fetuses, there is evidence that the mesonephric duct may have an inductive role in development of the paramesonephric or müllerian duct (8).

Development of the *metanephros* is initiated by the ureteric buds, which sprout from the distal mesonephric ducts; these buds extend cranially and penetrate the portion of the nephrogenic cord known as the *metanephric blastema.* The ureteric buds begin to branch sequentially, with each growing tip covered by metanephric blastema. The metanephric blastema ultimately form the renal functional units (the nephrons), whereas the ureteric buds become the collecting duct system of the kidneys (collecting tubules, minor and major calyces, renal pelvis) and the ureters. Although these primitive tissues differentiate along separate paths, they are interdependent on inductive influences from each other—neither can develop alone.

The kidneys initially lie in the pelvis but subsequently ascend to their permanent location, rotating almost 90 degrees in the process as the more caudal part of the embryo in effect grows away from them. Their blood supply, which first arises as branches of the middle sacral and common iliac arteries, comes from progressively higher branches of the aorta until the definitive renal arteries form; previous vessels then regress.

Bladder and Urethra

The cloaca forms as the result of dilation of the opening to the fetal exterior. The cloaca is partitioned by the mesenchymal urorectal septum into an anterior urogenital sinus and a posterior rectum. The bladder and urethra form from the most superior portion of the urogenital sinus, with surrounding mesenchyme contributing to their muscular and serosal layers. The remaining inferior urogenital sinus is known as the *phallic* or *definitive urogenital sinus.*

Concurrently, the distal mesonephric ducts and attached ureteric buds are incorporated into the posterior bladder wall in the area that will become the bladder trigone. As a result of the absorption process, the mesonephric duct ultimately opens independently into the urogenital sinus below the bladder neck.

The *allantois,* which is a vestigial diverticulum of the hindgut that extends into the umbilicus and is continuous with the bladder, loses its lumen and becomes the fibrous band known as the *urachus* or *median umbilical ligament.* In rare instances, the urachal lumen remains partially patent, with formation of urachal cysts, or completely patent, with the formation of a urinary fistula to the umbilicus.

Genital System

Although genetic sex is determined at fertilization, the early genital system is indistinguishable between the two sexes in the embryonic stage. This is known as the "indifferent stage" of genital development, during which both male and female fetuses have gonads with prominent cortical and medullary regions, dual sets of genital ducts, and external genitalia that appear similar. Clinically, **gender is not apparent until about the twelfth week of embryonic life and depends on the elaboration of testis-determining factor (TDY) and, subsequently, androgens by the male gonad.** Female development has been called the "basic developmental path of the human embryo," requiring not estrogen but the absence of testosterone.

Internal Reproductive Organs

The *primordial germ cells* migrate from the yolk sac through the mesentery of the hindgut to the posterior body wall mesenchyme at about the tenth thoracic level, which is the initial site of the future ovary (Figs. 5.9 and 5.10). Once the germ cells reach this area, they induce proliferation of cells in the adjacent mesonephros and celomic epithelium to form a pair of *genital ridges* medial to the mesonephros. The development of the gonad is absolutely dependent on this proliferation because these cells form a supporting aggregate of cells (the primitive sex cords) that invest the germ cells and without which the gonad would degenerate.

Müllerian Ducts The *paramesonephric* or *müllerian ducts* form lateral to the mesonephric ducts; they grow caudally and then medially to fuse in the midline. They contact the urogenital sinus in the region of the posterior urethra at a slight thickening known as the *sinusal tubercle.* Subsequent sexual development is controlled by the presence or absence of TDY, encoded on the Y chromosome and elaborated by the somatic sex cord cells. TDY results in the degeneration of the gonadal cortex and differentiation of the medullary region of the gonad into Sertoli cells.

The Sertoli cells secrete a glycoprotein known as *anti-müllerian hormone (AMH),* which causes regression of the paramesonephric duct system in the male embryo and is the likely signal for differentiation of Leydig cells from the surrounding mesenchyme. The Leydig cells produce testosterone and, with the converting enzyme 5α-reductase, dihydrotestosterone. Testosterone is responsible for evolution of the mesonephric duct system into the vas deferens, epididymis, ejaculatory ducts, and seminal vesicle; at puberty, testosterone leads to spermatogenesis and changes in primary and secondary sex characteristics. Dihydrotestosterone results in development of the male external genitalia and the prostate and bulbourethral glands. In the absence of TDY, the medulla regresses, and the cortical sex cords break up into isolated cell clusters (the primordial follicles).

The germ cells differentiate into oogonia and enter the first meiotic division as primary oocytes, at which point development is arrested until puberty. In the absence of AMH, the mesonephric duct system degenerates, although in at least one fourth of adult women (9), remnants may be found in the mesovarium (*epoophoron, paroophoron*) or along the lateral wall of the uterus or vagina (*Gartner duct cyst*).

The paramesonephric duct system then develops. The inferior fused portion becomes the *uterovaginal canal,* which later becomes the epithelium and glands of the uterus and the upper vagina. The endometrial stroma and myometrium differentiate from surrounding mesenchyme. The cranial unfused portions of the paramesonephric ducts open into the celomic (future peritoneal) cavity and become the *fallopian tubes.*

The fusion of the paramesonephric ducts brings together two folds of peritoneum, which become the broad ligament and divide the pelvic cavity into a posterior rectouterine and anterior vesicouterine pouch or cul-de-sac. Between the leaves of the broad ligament, mesenchyme proliferates and differentiates into loose areolar connective tissue and smooth muscle.

Vagina The *vagina* forms in the third month of embryonic life. While the uterovaginal canal is forming, the endodermal tissue of the sinusal tubercle begins to proliferate, forming a pair of *sinovaginal bulbs,* which become the inferior 20% of the vagina. The most inferior portion of the uterovaginal canal becomes occluded by a solid core of tissue (*the vaginal plate*), the origin of which is unclear. This tissue elongates over the subsequent 2 months and canalizes by a process of central desquamation, and the peripheral cells become the vaginal epithelium. The fibromuscular wall of the vagina originates from the mesoderm of the uterovaginal canal.

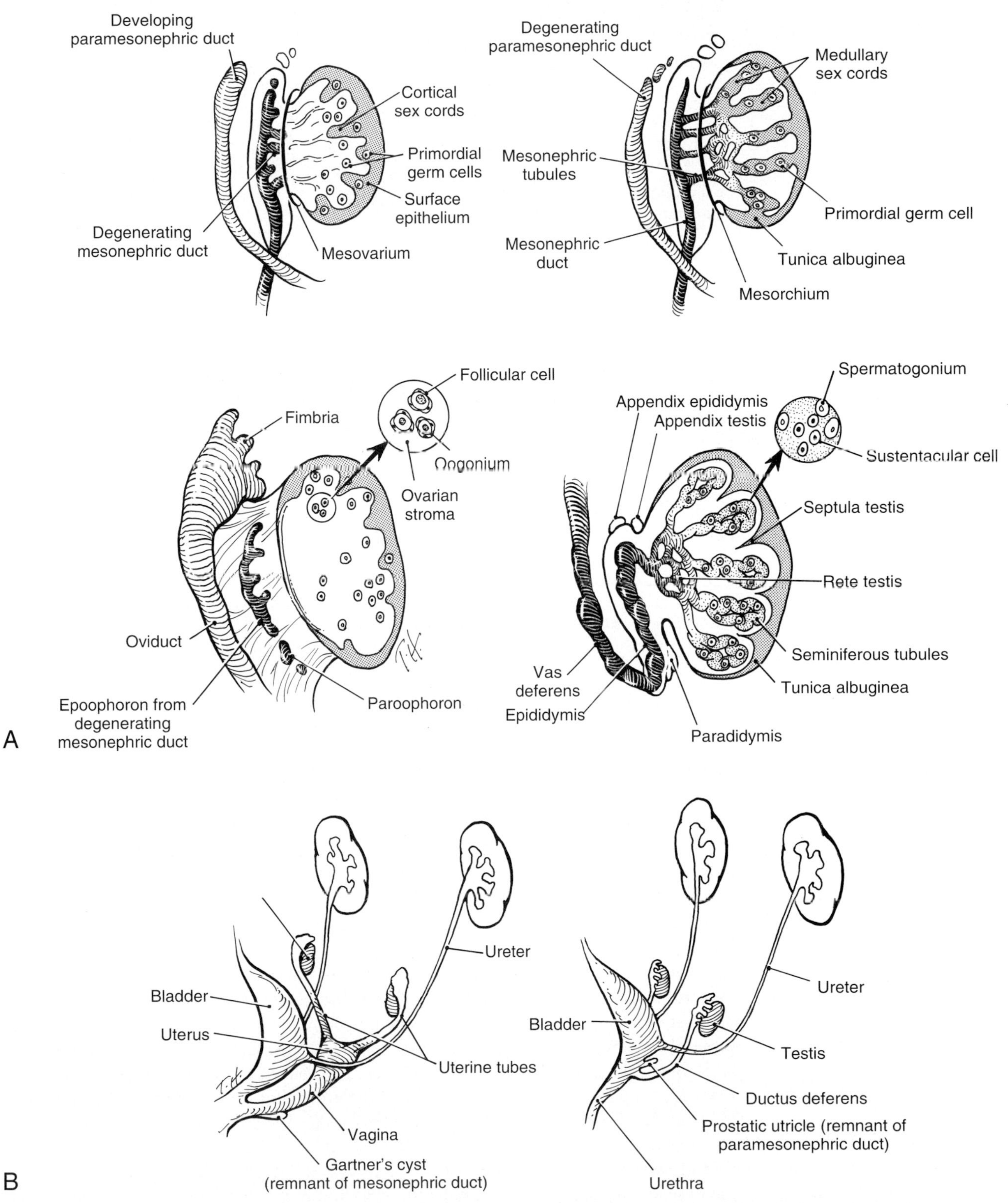

Figure 5.9 The comparative changes of the female and male during early embryonic development.

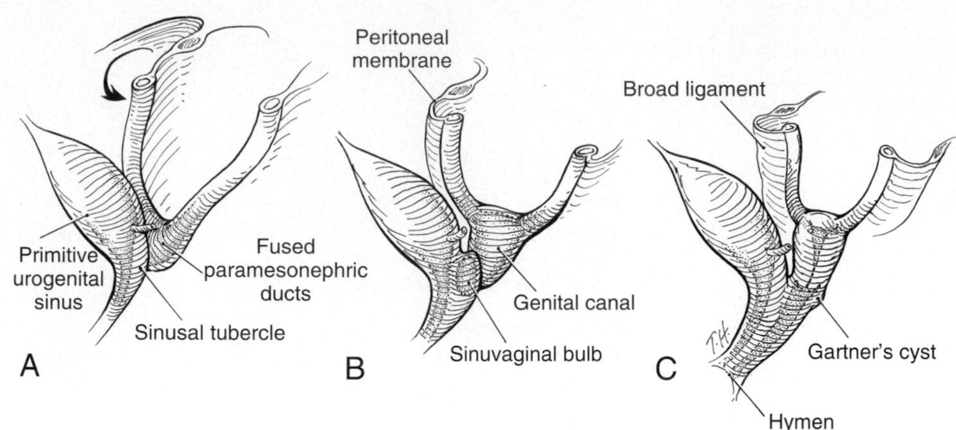

Figure 5.10 The embryonic development of the female genital tract. The formation of the uterus and vagina. **A:** The uterus and superior end of the vagina begin to form as the paramesonephric ducts fuse together near their attachment to the posterior wall of the primitive urogenital sinus. **B, C:** The ducts then zipper together in a superior direction between the third and fifth months. As the paramesonephric ducts are pulled away from the posterior body wall, they drag a fold of peritoneal membrane with them, forming the broad ligaments of the uterus. **A–C:** The inferior end of the vagina forms from the sinovaginal bulbs on the posterior wall of the primitive urogenital sinus.

Accessory Genital Glands The female accessory genital glands develop as outgrowths from the urethra (*paraurethral* or *Skene*) and the definitive urogenital sinus (*greater vestibular* or *Bartholin*). Although the ovaries first develop in the thoracic region, they ultimately arrive in the pelvis by a complicated process of descent. This descent *by differential growth* is under the control of a ligamentous cord called the *gubernaculum,* which is attached to the ovary superiorly and to the fascia in the region of the future labia majora inferiorly. The gubernaculum becomes attached to the paramesonephric ducts at their point of superior fusion so that it becomes divided into two separate structures. As the ovary and its mesentery (the mesovarium) are brought into the superior portion of the broad ligament, the more proximal part of the gubernaculum becomes the *ovarian ligament,* and the distal gubernaculum becomes the *round ligament.*

External Genitalia

Early in the fifth week of embryonic life, folds of tissue form on each side of the cloaca and meet anteriorly in the midline to form the genital tubercle (Fig. 5.11). With the division of the cloaca by the urorectal septum and consequent formation of the perineum, these cloacal folds are known anteriorly as the *urogenital folds* and posteriorly as the *anal folds.* The genital tubercle begins to enlarge, but in the female embryo, its growth gradually slows to become the clitoris, and the urogenital folds form the labia minora. In the male, the genital tubercle continues to grow to form the penis, and the urogenital folds are believed to fuse to enclose the penile urethra. Lateral to the urogenital folds, another pair of swellings develops, known in the indifferent stage as *labioscrotal swellings.* In the absence of androgens, they remain largely unfused to become the labia majora. The definitive urogenital sinus gives rise to the vaginal vestibule, into which open the urethra, vagina, and greater vestibular glands.

Clinical Correlations

Developmental abnormalities of the urinary and genital systems can be explained and understood by a consideration of female and male embryologic development. Because of

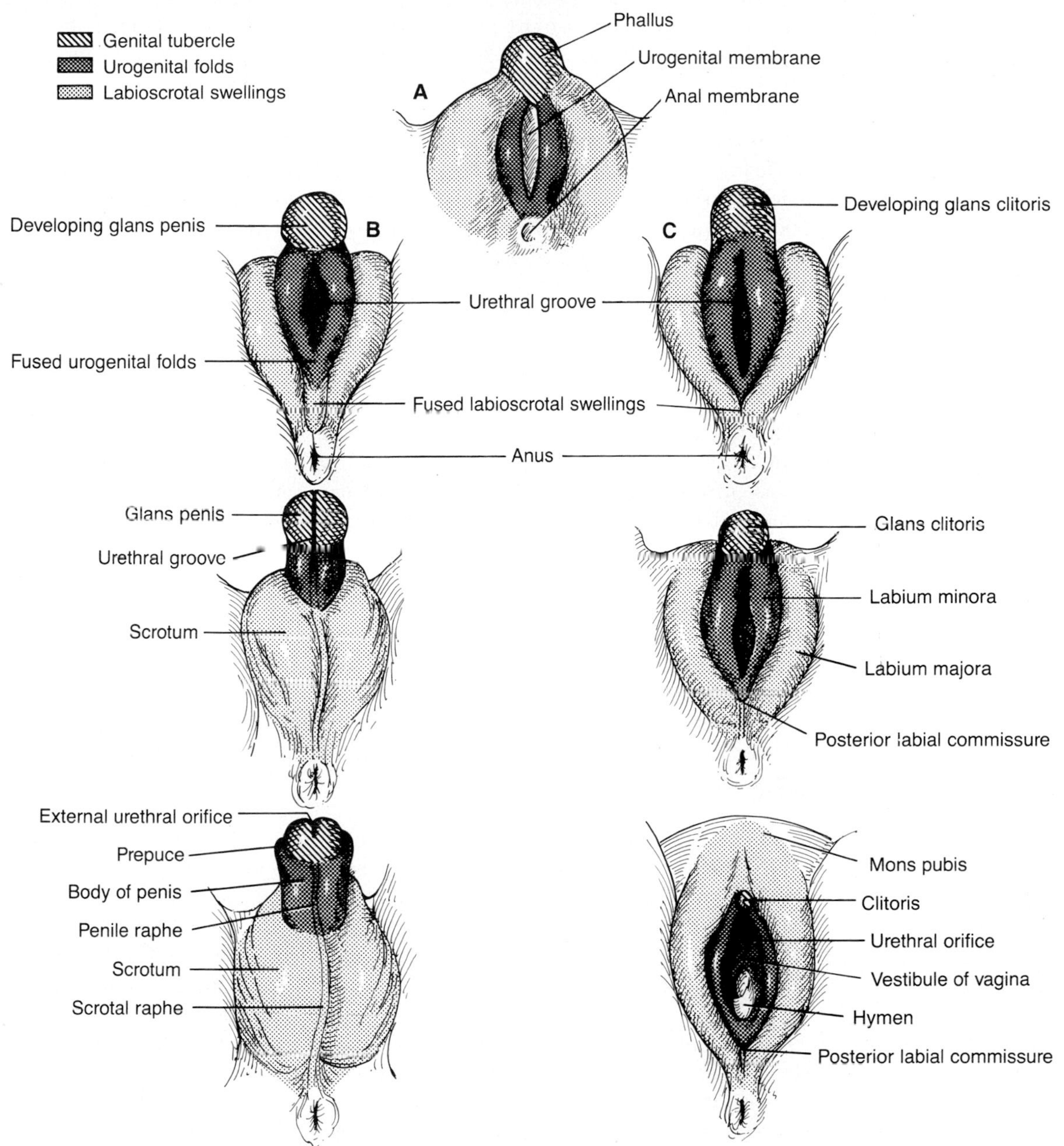

Figure 5.11 The comparative development of the female and male external genitalia. A: In both sexes, the development follows a uniform pattern through the seventh week and thereafter begins to differentiate. **B:** The male external genitalia. **C:** The female external genitalia.

the intertwined development of these two systems, it is easy to understand how abnormalities in one may be associated with abnormalities in the other (10).

Urinary System

Urinary tract anomalies arise from defects in the ureteric bud, the metanephric blastema, or their inductive interaction with each other.

Renal Agenesis Renal agenesis occurs when one or both ureteric buds fail to form or degenerate, and the metanephric blastema is therefore not induced to differentiate into nephrons. Bilateral renal agenesis is incompatible with postnatal survival, but infants with only one kidney usually survive, and the single kidney undergoes compensatory hypertrophy. Unilateral renal agenesis is often associated with absence or abnormality of fallopian tubes, uterus, or vagina—the paramesonephric duct derivatives.

Abnormalities of Renal Position Abnormalities of renal position result from disturbance in the normal ascent of the kidneys. A malrotated pelvic kidney is the most common result; a horseshoe kidney, in which the kidneys are fused across the midline, occurs in about 1 in 600 individuals and also has a final position lower than usual because its normal ascent is prevented by the root of the inferior mesenteric artery.

Duplication of the Upper Ureter and Renal Pelvis Duplication of the upper ureter and renal pelvis are relatively common and result from premature bifurcation of the ureteric bud. If two ureteric buds develop, there will be complete duplication of the collecting system. In this situation, one ureteric bud will open normally into the posterior bladder wall, and the second bud will be carried more distally within the mesonephric duct to form an ectopic ureteral orifice into the urethra, vagina, or vaginal vestibule; incontinence is the primary presenting symptom. Most of the aforementioned urinary abnormalities remain asymptomatic unless obstruction or infection supervenes. In that case, anomalous embryologic development must be included in the differential diagnosis.

Genital System

Because the early development of the genital system is similar in both sexes, congenital defects in sexual development, usually arising from a variety of chromosomal abnormalities, tend to present clinically with ambiguous external genitalia. These conditions are known as *intersex conditions* or *hermaphroditism* and are classified according to the histologic appearance of the gonads (see Chapter 24).

True Hermaphroditism **Individuals with true hermaphroditism have both ovarian and testicular tissue, most commonly as composite ovotestes but occasionally with an ovary on one side and a testis on the other.** In the latter case, a fallopian tube and single uterine horn may develop on the side with the ovary because of the absence of local AMH. True hermaphroditism is an extremely rare condition associated with chromosomal mosaicism, mutation, or abnormal cleavage involving the X and Y chromosomes.

Pseudohermaphroditism **In individuals with pseudohermaphroditism, the genetic sex indicates one gender, and the external genitalia has characteristics of the other gender.** Males with pseudohermaphroditism are genetic males with feminized external genitalia, most commonly manifesting as hypospadias (urethral opening on the ventral surface of the penis) or incomplete fusion of the urogenital or labioscrotal folds. Females with pseudohermaphroditism are genetic females with virilized external genitalia, including clitoral hypertrophy and some degree of fusion of the urogenital or labioscrotal folds. Both types of pseudohermaphroditism are caused either by abnormal levels of sex hormones or abnormalities in the sex hormone receptors.

Another major category of genital tract abnormalities involves various types of uterovaginal malformations (Fig. 5.12), which occur in 0.16% of women (12). These malformations are believed to result from one or more of the following situations:

1. Improper fusion of the paramesonephric ducts
2. Incomplete development of one paramesonephric duct
3. Failure of part of the paramesonephric duct on one or both sides to develop
4. Absent or incomplete canalization of the vaginal plate

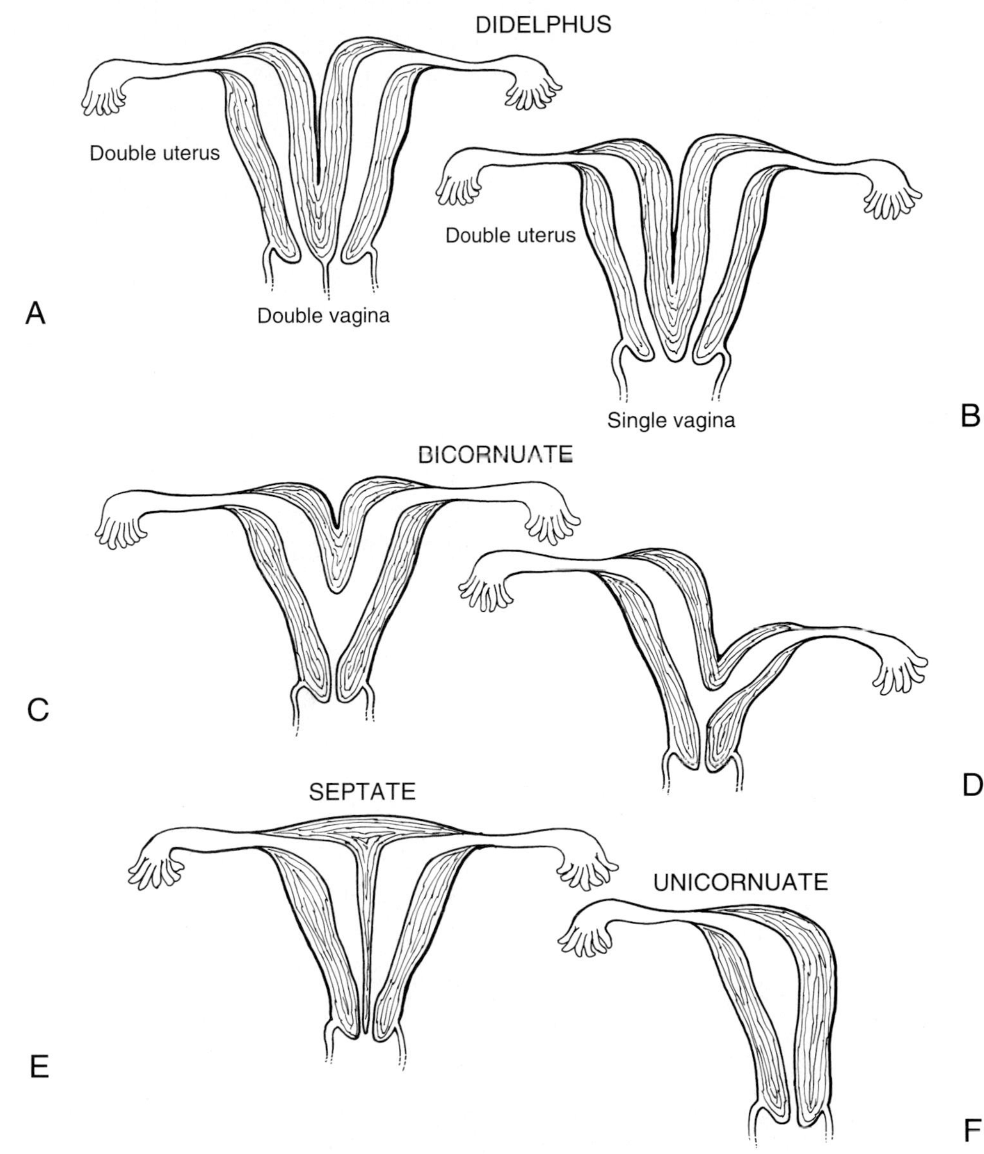

Figure 5.12 Types of congenital abnormalities. A: Double uterus (uterus didelphys) and double vagina. **B:** Double uterus with single vagina. **C:** Bicornuate uterus. **D:** Bicornuate uterus with a rudimentary left horn. **E:** Septate uterus. **F:** Unicornuate uterus.

Genital Structures

Vagina

A sagittal section of the female pelvis is presented in Fig. 5.13.

The vagina is a hollow fibromuscular tube extending from the vulvar vestibule to the uterus. In the dorsal lithotomy position, the vagina is directed posteriorly toward the sacrum, but its axis is almost horizontal in the upright position. It is attached at its upper end to the uterus just above the cervix. The spaces between the cervix and vagina are known as the *anterior, posterior,* and *lateral vaginal fornices.* Because the vagina is attached at a higher point posteriorly than anteriorly, the posterior vaginal wall is about 3 cm longer than the anterior wall.

The posterior vaginal fornix is separated from the posterior cul-de-sac and peritoneal cavity by the vaginal wall and peritoneum. This proximity is clinically useful, both diagnostically

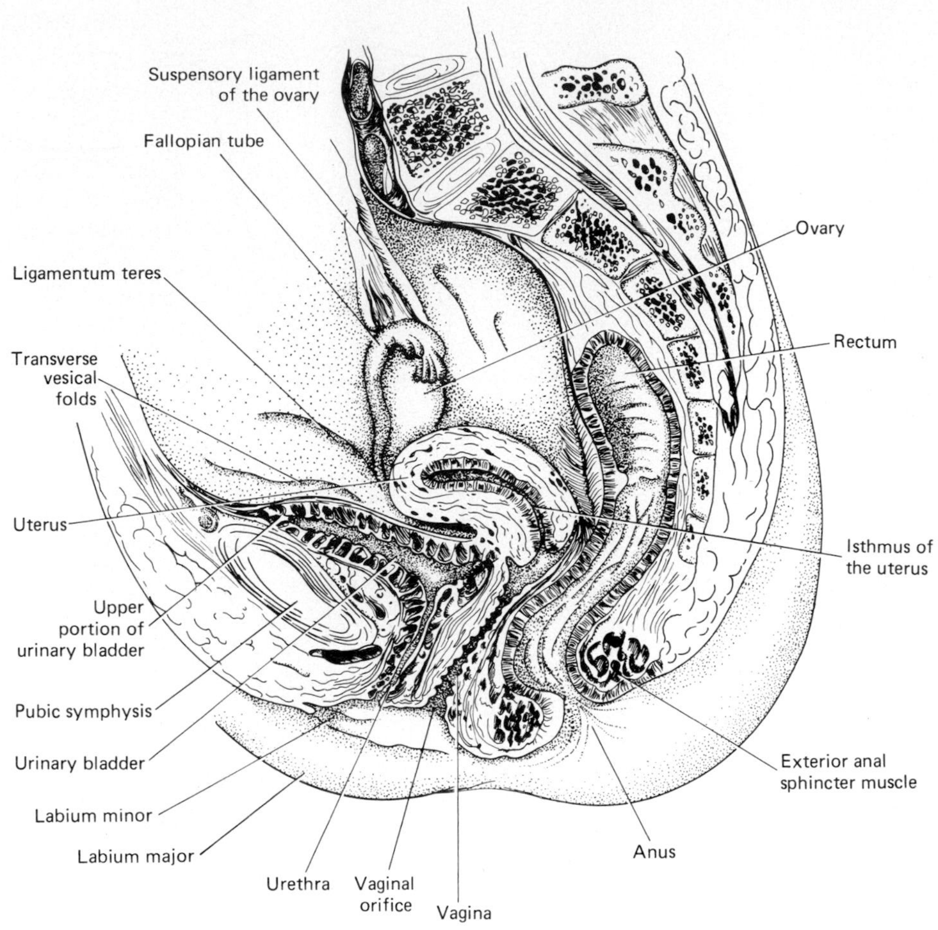

Figure 5.13 The pelvic viscera. A sagittal section of the female pelvis with the pelvic viscera and their relationships.

and therapeutically. *Culdocentesis, a technique in which a needle is inserted just posterior to the cervix through the vaginal wall into the peritoneal cavity, has been used to evaluate intraperitoneal hemorrhage (e.g., ruptured ectopic pregnancy, hemorrhagic corpus luteum, other intraabdominal bleeding), pus (e.g., pelvic inflammatory disease, ruptured intraabdominal abscess), or other intraabdominal fluid (e.g., ascites). Incision into the peritoneal cavity from this location in the vagina, known as a* posterior colpotomy, *can be used as an adjunct to laparoscopic excision of adnexal masses, with removal of the mass intact through the posterior vagina.*

The vagina is attached to the lateral pelvic wall with endopelvic fascial connections to the *arcus tendineus* (white line), which extends from the pubic bone to the ischial spine. This connection converts the vaginal lumen into a transverse slit with the anterior and posterior walls in apposition; the lateral space where the two walls meet is the vaginal sulcus. Lateral detachments of the vagina are recognized in some cystocele formation.

The opening of the vagina may be covered by a membrane or surrounded by a fold of connective tissue called the *hymen.* This tissue is usually replaced by irregular tissue tags later in life as sexual activity and childbirth occur. The lower vagina is somewhat constricted as it passes through the urogenital hiatus in the pelvic diaphragm; the upper vagina is more spacious. However, the entire vagina is characterized by its distensibility, which is most evident during childbirth.

The vagina is closely applied anteriorly to the urethra, bladder neck and trigonal region, and posterior bladder; posteriorly, the vagina lies in association with the perineal body, anal canal, lower rectum, and posterior cul-de-sac. It is separated from both the lower urinary and gastrointestinal tracts by their investing layers of fibromuscular elements known as the *endopelvic fascia.*

The vagina is composed of three layers:

1. **Mucosa**—nonkeratinized stratified squamous epithelium, without glands. Vaginal lubrication occurs by transudation primarily, with contributions from cervical and Bartholin gland secretions. The mucosa has a characteristic pattern of transverse ridges and furrows, known as *rugae.* It is hormonally sensitive, responding to stimulation by estrogen with proliferation and maturation. The mucosa is colonized by mixed bacterial flora with lactobacillus predominant; normal pH is 3.5 to 4.5.

2. **Muscularis**—contains connective tissue and smooth muscle, loosely arranged in inner circular and outer longitudinal layers.

3. **Adventitia**—consists of endopelvic fascia, adherent to the underlying muscularis.

Blood Supply The blood supply of the vagina includes the vaginal artery and branches from the uterine, middle rectal, and internal pudendal arteries.

Innervation The innervation of the vagina is as follows: the upper vagina—uterovaginal plexus; the distal vagina—pudendal nerve.

Uterus

The uterus is a fibromuscular organ usually divided into a lower cervix and an upper corpus or uterine body (Fig. 5.14).

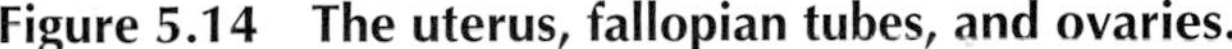

Figure 5.14 The uterus, fallopian tubes, and ovaries.

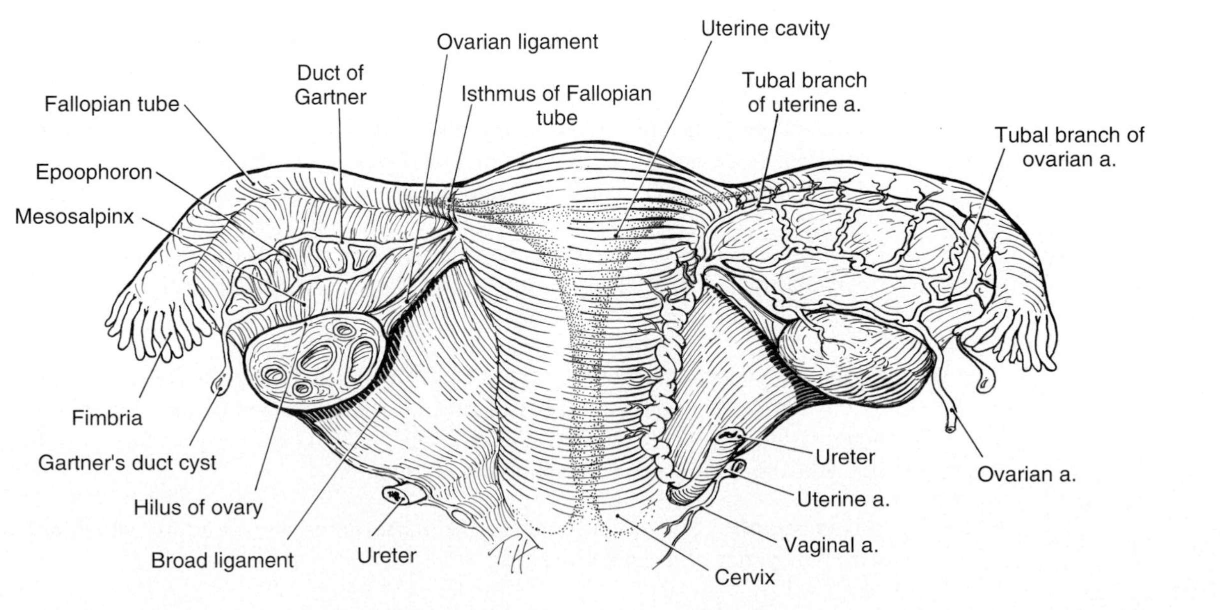

Cervix

The portion of cervix exposed to the vagina is the exocervix or portio vaginalis. It has a convex round surface with a circular or slitlike opening (the external os) into the endocervical canal. The endocervical canal is about 2 to 3 cm in length and opens proximally into the endometrial cavity at the internal os.

The cervical mucosa generally contains both stratified squamous epithelium, characteristic of the exocervix, and mucus-secreting columnar epithelium, characteristic of the endocervical canal. However, the intersection where these two epithelia meet—the squamocolumnar junction—is geographically variable and dependent on hormonal stimulation. It is this dynamic interface, the transformation zone, that is most vulnerable to the development of squamous neoplasia.

In early childhood, during pregnancy, or with oral contraceptive use, columnar epithelium may extend from the endocervical canal onto the exocervix, a condition known as *eversion* or *ectopy.* After menopause, the transformation zone usually recedes entirely into the endocervical canal.

Cervical mucus production is under hormonal influence. It varies from profuse, clear, and thin mucus around the time of ovulation to scant and thick mucus in the postovulatory phase of the cycle. Deep in the mucosa and submucosa, the cervix is composed of fibrous connective tissue and a small amount of smooth muscle in a circular arrangement.

Corpus

The body of the uterus varies in size and shape, depending on hormonal and childbearing status. **At birth, the cervix and corpus are about equal in size; in adult women, the corpus has grown to 2 to 3 times the size of the cervix.** The position of the uterus in relation to other pelvic structures is also variable and is generally described in terms of positioning—anterior, midposition, or posterior; flexion; and version. ***Flexion* is the angle between the long axis of the uterine corpus and the cervix, whereas *version* is the angle of the junction of the uterus with the upper vagina.** Occasionally, abnormal positioning may occur secondary to associated pelvic pathology, such as endometriosis or adhesions.

The uterine corpus is divided into several different regions. The area where the endocervical canal opens into the endometrial cavity is known as the *isthmus* or *lower uterine segment.* On each side of the upper uterine body, a funnel-shaped area receives the insertion of the fallopian tubes and is called the *uterine cornu*; the uterus above this area is the fundus.

The endometrial cavity is triangular in shape and represents the mucosal surface of the uterine corpus. The epithelium is columnar and gland forming with a specialized stroma. It undergoes cyclic structural and functional change during the reproductive years, with regular shedding of the superficial endometrium and regeneration from the basal layer.

The muscular layer of the uterus, the myometrium, consists of interlacing smooth muscle fibers and ranges in thickness from 1.5 to 2.5 cm. Some outer fibers are continuous with those of the tube and round ligament.

Peritoneum covers most of the corpus of the uterus and the posterior cervix and is known as the *serosa.* Laterally, the broad ligament, a double layer of peritoneum covering the neurovascular supply to the uterus, inserts into the cervix and corpus. Anteriorly, the bladder lies over the isthmic and cervical region of the uterus.

Blood Supply The blood supply to the uterus is the uterine artery, which anastomoses with the ovarian and vaginal arteries.

Innervation The nerve supply to the uterus is the uterovaginal plexus.

Fallopian Tubes

The fallopian tubes and ovaries collectively are referred to as the *adnexa.* The fallopian tubes are paired hollow structures representing the proximal unfused ends of the müllerian duct. They vary in length from 7 to 12 cm, and their function includes ovum pickup, provision of physical environment for conception, and transport and nourishment of the fertilized ovum.

The tubes are divided into several regions:

1. **Interstitial**—narrowest portion of the tube, lies within the uterine wall and forms the tubal ostia at the endometrial cavity.
2. **Isthmus**—narrow segment closest to the uterine wall.
3. **Ampulla**—larger diameter segment lateral to the isthmus.
4. **Fimbria (infundibulum)**—funnel-shaped abdominal ostia of the tubes, opening into the peritoneal cavity; this opening is fringed with numerous finger-like projections that provide a wide surface for ovum pickup. The fimbria ovarica is a connection between the end of the tube and ovary, bringing the two closer.

The tubal mucosa is ciliated columnar epithelium, which becomes progressively more architecturally complex as the fimbriated end is approached. The muscularis consists of an inner circular and outer longitudinal layer of smooth muscle. The tube is covered by peritoneum and, through its mesentery (mesosalpinx), which is situated dorsal to the round ligament, is connected to the upper margin of the broad ligament.

Blood Supply The vascular supply to the fallopian tubes is the uterine and ovarian arteries.

Innervation The innervation to the fallopian tubes is the uterovaginal plexus and the ovarian plexus.

Ovaries

The ovaries are paired gonadal structures that lie suspended between the pelvic wall and the uterus by the infundibulopelvic ligament laterally and the uteroovarian ligament medially. Inferiorly, the hilar surface of each ovary is attached to the broad ligament by its mesentery (mesovarium), which is dorsal to the mesosalpinx and fallopian tube. Primary neurovascular structures reach the ovary through the infundibulopelvic ligament and enter through the mesovarium. **The normal ovary varies in size, with measurements up to 5 × 3 × 3 cm.** Variation in dimension results from endogenous hormonal production, which varies with age and with each menstrual cycle. Exogenous substances, including oral contraceptives, gonadotropin-releasing hormone agonists, or ovulation-inducing medication, may either stimulate or suppress ovarian activity and, therefore, affect size.

Each ovary consists of a cortex and medulla and is covered by a single layer of flattened cuboidal to low columnar epithelium that is continuous with the peritoneum at the mesovarium. The cortex is composed of a specialized stroma and follicles in various stages of development or attrition. The medulla occupies a small portion of the ovary in its hilar region and is composed primarily of fibromuscular tissue and blood vessels.

Blood Supply The blood supply to the ovary is the ovarian artery, which anastomoses with the uterine artery.

Innervation The innervation to the ovary is the ovarian plexus and the uterovaginal plexus.

Urinary Tract

Ureters

The ureter is the urinary conduit leading from the kidney to the bladder; it measures about 25 cm in length and is totally retroperitoneal in location.

The lower half of each ureter traverses the pelvis after crossing the common iliac vessels at their bifurcation, just medial to the ovarian vessels. It descends into the pelvis adherent to the peritoneum of the lateral pelvic wall and the medial leaf of the broad ligament and enters the bladder base anterior to the upper vagina, traveling obliquely through the bladder wall to terminate in the bladder trigone.

The ureteral mucosa is a transitional epithelium. The muscularis consists of an inner longitudinal and outer circular layer of smooth muscle. A protective connective tissue sheath, which is adherent to the peritoneum, encloses the ureter.

Blood Supply The blood supply is variable, with contributions from the renal, ovarian, common iliac, internal iliac, uterine, and vesical arteries.

Innervation The innervation is through the ovarian plexus and the vesical plexus.

Bladder and Urethra

Bladder

The bladder is a hollow organ, spherically shaped when full, that stores urine. Its size varies with urine volume, normally reaching a maximum volume of at least 500 mL. The bladder is often divided into two areas, which are of physiologic significance:

1. The **base of the bladder** consists of the urinary trigone posteriorly and a thickened area of detrusor anteriorly. The three corners of the trigone are formed by the two ureteral orifices and the opening of the urethra into the bladder. The bladder base receives α-adrenergic sympathetic innervation and is the area responsible for maintaining continence.

2. The **dome of the bladder** is the remaining bladder area above the bladder base. It has parasympathetic innervation and is responsible for micturition.

The bladder is positioned posterior to the pubis and lower abdominal wall and anterior to the cervix, upper vagina, and part of the cardinal ligament. Laterally, it is bounded by the pelvic diaphragm and obturator internus muscle.

The bladder mucosa is transitional cell epithelium and the muscle wall (detrusor). Rather than being arranged in layers, it is composed of intermeshing muscle fibers.

Blood Supply The blood supply to the bladder is from the superior, middle, and inferior vesical arteries, with contribution from the uterine and vaginal vessels.

Innervation The innervation to the bladder is from the vesical plexus, with contribution from the uterovaginal plexus.

Urethra

The vesical neck is the region of the bladder that receives and incorporates the urethral lumen. The female urethra is about 3 to 4 cm in length and extends from the bladder to the vestibule, traveling just anterior to the vagina.

The urethra is lined by nonkeratinized squamous epithelium that is responsive to estrogen stimulation. Within the submucosa on the dorsal surface of the urethra are the paraurethral or Skene glands, which empty through ducts into the urethral lumen. Distally, these glands empty into the vestibule on either side of the external urethral orifice. Chronic infection of Skene glands, with obstruction of their ducts and cystic dilation, is believed to be an inciting factor in the development of suburethral diverticula.

The urethra contains an inner longitudinal layer of smooth muscle and outer, circularly oriented smooth muscle fibers. The inferior fascia of the urogenital diaphragm or perineal membrane begins at the junction of the middle and distal thirds of the urethra. Proximal to the middle and distal parts of the urethra, voluntary muscle fibers derived from the urogenital diaphragm intermix with the outer layer of smooth muscle, increasing urethral resistance and contributing to continence. At the level of the urogenital diaphragm, the skeletal muscle fibers leave the wall of the urethra to form the sphincter urethrae and deep transverse perineal muscles.

Blood Supply The vascular supply to the urethra is from the vesical and vaginal arteries and the internal pudendal branches.

Innervation The innervation to the urethra is from the vesical plexus and the pudendal nerve.

The lower urinary and genital tracts are intimately connected anatomically and functionally. In the midline, the bladder and proximal urethra can be dissected easily from the underlying lower uterine segment, cervix, and vagina through a loose avascular plane. The distal urethra is essentially inseparable from the vagina. Of surgical significance is the location of the bladder trigone immediately over the middle third of the vagina. Unrecognized injury to the bladder during pelvic surgery may result in development of a vesicovaginal fistula.

Fortunately, dissection to the level of the trigone is rarely required, and damage to this critical area is unusual. If dissection is carried too far laterally away from the midline, attachments between the bladder and cervix or vagina become much more dense and vascularized, resulting in increased blood loss and technical difficulty.

Lower Gastrointestinal Tract

Sigmoid Colon

The sigmoid colon begins its characteristic S-shaped curve as it enters the pelvis at the left pelvic brim (Fig. 5.15). The columnar mucosa and richly vascularized submucosa are surrounded by an inner circular layer of smooth muscle and three overlying longitudinal bands of muscle called *tenia coli.* A mesentery of varying length attaches the sigmoid to the posterior abdominal wall.

Blood Supply The blood supply to the sigmoid colon is from the sigmoid arteries.

Innervation The nerves to the sigmoid colon are derived from the inferior mesenteric plexus.

Rectum

The sigmoid colon loses its mesentery in the midsacral region and becomes the rectum about 15 to 20 cm above the anal opening. The rectum follows the curve of the lower sacrum and coccyx and becomes entirely retroperitoneal at the level of the rectouterine pouch or posterior cul-de-sac. It continues along the pelvic curve just posterior to the vagina until the level of the anal hiatus of the pelvic diaphragm, at which point it takes a sharp 90-degree turn posteriorly and becomes the anal canal, separated from the vagina by the perineal body.

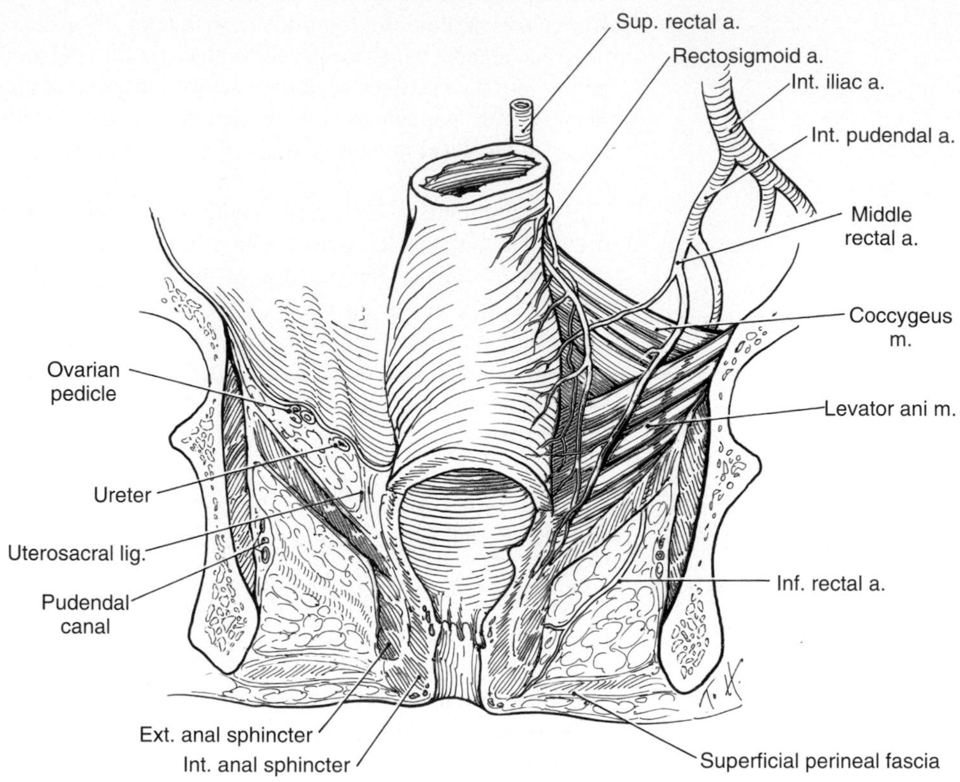

Figure 5.15 The rectosigmoid colon, its vascular supply, and muscular support. (Coronal view: peritoneum removed on right.)

The rectal mucosa is columnar epithelium characterized by three transverse folds that contain mucosa, submucosa, and the inner circular layer of smooth muscle. The tenia of the sigmoid wall broaden and fuse over the rectum to form a continuous longitudinal external layer of smooth muscle to the level of the anal canal.

Anal Canal

The anal canal begins at the level of the sharp turn in the direction of the distal colon and is 2 to 3 cm in length. At the anorectal junction, the mucosa changes to stratified squamous epithelium (the pectinate line), which continues until the termination of the anus at the anal verge, where there is a transition to perianal skin with typical skin appendages. It is surrounded by a thickened ring of circular muscle fibers that is a continuation of the circular muscle of the rectum, the internal anal sphincter. Its lower part is surrounded by bundles of striated muscle fibers, the external anal sphincter (12).

Fecal continence is primarily provided by the puborectalis muscle and the internal and external anal sphincters. The puborectalis surrounds the anal hiatus in the pelvic diaphragm and interdigitates posterior to the rectum to form a rectal sling. The external anal sphincter surrounds the terminal anal canal below the level of the levator ani.

The practicing gynecologist must be familiar with the lower gastrointestinal tract because of its anatomic proximity to the lower genital tract. This is particularly important during surgery of the vulva and vagina. Lack of attention to this proximity during repair of vaginal lacerations or episiotomies can lead to damage of the rectum and resulting fistula formation or injury to the external anal sphincter with development of fecal incontinence. Because of the avascular nature of the rectovaginal space, it is relatively easy to dissect the rectum from the vagina in the midline, which is routinely done in the repair of rectoceles.

Blood Supply The vascular supply to the rectum and anal canal is from the superior, middle, and inferior rectal arteries. The venous drainage is a complex submucosal plexus of vessels that, under conditions of increased intraabdominal pressure (pregnancy, pelvic mass, ascites), may dilate and become symptomatic with rectal bleeding or pain as hemorrhoids.

Innervation The nerve supply to the anal canal is from the middle rectal plexus, the inferior mesenteric plexus, and the pudendal nerve.

The Genital Tract and Its Relations

The genital tract is situated at the bottom of the intraabdominal cavity and is related to the intraperitoneal cavity and its contents, the retroperitoneal spaces, and the pelvic floor. Its access through the abdominal wall or the perineum requires a thorough knowledge of the anatomy of these areas and their relationships.

The Abdominal Wall

The anterior abdominal wall is bound superiorly by the xiphoid process and the costal cartilage of the seventh to tenth ribs and inferiorly by the iliac crest, anterosuperior iliac spine, inguinal ligament, and pubic bone. It consists of skin, muscle, fascia, and nerves and vessels.

Skin

The lower abdominal skin may exhibit striae, or "stretch marks," and increased pigmentation in the midline in parous women. The subcutaneous tissue contains a variable amount of fat.

Muscles

Five muscles and their aponeuroses contribute to the structure and strength of the anterolateral abdominal wall (Fig. 5.16; Table 5.7).

Fascia

Superficial Fascia

The superficial fascia consists of two layers:

1. **Camper fascia**—the most superficial layer, which contains a variable amount of fat and is continuous with the superficial fatty layer of the perineum
2. **Scarpa fascia**—a deeper membranous layer continuous in the perineum with Colles fascia (superficial perineal fascia) and with the deep fascia of the thigh (fascia lata).

Rectus Sheath

The aponeuroses of the external and internal oblique and the transversus abdominis combine to form a sheath for the rectus abdominis and pyramidalis, fusing medially in the midline at the linea alba and laterally at the semilunar line (Fig. 5.17). Above the arcuate line, the aponeurosis of the internal oblique muscle splits into anterior and posterior lamella (Fig. 5.17A). Below this line, all three layers are anterior to the body of the rectus muscle (Fig. 5.17B). The rectus is then covered posteriorly by the transversalis fascia, providing access to the muscle for the inferior epigastric vessels.

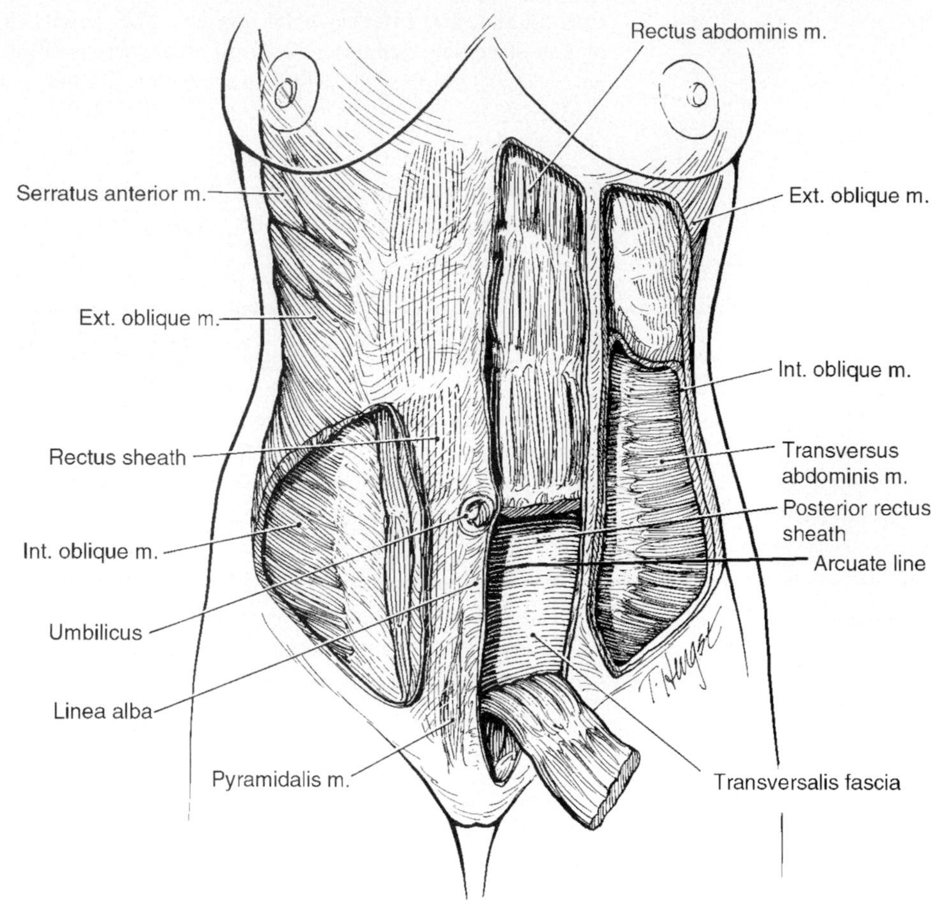

Figure 5.16 The abdominal wall muscles.

Transversalis Fascia and Endopelvic Fascia

The transversalis fascia is a firm membranous sheet on the internal surface of the transversus abdominis muscle that extends beyond the muscle and forms a fascia lining the entire abdominopelvic cavity. Like the peritoneum, it is divided into a parietal and a visceral component. It is continuous from side to side across the linea alba and covers the posterior aspect of the rectus abdominis muscle below the arcuate line. Superiorly, it becomes the inferior fascia of the diaphragm. Inferiorly, it is attached to the iliac crest, covers the iliac fascia and the obturator internus fascia, and extends downward and medially to form the superior fascia of the pelvic diaphragm.

Characteristically, the transversalis fascia continues along blood vessels and other structures leaving and entering the abdominopelvic cavity and contributes to the formation of the visceral (*endopelvic*) pelvic fascia (13). The pelvic fascia invests the pelvic organs and attaches them to the pelvic sidewalls, thereby playing a critical role in *pelvic support.* In the inguinal region, the fascial relationships result in the development of the inguinal canal, through which the round ligament exits into the perineum. The fascia is separated from the peritoneum by a layer of preperitoneal fat. Areas of fascial weaknesses or congenital or posttraumatic and surgical injuries result in herniation of the underlying structures through a defective abdominal wall. The incisions least likely to result in damage to the integrity and innervation of the abdominal wall muscles include a midline incision through the linea alba and a transverse incision through the recti muscle fibers that respects the integrity of its innervation (14).

Table 5.7.

Muscle	Origin	Insertion	Action
External oblique	Fleshy digitations from the outer surfaces of ribs 5–12	Fibers radiate inferiorly, anteriorly, and medially, in most cases ending in the aponeurosis of the external muscle and inserting into the anterior half of the iliac crest, the pubic tubercle, and the linea alba. The superficial inguinal ring is located above and lateral to the pubic tubercle at the end of a triangular cleft in the external oblique muscle, bordered by strong fibrous bands that transmit the round ligament	Compresses and supports abdominal viscera; flexes and rotates vertebral column
Internal oblique	Posterior layer of the thoracolumbar fascia, the anterior two thirds of the iliac crest, and the lateral two thirds of the inguinal ligament	Inferior border of ribs 10–12. The superior fibers of the aponeurosis split to enclose the rectus abdominus muscle and join at the linea alba above the arcuate line. The most inferior fibers join with those of the transverse abdomimis muscle to insert into the pubic crest and pecten pubis via the conjoint tendon	Compresses and supports abdominal viscera
Transversus abdominus	Inner aspect of the inferior six costal cartilages, the thoracolumbar fascia, the iliac crest, and the lateral one third of the inguinal ligament	Linea alba with the aponeurosis of the internal oblique, the pubic crest and the pecten pubis through the conjoint tendon	Compresses and supports abdominal viscera
Rectus abdominus	Superior pubic ramus and the ligaments of the symphysis pubis	Anterior surface of the xiphoid process and the cartilage of ribs 5–7	Tenses anterior abdominal wall and flexes trunk
Pyramidalis	Small triangular muscle contained within the rectus sheath, anterior to the lower part of the rectus muscle	On the linea alba, easily recognizable shape, used to locate the midline, particularly in a patient with previous abdominal surgery and scarring of the abdominal wall	Tenses the linea alba, insignificant in terms of function and is frequently absent

Nerves and Vessels

The tissues of the abdominal wall are innervated by the continuation of the inferior intercostal nerves T4 to T11 and the subcostal nerve T12. The inferior part of the abdominal wall is supplied by the first lumbar nerve through the iliohypogastric and the ilioinguinal nerves. The primary blood supply to the anterior lateral abdominal wall includes the following:

1. The **inferior epigastric and deep circumflex iliac arteries,** branches of the external iliac artery

2. The **superior epigastric artery,** a terminal branch of the internal thoracic artery

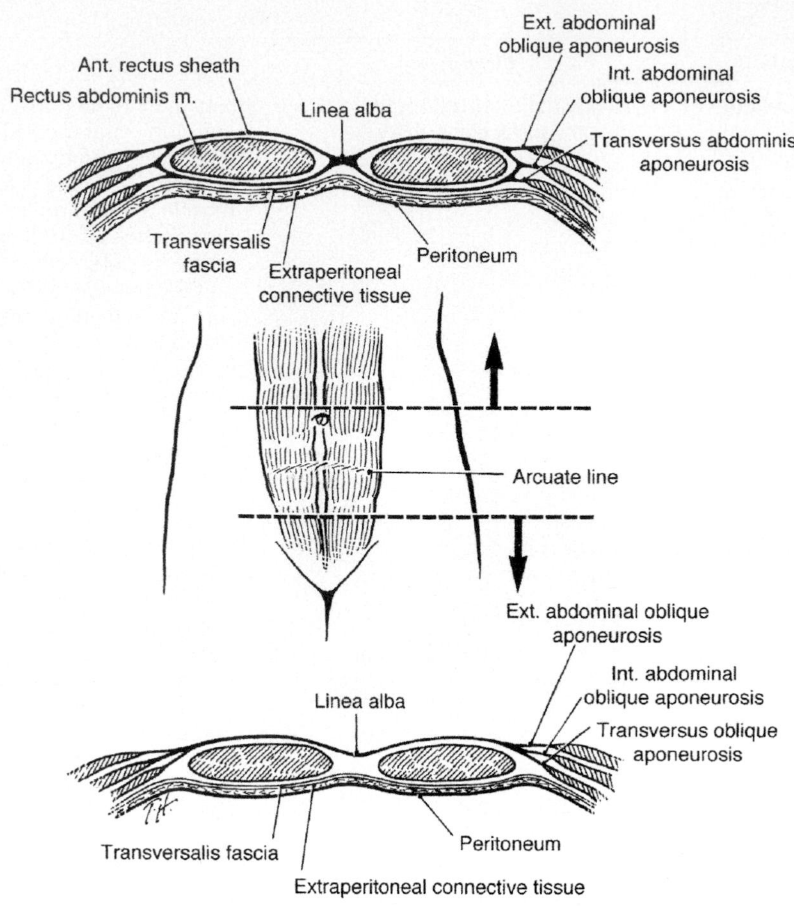

Figure 5.17 A transverse section of the rectus abdominis. The aponeurosis of the external and internal oblique and the transversus abdominis from the rectus abdominis. **A:** Above the arcuate line. **B:** Below the arcuate line.

The inferior epigastric artery runs superiorly in the transverse fascia to reach the arcuate line, where it enters the rectus sheath. It is vulnerable to damage with abdominal incisions in which the rectus muscle is completely or partially transected or with excessive lateral traction on the rectus. The deep circumflex artery runs on the deep aspect of the anterior abdominal wall parallel to the inguinal ligament and along the iliac crest between the transverse abdominis muscle and the internal oblique muscle. The superior epigastric vessels enter the rectus sheath superiorly just below the seventh costal cartilage.

The venous system drains into the saphenous vein, and the lymphatics drain to the axillary chain above the umbilicus and to the inguinal nodes below it. The subcutaneous tissues drain to the lumbar chain.

Perineum

The perineum is situated at the lower end of the trunk between the buttocks. Its bony boundaries include the lower margin of the pubic symphysis anteriorly, the tip of the coccyx posteriorly, and the ischial tuberosities laterally. These landmarks correspond to the boundaries of the pelvic outlet. The diamond shape of the perineum is customarily divided by an imaginary line joining the ischial tuberosities immediately in front of the anus, at the level of the perineal body, into an anterior urogenital and a posterior anal triangle (Fig. 5.18).

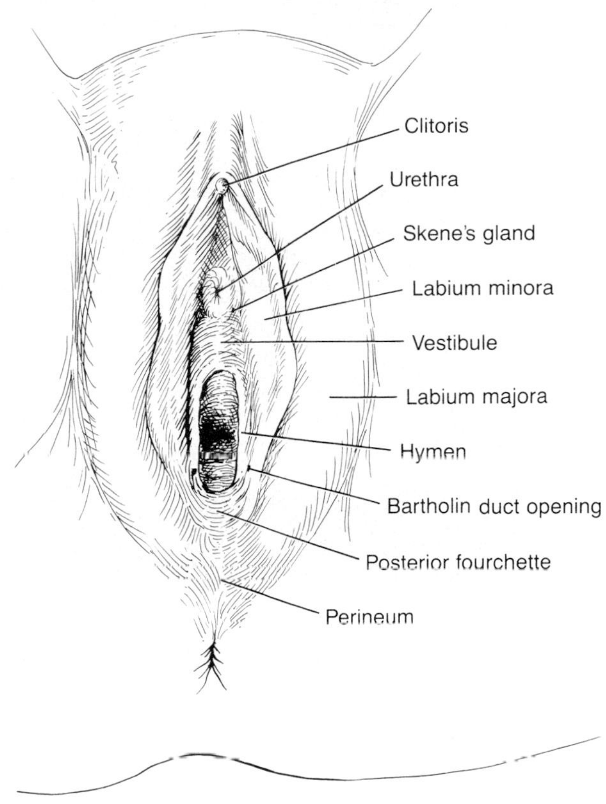

Figure 5.18 Vulva and perineum.

Urogenital Triangle

The urogenital triangle includes the external genital structures and the urethral opening (Fig. 5.18). These external structures cover the superficial and deep perineal compartments (Figs. 5.19 and 5.20) and are known as the *vulva.*

Vulva

Mons Pubis

The mons pubis is a triangular eminence in front of the pubic bones that consists of adipose tissue covered by hair-bearing skin up to its junction with the abdominal wall.

Labia Majora

The labia majora are a pair of fibroadipose folds of skin that extend from the mons pubis downward and backward to meet in the midline in front of the anus at the posterior fourchette. They include the terminal extension of the round ligament and occasionally a peritoneal diverticulum, the *canal of Nuck.* They are covered by skin with scattered hairs laterally and are rich in sebaceous, apocrine, and eccrine glands.

Labia Minora

The labia minora lie between the labia majora, with which they merge posteriorly and are separated into two folds as they approach the clitoris anteriorly. The anterior folds unite to form the prepuce or hood of the clitoris. The posterior folds form the frenulum of the clitoris as they attach to its inferior surface. The labia minora are covered by hairless skin overlying a fibroelastic stroma rich in neural and vascular elements. The area between the posterior labia minora forms the vestibule of the vagina.

Figure 5.19 Superficial perineal compartment.

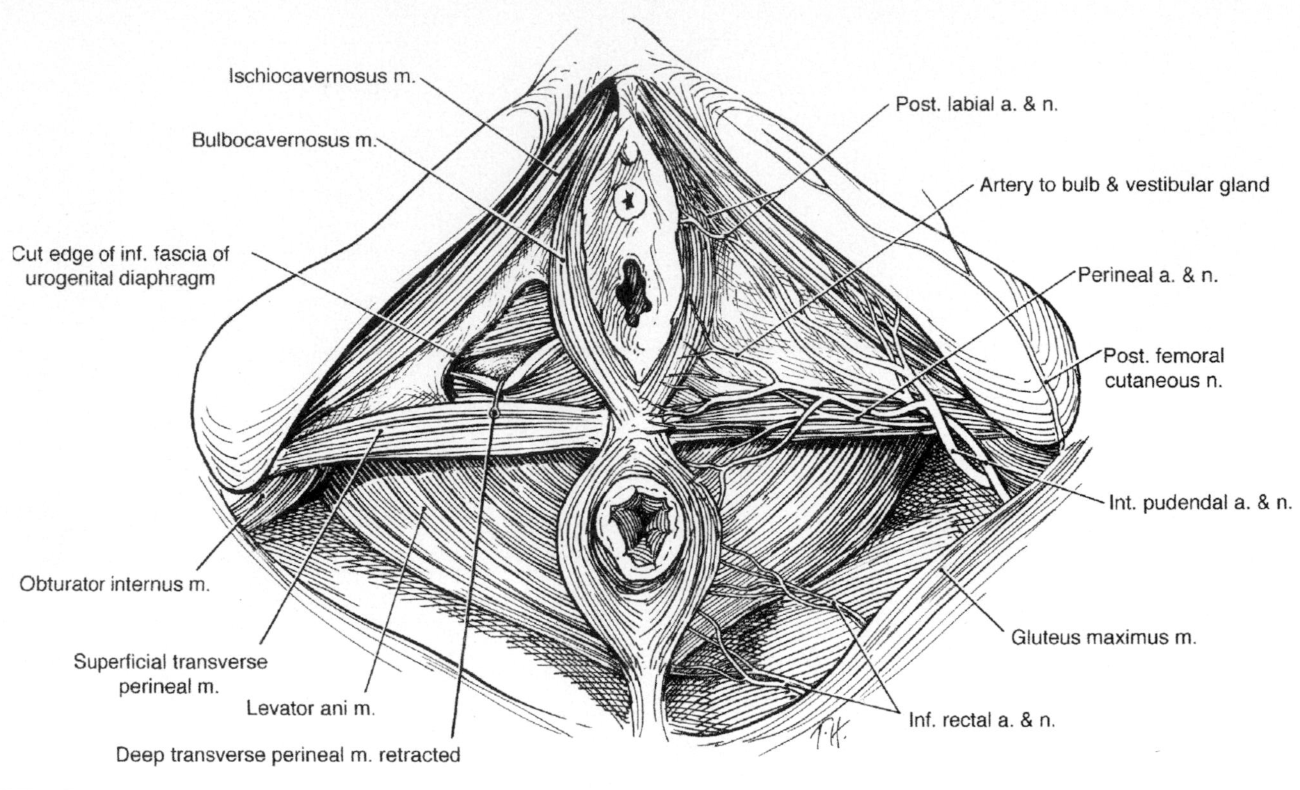

Figure 5.20 Deep perineal compartment

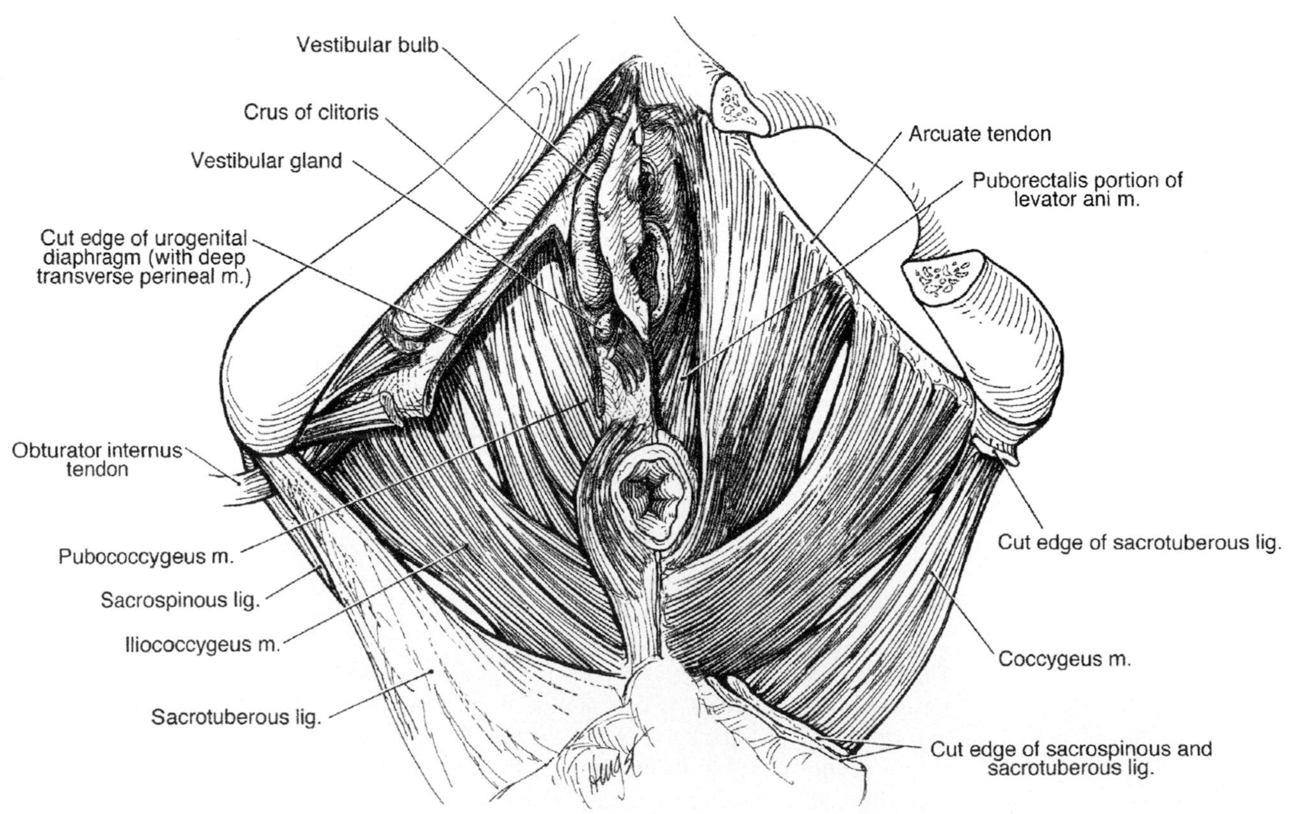

Clitoris

The clitoris is an erectile organ that is 2 to 3 cm in length. It consists of two crura and two corpora cavernosa and is covered by a sensitive rounded tubercle (the glans).

Vaginal Orifice

The vaginal orifice is surrounded by the hymen, a variable crescentic mucous membrane that is replaced by rounded caruncles after its rupture. The opening of the duct of the *greater vestibular (Bartholin) glands* is located on each side of the vestibule. Numerous lesser vestibular glands are also scattered posteriorly and between the urethral and vaginal orifices.

Urethral Orifice

The urethral orifice is immediately anterior to the vaginal orifice about 2 to 3 cm beneath the clitoris. The *Skene (paraurethral) gland* duct presents an opening on its posterior surface.

Superficial Perineal Compartment

The superficial perineal compartment lies between the superficial perineal fascia and the inferior fascia of the urogenital diaphragm (perineal membrane) (Fig. 5.19). The superficial perineal fascia has a superficial and deep component. The superficial layer is relatively thin and fatty and is continuous superiorly with the superficial fatty layer of the lower abdominal wall (*Camper fascia*). It continues laterally as the fatty layer of the thighs. The deep layer of the superficial perineal (*Colles*) fascia is continuous superiorly with the deep layer of the superficial abdominal fascia (*Scarpa fascia*), which attaches firmly to the ischiopubic rami and ischial tuberosities. The superficial perineal compartment is continuous superiorly with the superficial fascial spaces of the anterior abdominal wall, allowing spread of blood or infection along that route. Such spread is limited laterally by the ischiopubic rami, anteriorly by the transverse ligament of the perineum, and posteriorly by the superficial transverse perineal muscle. The superficial perineal compartment includes the following.

Erectile Bodies

The vestibular bulbs are 3-cm, highly vascular structures surrounding the vestibule and located under the bulbocavernosus muscle. The body of the clitoris is attached by two crura to the internal aspect of the ischiopubic rami. They are covered by the ischiocavernosus muscle.

Muscles

The muscles of the vulva are the ischiocavernosus, the bulbocavernosus, and superficial transverse perineal.

Ischiocavernosus

- Origin—ischial tuberosity
- Insertion—ischiopubic bone
- Action—compresses the crura and lowers the clitoris

Bulbocavernosus

- Origin—perineal body
- Insertion—posterior aspect of the clitoris; some fibers pass above the dorsal vein of the clitoris in a slinglike fashion
- Action—compresses the vestibular bulb and dorsal vein of the clitoris

Superficial Transverse Perineal

- Origin—ischial tuberosity
- Insertion—central perineal tendon
- Action—fixes the perineal body

Vestibular Glands

The vestibular glands are situated on either side of the vestibule under the posterior end of the vestibular bulb. They drain between the hymen and the labia minora. Their mucus secretion helps maintain adequate lubrication. Infection in these glands can result in an abscess.

Deep Perineal Compartment

The deep perineal compartment is a fascial space bound inferiorly by the perineal membrane and superiorly by a deep fascial layer that separates the urogenital diaphragm from the anterior recess of the ischiorectal fossa (Fig. 5.20). It is stretched across the anterior half of the pelvic outlet between the ischiopubic rami. The deep compartment may be directly continuous with the pelvic cavity superiorly (15). Indeed, the posterior pubourethral ligaments, functioning as winglike elevations of the fascia ascending from the pelvic floor to the posterior aspect of the symphysis pubis, provide a point of fixation to the urethra and support the concept of the continuity of the deep perineal compartment with the pelvic cavity.

The anterior pubourethral ligaments represent a similar elevation of the inferior fascia of the urogenital diaphragm and are joined by the intermediate pubourethral ligament, with the junction between the two fascial structures arcing under the pubic symphysis (16). The urogenital diaphragm includes the *sphincter urethrae (urogenital sphincter)* and the *deep transverse perineal (transversus vaginae)* muscle.

The sphincter urethrae (Fig. 5.21) is a continuous muscle fanning out as it develops proximally and distally, including the following:

1. The **external urethral sphincter**, which surrounds the middle third of the urethra
2. The **compressor urethrae**, arcing across the ventral side of the urethra
3. The **urethrovaginal sphincter**, which surrounds the ventral aspect of the urethra and terminates in the lateral vaginal wall

The deep transverse perineal muscle originates at the internal aspect of the ischial bone, parallels the muscle compressor urethrae, and attaches to the lateral vaginal wall along the perineal membrane.

There is a common reliance of the urinary and genital tracts on several interdependent structures for support. **The cardinal and uterosacral ligaments are condensations of endopelvic fascia that support the cervix and upper vagina over the levator plate. Laterally, endopelvic fascial condensations attach the midvagina to the pelvic walls at the arcus tendineus fascia pelvis anteriorly and the arcus tendineus levator ani posteriorly. The distal anterior vagina and urethra are anchored to the urogenital diaphragm, and the distal posterior vagina to the perineal body.**

Anteriorly, the pubourethral ligaments and pubovesical fascia and ligaments provide fixation and stabilization for the urethra and bladder. Posteriorly, they rely on the vagina and lower uterus for support. Partial resection or relaxation of the uterosacral ligaments often leads to relaxation of the genitourinary complex, resulting in the formation of a cystocele. Various

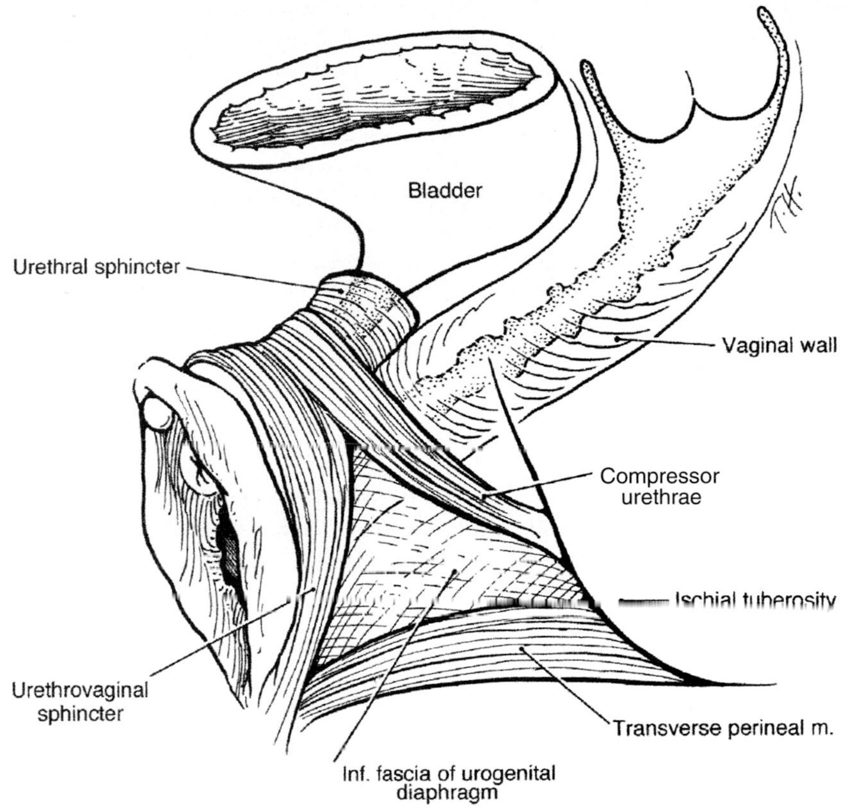

Figure 5.21 The complete urogenital sphincter musculature, bladder, and vagina.

types and degrees of genital tract prolapse or relaxation are almost always associated with similar findings in the bladder, urethra, or both.

Blood Supply The blood supply to the vulva is as follows:

1. External pudendal artery (from femoral artery), internal pudendal artery
2. Venous drainage—internal pudendal veins

The blood supply to the superficial and deep perineal compartments is as follows:

1. Internal pudendal artery, dorsal artery of the clitoris
2. Venous drainage—internal pudendal veins, which are richly anastomotic
3. Lymphatic drainage—internal iliac chain

Innervation The innervation to the vulva is from branches of the following nerves:

1. Ilioinguinal nerve
2. Genitofemoral nerve (genital branch)
3. Lateral femoral cutaneous nerve of the thigh (perineal branch)
4. Perineal nerve (branch of pudendal)

Superficial and deep perineal compartments are innervated by the perineal nerve.

Perineal Body

The perineal body or central perineal tendon is critical to the posterior support of the lower aspect of the anterior vaginal wall. It is a triangle-shaped structure separating the distal portion of the anal and vaginal canals that is formed by the convergence of the tendinous attachments of the bulbocavernosus, the external anal sphincter, and the superficial transverse perinei muscle. Its superior border represents the point of insertion of the *rectovaginal (Denonvilliers) fascia*, which extends to the underside of the peritoneum covering the cul-de-sac of Douglas, separating the anorectal from the urogenital compartment (17). The perineal body also plays an important anchoring role in the musculofascial support of the pelvic floor. It represents the central connection between the two layers of support of the pelvic floor—the pelvic and urogenital diaphragm. It also provides a posterior connection to the anococcygeal raphe. Thus, it is central to the definition of the bilevel support of the floor of the pelvis.

Anal Triangle

The anal triangle includes the lower end of the anal canal. The external anal sphincter surrounds the anal triangle, and the ischiorectal fossa is on each side.

Posteriorly, the *anococcygeal body* lies between the anus and the tip of the coccyx and consists of thick fibromuscular tissue (of levator ani and external anal sphincter origin) giving support to the lower part of the rectum and the anal canal.

The *external anal sphincter* forms a thick band of muscular fibers arranged in three layers running from the perineal body to the anococcygeal ligament. The subcutaneous fibers are thin and surround the anus and, without bony attachment, decussate in front of it. The superficial fibers sweep forward from the anococcygeal ligament, and the tip of the coccyx around the anus inserts into the perineal body. The deep fibers arise from the perineal body to encircle the lower half of the anal canal to form a true sphincter muscle, which fuses with the puborectalis portion of the levator ani.

The *ischiorectal fossa* is mainly occupied by fat and separates the ischium laterally from the median structures of the anal triangle. It is a fascia-lined space located between the perineal skin inferiorly and the pelvic diaphragm superiorly; it communicates with the contralateral ischiorectal fossa over the anococcygeal ligament. Superiorly, its apex is at the origin of the levator ani muscle from the obturator fascia. It is bound medially by the levator ani and the external sphincter with their fascial covering, laterally by the obturator internus muscle with its fascia, posteriorly by the sacrotuberous ligament and the lower border of the gluteus maximus muscle, and anteriorly by the base of the urogenital diaphragm. It is widest and deepest posteriorly and weakest medially. *Thus, an ischiorectal abscess should be drained without delay, or it will extend into the anal canal.* The cavity is filled with fat that cushions the anal canal and is traversed by many fibrous bands, vessels, and nerves, including the pudendal and the inferior rectal nerves. The perforating branch of S2 and S3 and the perineal branch of S4 also run through this space.

The *pudendal (Alcock) canal* is a tunnel formed by a splitting of the inferior portion of the obturator fascia running anteromedially from the ischial spine to the posterior edge of the urogenital diaphragm. It contains the pudendal artery, vein, and nerve in their traverse from the *pelvic* cavity to the perineum.

Blood Supply The blood supply to the anal triangle is from the inferior rectal (hemorrhoidal) artery and vein.

Innervation The innervation to the anal triangle is from the perineal branch of the fourth sacral nerve and the inferior rectal (hemorrhoidal) nerve.

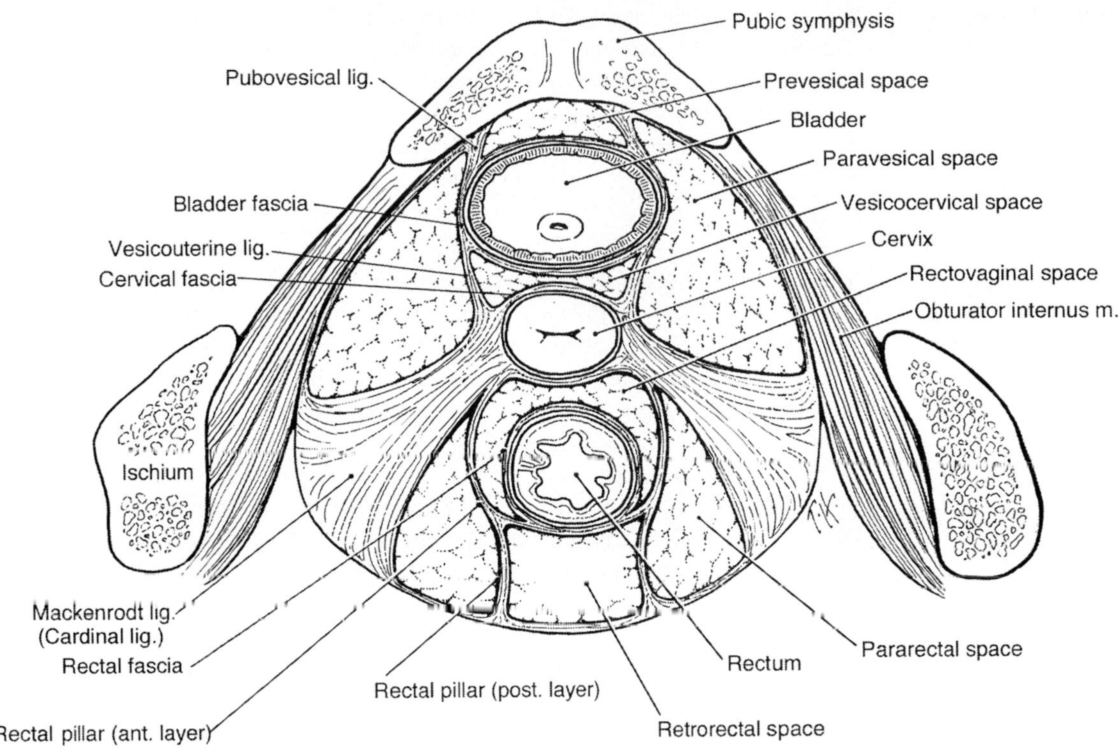

Figure 5.22 Schematic sectional drawing of the pelvis shows the firm connective tissue covering. The bladder, cervix, and rectum are surrounded by a connective tissue covering. The Mackenrodt ligament extends from the lateral cervix to the lateral abdominal pelvic wall. The vesicouterine ligament originating from the anterior edge of the Mackenrodt ligament leads to the covering of the bladder on the posterior side. The sagittal rectum column spreads both to the connective tissue of the rectum and the sacral vertebrae closely nestled against the back of the Mackenrodt ligament and lateral pelvic wall. Between the firm connective tissue bundles is loose connective tissue (paraspaces). (From Von Peham H, Amreich JA. *Gynaekologische Operationslehre.* Berlin: S Karger, 1930, with permission.)

Retroperitoneum and Retroperitoneal Spaces

The subperitoneal area of the true pelvis is partitioned into potential spaces by the various organs and their respective fascial coverings and by the selective thickenings of the endopelvic fascia into ligaments and septa (Fig. 5.22). It is imperative that surgeons operating in the pelvis be familiar with these spaces, which include the following:

Prevesical Space

The prevesical (Retzius) space is a fat-filled potential space bound anteriorly by the pubic bone, covered by the transversalis fascia, and extending to the umbilicus between the medial umbilical ligaments (obliterated umbilical arteries); posteriorly, the space extends to the anterior wall of the bladder. It is separated from the paravesical space by the ascending bladder septum (bladder pillars).

Upon entering the prevesical space, the pubourethral ligaments may be seen inserting the posterior aspect of the symphysis pubis as a thickened prolongation of the arcus tendineus fascia. With combined abdominal and vaginal bladder neck suspensory procedures, the point of entry is usually the Retzius space between the arcus tendineus and the pubourethral ligaments.

Paravesical Space

The paravesical spaces are fat filled and limited by the fascia of the obturator internus muscle and the pelvic diaphragm laterally, the bladder pillar medially, the endopelvic fascia inferiorly, and the lateral umbilical ligament superiorly.

Vesicovaginal Space

The vesicovaginal space is separated from the Retzius space by the endopelvic fascia. This space is limited anteriorly by the bladder wall (from the proximal urethra to the upper vagina), posteriorly by the anterior vaginal wall, and laterally by the bladder septa (selective thickenings of the endopelvic fascia inserting laterally into the arcus tendineus). *A tear in these fascial investments and thickenings medially, transversely, or laterally allows herniation and development of a cystocele.*

Rectovaginal Space

The rectovaginal space extends between the vagina and the rectum from the superior border of the perineal body to the underside of the rectouterine Douglas pouch. It is bound anteriorly by the rectovaginal septum (firmly adherent to the posterior aspect of the vagina), posteriorly by the anterior rectal wall, and laterally by the descending rectal septa separating the rectovaginal space from the pararectal space on each side. The rectovaginal septum represents a firm membranous transverse septum dividing the pelvis into rectal and urogenital compartments, allowing the independent function of the vagina and rectum and providing support for the rectum. It is fixed laterally to the pelvic sidewall by rectovaginal fascia (part of the endopelvic fascia) along a line extending from the posterior fourchette to the arcus tendineus fasciae pelvis, midway between the pubis and the ischial spine (18). An anterior rectocele often results from a defective *septum* or an avulsion of the septum from the perineal body. Reconstruction of the perineum is critical for the restoration of this important compartmental separation as well as for the support of the anterior vaginal wall (19). **Lateral detachment of the rectovaginal fascia from the pelvic sidewall may constitute a "pararectal" defect analogous to anterior paravaginal defects.**

Pararectal Space

The pararectal space is bound laterally by the levator ani, medially by the rectal pillars, and posteriorly above the ischial spine by the anterolateral aspect of the sacrum. It is separated from the retrorectal space by the posterior extension of the descending rectal septa.

Retrorectal Space

The retrorectal space is limited by the rectum anteriorly and the anterior aspect of the sacrum posteriorly. It communicates with the pararectal spaces laterally above the uterosacral ligaments and extends superiorly into the presacral space.

Presacral Space

The presacral space is the superior extension of the retrorectal space and is limited by the deep parietal peritoneum anteriorly and the anterior aspect of the sacrum posteriorly. It harbors the middle sacral vessels and the hypogastric plexi between the bifurcation of the aorta invested by loose areolar tissue. Presacral neurectomy requires a good familiarity and working knowledge of this space.

Peritoneal Cavity

The female pelvic organs lie at the bottom of the abdominopelvic cavity covered superiorly and posteriorly by the small and large bowel. Anteriorly, the uterine wall is in contact with the posterosuperior aspect of the bladder. The uterus is held in position by the following structures:

1. The **round ligaments** coursing inferolaterally toward the internal inguinal ring
2. The **uterosacral ligaments**, which provide support to the cervix and upper vagina and interdigitate with fibers from the cardinal ligament near the cervix
3. The **cardinal ligaments**, which provide support to the cervix and upper vagina and contribute to the support of the bladder

Anteriorly, the uterus is separated from the bladder by the vesicouterine pouch and from the rectum posteriorly by the rectouterine pouch or Douglas cul-de-sac. Laterally, the bilateral broad ligaments carry the neurovascular pedicles and their respective fascial coverings, attaching the uterus to the lateral pelvic sidewall.

The broad ligament is in contact inferiorly with the paravesical space, the obturator fossa, and the pelvic extension of the iliac fossa, to which it provides a peritoneal covering, and with the uterosacral ligament. Superiorly, it extends into the infundibulopelvic ligament.

Ureter

In its pelvic path, in the retroperitoneum, several relationships are of significance and identify areas of greatest vulnerability to injury of the ureter (Fig. 5.23):

1. The ovarian vessels cross over the ureter as it approaches the pelvic brim and lie in proximity just lateral to the ureter as it enters the pelvis.

2. As the ureter descends into the pelvis, it runs within the broad ligament just lateral to the uterosacral ligament, separating the uterosacral ligament from the mesosalpinx, mesovarium, and ovarian fossa.

3. At about the level of the ischial spine, the ureter crosses under the uterine artery in its course through the cardinal ligament; the ureter divides this area into the supraureteric parametrium surrounding the uterine vessels and the infraureteric paracervix molded around the vaginal vessels and extending posteriorly into the uterosacral ligament. In this location, the ureter lies 2 to 3 cm lateral to the cervix

Figure 5.23 The course of the ureter and its relationship to the sites of greatest vulnerability.

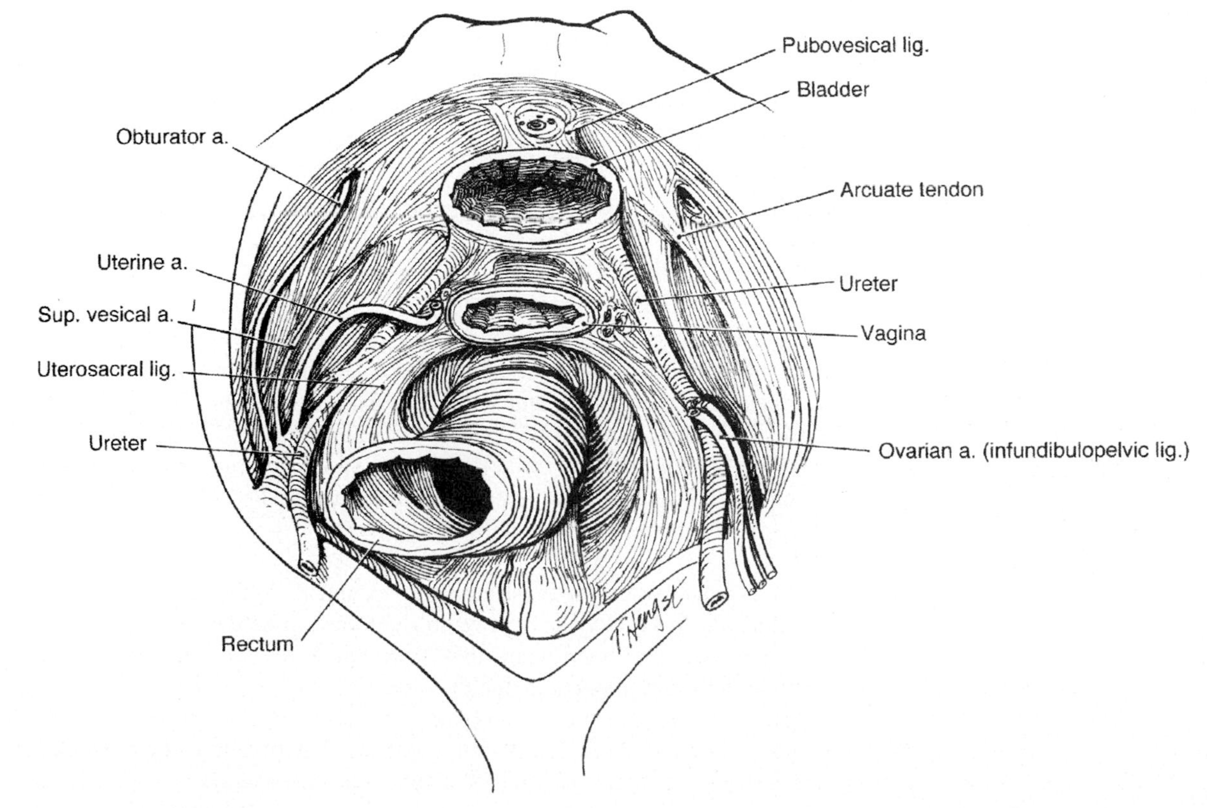

and in proximity to the insertion of the uterosacral ligament at the cervix. This proximity warrants caution when using the uterosacral ligament for vaginal vault suspension (20).

4. The ureter then turns medially to cross the anterior upper vagina as it traverses the bladder wall.

About 75% of all iatrogenic injuries to the ureter result from gynecologic procedures, most commonly abdominal hysterectomy (21). Distortions of pelvic anatomy, including adnexal masses, endometriosis, other pelvic adhesive disease, or fibroids, may increase susceptibility to injury by displacement or alteration of usual anatomy. **Even with severe intraperitoneal disease, however, the ureter can always be identified using a retroperitoneal approach and noting fundamental landmarks and relationships.**

Pelvic Floor

The pelvic floor includes all of the structures closing the pelvic outlet from the skin inferiorly to the peritoneum superiorly. It is commonly divided by the pelvic diaphragm into a pelvic and a perineal portion (22). The pelvic diaphragm is spread transversely in a hammock-like fashion across the true pelvis, with a central hiatus for the urethra, vagina, and rectum. Anatomically and physiologically, the pelvic diaphragm can be divided into two components—the internal and external components.

The *external component* originates from the arcus tendineus, extending from the pubic bone to the ischial spine. It gives rise to fibers of differing directions, including the *pubococcygeus,* the *iliococcygeus,* and the *coccygeus.*

The *internal component* originates from the pubic bone above and medial to the origins of the pubococcygeus and is smaller but thicker and stronger (22). Its fibers run in a sagittal direction and are divided into the following two portions.

Pubovaginalis The fibers of the pubovaginalis run in a perpendicular direction to the urethra, crossing the lateral vaginal wall at the junction of its lower one third and upper two thirds to insert into the perineal body. The intervening anterior interlevator space is covered by the urogenital diaphragm.

Puborectalis The superior fibers of the puborectalis sling around the rectum to the symphysis pubis; its inferior fibers insert into the lateral rectal wall between the internal and external sphincter.

The pelvic diaphragm is covered superiorly by fascia, which includes a parietal and a visceral component and is a continuation of the transversalis fascia (Fig. 5.24). The parietal fascia has areas of thickening (ligaments, septa) that provide reinforcement and fixation for the pelvic floor. The visceral *(endopelvic)* fascia extends medially to invest the pelvic viscera, resulting in a fascial covering to the bladder, vagina, uterus, and rectum. It becomes attenuated where the peritoneal covering is well defined and continues laterally with the pelvic cellular tissue and neurovascular pedicles.

Musculofascial elements (the hypogastric sheath) extend along the vessels originating from the internal iliac artery. Following these vessels to their respective organs, the hypogastric sheath extends perivascular investments that contribute to the formation of the endopelvic fascia so critical for the support of the pelvic organs.

Thus, the parietal fascia anchors the visceral fascia, which defines the relationship of the various viscera and provides them with significant fixation (uterosacral and cardinal ligaments), septation (vesicovaginal and rectovaginal), and definition of pelvic spaces (prevesical, vesicovaginal, rectovaginal, paravesical, pararectal, and retrorectal).

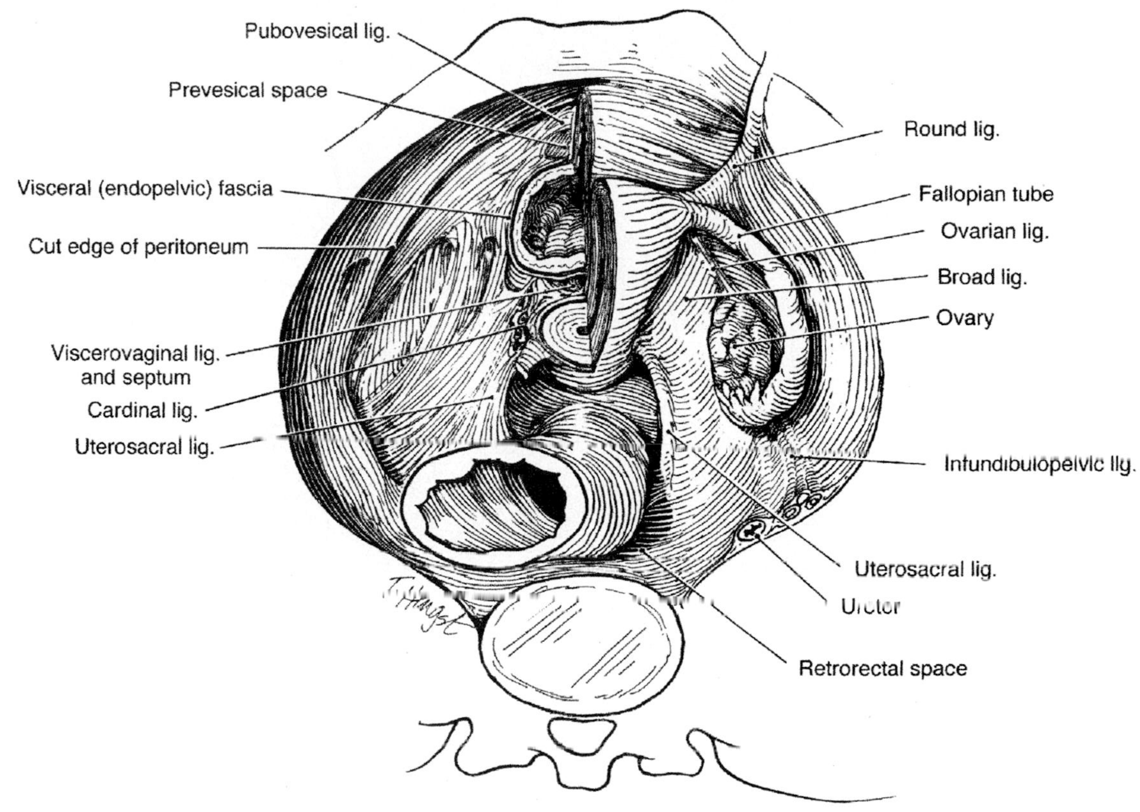

Figure 5.24 The fascial components of the pelvic diaphragm.

For its support, the pelvic floor relies on the complementary role of the pelvic diaphragm and its fascia resting on the perineal fibromuscular complex. It is composed of the perineal membrane (urogenital diaphragm) anteriorly, and the perineal body joined to the anococcygeal raphe by the external anal sphincter posteriorly. This double-layered arrangement, when intact, provides optimal support for the pelvic organs and counterbalances the forces pushing them downward with gravity and with any increase in intraabdominal pressure (Fig. 5.25).

Summary

Continuing review and education in anatomy are important for every pelvic surgeon. New surgical approaches are being developed to solve old problems and often require surgeons to revisit familiar anatomy from an unfamiliar perspective (e.g., through a laparoscope) or with a different understanding of complex anatomic relationships. Anatomic alterations secondary to disease, congenital variation, or intraoperative complications may make even familiar surgical territory suddenly seem foreign. All of these situations require surgeons to be perpetual students of anatomy, regardless of breadth or depth of experience.

Several strategies for continuing education in anatomy are suggested:

1. Review relevant anatomy before each surgical procedure.
2. Study the gynecologic literature on an ongoing basis—numerous publications have documented the evolution of newer concepts regarding anatomic issues such as pelvic support.

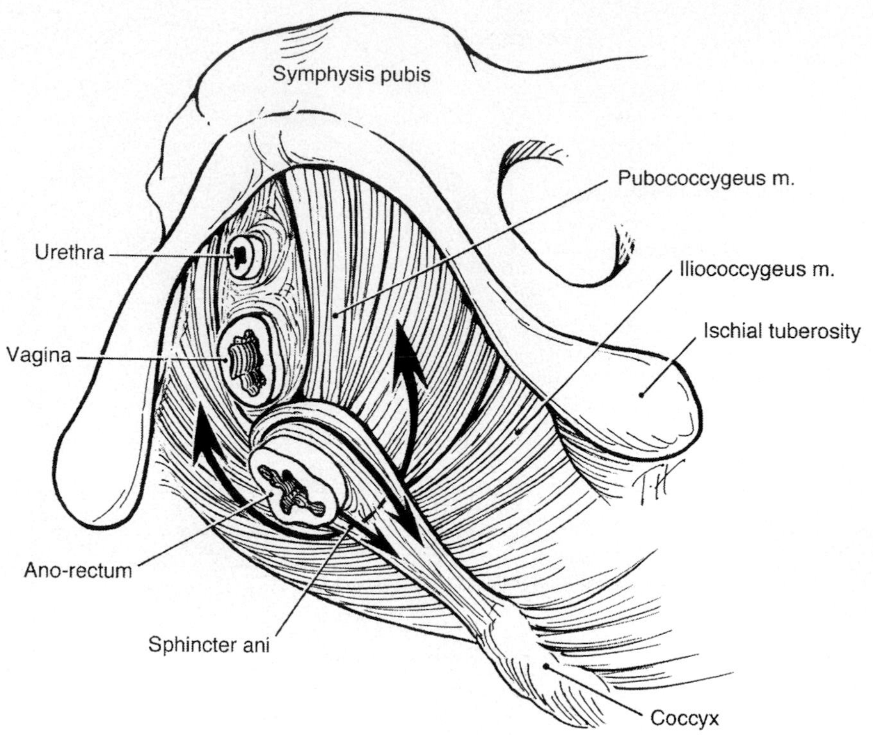

Figure 5.25 The double-layered muscular support of the pelvic diaphragm.

3. Operate with more experienced pelvic surgeons, particularly when incorporating new surgical procedures into practice.

4. Periodically dissect fresh or fixed cadaveric specimens; this practice can generally be arranged through local or regional anatomy boards or medical schools or by special arrangement at the time of autopsy.

References

1. **International Anatomical Nomenclature Committee.** *Nomina anatomica.* 6th ed. Edinburgh: Churchill Livingstone, 1989.

2. **Thompson JR, Gibbs JS, Genadry R, et al.** Anatomy of pelvic arteries adjacent to the sacrospinous ligament: importance of the coccygeal branch of the inferior gluteal artery. *Obstet Gynecol* 1999;94(6):973–977.

3. **Uhlenhuth E, Day EC, Smith RD, et al.** The visceral endopelvic fascia and the hypogastric sheath. *Surg Gynecol Obstet* 1948;86:9–28.

4. **Thompson JD, Rock WA, Wiskind A.** Control of pelvic hemorrhage: blood component therapy and hemorrhagic shock. In: **Thompson JD, Rock JA,** eds. *TeLinde's operative gynecology.* 7th ed. Philadelphia: JB Lippincott, 1991:151.

5. **Lee RB, Stone K, Magelssen D, et al.** Presacral neurectomy for chronic pelvic pain. *Obstet Gynecol* 1986;68:517–521.

6. **Polan ML, DeCherney A.** Presacral neurectomy for pelvic pain in infertility. *Fertil Steril* 1980;34:557–560.

7. **Vaughan ED Jr, Middleton GW.** Pertinent genitourinary embryology: review for the practicing urologist. *Urology* 1975;6:139–149.

8. **Byskov AG, Hoyer PE.** Embryology of mammalian gonads and ducts. In: **Knobil E, Neill JD,** eds. *The physiology of reproduction.* 2nd ed. New York: Raven, 1994:487.

9. **Arey LB.** The genital system. In: *Developmental anatomy.* 7th ed. Philadelphia: WB Saunders, 1974:315.

10. **Moore KL.** The urogenital system. In: *The developing human: clinically oriented embryology.* 3rd ed. Philadelphia: WB Saunders, 1982:255.

11. **Semmens JP.** Congenital anomalies of female genital tract: Functional classification based on review of 56 personal cases and 500 reported cases. *Obstet Gynecol* 1962;19:328–350.

12. **Lawson JO.** Pelvic anatomy. II. Anal canal and associated sphincters. *Ann R Coll Surg Engl* 1974;54:288–300.

13. **Curtis AH.** *A textbook of gynecology.* 4th ed. Philadelphia: WB Saunders, 1943.

14. **Moore KL.** *Clinically oriented anatomy.* 2nd ed. Baltimore: Williams & Wilkins, 1985.

15. **Oelrich TM.** The striated urogenital sphincter muscle in the female. *Anat Rec* 1983;205:223–232.

16. **Milley PS, Nichols DH.** The relationship between the pubo-urethral ligaments and the urogenital diaphragm in the human female. *Anat Rec* 1971;170:281.

17. **Uhlenhuth E, Wolfe WM, Smith EM, et al.** The rectovaginal septum. *Surg Gynecol Obstet* 1948;86:148–163.

18. **Leffler KS, Thompson JR, Cundiff GW, et al.** Attachment of the rectovaginal septum to the pelvic sidewall. *Am J Obstet Gynecol* 2001;185:41–43.

19. **Nichols DH, Randall CL.** Clinical pelvic anatomy of the living. In: *Vaginal surgery*. Baltimore: Williams & Wilkins, 1976:1.

20. **Buller JL, Thompson JR, Cundiff GW, et al.** Uterosacral ligament: description of anatomic relationships to optimize surgical safety. *Obstet Gynecol* 2001;97:873–879.

21. **Symmonds RE.** Urologic injuries: ureter. In: **Schaefer G, Graber EA,** eds. *Complications in obstetric and gynecologic surgery.* Philadelphia: Harper & Row, 1981:412.

22. **Lawson JO.** Pelvic anatomy. I. Pelvic floor muscles. *Ann R Coll Surg Engl* 1974;54:244–252.

6 Molecular Biology and Genetics

Vicki V. Baker
Otoniel Martínez-Maza
Jonathan S. Berek

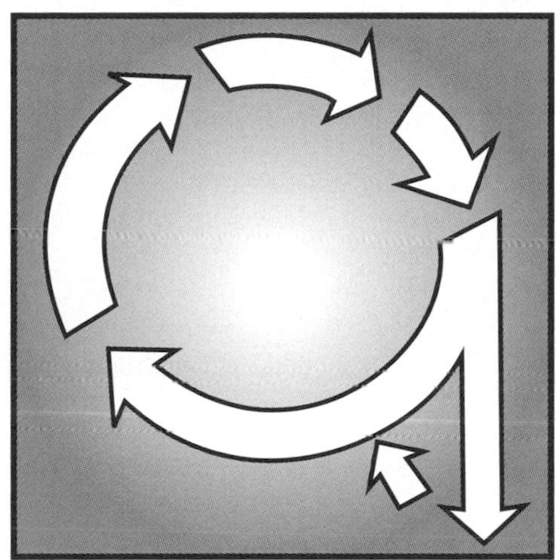

Significant scientific advances in molecular biology and genetics have occurred in the recent past. Completion of the human genome project, the emergence of new areas of investigation such as proteomics, and the development of new technologies for the manipulation of cells *ex vivo* are just some of the accomplishments that will have an impact on the specialty of obstetrics and gynecology. To place the significance of these advances in perspective, one must understand the basic concepts of molecular and cellular biology.

Normal cells are characterized by discrete metabolic, biochemical, and physiologic functions and responses. The observed functions and responses are influenced by the specific cell type and its genetic complement (Fig. 6.1). To orchestrate a coordinated and appropriate response, an external stimulus must be converted to an intracellular signal that is reliably transduced to the nucleus and then converted to specific genetic messages. Through these steps, extracellular signals prompt changes in cellular function, differentiation, and proliferation. Although specific cell types and tissues by definition exhibit unique functions and characteristics, there are also many aspects of cell biology and genetics that are common to all eukaryotic cells.

Cell Cycle

Normal Cell Cycle

The cell cycle and the factors that influence it are key to cell biology. Control of the cell cycle is the result of multiple levels of complex molecular regulation, most of which is incompletely understood. **Progression through the cell cycle occurs through four distinct phases: G_1, S, G_2, and M (Fig. 6.2). The duration of the cell cycle (e.g., the generation time) may be quite variable, although most human cells complete the cell cycle within approximately 24 hours. Variations in cell-cycle time reflect different durations of the G_1 phase.** With respect to the cell cycle, there are three subpopulations of cells:

1. ***Terminally differentiated cells*** cannot reenter the cell cycle.

Figure 6.1 External stimuli affect the cell, which has a specific coordinated response.

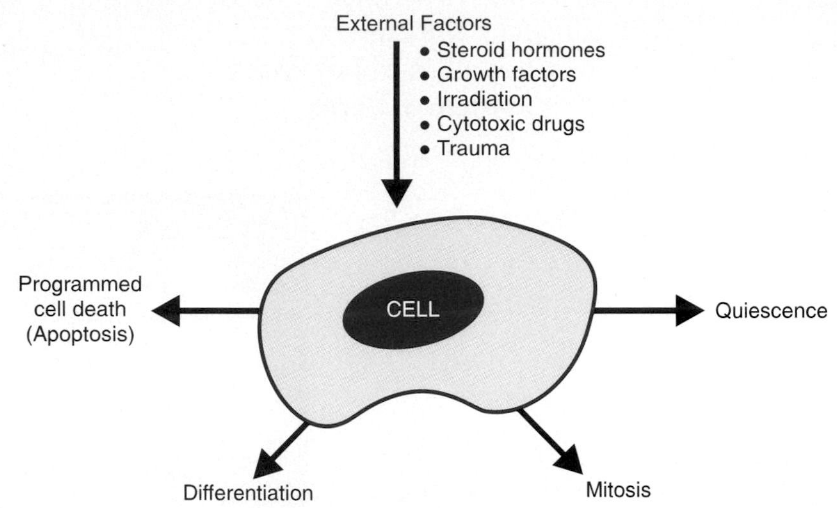

Figure 6.2 The cell cycle.

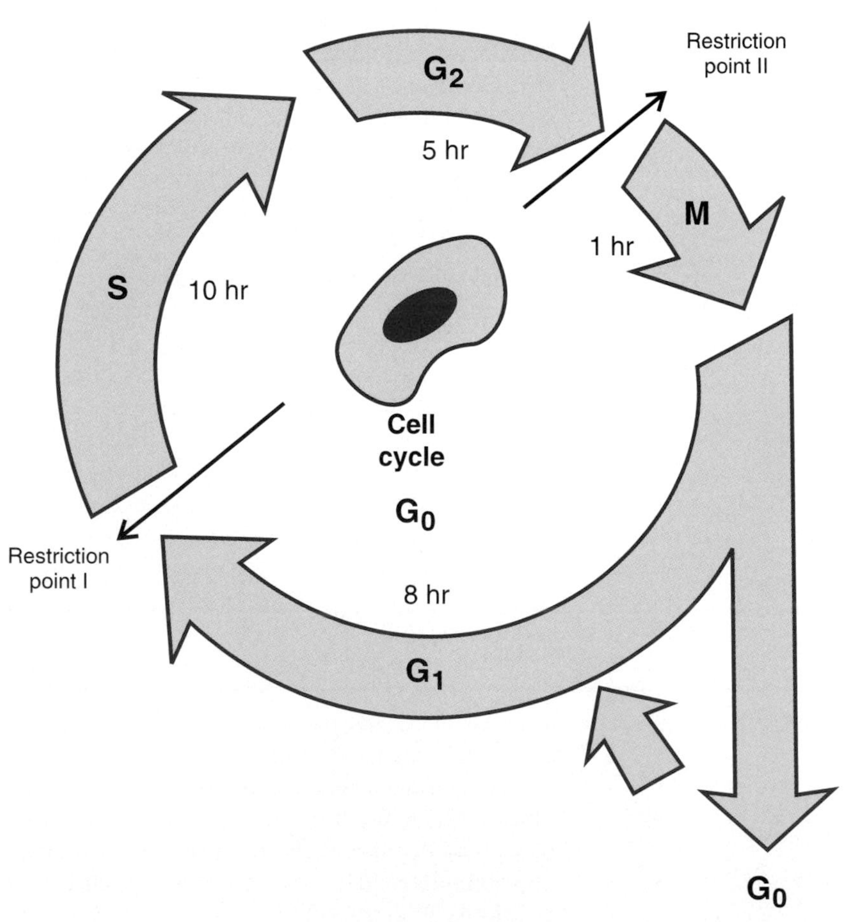

2. ***Quiescent (G_0) cells*** can enter the cell cycle if appropriately stimulated.

3. ***Dividing cells*** are currently in the cell cycle.

Red blood cells, striated muscle cells, uterine smooth muscle cells, and nerve cells are terminally differentiated. Other cells, such as fibroblasts, exist in the G_0 phase and are considered to be out of the cell cycle. These cells are stimulated to enter the cell cycle following exposure to specific stimuli, such as growth factors and steroid hormones. Dividing cells are found in the gastrointestinal tract, the skin, and the cervix.

G_1 Phase

In response to specific external stimuli, cells enter the cell cycle by moving from the G_0 phase into the G_1 phase. The G_1 phase of the cell cycle is characterized by diverse biosynthetic activities. The synthesis of enzymes and regulatory proteins necessary for DNA synthesis occurs during this phase. **Variation in the duration of the G_1 phase of the cell cycle, ranging from less than 8 hours to longer than 100 hours, accounts for the different generation times exhibited by different types of cells.**

S Phase

The nuclear DNA content of the cell is copied during the S phase of the cell cycle. It is not known what actually triggers the initiation of DNA synthesis, but once it begins, it proceeds as an "all-or-none" phenomenon. Upon completion of this phase, the DNA content of the cell is doubled.

G_2 Phase

RNA and protein synthesis occurs during the G_2 phase of the cell cycle. The burst of biosynthetic activity provides the metabolic substrates and enzymes to meet the metabolic requirements of the two daughter cells. Another important event that occurs during the G_2 phase of the cell cycle is repair of errors of DNA replication that may have occurred during the S phase. Failure to detect and correct these genetic errors can result in a broad spectrum of adverse consequences for the organism as well as the individual cell (1). Defects in the DNA repair mechanism have been associated with an increased incidence of cancer (2).

M Phase

During mitosis, or the M phase of the cell cycle, nuclear division occurs. During this phase, cellular DNA is equally distributed to each of the daughter cells. Mitosis provides a diploid (2n) DNA complement to each somatic daughter cell. Following mitosis, eukaryotic mammalian cells normally contain diploid DNA reflecting a karyotype that includes 44 somatic chromosomes and an XX or XY sex chromosome complement. Exceptions to the diploid cellular content include hepatocytes (4n) and the functional syncytium of the placenta.

Ploidy

Germ cells contain a haploid (1n) genetic complement after meiosis. After fertilization, a 46,XX or 46,XY diploid DNA complement is restored. Restoration of the normal cellular DNA content is crucial to normal function. Abnormalities of cellular DNA content cause distinct phenotypic abnormalities as exemplified by hydatidiform molar pregnancy (see Chapter 34). With complete hydatidiform mole, an oocyte without any nuclear genetic material (e.g., an empty ovum) is fertilized by one sperm. The haploid genetic content of the fertilized ovum is then duplicated and the diploid cellular DNA content is restored, resulting in a homozygous 46,XX gamete. Less often, a complete hydatidiform mole results from the fertilization of an empty ovum by two sperm, resulting in a heterozygous 46,XX or 46,XY gamete. In complete molar pregnancies, the nuclear DNA is paternally derived, embryonic structures do not develop, and trophoblast hyperplasia occurs. A partial hydatiform mole follows the fertilization of a haploid ovum by two sperm, resulting in a 69,XXX, 69,XXY, or 69,XYY karyotype. A partial mole contains paternal and maternal DNA, and both embryonic and placental development occur.

Both the 69,YYY karyotype and the 46,YY karyotype are incompatible with embryonic and placental development. These observations indicate the importance of the maternal genetic contribution, in general, and the X chromosome, in particular, to normal embryonic and placental development.

In addition to total cellular DNA content, the chromosome number is an important determinant of cellular function. Abnormalities of chromosome number, which are often the result of nondisjunction during meiosis, result in well-characterized clinical syndromes such as trisomy 21 (Down's syndrome), trisomy 18, and trisomy 13.

Nuclear division and the allocation of replicated DNA to the daughter cells is closely followed by cytoplasmic division (e.g., cytokinesis). Exceptions are hepatocytes and syncytiotrophoblasts, in which several nuclei exist in a common cytoplasm. After mitosis and completion of cellular division, the daughter cells continue in G_1, enter the G_0 phase, or undergo programmed cell death. The option that is pursued by the daughter cell has important implications for the integrity of the tissue and the organ.

Genetic Control of the Cell Cycle

Cellular proliferation must occur to balance normal cell loss and maintain tissue and organ integrity. This process requires the coordinated expression of many genes at discrete times during the cell cycle (3). To successfully complete the cell cycle, a number of cell division cycle *(cdc)* genes are activated. In addition, the cell must traverse two checkpoints, one at the G_1/S boundary and one at the G_2/M boundary (4,5). **The G_1/S boundary marks the point at which a cell commits to proliferation and the G_2/M boundary marks the point at which repair of any DNA damage must be completed (6,7).**

Cell Division Cycle Genes

Among the factors that regulate the cell cycle checkpoints, proteins encoded by the *cdc*2 family of genes and the cyclin proteins appear to play particularly important roles (8,9). **The accumulation and degradation of cyclins regulate the checkpoint at the G_1/S boundary.** It has been hypothesized that these proteins bind to specific chromosomal sites. When the chromosomal sites are fully occupied, a critical threshold is exceeded, the free intracellular concentration of cyclins increases, and the cell enters the S phase of the cycle. By an unknown mechanism, cyclins can also inhibit progression through the cell cycle in the presence of DNA damage.

The *p53* tumor suppressor gene also appears to participate in delay of the cell cycle in order for DNA repair to be completed. As an example, cells exposed to radiation therapy exhibit an S-phase arrest that is accompanied by increased expression of *p53*. This delay permits the repair of radiation-induced DNA damage. When the *p53* gene is mutated, the S-phase arrest that normally follows radiation therapy does not occur (10,11). A normal *p53* gene that is not mutated can be inactivated when human papillomavirus 16 E6 protein is present, and the S-phase arrest in response to ultraviolet-induced DNA damage does not occur (12).

Mitosis is initiated by activation of the *cdc* gene at the G_2/M checkpoint (13,14). The p34 cdc2 protein and specific cyclins form a complex heterodimer referred to as *mitosis-promoting factor (MPF),* which catalyzes protein phosphorylation and drives the cell into mitosis. Once the G_2/M checkpoint has been passed, the cell undergoes mitosis. In the presence of abnormally replicated chromosomes, progression past the G_2/M checkpoint does not occur.

Following cytoplasmic division, the daughter cells exit the cell cycle (e.g., enter the G_0 phase), continue in the G_1 phase of the cell cycle, or undergo programmed cell death.

Failure of the progeny cells to respond to the signals that regulate cellular proliferation at this point in the cell cycle is a fundamental characteristic of the neoplastic phenotype.

Apoptosis

The regulation and maintenance of normal tissue mass requires a balance between cell proliferation and programmed cell death, or *apoptosis*. When proliferation exceeds programmed cell death, the result is hyperplasia. When programmed cell death exceeds proliferation, the result is atrophy. Programmed cell death is a crucial concomitant of normal embryologic development. This mechanism accounts for deletion of the interdigital webs (15), palatal fusion (16), and development of the intestinal mucosa (17). Programmed cell death is also an important phenomenon in normal physiology (18). The reduction in the number of endometrial cells following alterations in steroid hormone levels during the menstrual cycle is, in part, a consequence of programmed cell death (19,20). In response to androgens, granulosa cells undergo programmed cell death (e.g., follicular atresia (21).

Programmed cell death, or apoptosis, is an energy-dependent, active process that is initiated by the expression of specific genes. It is a process distinct from cell necrosis, although both mechanisms result in a reduction in total cell number. In programmed cell death, cells shrink and undergo phagocytosis. Apoptosis is an energy-dependent process that results from the expression of specific genes. Conversely, in cell necrosis, groups of cells expand and lyse, and it is an energy-independent process that results from noxious stimuli. Programmed cell death is triggered by a variety of factors, including intracellular signals and exogenous stimuli such as radiation exposure, chemotherapy, and hormones. Cells undergoing programmed cell death may be identified on the basis of histologic, biochemical, and molecular biologic changes. Histologically, apoptotic cells exhibit cellular condensation and fragmentation of the nucleus. Biochemical correlates of impending programmed cell death include an increase in transglutaminase expression and fluxes in intracellular calcium concentration. The molecular mechanisms of programmed cell death are the subject of intense investigation (22,23).

Programmed cell death has recently emerged as an important factor in the growth of neoplasms. Historically, neoplastic growth has been characterized by uncontrolled cellular proliferation that resulted in a progressive increase in tumor burden. It is now recognized that **the increase in tumor burden associated with progressive disease reflects an imbalance between cell proliferation and cell death.** Cancer cells not only fail to respond to the normal signals to stop proliferating, but they may also fail to recognize the physiologic signals that trigger programmed cell death.

Modulation of Cell Growth and Function

The normal cell exhibits an orchestrated response to the changing extracellular environment. The three groups of substances that signal these extracellular changes are steroid hormones, growth factors, and cytokines. The capability to respond to these stimuli requires a cell surface recognition system, an intracellular signal transduction system, and a means to elicit the expression of specific genes in a coordinated fashion to affect changes in cell structure and function.

Oncogenes and Tumor Suppressor Genes

Among the genes that participate in cell growth and function, *protooncogenes* and *tumor suppressor genes* are particularly important (24–26). *Protooncogenes* encode growth factors, membrane and cytoplasmic receptors, proteins that play key roles in the intracellular signal transduction cascade, and nuclear DNA binding proteins (Table 6.1). More than 50 protooncogene products that contribute to growth regulation have been identified. As a group, protooncogenes exert positive effects upon cellular proliferation. In

Table 6.1. Protooncogenes

Protooncogenes	*Gene Product/Function*
	Growth factors
fgf-5	Fibroblast growth factor
sis	Platelet-derived growth factor beta
hst, int-2	
	Transmembrane receptors
erb-B	Epidermal growth factor (EGF) receptor
HER-2/*neu*	EGF-related receptor
fms	Colony-stimulating factor (CSF) receptor
kit	Stem cell receptor
trk	Nerve growth factor receptor
	Inner-membrane receptor
bcl-2	
Ha-*ras*, N-*ras*, N-*ras*	
fgr, lck, src, yes	
	Cytoplasmic messengers
crk	
cot, plm-1, *mos, raf/mil*	
	Nuclear DNA binding proteins
erb-B1	
jun, ets-1, *ets*-2, *fos, gil* 1, *rel, ski, vav*	
lyl-1, *maf, myb, myc*, L-*myc*, N-*myc, evi*-1	

Table 6.2. Tumor Suppressor Genes

p53	Mutated in as many as 50% of solid tumors
Rb	Deletions and mutations predispose to retinoblastoma
WT1	Mutations are correlated with Wilms' tumor
NF1	Neurofibromatosis gene
APC	Associated with colon cancer development in patients with familial adenomatous polyposis

contradistinction, *tumor suppressor genes* exert inhibitory regulatory effects on cellular proliferation (Table 6.2).

Steroid Hormones

Steroid hormones play crucial roles in reproductive biology as well as in general physiology. To mention only a few of their roles, steroid hormones influence pregnancy, phenotype, cardiovascular function, bone metabolism, and an individual's sense of general well-being. Steroid hormone action reflects the intracellular and genetic mechanisms that are necessary for the transduction of an extracellular signal to the nucleus to affect a physiologic response. Estrogen diffuses through the cell membrane and binds to estrogen receptors that are located in the nucleus. The receptor-steroid complex then binds to the DNA at specific sequences designated as *estrogen-response elements (EREs)*. These steroid-responsive elements are located near the promoter regions of genes that are regulated by estrogen (27). In the uterus, these interactions result in discrete changes in gene expression, protein synthesis, and cellular and tissue function (28). In any estrogen-responsive tissue, the estrogen receptor plays a pivotal role.

The estrogen receptor has been characterized in terms of its molecular biology, structure, function, and tissue distribution. As is the case for all hormone receptors, specificity of action is conferred by the ligand-binding and the DNA-binding domains (EREs). The role of hormone receptors in normal tissue and organ function, as well as their role in the cause and progression of clinically defined estrogen responsive neoplasms, is much more complicated than originally appreciated.

The estrogen receptor actually represents two distinct receptors, E_2R-α and E_2R-β that are encoded by different genes on different chromosomes. Both E_2R-α and E_2R-β bind estrogen and regulate transcription through interactions with EREs. These receptors exhibit different affinities and responsiveness not only to estrogen but also to *selective estrogen receptor modulators (SERMs).* Compared with E_2R-α, the E_2R-β receptor requires 5- to 10-fold higher concentrations of estradiol for maximal transcriptional activity. ***Tamoxifen* is a mixed agonist/antagonist for E_2R-α but it is a pure antagonist for E_2R-β.** The E_2R-β receptor is ubiquitously expressed in hormone-responsive tissues, whereas the expression of E_2R-α fluctuates in response to the hormonal milieu. The cellular and tissue effects of an estrogenic compound appear to reflect a dynamic interplay between the actions of these estrogen receptor isoforms. These observations underscore the complexity of estrogen interactions with both normal and neoplastic tissue.

Mutations of hormone receptors and their functional consequences illustrate their important contributions to normal physiology. For example, absence of E_2R-α in a male human has been reported (29). The clinical sequelae attributed to this mutation include incomplete epiphyseal closure, increased bone turnover, tall stature, and impaired glucose tolerance. The androgen insensitivity syndrome is caused by mutations of the androgen receptor (30). Mutations of the receptors for growth hormone and thyroid-stimulating hormone that result in a spectrum of phenotypic alterations have also been identified. It is speculated that mutations of hormone receptors may contribute to the progression of neoplastic disease and resistance to hormone therapy (31,32).

Growth Factors

Growth factors are polypeptides that are produced by a variety of cell types and exhibit a wide range of overlapping biochemical actions (23). Growth factors bind to high-affinity cell membrane receptors and trigger complex positive and negative signaling pathways that regulate cell proliferation and differentiation (33). **In general, growth factors exert positive or negative effects upon the cell cycle by influencing gene expression related to events that occur at the G_1/S cell cycle boundary** (34).

Because of their short half-life in the extracellular space, growth factors generally act over limited distances through autocrine or paracrine mechanisms. The autocrine mechanism of growth control involves the elaboration of a growth factor that acts on the cell that produced it. The paracrine mechanism of growth control involves the elaboration of a growth factor that acts on another cell in proximity.

More than 40 growth factors have been described. Those that appear to play important roles in female reproductive physiology are listed in Table 6.3. The biologic response of a cell to a specific growth factor depends on the cell type and the other stimuli that are concomitantly acting on the cell. Two growth factors acting in concert may produce a very different effect from either factor independently.

The regulation of ovarian function occurs through *autocrine, paracrine,* and *endocrine* mechanisms (35–41). The growth and differentiation of ovarian cells are particularly influenced by the insulin-like growth factors (IGF) (Fig. 6.3). The IGF amplify the actions of gonadotropin hormones on autocrine and paracrine growth factors found in the ovary. As an example, IGF-1 acts on granulosa cells to cause an increase in cyclic adenosine monophosphate (cAMP), progesterone, oxytocin, proteoglycans, and inhibin. Insulin-like growth factor 1 acts on theca cells to cause an increase in androgen production. The theca

Table 6.3. Growth Factors that Play Important Roles in Female Reproductive Physiology

Growth Factor	*Sources*	*Targets*	*Actions*
Platelet-derived growth factor (PDGF)	Placenta, platelets, preimplantation embryo, endothelial cells	Endothelial cells Trophoblasts	Mitogen
Epidermal growth factor (EGF)	Submaxillary gland, theca cells	Granulosa cells Endometrium, cervix	Mitogen
Transforming growth factor–alpha (TGF-alpha)	Embryo, placenta, theca cell, ovarian stromal cell	Placenta Granulosa cells	Mitogen
Transforming growth factor–beta (TGF-beta)	Embryo, theca cells	Endometrium Granulosa cells Theca cells	Mitogen
Insulin-like growth factor 1 (IGF-1)	Granulosa cells	Theca cells Granulosa cells	Mediates growth hormone activity
Insulin-like growth factor 2 (IGF-2)	Theca cells	Theca cells	Insulin-like effects
Fibroblast growth factor (FGF)	Granulosa cells	Granulosa cells	Angiogenic activity Mitogen

cells in turn produce tumor necrosis factor-α (TNF-α) and epidermal growth factor (EGF), both of which are also regulated by follicle-stimulating hormone (FSH). Epidermal growth factor acts on granulosa cells to stimulate mitogenesis. Insulin-like growth factor 2 is the principal growth factor found in follicular fluid although other factors, including IGF-1, TNF-α, TNF-β, and EGF, also play important roles. **Disruption of these autocrine and paracrine intraovarian pathways may be the basis of polycystic ovarian disease and disorders of ovulation.**

Transforming growth factor (TGF)-β activates intracytoplasmic serine threonine kinases and inhibits cells in the late G_1 phase of the cell cycle (41). It appears to play an important role in embryonic remodeling. Müllerian inhibiting substance (MIS), which is responsible for regression of the müllerian duct, is structurally and functionally related to TGF-β (42).

Transforming growth factor α is an EGF homologue that binds to the EGF receptor and acts as an autocrine factor in normal cells. Like EGF, TGF-α promotes entry of G_0 cells into the G_1 phase of the cell cycle. The role of growth factors in endometrial growth and function has been the subject of several reviews (36–41). Similar to the ovary, autocrine, paracrine, and endocrine mechanisms of control also occur in endometrial tissue.

Intracellular Signal Transduction

Growth factors trigger intracellular biochemical signals by binding to cell membrane receptors. In general, these membrane-bound receptors are *protein kinases* that convert an extracellular signal into an intracellular signal. The interaction between growth factor ligand and its receptor results in receptor dimerization, autophosphorylation, and tyrosine kinase activation. Activated receptors in turn phosphorylate substrates in the cytoplasm and trigger the intracellular signal transduction system (Fig. 6.4). The intracellular signal transduction system relies on serine threonine kinases, *src*-related kinases, and G proteins. Intracellular signals in turn activate nuclear effectors that regulate gene expression. **Many of the proteins that participate in the intracellular signal transduction**

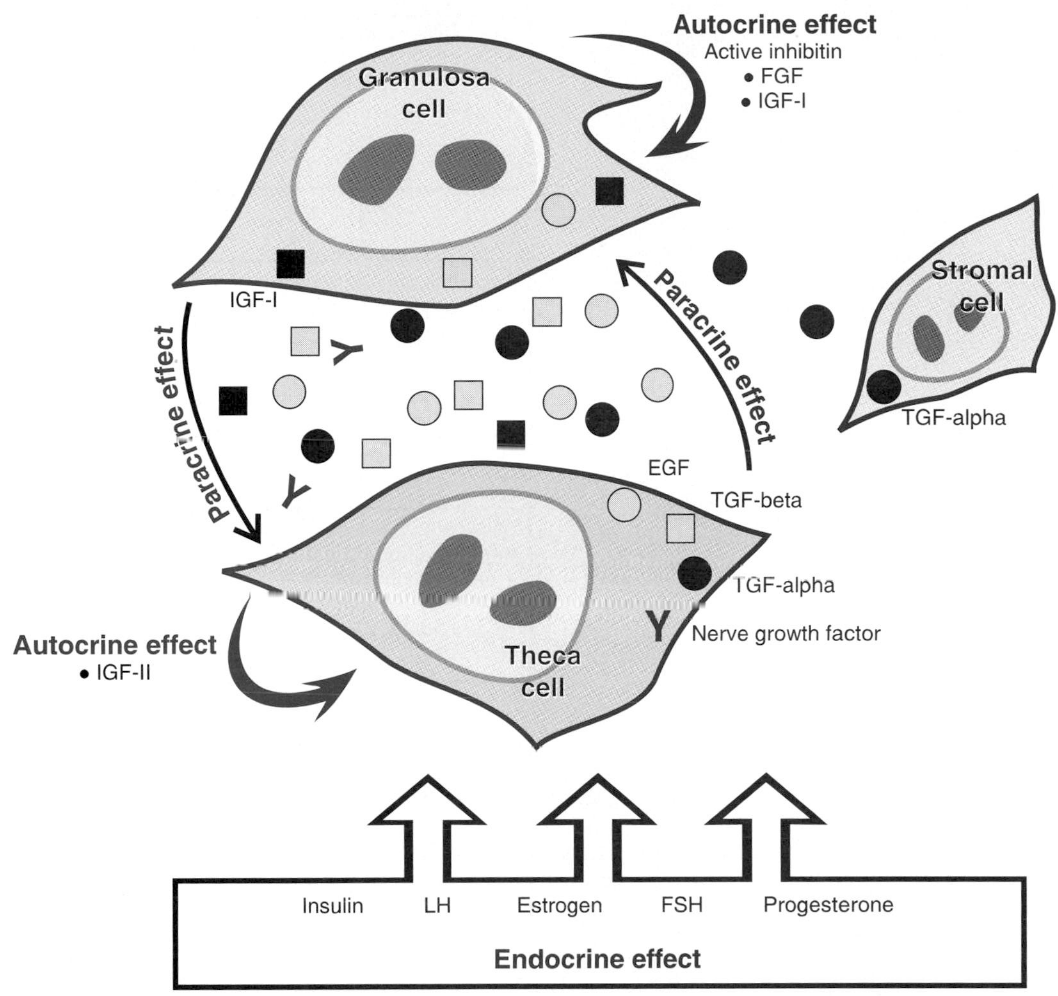

Figure 6.3 The regulation of ovarian function occurs through autocrine, paracrine, and endocrine mechanisms.

system are encoded by *protooncogenes* that are conveniently divided into subgroups based on their cellular location or enzymatic function (43,44) (Fig. 6.5).

The *raf* and *mos* protooncogenes encode proteins with serine threonine kinase activity. These kinases integrate signals originating at the cell membrane with those that are forwarded to the nucleus (45,46). Protein kinase C (PKC) is an important component of the second messenger system that exhibits serine threonine kinase activity. This enzyme plays a central role in phosphorylation, which is a general mechanism for activating and deactivating proteins. It also plays an important role in cell metabolism and division (47).

The Scr family of tyrosine kinases is related to PKC and includes protein products encoded by the *scr, yes, fgr, hck, lyn, fyn, lck, alt,* and *fps/fes* protooncogenes. These proteins bind to the inner cell membrane surface.

The *G proteins* are guanyl nucleotide-binding proteins. The heterotrimeric or large G proteins link receptor activation with effector proteins such as adenyl cyclase, which activates the cAMP-dependent, kinase-signaling cascade (48,49). The monomeric or small G proteins, encoded by the *ras* protooncogene family, are designated p21 and are particularly important regulators of mitogenic signals (50). The p21 Ras protein exhibits guanyl triphosphate (GTP) binding and GTPase activity. Hydrolysis of GTP to guanyl diphosphate (GDP) terminates p21 Ras activity. The p21 Ras protein influences the production

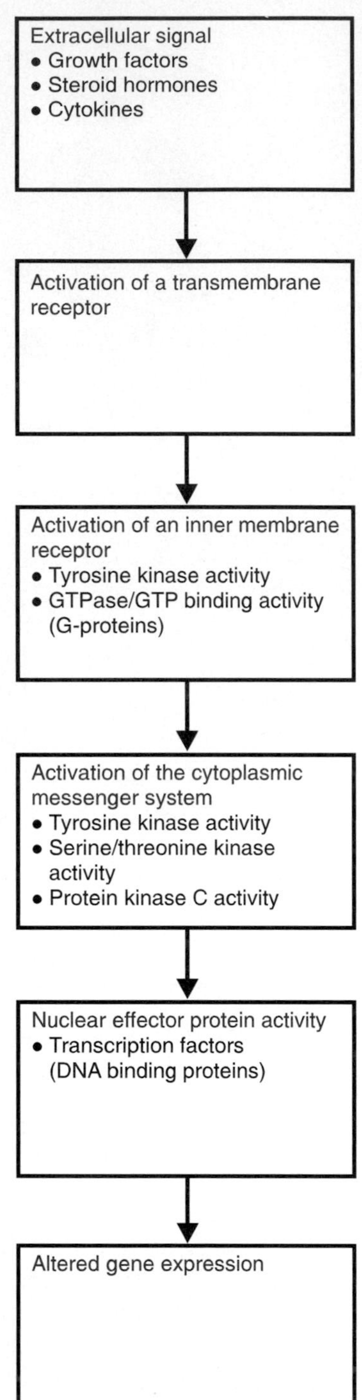

Figure 6.4 Pathways of intracellular signal transduction.

of deoxyguanosine (dG) and inositol phosphate (IP) 3, arachidonic acid production, and IP turnover.

Gene Expression

Regulation of genetic transcription and replication is crucial to the normal function of the daughter cells as well as the tissues and ultimately the organism. Transmission of external signals to the nucleus by way of the intracellular signal transduction cascade culminates in the transcription and translation of specific genes that ultimately affect the structure, function, and proliferation of the cell.

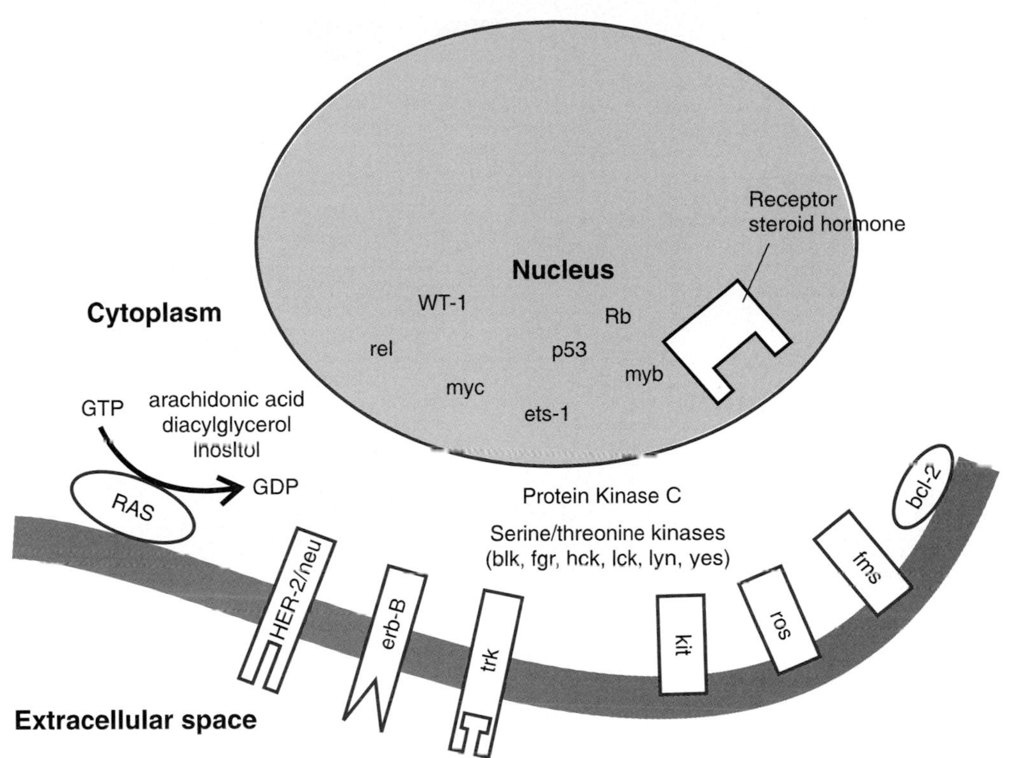

Figure 6.5 Protooncogenes are divided into subgroups based on their cellular location or enzymatic function.

The human genome project has resulted in the determination of the sequence of DNA of the entire human genome. With the completion of this project, it appears that the human genetic complement consists of approximately 30,000 genes. Sequencing the human genome is a major scientific achievement that opens the door for more detailed studies of structural and functional genomics. Structural genomics involves the study of three-dimensional structures of proteins based on their amino acid sequences. Functional genomics provides a way to correlate structure and function. Proteomics involves the identification and cataloging of all proteins used by a cell, and cytomics involves the study of cellular dynamics, including intracellular system regulation and response to external stimuli. Each of these areas of investigation requires an understanding of basic genetic alterations.

Gene replication, transcription, and translation are imperfect processes and the fidelity is less than 100% (51). Genetic errors may result in abnormal structure and function. Genomic alterations have been identified in premalignant, malignant, and benign neoplasms of the female genital tract (52–54).

In view of the critical roles that oncogenes and tumor suppressor genes play in the regulation of normal cell growth, it is understandable that mutations of these genes may causally contribute to the neoplastic phenotype. By convention, mutated protooncogenes are referred to as *c-oncogenes.* Mutations may occur by one of several mechanisms (Fig. 6.6).

Genetic abnormalities, such as amplification, point mutations, and deletions or rearrangements, are progressive in successive generations. One error tends to permit additional aberrations. A variety of genetic abnormalities have been associated with the neoplastic phenotype. The end result of the genetic abnormalities found in transformed cells is defective control of the cell cycle. Proliferation may be abnormally increased with inoperative normal constraints on cell growth, programmed cell death may fail to occur, or some combination of the two processes may exist.

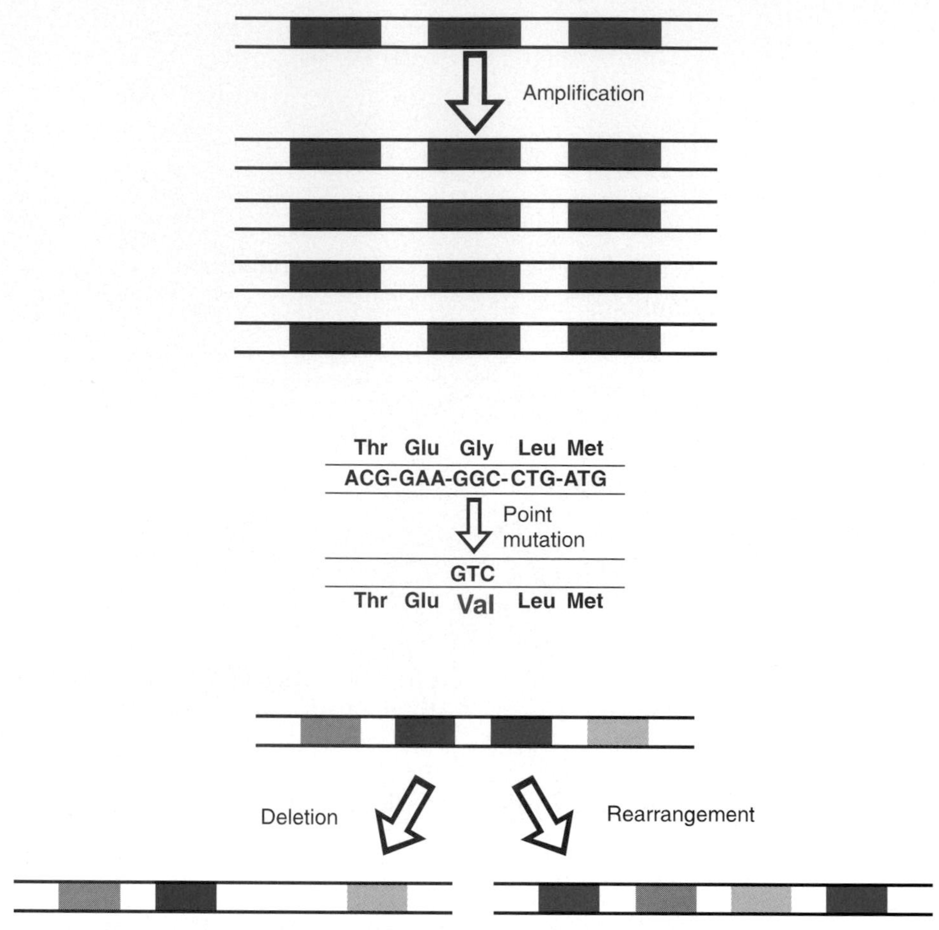

Figure 6.6 Genes can be amplified or undergo mutation, deletion, or rearrangement.

A single genetic mutation that causes cancer has not been identified. In fact, specific genetic mutations may not be as important as the accumulation of some critical number of mutations in a cell. Available data suggest that cancer results from the accumulation of mutations over time in several genes (55). From this perspective, exposure to factors that increase the likelihood of genetic mutations over time assumes importance in assessing cancer risk.

Amplification

Amplification refers to an increase in the copy number of a gene. Amplification results in enhanced gene expression by increasing the amount of template DNA that is available for transcription. Protooncogene amplification is a relatively common event in malignancies of the female genital tract.

Point Mutations

Point mutations of a gene, in which the codon sequence is altered, may result in altered gene action by qualitatively altering the gene product. The *ras* gene family is perhaps the best example of oncogene-encoded proteins that disrupt the intracellular signal transduction system following mutation. Transforming Ras proteins contain point mutations in critical codons (i.e., 11, 12, 59, 61) that reduce GTPase activity so that Ras is constitutively active in the GTP-bound form. Point mutations of the *p53* gene are the most common genetic mutation described in solid tumors. These mutations occur at preferential "hot spots" that coincide with the most highly conserved regions of the gene. Loss of normal *p53* gene activity removes one of the inhibitors of cell proliferation and also increases the likelihood that DNA damage may be successfully passed to daughter cells. Mutations of the *p53* gene occur in approximately 50% of ovarian cancers and 30% to 40% of endometrial cancers. In contrast, point mutations of *p53* are uncommon in cervical cancer. However, in cervical cancer, *p53* activity is often abnormal as a consequence of interactions between the p53 protein and the E6 protein encoded by the human papillomavirus.

As with *p53,* the *BRCA1* and *BRCA2* genes also play a role in DNA repair, and the activity of these genes may be altered by point mutations. Unlike the situation with *p53,* mutations of *BRCA1* and *BRCA2* do not occur at preferential positions. The "random" location of mutations coupled with the large size of these genes make genetic screening a complicated task. Mutations of the *BRCA1* and *BRCA2* genes may be associated with an increased risk of ovarian and breast cancer.

Deletions and Rearrangements

Deletions and rearrangements reflect gross changes in the DNA template that may result in the synthesis of a markedly altered protein product. As an example, deletion mutations of the EGF receptor affect tyrosine kinase activity. The mutated receptor is activated constitutively and transmits a signal to the cytoplasm for cellular proliferation in the absence of a bound ligand.

Immunology

The immune system plays an essential part in host defense and can respond to host cells that have undergone transformation to become neoplastic cells. These responses, whether natural or induced, can in some cases lead to tumor regression. As more is learned about the regulation of immune responses, new opportunities for novel immunotherapeutic approaches develop. Immunodiagnostic procedures using antitumor marker antibodies also show great promise as diagnostic and prognostic tools.

Immunologic Mechanisms

The human immune system has the potential to respond to abnormal or tumor cells in various ways. Some of these immune responses occur in an innate or antigen-nonspecific manner, whereas others are adaptive or antigen specific. Adaptive responses are specific to a given antigen and also establish a memory, allowing a more rapid and vigorous response to the same antigen in future encounters (55). Various innate and adaptive immune mechanisms are involved in responses to tumors, including cytotoxicity directed to tumor cells mediated by cytotoxic T cells, natural killer (NK) cells, macrophages, and antibody-dependent cytotoxicity mediated by complementation activation (56).

Adaptive or specific immune responses are made up of humoral and cellular responses. *Humoral immune responses* refer to the production of antibodies that are antigen reactive, soluble, bifunctional molecules composed of specific antigen-binding sites that react with foreign antigens. They are associated with a constant region that directs the biologic activities of the antibody, such as the binding of antibody molecules to cells, including phagocytic cells, or the activation of complement. *Cellular immune responses* are antigen-specific immune responses mediated directly by activated immune cells rather than by the production of antibodies. The distinction between humoral and cellular responses is historical and originates from the experimental observation that humoral immune function can be transferred by serum, whereas cellular immune function requires the transfer of cells. Most immune responses include both humoral and cellular components.

Several types of cells, including cells from both the myeloid and lymphoid lineages, make up the immune system. Specific humoral and cellular immune responses to foreign antigens involve the coordinated action of populations of lymphocytes operating in concert with each other and with phagocytic cells (macrophages). These cellular interactions include both direct cognate interactions involving cell-to-cell contact and cellular interactions involving the secretion of and response to cytokines or lymphokines. Lymphoid cells are found in lymphoid tissues, such as lymph nodes or spleen, or in the peripheral circulation. The cells that make up the immune system originate from stem cells in the bone marrow.

B Cells, Hormonal Immunity, and Monoclonal Antibodies

The cells that synthesize and secrete antibodies are B lymphocytes (56). Mature, antigen-responsive B cells develop from pre-B cells (committed B-cell progenitors) and differentiate to become plasma cells, which produce large quantities of antibodies. Pre-B cells originate from bone marrow stem cells in adults, after the rearrangement of immunoglobulin genes from their germ-cell configuration to that seen in B cells. Mature B cells express cell surface immunoglobulin molecules, which these cells use as their receptors for antigen.

Following interaction with antigen, and in the presence of appropriate cell–cell stimulatory signals and cytokines, mature B cells respond to become antibody-producing cells. Although the generation of antibodies directed to tumor cells is generally not thought to have a central role in antitumor immune responses, the production of monoclonal antibodies to tumor cell antigens has shown great potential for immunotherapy and tumor detection.

Kohler and Milstein developed monoclonal antibody technology more than 20 years ago, and there has been considerable interest in the use of monoclonal antibodies for detection and monitoring of tumors and for treatment (57). Monoclonal antibodies that react with tumor-associated antigens may provide new therapeutic agents for cancer. Immunotoxin-conjugated monoclonal antibodies directed to human ovarian adenocarcinoma antigens can induce tumor cell killing and can prolong survival in mice implanted with a human ovarian cancer cell line (58). However, many obstacles limit the clinical use of monoclonal antibodies, including tumor cell antigenic heterogeneity, modulation of tumor-associated antigens, and cross-reactivity of normal host and tumor-associated antigens. No unique tumor-specific antigens have been identified; all tumor antigens that have been identified to date are tumor-related antigens, which are expressed to a lesser extent by nonmalignant tissues. Because most monoclonal antibodies are murine, the host's immune system can also recognize and respond to these foreign mouse proteins. The use of the genetically engineered monoclonal antibodies composed of human-constant regions with specific antigen-reactive murine variable regions should result in reduced antigenicity to the host (58). This may help eliminate many of the problems associated with the use of murine monoclonal antibodies.

T Lymphocytes and Cellular Immunity

T lymphocytes have a central role in the generation of immune responses by acting as helper cells in both humoral and cellular immune responses and by acting as effector cells in cellular responses (55). T-cell precursors originate in bone marrow and move to the thymus, where they mature into functional T cells. During their thymic maturation, T cells learn to recognize antigen in the context of the *major histocompatibility complex (MHC)* type of the individual person. It also seems that self-responding T cells are removed during development in the thymus (54–56).

T cells can be distinguished from other types of lymphocytes by their cell surface phenotype based upon the pattern of expression of various molecules as well as by differences in their biologic functions. All mature T cells express certain cell surface molecules such as the cluster determinant 3 (CD3) molecular complex and the T-cell antigen receptor, which is found in close association with the CD3 complex. The availability of monoclonal antibody reagents specific for cell surface markers has led to great progress in understanding the organization of the immune system in recent years. Certainly, such monoclonal antibodies are of great value in monitoring the effects on the human immune system of experimental treatment with biologic response modifiers or cytokines.

T cells recognize antigen through the cell surface T-cell antigen receptor (TCR). The structure and molecular organization of this molecule are similar to those of antibody molecules, which are the B-cell receptors for antigen. During T-cell development, the T-cell receptor gene undergoes gene arrangements similar to those seen in B cells, but there are important differences between the antigen receptors on B cells and T cells. The T-cell receptor is not secreted, and its structure is somewhat different from that of antibody molecules. The way in which the B-cell and T-cell receptors interact with antigens is also quite different. T cells can respond to antigens only when these antigens are presented in association with MHC molecules on antigen-presenting cells. Effective antigen presentation involves the processing of antigen into small fragments of peptide within the antigen-presenting cell and the subsequent presentation of these fragments of antigen in association with MHC molecules expressed on the surface of the antigen-presenting cell. T cells can respond to antigen only when presented in this manner, unlike B cells, which can bind antigen directly, without processing and presentation by antigen-presenting cells (56).

There are two major subsets of mature T cells that are phenotypically and functionally distinct: *T helper/inducer cells,* which express the CD4 cell surface marker, and the *T suppressor/cytotoxic cells,* which express the CD8 marker. The expression of these markers is acquired during the passage of T cells through the thymus. CD4 T cells can provide help to B cells, resulting in the production of antibodies by B cells, and interact with antigen presented by antigen-presenting cells in association with MHC class II molecules. CD4 T cells can also act as helper cells for other T cells. CD8 T cells include cells that are cytotoxic (cells that can kill target cells bearing appropriate antigens), and they interact with antigen presented on target cells in association with MHC class I molecules. The CD8 T-cell subset also contains suppressor T cells. These T cells can inhibit the biologic functions of B cells or other T cells (56). Although the primary biologic role of *cytotoxic T cells (CTLs)* seems to be lysis of virus-infected autologous cells, cytotoxic immune T cells can mediate the lysis of tumor cells directly. Presumably, CTLs recognize antigens associated with MHC class I molecules on tumor cells through their antigen-specific T-cell receptor, setting off a series of events that ultimately results in the lysis of the target cell.

Monocytes and Macrophages

Monocytes and macrophages, which are myeloid cells, have important roles in both innate and adaptive immune responses; macrophages play a key part in the generation of immune receptors. T cells do not respond to foreign antigens unless those antigens are processed and presented by antigen-presenting cells. **Macrophages (and B cells) express MHC class II molecules and are effective antigen-presenting cells for CD4 T cells** (55). Helper-inducer (CD4) T cells that bear a T-cell receptor of appropriate antigen and self-specificity are activated by this antigen-presenting cell to provide help (various factors—lymphokines—that induce the activation of other lymphocytes). In addition to their role as antigen-presenting cells, macrophages play an important part in innate responses by ingesting and killing microorganisms. Activated macrophages, in addition to their many other functional capabilities, can act as cytotoxic, antitumor killer cells.

Natural Killer Cells

A third major population of lymphocytes includes NK cells (55). These cells do not consistently bear cell surface markers that are characteristic of T or B cells, although they can share certain cell surface molecules with other types of lymphocytes. Characteristically, NK cells have a large granular lymphocyte morphology (59).

Natural killer cells are effector cells in an innate type of immune response: the nonspecific killing of tumor cells and virus-infected cells. Therefore, **NK activity represents an innate form of immunity that does not require an adaptive, memory response for optimal biologic function, but the antitumor activity can be increased by exposure to several agents, particularly cytokines such as interleukin-2 (IL-2).**

Although NK cells can express certain cell surface receptors, particularly a receptor for the crystallizable fragment (Fc) portion of antibodies and other NK-associated markers, it seems that cells with NK function are phenotypically heterogeneous, at least when compared with T or B cells. The cells that can carry out antibody-dependent cellular cytotoxicity, or antibody-targeted cytotoxicity, seem to be NK-like cells. Antibody-dependent cellular cytotoxicity by NK-like cells has been shown to result in the lysis of tumor cells in vitro. The mechanisms of this tumor cell killing are not clearly understood, although close cellular contact between the effector cell and the target cell seems to be required.

Biologic Response Modifiers

Most immunotherapeutic agents used in the treatment of cancer have been nonspecific agents that, when introduced into the human system, elicit a generalized inflammatory reaction and immune response, probably mediated by the secretion of a range of cytokines by many different types of cells. These agents have diverse and broad biologic effects and are often referred to as immunomodulators or biologic response modifiers.

The response of a given patient to treatment with biologic response modifiers depends on the ability to react to treatment with a generalized immune response. It is possible that some elements of the immune response elicited by immunotherapeutic agents or biologic response modifiers may be counterproductive, possibly causing immune suppression, inducing the production of cytokines that enhance tumor growth, or inducing an unfavorable or inappropriate immune response.

Bacille Calmette-Guerin (BCG) vaccine has been widely used in many tumor systems, either systemically, by injection into the lesion, or by scarification (60). Occasionally, it has been mixed with whole irradiated tumor cells and injected into the patient as a vaccine. In a large series, intracutaneous injection of melanoma lesions with BCG resulted in some tumor regression in patients with cutaneous recurrence (61), but visceral or parenchymal metastatic disease is resistant to this treatment. Although there have been some preliminary observations about the use of BCG as an adjuvant in children with acute lymphocytic leukemia and with stage II melanoma, randomized studies have not shown any appreciable responses.

Cytokines, Lymphokines, and Immune Mediators

Many events in the generation of immune responses (as well as during the effector phase of immune responses) require or are enhanced by cytokines, which are soluble mediator molecules (Table 6.4) (62–82). Cytokines are pleiotropic, in that they have multiple biologic functions that depend on the type of target cell or its maturational state. Cytokines are also heterogeneous in the sense that most cytokines share little structural or amino acid homology. *Cytokines* (also called *monokines* if they are derived from monocytes, *lymphokines* if they are derived from lymphocytes, *interleukins* if they exert their actions on leukocytes, or *interferons* [IFNs] if they have antiviral effects) are produced by a wide variety of cell types and seem to have important roles in many biologic responses outside the immune response, such as hematopoiesis. They may also be involved in the pathophysiology of a wide range of diseases and show great potential as therapeutic agents in immunotherapy for cancer.

Although cytokines are a heterogeneous group of proteins, they share some characteristics. For instance, most cytokines are low- to intermediate-molecular-weight (10–60 kd) glycosylated secreted proteins. They are also involved in immunity and inflammation, are produced transiently and locally (they act in autocrine and paracrine rather than an endocrine manner), are extremely potent in small concentrations, and interact with high-affinity cellular receptors that are specific for each cytokine. The cell surface binding of cytokines by specific receptors results in signal transduction followed by changes in gene expression and, ultimately, by changes in cellular proliferation or altered cell behavior, or both. Their biologic actions overlap, and exposure of responsive cells to multiple cytokines can result in synergistic or antagonistic biologic effects.

Table 6.4. Sources, Target Cells, and Biological Activities of Cytokines Involved in Immune Responses

Cytokine	*Cellular Source*	*Target Cells*	*Biologic Effects*
IL-1	Monocytes and macrophages Tumor cells	T cells, B cells Neurons Endothelial cells	Costimulator Pyrogen
IL-2	T cells (T_H1)	T cells B cells NK cells	Growth Activation and antibody production Activation and growth
IL-3	T cells	Immature hemopoietic stem cells	Growth and differentiation
IL-4	T cells (T_H2)	B cells T cells	Activation and growth; isotype switch to IgE; increased MHC II expression Growth
IL-6	Monocytes and macrophages T cells, B cells Ovarian cancer cells Other tumors	B cells T cells Hepatocytes Stem cells Tumor cells	Differentiation, antibody production Costimulator Induction of acute-phase response Growth and differentiation Autocrine/paracrine growth and viability-enhancing factor
IL-10	T cells (T_H2) Monocytes and macrophages	T cells (T_H1) Monocytes and macrophages B cells	Inhibition of cytokine synthesis Inhibition of Ag presentation and cytokine production Activation
IL-12	Monocytes	NK cells, T cells (T_H1)	Induction
IFN-γ	T cells (T_H1) NK cells	Monocytes/macrophages NK cells, T cells, B cells	Activation Activation Enhances responses
TNF-α	Monocytes and macrophages T cells	Monocytes/macrophages T cells, B cells Neurons (hypothalamus) Endothelial cells Muscle and fat cells	Monokine production Costimulator Pyrogen Activation, inflammation Catabolism/cachexia

IL-1, interleukin-1; T_H1, type 1 T helper lymphocyte; NK cells, natural killer cells; T_H2, type 2 T helper lymphocyte; IgE, immunoglobulin E; MHCII, major histocompatibility complex class II; Ag, antigen; IFN, interferon; TNF, tumor necrosis factor.

From **Berek JS, Martinez-Maza O.** Immunology and immunotherapy. In: **Lawton FG, Neijt JP, Swenerton KD.** *Epithelial cancer of the ovary.* London: BMJ, 1995:224, with permission.

Interleukins

Many different cytokines are involved in immune responses, particularly the interleukins (IL-1, IL-2, IL-3, IL-4, IL-6, IL-7, IL-10, IL-11, and IL-12) (Table 6.4). The interleukins are heterogeneous and do not constitute a family of growth-related molecules.

Interleukin-1 Interleukin-1 has a wide range of biologic activities, including direct effects on several cells involved in immune responses (62–82). It is involved in fever and inflammatory responses and may play a role in the pathogenesis of several diseases, such as rheumatoid arthritis. There are two defined forms of IL-1, IL-1α and IL-1β, which have similar biologic activities. Interleukin-1 can be released as a soluble form or can be found as a cell-associated molecule on the cell surface of macrophages. The primary sources of IL-1 are macrophages, the phagocytic cells of the liver and spleen, some B cells, epithelial cells, certain brain cells, and the cells lining the synovial spaces. Interleukin-1 has a broad range of target cells and biologic activities, as do most lymphokines. A principal role of IL-1 is in the initiation of early events in immune responses (62,68).

Interleukin-2 Interleukin-2 is a lymphokine that was originally called *T-cell growth factor,* which indicates one of the major biologic activities of this molecule. Failure of T cells to produce IL-2 results in the absence of a T-cell immune response and a diminution of the antibody response. Natural human IL-2 is a 15-kd glycoprotein and is produced primarily by activated T cells. For IL-2 to exert its proliferation-inducing effects, it has to interact with a specific receptor for IL-2 on the surface of the target cell. The high-affinity receptor for IL-2 consists of two polypeptides, the α (75 kd) and β (55 kd) chains. After activation, T cells express greatly increased numbers of this high-affinity receptor for IL-2 and respond to IL-2 with increased proliferation. Stimulation of resting T cells with antigen presented in the context of self (antigen associated with an MHC molecule on the surface of an antigen-presenting cell) and with IL-1 therefore induces synthesis and secretion of IL-2. During this activation process, responding T cells undergo an alteration in their cell surface receptors, including the expression of cell surface receptors for IL-2. Continuing exposure to IL-2 leads to the proliferation of T cells bearing the IL-2 receptor, thereby serving as an activation and response-amplification stage in the generation of immune responses. Activated T cells not only respond to IL-2 but also produce IL-2. Interleukin-2 can therefore act in an autocrine manner (the cells producing the lymphokine then respond to it) or in a paracrine fashion (the IL-2 produced by a T cell is taken up and responded to by neighboring cells). Since its original description as a T-cell growth hormone, IL-2 has been shown to have various other immune functions, including the promotion of B-cell activation and maturation and activation of monocytes and NK cells. Interleukin-2 can also lead directly or indirectly to the stimulation of the production of interferon and other cytokines.

Interleukin-3 Interleukin-3, a factor that can increase the early differentiation of hematopoietic cells (82), may find a role in immunotherapy because of its ability to induce hematopoietic differentiation in people undergoing aggressive chemotherapeutic treatment or bone marrow transplantation.

Tumor necrosis factor α is a cytokine that can be directly cytotoxic for tumor cells, can increase immune cell–mediated cellular cytotoxicity, and can activate macrophages and induce secretion of monokines. Other biologic activities of TNF-α include the induction of cachexia, inflammation, and fever; it is an important mediator of endotoxic shock.

Interleukin-4, Interleukin-5, and Interleukin-6 B-lymphocyte activation and differentiation to immunoglobulin-secreting plasma cells are increased by cytokines produced by helper T lymphocytes or monocytes (Table 6.4) (55,56). Several cytokines originally described as B-cell stimulating factors (IL-4, IL-5, and IL-6) have additional biologic activities. For instance, IL-6 (a factor that can induce B-lymphocyte differentiation to immunoglobulin-secreting cells) is a pleiotropic cytokine with biologic activities that include the induction of cytotoxic T-lymphocyte differentiation, the induction of acute-phase reactant production by hepatocytes, and activity as a colony-stimulating factor for hematopoietic stem cell (63). Interleukin-6 is produced primarily by activated monocyte-macrophages and T lymphocytes. Interestingly, several types of tumor cells produce IL-6, and it has been proposed as an autocrine-paracrine growth factor for different types of neoplasms (64–69). It may prove to be an effective antitumor agent by virtue of its ability to enhance antitumor T-cell–mediated immune responsiveness (69,70).

Interleukin-8 and Interleukin-10 Interleukin-10, a 35- to 40-kd cytokine, also called *cytokine synthesis inhibitory factor* because of its activity as an inhibitor of cytokine production, is produced by a subset of CD4 cells, type 2 (T_H2) cells, and inhibits the cytokine production by another CD4 cell subset, type 1 (T_H1) cells (71). **T_H1 and T_H2 are two helper T-cell subpopulations that control the nature of an immune response by secreting a characteristic and mutually antagonistic set of cytokines: Clones of T_H1 produce IL-2 and IFN-α, while T_H2 clones produce IL-4, IL-5, IL-6, and IL-10** (72). A similar dichotomy between T_H1- and T_H2-type responses has been reported in humans (73,74). Human IL-10 inhibits the production of IFN-γ and other cytokines by human peripheral blood mononuclear cells (75) and by suppressing the release of cytokines (IL-1, IL-6, IL-8, and TNF-α) by activated monocytes (76–78). Interleukin-10 also downregulates class II MHC expression on monocytes, resulting in a strong reduction in the antigen-presenting capacity of these cells (78). Together, these observations support the concept that IL-10 has an important role as an immune-inhibitory cytokine.

Because epithelial cancers of the ovary usually remain confined to the peritoneal cavity, even in the advanced stages of the disease, it has been suggested that the growth of ovarian cancer intraperitoneally could be related to a local deficiency of antitumor immune effector mechanisms (79). Studies have shown that ascitic fluid from patients with ovarian cancer contained increased concentrations of IL-10 (80). Various other cytokines are also seen in ascitic fluid obtained from women with ovarian cancer including IL-6, IL-10, TNF-α, *granulocyte colony-stimulating factor (G-CSF),* and *granulocyte-macrophage colony-stimulating factor (GM-CSF)* (81). A similar pattern was seen in serum samples from women with ovarian cancer with elevations of IL-6 and IL-10. Preliminary results have revealed that ovarian cancer cells do not produce IL-10, so high concentrations of IL-10 could certainly result in a peritoneal environment characterized by immune unresponsiveness and promotion of tumor growth.

Interferons

There are three types of interferons: IFN-α, IFN-β, and IFN-γ (54,55,83). They can interfere with viral production in infected cells and have various effects on the immune system as well as direct antitumor effects. For instance, IFN-α, a cytokine produced by T lymphocytes, can affect immune function by increasing the induction of MHC molecule expression, increasing the activity of antigen-presenting cells, and thereby increasing T-lymphocyte activation.

Cytokines in Cancer Therapy

Cytokines are extraordinarily pleiotropic with a bewildering array of biologic activities, including some outside the immune system (54,55,63,69). Because some cytokines have direct or indirect antitumor and immune-enhancing effects, several of these factors have been used in the experimental treatment of cancer.

The precise roles of cytokines in antitumor responses have not been elucidated. Cytokines can exert antitumor effects by many different direct or indirect activities. It is possible that a single cytokine could increase tumor growth directly by acting as a growth factor, while at the same time increasing immune responses directed toward the tumor. The potential of cytokines to increase antitumor immune responses has been tested in experimental adoptive immunotherapy by exposing the patient's peripheral blood cells or tumor-infiltrating lymphocytes to cytokines such as IL-2 *in vitro,* thus generating activated cells with antitumor effects that can be given back to the patient (84–86). Some cytokines can also exert direct antitumor effects. Tumor necrosis factor can induce cell death in sensitive tumor cells.

The effects of cytokines on patients with cancer might be modulated by soluble receptors or blocking factors. For instance, blocking factors for TNF and for lymphotoxin were found in ascitic fluid from patients with ovarian cancer (87). Such factors could inhibit the cytolytic effects of TNF or lymphotoxin and should be taken into account in the design of clinical trials of intraperitoneal infusion of these cytokines.

Cytokines have growth-increasing effects on tumor cells in addition to inducing antitumor effects. They can act as autocrine or paracrine growth factors for human tumor cells, including those of nonlymphoid origin. For instance, IL-6 (which is produced by various types of human tumor cells) can act as a growth factor for human myeloma, Kaposi's sarcoma, renal carcinoma, and epithelial ovarian cancer cells (63–69).

Clearly, cytokines are of great potential value in the treatment of cancer, but because of their multiple, even conflicting biologic effects, a thorough understanding of cytokine biology is essential for their successful use (83–91).

Adoptive Immunotherapy

Recently, the *ex vivo* enhancement of antitumor immune cell responses, including the generation of lymphokine-activated killer (LAK) cells or the activation of tumor-infiltrating lymphocytes (TIL), has provided new immune system–based approaches for antitumor responses. The simultaneous treatment of patients with *ex vivo* activated autologous cells, along with IL-2, is the basis of adoptive immunotherapy, a form of experimental antitumor immunotherapy. In particular, adoptive immunotherapy with IL-2 can produce regression of tumor in various animals and human tumors, such as melanoma and renal cell carcinoma, when used in conjunction with the adoptive transfer of autologous LAK cells (84,85).

Exposure of peripheral blood monoclonal cells to cytokines *in vitro* (particularly IL-2) leads to the generation of cytotoxic effect cells called *LAK cells* (85). These cells are cytotoxic for various tumor cells, including those that are resistant to NK-cell– or T-cell–mediated lysis.

Experimental treatment of human subjects with autologous *ex vivo*-generated LAK cells and IL-2 has yielded tumor regression in some cases (84–88). This treatment has resulted in some complete responses (86); the combined response rate was 27% in 146 patients with cancer who were treated in two separate studies (88–90). The overall response rate to LAK treatment is low, however, and this type of adoptive immunotherapy causes high morbidity (90). It is also costly and impractical in most medical settings.

Much current experimental work is aimed at developing more efficient and practical applications of adoptive immunotherapy (91–97). One approach involves the *ex vivo* generation of immune effector cells from TILs, which are lymphocytes that are isolated from tumors and activated and expanded *in vitro* by exposure to IL-2. These cells are then administered to the patient with IL-2 (91,92). This approach is hampered by the need to expand a limited number of TILs *in vitro* to generate enough effector cells for treatment. Recently, attention has been directed toward the development of new methods for the generation of LAK cells or TILs, including methods that use cytokines other than IL-2 to stimulate these cells.

Another promising approach that has been explored in animal studies involves the targeting of activated T lymphocytes with a bifunctional monoclonal antibody that binds to the CD3–T-cell receptor complex (on the target tumor cell) (93). This approach has the potential advantage of allowing a large number of the activated lymphocytes to target their effects directly on tumor cells, thereby reducing the need to amplify a large number of effector cells from TILs. It also has the potential to avoid some of the side effects associated with LAK treatment, which is a more nonspecific form of adoptive immunotherapy.

Factors that Trigger Neoplasia

Cell biology is characterized by considerable redundancy and functional overlap, so that a defect in one mechanism does not invariably jeopardize the function of the cell. However, with a sufficient number of abnormalities in structure and function, normal cell function is jeopardized and uncontrolled cell growth or cell death results. Either end point may result from accumulated genetic mutations over time. Factors have been identified that enhance the likelihood of genetic mutations, jeopardize normal cell biology, and may increase the risk of cancer.

Increased Age

Increasing age is considered the single most important risk factor for the development of cancer (98). Cancer is diagnosed in as much as 50% of the population by 75 years of age (99). It has been suggested that the increasing risk of cancer with age reflects the accumulation of critical genetic mutations over time that ultimately culminate in neoplastic transformation. The basic premise of the multistep somatic mutation theory of carcinogenesis is that genetic or epigenetic alterations of numerous independent genes results in cancer. Factors that have been associated with an increased likelihood of cancer include exposure to exogenous mutagens, altered host immune function, and certain inherited genetic syndromes and disorders.

Environmental Factors

A mutagen is a compound that results in a genetic mutation. A number of environmental pollutants act as mutagens when tested *in vitro*. Environmental mutagens usually produce specific types of mutations that can be differentiated from spontaneous mutations. As an example, activated hydrocarbons tend to produce G · T transversions (100). A carcinogen is a compound that can produce cancer. It is important to recognize that all carcinogens are not mutagens and that all mutagens are not necessarily carcinogens.

Smoking

Cigarette smoking is perhaps the best known example of mutagen exposure that is associated with the development of lung cancer when the exposure is of sufficient duration and quantity in a susceptible individual. An association between cigarette smoking and cervical cancer has been recognized for decades. More recently, it has been determined that the mutagens in cigarette smoke are selectively concentrated in cervical mucus (52). It has been hypothesized that exposure of the proliferating epithelial cells of the transformation zone to cigarette smoke mutagens may increase the likelihood of DNA damage and subsequent cellular transformation.

Radiation

Radiation exposure can also be considered an environmental mutagen that increases the risk of cancer. This statement does not apply to exposure secondary to diagnostic radiology studies, which is not associated with an increased risk of cancer. Interestingly, the overall risk of radiation-induced cancer is approximately 10% greater in women than in men (101). This difference has been attributed to gender-specific cancers, including breast cancer. With respect to gynecology, radiation therapy for cervical cancer is associated with a small increase in the risk of colon cancer and thyroid cancer.

Radiation-induced cancer may be the result of sublethal DNA damage that is not repaired (101). Normally, radiation damage prompts an S-phase arrest so that DNA damage is repaired. This requires normal *p53* gene function. If DNA repair does not occur for some reason, the damaged DNA is propagated to daughter cells following mitosis. If a sufficient number of critical genes are mutated, cellular transformation may result.

Immune Function

Systemic immune dysfunction has been recognized as a risk factor for cancer for decades. The immunosuppressed renal transplant patient may have a 40-fold increased risk of cervical cancer (52). Patients infected with human immunodeficiency virus (HIV) who have a depressed CD4 cell count have been reported to be at increased risk of cervical dysplasia and invasive disease (96). Individuals who have undergone high-dose chemotherapy with stem cell support may be at increased risk of developing a variety of solid neoplasms. These examples illustrate the importance of immune function in host surveillance for transformed cells.

Another interesting example of altered immune function that may be related to the development of cervical dysplasia is the alteration in mucosal immune function that occurs in women who smoke cigarettes (52). The Langerhans cell population of the cervix is decreased in women who smoke. Langerhans cells are responsible for antigen processing. It is postulated that a reduction in these cells increases the likelihood of successful human papillomavirus infection of the cervix.

Diet

The role of diet in disease prevention and predisposition is widely recognized but poorly understood (96,99). Dietary fat intake has been correlated with the risk of colon and breast cancer. Fiber is considered protective against colon cancer. With respect to the female reproductive system, epidemiologic studies provide conflicting results. Deficiencies of folic acid and vitamins A and C have been associated with the development of cervical dysplasia and cervical cancer. Considerable research must be performed to clarify the impact of diet on cancer prevention and development.

References

1. **Taylor AM, McConville CM, Byrd PJ.** Cancer and DNA processing disorders. *Br Med Bull* 1994;50:708–717.
2. **Kraemer KH, Levy DD, Parris CN, et al.** Xeroderma pigmentosum and related disorders: examining the linkage between defective DNA repair and cancer. *J Invest Dermatol* 1994;103[Suppl 5]:96S–101S.
3. **Jacobs T.** Control of the cell cycle. *Dev Biol* 1992;153:1–15.
4. **Weinert T, Lydall D.** Cell cycle checkpoints, genetic instability and cancer. *Semin Cancer Biol* 1993;4:129–140.
5. **Fridovich-Keil JL, Hansen LJ, Keyomarsi K, et al.** Progression through the cell cycle: an overview. *Am Rev Respir Dis* 1990;142:53–56.
6. **Reddy GP.** Cell cycle: regulatory events in G1-S transition of mammalian cells. *J Cell Biochem* 1994;54:379–386.
7. **Hartwell LH, Weinert TA.** Checkpoints: controls that ensure the order of cell cycle events. *Science* 1989;246:629–634.
8. **Murray AW, Kirschner MW.** Dominoes and clocks: the union of two views of the cell cycle. *Science* 1989;246:614–621.
9. **Lee MG, Norbury CJ, Spurr NK, et al.** Regulated expression and phosphorylation of a possible mammalian cell-cycle control protein. *Nature* 1988;333:257–267.
10. **Kastan MB, Onyekwere O, Sidransky D, et al.** Participation of p53 protein in the cellular response to DNA damage. *Cancer Res* 1991;51:6304–6311.
11. **Kuerbitz SJ, Plunkett BS, Walsh WV, et al.** Wild type p53 is a cell cycle checkpoint determinant following irradiation. *Proc Natl Acad Sci U S A* 1992;89:7491–7495.
12. **Gu Z, Pim D, Labrecque S, et al.** DNA damage–induced p53-mediated transcription inhibited by human papillomavirus type 18 E6. *Oncogene* 1994;9:629–633.
13. **Morena S, Nurse P.** Substrates for p34cdc2: in vivo veritas? *Cell* 1990;61:549–551.
14. **Lewin B.** Driving the cell cycle: M-phase kinase, its partners, and substrates. *Cell* 1990;61:743–752.
15. **Hammar SP, Mottet NK.** Tetrazolium salt and electron microscopic studies of cellular degeneration and necrosis in the interdigital areas of the developing chick limb. *J Cell Sci* 1971;8:229–251.
16. **Farbman AI.** Electron microscopic study of palate fusion in mouse embryos. *Dev Biol* 1968;18:93–116.
17. **Harmon B, Bell L, Williams L.** An ultrasound study on the meconium corpuscles in rat foetal epithelium with particular reference to apoptosis. *Anat Embryol (Berl)* 1984;169:119–124.
18. **Cotter TG, Lennon SV, Glynn JG, et al.** Cell death via apoptosis and its relationship to growth, development, and differentiation of both tumor and normal cells. *Anticancer Res* 1990;10:1153–1160.
19. **Pollard JW, Pacey J, Cheng SUY, et al.** Estrogens and cell death in murine uterine luminal epithelium. *Cell Tissue Res* 1987;249:533–540.
20. **Nawaz S, Lynch MP, Galand P, et al.** Hormonal regulation of cell death in rabbit uterine epithelium. *Am J Pathol* 1987;127:51–59.
21. **Billig H, Furuta I, Hsueh AJW.** Estrogens inhibit and androgens enhance ovarian granulosa cell apoptosis. *Endocrinology* 1993;33:2204–2212.

22. **Williams GT, Smith CA.** Molecular regulation of apoptosis: genetic controls on cell death. *Cell* 1993;74:777–779.

23. **Vaux DL.** Toward an understanding of the molecular mechanisms of physiological cell death. *Proc Natl Acad Sci U S A* 1993;90:786–789.

24. **Baserga R, Porcu P, Sell C.** Oncogenes, growth factors, and control of the cell cycle. *Cancer Surv* 1993;16:201–213.

25. **Smith MR, Matthews NT, Jones KA, et al.** Biological actions of oncogenes. *Pharmacol Ther* 1993; 58:211–236.

26. **Studzinski GP.** Oncogenes, growth and the cell cycle: an overview. *Cell Tissue Kinet* 1989;22:405–424.

27. **Landers JP, Spelsberg TC.** New concepts in steroid hormone action: transcription factors, proto-oncogenes and the cascade model for steroid regulation of gene expression. *Crit Rev Eukaryot Gene Expr* 1993;2:19–63.

28. **Stancel GM, Baker VV, Hyder SM, et al.** Oncogenes and uterine function. In: **Milligan SR,** ed. *Oxf Rev Reprod Biol* 1993:1–42.

29. **Smith EP, Boyd J, Frank GR, et al.** Estrogen resistance caused by a mutation of the estrogen receptor gene in a man. *N Engl J Med* 1994;331:1056–1061.

30. **De Bellis A, Quigley CA, Marschke KB, et al.** Characterization of mutant androgen receptors causing partial androgen insensitivity syndrome. *J Clin Endocrinol Metab* 1994;78:513–522.

31. **Fuqua SA.** Estrogen receptor mutagenesis and hormone resistance. *Cancer* 1994;74:1026–1029.

32. **Osborne CK, Fuqua SA.** Mechanisms of tamoxifen resistance. *Breast Cancer Res Treat* 1994;32:49–55.

33. **Pusztal L, Lewis CE, Lorenzen J, et al.** Growth factors: regulation of normal and neoplastic growth. *J Pathol* 1993;169:191–201.

34. **Aaronson SA, Rubin JS, Finch PW, et al.** Growth factor regulated pathways in epithelial cell proliferation. *Am Rev Respir Dis* 1990;142:S7–S10.

35. **Giordano G, Barreca A, Minuto F.** Growth factors in the ovary. *J Endocrinol Invest* 1992;15:689 707.

36. **Baldi E, Bonaccorsi L, Finetti G, et al.** Platelet activating factor in human endometrium. *J Steroid Biochem Mol Biol* 1994;49:359–363.

37. **Gold LI, Saxena B, Mittal KR, et al.** Increased expression of transforming growth factor B isoforms and basic fibroblast growth factor in complex hyperplasia and adenocarcinoma of the endometrium: evidence for paracrine and autocrine action. *Cancer Res* 1994;54:2347–2358.

38. **Leake R, Carr L, Rinaldi F.** Autocrine and paracrine effects in the endometrium. *Ann N Y Acad Sci* 1991;622:145–148.

39. **Giudice LC.** Growth factors and growth modulators in human uterine endometrium: their potential relevance to reproductive medicine. *Fertil Steril* 1994;61:1–17.

40. **Murphy LJ.** Growth factors and steroid hormone action in endometrial cancer. *J Steroid Biochem Mol Biol* 1994;48:419–423.

41. **Laiho M, DeCaprio JA, Ludlow JW, et al.** Growth inhibition by TGF-β linked to suppression of retinoblastoma protein phosphorylation. *Cell* 1990;62:175–185.

42. **Cate RL, Donahoe PK, MacLaughlin DT.** Müllerian-inhibiting substance. In: **Sporn MB, Roberts AB,** eds. *Peptide growth factors and their receptors,* vol 2. Berlin: Springer-Verlag, 1990:179–210.

43. **Bates SE, Valverius EM, Ennis BW, et al.** Expression of the transforming growth factor α–epidermal growth factor receptor pathway in normal human breast epithelial cells. *Endocrinology* 1990;126:596–607.

44. **Hunter T.** Protein kinase classification. *Methods Enzymol* 1991;200:3–37.

45. **Ralph RK, Darkin-Rattray S, Schofield P.** Growth-related protein kinases. *Bioessays* 1990;12:121–123.

46. **Simon MI, Strathmann MP, Gautam N.** Diversity of G-proteins in signal transduction. *Science* 1991;252:802–808.

47. **Speigel AM.** G-proteins in cellular control. *Curr Opin Cell Biol* 1992;4:203–211.

48. **Hall A.** The cellular function of small GTP-binding proteins. *Science* 1990;249:635–640.

49. **Mendelsohn ML.** The somatic mutational component of human carcinogenesis. In: **Moolgavkar SH,** ed. *Scientific issues in quantitative cancer risk assessment.* New York: Birkhaeuser, Boston, 1990:22–31.

50. **Baker VV.** The molecular biology of endometrial cancer. *Clin Consult Obstet Gynecol* 1993;5:95–99.

51. **Baker VV.** The molecular genetics of epithelial ovarian cancer. *Clin Obstet Gynecol* 1994;21:25–40.

52. **Baker VV.** Update on the molecular carcinogenesis of cervix cancer. *Clin Consult Obstet Gynecol* 1995;7:86–93.

53. **Barrett JC.** Genetic and epigenetic mechanisms in carcinogenesis. In: **Barrett JD,** ed. *Mechanisms of environmental carcinogenesis,* vol 1. *Role of genetic and epigenetic changes.* Boca Raton: CRC Press, 1987:1–15.

54. **Abbas AK, Lictman AH, Pober JS.** *Cellular and molecular immunology.* Philadelphia: WB Saunders, 1991.

55. **Roitt I, Brostoff J, Male D.** *Immunology,* 2nd ed. London: Gower Medical Publishing, 1989.

56. **Boyer CM, Knapp RC, Bast RC Jr.** Biology and Immunology. In: **Berek JS, Hacker NF,** eds. *Practical gynecologic oncology,* 2nd ed. Baltimore: Williams & Wilkins, 1994:75–115.

57. **Kohler G, Milstein C.** Continuous cultures of fused cells secreting antibody of predefined specificity. *Nature* 1978;256:495–497.

58. **Ettenson D, Sheldon K, Marks A, et al.** Comparison of growth inhibition of a human ovarian adenocarcinoma cell line by free monoclonal antibodies and their corresponding antibody-recombinant ricin A chain immunotoxins. *Anticancer Res* 1988;8:833–838.

59. **Ortaldo JR, Herberman RB.** Heterogeneity of natural killer cells. *Annu Rev Immunol* 1984;2:359–394.

60. **Bast RC, Zbar B, Borsos T, et al.** BCG and cancer. *N Engl J Med* 1974;290:1413–1458.

61. **Borstein RS, Mastrangelo MJ, Sulit H.** Immunotherapy of melanoma with intralesional BCG. *Natl Cancer Inst Monogr* 1973;39:213–220.

62. **Di Giovine FS, Duff GW.** Interleukin 1: the first interleukin. *Immunol Today* 1990;11:13–20.

63. **Hirano T, Akira S, Taga T, et al.** Biological and clinical aspects of interleukin 6. *Immunol Today* 1990;11:443–449.

64. **Watson JM, Sensintaffar JL, Berek JS, et al.** Epithelial ovarian cancer cells constitutively produce interleukin-6 (IL-6). *Cancer Res* 1990;50:6959–6965.

65. **Berek JS, Chang C, Kaldi K, et al.** Serum interleukin-6 levels correlate with disease status in patients with epithelial ovarian cancer. *Am J Obstet Gynecol* 1991;164:1038–1043.

66. **Miles SA, Rezai AR, Salazar-Gonzalez JF, et al.** AIDS Kaposi's sarcoma-derived cells produce and respond to interleukin-6. *Proc Natl Acad Sci U S A* 1990;87:4068–4072.

67. **Miki S, Iwano M, Miki Y, et al.** Interleukin-6 (IL-6) functions as an in vitro autocrine growth factor in renal cell carcinomas. *FEB S Letters* 1989;250:607–610.

68. **Wu S, Rodabaugh K, Martínez-Maza O, et al.** Stimulation of ovarian tumor cell proliferation with monocyte products including interleukin-1, interleukin-6 and tumor necrosis factor-α. *Am J Obstet Gynecol* 1992;166:997–1007.

69. **Martínez-Maza O, Berek JS.** Interkeukin-6 and cancer therapy. *In Vivo* 911;5:583.

70. **Mule JJ, McIntosh JK, Jablons DM, et al.** Antitumor activity of recombinant interleukin-6 in mice. *J Exp Med* 1990;171:629–636.

71. **Fiorentino DF, Bond MW, Mosmann TR.** Two types of mouse helper T cells. IV. T_H2 clones secrete a factor that inhibits cytokine production by T_H1 clones. *J Exp Med* 1989;170:2081–2095.

72. **Mosmann TR, Moore KW.** The role IL-10 in crossregulation of T_H1 and T_H2 responses. *Immunol Today* 1991;12:A49–53.

73. **Del Prete GF, De Carli M, Ricci M, et al.** Helper activity for immunoglobulin synthesis of T helper type 1 (T_H1) and T_H2 human T cell clones: the help of T_H1 clones is limited by their cytolytic capacity. *J Exp Med* 1991;174:809–813.

74. **Romagnani S.** Human T_H1 and T_H2 subsets: doubt no more. *Immunol Today* 1991;12:256–257.

75. **Zlotnik A, Moore KW.** Interleukin-10. *Cytokine* 1991;3:366–371.

76. **Fiorentino DF, Zlotnik A, Mosmann TR, et al.** IL-10 inhibits cytokine production by activated macrophages. *J Immunol* 1991;147:3815–3822.

77. **Bogdan C, Vodovotz Y, Nathan C.** Macrophage deactivation by IL-10. *J Exp Med* 1991;174:1549–1555.

78. **de Waal Malefyt R, Abrams J, Bennett B, et al.** Interleukin-10 (IL-10) inhibits cytokine synthesis by human monocytes: an autoregulatory role of IL-10 produced by monocytes. *J Exp Med* 1991;174:1209–1220.

79. **Berek JS.** Epithelial ovarian cancer. In: **Berek JS, Hacker NF,** eds. *Practical gynecologic oncology,* 2nd ed. Baltimore: Williams & Wilkins, 1994:327–375.

80. **Gotlieb WH, Abrams JS, Watson JM, et al.** Presence of IL-10 in the ascites of patients with ovarian and other intraabdominal cancers. *Cytokine* 1992;4:385–390.

81. **Watson JM, Gotlieb WH, Abrams JH, et al.** Cytokine profiles in ascitic fluid from patients with ovarian cancer: relationship to levels of acute phase proteins and immunoglobulins, immunosuppression and tumor classification. *Proc Soc Gynecol Invest* 1993;186:8.

82. **Shrader JW.** The panspecific hemopoietin of activated T lymphocytes (interleukin-3). *Annu Rev Immunol* 1986;4:205–230.

83. **Golub SH.** Immunological and therapeutic effects of interferon treatment of cancer patients. *Clin Immunol Allergy* 1984;4:377–441.

84. **Rosenberg SA.** Immunotherapy of cancer by systemic administration of lymphoid cells plus interleukin-2. *J Biol Response Mod* 1984;3:501–511.

85. **Rosenberg SA, Lotze MT.** Cancer immunotherapy using interleukin-2 and interleukin-2–activated lymphocytes. *Annu Rev Immunol* 1986;4:681–709.

86. **Rosenberg SA, Lotze MT, Muul LM, et al.** Observations on the systemic administration of autologous lymphokine-activated killer cells and recombinant interleukin-2 to patients with metastatic cancer. *N Engl J Med* 1985;313:1485–1492.

87. **Cappuccini F, Yamamoto RS, DiSaia PJ, et al.** Identification of tumor necrosis factor and lymphotoxin blocking factor(s) in the ascites of patients with advanced and recurrent ovarian cancer. *Lymphokine Cytokine Res* 1991;10:225–229.

88. **Rosenberg SA, Lotze MT, Muul LM, et al.** A progress report on the treatment of 157 patients with advanced cancer using lymphokine-activated killer cells and interleukin-2 or high-dose interleukin-2 alone. *N Engl J Med* 1987;316:889–897.

89. **West WH, Tauer KW, Yannelli JR, et al.** Constant-infusion recombinant interleukin-2 in adoptive immunotherapy of advanced cancer. *N Engl J Med* 1987;316:898–905.

90. **Berek JS.** Intraperitoneal adoptive immunotherapy for peritoneal cancer. *J Clin Oncol* 1990;8:1610–1612.

91. **Topalian SL, Solomon D, Avis FP, et al.** Immunotherapy of patients with advanced cancer using tumor-infiltrating lymphocytes and recombinant interleukin-2: a pilot study. *J Clin Oncol* 1988;6:839–853.

92. **Lotzova E.** Role of human circulating and tumor-infiltrating lymphocytes in cancer defense and treatment. *Nat Immun* 1990;9:253–264.

93. **Garrido MA, Valdayo MJ, Winkler DF, et al.** Targeting human T lymphocytes with bispecific antibodies to react against human ovarian carcinoma cells growing in nu/nu mice. *Cancer Res* 1990;50:4227–4232.

94. **Bookman MA, Berek JS.** Biologic and immunologic therapy of ovarian cancer. *Hematol Oncol Clin North Am* 1992;6:941–965.

95. **Zighelboim J, Nio Y, Berek JS, et al.** Immunologic control of ovarian cancer. *Nat Immun* 1988;7:216–225.

96. **Berek JS, Martínez-Maza O, Montz FJ.** The immune system and gynecologic cancer. In: **Coppelson M, Tattersall M, Morrow CP,** eds. *Gynecologic Oncology.* Edinburgh: Churchill Livingstone, 1992:119.

97. **Berek JS, Lichtenstein AK, Knox RM, et al.** Synergistic effects of combination sequential immunotherapies in a murine ovarian cancer model. *Cancer Res* 1985;45:4215–4218.

98. **Newell GR, Spitz MR, Sider JG.** Cancer and age. *Semin Oncol* 1989;16:3–9.

99. **Yancik R.** *Perspectives on prevention and treatment of cancer in the elderly.* New York: Raven Press, 1983.

100. **Maher VM, Yang JL, Mah MC, et al.** Comparing the frequency of and spectra of mutations induced when an SV-40–based shuttle vector containing covalently bound residues of structurally-related carcinogens replicates in human cells. *Mutat Res* 1989;220:83–92.

101. **National Research Council.** *Health effects of exposure to low levels of ionizing radiation (BEIR V).* Washington, DC: National Academy Press, 1990.

7 Reproductive Physiology

Steven F. Palter
David L. Olive

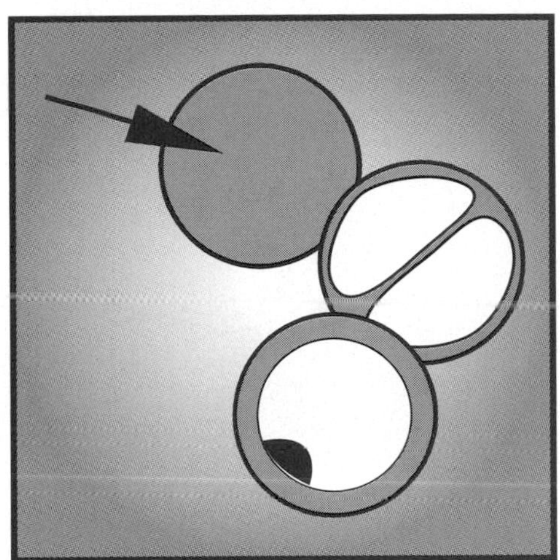

Neuroendocrinology

Neuroendocrinology represents facets of two traditional fields of medicine: endocrinology, which is the study of hormones (i.e., substances secreted into the bloodstream that have diverse actions at sites remote from the point of secretion), and neuroscience, which is the study of the action of neurons. The discovery of neurons that transmit impulses and secrete their products into the vascular system to function as hormones themselves, a process known as neurosecretion, demonstrates that the two systems are intimately linked. For instance, the menstrual cycle is regulated through the feedback of hormones on the neural tissue of the central nervous system (CNS).

Anatomy

Hypothalamus

The hypothalamus is a small neural structure situated at the base of the brain above the optic chiasm and below the third ventricle (Fig. 7.1). It is connected directly to the pituitary gland and is the part of the brain that is the source of many pituitary secretions. Anatomically, the hypothalamus is divided into three zones: periventricular (adjacent to the third ventricle), medial (primarily cell bodies), and lateral (primarily axonal). Each zone is further subdivided into structures known as nuclei, which represent locations of concentrations of similar types of neuronal cell bodies (Fig. 7.2).

The hypothalamus is not an isolated structure within the CNS; instead, it has multiple interconnections with other regions in the brain. In addition to the well-known pathways of hypothalamic output to the pituitary, there are numerous less well-characterized pathways of output to diverse regions of the brain, including the limbic system (amygdala and hippocampus), the thalamus, and the pons (1). Many of these pathways form feedback loops to areas supplying neural input to the hypothalamus.

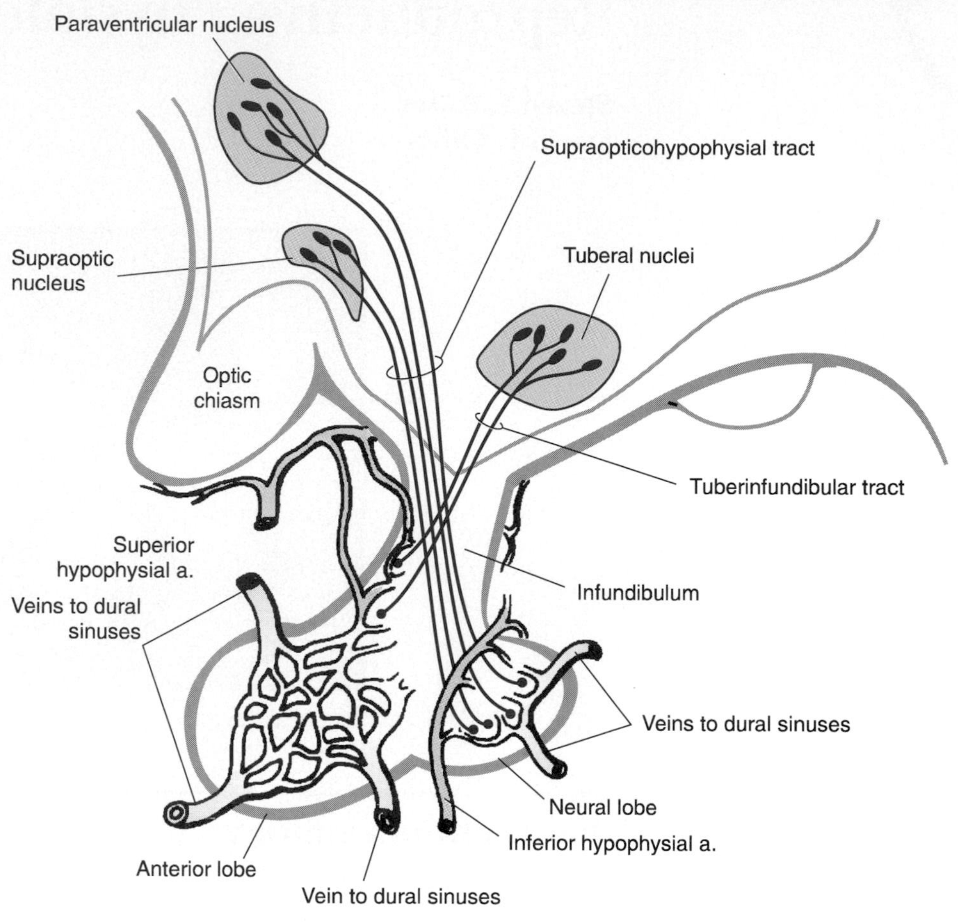

Figure 7.1 The hypothalamus and its neurologic connections to the pituitary.

Several levels of feedback to the hypothalamus exist and are known as the long, short, and ultrashort feedback loops. The long feedback loop is composed of endocrine input from circulating hormones, just as feedback of androgens and estrogens onto steroid receptors is present in the hypothalamus (2,3). Similarly, pituitary hormones may feed back to the hypothalamus and serve important regulatory functions in short-loop feedback. Finally, hypothalamic secretions may directly feed back to the hypothalamus, itself, in an ultrashort feedback loop.

The major secretory products of the hypothalamus are the pituitary-releasing factors (Fig. 7.3):

1. ***Gonadotropin-releasing hormone (GnRH),*** **which controls the secretion of** ***luteinizing hormone (LH)*** **and** ***follicle-stimulating hormone (FSH)***
2. ***Corticotropin-releasing hormone (CRH),*** **which controls the release of** ***adrenocorticotrophic hormone (ACTH)***
3. ***Growth hormone–releasing hormone (GHRH),*** **which regulates the release of** ***growth hormone (GH)***
4. ***Thyrotropin-releasing hormone (TRH),*** **which regulates the secretion of** ***thyroid-stimulating hormone (TSH).***

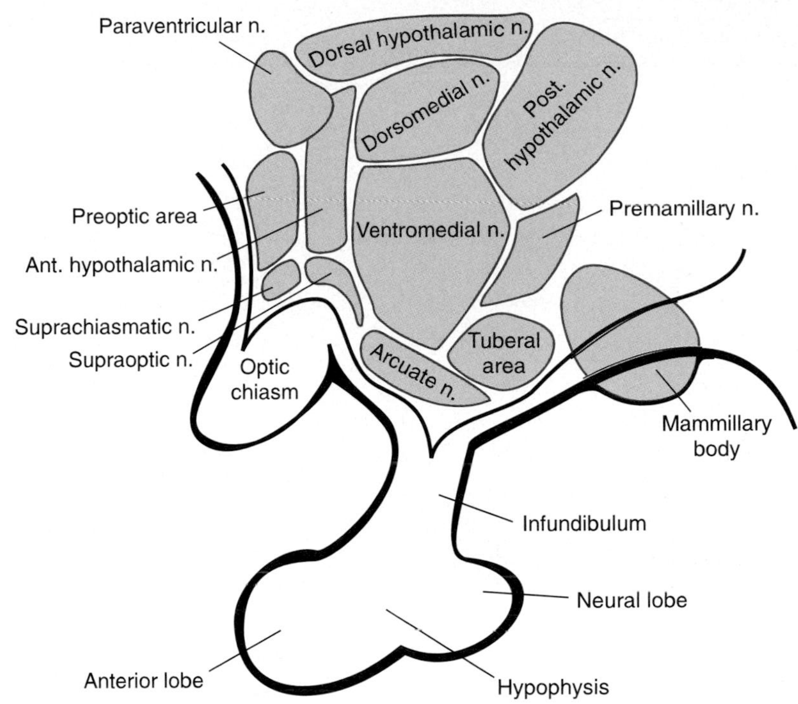

Figure 7.2 The neuronal cell bodies of the hypothalamus.

The hypothalamus is the source of all neurohypophyseal hormone production. The neural posterior pituitary can be viewed as a direct extension of the hypothalamus connected by the finger-like infundibular stalk. The discovery that the capillaries in the median eminence differ from those in other regions of the brain was a major one. Unlike the usual tight junctions that exist between adjacent capillary endothelial lining cells, the capillaries in this region are fenestrated in the same manner as capillaries outside the CNS. As a result, there is no blood-brain barrier in the median eminence.

Pituitary

The pituitary is divided into three regions or lobes: *anterior, intermediate,* and *posterior.* The *anterior pituitary (adenohypophysis)* is quite different structurally from the *posterior neural pituitary (neurohypophysis),* which is a direct physical extension of the hypothalamus. The adenohypophysis is derived embryologically from epidermal ectoderm from an infolding of Rathke's pouch. Therefore, it is not composed of neural tissue, as is the posterior pituitary, and does not have direct neural connections to the hypothalamus. Instead, a unique anatomic relationship exists that combines elements of neural production and endocrine secretion. The adenohypophysis itself has no direct arterial blood supply. Its major source of blood flow is also its source of hypothalamic input—the portal vessels. Blood flow in these portal vessels is primarily from the hypothalamus to the pituitary. Blood is supplied to the posterior pituitary via the superior, middle, and inferior hypophyseal arteries. In contrast, the anterior pituitary has no direct arterial blood supply. Instead, it receives blood via a rich capillary plexus of the portal vessels that originate in the median eminence of the hypothalamus and descend along the pituitary stalk. This pattern is not absolute, however, and retrograde blood flow has been demonstrated (4). This blood flow, combined with the location of the median eminence outside the blood-brain barrier, permits bidirectional feedback control between the two structures.

The specific secretory cells of the anterior pituitary have been classified based on their hematoxylin- and eosin-staining patterns. Acidophilic-staining cells primarily secrete GH and prolactin and, to a variable degree, ACTH (5). The gonadotropins are secreted by basophilic cells, and TSH is secreted by the neutral-staining chromophobes.

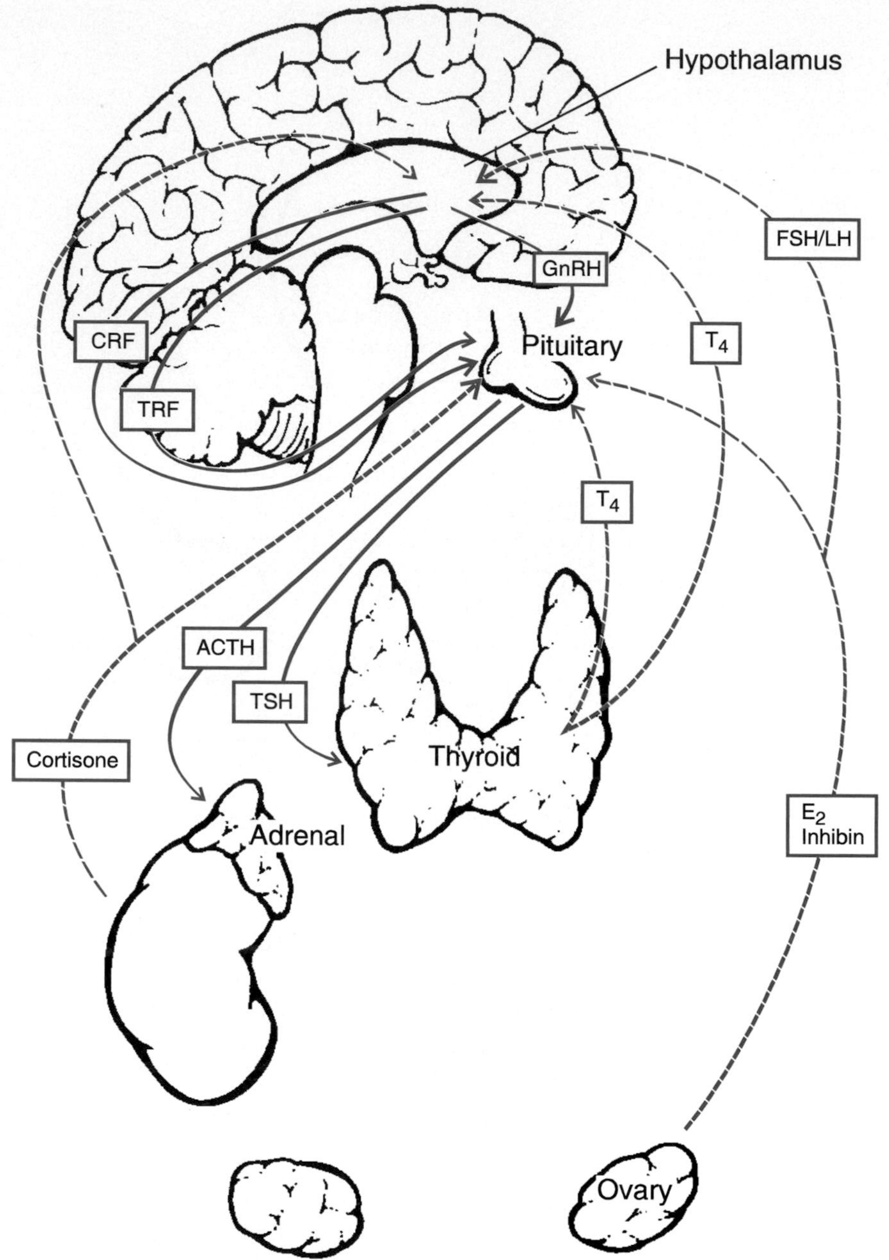

Figure 7.3 The hypothalamic secretory products function as pituitary releasing factors that control the endocrine function of the ovaries, the thyroid, and the adrenal glands.

Reproductive Hormone

Hypothalamus

Gonadotropin-releasing Hormone

Gonadotropin-releasing hormone (GnRH) (also called luteinizing hormone–releasing hormone, or LHRH) is the controlling factor for gonadotropin secretion (6). It is a decapeptide produced by neurons with cell bodies primarily in the arcuate nucleus of the hypothalamus (7–9) (Fig. 7.4). Embryologically, these neurons originate in the olfactory pit and then migrate to their adult locations (10). These GnRH-secreting neurons project axons that

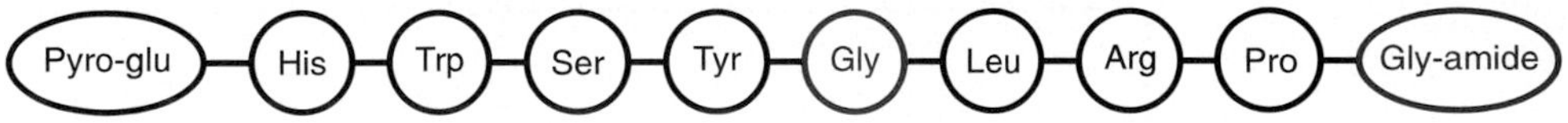

Pyro-glu — His — Trp — Ser — Tyr — Gly — Leu — Arg — Pro — Gly-amide

Figure 7.4 Gonadotropin-releasing hormone (GnRH) is a decapeptide.

terminate on the portal vessels at the median eminence where GnRH is secreted for delivery to the anterior pituitary. Less clear in function are multiple other secondary projections of GnRH neurons to locations within the CNS.

Pulsatile Secretion

GnRH is unique among releasing hormones in that it simultaneously regulates the secretion of two hormones—FSH and LH. It also is unique among the body's hormones because it must be secreted in a pulsatile fashion to be effective, and the pulsatile release of GnRH influences the release of the two gonadotropins (11–13). Using animals that had undergone electrical destruction of the arcuate nucleus and have no detectable levels of gonadotropins, a series of experiments were performed with varying dosages and intervals of GnRH infusion (13,14). Continual infusions did not result in gonadotropin secretion, whereas a pulsatile pattern led to physiologic secretion patterns and follicular growth. Continual exposure of the pituitary gonadotroph to GnRH results in a phenomenon called *downregulation,* through which the number of gonadotroph cell surface GnRH receptors is decreased (15). Similarly, intermittent exposure to GnRH will "upregulate" or "autoprime" the gonadotroph to increase its number of GnRH receptors (16). This allows the cell to have a greater response to subsequent GnRH exposure. Similar to the intrinsic electrical pacemaker cells of the heart, this action most likely represents an intrinsic property of the GnRH-secreting neuron, although it is subject to modulation by various neuronal and hormonal inputs to the hypothalamus.

The continual pulsatile secretion of GnRH is necessary because GnRH has an extremely short half-life (only 2 to 4 minutes) as a result of rapid proteolytic cleavage. The pulsatile secretion of GnRH varies in both frequency and amplitude throughout the menstrual cycle and is tightly regulated (17,18) (Fig. 7.5). The follicular phase is characterized by frequent, small-amplitude pulses of GnRH secretion. In the late follicular phase, there is an increase in both frequency and amplitude of pulses. During the luteal phase, however, there is a progressive lengthening of the interval between pulses as well as a decrease in the amplitude. This variation in pulse amplitude and frequency is directly responsible for the magnitude and relative proportions of gonadotropin secretion from the pituitary, although additional hormonal influences on the pituitary will modulate the GnRH effect.

Although GnRH is primarily involved in endocrine regulation of gonadotropin secretion from the pituitary, it is now apparent that this molecule has autocrine and paracrine functions throughout the body. The decapeptide is found in both neural and nonneural tissues; receptors are present in many extrapituitary structures, including the ovary and placenta. The role of GnRH in the extrapituitary sites remains to be fully elucidated.

Gonadotropin-releasing Hormone Agonists

Mechanism of Action Used clinically, GnRH agonists are modifications of the native molecule to either increase receptor affinity or decrease degradation (19). Their use, therefore, leads to a persistent activation of GnRH receptors, as if continuous GnRH exposure existed. As would be predicted by the constant GnRH infusion experiments, this leads to suppression of gonadotropin secretion. An initial release of gonadotropins followed by a profound suppression of secretion is observed. The initial release of gonadotropins represents the secretion of pituitary stores in response to receptor binding and activation. With

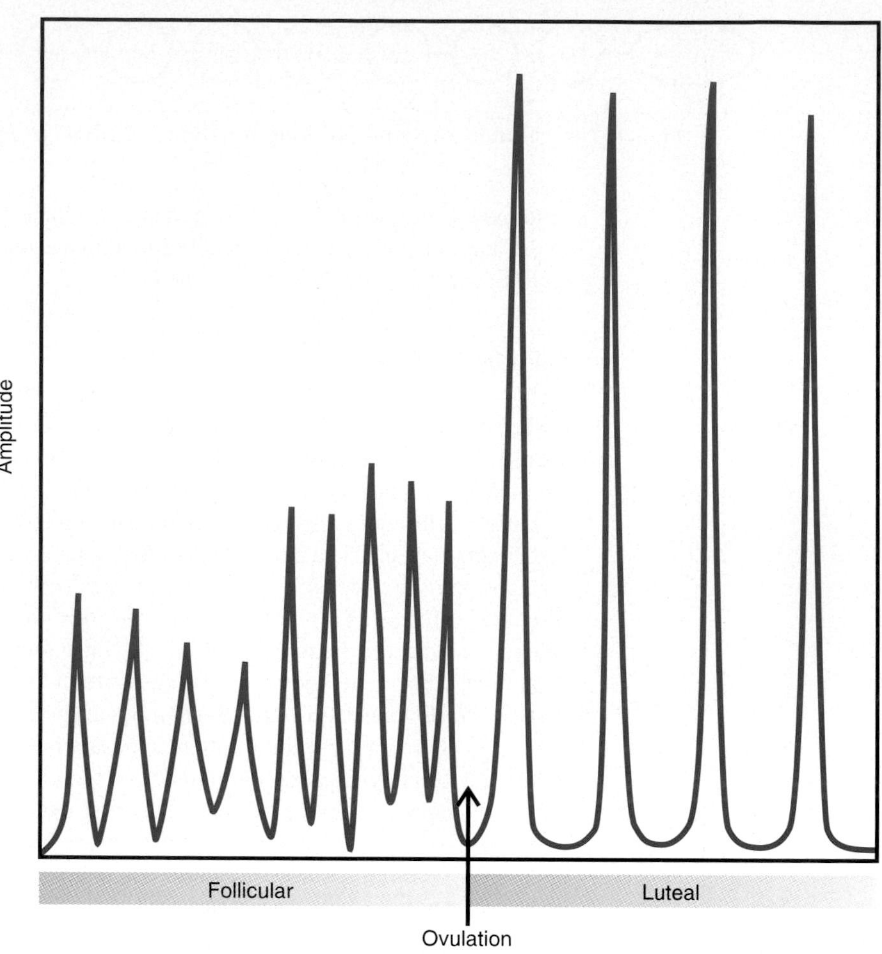

Figure 7.5 The pulsatile secretion of GnRH in the follicular and luteal phases of the cycle.

continued activation of the gonadotroph GnRH receptor, however, there is a downregulation effect and a decrease in the concentration of GnRH receptors. As a result, gonadotropin secretion decreases and sex steroid production falls to castrate levels (20).

Additional modification of the GnRH molecule results in an analogue that has no intrinsic activity but competes with GnRH for the same receptor site (21). These GnRH antagonists produce a competitive blockade of GnRH receptors, preventing stimulation by endogenous GnRH and causing an immediate fall in gonadotropin and sex steroid secretion (22). Compared with that of GnRH agonists, this action greatly reduces the time for therapy to become effective. Moreover, antagonists may not function solely as competitive inhibitors: recent evidence suggests they may also produce downregulation of GnRH receptors (23), further contributing to the loss of gonadotropin activity.

Structure—Agonists and Antagonists As a peptide hormone, GnRH is degraded by enzymatic cleavage of bonds between its amino acids. Pharmacologic alterations of the structure of GnRH have led to the creation of agonists and antagonists (Fig. 7.4). The primary sites of enzymatic cleavage are between amino acids 5 and 6, 6 and 7, and 9 and 10. Substitution of the position-6 amino acid glycine with large bulky amino acid analogues makes degradation more difficult and creates a form of GnRH with a relatively long half-life. Substitution at the carboxyl terminus produces a form of GnRH with increased receptor affinity. The resulting high affinity and slow degradation produces a molecule that mimics continuous exposure to native GnRH (19). Thus, as with constant GnRH exposure, downregulation occurs. GnRH agonists are now widely used to treat disorders that are dependent on ovarian hormones (20). They are used to control ovulation induction cycles and to treat precocious puberty, ovarian hyperandrogenism, leiomyomas, endometriosis, and hormonally dependent cancers. The development of GnRH antagonists proved more difficult, in that a molecule was needed that maintained the binding and degradation resistance of agonists but failed to activate the receptor. Early attempts involved modification of amino acids 1 and 2, as well as those previously utilized for agonists. Commercial antagonists currently have structural modifications at amino acids 1, 2, 3, 6, and 10. The treatment spectrum is expected to be similar to that of GnRH agonists.

Endogenous Opioids and Effects on GnRH The endogenous opioids are three related families of naturally occurring substances produced in the CNS that represent the natural ligands for the opioid receptors (24–26). There are three major classes of endogenous opioids, each derived from precursor molecules:

1. *Endorphins* are named for their endogenous morphine-like activity. These substances are produced in the hypothalamus from the precursor proopiomelanocortin (POMC) and have diverse activities, including regulation of temperature, appetite, mood, and behavior (27).

2. *Enkephalins* function primarily in regulation of the autonomic nervous system. Proenkephalin A is the precursor for the two enkephalins of primary importance: metenkephalin and leuenkephalin.

3. *Dynorphins* are endogenous opioids produced from the precursor proenkephalin B that serve a function similar to that of the endorphins.

The endogenous opioids play a significant role in the regulation of hypothalamic-pituitary function. Endorphins appear to inhibit GnRH release within the hypothalamus, resulting in inhibition of gonadotropin secretion (28). Ovarian sex steroids can increase the secretion of central endorphins, further depressing gonadotropin levels (29).

Endorphin levels vary significantly throughout the menstrual cycle, with peak levels in the luteal phase and a nadir during menses (30). This inherent variability, although helping to regulate gonadotropin levels, may contribute to cycle-specific symptoms experienced by ovulatory women. For example, the dysphoria experienced by some women in the premenstrual phase of the cycle may be related to a withdrawal of endogenous opiates (31).

Pituitary Hormone Secretion

Anterior Pituitary

The anterior pituitary is responsible for the secretion of the major hormone-releasing factors: FSH, LH, TSH, and ACTH, as well as GH and prolactin. Each hormone is released by a specific pituitary cell type.

Gonadotropins

The gonadotropins FSH and LH are produced by the anterior pituitary gonadotroph cells and are responsible for ovarian follicular stimulation. Structurally, there is great similarity between FSH and LH (Fig. 7.6). They are both glycoproteins that share identical α subunits and differ only in the structure of their β subunits, which confer receptor specificity (32,33). The synthesis of the β subunits is the rate-regulating step in gonadotropin biosynthesis (34). TSH and placental chorionic gonadotropin also share identical α subunits with the gonadotropins. There are several forms of each gonadotropin, which differ in carbohydrate content as a result of posttranslation modification. The degree of modification varies with steroid levels and is an important regulator of gonadotropin bioactivity.

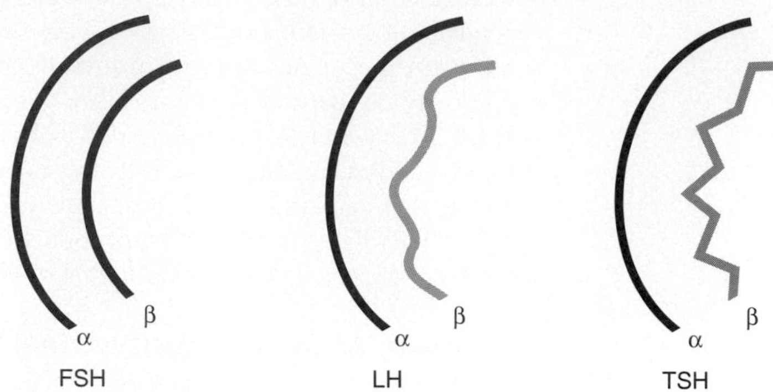

Figure 7.6 The structural similarity between FSH, LH, and TSH. The α subunits are identical and the β subunits differ.

Prolactin

***Prolactin,* a 198–amino acid polypeptide secreted by the anterior pituitary lactotroph, is the primary trophic factor responsible for the synthesis of milk by the breast** (35). Several forms of this hormone, which are named according to their size and bioactivity, are normally secreted (36). Prolactin production is under tonic inhibitory control by the hypothalamic secretion of dopamine (37). Therefore, disease states characterized by decreased dopamine secretion or any condition that interrupts transport of dopamine down the infundibular stalk to the pituitary gland will result in increased synthesis of prolactin. In this respect, prolactin is unique in comparison to all other pituitary hormones: it is predominantly under tonic inhibition, and release of control produces an increase in secretion. **Clinically, increased prolactin levels are associated with amenorrhea and galactorrhea, and hyperprolactinemia should be suspected in any individual with symptoms of either of these conditions.**

Although prolactin appears to be primarily under inhibitory control, many stimuli can elicit its release, including breast manipulation, drugs, stress, exercise, and certain foods. The existence of a releasing factor or factors for prolactin has been long hypothesized. Whereas such a factor has been identified in a variety of animal species, no physiologically significant releasing factor has been definitively identified in humans, although TRH appears to play this role to a large extent (38). Other hormones that may stimulate prolactin release include vasopressin, γ-aminobutyric acid (GABA), dopamine, β-endorphin, vasoactive intestinal peptide (VIP), epidermal growth factor, and angiotensin II (39,40). The relative contributions of these substances under normal conditions remain to be determined.

Thyroid-stimulating Hormone, Adrenocorticotropic Hormone, and Growth Hormone

The other hormones produced by the anterior pituitary are TSH, ACTH, and GH. Thyroid-stimulating hormone is secreted by the pituitary thyrotrophs in response to TRH. As with GnRH, TRH is synthesized primarily in the arcuate nucleus of the hypothalamus and is then secreted into the portal circulation for transport to the pituitary. In addition to stimulating TSH release, TRH is also a major stimulus for the release of prolactin. Thyroid-stimulating hormone stimulates release of T_3 and T_4 from the thyroid gland, which in turn has a negative feedback effect on pituitary TSH secretion. Abnormalities of thyroid secretion (both hyper- and hypothyroidism) are frequently associated with ovulatory dysfunction as a result of diverse actions on the hypothalamic-pituitary-ovarian axis (41).

ACTH is secreted by the anterior pituitary in response to another hypothalamic-releasing factor, CRH, and stimulates the release of adrenal glucocorticoids. Unlike the other anterior pituitary products, ACTH secretion has a diurnal variation with an early morning peak and a late evening nadir. As with the other pituitary hormones, ACTH secretion is negatively regulated by feedback from its primary end product, which in this case is cortisol.

The anterior pituitary hormone that is secreted in the greatest absolute amount is GH. It is secreted in response to the hypothalamic releasing factor, GHRH, as well as by thyroid hormone and glucocorticoids. This hormone is also secreted in a pulsatile fashion but with peak release occurring during sleep. In addition to its vital role in the stimulation of linear growth, GH plays a diverse role in physiologic hemostasis. The hormone has been shown to play a role in bone mitogenesis, CNS function (improved memory, cognition, and mood), body composition, breast development, and cardiovascular function. It also affects insulin regulation and acts anabolically. Growth hormone appears to have a role in the regulation of ovarian function, although the degree to which it serves this role in normal physiology is unclear (42).

Posterior Pituitary

Structure and Function

The posterior pituitary (neurohypophysis) is composed exclusively of neural tissue and is a direct extension of the hypothalamus. It lies directly adjacent to the adenohypophysis but is embryologically distinct, derived from an invagination of neuroectodermal tissue in the third ventricle. Axons in the posterior pituitary originate from neurons with cell bodies in two distinct regions of the hypothalamus, the supraoptic and paraventricular nuclei, named for their anatomic relationship to the optic chiasm and the third ventricle. Together these two nuclei comprise the hypothalamic magnocellular system. These neurons can secrete their synthetic products directly from axonal boutons into the general circulation to act as hormones. This is the mechanism of secretion of the hormones of the posterior pituitary, oxytocin and arginine vasopressin (AVP). Although this is the primary mode of release of these hormones, numerous other secondary pathways have been identified, including secretion into the portal circulation, intrahypothalamic secretion, and secretion into other regions of the CNS (43).

In addition to the established functions of oxytocin and vasopressin, several other diverse roles have been suggested in animal models. These include modulation of sexual activity and appetite, learning and memory consolidation, temperature regulation, and regulation of maternal behaviors (44). It remains to be seen which, if any, of these functions also exist in humans.

Oxytocin Oxytocin is a nine–amino acid peptide primarily produced by the paraventricular nucleus of the hypothalamus (Fig. 7.7). The primary function of this hormone in humans is the stimulation of two specific types of muscular contractions (Fig. 7.8). The first type, uterine muscular contraction, occurs during parturition. The second type of muscular contraction regulated by oxytocin is breast lactiferous duct myoepithelial contractions that occur during the milk letdown reflex. Oxytocin release may be stimulated by suckling, triggered by a signal from nipple stimulation transmitted via thoracic nerves to the spinal cord and then to the hypothalamus, where oxytocin is released in an episodic fashion (45).

Figure 7.7 Oxytocin and arginine-vasopressin (AVP) are nine–amino acid peptides produced by the hypothalamus. They differ in only two amino acids.

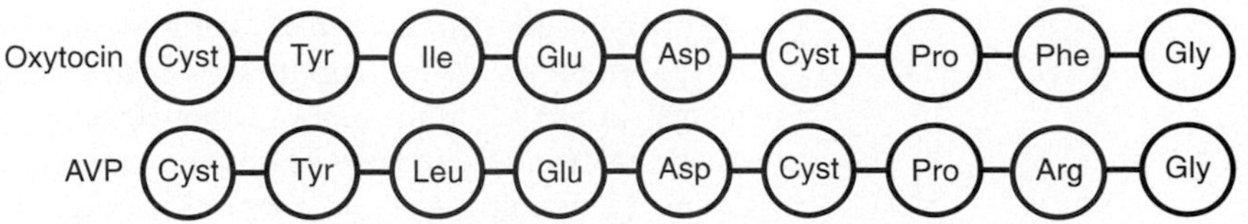

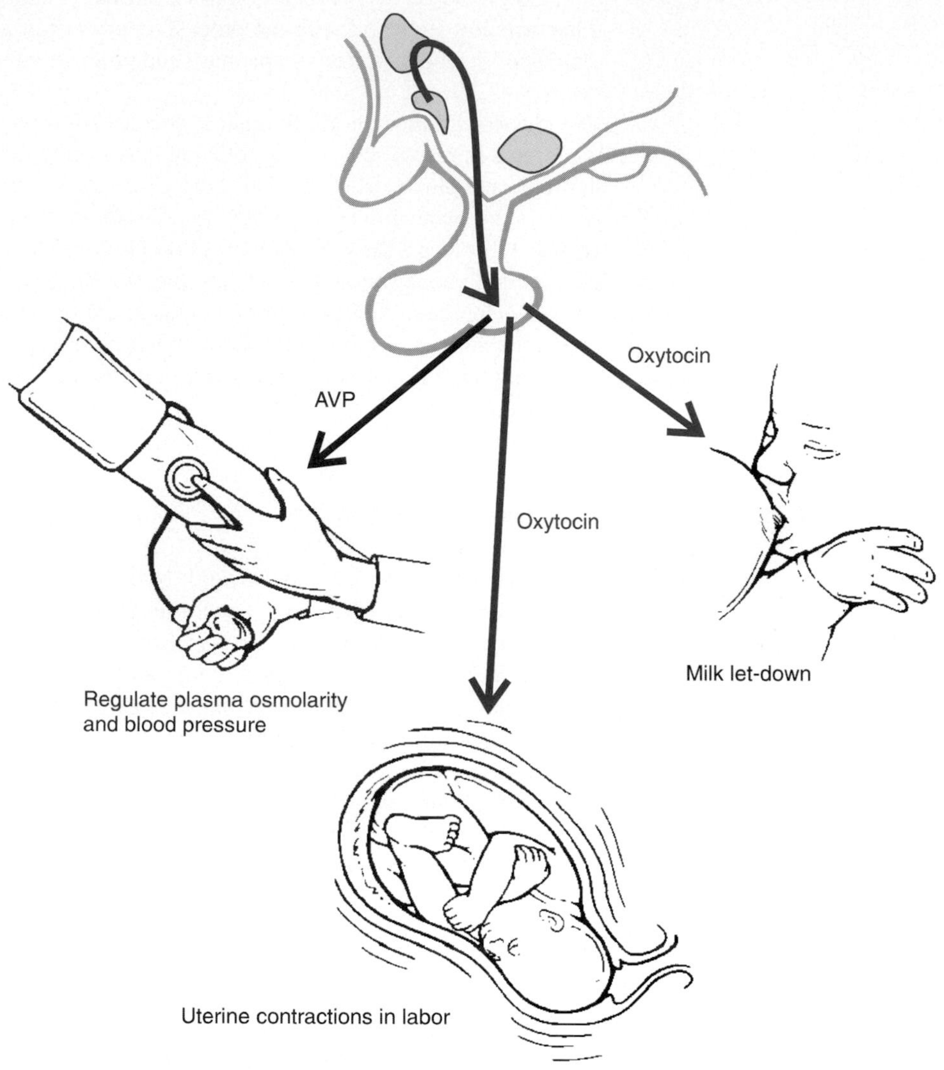

Figure 7.8 Oxytocin stimulates muscular contractions of the uterus during parturition and the breast lactiferous duct during the milk letdown reflex. Arginine-vasopressin (AVP) regulates circulating blood volume, pressure, and osmolality.

Oxytocin release also may be triggered by olfactory, auditory, and visual clues, and it may play a role in the conditioned reflex in nursing animals. Stimulation of the cervix and vagina can cause significant release of oxytocin, which may trigger reflex ovulation (the Ferguson reflex) in some species, although it is unclear to what extent this effect exists in humans.

Arginine-vasopressin AVP (also known as antidiuretic hormone, or ADH) is the second major secretory product of the posterior pituitary (Fig. 7.7). It is synthesized primarily by neurons with cell bodies in the supraoptic nuclei (Fig. 7.8). Its major function is the regulation of circulating blood volume, pressure, and osmolality (45). Specific receptors throughout the body can trigger the release of AVP. Osmoreceptors located in the hypothalamus sense changes in blood osmolality from a mean of 285 mOsm/kg. Baroceptors sense changes in blood pressure caused by alterations in blood volume and are peripherally located in the walls of the left atrium, carotid sinus, and aortic arch (46). These receptors can respond to changes in blood volume of more than 10%. In response to decreases in blood pressure or volume, AVP is released and causes arteriolar vasoconstriction and renal free-water conservation. This in turn leads to a decrease in blood osmolarity and an increase in blood pressure. Activation of the renal renin–angiotensin system can also activate AVP release.

Menstrual Cycle Physiology

In the normal menstrual cycle, there is an orderly cyclic hormone production and parallel proliferation of the uterine lining in preparation for implantation of the embryo. Disorders of the menstrual cycle and, likewise, disorders of menstrual physiology may lead to various pathologic states, including infertility, recurrent miscarriage, and malignancy.

Disorder of menstruation is one of the most frequent reasons women seek medical care (Table 7.1). Although helpful in formulating a diagnostic or therapeutic plan, specific abnormalities of menstrual flow are not directly related to specific defects.

Normal Menstrual Cycle

The normal human menstrual cycle can be divided into two segments: the ovarian cycle and the uterine cycle, based on the organ under examination. The ovarian cycle may be further divided into follicular and luteal phases, whereas the uterine cycle is divided into corresponding proliferative and secretory phases (Fig. 7.9). The phases of the ovarian cycle are characterized as follows:

1. **Follicular phase**—hormonal feedback promotes the orderly development of a single dominant follicle, which should be mature at midcycle and prepared for ovulation. The average length of the human follicular phase ranges from 10 to 14 days, and variability in this length is responsible for most variations in total cycle length.

2. **Luteal phase**—the time from ovulation to the onset of menses, with an average length of 14 days.

A normal menstrual cycle lasts from 21 to 35 days, with 2 to 6 days of flow and an average blood loss of 20 to 60 ml. However, studies of large numbers of women with normal menstrual cycles have shown that only approximately two-thirds of adult women have cycles lasting 21 to 35 days (47). The extremes of reproductive life (after menarche and perimenopause) are characterized by a higher percentage of anovulatory or irregularly timed cycles (48,49).

Hormonal Variations

The relative pattern of ovarian, uterine, and hormonal variation along the normal menstrual cycle is shown in Fig. 7.9.

Table 7.1. Definitions of Menstrual Cycle Irregularities

Oligomenorrhea	Infrequent, irregularly timed episodes of bleeding usually occurring at intervals of more than 35 days
Polymenorrhea	Frequent but regularly timed episodes of bleeding usually occurring at intervals of 21 days or less
Menorrhagia	Regularly timed episodes of bleeding that are excessive in amount (>80 ml) and duration of flow (>5 days)
Metrorrhagia	Irregularly timed bleeding
Menometrorrhagia	Excessive, prolonged bleeding that occurs at irregularly timed, frequent intervals
Hypomenorrhea	Regularly timed bleeding that is decreased in amount
Intermenstrual Bleeding	(usually not of an excessive amount) that occurs between bleeding otherwise normal menstrual cycles

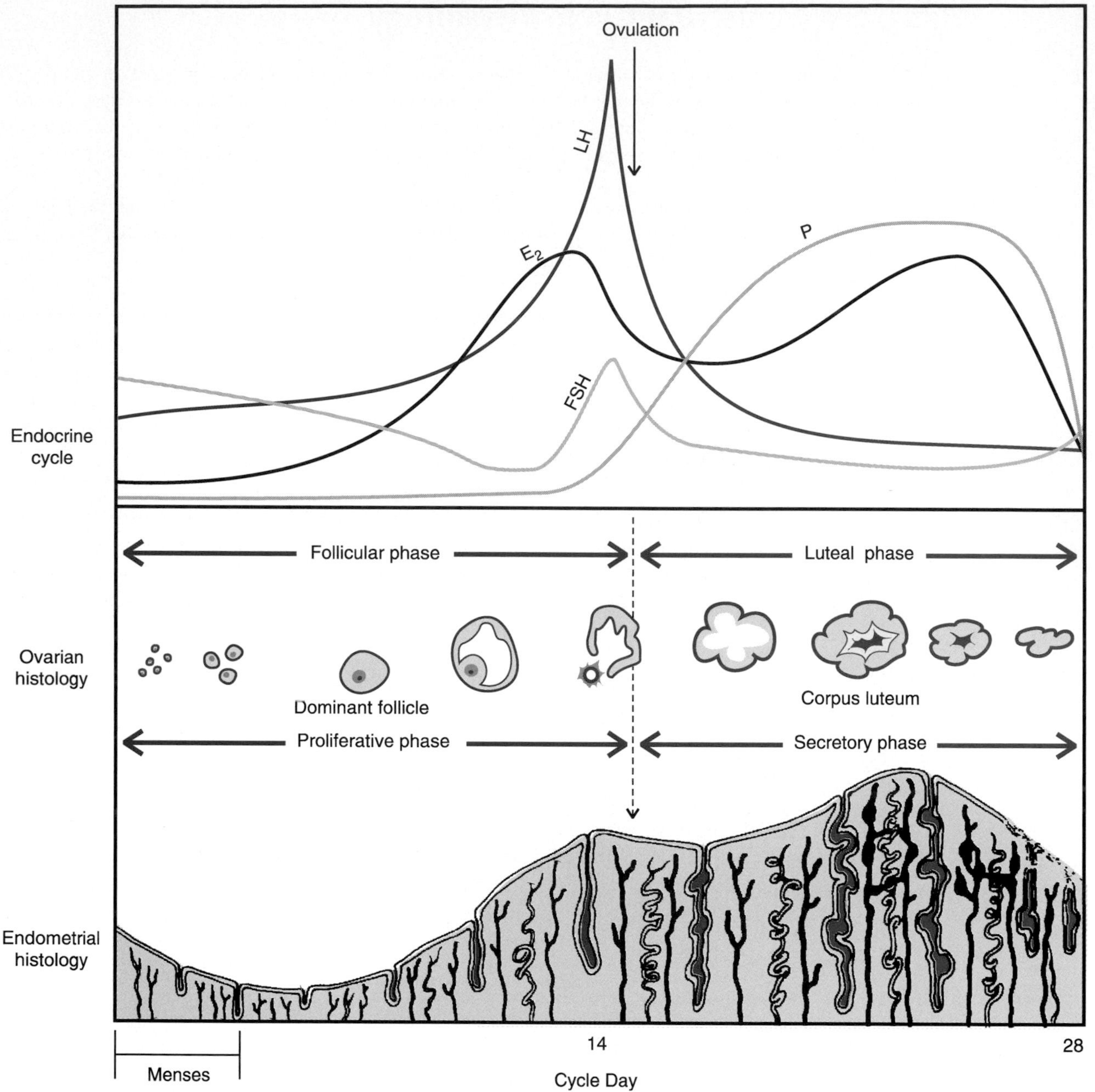

Figure 7.9 The menstrual cycle. The top panel shows the cyclic changes of FSH, LH, estradiol (E2), and progesterone (P) relative to the time of ovulation. The bottom panel correlates the ovarian cycle in the follicular and luteal phases and the endometrial cycle in the proliferative and secretory phases.

1. At the beginning of each monthly menstrual cycle, levels of gonadal steroids are low and have been decreasing since the end of the luteal phase of the previous cycle.

2. With the demise of the corpus luteum, FSH levels begin to rise and a cohort of growing follicles is recruited. These follicles each secrete increasing levels of estrogen as they grow in the follicular phase. This, in turn, is the stimulus for uterine endometrial proliferation.

3. Rising estrogen levels provide negative feedback on pituitary FSH secretion, which begins to wane by the midpoint of the follicular phase. Conversely, LH

initally decreases in response to rising estradiol levels, but late in the follicular phase the LH level is increased dramatically (biphasic response).

4. At the end of the follicular phase (just prior to ovulation), FSH-induced LH receptors are present on granulosa cells and, with LH stimulation, modulate the secretion of progesterone.

5. After a sufficient degree of estrogenic stimulation, the pituitary LH surge is triggered, which is the proximate cause of ovulation that occurs 24 to 36 hours later. Ovulation heralds the transition to the luteal-secretory phase.

6. The estrogen level decreases through the early luteal phase from just before ovulation until the midluteal phase, when it begins to rise again as a result of corpus luteum secretion.

7. Progesterone levels rise precipitously after ovulation and can be used as a presumptive sign that ovulation has occurred.

8. Both estrogen and progesterone levels remain elevated through the lifespan of the corpus luteum and then wane with its demise, thereby setting the stage for the next cycle.

Uterus

Cyclic Changes of the Endometrium

The cyclic histologic changes in the adult human endometrium were described by Noyes, Hertig, and Rock in 1950 (50) (Fig. 7.10). These changes proceed in an orderly fashion in response to cyclic hormonal production by the ovaries (Fig. 7.9). Histologic cycling of the endometrium can best be viewed in two parts: the endometrial glands and the surrounding stroma. The superficial two-thirds of the endometrium is the zone that proliferates and is ultimately shed with each cycle if pregnancy does not occur. This cycling portion of the endometrium is known as the *decidua functionalis* and is composed of a deeply situated intermediate zone (stratum spongiosum) and a superficial compact zone (stratum compactum). The *decidua basalis* is the deepest region of the endometrium. It does not undergo significant monthly proliferation but, instead, is the source of endometrial regeneration after each menses (51).

Proliferative Phase

By convention, the first day of vaginal bleeding is called day 1 of the menstrual cycle. After menses, the decidua basalis is composed of primordial glands and dense scant stroma in its location adjacent to the myometrium. The proliferative phase is characterized by progressive mitotic growth of the decidua functionalis in preparation for implantation of the embryo in response to rising circulating levels of estrogen (52). At the beginning of the proliferative phase, the endometrium is relatively thin (1 to 2 mm). The predominant change seen during this time is evolution of the initially straight, narrow, and short endometrial glands into longer, tortuous structures (53). Histologically, these proliferating glands have multiple mitotic cells, and their organization changes from a low columnar pattern in the early proliferative period to a pseudostratified pattern before ovulation. The stroma is a dense compact layer throughout this time. Vascular structures are infrequently seen.

Secretory Phase

In the typical 28-day cycle, ovulation occurs on cycle day 14. Within 48 to 72 hours following ovulation, the onset of progesterone secretion produces a shift in histologic appearance of the endometrium to the secretory phase, so named for the clear presence of eosinophilic protein-rich secretory products in the glandular lumen. In contrast to

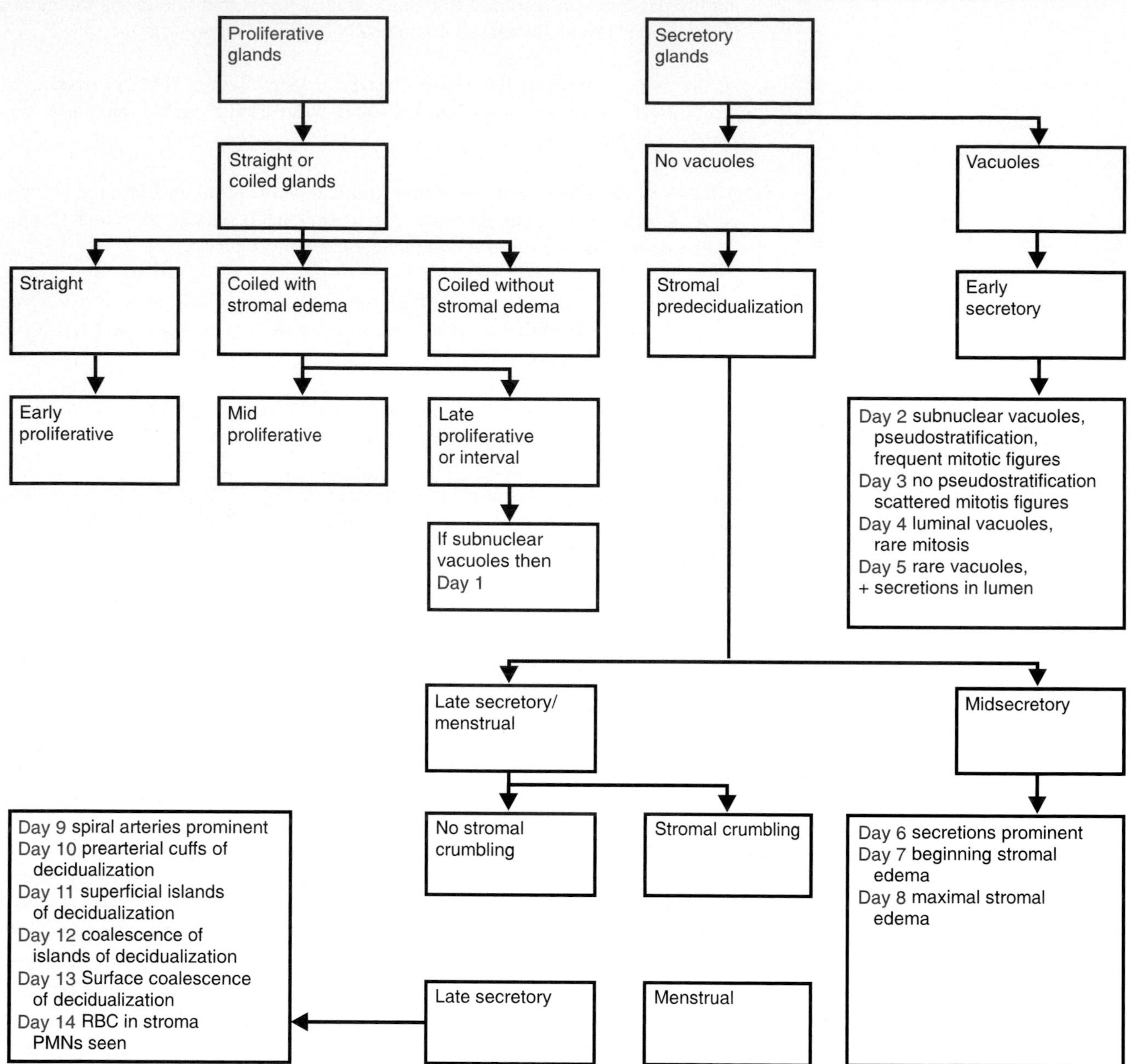

Figure 7.10 The histologic changes of the menstrual cycle. Endometrial biopsy can be used to determine the state of the endometrium corresponding to the day of the cycle.

the proliferative phase, the secretory phase of the menstrual cycle is characterized by the cellular effects of progesterone in addition to estrogen. In general, progesterone's effects are antagonistic to those of estrogen and there is a progressive decrease in the endometrial cell's estrogen receptor concentration. As a result, during the latter half of the cycle, there is an antagonism of estrogen-induced DNA synthesis and cellular mitosis (52).

During the secretory phase, the endometrial glands form characteristic periodic acid–Schiff positive–staining, glycogen-containing vacuoles. These vacuoles initially appear subnuclearly (by cycle day 16) and then progress toward the glandular lumen (50) (Fig. 7.10). The nuclei can be seen in the midportion of the cells by cycle day 17 and ultimately undergo apocrine secretion into the glandular lumen by cycle day 19 to 20. At postovulatory day 6 to 7, secretory activity of the glands is maximal and the endometrium is optimally prepared for implantation of the blastocyst.

The stroma of the secretory phase remains unchanged histologically until the seventh post-ovulatory day, when there is a progressive increase in edema. Coincident with maximal stromal edema in the late secretory phase, the spiral arteries become clearly visible and then progressively lengthen and coil during the remainder of the secretory phase. By day 24, an eosinophilic staining pattern, known as *cuffing,* is visible in the perivascular stroma. Eosinophilia then progresses to form islands in the stroma followed by areas of confluence. This staining pattern of the edematous stroma is termed *pseudodecidual* because of its similarity to the pattern that occurs in pregnancy. Approximately 2 days prior to menses, there is a dramatic increase in the number of polymorphonuclear lymphocytes that migrate from the vascular system. This leukocytic infiltration heralds the collapse of the endometrial stroma and the onset of the menstrual flow.

Menses

In the absence of implantation, glandular secretion ceases and an irregular breakdown of the decidua functionalis occurs. The result is a shedding of this layer of the endometrium, a process termed menses. It is the destruction of the corpus luteum and its production of estrogen and progesterone that is the proximate cause of the shedding. With withdrawal of sex steroids, there is a profound spiral artery vascular spasm that ultimately leads to endometrial ischemia. Simultaneously, there is a breakdown of lysosomes and a release of proteolytic enzymes, which further promote local tissue destruction. This layer of endometrium is then shed, leaving the decidua basalis as the source of subsequent endometrial growth. Prostaglandins are produced throughout the menstrual cycle and are at their highest concentration during menses (53). Prostaglandin $F_{2\alpha}$ ($PGF_{2\alpha}$) is a potent vasoconstrictor, causing further arteriolar vasospasm and endometrial ischemia. Prostaglandin $F_{2\alpha}$ also produces myometrial contractions that decrease local uterine wall blood flow and may serve to physically expel sloughing endometrial tissue from the uterus.

Dating the Endometrium

The precise nature of the histologic changes that occur in secretory endometrium relative to the LH surge allows the assessment of the "normalcy" of endometrial development (Fig. 7.9). By knowing when a patient is chronologically postovulatory, it is possible to obtain a sample of the endometrium by endometrial biopsy and determine whether the state of the endometrium corresponds to the phase of the cycle (Fig. 7.10). Any large discrepancy (more than 2-day lag time) is termed a luteal phase defect and has been linked to both failure of implantation and early pregnancy loss (54). To perform this diagnostic test, it is first critical to determine when ovulation occurs. Once the timing of ovulation has been established, investigators have traditionally chosen 10 to 12 days postovulation as the time for biopsy. However, endometrial sampling at the time of implantation (6 to 8 days postovulation) may be more accurate (55).

Simple hematoxylin and eosin (H&E) stain evaluation is a crude, insensitive, and frequently inaccurate method of assessing endometrial receptivity. Normal implantation requires a complex set of events, many being expressed as changes within the endometrium (56). These changes include expression of specific glycoproteins and adhesion molecules, production of cytokines, and variation in tissue enzyme levels (57). As the importance of each of these factors in implantation becomes clear, it will likely become possible to subject one or more endometrial biopsy samples to a complex variety of stains, thereby assessing the development of individual markers. Such complex screening, already used in other tissue systems, will allow a more precise diagnosis of endometrial dysfunction than the current general diagnosis of luteal phase defect.

Ovarian Follicular Development

The number of oocytes peaks in the fetus at 6 to 7 million by 20 weeks of gestation (58) (Fig. 7.11). Simultaneously (and peaking at the fifth month of gestation), atresia of the oogonia occurs, rapidly followed by follicular atresia. At birth, only 1 to 2 million oocytes remain in the ovaries, and at puberty, only 300,000 of the original 6 to 7 million oocytes

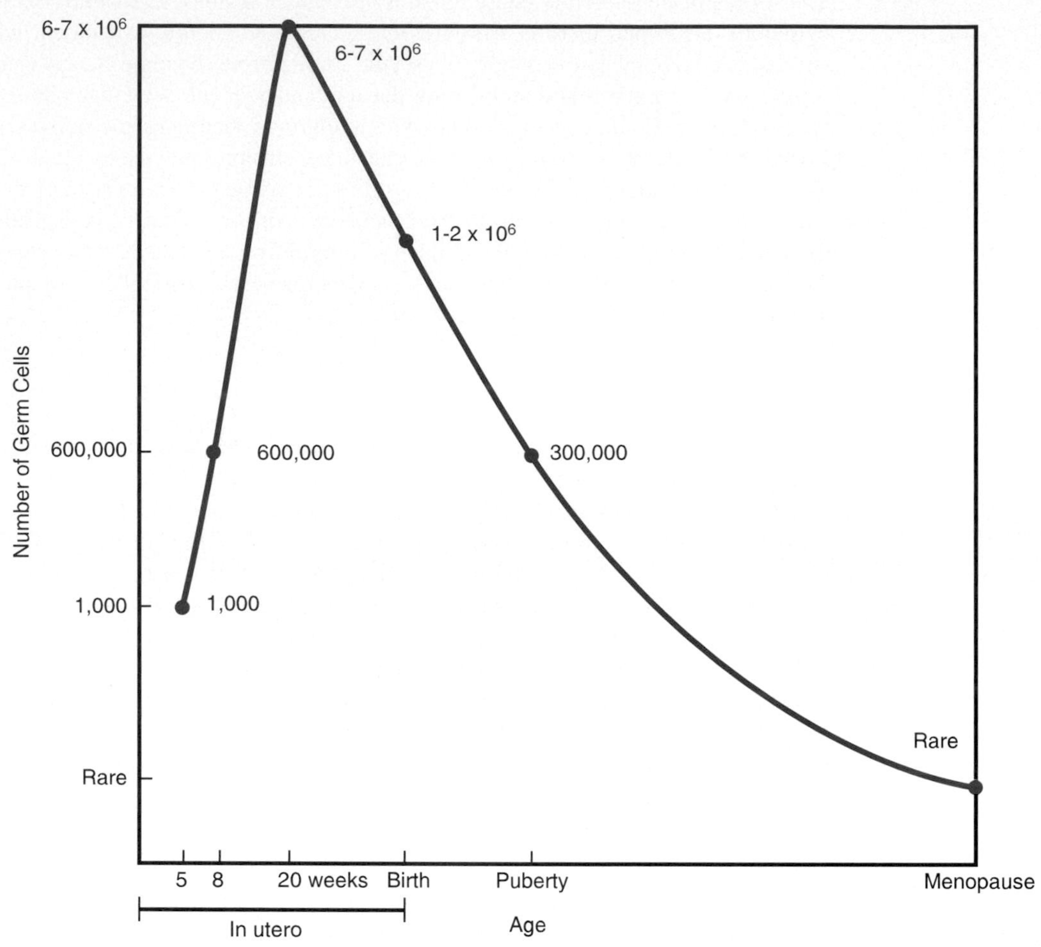

Figure 7.11 The number of oocytes in the ovary before and after birth and through menopause.

are available for ovulation (58,59). Of these, only 400 to 500 will ultimately be released during ovulation. By the time of menopause, the ovary will be composed primarily of dense stromal tissue with only rare interspersed oocytes remaining.

In humans, oogonial formation or mitosis does not occur postnatally. Because oocytes enter the diplotene resting stage of meiosis in the fetus and persist in this stage until ovulation, much of the deoxyribonucleic acid (DNA), proteins, and messenger ribonucleic acid (mRNA) necessary for development of the preimplantation embryo will have been synthesized by this stage. At the diplotene stage, a single layer of 8 to 10 granulosa cells surround the oogonia to form the primordial follicle. The oogonia that fail to become properly surrounded by granulosa cells undergo atresia (60).

Meiotic Arrest of Oocyte and Resumption

Meiosis* (the germ cell process of reduction division) is commonly divided into four phases: prophase, metaphase, anaphase, and telophase. The prophase of meiosis I is further divided into five stages: *leptotene, zygotene, pachytene, diplotene,* and *diakinesis.

Oogonia differ from spermatogonia in that only one final daughter cell (oocyte) forms from each precursor cell, with the excess genetic material discarded in three polar bodies. When the developing oogonia begin to enter meiotic prophase I, they are known as primary oocytes (61). This process begins at roughly 8 weeks of gestation. Only those oogonia that enter meiosis will survive the wave of atresia that sweeps the fetal ovary before birth. The oocytes arrested in prophase (in the late diplotene or "dictyate" stage) will remain so until the time of ovulation, when the process of meiosis resumes. The mechanism for this mitotic stasis is believed to be an oocyte maturation inhibitor (OMI) produced by granulosa cells (62). This inhibitor gains access to the oocyte via gap junctions connecting the oocyte and its surrounding cumulus of granulosa. With the midcycle LH surge, the gap junctions are disrupted, granulosa cells are no longer connected to the oocyte, and meiosis I is allowed to resume.

Follicular Development

Follicular development is a dynamic process that continues from menarche until menopause. The process is designed to allow the monthly recruitment of a cohort of follicles and, ultimately, to release a single mature dominant follicle during ovulation each month.

Primordial Follicles

The initial recruitment and growth of the primordial follicles is gonadotropin independent and affects a cohort over several months (63). However, the stimuli responsible for the recruitment of a specific cohort of follicles in each cycle are unknown. At the primordial follicle stage, shortly after initial recruitment, FSH assumes control of follicular differentiation and growth and allows a cohort of follicles to continue differentiation. This process signals the shift from gonadotropin-independent to gonadotropin-dependent growth. The first changes seen are growth of the oocyte and expansion of the single layer of follicular granulosa cells into a multilayer of cuboidal cells. The decline in luteal phase progesterone and inhibin production by the now-fading corpus luteum from the previous cycle allows the increase in FSH that stimulates this follicular growth (64).

Preantral Follicle

During the several days following the breakdown of the corpus luteum, growth of the cohort of follicles continues, driven by the stimulus of FSH. The enlarging oocyte then secretes a glycoprotein-rich substance, the zona pellucida, which separates it from the surrounding granulosa cells (except for the aforementioned gap junction). With transformation from a primordial to a preantral follicle, there is continued mitotic proliferation of the encompassing granulosa cells. Simultaneously, theca cells in the stroma bordering the granulosa cells proliferate. Both cell types function synergistically to produce estrogens that are secreted into the systemic circulation. At this stage of development, each of the seemingly identical cohort members must either be selected for dominance or undergo atresia. It is likely that the follicle destined to ovulate has been selected prior to this point, although the mechanism for selection remains obscure.

Two-cell Two-gonadotropin Theory

The fundamental tenet of follicular development is the two-cell two-gonadotropin theory (65–67) (Fig. 7.12). **This theory states that there is a subdivision and compartmentalization of steroid hormone synthesis activity in the developing follicle.** In general, most aromatase activity (for estrogen production) is in the granulosa cells (68). Aromatase activity is enhanced by FSH stimulation of specific receptors on these cells (69,70). However, granulosa cells lack several enzymes that occur earlier in the steroidogenic pathway and require androgens as a substrate for aromatization. Androgens, in turn, are synthesized primarily in response to stimulation by LH, and the theca cells possess most of the LH receptors at this stage (69,70). Therefore, a synergistic relationship must exist: LH stimulates the theca cells to produce androgens (primarily androstenedione) which, in turn, are transferred to the granulosa cells for FSH-stimulated aromatization into estrogens. These locally produced estrogens create a microenvironment within the follicle that is favorable for continued growth and nutrition (71). Both FSH and local estrogens serve to further stimulate estrogen production, FSH receptor synthesis and expression, and granulosa cell proliferation and differentiation.

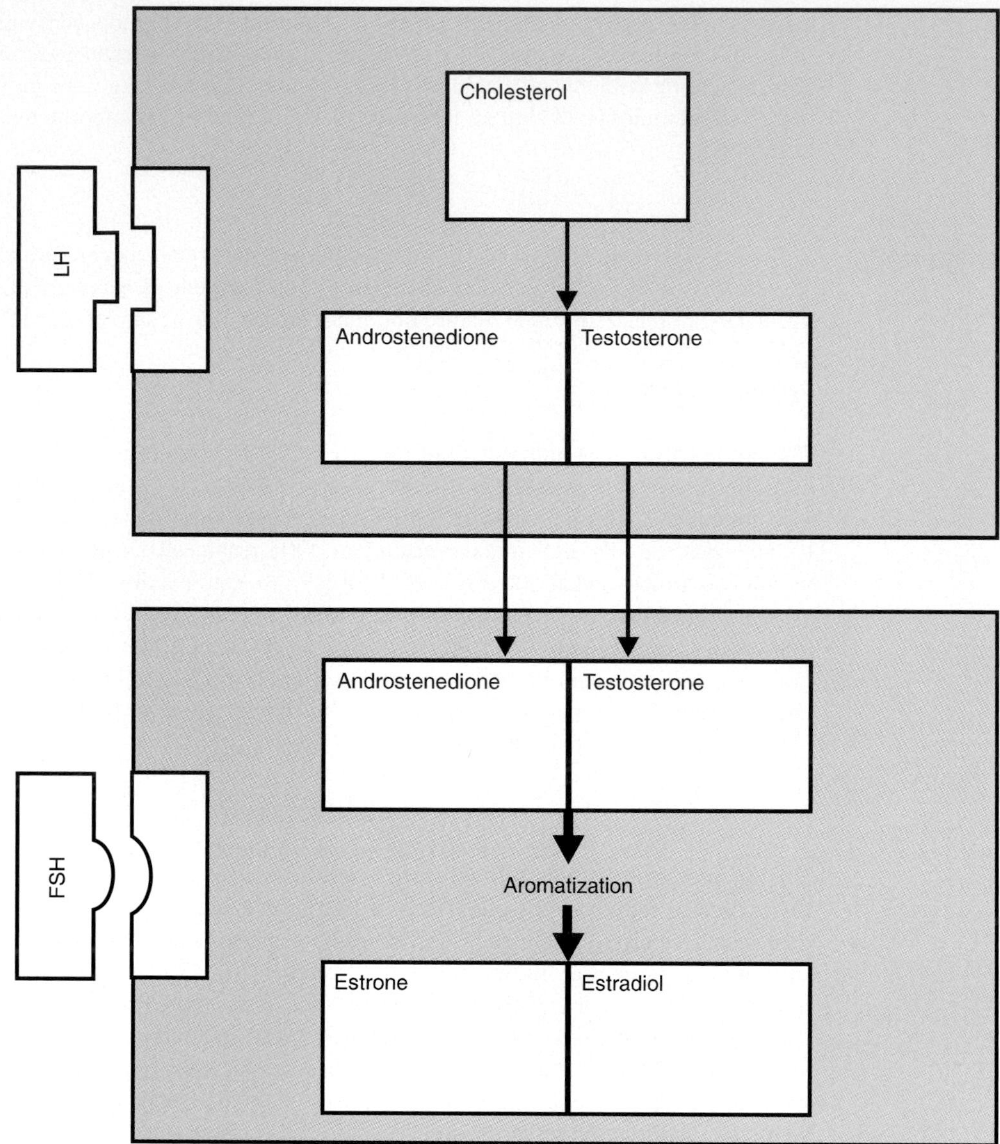

Figure 7.12 The two-cell two-gonadotropin theory of follicular development in which there is compartmentalization of steroid hormone synthesis in the developing follicle.

Androgens have two different regulatory roles in follicular development. At low concentrations (i.e., in the early preantral follicle), they serve to stimulate aromatase activity via specific receptors in granulosa cells. At higher levels of androgens, there is intense 5α-reductase activity that converts the androgens to forms that cannot be aromatized (65,72). This androgenic microenvironment inhibits the expression of FSH receptors on the granulosa cells, thereby inhibiting aromatase activity and setting the follicle on the path to atresia (73). Meanwhile, as the peripheral estrogen level rises, it negatively feeds back on the pituitary and hypothalamus to decrease circulating FSH levels (74). Increased ovarian production of inhibin further decreases FSH production at this point.

The falling FSH level that occurs with the progression of the follicular phase represents a threat to continued follicular growth. The resulting adverse environment can be withstood only by follicles with a selective advantage for binding the diminishing FSH molecules; that is, those with the greatest number of FSH receptors. The dominant follicle, therefore, can be perceived as the one with a richly estrogenic microenvironment and the most FSH receptors (75). As it grows and develops, the follicle continues to produce estrogen, which results in further lowering of the circulating FSH and creating a more adverse environment for competing follicles. This process continues until all members of the initial cohort have suffered atresia, with the exception of the single dominant follicle. The stage is then set for ovulation.

Preovulatory Follicle

Preovulatory follicles are characterized by a fluid-filled antrum that is composed of plasma with granulosa-cell secretions. The granulosa cells at this point have further differentiated into a heterogenous population. The oocyte remains connected to the follicle by a stalk of specialized granulosa known as the *cumulus oophorus.*

Rising estrogen levels have a negative feedback effect on FSH secretion. Conversely, LH undergoes biphasic regulation by circulating estrogens. At lower concentrations, estrogens inhibit LH secretion. At higher levels, however, estrogen enhances LH release. This stimulation requires a sustained high level of estrogen (200 pg/ml) for more than 48 hours (76). Once the rising estrogen level produces positive feedback, a substantial surge in LH secretion occurs. Concomitant to these events, the local estrogen-FSH interactions in the dominant follicle induce LH receptors on the granulosa cells. Thus, exposure to high levels of LH results in a specific response by the dominant follicle—the result is luteinization of the granulosa cells, production of progesterone, and initiation of ovulation. In general, ovulation will occur in the single mature, or Graafian, follicle 10 to 12 hours after the LH peak or 34 to 36 hours after the initial rise in midcycle LH (77–79).

The sex steroids are not the only gonadotropin regulators of follicular development. Two related granulosa cell–derived peptides have been identified that play opposing roles in pituitary feedback (80). The first of these, inhibin, is secreted in two forms: inhibin A and inhibin B. Inhibin B is secreted primarily in the follicular phase, and is stimulated by FSH (81), whereas inhibin A is mainly active in the luteal phase. Both forms act to inhibit FSH synthesis and release (82,83). The second peptide, activin, stimulates FSH release from the pituitary gland and potentiates its action in the ovary (84,85). It is likely that there are numerous other intraovarian regulators similar to inhibin and activin, each of which may play a key role in promoting the normal ovulatory process (86). Some of these include insulin-like growth factor (ILGF)-1, epidermal growth factor (EGF)/transforming growth factor (TGF)-α, TGF-β1, β-fibroblast growth factor (FGF), IL-1, TNF-α, OMI, and renin–angiotensin.

Ovulation

The midcycle LH surge is responsible for a dramatic increase in local concentrations of prostaglandins and proteolytic enzymes in the follicular wall (87). These substances progressively weaken the follicular wall and ultimately allow a perforation to form. Ovulation most likely represents a slow extrusion of the oocyte through this opening in the follicle rather than a rupture of the follicular structure (88). In fact, direct measurements of intrafollicular pressures have been recorded and have failed to demonstrate an explosive event.

Luteal Phase

Structure of Corpus Luteum **After ovulation, the remaining follicular shell is transformed into the primary regulator of the luteal phase—the corpus luteum.** Membranous granulosa cells remaining in the follicle begin to take up lipids and the characteristic yellow lutein pigment for which the structure is named. These cells are active secretory structures that produce progesterone, which supports the endometrium of the luteal phase. In addition, estrogen and inhibin A are produced in significant quantities. Unlike the process that occurs in the developing follicle, the basement membrane of the corpus luteum degenerates to allow proliferating blood vessels to invade the granulosa-luteal cells in response to secretion of angiogenic factors such as vascular endothelial growth factor (89). This angiogenic response allows large amounts of luteal hormones to enter the systemic circulation.

Hormonal Function and Regulation

The hormonal changes of the luteal phase are characterized by a series of negative feedback interactions designed to lead to regression of the corpus luteum if pregnancy does not occur. Corpus luteum steroids (estradiol and progesterone) provide negative central feedback and cause a decrease in FSH and LH secretion. Continued secretion of both steroids will decrease the stimuli for subsequent follicular recruitment. Similarly, luteal secretion of inhibin also potentiates FSH withdrawal. In the ovary, local production of progesterone inhibits the further development and recruitment of additional follicles.

Continued corpus luteum function depends on continued LH production. In the absence of this stimulation, the corpus luteum will invariably regress after 12 to 16 days and form the scarlike corpora albicans (90). The exact mechanism of luteolysis, however, is unclear and most likely also involves local paracrine factors. In the absence of pregnancy, the corpus luteum regresses, and estrogen and progesterone levels wane. This, in turn, removes central inhibition on gonadotropin secretion and allows FSH and LH levels to again rise and recruit another cohort of follicles.

If pregnancy does occur, placental human chorionic gonadotropin (hCG) will mimic LH action and continually stimulate the corpus luteum to secrete progesterone. Thus, successful implantation results in hormonal support to allow continued maintenance of the corpus luteum and the endometrium. Evidence from patients undergoing oocyte donation cycles has demonstrated that continued luteal function is essential to continuation of the pregnancy until approximately 5 weeks of gestation, when sufficient progesterone is produced by the developing placenta (91). This switch in the source of regulatory progesterone production is referred to as the luteal-placental shift.

Summary of Menstrual Cycle Regulation

Following is a summary of the regulation of the menstrual cycle:

1. GnRH is produced in the arcuate nucleus of the hypothalamus and secreted in a pulsatile fashion into the portal circulation, where it travels to the anterior pituitary.

2. Ovarian follicular development moves from a period of gonadotropin independence to a phase of FSH dependence.

3. As the corpus luteum of the previous cycle fades, luteal production of progesterone and inhibin A decreases, allowing FSH levels to rise.

4. In response to FSH stimulus, the follicles grow and differentiate and secrete increasing amounts of estrogen.

5. Estrogens stimulate growth and differentiation of the functional layer of the endometrium, which prepares for implantation. Estrogens work with FSH in stimulating follicular development.

6. The two-cell two-gonadotropin theory dictates that with LH stimulation the ovarian theca cells will produce androgens that are converted by the granulosa cells into estrogens under the stimulus of FSH.

7. Rising estrogen levels negatively feed back on the pituitary gland and hypothalamus and decrease the secretion of FSH.

8. The one follicle destined to ovulate each cycle is called the dominant follicle. It has relatively more FSH receptors and produces a larger concentration of estrogens than the follicles that will undergo atresia. It is able to continue to grow despite falling FSH levels.

9. Sustained high estrogen levels cause a surge in pituitary LH secretion that triggers ovulation, progesterone production, and the shift to the secretory, or luteal, phase.

10. Luteal function is dependent on the presence of LH. Without continued LH secretion, the corpus luteum will regress after 12 to 16 days.

11. If pregnancy occurs, the embryo secretes hCG, which mimics the action of LH by sustaining the corpus luteum. The corpus luteum continues to secrete progesterone and supports the secretory endometrium, allowing the pregnancy to continue to develop.

References

1. **Bloom FE.** Neuroendocrine mechanisms: cells and systems. In: **Yen SCC, Jaffe RB,** eds. *Reproductive endocrinology.* Philadelphia: WB Saunders, 1991:2–24.
2. **Simerly RB, Chang C, Muramatsu M, et al.** Distribution of androgen and estrogen receptor mRNA-containing cells in the rat brain: an in situ hybridization study. *J Comp Neurol* 1990;294:76–95.
3. **Brown TJ, Hochberg RB, Naftolin F.** Pubertal development of estrogen receptors in the rat brain. *Mol Cell Neurosci* 1994;5:475–483.
4. **Bergland RM, Page RB.** Can the pituitary secrete directly to the brain? Affirmative anatomic evidence. *Endocrinology* 1978;102:1325–1338.
5. **Duello TM, Halmi NS.** Ultrastructural-immunocytochemical localization of growth hormone and prolactin in human pituitaries. *J Clin Endocrinol Metab* 1979;49:189–196.
6. **Blackwell RE, Amoss M Jr, Vale W, et al.** Concomitant release of FSH and LH induced by native and synthetic LRF. *Am J Physiol* 1973;224:170–175.
7. **Krey LC, Butler WR, Knobil E.** Surgical disconnection of the medial basal hypothalamus and pituitary function in the rhesus monkey. I. Gonadotropin secretion. *Endocrinology* 1975;96:1073–1087.
8. **Plant TM, Krey LC, Moossy J, et al.** The arcuate nucleus and the control of the gonadotropin and prolactin secretion in the female rhesus monkey (Macaca mulatta). *Endocrinology* 1978;102:52–62.
9. **Amoss M, Burgus R, Blackwell RE, et al.** Purification, amino acid composition, and N-terminus of the hypothalamic luteinizing hormone releasing factor (LRF) of ovine origin. *Biochem Biophys Res Commun* 1971;44:205–210.
10. **Schwanzel-Fukuda M, Pfaff DW.** Origin of luteinizing hormone releasing hormone neurons. *Nature* 1989;338:161–164.
11. **Dierschke DJ, Bhattacharya AN, Atkinson LE, et al.** Circhoral oscillations of plasma LH levels in the ovariectomized rhesus monkey. *Endocrinology* 1970;87:850–853.
12. **Knobil E.** Neuroendocrine control of the menstrual cycle. *Recent Prog Horm Res* 1980;36:53–88.
13. **Belchetz PE, Plant TM, Nakai Y, et al.** Hypophyseal responses to continuous and intermittent delivery of hypothalamic gonadotropin-releasing hormone. *Science* 1978;202:631–633.
14. **Nakai Y, Plant TM, Hess DL, et al.** On the sites of the negative and positive feedback actions of estradiol and the control of gonadotropin secretion in the rhesus monkey. *Endocrinology* 1978;102:1008–1014.
15. **Rabin D, McNeil LW.** Pituitary and gonadal desensitization after continuous luteinizing hormone–releasing hormone infusion in normal females. *J Clin Endocrinol Metab*1980,51:873–876.
16. **Hoff JD, Lasley BL, Yen SSC.** Functional relationship between priming and releasing actions of luteinizing hormone–releasing hormone. *J Clin Endocrinol Metab* 1979;49:8–11.
17. **Soules MR, Steiner RA, Cohen NL, et al.** Nocturnal slowing of pulsatile luteinizing hormone secretion in women during the follicular phase of the menstrual cycle. *J Clin Endocrinol Metab* 1985;61:43–49.
18. **Filicori M, Santoro N, Marriam GR, et al.** Characterization of the physiological pattern of episodic gonadotropin secretion throughout the human menstrual cycle. *J Clin Endocrinol Metab* 1986;62:1136–1144.
19. **Karten MJ, Rivier JE.** Gonadotropin-releasing hormone analog design. Structure function studies towards the development of agonists and antagonists: rationale and perspective. *Endocr Rev* 1986;7:44–66.
20. **Conn PM, Crowley WF Jr.** Gonadotropin-releasing hormone and its analogs. *Annu Rev Med* 1994;45:391–405.
21. **Loy RA.** The pharmacology and potential applications of GnRH antagonists. *Curr Opin Obstet Gynecol* 1994;6:262–268.
22. **Schally AV.** LH-RH analogues. I. Their impact on reproductive medicine. *Gynecol Endocrinol* 1999;13:401–409.

23. **Halmos G, Schally AV, Pinski J, et al.** Down-regulation of pituitary receptors for luteinizing hormone–releasing hormone (LH-RH) in rats by LH-RH antagonist Cetrorelix. *Proc Natl Acad Sci U S A* 1996;93:2398–2402.

24. **Hughes J, Smith TW, Kosterlitz LH, et al.** Identification of two related pentapeptides from the brain with potent opiate agonist activity. *Nature* 1975;258:577–580.

25. **Howlett TA, Rees LH.** Endogenous opioid peptide and hypothalamo-pituitary function. *Annu Rev Physiol* 1986;48:527–536.

26. **Facchinetti F, Petraglia F, Genazzani AR.** Localization and expression of the three opioid systems. *Semin Reprod Endocrinol* 1987;5:103.

27. **Goldstein A.** Endorphins: physiology and clinical implications. *Ann N Y Acad Sci* 1978;311:49–58.

28. **Grossman A.** Opioid peptides and reproductive function. *Semin Reprod Endocrinol* 1987;5:115–124.

29. **Reid Rl, Hoff JD, Yen SSC, et al.** Effects of exogenous β-endorphin on pituitary hormone secretion and its disappearance rate in normal human subjects. *J Clin Endocrinol Metab* 1981;52:1179–1184.

30. **Gindoff PR, Ferin M.** Brain opioid peptides and menstrual cyclicity. *Semin Reprod Endocrinol* 1987;5:125–133.

31. **Halbreich U, Endicott J.** Possible involvement of endorphin withdrawal or imbalance in specific premenstrual syndromes and postpartum depression. *Med Hypotheses* 1981;7:1045–1058.

32. **Fiddes JC, Talmadge K.** Structure, expression and evolution of the genes for human glycoprotein hormones. *Recent Prog Horm Res* 1984;40:43–78.

33. **Vaitukaitis JL, Ross JT, Bourstein GD, et al.** Gonadotropins and their subunits: basic and clinical studies. *Recent Prog Horm Res* 1976;32:289–331.

34. **Lalloz MRA, Detta A, Clayton RN.** GnRH desensitization preferentially inhibits expression of the LH β-subunit gene in vivo. *Endocrinology* 1988;122:1689–1694.

35. **Brun del Re R, del Pozo E, de Grandi P, et al.** Prolactin inhibition and suppression of puerperal lactation by a Br-ergocriptine (CB 154): a comparison with estrogen. *Obstet Gynecol* 1973;41:884–890.

36. **Suh HK, Frantz AG.** Size heterogeneity of human prolactin in plasma and pituitary extracts. *J Clin Endocrinol Metab* 1974:39:928–935.

37. **MacLeod RM.** Influence of norepinephrine and catecholamine depletion agents synthesis in release of prolactin growth hormone. *Endocrinology* 1969;85:916–923.

38. **Vale W, Blackwell RE, Grant G, et al.** TRF and thyroid hormones on prolactin secretion by rat pituitary cell in vitro. *Endocrinology* 1973;93:26–33.

39. **Matsushita N, Kato Y, Shimatsu A, et al.** Effects of VIP, TRH, GABA and dopamine on prolactin release from superfused rat anterior pituitary cells. *Life Sci* 1983;32:1263–1269.

40. **Dufy-Barbe L, Rodriguez F, Arsaut J, et al.** Angiotensin-II stimulates prolactin release in the rhesus monkey. *Neuroendocrinology* 1982;35:242–247.

41. **Burrow GN.** The thyroid gland and reproduction. In: **Yen SCC, Jaffe RB,** eds. *Reproductive endocrinology.* Philadelphia: WB Saunders, 1991:555–575.

42. **Katz E, Ricciarelli E, Adashi EY.** The potential relevance of growth hormone to female reproductive physiology and pathophysiology. *Fertil Steril* 1993;59:8–34.

43. **Yen SCC.** The hypothalamic control of pituitary hormone secretion. In: **Yen SCC, Jaffe RB,** eds. *Reproductive endocrinology.* Philadelphia: WB Saunders, 1991:65–104.

44. **Insel TR.** Oxytocin and the neuroendocrine basis of affiliation. In: **Schulkin J,** ed. *Hormonally induced changes in mind and brain.* New York: Academic Press, 1993:225–251.

45. **McNeilly AS, Roinson CAF, Houston MJ, et al.** Release of oxytocin and PRL in response to suckling. *BMJ* 1983;286:257–259.

46. **Dunn FL, Brennan TJ, Nelson AE, et al.** The role of blood osmolality and volume in regulating vasopressin secretion in the rat. *J Clin Invest* 1973;52:3212–3219.

47. **Vollman RF.** The menstrual cycle. In: **Friedman E,** ed. *Major problems in obstetrics and gynecology.* Philadelphia: WB Saunders, 1977:1–193.

48. **Treloar AE, Boynton RE, Borghild GB, et al.** Variation of the human menstrual cycle through reproductive life. *Int J Fertil* 1967;12:77–126.

49. **Collett ME, Wertenberger GE, Fiske VM.** The effects of age upon the pattern of the menstrual cycle. *Fertil Steril* 1954;5:437–448.

50. **Noyes RW, Hertig AW, Rock J.** Dating the endometrial biopsy. *Fertil Steril* 1950;1:3–25.

51. **Flowers CE Jr, Wilbron WH.** Cellular mechanisms for endometrial conservation during menstrual bleeding. *Semin Reprod Endocrinol* 1984;2:307–341.

52. **Ferenczy A, Bertrand G, Gelfand MM.** Proliferation kinetics of human endometrium during the normal menstrual cycle. *Am J Obstet Gynecol* 1979;133:859–867.

53. **Schwarz BE.** The production and biologic effects of uterine prostaglandins. *Semin Reprod Endocrinol* 1983;1:189.

54. **Olive DL.** The prevalence and epidemiology of luteal-phase deficiency in normal and infertile women. *Clin Obstet Gynecol* 1991;34:157–166.

55. **Castelbaum AJ, Wheeler J, Coutifaris CB, et al.** Timing of the endometrial biopsy may be critical for the accurate diagnosis of luteal phase deficiency. *Fertil Steril* 1994;61:443–447.

56. **Ilesanmi AO, Hawkins DA, Lessey BA.** Immunohistochemical markers of uterine receptivity in the human endometrium. *Microsc Res Tech* 1993;25:208–222.

57. **Tabibzadeh S.** Human endometrium: an active site of cytokine production and action. *Endocr Rev* 1991;12:272–290.

58. **Peters H, Byskov AG, Grinsted J.** Follicular growth in fetal and prepubertal ovaries in humans and other primates. *J Clin Endocrinol Metab* 1978;7:469–485.

59. **Himelstein-Braw R, Byskov AG, Peters H, et al.** Follicular atresia in the infant human ovary. *J Reprod Fertil* 1976;46:55–59.

60. **Wassarman PM, Albertini DF.** The mammalian ovum. In: **Knobil E, Neill JD,** eds. *The physiology of reproduction.* New York: Raven Press, 1994:240–244.

61. **Gondos B, Bhiralcus P, Hobel CJ.** Ultrastructural observations on germ cells in human fetal ovaries. *Am J Obstet Gynecol* 1971;110:644–652.

62. **Tsafriri A, Dekel N, Bar-Ami S.** A role of oocyte maturation inhibitor in follicular regulation of oocyte maturation. *J Reprod Fertil* 1982;64:541–551.

63. **Halpin DMG, Jones A, Fink G, et al.** Post-natal ovarian follicle development in hypogonadal (HPG) and normal mice and associated changes in the hypothalamic-pituitary axis. *J Reprod Fertil* 1986;77:287–296.

64. **Vermesh M, Kletzky OA.** Longitudinal evaluation of the luteal phase and its transition into the follicular phase. *J Clin Endocrinol Metab* 1987;65:653–658.

65. **Erickson GF, Magoffin DA, Dyer CA, et al.** Ovarian androgen producing cells: a review of structure/function relationships. *Endocr Rev* 1985;6:371–399.

66. **Erickson GF.** An analysis of follicle development and ovum maturation. *Semin Reprod Endocrinol* 1986;46: 55–59.

67. **Halpin DMG, Jones A, Fink G, et al.** Post-natal ovarian follicle development in hypogonadal (HPG) and normal mice and associated changes in the hypothalamic-pituitary axis. *J Reprod Fertil* 1986;77:287–296.

68. **Ryan KJ, Petro Z.** Steroid biosynthesis of human ovarian granulosa and thecal cells. *J Clin Endocrinol Metab* 1966;26:46–52.

69. **Kobayashi M, Nakano R, Ooshima A.** Immunohistochemical localization of pituitary gonadotropin and gonadal steroids confirms the two cells two gonadotropins hypothesis of steroidogenesis in the human ovary. *J Endocrinol* 1990;126:483–488.

70. **Yamoto M, Shima K, Nakano R.** Gonadotropin receptors in human ovarian follicles and corpora lutea throughout the menstrual cycle. *Horm Res* 1992;37[Suppl 1]:5–11.

71. **Hseuh AJ, Adashi EY, Jones PB, et al.** Hormonal regulation of the differentiation of cultured ovarian granulosa cells. *Endocr Rev* 1984;5:76–127.

72. **McNatty KP, Makris A, Reinhold BN, et al.** Metabolism of androstenedione by human ovarian tissues in vitro with particular reference to reductase and aromatase activity. *Steroids* 1979;34:429–443.

73. **Hillier SG, Van Den Boogard AMJ, Reichert LE, et al.** Intraovarian sex steroid acute hormone interaction and the regulation of follicular maturation: aromatization of androgens by human granulosa cells in vitro. *J Clin Endocrinol Metab* 1980;50:640–647.

74. **Chappel SC, Resko JA, Norman RL, et al.** Studies on rhesus monkeys on the site where estrogen inhibits gonadotropins: delivery of 17 β-estradiol to the hypothalamus and pituitary gland. *J Clin Endocrinol Metab* 1981;52:1–8.

75. **Chabab A, Hedon B, Arnal F, et al.** Follicular steroids in relation to oocyte development in human ovarian stimulation protocols. *Hum Reprod* 1986;1:449–454.

76. **Young SR, Jaffe RB.** Strength-duration characteristics of estrogen effects on gonadotropin response to gonadotropin-releasing hormone in women: II. Effects of varying concentrations of estradiol. *J Clin Endocrinol Metab* 1976;42:432–442.

77. **Pauerstein CJ, Eddy CA, Croxatto HD, et al.** Temporal relationship of estrogen, progesterone, luteinizing hormone levels to ovulation in women and infra-human primates. *Am J Obstet Gynecol* 1978;130:876–886.

78. **World Health Organization Task Force Investigators.** Temporal relationship between ovulation and defined changes in the concentration of plasma estradiol-17β luteinizing hormone, follicle stimulating hormone and progesterone. *Am J Obstet Gynecol* 1980;138:383.

79. **Hoff JD, Quigley NE, Yen SSC.** Hormonal dynamics in mid-cycle: a re-evaluation. *J Clin Endocrinol Metab* 1983;57:792–796.

80. **Demura R, Suzuki T, Tajima S, et al.** Human plasma free activin and inhibin levels during the menstrual cycle. *J Clin Endocrinol Metab* 1993;76:1080–1082.

81. **Groome NP, Illingworth PG, O'Brien M, et al.** Measurement of dimeric inhibin B throughout the human menstrual cycle. *J Clin Endocrinol Metab* 1996;81:1401–1405.

82. **McLachlan RI, Robertson DM, Healy DL, et al.** Circulating immunoreactive inhibin levels during the normal human menstrual cycle. *J Clin Endocrinol Metab* 1987;65:954–961.

83. **Buckler HM, Healy DL, Burger HG.** Purified FSH stimulates inhibin production from the human ovary. *J Endocrinol* 1989;122:279–285.

84. **Ling N, Ying S, Ueno N, et al.** Pituitary FSH is released by heterodimer of the β-subunits from the two forms of inhibin. *Nature* 1986;321:779–782.

85. **Braden TD, Conn PM.** Activin-A stimulates the synthesis of gonadotropin-releasing hormone receptors. *Endocrinology* 1992;130:2101–2105.

86. **Adashi EY.** Putative intraovarian regulators. *Semin Reprod Endocrinol* 1988;7:1–100.

87. **Yoshimura Y, Santulli R, Atlas SJ, et al.** The effects of proteolytic enzymes on in vitro ovulation in the rabbit. *Am J Obstet Gynecol* 1987;157:468–475.

88. **Yoshimura Y, Wallach EE.** Studies on the mechanism(s) of mammalian ovulation. *Fertil Steril* 1987;47: 22–34.

89. **Anasti JN, Kalantaridou SN, Kimzey LM, et al.** Human follicle fluid vascular endothelial growth factor concentrations are correlated with luteinization in spontaneously developing follicles. *Hum Reprod* 1998;13:1144–1147.

90. **Lenton EA, Landgren B, Sexton L.** Normal variation in the length of the luteal phase of the menstrual cycle: identification of the short luteal phase. *Br J Obstet Gynaecol* 1994;91:685.

91. **Scott R, Navot D, Hung-Ching L, et al.** A human in vivo model for the luteal placental shift. *Fertil Steril* 1991;56:481–484.

SECTION

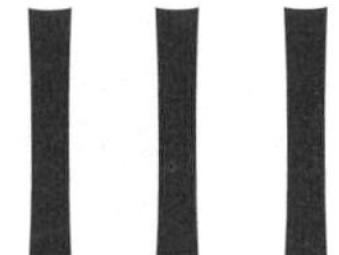

PREVENTIVE AND PRIMARY CARE

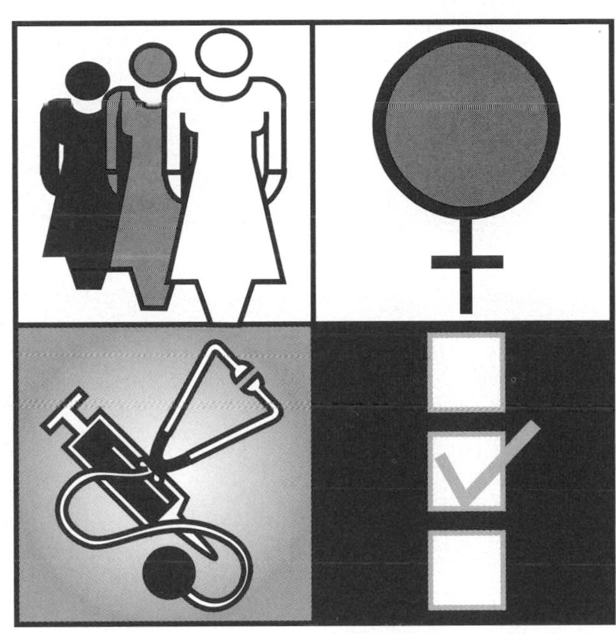

8 Preventive Health Care and Screening

Paula J. Adams Hillard

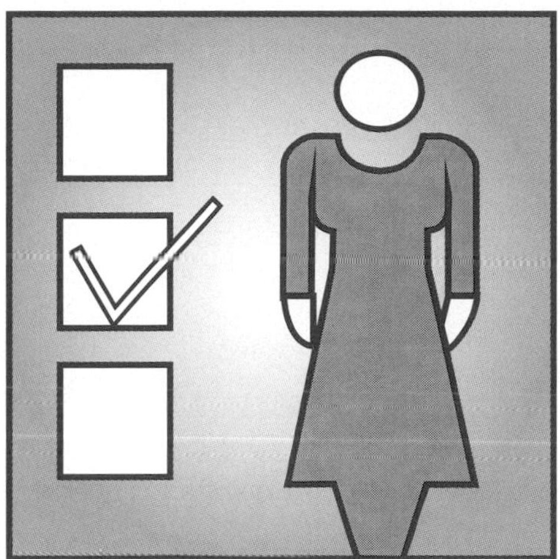

Although obstetrician-gynecologists traditionally focus on the management of illnesses and abnormal conditions, many provide care that is oriented toward health maintenance and prevention or early detection of disease. The value of preventive services is apparent in trends such as the reduced mortality rate from cervical cancer, in part resulting from the increased use of cervical cytology testing. Neonatal screening for phenylketonuria (PKU) and hypothyroidism are examples of effective mechanisms for prevention of mental retardation. Women often regard their gynecologist as their primary care provider; indeed, many women of reproductive age have had no other physician since childhood. In this role, some gynecologists include as a routine part of their practices screening for certain medical conditions, such as hypertension, diabetes mellitus, and thyroid disease, as well as management of those conditions in the absence of complications.

Some traditional aspects of gynecologic practice, such as family planning, can be considered preventive health care. Although hormone replacement therapy can be prescribed to relieve the relatively time-limited symptoms of menopause, it also offers long-term benefits in the prevention of osteoporosis. As primary care physicians, obstetrician-gynecologists provide ongoing care for women through all stages of their lives—from reproductive age to postmenopause. Preventive medical services encompass screening and counseling for a broad range of health behaviors and risks, including family planning, sexual practices, sexually transmitted diseases (STDs), smoking, alcohol and other drug use, diet, and exercise.

In recent years there has been increasing emphasis on women's health and gender-specific medicine. This has enabled obstetrician-gynecologists to become more knowledgeable about the pathophysiologic aspects of diseases in women and thus better equipped to manage them.

Gynecologist as Primary Care Provider

Primary preventive health care in obstetrics and gynecology has been defined as including the following elements (1):

1. The entry point to the health care system

2. Direct involvement in the patient's health care

3. Continuity in relationship between the physician and patient

4. Care managed with an awareness of the relationship of disease to the family structure

5. Dedication to long-term prevention and early detection of serious illness

6. Provision of general health care (i.e., concerned with diseases other than those of the reproductive tract)

7. Application of skill and judgment regarding consultation and referral, when required, for assurance of complete care by multiple health care providers

8. Availability on a 24-hour basis

In addition, the American College of Obstetricians and Gynecologists (ACOG) has outlined the components of primary preventive care as including the ability to (2):

1. Establish a physician-patient relationship that creates a health-promoting alliance, including helping patients to control their own health choices, to recognize the benefits of avoiding high-risk behavior, and to acquire the necessary attitudes and skills to change behaviors that place their health at risk.

2. Be familiar with the leading causes of death and morbidity within different age groups in order to incorporate a holistic approach to assessing patients' risks.

3. Apply the knowledge and skills needed to identify underlying problems, counsel patients, and educate patients, adapting to their individual needs, communication skills, age, race, sex, and socioeconomic status.

4. Encourage patient follow-up.

5. Incorporate a team approach to patient care, using the expertise of nurses, health educators, other allied health professionals, and relevant social services.

According to ACOG, primary care emphasizes health maintenance, preventive services, early detection of disease, availability of services, and continuity of care. The obstetrician-gynecologist often serves as a primary medical resource and counselor to the patient and her family for a wide range of medical conditions. However, all clinicians, regardless of the extent of their training, have limitations to their knowledge and skills and should seek consultation at appropriate times for the benefit of their patients in providing both reproductive and nonreproductive care (3).

Guidelines for primary and preventive services have been issued by a number of medical bodies (4,5): the American Academy of Family Physicians (6), the U.S. Preventive Services Task Force (7), and the American Medical Association (8). The guidelines from various organizations differ somewhat in their specifics, and a national guideline clearinghouse for evidence-based clinical practice guidelines, sponsored by the Agency for Healthcare Policy and Research, is available to provide comparisons between guidelines for a given medical condition or intervention (9). Books specific to the provision of primary health care by obstetrician-gynecologists are now available (10–16).

In 1998 in the United States, there were approximately 500 million visits by women to ambulatory medical care providers. Eighteen percent of the visits (76 million) were made to gynecologists (17). Forty-six percent of ambulatory visits were made by individuals between the ages of 15 and 44 years (17). The most frequently cited reason for an office visit to an obstetrician-gynecologist by women older than 15 years of age was routine prenatal examination. The second most frequently cited reason was general medical examination. For women in this age group, obstetrician-gynecologists provided more general medical examinations than general and family practitioners and internists combined. For women of reproductive age (15 to 44 years), gynecologists provided nearly 4 times as many general medical examinations than did general and family practitioners, and almost 12 times as many examinations as internists (18).

In a survey of practicing physicians who were asked to categorize themselves as a primary care physician, a specialist, or a consultant, nearly one-half of obstetricians and gynecologists (48%) considered themselves to be primary care providers (18). Gynecologists younger than 35 years of age, those in the South Atlantic census region, and those who were paid by hospitals and medical centers were more likely to consider themselves primary care providers. In a 1995 survey of those completing their residencies, 87% of the respondents believed that obstetrics and gynecology was primary care and 85% planned to practice accordingly after residency (19). However, only one-half of residency training directors support the inclusion of 6 months of primary care in the residency education program (20).

Obstetricians and gynecologists are less likely than other primary care physicians to refer their patients. Data compiled by the National Center for Health Statistics (NCHS) indicate that gynecologists had a referral rate of 4%, general internists 7.3%, and family and general practitioners 7.3% (21).

In 1993, ACOG commissioned a Gallup poll to assess how women viewed the care provided by their obstetrician-gynecologists (22). When compared with other physicians, obstetrician-gynecologists were more likely to perform cervical cytology testing, pelvic examination, and breast examination than were other physicians. Obstetrician-gynecologists were as likely as other physicians to have checked blood pressure and referred patients for mammography. When compared with other physicians, they were slightly less likely to have checked cholesterol levels. Obstetrician-gynecologists are somewhat more likely than other physicians to have discussed family planning, preconception issues, and STDs, including human immunodeficiency virus. Other physicians were more likely to discuss medication use than were obstetrician-gynecologists. Other physicians were as likely as obstetrician-gynecologists to have discussed diet and exercise, smoking, alcohol use, hormone replacement therapy, osteoporosis, emotional problems, illegal drug use, and physical abuse (22). More than one-half of all women who reported seeing an obstetrician-gynecologist considered him or her to be their primary physician. As expected, the percentage was highest among women aged 18 to 29 years (69%) and lowest among women older than 40 years (45%) (22).

Approaches to Preventive Care

Currently in health care, there is a shift from a focus on disease to a focus on prevention. Efforts are underway to promote effective screening measures that can have a beneficial effect on public and individual health. Following is a brief description of programs developed by ACOG, the U.S. Preventive Services Task Force, and the American Medical Association to provide guidelines for preventive care.

Guidelines for Primary and Preventive Care

The initial evaluation involves a complete history, physical examination, routine and indicated laboratory studies, evaluation and counseling, appropriate immunizations, and relevant interventions. Risk factors should be identified and arrangements should be made for

Table 8.1. Leading Causes of Death by Age Group

Ages 13–18 years

1. Motor vehicle accidents
2. Homicide
3. Suicide
4. Cancer
5. All other accidents and adverse effects
6. Diseases of the heart
7. Congenital anomalies
8. Chronic obstructive pulmonary diseases

Ages 19–39 years

1. Accidents and adverse effects
2. Cancer
3. Human immunodeficiency virus infection
4. Diseases of the heart
5. Homicide
6. Suicide
7. Cerebrovascular disease
8. Chronic liver disease and cirrhosis

Ages 40–64 years

1. Cancer
2. Diseases of the heart
3. Cerebrovascular diseases
4. Accidents and adverse effects
5. Chronic obstructive pulmonary disease
6. Diabetes mellitus
7. Chronic liver disease and cirrhosis
8. Pneumonia and influenza

Ages 65 years and older

1. Diseases of the heart
2. Cancer
3. Cerebrovascular disease
4. Chronic obstructive pulmonary diseases
5. Pneumonia and influenza
6. Diabetes mellitus
7. Accidents and adverse effects
8. Alzheimer's disease

From American College of Obstetricians and Gynecologists Committee on Gynecologic Practice. Primary and preventive care: periodic assessments Washington, DC: ACOG; 2000; Committee Opinion No. 246, with permission.

continuing care or referral, as needed. The leading causes of death and morbidity within different age groups are listed in Tables 8.1 and 8.2 (4). Subsequent care should follow a specific schedule, yearly or as appropriate based on the patient's needs and age. The ACOG recommendations for periodic evaluation, screening, and counseling by age groups are shown in Tables 8.3–8.6. These tables also include recommendations for patients who have high-risk factors that require targeted screening or treatment (7). High-risk factors are listed in Table 8.7. Recommendations for immunizations are included in Table 8.8.

Guide to Clinical Preventive Services

The U.S. Preventive Services Task Force, commissioned in 1984, was a 20-member non-governmental panel of experts in primary care medicine, epidemiology, and public health. Initial and subsequent reviews and recommendations are being revised and released (23). In 1976, a similar panel was convened in Canada—the Canadian Task Force on the Periodic Health Examination—which issued its report in 1979 (24). The charge of both panels was to develop recommendations for the appropriate use of preventive interventions based on a systematic review of evidence of clinical effectiveness.

Table 8.2. Leading Causes of Morbidity by Age Group

Ages 13–18 years
Acne
Asthma
Chlamydia
Depression
Dermatitis
Headaches
Infective, viral, and parasitic diseases
Influenza
Injuries
Nose, throat, ear, and upper respiratory infections
Sexual assault
Sexually transmitted diseases
Urinary tract infections
Ages 19–39 years
Asthma
Back symptoms
Breast disease
Deformity or orthopedic impairment
Depression
Diabetes
Gynecologic disorders
Headache or migraines
Hypertension
Infective, viral, and parasitic diseases
Influenza
Injuries
Nose, throat, ear, and upper respiratory infections
Sexual assault and domestic violence
Sexually transmitted diseases
Skin rash or dermatitis
Substance abuse
Urinary tract infections
Vaginitis
Ages 40–64 years
Arthritis or osteoarthritis
Asthma
Back symptoms
Breast disease
Cardiovascular disease
Carpal tunnel syndrome
Deformity or orthopedic impairment
Depression
Diabetes
Headache
Hypertension
Infective, viral, and parasitic diseases
Influenza
Injuries
Menopause
Nose, throat, and upper respiratory infections
Obesity
Skin conditions or dermatitis
Substance abuse
Urinary tract infections
Urinary tract (other conditions, including urinary incontinence)
Vision impairment

Table 8.2.—*continued*

Ages 65 years and older
Arthritis or osteoarthritis
Back symptoms
Breast cancer
Chronic obstructive pulmonary diseases
Cardiovascular disease
Deformity or orthopedic impairment
Degeneration of macula retinae and posterior pole
Diabetes
Hearing and vision impairment
Hypertension
Hypothyroidism and other thyroid disease
Influenza
Nose, throat, and upper respiratory infections
Osteoporosis
Skin lesions, dermatoses, dermatitis
Urinary tract infections
Urinary tract (other conditions, including urinary incontinence)
Vertigo

From American College of Obstetricians and Gynecologists Committee on Gynecologic Practice. Primary and preventive care: periodic assessments Washington, DC: ACOG; 2000; Committee Opinion No. 246, with permission.

Table 8.3. Periodic Assessment Ages 13–18 Years

Screening	***Evaluation and Counseling***
History	**Sexuality**
Reason for visit	Development
Health status: medical, surgical, family	High-risk behaviors
Dietary/nutrition assessment	Preventing unwanted/unintended pregnancy
Physical activity	—Postponing sexual involvement
Use of complementary and alternative medicine	—Contraceptive options
Tobacco, alcohol, other drug use	Sexually transmitted diseases
Abuse/neglect	—Partner selection
Sexual practices	—Barrier protection
Physical examination	**Fitness and nutrition**
Height	Dietary/nutrition assessment (including eating disorders)
Weight	Exercise: discussion of program
Blood pressure	Folic acid supplementation (0.4 mg/d)
Secondary sexual characteristics (Tanner staging)	Calcium intake
Pelvic examination (yearly when sexually active or beginning at age 18 years) Skin[a]	
Laboratory testing	**Psychosocial evaluation**
Periodic	
Pap testing (yearly when sexually active or beginning at age 18 years)	Interpersonal/family relationships

Table 8.3.—*continued*

	Sexual identity
	Personal goal development
	Behavioral/learning disorders
	Abuse/neglect
	Satisfactory school experience
	Peer relationships
High-risk groups [a]	**Cardiovascular risk factors**
Hemoglobin level assessment	Family history
Bacteriuria testing	Hypertension
Sexually transmitted disease testing	Dyslipidemia
Human immunodeficiency virus testing	Obesity
Genetic testing/counseling	Diabetes mellitus
Rubella titer assessment	
Tuberculosis skin testing	
Lipid profile assessment	
Fasting glucose testing	
Cholesterol testing	
Hepatitis C virus testing	
Colorectal cancer screening[b]	
	Health/risk behaviors
	Hygiene (including dental); fluoride supplementation
	Injury prevention
	—Safety belts and helmets
	—Recreational hazards
	—Firearms
	—Hearing
	Skin exposure to ultraviolet rays
	Suicide: depressive symptoms
	Tobacco, alcohol, other drug use

[a]See Table 8.7.
[b]Only for those with a family history of familial adenomatous polyposis or 8 years after the start of pancolitis. For a more detailed discussion of colorectal cancer screening, see **Byers T, Levin B, Rothenberger D, et al.** American Cancer Society guidelines for screening and surveillance for early detection of colorectal polyps and cancer: update 1997. American Cancer Society Detection and Treatment Advisory Group on Colorectal Cancer. *CA Cancer J Clin 1997*;47:154–160.
From American College of Obstetricians and Gynecologists Committee on Gynecologic Practice. Primary and preventive care: periodic assessments Washington, DC: ACOG; 2000; Committee Opinion No. 246, with permission.

The task force used several criteria for selecting conditions to evaluate, including the burden of suffering posed by a given condition, its prevalence (proportion of the population affected), and its incidence (number of new cases per year) (23). The task force reviewed only those preventive services that would be provided for asymptomatic individuals. Primary preventive measures are those that involve intervention before the disease develops, for example, quitting smoking, increasing physical activity, eating a healthy diet, quitting

Table 8.4. Periodic Assessment Ages 19–39 Years

Screening	*Evaluation and Counseling*
History	**Sexuality**
Reason for visit	High-risk behaviors
Health status: medical, surgical, family	Contraceptive options for prevention of unwanted pregnancy
Dietary/nutrition assessment	Preconceptional and genetic counseling for desired pregnancy
Physical activity	Sexually transmitted diseases
Use of complementary and alternative medicine	—Partner selection
Tobacco, alcohol, other drug use	—Barrier protection
Abuse/neglect	Sexual function
Sexual practices	
Urinary and fecal incontinence	
Physical examination	**Fitness and nutrition**
Height	Dietary/nutrition assessment
Weight	Exercise: discussion of program
Blood pressure	Folic acid supplementation (0.4 mg/d)
Neck: adenopathy, thyroid	Calcium intake
Breasts	
Abdomen	
Pelvic examination	
Skin[a]	
Laboratory testing	**Psychosocial evaluation**
Periodic	
Pap testing (physician and patient discretion after three consecutive normal tests if low risk)	Interpersonal/family relationships
	Domestic violence
	Work satisfaction
	Lifestyle/stress
	Sleep disorders
High-risk groups [a]	**Cardiovascular risk factors**
Hemoglobin level assessment	Family history
Bacteriuria testing	Hypertension
Mammography	Dyslipidemia
Fasting glucose testing	Obesity
Cholesterol testing	Diabetes mellitus
Sexually transmitted disease testing	Lifestyle
Human immunodeficiency virus testing	
Genetic testing/counseling	

Table 8.4.—*continued*

Rubella titer assessment	
Tuberculosis skin testing	
Lipid profile assessment	
Thyroid-stimulating hormone testing	
Colonoscopy	
Hepatitis C virus testing	
Colorectal cancer screening	
	Health/risk behaviors
	Hygiene (including dental)
	Injury prevention
	—Safety belts and helmets
	—Occupational hazards
	—Recreational hazards
	—Firearms
	—Hearing
	Breast self-examination
	Chemoprophylaxis for breast cancer (for high-risk women ages 35 years or older)[b]
	Skin exposure to ultraviolet rays
	Suicide: depressive symptoms
	Tobacco, alcohol, other drug use

[a]See Table 8.7.
[b]The decision to use tamoxifen should be individualized. For a more detailed discussion of risk assessment and chemoprevention therapy, see American College of Obstetricians and Gynecologists. Tamoxifen and the prevention of breast cancer in high-risk women. ACOG Committee Opinion 224. Washington, DC: ACOG, 1999.
From American College of Obstetricians and Gynecologists Committee on Gynecologic Practice. Primary and preventive care: periodic assessments Washington, DC: ACOG; 2000; Committee Opinion No. 246, with permission.

alcohol and other drug use, using seat belts, and receiving immunizations. Secondary preventive measures are those used to identify and treat asymptomatic persons who have risk factors or preclinical disease but in whom the disease itself has not become clinically apparent. Examples of secondary preventive measures are well known in gynecology: screening mammography and cervical cytology testing.

The Preventive Services Task Force analyzed the effectiveness of various screening measures and tests. For screening tests, they assessed the accuracy of the test, including its sensitivity, specificity, and positive and negative predictive values. The task force also reviewed the methodologic quality of the studies. Because the design of a study influences the interpretation of the data and the weight given to its results, the U.S. Preventive Services Task Force established a hierarchy of the types of studies available to assess the effectiveness of various interventions. This hierarchy is listed in Table 8.9. The strength of the task force's recommendations regarding the value of a screening or preventive intervention is based on the quality of the evidence available. In some circumstances, there is good evidence to recommend for or against an intervention, whereas in others, there is only fair or poor evidence regarding the effectiveness of an intervention. The strength of the task force's recommendations were graded according to a system used by the Canadian Task Force on the Periodic Health Examination (24) (Table 8.10).

Table 8.5. Periodic Assessment Ages 40–64 Years

Screening	*Evaluation and Counseling*
History	**Sexuality**[b]
Reason for visit	High-risk behaviors
Health status: medical, surgical, family	Contraceptive options for prevention of unwanted pregnancy
Dietary/nutrition assessment	Sexually transmitted diseases
Physical activity	—Partner selection
Use of complementary and alternative medicine	—Barrier protection
Tobacco, alcohol, other drug use	Sexual functioning
Abuse/neglect	
Sexual practices	
Urinary and fecal incontinence	
Physical examination	**Fitness and nutrition**
Height	Dietary/nutrition assessment
Weight	Exercise: discussion of program
Blood pressure	Folic acid supplementation (0.4 mg/d before age 50 years)
Oral cavity	Calcium intake
Neck: adenopathy, thyroid	
Breasts, axillae	
Abdomen	
Pelvic examination	
Skin[a]	
Laboratory testing	**Psychosocial evaluation**
Periodic	
Pap testing (physician and patient discretion after three consecutive normal tests if low risk)	Family relationships
Mammography (every 1–2 years until age 50 years, yearly beginning at age 50 years)	Domestic violence
Cholesterol testing (every 5 years beginning at age 45 years)	Work satisfaction
Yearly fecal occult blood testing plus flexible sigmoidoscopy every 5 years *or* colonoscopy every 10 years *or* double contrast barium enema (DCBE) every 5–10 years, with digital rectal examination performed at the time of each screening sigmoidoscopy, colonoscopy, or DCBE (beginning at age 50 years)	Retirement planning
Fasting glucose testing (every 3 years after age 45 years)	Lifestyle/stress
	Sleep disorders

Table 8.5.—*continued*

High-risk groups[a]	**Cardiovascular risk factors**
Hemoglobin level assessment	Family history
Bacteriuria testing	Hypertension
Fasting glucose testing	Dyslipidemia
Sexually transmitted disease testing	Obesity
Human immunodeficiency virus testing	Diabetes mellitus
Tuberculosis skin testing	Lifestyle
Lipid profile assessment	
Thyroid-stimulating hormone testing	
Colonoscopy	
Hepatitis C virus testing	
Colorectal cancer screening	
	Health/risk behaviors
	Hygiene (including dental)
	Hormone replacement therapy
	Injury prevention
	—Safety belts and helmets
	—Occupational hazards
	—Recreational hazards
	—Sports involvement
	—Firearms
	—Hearing
	Breast self-examination
	Chemoprophylaxis for breast cancer (for high-risk women)[c]
	Skin exposure to ultraviolet rays
	Suicide: depressive symptoms
	Tobacco, alcohol, other drug use

[a]See Table 8.7.
[b]Preconceptional and genetic counseling is appropriate for certain women in this age group.
[c]The decision to use tamoxifen should be individualized. For a more detailed discussion of risk assessment and chemoprevention therapy, see American College of Obstetricians and Gynecologists. Tamoxifen and the prevention of breast cancer in high-risk women. ACOG Committee Opinion 224. Washington, DC: ACOG, 1999.
From American College of Obstetricians and Gynecologists Committee on Gynecologic Practice. Primary and preventive care: periodic assessments Washington, DC: ACOG; 2000; Committee Opinion No. 246, with permission.

The U.S. Preventive Services Task Force drew a number of conclusions based on review of the data (7).

1. Interventions that address patients' personal health practices are vitally important.
2. The clinician and patient should share decision making.
3. Clinicians should be selective in ordering tests and providing preventive services.

Table 8.6. Periodic Assessment Age 65 Years and Older

Screening	*Evaluation and Counseling*
History	**Sexuality**
Reason for visit	Sexual functioning
Health status: medical, surgical, family	Sexual behaviors
Dietary/nutrition assessment	Sexually transmitted diseases
Physical activity	—Partner selection
Use of complementary and alternative medicine	—Barrier protection
Tobacco, alcohol, other drug use, and concurrent medication use	
Abuse/neglect	
Sexual practices	
Urinary and fecal incontinence	
Physical examination	**Fitness and nutrition**
Height	Dietary/nutrition assessment
Weight	Exercise: discussion of program
Blood pressure	Calcium intake
Oral cavity	
Neck: adenopathy, thyroid	
Breasts, axillae	
Abdomen	
Pelvic examination	
Skin[a]	
Laboratory testing	**Psychosocial evaluation**
Periodic	
Pap testing (physician and patient discretion after three consecutive normal tests if low risk)	Neglect/abuse
Urinalysis	Lifestyle/stress
Mammography	Depression/sleep disorders
Cholesterol testing (every 3–5 years before age 75 years)	Family relationships
Yearly fecal occult blood testing plus flexible sigmoidoscopy every 5 years *or* colonoscopy every 10 years *or* double contrast barium enema (DCBE) every 5–10 years, with digital rectal examination performed at the time of each screening sigmoidoscopy, colonoscopy, or DCBE	Work/retirement satisfaction
Fasting glucose testing (every 3 years after age 45 years)	
High-risk groups [a]	**Cardiovascular risk factors**
Hemoglobin level assessment	Hypertension
Sexually transmitted disease testing	Dyslipidemia
Human immunodeficiency virus testing	Obesity
Tuberculosis skin testing	Diabetes mellitus
Lipid profile assessment	Sedentary lifestyle

Table 8.6.— *continued*

Thyroid-stimulating hormone testing	
Colonoscopy	
Hepatitis C virus testing	
Colorectal cancer screening	
	Health/risk behaviors
	Hygiene (general and dental)
	Hormone replacement therapy
	Injury prevention
	—Safety belts and helmets
	—Prevention of falls
	—Occupational hazards
	—Recreational hazards
	—Firearms
	Visual acuity/glaucoma
	Hearing
	Breast self-examination
	Chemoprophylaxis for breast cancer (for high-risk women)[b]
	Skin exposure to ultraviolet rays
	Suicide: depressive symptoms
	Tobacco, alcohol, other drug use

[a]See Table 8.7.
[b]The decision to use tamoxifen should be individualized. For a more detailed discussion of risk assessment and chemoprevention therapy, see American College of Obstetricians and Gynecologists. Tamoxifen and the prevention of breast cancer in high-risk women. ACOG Committee Opinion 224. Washington, DC: ACOG, 1999.
From American College of Obstetricians and Gynecologists Committee on Gynecologic Practice. Primary and preventive care: periodic assessments Washington, DC: ACOG; 2000; Committee Opinion No. 246, with permission.

4. Clinicians must take every opportunity to deliver preventive services, especially to persons with limited access to care.

5. For some health problems, community-level interventions may be more effective than clinical preventive services.

The quality of clinical evidence also has been rated and published internationally by other medical groups using a rating system similar to that used by the U.S. Preventive Services Task Force (25). In one source, which is updated every 6 months and has a lag time of 5 to 9 months from search to publication, treatment effects are categorized as follows (25):

1. Beneficial

2. Likely to be beneficial

3. Trade-off between benefits and harms

4. Unknown effectiveness

Table 8.7. High-risk Factors

Intervention	*High-risk Factor*
Bacteriuria testing	Diabetes mellitus
Cholesterol testing	Familial lipid disorders; family history of premature coronary heart disease; history of coronary heart disease
Colorectal cancer screening[a]	Colorectal cancer or adenomatous polyps in first-degree relative younger than 60 years or in two or more first-degree relatives of any ages; family history of familial adenomatous polyposis or hereditary nonpolyposis colon cancer; history of colorectal cancer, adenomatous polyps, or inflammatory bowel disease
Fasting glucose testing	Obesity; first-degree relative with diabetes mellitus; member of a high-risk ethnic population (e.g., African American, Hispanic, Native American, Asian, Pacific Islander); have delivered a baby weighing more than 9 lb or history of gestational diabetes mellitus; hypertensive; high-density lipoprotein cholesterol level of at least 35 mg/dl; triglyceride level of at least 250 mg/dl; history of impaired glucose tolerance or impaired fasting glucose
Fluoride supplementation	Live in area with inadequate water fluoridation (<0.7 ppm)
Genetic testing/counseling	Exposure to teratogens; considering pregnancy at age 35 or older; patient, partner, or family member with history of genetic disorder or birth defect; African, Acadian, Eastern European Jewish, Mediterranean, or Southeast Asian ancestry
Hemoglobin level assessment	Caribbean, Latin American, Asian, Mediterranean, or African ancestry; history of excessive menstrual flow
Hepatitis A vaccination	International travelers; illegal drug users; people who work with nonhuman primates; chronic liver disease; clotting-factor disorders; sex partners of bisexual men; measles-, mumps-, and rubella nonimmune persons; food service workers; health care workers; day care workers
Hepatitis B vaccination	Intravenous drug users and their sexual contacts; recipients of clotting factor concentrates; occupational exposure to blood or blood products; patients and workers in dialysis units; persons with chronic renal or hepatic disease; household or sexual contact with hepatitis B virus carriers; history of sexual activity with multiple partners; history of sexual activity with sexually active homosexual or bisexual men; international travelers; residents and staff of institutions for the developmentally disabled and of correctional institutions
Hepatitis C virus (HCV) testing	History of injecting illegal drugs; recipients of clotting factor concentrates before 1987; chronic (long-term) hemodialysis; persistently abnormal alanine aminotransferase levels; recipient of blood from a donor who later tested positive for HCV infection; recipient of blood or blood-component transfusion or organ transplant before July 1992; occupational percutaneous or mucosal exposure to HCV-positive blood
Human immunodeficiency virus (HIV) testing	Seeking treatment for sexually transmitted diseases; drug use by injection; history of prostitution; past or present sexual partner who is HIV positive or bisexual or injects drugs; long-term residence or birth in an area with high prevalence of HIV infection; history of transfusion from 1978 to 1985; invasive cervical cancer; pregnancy. Offer to women seeking preconception care.

Table 8.7.—*continued*

Influenza vaccination	Anyone who wishes to reduce the chance of becoming ill with influenza; resident in long-term care facility; chronic cardiopulmonary disorders; metabolic diseases (e.g., diabetes mellitus, hemoglobinopathies, immunosuppression, renal dysfunction); health-care workers; day-care workers; pregnant women who will be in the second or third trimester during the epidemic season. Pregnant women with medical problems should be offered vaccination before the influenza season regardless of stage of pregnancy.
Lipid profile assessment	Elevated cholesterol level; history of parent or sibling with blood cholesterol of at least 240 mg/dl; first-degree relative with premature (<55 years of age for men, <65 years of age for women) coronary heart disease; diabetes mellitus; smoking habit
Mammography	Women who have had breast cancer or who have a first-degree relative (i.e., mother, sister, or daughter) or multiple other relatives who have a history of premenopausal breast or breast and ovarian cancer
Measles-mumps-rubella (MMR) vaccination	Adults born in 1957 or later should be offered vaccination (one dose of MMR) if there is no proof of immunity or documentation of a dose given after first birthday; persons vaccinated in 1963–1967 should be offered revaccination (2 doses); health care workers, students entering college, international travelers, and rubella-negative postpartum patients should be offered a second dose.
Pneumococcal vaccination	Chronic illness such as cardiovascular disease, pulmonary disease, diabetes mellitus, alcoholism, chronic liver disease, cerebrospinal fluid leaks, functional or anatomic asplenia; exposure to an environment where pneumococcal outbreaks have occurred; immunocompromised patients (e.g., HIV infection, hematologic or solid malignancies, chemotherapy, steroid therapy); pregnant patients with chronic illness. Revaccination after 5 years may be appropriate for certain high-risk groups.
Rubella titer assessment	Childbearing age and no evidence of immunity
Sexually transmitted disease (STD) testing	History of multiple sexual partners or a sexual partner with multiple contacts; sexual contact with persons with culture-proven STD; history of repeated episodes of STDs; attendance at clinics for STDs; routine screening for chlamydial and gonorrheal infection for all sexually active adolescents and other asymptomatic women at high risk for infection
Skin examination	Increased recreational or occupational exposure to sunlight; family or personal history of skin cancer; clinical evidence of precursor lesions
Thyroid-stimulating hormone testing	Strong family history of thyroid disease; autoimmune disease (evidence of subclinical hypothyroidism may be related to unfavorable lipid profiles)
Tuberculosis skin testing	Human immunodeficiency virus infection; close contact with persons known or suspected to have tuberculosis; medical risk factors known to increase risk of disease if infected; born in country with high tuberculosis prevalence; medically underserved; low income; alcoholism; intravenous drug use; resident of long-term care facility (e.g., correctional institutions, mental institutions, nursing homes and facilities); health professional working in high-risk health care facilities

Table 8.7.—*continued*

Varicella vaccination	All susceptible adults and adolescents, including health-care workers; household contacts of immunocompromised individuals; teachers; day care workers; residents and staff of institutional settings, colleges, prisons, or military installations; international travelers; nonpregnant women of childbearing age

[a]For a more detailed discussion of colorectal cancer screening, see **Byers T, Levin B, Rothenberger D, et al.** American Cancer Society guidelines for screening and surveillance for early detection of colorectal polyps and cancer: update 1997. American Cancer Society Detection and Treatment Advisory Group on Colorectal Cancer. *CA Cancer J Clin* 1997;47:154–160.

From American College of Obstetricians and Gynecologists Committee on Gynecologic Practice. Primary and preventive care: periodic assessments Washington, DC: ACOG; 2000; Committee Opinion No. 246, with permission.

Table 8.8. Immunizations

Ages 13–18 Years	*Ages 19–39 Years*	*Ages 40–64 Years*	*Age 65 Years and Older*
Periodic			
Tetanus-diphtheria booster (once between ages 11 years and 16 years) Hepatitis B vaccine (one series for those not previously immunized)	Tetanus-diphtheria booster (every 10 years)	Influenza vaccine (annually beginning at age 50 years) Tetanus-diphtheria booster (every 10 years)	Tetanus-diptheria booster (every 10 years) Influenza vaccine (annually) Pneumococcal vaccine (once)
High-risk groups[a]			
Influenza vaccine Hepatitis A vaccine Pneumococcal vaccine Measles-mumps-rubella vaccine Varicella vaccine	Measles-mumps-rubella vaccine Hepatitis A vaccine Hepatitis B vaccine Influenza vaccine Pneumococcal vaccine Varicella vaccine	Measles-mumps-rubella vaccine Hepatitis A vaccine Hepatitis B vaccine Influenza vaccine Pneumococcal vaccine Varicella vaccine	Hepatitis A vaccine Hepatitis B vaccine Varicella vaccine

[a]See Table 8.7.

From American College of Obstetricians and Gynecologists Committee on Gynecologic Practice. Primary and preventive care: periodic assessments Washington, DC: ACOG; 2000; Committee Opinion No. 246, with permission.

Table 8.9. Quality of Evidence—U.S. Preventive Services Task Force

I.	Evidence obtained from at least one properly designed randomized, controlled trial.
II-1.	Evidence obtained from well-designed controlled trials without randomization.
II-2.	Evidence obtained from well-designed cohort or case-control analytic studies, preferably from more than one center or research group.
II-3.	Evidence obtained from multiple time series with or without the intervention. Dramatic results in uncontrolled experiments (such as the results of the introduction of penicillin treatment in the 1940s) could also be regarded as this type of evidence.
III.	Opinions of respected authorities, based on clinical experience, descriptive studies, or reports of expert committees.

From **Canadian Task Force on the Periodic Health Examination.** The periodic health examination. *CMAJ* 1979;121:1193–254, with permission.

Table 8.10. The Task Force Graded the *Strength of Recommendations* for or Against Preventive Interventions as Follows

Strength of Recommendations
A: There is good evidence to support the recommendation that the condition be specifically considered in a periodic health examination.
B: There is fair evidence to support the recommendation that the condition be specifically considered in a periodic health examination.
C: There is insufficient evidence to recommend for or against the inclusion of the condition in a periodic health examination, but recommendations may be made on other grounds.
D: There is fair evidence to support the recommendation that the condition be excluded from consideration in a periodic health examination.
E: There is good evidence to support the recommendation that the condition be excluded from consideration in a periodic health examination.

U.S. Preventive Services Task Force. *Guide to Clinical Preventive Services,* 2nd ed. Baltimore: Williams & Wilkins, 1996.

5. Unlikely to be beneficial

6. Likely to be ineffective or harmful

Other international efforts to categorize the effectiveness of treatments include the Cochrane Library, which produces and publishes high-quality systematic reviews of controlled trials (26). The Cochrane Library provides searchable databases available online and through institutional purchase of licenses. Evidence-based guidelines are published in journals available in print and online, by discipline (i.e., medicine, mental health, and nursing).

Guidelines For Adolescent Preventive Services

Around the same time that clinicians were evaluating the primary health care needs of adults, clinicians who practice adolescent medicine (with backgrounds in pediatrics, internal medicine, family medicine, gynecology, nursing, psychology, nutrition, and other professions) recognized that the guidelines for adult and pediatric health services did not always fit the needs and health risks of adolescence. Neither the ACOG Guidelines for Primary Preventive Care (4) nor the U.S. Preventive Services Task Force recommendations (7) are sufficiently comprehensive or focused on this age group, although both documents include many important aspects of adolescent health care. The American Medical Association, with the assistance of a national scientific advisory board, developed the Guidelines for Adolescent Preventive Services (GAPS) in response to this perceived need for recommendations for delivering comprehensive adolescent preventive services (8,27).

Obstetrician-gynecologists typically see adolescents in crisis, to provide care for unintended pregnancies or STDs, including pelvic inflammatory disease. The need for preventing these crises is evident. The GAPS report extends the framework of services provided to adolescents. The impetus for developing GAPS was the belief that a fundamental change in the delivery of adolescent health services was necessary. Gynecologists could easily provide most, if not all, of the recommended services; annual preventive visits to a gynecologist might well lead to the prevention of gynecologic health problems. There are numerous opportunities for primary preventive care of adolescents in a gynecologist's office.

The GAPS report includes 24 recommendations (Table 8.11). These recommendations address the delivery of health care, focus on the use of health guidance to promote the health and well-being of adolescents and their families, promote the use of screening to identify conditions that occur relatively frequently in adolescents and cause significant suffering either during adolescence or later in life, and provide guidelines for immunizations for the primary prevention of specific infectious diseases (8).

Table 8.11. Guidelines for Adolescent Preventive Services

1.	From ages 11 to 21 years, all adolescents should have an annual routine health visit.
2.	Preventive services should be age and developmentally appropriate, and they should be sensitive to individual and sociocultural differences.
3.	Physicians should establish office policies regarding confidential care for adolescents and how parents will be involved in that care. These policies should be made clear to adolescent and the parents.
4.	Parents or other adult caregivers of adolescents should receive health guidance at least once during early adolescence, once during middle adolescence and, preferably, once during late adolescence.
5.	All adolescents should receive health guidance annually to promote a better understanding of their physical growth, psychosocial and psychosexual development, and the importance of becoming actively involved in decisions regarding their health care.
6.	All adolescents should receive health guidance annually to promote the reduction of injuries.
7.	All adolescents should receive health guidance annually about dietary habits, including the benefits of a healthy diet, ways to achieve a healthy diet, and safe weight management.
8.	All adolescents should receive health guidance annually about the benefits of exercise and should be encouraged to engage in safe exercise on a regular basis.
9.	All adolescents should receive health guidance annually regarding responsible sexual behaviors, including abstinence. Latex condoms to prevent sexually transmitted diseases (STDs) (including human immunodeficiency virus [HIV] infection) and appropriate methods of birth control should be made available with instructions on how to use them effectively.
10.	All adolescents should receive health guidance annually to promote avoidance of the use of tobacco, alcohol, abusable substances, and anabolic steroids.
11.	All adolescents should be screened annually for hypertension according to the protocol developed by the National Heart, Lung, and Blood Institute Second Task Force on Blood Pressure Control in Children (18).
12.	Selected adolescents should be screened to determine their risk of developing hyperlipidemia and adult coronary heart disease following the protocol by the Expert Panel on Blood Cholesterol Levels in Children and Adolescents (19).
13.	All adolescents should be screened annually for eating disorders and obesity by determining weight and stature and asking about body image and dieting patterns.
14.	All adolescents should be asked annually about their use of tobacco products, including cigarettes and smokeless tobacco.
15.	All adolescents should be asked annually about their use of alcohol and other abusable substances and about their use of over-the-counter or prescription drugs for nonmedical purposes, including anabolic steroids.
16.	All adolescents should be asked annually about involvement in sexual behaviors that may result in unintended pregnancies and STDs, including HIV infection.
17.	Sexually active adolescents should be screened for STDs.
18.	Adolescents at risk for HIV infection should be offered confidential HIV screening with the enzyme-linked immunosorbent assay and confirmatory testing.
19.	Female adolescents who are sexually active or any female 18 years of age or older should be screened annually for cervical cancer by use of a Papanicolaou (Pap) test.
20.	All adolescents should be asked annually about behaviors or emotions that indicate recurrent or severe depression or risk of suicide.
21.	All adolescents should be asked annually about a history of emotional, physical, and sexual abuse.
22.	All adolescents should be asked annually about learning or school problems.

Table 8.11.—*continued*

23. Adolescents should receive a tuberculin skin test if they have been exposed to active tuberculosis, have lived in a homeless shelter, have been incarcerated, have lived in or come from an area with a high prevalence of tuberculosis, or currently work in a health care setting.

24. All adolescents should receive prophylactic immunizations according to the guidelines established by the federally convened Advisory Committee on Immunization Practices: a bivalent tetanus-diphtheria vaccine 10 years after their previous diphtheria vaccination (usually 5 to 66 years old). All adolescents should receive a second trivalent measles-mumps-rubella vaccination, unless there is documentation of two vaccinations earlier during childhood. A measles-mumps-rubella vaccination should not be given to adolescents who are pregnant—susceptible adolescents who engage in high-risk behaviors should be vaccinated against hepatitis B virus. This includes adolescents who have had more than one sexual partner during the previous 6 months, have exchanged sex for drugs or money, are males who have engaged in sex with other males, or have used intravenous drugs. Widespread use of the hepatitis B vaccine is encouraged because risk factors are often not easily identifiable among adolescents.

From **Elster AB, Kuznets NJ.** *AMA Guidelines for adolescent preventive services (GAPS): recommendations and rationale.* Baltimore: Williams & Wilkins, 1994:1–191.

The GAPS recommendations stem from the conclusion that the current health threats to adolescents are predominantly behavioral rather than biomedical, that more of today's adolescents are involved in health behaviors with the potential for serious consequences, that today's adolescents are involved in health-risk behaviors at younger ages than previous generations, that many adolescents engage in multiple health-risk behaviors, and that most adolescents engage in at least some type of behavior that threatens their health and well-being (8). Gynecologists are in a good position to detect high-risk behaviors and to determine whether multiple risk-taking behaviors exist; for example, the early initiation of sexual activity and unsafe sexual practices are associated with substance use (28). Adolescents who are sexually active are much more likely to have used alcohol (6.3 times greater risk), 4 times more likely to have used drugs other than marijuana, and nearly 10 times more likely to have been a passenger in a motor vehicle with a driver who was using drugs than are adolescents who are not sexually active (29). Thus, by being aware of comorbidities, gynecologists can screen for these behaviors and potentially intervene before there are serious harmful health consequences.

ACOG has issued guidelines that build on the GAPS recommendations in recognition of the role that obstetrician-gynecologists potentially could play in providing preventive services for adolescents (5). These guidelines suggest an initial visit (not necessarily examination) to the obstetrician-gynecologist for health guidance, screening, and the provision of preventive health care service between the ages of 13 and 15 years (30) and subsequent annual preventive health care visits (5).

Counseling for Health Maintenance

During periodic assessments, patients should be counseled about preventive care depending on their age and risk factors. **Obesity, smoking, and alcohol abuse are associated with preventable problems that can have major long-term impacts on health.** Thus, patients should be counseled about smoking cessation and moderation in alcohol use and directed to appropriate community resources as necessary. Positive health behaviors, such as eating a healthy diet and engaging in regular exercise, should be reinforced. Adjustments may be necessary based on the presence of risk factors and the woman's current lifestyle and condition. Efforts should focus on weight control, cardiovascular fitness, and reduction of risk factors associated with cardiovascular disease and diabetes (30–33).

Nutrition

Patients should be given general nutritional information and referred to other professionals if they have special needs (34). Assessment of the patient's body mass index (weight [in

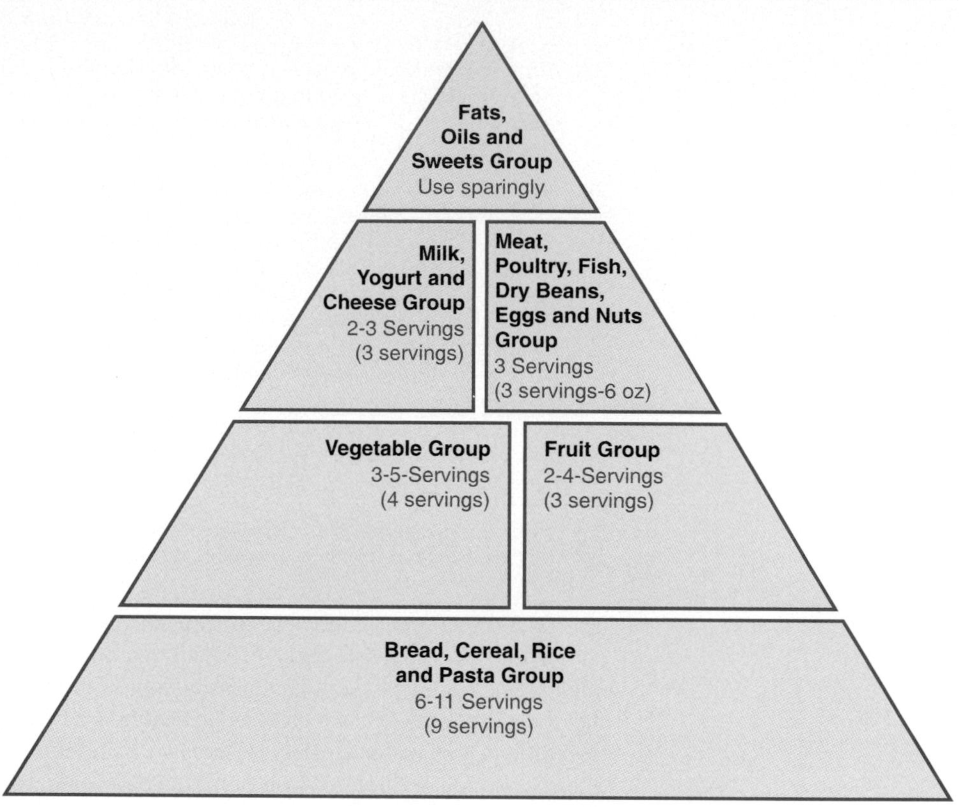

Figure 8.1 The Food Guide Pyramid. A Guide to Daily Food Choices. This is a guide to help men and nonpregnant women choose foods that will give them the nutrients they need. Because a pregnant woman needs extra calories, she should get at least the number of servings shown in parentheses after the standard servings.

kilograms] divided by height [in meters] squared [kilograms per square meter]) will give valuable information about the patient's nutritional status. Patients who are 20% above or below the normal range require evaluation and counseling and should be assessed for systemic disease or an eating disorder.

Central obesity—measured as waist-to-hip ratio—is a risk factor for coronary heart disease and some forms of cancer. When the waist-to-hip ratio exceeds 0.76, there is a greater relative risk of death from cancer or cardiovascular disease in women aged 55 to 69 years.

The Food Guide Pyramid developed by the U.S. Department of Agriculture helps women choose food from five groups to provide needed nutrients (Fig. 8.1) (35). The pyramid is based on the need to eat a variety of foods to get adequate energy, protein, vitamins, minerals, and fiber. The diet portrayed is high in vegetables, fruits, and grain products.

Fiber content of the diet is being studied for its potential role in the prevention of several disorders, particularly colon cancer. Currently, it is recommended that the average diet contain 20 to 30 g of fiber per day. Foods high in dietary fiber include whole-grain breads and cereals, green and yellow vegetables, citrus fruits, and some legumes.

Adequate calcium intake is important in the prevention of osteoporosis. A postmenopausal woman should ingest 1,500 mg/day. Adolescents require 1,300 mg/day. There is no evidence that moderate caffeine intake causes osteoporosis when calcium intake is inadequate. Because it is difficult to ingest an adequate amount of calcium daily in an average diet, supplements may be required.

The Centers for Disease Control and Prevention has recommended that women of reproductive age who are capable of becoming pregnant take supplemental folic acid (0.4 mg daily) to help prevent neural tube defects in their infants (36). Women who are contemplating pregnancy should be counseled about the risk of fetal neural tube defects and the role of folic acid in their prevention.

Following are some general nutritional guidelines for all women issued by the Committee on Diet and Health of the National Research Council (37):

1. **Total fat intake should be 30% of calories or less.** Saturated fatty acid intake should be less than 10% of calories, and the intake of cholesterol should be less than 300 mg daily.

2. **Every day, five or more servings of a combination of vegetables and fruits, especially green and yellow vegetables and citrus fruit, should be eaten.** The daily intake of starches and other complex carbohydrates should be increased by eating six or more servings of a combination of breads, cereals, and legumes.

3. **Protein should be maintained at moderate levels (<1.6 g/kg of body weight).**

4. **Total daily intake of salt should be limited to 6 g or less.**

5. **Vitamin-mineral supplement intake should not exceed the recommended dietary intake per day.**

Alcohol

Alcoholic beverages should be limited to less than 1 oz of absolute alcohol per day (equivalent to two cans of beer, two glasses of wine, or two average cocktails).

A simple device called the T-ACE questionnaire can be used to elicit information about alcohol use and identify problem drinkers (Table 8.12). Women should be questioned in a nonjudgmental fashion about their alcohol use and directed to counseling services as required.

Exercise

Exercise can help control or prevent hypertension, diabetes mellitus, hypercholesterolemia, and cardiovascular disease. Moderate exercise along with calcium supplementation and

Table 8.12. T-ACE Questionnaire

Do you have a drinking problem?	
Experts in treating alcohol abuse use the T-ACE questions below to help them find out whether a person has a drinking problem. These questions can also apply to other drugs.	
T	How many drinks does it take to make you feel high (Tolerance)?
A	Have people Annoyed you by criticizing your drinking?
C	Have you ever felt you ought to Cut down on your drinking?
E	Have you ever had a drink first thing in the morning to steady your nerves or get rid of a hangover (Eye opener)?
If your answer to the tolerance questions is more than two drinks, give yourself a score of 2. If you answer yes to any of the other questions, give yourself a score of 1 each. If your total score is 2 or more, you may have a drinking problem.	

From **Sokol RJ, Martier SS, Ager JW.** The T-ACE questions: practical prenatal detection of risk-drinking. *Am J Obstet Gynecol* 1989;160:865.

hormone replacement therapy can help retard bone loss in postmenopausal women (38). Exercise helps promote weight loss, strength and fitness, and stress reduction.

Before beginning an exercise program, patients should be examined to ensure that exercise will not pose a risk to their health. Women should be counseled about safety guidelines for exercise. Factors that should be considered in establishing an exercise program include medical limitations and selection of activities that promote health and enhance compliance. A variety of physical activities (e.g., gardening, raking leaves, walking to work, taking the stairs) can be incorporated easily into an individual's daily routine. Emphasis should be placed on regular physical activity (e.g., 30 min/d) rather than episodic vigorous exercise, especially in sedentary individuals (38). High-impact exercise is not necessary to achieve benefits, and it may be harmful. Regular low-impact or moderate aerobic exercise has been associated with improved long-term compliance and adequate health maintenance benefits.

Cardiovascular fitness can be evaluated by measurement of heart rate during exercise. As conditioning improves, the heart rate stabilizes at a fixed level. The heart rate at which conditioning will develop is called the target heart rate (38). **The formula for calculating the target heart rate is 220 minus the patient's age times 0.75.** For example, a 50-year-old woman would target her heart rate at 119 ($220 - 50 = 170 \times 0.75 = 119$).

Smoking Cessation

Smoking is a major cause of preventable illness, and every opportunity should be taken to encourage patients who smoke to quit. The effectiveness of smoking cessation programs varies, however, and numerous approaches have been used. The American Cancer Society suggests the following five-step approach:

1. Begin by obtaining a patient history of smoking habits and assessing the patient's motivation to stop smoking.
2. Give clear advice to stop smoking, emphasizing the benefits of cessation.
3. Set a specific goal (e.g., a realistic date to stop smoking).
4. Suggest cessation strategies.
5. Arrange a visit or phone call to monitor process.

Patient education about the benefits of smoking cessation, clear advice to quit smoking, and physician support improve smoking cessation rates, although 95% of smokers who successfully quit do so on their own. Self-help materials are available from the National Cancer Institute as well as community-based support groups and local chapters of the American Cancer Society and the American Lung Association. To aid in cessation, nicotine replacement therapy may be offered in the form of chewing gum or a transdermal patch. This should be prescribed only in conjunction with, not as a replacement for, ongoing visits for counseling and support.

References

1. **American College of Obstetricians and Gynecologists.** *Obstetrician-gynecologists: specialists in reproductive health care and primary physicians for women.* Washington DC: American College of Obstetricians and Gynecologists; 1986.
2. **American College of Obstetricians and Gynecologists.** *The obstetrician-gynecologist and primary-preventive health care.* Washington, DC: American College of Obstetricians and Gynecologists; 1993.
3. **American College of Obstetricians and Gynecologists, Committee on Primary Care.** *Delineation of obstetric-gynecologic primary care practice.* Washington, DC: American College of Obstetricians and Gynecologists; 1999; Report no 218.

4. **American College of Obstetricians and Gynecologists.** *Primary and preventive care: periodic assessments.* Washington, DC: American College of Obstetricians and Gynecologists; 2000; Committee Opinion no 246.

5. **American College of Obstetricians and Gynecologists.** *Primary and preventive health care for female adolescents.* Washington DC: American College of Obstetricians and Gynecologists; 1999; Education Bulletin no 254.

6. **American Academy of Family Physicians C.** *Age charts for periodic health examinations.* Kansas City, MO: American Academy of Family Physicians, 1990.

7. **U. S. Preventive Services Task Force.** *Guide to clinical preventive services,* 2nd ed. Baltimore, MD: Williams & Wilkins, 1996.

8. **Elster AB, Kuznets NJ.** *AMA guidelines for adolescent preventive services (gaps): recommendations and rationale.* Baltimore, MD: Williams & Wilkins, 1994.

9. **National Guideline Clearinghouse.** Agency for Healthcare Research and Quality, 2001. http://www.guideline.gov/index.asp

10. **Seltzer VL, Pearse WH.** *Women's primary health care: office practice and procedures,* 2nd ed. New York: McGraw-Hill, 2000.

11. **Sanfilippo JS, Smith RP.** *Primary care in obstetrics and gynecology: a handbook for clinicians.* New York: Springer, 1998.

12. **Thornton YS.** *Primary care for the obstetrician and gynecologist.* New York: Igaku-Shoin, 1997.

13. **Leppert PC, Howard FM.** *Primary care for women.* Philadelphia: Lippincott–Raven Publishers, 1997.

14. **Ling FW.** *Primary care in gynecology.* Baltimore: Williams & Wilkins, 1996.

15. **Nolan TE.** *Primary care for the obstetrician and gynecologist.* New York: Wiley-Liss, 1996.

16. **Carlson KJ, Eisenstat SA, Frigoletto AEFD, et al,** eds. *Primary care of women.* St. Louis: Mosby, 1995.

17. **Brett KM, Burt CW.** *Utilization of ambulatory medical care by women: United States, 1997–98. Vital and Health Statistics.* Atlanta, GA: US Centers for Disease Control; 2001; Report no 149, Series 13.

18. **Leader S, Perales PJ.** Provision of primary-preventive health care services by obstetrician-gynecologists. *Obstet Gynecol* 1995;85:391–395.

19. **Laube DW, Ling FW.** Primary care in obstetrics and gynecology resident education: a baseline survey of residents' perceptions and experiences. *Obstet Gynecol* 1999;94:632–636.

20. **Kuffel ME, Stovall DW, Kuffel TS, et al.** Reactions of residency directors to primary care requirements in obstetrics and gynecology training. *Obstet Gynecol* 1998;91:145–148.

21. **American College of Obstetricians and Gynecologists.** *Obstetrics and gynecology: primary care—a guide to communicating the lawmakers, the public, and patients.* Washington, DC: American College of Obstetricians and Gynecologists; 1993.

22. **The Gallop Organization.** *A Gallop study of women's attitudes toward the use of ob/gyn for primary care.* Washington, DC: American College of Obstetricians and Gynecologists; 1993.

23. **US Preventive Services Task Force.** *Guide to clinical preventive services,* 3rd ed. Baltimore: Williams & Wilkins, 2000–2002.

24. **Canadian Task Force on the Periodic Health Examination.** The periodic health examination. *CMAJ* 1979;121:1193–1254.

25. **Barton S,** ed. *Clinical evidence,* 5th ed. London: BMJ Publishing Group, 2001.

26. **The Cochrane Collaboration.** *The Cochrane Library.* 2001.

27. **American Medical Association.** *Guidelines for adolescent preventive services (GAPS).* Chicago, IL: American Medical Association; 1992.

28. **Zabin LS, Hardy JB, Smith EA, et al.** Substance use and its relation to sexual activity among inner-city adolescents. *J Adolesc Health Care* 1986;7:320–331.

29. **Orr DP, Beiter M, Ingersoll G.** Premature sexual activity as an indicator of psychosocial risk. *Pediatrics* 1991;87:141–147.

30. **American College of Obstetricians and Gynecologists.** *Guidelines for women's health care,* 2nd ed. Washington DC: American College of Obstetricians and Gynecologists; 2002.

31. **Uhari M, Nuutinen EM, Turtinen J, et al.** Blood pressure in children, adolescents and young adults. *Ann Med* 1991;23:47–51.

32. **Program NCE.** Report of the Expert Panel on Blood Cholesterol Levels in children and Adolescents. *Pediatrics* 1992;89[Suppl]:525–584.

33. **American College of Obstetricians and Gynecologists.** *Exercise and women.* Washington, DC: American College of Obstetricians and Gynecologists; 1992; Report no 173.

34. **American College of Obstetricians and Gynecologists.** *Nutrition and women.* Washington, DC: American College of Obstetricians and Gynecologists; 1996; Number 229.

35. **Center for Nutrition policy and promotion.** *The food guide pyramid.* US Department of Agriculture; 2000. http://www.health.gov/dietaryguidelines/dga2000/document/build.htm pyramid.

36. **CDC.** Recommendations for the use of folic acid to reduce the number of cases of spina bifida and other neural tube defects. *MMWR* 1992;41:1–17.

37. **National Research Council.** Subcommittee on the Tenth Edition of the RDAs, Food and Nutrition Board, Commission on Life Sciences. *Recommended dietary allowances,* 10th ed. Washington DC: National Academy Press; 1989.

38. **Bulletin AT.** *Women and exercise.* Washington DC: American College of Obstetricians and Gynecologists; 1992.

9 Primary Care in Gynecology

Dayton W. Daberkow II
Thomas E. Nolan

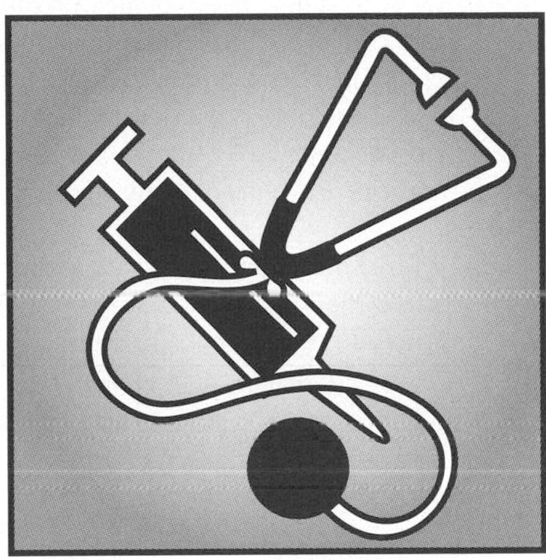

Gynecologists have become responsible for care that extends beyond diseases of the reproductive organs to include much of the general medical care of women. Broadening the spectrum of care places emphasis on the caring nature of the physician rather than the surgical or procedural aspects of the specialty. Early diagnosis and treatment of medical illnesses can have a major impact on a woman's health and is a key component of primary care. Although timely referral is important for complex and advanced disorders, the gynecologist initially may treat many conditions.

The gynecologist should provide screening and early intervention for certain conditions that commonly arise in the office setting or have a significant impact on women's health. Respiratory problems are the most common reasons patients seek care from a physician, so gynecologists should be aware of their pathophysiology. Cardiovascular disease has a significant impact on overall morbidity and is the main cause of death in women. Cardiovascular illness is associated with cigarette smoking, hypertension, hypercholesterolemia, and diabetes mellitus. These conditions are responsive to screening, behavior modification, and control to lower risk factors. A major cause of morbidity for women is thyroid disease; because of the interaction of hormones and the overall effect on the endocrine system, thyroid disease can be of special significance in women.

Respiratory Infections

Infections of the respiratory system can range from the common cold to life-threatening illness. Those who have risk factors should be counseled about preventive measures. Vaccines against flu and pneumonia should be offered as indicated (see Chapter 8, Table 8.7).

Sinusitis

A problem frequently encountered in women is self-diagnosed "sinus problems" (1). Many medical problems—headaches, dental pain, postnasal drainage, halitosis, and dyspepsia—may be related to sinus conditions. The sinuses are not an isolated organ, and diseases of the sinuses are often related to conditions that affect other portions of the respiratory system (i.e., the nose, bronchial tree, and lung) (2). The entire respiratory system may be infected by one particular virus or pathogen (the sinobronchial or sinopulmonary syndrome); however, the most prominent symptoms are usually produced in one anatomic area. Therefore, during the evaluation of complaints attributable to sinusitis, the presence of other infections should be investigated.

Exposure to multiple infectious and chemical agents or reaction to nervous, physical, emotional, or hormonal stimuli may cause an inflammatory response in the respiratory system (3). Systemic diseases such as connective tissue syndromes and malnutrition may contribute to chronic sinusitis. Environmental factors in the workplace and geographic conditions (e.g., cold and damp weather) may aggravate or accelerate the development of sinusitis. Factors to contributing the development of sinus disease include atmospheric pollutants, allergy, tobacco smoke, skeletal deformities, dental conditions, barotrauma from scuba diving or airline travel, and neoplasms.

Most infections begin with a viral agent in the nose or nasopharynx that causes inflammation that blocks the draining ostia. The location of the symptoms varies by anatomic site: maxillary sinus over the cheeks, ethmoid sinus across the nose, frontal sinus in the supraorbital area and sphenoid sinus to the vertex of the head. Viral agents impede the sweeping motion of cilia in the sinus and, in combination with edema from inflammation, lead to superinfection with bacteria. Common bacterial agents infecting sinuses are *Streptococcus pyogenes, Streptococcus pneumoniae, Haemophilus influenzae, Staphylococcus aureus,* and α-hemolytic streptococcus species. Gram-negative organisms are usually limited to compromised hosts in intensive care units. Chronic sinusitis develops from either inadequate drainage or compromised local defense mechanisms. The flora in chronic disease is usually polymicrobial, with mixed infections consisting of aerobic and anaerobic organisms.

Sinus ailments frequently occur in middle-aged individuals. Acute infection is usually located in the maxillary and frontal sinuses. Classically, infection in the maxillary sinus is due to obstruction of the ostia found in the medial wall of the nose. Fever, malaise, a vague headache, and pain in the maxillary teeth are early symptoms. Complaints of "fullness" in the face or exploding pressure behind the eyes are elicited. Pressure and percussion over the malar areas results in complaints of severe pain. Purulent exudates in the middle meatus of the nose or in the nasopharynx are commonly observed. **The five clinical findings of maxillary toothache, poor response to nasal decongestants, abnormal transillumination, a colored nasal discharge established by history or a colored nasal discharge on examination are the most useful clinical findings. When four or more features are present the likelihood of sinusitis is high, and when none is present sinusitis is highly unlikely** (4). Initial episodes of sinusitis do not require imaging studies, but when persistent infections occur, studies and referral are indicated. Therapy is usually empiric. Unless samples are obtained by direct needle drainage, cultures are of no value because it is impossible to avoid contamination by oropharyngeal flora.

Broad antibiotic therapy is necessary to cover common aerobes and anaerobes but should be limited to patients with acute pain and purulent discharge. For acute, uncomplicated sinus infections *amoxicillin* (500 mg 3 times a day) or *trimethoprim-sulfamethoxazole* (one tablet twice daily) remain the treatments of choice. *Amoxicillin* is inexpensive, penetrates the sinus tissues well, and can be discontinued and another antibiotic substituted if symptoms have not improved in 48 to 72 hours. If β-lactam resistance is likely, *amoxicillin-clavulanic acid* (875 mg twice daily), or *azithromycin* (5-day course once a day) may be used. Other second-line drugs include *cefuroxime* (250 mg twice daily), *ciprofloxacin* (500 mg twice daily), *clarithromycin* (500 mg twice daily), *levofloxacin* (500 mg once a day), and *loracarbef* (400 mg twice daily). The usual treatment course is 14 days, and patients should be informed that a relapse may occur if the full course of treatment is not completed. Systemic decongestants containing *pseudoephedrine* are useful in shrinking the obstructive ostia and promoting sinus drainage and ventilation. Topical decongestants should be used for no longer than 3 days, because prolonged use may lead to rebound vasodilation and worsening of symptoms. Mucolytic agents such as *guaifenesin* may help thin sinus secretions and promote drainage. Antihistamines should be avoided in acute sinusitis because their drying effects may lead to thickened secretions and poor drainage of the sinuses. Symptomatic therapies should include facial hot packs and analgesics. Improvement in symptoms should be apparent within 48 hours, but 10 days of therapy may be necessary for complete resolution. If symptoms do not respond, other classes of antibiotics should be used based on presumed microbial resistance. In difficult cases, referral to an otolaryngologist for sinus irrigation may be necessary.

Chronic sinusitis may result from repeated infections with inadequate drainage. The interval between infections becomes progressively shorter until there are no remissions. Symptoms are recurrent pain in the malar area or chronic postnasal drip. Chronic sinusitis is associated with chronic cough and laryngitis with intermittent acute infections. In the preantibiotic era, chronic sinusitis was the result of repeated acute sinusitis with incomplete resolution, whereas allergy currently is receiving greater attention as a possible cause. Surface ciliated epithelia are injured, resulting in impaired mucus removal. A vicious cycle of incomplete resolution of infection followed by reinfection and ending with the emergence of opportunistic organisms occurs. Swelling and edema of the mucosa, in conjunction with hypersecretion of mucus, lead to ductal obstruction and infection. Treatment is directed at the underlying etiology, either allergy control or aggressive management of infections. Resistant cases will require computed tomography (CT) and endoscopic surgery with polyp removal. Nasoantral window formation is radical surgery usually reserved for advanced conditions that do not respond to other forms of therapy.

Untreated, sinus infections may have serious consequences such as orbital cellulitis leading to orbital abscess, subperiosteal abscess formation of the facial bones, cavernous sinus thrombosis, and acute meningitis. Brain and dural abscesses are rare and usually are caused by direct spread of pathogens from a sinus. At present, CT scanning is the most accurate diagnostic tool. Aggressive surgical approaches used with broad-spectrum antibiotics are necessary for adequate drainage.

Otitis Media

Otitis media remains primarily a disease of children but may affect adults. Serous otitis media is usually secondary to a concurrent viral infection of the upper respiratory tract. In most cases, diagnosis reveals fluid behind the tympanic membrane. Therapy involves treatment of symptoms with antihistamines, decongestants, and glucocorticoids, but little data exist supporting use of these medications. Acute otitis media is usually caused by a bacterial infection; *Streptococcus pneumoniae* and *Haemophilus influenzae* are the pathogens most often involved. Symptoms include acute purulent otorrhea, fever, hearing loss, and leukocytosis (5). Physical examination of the ear will reveal a red, bulging, or perforated membrane. Indicated treatment is broad-spectrum antibiotics such as *amoxicillin-clavulanic acid, cefuroxime,* and *trimethoprim-sulfamethoxazole.* The role of antihistamines in treatment of otitis media is unclear.

Bronchitis

Acute bronchitis is an inflammatory condition of the tracheobronchial tree, most often caused by a viral infection and occurring in winter. Common cold viruses (rhinovirus and coronavirus), adenovirus, influenza virus and *Mycoplasma pneumoniae* (a nonviral pathogen) are the most common pathogens. Bacterial infections are less common and may occur as secondary pathogens. Cough, hoarseness, and fever are the usual initial symptoms. During the first 3 to 4 days, the symptoms of rhinitis and sore throat are prominent; however, coughing may last as long as 3 weeks. Unfortunately, the prolonged nature of these infections result in use of antibiotics to "clear up the infection." Sputum production is common and may be prolonged in cigarette smokers. Most serious bacterial infections occur in cigarette smokers because of damage to the lining of the upper respiratory tree and changes in the host flora.

Physical examination will demonstrate a variety of upper airway sounds, usually coarse rhonchi. Rales are usually not auscultated, and signs of consolidation and alveolar involvement are absent. During auscultation of the chest, signs of pneumonia such as fine rales, decreased breath sounds, and euphonia ("E to A changes") should be sought. If the findings of the physical examination are uncertain or if the patient's condition appears toxic, chest radiography should be performed to detect the presence of parenchymal disease. Paradoxically, as the initial acute syndrome subsides, sputum production may become more purulent. Sputum cultures are of limited value because of the polymicrobial nature of infections. In uncomplicated cases, the goal of treatment is symptomatic relief, whereas use of antibiotics is reserved for patients who have chest radiographic findings consistent with pneumonia. Cough is usually the most aggravating symptom and may be treated with antitussive preparations containing either dextromethorphan or codeine. The efficacy of expectorants has not been proved.

Chronic bronchitis is defined as the presence of a productive cough with excessive secretions for at least 3 months in a year for 2 consecutive years. Prevalence has been estimated to be between 10% to 25% of the adult population. In the past, incidence has been lower in women than men, but as the prevalence of cigarette smoking in women has increased, so has the incidence of bronchitis in women. Chronic bronchitis is usually classified as a form of chronic obstructive pulmonary disease (COPD). Other causes include chronic infections and environmental pathogens found in dust. The cardinal manifestation of disease is an incessant cough, usually in the morning, with expectoration of sputum. Because of frequent exacerbations and hospitalizations required, and the complexity of medical management, these patients should be referred to an internist for treatment.

Pneumonia

Pneumonia is defined as inflammation of the distal lung that includes terminal airways, alveolar spaces, and the interstitium. Pneumonia may have multiple causes, including viral and bacterial infections or aspiration. Aspiration pneumonia is usually the result of depressed awareness commonly associated with use of drugs, alcohol, or anesthesia. Viral pneumonias are caused by multiple infectious agents including influenza A or B, parainfluenza virus, or respiratory syncytial virus. Most viral syndromes are spread by aerosolization associated with coughing, sneezing, and even conversation. Incubation time is short, requiring only 1 to 3 days prior to the acute onset of fever, chills, headache, fatigue, and myalgia. Symptom intensity is directly related to intensity of the host febrile reaction. Pneumonia develops in only 1% of patients who have a viral syndrome, but mortality rates may reach 30% in immunocompromised individuals and the elderly. An additional risk is the development of secondary bacterial pneumonias after the initial viral insult. These infections are more common in elderly patients and may explain the high fatality rate associated with them in this group (6). Staphylococcal pneumonias, most commonly arising from a previous viral infection, are extremely lethal regardless of the patient's age. The best approach to viral pneumonia is prevention by immunization. Influenza and pneumonia immunization should be offered as indicated (see Chapter 8, Table 8.7). In epidemics, *amantadine* has been used to treat individuals who have not been vaccinated. Treatment is supportive with administration of antipyretics and fluids.

Bacterial pneumonia is classified as either nosocomial or community acquired. The classification determines the prognosis and choice of antibiotic therapy in many cases. Risk factors that contribute to mortality are chronic cardiopulmonary diseases, alcoholism, diabetes mellitus, renal failure, malignancy, and malnutrition. Prognostic features associated with poor outcome include greater than two-lobe involvement, respiratory rate greater than 30 breaths/minute on arrival in the health care center, severe hypoxemia (<60 mm Hg breathing room air), hypoalbuminemia, and septicemia (7). Pneumonia is a common cause of adult respiratory distress syndrome (ARDS), which has a mortality rate of between 50% to 70% (8).

Signs and symptoms of pneumonia vary depending on the infecting organism and the patient's immune status (9). In typical pneumonias, the patient appears toxic with high fever, rigors, productive cough, chills, or pleuritic chest pain. Chest radiographs will often disclose infiltrates. The following agents, listed in decreasing order, cause two-thirds of all bacterial pneumonias: *Streptococcus pneumoniae, Haemophilus influenzae, Klebsiella pneumoniae,* gram-negative organisms, and anaerobic bacteria. Atypical pneumonias are more insidious in onset; moderate fever is present without the characteristic rigors and chills. Additional symptoms include a nonproductive cough, headache, myalgias, and mild leukocytosis. Chest radiographic examination reveals a bronchopneumonia with a diffuse interstitial pattern ("bat wing distribution"); characteristically, the patient does not appear to be as ill as the radiographic findings suggest. Common causes of atypical pneumonia include viruses, *Mycoplasma pneumoniae, Legionella pneumophila, Chlamydia pneumoniae* (also called the TWAR agent), and other rare agents.

A strong index of suspicion is required to establish a diagnosis, especially in elderly and immunocompromised individuals, because of altered response mechanisms. This is even true with so-called *typical agents.* Subtle clues in the elderly include changes in mentation, confusion, and exacerbation of other illnesses. The febrile response may be entirely absent. Even in high-risk groups, an increased respiratory rate of greater than 25 breaths per minute remains the most reliable sign. In high-risk patients mortality is strongly correlated with the inability to mount normal defenses to the symptoms of fever, chills, and tachycardia.

Laboratory studies helpful in identifying community-acquired pneumonia are sputum Gram stain, sputum culture, and blood culture. An adequate sputum collection (defined as more than 25 neutrophils with less than 10 epithelial cells per low-powered field on microscopic examination) may be difficult to obtain. The assistance of respiratory therapists should be sought to obtain induced sputum. *Legionella pneumoniae* requires different laboratory techniques such as direct fluorescent antibody staining of organisms in the sputum or indirect serologic tests using enzyme-linked immunosorbent assay (ELISA) technology. *Mycoplasma pneumoniae* infection should be suspected in the presence of positive cold agglutinin findings and the appropriate clinical symptoms.

Therapy should be directed toward the responsible or most likely pathogen but, in many cases of pneumonia, the exact cause cannot be determined and empiric therapy should be initiated. Pneumonia that occurs without coexisting conditions such as heart disease, lung disease, renal insufficiency, liver disease, or other comorbid medical illnesses in patients who are $\leq$60 years of age should be treated on an outpatient basis with a macrolide such as *erythromycin* (500 mg four times a day). *Clarithromycin* (500 mg twice daily) or *azithromycin* (500 mg on day 1, followed by 250 mg once a day for 4 days) is preferred for smokers or those who are intolerant to *erythromycin. Doxycycline* (100 mg twice daily) may be used for patients who are allergic or intolerant to macrolides. Patients who have coexisting conditions, are $\geq$60 years of age, or both should be treated on an outpatient basis with a second-generation *cephalosporin* or β-lactam–β-lactamase inhibitor, like *amoxicillin-clavulanic acid,* with or without a macrolide if legionellosis is a concern.

The same protocol for outpatient therapy may be used for hospitalized patients except that a third-generation cephalosporin may be used (10). Hospitalization is usually necessary in patients who are very ill, elderly, or immunocompromised. Oxygen therapy and hydration, in addition to antibiotic therapy, should be initiated. The use of chest physiotherapy should be reserved for patients who have copious sputum or who have an ineffective cough. Patients may be switched to oral antibiotics when they are able to eat and drink, have negative blood cultures, a temperature $<38^\circ$C, a respiratory rate of $\leq$24 breaths per minute and a pulse rate of $\leq$100 beats per minute. Patients may be discharged when they fulfill the aforementioned criteria and their white blood cell count is 12×10^9 per liter, comorbid illnesses are stable, oxygen saturation is >90% on room air, or the patient has COPD with PO_2 >60 mm Hg and PCO_2 <45 mm Hg (11).

The pneumococcal vaccine should be given to women at high risk for pneumonia. All adults 65 years or older and people with special health problems such as heart or lung disease, alcoholism, kidney failure, diabetes mellitus, human immunodeficiency virus (HIV) infection, or certain types of cancer should be immunized (see Chapter 8, Table 8.7). Repeat vaccination is recommended 5 years after the first dose in high-risk groups. The vaccine is active against 23 types of pneumococcal strains and most people develop protection within 2 to 3 weeks of receiving the immunization.

The influenza vaccine should be given every fall to the following high-risk groups: individuals 50 years of age or older, individuals with serious long-term health problems like heart disease, lung disease, kidney disease, diabetes mellitus, immunosuppression secondary to long-term steroid or cancer therapy (see Chapter 8, Table 8.7), women who will be in their third trimester of pregnancy during the flu season (November through April), and anyone coming into close contact with people at risk of serious influenza, such as physicians, nurses, and family members. The best time for vaccination is October to mid-November. Antiviral agents should not be used as a substitute for vaccination but can be a useful adjunct. The four agents approved for use in the United States are *amantadine, rimantadine, zanamivir,* and *oseltamivir.* These medications should be given within 2 days of the onset of symptoms to shorten the duration of uncomplicated illness caused by influenza (12).

Cardiovascular Disease

The risk factors for coronary artery disease are presented in Table 9.1. Central to treating cardiovascular disease is the control of contributing diseases and risk factors (Table 9.2). Aerobic exercise protects against cardiovascular disease (13). Additional aspects of prevention of myocardial disease, renal disease, and stroke include control of hypertension, identification and control of diabetes mellitus and obesity, and control of dietary fats, especially cholesterol, in susceptible individuals (Fig. 9.1). The presence or absence of target-organ damage shown in Table 9.3 also determines the risk for coronary artery disease in hypertensive patients.

Hypertension

The relationship between hypertension and cardiovascular events such as stroke, coronary artery disease, congestive heart disease, and renal disease is well known. More than 50 million people in the United States have hypertension and it is found in 15% of the population between the ages of 18 and 74 years. The incidence increases with age and varies with race. After age 50, women have a higher incidence of hypertension than males; however, this may be a confounding variable related to the overall mortality of men at an earlier age (14). Over 60% of those 60 years and older can be classified as hypertensive (15). The contribution of hypertension to overall cardiovascular morbidity and mortality in

Table 9.1. Major Risk Factors for Coronary Artery Disease

Age >60
Diabetes mellitus
Smoking
Dyslipidemia
Gender (men and postmenopausal women)
Family history of cardiovascular disease (men <55 y; women <65 y)

Adapted from *The Sixth Report of the Joint National Committee on Prevention, Detection, Evaluation, and Treatment of High Blood Pressure (JNC VI).* Bethesda, MD: National Institutes of Health, National Heart, Lung, and Blood Institute; 1997; NIH publication 99-4080.

Table 9.2. Lifestyle Adjustment for Cardiovascular Risk Reduction and Hypertensive Therapy

Weight reduction if overweight
Limit alcohol use to less than 1 ounce of absolute alcohol per day (2 beers, 10 ounces of wine, 2 ounces of 100-proof whiskey)
Regular aerobic exercise (30–45 minutes fast walking 3 times/week)
Decrease salt intake to less than 2.4 grams per day
Stop cigarette smoking
Reduce dietary saturated fat and cholesterol
Maintain adequate intake of calcium, potassium, and magnesium
If diabetic, control glucose

From ***The Sixth Report of the Joint National Committee on Prevention, Detection, Evaluation, and Treatment of High Blood Pressure (JNC VI).*** Bethesda, MD: National Institutes of Health, National Heart, Lung, and Blood Institute; 1997; NIH publication 99-4080, with permission.

women has been thought to be less important than in males, but this may reflect the relative absence of research done with women. Recognition and treatment of hypertension may decrease the development of renal and cardiac disease.

Epidemiology

The incidence of hypertension is twice as high in African Americans than in whites. Geographic variations are present: there is a higher prevalence of hypertension and stroke in the southeastern United States, regardless of race (16). One multicenter study confirmed that there is an increased incidence of hypertension, not only in African Americans, but also in those with lower levels of education (17). Preventive measures can be most effective in those at highest risk, such as African American women and individuals from the lowest socioeconomic levels (17). The influence of genetic predisposition is poorly understood. Studies of women have been limited to those that determine side effects of medication and the impact of certain medications on long-term lipid status (14).

Figure 9.1 Disease and risk factors contributing to cardiovascular disease.

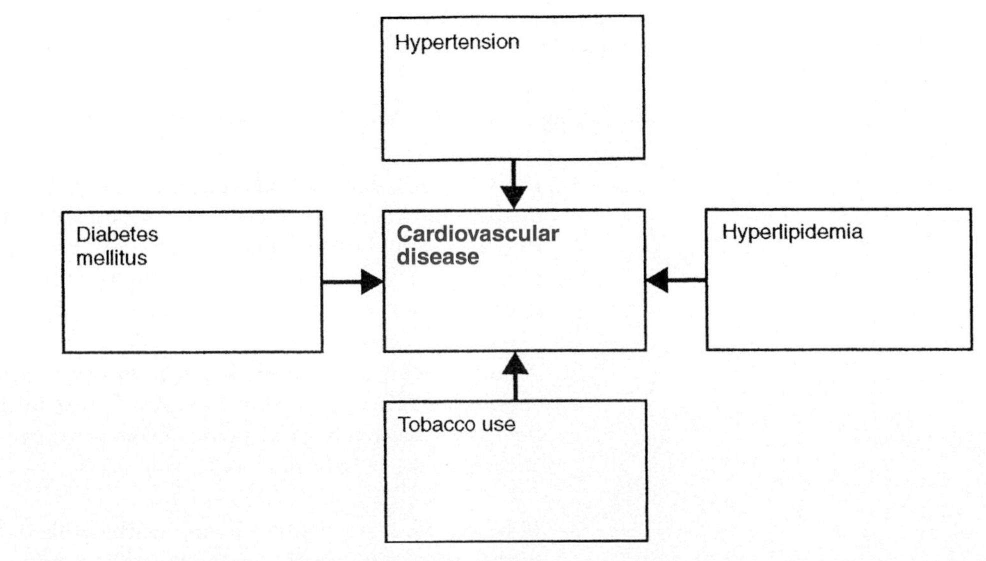

Table 9.3. Target-organ Damage and Clinical Cardiovascular Disease

Stroke or transient ischemic attacks
Hypertensive retinopathy
Heart disease
Angina or prior myocardial infarction
Congestive heart failure
Prior coronary revascularization
Left ventricular hypertrophy
Nephropathy
Peripheral arterial disease

From *The Sixth Report of the Joint National Committee on Prevention, Detection, Evaluation, and Treatment of High Blood Pressure (JNC VI).* Bethesda, MD; National Institutes of Health, National Heart, Lung, and Blood Institute; 1997; NIH publication 99-4080, with permission.

Classically, hypertension is defined as blood pressure levels higher than 140/90 when measured on two separate occasions. However, therapy may be indicated only for individuals at high risk. Individuals at low risk, such as white women with no other risk factors, may benefit from lifestyle modification only (17). Elevation of systolic blood pressure in middle-aged and elderly patients was once considered innocuous; however, recent studies suggest that control of systolic blood pressure is more important than control of diastolic blood pressure (18). Life insurance risk tables indicate that when blood pressure is controlled to lower than 140/90, normal survival occurs over a 10- to 20-year follow-up period, regardless of gender. **Recommendations for treatment of hypertension are based on sustained blood pressure levels higher than 140/90.**

Most individuals (>95%) with hypertension have primary or essential hypertension (cause unknown), whereas less than 5% have secondary hypertension resulting from another disorder. Key factors should be determined in the history and physical examination. The presence of prior elevated readings, previous use of antihypertensive agents, a family history of death from cardiovascular disease prior to age 55, and excessive alcohol and sodium use constitute important historical information. Lifestyle modification is increasingly important in the therapy of hypertension; thus, a detailed history of diet and physical activity should be obtained (19). Baseline laboratory evaluations to rule out reversible causes of hypertension (secondary hypertension) are listed in Table 9.4. Diagnosis and management are based on the classification of blood pressure readings in Table 9.5. In addition, patients are stratified into three different risk groups for therapeutic decision making (Table 9.6).

Following are general guidelines in assessing individuals for therapy:

1. **Patients with high normal readings (systolic blood pressure 130 to 139 mm Hg or diastolic blood pressures 85 to 89 mm Hg) are at high risk for developing hypertension.** They should be monitored yearly, and consideration should be given to nonpharmacologic interventions (20). A scheme for the treatment of uncomplicated hypertension is found in Fig. 9.2.

2. **A single elevated diastolic blood pressure reading of less than 100 mm Hg should be rechecked within 2 months before initiating therapy.** In 33% of patients, elevated readings will spontaneously resolve during the observation period because of so-called *white-coat hypertension.*

3. **If blood pressure control is not easily achieved, systolic blood pressure is higher than 180 mm Hg, or the diastolic reading is higher than 110 mm Hg,**

Table 9.4. Laboratory Tests and Procedures Recommended in the Evaluation of Uncomplicated Hypertension[a]

Urinalysis
Complete blood count
Potassium, sodium, creatinine
Fasting glucose
Total cholesterol, high-density lipoprotein cholesterol
12-lead electrocardiogram

[a]If any of the above are abnormal, consultation or referral to an internist is indicated.
Adapted from ***The Sixth Report of the Joint National Committee on Prevention, Detection, Evaluation, and Treatment of High Blood Pressure (JNC VI).*** Bethesda, MD: National Institutes of Health, National Heart, Lung, and Blood Institute; 1997; NIH publication 99-4080.

Table 9.5. Blood Pressure Classification (Adults 18 years and Older)

Category	*Systolic BP (mm Hg)*	*Diastolic BP (mm Hg)*
Optimal	<120	<80
Normal	<130	<85
High normal	130–139	85–89
Hypertension	—	—
Stage 1	140–159	90–99
Stage 2	160–179	100–109
Stage 3	≥180	≥110

BP, blood pressure.
Adapted from ***The Sixth Report of the Joint National Committee on Prevention, Detection, Evaluation, and Treatment of High Blood Pressure (JNC VI).*** Bethesda, MD: National Institutes of Health, National Heart, Lung, and Blood Institute; 1997; NIH publication 99-4080.

Table 9.6. JNC Blood Pressure Risk Group Stratification

Risk Group A:	No major risk factors and no target-organ damage or clinical cardiovascular disease.
Risk Group B:	At least one major risk factor, not including diabetes; no target-organ damage or clinical cardiovascular disease.
Risk Group C:	Any target-organ damage, clinical cardiovascular disease, or diabetes, with or without other risk factors.

JNC, Joint National Commission.
Adapted from ***The Sixth Report of the Joint National Committee on Prevention, Detection, Evaluation, and Treatment of High Blood Pressure (JNC VI).*** Bethesda, MD: National Institutes of Health, National Heart, Lung, and Blood Institute; 1997; NIH publication 99-4080.

referral to an internist is recommended. Referral also is indicated if secondary hypertension is suspected or evidence of end-organ damage (renal insufficiency or congestive heart failure) is detected.

Measurement of Blood Pressure

An often overlooked but essential variable in the evaluation of hypertension is the method used to obtain measurements and the need to standardize measurements (22). Ambulatory

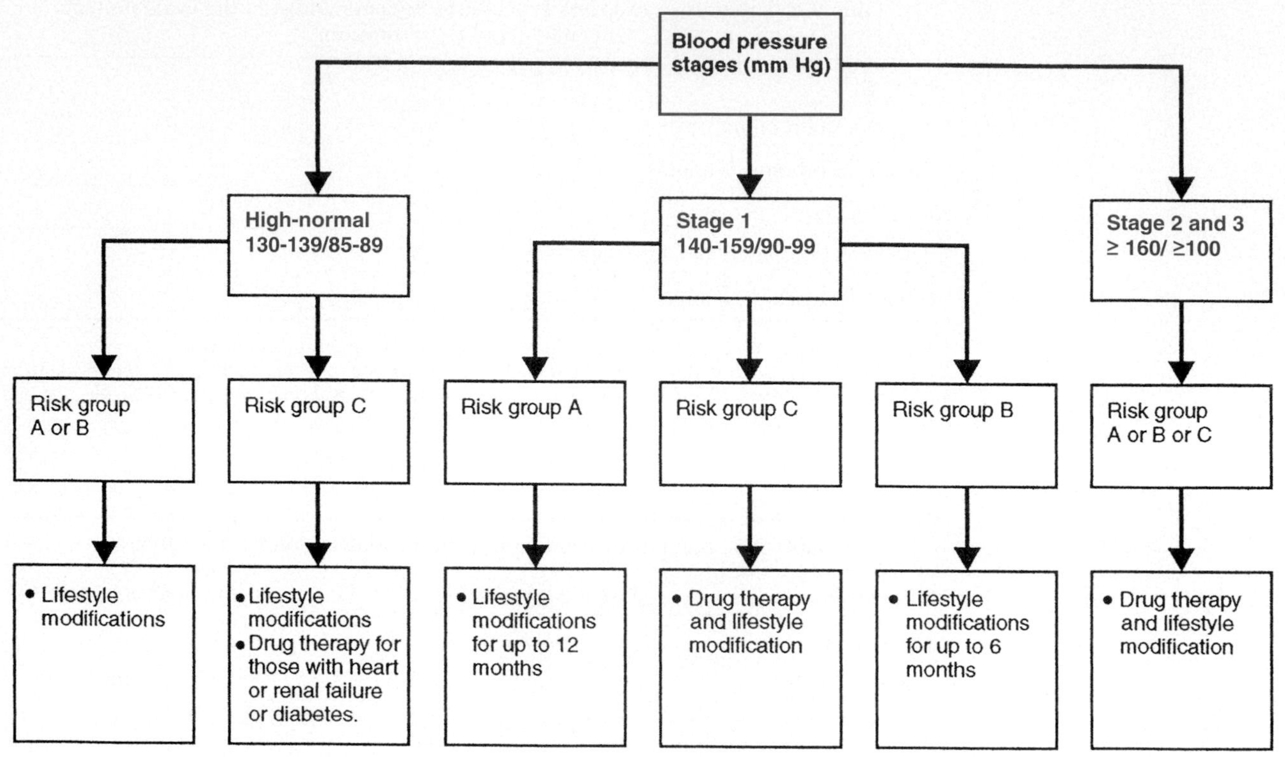

Figure 9.2 Algorithm for the treatment of uncomplicated hypertension. See Table 9.6 for definitions of Risk Group A, B, and C. (Modified from The Sixth Report of the Joint National Committee on Prevention, Detection, Evaluation, and Treatment of High Blood Pressure (JNC VI). Bethesda, MD: National Institutes of Health, National Heart, Lung, and Blood Institute; 1997; NIH publication 99-4080.)

or home monitoring devices, which are becoming less expensive and more reliable, may be appropriate for use by patients who have repeated normal measures outside of the office. In most patients, readings done in the office are all that is necessary to adequately diagnose and monitor hypertension and eliminate problems arising from unreliable commercial devices and patient interpretation skills.

Protocols for measurement of blood pressure should be standardized. The patient should be allowed to rest for 5 minutes in a seated position and the right arm used for measurements (for unknown reasons, the right arm has higher readings). The cuff should be applied 20 mm above the bend of the elbow and the arm positioned parallel to the floor. The cuff should be inflated to 30 mm Hg above the disappearance of the brachial pulse, or 220 mm Hg. The cuff should be deflated slowly at a rate no more than 2 mm Hg per second.

The cuff size is important. Most cuffs are marked with "normal limits" for the relative size they can accommodate. The most common clinical problem encountered is small cuffs used for obese patients, resulting in so-called *cuff hypertension.* Phase IV Korotkoff's sounds are described as the point when pulsations are muffled, while phase V is complete disappearance. Most experts in hypertension advocate the use of phase V Korotkoff sounds, but phase IV sounds may be used in special circumstances, with the reason documented.

The use of automated devices may help eliminate discrepancies in measurements. Regardless of the method or device used, two measurements should be obtained with less than a 10 mm Hg disparity to be judged adequate. When repeated measures are performed, there should be a 2-minute rest period between readings. Blood pressure has a diurnal pattern, so determinations preferably should be done at the same time of day. Ambulatory monitoring is not cost effective in all patients but should be used in some situations, mainly to evaluate resistance to therapy, to detect white-coat hypertension, and to assess whether syncopal episodes are related to hypotension or episodic hypertension (23).

Therapy

The definition of what constitutes systolic hypertension requiring treatment has been contested for years. **Patients with systolic blood pressure higher than 160 mm Hg benefit from antihypertensive therapy regardless of their diastolic pressures** (21). Middle-aged to elderly patients treated for systolic hypertension have a significant decrease in cerebral vascular accidents and coronary artery disease.

Lifestyle modification should be initiated for patients with systolic blood pressures greater than 130 mm Hg but less than 160 mm Hg or diastolic blood pressures greater than 85 mm Hg but less than 100 mm Hg and belonging to risk groups A or B (Fig. 9.2).

Nonpharmacologic interventions or lifestyle modification should be attempted prior to initiation of medication unless the systolic blood pressure exceeds 159 mm Hg, the diastolic blood pressure exceeds 99 mm Hg, or the systolic blood pressure exceeds 139 mm Hg or diastolic blood pressure exceeds 89 mm Hg and the patient has any target-organ damage or diabetes mellitus with or without any other risk factors. Drug therapy should also be initiated for systolic blood pressure higher than 130 mm Hg or diastolic blood pressure higher than 85 mm Hg in those with heart failure, diabetes mellitus, or renal failure (Fig. 9.2). An important element in lifestyle modifications is to modify all contributors to cardiovascular disease. Weight loss in obese patients, especially in individuals with truncal and abdominal obesity, can prevent the development of atherosclerosis (24). A loss of just 10 pounds has been reported to lower blood pressure (25). Patients should be advised to eliminate excess salt in their diets, specifically certain food groups that are high in sodium such as canned goods, snack food, pork products, and soy sauce. Reducing salt intake to 3 grams per day would decrease annual mortality by 70,000 deaths (26). Intake of cholesterol and fat should be limited. Following an exercise program, losing weight, and limiting alcohol intake to no more than 2 drinks per day contributes to overall cardiovascular health. Aerobic exercise alone may prevent hypertension in 20% to 50% of normotensive individuals (27).

The goal of therapy is to lower blood pressure into the normal range, a systolic reading less than 130 mm Hg and a diastolic reading less than 85 mm Hg. If lifestyle modifications are not sufficient to control blood pressure, pharmacologic intervention is indicated. The number of antihypertensive medications has exploded over the past decade. Currently, only diuretics and β-blocking agents have been proved to reduce mortality and morbidity (28).

Diuretics

The most commonly used medication for initial blood pressure reduction is *hydrochlorthiazide.* The mechanism of action is to reduce plasma and extracellular fluid volume. This lowering of volume is thought to decrease peripheral resistance. Cardiac output initially decreases and then normalizes. The important long-term effect is a slight decrease in extracellular fluid volume. The maximal therapeutic dose of thiazide should be 25 mg rather than the commonly used 50 mg. The benefit of higher doses is eliminated by the corresponding increase in side effects. Potassium-sparing diuretics *(spironolactone, triamterene,* or *amiloride)* are usually available in fixed doses and should be prescribed to prevent hypokalemia. Potassium supplementation is less effective than the use of potassium-sparing agents. Thiazide diuretics are best used in patients with creatinine levels less than 2.5 g/L. Loop diuretics *(furosemide)* work better than thiazide diuretics at lower glomerular filtration rates and higher serum creatinine levels. Control of hypertension with concurrent renal insufficiency is difficult and is probably best handled by an internist or nephrologist. Thiazides and loop diuretics should not be used concurrently because they cause profound diuresis, which may lead to renal impairment. Concurrent use of nonsteroidal antiinflammatory drugs

(NSAIDs) limits the effectiveness of thiazides. Other side effects, which further limit the usefulness of thiazide diuretics, include hyperuricemia, which may contribute to acute gout attacks, glucose intolerance, and hyperlipidemias (29). The metabolic side effects of these drugs have limited their popularity recently.

Adrenergic Inhibitors

β-Blockers have been used extensively for years as antihypertensive agents. The mechanism of action is decreasing cardiac output and plasma renin activity with some increase in total peripheral resistance. As a class, they are an excellent source of first-line therapy, especially for migraine sufferers. The original formulation, *propranolol,* was highly lipid soluble, which contributed to bothersome side effects such as depression, sleep disturbances (nightmares in the elderly), and constipation in higher doses. Formulations such as *atenolol* are water soluble, are β_1 selective, and have fewer side effects. At higher doses, however, β_2 effects emerge. Despite speculation that β_1-selective agents may be safe in asthmatics, they should never be used in these patients. Additional advantages of water-soluble agents are longer half-lives and reduced dosing schedules, which improve compliance. Metabolic changes, similar to those of thiazide diuretics, have reduced the popularity of these drugs. These side effects include an increase in triglyceride levels, a decrease in high-density lipoprotein (HDL) cholesterol levels, and blunting of adrenergic release in response to hypoglycemia. These metabolic problems far outweigh the benefits in patients with diabetes mellitus (30). NSAIDs may also decrease the effectiveness of β-blockers. Additional contraindications are COPD, sick sinus syndrome, or any bradyarrhythmia. A popular use of β-blockers is for treatment of angina and myocardial infarctions. If these drugs are acutely withdrawn, however, a rebound phenomenon of ischemia may occur, leading to acute myocardial infarction. β-Blockers continue to be useful, despite these potential problems, especially to counteract reflex tachycardia common with smooth muscle–relaxing drugs.

α_1-Adrenergic drugs became popular in males because they have minimal effects on potency and a unique relationship to lipids. Interestingly, they may contribute to stress urinary incontinence in women as a result of altered urethral tone (31). As single agents, they decrease total cholesterol and low-density lipoprotein (LDL) cholesterol while increasing HDL cholesterol levels, in contrast to the metabolic effects of β-blockers. Mode of action is to promote vascular relaxation by blocking postganglionic norepinephrine vasoconstriction in the peripheral vascular smooth muscle. *Prazosin* and *doxazosin* are currently the most popular preparations available in this class. A serious side effect of these drugs, most commonly described in the elderly, is called the *first-dose effect.* In susceptible individuals, severe orthostasis was reported when therapy was initiated, but it subsided after several days. In combination with diuretics, hypotension may be further exacerbated. Therapy should begin with small bedtime doses followed by incremental increases. Other side effects, which may limit usefulness in some patients, include tachycardia, weakness, dizziness, and mild fluid retention.

Angiotensin-converting Enzyme Inhibitors

Angiotensin-converting enzyme inhibitors (ACE inhibitors) have rapidly become a first-line drug in the treatment of hypertension. Their rapid rise in popularity is due to the introduction of new formulations that allow for once- or twice-daily dosing with a good therapeutic response. There are relatively few side effects; chronic cough is the most worrisome and is the most common cause of discontinuing therapy for this group of drugs. Other side effects are occasional first-dose hypotension and blood dyscrasias. Occasionally patients will suffer from rashes, loss of taste, fatigue, or headaches. Because use is strictly contraindicated during pregnancy, other agents should be considered for women who could become pregnant. ACE inhibitors can be used in combination with other agents, including diuretics, calcium-channel antagonists, and β-blockers. In contrast to β-blockers, these medications can be used in patients with asthma, COPD, depression, and diabetes or peripheral vascular disease. For unknown reasons, they are less effective in African Americans unless a diuretic is used concomitantly. Combined with diuretics, the effectiveness of both drugs increases, but hypovolemia may result. If renal failure is present, hyperkalemia may result from potassium supplementation and altered tubular metabolism. Any NSAID, including *aspirin,* may decrease the antihypertensive effectiveness.

Angiotensin Receptor Antagonists

Angiotensin receptor antagonists such as *losartan* and *valsartan* are drugs that interfere with the binding of angiotensin-II to AT-I receptors. They are as effective as ACE inhibitors in lowering blood pressure without causing the side effect of coughing. Their efficacy in protecting the heart and kidney, similar to ACE inhibitors, remains to be established.

Calcium-channel Blockers

Calcium-channel blockers have been a major therapeutic breakthrough for patients with coronary artery disease and have been found to be effective in patients with hypertension and peripheral vascular disease. The mechanism of action is to block calcium movement across smooth muscle, therefore promoting vessel wall relaxation. Calcium-channel blockers are especially useful in treating concurrent hypertension and coronary artery disease. Additionally, these drugs have been shown to be particularly effective in the elderly and African Americans. Side effects noted include headache, dizziness, constipation, and peripheral edema. The introduction of long-acting calcium-channel blockers has made these preparations more amenable for use in hypertension. Heart failure or conduction disturbances are relative contraindications for use of these drugs.

Direct Vasodilators

Hydralazine is a potent vasodilator used for years in obstetrics for severe hypertension associated with preeclampsia and eclampsia. The mechanism of action is direct relaxation of vascular smooth muscle, primarily arterial. Major side effects include headaches, tachycardia, and fluid (sodium) retention that may result in paradoxical hypertension. Several combinations have been used to counter the side effects and enhance antihypertensive effects. Diuretics may be added to reverse fluid retention caused by sodium retention. When used in combination with β-blockers, tachycardia and headaches may be controlled without compromising the objective of lowering blood pressure. Drug-induced lupus erythematosus has been widely stated as a potential side effect but is rare in normal therapeutic doses of 25 to 50 mg three times per day. *Minoxidil* is another extremely potent drug in this class, but it is of limited use to the gynecologist due to its side effects in women (beard growth). Because of *minoxidil's* potency, only experienced practitioners should use it.

Central-acting Agents

Central-acting agents *(methyldopa* and *clonidine)* have long been used in obstetrics. The mechanism of action is to inhibit the sympathetic nervous system, resulting in peripheral vascular relaxation. The popularity of this group of drugs has been limited by side effects such as taste disorders and dry mouth, as well as the need for frequent dosing (except for the transdermal form of clonidine). Sudden withdrawal of clonidine may precipitate a hypertensive crisis and induce angina. The clonidine withdrawal syndrome is more likely with concomitant use of β-blockers. Compliance is always a major issue in patient care, and side effects can have a major impact. With the introduction of new classes of drugs with improved efficacy and reduced side effects, the use of medications in this class is expected to decline.

Monitoring Therapy

For patients with slightly elevated blood pressure who are being managed with lifestyle modification, blood pressure readings should be monitored frequently by a professional nurse, the patient, or medical office staff at 1- to 2-week intervals. If the patient has other diseases (i.e., cardiovascular or renal), therapy should be initiated earlier and should be directed to the target organ. If lifestyle modification alone is successful, close monitoring is necessary at 3- to 6-month intervals. When lifestyle modification is unsuccessful, blood pressure medication should be administered to decrease target organ disease.

When beginning therapy, concurrent medical conditions that can be treated with a common agent should be considered. Gender, as a consideration in choosing an antihypertensive agent, has been found unimportant. Concurrent diseases that are important include (a) migraine headaches, for which β-blockers or calcium-channel blockers may be the best choice, (b) diabetes mellitus, for which ACE inhibitors should be used, and (c) patients who have had myocardial infarctions who should receive β-blockers because they reduce the risk for sudden death and recurrent myocardial infarctions. In addition, African Americans are noted to respond better to a combination of diuretics and calcium-channel blockers.

Once antihypertensive medications are initiated, monitoring should be frequent. Selected agents and dosages for therapy are found in Table 9.7 and are not meant to be all-inclusive. Patients capable of home blood pressure monitoring should be encouraged to measure blood pressure at the same time twice weekly (32) and maintain a log for physician review of effectiveness of therapy. Once medications are begun, a return appointment should be scheduled in 2 to 4 weeks to monitor effectiveness and side effects. Where possible, single agents (monotherapy) should be used to improve compliance. Monotherapy should control 50% to 60% of patients with mild-to-moderate hypertension. If initial doses are ineffective, then a higher dose should be used prior to changing agents. If resistance to therapy continues, then a different class may be started or a second drug should be added.

If intolerable side effects develop, a different class of medications should be started and monitored. In the past, step therapy was used, starting with thiazides, followed by the addition of β-blockers, and finally followed by vasodilator drugs. The newer drugs (ACE inhibitors, postadrenergic ganglionic blockers, and calcium-channel blockers) are more potent, have longer half-lives, and may be used as single agents. Patients whose blood pressure is difficult to control with monotherapy should be considered for referral. Causes of resistance to therapy include diseases and secondary causes of hypertension missed during the initial evaluation, unrecognized early end-stage disease, and poor compliance.

Table 9.7. Selected Medications and Dosage for Control of Essential Hypertension

Medication (Class)	*Normal Daily Dosage (mg/day) and Interval*	*Dispensing Unit (mg)*
ACE inhibitors		
Enalapril	5–40 (qd, bid)	2.5, 5, 10, 20
Captopril	12.5–150 (bid, tid)	12.5, 25, 50, 100
Calcium channel blockers		
Verapamil, sustained release	120–480 (qd)	120, 180, 240, 360
Diltiazem, sustained release	120–240 (bid)	60, 90, 120
α-Blockers		
Terazosin	1–20 (qd)	1, 2, 5, 10
Mixed α-and β-blockers		
Labetalol	200–800 (bid)	100, 200, 300
Diuretics		
Hydrochlorothiazide	12.5–50 (qd)	25, 50
Triamterene (potassium-sparing)	50–100 (bid)	50, 100
β-Blockers		
Propranolol (lipid soluble)	60–160 (qd)	60, 80, 120, 160
Atenolol (water soluble)	50–100 (qd)	50, 100
Angiotensin receptor antagonists		
Losartan	25–100 (qd)	25, 50, 100

ACE, angiotensin-converting enzyme.

Patients with evidence of target-organ disease should also be considered for transfer or referral to the appropriate specialist for more intensive diagnostic workup and therapy.

Cholesterol

It has been stated that cholesterol is the most highly decorated small molecule in biology (33). The dietary influence of cholesterol on atherosclerosis and its relationship to hypertension and cardiovascular events (myocardial infarction and stroke) has been widely debated in both the scientific and lay communities (34). The controversy centers on the influence of dietary cholesterol in risk assessment and prevention of cardiovascular disease (35). Many assume that all cholesterol and fat in the diet have negative health consequences. Furthermore, cholesterol metabolism is complex and our understanding in some cases is extrapolated from animal models. The role of cholesterol testing (who, when, and at what age) is hotly debated among health care professionals. Cholesterol testing is fraught with multiple variables that affect results. The purpose of the following discussion is to identify patients at risk for complications of hypercholesterolemia and better understand overall metabolism and therapy.

Terms and Definitions

Exclusively LDL and HDL cholesterol do not determine cholesterol metabolism, despite popular discussion. Cholesterol is usually found in an esterized form with various proteins and glycerides that characterize the stage of metabolism. The following components are important lipid particles in cholesterol metabolism.

Chylomicrons These are large lipoprotein particles that consist of dietary triglycerides and cholesterol. Chylomicrons are secreted in the intestinal lumen, absorbed in the lymph, and then passed into general circulation. In adipose tissue and skeletal muscle, they adhere to binding sites on the capillary wall and are metabolized for energy production.

Lipoprotein Particle A lipoprotein particle is made from three major components. The core consists of nonpolar lipids (triglycerides and cholesterol esters) that are present in varying amounts, depending on which stage of the metabolic pathway they are found. Surrounding the nonpolar core is a surface coat of phospholipids that is made of apoproteins and structural proteins.

Apoprotein Attached to all lipoprotein particles is an apoprotein. This is a specific recognition protein exposed at the surface of a lipoprotein particle. Apoproteins have specific receptors and demarcate the stage of cholesterol metabolism. Certain apoproteins are associated with specific types of cholesterol. For example, apoprotein A-I and apoprotein A-II are associated with HDL cholesterol, the so-called *scavenger cholesterol.* Apoprotein C-II has additional activity as a cofactor for lipoprotein lipase.

Lipoprotein Class Lipoprotein particles are separated into five classes that are dependent on physical characteristics. Lipoprotein classes are determined by the separation of lipids in an electrophoretic field; however, *in vivo* they are in a continuum. The various cholesterol metabolites are separated by density. As lipoprotein particles are metabolized and lipids are removed for energy production, they become denser. Additionally, attached apoproteins are modified as cholesterol moves from the so-called *exogenous pathway* (dietary) to the *endogenous pathway* (postabsorption and metabolized by the liver).

Subdivisions of the lipoprotein classes are described below and summarized in Fig. 9.3.

Prehepatic Metabolites

Chylomicrons and Remnants These metabolites are composed of major lipids and apoproteins of the A, B-48, C, and E classes. Their density is 1.006 g/ml. As expected, these are large particles made up of dietary cholesterol molecules that are absorbed with triglycerides.

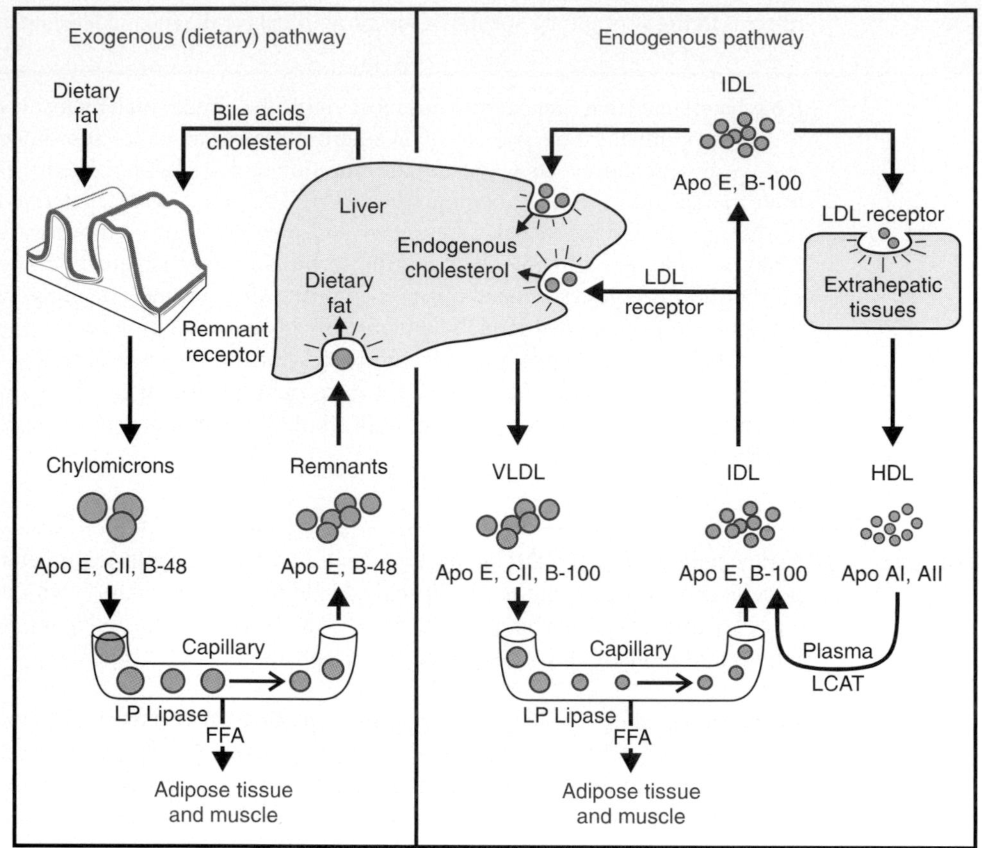

Figure 9.3 Metabolic pathways for lipid metabolism.

Posthepatic Metabolites

Very-low-density Lipoprotein These metabolites are transient remnants found after initial liver metabolism and comprise only 10% to 15% of cholesterol particles. Very-low-density lipoproteins (VLDLs) consist of endogenously synthesized triglycerides with a density of 1.006 g/ml. The diameter is considerably smaller than that of the chylomicrons, ranging from 300 to 800 nm.

Intermediate-density Lipoprotein (IDL) The major lipids in this group consist of cholesterol esters that are posthepatic remnants but are derived from dietary sources. Associated apoproteins are B-100, C-III, and E. Apoprotein B-48 is lost after the initial hepatic metabolism and B-100 is substituted. Apoprotein E, which is a liver recognition apoprotein, is found only in VLDLs and intermediate-density lipoproteins (IDL). IDL metabolites are transient lipoproteins and are measured only in certain pathologic conditions. The density is 1.019 g/ml with a diameter of 250 nm—a very significant drop in diameter from 800 nm found in the VLDL.

LDL Cholesterol The major lipid in this group is the cholesterol ester and is associated with B-100 apoprotein. LDL cholesterol accounts for approximately 60% to 70% of total cholesterol. Elevated levels of LDL cholesterol have been associated with increased rates of myocardial infarction in women over 65 years of age. There is a structural class called LDL(a′) that is associated with myocardial infarction. Several families have been described with structurally abnormal B-100 apoprotein and are at high risk for myocardial infarction due to lipid buildup and premature atherosclerosis (36). Density ranges from 1.019 to 1.063, with a diameter of 180 to 280 nm.

HDL Cholesterol This is composed of cholesterol esters with apoproteins A-I and A-II. These particles account for 20% to 30% of total cholesterol and are the densest, with a weight of 1.063 to 1.120 g/ml. The diameter of this group of proteins is 50 to 120 nm.

Metabolism

Cholesterol metabolism is divided into two pathways. The first pathway is the exogenous pathway derived from dietary sources. The second pathway is called the endogenous pathway or the lipid transport pathway. Individual variations exist in the ability to metabolize cholesterol, with patients classified as normals, hyporesponders, and hyperresponders (37). Hyporesponders may be given cholesterol-loaded diets with no effect on serum cholesterol measurements. The hyperresponder, in contrast, has high serum cholesterol levels, regardless of dietary intake. Explanations of differences are well described in animal models but not in humans.

Once a meal is eaten, cholesterol is transported as dietary fat. The average American diet contains approximately 100 grams of triglyceride and approximately 1 gram of cholesterol daily. Dietary fats are saponified in the intestinal lumen by pancreatic lipases and synthesized into chylomicrons that are first absorbed by active transport into intestinal lymph and then into the general circulation. Capillaries in the adipose tissue and skeletal muscle are able to incorporate triglycerides and fats by the action of lipoprotein lipase. As schematically depicted in Fig. 9.3, metabolic utilization may occur during either phase of metabolism (e.g., dietary or endogenous). During absorption and synthesis of chylomicrons, *apoproteins* are incorporated. Apoprotein C-II is important as a cofactor to activate lipoprotein lipase, which enzymatically liberates fatty acids (for energy) and monoglycerides. These fatty acids may enter endothelial, adipose, or muscle cells, where they are either oxidized into active metabolic products or reesterified to triglycerides.

Triglycerides are found in the core lipoprotein particles and are removed through the capillary endothelium and the chylomicron. Predominant apoproteins are B-48 or B-100 and E apoproteins. When chylomicron synthesis occurs in the intestine, the primary B apoprotein is B-48; upon leaving adipose cells, muscle cells, or the liver the second B apoprotein, or B-100, is substituted. Abnormal forms of B-100 are associated with premature cardiovascular disease and are currently used as genetic markers in research laboratories (38). Another apoprotein added during cellular metabolism is apoprotein E. Apoprotein E plays an important role in liver recognition of chylomicron remnants. Theories suggest that hypo- and hyperresponders to dietary cholesterol may be secondary to the liver's ability to recognize and metabolize apoprotein E (39). In the animal model, populations with large numbers of liver receptors for apoprotein E easily metabolize cholesterol and are labeled hyporesponders. Individuals with a reduced number of apoprotein E receptors are unable to metabolize cholesterol as readily, which increases the number of lipid particles in their blood. These individuals are labeled hyperresponders. Despite dietary cholesterol modification, these individuals continue to have high serum cholesterol levels.

After metabolic degradation of dietary chylomicrons, apoprotein substitution occurs and liver metabolism of cholesterol esters begins. Lipid transport is now in the endogenous pathway. Carbohydrates are synthesized to fatty acids and esterified with glycerol to form triglycerides. These newly formed triglycerides are not of dietary origin and are placed in the core of VLDLs. VLDL particles are relatively large and carry 5 to 10 times more triglyceride than cholesterol esters with apoprotein B-100. Hypertriglyceridemia is an independent risk factor for cardiovascular disease (40). The relationship between hypertriglyceridemia and cardiovascular disease is well known but poorly defined.

VLDL particles are transported to tissue capillaries, where they are broken down to usable fuels, monoglycerides, and fatty acids. Apoproteins C and E are still present within this lipoprotein particle. After metabolic enzymatic degradation in the peripheral tissues, the IDLs remain. IDLs are either catabolized in the liver by binding to LDL receptors or are modified in the peripheral tissues. As noted above, they are associated with apoprotein E receptors, the liver recognition receptors. During the transformation from IDL to LDL cholesterol, all apoproteins are removed, except apoprotein B-100. The LDL cholesterol, or the so-called *high-risk cholesterol,* is found in high circulating levels.

Despite the negative connotation of LDL cholesterol in cardiovascular research, it is a very important cellular metabolite that is a precursor for adrenocortical cells, lymphocytes, and renal cells. LDL receptors on cell surfaces allow for LDL cholesterol incorporation into cellular metabolism. In target cells, these lipid particles are hydrolyzed to form cholesterol for use in membrane synthesis and as precursors for steroid hormones (such as estrogen and progesterone). Once the cell has incorporated the necessary cholesterol, the cell surface receptor reforms limiting further absorption. The liver uses the LDL cholesterol for bile acids synthesis and free cholesterol, which is secreted into the bile. In the normal human, 70% to 80% of LDL is removed from the plasma each day and secreted in the bile by utilization of the LDL receptor pathway.

The final metabolic pathway is the transformation of HDL cholesterol in extrahepatic tissue. HDL cholesterol carries the plasma enzyme lecithin cholesterol acyltransferase (LCAT). LCAT allows HDL cholesterol to resynthesize lipids to VLDL cholesterol and recycle the lipid cascade. The fate of newly synthesized VLDL cholesterol is the same as absorbed VLDL and it eventually becomes LDL cholesterol. HDL cholesterol acts as a "scavenger" and therefore reverses the deposit of cholesterol into tissues. There is good evidence that HDL cholesterol is responsible for the reversal of atherosclerotic changes in vessels, hence the term *the good cholesterol.* (41,42).

Hyperlipoproteinemia

When cholesterol is measured, various fractions are reported. Plasma cholesterol or total cholesterol consists of cholesterol and unesterified cholesterol fractions. If triglycerides are analyzed in conjunction with cholesterol, then assumptions can be made concerning which metabolic pathway may be abnormal. The elevation of both total cholesterol and triglyceride levels signifies a problem with chylomicrons and VLDL synthesis. If the triglyceride-to-cholesterol ratio is greater than 5:1, then the predominant fractions are chylomicrons and VLDL. When the triglycerides-to-cholesterol ratio is less than 5:1, then the problems exist in the VLDL and LDL fractions. Establishing a "normal population" and then setting various limits at the 10th and 90th percentiles define hyperlipoproteinemias. A recent standard for women sets the 80th percentile for cholesterol at 240 mg/dl and the 50th percentile at 200 mg/dl (Table 9.8). Researchers continue to argue that populations vary and may have different cutoff limits depending on the amount of fat versus vegetable and fiber consumption within the diet (43).

Laboratory Testing

The consensus of most researchers is that office laboratory analyses of total cholesterol are virtually worthless as an accurate measure of cholesterol. The measurement techniques are extremely variable. In well-controlled studies, it has been shown that the variation in readings is large (44). Therefore, despite their popularity, they are totally inadequate for either screening or monitoring treatment of patients with hypercholesterolemia.

There are multiple environmental causes of variation in cholesterol measurements (45). Major sources of variation within individuals include diet, obesity, smoking, ethanol intake, and the effects of exercise. Other clinical conditions that affect cholesterol measurements include hypothyroidism, diabetes mellitus, acute or recent myocardial infarction, and recent weight changes. Other variables include the fasting state, position while the sample is drawn, and the use and duration of venous occlusion. Anticoagulants and storage and shipping conditions also can alter lipoprotein measurements (46).

Intraperson variation has been well described. If a single individual has total cholesterol measured 4 times during the day, the variation is 2.5%. If retested within 1 month, on a

Table 9.8. Initial Classification Based on the Total Cholesterol and HDL Cholesterol Levels

	Initial Classification
Total cholesterol	
<200 mg/dl	Desirable blood cholesterol
200–239 mg/dl	Borderline high blood cholesterol
≥240 mg/dl	High blood cholesterol
HDL cholesterol	
<35 mg/dl	Low HDL cholesterol
Triglycerides	
<200 mg/dl	Normal
200–400 mg/dl	Borderline high
400–1000 mg/dl	High
>1000 mg/dl	Very high

HDL, high-density lipoproteins.
Adapted from The Second Report of the National Cholesterol Education Program (NCEP) Expert Panel on the Detection, Evaluation, and Treatment of High Blood Cholesterol in Adults. *JAMA* 1993;269: 3015–3023.

twice-weekly basis, the coefficient of variation increases to 4.8%. Monthly measurements over 1 year may result in a variation as high as 6.1%. Therefore, for accurate standardization, at least two and preferably four specimens taken 1 month apart should be collected in the same dietary state in order for a lipid value to be considered accurate.

Age and sex contribute to variations in total cholesterol measurements. Before age 50, women have lower lipid values than men; after age 50, lipid values increase. Exogenous oral conjugated estrogens are thought to contribute to this effect. The genetic basis for interperson variability is thought to be mediated by apolipoprotein receptors.

Seasonal variation also occurs. In December or January, lipid samples taken were found to be approximately 2.5% higher than those measured in June or July. LDL cholesterol and total cholesterol were higher, with no significant variation found for HDL cholesterol. The index population was found to weigh approximately 6% more in December and January than in June or July, which may account for the differences.

The effect of diet and obesity has been well studied. Some researchers felt this effect may be related to hypo- and hyperresponder status. However, weight reduction in an obese individual generally affects the triglyceride level, which may decrease as much as 40%. Total cholesterol and LDL cholesterol levels decrease less than 10% with diet changes; however, HDL cholesterol levels increase approximately 10%. Weight gain negates any benefit from prior weight loss. Therefore, accuracy of lipid measurements depends on the stability of the patient's weight.

Alcohol and cigarette smoking are well-known modifiers of cholesterol levels. Moderate sustained alcohol intake is noted to increase HDL cholesterol and decrease LDL cholesterol levels; however, there is a complementary increase in triglyceride levels. Alcohol has a protective effect when taken in moderation (defined as approximately 2 ounces of absolute alcohol per day), but this effect is negated with higher quantities. The increase in HDL cholesterol levels is in the HDL_3 fraction, important in the scavenger mechanism of removing LDL cholesterol. Smoking has the opposite effect, by increasing LDL cholesterol and triglyceride levels and decreasing HDL cholesterol levels. The HDL_3 fraction decreases with cigarette smoking. The critical number of cigarettes smoked is 15 to 20 per day, regardless of sex. Caffeine has a mixed effect on lipoprotein measurements but should be avoided in the 12 hours prior to blood collection.

Exercise is an important variable in overall risk management for heart disease. Federal agencies have recognized that moderate levels of exercise are as important in overall cardiovascular health as control of hypertension and cessation of cigarette smoking. Strenuous exercise lowers the concentrations of triglycerides and LDL and increases HDL in the serum. To obtain accurate measurements, vigorous exercise should not be performed within 12 hours of obtaining blood samples.

Because of the diurnal variation of blood triglyceride levels, blood samples should be collected in the morning after a 12-hour fast. Excessive quantities of water should not be consumed before the blood is drawn. The patient should be sitting quietly for approximately 15 minutes prior to the blood draw. Patients who were placed in the supine position for 30 minutes and then required to stand for 30 minutes had a 9% increase in total cholesterol, LDL cholesterol, and VLDL cholesterol fractions, while the HDL cholesterol increased by 10% and triglyceride levels increased by 12%. Additionally, if the tourniquet time is more than 5 minutes, causing vascular stasis, all measurements increase by 10% to 15%. After even 2 minutes of venous occlusion, serum cholesterol increases can be 2% to 5%. Therefore, collection of the cholesterol sample should be done first if multiple blood samples are required. Finger-stick samples are approximately 8.5% lower for all component measurements than venous blood due to contamination from interstitial and lymph fluids.

Collection tube anticoagulants may have a profound effect on lipoproteins. The total cholesterol level has been observed to change depending on the anticoagulant used: ethylenediaminetetraacetic acid (EDTA) increases measurements by 3%, oxalate increases by 9%, citrate increases by 14%, and fluoride by 18%. EDTA is considered the standard anticoagulant for cholesterol measurement. If cholesterol measurements cannot be run in a reasonable time, the samples may be stored at 0°C for up to 4 days, at −20°C for 6 months, or at −50° to −80°C indefinitely. Specimens transported by mail should be placed on dry ice.

One of the most important aspects of overall standardization of lipoprotein measurements is the laboratory used. Currently, laboratory levels should be within ±5% of CDC standards for lipoprotein measurements. Approximately 80% of laboratories in one study met this criteria (47). Therefore, to accurately assess cholesterol values, the clinician should be knowledgeable about the laboratory used. It may be useful to consult with the clinical pathologist of a hospital to determine if the laboratory complies with CDC standards for cholesterol and lipoprotein measurements.

Disease States and Medication Effects

Certain disease states and medications have an impact on cholesterol measurements. As noted previously, diuretics and propranolol increase triglyceride and decrease HDL cholesterol levels. Diuretics may also increase total cholesterol levels. Patients with diabetes mellitus, especially those with poor control, may have very high levels of triglycerides, LDL cholesterol, and decreased HDL cholesterol. This may explain why they are prone to cardiovascular diseases. Diabetics under "tight" control generally have improved lipoprotein levels.

Pregnancy is associated with decreased total serum cholesterol in the first trimester with continuous increases of all fractions over the second and third trimesters (48). The LDL and triglyceride concentrations are the lipoproteins most affected by pregnancy. Limited studies have been done on standardization of lipid levels in pregnancy. Because of the short span, interventions would be of little clinical significance. Lastly, patients with hypothyroidism are also noted to have increased levels of total cholesterol and LDL cholesterol.

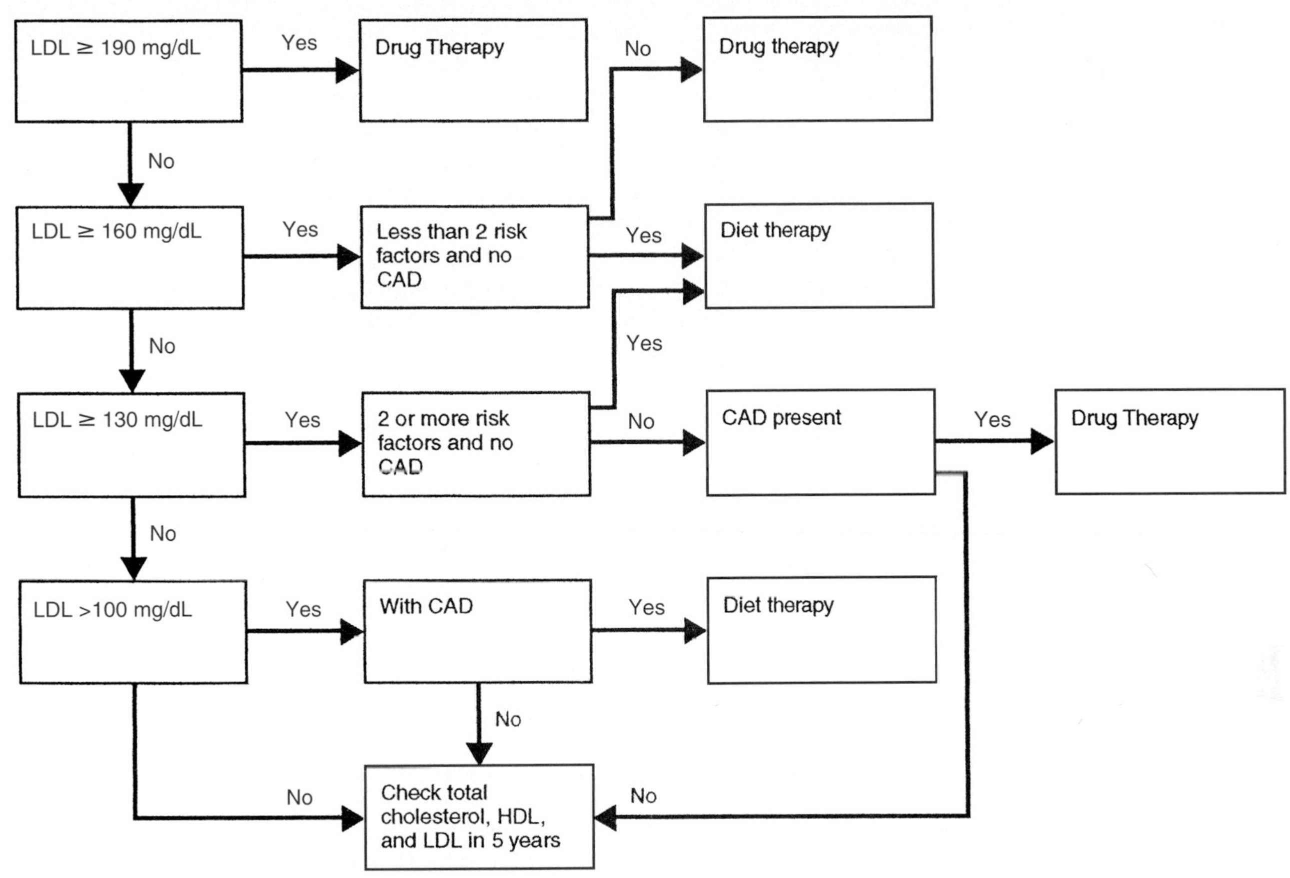

Figure 9.4 Treatment decisions based on the LDL cholesterol level. (Adapted from the Second Report of the National Cholesterol Education Program (NCEP) Expert Panel on the Detection, Evaluation, and Treatment of High Blood Cholesterol in Adults. *JAMA* 1993;269:3015–3023.)

Management

Once hyperlipidemia is confirmed on at least two separate occasions, secondary causes should be diagnosed or excluded by taking a detailed medical and drug history, measuring serum creatinine and fasting glucose levels, and performing thyroid and liver function tests. For obese patients, diet and weight loss is the first level of therapy. Figure 9.4 shows a suggested algorithm for cholesterol control based on the LDL level. Cholesterol- and fat-lowering diets abound in most bookstores and allow the patient to choose a diet she will best follow. The role of exercise and cigarette cessation should be stressed to all patients. Patients with family history of cardiovascular disease (history of premature coronary artery problems and strokes) should be tested and started on conservative programs when they are in their twenties. After 3 to 6 months, if the LDL cholesterol level remains above 160 mg/dl, or above 130 mg/dl with risk factors, medical therapy should be initiated. Since the second report of the Adult Treatment Panel of the National Cholesterol Education Program (NCEP ATP II) was published in 1993, evidence from recent clinical trials has suggested a lower treatment threshold for patients with established coronary artery disease.

The bile acid–binding resins cholestyramine and colestipol were the mainstay of therapy for years but are associated with constipation, bloating, nausea, and heartburn. These agents also may interfere with the absorption of many drugs, which has limited their usefulness. *Nicotinic acid* (500 mg 3 times a day) decreases triglyceride, LDL, and lipoprotein(a) levels and increases HDL levels more than any other drug. However, flushing, pruritus, and gastrointestinal distress are a few of the adverse effects of nicotinic acid. Starting at a low dose and pretreating with *aspirin* (325 mg) or *ibuprofen* (200 mg) can minimize the facial flushing. Fibric acid derivatives like clofibrate and gemfibrozil are used mainly to lower triglycerides and increase HDL but may increase LDL levels in some patients. The 3-hydroxy-3-methylglutaryl coenzyme A (HMG CoA) reductase inhibitors ("statins") include *atorvastatin, fluvastatin, lovastatin, pravastatin,* and *simvastatin.* These medicines inhibit HMG-CoA reductase, the enzyme that catalyzes the rate-limiting step in cholesterol synthesis. Several clinical trials have shown that *pravastatin, simvastatin,* and *lovastatin* have a beneficial effect in cardiovascular disease. Statins are generally better tolerated than other lipid-lowering drugs, but severe myalgias, muscle weakness with increases in creatine phosphokinase levels, and rarely rhabdomyolysis leading to renal failure have been reported. Symptomatic hepatitis is rare, but serum glutamic oxaloacetic transaminases should be measured 6 and 12 weeks after initiation of therapy, and semiannually once therapeutic levels are reached. The usual daily starting doses for the statin drugs are the following: *atorvastatin* (10 mg), *fluvastatin* (20 mg), *lovastatin* (20 mg), *pravastatin* (20 mg), and *simvastatin* (20 mg) (49).

Diabetes Mellitus

Diabetes mellitus (DM) is a chronic disorder of altered carbohydrate, protein, and fat metabolism from a deficiency in the secretion or function of insulin. The disease is defined by either fasting hyperglycemia or elevated plasma glucose levels after an oral glucose tolerance test (OGTT). The major complications of DM are primarily vascular and metabolic complications. Only 50% of an estimated 13 million Americans with DM have been diagnosed. The prevalence of DM is higher in women and certain ethnic groups, although a background rate in the general population is 2.5% (50). Risk factors for DM are (a) age greater than 45 years, (b) adiposity or obesity, (c) a family history of diabetes, (d) race and ethnicity, (e) hypertension (140/90 or greater), (f) HDL cholesterol less than or equal to 35 mg/dl with or without a triglyceride level greater than or equal to 250 mg/dl, and (g) history of gestational diabetes or delivery of baby over 9 pounds. Lifestyle may be the most important variable for type 2 diabetes, as discussed below. Major complications of DM include blindness, renal disease, gangrene of an extremity, heart disease, and stroke. Diabetes is one of the four major risk factors for cardiovascular disease (51).

Classification

In January of 1999, the Expert Committee on the Diagnosis and Classification of Diabetes Mellitus published a report revising the system that had been in use since 1979 (52). The goal of the revision is to provide guidelines for nomenclature and testing that may reduce diagnostic confusion and improve patient well-being (Table 9.9). The terms insulin-dependent diabetes mellitus (IDDM) and non–insulin-dependent diabetes mellitus (NIDDM) should be eliminated to reduce confusion regarding the meaning of each of these categories. These terms should be replaced by the designations of type 1 and type 2 diabetes mellitus.

Type 1 Diabetes Mellitus

The major metabolic disturbance of type 1 diabetes is the absence of insulin from destruction of β cells in the pancreas. Insulin is necessary for glucose metabolism and cellular respiration. When insulin is absent, ketosis results. The cause of type 1 diabetes is unknown; however, data suggest an autoimmune factor from either a viral infection or toxic components in the environment. Studies in the past decade have shown a correlation between many autoimmune diseases and the human leukocyte antigens (HLA).

Insulin-sensitive tissues (muscle, liver, and fat) fail to metabolize glucose efficiently in the absence of insulin. In uncontrolled type 1 diabetes, additional excess of counterregulatory hormones (cortisol, catecholamines, and glucagon) contributes to further metabolic dysfunction. In the absence of adequate amounts of insulin, increasing breakdown products of muscle (amino acid proteolysis), fat (fatty acid lipolysis), and glycogen (glucose glycogenolysis) are recognized. Additionally, there is an increase in glucose production

Table 9.9. Classification of Diabetes Mellitus
1. Type 1 diabetes (characterized by pancreatic destruction leading to insulin deficiency)
A. Idiopathic
B. Immune mediated
2. Type 2 diabetes (a combination of insulin resistance and some degree of inadequate insulin secretion)
3. Other types of diabetes
A. Impaired glucose tolerance (IGT)
B. Endocrinopathies (Cushing's syndrome, acromegaly, pheochromocytoma, hyperaldosteronism)
C. Drug- or chemical-induced
D. Diseases of the exocrine pancreas (pancreatitis, neoplasia)
E. Infections
F. Genetic defects of β-cell function and insulin action
G. Gestational diabetes mellitus

Adapted from The Expert Committee on the Diagnosis and Classification of Diabetes Mellitus. Report of the Expert Committee on the Diagnosis and Classification of Diabetes Mellitus. *Diabetes Care* 2000;23: S4–S42.

from noncarbohydrate precursors from gluconeogenesis and ketogenesis in the liver. If not promptly treated, severe metabolic decompensation (i.e., diabetic ketoacidosis [DKA]) will occur and may lead to death.

Type 2 Diabetes Mellitus

Type 2 diabetes mellitus is a heterogeneous form of diabetes that commonly occurs in older age groups (>40 years), and is more frequently noted to have familial tendency than type 1 diabetes. In contrast to an absence of insulin that occurs with type 1 diabetes, altered metabolism of insulin occurs in type 2 diabetes, resulting in insulin resistance. This condition is characterized by impaired glucose uptake in target tissues. A compensatory increase in insulin secretion results, with higher-than-normal circulating insulin levels (53). Obesity is present in 85% of affected patients. The cause of type 2 diabetes is unknown, but defects in both the secretion and action of insulin are suspected.

Many patients diagnosed with type 2 diabetes at an early age eventually exhaust endogenous pancreatic insulin and require injected insulin. When under severe stress, such as infection or surgery, they may develop DKA, or a hyperglycemic hyperosmolar nonketotic state (HHNS). Risk factors for type 2 diabetes include ethnicity, obesity, strong family history of DM, sedentary lifestyle, impaired glucose tolerance, upper body adiposity, history of gestational diabetes, and hyperinsulinemia. The presence of risk factors strongly influences the development of type 2 diabetes in susceptible populations.

Diagnosis

Three methods are available to diagnose diabetes mellitus in nonpregnant adults:

1. A single fasting blood glucose greater than or equal to 126 mg/dl on two separate occasions;

2. A random blood glucose equal to or above 200 mg/dl in an individual with classic signs and symptoms of diabetes (polydipsia, polyuria, polyphagia, and weight loss); and

3. A 2-hour OGTT (fasting sample, 60- and 120-minute samples) after a 75-gram load of glucose.

A 2-hour OGTT should not be performed if the first two criteria are present.

Diagnostic criteria for impaired glucose intolerance (IGT) testing are a fasting glucose ≥110 mg/dl but <126 mg/dl.

The 2-hour OGTT should be performed under the following conditions:

1. A 10-hour fast precedes morning testing.
2. The patient should sit throughout the procedure.
3. No smoking is permitted during the test interval.
4. Caffeinated beverages should not be consumed.
5. More than 150 grams of carbohydrates should be ingested for 3 days prior to the test.
6. No drugs should be taken prior to the test.
7. The patient should not be bedridden or under stress.

Patients should be considered for diabetes mellitus testing if the following factors are present:

- Age ≥45 years (repeat at 3-year intervals)
- Classic signs and symptoms of diabetes (i.e., polyuria, polydipsia, polyphagia, and weight loss)
- Ethnic groups at high risk (Pacific Islanders, Native Americans, African Americans, Hispanic Americans, Asian Americans)
- Obesity
- First-degree relative with diabetes
- Gestational diabetes or birth of a baby over 9 pounds
- Hypertension (≥140/90)
- HDL cholesterol levels ≤35 mg/dl or triglyeride level ≥250 mg/dl
- Impaired glucose tolerance based on previous testing

Assessment of Glycemic Control

The only acceptable method for assessment of glycemic control is by determination of blood glucose by the direct enzymatic method and not by urine values. Urine values have been proven not to reflect current blood values. In the past decade multiple adequate techniques using test strips and meters have been introduced. These machines work well but reflect whole blood determinations, not serum values. Upgrades of testing strips (in which blood does not need to be wiped away) and glucometers with memory storage have made home glucose monitoring more reliable. Urine tapes to test for ketones are useful and quick methods for assessing ketosis. If the urine is consistently positive for ketones and blood glucose values remain above 300 mg/dl, the patient should seek medical advice. Physician treatment guidelines are in Table 9.10 and patient guidelines in Table 9.11. A 10-year multicenter study for diabetes control and complication trial (DCCT) performed under the auspices of the National Institutes of Health (NIH) showed a marked reduction (40% to 50%) in complications of neuropathy, retinopathy, and nephropathy when patients with type 1 diabetes mellitus received intensive therapy (accomplished by a team approach) as compared with those who received standard therapy.

Table 9.10. Physician Guidelines in the Therapy of Diabetes Mellitus

• Establish diagnosis and classify type of diabetes mellitus (DM).
• The oral glucose tolerance test (OGTT) is not recommended for routine clinical use because of its higher cost, time requirement, and limited reproducibility.
• Initiate diabetes education classes to learn blood glucose monitoring and diabetic medications, to learn signs and symptoms and complications, and to learn how to manage sick days.
• Place patient on ADA diet with appropriate caloric, sodium, and lipid restrictions.
• Establish cardiac risk factors, evaluate for baseline kidney function (serum creatinine, urine for microalbuminuria).
• If neuropathy is present, refer to a neurologist.
• Establish extent of funduscopic lesion (refer to ophthalmologist as needed).
• Check feet and toenails at each visit.
• Patient to use finger-stick blood glucose for daily diabetic control.
• Follow chronic glycemic control by HbA_{1c} every 2 to 3 months in the office.
• Initial general health evaluation should consist of a complete history and physical examination and the following laboratory tests: CBC with differential, chemistry profile, fasting lipid profile, urinalysis, thyroid function tests, urine for microalbuminuria and ECG (baseline at age 40 or older, repeat yearly).
• Oral hypoglycemic agents (OHA) like the sulfonylureas may be considered if fasting blood glucose does not decline or increase, if the patient has had diabetes for less than 10 years, does not have severe hepatic or renal disease, and is not pregnant or allergic to sulfa drugs.
• While on oral hypoglycemic agents, check the HbA_{1c} every 3 months.
• If the HbA_{1c} is <7% or the postprandial glucose is <200 mg/dl, omit the oral hypoglycemic agents, place on diet therapy alone, and follow every 3 months.
• If the fasting serum glucose is >200 mg/dl consistently or the HbA_{1c} is over 10%, consider starting insulin and referring the patient to an internist.
• Administer the flu vaccine every fall and the pneumococcal vaccine every 6 years.

ADA, American Diabetic Association; HgA_{1c}, hemoglobin A_{1c}; CBC, complete blood count; ECG, electrocardiogram; FSG, fasting serum glucose.
Adapted from The Expert Committee on the Diagnosis and Classification of Diabetes Mellitus. Report of the Expert Committee on the Diagnosis and Classification of Diabetes Mellitus. *Diabetes Care* 2000;23:S4–S42.

Table 9.11. Patient Guidelines for Treatment of Type 2 Diabetes

• Initiate an ADA reducing diet (50% CHO, 30% fat, 20% protein, high fiber) with three meals a day.
• Maintain ideal body weight or reduce weight by 5% to 15% in 3 months if obese.
• Modify risk factors (smoking, exercise, fat intake).
• Check fasting blood glucose by finger stick daily for 2 months. If FBG declines, no other therapy is needed. If FBG does not decline or increases, use of an oral hypoglycemic agent may be considered.

ADA, American Diabetic Association; CHO, carbohydrate; FBG, fasting blood glucose.
Adapted from The Expert Committee on the Diagnosis and Classification of Diabetes Mellitus. Report of the Expert Committee on the Diagnosis and Classification of Diabetes Mellitus. *Diabetes Care* 2000;23:S4–S42.

Treatment of Type 2 Diabetes Mellitus

Diet is the most important component of diabetes mellitus management and usually the hardest way to achieve control. Three major strategies are used: weight loss, low

Table 9.12. Commonly Used Oral Hypoglycemic Agents

OHA	*Trade Name*	*Daily Dose*	*Duration of Action (hrs)*
Tolbutamide	*Orinase*	750 mg–3.0 g in divided doses	6–12
Tolazamide	*Tolinase*	200–1000 mg in divided doses	12–24
Acetohexamide	*Dymelor*	250–1500 mg in a single dose	12–24
Chlorpropamide	*Diabinese*	100–500 mg in a single dose	up to 60
Glyburide	*Micronase, DiaBeta*	2.5–20 mg variable dose	10–24
Glipizide	*Glucotrol*	2.5–40 mg variable dose	3–8
Metformin	*Glucophage*	500 mg–2.5 grams in 2 or 3 divided doses	6–12

OHA, oral hypoglycemic agent.

fat diet (<30% of calories from fat), and physical exercise. Obese patients should reduce their weight to ideal body weight. Metabolic advantages of weight reduction are improved lipid profile and improved glucose control secondary to increased insulin sensitivity and decreased insulin resistance. The greater the weight loss, the greater the improvement in lipid disorders. Physical exercise promotes weight loss and improves insulin sensitivity and dyslipidemia in those who are in high-risk groups for cardiovascular and microvascular diseases (54).

Oral hypoglycemic agents (OHAs) are recommended for many type 2 diabetic patients (55). First- and second-generation sulfonylureas are currently the only agents approved by the FDA. Other classes of drugs like biguanides, thiazolidinediones, and α-glucosidase inhibitors have recently been introduced which have different effects in patients with type 2 diabetes than sulfonylureas. Currently available sulfonylurea formulations and biguanides are listed in Table 9.12. The mode of action of sulfonylureas is based on two different mechanisms, (a) enhanced insulin secretion from the pancreas, and (b) an extrapancreatic effect which is poorly understood. Endogenous insulin secretion (as measured by C peptide) is necessary for OHAs to work. Additionally, if the fasting blood glucose in a patient on an adequate diabetic diet is greater than 250 mg/dl, there is little effect. OHAs fail to control glucose in 3% to 5% of patients annually. Frequent evaluation to monitor control (every 3 months) is important. If glucose levels cannot be controlled with oral hypoglycemic agents like sulfonylureas, then *insulin, metformin* (a biguanide), or an α-glucosidase inhibitor should be started and referral should be considered because of the increased rate of complications experienced by this group.

Thyroid Diseases

Thyroid disorders are more common in women and some families, although the exact inheritance is unknown (56). **In geriatric populations, the incidence may be as high as 5%** (57). Unfortunately, the laboratory diagnosis of thyroid disease can be difficult because of altered hormonal states such as pregnancy and exogenous hormones. Thyroid hormones act in target tissues by binding to nuclear receptors, which induce changes in gene expression (58). Extrathyroidal conversion of thyroxine (T_4) to triiodothyronine (T_3) takes place in target tissue. T_3 binds the nuclear receptor with higher affinity than T_4, which makes T_3 more biologically active. Pituitary thyroid-stimulating hormone (TSH) and hypothalamic thyrotropin-releasing hormone (TRH) regulate hormone production and thyroid growth by normal feedback physiology. Thyroid-stimulating immunoglobulins (TSIs), once known as long-acting thyroid stimulator (LATS), bind to the TSH receptor that results in hyperthyroid Graves' disease.

Plasma proteins bind over 99% of circulating T_4 and T_3, predominately to thyroxine-binding globulin (TBG), and the remaining 1% of thyroid hormones are free. Free levels of thyroid hormones remain constant despite physiologic or pharmacologic alterations. Regardless of total serum protein levels, active thyroid hormone remains stable. In healthy women, transitions from puberty to menopause do not alter free thyroid hormone concentrations. Excess endogenous or exogenous sources of estrogen increase TBG plasma concentration by decreasing hepatic clearance. Androgens (especially testosterone) and corticosteroids have the opposite effect by increasing hepatic TBG clearance.

Thyroid function tests may be misleading in women receiving exogenous sources of estrogen because of altered binding characteristics. In euthyroid individuals, elevations of thyroid hormone concentrations arise from three mechanisms, (a) increased protein binding because of altered albumin and estrogen states, (b) decreased peripheral conversion of T_4 to T_3, or (c) rarely occurring congenital tissue resistance to thyroid hormones. The most common alteration in laboratory findings is due to altered estrogen states (hormonal replacement therapy, pregnancy), which complicate interpretation of thyroid function studies. Most laboratories compensate by reporting a free T_4 index or a "T_7" which mathematically corrects for physiologic alterations. If a question arises, consultation with the clinical pathologist should be sought.

Hypothyroidism

Overt hypothyroidism occurs in 2% of women, and at least an additional 5% develop subclinical hypothyroidism. This is especially true in the elderly in whom many of the signs and symptoms are subtle. The principal cause of hypothyroidism is autoimmune thyroiditis (Hashimoto's thyroiditis). A familial predisposition is observed in many cases, but the specific genetic or environmental trigger is unknown. The incidence of autoimmune thyroiditis increases with age, affecting up to 15% of women over 65 years of age. Many have subclinical hypothyroidism that is defined as an elevated serum TSH concentration with a normal serum free T_4 level. Thyroid replacement therapy usually reverses this condition. Autoimmune thyroiditis may be associated with other endocrine (e.g., type 1 diabetes, primary ovarian failure, adrenal insufficiency, and hypoparathyroidism) and nonendocrine disorders (e.g., vitiligo and pernicious anemia) (59). Therefore, when autoimmune diseases are present, there should be a high degree of suspicion for concurrent thyroid disorders. Iatrogenic causes of hypothyroidism occur after surgical removal or radioactive iodine therapy for hyperthyroidism or thyroid cancer. Forty years ago, radiation was used to treat acne and other dermatologic disorders; these patients have an increased risk of thyroid cancer and require close monitoring. Hypothyroidism rarely occurs secondary to pituitary or hypothalamic diseases from TSH or TRH deficiency but must be considered if symptoms occur after neurosurgical procedures.

Clinical Features

Manifestations of hypothyroidism include a broad range of signs and symptoms including fatigue, lethargy, cold intolerance, nightmares, dry skin, hair loss, constipation, periorbital carotene deposition (causing a yellow discoloration), carpal tunnel syndrome, and weight gain (usually less than 5 to 10 kg). Menstrual dysfunction is common, either as menorrhagia or amenorrhea. Infertility may arise from anovulation, but exogenous thyroid hormone is not useful for women who are anovulatory and euthyroid. Empiric use of thyroid extract, common many years ago, should be discouraged. Common neuropsychiatric symptoms that may be early signs of hypothyroidism include depression, irritability, impaired memory, and dementia in the elderly.

Hypothyroidism is not a cause of premenstrual syndrome (PMS), but worsening PMS may be a subtle manifestation of hypothyroidism (60). Hypothyroidism may cause precocious or delayed puberty. Hyperprolactinemia and galactorrhea are unusual manifestations of hypothyroidism; however, assessment of thyroid function should be considered. A TSH level should be obtained in cases of amenorrhea, galactorrhea, and hyperprolactinemia to distinguish primary hypothyroidism from a prolactin-secreting pituitary adenoma.

Diagnosis

Hypothyroidism should always be confirmed with laboratory studies. Primary hypothyroidism is characterized by the combination of an elevated serum TSH with a low serum free T_4 or free T_4 index. Autoimmune thyroiditis can be confirmed by the presence of serum antithyroid peroxidase (formerly referred to as antimicrosomal) antibodies. Central hypothyroidism, although rare, is distinguished by a low or low-normal serum free T_4 with either a low or inappropriately normal serum TSH concentration.

Therapy

L-thyroxine (T_4) is the treatment of choice for hypothyroidism and is available as levothyroxine (Synthroid or Levothroid) (61). The mode of action is by conversion of T_4 to T_3 in peripheral tissues. A parenteral formulation is available but seldom needed because of the long half-life (7 days) of oral preparations. Absorption may be poor when taken in combination with aluminum hydroxide (common in antacids), cholestyramine, ferrous sulfate, or sucralfate because of binding or chelation. The usual T_4 requirement is weight-related (approximately 1.6 μg/kg) but decreases for the elderly. Normal daily dosage is 0.1 to 0.15 mg, but should be adjusted to maintain TSH levels within the normal range.

In the early 1980s, many clinicians thought that by increasing the serum T_4 to mildly elevated levels that conversion of T_4 to T_3 would be enhanced. Subsequent data has proven that even with a mild increase of T_4 there was associated cortical bone loss and atrial fibrillation, particularly in older women (62). A low initial T_4 dose (0.025 mg/day) should be initiated in patients with known or suspected coronary artery disease. Rapid replacement may worsen angina and, in some cases, induce myocardial infarction.

Hyperthyroidism

Hyperthyroidism affects 2% of women during their lifetimes, most often during their childbearing years. Graves' disease represents the most common disorder; it is associated with orbital inflammation causing the classic exophthalmus associated with the disease, and a characteristic dermopathy, pretibial myxedema. The cause of Graves' disease in genetically susceptible women is unknown. Autonomously functioning benign thyroid neoplasias are less common causes of hyperthyroidism and are associated with toxic adenomas and toxic multinodular goiters. Transient thyrotoxicosis may be the result of unregulated glandular release of thyroid hormone in postpartum (painless, silent, or lymphocytic) thyroiditis and subacute (painful) thyroiditis. Other rare causes of thyroid overactivity include: human chorionic gonadotropin (hCG)–secreting choriocarcinoma, TSH-secreting pituitary adenoma, and struma ovarii. Factitious ingestion or iatrogenic overprescribing should be considered in patients with eating disorders.

Clinical Features

Symptoms of thyrotoxicosis include fatigue, diarrhea, heat intolerance, palpitations, dyspnea, nervousness, and weight loss. In young patients there may be paradoxical weight gain from an increased appetite. Thyrotoxicosis may cause vomiting in pregnant women that may be confused with hyperemesis gravidarum (63). Tachycardia, lid lag, tremor, proximal muscle weakness, and warm, moist skin are classic physical findings on examination. The most dramatic physical changes are ophthalmologic and include lid retraction, periorbital edema, and proptosis. These eye findings, however, occur in less than one-third of women. In elderly adults, symptoms are often more subtle with presentations of unexplained weight loss, atrial fibrillation, or new-onset angina pectoris (64). Menstrual abnormalities span from regular menses to light flow, to anovulatory menses and associated infertility. Goiter is common in younger women with Graves' disease but may be absent in older women. Toxic nodular goiter is associated with nonhomogeneous glandular enlargement, while in subacute thyroiditis the gland is tender, hard, and enlarged.

Diagnosis

Most thyrotoxic patients have elevated total and free T_4 and T_3 (measured by radioimmune assay [RIA]) concentrations. In thyrotoxicosis, serum TSH concentrations are virtually undetectable, even with very sensitive assays (sensitivity measured to 0.1 units). Sensitive serum TSH measurements may aid in the diagnosis of hyperthyroidism. Radioiodine uptake scans are useful in the differential diagnosis of established hyperthyroidism. Scans with homogeneous uptake of radioactive iodine are suggestive of Graves' disease, while those with a heterogeneous tracer uptake are suggestive of a diagnosis of toxic nodular goiter. In distinction, thyroiditis and medication-induced thyrotoxicosis are associated with diminished glandular radioisotope concentration.

Therapy

Antithyroid medications, either *propylthiouracil (PTU)* (50 to 300 mg every 6 to 8 hours) or *methimazole* (10 to 30 mg per day) are initial therapies used. After metabolic control is obtained, definitive therapy is obtained by thyroid ablation with radioiodine. This results in permanent hypothyroidism. Both antithyroid drugs block thyroid hormone biosynthesis and may have additional immunosuppressive effects on the gland. The primary difference in oral medications is that PTU partially inhibits extrathyroidal T_4-to-T_3 conversion, while methimazole does not. However, methimazole has a longer half-life and permits single-daily dosing that may encourage compliance. Euthyroidism is typically restored in 3 to 10 weeks, and treatment with oral antithyroid agents is continued for 6 to 24 months, unless total ablation with radioiodine or surgical resection is performed. Surgery has become less popular, because it is invasive and may result in inadvertent parathyroid removal that commits the patient to lifelong calcium therapy.

The relapse rate with oral antithyroid medications is 50% over a lifetime. Lifelong follow-up is important when medical therapy is used solely because of the high relapse rate. Both medications have infrequent (5%) minor side effects that include fever, rash, or arthralgias. Major toxicity is rare ($<1\%$) and includes hepatitis, vasculitis, and agranulocytosis. Agranulocytosis is not predictable by periodic complete blood counts; therefore, patients who have sore throats or fevers should stop the medication and call their physicians immediately.

Therapy with iodine-131 provides a permanent cure of hyperthyroidism in 70% to 80% of patients. The principal drawback to radioactive iodine therapy is the high rate of postablative hypothyroidism, which occurs in at least 50% of patients immediately posttherapy, with additional cases developing at a rate of 2% to 3% per year.

Based on the assumption that hypothyroidism will develop, patients should be given lifetime thyroid replacement. β-Adrenergic blocking agents such as propranolol are useful adjunctive therapy for control of sympathomimetic symptoms such as tachycardia (65). An additional benefit of β-blockers is the blocking of peripheral conversion of T_4 to T_3. In rare cases of thyroid storm, PTU, β-blockers, glucocorticoids, and high-dose iodine preparations (SSKI, or intravenous sodium iodide) should be started immediately, and referral to an intensive care unit is advisable.

Thyroid Nodules and Cancer

Thyroid nodules are common and found on physical examination in up to 5% of patients. Nodules may be demonstrated ultrasonographically in as many as 30% of unselected patients. Most nodules, when discovered, are asymptomatic and benign; however, malignancy and hyperthyroidism must be excluded. Irradiation in childhood, regardless of dose, is associated with a higher risk of malignancy. Virtually all nodules require histologic evaluation. In the past decade, this is accomplished by fine-needle aspiration (FNA) biopsy rather than open surgical biopsy. Thyroid function tests should be performed prior to FNA, and if the results are abnormal the underlying disease should be treated. In many cases, the nodule will regress during therapy and eliminate the need for FNA. Nodules that persist after treatment should undergo biopsy. Because most nodules are "cold" on scanning, it is more cost effective to proceed with tissue sampling rather than scanning. Biopsy is successful and provides a diagnosis in 95% of cases; however, in the 5% without diagnosis, surgical biopsy is necessary. Only 20% of surgical biopsies of an "indeterminate aspiration" are found to be malignant (66).

Papillary thyroid carcinoma is the most common malignancy, found in 75% of cases. Patients who are less than 50 years of age with a primary tumor of less than 4 centimeters when discovered, even with associated cervical lymph node metastasis, usually are cured. Anaplastic tumors in the elderly have a poor prognosis and progress rapidly despite therapy. Radioiodine therapy or surgical ablation are the most common methods of therapy. After therapy, the patient should be placed on lifetime suppression and monitored by assessment of TBG levels.

References

1. **Evans FO, Sydnor JB, Moore WEC, et al.** Sinusitis of maxillary antrum. *N Eng J Med* 1975;293:735–739.
2. **Slavin RG.** Sinopulmonary relationships. *Am J Otolaryngol* 1994;15:18–25.
3. **Mabry RL.** Allergic rhinosinusitis. In: **Bailey BJ,** ed. *Head and neck surgery otolaryngology.* Philadelphia: JB Lippincott, 1993:290–301.
4. **Williams JN, Simel DL.** Does this patient have sinusitis? Diagnosing acute sinusitis by history and physical examination. *JAMA* 1993;270:1242–1246.
5. **Ruben RJ, Bagger-Sjoback D, Downs MP, et al.** Recent advances in otitis media. Complications and sequelae. *Ann Otol Rhinol Laryngol Suppl* 1989;139:46–55.
6. **Douglas RG Jr.** Prophylaxis and treatment of influenza. *N Engl J Med* 1990;322:443–450.
7. **Woodhead MA, MacFarlane JT, McCraken JS, et al.** Prospective study of the etiology and outcome of pneumonia in the community. *Lancet* 1987;671–674.
8. **Nolan TE, Hankins GDV.** Adult respiratory distress. In: **Pastorek,** ed. *Infectious disease in obstetrics and gynecology.* Rockville, MD: Aspen Publications, 1994:197–206.
9. **Farr BM, Kaiser DL, Harrison BD, et al.** Prediction of microbial etiology at admission to hospital for pneumonia from the presenting clinical features. *Thorax* 1989;44:1031–1035.
10. **Niederman MS, Bass JB, Campbell GD, et al.** American Thoracic Society guidelines for the initial management of adults with community-acquired pneumonia: diagnosis, assessment of severity, and initial antimicrobial therapy. *Am Rev Respir Dis* 1993;148:1418–1426.
11. **Marrie TJ, Lau CY, Wheeler SL, et al.** A controlled trial of a critical pathway for treatment of community-acquired pneumonia. *JAMA* 2000;283:749–755.
12. **Centers for Disease Control and Prevention.** Prevention and control of influenza: recommendations of the Advisory Committee on Immunization Practices (ACIP). *MMWR* 2000;49:1–38.
13. **Blair SN, Kohl HW III, Pafferbarger RS Jr, et al.** Physical fitness and all-cause mortality. *JAMA* 1989;262:2395–2401.
14. **Anastos K, Charney P, Charon RA, et al.** Hypertension in women: what is really known. *Ann Int Med* 1991;115:287–293.
15. **The Sixth Report of the Joint National Committee on the Prevention, Detection, Evaluation, and Treatment of High Blood Pressure (JNC VI).** *Arch Intern Med* 1997;157:2413–2445.
16. **Roccella EJ, Lenfant C.** Regional and racial differences among stroke victims in the United States. *Clin Cardiol* 1989;12:IV4–8.
17. **Moorman PG, Hames CG, Tyroler HA.** Socioeconomic status and morbidity and mortality in hypertensive blacks. *Cardiovasc Clin* 1991;21:179–194.
18. **Stamler J, Stamler R, Neaton JD.** Blood pressure, systolic and diastolic, and cardiovascular risks. *Arch Intern Med* 1993;153:598–615.
19. **Preuss HG.** Nutrition and diseases of women: cardiovascular disorders. *J Am Coll Nutr* 1993;12:417–425.
20. **Stamler R, Stamler J, Gosch FC, et al.** Primary prevention of hypertension by nutritionally hygienic means: final report of a randomized, controlled trial. *JAMA* 1989;262:1801–1807.
21. **SHEP Cooperative Research Group.** Prevention of stroke by antihypertensive drug treatment in older persons with isolated systolic hypertension. *JAMA* 1991;265:3255–3264.
22. **American Society of Hypertension.** Recommendations for routine blood pressure measurement by indirect cuff sphygmomanometry. *Am J Hypertens* 1992;5:207–209.

23. **The National High Blood Pressure Education Program Working Group Report on Ambulatory Blood Pressure Monitoring.** *Arch Intern Med* 1990;150:2270–2280.

24. **Selby JV, Friedman GD, Quensenberry CP Jr.** Precursors of essential hypertension: the role of body fat distribution pattern. *Am J Epidemiol* 1989;129:43–53.

25. **Schotte DE, Stunkard AJ.** The effects of weight reduction on blood pressure in 301 obese patients. *Arch Intern Med* 1990;150:1701–1704.

26. **Law MR, Frost CD, Wald NJ.** By how much does dietary salt reduction lower blood pressure? Analysis of data from trials of salt reduction. *BMJ* 1991;302:819–824.

27. **Blair SN, Goodyear NN, Gibbons LW, et al.** Physical fitness and incidence of hypertension in healthy normotensive men and women. *JAMA* 1989;262:2395–2401.

28. **Alderman MH.** Which antihypertensive drugs first—and why! *JAMA* 1992;267:2786–2787.

29. **Freis ED.** Critique of the clinical importance of diuretic-induced hypokalemia and elevated cholesterol level. *Arch Intern Med* 1989;149:2640–2648.

30. **Garber AJ.** Effective treatment of hypertension in patients with diabetes mellitus. *Clin Cardiol* 1992;15:715–719.

31. **Dwyer PL, Teele JS.** Prazosin: a neglected cause of genuine stress incontinence. *Obstet Gynecol* 1992;79:117–121.

32. **National High Blood Pressure Education Program Working Group Report on Ambulatory Blood Pressure Monitoring.** *Arch Intern Med* 1990;150:2270–2280.

33. **Brown MS, Goldstein JL.** A receptor-mediated pathway for cholesterol homeostasis. *Science* 1986;232:34–47.

34. **Smith GD, Pekkanen J.** Should there be a moratorium on the use of cholesterol lowering drugs? *BMJ* 1992;304:431–434.

35. **Boyd NF, Cousins M, Beaton M, et al.** Quantitative changes in dietary fat intake and serum cholesterol in women: results from a randomized controlled trial. *Am J Clin Nutr* 1990;52:470–476.

36. **Ladias JAA, Kwiterovich PO, Smith HH, et al.** Apolipoprotein B-100 Hopkins (Arginin 4019-Tryptophan). *JAMA* 1989;262:1980–1988.

37. **Katan MB, Beynen AC.** Characteristics of human hypo- and hyperresponders to dietary cholesterol. *Am J Epidemiol* 1987;125:387–399.

38. **Rauh G, Keller C, Kormann B, et al.** Familial defective apolipoprotein B-100: clinical characteristics of 54 cases. *Atherosclerosis* 1992;92:233–241.

39. **Mahley RW, Weisgraber KH, Innerarity TL, et al.** Genetic defects in lipoprotein metabolism. *JAMA* 1991;265:78–83.

40. **Avins, AL, Haber RJ, Hulley SB.** The status of hypertriglyceridemia as a risk factor for coronary heart disease. *Clin Laboratory Med* 1989;9:153–168.

41. **Goldbourt U, Holtzman E, Neufeld HN.** Total and high-density lipoprotein cholesterol in the serum and risk of mortality: evidence of a threshold effect. *BMJ* 1987;290:1239–1243.

42. **Gordon DJ, Rifkind BM.** High-density lipoprotein—the clinical implications of recent studies. *N Engl J Med* 1989;321:1311–1316.

43. **Ramsey LE, Yeo WW, Jackson PR.** Dietary reduction of serum cholesterol concentration: time to think again. *BMJ* 1991;303:953–957.

44. **Naughton MJ, Luepker RV, Strickland D.** The accuracy of portable cholesterol analyzers in public screening programs. *JAMA* 1990;263:1213–1217.

45. **Irwig L, Glasziou P, Wilson A, et al.** Estimating an individual's true cholesterol level and response to intervention. *JAMA* 1991;266:1678–1685.

46. **Cooper GR, Myers GL, Smith SJ, et al.** Standardization of lipid, lipoprotein, and porkipoprotein measurements. *Clin Chem* 1988;34:B95–B105.

47. **McManus BM, Toth AB, Engel JA, et al.** Progress in lipid reporting practices and reliability of cholesterol measurement in clinical laboratories in Nebraska. *JAMA* 1989;262:83–88.

48. **van Stiphout WAHJ, Hofman A, de Bruijn AM.** Serum lipids in young women before, during, and after pregnancy. *Am J Epidemiol* 1987;126:922–928.

49. **Abramowicz M, Rizack MA, et al.** Choice of lipid-lowering drugs. *Med Lett* 1998;40:117–122.

50. **Centers for Disease Control and Prevention.** *Diabetes surveillance, 1993.* Washington DC: US Department of Health and Human Services, Public Health Service; 1993.

51. **Jarrett RJ.** Risk factors for coronary heart disease in diabetes mellitus. *Diabetes* 1992;41[Suppl 2]:1–3.

52. **The Expert Committee on the Diagnosis and Classification of Diabetes Mellitus.** Report of the Expert Committee on the Diagnosis and Classification of Diabetes Mellitus. *Diabetes Care* 2000;23:S4–S42.

53. **Bogardus C, Lilloja S, Howard VV, et al.** Relationships between insulin secretion, insulin action, and fasting plasma glucose concentration in non-diabetic and non–insulin-dependent diabetic subjects. *J Clin Invest* 1984;74:1238–1246.

54. **Wood PD, Stefanick ML, Williams PT, et al.** The effects on plasma lipoproteins of a prudent weight-reducing diet, with or without exercise, in overweight men and women. *N Engl J Med* 1991;325:461–466.

55. **Tal A.** Oral hypoglycemic agents in the treatment of type II diabetes. *Am Fam Physician* 1993;43:1089–1095.

56. **Tunbridge WM, Evered DC, Hall R, et al.** The spectrum of thyroid disease in a community: the Whickham survey. *Clin Endocrinol (Oxf)* 1977;7:481–493.

57. **Helfand M, Crapo LM.** Screening for thyroid disease. *Ann Intern Med* 1990;112:840–849.

58. **Brent GA, Moore DD, Larsen RP.** Thyroid hormone regulation of gene expression. *Annu Rev Physiol* 1991;53:17–35.

59. **Volpé R.** Autoimmunity causing thyroid dysfunction. *Endocrinol Metab Clin North Am* 1991;20:565–587.

60. **Schmidt PJ, Grover GN, Roy-Byrne PP, et al.** Thyroid function in women with premenstrual syndrome. *J Clin Endocrinol Metab* 1993;76:671–674.

61. **Mandel SJ, Brent GA, Larsen PR.** Levothyroxine therapy in patients with thyroid disease. *Ann Intern Med* 1993;119:492–502.

62. **Schneider DL, Barrett-Connor EL, Morton DJ.** Thyroid hormone use and bone mineral density in elderly women. Effects of estrogen. *JAMA* 1994;271:1245–1249.

63. **Mori M, Amino N, Tamaki H, et al.** Morning sickness and thyroid function in normal pregnancy. *Obstet Gynecol* 1988;72:355–359.

64. **Siebers MJ, Drinka PJ, Vergauwen C.** Hyperthyroidism as a cause of atrial fibrillation in long-term care. *Arch Intern Med* 1992;152:2063–2064.

65. **Zonszein J, Santangelo RP, Mackin JF, et al.** Propranolol therapy in thyrotoxicosis. *Am J Med* 1979;66:411–416.

66. **McHenry CR, Walfish PG, Rosen IB.** Non-diagnostic fine needle aspiration biopsy: a dilemma in management of nodular thyroid disease. *Am Surgeon* 1993;59:415–419.

67. **The Sixth Report of the Joint National Committee on Prevention, Detection, Evaluation, and Treatment of High Blood Pressure (JNC VI).** Bethesda, MD: National Institutes of Health, National Heart, Lung, and Blood Institute; 1997; NIH publication 99-4080.

68. **Second Report of the National Cholesterol Education Program (NCEP) Expert Panel on the Detection, Evaluation, and Treatment of High Blood Cholesterol in Adults.** *JAMA* 1993;269:3015–3023.

Novak's Gynecology, 13th Edition. Edited by J.S. Berek. Lippincott Williams & Wilkins, Philadelphia © 2002.

10 Family Planning

Phillip G. Stubblefield

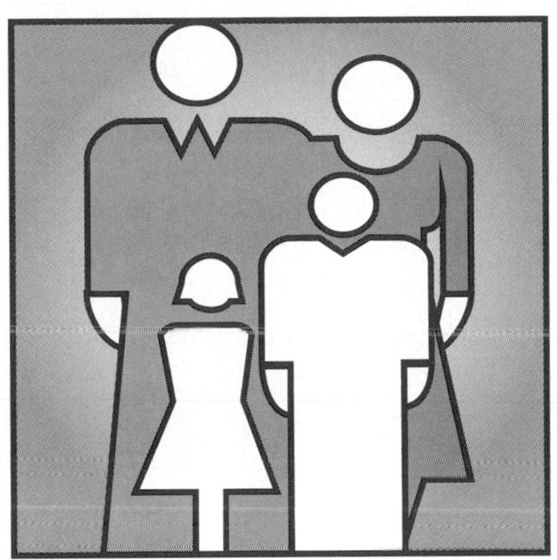

The history of contraception is a long one; however, the voluntary control of fertility is even more important in modern society (1). With each woman expected to have no more than one or two children, most of the reproductive years are spent trying to avoid pregnancy. Effective control of reproduction is essential to a woman's ability to accomplish her individual goals. From a larger perspective, the rapid growth of the human population in this century threatens the survival of all. At its present rate, the population of the world will double in 47 years and that of many of the poorer countries of the world will double in about 20 years (2) (Fig. 10.1). For the individual and for the planet, reproductive health requires careful use of effective means to prevent both pregnancy and sexually transmitted diseases (STDs) (3).

From puberty until menopause, women are faced with concerns about childbearing or its avoidance: the only options are sexual abstinence, contraception, or pregnancy. The contraceptive choices made by American couples in 1995, when the last national fertility survey was conducted by the U.S. government from a large national probability sample, are shown in Table 10.1 (4). For couples older than 35 years of age, sterilization is the number one choice. For younger couples, oral contraceptives (OCs) are the most used method, and the condom ranks second. Although use of contraception is high, a significant proportion of sexually active couples do not use contraception: 5.2% in the 1995 National Fertility Survey (4). The percentage of women using no contraception is highest among the youngest group (i.e., adolescents).

It is estimated that 49% of births in the United States in 1994 were unintended, and that by 45 years of age, 43% of women will have at least one induced abortion (5). Abortion is an obvious indicator of unplanned pregnancy. Abortion ratios by age group indicate that the use of abortion is greatest for the youngest women and least for women in their late 20s and early 30s (Fig. 10.2). Use increases again as women become older. Young people are much more likely to experience contraceptive failure because their fertility is greater than that of older women and because they are more likely to have intercourse without contraception. The effect of age on pregnancy rates with different contraceptive methods is shown in Figure 10.3.

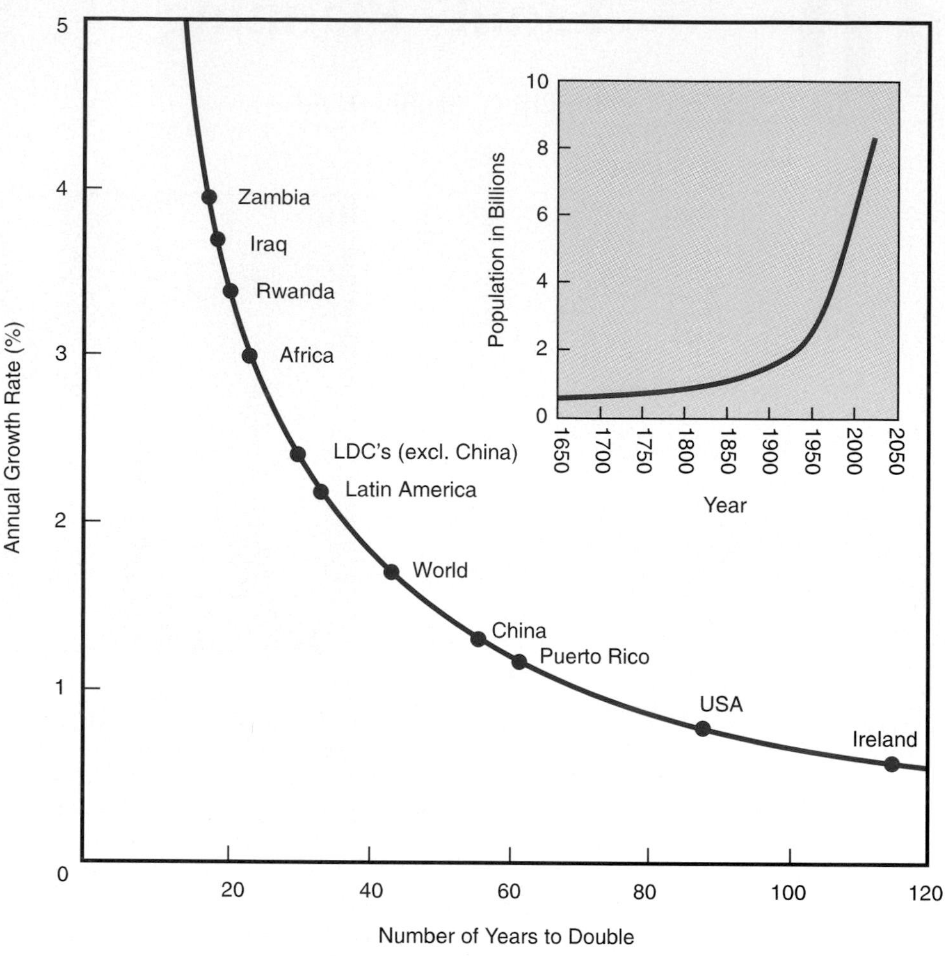

Figure 10.1 Doubling time at different rates of population growth, with representative countries, and world population growth curve. (From **Hatcher RA, Trussell J, Stewart F, et al.** *Contraceptive technology.* 17th ed. New York: Ardent Media, 1998:768, with permission.)

Efficacy of Contraception

Factors affecting whether pregnancy will occur include the fecundity of both partners, the timing of intercourse in relation to the time of ovulation, the method of contraception used, the intrinsic effectiveness of the contraceptive method, and the correct use of the method. It is impossible to assess the effectiveness of a contraceptive method in isolation from the other factors. The best way to assess effectiveness is long-term evaluation of a group of sexually active women using a particular method for a specified period to observe how frequently pregnancy occurs. **A pregnancy rate per 100 women per year can be calculated using the Pearl formula (dividing the number of pregnancies by the total number of months contributed by all couples, and then multiplying the quotient by 1,200).** With most methods, pregnancy rates decrease with time as the more fertile or less careful couples become pregnant and drop out. More accurate information is provided by the life-table method, which calculates the probability of pregnancy in successive months, which are then added over a given interval. Problems relate to which pregnancies are counted: those occurring among all couples or those in women the investigators deem to have used the method correctly. Because of this complexity, rates of pregnancy with different methods are best calculated by reporting two different rates derived from multiple studies (i.e., the lowest rate) and the usual rate as shown in Table 10.2.

Table 10.1. Percentage Distribution of Contraceptive Users Aged 15–44 Years, by Current Method, 1982–1995

Method	*1982*	*1988*	*1995*
Sterilization	34.1	39.2	38.6
Female	23.2	27.5	27.7
Male	10.9	11.7	10.9
Pill	28.0	30.7	26.9
Implant	NA	NA	1.3
Injectable	NA	NA	3.0
Intrauterine device	7.1	2.0	0.8
Diaphragm	8.1	5.7	1.9
Male condom	12.0	14.6	20.4
Foam	2.4	1.1	0.4
Periodic abstinence	3.9	2.3	2.3
Withdrawal	2.0	2.2	3.0
Other	2.5	2.1	1.3
Total no. of women	30,142,000	34,912,000	38,663,000

NA, not applicable.
From **Piccinino LJ, Mosher WD.** Trends in contraceptive use in the United States: 1982–1995. *Fam Plann Perspect* 1998;30:4–10, 46, with permission.

Safety

Some contraceptive methods have associated health risks; areas of concern are listed in Table 10.3. All of the methods are safer than the alternative (pregnancy with birth), with the possible exception of OC use by cigarette smokers older than 35 years of age (6). Most methods provide noncontraceptive health benefits in addition to contraception. Oral contraceptives reduce the risk for ovarian and endometrial cancer and ectopic pregnancy. Barrier methods and spermicides provide some protection against STDs, cervical cancer, and tubal infertility.

Cost

Some methods, such as intrauterine devices (IUDs) and subdermal implants, require an expensive initial investment but provide prolonged protection for a low annual cost. The results of a complex cost analysis based on the cost of the method plus the cost of pregnancy if the method fails are shown in Table 10.4. Sterilization and the long-acting methods are least expensive over the long term (7).

Nonhormonal Methods

Coitus Interruptus

Coitus interruptus is withdrawal of the penis from the vagina before ejaculation. This method, along with induced abortion and late marriage, is believed to account for most of the decline in fertility of preindustrial Europe (8). Coitus interruptus remains a very important means of fertility control in the Third World. This method has obvious advantages: immediate availability and no cost. Theoretically, the risk for STDs should be reduced, although this has not been studied. The Oxford Study reported a failure rate of 6.7 per 100 woman-years for this method (9). The penis must be completely withdrawn both from the vagina and from the external genitalia because pregnancy has occurred from ejaculation on the female external genitalia without penetration.

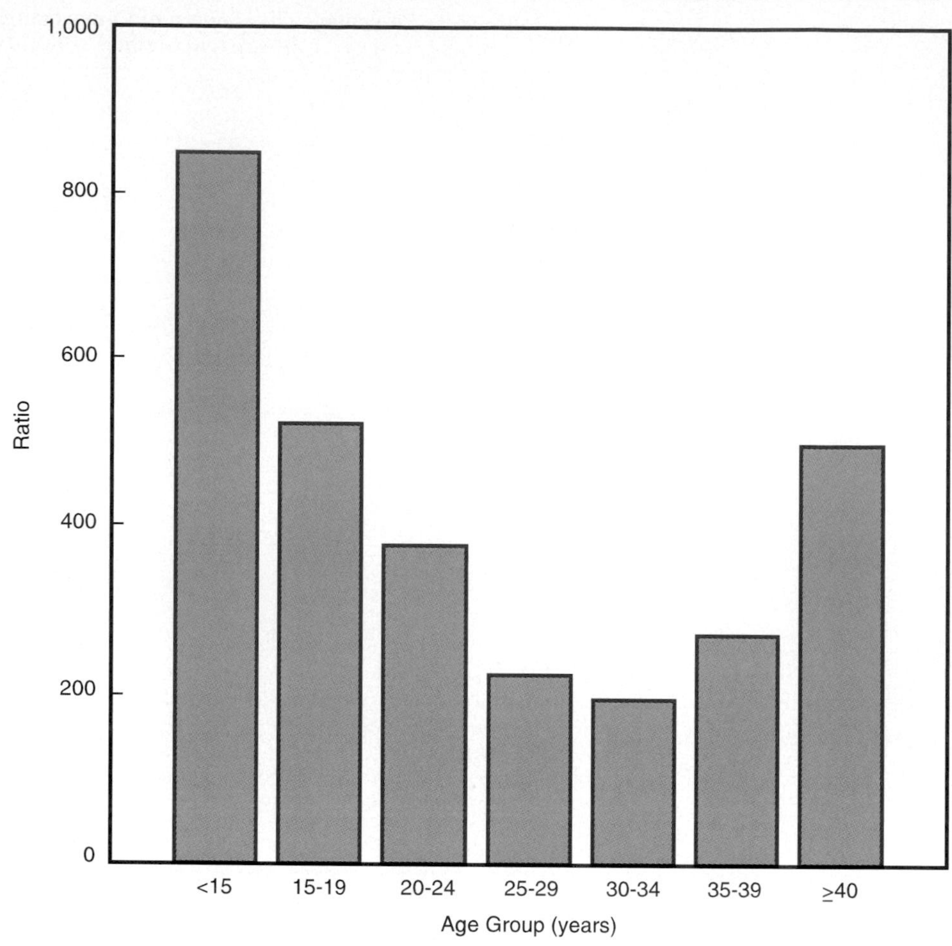

Figure 10.2 Abortion ratios, by age groups—United States, 1997. Ratio of induced abortions per 1,000 live births. [From **Koonin LM, Strauss LT, Chrisman CE, et al.** Abortion surveillance, 1997. *MMWR Morb Mortal Wkly Rep* 2000;49(No. SS-11):14, with permission.]

Lactation Amenorrhea

Ovulation is suppressed during lactation. The suckling of the infant elevates prolactin levels and reduces gonadotropin-releasing hormone (GnRH) from the hypothalamus, reducing luteinizing hormone (LH) release so that follicular maturation is inhibited (10). The duration of this suppression is variable and is influenced by the frequency and duration of nursing, length of time since birth, and probably by the mother's nutritional status. Even with continued nursing, ovulation eventually returns but is unlikely before 6 months, especially if the woman is amenorrheic and is fully breast feeding with no supplemental foods given to the infant (11). If pregnancy is to be delayed, another method of contraception should be used from 6 months after birth, when menstruation resumes, or when supplemental feeding is instituted. The risk for breast cancer may be reduced in women who have lactated, but whether this apparent benefit exists independent of early first pregnancy is not clear.

Combination OCs are generally not advised during lactation because they reduce the amount of milk produced by some women, although they can be used once milk production is established. Hormonal methods without estrogen can be used. These include progestin-only OCs, implants, and injectable contraception, none of which decreases milk production. Barrier methods, spermicides, and IUDs are also good options for nursing mothers (12).

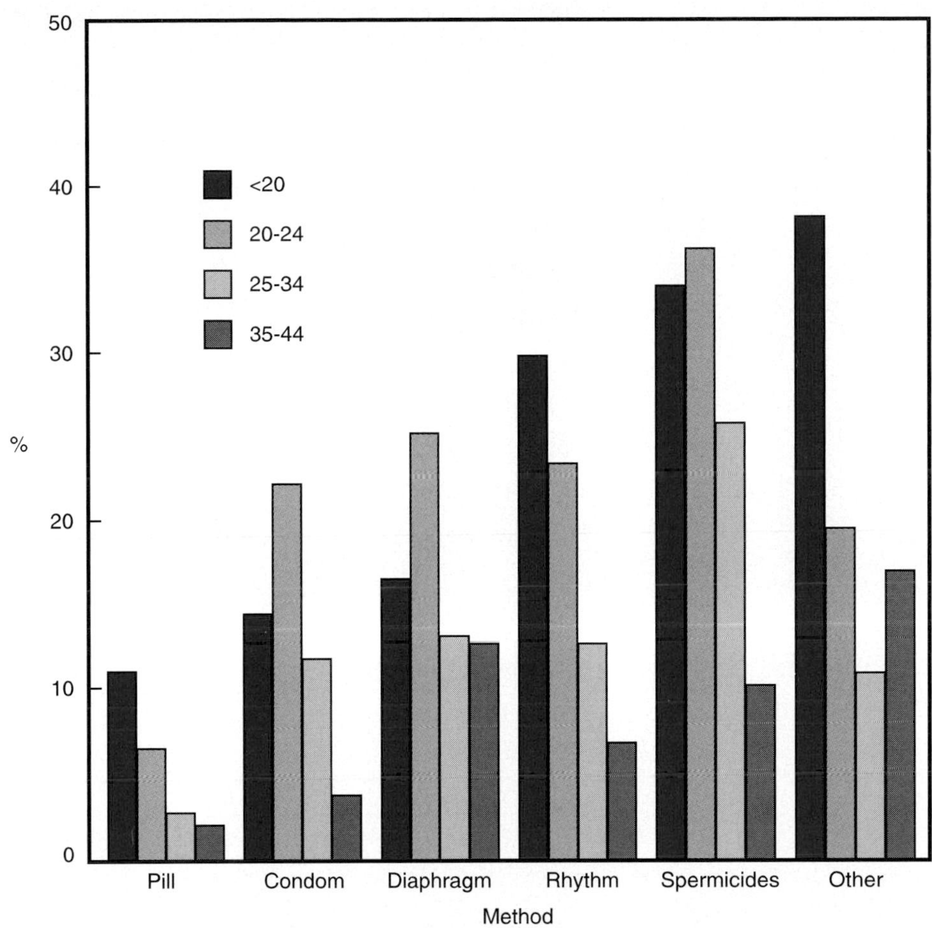

Figure 10.3 Percentage of women experiencing an accidental pregnancy, in the first 2 years of use, according to method, combined 1988 and 1995 National Survey of Family Growth. [From **Ranjit N, Bankole A, Forrest JD, et al.** Contraception failure in the first two years of use: differences across socioeconomic subgroups. *Fam Plann Perspect* 2001;33:25 (Table 6), with permission.]

Periodic Abstinence or Natural Family Planning

With periodic abstinence methods, couples attempt to avoid intercourse during the fertile period around the time of ovulation. A variety of methods are available: the calendar method, the mucus method (Billings or ovulation method), and the symptothermal method, which is a combination of the first two methods. The calendar method is the least effective. With the mucus method, the woman attempts to predict the fertile period by feeling the cervical mucus with her fingers. Under estrogen influence, the mucus increases in quantity and becomes progressively more slippery and elastic until a peak day is reached. Thereafter, the mucus becomes scant and dry under the influence of progesterone until onset of the next menses. Intercourse may be allowed during the "dry days" immediately after menses until mucus is detected. Thereafter, the couple must abstain until the fourth day after the "peak" day.

In the symptothermal method, the first day of abstinence is predicted either from the calendar, by subtracting 21 from the length of the shortest menstrual cycle in the preceding 6 months, or the first day mucus is detected, whichever comes first. The end of the fertile period is predicted by use of basal body temperature. The woman takes her temperature every morning and resumes intercourse 3 days after the thermal shift, the rise in body temperature that signals that the corpus luteum is producing progesterone and that ovulation has occurred.

Table 10.2. Percentage of Women Experiencing a Contraceptive Failure During the First Year of Use and the Percentage Continuing Use at the End of the First Year

	Women Experiencing Accidental Pregnancy within the First Year of Use (%)		*Women Continuing Use at 1 Year (%)*
Method	*Typical Use*	*Perfect Use*	
Chance	85	85	
Spermicides	21	6	43
Periodic abstinence			67
Calendar		9	
Ovulation method		3	
Symptothermal		2	
Postovulation		1	
Withdrawal	19	4	
Cap			
Parous women	36	26	45
Nulliparous women	18	9	58
Diaphragm	18	6	58
Condom			
Female (Reality)	21	5	56
Male	12	3	63
Pill	3		72
Progestin only		0.5	
Combined		0.1	
Intrauterine device			
Progesterone T	2.0	1.5	81
Copper T380A	0.8	0.6	78
Levonorgestrel T20	0.1	0.1	81
DepoProvera	0.3	0.3	70
Norplant[a]	0.3	0.3	85
Female sterilization	0.4	0.4	100
Male sterilization	0.15	0.10	100

[a] Cumulative 5-year pregnancy rate for pliable tubing, divided by 5.
From **Hatcher RA, Trussell J, Stewart F, et al.** *Contraceptive technology.* 16th ed. New York: Irvington Publishers Inc., 1994:113, with permission.

Efficacy

The ovulation method was evaluated by the World Health Organization in a five-country study. Women who successfully completed three monthly cycles of teaching were then enrolled in a 13-cycle efficacy study. Trussell and Grummer-Strawn calculated a 3.1% probability of pregnancy in 1 year for the small proportion of couples who used the method perfectly and 86.4% probability of pregnancy for the rest (13). Because sperm may survive several days in the female genital tract, even a week's abstinence around the time of actual ovulation offers no guarantee against pregnancy. Also, ovulation can occur even in the

Table 10.3. Overview of Contraceptive Methods

Method	*Advantages*	*Disadvantages*	*Risks*	*Noncontraceptive Benefits*
Coitus interruptus	Available, free	Depends on male control	Pregnancy	?Decreased STD risk
Lactation	Available, free	Unreliable duration of effect	Pregnancy	?Decreased breast cancer
Periodic abstinence	Available, free	Complex methodology; motivation is essential	Pregnancy	None
Condoms	Available, no prescription needed	Motivation is essential; must be used each time; depends on male	Pregnancy	Proven to decrease STDs and cervical cancer
Spermicides	Available, no prescription needed	Must be used each time	Pregnancy	Some decrease in STDs
Diaphragm/cap	Nonhormonal	Must be used each time; fitting required	Pregnancy, cystitis	Proven to decrease STDs and cervical cancer
IUD T380A	High efficacy for 10 years, unrelated to coitus	Initial cost; skilled inserter; pain and bleeding	Initial mild risk for PID and septic abortion	None
Levo-Norgestrel T	High efficacy for 5 years; unrelated to coitus	Initial cost; skilled inserter; amenorrhea for some	Initial mild risk for PID and septic abortion	Reduced bleeding; can be used to treat menorrhagia
Progestasert	Reasonable efficacy	Initial cost; skilled inserter; replace every year	Initial mild risk for PID, ectopic pregnancy	Reduced dysmenorrhea and menstrual blood loss
Oral contraceptives	High efficacy	Motivation to take daily; cost	Thrombosis; older smokers have increased risk of MI and stroke	Many benefits (see text)
DMPA	High efficacy, convenience	Injection required; bleeding pattern	Probably none	Many (see text)
Monthly injectable	High efficacy, convenience	Monthly injection	Probably same as orals	Probably same as orals
Implants	High efficacy, convenience	Surgical insertion and removal; initial cost; bleeding pattern	Functional cysts	Unknown
Postcoital hormones	Moderate efficacy	Frequent use disrupts menses; nausea	None	Unknown

STDs, sexually transmitted diseases; IUD, intrauterine device; PID, pelvic inflammatory disease; MI, myocardial infarction; DMPA, depomedroxyprogesterone acetate.

absence of menstruation. Pregnancies have occurred after a single act of coitus 7 days before apparent ovulation indicated by basal body temperature. Vaginal infections increase vaginal discharge, complicating the use of the method.

Accurate advance prediction of the time of ovulation would greatly facilitate both the use and efficacy of periodic abstinence. Devices that combine an electronic thermometer with small computers are being explored in an effort to improve the accuracy of basal body temperature as a predictor of the fertile phase (14). Home monitoring of estrogen provides 4 or more days' warning before ovulation and allows intercourse to be resumed 1 to 3 days after ovulation (15). Another approach is the identification of microcrystals in saliva as an indication of approaching ovulation (16).

The technique of insertion is as follows:

1. **The cervix is exposed with a speculum.** The vaginal vault and cervix are cleansed with a bacteriocidal solution, such as an iodine-containing solution.

2. **The uterine cavity should be measured with a uterine sound.** The depth of the cavity should measure at least 6 cm from the external os. A smaller uterus is not likely to tolerate currently available IUDs.

3. **A paracervical block** with 10 mL of 1% *lidocaine* mixed with *atropine* (0.5 mg) can be used to avoid vasovagal syncope and minimize discomfort. In some women, serious cardiac arrhythmia can occur with cervical stimulation and can be avoided by these measures.

4. **Use of a tenaculum for insertion is mandatory to prevent perforation.** The cervix is grasped with a tenaculum and gently pulled downward to straighten the angle between the cervical canal and the uterine cavity. The IUD, previously loaded into its inserter, is then gently introduced through the cervical canal.

5. **With the *ParaGard* and the *Progestasert,* the outer sheath of the inserter is withdrawn a short distance to release the arms of the T and is then gently pushed inward again to elevate the now-opened T against the fundus** (71). The outer sheath and the inner stylet of the inserter are withdrawn, and the strings are cut to project about 2 cm from the external cervical os.

6. **With the *Mirena* IUD, insertion is somewhat different. The inserter tube loaded with the IUD is introduced into the uterus until the preset sliding flange on the inserter is 1.5 to 2 cm from the external os of the cervix.** The arms of the T device are then released upward into the uterine cavity, and the inserter is pushed up under them to elevate the IUD up against the uterine fundus.

Intrauterine Devices in Pregnancy

A woman with an IUD in place who has amenorrhea should have a pregnancy test and pelvic examination. If an intrauterine pregnancy is diagnosed and the IUD strings are visible, the IUD should be removed as soon as possible in order to prevent later septic abortion, premature rupture of the membranes, and premature birth (72). When the strings of the IUD are not visible, an ultrasound examination should be performed to localize the IUD and determine whether expulsion has occurred. If the IUD is present, there are three options for management:

1. Therapeutic abortion

2. Ultrasound-guided intrauterine removal of the IUD

3. Continuation of the pregnancy with the device left in place

If the patient wishes to continue the pregnancy, ultrasound evaluation of the location of the IUD is advised (73). If the IUD is not in a fundal location, ultrasound-guided removal using small alligator forceps is advised. If the location is fundal, the IUD should be left in place. If pregnancy continues with an IUD in place, the patient must be warned of the symptoms of intrauterine infection and should be cautioned to seek care promptly for fever or flulike symptoms, abdominal cramping, or bleeding. At the earliest sign of infection, high-dose intravenous antibiotic therapy should be given and the pregnancy evacuated promptly.

Duration of Use

Annual rates of pregnancy, expulsions, and medical removals decrease with each year of use (74,75). Therefore, a woman who has had no problem by year 5, for example, is very unlikely to experience problems in the subsequent years. As noted, the *Progestasert* should be replaced at the end of 1 year, but the *copper T380A* is approved for 10 years and the *levonorgestrel T* for 5 years. Actinomyces can be detected by cervical cytology. Should actinomyces-like particles be found, removal of the IUD and treatment with oral penicillin is recommended.

Choice of Devices

Of the three IUDs approved in the United States, the *copper T380A* and *levonorgestrel T* are preferred. They provide protection for many years, have remarkably low pregnancy rates, and reduce risk for ectopic pregnancy substantially. The *Progestasert* must be replaced annually, theoretically exposing the patient to some risk for infection with each insertion, and increasing cost markedly. It is less effective and increases the risk for ectopic pregnancy slightly. Both the *Progestasert* and *Mirena IUDs* reduce the amount of menstrual bleeding and dysmenorrhea. The *copper T380A* can be expected to increase menstrual bleeding.

Hormonal Contraception

Hormonal contraceptives are female sex steroids, synthetic estrogen and synthetic progesterone (progestin), or progestin only. They can be administered in the form of OCs, implants, and injectables.

The most widely used hormonal contraceptive is the combination OC. Combination OCs can be monophasic, with the same dose of estrogen and progestin administered each day, or multiphasic, in which varying doses of steroids are given through a 21-day cycle. Typically, they are administered for 21 days beginning on the Sunday after a menstrual period, then discontinued for 7 days to allow for withdrawal bleeding that mimics the normal menstrual cycle. The 28-day version provides placebo tablets for the last 7 days of the cycle so the user simply takes one pill a day and starts a new pack as soon as the first pack is completed. Progestin-only formulations contain no estrogen. These are taken every day without interruption. Other forms of hormonal contraception include injectable progestins and estrogen-progestin combinations, subdermal implants releasing progestin, and the experimental vaginal rings that release either estrogen-progestin or progestin alone.

Silastic rings worn in the vagina release steroid hormones that are absorbed at a constant rate, allowing contraception with blood levels of steroids well below the peak levels that are seen with OCs. Rings containing levonorgestrel or combinations of levonorgestrel and estrogens are being studied (76).

Steroid Hormone Action

Sex steroids were originally defined by their biologic activity. They are characterized by their affinity for specific estrogen, progesterone, or androgen receptors as well as by their biologic effects in different systems (74). Steroids are rapidly absorbed in the gut but go directly into the liver through the portal circulation, where they are rapidly metabolized and inactivated. Therefore, large doses of steroids are required when they are administered orally. The addition of the ethinyl group to carbon-17 of the steroid molecule hinders degradation by the liver enzyme 17-hydroxysteroid dehydrogenase.

Progestins

Progestins are synthetic compounds that mimic the effect of natural progesterone but differ from it structurally (Fig. 10.8). There are three classes: the estranes and gonanes, which

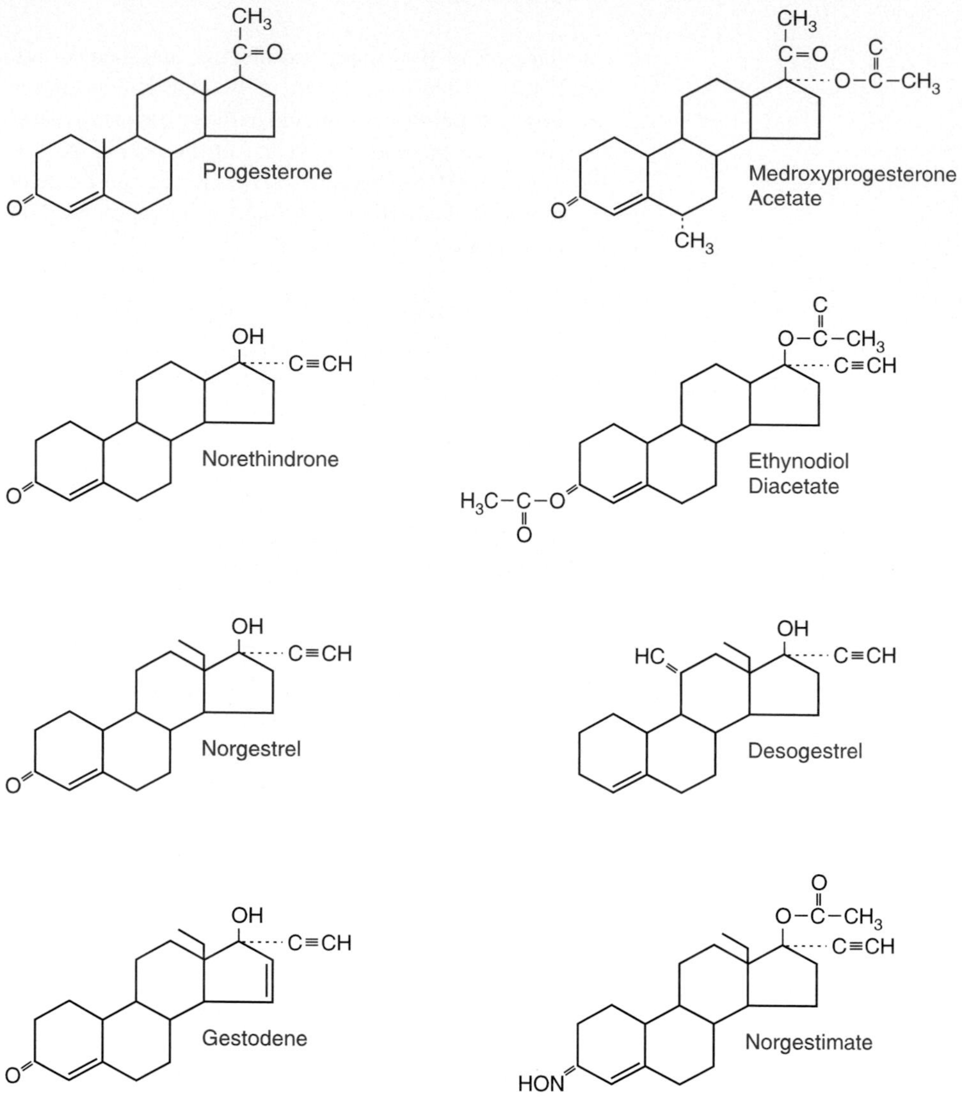

Figure 10.8 Progestins of interest for contraception. (From **Copeland LJ, Jarrell JF.** *Textbook of gynecology.* 2nd ed. Philadelphia: WB Saunders, 2000:303, with permission.)

are 19-nor progestins and are structurally similar to testosterone but lacking a carbon at position 19, and the pregnane or 17-acetoxy compounds, which are structurally similar to progesterone. Only the estrane and gonane compounds are used in oral contraceptives in the United States, but *medroxyprogesterone acetate* (*Provera*), one of the pregnane compounds, is the major injectable progestin. The progestins differ from each other in their affinities for estrogen, androgen, and progesterone receptors; their ability to inhibit ovulation; and their ability to substitute for progesterone and antagonize estrogen. Some are directly bound to the receptor (levonorgestrel, norethindrone), whereas others require bioactivation as, for example, desogestrel, which is converted in the body to its active metabolite, 3-keto-desogestrel. The 17-acetoxy progestins (e.g., *medroxyprogesterone acetate*) are bound by the progesterone receptor. *Norgestrel* exists as two stereoisomers, identified as dextronorgestrel and levonorgestrel. Only levonorgestrel is biologically active. Three newer progestins (*norgestimate, desogestrel,* and *gestodene*) are viewed as more "selective" than the other 19-nor progestins, in that they have little or no androgenic effect at doses that inhibit ovulation(78). The FDA has approved norgestimate- and desogestrel-containing OCs, and *gestodene* is available in Europe. *Gestodene* is a derivative of levonorgestrel that is more potent than the other preparations (i.e., very little of it is required for antifertility effects). Androgenic potency is considered undesirable because of the adverse effect of androgen and androgenic progestins on lipid and glucose metabolism. Androgenic progestins reduce levels of circulating high-density lipoprotein (HDL), elevate low-density lipoprotein (LDL), and adversely effect glucose tolerance in a dose-dependent fashion (79).

Estrogens

In the United States, OCs contain either of two estrogens: *mestranol* or *ethinyl estradiol (EE)*. *Mestranol* is *EE* with an extra methyl group. It requires bioactivation in the liver, where the methyl group is cleaved, releasing the active agent, *EE*. **OCs with 35 μg of *EE* provide the same blood levels of hormone as do OCs containing 50 μg of *mestranol*** (80).

Antifertility Effects

Combination Oral Contraceptives

Ovulation can be inhibited by oral estrogen or by oral progestin alone, but large doses are required. Pharmacologic synergism is exhibited when the two hormones are combined and ovulation is suppressed at a much lower dose of each agent. Combination OCs suppress basal follicle-stimulating hormone (FSH) and LH. Oral contraceptives diminish the ability of the pituitary gland to synthesize gonadotropins when it is stimulated by the hypothalamic gonadotropin-releasing hormone (GnRH) (81). Ovarian follicles do not mature, little estradiol is produced, and there is no midcycle LH surge. Ovulation does not occur, the corpus luteum does not form, and progesterone is not produced. This blockade of ovulation is dose related. Newer low-dose OCs do not provide as dense a block and allow somewhat higher base-line FSH and LH levels than higher-dose formulations (82). This makes ovulation somewhat more likely to occur if pills are missed or if the patient takes another medication that interferes with OC action.

Progestin-only Preparations

The mode of action of progestin-only contraceptives depends very much on the dose of the compound (83). At low blood levels of progestin, ovulation will occur part of the time. With the progestin-only "minipill," which supplies 0.3 mg of *norethindrone* per day (*Micronor*), 40% of cycles are ovulatory, 25% have inadequate luteal function, 18% have follicular maturation without ovulation, and 18% have complete suppression of follicle development. At moderate blood levels of progestin, normal basal levels of FSH and LH are present, and some follicle maturation may occur. Estradiol production is present, and the surge of estradiol that would normally trigger pituitary release of LH occurs; there is no answering LH surge, however, and hence no ovulation. At higher blood levels of progestin, basal FSH is reduced, and there is less follicular activity, less estradiol production, and no LH surge.

Hormonal Implants

With the subdermal implant that releases *levonorgestrel* (*Norplant*), there is some follicular maturation and estrogen production, but LH peak levels are low and ovulation is often inhibited. In the first year of use, ovulation is believed to occur in about 20% of cycles. The proportion of ovulatory cycles increases with time, probably as a result of the decline in hormone release. By the fourth year of use, 41% of cycles are ovulatory. The mechanisms of contraception with low-dose progestins are believed to include effects on the cervical mucus, endometrium, and tubal motility. The scant, dry cervical mucus in women using these preparations inhibits sperm migration into the upper tract. Progestins decrease nuclear estrogen receptor levels, decrease progesterone receptors, and induce activity of the enzyme 17-hydroxysteroid dehydrogenase that metabolizes natural estradiol 17β (84).

The sustained release offered by contraceptive implants allows for highly effective contraception at relatively low blood levels of the steroid. Figure 10.9 depicts expected steroid blood levels with implants, injectables, and oral contraceptives. An additional mechanism for contraception has been discovered with the antiprogesterone *mefipristone (RU486)*. In the normal cycle, there is a small amount of progesterone production from the follicle just

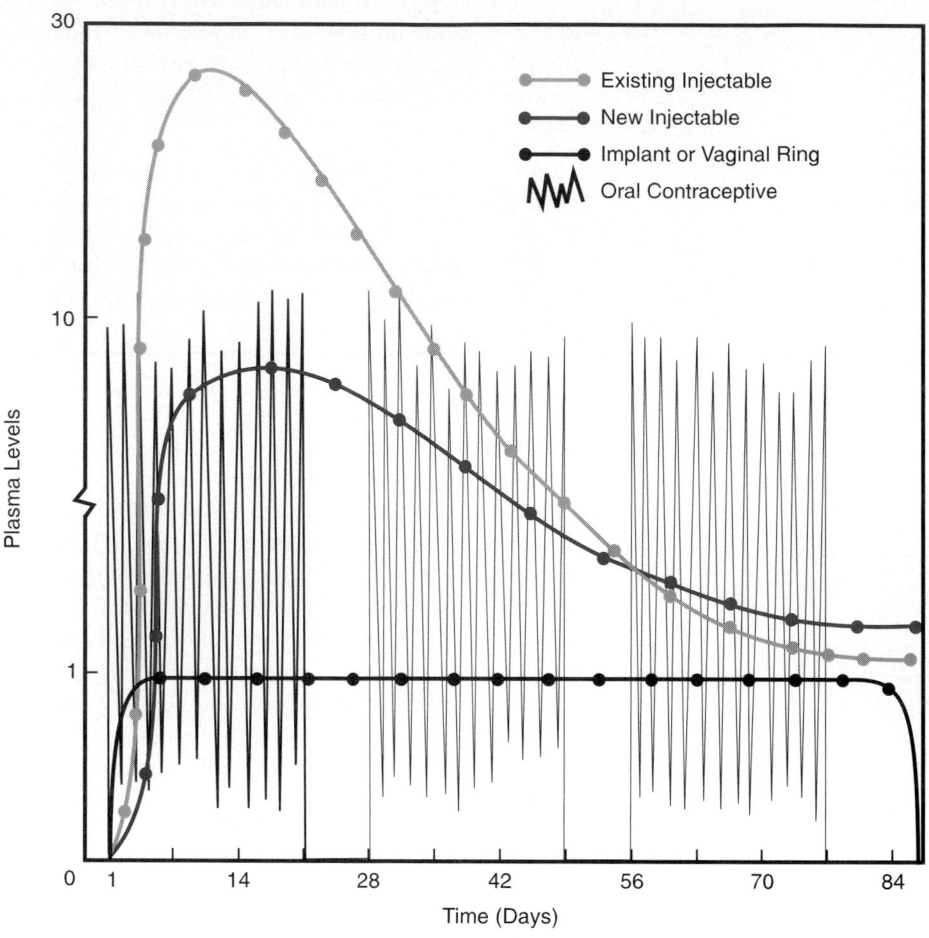

Figure 10.9 Schematic representation of the expected pharmacokinetic profiles of progestogens administered in different formulations. (From **Landgren BM.** Mechanism of action of gestagens. *Int J Gynecol Obstet* 1990;32:95–110, with permission.)

before ovulation. This progesterone appears essential to ovulation, because if the antiprogesterone is given before ovulation, it can be delayed for several days (84,85).

Oral Contraceptives

When used consistently, combination OCs have pregnancy rates as low as two to three per 1,000 women per year. Progestin-only OCs are less effective, with best results of three to four pregnancies per 100 woman-years. Both methods have the potential for user error; therefore, there may be a 10-fold difference between the best results and results in typical users for pregnancy prevention. Injectable progestins and implants are much less subject to user error. The difference between the best results and results in typical users is small and is comparable to pregnancy rates after tubal sterilization (Table 10.2).

Metabolic Effects and Safety

Venous Thrombosis Older studies linked OC use to venous thrombosis and embolism, cerebral vascular accidents, and heart attack (86,87). More recent studies have found a much lower risk (88). Rereading of the older literature on venous thrombosis reveals that absolute risk was strongly determined by other very obvious predisposing causes of thrombosis that are now considered contraindications to OC use: previous thrombosis, preexisting vascular disease, coronary artery disease, leukemia, cancer, and serious trauma (89).

Normally, the coagulation system maintains a dynamic balance of procoagulant and anticoagulant systems in the blood. Estrogens affect both systems in a dose-related fashion.

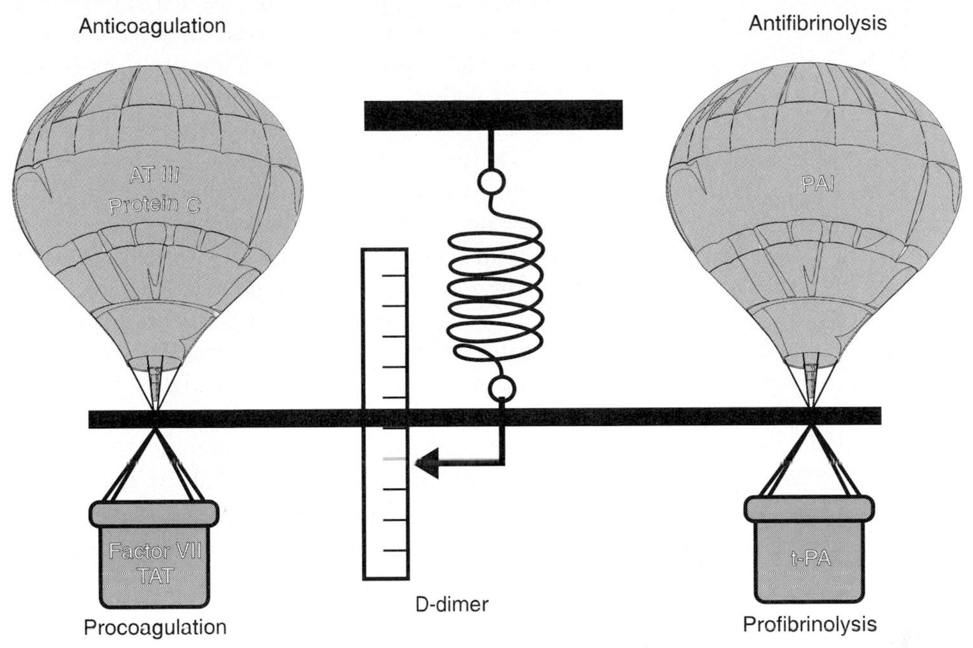

Figure 10.10 Dynamic balance of hemostasis. (From **Winkler UH, Buhler K, Schlinder AE.** The dynamic balance of hemostasis: implications for the risk of oral contraceptive use. In: **Runnebaum B, Rabe T, Kissel L,** eds. *Female contraception and male fertility regulation.* Advances in Gynecological and Obstetric Research Series. Confort, England: Parthenon Publishing Group, 1991:85–92, with permission.)

For most women, fibrinolysis (anticoagulation) is increased as much as coagulation, maintaining the dynamic balance at increased levels of production and destruction of fibrinogen (90,91) (Fig. 10.10). Current low-dose OCs have less measurable effect on the coagulation system, and fibrinolytic factors increase at the same rate as procoagulant factors (92,93). The lower estrogen dose (30 to 35 μg *EE*) reduces the risk for a thromboembolic event when compared with higher-dose (50 μg estrogen) OCs (94) (Table 10.5). Theoretically, thrombosis risk should be still less with current OCs containing only 20 μg of *EE,* but this has not been demonstrated. Smokers taking low-dose OCs demonstrate more marked activation of the coagulation system than nonsmokers—shortening of the prothrombin time, increased fibrinogen levels, and decreased antithrombin III—but also have increased fibrinolysis as measured by plasminogen activity (94).

The absolute risk for thrombosis in OC users taking pills containing 30 to 35 μg *EE* is 3 per 10,000 per year, compared with 1 per 10,000 reproductive-aged women not using OCs and 6 per 10,000 in pregnancy (95). **Thrombosis risk is apparent by 4 months after starting estrogen-containing OCs and does not increase further with continued use. Risk is highest during the first year of use** (96).

Table 10.5. Oral Contraceptive Estrogen Dose and Risk for Deep Vein Thrombosis

Estrogen (dose)	*(Rate/10,000 person years)*	*Relative Risk (all cases)*	*Relative Risk (proven diagnosis)*
<50 μg	4.2	1.0	1.0[a]
50 μg	7.0	1.5	2.0 (0.0–4.0)
>50 μg	10.0	1.7	3.2 (2.4–4.3)

[a] Base line risk used to calculate risk for higher doses.

From **Gerstman BB, Piper JM, Tomita DK, et al.** Oral contraceptive dose and the risk of deep venous thrombosis. *Am J Epidemiol* 1991;133:32–37, with permission.

Thrombophilia Changes in the coagulation system are detectable in all women, even those taking lower-dose OCs; however, some are genetically predisposed to thrombosis when challenged by pregnancy or administration of exogenous estrogen. Bloemenkamp and colleagues studied hemostatic variables in women given low-dose OCs who had previous thrombosis with OCs and compared them with women with no thrombosis (97). Women known to have inherited thrombophilic disorders were excluded. Both groups of women had significant changes in clotting factors: increased factor VII, factor VIII, and protein C, and a decrease in antithrombin, activated protein C sensitivity ratio, and protein S. However, the women with a history of thrombosis who were taking OCs had more pronounced changes. They were "high hemostatic responders" when exposed to OCs. Women with inherited deficiencies of antithrombin III, protein C, or protein S are at very high risk for thrombosis with pregnancy or estrogen therapy, but they make up a very small proportion of potential OC users. A much more common variation has been identified, factor V Leiden. This genetic variation exists in 3% to 5% of the white population. It codes for a one amino acid mutation in the factor V protein, inhibiting cleavage of the protein by activated protein C, an essential step in maintaining the balance between coagulation and fibrinolysis (98). A study of risk for a first thromboembolic episode among women using OCs found it to be 2.2 per 10,000 woman-years for women without the factor V mutation and 27.7 per 10,000 woman-years for women with the mutation (99). In women homozygous or heterozygous for factor V Leiden who do not use OCs, the risk is estimated to be 4.9 per 10,000 woman-years. The effect of estrogen dose was not examined. Cigarette smoking did not affect this risk. There are pronounced ethnic differences in the presence of this mutation. The Leiden allele is found in 5% of whites but is rare in Africans, Asians, Amerindians, Eskimos, and Polynesians (100). A similar mutation is found in the prothrombin gene at position 20210 and is described as prothrombin G20210A. It is found in 3% of a European population and is also strongly associated with venous thrombosis in women taking OCs (101).

Pregnancy is an even greater challenge for women with inherited defects of anticoagulation (102). A woman who sustains a venous event while using OCs should be evaluated thoroughly after she has recovered. Assessment should include measurement of antithrombin III, protein C, and protein S levels, resistance to activated protein C, genetic testing for factor V Leiden mutation and the prothrombin G20210A mutation, and testing for antiphospholipid antibody. It should not be assumed that OCs are the unique cause of the thrombotic episode.

Vandenbroucke and colleagues have explored the issue of routine screening for factor V Leiden (103). They conclude that routine screening of OC patients is not justified because effective contraception would be denied to 5% of white women, while preventing only a small number of fatal pulmonary emboli. Furthermore, if pregnant women were screened and those who screened positive were then treated with heparin, the number of cases of fatal bleeding might equal or exceed the number of fatal pulmonary emboli (104). Screening based on personal or family history of deep vein thrombosis before starting OCs or at the first antenatal visit was considered worthwhile.

Several studies have found a modest increased risk for venous thrombosis when users of OCs containing newer agents (i.e., *progestins, desogestrel,* or gestodene) were compared with users of older progestins (105). Physiologically, this was hard to understand because the estrogen and its dose are the same, and a 1993 review of *desogestrel*-containing OCs had found only minimal changes in coagulation and fibrinolysis (106). Lewis and colleagues have concluded that the biases "attrition of susceptibles" and "adverse selection" explain the apparent increase in thrombosis. Most cases of venous thrombosis attributable to OCs occur during the initial months of use (107). Hence, comparing new users to women already taking OCs for some time without incident will demonstrate an apparent increase with the new product that is artificial. Also, physicians may presume that newer drugs are safer, and prescribe them selectively for women with risk factors. Analysis of data from a large European study of thrombosis with different OCs has shown that apparent risk for thrombosis was lowest with the first low-dose pills introduced and highest with

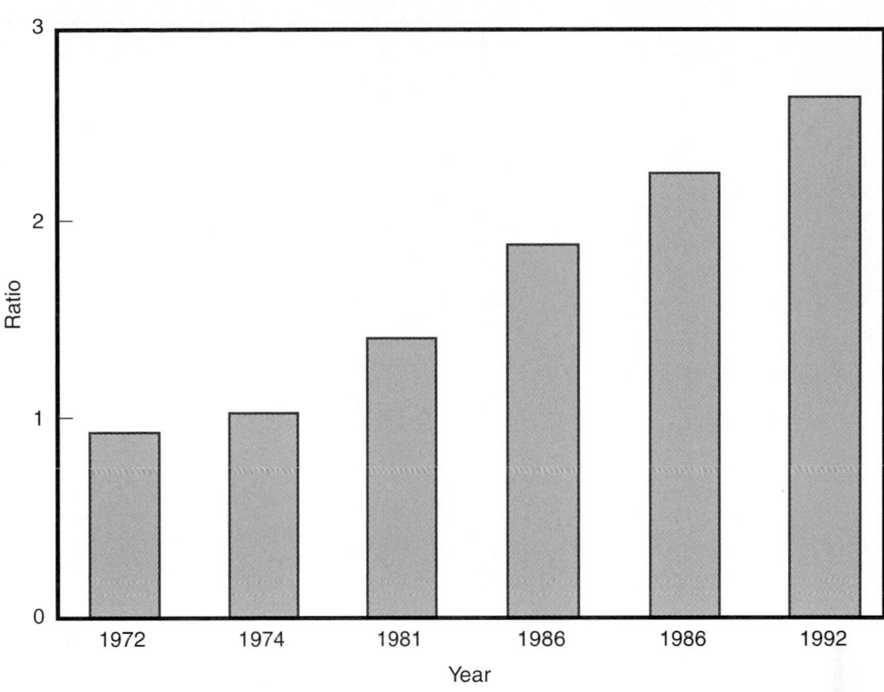

Figure 10.11 Risk ratios of oral contraceptives for thrombosis by year of market introduction for women aged 25 to 44 years. LNG, levonorgestrel with 30 μg ethinyl estradiol; GES, gestodene with 30 μg ethinyl estradiol; NORG, norgestimate with 35 μg of ethinyl estradiol; DES20, desogestrel with 20 μg of ethinyl estradiol. (From **Lewis MA, Heinemann LAJ, MacRae KD, et al.** The increased risk of venous thrombosis and the use of third generation progestagens: role of bias in observational research. *Contraception* 1996;54:5–13, with permission.)

those recently introduced, even though the newest pill had the lowest estrogen dose (105) (Fig. 10.11).

Ischemic Heart Disease Ischemic heart disease and stroke were the major causes of death blamed on OC use in the past. It is now known that the principal determinants of risk are advancing age and cigarette smoking (108). With the higher-dose OCs used in the 1980s, smoking had a profound effect on risk. Women smoking 25 or more cigarettes per day had a 30-fold increased risk for myocardial infarction if they used OCs, compared with nonsmokers not using OCs (109) (Fig. 10.12). Use of OCs is now much safer because most women are taking low-dose pills and because physicians prescribe selectively, excluding women with major cardiovascular risk factors. A very large U.S. study confirms the safety of OCs as currently prescribed. A total of 187 women aged 15 to 44 years with confirmed myocardial infarction were identified during 3.6 million woman-years of observation in the Kaiser Permanente Medical Care Program in California between 1991 and 1994. This is a rate of 3.2 per 100,000 woman-years (110). Nearly all current users took OCs with less than 50 μg of *EE.* After adjusting for age, illness, smoking, ethnicity, and body mass index, risk for myocardial infarction was not increased [odds ratio (OR), 1.14; 95% confidence interval (CI), 0.27 to 4.72]. Of heart attack victims, 61% were smokers; only 7.7% were current OC users. In a later study, the same investigators pooled results from the California study with a similar study from Washington State. The results were the same. Current users of low-dose OCs had no increased risk for myocardial infarction, after adjustment for major risk factors and sociodemographic factors (111). That past use of OCs does not increase risk for myocardial infarction later has already been clearly established (112).

One study of so-called third-generation OCs found that women using OCs containing the new progestins desogestrel or gestodene are less likely to have myocardial infarction than

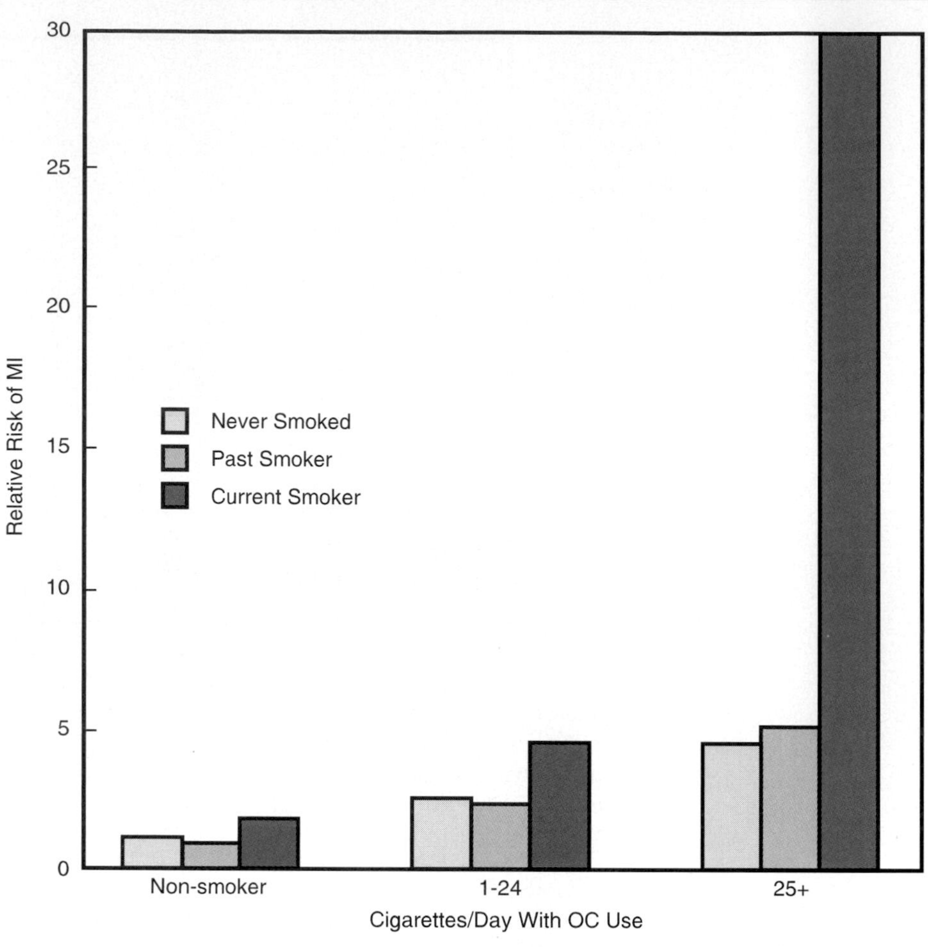

Figure 10.12 Risk for myocardial infarction in women younger than 50 years of age: effect of oral contraceptives and smoking. (From **Rosenberg L, Kaufman DW, Helmrich SP, et al.** Myocardial infarction and cigarette smoking in women younger than 50 years of age. *JAMA* 1985;253:2965–2969, with permission.)

women who use OCs with similar estrogen doses (113). Myocardial infarction risk was strongly increased among smokers, even after adjustment for OC use, but smokers who used OCs with the new progestins were less likely to have myocardial infarction than smokers who used the older OCs (113). These findings are biologically plausible based on the beneficial effect on lipids of OCs containing the new progestins.

Oral Contraceptives and Stroke In the 1970s, OC use appeared to be linked to risk for both hemorrhagic and thrombotic stroke, but these studies failed to take into consideration preexisting risk factors (114). Although a rare form of cerebrovascular insufficiency, moyamoya disease, is clearly linked to OC use (115), new information shows no risk for women who are otherwise healthy and who use currently available low-dose pills. Petitti and colleagues identified all Kaiser Permanente Medical Care Program patients aged 15 to 44 years who sustained fatal or nonfatal stroke in California from 1991 to 1994 (116). Hypertension, diabetes, obesity, current cigarette smoking, and black race were strongly associated with stroke risk, but neither current nor past OC use was associated with stroke in this study. A World Health Organization (WHO) study of cases from 1989 to 1993 from 17 countries in Europe and the developing world included women on higher-dose OCs as well as low-dose OCs. European women using low-dose OCs had no increased risk for either type of stroke, thrombotic or hemorrhagic. Those on higher-dose OCs did have measurable risk (117,118). Women in developing countries had an apparent modest increase in risk, but this finding was attributed to undetected existing risk factors. Another study from Europe found less stroke risk from low-dose pills than from older higher-dose pills, and that risk was less if the patient's blood pressure was checked before starting OCs. The authors concluded that a small risk from low-dose OCs could be controlled if women with hypertension were not given OCs (119).

Smokers and women with hypertension and diabetes are clearly at increased risk for cardiovascular disease whether or not they use oral contraceptives. The important question is whether risk is further increased if they use low-dose OCs, and if so, by how much. The World Health Organization study described previously provides some insight: Smokers taking OCs had 7 times the risk for ischemic (thrombotic) stroke when compared with smokers who did not use OCs, and hypertensive women had 10-fold increased risk if they took OCs, but a 5-fold risk if they did not (117). Similarly, Lidegaard reported from Denmark that diabetic women had a 5-fold increase risk for stroke, which increased to 10-fold if they took OCs (120). Unfortunately, Lidegaard's data were not limited to low-estrogen OCs. The data suggest that although risk is primarily determined by the predisposing condition—hypertension, diabetes, or cigarette smoking—the risk can be magnified by OC use, even when the OCs are low dose. The current U.S. practice of limiting OC use by women older than 35 years of age to nonsmokers without other vascular disease risk factors is prudent.

Blood Pressure Oral contraceptives have a dose-related effect on blood pressure. With the older high-dose pills, as many as 5% of patients could be expected to have blood pressure levels of higher than 140/90 mm Hg. The mechanism is believed to be an estrogen-induced increase in renin substrate in susceptible individuals. Current low-dose pills have minimal blood pressure effects, but surveillance of blood pressure is still advised to detect the occasional idiosyncratic response.

Glucose Metabolism Oral estrogen alone has no adverse effect on glucose metabolism, but progestins exhibit insulin antagonism (121). Older OC formulations with higher doses of progestins produced abnormal glucose tolerance tests with elevated insulin levels in the average patient. The effect on glucose metabolism, similar to the effect on lipids, is related to androgenic potency of the progestin and to its dose (7972).

Lipid Metabolism Higher-dose OCs could have significant adverse effects on lipids (122). Androgens and estrogens have competing effects on hepatic lipase, a liver enzyme critical to lipid metabolism. Estrogens depress LDL and elevate HDL, which are changes that can be expected to reduce the risk for atherosclerosis (123). Androgens and androgenic progestins can antagonize these beneficial changes, reducing HDL and elevating LDL levels. Estrogens elevate triglyceride levels. Low-dose formulations have minimal adverse effect on lipids (124), and the newer formulations (with desogestrel and norgestimate as the progestin) produce potentially beneficial changes by elevating HDL and lowering LDL (79) (Fig. 10.13). Although average values of a large group show only small lipid changes with current OCs, an occasional patient may have exaggerated effects. Women whose lipid values are higher than the mean before treatment are more likely to experience abnormalities during treatment (124).

Other Metabolic Effects Oral contraceptives can produce changes in a broad variety of proteins synthesized by the liver. The estrogen in OCs increases circulating-thyroid-binding globulin, thereby affecting tests of thyroid function that are based on binding, increasing total thyroxine (T_4), and decreasing triiodothyronine (T_3) resin uptake. The results of actual thyroid function tests, as measured by free T_4 and radioiodine tests, are normal (125).

Oral Contraceptives and Neoplasia

Endometrial Cancer and Ovarian Cancer **Combination OCs reduce the risk for subsequent endometrial cancer and ovarian cancer** (126,127). **A recent study found that as little as 1 year of OC use was protective (OR, 0.57; 95% CI, 0.87 to 1.03), and**

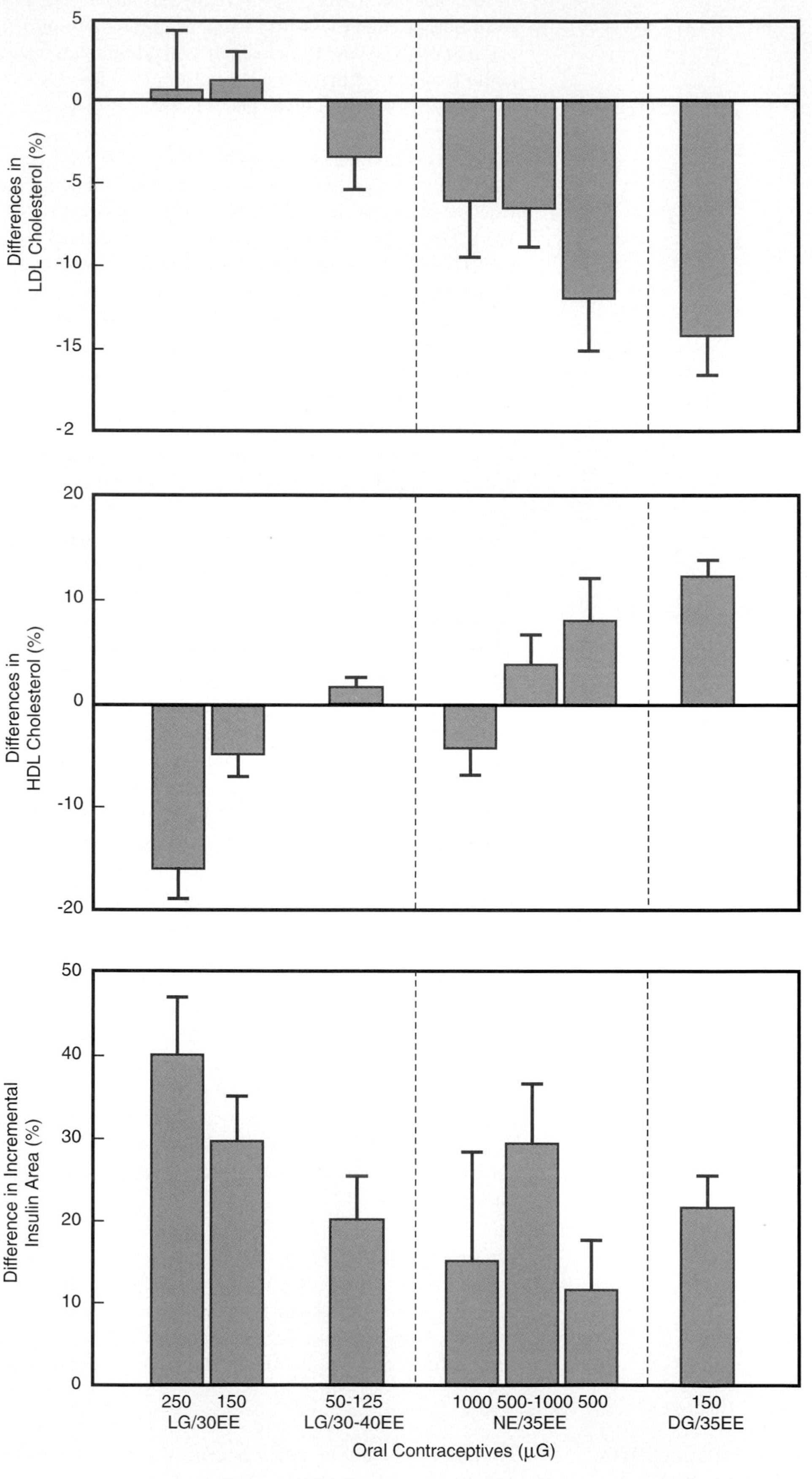
Differences in LDL Cholesterol (%)
5
0
-5
-10
-15
-2
Differences in HDL Cholesterol (%)
20
10
0
-10
-20
Difference in Incremental Insulin Area (%)
50
40
30
20
10
0
250 150
LG/30EE
50-125
LG/30-40EE
1000 500-1000 500
NE/35EE
150
DG/35EE
Oral Contraceptives (µG)

continued use reduced risk by 7% per year. Benefit persisted for 15 years after last use, with little diminution (128). **A 50% reduction in ovarian cancer risk was observed for women who took OCs for 3 to 4 years, and an 80% reduction was seen with 10 or more years of use.** There was some benefit from as little as 3 to 11 months of use. The benefit continues for at least 15 years since last use, and it does not diminish even at 15 years from use (126). National vital statistics data from England support these observations. Ovarian cancer mortality is declining in England and Wales in women younger than 55 years of age, and this decline has been attributed to OC use (129). Use of OCs after 1980, when low-dose pills predominated, provides protection equivalent to older, higher-dose OCs (130).

Two years of OC use reduces the risk for subsequent endometrial cancer by 40%, and 4 or more years of use reduces the risk by 60% (127).

Cervical Cancer There may be a weak association between OC use and squamous cancer of the cervix. Important risk factors are early sexual intercourse and exposure to human papillomavirus (131). Women who have used OCs typically started sexual relations at younger ages than women who have not used OCs and, in some studies, report having had more partners. These factors also increase one's chance of acquiring human papillomavirus (HPV), the most important risk factor for cervical cancer. Because barrier contraceptives reduce the risk for cervical cancer, use of alternative choices for contraception can compound the difficulty in establishing an association with OC use alone. The presence of HPV types 16 or 18 is associated with a 50-fold increase in risk for preneoplastic lesions of the cervix (132). **If a woman already has HPV, OC use does not further increase her risk for cervical neoplasia, but among women who are HPV negative, OC use doubles the risk of having such a lesion.** This apparent adverse effect could be explained entirely by OC users being less likely to use barrier contraception.

Adenocarcinomas of the cervix are rare, but they are not as easily detected as other lesions by screening cervical cytology, and the incidence appears to be increasing. A 1994 study found a doubling of risk for adenocarcinoma with OC use that increased with duration of use, reaching a relative risk of 4.4 if total use of OCs exceeded 12 years (133). The results of this study were adjusted for history of genital warts, number of sexual partners, and age at first intercourse. Because adenocarcinoma of the cervix is rare, absolute risk is low. If this apparent association were real, the cumulative risk of long-term OC use to 55 years of age would be about 1 in 1,000 patients (134).

Use of OCs is, at most, a minor factor in causation of cervical cancer; however, women who have used OCs should have annual Papanicolaou (Pap) tests. To reduce risk, women who are not in mutually monogamous relationships should be advised to use barrier methods in addition to hormonal contraception.

Breast Cancer There is a large volume of conflicting literature on the relationship between OC use and breast cancer. Generally, no increase in overall risk is found from OC use, but some studies have found that risk may increase in women who used OCs before their first term pregnancy (135) or who used OCs for many years, who are nulligravid, who

Figure 10.13 Percentage differences in HDL and LDL cholesterol levels and in the incremental area for insulin in response to the oral glucose tolerance test (OGTT) between women taking one of seven combination oral contraceptives and those not taking oral contraceptives. The T bars indicate 1 standard deviation, and the double daggers ($p < 0.05$) indicate significant differences between users and nonusers in the mean values for the principal metabolic variables. EE, ethinyl estradiol; LG, levonorgestrel; NE, norethindrone; DG, desogestrel. (From **Godsland IF, Crook D, Simpson R, et al.** The effects of different formulations of oral contraceptive agents on lipid and carbohydrate metabolism. *N Engl J Med* 1990;323:1375–1382, with permission.)

are young at the time of diagnosis, and who continue using OCs in their 40s (136). A large British study found a small but statistically stable increase in breast cancer diagnosed before 36 years of age among OC users, but that risk was less for OCs with less than 50 μg of estrogen. Progestin-only OCs appeared to have a protective effect. Significantly, OC users who developed breast cancer were more likely to be diagnosed in early stages and were less likely to have lymph node involvement than were controls (136). Women with a family history of breast cancer were not found at increased risk with OC use in one study (137). Some of the findings are difficult to interpret; for example, risk does not increase with prolonged exposure. This finding would not be expected if OCs were truly causal (137).

The best information to date comes from a metaanalysis of 54 studies of breast cancer and hormonal contraceptives. The Collaborative Group on Hormonal Factors in Breast Cancer reanalyzed data on 53,297 women with breast cancer and 100,239 controls from 25 countries, representing about 90% of the epidemiologic data available worldwide (138). Current use of OCs was associated with a very small but statistically stable 24% increased risk [relative risk (RR), 1.24; 95% CI, 1.15 to 1.33]. The risk fell rapidly after discontinuation, to 16% 1 to 4 years after stopping and to 7% 5 to 9 years after stopping. Risk disappeared 10 years after cessation (RR, 1.01; 95% CI, 0.96 to 1.05). Breast cancers diagnosed while women were taking OCs were less advanced clinically than those in women who had never used OCs. Results did not differ in any important way by ethnic group, reproductive history, or family history. There was a greater risk in women who started OC use before 20 years of age relative to women who started OCs later, but because breast cancer is so rare before 20 years of age, there was no increase in actual numbers of breast cancer cases among women who started use of OCs at a young age. A term pregnancy also causes a short-term increase in breast cancer risk, thought to be from the growth-enhancing effects of estrogen, but there is a longer-term reduction in risk, perhaps the result of pregnancy-induced terminal differentiation of breast cells (139). The effects of OCs may be the same and may promote growth of existing cancers, leading to their presentation and diagnosis at an earlier age, rather than actually causing cancers to form. Most breast cancers are seen after 50 years of age, and only now are large numbers of women with OC exposure entering this age group. At present the risk, if it is increased, is small, and is not present 10 years after cessation of use. Reassurance is provided by a 1999 Swedish study that compared 3,016 women aged 50 to 74 years who had invasive breast cancer with 3,263 controls of the same age. No relation between past use of OCs and breast cancer was found (140).

In the Collaborative Group's study, oral contraceptive use by women with a first-degree relative who had breast cancer did not increase risk regardless of the duration of use before first-term pregnancy (138). In contrast, a recent historical cohort study of 426 families with breast cancer found that sisters and daughters of women with breast cancer had a threefold increase risk for breast cancer if they had used OCs before 1975. Granddaughters and nieces or women who married into the families had no increased risk. There were too few cases among women who used the lower-dose OCs available after 1975 to determine whether there is risk (141).

Liver Tumors OCs have been implicated as a cause of benign adenomas of the liver. These hormonally responsive tumors can cause fatal hemorrhage. They usually regress when OC use is discontinued; risk is related to prolonged use (142). There is a strong correlation between OC use and hepatocellular adenoma. Fortunately, the tumors are rare; about 30 cases per 1,000,000 users per year have been predicted with older formulations. Presumably, newer low-dose products pose less risk. A link to hepatic carcinoma has been proposed, but a large study from six countries in Europe found no association between use of OCs and subsequent liver cancer (143).

Health Benefits of Oral Contraceptives

OCs have important health benefits (Table 10.6). As noted earlier, OC use produces strong and lasting reduced risk for endometrial and ovarian cancer. In addition, protection has been

Table 10.6. Noncontraceptive Benefits of Oral Contraception
Clearly established benefits
Reduced ovarian cancer
Reduced endometrial cancer
Reduced ectopic pregnancy
Reduced benign breast disease
Reduced functional ovarian cysts
Reduced uterine fibroids
Less dysmenorrhea
Less anemia
Regular menstrual cycle
Reduced pelvic inflammatory disease
Reduced risk of colon cancer
Less clearly established benefits
Fewer new cases of rheumatoid arthritis
Less osteopenia
Less endometriosis
Less atherosclerosis

From **Stubblefield PG.** Health benefits beyond contraception. *Int J Fertil* 1994;39(Suppl 3):132–138, with permission.

found for women with known hereditary ovarian cancer. Any past use of OCs conferred a 50% reduction in ovarian cancer risk when women with this history who took OCs were compared with their sisters as controls (OR, 0.5; 95% CI, 0.3 to 0.8). Protection increased with increasing duration of use (144). The mechanism of action of OCs in the prevention of ovarian cancer is unknown but may involve selective induction of apoptosis (programmed cell death). Macaques treated with *EE* plus *levonorgestrel* or *levonorgestrel* alone showed an increase in the proportion of ovarian epithelial cells in apoptosis in comparison with animals fed a diet containing no hormones (145).

Chlamydial colonization of the cervix appears more likely in OC users than in nonusers but, despite this, there is a 40% to 50% reduction in risk for chlamydial PID (146). Combination OCs confer marked reduction in risk for ectopic pregnancy, although the progestin-only OCs appear to increase risk.

Other documented benefits of OC use include a significant reduction in the need for biopsies for benign breast disease and surgery for ovarian cysts. Use of OCs also helps relieve dysmenorrhea and associated anemia from menstrual blood loss (147). All combination OCs offer some protection from functional ovarian cysts, but multiphasic preparations offer less protection than other forms of combination OCs (148). If progestin-only OCs are truly protective against breast cancer, the *levonorgestrel* implants also could be expected to confer this benefit.

There is growing evidence that OC use is also protective against colon cancer. A case-control study in Italy comparing women with colon cancer with controls found a 37% reduction in colon cancer and a 34% reduction in rectal cancer (colon cancer OR, 0.63, 95% CI 0.45 to 0.87; rectal cancer OR, 0.66, 95% CI 0.43 to 1.01). Longer use produced more protection against colon cancer (149). Results of the U.S. Nurses Health Study also disclosed some degree of protection. Women who had used OCs for 96 months or more had a 40% lower risk for colorectal cancer (RR, 0.60; 95% CI, 1.15 to 2.14) (150). The mechanism of protection has not been identified.

Fertility after OC Use **After discontinuing OCs, return of ovulatory cycles may be delayed for a few months. Women who have amenorrhea more than 6 months after discontinuation of OCs should undergo a full evaluation because of the risk for prolactin-producing pituitary tumors.** This risk is not related to OC use but rather to the probability that the slow-growing tumor was already present and produced menstrual irregularity, prompting the patient to take OCs (151).

Sexuality In a study that recorded all episodes of female-initiated sexual behavior throughout the menstrual cycle, an increase in sexual activity at the time of ovulation was noted. This increase was not present in women who were taking OCs (152).

Teratogenicity A metaanalysis of 12 prospective studies, including 6,102 women who used OCs and 85,167 women who did not, revealed no increase in overall risk for malformation, congenital heart defects, or limb reduction defects with the use of OCs (153). Progestins have been used to prevent miscarriage. A large study compared women showing signs of threatened abortion who were treated with progestins (primarily medroxyprogesterone acetate) with women who were not treated. The rate of malformation was the same among the 1,146 exposed infants as among the 1,608 unexposed infants (154). Conversely, estrogens taken in high doses in pregnancy can induce vaginal cancer in exposed female offspring *in utero.*

Interaction of Oral Contraceptives with Other Drugs

Some drugs reduce the effectiveness of oral contraceptives (e.g., rifampin); conversely, OCs can augment or reduce the effectiveness of other drugs (e.g., benzodiazepines). Phenytoin, phenobarbital, and rifampin induce synthesis of cytochrome P450 enzymes in the liver and reduce plasma levels of *EE* in women taking OCs, which may cause contraceptive failure (155). The antifungal agents *griseofulvin, ketoconazole,* and *itraconazole* also induce these hepatic enzymes and may reduce OC efficacy (156). *Ampicillin* and *tetracycline* have been implicated in numerous case reports of OC failure. They kill gut bacteria (primarily clostridia) that are responsible for hydrolysis of steroid glucuronides in the intestine, which allows reabsorption of the steroid through the enterohepatic circulation. In human studies, however, it has not been possible to demonstrate reduced plasma levels of *EE.* Although women taking OCs who will be treated with antibiotics are commonly advised to use condoms as well, controlled studies of OC users have found no difference in pregnancy rates with exposure to penicillins, cephalosporins, and tetracyclines (157).

Certain drugs actually appear to increase plasma levels of contraceptive steroids. Ascorbic acid (vitamin C) and *acetaminophen* may elevate plasma EE.

An example of OCs affecting the metabolism of other drugs is seen with *diazepam* and related compounds. OCs reduce the metabolic clearance and increase the half-life of those benzodiazepines that are metabolized primarily by oxidation: *chlordiazepoxide, alprazolam, diazepam,* and *nitrazepam. Caffeine* and *theophylline* are metabolized in the liver by two of the P450 isozymes, and their clearance is also reduced in OC users. *Cyclosporine* is hydroxylated by another of the P450 isozymes, and its plasma concentrations are increased by OCs. Plasma levels of some analgesic drugs are decreased in OC users. *Salicyclic acid* and *morphine* clearances are enhanced by OC use; therefore, higher doses could be needed for adequate therapeutic effect. Clearance of *ethanol* may be reduced in OC users (158).

Oral Contraceptives and Clinical Chemistry Alterations

Oral contraceptives have the potential to alter a number of clinical laboratory tests as a result of estrogen-induced changes in hepatic synthesis; however, a large study comparing OC users to pregnant and nonpregnant controls found minimal changes (158). Hormone users took a variety of OCs containing 50 to 100 μg of estrogen, higher doses than are used today. Compared with nonpregnant women who were not using OCs, the OC users had an increase in T_4 that is explained by increased circulating thyroid-binding protein, no change in creatinine, a slight reduction in mean fasting glucose values, a reduction in total bilirubin, a modest reduction in serum glutamic oxaloacetic transaminase, a decrease in alkaline phosphatase, and no change in globulin.

Choice of Oral Contraceptives

The oral contraceptives currently available in the United States are listed in Table 10.7. With the introduction of OCs containing the new progestins, new preparations with 20 μg of *EE,* new variations of multiphasic preparations, plus branded generic formulations of older OCs, an array of choices are possible.

The lowest-dose OCs all contain the same amount of the same estrogen, 20 μg of *EE.* However, the progestins differ: *norethindrone acetate, levonorgestrel, desogestrel,* or *norgestimate* (Table 10.7). The first 20-μg *EE* OC (*LoEstrin 1-20*) contained 1 mg *norethindrone* acetate. A comparison of this OC to a triphasic OC with 35 μg of *EE* and *norgestimate* (NGM) (*Ortho Tri-Cylen*) found considerable more breakthrough bleeding and spotting and more episodes of missed menses with the 20-μg *norethindrone acetate/EE* than with the higher-estrogen OC containing *norgestimate.* There was no difference in compliance, discontinuation rates, or adverse events (159). In a three-way trial, the 35-μg *NGM/EE* triphasic OC (*Ortho Tri-Cyclen*) was compared with two new 20-μg *EE* pills, one containing 100 μg of *levonorgestrel* (*Allese*), the other containing 150 μg *desogestrel,* followed by 2 hormone-free days then 5 days of 10 μg *EE* per day (*Mircette*) (160). Contraceptive efficacy was not significantly different. Women starting on OCs had more breakthrough bleeding and bleeding in the second half of the cycle with *Allese* than with the other two OCs in the first two cycles, but thereafter there was little difference, except that *Mircette* users had more breakthrough bleeding in cycle 4. Women taking *Tri-Cyclen* consistently experienced more frequent estrogenic side effects of bloating, breast tenderness, and nausea than did women on either 20-μg *EE* OC. These authors concluded that for the specific OCs evaluated, changing to the lowest estrogen dose was beneficial.

For the average patient, the first choice of preparation for contraceptive purposes is a low-estrogen OC (20 to 35 μg of *EE*) or a very low-estrogen OC (20 μg *EE*).

1. Breakthrough bleeding and spotting are common at first and generally improve with time. If the problem persists, it may be relieved by changing from a multiphasic to monophasic version at the same estrogen level.
2. If bleeding remains a problem, a temporary increase in estrogen should be tried: 20 μg of *EE* daily for 7 days while continuing the OC (161).

Side effects—nausea, breast tenderness, mood changes, and weight gain—are less common with current formulations than with previous OCs and usually resolve after the first few cycles.

1. If symptoms persist, the lowest-dose highly effective formulations could be tried: those containing only 20 μg of *EE.*
2. In patients who have persistent breast tenderness, the type of OC could be changed to one with more progestin activity, for example, the 20- to 30-μg *EE* pills that contain *levonorgestrel.* High-potency progestin OCs produce fewer breast symptoms (162).
3. Nausea is generally related to the estrogen component, and changing to the 20-μg *EE* preparation may be beneficial.

Table 10.7. Composition of Oral Contraceptives in Current Use in the United States, 2001

Trade Name[a]	*Progestin*	*Estrogen*
Progestin-only		
Micronor (NorQD)	NE 350 μg	none
Ovrette	d,l-NG 75 μg	none
Combination-monophasic		
Norlestrin	NEA 2.5 mg	EE 50 μg
Norlestrin-1	NEA 1.0 mg	EE 50 μg
Loestrin 1.5/30	NEA 1.5 mg	EE 30 μg
Ovral	d,l-NG 0.5 mg	EE 50 μg
Lo Ovral	d,l-NG 0.3 mg	EE 30 μg
Nordette (Levlen, *Levora* 0.15/30)	levo NG 0.15 mg	EE 30 μg
Orthonovum 1/50 (*Norinyl* 1/50, *Necon* 1/50, *Nelova* 1/50 M)	NE 1.0 mg	ME 50 μg
Ovcon 50	NE 1.0 mg	EE 50 μg
Orthonovum 1/35 (*Norinyl* 1/35, *Necon* 1/35, *Nelova* 1/35E)	NE 1.0 mg	EE 35 μg
Modicon (*Brevicon, Necon* 0.5/35, *Nelova* 0.5/35E)	NE 0.5 mg	EE 35 μg
Ovcon 35	NE 0.4 mg	EE 35 μg
Demulen 1/50 (*Zovia* 1/50E)	ED 1.0 mg	EE 50 μg
Demulen 1/35 (*Zovia* 1/35E)	ED 1.0 mg	EE 35 μg
Desogen (*Orthocept*)	Deso 0.15 mg	EE 30 μg
OrthoCyclen	Norg 0.25 mg	EE 35 μg
Loestrin 1/20	NEA 1.0 mg	EE 20 μg
Alesse (*Levlite*)	levoNG 0.10 mg	EE 20 μg
Multiphasic		
Orthonovum 10/11 (*Neocon* 10/11, *Nelova* 10/11)		
NE 0.5 mg and *EE* 35 μg (first 10 days)		
NE 1.0 mg and *EE* 35 μg (next 11 days)		
Orthonovum 7/7/7 NE .5 mg and *EE* 35 μg (first 7 days)		
NE 0.75 mg and *EE* 35 μg (next 7 days)		
NE 1.0 mg and *EE* 35 μg (last 7 days)		
Triphasil (*TriLlevlen, Trivora*)		
Levo NG 0.050 mg and *EE* 30 μg (first 6 days)		
Levo NG 0.075 mg and *EE* 40 μg (next 5 days)		
Levo NG 0.125 mg and *EE* 30 μg (last 10 days)		
Tri-Norinyl		
NE 0.5 mg and *EE* 35 μg (first 7 days)		
NE 1.0 mg and *EE* 35 μg (next 9 days)		
NE 0.5 mg and *EE* 35 μg (next 5 days)		

Table 10.7.—*continued*

OrthoTri-Cyclen
Norg 0.18 mg and EE 35 μg (first 7 days)
Norg 0.215 mg and EE 35 μg (next 7 days)
Norg 0.250 mg and EE 35 μg (next 7 days)
Estrostep
NEA 1.0 mg and EE 20 μg (first 5 days)
NEA 1.0 mg and EE 30 μg (next 7 days)
NEA 1.0 mg and EE 35 μg (next 9 days)
Mircette
Deso 0.15 mg and EE 20 μg (first 21 days)
Placebo and placebo (next 2 days)
Placebo and EE 10 μg (next 5 days)

[a] Trade names are used for ease of identification. A second or third, identical formulation by a different manufacturer is identified in parenthesis. Most formulations are available either as a 21-day or 28-day package. The 28-day package has 7 placebo tablets. Some formulations add iron, usually ferrous fumarate, to each of the 7 placebo tablets in a 28-day package.E
EE, ethinyl estradiol; ME, mestranol; NE, norethindrone; NEA, norethindrone acetate; ED, ethynodiol diacetate; d,l-NG, d,l-norgestrel; levoNG, levonorgestrel; Deso, desogestrel; Norg, norgestimate.

Injectable Hormonal Contraceptives

Depomedroxyprogesterone Acetate

Depomedroxyprogesterone acetate (*DMPA*), a suspension of microcrystals of a synthetic progestin, was approved for contraception in 1992. A single 150-mg intramuscular dose will suppress ovulation in most women for 14 weeks or longer (163). The regimen of 150 mg every 3 months is highly effective, producing pregnancy rates of about 0.3 per 100 women per year. Probably because of the high blood levels of the progestin, efficacy appears not to be reduced by administration of other drugs and is not dependent on the patient's weight. Women treated with *DMPA* experience disruption of the menstrual cycle and have initial spotting and bleeding at irregular intervals. Eventually, total amenorrhea develops in most women who take *DMPA*; with continued administration, amenorrhea develops in 50% of women by 1 year and in 80% by 3 years (Fig. 10.14). Persistent irregular bleeding is treated by adding low-dose estrogen temporarily; for example, conjugated estrogens, 1.25 mg per day, can be given for 10 to 21 days at a time. *DMPA* persists in the body for several months in women who have used it for long-term contraception, and return to fertility may be delayed. In a large study, however, 70% of former users desiring pregnancy conceived within 12 months, and 90% conceived within 24 months (164).

Safety

Long-term users of *DMPA* may have lower bone density than nonusers, probably reflecting reduced estrogen levels; however, this effect has not been associated with increased fractures (165). Other investigators have not detected bone loss during 3 years or more of *DMPA* use (166). A small study comparing *DMPA* to implant or OC users found that *DMPA* blocked the usual rapid increase in bone density normally seen in adolescents (167). This may suggest that *DMPA* may be less desirable for young adolescents. The effect of *DMPA* on plasma lipids has been inconsistent; in general, *DMPA* users appear to have reduced total cholesterol and triglycerides, slight reduction in HDL cholesterol, and no change

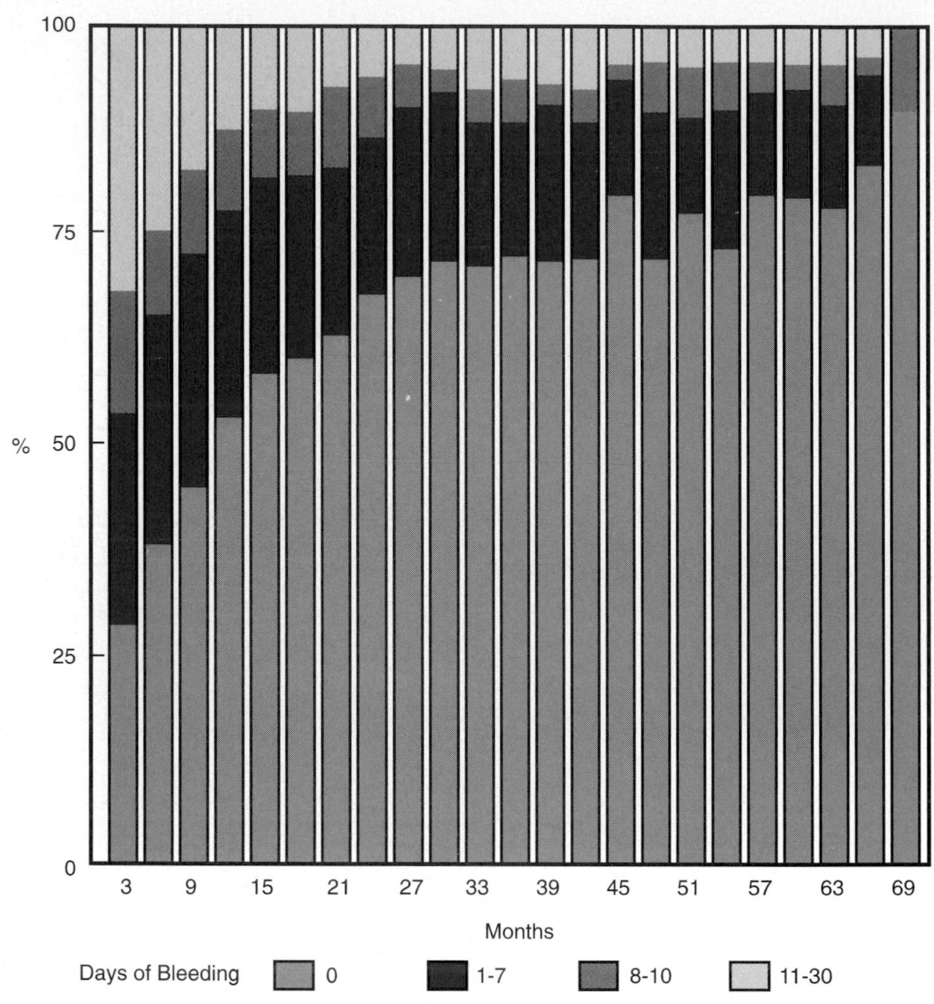

Figure 10.14 Bleeding pattern and duration of use of depomedroxyprogesterone acetate (DMPA): percentage of women who have bleeding, spotting, or amenorrhea while taking DMPA 150 mg every 3 months. (From **Schwallie PC, Assenzo JR.** Contraceptive use-efficacy study utilizing *medroxyprogesterone acetate* administered as an intramuscular injection once every 90 days. *Fertil Steril* 1973;24:331–339, with permission.)

or slight increase in LDL cholesterol, all of which are consistent with a reduction in circulating estrogen levels. In some studies, the decrease in HDL and increase in LDL are statistically significant, although the values remain within normal ranges (168). The use of *DMPA* has not been associated with myocardial infarction. Glucose tolerance tests disclose a small elevation of glucose in *DMPA* users. There is no change in hemostatic parameters, with the exception that antithrombin III levels are sometimes found to be reduced with chronic therapy (168). *DMPA* has not been linked to thrombotic episodes in women of reproductive age. However, thrombotic episodes have occurred in elderly women with advanced cancer who were treated with a variety of agents, including *DMPA* and *tamoxifen* (169,170). Such patients are at high risk for thrombosis regardless of the use of *DMPA*. Women taking *DMPA* appear to experience a weight gain of 2 to 3 pounds more than nonusers over several years. Its use has not been associated with teratogenesis. It is safe for use by lactating women and, as with other progestin-only hormonal methods, appears to increase milk production. *DMPA* has not been associated with affective disorders or mood changes, although the data are limited (171,172).

Benefits

DMPA appears to have many of the noncontraceptive benefits of combination oral contraceptives. Decreases in anemia, PID, ectopic pregnancy, and endometrial cancer have been reported (173). No association between *DMPA* and cervical cancer has been demonstrated (174). Ovarian cancer has been found to be unrelated to the use of *DMPA* (175). The risk for breast cancer diagnosis during the first 4 years of use appears to be slightly increased, but there is no relation to long-term use and no overall increase in breast cancer risk; hence, any causal relationship between *DMPA* and breast cancer is unlikely (176).

Once-a-Month Injectable

A once-a-month injectable containing only 25 mg of *DMPA* in combination with 5 mg of the long-acting estrogen, estradiol cypionate, has recently become available in the United States after extensive use in developing countries. Originally developed by the World Health Organization, it is described as *CycloFem* or *CycloProvera* in the literature, and is marketed in the United States as *Lunelle* (177). Given once a month, this combination produces excellent contraceptive effects. Monthly withdrawal bleeding is like a normal menses, leading to high continuation rates (178).

Subdermal Implants

The *levonorgestrel* implant (*Norplant*) consists of six rods, each measuring 34 mm in length and 2.4 mm in outside diameter and containing 36 mg of the progestin *levonorgestrel* (179–186). About 80 mg/d is released during the first 6 to 12 months after insertion. The release rate then gradually declines to 30 to 35 mg/d. Blood levels of the steroid are about 0.35 ng/mL at 6 months and remain above 0.25 ng/mL for 5 years. Plasma levels less than 0.20 ng/mL result in higher pregnancy rates. The level of progestin present for implant users produces very effective contraception; the total number of pregnancies over 5 years is only 1 in 100 (180). The progestin blocks the LH surge necessary for ovulation, so that over 5 years, only about one third of cycles are ovulatory. In response to the progestin, the cervical mucus becomes scant and thick and does not allow sperm penetration. An older, thicker-walled version of the implants was studied in the United States and had less contraceptive efficacy for women weighing 70 kg or more. Current devices have a pliable, less dense wall, and the release rate of *levonorgestrel* is 15% higher than with earlier versions, so that weight is less of a problem (Table 10.8). Some advise that in obese women, the implants should be replaced after 3 years in order to maintain a high level of pregnancy protection.

A two-rod version of *Norplant, Norplant II,* has undergone extensive testing. It is as effective as *Norplant* and is easier to insert and remove (185). Single-rod systems containing a new progestin, 3-keto-desogestrel (*Implanon*) are in the final phase of U.S. trials. In preliminary studies, Implanon appeared to be even more effective than *Norplant* (186). It is intended for 3 years of use.

Table 10.8. Pregnancy Rates with Norplant: Gross Cumulative Pregnancy Rates at 5 Years by Patient's Weight and Type of Tubing

Weight at Insertion (kg)	*No. of Patients*	*Total*	*Pliable Tubing*	*Rigid Tubing*
<50	552	0.2	0	0.3
50–59	1,041	3.5	2.0	4.3
60–69	585	3.5	1.5	4.5
>70	309	7.6	2.4	9.3
Total	2,469	3.5	1.6	4.9

From **Darney PD.** Hormonal implants: contraception for a new century. *Am J Obstet Gynecol* 1994;170: 1536–1543, with permission.

Bleeding Patterns

The implant produces endometrial atrophy. The normal menstrual cycle is disrupted, resulting in a range of possible bleeding patterns, from reasonably regular monthly bleeding, to frequent spotting and almost daily bleeding, to complete amenorrhea. The bleeding pattern changes over time and eventually tends to become more like a normal menstrual pattern. Women who have monthly bleeding are more likely to be ovulating and should be evaluated for pregnancy if they become amenorrheic. Irregular bleeding and spotting can be treated with low-dose oral estrogen, low-dose oral *levonorgestrel,* or *ibuprofen* (179). Implants have no adverse effect on lactation and can be used by lactating women. Their effects are immediately reversed by removing the implants, and the return to fertility is generally prompt.

Metabolic Effects

Implants do not alter glucose metabolism. There are minimal lipid changes. Total cholesterol and triglycerides are reduced, and there is either no change or minimal decrease in HDL, but the same ratio of total cholesterol to HDL is maintained. Therefore, it is very unlikely that implants promote development of atherosclerosis (180). Implants have no adverse effect on bone density. A cross-sectional comparison of long-term implant users with IUD-wearing women found no differences in bone density as assessed by dual-energy x-ray absorptiometry (181).

Adverse Events and Side Effects

Irregular bleeding and headache are the main reasons given for discontinuing use of implants. Side effects that are occasionally reported include acne, weight gain or loss, mastalgia, mood change, depression, hyperpigmentation over the implants, hirsutism, and galactorrhea. Symptomatic functional cysts occasionally occur. These usually resolve spontaneously over a few weeks without surgery. If pregnancy occurs, the probability of it being ectopic is increased compared with conceptions in other women; however, because pregnancy is so rare in women using implants, the total rate of ectopic pregnancies (0.28 per 1,000 woman-years) is well below that of the U.S. population (180). Serious side effects resulting in hospitalization or disability reported to the FDA from 1991 to 1993 included 24 women with infection at the implantation site, 14 with difficulties in removing the capsules, 14 with stroke, 3 with thrombotic thrombocytopenic purpura, 6 with thrombocytopenia, and 29 with pseudotumor cerebri (182). The rate of occurrence of these illnesses did not exceed that expected in women in the reproductive years, and no causal connection was implied. The hospitalizations from problems of insertion and removal can be totally prevented by using proper technique with these procedures (183).

Insertion

Implants are inserted just beneath the skin of the inner surface of the upper arm using a 10-gauge trocar as an inserter. Insertion is readily accomplished in a few minutes with local anesthesia. It is important to place the trocar just beneath the skin, inserted parallel to the skin, all the way to the second mark on the trocar before loading the rod for insertion. In this way, the rods are inserted without tension and will not migrate. Difficult removals generally are the result of poor insertion technique. Removal of implants can be time consuming. The end of the rod should be manipulated into a small incision in the skin, using a scalpel to nick the fibrous sheath that forms around the rod and then pushing it out with finger pressure (183). With the Emory technique, a somewhat longer (10-mm) incision is used, and hemostat forceps are used to disrupt the fibrous capsule around the ends of all of the implants before removal with an instrument (180). With the "U" technique, an incision is made over the midportion of the middle implant, and a special grasping forceps developed for vasectomy procedures is advanced subcutaneously to grasp the midportion of each rod and extract it (184).

Emergency Contraception

Implantation of the fertilized ovum is believed to occur on the sixth day after fertilization. This interval provides an opportunity to prevent pregnancy even after fertilization occurs. This can be accomplished using hormonal agents singly or in combination, or IUDs.

Estrogens

High-dose estrogen taken within 72 hours of coitus prevents pregnancy. The mechanism of action of postcoital estrogen use may involve altered tubal motility, interference with corpus luteum function mediated by prostaglandins, or alteration of the endometrium. In an analysis of more than 3,000 women treated after coitus with 5 mg of *EE* daily for 5 days, the pregnancy rate was 0.15% (187).

Estrogen and Progestin in Combination

High-dose estrogen has largely replaced the combination of *EE* 0.200 mg and *levonorgestrel* 2 mg (2 *Ovral* tablets followed by 2 more tablets 12 hours later), as first described by Yuzpe (188). The average pregnancy rate with this method is 1.8%, but it is 1.2% if treatment is started within 12 hours of intercourse (189). Nausea and vomiting are common with both regimens, and an antiemetic is usually prescribed. A comparable dosing of *EE* and *levonorgestrel* is provided by taking 4 tablets of *LoOvral, Nordette, Levlen, Triphasil,* or *TriLevlen,* or 5 tablets of *Allese,* instead of 2 tablets of *Ovral.* A kit containing four tablets, each containing 50 μg of *EE* and 250 μg of *levonorgestrel,* is marketed in the United States under the name *Preven* specifically for emergency contraception.

Levonorgestrel Alone

A new and better alternative for emergency contraception is using *levonorgestrel* alone, 0.75 mg initially, followed by another 0.75 mg 12 hours later. This preparation is sold in the United States as Plan B. The World Health Organization carried out a randomized trial with 1998 women assigned to the Yuzpe method or to levonorgestrel alone, started within 72 hours of intercourse. The pregnancy rate was 3.2% with the Yuzpe method, and only 1.1% with *levonorgestrel* alone (RR for pregnancy, 0.32; 95% CI, 0.18 to 0.70). Nausea and vomiting occurred much less frequently with *levonorgestrel* alone (23.1% versus 50.5%, and 5.6% versus 18.8%) (190). The efficacy of both methods declines as time increases since intercourse. Even after 49 to 72 hours, however, the pregnancy rate with the *levonorgestrel* treatment was only 2.7%, and it is likely that considerable efficacy would be found beyond 72 hours (Fig. 10.15). Because of greater efficacy and less nausea, *levonorgestrel* used alone appears to be the best hormonal method for emergency contraception currently available in the United States.

Copper Intrauterine Device

Postcoital insertion of a copper IUD within 72 hours appears to be even more effective than steroids (191). In 879 patients treated with an IUD, only one pregnancy occurred (187). No pregnancies occurred during the first month after insertion of copper IUDs as long as 7 days after coitus. It is likely that the *levonorgestrel* IUD would also work for this purpose, but there are as yet no studies of its use after coitus.

Danazol

A weak androgen, danazol has also been used for emergency contraception. The pregnancy rate was 2% among 998 women (187). In general, the oral contraceptive preparations are more desirable because they are less costly and have fewer side effects.

Mifepristone

The antiprogesterone *mifepristone* (*RU486*) is also highly effective for postcoital contraception and appears to have no significant side effects. A three-way trial of the Yuzpe method—*danazol,* 600 mg repeated after 12 hours, and *mifepristone,* 600 mg as a single dose, yielded pregnancy rates of 2.62, 4.66, and 0%, respectively (192). Much lower does

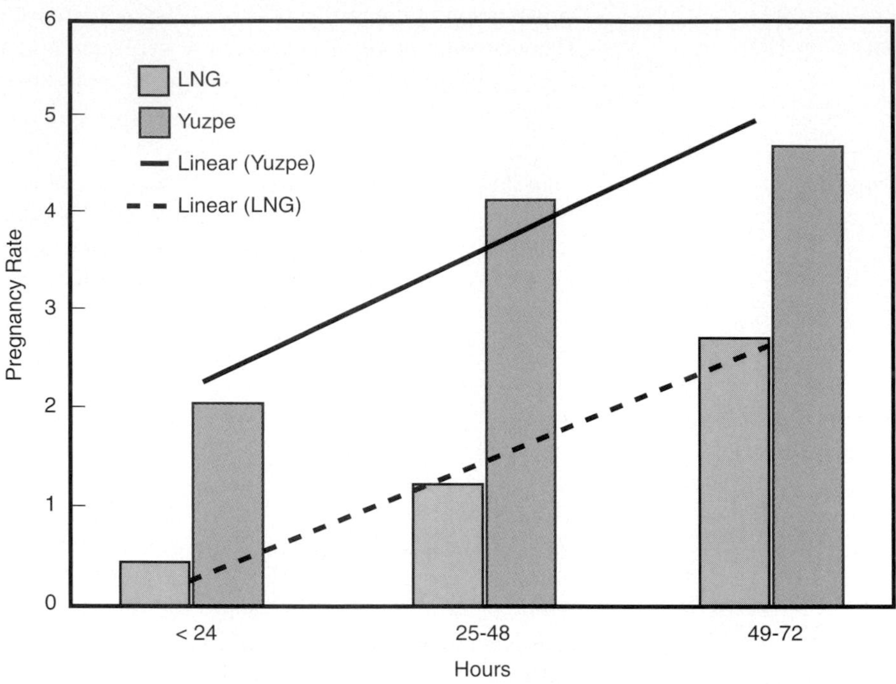

Figure 10.15 Emergency contraception: pregnancy rates by treatment group and time since unprotected coitus. LNG is levonorgestrel, 0.75 mg × 2. Yuzpe method is ethinyl estradiol, 0.100 mg plus levonorgestrel 0.50 mg × 2, 12 hours later. [From **Anon.** Randomized controlled trial of levonorgestrel versus the Yuzpe regimen of combined oral contraceptives for emergency contraception. Task Force on Postovulatory Methods of Fertility Regulation. *Lancet* 1998;352:430 (modified from Table 3), with permission.)

of mifepristone have been studied. Doses as low as 10 mg are effective (193). *Mifepristone* is also highly effective in inducing menstruation when taken on day 27 of the menstrual cycle, well beyond the 72-hour window usually considered for postcoital contraception. Of 62 women treated in this fashion, only 1 conceived (187).

Contraception for Women with Chronic Illness

Women with chronic illness may present special problems that should be considered in the choice of a method of contraception. The illness may make pregnancy more complicated and dangerous for these women, thus making effective contraception all the more important. Some common conditions and considerations about contraception are listed in Table 10.9.

Hormonal Contraception for Men

The same negative feedback of sex steroids that can block ovulation in women will also suppress spermatogenesis in men, but it will produce loss of libido and potentially extinguish sexual performance. Replacement testosterone therapy restores libido and performance without restoring spermatogenesis. The principle was first demonstrated in 1974 using oral estrogen and methyl testosterone (194). Testosterone alone suppresses pituitary release of LH and FSH to very low levels and depresses or abolishes spermatogenesis, whereas the testosterone in systemic circulation maintains normal sexual behavior and body habitus. Weekly doses of 200 mg achieved azoospermia in only 40% to 70% of white men; the rest became oligospermic (195). Pregnancy has occurred in partners of androgen-treated oligospermic men with sperm counts as low as 3 million/mL (196). Asian men may be treated more effectively than white men. In a study of seven Indonesian men, 100 mg of testosterone weekly produced azoospermia in all of them (197). Combinations of *DMPA*

Table 10.9. Contraception for Women with Chronic Illness

Psychiatric disorders

- Oral contraceptives, implants, DMPA, and copper IUD are good choices.
- Use of barrier methods should be encouraged to decrease risk for STDs.

Coagulation disorders

- Hemorrhagic disorders: OCs may be indicated to prevent hemorrhagic ovarian cysts and menstrual hemorrhage.
- Thrombotic disorders: avoid estrogen-containing OCs.

Dyslipidemia

- May use low-dose OCs if lipid abnormality successfully managed by diet or drug therapy, but lipids should be monitored at 3–6 months.
- Avoid OCs if triglycerides are elevated.
- Select less androgenic OCs.
- Progestin-only OCs, *DMPA,* and IUDs are acceptable.

Hypertension

- Young women with no other risk factors with well-controlled hypertension may use low-dose OCs under close supervision.
- Older women, smokers, and those with poorly controlled hypertension should probably avoid combination OCs.
- *DMPA, Norplant,* IUDs, and progestin-only OCs are good alternatives.

Diabetes

- Young diabetic women without vascular disease can use low-dose OCs.
- Older women or women with vascular disease probably should not use combination OCs.
- DMPA, Norplant, IUDs, and progestin-only OCs are good alternatives.

Headache

- Migraine without aura, without neurologic symptoms, does not rule out OCs if use is closely supervised.
- Norplant and DMPA may be used safely.

Epilepsy

- OCs do not increase the risk for seizure, but antiseizure drugs reduce efficacy of OCs and Norplant.
- OCs with 50 μg estrogen can be used, as can *DMPA*. IUDs are not contraindicated.

DMPA, depomedroxyprogesterone acetate; IUD, intrauterine device; OCs, oral contraceptives.
From **Association of Reproductive Health Professionals.** *Clinical challenges in contraception: a program on women with special medical conditions.* Clinical Proceedings. Washington, DC: ARHP, 1994.

and androgen have been widely studied but also fail to achieve 100% sperm suppression in white men (198). Current interest is in using GnRH analogues to suppress spermatogenesis, with long-acting androgens used for replacement. One of these regimens will likely prove clinically useful, but at present, costs are high, and long-term safety remains to be established. Adverse lipid changes have been noted with *DMPA* and androgen combinations, raising concern about vascular disease with prolonged use. Liver cancer is a concern with long-term androgen therapy (199).

Sterilization

Surgical sterilization is the most common method of fertility control used by couples in the United States (4). Laparoscopic techniques for women and vasectomy for men are safe and readily available throughout the United States. The mean age at sterilization is 30 years. Age younger than 30 years when sterilized and divorce and remarriage are predictors of sterilization regret, which may lead to a request for reversal of sterilization (200).

Female Sterilization

Hysterectomy is no longer considered for sterilization because morbidity and mortality are too high in comparison with tubal sterilization. Four procedures are common in the United States.

1. Tubal sterilization at the time of laparotomy for a cesarean delivery or other abdominal operation
2. Postpartum minilaparotomy soon after vaginal delivery
3. Interval minilaparotomy
4. Laparoscopy

Vaginal tubal sterilization, which has been associated with occasional pelvic abscess, is rarely performed in the United States.

Postpartum tubal sterilization at the time of cesarean delivery adds no risk, other than a slight prolongation of operating time; however, cesarean birth has more risk than vaginal birth, and planned sterilization should not influence the decision to perform a cesarean delivery. Sterilization is no more likely to fail if done with a cesarean delivery than at other times (201).

Postpartum minilaparotomy can be performed in the immediate postpartum state. The uterus is enlarged, and the fallopian tubes lie in the midabdomen, easily accessible through a small, 3- to 4-cm subumbilical incision.

Interval minilaparotomy, first described by Uchida (202), was rediscovered and popularized in the early 1970s in response to the increased demand for sterilization procedures as a simpler alternative to laparoscopy. In the nongravid state, the uterus and tubes lie deep in the pelvis. A short transverse suprapubic incision is made, and the uterus and tubes are then elevated upward, just beneath the incision by use of a uterine-elevating probe placed into the uterine cavity through the vagina. Interval minilaparotomy is usually performed as an outpatient procedure and can be accomplished readily with local anesthesia and conscious sedation.

Surgical Technique

The tubal lesion usually elected is the Pomeroy or modified Pomeroy technique (Fig. 10.16). In the classic Pomeroy procedure, a loop of tube is excised after ligating the base of the loop with a single absorbable suture. A modification of the procedure is excision of the midportion of the tube after ligation of the segment with two separate absorbable sutures. This modified procedure has several names: *partial salpingectomy, Parkland Hospital technique, separate sutures technique,* and *modified Pomeroy.* In the Madlener technique, now abandoned because of too many failures, a loop of tube is crushed by cross-clamping its base, ligated with permanent suture, and then excised. Pomeroy and partial salpingectomy procedures have failure rates of 1 to 4 per 1,000 cases (201). In contrast, pregnancy is almost unheard of after tubal sterilization by the Irving or Uchida methods (201,202). In the Irving method, the midportion of the tube is excised, and the proximal stump of each tube is turned back and led into a small stab wound in the wall of the uterus and sutured in place, creating a blind loop (203). With the Uchida method, a saline-*epinephrine* solution (1:1,000) is injected beneath the mucosa of the midportion of the tube, separating the mucosa from the underlying tube. The mucosa is incised along the antimesenteric border of the tube, and a tubal segment is excised under traction so that the ligated proximal stump will retract beneath the mucosa when released. The mucosa is then closed with sutures, burying the proximal stump and separating it from the distal stump. In Uchida's personal series of more than 20,000 cases, there were no pregnancies (202).

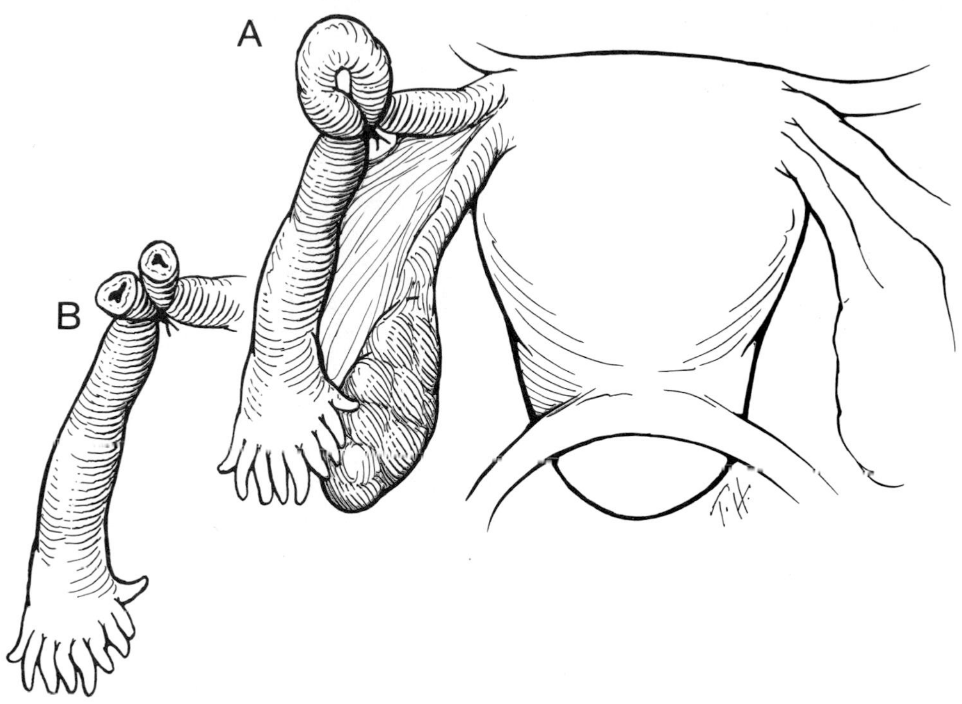

Figure 10.16 Pomeroy technique for tubal sterilization.

Laparoscopy

In the standard laparoscopy technique, the abdomen is inflated with a gas (carbon dioxide or nitrous oxide) through a special needle inserted at the lower margin of the umbilicus (204). A hollow sheath containing a pointed trocar is then pushed through the abdominal wall at the same location; the trocar is removed; and the laparoscope is inserted into the abdominal cavity through the sheath to visualize the pelvic organs. A second, smaller trocar is inserted in the suprapubic region to allow the insertion of special grasping forceps. Alternatively, an operating laparoscope that has a channel for the instruments can be used; thus, the procedure can be performed through a single small incision. Laparoscopic sterilization is usually performed in the hospital under general anesthesia but can be performed under local anesthesia with conscious sedation. Overnight hospitalization for laparoscopy is rarely needed.

Open Laparoscopy Standard laparoscopy carries with it a small but definite risk for injury to major blood vessels with insertion of the sharp trocar. With the alternative technique of open laparoscopy, neither needle nor sharp trocar is used; instead, the peritoneal cavity is opened directly through an incision at the lower edge of the umbilicus (205). A special funnel-shaped sleeve, the Hasson cannula, is then inserted, and the laparoscope is introduced through it.

Techniques of Laparoscopic Sterilization Sterilization is accomplished by any of four techniques: bipolar electrical coagulation, application of a small Silastic rubber band (Falope ring) (206), the plastic and metal Hulka clip (204), or the Filshie clip (207). The Filshie clip is new to the United States, although it has been used extensively in the United Kingdom and Canada (208). It is a hinged device made of titanium with a liner of silicone rubber tubing. In the bipolar electrocoagulation technique, the midisthmic portion of the tube and adjacent mesosalpinx are grasped with special bipolar forceps, and radiofrequency electric current is applied to three adjacent areas, coagulating 3 cm of tube (Fig. 10.17). The tube alone is then recoagulated in the same places. The radiofrequency generator must deliver at least 25 watts into a 100-ohm resistance at the probe tips to ensure coagulation of the complete

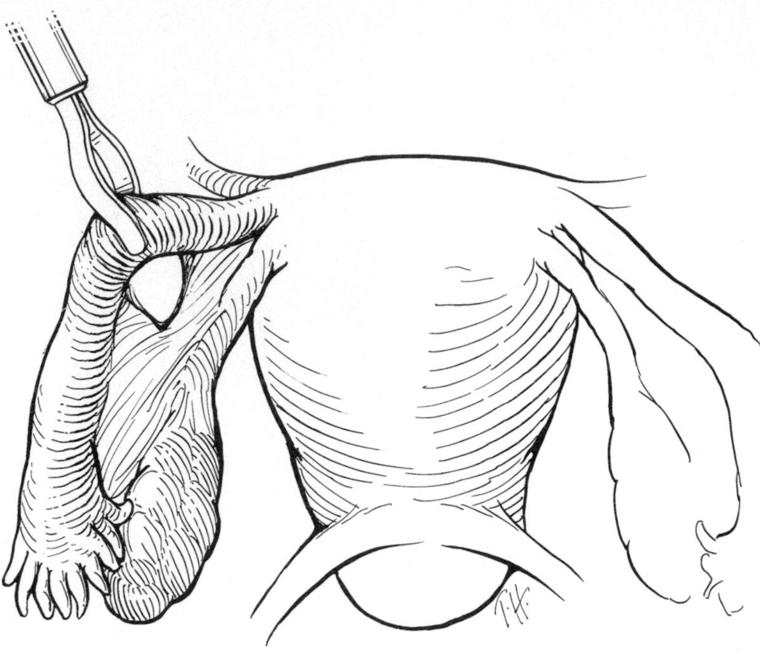

Figure 10.17 Technique for bipolar electrocoagulation tubal sterilization.

thickness of the fallopian tube and not just the outer layer; otherwise, the sterilization will fail (209). To apply the Falope ring, the midisthmic portion of the tube is grasped, with tongs advanced through a cylindrical probe that has the ring stretched around it. A loop of tube is pulled back into the probe, and the outer cylinder is advanced, releasing the Silastic ring around the base of the loop of tube, producing ischemic necrosis (Fig. 10.18). If the tube cannot be pulled easily into the applicator, the operator should stop and change to electrical coagulation rather than persist and risk lacerating the tube with the Falope ring applicator. The banded tube must be inspected at close range through the laparoscope to demonstrate that the full thickness of the tube has been pulled through the Falope ring. The Hulka clip is also placed across the midisthmus, ensuring that the applicator is at right angles to the tube and that the tube is completely contained within the clip before the clip is closed. The Filshie clip (Fig. 10.19) is also placed at right angles across the midisthmus, taking care that the anvil of the posterior jaw can be visualized through the mesosalpinx beyond the tube to ensure that the complete thickness of the tube is completely within the jaws of the clip before it is closed.

The electric and band or clip techniques each have advantages and disadvantages. Bipolar coagulation can be used with any fallopian tube. The Falope ring and Hulka and Filshie clips cannot be applied if the tube is thickened from previous salpingitis. There is more pain during the first several hours after Falope ring application. This can be prevented by bathing the tubes with a few milliliters of 2% lidocaine just before ring placement. Failures of the Falope ring or the clips generally result from misapplication, and pregnancy, if it occurs, is usually intrauterine. After bipolar sterilization, pregnancy may result from tuboperitoneal fistula and is ectopic in more than 50% of cases. If inadequate electrical energy is used, a thin band of fallopian tube remains that contains the intact lumen and allows intrauterine pregnancy to occur. Thermocoagulation, the use of heat probes rather than electrical current, is employed extensively in Germany for laparoscopic tubal sterilization but has had little use in the United States.

Risks of Tubal Sterilization

Tubal sterilization is remarkably safe. In 1983, the total complication rate in a large series from several institutions was 1.7 per 100 (210). Complications were increased by use of

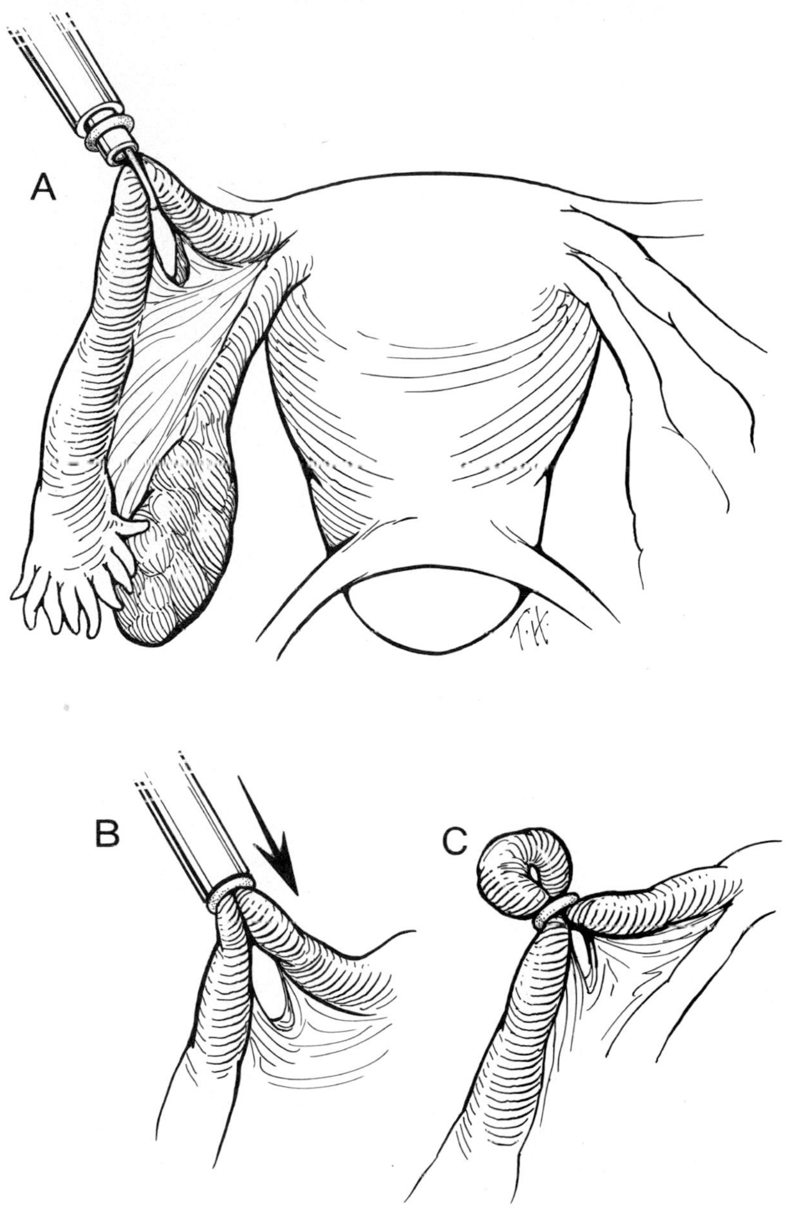

Figure 10.18 Placement of the Falope ring for tubal sterilization.

general anesthesia, previous pelvic or abdominal surgery, history of PID, obesity, and diabetes mellitus. The most common significant complication was unintended laparotomy for sterilization after intraabdominal adhesions were found. In another series, 2,827 laparoscopic sterilizations were performed with the Silastic band using local anesthesia and intravenous sedation. Only four cases could not be completed (a technical failure rate of 0.14%), and laparotomy was not needed (211). Rarely, salpingitis can occur as a complication of the surgery. This occurs more often with electric coagulation than nonelectric techniques. From 1977 until 1981, there were four deaths per 100,000 procedures in the United States, less than the risk of one pregnancy; almost half of the deaths were from complications of general anesthesia, usually related to the use of mask ventilation (212). The last U.S. national study was of sterilizations performed in 1979 to 1980. There were a total of 9 to 10 deaths per 100,000 sterilizations, but only 1 to 2 per 100,000 were attributed to the sterilization procedure alone (213). When general anesthesia is used for laparoscopy, endotracheal intubation is mandatory because the pneumoperitoneum increases the risk for aspiration. International data from the Association for Voluntary Surgical Contraception

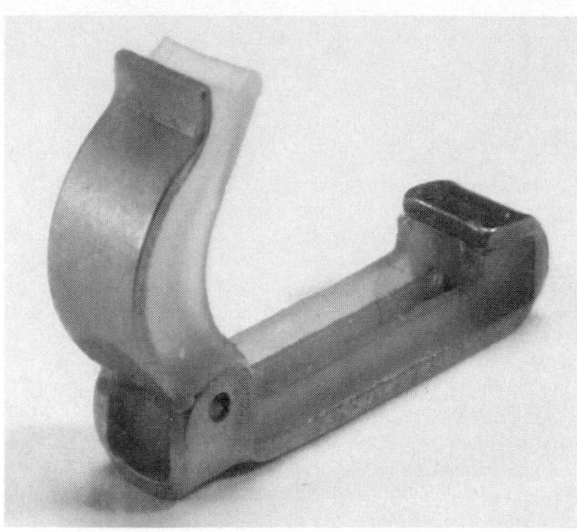

Figure 10.19 Filshie clip for tubal sterilization.

show a similar record of safety from Third World programs: 4.7 deaths per 100,000 female sterilizations and 0.5 per 100,000 vasectomies (214).

Family Health International has reported large randomized multicenter trials of the different means for tubal sterilization. The Filshie and Hulka clips were compared in two trials. A total of 2,126 women were studied, of which 878 had either clip placed by minilaparotomy and 1,248 had either clip placed by laparoscopy, and were then evaluated at up to 24 months (215). Pregnancy rates were 1.1 per 1,000 women with the Filshie clip and 6.9 per 1,000 with the Hulka clip at 12 months, a difference in rates that was close to statistically significant ($p = 0.06$). This same group compared the Filshie clip to the Silastic tubal ring in a similar study with a total of 2,746 women, of which 915 had the devices placed at minilaparotomy and 1,831 had laparoscopy (216). Pregnancy rates at 12 months were the same for the Filshie clip and the tubal ring: 1.7 per 1,000 women. The ring was judged more difficult to apply, but three women spontaneously expelled the Filshie clip during the 12 months of follow-up.

Benefits of Tubal Sterilization

In addition to providing excellent contraception, tubal ligation is associated with reduced risk for ovarian cancer that persists for as long as 20 years after surgery (217).

Sterilization Failure

Many "failures" occur during the first month after laparoscopy and are the result of a pregnancy already begun when the sterilization was performed. Contraception should be continued until the day of surgery, and a sensitive pregnancy test should be routinely performed on the day of surgery. Because implantation does not occur until 6 days after conception, however, a woman could conceive just before her surgery and there would be no way to detect it. Scheduling sterilization early in the menstrual cycle obviates the problem but adds to the logistic difficulty. Another cause of failure is the presence of anatomic abnormalities, usually adhesions surrounding and obscuring one or both tubes. An experienced laparoscopic surgeon with proper instruments can usually lyse the adhesions, restore normal anatomic relations, and positively identify the tube. In some circumstances, however, successful sterilization will not be possible by laparoscopy, and the surgeon must know before surgery whether the patient is prepared to undergo laparotomy, if necessary, to accomplish sterilization.

Most studies of sterilization failure are short term. The Centers for Disease Control and Prevention's Collaborative Review of Sterilization (CREST) reported on a cohort of 10,685 women sterilized between 1978 and 1986 at any of 16 participating centers in the United States who were followed from 8 to 14 years (218). The true failure rates for 10 years

Table 10.10. Ten-year Life-table Cumulative Probability of Pregnancy per 1,000 Procedures with Different Methods of Tubal Sterilization, United States, 1978–1986.

Method	
Unipolar coagulation	7.5
Postpartum partial salpingectomy	7.5
Silastic band (Falope or Yoon)	17.7
Interval partial salpingectomy	20.1
Bipolar coagulation	24.8
Hulka-Clemens clip	36.5
Total: all methods	18.5

From **Peterson HB, Xia Z, Hughes JM, et al.** The risk of pregnancy after tubal sterilization: findings from the U.S. Collaborative Review of Sterilization. *Am J Obstet Gynecol* 1996;174:1164 (Table II) (184), with permission.

obtained by the life-table method are given in Table 10.10. Pregnancies resulting from sterilization during the luteal phase of the cycle in which the surgery was performed were excluded. Thirty-three percent of all remaining pregnancies were ectopic. The most effective methods at 10 years were unipolar coagulation at laparoscopy and postpartum partial salpingectomy, generally a modified Pomeroy procedure. Bipolar tubal coagulation and the Hulka-Clemens clip were least effective. Younger women had higher risk for failure, as would be expected because of their greater fecundity.

Over the years since the CREST study began, sterilization by unipolar electrosurgery was abandoned because of risk for bowel burns and was replaced with bipolar electrosurgery or the nonelectric methods (tubal ring, Hulka-Clemens clip, and more recently, the Filshie clip). An important later analysis of the CREST data found that bipolar sterilization could have a very low long-term failure rate if an adequate portion of the tube is coagulated. CREST study subjects who were sterilized with bipolar electrosurgery in 1985 to 1987 had lower failure rates than those sterilized earlier (1978 to 1985). The important difference was in the technique of application of the electric energy to the tubes. Women whose bipolar procedure involved coagulation at three sites or more had low 5-year failure rates (3.2 per 1,000 procedures), whereas women who had fewer than three sites of tubal coagulation had a 5-year failure rate of 12.9 per 1,000 ($p = 0.01$) (219).

Reversal of Sterilization

Reversal of sterilization is more successful after mechanical occlusion than after electrocoagulation because the latter method destroys much more of the tube. With modern microsurgical techniques and an isthmus-to-isthmus anastomosis, pregnancy follows in about 75% of cases (220). A substantial risk for ectopic pregnancy exists after reversal.

Late Sequelae of Tubal Sterilization

Increased menstrual irregularity and pain have been attributed to previous tubal sterilization. In patients who underwent the older laparoscopy technique with unipolar electrical destruction of a major portion of the tube, these concerns may be warranted (221). Study of the problem is complicated by the facts that many women develop these symptoms even though they have not had tubal surgery, and OCs reduce pain and create an artificially normal menstrual cycle. Therefore, women who discontinued OC use concurrent with tubal sterilization will experience more dysmenorrhea, which is entirely unrelated to the sterilization. The best answer presently available also comes from the CREST study (222). A total of 9,514 women who had undergone tubal sterilization were compared with 573 women whose partners had undergone vasectomy. Both groups were followed up to 5 years with annual standardized telephone interviews. Women who had undergone tubal sterilization were no more likely to report persistent changes in intermenstrual bleeding or length of the menstrual cycle than women whose partners had vasectomy. The sterilized women, in fact, reported decreases in days of bleeding, amount of bleeding, and menstrual pain but were slightly more likely to report cycle irregularity (OR, 1.6; 95% CI, 1.1 to 2.3). Hence, this study found no evidence to support the existence of a posttubal ligation syndrome.

Vasectomy

Vasectomy, excision of a portion of the vas deferens, is readily accomplished with local anesthesia in an office setting. It does not decrease sexual performance (223). The basic technique is to palpate the vas through the scrotum, grasp it with fingers or atraumatic forceps, make a small incision over the vas, and pull a loop of the vas into the incision. A small segment is removed, and then a needle electrode is used to coagulate the lumen of both ends. Improved techniques include the no-scalpel vasectomy, in which the pointed end of the forceps is used to puncture the skin over the vas. This small variation reduces the chance of bleeding and avoids the need to suture the incision. Another variation is the open-ended vasectomy, in which only the abdominal end of the severed vas is coagulated while the testicular end is left open. This is believed to prevent congestive epididymitis (224).

Reversibility

Vasectomy must be regarded as a permanent means of sterilization; however, with microsurgical techniques, vasovasostomy will result in pregnancy about half the time. The longer the interval since vasectomy, the poorer the chance of reversal.

Safety

Operative complications include scrotal hematomas, wound infection, and epididymitis, but serious sequelae are rare. There have been no reports of deaths from vasectomy in the United States in many years, and the death rate in a large Third World series was only 0.5 per 100,000. Studies of vasectomized monkeys showed accelerated atherosclerosis, but several large-scale human studies have found no connection between vasectomy and vascular disease (225,226). Concerns about long-term safety recurred with the report of a possible association between prostate cancer and vasectomy (227). Prostate cancer is largely a disease of the Western world and is strongly linked to dietary animal fat, family history, and race (228). In the West, it is more common in men of African American ancestry and rare in men of Asian descent. Recent studies are reassuring. A large multiethnic case-control study from the United States and Canada compared 1,642 men with prostate cancer to 1,636 controls and found no overall association (OR, 1.1; 95% CI, 0.83 to 1.3) (229). Older reports may reflect bias, perhaps that higher-status men, with diets higher in animal fat, were more likely than lower-status men to choose vasectomy.

Abortion

Given the desire in developed countries to limit families to one or two children and the efficacy of contraception in general use, it is extremely likely that any normal couple will experience at least one unwanted pregnancy at some time during their reproductive years. In Third World countries, desired family size is larger, but access to effective contraception is limited. As a result, abortion is common. Worldwide, about 26 to 31 million legal abortions and an estimated 10 to 22 million clandestine abortions are performed every year (230). Where abortion is legal, it is generaliy reasonably safe; where it is illegal, complications are common, and about 150,000 women die every year from these complications (231). Societies cannot prevent abortion, but they can determine whether it will be illegal and dangerous or legal and safe. Many countries in which abortion is completely illegal have very high rates of clandestine abortion. Abortion rates in representative countries are given in Table 10.11 (232).

Death from illegal abortion was once common in the United States. In the 1940s, more than 1,000 women died each year of complications from abortion (233). In 1992, the last year

Table 10.11. Rates of Induced Abortion in Representative Countries, 1985–1991 per 1,000 Women Aged 15–44 Years

Legal Abortion[a]		*Illegal Abortion*[b]	
Netherlands, 1986	5.3	Brazil, 1991	36.5
Canada, 1985	12.0	Columbia, 1989	32.7
England/Wales, 1987	14.2	Chile, 1990	45.4
United States, 1985	28.0	Mexico, 1990	22.3
Cuba, 1988	58.0	Peru, 1990	51.9
Former USSR, 1987	181.0	Dominican Republic	43.7

[a] From **Henshaw SK, Morrow E.** Induced abortion: a world review. *Fam Plann Perspect* 1990;22:76–120, with permission.
[b] From **The Alan Guttmacher Institute.** *Aborto clandestino: Un realidad Latinoamericana.* New York: The Alan Guttmacher Institute, 1994:24, with permission.

for which complete data are available, there were 17 deaths from spontaneous abortion, 10 deaths from legally induced abortion, and no deaths from illegal abortion (abortion induced by a nonprofessional) in the entire United States. (234). The American Medical Association's Council on Scientific Affairs has reviewed the impact of legal abortion and attributes the decline in deaths during this century to the introduction of antibiotics to treat sepsis; the widespread use of effective contraception beginning in the 1960s, which reduced the number of unwanted pregnancies; and, more recently, the shift from illegal to legal abortion (235). Much of the continued decline in non–abortion-related maternal mortality of recent years can be attributed to choice of legal abortion by women at high risk for pregnancy mortality. The United States has a serious problem with teenage pregnancy. Without legal abortion, there would be almost twice as many teenage births each year.

The number of abortions reported each year in the United States—1,186,039 in 1997 according to the Centers for Disease Control and Prevention—has been decreasing since 1990. In 1997, the national abortion ratio was 306 abortions for every 1,000 live births, and the national abortion rate was 20 per 1,000 women aged 15 to 44 years (236). Most women who obtain abortions are unmarried (79% in 1997), and the ratio of abortions to live births is 9 times higher for unmarried women than for married women. Use of abortion varies markedly with age. In 1997, 20% of women obtaining abortions were 19 years of age or younger, and 51.8% were 24 years of age or younger. In 1997, the last year for which detailed information is available, the abortion ratio for women younger than 15 years of age was 729 per 1,000 live births, almost as many abortions as births (Fig. 10.2). The lowest abortion ratio, 161 per 1,000 live births, is for women aged 30 to 34 years. Legal abortion rates and ratios reached their highest in the early 1980s as they replaced illegal abortions, and both have declined since, especially for the youngest women (Fig. 10.20) (16).

Regardless of personal feelings about the ethics of interrupting pregnancy, health professionals have a duty to know the medical facts about abortion and to share them with their patients (237). Providers are not required to perform abortions against their ethical principles, but they have a duty to help patients assess pregnancy risks and to make appropriate referrals.

Safety Issues

The risk for death from legal abortion was 0.7 per 100,000 induced abortions in 1996 (234). In contrast, total maternal mortality is about 7 or 8 per 100,000 live births. The risk for death from legal abortion before 16 weeks is 10-fold less than that from continuing the pregnancy to delivery. As shown in Table 10.12, the risk for death increases with gestational age (238). For individual women with high-risk conditions (e.g., cyanotic

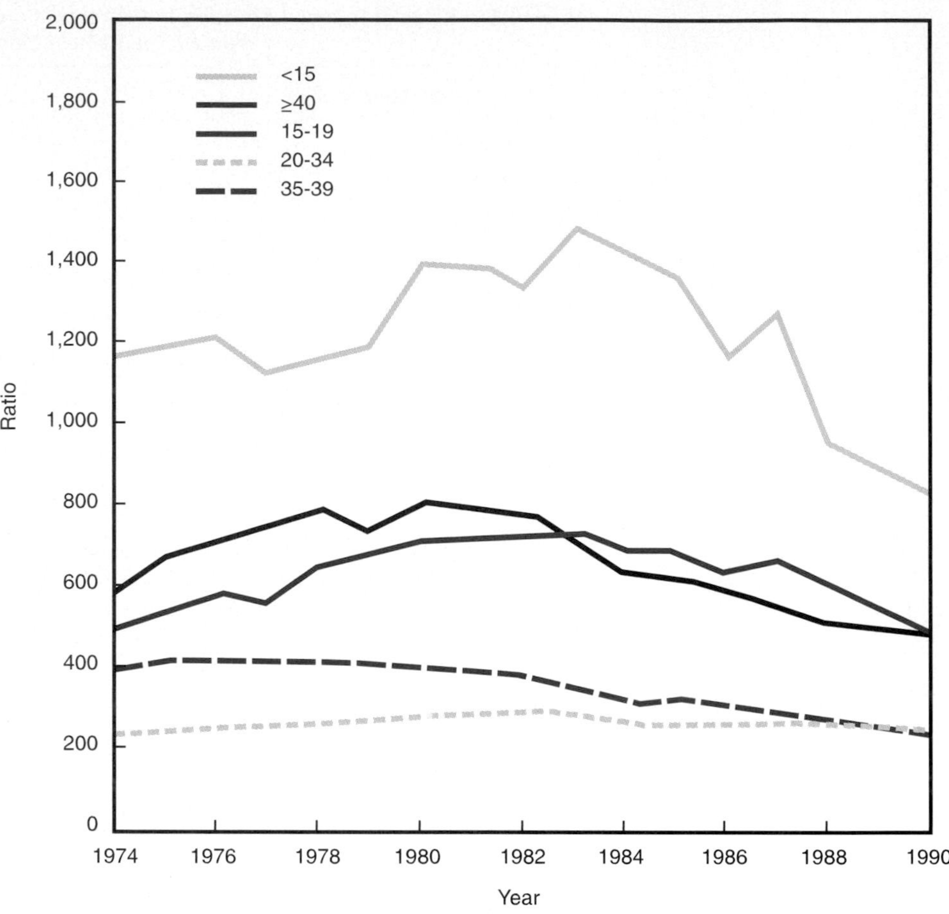

Figure 10.20 Abortion ratios, by age group and by year, United States, 1974–1997. Ratio equals induced abortions per 1,000 live births. [From **Koonin LM, Strauss LT, Chrisman CE, et al.** Abortion surveillance, 1997. *MMWR Morb Mortal Wkly Rep* 2000,49(SS-11):14, with permission.]

heart disease), even late abortion is a safer alternative to birth. Because of the availability of low-cost, out-of-hospital first-trimester abortion, 88% of legal abortions are performed during the first trimester (before 13 weeks of amenorrhea), when abortion is the safest (238). The type of procedure is another determinant of risk. First-trimester abortions are virtually all performed by vacuum curettage; however, in the midtrimester, a variety of techniques can be used. Risk for death from abortion by the various techniques at different gestational ages is given in Table 10.13. The data clearly show the greater safety of instrumental evacuation of the uterus [dilation and evacuation (D & E)] performed in the early midtrimester. Another determinant of risk is anesthesia. Use of general anesthesia increases the risk for perforation of the uterus, visceral injury, hemorrhage, hysterectomy, and death (239). The preferred alternative is paracervical block with local anesthetic, augmented with conscious sedation when needed.

Techniques for Abortion

Most abortions are performed by vacuum curettage. Early procedures (5 to 7 weeks from beginning of last normal menses) can be readily performed in an office setting using simple instruments: a 5- to 6-mm flexible plastic cannula and a modified 50-mL plastic syringe as vacuum source (240). After 7 weeks, somewhat larger rigid plastic cannulas (8 to 12 mm in diameter) are generally used, depending on gestational age, with an electric pump as the vacuum source. Most abortions in the United States are performed outside of hospitals, usually in freestanding specialty clinics, at a cost far below that of hospital services. General anesthesia is unnecessary. Adequate pain relief is provided by infiltrating the cervix

Table 10.12. Death to Case Rates for Legal Abortion Mortality by Weeks of Gestation, United States, 1972–1987

Weeks of Gestation	*Deaths*	*Abortions*	*Rate*[a]	*Relative Risk*
≤8	33	8,673,759	0.4	1.0
9–10	39	4,847,321	0.8	2.1
11–12	33	2,360,768	1.4	3.7
13–15	28	962,185	2.9	7.7
16–20	74	794,093	9.3	24.5
≥21	21	175,395	12.0	31.5

[a] Legal abortion deaths per 100,000 procedures; excludes deaths from ectopic pregnancies or pregnancy with gestation length unknown.
From **Lawson HW, Frye A, Atrash HK, et al.** Abortion mortality, United States, 1972–1987. *Am J Obstet Gynecol* 1994;171:1365–1372, with permission.

with local anesthetic, augmented with intravenous sedatives and analgesics for conscious sedation (241).

Medical Means for Abortion

Mifepristone (*RU486*), an analogue of the progestin *norethindrone,* has strong affinity for the progesterone receptor but acts as an antagonist, blocking the effect of natural progesterone. Given alone, the drug was moderately effective in causing abortion of early pregnancy; however, the combination of *mifepristone* with a low dose of prostaglandin proved very effective. In a series of almost 17,000 cases, 600 mg of *mifepristone* orally followed in 36 to 48 hours by either *sulprostone* or *gemeprost* produced complete abortion in 95% of cases (242). The only significant complications of this method to date have been three myocardial infarctions, with one death. All three myocardial infarctions occurred in women older than 35 years of age who were heavy smokers and occurred at the time of administration of *sulprostone,* a prostaglandin E_2 analogue (243). No myocardial infarctions have occurred with the prostaglandin E_1 analogue *gemeprost. Misoprostol,* another prostaglandin E_1 analogue, seems to have fewer side effects and a greater margin of safety than *sulprostone.* It is very effective when combined with *mifepristone* and is the prostaglandin used with *mifepristone* in the United States (244).

The 600-mg dose of *mifepristone* used initially is actually far more than needed. Several investigators have shown that a 200-mg dose is equally effective (245–248). Initially, *misoprostol* was given orally, but the vaginal route of administration is more effective, probably because it provides sustained blood levels of the drug over several hours (249).

Table 10.13. Death to Case Rates for Legal Abortions by Type of Procedure and Weeks of Gestation, United States, 1974–1987[a]

Procedure	*≤8*	*9–10*	*11–12*	*13–15*	*16–20*	*≥21*
Vacuum curettage[b]	0.3	0.7	1.1	—	—	—
Dilation and evacuation	—	—	—	2.0	6.5	11.9
Instillation[c]	—	—	—	3.8	7.9	10.3
Hysterectomy, hysterotomy	18.3	30.0	41.2	28.1	103.4	274.3

[a] Legal induced abortion deaths per 100,000 legal induced abortions.
[b] Includes all suction and sharp curettage procedures.
[c] Includes all instillation methods (saline, prostaglandin).
From **Lawson HW, Frye A, Atrash HK, et al.** Abortion mortality, United States, 1972–1987. *Am J Obstet Gynecol* 1994;171:1365–1372, with permission.

The combination of 200 mg *mifepristone* orally followed by 800 μg of vaginal *misoprostol* produced complete abortion in 98% of women treated, after up to 63 days of amenorrhea, and appears to be the regimen of choice (246). *Misoprostol* can be given 1 to 3 days after the *mifepristone* with no loss of efficacy (248). Initially, patients returned to the clinics to receive *misoprostol* and remained on site for several hours. Half or more expel the pregnancy within 4 to 5 hours after *misoprostol* is given. However, it has been shown that patients may safely be given the *misoprostol* for self-administration at home (250).

Methotrexate and Misoprostol

The antifolate *methotrexate* provides another medical approach to pregnancy termination. Widely used to treat ectopic pregnancies without surgery (251), it can also be used with intrauterine gestations. *Methotrexate,* 50 mg/M^2 given intramuscularly, followed by *misoprostol,* 800 mg inserted vaginally, produced abortion in six pregnancies up to 56 days from the last menstrual period (252). *Methotrexate* used alone without the *misoprostol* is also successful, although bleeding does not begin until an average of 24 days after treatment (253). In a large multicenter trial, 53% of patients aborted after the first dose of *misoprostol* and an additional 15% after the second dose. A total of 92% had successful abortion by 35 days after the initial *methotrexate* injection (254). The *methotrexate-misoprostol* regimen takes longer than *mifepristone-methotrexate* and is not as effective, but it is much less expensive. *Methotrexate* is usually given as an intramuscular injection, but a 50-mg oral dose is equally effective (255).

Second-trimester Abortion

Most legal abortions are performed before 13 menstrual weeks. Abortions performed after 13 weeks include those done because of fetal defects, medical or psychiatric illness that had not manifested earlier in pregnancy, and changed social circumstances, such as abandonment by the spouse. Young age is the single greatest factor determining the need for late abortion. In 1997, 24.9% of abortions for women younger than 15 years of age were midtrimester, whereas 16.8% of abortions for women 15 to 19 years of age and only 9.3% of abortions for women 30 to 34 years of age were performed after 12 weeks of gestation (236). These proportions have changed little in a decade.

Dilation and Evacuation

D & E is the most commonly used method of midtrimester abortion in the United States (236). Typically, the cervix is prepared by insertion of hygroscopic dilators, stems of the seaweed *Laminaria japonicum* (laminaria). Placed in the cervical canal as small sticks, these devices take up water from the cervix and swell, triggering dilation. When these are removed the following day, sufficient cervical dilation is accomplished to allow insertion of strong forceps and a large-bore vacuum cannula to extract the fetus and placenta (256,257). Ultrasound guidance during the procedure is helpful (258). For more advanced procedures, sequential insertion of laminaria over 2 or more days is practiced, in order to achieve a greater degree of cervical dilation (259). At the end of the midtrimester, procedures that combine serial multiple laminaria dilation of the cervix with intrafetal injection of digoxin, induction of labor, and assisted expulsion of the fetus are used (260).

Labor-induction Methods

Hypertonic Solutions Amnioinfusion of hypertonic saline is historically important as one of the oldest labor-induction methods for abortion. Saline has serious hazards: cardiovascular collapse, pulmonary and cerebral edema, and renal failure occur if the solution is injected intravenously. All patients are at risk for serious disseminated intravascular coagulopathy (261). However, attention to proper technique for amnioinfusion, with the saline instilled by gravity flow through connecting tubing from a single-dose bottle under ultrasound guidance, reduces the frequency of such mishaps. Hypertonic urea is safer than saline. It is combined with low doses of prostaglandin to increase efficacy and shorten the interval from injection to abortion.

Prostaglandins Prostaglandins, oxygenated metabolites of C_{20} carboxylic acid, are found naturally in most biologic tissues, where they act as modulators of cell function. They act through specific receptors of the G-protein family that are coupled to a variety of intracellular signal mechanisms, which may stimulate or inhibit adenyl cyclase, or phosphatidylinositol (262). Prostaglandins of the E and F series can cause uterine contraction at any stage of gestation. These agents can be given by intraamniotic infusion, by intramuscular injection, or by vaginal suppository. The 15 methyl analogues of prostaglandin $F_{2\alpha}$ (*carboprost*) and prostaglandin E_2 (*dinoprostone*) are highly effective but frequently produce side effects of vomiting and diarrhea. Vaginal *misoprostol* (200 μg every 2 hours) has been shown to be as effective as *dinoprost* suppositories (20 mg every 3 hours) in patients with fetal death or intact pregnancy at 12 to 22 weeks of gestation (263). In this study, patients with a living fetus were treated with ultrasound-guided intracardiac injection of potassium chloride to ensure fetal death before administration of misoprostol. *Misoprostol*-treated patients experienced fewer side effects of fever, uterine pain, vomiting, and diarrhea. *Misoprostol* was much less expensive and easier to administer. A comparison of 200-, 400-, and 600-μg doses of misoprostol at 12-hour intervals produced rates of abortion of 70.6%, 82%, and 96%, respectively, within 48 hours; however, the side effects of vomiting, diarrhea, and fever increased with increasing dose (264). Doses as high as 400 μg vaginally every 3 hours have been used (265), but caution is needed because there is risk for uterine rupture with higher doses used in the later midtrimester. More investigation is needed to determine the ideal dosage; one regimen is 400 μg of *misoprostol* at 6-hour intervals.

There is also interest in midtrimester abortion induced with combinations of *mifepristone* and *misoprostol*. Pretreatment with mifepristone would undoubtedly increase the effect of *misoprostol,* reducing the necessary dose of the second drug. A French protocol used 600 μg of *mifepristone,* followed at 26 hours with placement of laminaria into the cervix, after which *misoprostol* was administered. The method was highly effective, with very short time intervals from the onset of *misoprostol* administration to abortion; however, one case of uterine rupture occurred in a patient with a uterine scar (266).

About one third of patients treated with 20-mg doses of *dinoprostone* have a temperature elevation of 1°C or more. This phenomenon is not seen with *carboprost tromethamine,* which slightly reduced body temperature. The effect of *misoprostol* on body temperature is dose related; generally, there is no effect at 200 μg given every 12 hours, but the effect increases as the dose increases and intervals are shortened.

Transient fetal survival can be a problem with all prostaglandin methods used in the midtrimester. To prevent this problem, and to shorten the interval to abortion and avoid failed abortion, many centers use a fetal intracardiac injection of potassium chloride (3 mL of a 2-mmol solution) or 1.5 mg of *digoxin.* Others perform amniocentesis and inject a small volume of intraamniotic hypertonic saline (60 mL of a 23% solution).

Retained placenta is common with all prostaglandin abortions. Instrumental extraction is necessary in about half of cases.

Oxytocin in very high doses is as effective as dinoprostone at 17 to 24 weeks of pregnancy (267). Patients initially receive an infusion of 50 units of *oxytocin* in 500 mL of 5% dextrose and normal saline over 3 hours, 1 hour of no *oxytocin,* followed by a 100-unit, 500-mL solution over 3 hours, another hour of rest, and then a 150-unit, 500-mL solution over 3 hours, alternating 3 hours of *oxytocin* with 1 hour of rest. The *oxytocin* is increased by 50 units in each successive period until a final concentration of 300 units per 500 mL has been reached.

Complications The labor-induction methods share common hazards: failure of the primary procedure to produce abortion within a reasonable time, incomplete abortion, retained placenta, hemorrhage, infection, and embolic phenomena. Failed abortion can lead to serious infection and continued blood loss. If fetal expulsion has not occurred after 24 to 36 hours, consideration should be given to a D & E procedure.

Selective Reduction

Multifetal pregnancies are at risk for extremely premature birth, with major neonatal complications resulting. To prevent this, selective reduction of higher-order multiple gestation to twins is often practiced. In a series of 463 pregnancies treated with ultrasound-guided fetal intracardiac injection of potassium chloride (0.2 to 0.4 mL of a 2-mmol solution in the first trimester, 0.5 to 3.0 mL in the second trimester), 83% of the surviving fetuses delivered at 33 weeks or later (268). Another indication for selective reduction is one anomalous fetus of a multifetal gestation. A 1999 series reported 402 patients treated as described for this indication (269). Rates of pregnancy loss after the procedure by gestational age at the time of procedure were 5.4% at 9 to 12 weeks, 8.7% at 13 to 18 weeks, 6.8% at 19 to 24 weeks, and 9.1% at 25 weeks or more. No maternal coagulopathy occurred, and no ischemic damages or coagulopathies were seen in the surviving neonates. Selective induction should not be attempted with monoamniotic twins or with twin–twin transfusion syndrome because of the possibility of embolic phenomena and infarction in the surviving twin. Maternal serum α-fetoprotein remains elevated into the second trimester after first-trimester procedures.

Induced Abortion and Subsequent Reproduction

Legal abortion, as currently practiced in the United States, has no measurable adverse effect on later reproduction (270). Even two or more induced abortions have no detectable adverse effect (271). Abortion as practiced in the United States is not associated with low birth weight, premature birth, or increased perinatal loss (272). Concerns about infertility as a result of induced abortion are unfounded, except for the rare severe complication managed by hysterectomy (273). The lack of adverse effects on later pregnancy probably reflects the safety of current abortion technology in the United States.

The Future

Contraceptive development is extremely slow in the United States because of the legal climate, the great cost of meeting regulatory requirements, and the low priority given this area by the medical community. On the international scene, a number of new approaches to contraception are in development. The two-rod version of *Norplant* (*Norplant II*) should soon be available. *Levonorgestrel* in a biodegradable rod of *caprolactone* that does not require removal is currently being tested, as is the single-rod implant releasing *3-keto-desogestrel*.

The *GyneFix,* a frameless copper IUD now available in Europe, consists of a surgical suture with small copper cylinders crimped to it. The knot on the proximal end of the suture is pushed 1 cm into the uterine wall with a special inserter. Comparative trials have found it more effective than the *copper T380A* and to have fewer expulsions and fewer removals for pain and bleeding (274). It is of considerable interest for these reasons and also because of excellent retention after postaortal insertion.

Silastic vaginal rings releasing either progestin or progestin-estrogen combinations have been studied for years and are now undergoing field trials in a number of countries. A patch for transdermal release of estrogen and progestin for contraception is being tested in the United States. Both of these methods for steroid delivery have the advantage of greater ease of compliance for the user. There is great interest in developing compounds that could be used as a vaginal contraceptive and that would be protective against HIV. One such compound is a phenyl phosphate derivative of *zidovudine.* It has both spermicidal and antiretroviral activity and has proved nontoxic in short-term trials in mice (275).

Current methods of tubal sterilization require abdominal surgery. To meet the coming demand for vast numbers of sterilizations worldwide, easier means must be devised. Considerable effort has gone into developing transuterine methods of female sterilization that would avoid the need to open the abdominal cavity to gain access to the fallopian tubes. Hysteroscopy with tubal cannulation and electrofulguration or the injection of Silastic that forms in place into tubal plugs have been explored and largely abandoned (276). A simpler option is placement of quinine pellets in the uterus through an IUD inserter. It has been known for years that intrauterine quinine can produce sclerosis of the proximal fallopian tube. This method has recently been rediscovered and is being seriously explored. A pellet containing 252 mg of quinacrine is inserted into the uterus during the proliferative phase of the cycle and again 1 month later. In a large trial, the 1-year pregnancy rate for 9,461 women who received two doses was 2.63 per 100 woman-years. The rate of ectopic pregnancy was 0.89 per 1,000 woman-years (277).

Immunologic contraception-sterilization has been pursued for many years. Talwar and colleagues in India have worked for many years toward vaccination against human chorionic gonadotropin (hCG) and have performed trials in humans (278). Another area of interest is in vaccinating men or women against specific sperm antigens and the zona pellucida (279).

Chinese researchers have developed a method of percutaneous occlusion of the vas that has been used in more than 100,000 men, is effective, and appears to be reversible. Polyurethane elastomer is injected into the vas, where it solidifies and forms a plug, providing an effective block to sperm. The plugs are removed using local anesthesia, and fertility returns in most cases after as long as 4 years with the plugs *in situ* (280). *Gossypol,* an extract of cottonseed, was evaluated in China as a male contraceptive but abandoned because of problems with hypokalemia in users. When *gossypol* was reevaluated in a multinational study, hypokalemia was not a problem. Of 134 men treated, 65% had sperm counts less than 1 million/mL. About half of men followed more than 1 year after treatment recovered to a normal sperm count. *Gossypol* may be an alternative to vasectomy (281).

References

1. **Haymes NE.** *Medical history of contraception.* New York: Gamut Press, 1963.
2. **Hatcher RA, Trussell J, Stewart F, et al.** *Contraceptive technology.* 17th ed. New York: Ardent Media, 1998:767.
3. **Cates W Jr.** Family planning, sexually transmitted diseases and contraceptive choice: a literature update: part I. *Fam Plann Perspect* 1992;24:75–84.
4. **Piccinino LJ, Mosher WD.** Trends in contraceptive use in the United States: 1982–1995. *Fam Plann Perspect* 1998;30:4–10.
5. **Henshaw SK.** Unintended pregnancy in the United States. *Fam Plann Perspect* 1998;30:24–29.
6. **Ory HW.** Mortality associated with fertility and fertility control: 1983. *Fam Plann Perspect* 1983;15:57–63.
7. **Ashraf T, Arnold SB, Maxfield M.** Cost effectiveness of levonorgestrel subdermal implants: comparison with other contraceptive methods available in the United States. *J Reprod Med* 1994;39:791–798.
8. **Potts M.** Coitus interruptus. In: **Corson SL, Derman RJ, Tyrer L,** eds. *Fertility control.* Boston: Little, Brown, 1985:299–306.
9. **Vessey M, Lawless M, Yeates D.** Efficacy of different contraceptive methods. *Lancet* 1982;1:841–843.
10. **McNeilly AS.** Suckling and the control of gonadotropin secretion. In: **Knobil E, Neil JD, Ewing LI, et al,** eds. *The physiology of reproduction.* New York: Raven Press, 1988:2323–2349.
11. **Short RV, Lewis PR, Renfree MB, et al.** Contraceptive effects of extended lactational amenorrhoea: beyond the Bellagio Consensus. *Lancet* 1991:337:715–717.
12. **Saarikoski S.** Contraception during lactation. *Ann Med* 1993;25:181–184.
13. **Trussell J, Grummer-Strawn L.** Contraceptive failure of the ovulation method of periodic abstinence. *Fam Plann Perspect* 1990;22:65–75.
14. **Flynn A, Pulcrano J, Spieler, J.** An evaluation of the Bioself 110 electronic fertility indicator as a contraceptive aid. *Contraception* 1991;44:125–139.

15. **Brown JB, Holmes J, Barker G.** Use of the Home Ovarian Monitor in pregnancy avoidance. *Am J Obstet Gynecol* 1991;165:2008–2011.

16. **Rotta L, Matechova E, Cerny M, et al.** Determination of the fertile period during the menstrual cycle in women by monitoring changes in crystallization of saliva with the PC2000 IMPCON minimicroscope. Cesk Gynekol 1992;57:340–352.

17. **Guerrero R, Rojas OI.** Spontaneous abortion and aging of human ova and spermatozoa. *N Engl J Med* 1975;293.

18. **Labbock MH, Queenan JT.** The use of periodic abstinence for family planning. *Clin Obstet Gynecol* 1989;32:387–402.

19. **Potts M, McDevitt J.** A use-effectiveness trial of spermicidally lubricated condoms. *Contraception* 1975;11:701–710.

20. **Grady WR, Tanfer K.** Condom breakage and slippage among men in the United States. *Fam Plann Perspect* 1994;26:107–112.

21. **Voeller B, Coulson AH, Bernstein GS, et al.** Mineral oil lubricant causes rapid deteriorization of latex condoms. *Contraception* 1989;39:95–102.

22. **Stone KM, Grimes DA, Magder LS.** Personal protection against sexually transmitted diseases. *Am J Obstet Gynecol* 1986;155:180–188.

23. **Kelaghan J, Rubin GL, Ory HW, et al.** Barrier-method contraceptives and pelvic inflammatory disease. *JAMA* 1982;248:184–187.

24. **Cramer DW, Goldman MB, Schiff I, et al.** The relationship of tubal infertility to barrier method and oral contraceptive use. *JAMA* 1987;257:2246–2250.

25. **Connell EB.** Barrier contraceptives. *Clin Obstet Gynecol* 1989;32:377–386.

26. **Judson FN, Ehret JM, Bodin GF, et al.** In vitro evaluations of condoms with and without nonoxynol 9 as physical and chemical barrier against Chlamydia trachomatis, herpes simplex virus type 2 and human immunodeficiency virus. *Sex Transm Dis* 1989;16:251–256.

27. **Fischl MA, Dickinson GM, Scott GB, et al.** Evaluation of heterosexual partners, children, and household contacts of adults with AIDS. *JAMA* 1987;257:640–644.

28. **deVincenzi I.** A longitudinal study of human immunodeficiency virus transmission by heterosexual partners. European Study Group on Heterosexual Transmission of HIV. *N Engl J Med* 1994;331:341–346.

29. **Zekeng L, Feldblum PJ, Oliver RM, et al.** Barrier contraceptive use and HIV infection among high-risk women in Cameroon. *AIDS* 1993;7:725–731.

30. **Harris RW, Brinton LA, Cowdell RH, et al.** Characteristics of women with dysplasia or carcinoma in situ of the cervix uteri. *Br J Cancer* 1980;42:359–369.

31. **Parazzini F, Negri E, La Vecchia C, et al.** Barrier methods of contraception and the risk of cervical neoplasia. *Contraception* 1989;40:519–530.

32. **Blank A.** Latex condoms lubricated with nonoxynol-9 may increase release of latex protein that may trigger latex hypersensitivity. Research reports from the NICHD. National Institute of Child Health and Development MSC 2425.

33. **Trussel J, Sturgen K, Strickler J, et al.** Comparative efficacy of the female condom and other barrier methods. *Fam Plann Perspect* 1994;26:66–72.

34. **Soper DE, Brockwell NJ, Dalton HP.** Evaluation of the effects of a female condom on the female genital tract. *Contraception* 1991;44:21–29.

35. **Johnson V, Masters WH.** Intravaginal contraceptive study. Phase II. Physiology. *West J Surg Obstet Gynecol* 1963;71:144–153.

36. **Jones BM, Eley A, Hicks DA, et al.** Comparison of the influence of spermicidal and non-spermicidal contraception on bacterial vaginosis, candidal infection and inflammation of the vagina- a preliminary study. *Int J STD AIDS* 1994;5:362–364.

37. **Malyk B.** *Nonoxynol-9: evaluation of vaginal absorption in humans.* Raritan, NJ: Ortho Pharmaceutical, 1983.

38. **Linn S, Schoenbaum SC, Monson RR, et al.** Lack of association between contraceptive usage and congenital malformation in offspring. *Am J Obstet Gynecol* 1983;147:923–928.

39. **Harlap S, Shiono PH, Ramcharon S, et al.** Chromosomal abnormalities in the Kaiser-Permanente birth defects study, with special reference to contraceptive use around the time of conception. *Teratology* 1985;31:381–387.

40. **Hooton TM, Hillier S, Johnson C, et al.** Esherichia coli bacteriuria and contraceptive method. *JAMA* 1991;265:64–69.

41. **Bounds W, Guillebaud J, Dominik R, et al.** The diaphragm with and without spermicide: a randomized comparative trial. *J Reprod Med* 1995;40:764–774.

42. **Ferreira AE, Araujo MJ, Regina CH, et al.** Effectiveness of the diaphragm, used continuously without spermicide. *Contraception* 1993;48:29–35.

43. **Hooton TM, Scholes D, Huges JP, et al.** A prospective study of risk factors for symptomatic urinary tract infection in young women. *N Engl J Med* 1996;335:468–474.

44. **Davis JP, Chesney J, Wand PJ, et al.** Toxic shock syndrome: epidemiologic features, recurrence, risk factors and prevention. *N Engl J Med* 1980;303:1429–1435.

45. **Koch JP.** The Prentiff contraceptive cervical cap: a contemporary study of its clinical safety and effectiveness. *Contraception* 1982;25:135–139.

46. **Richwald MA, Greenland S, Gerber MM, et al.** Effectiveness of the cavity rim cervical cap: results of a large clinical study. *Obstet Gynecol* 1989;74:143–148.

47. **Trussell J, Strickler J, Vaughan B.** Contraceptive efficacy of the diaphragm, the sponge and the cervical cap. *Fam Plann Perspect* 1993;25:100–105.

48. **Shihata AA, Gollub E.** Acceptability of a new intravaginal barrier contraceptive device (Femcap). *Contraception* 1992;46:511–519.

49. **Sivin I, Stern J.** Health during prolonged use of levonorgestrel 20 micrograms/d and the copper TCu 380A intrauterine contraceptive devices: a multicenter study. *Fertil Steril* 1994;61:70–77.

50. **Centers for Disease Control.** Leads from MMWR 1984:33(4). *JAMA* 1984;251:1015.

51. **El Badrawi HH, Hafez ES, Barnhart MI, et al.** Ultrastructural changes in human endometrium with copper and nonmedicated IUD's in utero. *Fertil Steril* 1981;36:41–49.

52. **Umapathysivam K, Jones WR.** Effects of contraceptive agents on the biochemical and protein composition of human endometrium. *Contraception* 1980;22:425–440.

53. **Habashi M, Sahwi S, Gawish S, et al.** Effect of Lippes Loop on sperm recovery from human fallopian tubes. *Contraception* 1980;22:549–555.

54. **Alvarez F, Guiloff E, Brache V, et al.** New insights on the mode of action of intrauterine devices in women. *Fertil Steril* 1989;49:768–773.

55. **Segal S, Alvarez-Sanchez F, Adejeuwon CA, et al.** Absence of chorionic gonadotropin in sera of women who use intrauterine devices. *Fertil Steril* 1985;44:214–218.

56. **Anon.** Long term reversible contraception. Twelve years experience with the TCU380A and TCU220C. *Contraception* 1997;56:341–352.

57. **Irvine GA, Campbell-Brown MB, Lumsden MA, et al.** Randomized comparative trial of the levonorgestrel intrauterine system and norethisterone for treatment of idiopathic menorrhagia. *Br J Obstet Gynaecol* 1998;10:592–598.

58. **Burkeman RT, the Women's Health Study.** Association between intrauterine devices and pelvic inflammatory disease. *Obstet Gynecol* 1981;57:269–276.

59. **Farley TMM, Rosenberg MJ, Rowe PJ, et al.** Intrauterine devices and pelvic inflammatory disease: an international perspective. *Lancet* 1992;339:785–788.

60. **Lee NC, Rubin GL, Borucki R.** The intrauterine device and pelvic inflammatory disease revisited: new results from the Women's Health Study. *Obstet Gynecol* 1988;72:721–726.

61. **Kriplani A, Buckshee K, Relan S, et al.** Forgotten intrauterine device leading to actinomycotic pyometra, 13 years after menopause. *Eur J Obstet Gynecol Reprod Biol* 1994;53:215–216.

62. **Ory HW, for the Women's Health Study.** Ectopic pregnancy and intrauterine contraceptive devices: new perspectives. *Obstet Gynecol* 1981;57:137–140.

63. **Snowden R.** The Progestasert and ectopic pregnancy. *BMJ* 1977;1:1600–1601.

64. **Rossing MA, Daling JR, Voigt LF, et al.** Current use of an intrauterine device and the risk of tubal pregnancy. *Epidemiology* 1993;4:252–258.

65. **Cramer DW, Schiff I, Schoenbaum SC.** Tubal infertility and the intrauterine device. *N Engl J Med* 1985;312:941–947.

66. **Daling JR, Weiss N, Metch BJ.** Primary tubal infertility in relation to the use of an intrauterine device. *N Engl J Med* 1985;312:937–941.

67. **Grimes DA.** The intrauterine device, pelvic inflammatory disease, and infertility: the confusion between hypothesis and knowledge. *Fertil Steril* 1992;58:670–673.

68. **Vessey M, Doll R, Peto R, et al.** A long term follow up study of women using different methods of contraception—an interim report. *J Biosoc Sci* 1974;8:373–420.

69. **Walsh T, Grimes D, Frezieres R, et al.** Randomized trial of prophylactic antibiotics before insertion of intrauterine devices. *Lancet* 1998;351:1005–1008.

70. **White MK, Ory HW, Rooks JB, et al.** Intrauterine device termination rates and the menstrual cycle day of insertion. *Obstet Gynecol* 1980;55:220–224.

71. **Burnhill MS.** Intrauterine contraception. In: **Carson SL, Derman RJ, Tyrer LB,** eds. *Fertility control.* Boston: Little, Brown, 1985:272–288.

72. **Tatum HJ, Schmidt FH, Jain AK.** Management and outcome of pregnancies associated with copper-T intrauterine contraceptive device. *Am J Obstet Gynecol* 1976;126:869–877.

73. **Stubblefield PG, Fuller AF, Foster SG.** Ultrasound guided intrauterine removal of intrauterine contraceptive device in pregnancy. *Obstet Gynecol* 1988;72:961–964.

74. **Tietze C, Lewit S.** Evaluation of intrauterine devices: ninth progress report of the Cooperative Statistical Program. *Stud Fam Plann* 1970;1:1–40.

75. **Lippes J, Zielezny M.** The loop decade. *Mt Sinai J Med* 1975;4:353–356.

76. **Mishell DR Jr.** Vaginal contraceptive rings. *Ann Med* 1993;25:191–197.

77. **Spelsberg TC, Rories C, Rejman JJ.** Steroid action on gene expression: possible roles of regulatory genes and nuclear acceptor sites. *Biol Reprod* 1989;40:54–69.

78. **Phillips A.** The selectivity of a new progestin. *Acta Obstet Gynecol Scand* 1990;152[Suppl]:21–24.

79. **Godsland IF, Crook D, Simpson R, et al.** The effects of different formulations of oral contraceptive agents on lipids and carbohydrate metabolism. *N Engl J Med* 1990;323:1375–1381.

80. **Brody SA, Turkes A, Goldzieher JW.** Pharmacokinetics of three bioequivalent norethindrone/mestranol-50 mcg and three norethindrone/ethinyl estradiol-35 mg formulations: are "low dose" pills really lower? *Contraception* 1989;40:269–284.

81. **Dericks-Tan JSE, Kock P, Taubert HD.** Synthesis and release of gonadotropins: effect of an oral contraceptive. *Obstet Gynecol* 1983;62:687–690.

82. **Gaspard UJ, Dubois M, Gillain D, et al.** Ovarian function is effectively inhibited by a low dose triphasic oral contraceptive containing ethinyl estradiol and levonorgestrel. *Contraception* 1984;29:305–318.

83. **Landgren BM.** Mechanism of action of gestagens. *Int J Gynaecol Obstet* 1990;32:95–110.

84. **Luukkainen T, Heikinheimo O, Haukkamaa M, et al.** Inhibition of folliculogenesis and ovulation by the antiprogesterone RU 486. *Fertil Steril* 1988;49:961–963.

85. **Van Uem JF, Hsiu JG, Chillik CF, et al.** Contraceptive potential of RU486 by ovulation inhibition. I. Pituitary versus ovarian action with blockade of estrogen-induced endometrial proliferation. *Contraception* 1989;40:171–184.

86. **Stadel BV.** Oral contraceptives and cardiovascular disease: part I. *N Engl J Med* 1981;305:612–618.

87. **Stadel BV.** Oral contraceptives and cardiovascular disease: part II. *N Engl J Med* 1981;305:672–678.

88. **Porter JB, Hunter JR, Jick H, et al.** Oral contraceptives and nonfatal vascular disease. *Obstet Gynecol* 1985;66:1–4.

89. **Maguire MG, Tonascia J, Sartwell PE, et al.** Increased risk of thrombosis due to oral contraceptives: a further report. *Am J Epidemiol* 1979;110:188–195.

90. **Ambrus JL, Mink IB, Courey NG, et al.** Progestational agents and blood coagulation. VII. Thromboembolic and other complications of oral contraceptive therapy in relationship to pretreatment levels of blood coagulation factors: summary report of a ten year study. *Am J Obstet Gynecol* 1976;125:1057–1062.

91. **Winkler UH, Buhler K, Schindler AE.** The dynamic balance of hemostasis: implications for the risk of oral contraceptive use. In: **Runnebaum B, Rabe T, Kissel L,** eds. *Female contraception and male fertility regulation.* Advances in Gynecological and Obstetric Research Series. Confort, England: Parthenon Publishing Group, 1991:85–92.

92. **Notelovitz M, Kitchens CS, Coone L, et al.** Low dose oral contraceptive usage and coagulation. *Am J Obstet Gynecol* 1981;141:71–75.

93. **Notelovitz M, Levenson I, McKenzie L, et al.** The effects of low dose oral contraceptives on coagulation and fibrinolysis in two high risk populations: young female smokers and older premenopausal women. *Am J Obstet Gynecol* 1985;152:995–1000.

94. **Gerstman BB, Piper JM, Tomita DK, et al.** Oral contraceptive dose and the risk of deep venous thromboembolic disease. *Am J Epidemiol* 1991;133:32–37.

95. **Farmer RDT, Preston TD.** The risk of venous thromboembolism associated with low oestrogen oral contraceptives. *J Obstet Gynecol* 1995;15:195–200.

96. **Sazelenko JK, Nace MC, Alving B.** Women with thrombophilia: assessing the risks for thrombosis with oral contraceptives or hormone replacement therapy. *Semin Thromb Hemost* 1998;24[Suppl]1:33–39.

97. **Bloemenkamp KW, Rosendaal, FR, Helmerhorst FM, et al.** Hemostatic effects of oral contraceptives in women who developed deep-vein thrombosis while using oral contraceptives. *Thromb Haemost* 1998;80:382–387.

98. **Bertina RM, Koeleman BP, Koster T, et al.** Mutation in blood coagulation factor V associated with resistance to activated protein C. *Nature* 1994;369:64–67.

99. **Vandenbroucke JP, Koster T, Briet E, et al.** Increased risk of venous thrombosis in oral contraceptive users who are carriers of factor V Leiden mutation. *Lancet* 1994;344:1453–1457.

100. **DeStefano V, Chiusolo P, Paciaroni K, et al.** Epidemiology of factor V Leiden: clinical implications. *Semin Thromb Hemost* 1998;24:367–379.

101. **Martinelli I, Sacchi E, Landi G, et al.** High risk of cerebral vein thrombosis in carriers of a prothrombin gene mutation and in users of oral contraceptives. *N Engl J Med* 1988;338:1793–1797.

102. **Trauscht-Van-Horn JJ, Capeless EL, Easterling TR, et al.** Pregnancy loss and thrombosis with protein C deficiency. *Am J Obstet Gynecol* 1992;167:968–972.

103. **Vandenbroucke JP, van der Meer FJM, Helmerhorst FM, et al.** Factor V Leiden: should we screen oral contraceptive users and pregnant women? *Br Med J* 1996;313:1127–1130.

104. **Vandenbroucke JP, van der Meer FJM, Helmerhorst FM, et al.** Factor V Leiden: should we screen oral contraceptive users and pregnant women? *Br Med J* 1996;313:1129.

105. **Lewis MA, Heinemann LAJ, MacRae KD, et al.** The increased risk of venous thromboembolism and the use of third generation progestagens: role of bias in observational research. *Contraception* 1996;54:5–13.

106. **Stubblefield PG.** The effects on hemostasis of oral contraceptives containing desogestrel. *Am J Obstet Gynecol* 1993;168:1047–1052.

107. **World Health Organization Collaborative Study of Cardiovascular Disease and Steroid Hormone Contraception.** Venous thromboembolic disease and combined oral contraceptives: results of international multicenter case-control study. *Lancet* 1995;346:1575–1582.

108. **Mant D, Villard-Mackintosh L, Vessey MP, et al.** Myocardial infarction and angina pectoris in young women. *J Epidemiol Community Health* 1987;41:215–219.

109. **Rosenberg L, Kaufman DW, Helmrich SP, et al.** Myocardial infarction and cigarette smoking in women younger than 50 years of age. *JAMA* 1985;253:2965–2969.

110. **Sidney S, Petitt DB, Quesenberry CP, et al.** Myocardial infarction in users of low dose oral contraceptives. *Obstet Gynecol* 1996;88:939–944.

111. **Sidney S, Siscovick DS, Petitti DB, et al.** Myocardial infarction and use of low dose oral contraceptives: a pooled analysis of 2 U.S. studies. *Circulation* 1998;98:1058–1063.

112. **Stampfer MJ, Willett WC, Colditz GA, et al.** A prospective study of past use of oral contraceptive agents and risk of cardiovascular diseases. *N Engl J Med* 1988;319:1313–1317.

113. **Lewis MA, Heinemann LA, Spitzer WO, et al.** The use of oral contraceptives and the occurrence of acute myocardial infarction in young women. Results from the Transnational Study of Oral Contraceptives and the Health of Young Women. *Contraception* 1997;56:129–140.

114. **Vessey MP, Lawless M, Yeates D.** Oral contraceptives and stroke: findings in a large prospective study. *BMJ* 1984;289:530–531.

115. **Bruno A, Adams HP, Biller J, et al.** Cerebral infarction due to moyamoya disease in young adults. *Stroke* 1988;19:826–831.

116. **Petitti DB, Sidney S, Bernstien A, et al.** Stroke in users of low dose oral contraceptives. *N Engl J Med* 1996;335:8–15.

117. **World Health Organization Collaborative Study of Cardiovascular Disease and Steroid hormone Contraception.** Ischaemic stroke and combined oral contraceptives: results of an international, multicenter, case control study. *Lancet* 1996;348:505–510.

118. **World Health Organization Collaborative Study of Cardiovascular Disease and Steroid hormone Contraception.** Hemorrhagic stroke, overall stroke risk, and combined oral contraceptives: results of an international, multicenter, case control study. *Lancet* 1996;348:505–510.

119. **Heinemann LA, Lewis MA, Thorogood M, et al.** Case control study of oral contraceptives and risk of thromboembolic stroke: results from international study on oral contraceptives and health of young women. *BMJ* 1997;315:1502–1508.

120. **Lidegaard O.** Oral contraceptives, pregnancy and the risk of cerebral thromboembolism: the influence of diabetes, hypertension, migraine and previous thromboembolic disease. *Br J Obstet Gynecol* 1995;102: 153–159.

121. **Spellacy WN, Buhi WC, Birk SA.** The effect of estrogens on carbohydrate metabolism: glucose, insulin, and growth hormone studies on 171 women ingesting Premarin, mestranol and ethinyl estradiol for six months. *Am J Obstet Gynecol* 1972;114:378–392.

122. **Lipson A, Stoy DB, La Rosa JC, et al.** Progestins and oral contraceptive-induced lipoprotein changes: a prospective study. *Contraception* 1986;34:121–134.

123. **Knopp RH.** Cardiovascular effects of endogenous and exogenous sex hormones over a woman's lifetime. *Am J Obstet Gynecol* 1988;158:1630–1643.

124. **Burkman RT, Zacur HA, Kimball AW, et al.** Oral contraceptives and lipids and lipoproteins. II. Relationship to plasma steroid levels and outlier status. *Contraception* 1989;40:675–689.

125. **Mishell DR Jr, Colodyn SZ, Swanson LA.** The effect of an oral contraceptive on tests of thyroid function. *Fertil Steril* 1969;20:335–339.

126. **Centers for Disease Control Cancer and Steroid Hormone Study.** Oral contraceptive use and the risk of ovarian cancer. *JAMA* 1983;249:1596–1599.

127. **Centers for Disease Control Cancer and Steroid Hormone Study.** Oral contraceptive use and the risk of endometrial cancer. *JAMA* 1983;249:1600–1604.

128. **Siskind V, Green A, Bain C, et al.** Beyond ovulation: oral contraceptives and epithelial ovarian cancer. *Epidemiol* 2000;11;106–110.

129. **Villard-Mackintosh L, Vessey MP, Jones L.** The effects of oral contraceptives and parity on ovarian cancer trends in women under 55 years of age. *Br J Obstet Gynaecol* 1989;96:783–788.

130. **Ness RB, Grisso JA, Klapper J, et al.** Risk of ovarian cancer in relation to estrogen and progestin dose and use characteristics of oral contraceptives. *Am J Epidemiol* 2000;152:233–241.

131. **Swann SH, Petitti DB.** A review of problems of bias and confounding in epidemiologic studies of cervical neoplasia and oral contraceptive use. *Am J Epidemiol* 1982;115:10–18.

132. **Schiffman MH, Bauer HM, Hoover RN, et al.** Epidemiologic evidence showing that human papilloma virus infection causes most cervical intraepithelial neoplasia. *J Natl Cancer Inst* 1993;85:958–964.

133. **Ursin G, Peters RK, Henderson BE, et al.** Oral contraceptive use and adenocarcinoma of cervix. *Lancet* 1994;344:1390–1394.

134. **Chilvers C.** Oral contraceptives and cancer. *Lancet* 1994;344:1378–1379.

135. **U.K. National Case-Controlled Study Group.** Oral contraceptive use and breast cancer risk in young women. *Lancet* 1989;1:973–982.

136. **Caygill CP, Hill MJ.** Oral contraceptives and breast cancer. *Lancet* 1989;1:1258–1260.

137. **Schlesselman JJ.** Cancer of the breast and reproductive tract in relation to use of oral contraceptives. *Contraception* 1989;40:1–38.

138. **Collaborative Group on Hormonal Factors in Breast Cancer.** Breast cancer and hormonal contraceptives: collaborative reanalysis of individual data on 53,297 women with breast cancer and 100,239 women without breast cancer from 54 epidemiologic studies. *Lancet* 1996;347:1713–1727.

139. **Melbye M, Wohlfahrt J, Olsen JH, et al.** Induced abortion and the risk of breast cancer. *N Engl J Med* 1997;336:81–85.

140. **Magnusson CM, Persson IR, Baron JA, et al.** The role of reproductive factors and use of oral contraceptives in the aetiology of breast cancer in women aged 50-74 years. *Int J Cancer* 1999;80:231–236.

141. **Grabrick DM, Hartmann LC, Cerhan JR, et al.** Risk of breast cancer with oral contraceptive use in women with a family history of breast cancer. *JAMA* 2000;284:1791–1798.

142. **Rooks JB, Ory HW, Ishak KG, et al.** Epidemiology of hepatocellular adenoma: the role of oral contraceptive use. *JAMA* 1979;262:644–648.

143. **Anon.** Oral contraceptives and liver cancer. Results from the Multicentre International Liver Tumor Study (MILTS). *Contraception* 1997;56:275–284.

144. **Narod SA, Risch H, Moslehi R, et al.** Oral contraceptives and the risk of hereditary ovarian cancer. Hereditary Ovarian Cancer Clinical Study Group. *N Engl J Med* 1998;339:424–428.

145. **Rodriguez GC, Walmer DK, Cline M, et al.** Effect of progestin on the ovarian epithelium of macaques: cancer prevention through apoptosis. *J Soc Gynecol Invest* 1998;5:271–276.

146. **Wolner-Hanssen P, Eschenbach DA, Paavonen J, et al.** Decreased risk of symptomatic chlamydial pelvic inflammatory disease associated with oral contraceptives. *JAMA* 1990;263:54–59.

147. **Vessey M, Doll R, Peto R, et al.** A long term follow up study of women using different methods of contraception an interim report. *J Biosoc Sci* 1974;8:373–427.

148. **Lanes SF, Birmann B, Walker AM, et al.** Oral contraceptive type and functional ovarian cysts. *Am J Obstet Gynecol* 1992;166:956–961.

149. **Fernandez E, La Vecchia C, Franceschi S, et al.** Oral contraceptives and risk of colorectal cancer. *Epidemiology* 1998;9:295–300.

150. **Martinez ME, Grodstein F, Giovannucci E, et al.** A prospective study of reproductive factors, oral contraceptive use and risk of colorectal cancer. *Cancer Epidemiol Biomarkers Prev* 1997;6:1–5.

151. **Shy KK, McTiernan AM, Daling JR, et al.** Oral contraceptive use and the occurrence of pituitary prolactinoma. *JAMA* 1983;249:2204–2207.

152. **Adams DB, Gold AR, Burt AD.** Rise in female initiated sexual activity at ovulation and its suppression by oral contraceptives. *N Engl J Med* 1978;299:1145–1150.

153. **Bracken MP.** Oral contraception and congenital malformations in offspring: a review and meta-analysis of the prospective studies. *Obstet Gynecol* 1990;76:552–557.

154. **Katz Z, Lancet M, Skornik J, et al.** Teratogenicity of progestogens given during the first trimester of pregnancy. *Obstet Gynecol* 1985;65:775–780.

155. **Back DJ, Orme ML'E.** Pharmacokinetic drug interactions with oral contraceptives. *Clin Pharmacokinet* 1990;18:472–484.

156. **Geurts TBP, Goorissen EM, Sitsen JMA.** *Summary of drug interactions with oral contraceptives*. London: Parthenon Publishing, 1993:64–81.

157. **Helms SE, Bredle DL, Zajic J, et al.** Oral contraceptive failure rates and oral antibiotics. *J Am Acad Dermatol* 1997;36:705–710.

158. **Knopp RH, Bergelin RO, Wahl PW, et al.** Clinical chemistry alterations in pregnancy and with oral contraceptive use. *Obstet Gynecol* 1985;66:682–690.

159. **Sulak P, Lippman J, Siu C, et al.** Clinical comparison of triphasic norgestimate/35 micrograms ethinyl estradiol and monophasic norethindrone acetate/20 micrograms ethinyl estradiol: cycle control, lipid effects and user satisfaction. *Contraception* 1999;59:161–166.

160. **Rosenberg MJ, Meyers A, Roy V.** Efficacy, cycle control and side effects of low and lower-dose oral contraceptives: a randomized trial of 20 microgram and 35 microgram estrogen preparations. *Contraception* 1999;60:321–329.

161. **Speroff L.** A brief for low-dose pills. *Contemp Ob/Gyn* 1981;17:27–32.

162. **Kay CR.** The happiness pill. *J R Coll Gen Pract* 1980;30:8–10.

163. **Kaunitz AM.** Long-acting injectable contraception with depot medroxyprogesterone acetate. *Am J Obstet Gynecol* 1994;170:1543–1549.

164. **Pardthaisong T.** Return of fertility after use of the injectable contraceptive Depo-Provera: updated analysis. *J Biosoc Sci* 1984;16:23–34.

165. **Cundy T, Reid OR, Roberts H.** Bone density in women receiving depot medroxyprogesterone acetate for contraception. *BMJ* 1991;303:13–16.

166. **Taneepanichskul S, Intaraprasert S, Theppisai U, et al.** Bone mineral density during long-term treatment with Norplant implants and depot medroxyprogesterone acetate. *Contraception* 1997;56:153–155.

167. **Cromer BA, Blair JM, Mahan JD, et al.** A prospective comparison of bone density in adolescent girls receiving depot medroxyprogesterone acetate (Depo-Provera), levonorgestrel (Norplant), or oral contraceptives. *J Pediatr* 1996;129:671–676.

168. **Fahmy K, Khairy M, Allam G, et al.** Effect of depo-medroxyprogesterone acetate on coagulation factors and serum lipids in Egyptian women. *Contraception* 1991;44:431–434.

169. **Okada Y, Horikawa K.** A case of phlebothrombosis of lower extremity and pulmonary embolism due to progesterone. *Kokyu To Junkan* 1992;40:819–822.

170. **Ishizaki T, Itoh R, Yasuda J, et al.** Effect of high dose medroxyprogesterone acetate on coagulative and fibrinolytic factors in patients with gynecological cancers. *Gan To Kagaku Ryoho* 1992;19:837–842.

171. **Westoff C.** Depot medroxyprogesterone acetate contraception: metabolic parameters and mood changes. *J Reprod Med* 1996;41:401–406.

172. **Westhoff C, Wieland D, Tiezzi L.** Depression in users of depo-medroxyprogesterone acetate. *Contraception* 1995;51:351–354.

173. **Kaunitz AM, Rosenfield A.** Injectable contraception with depot medroxyprogesterone acetate: current status. *Drugs* 1993;45:857–865.

174. **La Vecchia C.** Depot-medroxyprogesterone acetate, other injectable contraceptives, and cervical cancer. *Contraception* 1994;49:223–229.

175. **World Health Organization.** Depot medroxyprogesterone acetate (DMPA) and the risk of epithelial ovarian cancer. The WHO Collaborative Study of Neoplasia and Steroid Contraceptives. *Int J Cancer* 1991;49:191–195.

176. **Chilvers C.** Breast cancer and depot-medroxyprogesterone acetate: a review. *Contraception* 1994;49:211–222.

177. **Guo-wei S.** Pharmacodynamic effects of once a month combined injectable contraceptives. *Contraception* 1994;49:361–385.

178. **Kaunitz AM, Garceau RJ, Cromie MA,** for the Lunelle Study Group. Comparative safety, efficacy and cycle control of Lunelle× monthly contraceptive injection (medroxyprogesterone acetate and estradiol cypionate injectable suspension) and Ortho-Novum 7/7/7 orql contraceptive (Norethindrone/ethinyl estradiol triphasic). *Contraception* 1999;60:179–187.

179. **Speroff L, Darney PD.** *A clinical guide for contraception.* Baltimore: Williams & Wilkins, 1992: 117–156.

180. **Darney PD.** Hormonal implants: contraception for a new century. *Am J Obstet Gynecol* 1994;170:1536–1543.

181. **Intaraprasert S, Taneepanichskul S, Theppisai U, et al.** Bone density in women receiving Norplant implants for contraception. *J Med Assoc Thailand* 1997;80:738–741.

182. **Wysowski DW, Green L.** Serious adverse events in Norplant users reported to the Food and Drug Administration's MedWatch Spontaneous Reporting System. *Obstet Gynecol* 1995;86:154–155.

183. **Speroff L, Darney PD.** *A clinical guide for contraception.* 3rd ed. Philadelphia: Lippincott Williams & Wilkins, 2001:169–187.

184. **Praptohardjo U, Wibowo S.** The "U" technique: a new method for Norplants implant removal. *Contraception* 1993;48:526.

185. **Gao J, Wang SL, Wu SC, et al.** Comparison of the clinical performance, contraceptive efficacy and acceptability of levonorgestrel releasing IUD, and Norplant 2 implants in China. *Contraception* 1990;41:485–494.

186. **Davies GC, Li XF, Newton JR, et al.** Release characteristics, ovarian activity and menstrual bleeding pattern with a single contraceptive implant releasing 3 keto desogestrel. *Contraception* 1993;47:251–261.

187. **Haspells AA.** Emergency contraception: a review. *Contraception* 1994;50:101–108.

188. **Yuzpe AA.** Postcoital contraception. *Clin Obstet Gynecol* 1984;11:787–797.

189. **Kane LA, Sparrow MJ.** Postcoital contraception: a family planning study. *N Z Med J* 1989;102:151–153.

190. **Anon.** Randomized controlled trial of levonorgestrel versus the Yuzpe regimen of combined oral contraceptives for emergency contraception. Task Force on Postovulatory Methods of Fertility Regulation. *Lancet* 1998;352:428–433.

191. **Lippes J, Malik T, Tautum HJ.** The postcoital copper-T. *Adv Plann Parent* 1976;11:24–29.

192. **Webb AMC, Russell J, Elstein M.** Comparison of Yuszpe regimen, Danazol and Mifepristone (RU486) in oral postcoital contraception. *BMJ* 1992;305:927–931.

193. **Ho PC.** Emergency contraception: methods and efficacy. *Curr Opin Obstet Gynecol* 2000;12;175–179.

194. **Briggs MH, Briggs M.** Oral contraceptives for men. *Nature* 1974;252:585–586.

195. **Wallace EM, Gow SM, Wu FC.** Comparison between testosterone enanthate-induced azoospermia and oligozoospermia in a male contraceptive study. I. Plasma luteinizing hormone, follicle stimulating hormone, testosterone, estradiol, and inhibin concentrations. *J Clin Endocrinol Metab* 1993;77:290–293.

196. **Wallace EM, Aitken RJ, Wu FC.** Residual sperm function in oligozoospermia induced by testosterone enanthate administered as a potential steroid male contraceptive. *Int J Androl* 1992;15:416–424.

197. **Arsyad KM.** Sperm function in Indonesian men treated with testosterone enanthate. *Int J Androl* 1993;16:355–361.

198. **Swerdloff RS, Wang C, Bhasin S.** Developments in the control of testicular function. *Baillieres Clin Endocrinol Metab* 1992;6:451–483.

199. **Murad F, Haynes RC.** Androgens and anabolic steroids. In: **Gilman AG, Goodman LS, Gilman A,** eds. *Goodman and Gilman's the pharmacological basis of therapeutics.* 6th ed. New York: MacMillan, 1980:1448–1465.

200. **Marcil-Gratton N.** Sterilization regret among women in metropolitan Montreal. *Fam Plann Perspect* 1988;20:222–227.

201. **Shepard MK.** Female contraceptive sterilization. *Obstet Gynecol Surv* 1974;29:739–787.

202. **Uchida H.** Uchida tubal sterilization. *Am J Obstet Gynecol* 1975;121:153–159.

203. **Irving FC.** A new method of insuring sterility following cesarean section. *Am J Obstet Gynecol* 1924;8:335–337.

204. **Hulka JF.** Methods of female sterilization. In: **Nichols DH,** ed. *Gynecologic and obstetric surgery.* St. Louis: Mosby, 1993:640–651.

205. **Hasson HM.** Open laparosocopy. In: **Zatuchni GI, Daly MJ, Sciarra JJ,** eds. *Gynecology and obstetrics.* Vol. 6. Philadelphia: Harper & Row, 1982:1–8.

206. **Yoon IB, King TM, Parmley TH.** A two-year experience with the Falope ring sterilization procedure. *Am J Obstet Gynecol* 1977;127:109–112.

207. **Filshie GM, Pogmore JR, Dutton AG, et al.** The titanium/silicone rubber clip for female sterilization. *Br J Obstet Gynaecol* 1981;88:655–662.

208. **Penfield AJ.** The Filshie clip for female sterilization: a review of world experience. *Am J Obstet Gynecol* 2000;182:485–489.

209. **Soderstrom RM, Levy BS, Engel T.** Reducing bipolar sterilization failures. *Obstet Gynecol* 1989;74:60–63.

210. **DeStefano F, Greenspan JR, Dicker RC, et al.** Complications of interval laparoscopic tubal sterilization. *Obstet Gynecol* 1983;61:153–158.

211. **Poindexter AN, Abdul-Malak M, Fast JE.** Laparoscopic tubal sterilization under local anesthesia. *Obstet Gynecol* 1990;75:5–8.

212. **Peterson HB, DeStefano F, Rubin GL, et al.** Deaths attributable to tubal sterilization in the United States, 1977–1981. *Am J Obstet Gynecol* 1983;146:131–136.

213. **Escobedo LG, Peterson HB, Grubb GS, et al.** Case-fatality rates for tubal sterilization in U.S. hospitals, 1979–80. *Am J Obstet Gynecol* 1989;160:147–150.

214. **Khairullah Z, Huber DH, Gonzales B.** Declining mortality in international sterilization services. *Int J Gynaecol Obstet* 1992;39:41–50.

215. **Dominik R, Gates D, Sokal D, et al.** Two randomized controlled trials comparing the Hulka and Filshie clips for tubal sterilization. *Contraception* 2000;62:169–175.

216. **Sokal D, Gates D, Amatya R, et al.** Two randomized controlled trials comparing the tubal ring and Filshie clip for tubal sterilization. *Fertil Steril* 2000;74:525–533.

217. **Ness RB, Grisso JA, Cottreau C, et al.** Factors related to inflammation of the ovarian epithelium and risk of ovarian cancer. *Epidemiology* 2000;11:111–117.

218. **Peterson HB, Xia Z, Hughes JM, et al.** The risk of pregnancy after tubal sterilization: findings from the U.S. Collaborative Review of Sterilization. *Am J Obstet Gynecol* 1996;174:1161–1168

219. **Peterson HB, Xia Z, Wilcox LS, et al.** Pregnancy after tubal sterilization with bipolar electrocoagulation. *Obstet Gynecol* 1999;94:163–167.

220. **Corson SL.** Female sterilization reversal. In: **Corson SL, Derman RJ, Tyrer LB,** eds. *Fertility control.* Boston: Little, Brown, 1985:107–118.

221. **Neil JR, Hammond GT, Noble AD, et al.** Late complications of sterilization by laparoscopy and tubal ligation: a controlled study. *Lancet* 1975;2:669–671.

222. **Peterson HB, Jeng G, Folger SG, et al.** The risk of menstrual abnormalities after tubal sterilization. *N Engl J Med* 2000;343:1681–1687.

223. **Liskin LS, Pile JM, Quillin WF.** Vasectomy—safe and simple. Baltimore, population information program. *Popul Rep D* 1983;11(5):62–99.

224. **Hatcher RA, Trussell J, Stewart F, et al.** *Contraceptive technology.* 17th ed. New York: Ardent Media, 1998:567.

225. **Walker AM, Jick H, Hunter JR, et al.** Vasectomy and non-fatal myocardial infarction. *Lancet* 1981;1(8210):13–15.

226. **Goldacre MJ, Holford TR, Vessey MP.** Cardiovascular disease and vasectomy. *N Engl J Med* 1982;308:805–808.

227. **Rosenberg L, Palmer JR, Zauber AG, et al.** Vasectomy and the risk of prostate cancer. *Am J Epidemiol* 1990;132;1051–1055.

228. **Key T.** Risk factors for prostatic cancer. *Cancer Surv* 1995;23:63.

229. **John EM, Whittemore AS, Wu AH, et al.** Vasectomy and prostate cancer: results from a multiethnic case-control study. *J Natl Cancer Inst* 1995;87:62-t.

230. **Henshaw SK, Morrow E.** Induced abortion: a world review. *Fam Plann Perspect* 1990;22:76–120.

231. **Mahler H.** The safe motherhood initiative: a call to action. *Lancet* 1987;1:668–670.

232. **Alan Guttmacher Institute.** Aborto Clandestino: Una Realidad Latinoamericana. New York: The Alan Guttmacher Institute, 1994.

233. **Cates W Jr, Rochat RW.** Illegal abortions in the United States: 1972–1974. *Fam Plann Perspect* 1976;8: 86–92.

234. **Koonin LM, Strauss LT, Chrisman CE, et al.** Abortion surveillance—United States, 1996. In: CDC Surveillance Summaries, July 30, 1999. *MMWR Morb Mortal Wkly Rep* 1999;48(No. SS-4):42.

235. **Council on Scientific Affairs, American Medical Association.** Induced termination of pregnancy before and after Roe v Wade: trends in the mortality and morbidity of women. *JAMA* 1992;268:3231–3239.

236. **Koonin LM, Strauss LT, Chrisman CE, et al.** Abortion surveillance—United States, 1997. In: CDC Surveillance Summaries, Dec 8, 2000. *MMWR Morb Mortal Wkly Rep* 2000;49(No. SS-11):1–43.

237. **Susser M.** Induced abortion and health as a value. *Am J Public Health* 1992;82:1323–1324.

238. **Lawson HW, Frye A, Atrash HK, et al.** Abortion mortality, United States, 1972–1987. *Am J Obstet Gynecol* 1994;171:1365–1372.

239. **Atrash HK, Cheek TG, Hogue CJ.** Legal abortion mortality and general anesthesia. *Am J Obstet Gynecol* 1988;158:420–424.

240. **Karman H, Potts M.** Very early abortion using syringe as vacuum source. *Lancet* 1972;1:1051–1052.

241. **Stubblefield PG.** Control of pain for women undergoing abortion. *Int J Gynaecol Obstet* 1989;3[Suppl]:131–140.

242. **Ulmann A, Silvestre L, Chemama L, et al.** Medical termination of early pregnancy with mifepristpone (RU486) followed by a prostaglandin analogue: study in 16,639 women. *Acta Obstet Gynecol Scand* 1992;71:278–283.

243. **Anonymous.** A death associated with mifepristone/sulprostone. *Lancet* 1991:337:969–970.

244. **Peyron R, Aubeny E, Targosz V, et al.** Early termination of pregnancy with mifeprisone (RU486) and the orally active prostaglandin misoprostol. *N Engl J Med* 1993;328:1509–1513.

245. **McKinley C, Thong KJ, Baird DT.** The effect of dose of mifepristone and gestation on the efficacy of medical abortion with mifepristone and misoprostol. *Hum Reprod* 1993;8:1502–1505.

246. **Ashok PW, Penney GC, Flett GM, et al.** An effective regimen for early medical abortion: a report of 2000 consecutive cases. *Hum Reprod* 1998;13:2962–2965.

247. **Schaff EA, Eisinger SH, Stadalius LS, et al.** Low dose mifepristone 200 mg and vaginal misoprostol for abortion. *Contraception* 1999;59:1–6.

248. **Schaff EA, Fielding SL, Westoff C, et al.** Vaginal misoprostol administered 1,2 or 3 days after mifepristone for early medical abortion: a randomized trial. *JAMA* 2000;84:1948–1953.

249. **Goldberg AB, Greenberg BS, Darney PD.** Misoprostol and pregnancy. *N Engl J Med* 2001;344:38–47.

250. **Schaff EA, Stadalius LS, Eisinger SH, et al.** Vaginal misoprostol administered at home after mifepristone (RU486) for abortion. *J Fam Pract* 1997;44:353–360.

251. **Stovall TG, Ling FW.** Single dose methotrexate: an expanded clinical trial. *Am J Obstet Gynecol* 1993;168:1759–1765.

252. **Creinin MD, Darney PD.** Methotrexate and misoprostol for early abortion. *Contraception* 1993;48:339–348.

253. **Creinin MD, Darney PD.** Methotrexate for abortion at #42 days gestation. *Contraception* 1993;48:519–525.

254. **Creinin MD, Vittinghoff E, Keder L, et al.** Methotrexate and misoprostol for early abortion: a multicenter trial. I. Safety and efficacy. *Contraception* 1996;53:321–327.

255. **Creinin MD.** Oral methotrexate and vaginal misoprostol for early abortion. *Contraception* 1996;54:15–18.

256. **Stubblefield PG.** First and second trimester abortion. In **Nichols DH, Clarke-Pearse DL,** eds. *Gynecologic, obstetric and related surgery.* 2nd ed. St. Louis: Mosby, 2000:1033–1045.

257. **Haskell WM, Easterling TR, Lichtenberg ES.** Surgical abortion after the first trimester. In: **Paul M, Lichtenberg ES, Borgatta L, et al,** eds. *A clinician's guide to medical and surgical abortion.* New York: Churchill Livingstone, 1999:123–138.

258. **Darney PD, Sweet RL.** Routine intra-operative ultrasonography for second trimester abortion reduced incidence of uterine perforation. *J Ultrasound Med* 1989;8:71–75.

259. **Hern WM.** *Abortion practice.* Philadelphia: JB Lippincott, 1984.

260. **Hern WM, Xen C, Ferguson RA, et al.** Outpatient abortion for fetal anomaly and fetal death from 15–34 menstrual weeks gestation: techniques and clinical management. *Obstet Gynecol* 1993;81:301–306.

261. **Binkin NJ, Schulz KF, Grimes DA, et al.** Urea-prostaglandin versus hypertonic saline for instillation abortion. *Am J Obstet Gynecol* 1983;146:947–952.

262. **Negishi M, Sugimoto YL, Ichikawa A.** Prostanoid receptors and their biological actions. *Prog Lipid Res* 1993;32:417–434.

263. **Jain JK, Mishell DR.** A comparison of intravaginal misoprostol with prostaglandin E_2 for termination of second trimester pregnancy. *N Engl J Med* 1994;331:290–293.

264. **Herabutya Y, O-Prasertwawat P.** Second trimester abortion using intravaginal misoprostol. *Int J Gynecol Obstet* 1998;60:161–165.

265. **Wong KS, Ngai CS, Wong AY, et al.** Vaginal misoprostol compared with vaginal gemeprost in termination of second trimester pregnancy: a randomized trial. *Contraception* 1998;57:207–210.

266. **Hoffer MC, Charlier C, Giacalone PL, et al.** Evaluation de l'association RU486: laminaires-anesthesie peridural dans les interruptions de grossesse de 2e et 3e trimester. *J Gynecol Obstet Biol Reprod (Paris)* 1998;27:83–86.

267. **Winkler CL, Gray SE, Hauth JC, et al.** Mid-second-trimester labor induction: concentrated oxytocin compared with prostaglandin E_2 suppositories. *Obstet Gynecol* 1991;77:297–300.

268. **Evans MI, Dommergues M, Wapner RJ, et al.** Efficacy of transabdominal multifetal pregnancy reduction: collaborative experience among the world's largest centers. *Obstet Gynecol* 1993:82:61–66.

269. **Evans MI, Goldberg JD, Horenstein J, et al.** Selective termination for structural, chromosomal and mendelian anomalies: international experience. *Am J Obstet Gynecol* 1999;82:61–66.

270. **Hogue CJR, Cates W Jr, Tietze C.** The effects of induced abortion on subsequent reproduction. *Epidemiol Rev* 1982;4:66–94.

271. **Chung CS, Steinhoff PG, Smith RG, et al.** The effects of induced abortion on subsequent reproductive function and pregnancy. In: *Papers of the East-West Population Institute.* Honolulu: East-West Institute, 1983;86.

272. **Linn S, Schoenbaum SC, Monson RR, et al.** The relationship between induced abortion and outcome of subsequent pregnancies. *Am J Obstet Gynecol* 1983;146:136–140.

273. **Stubblefield PG, Monson RR, Schoenbaum SC, et al.** Fertility after induced abortion: a prospective follow-up study. *Obstet Gynecol* 1984;63:186–193.

274. **Wu S, Hu J, Wildemeersch D.** Performance of the frameless GyneFix and theTCU380A IUDs in a three year multicenter randomized comparative trial in parous women. *Contraception* 2000;61:91–98.

275. **D'Cruz O.** Evaluation of subchronic (13 weeks) and reproductive toxicity potential of intravaginal gel: microemulsion formulation of a dual function phenyl phosphate derivative of bromo-methoxy zidovudine (Compound WHI-05) in B(6)C(3)F(1) mice. *Contraception* 2000;61:69–76.

276. **Thatcher SS.** Hysteroscopic sterilization. *Obstet Gynecol Clin North Am* 1988;15:51–59.

277. **Hieu DT, Tan TT, Tan DN, et al.** 33,781 Cases of non-surgical female sterilization with quinacrine pellets in Vietnam. *Lancet* 1993;342:213–217.

278. **Talwar GP, Singh O, Pal R, et al.** A birth control vaccine is on the horizon for family planning. *Ann Med* 1993;25:207–212.

279. **Aitken RJ, Peterson M, Koothan PT.** Contraceptive vaccines. *Br Med Bull* 1993;49:88–99.

280. **Zhao SC.** Vas deferens occlusion by percutaneous injection of polyurethane elastomer plugs: clinical experience and reversibility. *Contraception* 1990;41:453–459.

281. **Coutinho EM, Athaycde C, Alta G, et al.** Gossypol blood levels and inhibition of spermatogenesis in men taking gossypol as a contraceptive: a multicenter, international dose finding study. *Contraception* 2000;61:61–67.

11 Sexuality, Sexual Dysfunction, and Sexual Assault

David A. Baram

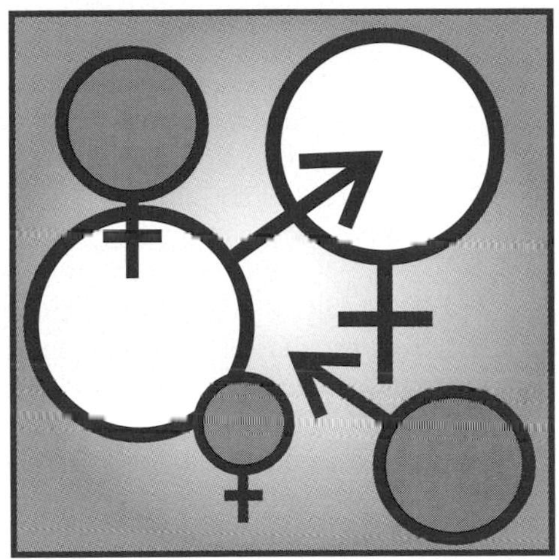

Sexuality is an important and integral part of every woman's life. Questions and concerns about sexuality span a woman's entire lifetime, from questions about puberty to concerns about change in sexual function with menopause and aging. The obstetrician-gynecologist, as a primary health care provider for women, should include a sexual history as a routine part of a woman's periodic health assessment.

Concerns about sexuality and sexual dysfunction are common in the general population. Surveys have found that almost two thirds of the women questioned had concerns about their sexuality (1–5). One third of women lacked interest in sex, 20% said sex was not always pleasurable, 15% experienced pain with intercourse, up to 50% experienced difficulty becoming aroused, 50% noted difficulty reaching orgasm, and up to 25% were unable to experience orgasm.

In addition, obstetrician-gynecologists should routinely inquire about a history of childhood sexual abuse or adult sexual assault because these experiences are common and often have a lasting and profound effect on a woman's mental and sexual function as well as her general health and well-being. One of eight American women will be forcibly raped during her lifetime (6), and nearly half of women in the United States report some type of contact sexual victimization (7). Fifty percent of American women report uninvited sexual attention in the workplace (7).

Despite the importance of these issues to their health care, many women find it difficult to talk to their physicians about sexual concerns, and many physicians are uncomfortable discussing sexual issues with their patients (8). In a recent survey, 71% of adults said they thought their doctor would dismiss any concerns about sexual problems they might bring up, and 68% said they were afraid that discussing sexuality would embarrass their physician (9). **Surveys of primary care physicians reveal that fewer than half ask their new patients about sexual practices and concerns and that many physicians make incorrect assumptions about their patients' sexual activity based on marital status, profession, age, race, or socioeconomic status** (10,11).

Sexuality

Physicians may be concerned that patients will be offended by questions about their sexual practices or may believe that little useful information will be gained by asking patients about sexual concerns or a history of sexual assault. In addition, some physicians may have anxiety about their perceived inability to treat sexual concerns, may believe that they have too little time to obtain a sexual history, may be distressed by their patient's history of sexually related violence, or may experience personal discomfort when discussing sexual matters with their patients (12). However, surveys of patients reveal that they expect their physician to be able to address sex-related concerns and believe it is appropriate for questions about sexuality to be included as a routine part of the gynecologic history (8). Not asking about sexuality suggests to the patient that sexuality is not important and is not to be discussed. Furthermore, not discussing sexual abuse implies that sexual assault has no long-term consequences.

Physicians will feel more comfortable talking to their patients about sex if they have an understanding of the normal sexual response and know how to approach the evaluation and treatment of common sexual dysfunctions. **Asking about sexual concerns gives physicians an opportunity to educate patients about the risk for sexually transmitted infections (STIs), counsel patients about safe sex practices, evaluate patients' needs for contraception, and dispel sexual myths and misconceptions. Furthermore, patients are given permission to address sexual issues in a professional, confidential, and nonjudgmental setting** (13). Even if patients are initially uncomfortable discussing these sensitive and private issues, they know that their physician will be receptive if they want to discuss sexual concerns in the future.

When taking a sexual history, it is important to allow patients to feel comfortable and safe (14). The physician's personal values and potential biases should be left out of the discussion. Physicians should use a private location for the interview and let the patient know that the conversation will be confidential. Good listening skills and attention to nonverbal cues are helpful. It is important to use straightforward language that the patient can understand and acknowledge that many people find it difficult to discuss sensitive and intimate issues. Most sexual concerns can be resolved by providing factual information, reassurance, and appropriate medical intervention. Only a few open-ended questions are required to elicit a basic sexual history from patients. These questions should be a part of the medical history taken during a routine examination and can be obtained in either a face-to-face interview or in a written history the patient completes before seeing the physician (12,15):

"Are you currently sexually active?" "With men, women, or both?"
"Are you or your partner having any sexual difficulties?"
"Has there been any change in your sexual activity?"
"Have you ever experienced any unwanted or harmful touching or sexual activity?"

If a positive response is elicited by any of these questions, further evaluation of the patient may be warranted. Follow-up questions might include:

"Are you having difficulty initiating a sexual encounter or becoming aroused when you want to be sexual?"
"Do you experience as much arousal as you would like?"
"Do you experience vaginal dryness during intercourse?"
"Do you have orgasms when you want to?"
"Are you satisfied with your sexual relationship?"
"Do you have pain with intercourse?"
"Has this difficulty always been present, or is it new to you?"
"Have you had this difficulty with all of your partners or just with the current one?"
"Is the difficulty always there or just some of the time?"

"Does anything make it better or worse?"
"How much of a concern is this for you and your partner?"
"Do you have any idea what may have caused your sexual difficulty?"
"Have you received any treatment for this difficulty?"
"What are your expectations and goals for treatment?"

Further inquiries about specific sexual dysfunction or the sequelae of sexual abuse can be addressed when appropriate, and the patient can be referred for psychological counseling or sex therapy when necessary (16).

Sexual Practices

Two recent comprehensive surveys provide an interesting and useful description of the sexual behavior of Americans (2,3,17). Sexual activity among adolescents in the United States has increased significantly during the past 20 years. The average age for first intercourse in both men and women is 16 years. By 19 years of age, 66% to 75% of women and 79% to 86% of men will have had intercourse. Most young men and women have multiple, serial sexual partners. They use condoms infrequently and inconsistently, thus exposing themselves to STIs and unintended pregnancy. A survey of American men and women between the ages of 18 and 59 years revealed the following findings (2):

- Most men and women are satisfied with their sex lives, even those who rarely have sex. Among married men and women, 87% reported that they were satisfied with their sexual relationship.
- Sexual dysfunction was reported in 43% of women and was more likely in women with poor physical and emotional health, unmarried women, younger women, uneducated women, women who had experienced sexual victimization, women who were sexually inexperienced, and women with negative experiences in prior sexual relationships (3).
- Women have sex with a partner from a few times per month (47%), to 2 to 3 times per week (32%), to 4 or more times per week (7%). Twelve percent of women have sex a few times per year, and 3% have never been sexually active.
- The most appealing sexual activity for both men and women is vaginal intercourse. Watching their partner undress and receiving and giving oral sex were also considered very pleasurable.
- Most Americans are monogamous. Of married men and women, 75% and 85%, respectively, said they had never been unfaithful.
- There may be fewer homosexuals than previously believed—2.7% of men and 1.3% of women had a homosexual partner in the past year. Since puberty, 7.1% of men and 3.8% of women had same-gender sexual partners.
- Twenty-two percent of women said they had been forced to do something sexual, usually by someone they loved, but only 3% of men admitted to forcing themselves on a woman. Perhaps men and women have different ideas about what constitutes sexual coercion.

The Sexual Response Cycle

The sexual response cycle in women is mediated by the complex interplay of psychological, environmental, and physiologic (hormonal, vascular, muscular, and neurologic) factors. The initial phase of the sexual response cycle is interest and desire, followed by the four successive phases originally described by Masters and Johnson (18): arousal, plateau, orgasm, and resolution. There is wide variability in the way women respond sexually, and each phase can be affected by aging, illness, medication, alcohol, illicit drugs, and relationship factors.

An attempt has been made to redefine the linear progression of sexual response described by Masters and Johnson. The Basson model postulates that the sexual cycle in women is cyclical rather than linear and that arousal and desire are interchangeable (19,20). In this model, the starting point for sexuality is the desire for intimacy and closeness rather then a need for physical sexual release. Many women are satisfied with an intimate encounter that does not necessarily include intercourse or orgasm.

For most women, the clitoris is the most sexually sensitive part of their anatomy, and stimulation of the clitoris produces the greatest sexual arousal and the most intense orgasms. Other sexually sensitive areas are the nipples, breasts, labia, and, to a lesser extent, the vagina. Although the lower third of the vagina is responsive to touch, the upper two thirds of the vagina is sensitive primarily to pressure.

There has been speculation about the existence of a *G spot* (named after Ernest Graefenberg, who first described it in 1944), an area of the vagina located anteriorly midway between the symphysis pubis and the cervix that is believed to be exquisitely sensitive to deep pressure. This area, believed to be similar to the male prostate, has been described as glandular tissue capable of secreting prostatic acid phosphatase into the urethra, sometimes in such copious amounts that women seem to ejaculate during orgasm. However, analysis of the fluid "ejaculate" has proved that it is probably urine, not prostatic fluid. It is not uncommon for women who are normally continent to leak urine during orgasm. These women should be reassured that this is a common phenomenon and does not require medical intervention.

Desire Phase

Sexual desire is the motivation and the inclination to be sexual. It is a "subjective feeling state" that may be triggered by both internal (fantasy) and external (an interested partner) sexual cues and is dependent on adequate neuroendocrine functioning (20). The sensation of desire is under the influence of dopamine-sensitive excitatory centers located in the limbic system. Testosterone is responsible for desire and arousal in both men and women. Drive is the biologic component of desire and is characterized by sexual thoughts, erotic interest in others, genital tingling, and seeking out of sexual activity (20). Desire is influenced by sexual orientation, preferences, psychological mindset, beliefs and values, expectations, willingness to behave sexually, and environmental setting.

Arousal (Excitement) Phase

The arousal (excitement) phase is mediated by the parasympathetic nervous system and is characterized by erotic feelings and the appearance of vaginal lubrication. Sexual arousal increases blood flow to the vagina, and the resulting vasocongestion and changes in capillary permeability create a condition that increases the capillary filtration fraction. The filtered capillary fluid transudates between the intercellular spaces of the vaginal epithelium, causing droplets of fluid to form on the walls of the vagina. In addition to feelings of sexual tension, sexually excited women experience tachycardia, rapid breathing, an elevation in blood pressure, a generalized feeling of warmth, breast engorgement, generalized muscle tension (myotonia), nipple erection, mottling of the skin, and a maculopapular erythematous rash ("sex flush") over the chest and breasts. During this phase, the clitoris and labia become swollen; the vagina lengthens, distends, and dilates; and the uterus elevates out of the pelvis (18,20). During the latter stages of arousal, sexual tension and erotic feelings intensify, and vasocongestion reaches maximum intensity (plateau). The skin becomes more mottled, the breasts become more engorged, and the nipples become more erect. The labia become more swollen and turn dark red, and the lower third of the vagina swells and thickens to form the "orgasmic platform" (18,20). The clitoris becomes more swollen and elevates to lie nearer the symphysis pubis. The uterus elevates fully out of the pelvis. With adequate sexual stimulation, women reach the point of orgasmic inevitability (threshold point).

Orgasm Phase

Orgasm is a myotonic response mediated by the sympathetic nervous system. It is experienced as a sudden release of the tension that has built up during the arousal. Orgasm is the most intensely pleasurable of the sexual sensations. It consists of multiple (3 to 15)

0.8-second reflex rhythmic contractions of the muscles (pubococcygeal) surrounding the vagina, perineum, anus, and orgasmic platform. Uterine contractions are also experienced by many women during orgasm (18). Thus, some women describe the sensation of an orgasm as different after hysterectomy. Many women who are orgasmic prefer to have orgasms before intercourse, during the time when clitoral stimulation is most intense. Unlike men, who are relatively unresponsive to sexual stimulation after orgasm (refractory period), women are potentially multiorgasmic and capable of experiencing more than one orgasm during a single sexual cycle. Thus, they can experience orgasms both before and during intercourse if adequate clitoral stimulation is provided.

Resolution Phase

Following the sudden release of sexual tension brought about by orgasm, women experience a feeling of relaxation and well-being. The physiologic changes that took place during arousal are reversed, and the body returns to a resting state. Complete uterine descent, detumescence of the clitoris and orgasmic platform, and decongestion of the vagina and labia takes about 5 to 10 minutes.

Factors Affecting Sexual Response

Aging

Aging and the cessation of ovarian function accompanying menopause have a significant effect on the sexual response cycle of women. **Sexual desire and the frequency of intercourse decrease gradually as women age, although women retain interest in sex and continue to have the potential for sexual pleasure for their entire lives.** The need for closeness, love, and intimacy does not change with age. The way women function sexually as they grow older is largely dependent on health status, partner availability, and how frequently they had sex and how much they enjoyed sex when they were younger (21). Results of a study of healthy men and women aged 80 to 101 years living in retirement communities indicated that these elderly people were still very sexually active (22). Sexual touching and caressing, followed by masturbation and then intercourse, were the most common sexual activities in this population.

Anatomic changes that accompany aging are noted in Table 11.1. These changes predispose women to more frequent episodes of vulvovaginitis and urinary tract infections that, along with decreased vaginal lubrication, may cause dyspareunia. The effects of aging on sexual physiology are noted in Table 11.2. Women who remain coitally active after menopause have less vulvar and vaginal atrophy than abstinent women (23). Illnesses that accompany aging may also have an impact on sexual function. Arteriosclerosis may decrease vaginal blood flow and cause decreased arousal, lubrication, and orgasmic intensity. Chronic obstructive pulmonary disease may cause lowered testosterone levels, impairing sexual desire. Pain from an arthritic hip may make it difficult for a woman to find a comfortable position for intercourse.

Several psychosocial factors may influence an older woman's sexual activity. Older women may lack a sexual partner, or their partner may develop erectile dysfunction. The couple may have had an unsatisfactory sexual relationship earlier in life and may not be able to negotiate the changes and possible sexual dysfunctions that can come with aging. Couples may find that they can no longer function sexually as they did in the past and are unable to make the transition or adapt to a new (noncoital) way of lovemaking. Other factors include privacy issues (such as living in a nursing home), reluctance to masturbate, and the negative attitudes of society toward sexuality in older women (23). Aging men and women may experience performance anxiety as they enter into new relationships (24–26). As women age, many tend to be less fit. Improved physical fitness is positively related to the frequency of sexual intimacy, which in turn is related to longevity (26). Suggestions for aging patients might include taking a warm bath before lovemaking to loosen stiff joints, making love in

Table 11.1. Anatomic Changes of Aging
Reduced pubic hair
Loss of fat and subcutaneous tissue from the mons pubis
Reduced vaginal size
Thinning of vaginal walls
Decreased elasticity of vaginal walls
Shrinkage of the labia majora
Thinning of the labia minora
Decreased clitoral sensitivity
Decreased clitoral size
Reduced uterine size
Cervical atrophy
Reduced ovarian size and weight
Reduced perineal muscle tone
Thinner orgasmic platform
Breast atrophy
Decreased breast engorgement during arousal
Sensory changes in the nipple and areola

From **Meston CM.** Aging and sexuality. *West J Med* 1997;167:285–290, with permission.

the morning when the couple is less fatigued, and experimenting with oral or manual sexual stimulation to orgasm without having intercourse.

Management of sexual difficulties in older women should include estrogen or testosterone supplementation (27–29). Local or systemic estrogen supplementation can alleviate vaginal dryness, urinary tract symptoms, and dyspareunia. Estrogen replacement restores vaginal cells, decreases pH, and increases vaginal blood flow, thus alleviating vaginal dryness, urinary tract symptoms, and dyspareunia. Estrogen replacement also seems to benefit sexual desire, sexual fantasy, arousal, sexual enjoyment, and orgasmic frequency in postmenopausal women (27). In addition, estrogen supplementation improves insomnia, hot flushes, and other menopausal symptoms (e.g., sense of well-being) that may interfere with sexual function. The addition of progesterone to the hormone replacement therapy regimen partially

Table 11.2. Sexual Physiology—Effects of Aging
Decreased sexual desire
Increased time required to become sexually aroused
Longer time needed to lubricate
Production of less vaginal lubrication
Less intense orgasms
Increased need for stimulation to become orgasmic
No change in the ability to have orgasms
Less likely to be multiorgasmic

From **Mooradian AD, Greiff V.** Sexuality in older women. *Arch Intern Med* 1990;150:1033–1038, with permission.

opposes the beneficial effects of estrogen by decreasing vaginal blood flow (27). Estrogen supplementation also decreases free testosterone levels by nearly 50% by increasing levels of sex hormone–binding globulin, thus decreasing free testosterone levels (29,31).

Testosterone levels gradually decrease in women as they age (29). Testosterone supplementation, either alone or in combination with estrogen, has been demonstrated to improve libido, arousal, sexual responsiveness, frequency of sexual fantasies and dreams, clitoral sensitivity, and frequency of orgasm in women who are testosterone deficient (<30 ng/mL) from surgical or natural menopause. In addition, restoration of normal testosterone levels can benefit muscle tone, physical energy, mood, sense of well-being, and genital atrophy not responsive to estrogen supplementation (27,32). Side effects of testosterone include acne, hirsutism, deepening of the voice, clitoromegaly, hepatotoxicity, alopecia, and undesirable changes in lipoprotein levels. Patients taking androgens should be prescribed the lowest effective dose of medication and carefully monitored for side effects.

Sildenafil, effective for treating erectile dysfunction in men, has been investigated for the treatment of sexual dysfunction in women (33,34). One study demonstrated the effectiveness of sildenafil in reversing female sexual dysfunction induced by selective serotonin reuptake inhibitors (SSRIs) (34). Another study failed to demonstrate any improvement in sexual function in postmenopausal women but did note improvement in vaginal lubrication and clitoral sensitivity. The effectiveness of sildenafil and other recently developed pharmacologic agents in the treatment of sexual dysfunction in women has yet to be documented.

The sexual expectations of the aging patient and her partner and an assessment of their current level of sexual functioning should also be evaluated. Myths they may have heard about sexuality in the elderly should be dispelled. If the couple is interested in retaining sexual function, they should be instructed in alternative forms of sexual expression and ways of alleviating discomfort. However, aging patients may have difficulty changing their sexual expectations and ways of making love. They may not easily adapt to change and may resist reevaluating long-held sexual beliefs, attitudes, behavior, and gender roles.

Drugs

A variety of prescription and nonprescription medications, including alcohol and illicit drugs, can alter the normal sexual response (35–39) (Table 11.3). The patient's use of these drugs should be assessed as part of the medical history, and adjustments in dosage or formulation may be suggested, if appropriate. With some medications, like the SSRIs, it may be appropriate to suggest a short medication holiday to allow for temporary return of sexual function.

Illness

Both acute (e.g., myocardial infarction) and chronic (e.g., chronic renal disease or arthritis) illnesses can create depression, a distorted body image, physical discomfort, and disturbances in the hormonal, vascular, and neurologic integrity needed for sexual functioning (40). Neurologic disorders that impair sexual functioning include multiple sclerosis, alcoholic neuropathy, and spinal cord injury. Endocrine and metabolic disorders, such as diabetes mellitus, hyperprolactinemia, testosterone deficiency, estrogen deficiency states, and hypothyroidism can affect the sexual response.

Infertility evaluation and treatment can have a significant effect on a woman's body image and feelings of self-worth and self-esteem. Infertility may cause her to feel depressed, helpless, hopeless, unattractive, and sexually undesirable. The loss of sexual spontaneity, a goal-directed approach to sex, and the need for scheduled intercourse may lead to sexual dysfunction and relationship difficulties (41).

Breast cancer diagnosis and treatment can affect sexuality (42,43). However, most women cope well with the stress of treatment and do not develop major psychiatric disorders

Table 11.3. Drugs that Can Interfere with Sexual Functioning
Antihypertensives
Thiazide diuretics
Antidepressants
Lithium
Antipsychotics
Antihistamines
Barbiturates
Narcotics
Benzodiazepines
Hallucinogens
Amphetamines
Cocaine
Oral contraceptives
Anticonvulsants
Cimetidine
Danazol
Digoxin
Levodopa

or significant sexual dysfunction. A number of studies have compared women who undergo mastectomies with women who have conservative surgery (lumpectomy) with breast conservation. These studies have revealed little difference between the two groups in postoperative marital satisfaction, psychological adjustment, frequency of sex, or incidence of sexual dysfunction. The frequency of breast stimulation with sexual activity does decrease after mastectomy (18), and many men and women avoid looking at the surgical scar. Women who undergo lumpectomy have more positive feelings about their bodies, especially their appearance in the nude, than do women who have mastectomies (44). The strongest predictor of postcancer sexual satisfaction is not the extent of the surgery but rather the woman's overall psychological health, relationship satisfaction, and precancer level of sexual functioning (45). Interestingly, many women report that their physicians did not discuss the impact of breast surgery on sexuality before their operations took place.

Common gynecologic procedures, performed for either benign or malignant conditions, can significantly affect a woman's body image, feelings of self-worth and self-esteem, and psychosexual function (46–48). In premenopausal women, an oophorectomy can have a deleterious effect on sexual desire and feelings of sexual arousal.

Concern about sexual functioning following hysterectomy is often the most common preoperative anxiety experienced by patients (49). **A number of studies have shown that abdominal hysterectomy does not have an adverse effect on sexual functioning if the vagina is not shortened excessively and if the ovaries are preserved** (50,51). Many women report a decrease in dyspareunia, an increase in frequency and strength of orgasms, and an increase in libido and frequency of intercourse following hysterectomy for benign disease (49). Some gynecologists prefer to perform supracervical hysterectomies in an effort to preserve full sexual function; however, there are inadequate data to support that this practice is effective for this purpose.

Women who undergo surgery for gynecologic cancer experience more sexual dysfunction (inhibited sexual desire, decreased arousal, dyspareunia, and anorgasmia) and are less sexually active than healthy women of the same age (52,53). Dyspareunia may be related to a decrease in vaginal lubrication secondary to surgical menopause or to vaginal shortening and scarring from radiation therapy. Some patients, especially those with cervical cancer, may worry that resumption of sexual activity may provoke a recurrence of their disease (54). Among patients with gynecologic cancer, sexual activity following treatment does not seem related to the type of cancer or the stage of the disease.

Physicians should discuss sexual concerns with the patient and her partner before surgery, attempt to dispel myths and misconceptions, and continue to offer counseling to patients after treatment. Specific technical advice (the use of water-based lubricating jelly, noncoital sexual activity for patients with severe dyspareunia, the use of vaginal dilators, and Kegel exercises) should also be provided. Women who function well sexually before surgery and have a positive self-image will be better able to cope with the sexual difficulties caused by gynecologic cancer treatment than women with poor precancer sexual adjustment (53).

The physical, emotional, and economic stresses of pregnancy often affect a couple's sexual and marital relationship (55–58). Sexual attitudes and behavior during pregnancy are influenced by sexual value systems, folklore (taboos), religious beliefs, physical changes, and arbitrary medical restrictions. In a pregnancy uncomplicated by preterm labor, antepartum bleeding, or an incompetent cervix, there is no evidence that intercourse increases the risk for pregnancy complications.

Pregnancy-related alterations in sexual response include breast tenderness, a feeling of fullness in the labia and vagina, possible bleeding from the cervix with intercourse, and uterine contractions with orgasm (56,57). Pregnant women may find it difficult to feel sexual when they perceive themselves as unattractive or when they are fatigued, nauseated, or uncomfortable. Both partners may be afraid that intercourse may precipitate preterm labor, rupture the membranes, or harm the fetus. Increasing abdominal size may make the couple's usual positions for lovemaking awkward and uncomfortable.

Most women and men experience a longitudinal decrease in sexual desire, frequency of orgasm, sexual satisfaction, and frequency of intercourse as pregnancy progresses. Sexual satisfaction in pregnancy is closely correlated with feeling happy about the pregnancy, feeling attractive, and experiencing orgasm with lovemaking. Toward the end of the third trimester, there is a significant increase in physical discomfort and concerns about labor and delivery and the health of the child. At this time, many couples decrease sexual activity or become abstinent. However, the need for closeness, emotional support, and nurturing during late pregnancy can continue to be met with touching, caressing, holding, and noncoital lovemaking.

After delivery, many women experience fatigue, weakness, vaginal bleeding and discharge, perineal discomfort, hemorrhoids, sore breasts, and decreased vaginal lubrication and dyspareunia secondary to decreased estrogen levels. Women may be hesitant to resume having intercourse because of lack of sexual desire, fear of vaginal injury or infection, physical discomfort, fear of waking the baby, decreased sense of attractiveness, change in body image, or postpartum depression. Compared with women who bottle feed, women who breast feed are more likely to experience decreased sexual desire and dyspareunia as a result of lower testosterone and estrogen levels. Although many couples begin to have intercourse 6 to 8 weeks after delivery, many couples may wait as long as a year to resume their prepregnancy level of intimacy.

Physicians can help their patients by acknowledging and discussing the normal fluctuations in sexual desire and frequency of intercourse that occur during and after pregnancy. Couples should be encouraged to continue their usual patterns of lovemaking during pregnancy as long they are emotionally and physically comfortable and there are no contraindications to intercourse.

Sexual Dysfunction

Types of sexual dysfunctions include (59,60):

1. Sexual desire disorders (hypoactive or inhibited sexual desire and sexual aversion)
2. Sexual arousal disorders
3. Orgasmic disorders
4. Sexual pain disorders (vaginismus, dyspareunia, and noncoital sexual pain)
5. Sexual disorders resulting from general medical conditions and substance abuse

Each disorder can be further classified as either (59):

1. Lifelong or acquired (after a period of normal sexual functioning)
2. Generalized (i.e., not limited to a specific partner or situation) or situational
3. Caused by psychological or medical factors

When evaluating patients with sexual dysfunction, it is important to obtain the following information (60–62):

1. A specific description of the dysfunction and an analysis of current sexual functioning
2. When the dysfunction began and how it progressed over time
3. Any precipitating factors
4. The patient's theory about what caused the dysfunction
5. What effect the dysfunction has had on her relationship
6. Past treatment and outcomes
7. Expectations and goals for treatment
8. Understanding of sexual physiology and sexual behavior
9. Any myths or misinformation

Although many physicians have some anxiety about discussing sexual issues with their patients and believe that they lack the basic skills to provide sexual counseling, most sexual concerns can be treated by the general gynecologist. **The PLISSIT model is a useful sexual counseling and therapy method consisting of four levels of therapeutic intervention** (63). Using the first three levels of this model, 80% to 90% of sexual concerns can be addressed (61). The PLISSIT model is as follows:

1. **P**ermission validates the patient's feelings and gives her permission to address her sexual concerns.
2. **L**imited **I**nformation provides the patient with information about sexual physiology and behavior.

3. **S**pecific **S**uggestions involve specific reeducation regarding the patient's sexual attitudes and practices.

4. Referral for **I**ntensive **T**herapy is reserved for those patients who do not respond to the first three levels of intervention and who may require intensive individual or couple therapy.

As an example of a specific suggestion, a woman with primary anorgasmia is first given permission to look at her genitalia and touch her clitoris. She is then given limited information about genital anatomy and the physiology of the sexual response. Specific suggestions are then offered about using fantasy and directed masturbation, encouraging her to make use of self-help books (64). Patients who have been sexually abused or who have significant anxiety or depression, sexual aversion, or significant marital dysfunction should be referred to a therapist who specializes in these areas.

Hypoactive Sexual Desire Disorder

Hypoactive sexual desire disorder (HSDD) is a recurrent deficiency or absence of sexual fantasies or thoughts or desire for sexual activity causing marked distress and interpersonal difficulty (65,66). Patients with HSDD have little interest in seeking sexual stimuli but often retain the ability to become sexually aroused and experience orgasm if they are approached sexually by their partner. This disorder usually develops in adulthood, often after a period of adequate sexual interest and functioning. HSDD is the most common sexual dysfunction in both women and men and is the most difficult to treat (67,68). It often is accompanied by another sexual disorder, such as dyspareunia or anorgasmia. Some individuals may experience sexual aversion, a complete avoidance of all sexual activity with a partner (59).

Physiologic causes of HSDD include medications (Table 11.3), chronic medical illnesses, depression, stress, substance abuse, aging, and hormonal alterations (36,69). Serum testosterone and prolactin levels should be evaluated in any patient presenting with the recent onset of HSDD because elevated prolactin levels (from a pituitary adenoma) or low testosterone levels (sometimes following natural or surgical menopause) could be responsible. Some postmenopausal patients who experience dyspareunia secondary to vaginal atrophy may avoid intercourse. This condition will resolve with systemic or vaginal estrogen replacement therapy. Some women with HSDD benefit from testosterone supplementation.

Individual causes of HSDD include religious orthodoxy, anhedonic or obsessive-compulsive personality (these patients may lack the capacity for play and find it difficult to display emotion and let themselves go), masked sexual deviation (e.g., transvestism), fear of pregnancy or STIs, and object choice issues (i.e., the patient may be a homosexual trying to function sexually in a heterosexual relationship).

Some individuals experience an unconscious and involuntary suppression of sexual desire and actively avoid sexual situations. They may suppress their desire by evoking negative thoughts or by allowing spontaneously emerging negative thoughts to intrude when they have a sexual opportunity (antifantasies) (65). Sexual desire can also be inhibited by performance anxiety, negative body image, chronic stress, low self-esteem, depression, the anticipation of an unpleasant sexual experience, fear of intimacy, or residual guilt about sex and pleasure. Women who have been sexually abused as children or sexually assaulted as adults may experience sexual avoidance or aversion. Some patients may fear loss of control over their sexual feelings and, therefore, may suppress them completely. If a patient is experiencing another form of sexual dysfunction, such as dyspareunia or anorgasmia, she may also be experiencing HSDD (65).

The way a couple functions sexually is often a good barometer of how things are going in the rest of the relationship. Therefore, whenever a woman presents with sexual concerns or sexual dysfunction, it is important to inquire about the relationship in general. If significant relationship problems exist in addition to sexual concerns, the couple should be referred for counseling. Relationship causes of HSDD include lack of sexual attraction for the partner (due to factors such as poor hygiene), poor lovemaking skills, sexual inexperience of one or both partners, marital conflict, lack of commitment, or discomfort with physical closeness owing to distrust of the partner or a sense of vulnerability. Some couples experience sexual difficulties because of differences in feelings regarding how close one partner would like to be to the other. One partner may want to be very close, whereas the other desires more distance (70). Couples may be sexually incompatible, with one partner making sexual demands the other is unable or unwilling to accommodate. Couples may have difficulty with the timing or the way they initiate sexual activity, or they may have incompatible or very different levels of sexual desire (71). Spouse abuse, financial problems, concerns about children, and marital power and control issues can significantly affect the way a couple functions sexually. It is difficult for anyone to feel sexual if they feel unloved or are depressed, overwhelmed with career and household responsibilities, unhappy about their relationship, or afraid of or angry with their partner.

Treatment of patients with HSDD may require both individual therapy and relationship counseling. Insight-oriented psychotherapy may allow the patient to identify the negative feelings that inhibit her erotic impulses and to gain insight into the underlying causes of her low sexual desire (69). Individual "homework" assignments include identifying erotic feelings, body awareness exercises, reading about human sexuality and sexual techniques, and fantasy training (72). In addition, the couple may benefit from learning how to perform structured sexual exercises known as *sensate focus exercises* (73). These behavior-modification exercises are designed to reduce sexual anxiety and to provide the couple with a nondemanding, nonthreatening, and reassuring environment in which they can address performance anxiety, sexual communication issues, and lack of sexual experience and knowledge.

Meeting with a couple for a few sessions to assess their sexual knowledge, attitudes, and practices is often beneficial. Many of the sexual problems couples encounter are due to a knowledge or experience deficit, sexual misconceptions, or the inability of the couple to communicate about what they would like to give and to receive in the sexual part of their relationship. Brief counseling and education by the obstetrician-gynecologist regarding the sexual response cycle and encouragement to communicate openly and honestly are often all that is needed to help couples achieve a fulfilling sexual relationship.

Arousal phase disorders, in which women experience sexual desire and orgasm but lack vaginal lubrication and other signs of sexual stimulation, are relatively rare. Lack of lubrication may lead to dyspareunia and eventually may impair a woman's subjective sense of arousal and pleasure. These women may benefit from the use of intravaginal lubricants, estrogen replacement therapy, or both.

Orgasmic Dysfunction

Orgasmic dysfunction in women is characterized by persistent or recurrent delay in or absence of orgasm following a normal sexual excitement phase, resulting in distress or interpersonal difficulty. Orgasmic dysfunction is more prevalent in younger and less sexually experienced women. Primary (lifelong) anorgasmia is found in about 5% to 10% of women (68) and is more common than secondary (acquired) anorgasmia. Some women develop secondary anorgasmia owing to relationship problems, depression, substance abuse, prescription medication (e.g., fluoxetine, SSRIs), chronic medical illness (e.g., diabetes), estrogen deficiency, or neurologic disorders (e.g., multiple sclerosis) (59). Many women who are orgasmic with masturbation and during noncoital sex may be distressed because they are not orgasmic during intercourse, do not have multiple orgasms or an orgasm with every sexual encounter, or do not have an orgasm at the same time as their partner. Surveys of sexual behavior demonstrate, however, that most couples do not experience orgasm simultaneously and that many women are more likely to be orgasmic during foreplay, when they receive more direct and intense clitoral stimulation, than during intercourse (68).

The most common psychological cause of anorgasmia is obsessive self-observation and monitoring during the arousal phase, often accompanied by anxiety and distracting, negative, and self-defeating thoughts (74,75). A woman with orgasmic dysfunction may be so busy monitoring her own and her partner's response and so concerned about "failing" that she is unable to relax enough to allow her natural reflexes to take over and trigger an orgasm (69,76). Masters and Johnson call this form of performance anxiety "spectatoring" (73). Inhibited orgasm may be related to a history of sexual abuse, negative feelings toward sexuality, relationship problems, an inattentive partner, ineffective sexual technique, low self-esteem, poor body image, or fear of losing control (75).

Numerous programs have been proposed for the treatment of orgasmic dysfunction (75). Approaches include evaluation and treatment of medical and psychiatric disorders (including substance abuse), sex education, communication and sexual skills training, marital therapy, group therapy, erotic fantasy, and counseling to reduce sexual anxiety and performance anxiety.

The most effective treatment for primary anorgasmia is employing a program of directed masturbation accompanied by erotic fantasy. Success rates of 80% to 90% have been reported using this technique (76). Several excellent self-help books are available to help women learn how to become orgasmic through masturbation (64,77). These self-help books instruct women how to increase their self-awareness by exploring their genital area in a nondemanding way. Once a woman has identified the most sensitive and pleasurable parts of her body, she can manually stimulate her clitoris and other erogenous areas while incorporating erotic fantasy until she reaches orgasm. A vibrator may be useful if the patient is unable to have an orgasm without one. Once the patient has experienced orgasm through masturbation, she may want to teach the technique to her partner, showing him how and where she likes to be touched during lovemaking. Manual stimulation of the clitoris by the woman or her partner while having intercourse (the bridge technique) may help women become orgasmic during intercourse.

Sexual Pain Disorder

Vaginismus

Vaginismus is the recurrent or persistent involuntary contraction of the perineal muscles surrounding the outer third of the vagina when vaginal penetration with a penis, finger, tampon, or speculum is attempted (59). Vaginismus is an involuntary reflex precipitated by real or imagined attempts at vaginal penetration. It can be global, in which the woman is unable to place anything inside her vagina, or situational, in which she is able to use a tampon and can tolerate a pelvic examination but cannot have intercourse. Many women with vaginismus have normal sexual desire, experience vaginal lubrication, and are orgasmic but are unable to have intercourse. Vaginismus can be primary, in which the woman has never been able to have intercourse, or secondary, which is often due to acquired dyspareunia. Some couples may cope with this difficulty for years before they seek help. They usually seek treatment because they desire children or decide they would like to consummate their relationship. Vaginismus is relatively rare, affecting about 1% of women (68).

Vaginismus can be a conditioned response to an unpleasant experience such as past sexual trauma or abuse, a painful first pelvic examination, or a painful first attempt at intercourse. It may occur secondary to religious orthodoxy, negative sexual upbringing, or sexual orientation concerns (78,79). Many women with vaginismus have an extreme fear of penetration and misconceptions about their anatomy and about the size of their vagina. They may believe that their vagina is too small to accommodate a tampon or penis and that great physical harm will result from placing anything inside the vagina.

Although medical conditions are rarely the cause of vaginismus, conditions such as endometriosis, chronic pelvic inflammatory disease, partially imperforate hymen, and vaginal stenosis must be ruled out by a careful pelvic examination. The pelvic examination, which should be performed, if possible, in the presence of the woman's partner, allows the physician to help educate the couple about normal female anatomy and may help dispel misconceptions about the size of the introitus and vagina. Providing the patient with a mirror to observe the examination is helpful. Because the etiology of vaginismus is usually psychophysiologic, patients with this condition should not have surgery to "enlarge" their introitus unless they have a partially imperforate hymen or other valid indication for surgery.

Treatment of vaginismus is directed toward extinguishing the conditioned involuntary vaginal spasm. This can be accomplished by the following:

1. Help the woman become more familiar with her anatomy and more comfortable with her sexuality.

2. Teach her techniques to help her relax when she anticipates vaginal penetration.

3. Instruct her in the use of Kegel exercises in order to gain control over the muscles surrounding her introitus.

4. Instruct her how to use graduated rubber dilators (fingers can also be used as dilators).

The protocol for use of the dilators is explained to the patient while she is in the office, but the actual placement of the dilators is done by the patient when she is at home. It is important for the patient to maintain total control over the use the dilators and to use them in an environment that is comfortable and safe. The dilators should be covered with a warm, water-soluble lubricant. She should initially try to place the dilators (or her finger) in her vagina when she is alone and relaxed. If she is unable to relax enough to place to the smallest dilator in her vagina, she may be able to reduce her anxiety by learning relaxation or self-hypnosis techniques. Medications, such as *propranolol* or *alprazolam,* may also help reduce anxiety. Once the patient has been able to place the smallest dilator in her vagina, she can progressively insert the larger dilators, practicing Kegel exercises while the dilators are in place. When she is comfortable inserting the larger dilators, she can teach her partner how to place the dilators in her vagina while she maintains control over how quickly and deeply the dilators are placed. She may then be ready to proceed to intercourse. Again, this must be under her control, with her sitting or kneeling over her partner and inserting his penis herself. Most couples (90%) who follow this protocol are successful and able to have intercourse.

Dyspareunia

Dyspareunia ("difficult mating") is genital pain that occurs before, during, or after intercourse in the absence of vaginismus. The repeated experience of pain during intercourse can cause marked distress, anxiety, and interpersonal difficulties, leading to anticipation of a negative sexual experience and eventually to sexual avoidance (59). As with other forms of sexual dysfunction, dyspareunia can be generalized or situational, lifelong or acquired. Secondary dyspareunia occurs, on the average, about 10 years after the onset of sexual activity. **Dyspareunia is one of the most common sexual dysfunctions seen by gynecologists and is estimated to affect about two thirds of women during their lifetime** (80,81). Women with dyspareunia usually discuss the pain with their sexual partner, but fewer than half of these women consult a physician. Because dyspareunia is a psychophysiologic condition, both psychological and physical factors must be considered in patient assessment. Many women with dyspareunia report more physical symptoms, psychological distress, and relationship issues than women who do not have pain during intercourse (82).

A careful history should be directed toward a complete chronology of the discomfort, an assessment of the impact of the dyspareunia on the patient and her partner, and any prior attempts to treat the condition (78–80). The patient should be asked about the specific location of the pain, when in the course of lovemaking the pain occurs, how long the pain lasts, the nature and quality of the pain, what factors relieve or aggravate the discomfort, and the severity of the pain. It is useful to ask the patient her theory about how the pain began and to assess her expectations and goals for treatment. Patients should be carefully asked about a history of childhood sexual or physical abuse or adult sexual assault because these situations may be associated with dyspareunia. Patients who are anxious about sexuality because of sexual misconceptions, guilt, fear of pregnancy or STIs, or prior unpleasant sexual experiences may be unable to relax during lovemaking, leading to impaired arousal and lubrication.

During the physical examination, attempts should be made to identify any organic factors contributing to the discomfort. Physiologic changes that take place during sexual arousal may account for pain that is present during intercourse but absent at other times, such as during a routine pelvic examination. Examples are Bartholin gland cysts, which swell during intercourse, and adhesive bands that form between portions of the hymenal ring only during arousal (78).

Causes of pain on stimulation of the external genitalia include chronic vulvitis and clitoral irritation and hypersensitivity. Pain at the introitus caused by penile entry can be caused by a rigid hymenal ring; scar tissue in an episiotomy repair; a müllerian abnormality; and vaginitis caused by one of the many common vaginal pathogens, such as *Candida, Trichomonas,* or *Gardnerella* species, or by irritation from over-the-counter vaginal sprays, douches, or contraceptive devices. Other causes include Bartholin gland inflammation, radiation vaginitis, infection with human papillomavirus, urethral syndrome, cystitis, vaginal trauma, chronic constipation, or proctitis. Vaginal infection is the most common cause of successfully treated dyspareunia (81). Another common cause of dyspareunia is friction due to inadequate sexual arousal. This situation can be resolved by counseling the couple to spend more time with foreplay, ensuring that the woman has adequate lubrication before intercourse. Use of a water-soluble lubricant (e.g., *Astroglide*) is also helpful. Vaginal atrophy resulting from hypoestrogenic states (menopause and lactation) can be treated with systemic or vaginal estrogen replacement.

Vulvar vestibulitis syndrome is a constellation of symptoms consisting of severe pain or burning on touching the vestibule and attempting vaginal entry (83). Women with vulvar vestibulitis report difficulty with sexual arousal, decreased lubrication, dyspareunia, and negative emotions during sexual encounters (84,85). On examination, diffuse or focal vulvar erythema is noted around the orifices of Bartholin, Skene, periurethral, or vestibular glands. This syndrome may be caused by an infection (subclinical human papillomavirus, bacterial vaginosis, or chronic candidiasis), irritants (soaps, detergents, douches, vaginal sprays), or altered vaginal pH secondary to a decrease in lactobacilli. Vulvar vestibulitis may be secondary to treatment of human papillomavirus with podophyllin, trichloroacetic acid, or laser.

The treatment of vulvar vestibulitis syndrome is empirical because the cause is unknown (83). A comprehensive multimodality approach may be necessary, as outlined in Chapter 14. Associated infections should be treated, vulvovaginal irritants should be eliminated, and surgery (vestibulectomy with vaginal advancement) should be reserved for patients with severe dyspareunia who have not responded to conservative management (83).

Causes of midvaginal pain include a congenitally shortened vagina, interstitial cystitis, and urethritis. Pain with orgasm may be associated with uterine contractions. Dyspareunia with deep vaginal penetration can be associated with inadequate vaginal lengthening and lubrication secondary to inadequate sexual arousal, chronic pelvic inflammatory disease, endometriosis, a fixed retroverted uterus, a pelvic mass, an enlarged uterus as a result of

Table 11.4. Assessment of Dyspareunia
Behavior: Faulty technique
Affect: Guilt, anger, fear, and shame
Sensation: Where is the pain?
Imagery: Do intrusive thoughts or negative images disrupt sexual enjoyment?
Cognition: Are there dysfunctional beliefs or misinformation that play a role in undermining sexual participation?
Interpersonal: How do the partners communicate and relate in both sexual and nonsexual settings?
Drugs: Is the patient on any medication that would diminish vaginal lubrication?

From **Lazarus AA.** Dyspareunia: a multimodal psychotherapeutic perspective. In: **Leiblum SR, Rosen RC,** eds. *Principles and practice of sex therapy,* 2nd ed. New York: The Guilford Press, 1989:89–112, with permission.

myomas or adenomyosis, inflammatory bowel disease, irritable bowel syndrome, or pelvic relaxation (80).

Psychological factors contributing to dyspareunia include:

1. *Developmental factors* (e.g., an upbringing that invested sex with guilt and shame)
2. *Traumatic factors* (e.g., childhood sexual abuse or other sexual assault)
3. *Relationship factors* (e.g., anger or resentment toward a sexual partner)

Lazarus uses the mnemonic BASIC ID to describe his multimodal approach to the assessment of dyspareunia (84). This approach addresses the issues noted in Table 11.4.

Sexual Assault

Sexual assault of children and adult women has reached epidemic proportions in the United States and is the fastest growing, most frequently committed, and most underreported crime (86–88). Sexual assault is a crime of violence and aggression, not passion, and encompasses a continuum of sexual activity that ranges from sexual coercion to contact abuse (unwanted kissing, touching, or fondling) to forcible rape. In a survey of female family practice patients, 47% reported some type of contact sexual victimization during their lifetime. Twenty-five percent reported attempted rape, and 13% had been forcibly raped, many as children (7,89). Among battered women, about 35% experience marital rape as an element of their repetitive abuse. Spousal rape is infrequently reported because of fear of retribution and economic dependency (90). **The terms *sexual abuse survivor* and *assault survivor* are preferable to *victim*.**

Childhood Sexual Abuse

Childhood sexual abuse has a profound and potentially lifelong effect on the survivor. Although most cases of childhood sexual abuse are not reported by the survivor or her family, it is estimated that as many as one third of adult women were sexually abused as children. Childhood sexual abuse is often accompanied by another type of household dysfunction, such as physical abuse, violence against other family members, or substance abuse by parental figures (88). Younger children are more often exposed to genital fondling or noncontact abuse (exhibitionism, forced observation of masturbation, or posing in child pornography), and children older than 10 years of age are more likely to be forced to have intercourse or oral sex (91). As children age, they are more likely to experience sexual abuse outside the home and more likely to be victimized by strangers. As adolescents, women survivors of childhood sexual abuse are at risk for early unplanned pregnancy, STIs, prostitution, antisocial behavior, running away from home, lying, stealing, eating disorders, and multiple somatic symptoms. These women are more likely to engage in health risk behaviors such as smoking, substance abuse, and early sexual activity with multiple partners (92). They may be less likely to use contraception. Survivors often avoid pelvic examinations and are less likely to have Papanicolaou (Pap) tests because of the association between vaginal examinations and pain. They often receive inadequate prenatal care and are more likely than women who have not been abused to experience suicidal ideation and depression and to deliver smaller and less mature babies (88).

Obstetrician-gynecologists can assist their sexual assault patients by validating their feelings and concerns and giving them control over their examination. It is important to ask the patient for permission to perform the examination, give her the opportunity to have an advocate in the room with her, and let her know that she has the right to stop the examination at any time (88).

Survivors may be unable to trust or establish rapport with adults. Some women blame themselves for the abuse and come to believe that they are not entitled to assistance from others. Thus, they risk continuing to enter abusive relationships. Women survivors of childhood sexual abuse often develop feelings of powerlessness and helplessness and may become chronically depressed. There is a high incidence of self-destructive behavior, including suicide and deliberate self-harm, such as cutting or burning themselves (88,93,94). The most extreme mental health symptoms in assault survivors are associated with the onset of abuse at an early age, frequent abuse over a long period, use of force, or abuse by a parent. Survivors are also at risk for becoming victimized again later in life (95). Fifty percent of women who report being abused as children are abused again as adults. Women who are sexually abused as children carry the effects of abuse into adulthood. As adults, they have the same level of physical symptoms and psychological distress as women who do not report childhood sexual abuse but are currently experiencing sexual or physical abuse (96).

Women who have been sexually abused as children or sexually assaulted as adults often experience sexual dysfunction and difficulty with intimate relationships and parenting (97). Chronic sexual concerns may include fear of intimate relationships, lack of sexual enjoyment, difficulty with desire and arousal, and anorgasmia. Compared with women who have not been sexually assaulted, they are more likely to experience depression, suicide attempts, chronic anxiety, anger, substance abuse problems, dissociative personality disorder, borderline personality disorder, fatigue, low self-esteem, feelings of guilt and self-blame, and sleep disturbance (96,98,99). They often experience social isolation, phobias, feelings of vulnerability, fear, humiliation, grief, and loss of control (6,100). Survivors of sexual assault represent a disproportionate number of patients with chronic headaches and chronic pelvic pain (they have a lower pain threshold) and are more likely to have somatic symptoms that do not respond to routine medical treatment (99,101). Women with common gynecologic symptoms, such as dysmenorrhea, menorrhagia, and sexual dysfunction, are much more likely to have a history of sexual assault (102). If they have been forced to perform oral sex, they may have a dental phobia and avoid preventive dental care.

Survivors may develop posttraumatic stress disorder (PTSD), defined as development of characteristic symptoms following a psychologically traumatic event outside of normal human experience. Symptoms of PTSD include blunting of affect, denial of symptoms, intrusive reexperiencing of the incident, avoidance of stimuli associated with the assault, and intense psychological distress and agitation in response to reminders of the event (86,93). Women affected by PTSD are more likely to commit suicide. The cognitive sequelae include flashbacks, nightmares, disturbances in perception, memory loss, and dissociative experiences (103). These women may not be able to tolerate pelvic examinations and may avoid seeking routine gynecologic care because these examinations may remind them of the sexual abuse they experienced as children. However, they are more likely to use the medical care system for nongynecologic concerns (104). Women with PTSD are at greater risk for being overweight and having gastrointestinal disturbances (92).

Rape

Although the legal definition of sexual assault may vary from state to state, most definitions of rape include:

1. The use of physical force, deception, intimidation, or the threat of bodily harm
2. Lack of consent or inability to give consent because the survivor is very young or very old, impaired by alcohol or drug use, unconsciousness, or mentally or physically impaired
3. Oral, vaginal, or rectal penetration with a penis, finger, or object

The National Women's Study provides the best statistics available about the incidence of forcible rape in the United States (6). This study revealed that 13%, or one of eight adult women, are survivors of at least one completed rape during their lifetime. Of the women they surveyed, 0.7% had been raped during the past year, equaling an estimated 683,000 adult women who were raped during a 12-month period. Of the women surveyed, 39% were raped more than once. Most disturbing, however, is the finding that most rapes occurred during childhood and adolescence; 29% of all forcible rapes occurred when the survivor was younger than 11 years of age, and 32% occurred between the ages of 11 and 17 years. Indeed, "rape in America is a tragedy of youth" (6). Twenty-two percent of rapes occurred between the ages of 18 and 24 years, 7% between the ages of 25 and 29 years, and only 6% occurred when the survivor was older than 30 years of age.

There are many myths about rape. Perhaps the most common is that women are raped by strangers. In fact, only about 20% to 25% of women are raped by someone they do not know. Most women are raped by a relative or acquaintance (9% by husbands or ex-husbands, 11% by fathers or stepfathers, 10% by boyfriends or ex-boyfriends, 16% by other relatives, and 29% by other nonrelatives) (6). Although acquaintance rape may seem to be less traumatic than stranger rape, survivors of acquaintance rape often take longer to recover. Another common misconception about rape is that most survivors sustain serious physical injury. Seventy percent of rape survivors report no physical injury, and only 4% sustain serious injury. Serious injury is rare, although almost half of the rape survivors report being fearful of serious injury or death during the assault (6). The most common injuries from a sexual assault are vaginal lacerations resulting in bleeding and pain. Intraperitoneal extension of a vaginal laceration or damage to the anal mucosa is rare (105). Common nongenital injuries in survivors include cuts, bruises, scratches, broken bones and teeth, and knife or gunshot wounds (106). About 0.1% of sexual assaults result in death. Common causes of death during a sexual assault include mechanical asphyxiation, trauma, lacerations, drowning, and gunshot wounds (105).

There are at least four types of rapists (107):

1. ***Opportunist rapists* (30%) exhibit no anger toward the women they assault and usually use little or no force.** These rapes are impulsive and may occur in the context of an existing relationship ("date" or acquaintance rape). The highest incidence of acquaintance rape is among women in the twelfth grade of high school and in the first year of college (108). Up to half of college women report date rape. Many of these women may have been unable to give consent because of impairment by alcohol or rohypnol, the "date rape drug." Date rape may have even greater psychological consequences than rape by a stranger because it involves a violation of trust (105).

2. ***Anger rapists* (40%) usually batter the survivor and use more physical force than is necessary to overpower her.** This type of sexual assault is episodic, impulsive, and spontaneous. An anger rapist often physically assaults his victim, sexually assaults her, and forces her to perform degrading acts. The rapist is angry or depressed and is often seeking retribution—for perceived wrongs or injustices he imagines have been done to him by others, especially women. He may victimize the very young or the very old.

3. ***Power rapists* (25%) do not intend to *physically* harm their victim but rather to possess or control her in order to gain sexual gratification.** However, a power rapist may use force or the threat of force to overcome his victim. These assaults are premeditated and repetitive, and they may increase in aggression over time. The rapist is usually anxious and may give orders to his victim, ask her personal questions, or inquire about her response during the assault. This assault may occur over an extended period while the victim is held captive. These rapists are insecure about their virility and are trying to compensate for their feelings of inadequacy and low self-esteem.

4. ***Sadistic rapists* (5%) become sexually excited by inflicting pain on their victim.** These rapists may have a thought disorder and often exhibit other forms of psychopathology. This type of assault is calculated and planned. The victim is often a stranger. The rape may involve bondage, torture, or bizarre acts and may occur over an extended period of time. The survivor often suffers both genital and nongenital injuries and may be murdered or mutilated. Other rapists may act out of impulse, as when they encounter a victim during the course of another crime such as burglary. Some rapists believe they are entitled to their victim, as in acquaintance rape or father–daughter incest (86). A consistent finding among all types of rapists is a lack of empathy for the survivor.

Even when sexual assaults are reported (only 16% of rapes are ever reported to the police), few rapists are arrested, and even fewer are brought to trial and convicted. Fewer than 1% of rapists ever serve a prison term (107). Many women do not report the assault to the police because they are concerned about their name being disclosed by the news media, fear retaliation from the perpetrator, are afraid they will not be believed, or do not trust the judicial process.

Only 17% of rape survivors seek medical attention after an assault. Many rape survivors do not inform their physicians about the assault and may never volunteer information about the assault unless they are directly asked. Therefore, when obtaining a medical history, physicians should routinely ask, "Has anyone ever forced you to have sexual relations when you did not want to?"

Effects of Rape

Following sexual assault, women have many concerns, including pregnancy, STIs (including human immunodeficiency virus [HIV] infection), being blamed for the assault, having their name made public, and having their family and friends find out about the assault. The initial reactions to sexual assault may be shock, numbness, withdrawal, and possibly denial. It is difficult to predict how any assaulted individual will react. Despite their recent trauma, women presenting for medical care may appear calm and detached.

The *rape trauma syndrome* is a constellation of physical and psychological symptoms, including fear, helplessness, disbelief, shock, guilt, humiliation, embarrassment, anger, and self-blame. The acute, or disorganization, phase of the syndrome lasts from days to weeks. Survivors may experience intrusive memories of the assault, blunting of affect, and hypersensitivity to environmental stimuli. They are anxious, do not feel safe, have difficulty sleeping and eating, and experience nightmares and a variety of somatic symptoms (86,109,110). They may fear that their assailant will return to retaliate or rape them again.

In the weeks to months following the sexual assault, survivors often return to normal activities and routines. They may appear to have dealt successfully with the assault, but they may be repressing strong feelings of anger, fear, guilt, and embarrassment. In the months following the assault, survivors begin the process of integration and resolution. During this phase, they begin to accept the assault as part of their life experience, and somatic and emotional symptoms may decrease progressively in severity. However, the sequelae of rape are often persistent and long-lasting (93). Over the long-term, survivors may have difficulty with work and with family relationships. Disruption of existing relationships is not uncommon. Nearly half of the survivors lose their jobs or are forced to quit in the year following the rape, and half change their place of residency (100).

Examination and Treatment

The responsibilities of physicians providing immediate treatment for sexual assault survivors are listed in Table 11.5. **Because of the legal ramifications, consent must be obtained from the patient before obtaining the history, performing the physical examination, and collecting evidence. Documentation of the handling of specimens is especially important, and the "chain of evidence" for collected material must be carefully maintained. Everyone who handles the evidence must sign for it and hand it directly to the next person in the chain. The patient should be interviewed in a quiet and supportive environment by an examiner who is objective and nonjudgmental. Support personnel and patient advocates, such as family, friends, or, if available, a counselor from a rape crisis service, should be encouraged to accompany the patient. It is important not to leave the survivor alone and to give her as much control as possible over the examination.** In order to provide useful forensic information, the examination should be performed as soon as possible after the incident occurred.

The history should include the following information:

1. A general medical history and a gynecologic history, including last menstrual period, prior pregnancies, past gynecologic infections, tetanus status, history of liver disease, thrombosis or hypertension (possible contraindications to pregnancy prophylaxis with estrogens), contraceptive use, prior sexual assault, and last voluntary intercourse before the assault.

2. It is important to ascertain whether the survivor bathed, douched, used a tampon, urinated, defecated, brushed her teeth, or changed her clothes after the assault.

Table 11.5. Physician Responsibilities in Treating Sexual Assault Survivors

1. Obtaining an accurate gynecologic history, including a recording of the sexual assault
2. Assessing, documenting, and treating physical injuries
3. Obtaining appropriate cultures (including samples for forensic tests), treating any existing infection, and providing prophylaxis for sexually transmitted diseases
4. Providing therapy to prevent unwanted pregnancy
5. Providing counseling for the patient and her partner and/or family
6. Arranging for follow-up medical care and counseling
7. Reporting to legal authorities as required by state law

From **American College of Obstetricians and Gynecologists.** *Sexual assault. Technical bulletin.* Washington, DC: ACOG, 1997:242, with permission.

3. A detailed description of the sexual assault should be obtained, including the date and time of the assault, number of assailants, use of weapons, threats, and restraints, and any physical injuries that may have occurred.

4. A detailed description of the type of sexual contact must be obtained, including whether vaginal, oral, or anal contact or penetration occurred, whether the assailant used a condom, and whether there were other possible sites of ejaculation, such as the hands, clothes, or hair of the survivor.

5. The emotional state of the survivor should be observed and recorded.

The survivor should undress while standing on clean examination table paper in order to catch any hair or fibers falling from her clothing. All of her clothing should be placed in individually labeled paper bags, sealed, and given to the proper authorities. Wet or damp clothing should be air dried before packaging. During the physical examination, the degree of injury to the survivor should be assessed, and any injuries should be documented for use as evidence. The nature, size, and location of all injuries should be carefully documented, using photographs or drawings if possible. Nongenital injuries occur in 20% to 50% of all rapes (111). The most common injuries are bruises and abrasions of the head, neck, and arms (86) and genital injuries accompanied by bleeding and pain. The most common genital findings are erythema and small tears of the vulva, perineum, and introitus. There may be bleeding, mucosal tears, erythema, or a hematoma noted around the rectum if penetration has occurred. Identification of small lacerations of the genitalia or rectum may be aided by colposcopy or by staining with toluidine blue (112). Bite marks are not uncommon and frequently are found on the breasts or genitalia. Foreign bodies may be found in the vagina, rectum, or urethra. If oral penetration has taken place, injuries of the mouth and pharynx may occur (113).

Evidence must be properly collected for legal purposes as follows:

1. Examination of the patient with a Wood light may help identify semen, which will fluoresce blue-green to orange. Areas of fluorescence should be swabbed with a cotton-tipped applicator moistened with sterile water. Swabs of the vagina, mouth, and rectum may be obtained to test for the presence of sperm or semen.

2. A Pap test may also be useful to document the presence of sperm.

3. A sample of the vaginal secretions should be obtained for examination for motile sperm, semen, or pathogens. Motile sperm in the vagina indicate ejaculation within 6 hours. Nonmotile sperm can be found in the cervical mucus for as long as 1 week. If ejaculation has occurred in the mouth, seminal fluid will be rapidly destroyed by salivary enzymes (105).

4. Vaginal secretions should also be collected to test for the presence of seminal contents, including acid phosphatase, p30 protein (specific to the prostate), seminal vesicle–specific antigen, and ABO antigens, and for DNA fingerprinting (88).

5. The survivor's pubic hair should be combed over a sheet of paper in an attempt to obtain pubic hair from the assailant.

6. Fingernail scrapings from the survivor should be collected and evaluated for evidence of the assailant's blood, hair, or skin. This evidence may also be used for DNA fingerprinting.

7. Saliva should be collected from the survivor to document whether she is a secretor of major blood group antigens (80% of the population are secretors). If the patient is not a secretor and blood group antigens are found in vaginal washings, the

Table 11.6. Laboratory Studies in the Evaluation of Sexually Assaulted Adults

Cultures of the cervix, mouth, and rectum for:
Neisseria gonorrhoeae
Chlamydia trachomatis
Herpes simplex
Serologic test for syphilis
Wet prep for trichomonas
Hepatitis B surface antigen
Human immunodeficiency virus antibody
Pregnancy test

antigens are probably from the semen of the assailant (88). Laboratory tests that should be performed on all sexual assault survivors are listed in Table 11.6.

Treatment of sexual assault survivors should be directed to prevention of possible pregnancy and provision of prophylactic treatment for STIs. About 5% of fertile rape survivors will become pregnant as a result of the rape (114). Options include (a) awaiting the next expected menses; (b) repeating the serum pregnancy test in 1 to 2 weeks; and (c) using emergency (postcoital) contraception. If the patient desires emergency contraception, a preexisting pregnancy can usually be ruled out by performing a sensitive human chorionic gonadotropin assay. Pregnancy prophylaxis can be provided by several different regimens (115) (see also Chapter 10):

1. Immediate administration of two tablets of a combination oral contraceptive (each containing 50 μg of *ethinyl estradiol* and 0.5 mg *norgestrel,* i.e., *Ovral* birth control pills) followed by two more tablets 12 hours later
2. Four tablets of a combination birth control pill containing 35 μg of *ethinyl estradiol* and a progesterone followed by four more tablets 12 hours later
3. Administration of one tablet containing 0.75 mg of *levonorgestrel* followed by a second tablet 12 hours later (Plan B)
4. Placement of a copper-containing intrauterine device
5. *Mifepristone* as a single 600-mg dose

These regimens are highly effective if administered within 72 hours after the sexual assault. Some investigators believe that emergency contraception can be effective up to 5 days after unprotected intercourse (88). However, the sooner the medications are taken, the more effective they are. Some patients experience nausea and vomiting when given postcoital contraception; these symptoms can be controlled with an antiemetic agent such as promethazine (12.5 mg every 4 to 6 hours). Emergency contraception has a small failure rate and potential teratogenicity, which should be discussed with the patient (116). Most women who take emergency contraception experience their next menstrual period within 3 days of the expected date.

The risk for acquiring an STI from a rape is difficult to assess because the prevalence of preexisting STIs is high (43%) in rape survivors (117,118). However, it is estimated that the risk for acquiring STIs from a sexual assault is as follows: gonorrhea, 6% to 12%; trichomonas, 12%; chlamydia, 2% to 12%; syphilis, 5%.

1. Because it is difficult to differentiate between a preexisting STI and a newly contracted STI attributable to a sexual assault, prophylaxis for STIs should be offered to all survivors. This is especially important because most sexual assault patients do not return for follow-up appointments (110). STI prophylaxis should cover infections with *Neisseria gonorrhoeae, Chlamydia trachomatis,* trichomonas, and incubating syphilis. Current recommendations include (118,119):
   a. *Ceftriaxone,* 250 mg intramuscularly (if the patient is allergic to cephalosporins, *spectinomycin,* 2 g intramuscularly, or *ciprofloxacin,* 500 mg orally, may be used), PLUS:
   b. A single dose of 2 gm of *metronidazole* orally, PLUS:
   c. A single dose of 1 gm of *azithromycin* orally or 100 mg of *doxycycline* orally twice a day for 7 days (if the patient is pregnant at the time of the assault, *erythromycin* may be substituted for *doxycycline*)

2. Hepatitis B vaccination should be offered if the sexual assault survivor has experienced vaginal, oral, or anal penetration. Hepatitis B is 20 times more infectious than HIV during intercourse (88). Vaccination is recommended at the time of the initial evaluation. Subsequent doses are provided 1 month and 6 months after the first dose is administered. It is not necessary to treat the patient with hepatitis B immune globulin (HBIG) (119).

3. Tetanus prophylaxis (5 mL intramuscularly) should also be administered if indicated.

4. If prophylactic treatment for gonorrhea, chlamydia, and trichomonas is not given, the patient should return for repeat testing in 2 weeks. If the initial test results were negative, repeat serologic tests for syphilis, hepatitis B, and HIV should be performed at 6, 12, and 24 weeks after the assault.

5. HIV conversion through sexual assault, although reported, is low and similar to conversion from occupational exposure (<0.1%). The probability of transmission depends on the type of assault, presence of trauma, site of ejaculation, HIV viral load in the ejaculate, and presence of a concomitant STI in the patient (111). At present, no recommendation can be made regarding the use of antiretroviral prophylaxis for HIV in sexual assault survivors. Factors to consider when discussing HIV prophylaxis with patients include the likelihood of exposure to the virus, the risks and benefits of treatment, the interval between the sexual assault and the initiation of therapy, and the patient's desire to be treated. Patients should be aware that the efficacy of prophylactic treatment for HIV is unknown and that they will have to be carefully monitored if they initiate treatment with antiretroviral medication.

6. Ongoing supportive counseling for the patient should be arranged, and the patient should be referred to a sexual assault center or a therapist who specializes in the treatment of sexual assault survivors.

References

1. **Frank E, Anderson C, Rubinstein D.** Frequency of sexual dysfunction in "normal" couples. *N Engl J Med* 1978;299:111–115.

2. **Michael RT, Gagnon JH, Laumann EO, et al.** *Sex in America.* Boston: Little, Brown, 1994.

3. **Laumann EO, Paik A, Rosen RC.** Sexual dysfunction in the United States. *JAMA* 1999;281:537–544.

4. **Kohn II, Kaplan SA.** Female sexual dysfunction: what is known and what can be done. *Contemp Obstet Gynecol* 2000;45:25–46.

5. **Francoeur RT, Kock PT, Weis DL.** *Sexuality in America: understanding our sexual values and behavior.* New York: Continuum, 1998.

6. **Kilpatrick DG, Edmunds CN, Seymour AK.** *Rape in America.* New York: National Victim Center, 1992.

7. **Walch AG, Broadhead WE.** Prevalence of lifetime sexual victimization among female patients. *J Fam Pract* 1992;35:511–516.

8. **Ende J, Rockwell S, Glasgow M.** The sexual history in general medical practice. *Arch Intern Med* 1984;144:558–561.

9. **Marwick C.** Survey says patients expect little physician help on sex. *JAMA* 1999;281:2173–2174.

10. **Hunt AD, Litt IF, Loebner M.** Obtaining a sexual history from adolescent girls. *J Adolesc Health* 1988;9:52–54.

11. **Bowman M.** The new sexual history: inquiring about sexual practices. *Am Fam Physician* 1989;40:82–83.

12. **Bachman GA, Leiblum SR, Grill J.** Brief sexual inquiry in gynecologic practice. *Obstet Gynecol* 1989;73:425–427.

13. **Stevenson RWD, Szasz G, Maurice WL, Miles JE.** How to become comfortable talking about sex to your patients. *Can Med Assoc J* 1983;128:797–800.

14. **Risen CB.** A guide to taking a sexual history. *Psychiatric Clin North Am* 1995;150:1033–1038.

15. **Andrews WC.** Approaches to taking a sexual history. *J Women's Health and Gender-Based Medicine* 2000;9(Suppl 1):S21–S24.

16. **Reamy K.** Sexual counseling for the nontherapist. *Clin Obstet Gynecol* 1984;27:781–788.

17. **Seidman SN, Rieder RO.** A review of sexual behavior in the United States. *Am J Psychiatry* 1994;151:330–341.

18. **Masters WH, Johnson VE.** *Human sexual response.* Boston: Little, Brown, 1966.

19. **Basson R.** The female sexual response: a different model. *J Sex Marital Ther* 2000;26:51–65.

20. **Leiblum SR.** Redefining female sexual response. *Contemp Obstet Gynecol* 2000;45:120–126.

21. **Mooradian AD, Greiff V.** Sexuality in older women. *Arch Intern Med* 1990;150:1033–1038.

22. **Bretschneider JG, McCoy NL.** Sexual interest and behavior in healthy 80- to 102-year-olds. *Arch Sex Behav* 1988;17:109–129.

23. **Bachmann GA.** Sexual issues at menopause. *Ann N Y Acad Sci* 1990;592:87–94.

24. **Meston CM.** Aging and sexuality. *West J Med* 1997;167:285–290.

25. **Kingsberg SA.** The psychological impact of aging on sexuality and relationships. *J Womens Health Gender Med* 2000;9(Suppl 1):S33–S38.

26. **Bortz WM, Wallace DH.** Physical fitness, aging, and sexuality. *West J Med* 1999;170:167–169.

27. **Sarrel PM.** Effects of hormone replacement therapy on sexual psychophysiology and behavior in post-menopause. *J Womens Health Gender Med* 2000;9(Suppl 1):S25–S32.

28. **Redman GR.** Hormones and sexual function. *Int J Fertil* 1999;44:193–197.

29. **DeCherney AH.** Hormone receptors and sexuality in the human female. *J Women Health Gender Med* 2000;9(Suppl 1):S9–S13.

30. **Casson PR, Elkind-Hirsch KE, Buster JE, et al.** Effect of postmenopausal estrogen replacement on circulating androgens. *Obstet Gynecol* 1997;90:995–998.

31. **American College of Obstetricians and Gynecologists.** *Androgen treatment of decreased libido. Technical bulletin.* Washington, DC: ACOG, 2000:244.

32. **Shifren JL, Braunstein GD, Simon JA, et al.** Transdermal testosterone treatment in women with impaired sexual function after oophorectomy. *N Engl J Med* 2000;343:682–688.

33. **Kaplan SA, Reis RB, Kohn IJ, et al.** Safety and efficacy of sildenafil in postmenopausal women with sexual dysfunction. *Urology* 1999;53:481–486.

34. **Shen WW, Urosevich Z, Clayton DO.** Sildenafil in the treatment of female sexual dysfunction induced by selective serotonin reuptake inhibitors. *J Reprod Med* 1999;44:535-542.

35. Drugs that cause sexual dysfunction: an update. *Med Lett Drugs Ther* 1992;34:73–78.

36. **Kaplan HS.** *The evaluation of sexual disorders: psychological and medical aspects.* New York: Brunner/Mazel, 1983.

37. **Buffum J.** Prescription drugs and sexual function. *Psychiatr Med* 1992;10:181–198.

38. **Finger WW, Lund M, Slagle MA.** Medications that may contribute to sexual disorders. *J Fam Pract* 1997;44:33–43.

39. **Crenshaw TL, Goldberg JP.** *Sexual pharmacology: drugs that affect sexual functioning.* New York: WW Norton, 1996.

40. **Wincze JP, Carey MP.** *Sexual dysfunction.* New York: Guilford Press, 1991.

41. **Keye WR.** Psychosexual responses to infertility. *Clin Obstet Gynecol* 1984;27:760–766.

42. **Ganz PA, Rowland JH, Desmond K, et al.** Life after breast cancer: understanding women's health-related quality of life and sexual functioning. *J Clin Oncol* 1998;16:501–514.

43. **Schover LR, Yetman RJ, Tuason LJ, et al.** Partial mastectomy and breast reconstruction: a comparison of their effects on psychosocial adjustment, body image, and sexuality. *Cancer* 1995;75:54–64.

44. **Schover LR.** The impact of breast cancer of sexuality, body image, and intimate relationships. *CA Cancer J Clin* 1991;41:112–120.

45. **Schover LR, Jensen SB.** *Sexuality and chronic illness: a comprehensive approach.* New York: Guilford Press, 1988.

46. **Bachman GA.** Psychosexual aspects of hysterectomy. *Womens Health Issues* 1990;1:41–49.

47. **Nathorst-Boos J, von Schoultz B.** Psychological reactions and sexual life after hysterectomy with and without oophorectomy. *Gynecol Obstet Invest* 1992;34:97–101.

48. **Bellarose SB, Yitzchak MB.** Body image and sexuality in oophorectomized women. *Arch Sex Behav* 1993;5:435–459.

49. **Rhodes JC, Kjerulff KH, Langenberg PW, et al.** Hysterectomy and sexual functioning. *JAMA* 1999;282:1934–1941.

50. **Virtanen H, Makinen J, Tenho T, et al.** Effects of abdominal hysterectomy on urinary and sexual symptoms. *Br J Urol* 1993;72:868–872.

51. **Helmstrom L, Lundberg PO, Sorbom D, et al.** Sexuality after hysterectomy: a factor analysis of women's sexual lives before and after subtotal hysterectomy. *Obstet Gynecol* 1993;81:357–362.

52. **Thranov I, Klee M.** Sexuality among gynecologic cancer patients: a cross-sectional study. *Gynecol Oncol* 1994;52:14–19.

53. **Anderson BL.** Yes, there are sexual problems. Now, what can we do about them? *Gynecol Oncol* 1994;52:10–13.

54. **Cull A, Cowie VJ, Farquharson DIM, et al.** Early stage cervical cancer: psychosocial and sexual outcomes of treatment. *Br J Cancer* 1993;68:216–220.

55. **Barrett G, Pendry E, Peacock J, et al.** Sexual function after childbirth: women's experiences, persistent morbidity, and lack of professional recognition. *Br J Obstet Gyn* 1997;104:330–335.

56. **Bogren LY.** Changes in sexuality in women and men during pregnancy. *Arch Sex Behav* 1991;20:35–45.

57. **Reamy K, White SE, Daniell WC, et al.** Sexuality and pregnancy: a prospective study. *J Reprod Med* 1982;27:321–327.

58. **Dameron GW.** Helping couples cope with sexual changes pregnancy brings. *Contemp Obstet Gynecol* 1983;21:23–35.

59. **American Psychiatric Association.** *Diagnostic and statistical manual of mental disorders,* (4th ed). Washington, DC: American Psychiatric Association, 1994.

60. **Basson R, Berman J, Burnett A, et al.** Report on the international consensus development conference on female sexual dysfunction: definitions and classifications. *J Urol* 2000;163:888–893.

61. **Franger AL.** Taking a sexual history and managing common sexual problems. *J Reprod Med* 1988;33:639–643.

62. **Heiman J, Meston CM.** Evaluating sexual dysfunction in women. *Clin Obstet Gynecol* 1997;40:616–629.

63. **Pion R, Annon J.** The office management of sexual problems: brief therapy approaches. *J Reprod Med* 1975;15:127–144.

64. **Heiman JR, LoPiccolo J.** *Becoming orgasmic: a sexual and personal growth program for women,* (2nd ed). New York: Simon and Schuster, 1988.

65. **Leiblum SR, Rosen RC.** *Sexual desire disorders.* New York: The Guilford Press, 1988.

66. **Rosen RC, Leiblum SR.** Treatment of sexual disorders in the 1990s: an integrated approach. *J Consult Clin Psychol* 1995;63:887–890.

67. **Hawton K, Catalan J, Fagg J.** Low sexual desire: sex therapy results and prognostic factors. *Behav Res Ther* 1991;29:217–224.

68. **Spector IP, Carey MP.** Incidence and prevalence of the sexual dysfunctions: a critical review of the empirical literature. *Arch Sex Behav* 1990;19:389–408.

69. **Kaplan HS.** *Disorders of sexual desire and other new concepts and techniques in sex therapy.* New York: Brunner/Mazel, 1979.

70. **Lazarus AA.** A multimodal perspective on problems of sexual desire. In: **Leiblum SR, Rosen RC**, eds. *Sexual desire disorders.* New York: The Guilford Press, 1988:145–167.

71. **Levine SB.** Intrapsychic and individual aspects of sexual desire. In: **Leiblum SR, Rosen RC**, eds. *Sexual desire disorders.* New York: The Guilford Press, 1988:21–44.

72. **LoPiccolo J, Friedman JM.** Broad-spectrum treatment of low sexual desire: integration of cognitive, behavioral, and systemic therapy. In: **Leiblum SR, Rosen RC**, eds. *Sexual desire disorders.* New York: The Guilford Press, 1988:107–144.

73. **Masters WH, Johnson VE.** *Human sexual inadequacy.* New York: Bantam Books, 1970.

74. **Wincze JP, Carey MP.** *Sexual dysfunction: a guide for assessment and treatment.* New York: The Guilford Press, 1991.

75. **McCabe MP, Delaney SM.** An evaluation of therapeutic programs for the treatment of secondary inorgasmia in women. *Arch Sexual Behav* 1992;21:69–89.

76. **Heiman JR, Grafton-Becker V.** Orgasmic disorders in women. In: **Leiblum SR, Rosen RC,** eds. *Principles and practice of sex therapy,* 2nd ed. New York: The Guilford Press, 1989:51–88.

77. **Barbach L.** *For yourself: the fulfillment of female sexuality.* New York, Signet, 2000.

78. **Steege J.** Dyspareunia and vaginismus. *Clin Obstet Gynecol* 1984;27:750–759.

79. **Lamont J.** Vaginismus. *Am J Obstet Gynecol* 1978;131:632–638.

80. **Steege JF, Ling FW.** Dyspareunia. *Obstet Gynecol Clin North Am* 1993;20:779–793.

81. **Glatt AE, Zinner SH, McCormack WM.** The prevalence of dyspareunia. *Obstet Gynecol* 1990;75: 433–436.

82. **Meana M, Binik YM, Khalife S, et al.** Biopsychosocial profile of women with dyspareunia. *Obstet Gynecol* 1997;90:583–589.

83. **Marinoff SC, Turner MLC.** Vulvar vestibulitis syndrome: an overview. *Am J Obstet Gynecol* 1991;165:1228–1233.

84. **Lazarus AA.** Dyspareunia: a multimodal psychotherapeutic perspective. In: **Leiblum SR, Rosen RC**, eds. *Principles and practice of sex therapy,* 2nd ed. New York: The Guilford Press, 1989:89–112.

85. **Van Lankveld JJDM, Weijenborg PThM, Ter Kuile MM.** Psychologic profiles of and sexual function in women with vulvar vestibulitis and their partners. *Obstet Gycolol* 1996;88:65–70.

86. **Dunn SFM, Gilchrist VJ.** Sexual assault. *Prim Care* 1993;20:359–373.

87. **Sorenson SB, Stein JA, Siegel JM, et al.** The prevalence of adult sexual assault. *Am J Epidemiol* 1987;126:1154–1164.

88. **American College of Obstetrics and Gynecology.** *Sexual assault. Technical bulletin.* Washington, DC: ACOG, 1997:242.

89. **McGrath ME, Hogan JW, Peipert JF.** A prevalence survey of abuse and screening for abuse in urgent care patients. *Obstet Gynecol* 1998;91:511–514.

90. **DeLahunta EA, Baram DA.** Sexual assault. *Clin Obstet Gynecol* 1997;40:648-60.

91. **Bachman GA, Moeller TP, Bennet J.** Childhood sexual abuse and the consequences in adult women. *Obstet Gynecol* 1988;71:631–642.

92. **Springs FE, Friedrich WN.** Health risk behaviors and medical sequelae of childhood sexual abuse. *Mayo Clin Proc* 1992;67:527–532.

93. **Council on Scientific Affairs, American Medical Association.** Violence against women: relevance for medical practitioners. *JAMA* 1992;267:3184–3189.

94. **Wyatt GE, Guthrie D, Notgrass CM.** Differential effects of women's child sexual abuse and subsequent sexual revictimization. *J Consult Clin Psychol* 1992;60:167–173.

95. **Polit DF, White CM, Morton TD.** Child sexual abuse and premarital intercourse among high-risk adolescents. *J Adolesc Health* 1990;11:231–234.

96. **McCauley J, Kern DE, Kolodner K, et al.** Clinical characteristics of women with a history of childhood abuse: unhealed wounds. *JAMA* 1997;277:1362–1368.

97. **Mackey TF, Hacker SS, Weissfeld LA, et al.** Comparative effects of sexual assault on sexual functioning of child sexual abuse survivors and others. *Issues Mental Health Nurs* 1991;12:89–112.

98. **Laws A.** Does a history of sexual abuse in childhood play a role in women's medical problems? A review. *J Womens Health* 1993;2:165–172.

99. **American College of Obstetricians and Gynecologists.** *Adult manifestations of childhood sexual abuse. Technical bulletin.* Washington, DC: ACOG, 2000:259.

100. **Ellis E, Atkeson B, Calhoun K.** An assessment of long term reaction to rape. *J Abnorm Psychol* 1981;90:263–266.

101. **Walling MK, Reiter RC, O'Hara MW, et al.** Abuse history and chronic pain in women. 1. Prevalences of sexual abuse and physical abuse. *Obstet Gynecol* 1994;84:193–199.

102. **Golding JM, Wilsnack SC, Learman LA.** Prevalence of sexual assault history among women with common gynecologic symptoms. *Am J Obstet Gynecol* 1998;179:1013–1019.

103. **Hendricks-Matthews MK.** Survivors of abuse. *Prim Care* 1993;20:391–406.

104. **Felitti VJ.** Long-term medical consequences of incest, rape, and molestation. *South Med J* 1991;84:328–331.

105. **Hampton HL.** Care of the women who has been raped. *N Engl J Med* 1995;332:234–237.

106. **Linden JA.** Sexual assault. *Emerg Med Clin North Am* 1999;17:685–697.

107. **Groth AN.** *Men who rape: the psychology of the offender.* New York: Plenum Press, 1979.

108. **Bechtel K, Podrazik M.** Evaluation of the adolescent rape victim. *Pediatr Clin North Am* 1999;46:809–822.

109. **Burgess A, Holmstrom L.** Rape trauma syndrome. *Am J Psychol* 1974;131:981–986.

110. **Holmes MM, Resnick HS, Frampton D.** Follow-up of sexual assault victims. *Am J Obstet Gynecol* 1998;179:336–342.

111. **Geist F.** Sexually related trauma. *Emerg Med Clin North Am* 1988;6:439–466.

112. **Slaughter L, Brown CRV, Crowley S, et al.** Patterns of genital injury in female sexual assault victims. *Am J Obstet Gynecol* 1997;176:609–616.

113. **Dupre AR, Hampton HL, Morrison H, et al.** Sexual assault. *Obstet Gynecol Surv* 1993;48:640–647.

114. **Beckmann CR, Groetzinger LL.** Treating sexual assault victims: a protocol for health professionals. *Female Patient* 1989;14:78–83.

115. **Glasier A.** Emergency postcoital contraception. *N Engl J Med* 1997;337:1058–1064.

116. **Beebe DK.** Emergency management of the adult female rape victim. *Am Fam Physician* 1991;43:2041–2046.

117. **Jenny C, Hooton TM, Bowers A, et al.** Sexually transmitted diseases in victims of rape. *N Engl J Med* 1990;322:713–716.

118. **Reynolds MW, Peipert JF, Collins B.** Epidemiologic issues of sexually transmitted diseases in sexual assault victims. *Obstet Gynecol Surv* 2000;55:51–57.

119. **Centers for Disease Control and Prevention.** 1998 Guidelines for sexually transmitted diseases. *Morb Mortal Wkly Rep* 1998;January 23:47.s

Novak's Gynecology, 13th Edition. Edited by J.S. Berek. Lippincott Williams & Wilkins, Philadelphia © 2002.

12 Common Psychiatric Problems

Nada L. Stotland

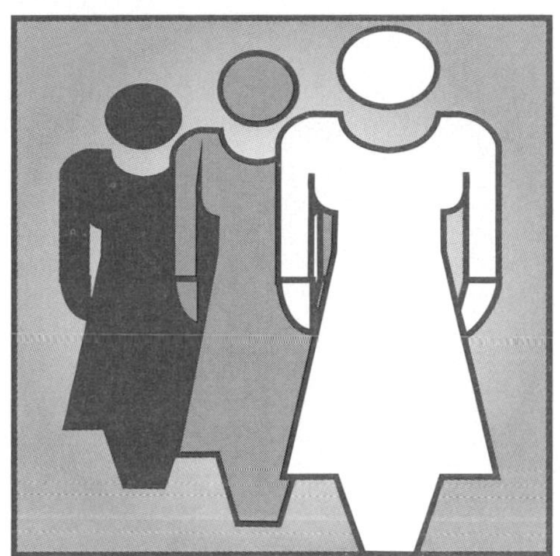

Psychiatric problems are a central or complicating factor in most outpatient visits (1,2). Psychiatric diagnoses are extremely common and account for considerable morbidity and mortality in the general population (3). Despite this, however, psychiatric disorders are often undiagnosed or misdiagnosed in the medical setting (4–7). Clinical depression affects up to one-fourth of women during their lives (8–10), but an estimated 80% of the cases are neither diagnosed nor treated (11). More than one-half of the patients who commit suicide have seen a nonpsychiatric physician during the previous 3 months (12).

Many gynecologists feel uncomfortable diagnosing and treating psychiatric illnesses for a variety of reasons. The practice of gynecology has many demands, and the care of these patients requires a commitment. Patients with psychological problems can evoke negative reactions in physicians (Table 12.1). In the past, gynecologists have found it difficult to use psychiatric diagnostic systems that were based on theories of unconscious motivation and conflict. New systems for the diagnosis of psychiatric disorders are reliable and valid and can be systematically applied, and treatments are specific and effective (8). By incorporating these management strategies into practice, gynecologists can play a major role in improving the health and well-being of their patients.

Psychiatric Assessment

In the past, psychiatric diagnosis was based partially on hypotheses about a patient's unconscious psychological conflicts (13). Current psychiatric diagnosis, as codified in the Diagnostic and Statistical Manual of Mental Disorders, Fourth Edition (DSM IV), produced and published by the American Psychiatric Association, is based on empirical, valid, and reliable evidence (8). Use of the DSM IV yields reliability comparable to that of diagnostic systems in other areas of medicine. DSM IV diagnoses are also strongly correlated with response to treatment. The criteria in DSM IV are the basis for the diagnostic entities described in this chapter. A new edition, DSM IV TR, differs only in the text explaining some of the diagnoses, and not in the diagnostic criteria themselves (9). DSM IV PC is a special edition designed for the primary care provider. This volume is organized by initial

Table 12.1. Practitioners' Negative Reactions Toward Patients with Psychiatric Problems

1. Social stigma attached to psychiatric diagnoses, patients, and practitioners.
2. Belief that individuals with psychiatric disorders are weak, unmotivated, manipulative, or defective.
3. Belief that the criteria for psychiatric diagnoses are intuitive rather than empirical.
4. Belief that psychiatric treatments are ineffective and unsupported by medical evidence.
5. Fear that patients with psychiatric problems will demand and consume inordinate and limitless time from a medical practice.
6. Precipitation in others, including doctors, of feelings that are complementary to the strong and unpleasant emotions experienced by patients with psychiatric disorders.
7. Gynecologists' own uncertainty about their skills at psychiatric diagnosis, referral, and treatment.
8. Failure to view psychiatric problems as legitimate grounds for medical attention.

signs and symptoms rather than psychiatric categories and uses algorithms and decision trees to facilitate the diagnostic process. Accurate diagnosis is absolutely critical to successful management, whether provided by the gynecologist or through referral to a mental health expert.

Approach to the Patient

Although diagnostic criteria list signs and symptoms, the interaction with a patient should not be reduced to a series of rapid-fire questions and answers. **A wealth of valuable information can be obtained from the patient's spontaneous description of her concerns and from her responses to the physician's open-ended questions.** A patient who is encouraged to speak for several minutes before being asked to respond to specific questions will reveal information that is useful, even vital, to her care: a thought disorder, a predominant mood, abnormally high anxiety, a personality style or disorder, and attitudes towards her diagnosis and treatment. Such information may emerge only much later, or not at all, in a question-and-answer format (15,18). It is critical that the gynecologist neither jumps to diagnostic conclusions nor proceeds directly to therapeutic interventions. One study revealed that many primary care physicians, feeling that they had too little time or training to assess psychological symptoms, tended to minimize verbal interactions with patients and to rely on the prescription of psychotropic medications (14). It is not necessary, however, for the physician and the other patients awaiting care to be held hostage by the overly talkative patient. The clinician can tell the patient with multiple, detailed complaints how much time is available for the current appointment, invite her to focus on her most pressing problem, and offer a future appointment to continue the account.

Psychiatric Referral

Many gynecologists consider referral to a mental health professional, particularly a psychiatrist, to be a delicate matter. The first question is when to refer. Most mild psychiatric disorders are treated by nonpsychiatric physicians (17). Most antidepressants and anxiolytics are prescribed by nonpsychiatric physicians. At the same time, however, most cases of psychiatric disorder are overlooked, misdiagnosed, or mistreated in primary care practice. The following factors determine the decision to refer:

- The nature and severity of the patient's disorder
- The expertise of the gynecologist
- The time available in the gynecologic practice
- The patient's preference
- The gynecologist's degree of comfort with the patient and the disorder
- The availability of mental health professionals.

Patients who are suicidal, homicidal, or acutely psychotic should be seen by a psychiatrist. Patients should also be referred for evaluation when the psychiatric diagnosis is not clear and when they fail to respond to initial treatment. For many patients, the gynecologist can resume the responsibility for ongoing care after an initial or periodic assessment by a psychiatrist.

How to Refer?

Some clinicians fear that patients will be insulted, alienated, or alarmed by a psychiatric referral. Techniques that decrease the discomfort of the gynecologist and patient and enhance the likelihood of a successful referral are discussed below (19).

The referral should be explained on the basis of the patient's own signs, symptoms, and distress. For a patient suffering from clinical depression, this might be her difficulty sleeping, her loss of appetite, or her lack of energy. For a patient with an anxiety disorder, it might be her palpitations, shortness of breath, or nervousness. For a patient with mild Alzheimer's disease, it might be forgetfulness or frightening episodes, in which she finds herself in a neighborhood she does not recognize. The advent of treatments that may slow the dementing process makes these referrals easier as well.

When somatizing (psychosomatic) disorder is suspected, the gynecologist should emphasize the difficulty of living with symptoms without definitive diagnosis and treatment, rather than the physician's hypothesis that the symptoms have a psychological basis:

1. "It is very stressful to be suffering while we can't pinpoint the problem. I would like you to see one of our staff who specializes in helping people cope with these difficult situations."
2. "It must be difficult to function when you have been so sickly all your life, have seen so many doctors, have had so many diagnostic tests and medical treatments, and still don't have an answer or feel well."

It is counterproductive to convey the idea that, because the diagnostic process has not revealed a specific disorder, the problem must be "in the patient's head." It is never possible to rule out an organic cause with absolute certainty.

Many physicians fear that questioning patients about suicide or homicide will provoke these behaviors. The opposite is the case (12). An open discussion of impulses to hurt oneself or someone else helps the patient to regain control, recognize the need for mental health care, or agree to emergency interventions such as psychiatric hospitalization, while avoiding the subject intensifies the patient's feelings of isolation. The management of suicidality is addressed in the section on mood disorders.

The possibility of psychosis need not be avoided, either. Most psychotic patients have had previous experience with psychiatric referral. Their psychotic symptoms are often distressing, and they can generally discuss hallucinations and delusions quite matter-of-factly. The rare patient who comes to a gynecologist with a first episode of acute psychosis is likely to be frightened by her symptoms and willing to accept expert consultation.

Despite increasing public sophistication about mental illnesses and psychiatric care, some patients believe that any mention of mental health intervention implies either that they are "crazy" or that the referring physician is convinced that their physical symptoms are imaginary or feigned. The gynecologist may wish to state explicitly that this is not the case. Again, making the real reason for the referral clear and founded in signs and symptoms obvious to the patient will nearly always allay anxiety over a psychiatric referral.

It is not acceptable to refer a patient to a psychiatrist without informing and asking her in advance unless she is acutely psychotic, functionally incompetent, or in the throes of a suicidal or homicidal emergency. Even under those circumstances, it is highly preferable to be straightforward. A referral that begins with an unexpected clinical encounter with a psychiatrist is unfair to the psychiatrist and the patient and is unlikely to result in a satisfactory collaboration.

In order to address any concern a patient may have that a mental health referral is an indication of the gynecologist's disdain or disinterest, and in the interest of good patient care in general, the referring gynecologist should make it clear to the patient that he or she will remain involved in her care. The mental health professional should be introduced as an integral member of the health care team, and the gynecologist should ask the patient to call after the mental health appointment to report on how it went and to make a follow-up appointment with the gynecologist.

Where to Refer: Which Mental Health Professional?

Mental disorders are treated by social workers, psychologists, members of the clergy (often the first to be consulted), and various kinds of counselors as well as by psychiatrists. The distinctions among mental health professionals are not generally well known or understood by the lay public. The criteria for membership in each profession can vary from place to place and institution to institution. Social workers and psychologists can be educated at the bachelor's, master's, or doctoral level. In some states, licensure is required; generally, social workers require a master's degree and psychologists a doctoral degree, as well as supervised clinical experience, to qualify. The category of counselor includes a wide variety of practitioners, including marriage counselors, pastoral counselors, school counselors, family counselors, and others. The training of social workers may focus on social policy, institutional work, the psychosocial aspects of medical illness, or individual psychotherapy.

Practitioners of all these disciplines may or may not be trained in psychotherapy. For symptoms not meeting criteria for a major psychiatric disorder, in a patient who is able to eat, sleep, and carry out her duties, supportive psychotherapy provided by an trained mental health professional may suffice. Doctoral-level psychologists and neuropsychologists can also perform testing that can be diagnostically helpful, especially in identifying and localizing brain pathology and in defining intelligence levels. Undiagnosed cognitive deficits may contribute to noncompliance with gynecologic care as well as other problems.

Trained social workers are often knowledgeable about community resources for patients and their families and about the impact of gynecologic diseases and treatments on them. Self-help or professionally led therapy groups can be helpful for patients reacting to gynecologic problems such as infertility or malignancy. Participation in a supportive group lengthens the survival time and improves the quality of life for some patients with cancer (20–25).

Psychiatrists are the only medically trained mental health professionals. They are particularly important with diagnostic dilemmas, especially when there is a question of psychological or behavioral manifestations of medical illness and pharmacologic treatment, and when a medical understanding of the gynecologic condition and treatment is necessary for clinical care. Of all mental health professionals, only psychiatrists can prescribe psychoactive medications and other biologic interventions as well as psychotherapies. Psychiatrists treat the most seriously ill patients and take responsibility for psychiatric emergencies.

In light of frequent occurrence of psychiatric problems in gynecologic practice, it is worthwhile for the gynecologist to develop an ongoing relationship with one or more local mental health professionals. The state psychiatric society may have a list of subspecialists in "consultation liaison" psychiatry. The availability of familiar and trusted resources enhances the likelihood that problems will be identified and addressed. It is also important to keep up-to-date information on local suicide prevention and other kinds of hot lines and resources for battered women and for mothers who may pose a danger to their children.

Specific Disorders

Whenever a patient's thinking, emotions, or behaviors cause concern, the gynecologist should first consider a nonpsychiatric medical disorder and a reaction to prescribed or illicit drugs. Psychiatric disorders frequently coexist with these conditions as well.

Mood Disorders

Definitions and Diagnostic Criteria

Mood is the emotional coloration of a person's experience. Mood may be pathologically elevated (mania) or lowered (depression) or may alternate between the two (bipolar or manic-depressive disorder) (26). Mood disorders are frequently confused with the inevitable ups and downs of everyday life, such as the reactions to difficult situations, including gynecologic conditions. Because of this confusion, both patients and their loved ones become frustrated when well-meaning attempts to reason with them, distract them, or do thoughtful things for them fail to influence their protractedly disturbed moods.

Mania

Mania is characterized by:

1. Elevated mood, with euphoria or without irritability
2. Grandiosity
3. Pressured, speeded-up speech, and physical activity
4. Increased energy
5. Decreased sleep
6. Reckless and potentially damaging behaviors, such as wild expenditures and promiscuity.

Mania can be acute or subacute (hypomania). Hypomania can produce self-confidence, ebullience, energy, and productivity that are the envy of others, and the patient is very reluctant to relinquish this mood for treatment and return to normal. It can therefore be particularly difficult to arrest the condition before it progresses to full-blown mania. Acute mania is a life-threatening condition; without treatment, patients literally exhaust themselves with frantic activity in the absence of adequate nutrition and rest.

Depression

The overall lifetime prevalence of affective disorders is 8.3%; the 6-month prevalence is 5.8%. During the reproductive years, depression is 2 to 3 times more common in women than in men (27–29). The highest incidence of depression is in the age group of 25 to 44 years, but depression occurs in every age group, from toddlers to the aged. Women have a lifetime risk of 10% to 25% and a point prevalence of 5% to 9% (30–32). Depression is the single most common reason for psychiatric hospitalization in the United States. As many as 15% of individuals with severe depressive disorders are successful in committing suicide. Depression is a recurrent disorder; of those who experience a major depressive episode, 50% have a second one. Of these, 70% have a third, and the incidence continues to increase with each subsequent episode. It is difficult to know whether the incidence of depression has increased over the years recently; diagnostic criteria in the past were vague and very different from those used in DSM III and IV. There is no evidence that employment outside the home increases women's vulnerability to depression, although the need to carry out multiple roles in the absence of adequate social support can be stressful (33–36).

Depression is characterized by:

1. Sad mood or irritability
2. Hopelessness
3. Helplessness
4. Decreased ability to concentrate
5. Decreased energy
6. Interference with sleep, generally with early awakening, inability to return to sleep, and failure to feel rested; in atypical cases, with increased sleep
7. Decreased appetite and weight; in atypical cases, increased food intake
8. Withdrawal from social relationships
9. Inability to enjoy previously gratifying activities
10. Loss of libido
11. Guilt
12. Psychomotor retardation or agitation
13. Thoughts of death or suicide.

The patient who has five or more of the signs and symptoms of depression for most of each day for weeks or more has a clinical depression. Depression may be acute or chronic (dysthymic disorder). Depression can be caused by genetic, neurophysiologic, and environmental factors. Trauma in early life plays a role. Serotonin is a major mediator. Changes appear on magnetic resonance imaging, and are reversed with effective treatment or spontaneous recovery. The average duration of a major depressive episode is approximately 9 months.

Depression may be precipitated by an adverse life event such as an interpersonal loss, economic reversal, or serious illness (37,38). When there is an identifiable precipitant, there is a danger that the depression will be written off as the inevitable reaction to the event rather than considered properly as a complication, like infection or pneumonia, requiring active treatment. When a patient's symptoms meet criteria for the diagnosis, treating the depression will make her much more able to cope with the precipitating situation. Co-occurring gynecologic or other medical illness can cause signs and symptoms similar to those of depression—loss of energy, sleep, and appetite—but does not cause guilt, hopelessness, or helplessness (16).

Gynecologic Issues

The incidence of depression peaks, and the gender difference prevails, during the reproductive years, which has provoked study of both psychosocial and biologic factors. There may be a subgroup of women who are vulnerable, not to absolute circulating hormone levels, but to hormonal changes. These women experience severe premenstrual mood symptoms, postpartum depression and, possibly, depression in association with hormonal influences such as hormonal contraceptive methods, menopause, and hormone treatments.

Premenstrual Syndrome

Depending on the methodology used to gather the data, many women, perhaps a majority, experience mood and behavioral changes associated with the menstrual cycle, and many women seek care for self-diagnosed PMS, or premenstrual syndrome. **Perhaps 3% to 5% of menstruating women suffer from symptoms so marked that they qualify for a diagnosis of premenstrual dysphoric disorder (PMDD).** These categories have been the subject of many debates. In the United States, the prevalence of attitudes linking the menstrual cycle to adverse mood and behavioral changes is so high that it skews women's perceptions, the way they report symptoms to researchers, and the factors to which they attribute negative feelings. No specific hormone levels or markers are associated with premenstrual symptoms (39).

Most women who seek care for PMS have symptoms not related to the timing of the menstrual cycle (40,41). Therefore careful assessment is essential. Before the diagnosis of PMS or PMDD can be determined, a woman must record symptom ratings daily for at least two full cycles. Records of emotions and behaviors should be kept separate from menstrual records to avoid confounding patients' perceptions. At the same time, the patient must be screened for other psychiatric disorders, including depression, personality disorders, and domestic abuse.

While the evaluation proceeds, the clinician can recommend a number of lifestyle changes that have proved effective in milder cases. These include:

- Elimination of caffeine from the diet
- Smoking cessation
- Regular exercise
- Regular meals and a nutritious diet
- Adequate sleep
- Stress reduction.

Stress reduction can be accomplished by reducing or delegating responsibilities, insofar as that is possible, and devoting part of every day to relaxation techniques such as yoga. Still, many women experience stresses they cannot reduce: responsibility for the care of children and aging relatives, running a household, and employment often must be balanced.

The selective *serotonin reuptake inhibitors (SSRIs)* have proven effective for PMDD in clinical trials. As of this writing, fluoxetine has received U.S. Food and Drug Administration (FDA) approval for this indication, and other SSRIs are in the midst of the approval process (42–45). Although SSRIs and all other antidepressants require about 2 weeks of daily administration to achieve therapeutic effect, it appears that fluoxetine is effective for PMDD when taken in the usual daily doses for just the 1 to 2 weeks preceding menstruation. The medication has been packaged for this specific indication and dosage regimen. It is thought that the mode of action of SSRIs when used in this fashion is different from that which alleviates major depression. Other medications used for the treatment of PMS are shown in Table 12.2.

Other Reproductive Events

Infertility is described by most women undergoing treatment as the most stressful event of their lives. Each unsuccessful treatment is experienced as the loss of a hoped-for pregnancy. The loss or a fetus or newborn induces grief, which entails some of the same symptoms as depression. Patients should not be pressed to "put the loss behind them" or expected to be "over it" within several months. Some feelings of sadness may persist for years. However,

Table 12.2. Scientific Basis of Selected Medications Used to Treat PMS

Treatment	Scientific Basis	Advantages	Disadvantages	Notes
Alprazolam	Several double-blind, placebo-controlled, randomized crossover studies. Results were mixed. Placebo was as effective as alprazolam in some studies.	Oral medication appears to be more effective in alleviating depression and anxiety symptoms than physical symptoms.	Potential for dependence, requires tapering; drowsiness reported by many subjects; long-term effects unknown; safety during pregnancy unknown.	The studies involved highly selective groups of women. There was a high dropout rate in one of the positive studies. In one study that found alprazolam effective, 87% of the women had a history of major depression or an anxiety disorder. Different doses were used in the studies (0.75–2.25 mg); the standard effective dosage is unknown.
Fluoxetine (Prozac)	Several double-blind, randomized, placebo-controlled, crossover trials. All found fluoxetine effective.	Well tolerated; single daily oral dose. Significant decrease in psychic and behavioral symptoms.	Long-term effects unknown. Safety during pregnancy unknown. Appears less effective in controlling physical symptoms.	Trials involved very small, highly select groups of women. Duration of treatment did not exceed 3 months. All trials used 20 mg orally daily.
Gonadotropin-releasing hormone agonist	Several small, double-blind, randomized, placebo-controlled, crossover trials. Most patients experienced improvement.	Rapidly reversible; many patients report being virtually symptom-free during therapy.	Produces pseudomenopause; expensive; risk for osteoporosis, hypoestrogenic symptoms. Usually given for only short periods of time.	An add-back regimen of estrogen-progestin in addition to gonadotropin-releasing hormone agonist has been reported. If replicated, it may have potential for an effective, long-term treatment for premenstrual syndrome.
Spironolactone	Several double-blind, randomized, placebo-controlled trials. Mixed results.	May alleviate bloating and improve symptoms related to mood. Oral medication taken once or twice a day. Nonaddictive.	Effectiveness not proven consistently across studies.	Spironolactone is the only diuretic that has shown effectiveness in treating premenstrual syndrome in controlled, randomized trials. Method of action may be antiandrogen properties.
Vitamin B_6	Ten randomized double-blind trials. About one-third of the trials reported positive results, one-third reported negative results, and one-third reported ambiguous results.	—	No conclusive evidence that vitamin B_6 is more effective than placebo.	Doses ranged from 50 to 500 mg. Only one study involved more than 40 subjects. The large multicenter trial (N = 204) reported similar results for placebo and vitamin B_6.

PMS; premenstrual syndrome.
From **The American College of Obstetricians and Gynecologists.** *Committee Opinion.* Washington, DC: ACOG, 1995, with permission.

their sleep, appetite, and other vital functions and behaviors should begin to improve after a few weeks (37). Depression can complicate grief and should be treated. There is no evidence that induced abortion increases the incidence of clinical depression.

Peripartum Depression

The incidence of depression does not decrease during pregnancy and increases to approximately 10% postpartum. It must be distinguished from the transitory, self-limited, and very common "baby blues." Mild cases can be managed with psychotherapy. Moderate-to-severe cases may require antidepressant medications. Although no agent can be declared perfectly safe for use during pregnancy and lactation, the older SSRI agents have been well studied, yielding little or no evidence of adverse effects on the fetus or nursing infant (46,47). Medication should not be stopped arbitrarily, nor breast feeding prohibited.

Menopause

Although menopause was assumed for many years to be associated with an increased incidence of depression, this assumption has not been borne out in empirical studies. Whereas some patients are upset by their loss of fertility, others find menopause liberating (48,49). Patients who have suffered PMS or postpartum depression may, however, be vulnerable. Patients with depression at the time of menopause should be assessed for psychosocial precipitants and domestic abuse.

Depression in elderly patients can cause a pseudodementia, characterized by decreased activity and interest and what appears to be forgetfulness. Unlike patients with organically based dementia, these patients report memory loss rather than trying to compensate and cover up for it.

Approach to the Patient

The severity of depression is determined by the patient's emotional pain and the degree of interference with her normal functioning. Depression is an agonizingly painful but readily diagnosable and treatable disease (3). Nevertheless, it shares the stigma of all psychiatric disorders. Patients and their families often attribute the signs and symptoms of depression to life circumstances or to a medical condition, either diagnosed or undiagnosed. The persistence of symptoms in the face of a pleasant life situation or the failure of the patient to respond to attempts at cheering, such as changes of scene, often exacerbate suffering by provoking guilt in the patient and frustration in her significant others. Patients are more likely to report low energy and general malaise than depressed mood. Even patients with moderately severe depression can continue to function and can appear not only normal, but cheerful. The only way to rule out depression is by following the diagnostic criteria (26).

Management

Both antidepressant medication and psychotherapy are effective treatments for depression. There is evidence that a combination of the two produces the best outcomes. There are many forms of psychotherapy. Those that have been specifically studied for efficacy in the treatment of depression are cognitive-behavioral therapy and interpersonal therapy. These forms of therapy are focused on present thoughts, feelings, relationships, and behaviors. They proceed for a set number of sessions, usually no more than 16 weekly sessions, in a prescribed, predetermined direction (50). Supportive and psychodynamic psychotherapy are less clearly defined and studied modalities that also may be of help.

It is especially important for the patient to have ample opportunity to work out her feelings about having a psychiatric disorder, understand how it has affected her life, and feel comfortable about taking any medication prescribed. Patients often attribute depression to weakness or laziness, and they often confuse antidepressants with stimulants and other psychoactive drugs. It is useful to provide the patient with written material about depression so that she can review it and explain the diagnosis to her family and friends.

The types and characteristics of antidepressants are in Table 12.3. All of these agents have comparable therapeutic efficacy and all require at least 2 to 4 weeks to take full effect. It is not yet possible to identify which patients will respond best to which medications; responses vary on an individual basis, even within the same class of medications. The choice of antidepressant, therefore, is based on side effects, dosage schedule, cost, and familiarity of the physician (Table 12.4). Patients tend to respond to medications that have worked for them in the past and to those that have worked for depressed family members. It is essential to continue active management until the patient has not only responded but has returned to her premorbid level of mood and function. If she does not recover completely, she should be referred to a psychiatrist (51).

Table 12.3. Pharmacology of Antidepressant Medications

Drug	Therapeutic Dosage Range (mg/day)	Average (range) of Elimination Half-lives (hours)[a]	Potentially Fatal Drug Interactions
Tricyclics			
Amitriptyline (Elavil, Endep)	75–300	24 (16–46)	Antiarrhythmics, MAO inhibitors
Clomipramine (Anafranil)	75–300	24 (20–40)	Antiarrhythmics, MAO inhibitors
Desipramine (Norpramin, Pertofrane)	75–300	18 (12–50)	Antiarrhythmics, MAO inhibitors
Doxepin (Adapin, Sinequan)	75–300	17 (10–47)	Antiarrhythmics, MAO inhibitors
Imipramine (Janimine, Tofranil)	75–300	22 (12–34)	Antiarrhythmics, MAO inhibitors
Nortiptyline (Aventyl, Pamelor)	40–200	26 (18–88)	Antiarrhythmics, MAO inhibitors
Protriptyline (Vivactil)	20–60	76 (54–124)	Antiarrhythmics, MAO inhibitors
Trimipramine (Surmontil)	75–300	12 (8–30)	Antiarrhythmics, MAO inhibitors
Heterocyclics			
Amoxapine (Asendin)	100–600	10 (8–14)	MAO inhibitors
Bupropion (Wellbutrin)	225–450	14 (8–24)	MAO inhibitors (possibly)
Maprotiline (Ludiomil)	100–225	43 (27–58)	MAO inhibitors
Trazodone (Desyrel)	150–600	8 (4–14)	—
Selective serotin reuptake inhibitors			
Fluoxetine (Prozac)	10–40	168 (72–360)[b]	MAO inhibitors
Paroxetine (Paxil)	20–50	24 (3–65)	MAO inhibitors[c]
Sertraline (Zoloft)	50–150	24 (10–30)	MAO inhibitors[c]
Monoamine oxidase inhibitors (MAO inhibitors)[d]			
Isocarboxazid (Marplan)	30–50	Unknown	For all three MAO inhibitors: vasoconstrictors,[e] decongestants,[e] meperidine, and possibly other narcotics
Phenelzine (Nardil)	45–90	2 (1.5–4.0)	
Tranylcypromine (Parnate)	20–60	2 (1.5–3.0)	

[a] Half-lives are affected by age, sex, race, concurrent medications, and length of drug exposure.
[b] Includes both fluoxetine and norfluoxetine.
[c] By extrapolation from fluoxetine data.
[d] MAO inhibition lasts longer (7 days) than drug half-life.
[e] Including pseudoephedrine, phenylephrine, phenylpropanolamine, epinephrine, norepinephrine, and others.
From **Depression Guideline Panel.** *Depression in primary care: detection, diagnosis, and treatment.* Quick reference guide for clinicians, No. 5. Rockville, MD: U.S. Department of Health and Human Services, Public Health Service, Agency for Health Care Policy and Research; 1993:15; AHCPR pub no 93-0552, with permission.

Tricyclic antidepressants are the oldest and least expensive antidepressants. They all have significant anticholinergic side effects that may be problematic in medically ill and elderly patients. They are associated with some slowing of intracardiac conduction, but this side effect can be tolerated and managed in all but a few patients, and can be therapeutic for those with hyperconductibility. Tricyclic antidepressants should be taken in divided doses through the day, although bedtime dosing may help patients who have difficulty sleeping. Some tricyclics, such as *nortriptyline,* have "therapeutic windows"—blood levels above or below which they are not effective—that must be monitored. The average dose for tricyclics is 225 mg/day in divided doses. The most important drawback of tricyclics is their lethality in overdose, especially because they are used with patients already at risk for suicide. In the rare event that that they must be used by a potentially suicidal patient, the patient must be given only a few pills at a time.

Monoamine oxidase (MAO) inhibitors are especially effective for atypical depression. They require dietary restrictions and can be used only in patients who are able to understand and comply with those restrictions in order to avoid hypertensive crises.

Table 12.4. Side-Effect Profiles of Antidepressant Medications

	Side Effect[a]						
		Central Nervous System		Cardiovascular			
	Anticholinergic[b]	*Drowsiness*	*Insomnia/ Agitation*	*Orthostatic Hypotension*	*Cardiac Arrhythmia*	*Gastrointestinal Distress*	*Weight Gain (over 6 kg)*
Amitriptyline	4+	4+	0	4+	3+	0	4+
Desipramine	1+	1+	1+	2+	2+	0	1+
Doxepin	3+	4+	0	2+	2+	0	3+
Imipramine	3+	3+	1+	4+	3+	1+	3+
Nortriptyline	1+	1+	0	2+	2+	0	1+
Protriptyline	2+	1+	1+	2+	2+	0	0
Trimipramine	1+	4+	0	2+	2+	0	3+
Amoxapine	2+	2+	2+	2+	3+	0	1+
Maprotiline	2+	4+	0	0	1+	0	2+
Trazodone	0	4+	0	1+	1+	1+	1+
Bupropion	0	0	2+	0	1+	1+	0
Fluoxetine	0	0	2+	0	0	3+	0
Paroxetine	0	0	2+	0	0	3+	0
Sertraline	0	0	2+	0	0	3+	0
Monoamine oxidase inhibitors	1	1+	2+	2+	0	1+	2+

[a] Numerals indicate the likehood of side effect occurring ranging from 0 for absent or rare to 4+ for relatively common.
[b] Dry mouth, blurred vision, urinary hesitancy, constipation.
From **Depression Guideline Panel.** *Depression in primary care: detection, diagnosis, and treatment.* Quick reference guide for clinicians, No. 5. Rockville, MD: U.S. Department of Health and Human Services, Public Health Service, Agency for Health Care Policy and Research; 1993:14; AHCPR pub no 93-0553, with permission.

SSRIs pose few risks of medical or suicidal complications. Side effects include anxiety, tremor, headache, and gastrointestinal upset (either diarrhea or constipation), and usually abate within a few days of the onset of treatment. A more serious side effect is loss of libido and interference with orgasm (52). Patients may be reluctant to report this side effect, but it may be the reason they discontinue treatment. Some women are willing to accept this side effect because it is an acceptable price to pay for recovery and because depression interferes with their sexual functioning anyway. Female patients are frequently concerned about weight gain. In one study, it appeared that a weight gain of 5 to 7 pounds may be expected. It is difficult to know, however, whether the weight gain is a result of the medication alone or whether it results from improved appetite associated with recovery from depression. This concern should be brought into the open; patients may be advised to watch their diets carefully while taking the medication.

SSRIs are administered in a once-a-day regimen, with little need for dosage adjustments in most cases. It is important to continue treatment until the patient is fully recovered. SSRIs have long half-lives, so occasional missed doses do not constitute a problem. There is an SSRI withdrawal syndrome, however, and patients should be cautioned not to discontinue their medication without consulting the physician, and only then by gradually decreasing the dose. SSRIs are considerably more expensive than tricyclic antidepressants. They were not initially tested in older women, but several are under consideration by the FDA for administration to this age group (53).

Atypical Agents

Medications considered atypical include *venlafaxine* (54–56), *lithium* salts, and anticonvulsants, which are effective mood stabilizers used for bipolar disorders (57,58), and *bupropion.*

Bupropion must be taken twice a day. It lowers the seizure threshold significantly more than other antidepressants. It is used, under a special trade name, for smoking cessation, and thus is particularly useful for depressed smokers. *Bupropion* seems to cause fewer sexual side effects than the SSRIs and may decrease these side effects when added to an SSRI regimen.

Suicide

The most critical issue in the assessment and referral of depressed patients is the possibility of suicide. Risk factors for suicide include:

- Depression
- Recent losses
- Previous suicide attempts, even if seemingly not serious
- Impulsivity
- Concurrent alcohol or substance abuse
- Current or past physical or sexual abuse
- Family history of suicide
- A plan to commit suicide
- The means to carry out the plan.

Women attempt suicide more frequently than men, but men complete the act more frequently than women (59,60). This is probably due, at least in the past, to men's use of more drastic or irreversible means, such as firearms, while women tend to overdose and can be treated if discovered.

The association between unsuccessful past self-destructive behavior and successful suicide is counterintuitive. It would seem that someone who had repeatedly made suicidal gestures is more interested in the responses of others than in ending her life. However, past attempts or gestures increase the risk of completed suicide, and expressed suicidality in such patients cannot be dismissed. Most people who commit suicide have consulted a nonpsychiatric physician within the prior month. All clinicians must be prepared to discuss the possibility of suicide with their patients.

Inquiry about suicidal ideation and behavior is an inherent part of every mental status examination and is mandatory for every patient with past or current depression or evidence of self-destructive behavior. It follows from discussion of difficulties in the patient's life or mood, or the physician can open the subject by mentioning that almost everyone has thoughts of death at one time or another. Most patients will immediately volunteer that they have had such thoughts and that they have no intention of acting on them. They will often add the reasons: they have too much to look forward to, it is against their religion, it would hurt their family.

It is important to distinguish between the wish to be dead and the intention to kill oneself. In the context of a trusting doctor-patient relationship, patients will nearly always tell the truth about their feelings. A patient in a painful life situation—a chronic, painful, or terminal medical condition, the birth of a severely damaged child, or a grievous loss—may express a wish to die, and even refuse recommended medical care, but emphatically disavow any intention of actively harming herself.

If the patient has previously engaged in self-destructive behavior impulsively, without a plan or warning, it is wise to consult a psychiatrist. If a patient is actively contemplating suicide, she must see a psychiatrist immediately. Other mental health professionals may be helpful but are less likely to have dealt extensively with and assumed responsibility for suicidal patients, to be able to determine whether the patient should be hospitalized, and to have admitting privileges. Until she is in the physical presence of a psychiatrist, or in a safe environment such as a hospital emergency room, a suicidal patient should be observed and protected at all times—every second—whether she is in the consulting room or the bathroom. The staff member assigned to remain with her may not leave to make a telephone call, go to the bathroom, or get a cup of coffee. Family members may offer to monitor the patient, and can sometimes be effective, but the health care professional is responsible for ensuring that they understand these necessities. It is better to risk inconvenience and possible embarrassment to both the gynecologist and the patient than to risk a fatal outcome. Once suicide is a possibility, only a psychiatrist can make the decision that a patient is safe (33).

Psychiatric referral can also be useful in less dramatic cases: when the gynecologist lacks experience or is overloaded with other needy patients, when a first trial of treatment is unsuccessful or there is uncertainty about the diagnosis when domestic violence or substance abuse may be present, and when the depression is recurrent.

Anxiety Disorders

Diagnosis

Anxiety is a sense of dread without objective cause for fear, accompanied by the usual physical concomitants of fear. Although every human being has anxious feelings from time to time, anxiety disorders are anxiety to the point of pathology: genuine painful, disabling diseases. The anxiety disorders include generalized anxiety disorder, panic disorder, agoraphobia, specific phobias, obsessive-compulsive disorder, and posttraumatic stress disorder (61,62).

Generalized anxiety disorder is a condition in which anxiety pervades every aspect of a patient's life. She suffers from restlessness, easy fatigability, difficulty concentrating, irritability, muscle tension, and sleep disturbances. Whereas depressed patients fall asleep more or less normally and then awaken earlier than intended, anxious patients have difficulty falling asleep.

Panic disorder is characterized by panic attacks: acute periods, generally lasting about 15 minutes, with intense fear and at least four of the following symptoms:

- Palpitations
- Diaphoresis
- Trembling
- Shortness of breath
- A choking sensation
- Chest discomfort
- Gastrointestinal distress
- Lightheadedness
- A sense of unreality
- Fear of going crazy or dying
- Paresthesias
- Chills or hot flushes.

The attacks can recur without specific precipitating events. The patient is preoccupied with them and makes behavioral changes she hopes will avert future attacks: avoiding specific situations, assuring herself there is an escape route from certain situations, or refusing to be alone.

The symptoms of panic attacks are often confused with the symptoms of cardiac or pulmonary disease. They lead to many fruitless trips to the emergency department and to costly, even invasive, medical investigations. A careful history can establish the correct diagnosis in most cases.

***Agoraphobia* is the avoidance of situations in which the patient fears she may be trapped, such as the center of a row in the theater or driving over a bridge.** She fears that such a situation will trigger a panic attack. Agoraphobia and panic disorder can occur separately or together.

***Specific phobias* are irrational fears of certain objects or situations, although the patient recognizes that the object or situation poses no real danger.** Of particular concern in gynecology are fear of needles and fear of vomiting. Social phobia causes the patient to fear and avoid situations in which the patient fears she will be observed by others in a humiliating light. Patients may alter their lives to avoid these anxieties, interfering with their interpersonal relationships and their ability to carry out their responsibilities, or they may manage to carry on despite considerable psychological pain.

***Obsessive-compulsive disorder* is characterized by obsessions: recurrent impulses, images, or thoughts that the patient recognizes as her own, dislikes, and cannot control, or compulsions: intrusive, repetitive behaviors that the patient feels she must perform in order to prevent some dire consequence.** The disorder can be mild or totally crippling; in one-half of the cases it becomes chronic. This disorder is classified as an anxiety disorder because the obsessions are anxiety-provoking, and the compulsions are performed in order to avoid overwhelming anxiety.

***Posttraumatic stress disorder (PTSD)* is the result of exposure to an event that threatens the life or safety of the patient or others.** At the time of the trauma, the patient experiences horror, terror, or a sense of helplessness. Afterward, the patient may lose conscious memory of all or part of the event, avoid situations reminiscent of it, and become acutely distressed when she cannot avoid them. She feels numb and detached, without a sense of the future. She is hyperarousable and irritable and experiences difficulty sleeping and concentrating. She reexperiences the event in nightmares, flashbacks, and intrusive thoughts.

Epidemiology

Panic disorder without agoraphobia is twice as common in women as it is in men; panic disorder with agoraphobia is 3 times more common in women. Onset is generally in young adulthood, often following a stressful event. The lifetime prevalence is 1.5% to 3.5%; the 1-year prevalence is 1% to 2%. A substantial percentage of patients experience depressive episodes as well. Phobias are somewhat more common in women, depending on the object of the phobia. The 1-year prevalence is 9%, and the lifetime prevalence is 10% to 11%. Obsessive-compulsive disorder is equally common in women and men, with evidence of familial transmission. Prevalences are 2.5% for lifetime and 1.5% to 2.1% for 1 year. Posttraumatic stress disorder has a lifetime prevalence of 1% to 14%; victims of violence (including child abuse and wife battering) and war are at increased risk.

Assessment

Given the relationship between anxiety disorders and traumatic experiences, the presence of signs and symptoms of anxiety disorders should trigger inquiries about abuse. It is important to know how long the patient has suffered from the disorder, what previous attempts have been made to diagnose and treat it, and the effect is has had on her psychological development, life choices, lifestyle, and relationships. In some cases, the entire family will have organized their schedules and activities around the patient's symptoms and limitations; they may not volunteer this information.

Management

Treatment should not be limited to antianxiety medications. Managing, even tolerating, patient anxiety is an anxiety-provoking process; anxiety is contagious, and raises the specter of unlimited demands on the gynecologist's time and energy. Prescribing medication is a familiar and comfortable, if not optimal, way to end a medical interview. The overprescription of benzodiazepines has become a cause for medical and media concern. It is useful to defer the administration of anxiolytics until the impact of the physician's support and interest can be assessed (63). Treatment should address the effects on the patient's life and family as well as the signs and symptoms of the specific disease (64).

Benzodiazepines are most useful in acute situations. Use can quickly become chronic, with escalating dosages, diminishing therapeutic effects, and increasing demands on the physician. So many women are taking benzodiazepines, and taking them for granted, that they forget to include them in their medical histories. Patients admitted to the hospital may suffer unrecognized withdrawal symptoms, complicating their treatment, or may continue to take medications from a personal supply without informing the medical staff. For chronic anxiety and many cases of acute anxiety, there are highly effective and safer approaches.

It is important to ascertain the source of anxiety or obsessiveness. Many patients and their families are anxious because of misinformation or misunderstanding about a medical problem or treatment. Few patients can absorb all the information about significant gynecologic conditions at a single visit, but most feel that asking questions will burden the physician or make them look stupid. Patients also suffer anxiety when there is disagreement among family members or medical staff about the diagnosis or recommended treatment. Many patients dread certain aspects of care, sometimes on the basis of past experience or outdated information. A simple explanation or alteration in procedure can alleviate the anxiety. For example, a reassuring family member or friend can be allowed to stay with the patient during a diagnostic test, sedation can be administered orally or by inhalation before an intravenous line is inserted, or the patient can be allowed control over her own analgesia.

Behavioral interventions are extremely useful in managing anxiety without problematic side effects. They include hypnosis, desensitization, and relaxation techniques (65–69). Whereas the use of prescribed medications fosters the patient's dependence, these techniques provide her with tools to cope with her own anxiety. Specialists in behavioral medicine, usually psychologists, are expert in these techniques. Interested gynecologists can master some of them as well.

It is easy to be trapped into a cat-and-mouse game with an anxious and needy patient. Faced with an obsessional or anxious, talkative, and needy patient in the midst of bedside rounds, clinic, or office hours, the clinician can develop a pattern of avoidance, sometimes alternating with overindulgence stemming from feelings of guilt. This kind of behavior results in sporadic, unpredictable reinforcement of the patient's symptoms and demands for attention and is very likely to increase them. Attempting to escape by appearing distracted or harassed, or yielding with despair to the destruction of the day's schedule and the care of other patients, simply heightens the patient's anxiety.

It is preferable to develop a prospective approach. Gynecologists tend to underrate the power of their personal interactions with patients and their own ability to structure and limit those interactions appropriately. The patient should be informed of the time available and asked to focus on her most important problem, with other problems to be discussed at future, scheduled appointments. Instead of scheduling appointments and returning telephone calls grudgingly, in response to patient demands, the gynecologist should inform the patient that her condition requires regular, brief, scheduled visits. If she has been contacting the office more often than visits can reasonably be scheduled, she should be asked to call between visits, at prearranged times, to advise the staff of her progress. There are useful self-help groups for patients with various psychiatric conditions, and their families. Groups focused on victimization can validate patients' experiences and pain and help them build new lives, but they can also interfere with their motivation to find other ways to identify themselves and obtain gratification.

Medication does have a place in the management of anxiety disorders (70–72). Table 12.5 describes many of these agents. Sertraline recently received FDA approval for the treatment of PTSD, and other selective serotonin reuptake inhibitors are effective for other anxiety

Table 12.5. Compounds Used for Anxiety

Medication	Trade Name	Rate of Absorption[a]	Half-Life[b]	Active Long-Acting Metabolite	Comments
Benzodiazepines					
					Metabolism of benzodiazepines is inhibited by cimetidine, disulfiram, isoniazid, and oral contraceptives. Metabolism of benzodiazepines is enhanced by rifampin.
Alprazolam	*Xanax*	Intermediate	Intermediate	No	Preferred in elderly patients or patients with poor hepatic functions.
Chlordiazepoxide	*Librium,* others	Intermediate	Intermediate	Yes	
Clonazepam	*Klonopin*	Long	Long	No	
Clorazepate	*Tranxene,* others	Short	Short	Yes	
Diazepam	*Valium,* others	Short	Long	Yes	Half-life increased 3 or 4 times in elderly patients.
Lorazepam	*Ativan,* others	Intermediate	Intermediate	No	Preferred in elderly patients or patients with poor hepatic function.
Oxazepam	*Serax*	Long	Intermediate	No	Preferred in elderly patients or patients with poor hepatic function.
Prazepam	*Centrax*	Long	Short	Yes	
Atypical agent					
Buspirone	*BuSpar*	—	—	—	Not effective in panic disorder, little sedation, little risk of dependence or tolerance.

[a] Long ≥2 hours; Intermediate = 1–2 hours; Short ≤1 hour.
[b] Long >20 hours; Intermediate = 6–20 hours; Short <6 hours.
From **Gilman AG, Rall TW, Nies AS, et al.** *The pharmacological basis of therapeutics,* 8th ed. New York: McGraw-Hill, 1990.
From **Stotland NL.** Psychiatric and psychosocial issues in primary care for women. In: **Seltzer VL, Pearse WH,** eds. *Women's primary health care: office practice and procedures.* New York: McGraw-Hill, 1995.

disorders as well. Benzodiazepines are effective when taken for acute anxiety or during relatively brief, time-limited (several days) stressful situations. The specific agent should be chosen on the basis of onset of action and half-life. The patient must be admonished to avoid concomitant use of alcohol and to exercise extreme care about driving or engaging in other activities requiring attention, concentration, and coordination.

Patients who fail to respond to a trial of office counseling or medication, who are unable to fulfill their responsibilities, who exhaust the patience and resources of significant others, who pose a diagnostic dilemma, who consume inordinate quantities of medical resources, or whose symptoms are becoming increasingly worse should be evaluated by a psychiatrist.

Somatizing Disorders

Definitions

Somatizing disorders are those in which psychological conflicts are expressed in the form of physical symptoms. There is a spectrum of somatizing disorders based on the degree to which the patient is consciously aware of or responsible for the onset of the symptoms. The spectrum ranges from the deliberate malingerer to the so-called *hysteric,* who is completely unaware of the link between her psyche and her physical symptom (73).

Malingering

Malingering is the deliberate mimicking of signs and symptoms of physical or mental illness in order to achieve a tangible personal gain, such as exemption from dangerous military duties or exoneration from criminal responsibility. Factitious disorder, or *Munchausen syndrome,* is a related but poorly understood condition in which the patient actively causes physical damage to herself or feigns somatic symptoms that result in repeated hospital admissions and painful, dangerous, invasive diagnostic and therapeutic procedures. These patients introduce feces or purulent material into wounds or intravenous lines, inject themselves with insulin, or produce hemorrhages.

Significant iatrogenic conditions, such as adhesions from surgery or Cushing's syndrome from the administration of steroids, may develop. These patients are initially engaging but eventually frustrate the staff. When the staff becomes suspicious and calls for a psychiatric consultation, the patient generally flees, only to reappear in another medical facility. As a result, there are little data about the etiology, incidence, and management of this condition. Often these patients are medically sophisticated because they or their family members have had some kind of medical training, as well as knowledge gained during previous hospitalizations. Mothers may enact this disorder through their children, by deliberately making them ill; this is called *Munchausen's by proxy.* Declaring that the patient "only wants attention" is not helpful. Most people want attention, but very few are willing to go to these lengths to get it.

Somatization Disorder

***Somatization disorder* consists of multiple physical symptoms for which adequate medical bases cannot be established, with these symptoms leading either to numerous medical visits or to impairment in the patient's performance of her responsibilities.** The disorder must begin before age 30 and continue for many years after. The diagnosis requires symptoms of pain related to at least four different anatomic sites or physiologic functions, two gastrointestinal symptoms, one sexual or reproductive symptom and one pseudoneurologic symptom or deficit other than pain (seizures, paresis). The patient's perception is that she is "sickly." She responds accurately to questions about her past symptoms and treatments but may not volunteer information about them unless she is asked.

Conversion Disorder

Conversion disorder* is the condition formerly called *hysteria. The patient loses a voluntary motor or sensory function that cannot be explained by medical illness, that is not deliberately produced by the patient, and that appears to be related to psychological stress or conflict. The prognosis is directly related to the length of time from onset to diagnosis and treatment (74–77).

***Pain disorder* is a conversion condition with pain as the only symptom.**

***Body dysmorphic disorder* is preoccupation with a trivial or imagined defect in bodily appearance, a preoccupation that is not alleviated by the many medical and surgical treatments on which the patient insists.** The gynecologist should hesitate to refer such a patient to a plastic surgeon, although plastic surgeons are quite familiar with the condition.

***Hypochondriasis* is not a matter of particular numbers or types of symptoms. It is a patient's (nonpsychotic) conviction or fear that she suffers from a serious disease.**

Epidemiology

Somatization is believed to be the most common and most difficult set of psychological conditions in office practice. It has been estimated that 60% to 80% of the general population experiences one or more somatic symptoms in a given week. Somatization disorder occurs almost exclusively in women; menstrual complaints may be an early sign. Lifetime prevalence in women is 0.2% to 2.0%. Conversion disorder is 2 to 10 times more frequent in women than in men (there is no gender difference in children), and it is more common in rural and disadvantaged populations with little medical sophistication. Conversion disorder may develop into somatization disorder. Reported rates of somatization disorder range from 11 to 300 per 100,000. Pain disorder is extremely common in both genders. Hypochondriasis is equally distributed between men and women; prevalence in general medical practice is estimated to be 4% to 9%. There are few statistics about body dysmorphic disorder, but it seems to be equally distributed between men and women, with an average age of onset of about 30 years.

Assessment

Most somatizing disorders are chronic. The goal of treatment in primary care is not to eliminate all the somatic symptoms but to help the patient cope with them with as little effect on her relationships and responsibilities as possible. Because patients often seek care simultaneously or sequentially from several physicians, it is crucial to ask about all past and current diagnostic procedures, diagnoses, treatments, and responses. Her level of function over the years is also important; prognosis is inversely related to chronicity. The gynecologist needs to know what the patient believes is wrong with her and what she believes she needs in the way of diagnostic and therapeutic interventions.

Management

The management of somatizing disorders is focused on the avoidance of unnecessary medical interventions, iatrogenic medical or psychological complications, and disability. Unfortunately, it is never possible to definitively rule out all possible medical causes. The literature is full of case presentations of patients with multiple sclerosis, brain tumors, and intermittently flaring infections, labeled for years as neurotic before the condition was diagnosed correctly. Patients who for years have had benign gastrointestinal symptoms can get appendicitis.

Patients who have a somatizing disorder often approach each new clinician as the one who, unlike the incompetent and insensitive physicians she has consulted in the past, will finally get to the bottom of her troubles and allow her to live the perfect life that her symptoms have denied her. The gynecologist must not get caught up in these expectations but rather remind the patient that symptoms that have resisted diagnosis and treatment for many years are likely to be challenging ones.

As with anxious patients, it is important not to structure the doctor-patient relationship so that the patient receives attention inconsistently and only in response to escalating symptoms and demands. It is best to schedule frequent, brief office visits during which the clinician allots a small amount of time to listen to and sympathize with the patient's somatic complaints and spends the bulk of the time reinforcing the patient's efforts to function despite her symptoms. Family members should be encouraged to facilitate function rather than invalidism.

It is often tempting to unmask patently psychologically based symptoms by tricking the patient: shouting "Fire!" in the vicinity of a "paralyzed" patient, searching the patient's hospital room or belongings for paraphernalia used to cause symptoms, documenting the patient's behavior when she does not realize she is being observed. Some of these attempts are useful diagnostically, but not therapeutically, and some (searches) are unethical and illegal. Humiliating a frustrating patient may be momentarily gratifying, and may force her to relinquish a symptom, at least temporarily. She may seek care elsewhere, relieving the original treatment team but exacerbating her dysfunction, distrust, and demands on the health care system as a whole.

Patients with conversion, somatization, and hypochondriacal disorders often benefit from prescriptive behavioral regimens aimed at saving face and improving function. It was once believed that a patient so relieved of one symptom would soon substitute another, but this assumption has not been confirmed by empirical evidence. The behavioral regimen should consist of health-promoting activities relevant to the target symptoms, planned in a step-wise progression, and recommended with reasonable medical conviction and authority. For example, the patient with psychogenic difficulty swallowing should be advised to drink only clear liquids, at specified intervals, for a specified number of days, and then go on similarly to full liquids, purees, soft foods, and finally a regular diet. The patient with difficulties in the extremities can undertake an exercise regimen. The patient's preoccupation with her symptoms can be channeled into documentation of her progress in a log that she brings to her medical appointments. She should be advised not to dwell on her symptoms apart from this important notation.

It is critical to remember that patients with somatic complaints due to depression, posttraumatic stress disorder and other anxiety disorders, and domestic violence frequently seek care from gynecologists. In the case of domestic violence, the gynecologist is often the only human contact the abuser allows the patient outside the domestic situation (78–80). These possibilities must be ruled out before care is directed to symptom management.

There is considerable cross-cultural variation in the extent to which feelings and psychological conflicts are somatized. In many Asian cultures, for example, complaints about problems with feelings, behaviors, and interpersonal relationships are almost unheard of; these problems are expressed, diagnosed, and treated somatically. On the other hand, some very sophisticated and psychologically informed patients in the West may dismiss serious somatic signs and symptoms as indications of psychological conflict.

Referral

Patients with somatizing disorders may resist mental health referral more adamantly than any other single class of patients. Focused as they are on physical symptoms, these patients can regard referral as a message that their complaints are not being taken seriously and as a sign of contempt and rejection by the gynecologist. It is particularly useful with these patients to emphasize that distinctions between mind and body are artificial. The brain is part of the body. Our language expresses this synthesis; anxiety causes "butterflies in the stomach," aggravation "gives us a headache," and unwelcome news "gives us a heart attack."

The referral should be framed as support for the patient's suffering rather than as a statement that her problems are "all in her head." The mental health professional should be introduced as a member of the medical team. Some medical institutions have dedicated psychiatric consultation, medical psychiatry, or behavioral medicine services offering expertise in the psychological complications of disease and in somatization. Because so-called *somatic* and *psychological* symptoms often coexist and interact, the gynecologist should work in collaboration with the mental health professional.

Personality Disorders

Personality disorders are pervasive, lifelong, maladaptive patterns of perception and behavior. Patients with personality disorders do not consider themselves symptomatic, but as treated unfairly by circumstances and other people. They view their own behaviors, which can wreak havoc in the health care setting as well as in patients' lives, as normal, expectable, inevitable reactions to these perceived circumstances. To make matters worse, their behaviors tend to provoke in others the very responses that confirm their expectations. For example, a patient who is convinced that people always abandon her clings desperately to others, eventually driving them away.

Personality disorders are organized into clusters in DSM IV. Patients often manifest characteristics of several disorders within a cluster and between clusters.

Cluster A
Paranoid personality disorder
Schizoid personality disorder
Schizotypal personality disorder
Cluster B
Narcissistic personality disorder
Histrionic personality disorder
Borderline personality disorder
Antisocial personality disorder
Cluster C
Avoidant personality disorder
Dependent personality disorder
Obsessive-compulsive personality disorder

Individuals with Cluster A disorders are isolated, suspicious, detached, and odd. Narcissistic patients are grandiose, arrogant, envious, and entitled. Histrionic individuals are flamboyant and provocative. Antisocial patients disregard laws and rules of common decency toward others. Borderline personality disorder causes patients to have difficulty controlling their impulses and maintaining stable moods and relationships. They also engage in self-destructive behaviors. They fluctuate between overvaluation and castigation of the same person, or direct these feelings alternately between one person and another. When this happens on a gynecology service or in the office, it can precipitate significant tensions among the staff. Recent research reveals that many women who have been abused are diagnosed as borderline when posttraumatic stress disorder more accurately fits their symptoms. *Posttraumatic stress disorder* is a less stigmatizing and more treatable condition than abuse.

Epidemiology

Lifetime prevalence of personality disorders as a group is 2.5%. Cluster A disorders are more common in males. Within Cluster B, 75% of cases are female; the prevalence in the general population is 2%. Personality disorders such as narcissistic personality are more common in the clinical population than in the general population. Among cluster C disorders, dependent personality is one of the most frequently diagnosed. Obsessive-compulsive personality is twice as common in males as in females. It is important to distinguish the personality disorder from the symptomatic obsessive-compulsive disorder. There is a strong association between personality disorders and a history of childhood abuse. The possibility of an ongoing abusive situation should be considered as well.

Assessment

The impact of personality disorders ranges widely. At one end of the spectrum, the disorder is an exaggerated personality style. At the other end of the spectrum, the individual suffers terrible emotional pain and is unable to function in work roles or relationships, spending significant periods of time in psychiatric hospitals. As the definition implies, the patient will not seek treatment for the signs and symptoms listed in the diagnostic criteria but instead will have complaints about her treatment by others, their responses to her, and the unfairness and difficulties of life in general. Taking the history, the clinician should frame questions in those same terms: how long have these troubles gone on, and how much do they interfere with her ability to work and relate to others? Personality disorders do not bring patients to gynecologists' offices directly, but they greatly complicate things once patients arrive there.

Management

It generally requires intense and lengthy psychotherapy to effect significant improvement in patients who have personality disorders. The challenge in the gynecology setting is to minimize contention and drain on medical staff while maximizing the likelihood of effective diagnosis and treatment of the patient's medical problems. The most helpful single step is the identification of the personality disorder. Diagnosis enables the gynecologist to recognize the reasons for a patient's problem behaviors, to avoid becoming entangled in fruitless interactions with the patient, and to set limits on her demands that are neither withholding nor overindulgent.

There is increasing evidence that psychotropic medications are useful for personality disorders. Treatment should be provided in consultation with a psychiatrist. The patient's ability to use the medication properly is compromised by impulsivity, self-destructive tendencies, and unstable relationships. Low doses of major tranquilizers are sometimes helpful, especially when the patient has brief psychotic episodes. Minor tranquilizers pose significant risk of habituation, overdose, and physical and psychological habituation. They can be prescribed for temporary stresses, but only in a quantity sufficient for several days and with no refill allowed. At the same time, some patients' anxiety, demands, and power struggles are eased when they are given control over their own use of medication. Such an approach requires enough familiarity with the patient to ensure her safety.

Because the patient with a personality disorder attributes her problems to others, her symptoms cannot be adduced as reasons for psychiatric referral, but her suffering can be. If a diagnosis of a personality disorder is noted in the patient's chart or on insurance forms, it is essential that she be so informed. It is useful to review the DSM IV criteria with her so that she understands the basis for the diagnosis.

Adjustment Disorders

Definitions

Adjustment disorders are temporary, self-limited responses to life stressors that are part of the normative range of human experience (unlike those that precipitate post-traumatic stress disorder). The patient has mood or anxiety symptoms that are sufficient to lead her to seek medical care but that do not meet criteria of sufficient quantity or quality to qualify for psychiatric diagnosis. The diagnosis requires an identifiable stressor, onset within 3 months after the stress begins, and spontaneous resolution within 6 months after the stressor ends. Obviously the latter cannot be determined until the symptoms resolve—but they do rule out the disorder if the symptoms persist beyond that time (81,82).

Adjustment disorders can be distinguished from normal grieving. Grieving produces symptoms similar to those of depression. Interference with function does not persist, but some degree of sadness and preoccupation with the lost loved one often goes on for months and years.

Epidemiology

Adjustment disorders affect males and females equally. Approximately 5% to 20% of patients in outpatient mental health treatment suffer from adjustment disorders. There is little literature on the subject; one study reported a 2.3% prevalence among a sample of patients receiving care in a walk-in general health clinic.

Management

Patients with adjustment disorders can be treated effectively with brief counseling in the primary care setting. The counseling can be provided by the gynecologist or by a nurse clinician, social worker, or psychologist, preferably a member of the office or hospital staff who is familiar with the gynecologist and the practice. The medical setting is sometimes the only one where the patient can vent her feelings and think through her situation. Counseling is aimed at facilitating the patient's own coping skills and helping her to make autonomous decisions about her situation. The gynecologist should follow the patient's progress and facilitate referral to a psychiatrist if symptoms do not resolve.

Eating Disorders

Definitions

Preoccupation with thinness, sometimes to the point of pathology, is a major problem for women in North America. Only a small number of women profess to be satisfied with their weights and body shapes. Nearly all admit to current or recent attempts to limit food intake. Physicians often share social prejudices against overweight patients and can easily exacerbate patients' concerns by making chance comments.

***Anorexia nervosa* is characterized by severe restrictions on food intake, often accompanied by excessive physical exercise and the use of diuretics or laxatives.** Clinical features include menstrual irregularities or amenorrhea, intense, irrational fear of becoming fat, preoccupation with body weight as an indicator of self-worth, and inability to acknowledge the realities and dangers of the condition. Some patients approach gynecologists for care of infertility (83).

***Bulimia* is characterized by eating binges followed by self-induced vomiting or purging.** Patients' weights may be normal or somewhat more. Patients have drastically low self-esteem, and the condition is frequently comorbid with depression (84).

***Obesity* is an increasingly frequent health problem, with little evidence that any non-surgical approach is effective over time.** Sensible eating should be encouraged, and fad or crash diets are medically and psychologically counterproductive (85).

Epidemiology

More than 90% of cases of anorexia and bulimia occur in females. The prevalence is 0.5% to 1.0% in late adolescence and 1% to 3% in early adulthood. There is some evidence of familial transmission.

Assessment

The clinician treating the anorexic patient needs to know how much insight she has into her problem and to assess her mood, relationships, and general level of function. Anorexia poses significant risks of severe metabolic complications and death, often from cardiac consequences of electrolyte abnormalities. Thorough physical and laboratory examination is critical; immediate hospitalization may be necessary.

Management

Patients with anorexia or bulimia should be treated by mental health professionals, preferably subspecialists in this area. The conditions are highly refractory to treatment; patients can resort to elaborate subterfuges to conceal their failure to eat and gain weight. Antidepressant medication is sometimes helpful. Amenorrheic patients should not be treated with ovulation induction. Evaluation for osteopenia and osteoporosis is necessary.

Psychotic Disorders

Definitions

Psychotic disorders are characterized by major distortions of thinking and behavior. They include schizophrenia, schizophreniform disorders, schizoaffective disorders, delusional disorders, and brief psychotic disorders. General medical and toxic conditions must be ruled out. Distinctions between the disorders are based on symptoms, time course, severity, and associated affective symptoms. **The hallmark of psychosis is the presence of delusions or hallucinations.** Hallucinations are sensory perceptions in the absence of external sensory stimuli. Delusions are bizarre beliefs about the nature of motivation of external events. Because there is no reliable definition of "bizarre," the diagnostician working with a patient from an unfamiliar culture must determine whether a given belief is normal in that culture. Delusions and hallucinations are the "positive symptoms" of schizophrenia.

The "negative symptoms" include apathy and loss of connection to others and to interests. The negative symptoms may be more disabling than the positive.

Epidemiology

Schizophrenia occurs in approximately 1% of the population worldwide (86). Onset is in the late teens to mid-30s. Women succumb later and have more prominent mood symptoms and a better prognosis than men. The risk is 10 times greater for first-degree biologic relatives and for individuals of low socioeconomic status. It is unclear whether indigent status is a precipitating stress or a result of psychotic illness.

Assessment

There is wide variability in the functional impact of psychotic disorders. Patients must not be assumed to be incompetent to make medical decision or lead independent lives, especially if they comply with treatment. Patients must be asked specifically about their living situations and coping skills. When psychotic women have responsibility for the care of children, their ability to do so should be assessed in consultation with a mental health expert. Motherhood and child custody are exceedingly sensitive matters for these vulnerable patients.

A relentlessly downhill course is not inevitable; remissions and recovery can occur. Therefore, the patient's mental status must be examined. Under the pressures of a busy medical setting, psychotic illnesses can be overlooked, only to erupt in the labor room, operating room, or recovery room. Patients who believe that conspiracies or Martians are responsible for their symptoms can answer yes-or-no questions without revealing their delusions. Open-ended questions are more useful (87).

Sensationalized media accounts of violent crimes committed by psychotic patients exacerbate public misconceptions about these diseases. Statistically, individuals with psychoses are more likely to be victims than perpetrators of crime. Untreated patients, especially when under the influence of alcohol or other substances, are at somewhat increased risk of violent behavior.

Management

Psychotic illnesses are nearly always managed by psychiatrists. However, a primary care practitioner can readily assume responsibility, in consultation with a psychiatrist, for a stable patient who complies with treatment. When a patient expresses delusions, the clinician may indicate that he or she does not share them, but should not debate with the patient (88–90). It is important to concentrate on the patient's strengths. She can easily be humiliated by thoughtless epithets or behaviors that betray the expectation of violence or incompetence. Patients with severe cases must be treated with an integrated system of social services, family support, rehabilitation, general medical care, psychotherapy, and psychopharmacology. In the process of referral to a mental health professional, the primary clinician should be clear, matter-of-fact, open, and confident of the possibility of successful treatment (91).

References

1. **Schurman RA, Kramer PD, Mitchell JB.** The hidden mental health network: treatment of mental illness by nonpsychiatrist physicians. *Arch Gen Psychiatry* 1985;42:89–94.
2. **Dubovsky SL.** *Psychotherapeutics in primary care.* New York: Grune & Stratton, 1981.
3. **Berndt ER, Koran LM, Finkelstein SN, et al.** Lost human capital from early-onset chronic depression. *Am J Psychiatry* 2000;157:940–947.
4. **Smith I, Adkins S, Walton J.** *Pharmaceuticals: therapeutic review.* New York: Shearson, Lehman, Hutton International Research, 1988.
5. **Pierce C.** Failure to spot mental illness in primary care is a global problem. *Clin Psych News* 1993;21:5.
6. **Margolis RL.** Nonpsychiatric house staff frequently misdiagnose psychiatric disorders in general hospital inpatients. *Psychosomatics* 1994;35:485–491.
7. **Perez-Stable EJ, Miranda J, Munoz RF, et al.** Depression in medical outpatients: underrecognition and misdiagnosis. *Arch Intern Med* 1990;150:1083–1088.

8. **American Psychiatric Association.** *Diagnostic and statistical manual of mental disorders,* 4th ed. Washington, DC: American Psychiatric Press, 1994.

9. **American Psychiatric Association.** *Diagnostic and statistical manual of mental disorders,* 4th ed. Text Revision. Washington, DC, American Psychiatric Association, 2000.

10. **Depression Guideline Panel.** *Depression in primary care: vol 1, detection and diagnosis.* Rockville, MD: US Department of Health and Human Services, Public Health Service, Agency for Health Care Policy and Research; 1993; Clinical practice guideline no 5. AHCPR publication no 93-0550.

11. **Cassem NH.** Depression. In: **Cassem NH,** ed. *Massachusetts General Hospital handbook of general hospital psychiatry.* St. Louis: Mosby Year Book, 1991:237–268.

12. **Murphy GE.** The physician's responsibility for suicide. II: Errors of omission. *Ann Intern Med* 1975;82:305–309.

13. **Veith I.** *Hysteria: the history of a disease.* Chicago: University of Chicago Press, 1965.

14. **Orleans CT, George LK, Houpt JL, et al.** How primary care physicians treat psychiatric disorders: a national survey of family practitioners. *Am J Psychiatry* 1985;142:52–57.

15. **Beckman HB, Frankel RM.** The effect of physician behavior on the collection of data. *Ann Intern Med* 1984;101:692–696.

16. **McGrath E, Keita GP, Strickland BR, et al.** Women and depression: risk factors and treatment issues. Final report of the American Psychological Association's National Task Force on Women and Depression. Washington, DC: American Psychological Association, 1990.

17. **Dubovsky SL, Weissberg MP.** *Clinical psychiatry in primary care,* 3rd ed. Baltimore: Williams & Wilkins, 1986.

18. **Scheiber SC.** The psychiatric interview, psychiatric history, and mental status examination. In: **Hales RE, Yudofsky SC, Talbott JA,** eds. *Textbook of psychiatry,* 2nd ed. Washington, DC: The American Psychiatric Press, 1994:187–219.

19. **Stotland NL, Garrick TR.** *Manual of psychiatric consultation.* Washington, DC: American Psychiatric Press, 1990.

20. **Spiegel D, Bloom JR, Kraemer HL, et al.** Effect of psychosocial treatment on survival of patients with metastatic breast cancer. *Lancet* 1989;2:888–891.

21. **Fawzy FI, Cousins NI, Fawzy NW, et al.** A structured psychiatric intervention for cancer patients. I: Changes over time in methods of coping and affective disturbance. *Arch Gen Psychiatry* 1990;47:720–725.

22. **Cunningham AJ, Edmonds CV, Jenkins GP, et al.** A randomized controlled trial of the effects of group psychological therapy on survival in women with metastatic breast cancer. *Psychooncology* 1998;7:508–517.

23. **Maunsell E, Brisson J, Deschênes L.** Social support and survival among women with breast cancer. *Cancer* 1995;76:631–637.

24. **Gellert GA, Maxwell RM, Siegel BS.** Survival of breast cancer patients receiving adjunctive psychosocial support therapy: a 10-year follow-up study. *J Clin Oncol* 1993;11:66–69.

25. **Blake-Mortimer J, Gore-Felton C, Kimerling R, et al.** Improving the quality and quantity of life among patients with cancer: a review of the effectiveness of group psychotherapy. *Eur J Cancer* 1999;35:1581–1586.

26. **Jefferson JW, Greist JH.** Mood disorders. In: **Hales RE, Yudofsky SC, Talbott JA,** eds. *Textbook of psychiatry,* 2nd ed. Washington, DC: American Psychiatric Press, 1994:465–494.

27. **Goldman N, Ravid R.** Community surveys: sex differences in mental illness. In: **Guttentag M, Salasin S, Belle D,** eds. *The mental health of women.* New York: Academic Press, 1980.

28. **Nolen-Hoeksema S.** *Sex differences in depression.* Stanford, CA: Stanford University Press, 1990.

29. **Weissman MM, Leaf PJ, Holzer CE, et al.** The epidemiology of depression: an update on sex differences in rates. *J Affect Disord* 1984;7:179–188.

30. **Regier DA, Boyd JK, Burke JD Jr, et al.** One-month prevalence of mental disorders in the United States—based on five Epidemiologic Catchment Area sites. *Arch Gen Psychiatry* 1988;45:977–985.

31. **Robins LN, Helzer JE, Weissman MN, et al.** Lifetime prevalence of specific psychiatric disorders in three sites. *Arch Gen Psychiatry* 1984;41:949–958.

32. **Boyd JH, Weissman MM.** Epidemiology of affective disorders: a reexamination and future directions. *Arch Gen Psychiatry* 1981;38:1039–1046.

33. **Sainsbury P.** Depression, suicide, and suicide prevention. In: **Baltimore RA,** ed. *Suicide.* Baltimore: Williams & Wilkins, 1990:17–38.

34. **Perlin LI.** Sex roles and depression. In: **Datan N, Ginsberg L,** eds. *Life-span developmental psychology: normative life crises.* New York: Academic Press, 1975:191–207.

35. **Radloff LS.** Sex differences in depression: the effects of occupation and marital status. *Sex Roles* 1975;1:249–265.

36. **Roberts RE, O'Keefe SJ.** Sex differences in depression reexamined. *J Health Soc Behav* 1981;22:394–399.

37. **Swanson KM.** Predicting depressive symptoms after miscarriage: a path analysis based on the Lazarus paradigm. *J Women's Health & Gender-based Med* 2000;9:191–206.

38. **Dugan E, Cohen SJ, Bland DR, et al.** The association of depressive symptoms and urinary incontinence among older adults. *J Am Geriatr Soc* 2000;48:413–416.

39. **Hamilton JA, Parry BL, Blumenthal SL.** The menstrual cycle in context: I. Affective syndromes associated with reproductive hormonal changes. *J Clin Psych* 1988;49:474–480.

40. **Jensvold MF.** Psychiatric aspects of the menstrual cycle. In: **Stewart DE, Stotland NL,** eds. *Psychological aspects of women's health care.* Washington, DC: American Psychiatric Press, 1993:165–192.

41. **Bailey JW, Cohen LS.** Prevalence of mood and anxiety disorders in women who seek treatment for premenstrual syndrome. *J Women's Health & Gender-based Med* 1999;8:1181–1184.

42. **Pearlstein TB, Halbreich U, Batzar ED, et al.** Psychosocial functioning in women with premenstrual dysphoric disorder before and after treatment with sertraline or placebo. *J Clin Psychiatry* 2000;61:101–109.

43. **Freeman EW, Rickels K, Sondheimer SJ, et al.** Differential response to antidepressants in women with premenstrual syndrome/premenstrual dysphoric disorder: a randomized controlled trial. *Arch Gen Psychiatry* 1999;56:932–939.

44. **Romano S, Judge R, Dillon J, et al.** The role of fluoxetine in the treatment of premenstrual dysphoric disorder. *Clin Ther* 1999;21:615–633.

45. **Young SA, Hurt PH, Benedek DM, et al.** Treatment of premenstrual dysphoric disorder with sertraline during the luteal phase: a randomized, double-blind, placebo-controlled crossover trial. *J Clin Psych* 1998;59:76–80.

46. **Iqbal MM.** Effects of antidepressants during pregnancy and lactation. *Ann Clin Psychiatry* 1999;11:237–256.

47. **Wisner KL, Gelenberg AJ, Leonard H, et al.** Pharmacologic treatment of depression during pregnancy. *JAMA* 1999;282:1264–1269.

48. **McKinlay JB, McKinlay SM, Brambilla DJ.** Health status and utilization behavior associated with menopause. *Am J Epidemiol* 1987;125:110–121.

49. **Hamilton JA.** Psychobiology in context: reproductive-related events in men's and women's lives (review of motherhood and mental illness). *Contemp Psych* 1984;3:12–16.

50. **Wright JK, Beck AT.** Cognitive therapy. In: **Hales RE, Yudofsky SC, Talbott JA,** eds. *Textbook of psychiatry,* 2nd ed. Washington, DC: American Psychiatric Press, 1994:1083–1114.

51. **Druss BG, Hoff RA, Rosenheck RA.** Underuse of antidepressants in major depression: prevalence and correlates in a national sample of young adults. *J Clin Psychiatry* 2000;61:234–237.

52. **Kennedy SH, Eisfeld BS, Dickens SE, et al.** Meeting of the American Psychiatric Association. 152nd, May, 1999, Washington, DC, US. Antidepressant-induced sexual dysfunction during treatment with moclobemide, paroxetine, sertraline, and venlafaxine. *J Clin Psychiatry* 2000;61:276–281.

53. **Masand PS, Gupta S.** Selective serotonin-reuptake inhibitors: an update. *Harvard Rev Psychiatry* 1999;7:69–84.

54. **Kent JM.** SNaRIs, NaSSAs, and NaRIs: new agents for the treatment of depression. *Lancet* 2000;355:911–918.

55. **Montgomery SA.** New developments in the treatment of depression. *J Clin Psychiatry* 1999;60[Suppl 14]: 10–15.

56. **Horst WD, Preskorn SH.** Mechanisms of action and clinical characteristics of three atypical antidepressants: venlafaxine, nefazodone, bupropion. *J Affect Disord* 1998;51:237–254.

57. **Goodwin FK, Jamison KR.** Medical treatment of acute bipolar depression. In: **Goodwin FK, Jamison KR,** eds. *Manic-depressive illness.* New York: Oxford University Press, 1990:630–664.

58. **Goodwin FK, Jamison KR.** Medical treatment of manic episodes. In: **Goodwin FK, Jamison KR,** eds. *Manic-depressive illness.* New York: Oxford University Press, 1990:603–629.

59. **Klerman GL.** Clinical epidemiology of suicide. *J Clin Psychiatry* 987;48[Suppl]:33–38.

60. **Buda M, Tsuang MT.** The epidemiology of suicide: implications for clinical practice. In: **Blumenthal SJ, Kupfer DJ,** eds. *Suicide over the life cycle: risk factors, assessment, and treatment of suicidal patients.* Washington, DC: American Psychiatric Press, 1990:17–38.

61. **Rosenbaum JF, Pollack MH.** Anxiety. In: **Cassem NH,** ed. *Massachusetts General Hospital handbook of general hospital psychiatry.* St Louis: Mosby Year Book, 1991:159–190.

62. **Hollander E, Simeon D, Gorman JM.** Anxiety disorders. In: **Hales RE, Yudofsky SC, Talbott JA,** eds. *Textbook of psychiatry,* 2nd ed. Washington, DC: American Psychiatric Press, 1994:495–564.

63. **Baldessrini RJ.** Drugs and the treatment of psychiatric disorders. In: **Gilman AG, Rall TW, Nies AS, et al,** eds. *Goodman and Gilman's the pharmacological basis of therapeutics,* 8th ed. New York: Pergamon Press, 1990:383–435.

64. **Bakish D.** The patient with comorbid depression and anxiety: the unmet need. *J Clin Psychiatry* 1999;60 [Suppl 6]:20–24.

65. **Barlow DH, Craske MG, Cerny JA, et al.** Behavioral treatment of panic disorder. *Behav Ther* 1989;20:261–282.

66. **Foa EB, Steketee G, Grayson JB, et al.** Deliberate exposure and blocking of obsessive-compulsive rituals: immediate and long-term effects. *Behav Ther* 1984;15:450–472.

67. **Cooper NA, Clum GA.** Imaginal flooding as a supplementary treatment for PTSD in combat veterans: a controlled study. *Behav Ther* 1989;20:381–391.

68. **Butler G.** Issues in the application of cognitive and behavioral strategies to the treatment of social phobia. *Clin Psychol Rev* 1989;9:91–106.

69. **Craske MG, Brown TA, Barlow DH.** Behavioral treatment of panic disorder: a two-year followup. *Behav Ther* 1991;22:289–304.

70. **Roy-Byrne PP, Cowley DS.** *Benzodiazepines in clinical practice: risks and benefits.* Washington, DC: American Psychiatric Press, 1991.

71. **Jenike MA, Baer L, Summergrad P, et al.** Obsessive-compulsive disorder: a double-blind, placebo-controlled trial of clomipramine in 27 patients. *Am J Psychol* 1989;146:1328–1330.

72. **Jenike MA, Baer L.** An open trial of buspirone in obsessive-compulsive disorder. *Am J Psychol* 1988;145: 1285–1286.

73. **Cassem NH, Barsky AJ.** Functional symptoms and somatoform disorders. In: **Cassem NH,** ed. *Massachusetts General Hospital handbook of general hospital psychiatry.* St Louis: Mosby Year Book, 1991:131–157.

74. **Ford CV, Folks DG.** Conversion disorders: an overview. *Psychosomatics* 985;26:371–377, 380–383.

75. **Ljundberg L.** Hysteria: clinical, prognostic, and genetic study. *Acta Psychol Scand* 1957;32[Suppl]:1–162.

76. **Stefansson JH, Messina JA, Meyerowitz S.** Hysterical neurosis, conversion type: clinical and epidemiological considerations. *Acta Psychol Scand* 1976;59:119–138.

77. **Toone BK.** Disorders of hysterical conversion. In: **Bass C,** ed. *Physical symptoms and psychological illness.* London: Blackwell Science, 1990:207–234.

78. **Koss MP.** The women's mental health research agenda: violence against women. *Am Psychol* 1990;45: 257–263.

79. **Bryer JB, Nelson BA, Miller JB, et al.** Childhood sexual and physical abuse as factors in adult psychiatric illness. *Am J Psychol* 1987;114:1426–1430.

80. **Warshaw C.** Women and violence. In: **Stotland NL, Stewart DE,** eds. *Psychological aspects of women's health care,* 2nd ed. Washington, DC: American Psychiatric Press, 2001:477–548.

81. **Andreasen NC, Wasek P.** Adjustment disorders in adolescents and adults. *Arch Gen Psychiatry* 1980;37: 1166–1170.

82. **Fabrega H Jr, Mezzich JE, Mezzich AC.** Adjustment disorder as a marginal or transitional illness category in DSM-III. *Arch Gen Psychol* 1987;44:567–572.

83. **Strober M, Morell W, Burroughs J, et al.** A controlled family study of anorexia nervosa. *J Psych Res* 1985;19:329–346.

84. **Stewart DE, Robinson GE.** Eating disorders and reproduction. In: **Stotland NL, Stewart DE,** eds. *Psychological aspects of women's health care,* 2nd ed. Washington, DC: American Psychiatric Press, 2001:411–456.

85. **VanItallie TB.** Health implications of overweight and obesity in the United States. *Ann Intern Med* 1985;103: 983–1038.

86. **Von Korff M, Nestadt G, Romanoski A, et al.** Prevalence of treated and untreated DSM-III schizophrenia: results of a two-stage community survey. *J Nerv Ment Dis* 1985;173:577–581.

87. **Goff DC, Manschreck TC, Groves JE.** Psychotic patients. In: **Cassem NH,** ed. *Massachusetts General Hospital handbook of general hospital psychiatry* St. Louis: Mosby Year Book, 1991:217–236.

88. **Black DW, Andreasen NC.** Schizophrenia, schizophreniform disorder, and delusional (paranoid) disorder. In: **Hales RE, Yudofsky SC, Talbott JA,** eds. *Textbook of psychiatry,* 2nd ed. Washington, DC: American Psychiatric Press, 1994:411–463.

89. **Beiser M, Iacono WG.** Update on the epidemiology of schizophrenia. *Can J Psychiatry* 1990;35:657–668.

90. **Michels R, Marzuk PM.** Progress in psychiatry. *N Engl J Med* 1993;329:552–560.

91. **Stotland NL.** Psychiatric and psychosocial issues in primary care for women. In: **Seltzer VL, Pearse WH,** eds. *Women's primary health care: office practice and procedures.* New York: McGraw-Hill, 1995.

Novak's Gynecology, 13th Edition. Edited by J.S. Berek. Lippincott Williams & Wilkins, Philadelphia © 2002.

SECTION

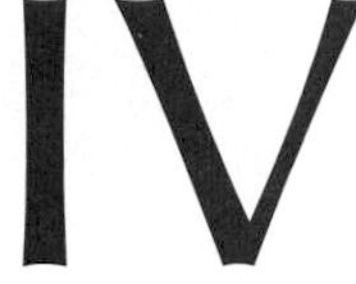

IV GENERAL GYNECOLOGY

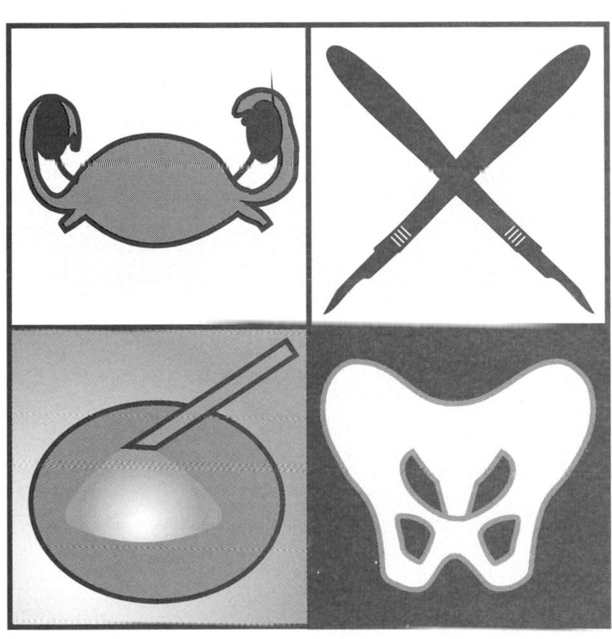

13 Benign Diseases of the Female Reproductive Tract: Symptoms and Signs

Paula J. Adams Hillard

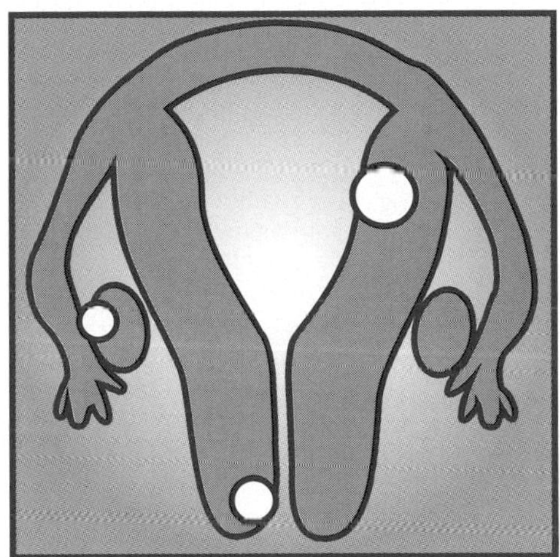

Benign conditions of the female genital tract include lesions of the uterine corpus and cervix, ovaries and fallopian tubes, and the vagina and vulva. A classification of the benign lesions of the vulva, vagina, and cervix appears in Table 13.1. Leiomyoma, polyps, and hyperplasia are the most common benign conditions of the uterus in adult women. Benign tumors of the ovaries are listed in Table 13.2.

Common gynecologic problems include abnormal bleeding, a pelvic mass, and vulvovaginal symptoms. The causes of vaginal bleeding and a pelvic mass vary by age group (Table 13.3). For each age group, the most common causes of these problems are described, along with techniques of diagnosis and principles of management. Malignant diseases are presented in Chapters 30 through 35.

Abnormal Bleeding

Prepubertal Age Group

To appropriately evaluate a young girl with vaginal bleeding, the events of puberty must be understood (1,2). The hormonal changes that control the cyclic functioning of the hypothalamic–pituitary–ovarian axis are described in Chapter 7. An understanding of the normal sequence and timing of these events is critical to an appropriate assessment of a girl at the onset of bleeding (see Chapter 23).

Differential Diagnosis

Slight vaginal bleeding can occur within the first few days of life because of withdrawal from the high level of maternal estrogens. New mothers of female infants should be informed of this possibility in an effort to preclude unnecessary anxiety. After the neonatal period, a number of causes of bleeding should be considered in this age group (Table 13.4). Menses rarely occurs before breast budding (3,4). Vaginal bleeding in the absence of secondary sexual characteristics should be evaluated carefully.

Table 13.1. Classification of Benign Conditions of the Vulva, Vagina, and Cervix

Vulva
Skin conditions
Pigmented lesions
Tumors and cysts
Ulcers
Nonneoplastic epithelial disorders
Vagina
Embryonic origin
Mesonephric, paramesonephric, and urogenital sinus cysts
Adenosis (related to diethylstilbestrol)
Vaginal septa or duplications
Disorders of pelvic support
Anterior vaginal prolapse
Cystourethrocele
Cystocele
Apical vaginal prolapse
Uterovaginal
Vaginal vault
Posterior vaginal prolapse
Enterocele
Rectocele
Other
Condyloma
Urethral diverticula
Fibroepithelial polyp
Vaginal endometriosis
Cervix
Infectious
Condyloma
Herpes simplex virus ulceration
Chlamydial cervicitis
Other cervicitis
Other
Endocervical polyps
Nabothian cysts
Columnar epithelium eversion

The causes of bleeding in this age group range from the medically mundane to malignancies that may be life-threatening. The source of the bleeding is sometimes difficult to identify, and parents who observe blood in a child's diapers or panties may be unsure of the source. Pediatricians will usually look for urinary causes of bleeding, and gastrointestinal factors should also be considered.

Vulvar Lesions Vulvar irritation can lead to pruritus with excoriation, maceration of the vulvar skin, or fissures that can bleed. Other visible external causes of bleeding in this age group include urethral prolapse, condylomas, or molluscum contagiosum. Urethral prolapse can present acutely with a tender mass that may be friable or bleed slightly; it occurs more commonly in African American girls. It may be confused with a vaginal mass. The classic presentation is a mass symmetrically surrounding the urethra. This condition can be managed medically with the application of topical estrogens (5). The presence of a condyloma should prompt questioning about abuse, although it has been suggested that a condyloma that appears during the first 2 years of life may have been acquired perinatally from a mother with human papillomavirus infection (6,7). Excoriation and hemorrhage into the skin can cause external bleeding.

Foreign Body A foreign body in the vagina is a common cause of vaginal discharge, which may appear purulent or bloody. Young children explore all orifices and may place all

Table 13.2. Benign Ovarian Tumors

Functional
Follicular Corpus luteum Theca lutein
Inflammatory
Tuboovarian abscess or complex
Neoplastic
Germ cell Benign cystic teratoma Other and mixed
Epithelial
Serous cystadenoma Mucinous cystadenoma Fibroma Cystadenofibroma Brenner tumor Mixed tumor
Other
Endometrioma

varieties of small objects inside their vaginas (Fig. 13.1). An object, such as a small plastic toy, can sometimes be palpated on rectal examination. The most common foreign bodies are small pieces of toilet paper that find their way into the vagina (8). One recent study suggests that the presence of vaginal foreign bodies may be a marker for sexual abuse; although this is by no means always the case, the possibility of abuse should be kept in mind in examining any child with vulvovaginal symptoms (9).

Precocious Puberty Precocious puberty (see Chapter 23) occasionally is marked by vaginal bleeding in the absence of other secondary sexual characteristics, although it is more common for the onset of breast budding or pubic hair growth to occur before vaginal bleeding. Although a large observational study suggests that the onset of pubertal changes—breast budding and pubic hair—may occur earlier than had originally been thought, the onset of menarche before age 8 is sufficiently early to warrant evaluation for precocious puberty (2).

Trauma Trauma can be a cause of genital bleeding. **A careful history should be obtained from one or both parents or caretakers and the child herself, because trauma caused by sexual abuse is often not recognized.** Physical findings that are inconsistent with the description of the alleged accident should prompt consideration of abuse and appropriate consultation or referral to an experienced social worker or sexual abuse team. **There is a mandatory legal obligation to report suspected child physical abuse in all states;** most states specifically require reporting child sexual abuse as well, but even in those that do not, the laws are broad enough to encompass sexual abuse implicitly (10). Even the suspicion of sexual abuse requires notification. In general, straddle injuries affect the vulvar area, whereas penetrating injuries with lesions of the fourchette or lesions that extend through the hymenal ring are less likely to occur as a result of accidental trauma (Fig. 13.2) (11).

The medical evaluation of suspected child sexual abuse is best managed by individuals who have experience in assessing the physical findings, laboratory results,

Table 13.3. Causes of Bleeding and Pelvic Mass By Approximate Frequency and Age Group

Causes of bleeding by approximate frequency and age group

—	*Prepubertal*	*Adolescent*	*Reproductive*	*Perimenopausal*	*Postmenopausal*
—	Vulvovaginitis	Anovulation	Exogenous hormone use	Anovulation	Exogenous hormone use
—	Vaginal foreign body	Exogenous hormone use	Pregnancy	Fibroids	Endometrial lesions, including cancer
—	Precocious puberty	Pregnancy	Anovulation	Cervical and endometrial polyps	Atrophic vaginitis
—	Tumor	Coagulopathy	Fibroids	Thyroid dysfunction	Other tumor—vulvar, vaginal, cervical
—	—	—	Cervical and endometrial polyps	—	—
—	—	—	Thyroid dysfunction	—	—

Causes of pelvic mass by approximate frequency and age group

Infancy	*Prepubertal*	*Adolescent*	*Reproductive*	*Perimenopausal*	*Postmenopausal*
Functional cyst	Functional cyst	Functional cyst	Functional cyst	Fibroids	Ovarian tumor (malignant or benign)
Germ cell tumor	Germ cell tumor	Pregnancy	Pregnancy	Epithelial ovarian tumor	Functional cyst
—	—	Dermoid/other germ cell tumors	Uterine fibroids	Functional cyst	Bowel, malignant tumor or inflammatory
—	—	Obstructing vaginal or uterine anomalies	Epithelial ovarian tumor	—	Metastases
—	—	Epithelial ovarian tumor	—	—	—

and the children's statements and behaviors. Genital findings have been described as follows (12):

1. Normal or unrelated to abuse
2. Nonspecific for abuse
3. Concerning for abuse
4. Clear evidence of blunt force or penetrating trauma.

The overall classification of the likelihood for abuse can be categorized as follows (12):

1. No evidence of abuse
2. Possible abuse
3. Probable abuse
4. Definitive evidence of abuse or penetrating trauma.

Table 13.4. Causes of Vaginal Bleeding in Prepubertal Girls

Vulvar and external
Vulvitis with excoriation
Trauma (e.g., straddle injury)
Lichen sclerosus
Condylomas
Molluscum contagiosum
Urethral prolapse
Vaginal
Vaginitis
Vaginal foreign body
Trauma (abuse, penetration)
Vaginal tumor
Uterine
Precocious puberty
Ovarian tumor
Granulosa cell tumor
Germ cell tumor
Exogenous estrogens
Topical
Enteral

Most cases of child sexual abuse do not come to light with an acute injury and instead are associated with normal or nonspecific genital findings (13,14). Forms of abuse such as fondling or digital penetration may not result in lasting visible genital lesions.

Other Causes Other serious but rare causes of true vaginal bleeding include vaginal tumors. The most common tumor in the prepubertal age group is a rhabdomyosarcoma

Figure 13.1 Foreign body (plastic toy) in the vagina of an 8-year-old girl.

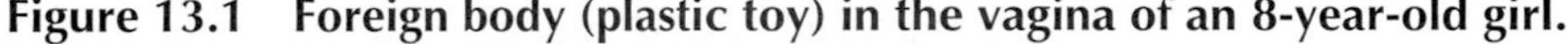

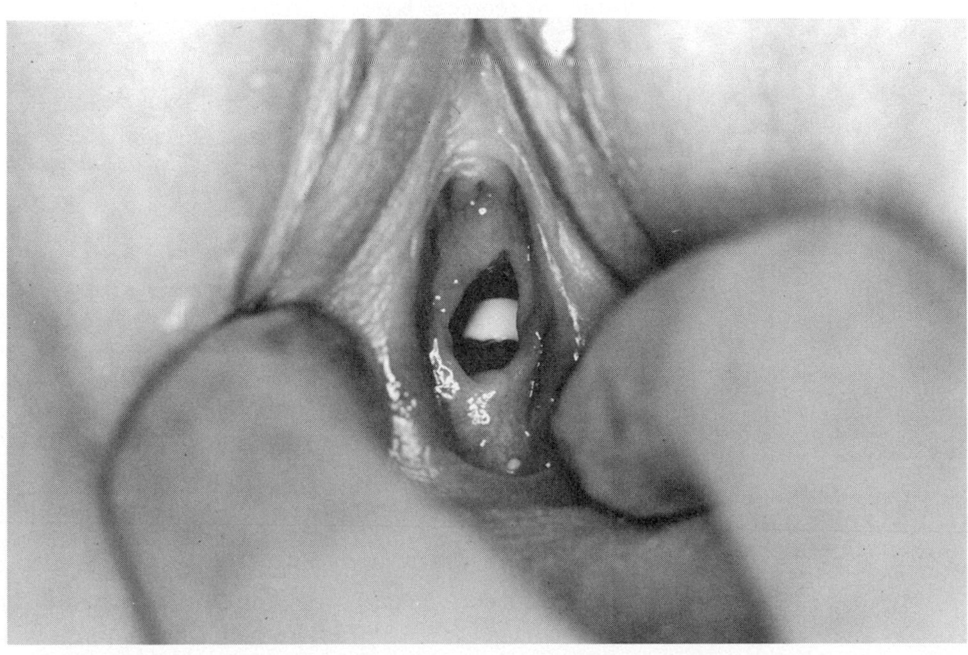

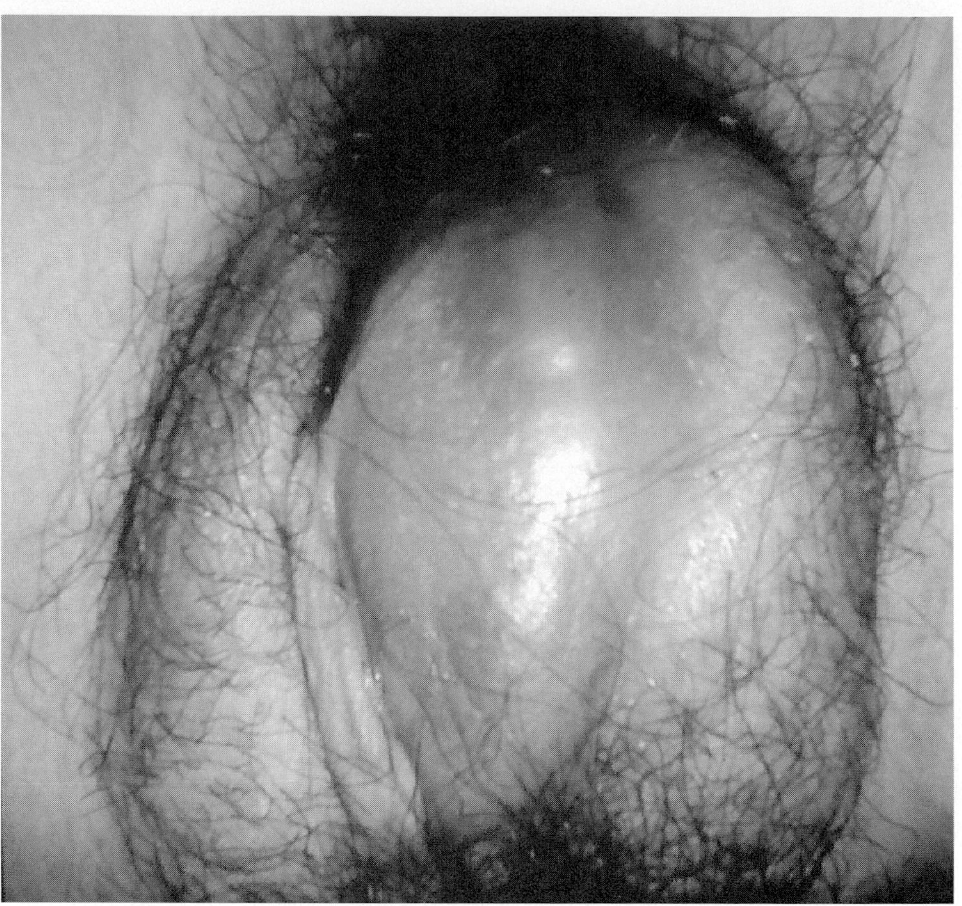

Figure 13.2 Straddle injury—vulvar hematoma in a 13-year-old girl.

(sarcoma botryoides), which is associated with bleeding and a grapelike clustered mass (Chapter 31). Other forms of vaginal tumor are also rare but should be ruled out if no other obvious source of bleeding is found externally.

Hormonally active ovarian tumors can lead to endometrial proliferation and bleeding. Exogenously administered estrogens can result in bleeding. This can be caused by the prolonged use of topical estrogens prescribed as therapy for vulvovaginitis or labial adhesions or can result from accidental ingestion of prescription estrogens.

Diagnosis

A careful examination is indicated when a child makes genital complaints. The technique of examining the prepubertal child is described in Chapter 1. **If no obvious cause of bleeding is visible externally or within the distal vagina, an examination can be performed using anesthesia and an endoscope to completely visualize the vagina and cervix. This exam is best performed by a clinician with experience in pediatric and adolescent gynecology.**

If an ovarian or vaginal mass is suspected, a pelvic ultrasonographic examination can provide useful information. The appearance of the ovaries (normal prepubertal size and volume, follicular development, cystic or solid) can be noted, as well as the size and configuration of the uterus. **The prepubertal uterus has a distinctive appearance, with equal proportions of cervix and fundus and a size of approximately 2 to 3.5 cm in length and**

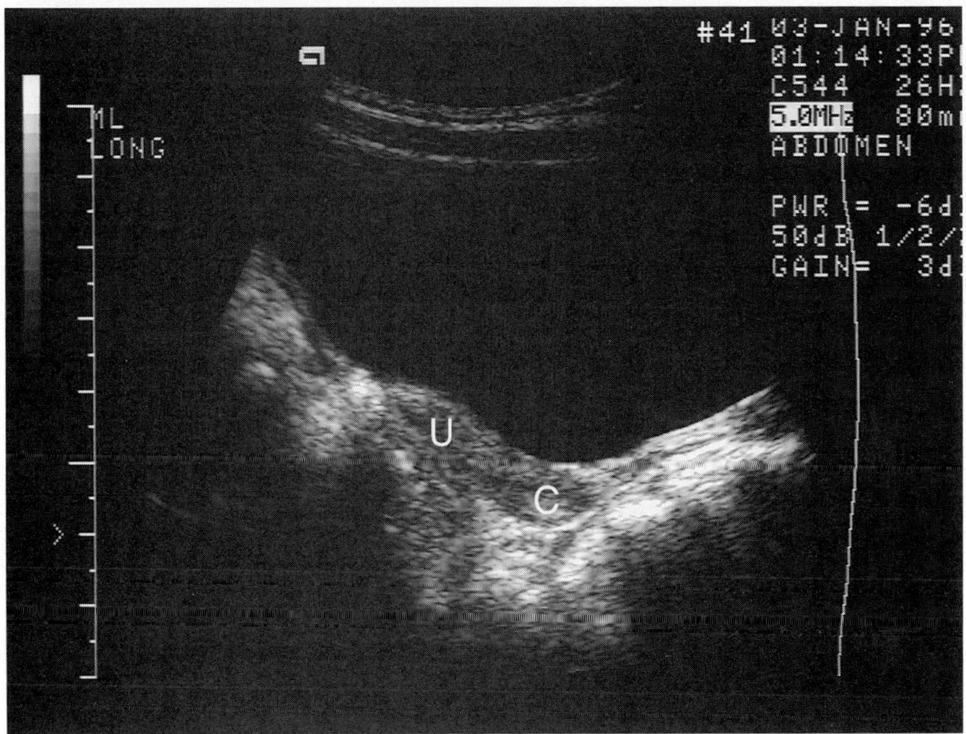

Figure 13.3 Pelvic ultrasound (transabdominal) of a premenarchal 10-year-old girl. *U,* uterine corpus; *C,* cervix. Note that the body of the uterus is about the same size as the cervix.

0.5 to 1 cm in width (Fig. 13.3). The fundus enlarges with estrogen stimulation. An ultrasonographic examination should be the first imaging study performed; more sophisticated imaging techniques such as magnetic resonance imaging (MRI) or computed tomography (CT) scanning are rarely indicated.

Management

The management of bleeding in the prepubertal age group is directed toward the cause of bleeding. If bloody discharge believed to be due to nonspecific vulvovaginitis persists despite therapy, further evaluation to rule out the presence of a foreign body may be necessary. Skin lesions (chronic irritation) and lichen sclerosus may be difficult or frustrating to manage but can be treated with a course of topical steroids; lichen sclerosus often requires ongoing maintenance therapy. **Vaginal and ovarian tumors should be managed in consultation with a gynecologic oncologist.**

Adolescence

To assess vaginal bleeding during adolescence, it is necessary to have an understanding of the range of normal menstrual cycles (see Chapter 7). **During the first 2 years after menarche, most cycles are anovulatory.** Despite this, they are somewhat regular, within a range of approximately 21 to 40 days (15–17). In more than one-fourth of girls, a pattern of plus or minus 10 days and a cycle length of 21 to approximately 42 days are established within the first three cycles; in one-half of girls, the pattern is established by the seventh cycle; and in two-thirds of girls, such a pattern is established within 2 years of menarche (17).

Normal Menses

The mean duration of menses is 4.7 days; 89% of cycles last ≤7 days. The average blood loss per cycle is 35 ml (18), **and the major component of menstrual discharge is endometrial tissue. Recurrent bleeding in excess of 80 ml/cycle results in anemia.**

Quantitative information about the volume of menstrual blood loss is of little clinical use, however. The common clinical practice of asking how many pads or tampons are soaked on a heavy day or per cycle can give a rough approximation of blood loss (3 to 5 pads per day is typical). Individual variations in fastidiousness, lack of familiarity with the volume of blood loss other than one's own, and errors in estimation or recollection result in inaccuracies in estimations of menstrual volume. One study found that one-third of individuals who estimated their cycles to be moderate or light had bleeding in excess of 80 ml/cycle, whereas nearly one-half of those who described the bleeding as heavy had flow less than 80 ml/cycle (19). In addition, the amount of menstrual blood contained in each tampon or pad may vary both within brands as well as from one brand to another (20).

The transition from anovulatory to ovulatory cycles takes place during the first several years after menarche. It results from the so-called *maturation of the hypothalamic–pituitary–ovarian axis,* characterized by positive feedback mechanisms in which a rising estrogen level triggers a surge of luteinizing hormone and ovulation. **Most adolescents have ovulatory cycles by the end of their second year of menstruation, although most cycles (even anovulatory ones) remain within a rather narrow range of approximately 21 to 42 days.**

Cycles that are longer than 42 days, cycles that are shorter than 21 days, and bleeding that lasts more than 7 days should be considered out of the ordinary, particularly after the first 2 years from the onset of menarche. The variability in cycle length is greater during adolescence than adulthood; thus, greater irregularity is acceptable if significant anemia or hemorrhage is not present. However, consideration should be given to an evaluation of possible causes of abnormal menses (particularly underlying causes of anovulation such as androgen excess syndromes) for girls whose cycles are consistently outside normal ranges (21) or whose cycles were previously regular and become irregular.

Differential Diagnosis

Anovulation **Anovulatory bleeding can be too frequent, prolonged, or heavy, particularly after a long interval of amenorrhea.** The physiology of this phenomenon relates to a failure of the feedback mechanism in which rising estrogen levels result in a decline in follicle-stimulating hormone (FSH) with subsequent decline of estrogen levels. In anovulatory cycles, estrogen secretion continues, resulting in endometrial proliferation with subsequent unstable growth and incomplete shedding. The clinical result is irregular, prolonged, and heavy bleeding. Conditions that are associated with anovulation are listed in Table 13.5 and more fully discussed in Chapters 24, 25, and 27.

Studies of adolescent menses show differences in rates of ovulation based on the number of months or years postmenarche. **The younger the age at menarche, the sooner regular ovulation is established.** In one study, the time from menarche until 50% of the cycles were ovulatory was 1 year for girls whose menarche occurred when they were younger than 12 years of age, 3 years for girls whose menarche occurred between 12 and 12.9 years of age, and 4.5 years for girls whose menarche occurred at 13 years of age or older (22).

Pregnancy-related Bleeding **The possibility of pregnancy must be considered when an adolescent seeks treatment for abnormal bleeding.** Bleeding in pregnancy can be associated with a spontaneous abortion, ectopic pregnancy, or other pregnancy-related complications such as a molar pregnancy. In the United States, 50% of 17-year-old females have had sexual intercourse (23). Issues of confidentiality for adolescent health care are addressed in Chapter 1.

Table 13.5. Conditions Associated with Anovulation and Abnormal Bleeding

Eating disorders Anorexia nervosa Bulimia nervosa
Excessive physical exercise
Chronic illness
Alcohol and other drug abuse
Stress
Thyroid disease Hypothyroidism Hyperthyroidism
Diabetes mellitus
Androgen excess syndromes

Exogenous Hormones The cause of abnormal bleeding that is experienced while an individual is taking exogenous hormones usually is very different from bleeding that occurs without hormonal manipulation (24). **Oral contraceptive use is associated with breakthrough bleeding, which occurs in as many as 30% to 40% of individuals during the first cycle of combination pill use. In addition, irregular bleeding can result from missed pills** (25,26). Strict compliance with correct and consistent pill taking is difficult for many individuals who take oral contraceptives; one study reported that only 40% of women took a pill every day (27). Other studies suggest that adolescents have an even more difficult time taking oral contraceptives, missing an average of three pills per month (28). With this many missed pills, it is not surprising that some individuals experience irregular bleeding. The solution is to emphasize consistent pill taking; if the individual is unable to comply with daily pill use, perhaps an alternative contraceptive method may be preferable.

Other methods of contraception can also produce irregular bleeding. Irregular bleeding occurs frequently in users of *depomedroxyprogesterone acetate* (*DMPA*), although at the end of 1 year, more than 50% of users will be amenorrheic (29). The implantable subdermal *levonorgestrel* implant also is associated with relatively high rates of irregular and unpredictable bleeding (30). Other contraceptive methods, including the monthly injectable combination contraceptive and the progestin-containing intrauterine system are associated with irregular bleeding in the first few months of use (31,32). Although the mechanism of bleeding associated with these hormonal methods is not well established, many believe that bleeding occurs from an atrophic endometrium, suggesting options for therapy (24). However, it should not be assumed that any bleeding occurring while an individual is using a hormonal method of contraception is caused by that method. Other local causes of bleeding, such as cervicitis or endometritis, also can occur during hormone therapy (33).

Hematologic Abnormalities In the adolescent age group, the possibility of a hematologic cause of abnormal bleeding must be considered. One classic study reviewed all patient visits of adolescents to an emergency room with the complaint of excessive or abnormal bleeding (Fig. 13.4) (34). The most common coagulation abnormality diagnosed was idiopathic thrombocytopenic purpura, followed by von Willebrand's disease. **Adolescents who have severe menorrhagia, especially at menarche, should be screened for coagulation abnormalities, including von Willebrand's disease.**

Infections Irregular or postcoital bleeding can be associated with chlamydial cervicitis. **Adolescents have the highest rates of chlamydial infections of any age group, and screening for chlamydia should be performed routinely among sexually active teens** (35).

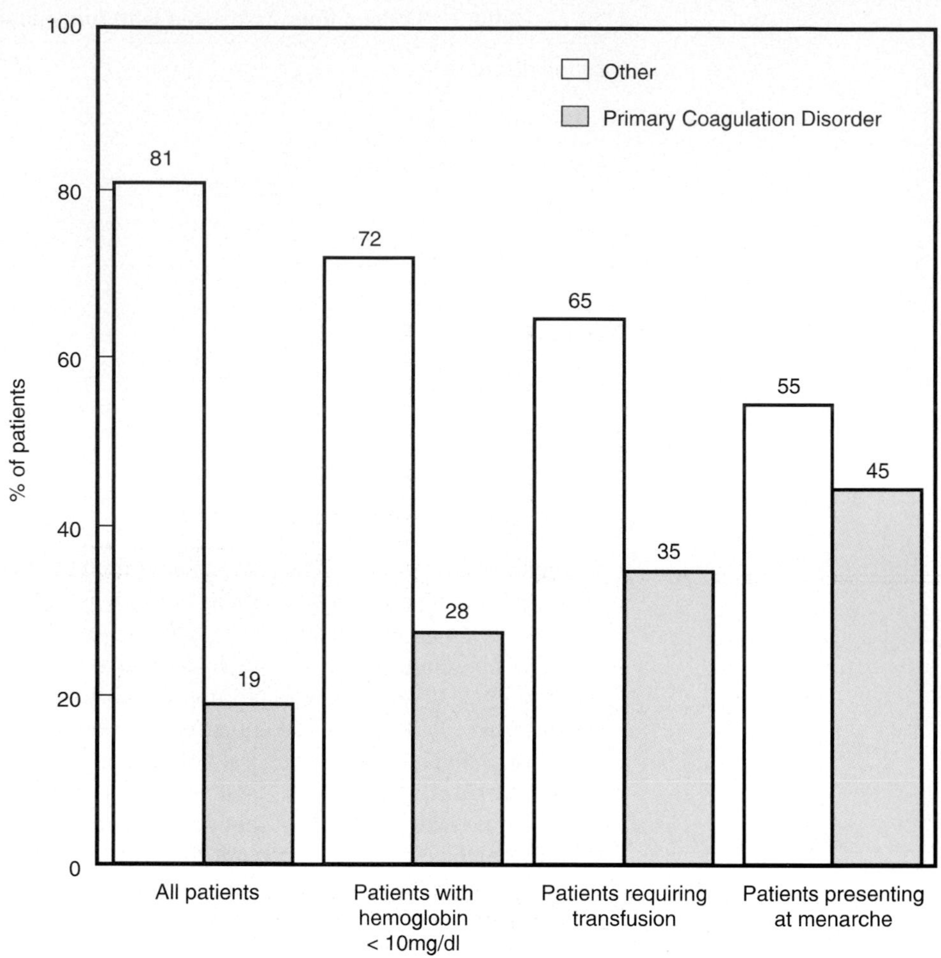

Figure 13.4 Etiology of menorrhagia in adolescents. (From **Classens AE, Cowell CA.** Acute adolescent menorrhagia. *Am J Obstet Gynecol* 1981;139:277–280, with permission.)

Menorrhagia can be the initial sign for patients infected with sexually transmissible organisms. Adolescents have the highest rates of pelvic inflammatory disease (PID) of any age group when only sexually experienced individuals are considered (36) (see Chapter 15).

Other Endocrine or Systemic Problems Abnormal bleeding can be associated with thyroid dysfunction. Signs and symptoms of thyroid disease can be somewhat subtle in teens (Chapter 25). Hepatic dysfunction should be considered, because it can lead to abnormalities in clotting factor production.

Polycystic ovarian syndrome (PCOS) can occur during adolescence, and manifestations of excess androgen effect (hirsutism, acne) should prompt evaluation (37). **Androgen disorders occur in about 5% to 10% of women, making them the most common endocrine disorders in women** (Chapter 25). Classic PCOS, functional ovarian hyperandrogenism, or partial late-onset congenital adrenal hyperplasia all can occur in adolescence (38). **These disorders are often overlooked, unrecognized, or untreated.** Women with even mild disorders are candidates for intervention. These disorders may be a harbinger of diabetes, endometrial cancer, and cerebrovascular disease. **Acne, hirsutism and menstrual irregularities are often dismissed as normal during adolescence but may be manifestations of hyperandrogenism** (39). If an androgen abnormality is not treated, it is likely to persist beyond adolescence. Obesity, hirsutism, and acne should be evaluated to minimize the

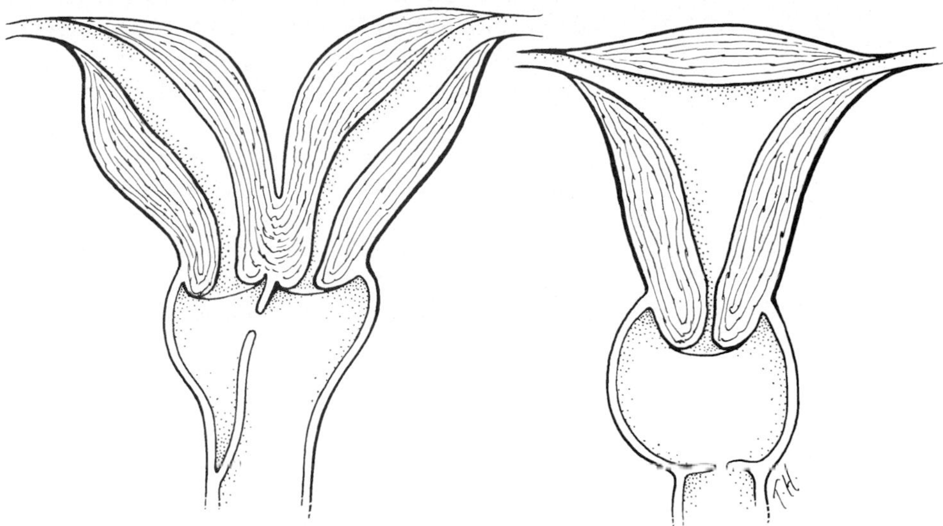

Figure 13.5 The types of obstructive or partially obstructive genital anomalies that can occur during adolescence.

significant psychosocial costs (40). Androgenic changes are partially reversible if detected early and managed appropriately. Behavioral changes (diet and exercise) are desirable. Signs of insulin resistance (acanthosis nigricans) should also be evaluated and managed appropriately.

Anatomic Causes Obstructive or partially obstructive genital anomalies typically present during adolescence. Müllerian abnormalities, such as obstructing longitudinal vaginal septa or uterus didelphis, can cause hematocolpos or hematometra. If these obstructing anomalies have or develop a small outlet, the sign may be of persistent dark brownish discharge (old blood) rather than or in addition to a pelvic mass. Many varieties of uterine and vaginal anomalies exist and should be managed by or in consultation with clinicians who have sufficient experience and expertise with these anomalies. Fig. 13.5 illustrates situations in which abnormal bleeding can occur as a result of obstructing septa.

Diagnosis

Any adolescent with abnormal bleeding should undergo sensitive pregnancy testing, regardless of whether she states that she has had intercourse. The medical consequences of failing to diagnose a pregnancy are too severe to risk missing the diagnosis. Complications of pregnancy should then be managed accordingly.

Laboratory Testing In addition to a pregnancy test, laboratory testing should include a complete blood count with platelets, coagulation studies, and bleeding time. Thyroid studies also may be appropriate. A complete pelvic examination is appropriate if the patient has been sexually active, is having severe pain, or an anomaly is suspected. Cultures for gonorrhea and testing for chlamydia infection are appropriate if the patient has been sexually active. Some young teens who have a history that is classic for anovulation, who deny sexual activity, and who agree to return for follow-up evaluation may be managed with a limited gynecologic examination and pelvic ultrasonography.

Imaging Studies If the pregnancy test is positive, pelvic imaging using ultrasonography may be necessary to confirm a viable intrauterine pregnancy and rule out a spontaneous abortion or ectopic pregnancy. If a pelvic mass is suspected on examination, or if the examination is inadequate (more likely to be the case in an adolescent than an older woman) and additional information is required, pelvic ultrasonography may be helpful. **Although transvaginal ultrasonographic examination can be more helpful than transabdominal**

ultrasonography in ascertaining details of pelvic anatomy, the use of the vaginal probe may not be possible in a young girl or one who has not used tampons or had intercourse. Direct communication between the clinician and the radiologist can be helpful in identifying candidates for transvaginal ultrasonographic examination.

Other imaging studies are not indicated as initial testing but may be helpful in selected instances. If a pelvic ultrasonographic examination does not lead to clarification of the anatomy when vaginal septa, uterine septa, uterine duplication, or vaginal agenesis are suspected, MRI can be helpful in delineating anatomic abnormalities. It has been suggested that this imaging technique may replace laparoscopy in the evaluation of uterine and vaginal developmental anomalies (41). CT scanning may be helpful in detecting nongenital intraabdominal abnormalities.

Management

Management of bleeding abnormalities related to pregnancy, thyroid dysfunction, hepatic abnormalities, hematologic abnormalities, or androgen excess syndromes should be directed to treating the underlying condition. Oral contraceptives can be extremely helpful in managing androgen excess syndromes. After specific diagnoses have been ruled out by appropriate laboratory testing, anovulation or dysfunctional bleeding becomes the diagnosis of exclusion.

Anovulation: Mild Bleeding

Adolescents who have mildly abnormal bleeding, as defined by adequate hemoglobin levels and minimal disruption of daily activities, are best treated with frequent reassurance, close follow-up, and supplemental iron. If the patient has been bleeding heavily or for a prolonged interval, however, an apparent decrease in the bleeding does not necessarily mean that therapy is not required. This type of on-again, off-again bleeding characterizes anovulatory bleeding and is likely to continue in the absence of therapy.

A patient who is mildly anemic will benefit from hormone therapy. If the patient is not bleeding at the time of evaluation, a combination low-dose oral contraceptive can be prescribed to be used in the manner in which it is used for contraception (21 days of hormonally active pills, followed by 7 days of placebo, during which time withdrawal bleeding is expected). If the patient is not sexually active, she should be reevaluated after three to six cycles to determine if she desires to continue this regimen. Parents may sometimes object to the use of oral contraceptives if their daughter is not sexually active (or if they believe her not to be or even if they would like her not to be). These objections are frequently based on misconceptions about the potential risks of the pill and can be overcome by careful explanation of the pill's role as medical therapy. If the medication is discontinued when the young woman is not sexually active and she subsequently becomes sexually active and requires contraception, it may be difficult to explain the reinstitution of oral contraceptives to the parents. Consideration can certainly be given to continuing the pill, and parents should be reassured that there are no medical risks associated with prolonged use.

Sometimes, providing parents with accurate information about the safety of oral contraceptives, emphasizing that currently available oral contraceptive preparations contain lower doses of estrogens and progestins than those used in the 1960s and 1970s, and emphasizing the hormonal rather than contraceptive function, may not be persuasive. In such cases, cyclic progestins are an alternative. ***Medroxyprogesterone acetate*, 5 to 10 mg/day for 10 to 13 days every 1 to 2 months, prevents excessive endometrial buildup and irregular shedding caused by unopposed estrogen stimulation.** This therapy also should be reevaluated regularly and accompanied by oral administration of iron. Eventual maturation of the hypothalamic–pituitary–ovarian axis usually will result in the establishment of regular menses unless there are underlying conditions such as hyperandrogenism. Individuals may choose to continue oral contraceptives for contraception or their noncontraceptive benefits (improvement of acne, decreased dysmenorrhea, and lighter, more regular menstrual flow).

Acute Bleeding: Moderate

Patients who are bleeding acutely but who are stable and do not require hospital admission will require doses of hormones that are much higher than those in oral contraceptives. An effective regimen is the use of combination monophasic oral contraceptives (every 6 hours for 4 to 7 days). After that time, the dose should be tapered or stopped to allow withdrawal flow. With this therapy, the patient and her parents should be given specific written and verbal instructions warning them about the potential side effects of high-dose hormone therapy—nausea, breast tenderness, and breakthrough bleeding. The patient should be instructed to call with any concerns rather than discontinue the pills, and she must understand that stopping the prescribed regimen may result in a recurrence of heavy bleeding.

Both the patient and her mother should be warned to expect heavy withdrawal flow for the first period. It will be controlled by the institution of combination low-dose oral contraceptive therapy given once daily and continued for three to six cycles to allow regular withdrawal flow. If the patient is not sexually active, the pill may be discontinued and the menstrual cycles may be reassessed.

Acute Bleeding: Emergency Management

The decision to hospitalize a patient depends on the rate of current bleeding and the severity of any existing anemia. The actual acute blood loss may not adequately be reflected in the initial blood count but will be revealed with serial hemoglobin assessments. The cause of acute menorrhagia may be a primary coagulation disorder (34), **so measurements of coagulation and hemostasis, including bleeding time, should be performed for any adolescent patients with acute menorrhagia.** Von Willebrand's disease, platelet disorders, or hematologic malignancies can all cause menorrhagia. Depending on the patient's level of hemodynamic stability or compromise, a blood sample can be analyzed for type and screen. The decision to transfuse must be considered carefully, and the benefits and risks should be discussed with the adolescent and her parents. Generally, there is no need for transfusion unless the patient is hemodynamically unstable.

In patients who, by exclusion, have been diagnosed as having dysfunctional bleeding, hormone therapy usually makes it possible to avoid surgical intervention (dilation and curettage [D & C], operative hysteroscopy, or laparoscopy). A patient who has been hospitalized for severe bleeding requires aggressive management as follows:

1. **After stabilization, when appropriate laboratory assessment and an examination have established a working diagnosis of anovulation; hormonal management will usually control bleeding.**

2. **Conjugated estrogens, either 25 to 40 mg given intravenously every 6 hours or 2.5 mg given orally every 6 hours, will usually be effective.**

3. **If estrogens are not effective, the patient should be reevaluated, and the diagnosis should be reassessed.** The failure of hormonal management suggests that a local cause of bleeding is more likely. In this event, consideration should be given to a pelvic ultrasonographic examination to determine any unusual causes of bleeding (such as uterine leiomyomas or endometrial hyperplasia) and to assess the presence of intrauterine clots that may impair uterine contractility and prolong the bleeding episode.

4. **If intrauterine clots are detected, evacuation of the clots (suction curettage or D & C) is indicated.** Although a D & C will provide effective immediate control of the bleeding, it is unusual to reach this step in adolescents.

More drastic forms of treatment other than a D & C (such as ablation of the endometrium by laser or rollerball devices) are considered inappropriate for adolescents because of concerns about future fertility.

If intravenous or oral administration of estrogen controls the bleeding, oral progestin therapy should be instituted and continued for several days to stabilize the endometrium. This therapy can be accomplished by using a combination oral contraceptive, usually one with 30 to 35 μg of estrogen, or by using the tapering regimen previously described. The medication can be tapered and ultimately stopped to allow withdrawal bleeding. Low-dose combination oral contraception should be continued for three to six cycles, or longer if desired, to provide normal menstrual cycles.

In general, the prognosis for regular ovulatory cycles and subsequent normal fertility in young women who experience an episode of abnormal bleeding is good, particularly for patients who develop abnormal bleeding as a result of anovulation within the first years after menarche and in whom there are no signs of other specific conditions. Some girls, including those in whom there is an underlying medical cause, such as polycystic ovary syndrome, will continue to have abnormal bleeding into middle and late adolescence and adulthood and will benefit from the ongoing use of oral contraceptives to manage hirsutism, acne, and irregular periods. Ovulation induction may be necessary to achieve fertility in these individuals. Girls with coagulopathies may also benefit from ongoing oral contraceptive use.

Long-term Hormonal Suppression

For patients with underlying medical conditions, such as coagulopathies or a malignancy requiring chemotherapy, long-term therapeutic amenorrhea with menstrual suppression using the following regimens may be necessary:

1. Progestins, such as oral *norethindrone, norethindrone acetate,* or *medroxyprogesterone acetate,* on a continuous daily basis

2. Continuous (noncyclic) combination regimens of oral estrogen and progestins (birth control pills) that do not include a withdrawal bleeding–placebo week

3. Depot formulations of progestins (*DMPA*), with or without concurrent estrogens

4. Gonadotropin-releasing hormone (GnRH) analogs with or without estrogen add-back therapy.

The choice of regimen depends on any contraindications (such as active liver disease precluding the use of estrogens) and the clinician's experience. Although the goal of these long-term suppressive therapies is amenorrhea, all of these regimens may be accompanied by breakthrough bleeding. They require regular follow-up visits and continued patient encouragement. Occasional episodes of spotting and mild breakthrough bleeding that do not result in a lowered hemoglobin level may be managed expectantly. When breakthrough bleeding affects the hemoglobin level, it should be evaluated with respect to the underlying disease. For example, in a patient with underlying platelet dysfunction, breakthrough bleeding may reflect a lowered platelet count. Bleeding in a patient with hepatic disease may reflect worsening hepatic function. Supplemental low-dose estrogen can be helpful in the management of excessive breakthrough bleeding that has no specific cause other than the hormone therapy.

Reproductive Age Group

Normal Menses

Beyond the first 1 to 2 years after menarche, menstrual cycles generally conform to a cycle length of 21 to 35 days, with a duration of less than 7 days of menstrual flow. As a woman approaches menopause, cycle length becomes more irregular as more cycles become anovulatory. Although the most frequent cause of irregular bleeding is hormonal, other causes occur more often during the adolescent years. Pregnancy-related bleeding (spontaneous abortion, ectopic pregnancy) should always be considered, and a pregnancy test should always be obtained as part of the evaluation of abnormal bleeding. Although a variety of terms have been used to describe abnormal menses (Table 13.6), accurate characterization of the bleeding based on recorded records (preferably charted prospectively) may be more important than the use of the specific term.

Dysfunctional Uterine Bleeding **The term *dysfunctional uterine bleeding* has been used to describe abnormal bleeding for which no specific cause has been found. It most often implies a mechanism of anovulation, although not all bleeding that is outside the normal range (either in cycle length or duration) is anovulatory. The term is a diagnosis of exclusion, which is probably more confusing than enlightening.**

Most anovulatory bleeding is a result of what has been termed *estrogen breakthrough.* In the absence of ovulation and the production of progesterone, the endometrium responds to estrogen stimulation with proliferation. This endometrial growth without periodic shedding results in eventual breakdown of the fragile endometrial tissue. Healing within the endometrium is irregular and dyssynchronous. Relatively low levels of estrogen stimulation will result in irregular and prolonged bleeding, whereas higher sustained levels result in episodes of amenorrhea followed by acute, heavy bleeding.

Pregnancy-related Bleeding Spontaneous abortion can be associated with excessive or prolonged bleeding. In the United States, more than 50% of pregnancies are unintended (42), and 10% of women are at risk for unintended pregnancy but use no method of contraception. About one-half of unintended pregnancies are a result of nonuse of contraception; however, the other one-half are contraceptive failures (43). Unintended pregnancies are most likely to occur among adolescents and women over 40 years of age (Chapter 10). A woman may be unaware that she has conceived and may seek care because of abnormal bleeding. If an ectopic pregnancy is ruled out, the management of spontaneous abortion may include either observation, if the bleeding is not excessive, or curettage or D & C, depending on the clinician's judgment and the patient's preference (44–46).

Exogenous Hormones Irregular bleeding that occurs while a woman is using contraceptive hormones should be considered in a different context than bleeding that occurs in the absence of exogenous hormone use. Breakthrough bleeding during the first 1 to 3 months

Table 13.6. Abnormal Menses—Terminology

Term	*Interval*	*Duration*	*Amount*
Menorrhagia	Regular	Prolonged	Excessive
Metrorrhagia	Irregular	±Prolonged	Normal
Menometrorrhagia	Irregular	Prolonged	Excessive
Hypermenorrhea	Regular	Normal	Excessive
Hypomenorrhea	Regular	Normal or less	Less
Oligomenorrhea	Infrequent or irregular	Variable	Scanty

of oral contraceptive use occurs in up to 30% to 40% of users and should almost always be managed expectantly with reassurance, because the frequency of breakthrough bleeding decreases with each subsequent month of use (25). Irregular bleeding can also result from inconsistent pill taking (47–49).

Not all bleeding that occurs while an individual is taking oral contraceptives is a consequence of hormonal factors. In one study, women who experienced irregular bleeding while taking oral contraceptives were found to have a higher frequency of chlamydia infection (33).

Irregular bleeding is almost invariably present during the first year of use of both the subdermal implant *levonorgestrel* and *DMPA* (29,30). Because irregular bleeding is so often present with these two methods of contraception, counseling prior to their use is imperative. Women who do not believe that they can cope with irregular, unpredictable bleeding may not be good candidates for these methods. As with oral contraceptives, the possibility of nonhormonal causes of bleeding (e.g., chlamydial cervicitis) should be considered. When an individual is using one of these methods, reassurance and counseling should be provided. The exact mechanism of irregular bleeding associated with progestin-only methods is not well established but may be related to incomplete suppression of follicular activity with periodic elevations of estradiol (24). The additional oral use of estrogen has been reported to improve bleeding with both *DMPA* and the subdermal *levonorgestrel* (29,50,51). Combination oral contraceptives have also been used in patients with the subdermal *levonorgestrel* implants. For a patient who is considering removal of the implants because of irregular bleeding and who may choose an oral contraceptive as an alternative, the use of combination pills can allow both the clinician and the patient to assess the patient's tolerance of and compliance with oral contraceptive therapy. The use of nonsteroidal antiinflammatory drugs (NSAIDs) has been shown to result in decreased bleeding (50).

Endocrine Causes Both hypothyroidism and hyperthyroidism can be associated with abnormal bleeding. With hypothyroidism, menstrual abnormalities including menorrhagia are common (Chapter 25). The most common cause of thyroid hyperfunctioning in premenopausal women is Graves' disease, which occurs 4 to 5 times more often in women than men. Hyperthyroidism can result in oligomenorrhea or amenorrhea, and it can also lead to elevated levels of plasma estrogen (52).

Diabetes mellitus can be associated with anovulation, obesity, insulin resistance, and androgen excess. Androgen disorders are very common among women of reproductive age and should be evaluated and managed. Because androgen disorders are associated with significant cardiovascular disease, the condition should be diagnosed promptly. This condition becomes more immediately of concern in older women of reproductive age. Management of bleeding disorders associated with androgen excess consists of an appropriate diagnostic evaluation followed by the use of oral contraceptives (in the absence of significant contraindications), coupled with dietary and exercise modification.

Anatomic Causes **Anatomic causes of abnormal bleeding in women of reproductive age occur more frequently than in women in other age groups. Uterine leiomyomas occur in as many as one-half of all women older than 35 years of age and are the most common tumors of the genital tract** (53). **Although they are asymptomatic in many or even most women, they have been estimated to be clinically significant in at least 25% of the American female population of reproductive age. They are more common in African American women and have been associated with obesity** (54,55). **The mechanism of abnormal bleeding related to leiomyomas is not well established.** Several theories have been postulated, including dysregulation of a number of growth factors that regulate angiogenesis in a uterus in which leiomyomas are present. Growth factors that are currently being investigated for their role in the process of abnormal bleeding associated with leiomyomas include basic fibroblast growth factor, vascular endothelial growth factor, heparin-binding epidermal growth factor, platelet-derived growth factor, transforming growth factor-β, parathyroid hormone-related protein, and prolactin (56).

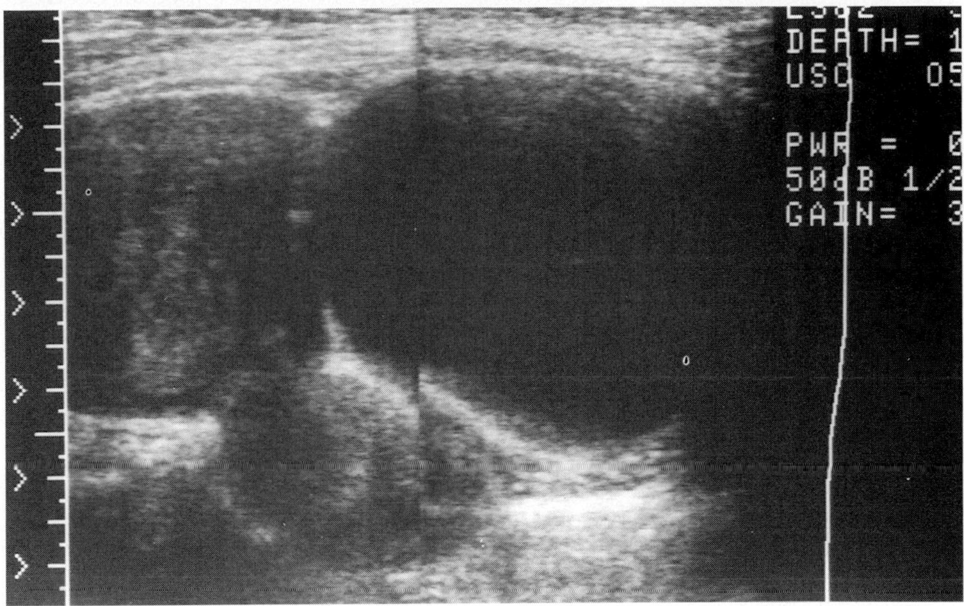

Figure 13.6 Transvaginal pelvic ultrasound demonstrating multiple uterine leiomyomas.

Diagnosis is based on the characteristic finding of an irregularly enlarged uterus. The size and location of the usually multiple leiomyomas can be confirmed and documented with pelvic ultrasonography (Fig. 13.6). If the examination is adequate and symptoms are absent, ultrasonography is not always necessary unless an ovarian mass cannot be excluded.

Endometrial polyps are a cause of intermenstrual bleeding, irregular bleeding, and menorrhagia. The diagnosis is based on either visualization with hysteroscopy or sonohysteroscopy, or on the microscopic assessment of tissue obtained by a biopsy done in the office or a curettage specimen. Abnormal bleeding, either intermenstrual or postcoital, can be caused by cervical lesions. Bleeding can also result from endocervical polyps and infectious cervical lesions, such as condylomas, herpes simplex virus ulcerations, chlamydial cervicitis, or cervicitis caused by other organisms. Other benign cervical lesions, such as wide eversion of endocervical columnar epithelium or Nabothian cysts, may be noted on examination but rarely cause symptoms.

Coagulopathies and Other Hematologic Causes The presence of excessively heavy menses should prompt an evaluation of hematologic status. A complete blood count will be helpful in detecting anemia, significant problems such as leukemia, or disorders associated with thrombocytopenia. Abnormal liver function, which can be seen with alcoholism or other chronic liver diseases, results in inadequate production of clotting factors and can lead to excessive menstrual bleeding. Coagulation abnormalities such as von Willebrand's disease can have a variable clinical picture and may escape diagnosis until the reproductive years (57,58). Oral contraceptives, which increase the level of factor VIII, can be helpful and newer therapies, including desmopressin acetate, may be necessary, particularly before surgical procedures are performed.

Infectious Causes Women with cervicitis, particularly chlamydial cervicitis, can experience irregular bleeding and postcoital spotting (see Chapter 15). Therefore, cervical testing for chlamydia should be considered, especially for sexually active adolescents, women in their twenties, and women who are not in a monogamous relationship. Endometritis can cause excessive menstrual flow. Thus, a woman who seeks treatment for menorrhagia and increased menstrual pain and has a history of light-to-moderate previous menstrual flow may have an upper genital tract infection or PID (endometritis, salpingitis, oophoritis).

Occasionally, chronic endometritis will be diagnosed when an endometrial biopsy is obtained for evaluation of abnormal bleeding in a patient without specific risk factors for PID.

Neoplasia Abnormal bleeding is the most frequent symptom of women with invasive cervical cancer. An obvious cervical lesion should be evaluated by biopsy, because the results of a Papanicolaou (Pap) test may be falsely negative with invasive lesions as a result of tumor necrosis. Unopposed estrogen has been associated with a variety of abnormalities of the endometrium, from cystic hyperplasia to adenomatous hyperplasia, hyperplasia with cytologic atypia, and invasive carcinoma. **Endometrial hyperplasia, hyperplasia with atypia, and invasive endometrial cancer can be diagnosed by endometrial sampling or D & C. Such sampling is mandatory in the evaluation of abnormal bleeding in women older than 35 to 40 years of age, obese women, and those with a history of anovulation.** Although vaginal neoplasia is uncommon, the vagina should be evaluated carefully when there is abnormal bleeding. This includes attention to all surfaces of the vagina, including anterior and posterior areas that may be obscured by the vaginal speculum on examination.

Diagnosis

For all women, the evaluation of excessive and abnormal menses includes a thorough medical and gynecologic history, the exclusion of pregnancy, and a careful gynecologic examination. For women of normal weight between the ages of approximately 20 and 35 years who do not have clear risk factors for sexually transmitted diseases (STDs), who have no signs of androgen excess, who are not using exogenous hormones, and who have no other findings on examination, management may be based on a clinical diagnosis.

Laboratory Studies In any patients with excessive bleeding, an objective measurement of hematologic status should be performed with a complete blood count to detect anemia or thrombocytopenia. A pregnancy test should be performed to rule out pregnancy-related problems. In addition, because of the possibility of a primary coagulation problem, screening coagulation studies such as a prothrombin time and partial thromboplastin time should be considered; an assessment of bleeding time may help diagnose von Willebrand's disease, although if this diagnosis is strongly suspected further testing may be necessary (59).

Imaging Studies **Women with abnormal bleeding who have a history consistent with chronic anovulation, who are obese, or who are older than 35 to 40 years of age require further evaluation.** A pelvic ultrasonographic examination may be helpful in delineating anatomic abnormalities if the examination results are suboptimal or if an ovarian mass is suspected. A pelvic ultrasonographic examination is the best technique for evaluating the uterine contour, endometrial thickness, and ovarian structure. Ultrasonography is particularly valuable in determining whether a pelvic mass is cystic or solid. The use of a vaginal probe transducer allows assessment of endometrial and ovarian disorders, particularly in women who are obese. Sonohysterography involves the infusion of saline into the uterine cavity during transvaginal ultrasonography. This technique has been reported to be especially helpful in visualizing intrauterine problems such as polyps (60). Transvaginal ultrasonography alone has also been reported to have value in differentiating benign polyps from malignant lesions. Although these techniques are helpful in visualizing intrauterine pathology, histologic evaluation is required to rule out malignancy (61). Other techniques, such as CT scanning and MRI, are not as helpful in the initial evaluation and should be reserved for specific indications, such as exploring the possibility of other intraabdominal disorders or adenopathy. Contrast-enhanced MRI shows promise for staging endometrial cancer (62).

Endometrial Sampling **Endometrial sampling should be performed to evaluate abnormal bleeding in women who are at risk for endometrial polyps, hyperplasia, or carcinoma. The technique of D & C, which in the past was used extensively for the evaluation of abnormal bleeding, has been replaced largely by endometrial biopsy in**

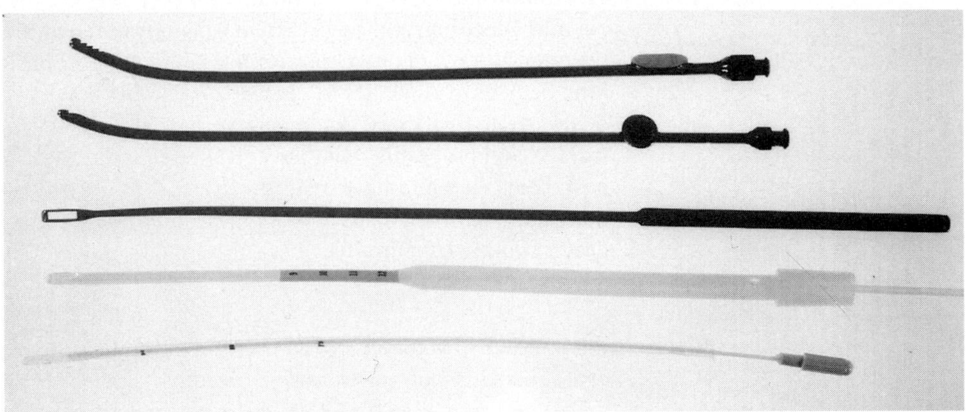

Figure 13.7 Devices used for sampling endometrium. From top to bottom: serrated Novak, Novak, Kevorkian, Explora (Mylex), and Pipelle (Unimar). (From **Berek JS, Hacker NF.** *Practical gynecologic oncology,* 3rd ed. Baltimore: Lippincott Williams & Wilkins, 2000:408, with permission.)

the office. The classic study in which a D & C was performed before hysterectomy with the conclusion that less than one-half of the endometrium was sampled in more than one-half of the patients has led to questioning the use of D & C for endometrial diagnosis (63,64).

It has been argued that there is no longer a place for a "blind" D & C, because hysteroscopy can direct a biopsy to a specific area of the uterus (65). **In most cases, however, endometrial biopsy done in the office can be performed instead of a D & C.** Indications for a hysteroscopy with endometrial sampling include the following:

1. Cervical stenosis precluding adequate endometrial biopsy
2. Patient intolerance of endometrial biopsy
3. Anatomic factors (e.g., massive obesity) precluding adequate endometrial biopsy
4. The presence of abnormal bleeding in a patient who is undergoing another surgical procedure performed with general anesthesia.

A number of devices are designed for endometrial sampling (Fig. 13.7), including an inexpensive disposable flexible plastic sheath with an internal plunger that allows tissue aspiration, disposable plastic cannulae of varying diameters that attach to a manually locking syringe that allows the establishment of a vacuum, and cannulae (both rigid metal and plastic) with tissue traps that attach to an electric vacuum pump. Several studies comparing the adequacy of sampling using these devices with D & C have shown a comparable ability to detect abnormalities. It should be noted that these devices are designed to obtain a tissue sample rather than a cytologic washing. Devices designed to obtain an endometrial sample for assessment of cytology are also available; they have been shown to detect invasive cancer as well as D & C but to have a lower sensitivity for detecting premalignant lesions.

Management

Nonsurgical Management Most bleeding problems, including anovulatory bleeding can be managed nonsurgically (66). Treatment with NSAIDs such as *ibuprofen* and *mefenamic* acid has been shown to decrease menstrual flow by 30% to 50% (67). Antifibrinolytics, currently not available for use in the United States, have been shown to be effective in reducing menstrual blood loss (68,69). *Levonorgestrel*-containing intrauterine devices also have been shown to reduce menstrual blood loss (70).

Hormonal management of abnormal bleeding frequently can control excessive or irregular bleeding. Although there is a paucity of randomized controlled trials demonstrating the effectiveness of oral contraceptives in reducing menstrual flow, oral contraceptives have long been used clinically to decrease menstrual flow (71,72). Although this effect was first demonstrated with oral contraceptive formulations that contained higher doses of both estrogens and progestins than the agents used today, low-dose combined oral contraceptives have been shown to have a similar effect (73). Low-dose oral contraceptives may be used during the perimenopausal years in healthy nonsmoking women who have no major cardiovascular risk factors. The benefits of menstrual regulation in such women often override the potential risks.

For patients in whom estrogen use is contraindicated, progestins, both oral and parenteral, can be used to control excessive bleeding. Cyclic oral *medroxyprogesterone acetate,* administered from days 5 to 26 of the cycle, results in a reduction of menstrual flow, although it is less effective than the progestin-containing intrauterine device (70). The benefits to the patient with oligomenorrhea and anovulation include a regular flow and the prevention of long intervals of amenorrhea, which may end in unpredictable, profuse bleeding. This therapy reduces the risk of hyperplasia resulting from persistent, unopposed estrogen stimulation of the endometrium. Depot formulations of *medroxyprogesterone acetate* also have been used to establish amenorrhea in women at risk of excessive bleeding.

In Europe, the intrauterine device containing norgestrel has long been used therapeutically to deliver progestin locally to the endometrium in women with abnormal bleeding who have been diagnosed with dysfunctional uterine bleeding (74). This device was approved for use in the United States in 2000, and its use has been suggested as a cost-effective alternative to hysterectomy for excessive bleeding (75).

Surgical Therapy **The surgical management of abnormal bleeding should be reserved for situations in which medical therapy has been unsuccessful or is contraindicated. The D & C, although sometimes appropriate as a diagnostic technique, is questionable as a therapeutic modality.** One study reported a measured reduction in menstrual blood loss for the first menstrual period only (76). Other studies have suggested a longer-lasting benefit (77).

The surgical options range from hysteroscopy with resection of submucous leiomyomas to laparoscopic techniques of myomectomy to uterine artery embolization to endometrial ablation (Chapter 21) to hysterectomy (Chapter 22). The choice of procedure depends on the cause of the bleeding. The assessment of the relative advances, risks, benefits, complications, and indications of these procedures is a subject of ongoing clinical research (78,79). The proposed advantages of techniques other than hysterectomy include a shorter recovery time and less early morbidity. However, symptoms can recur or persist; repeat procedures or subsequent hysterectomy may be required if conservative options are chosen. Quality of life outcomes should be assessed, and current studies do not indicate there is a definitive management advantage to any particular technique (80,81).

Much has been written about the psychologic sequelae of hysterectomy, and some of the aforementioned surgical techniques have been developed in an effort to provide less drastic management options. Most well-controlled recent studies have suggested that, in the absence of preexisting psychopathology, indicated but elective surgical procedures for hysterectomy have few, if any, significant psychologic sequelae (including depression) (82) (Chapter 12).

Postmenopausal Women

Differential Diagnosis

The causes of postmenopausal bleeding and the percentage of patients who seek treatment for different conditions are presented in Table 13.7.

Table 13.7. Etiology of Postmenopausal Bleeding

Factor	Approximate Percentage
Exogenous estrogens	30
Atrophic endometritis/vaginitis	30
Endometrial cancer	15
Endometrial or cervical polyps	10
Endometrial hyperplasia	5
Miscellaneous (e.g., cervical cancer, uterine sarcoma, urethral caruncle, trauma)	10

From **Hacker NF, Moore JG.** *Essentials of obstetrics and gynecology,* 3rd ed. Philadelphia: WB Saunders, 1998:635, with permission.

Benign Disorders Women who are taking hormone replacement therapy during menopause may be using a variety of hormonal regimens that can result in bleeding (see Chapter 29). In the classic sequential method of administration, estrogens are given for the first 25 days of each month. A progestin, often 5 to 10 mg/day of *medroxyprogesterone acetate,* is added to the last 10 to 13 days of this regimen in an effort to reduce the risk of endometrial hyperplasia and neoplasia. Most women who take these hormones in this way will experience withdrawal bleeding, which is perceived by the patient as a menstrual period. Although the incidence of withdrawal bleeding does decline somewhat with age and duration of therapy, more than 50% of women continue to experience bleeding after 65 years of age.

Because some women become symptomatic during the days when they are not taking estrogens, as in the previously described regimen, many clinicians have modified this regimen to include continuous (every day) estrogen therapy. In addition, studies have assessed endometrial response to varying durations of progestin regimens; longer duration of therapy is associated with a lower risk of hyperplasia. It has been suggested that endometrial sampling is indicated for any bleeding that occurs beyond the expected time of withdrawal following cyclic progestin therapy. **A significant change in withdrawal bleeding (e.g., absence of withdrawal bleeding for several months followed by resumption of bleeding or a marked increase in the amount of bleeding) should prompt endometrial sampling.**

Patient compliance has been a significant issue with hormone replacement therapy. Missed doses of medication and failure to take the medication in the prescribed fashion can lead to irregular bleeding or spotting that is benign in origin but that can result in patient dissatisfaction (83).

The primary problems that women report with hormone replacement therapy include vaginal bleeding and weight gain. The use of a continuous low-dose combined regimen has the advantage that, for many women, bleeding will ultimately cease after a period of several months during which irregular and unpredictable bleeding may occur (84). Some women are unable to tolerate these initial months of irregular bleeding. The risk of endometrial hyperplasia or neoplasia with this regimen appears to be low.

Other benign causes of bleeding include atrophic vaginitis and cervical polyps, which may become apparent as postcoital bleeding or spotting. Women who experience bleeding after menopause may attempt to minimize the extent of the problem; they may describe only "spotting" or "pink or brownish discharge." However, any indication of bleeding or spotting should be evaluated. In the absence of hormone therapy, any bleeding after menopause (classically defined as absence of menses for 1 year) should prompt evaluation with endometrial sampling. At least one-fourth of postmenopausal women with bleeding have a neoplastic lesion.

Endometrial polyps and other abnormalities can be seen in women who are taking tamoxifen. These polyps can be benign, although they must be distinguished from endometrial malignancies, which may also occur with this medication.

Neoplasia Endometrial, cervical, and ovarian malignancies must be ruled out in cases of postmenopausal bleeding. **A Pap test is essential when postmenopausal bleeding is noted, although the Pap test is an insensitive diagnostic test for detecting endometrial cancer.** The Pap test results are negative in some cases of invasive cervical carcinoma because of tumor necrosis.

Cervical malignancy is diagnosed by cervical biopsy of grossly visible lesions and colposcopically directed biopsy for women with abnormal Pap test results (Chapter 16). Functional ovarian tumors may produce estrogen and lead to endometrial hyperplasia or carcinoma, which may cause bleeding.

Diagnosis

Pelvic examination to detect local lesions and a Pap test to assess cytology are essential first steps in finding the cause of postmenopausal bleeding. Endometrial sampling, through office biopsy, hysteroscopy, or D & C, is usually considered essential. Pelvic ultrasonographic examination and, in particular, vaginal ultrasonography or sonohysterography can suggest the cause of bleeding. Initial biopsy done in the office is more cost effective than D & C, surgery, or observation alone (85). The cost effectiveness of other screening strategies, including transvaginal ultrasonography or sonohysterography, has not been well studied. It has been suggested that an endometrial thickness of less than 6 mm (4 to 5 mm in some reports) measured by transvaginal ultrasonography is unlikely to indicate endometrial cancer.

Management

The management of atrophic vaginitis includes topical or systemic use of estrogens after other causes of abnormal bleeding have been excluded. Cervical polyps can easily be removed in the office.

Endometrial Hyperplasia The terminology that has been used to describe endometrial hyperplasia is confusing, and the clinician must consult with the pathologist to ensure an understanding of the diagnosis. **The following lesions are considered to be benign: *anovulatory, proliferative, cystic glandular hyperplasia, simple cystic hyperplasia*** (Fig. 13.8), ***simple hyperplasia, and adenomatous hyperplasia without atypia.* These terms reflect and describe an exaggerated proliferative response of the endometrium. In most cases, benign endometrial hyperplasia is resolved with D & C or progestin therapy.** Repeat surveillance with endometrial biopsy may be warranted.

The presence of atypia with abnormal proliferation, including features of back-to-back crowding of the glands, with epithelial activity demonstrated by papillary projections into the glands, is associated with an increased risk of progression to endometrial carcinoma (Fig. 13.9). These architectural abnormalities may be associated with individual cellular atypia (enlarged, irregular nuclei, chromatin clumping, and prominent nucleoli). The presence of mitotic activity also can be variable.

The management of endometrial hyperplasia rests on an understanding of the natural history of the lesion involved. In one study, only 2% of 122 patients with hyperplasia without cytologic atypia progressed to carcinoma, whereas 23% of those with atypical hyperplasia subsequently developed carcinoma (86). Architectural complexity and crowding appears to place patients at greater risk for progression than does the presence of cytologic atypia alone.

These data suggest that most women with endometrial hyperplasia will respond to progestin therapy and are not at increased risk of developing cancer. Patients who do

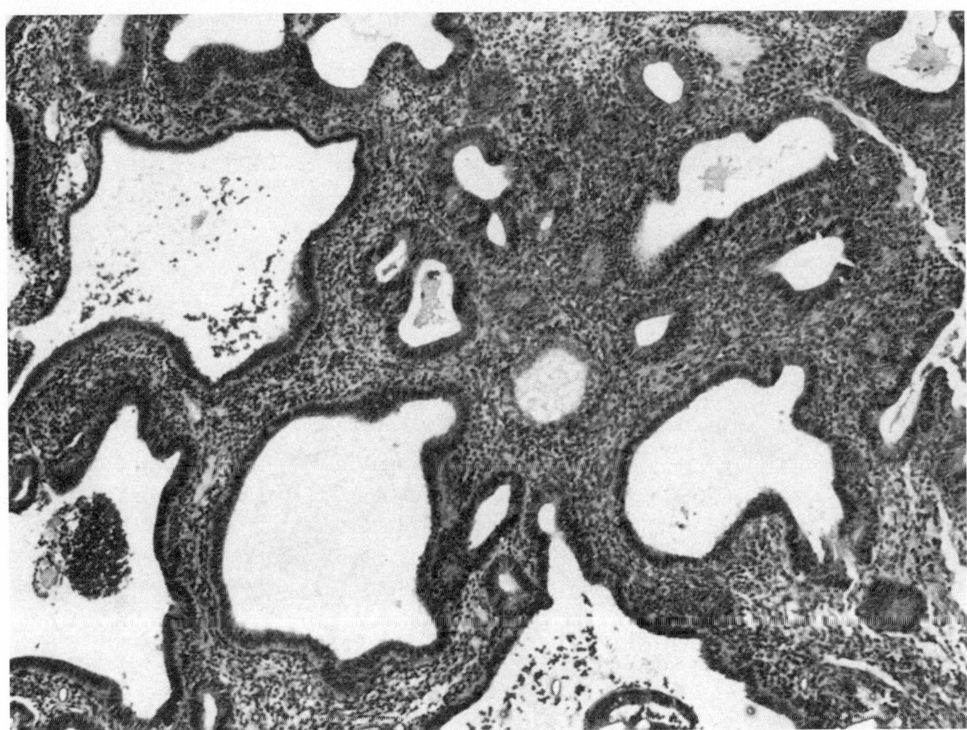

Figure 13.8 Simple cystic hyperplasia of the endometrium. The normal tabular pattern is replaced by cystically dilated proliferative endometrial glands. (From **Berek JS, Hacker NF.** *Practical gynecologic oncology,* 2nd ed. Baltimore: Lippincott Williams & Wilkins, 1994:126, with permission.)

not respond are at a significantly increased risk of progressing to invasive cancer and should be advised to have a hysterectomy. Patients who are unlikely to respond can be identified on the basis of cytologic atypia. A suggested scheme of management is outlined in Fig. 13.10. This treatment is discussed in more detail in Chapter 30.

Pelvic Mass

The probable causes of a pelvic mass found on physical examination or through radiologic studies are vastly different in a prepubertal child than they are during adolescence or during the postmenopausal years (Table 13.3). A pelvic mass may be gynecologic in origin or it may arise from the urinary tract or bowel. The gynecologic causes of a pelvic mass may be uterine, adnexal, or more specifically ovarian.

Prepubertal Age Group

Differential Diagnosis

Fewer than 5% of ovarian malignancies occur in children and adolescents. Ovarian tumors account for approximately 1% of all tumors in these age groups. Germ cell tumors make up one-half to two-thirds of ovarian neoplasms in individuals younger than 20 years of age. A review of studies conducted from 1940 until 1975 concluded that 35% of all ovarian neoplasms occurring during childhood and adolescence were malignant (87). **In girls younger than 9 years of age, approximately 80% of the ovarian neoplasms were found to be malignant** (88,89). Germ cell tumors account for approximately 60% of ovarian neoplasms in children and adolescents compared with 20% of these tumors in

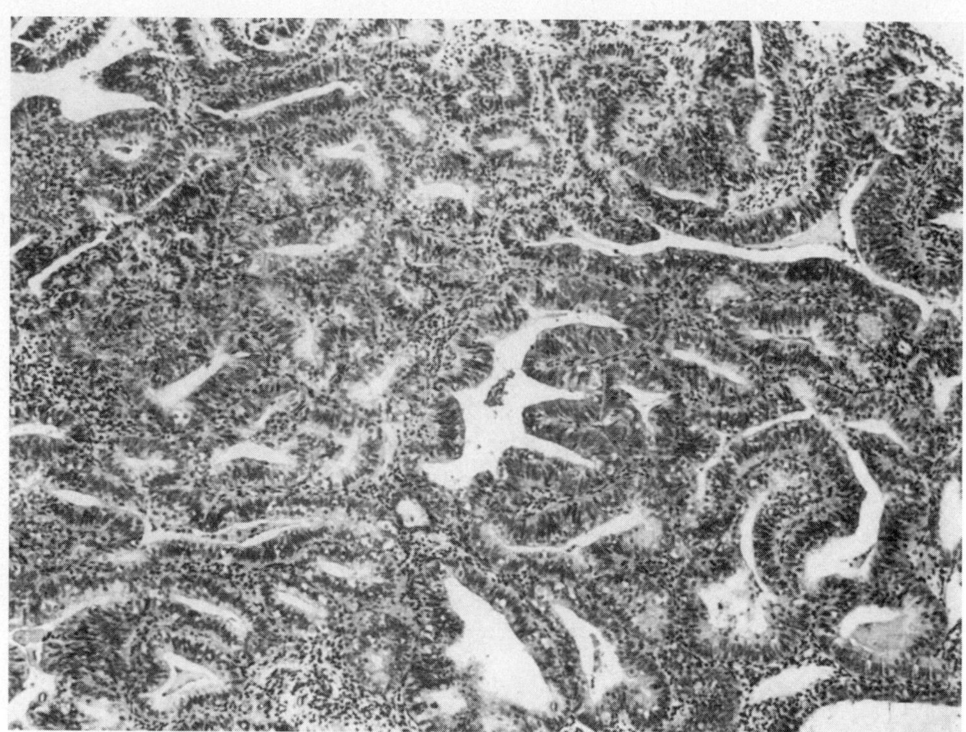

Figure 13.9 Aypical hyperplasia (complex hyperplasia with severe nuclear atypia). The proliferative endometrial glands reveal considerable crowding and papillary infoldings. The endometrial stroma, although markedly diminished, can still be recognized between the glands. (From **Berek JS, Hacker NF.** *Practical gynecologic oncology,* 2nd ed. Baltimore: Lippincott Williams & Wilkins, 1994:127, with permission.)

adults (87). Epithelial neoplasms are rare in the prepubertal age group; thus, data usually are reported from referral centers. However, some reports include only neoplastic masses, whereas others include nonneoplastic masses; some series combine data from prepubertal and adolescent girls. One community survey of ovarian masses revealed that the frequency of malignancy was much lower than previously reported; of all ovarian masses confirmed surgically in childhood and adolescence, only 6% of masses were malignant neoplasms, and only 10% of neoplasms were malignant (90). Surgical decision making clearly influences the statistics on incidence; the surgical excision of functional masses that would resolve in time inflates the percentage of benign masses. In one series, nonneoplastic masses in young women and girls younger than 20 years of age constituted two-thirds of the total (91). Even in girls younger than 10 years of age, 60% of the masses were nonneoplastic, and two-thirds of the neoplastic masses were benign. Functional, follicular cysts can occur in fetuses, newborns, and prepubertal children. They may be associated with sexual precocity.

Abdominal or pelvic pain is one of the most frequent initial symptoms. In a prepubertal child, a pelvic mass very quickly becomes abdominal in location as it enlarges because of the small size of the pelvic cavity. The diagnosis of ovarian masses in the prepubertal age group is difficult because of the rarity of the condition (and therefore a low index of suspicion), because many symptoms are nonspecific, and acute symptoms are more likely to be attributed to more common entities such as appendicitis. Abdominal palpation and bimanual rectoabdominal examination are important in any child who has nonspecific abdominal or pelvic complaints. An ovarian mass that is abdominal in location can be confused with other abdominal masses occurring in children, such as Wilms' tumor or neuroblastoma. Acute pain is often associated with torsion. The ovarian ligament becomes elongated as a result of the abdominal location of these tumors, thus creating a predisposition to torsion.

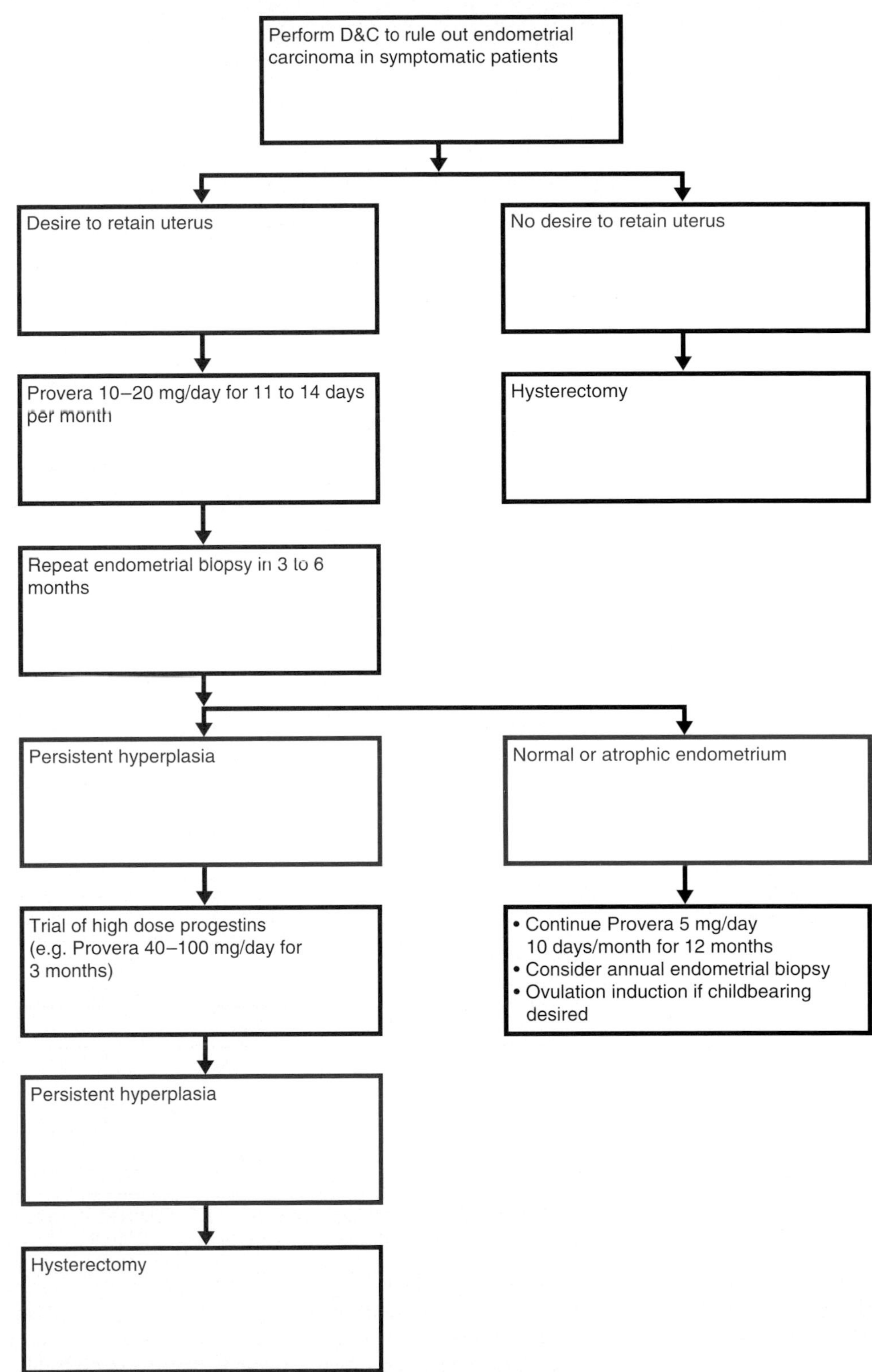

Figure 13.10 Management of endometrial hyperplasia. (From **Berek JS, Hacker NF.** *Practical gynecologic oncology,* 3rd ed. Baltimore: Lippincott Williams & Wilkins, 2000:422, with permission.)

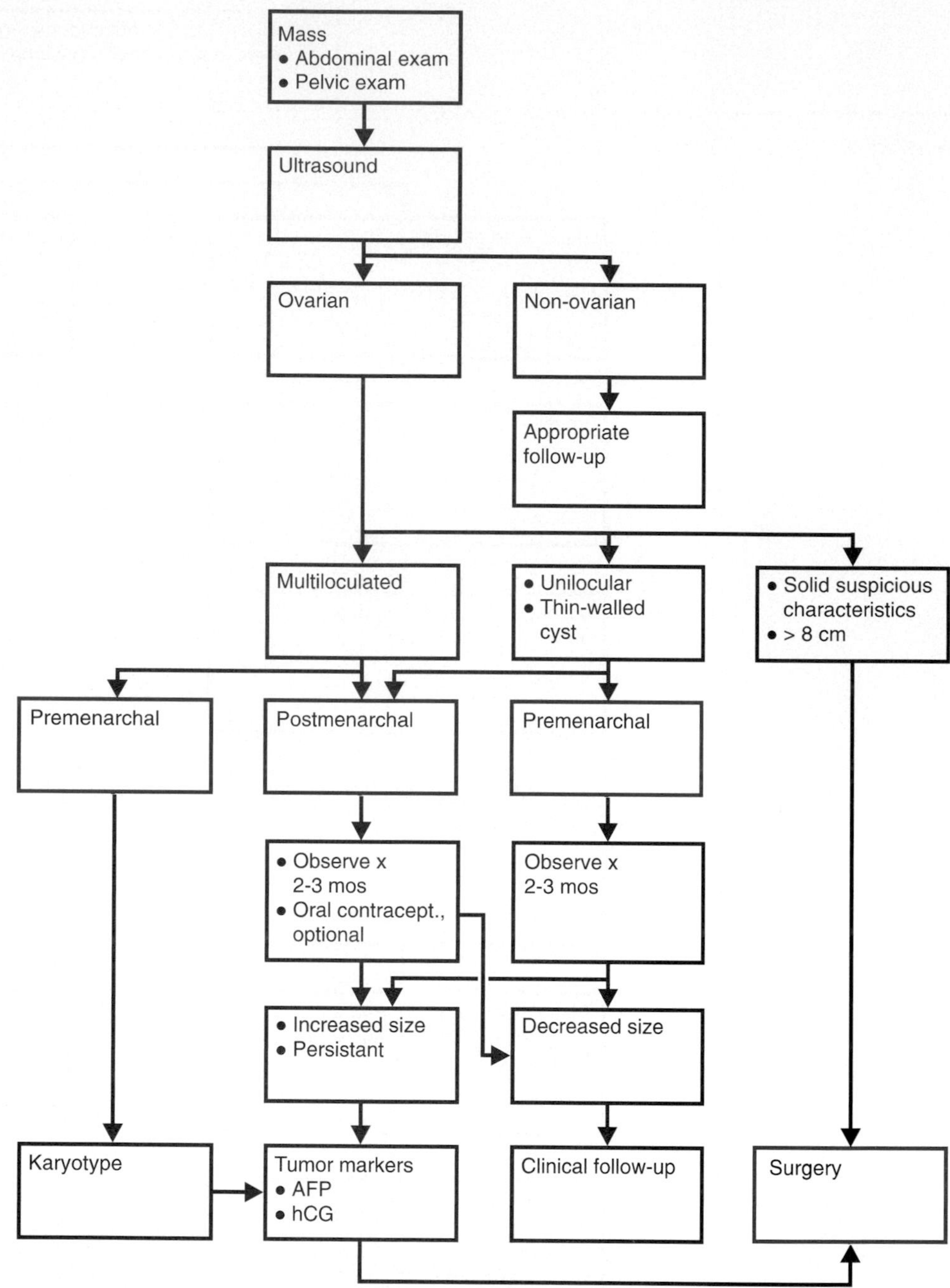

Figure 13.11 Management of pelvic masses in premenarchal and adolescent girls.

Diagnosis and Management

In recent years, ultrasonography has become an excellent tool for predicting the presence of a simple ovarian cyst. Figure 13.11 outlines a plan of management for pelvic masses in the prepubertal age group. **Unilocular cysts are virtually always benign and will regress in 3 to 6 months; thus, they do not require surgical management with oophorectomy or oophorocystectomy.** Close observation is recommended, although there is a risk of ovarian torsion that must be discussed with the child's parents. Recurrence rates after cyst aspiration (either ultrasonographically guided or with laparoscopy) may be as high as 50%. Attention must be paid to long-term effects on endocrine functioning as well as future fertility; preservation of ovarian tissue is a priority for patients with benign tumors. **Premature surgical therapy for a functional ovarian mass can result in ovarian and tubal adhesions that can affect future fertility.**

Additional imaging studies, such as CT scanning, MRI, or Doppler flow studies, may be helpful in establishing the diagnosis (92). Because the risk of a germ cell tumor is high, the finding of a solid component mandates surgical assessment (93).

Adolescent Age Group

Differential Diagnosis

Ovarian Masses

Many series report ovarian tumors occurring in both children and adolescents. Some reports divide their findings by age group, although this is less helpful than a division by pubertal development. The clinician's response to a pelvic or abdominal mass varies in relation to the patient's pubertal status, because the likelihood of functional masses increases after menarche. **The risk of malignant neoplasms is lower among adolescents than among younger children. Epithelial neoplasms occur with increasing frequency with age. Germ cell tumors are the most common tumors of the first decade of life but occur less frequently during adolescence** (Chapter 32). **Mature cystic teratoma is the most frequent neoplastic tumor of children and adolescents, accounting for more than one-half of ovarian neoplasms in women younger than 20 years of age** (94).

It is well established that neoplasia can arise in dysgenetic gonads. Malignant tumors have been found in about 25% of dysgenetic gonads of patients with a Y chromosome (95). Gonadectomy is recommended for patients with XY gonadal dysgenesis or its mosaic variations (96).

Functional ovarian cysts occur frequently in adolescence. They may be an incidental finding on examination or may be associated with pain caused by torsion, leakage, or rupture. Endometriosis is less common during adolescence than in adulthood, although it can occur during adolescence. In series of adolescents referred with chronic pain, 50% to 65% have been found to have endometriosis (97). Although endometriosis can occur in young women with obstructive genital anomalies (presumably as a result of retrograde menstruation), most adolescents with endometriosis do not have associated obstructive anomalies (98). In young women, endometriosis may have an atypical appearance, with nonpigmented or vesicular lesions, peritoneal windows, and puckering.

Uterine Masses

Other causes of pelvic masses, such as uterine abnormalities, are rare in adolescence. Uterine leiomyomas are not commonly seen in this age group. Obstructive uterovaginal anomalies occur during adolescence, at the time of menarche, or shortly thereafter. The diagnosis is frequently neither suspected nor delayed, particularly when the patient is seen by a general surgeon (99). A wide range of anomalies can be seen, from imperforate hymen to transverse vaginal septa, to vaginal agenesis with a normal uterus and functional endometrium, vaginal duplications with obstructing longitudinal septa, and obstructed uterine horns. Patients may seek treatment for cyclic pain, amenorrhea, vaginal discharge, or an abdominal, pelvic, or vaginal mass (Fig. 13.5). A hematocolpos, hematometra, or both frequently will be present, and the resulting mass can be quite large.

Inflammatory Masses

Adolescents have the highest rates of PID of any age group, if one considers only individuals at risk for STD (i.e., those who have had sexual intercourse) (36). Thus, an adolescent who has pelvic pain may be found to have an inflammatory mass. The diagnosis of PID is primarily a clinical one based on the presence of lower abdominal, pelvic, and adnexal tenderness; cervical motion tenderness; a mucopurulent discharge; and the signs of elevated temperature, white blood cell count, or sedimentation rate (Chapter 15). PID is clearly associated with the risks of acquiring STD, and methods of contraception may either decrease the risk (oral contraceptives, male latex condoms) or increase it (the intrauterine device in the interval immediately after insertion) (100,101). Inflammatory masses may consist of a tuboovarian complex (a mass consisting of matted bowel, tube, and ovary), tuboovarian abscess (a mass consisting primarily of an abscess cavity within an anatomically defined structure such as the ovary), pyosalpinx or, chronically, hydrosalpinx.

Pregnancy

In adolescents, pregnancy should always be considered as a cause of a pelvic mass. In the United States, more than 50% of adolescent young women have experienced sexual intercourse by 17 years of age (23). Most pregnancies in adolescents are unintended; 82% of pregnancies in adolescents under age 15, 83% in women aged 15 to 17, and 75% of pregnancies in women aged 18 to 19 are unintended (42). Adolescents may be more likely than adults to deny the possibility of pregnancy because of wishful thinking, anxiety about discovery by parents or peers, or unfamiliarity with menstrual cycles and information about fertility. Ectopic pregnancies may cause pelvic pain and an adnexal mass. With the availability of quantitative measurements of β-human chorionic gonadotropin (hCG), more ectopic pregnancies are being discovered before rupture, allowing conservative management with laparoscopic surgery or medical therapy with *methotrexate* (Chapter 17). The risk of ectopic pregnancy varies by method of contraception; users of no contraception have the highest risk, whereas oral contraceptive users have the lowest risk (102). As in older patients, paraovarian cysts and nongynecologic masses can appear as a pelvic or abdominal mass in adolescents.

Diagnosis

A history and pelvic examination are critical in the diagnosis of a pelvic mass. Considerations in adolescents include the anxiety associated with a first pelvic examination, as well as issues of confidentiality related to questions of sexual activity. Techniques for history taking and the performance of the first examination are discussed in Chapter 1.

Laboratory studies should always include a pregnancy test (regardless of stated sexual activity), and a complete blood count may be helpful in diagnosing inflammatory masses. Tumor markers, including α-fetoprotein and hCG, may be elaborated by germ cell tumors and can be useful in preoperative diagnosis as well as follow-up (Chapter 32).

As in all age groups, the primary diagnostic technique for evaluating pelvic masses in adolescents is ultrasonography. Although transvaginal ultrasonographic examinations may provide more detail than transabdominal ultrasonography, particularly for inflammatory masses, a transvaginal examination may not be well tolerated by adolescents (103). For cases in which the ultrasonographic examination is inconclusive, CT or MRI may be helpful. An accurate preoperative assessment of anatomy is critical, particularly in cases of uterovaginal malformations. MRI can be useful for evaluating this group of rare anomalies (104,105). Some sort of imaging technique should be used in evaluating adolescents who come in with abdominal pain, because an unexpected finding of a complex uterine or vaginal anomaly requires careful surgical planning and decision making.

Management

The management of masses in adolescents depends on the suspected diagnosis as well as the initial complaint. Figure 13.11 outlines a plan of management for pelvic masses in adolescents. **Asymptomatic unilocular cystic masses are best managed conservatively, because the likelihood of malignancy is low. If surgical management is required based on symptoms or uncertainty of diagnosis, attention should be paid to minimizing the risks of subsequent infertility resulting from pelvic adhesions. In addition, every effort should be made to conserve ovarian tissue. In the presence of a malignant unilateral ovarian mass, management may include unilateral oophorectomy rather than more**

radical surgery, even if the ovarian tumor has metastasized (Chapter 32). **Analysis of frozen sections may not be reliable. In general, conservative surgery is appropriate; further surgery can be performed, if necessary, after an adequate histologic evaluation of the ovarian tumor.**

Some surgeons advocate the use of laparoscopy in the management of suspected acute PID to confirm the diagnosis, and to perform irrigation, lysis of adhesions, drainage and irrigation of unilateral or bilateral pyosalpinx or tuboovarian abscess, or extirpation of significant disease (106,107). While symptoms persist in a patient with the clinical diagnosis of PID or tuboovarian abscess, laparoscopy should be considered to confirm the diagnosis. A clinical diagnosis may be incorrect in up to one-third of patients (108). The surgical management of inflammatory masses is rarely necessary in adolescents, except to treat rupture of tuboovarian abscess or failure of medical management with broad-spectrum antibiotics (Chapter 15). Conservative, unilateral adnexectomy usually can be performed in these situations, rather than a pelvic clean-out, maintaining reproductive potential. Percutaneous drainage, transvaginal ultrasonographic drainage, and laparoscopic management of tuboovarian abscesses are becoming more popular, although, as with the laparoscopic management of ovarian masses, the surgeon's skill and experience are critical and prospective studies are lacking (109). Laparoscopic management has been associated with a risk of major complications, including bowel obstruction and bowel or vessel injury (110).

Reproductive Age Group

Conditions diagnosed as a pelvic mass in women of reproductive age are presented in Table 13.8.

Table 13.8. Conditions Diagnosed as a Pelvic Mass in Women of Reproductive Age

Full urinary bladder
Urachal cyst
Sharply anteflexed or retroflexed uterus
Pregnancy (with or without concomitant leiomyomas) Intrauterine Tubal Abdominal
Ovarian or adnexal masses Functional cysts Inflammatory masses Tuboovarian complex Diverticular abscess Appendiceal abscess Matted bowel and omentum Peritoneal cyst Stool in sigmoid Neoplastic tumors Benign Malignant
Paraovarian or paratubal cysts
Intraligamentous myomas
Less common conditions that must be excluded: Pelvic kidney Carcinoma of the colon, rectum, appendix Carcinoma of the fallopian tube Retroperitoneal tumors (anterior sacral meningocele) Uterine sarcoma or other malignant tumors

Differential Diagnosis

It is difficult to determine the frequency of diagnoses of pelvic mass in women of reproductive age, because many pelvic masses are not ultimately treated with surgery. Nonovarian or nongynecologic conditions may be confused with an ovarian or uterine mass (Table 13.8). There are series in which the frequency of masses found at laparotomy is reviewed, although the varying indications for surgery, indications for referral, type of practice (gynecologic oncology versus general gynecology), and patient populations (a higher percentage of African Americans with uterine leiomyomas, for example) will affect the percentages. Benign masses, such as functional ovarian cysts, will often not require surgery.

Age is an important determinant of the likelihood of malignancy. In one series of women who underwent laparotomy for pelvic mass, malignancy was seen in only 10% of those younger than 30 years of age, and most of these tumors had low malignant potential (111). The most common tumors found during laparotomy for pelvic mass are mature cystic teratomas or dermoids (seen in one-third of women younger than 30 years of age) and endometriomas (approximately one-fourth of women 31 to 49 years of age) (111).

Uterine Masses

Uterine leiomyomas, also known as myomas or fibroids, are by far the most common benign uterine tumors. Other benign uterine growths, such as uterine vascular tumors, are rare. Uterine leiomyomas are usually diagnosed on physical examination. They may be subserosal, intramucosal, or submucosal in location within the uterus or located in the cervix, in the broad ligament, or on a pedicle (Fig. 13.12). They are estimated to be present in at least 20% of all women of reproductive age and may be discovered incidentally during routine annual examination. Leiomyomas are more common in African American than in white women. Asymptomatic fibroids may be present in 40% to 50% of women older than 35 years of

Figure 13.12 Uterine leiomyomas in various anatomic locations. (From **Hacker NF, Moore JG.** *Essentials of obstetrics and gynecology,* 3rd ed. Philadelphia: WB Saunders, 1998:413, with permission.)

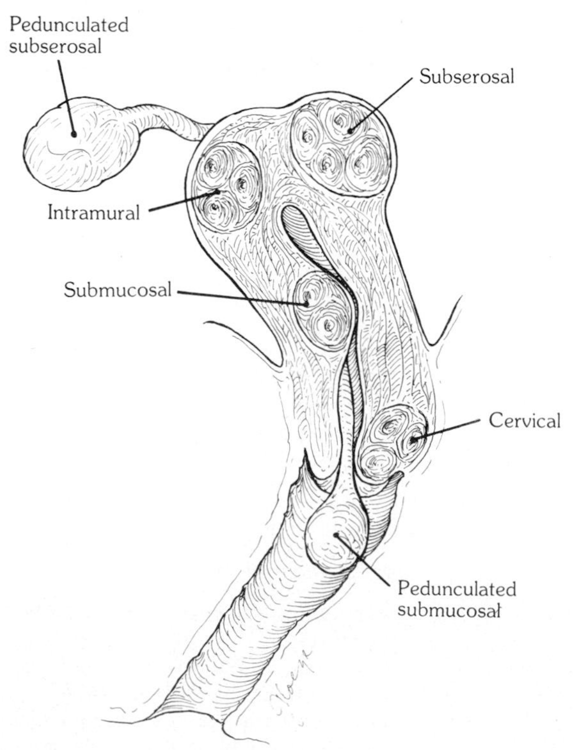

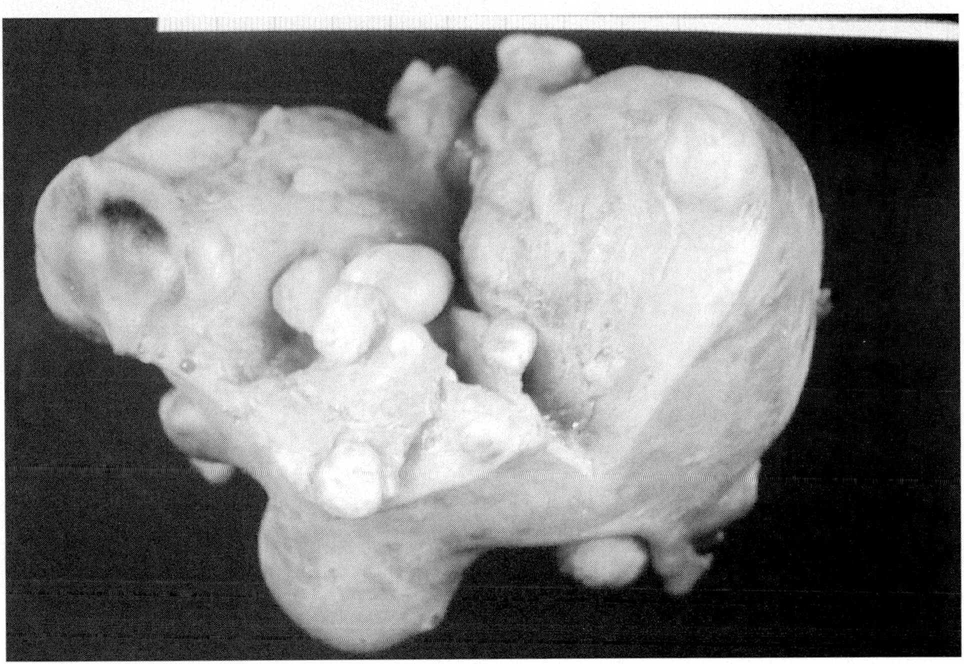

Figure 13.13 Multiple uterine leiomyomas.

age (55). They may occur singly but often are multiple. They may cause a range of symptoms, from abnormal bleeding to pelvic pressure, which may lead to the diagnosis. Fewer than one-half of uterine leiomyomas are estimated to produce symptoms, however (112).

The cause of uterine leiomyomas is unknown. Several studies have suggested that each leiomyoma arises from a single neoplastic cell within the smooth muscle of the myometrium (113). There appears to be an increased familial incidence (55). Hormonal responsiveness and binding has been demonstrated *in vitro.* Fibroids have the potential to enlarge during pregnancy as well as to regress after menopause.

Grossly, fibroids are discrete nodular tumors that vary in size and number (Fig. 13.13). They may be microscopic or huge (a uterine weight of 74 lb has been reported). They may cause symmetric uterine enlargement or they may distort the uterine contour significantly. The consistency of an individual leiomyoma varies from hard and stony (as with a calcified leiomyoma) to soft (as with cystic degeneration), although the usual consistency is described as firm or rubbery. Although they do not have a true capsule, the margins of the tumor are blunt, noninfiltrating, and pushing, and are usually separated from the myometrium by a pseudocapsule of connective tissue, which allows easy enucleation at the time of surgery. There is usually one major blood vessel supplying each tumor. The cut surface is characteristically whorled.

Degenerative changes are reported in approximately two-thirds of all specimens (114). Leiomyomas, with an increased number of mitotic figures, may occur in various forms: (a) during pregnancy or in women taking progestational agents, (b) with necrosis, and (c) as a ***smooth muscle tumor of uncertain malignant potential*** **(defined as having 5 to 9 mitoses per 10 high-power fields (hpf) that do not demonstrate nuclear atypia or giant cells, or with a lower mitotic count (2 to 4 mitoses/10 hpf) that does demonstrate atypical nuclear features or giant cells).** Studies suggest that malignant degeneration of a preexisting leiomyoma is extremely uncommon, occurring in less than 0.5% (115).

Leiomyosarcoma is a rare malignant neoplasm composed of cells that have smooth muscle differentiation (Chapter 30). The typical patient with leiomyosarcoma is in her mid-50s and seeks treatment for abnormal bleeding. In most cases, diagnoses are determined (postoperatively) after microscopic examination of a uterus removed because of suspected leiomyomas. **Sarcomas that have a malignant behavior have ≥10 mitoses/hpf.**

Uterine fibroids are frequently diagnosed on the basis of clinical findings of an enlarged, irregular uterus on pelvic examination. They are also frequently noted on ultrasonography obtained for a variety of indications and may be an incidental finding. However, any pelvic tumor potentially can be confused with an enlarged uterus.

The most common initial symptom associated with fibroids, and the one that most frequently leads to surgical intervention, is menorrhagia. Chronic pelvic pain may also be present. Pain may be characterized as dysmenorrhea, dyspareunia, or pelvic pressure (Chapter 14). Acute pain may result from torsion of a pedunculated leiomyoma or infarction and degeneration. The following urinary symptoms may be present:

1. Frequency, which may result from extrinsic pressure on the bladder.

2. Partial ureteral obstruction may be caused by pressure from large tumors at the pelvic brim. Reports suggest some degree of ureteral obstruction in 30% to 70% of tumors above the pelvic brim. Ureteral compression is 3 to 4 times more common on the right, because the left ureter is protected by the sigmoid colon.

3. Rarely, complete urethral obstruction, resulting from elevation of the base of the bladder by the cervical or lower uterine leiomyoma with impingement on the region of the internal sphincter, may occur.

Leiomyomas are an infrequent primary cause of infertility and have been reported as a sole cause in only a small percentage of infertile patients (116). One review of myomectomies performed for all indications noted a history of infertility in 27% of women (112). Pregnancy loss or complications can occur in women with leiomyomas, although most patients have uncomplicated pregnancies and deliveries. One study calculated a 10% rate of pregnancy complications in women with fibroids (117). **Although growth of leiomyomas may occur with pregnancy, no demonstrable change in size (based on serial ultrasonographic examination) has been noted in 70% to 80% of patients** (118,119). The risk of pregnancy complications is influenced by both myoma location and size (120).

The following symptoms may infrequently be associated with leiomyomas:

1. Rectosigmoid compression, with constipation or intestinal obstruction

2. Prolapse of a pedunculated submucous tumor through the cervix, with associated symptoms of severe cramping and subsequent ulceration and infection (uterine inversion has also been reported)

3. Venous stasis of the lower extremities and possible thrombophlebitis secondary to pelvic compression

4. Polycythemia

5. Ascites.

Ovarian Masses

During the reproductive years, the most common ovarian masses are benign. About two-thirds of ovarian tumors are encountered during the reproductive years. Most ovarian tumors (80% to 85%) are benign, and two-thirds of these occur in women between 20 and 44 years of age. **The chance that a primary ovarian tumor is malignant in a patient younger**

than 45 years of age is less than 1 in 15. Most tumors produce few or only mild, nonspecific symptoms. The most common symptoms include abdominal distension, abdominal pain or discomfort, lower abdominal pressure sensation, and urinary or gastrointestinal symptoms. If the tumor is hormonally active, symptoms of hormonal imbalance, such as vaginal bleeding related to estrogen production, may be present. Acute pain may occur with adnexal torsion, cyst rupture, or bleeding into a cyst. Pelvic findings in patients with benign and malignant tumors differ. Masses that are unilateral, cystic, mobile, and smooth are most likely to be benign, whereas those that are bilateral, solid, fixed, irregular, and associated with ascites, *cul-de-sac* nodules, and a rapid rate of growth are more likely to be malignant.

In terms of assessing ovarian masses, the distribution of primary ovarian neoplasms by decade of life can be helpful (121). Ovarian masses in women of reproductive age are most likely to be benign, but the possibility of malignancy must be considered (Fig. 13.14).

Nonneoplastic Ovarian Masses **Functional ovarian cysts include follicular cysts, corpus luteum cysts, and theca lutein cysts. All are benign and usually do not cause symptoms or require surgical management.** The annual rate of hospitalization for functional ovarian cysts has been estimated to be as high as 500 per 100,000 woman-years in the United States, although little is known about the epidemiology of the condition (122). **The most common functional cyst is the follicular cyst, which is rarely larger than 8 cm.** A cystic follicle can be defined as a follicular cyst when its diameter is greater than 3 cm. These cysts are usually found incidental to pelvic examination, although they may rupture, causing pain and peritoneal signs (Fig. 13.15). They usually resolve in 4 to 8 weeks.

Corpus luteum cysts are less common than follicular cysts. Corpus luteum cysts may rupture, leading to a hemoperitoneum and requiring surgical management (Fig. 13.16). Patients taking anticoagulant therapy are at particular risk for rupture. Rupture of these cysts occurs more often on the right side and may occur during intercourse. Most ruptures occur on cycle days 20 to 26 (123).

Theca lutein cysts are the least common of functional ovarian cysts. They are usually bilateral and occur with pregnancy, including molar pregnancies. They may be associated with multiple gestations, molar pregnancies, choriocarcinoma, diabetes, Rh sensitization, clomiphene citrate use, human menopausal gonadotropin–human chorionic gonadotropin ovulation induction, and the use of GnRH analogs. Theca lutein cysts may be quite large (up to 30 cm), are multicystic, and regress spontaneously (124,125).

Combination monophasic oral contraceptive therapy has been reported to markedly reduce the risk of functional ovarian cysts (126). It appears that, in comparison with previously available higher-dose pills, the effect of cyst suppression with current low-dose oral contraceptives is attenuated (127,128). Most studies have suggested that the use of triphasic oral contraceptives is not associated with an appreciable increased risk of functional ovarian cysts (129). It has been suggested that smokers have as much as a twofold increased risk of developing ovarian cysts, although other studies have not found smoking to be a risk factor (130,131).

Other Benign Masses Women with endometriosis may develop ovarian endometriomas ("chocolate" cysts), which can enlarge to 6 to 8 cm in size. A mass that does not resolve with observation may be an endometrioma (Chapter 26).

Although enlarged, polycystic ovaries were originally considered the *sine qua non* of PCOS, polycystic ovaries probably represent a final common phenotype of a wide variety of causes; they are not always present with other features of the syndrome. The prevalence of PCOS among the general population depends on the diagnostic criteria used. In one study, 257 volunteers were examined with ultrasonography; 22% were found to have polycystic ovaries (132). The finding of bilateral generously sized ovaries on examination or polycystic ovaries on ultrasonographic examination should prompt evaluation for the full-blown syndrome,

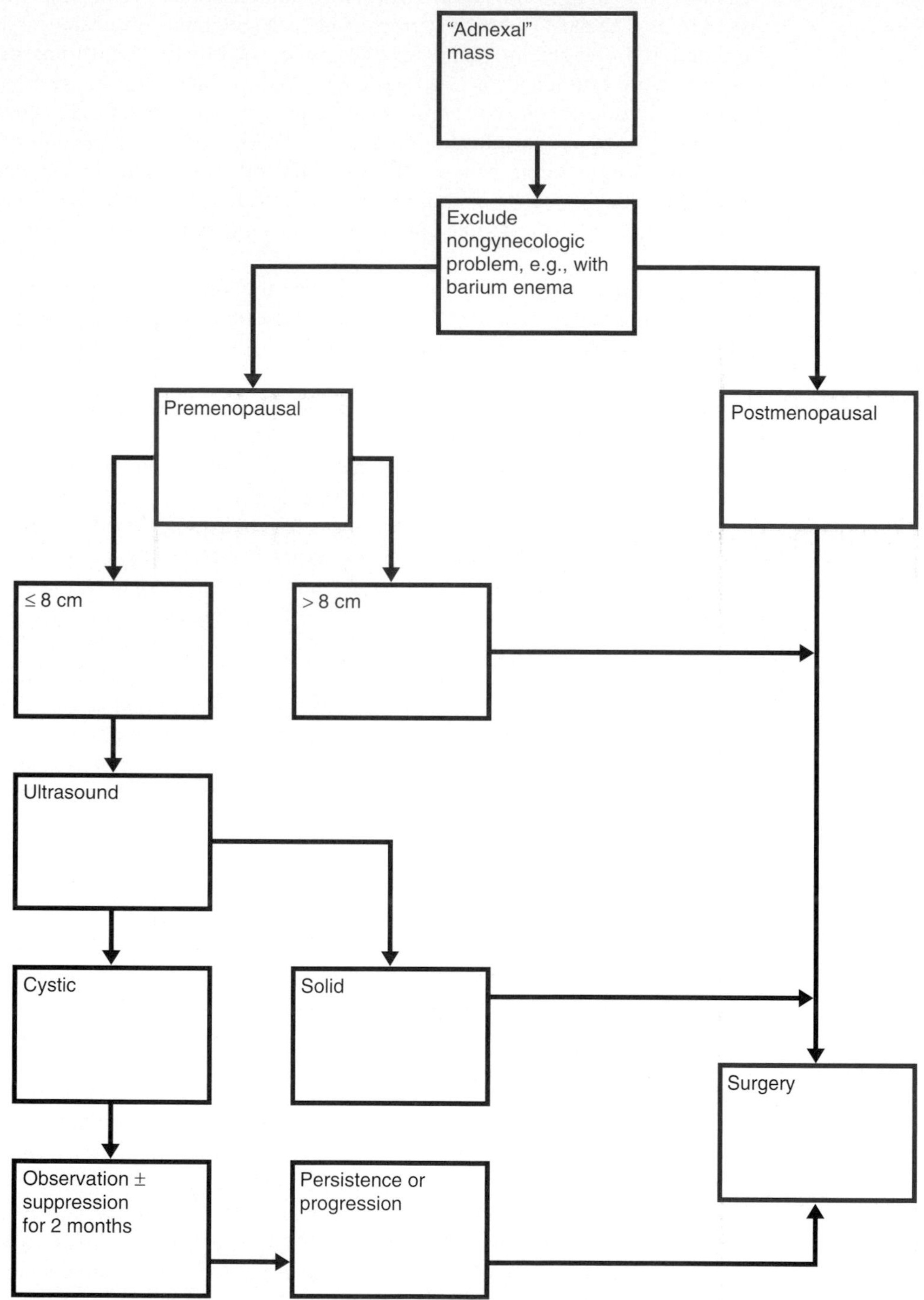

Figure 13.14 Preoperative evaluation of the patient with an adnexal mass. (From **Berek JS, Hacker NF.** *Practical gynecologic oncology,* 3rd ed. Baltimore: Lippincott Williams & Wilkins, 2000:465.)

which includes hyperandrogenism and chronic anovulation as well as polycystic ovaries. Therapy for PCOS is medical and generally not surgical.

Neoplastic Masses **More than 80% of benign cystic teratomas (dermoid cysts) occur during the reproductive years, although dermoid cysts have a wider age distribution than other ovarian germ cell tumors** (133). Histologically, benign cystic teratomas have an admixture of elements (Fig. 13.17). In one study of ovarian masses that were surgically excised, dermoid cysts represented 62% of all ovarian neoplasms in women younger than 40 years of age (121). Malignant transformation occurs in less than 2% of dermoid cysts

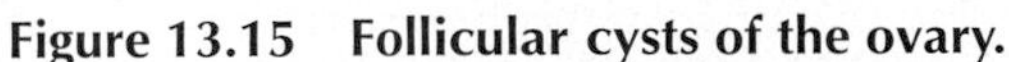

Figure 13.15 Follicular cysts of the ovary.

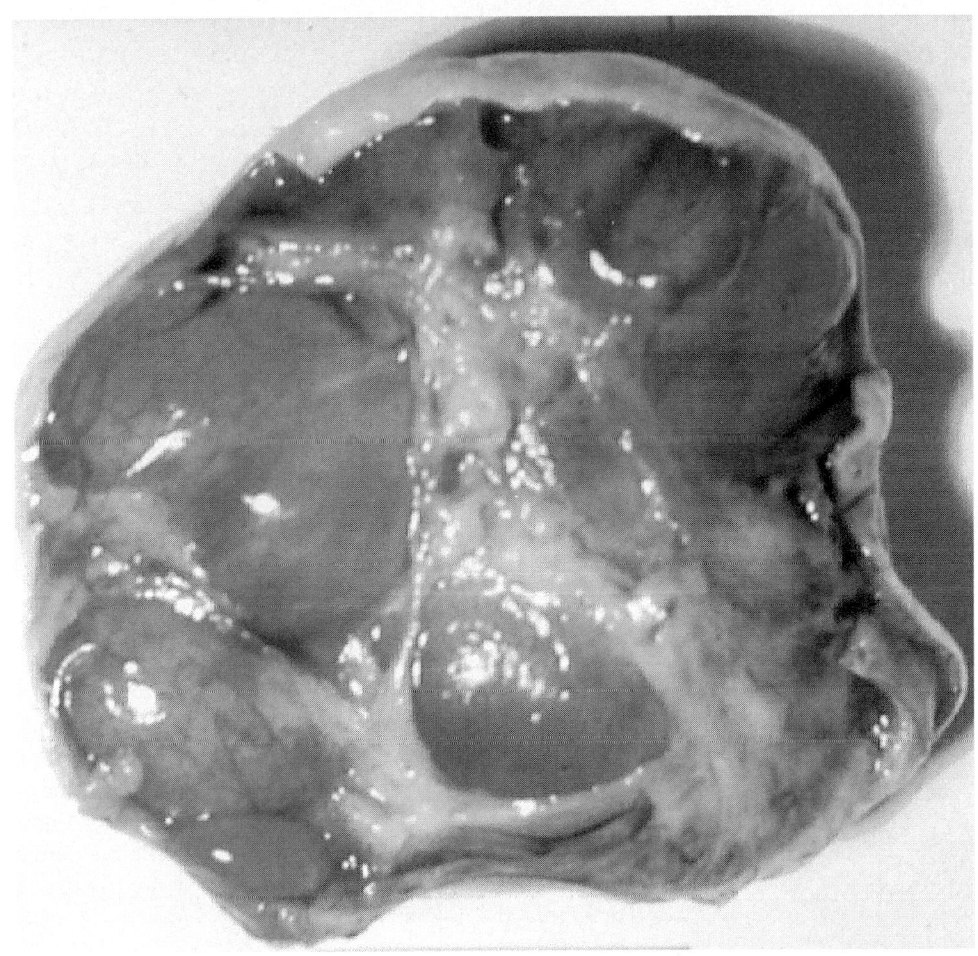

Figure 13.16 Corpus luteum cyst of the ovary. The left ovary is normal and the right ovary has a ruptured hemorrhagic corpus luteum cyst.

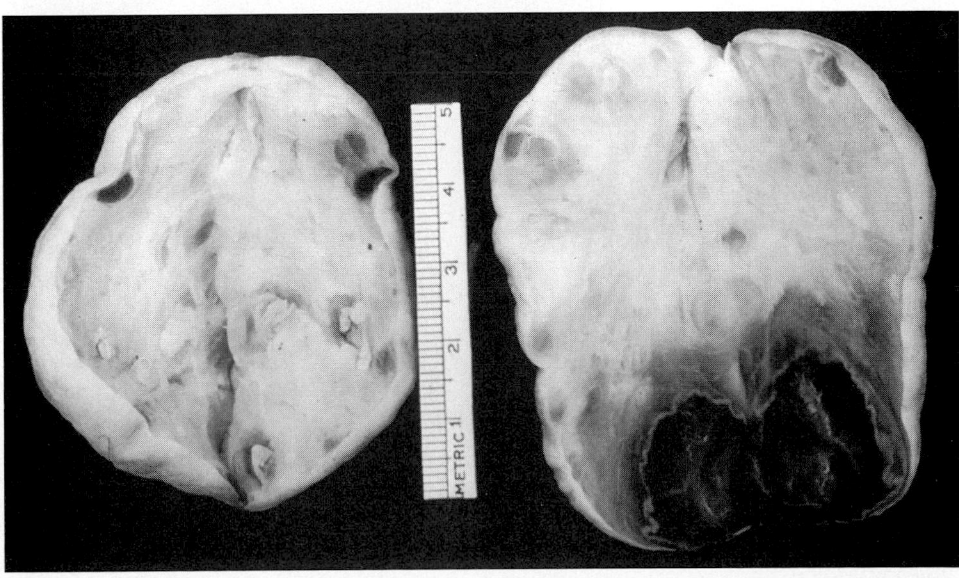

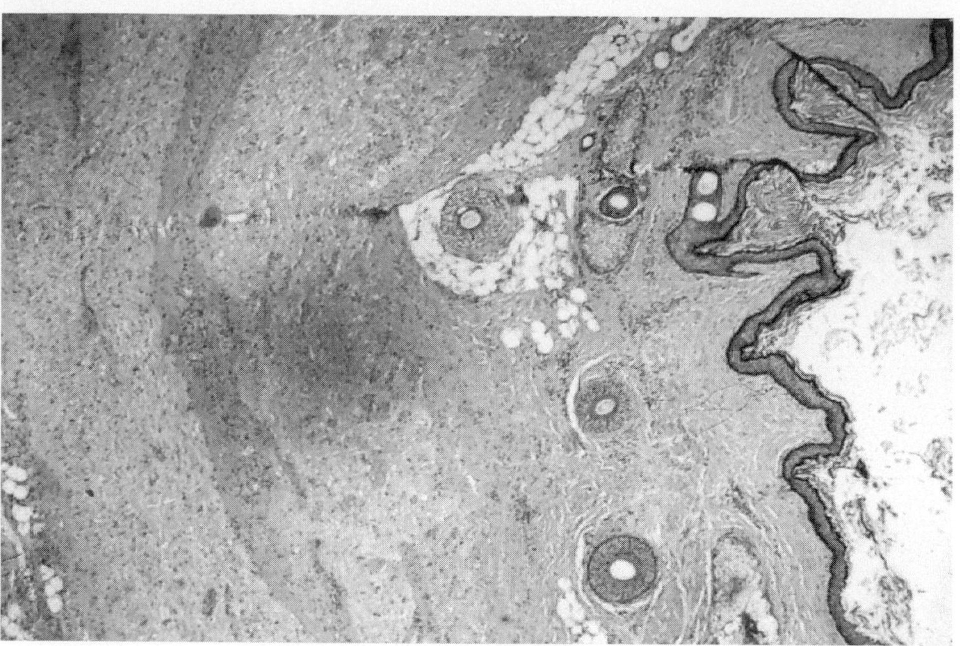

Figure 13.17 Histologic appearance of a mature cystic teratoma of the ovary.

in women of all ages; most cases occur in women older than 40 years of age. The risk of torsion with dermoid cysts is approximately 15%, and it occurs more frequently than with ovarian tumors in general, perhaps because the high-fat content of most dermoid cysts, allowing them to float within the abdominal and pelvic cavity (Fig. 13.18). As a result of this fat content, on pelvic examination, a dermoid cyst frequently is described as anterior in location. They are bilateral in approximately 10% of cases, although many have advanced the argument against bivalving a normal-appearing contralateral ovary because

Figure 13.18 Mature cystic teratoma (dermoid cyst) of the ovary associated with adnexal torsion.

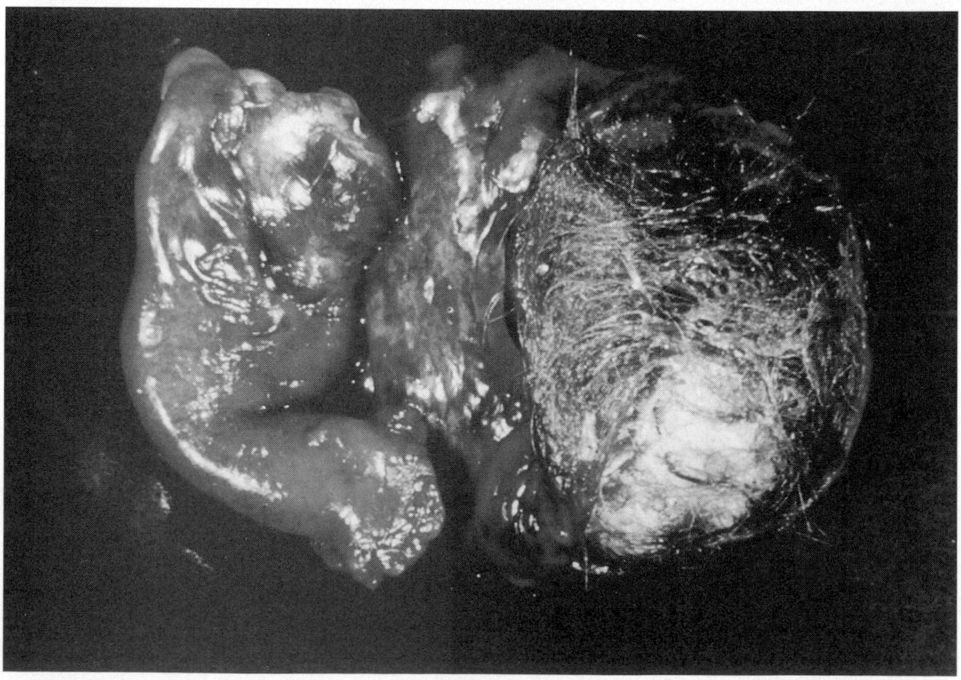

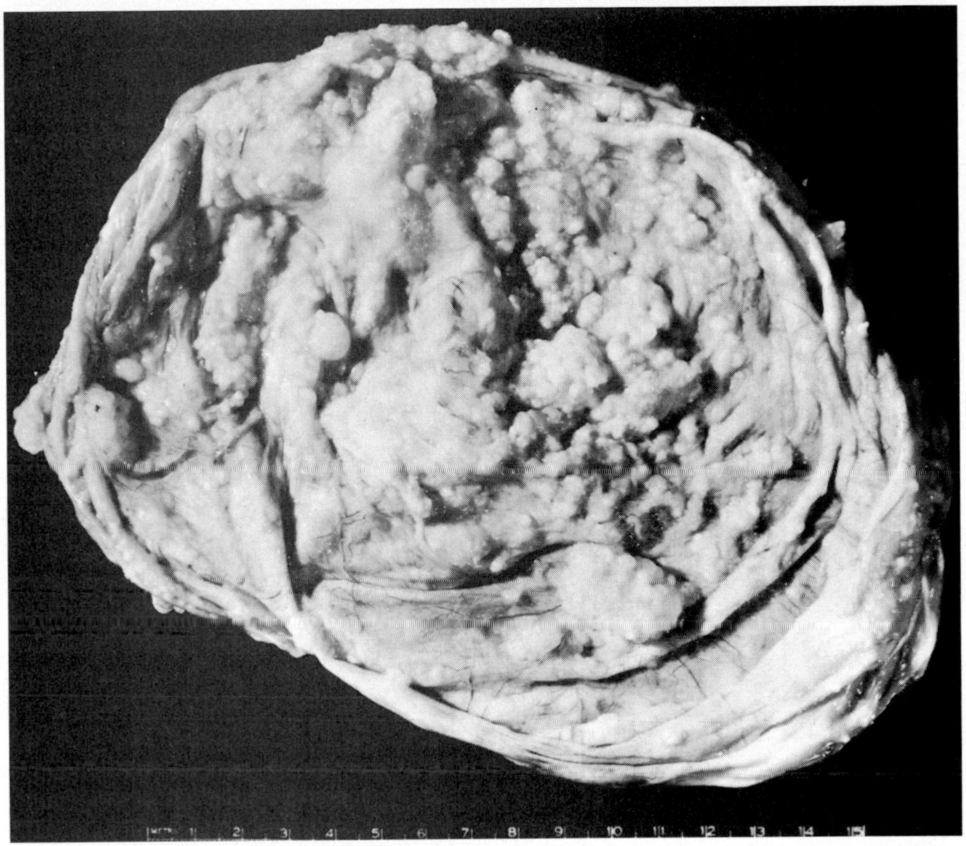

Figure 13.19 Gross appearance of a multilocular serous cystadenoma of the ovary. (From **Scully RE.** Atlas of tumor pathology. Tumors of the ovary, maldeveloped gonads, fallopian tube, and broad ligament. Washington, DC: Armed Forces Institute of Pathology; 1998:54; Fascicle 23, with permission.)

of the risk of adhesions, which may result in infertility. **An ovarian cystectomy is almost always possible, even if it appears that only a small amount of ovarian tissue remains.** Preserving a small amount of ovarian cortex in a young patient with a benign lesion is preferable to the loss of the entire ovary (134). Laparoscopic cystectomy is often possible, and intraoperative spill of tumor contents is rarely a cause of complications (135,136).

The risk of epithelial tumors increases with age. Although serous cystadenomas are often considered the more common benign neoplasm, in one study, benign cystic teratomas represented 66% of benign tumors in women younger than 50 years of age; serous tumors accounted for only 20% (121). **Serous tumors are generally benign; 5% to 10% have borderline malignant potential and 20% to 25% are malignant.** Serous cystadenomas are often multilocular, sometimes with papillary components (Fig. 13.19). The surface epithelial cells secrete serous fluid, resulting in a watery cyst content. Psammoma bodies, which are areas of fine calcific granulation, may be scattered within the tumor and are visible on radiograph. A frozen section is necessary to distinguish between benign (Fig. 13.20), borderline, and malignant serous tumors, because gross examination alone cannot make this distinction. Mucinous ovarian tumors may grow to large dimensions (Fig. 13.21). Benign mucinous tumors typically have a lobulated, smooth surface, are multilocular, and may be bilateral in up to 10% of cases. Mucoid material is present within the cystic loculations (Fig. 13.22). **Five to ten percent of mucinous ovarian tumors are malignant.** They may be difficult to distinguish histologically from metastatic gastrointestinal malignancies. Other benign ovarian tumors include fibromas (Fig. 13.23) (a focus of stromal cells), Brenner tumors (Fig. 13.24) (which appear grossly similar to fibromas and which are frequently found incidentally), and mixed forms of tumors such as the cystadenofibroma.

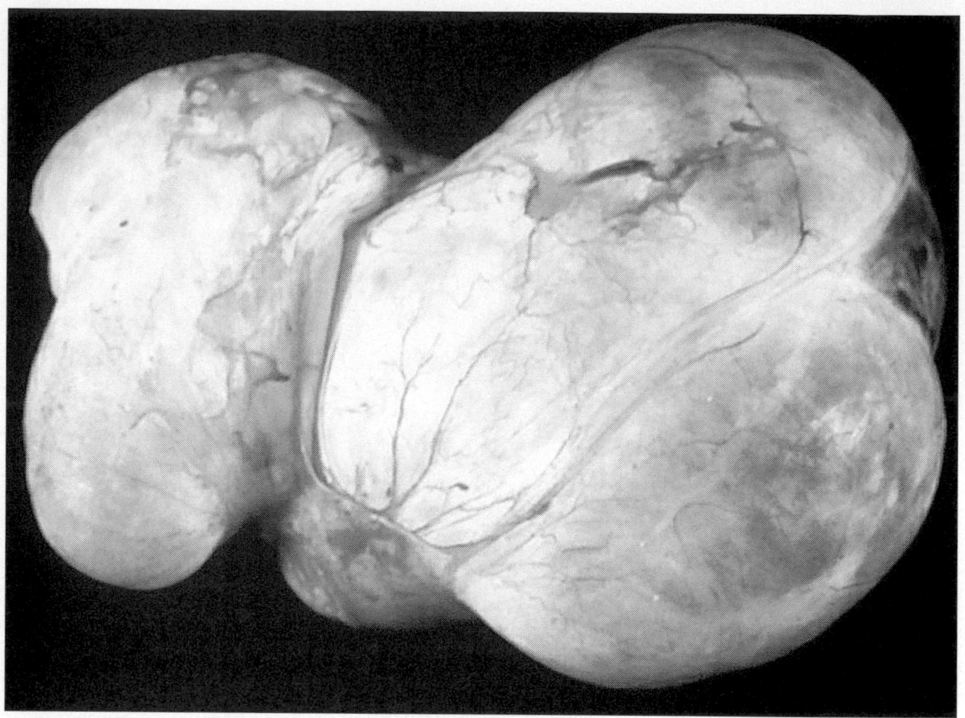

Figure 13.20 Benign serous papillary cystadenoma of the ovary.

Other Adnexal Masses

Masses that include the fallopian tube are related primarily to inflammatory causes in this age group. A tuboovarian abscess can be present in association with PID (Chapter 15). In addition, a complex inflammatory mass consisting of bowel, tube, and ovary may be present

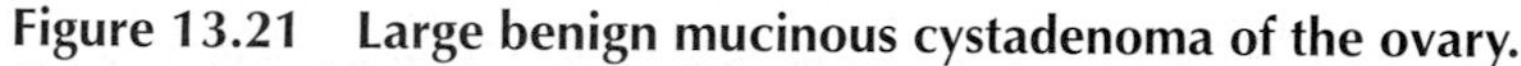

Figure 13.21 Large benign mucinous cystadenoma of the ovary.

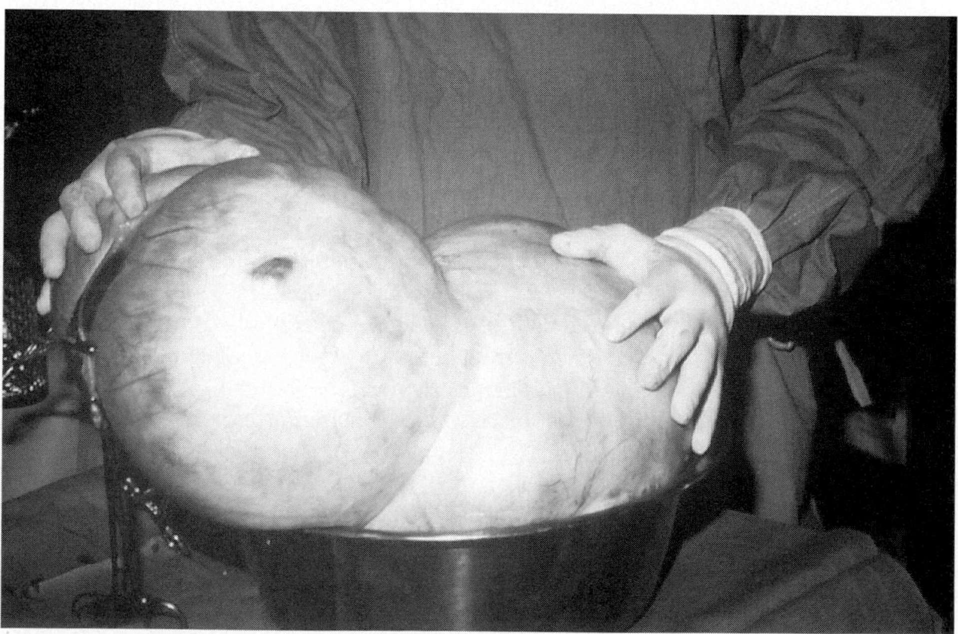

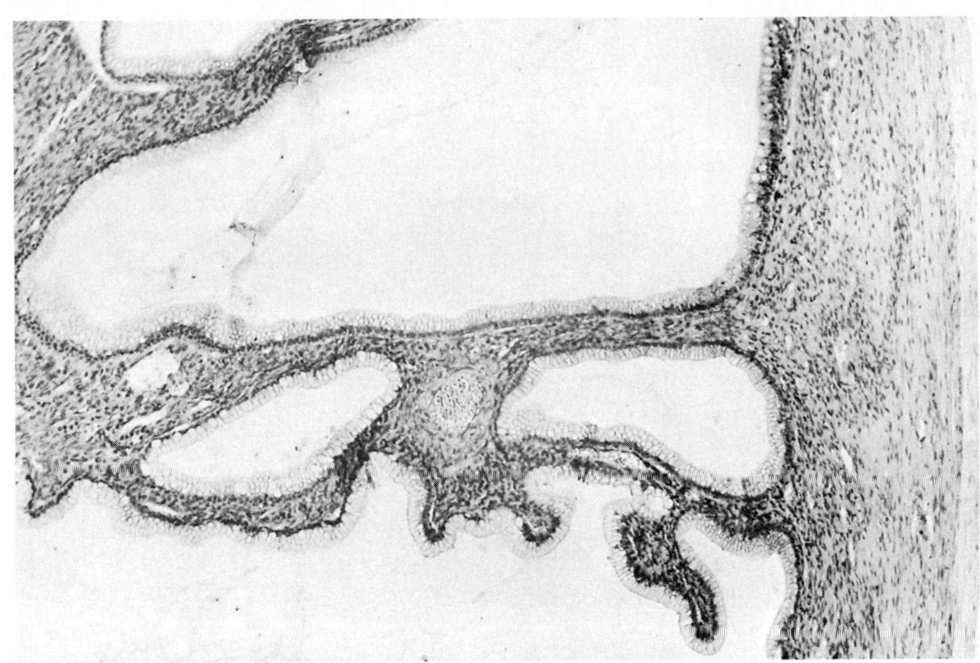

Figure 13.22 Histologic appearance of mucinous cystadenoma of the ovary. (From **Scully RE:** *Tumors of the ovary and maldeveloped gonads.* Washington, DC: Armed Forces Institute of Pathology, 1979:83, with permission.)

without a large abscess cavity. Ectopic pregnancies can occur in the reproductive age group and must be excluded when a patient presents with pain, a positive pregnancy test, and an adnexal mass (Chapter 17). Paraovarian cysts may be noted either on examination or on imaging studies. In many instances, a normal ipsilateral ovary can be visualized using ultrasonography. The frequency of malignancy in paraovarian tumors is quite low, although one review reported malignancy in 2% of patients (137).

Figure 13.23 Ovarian fibroma that was removed from a patient with ascites and a right pleural effusion (Meigs' syndrome).

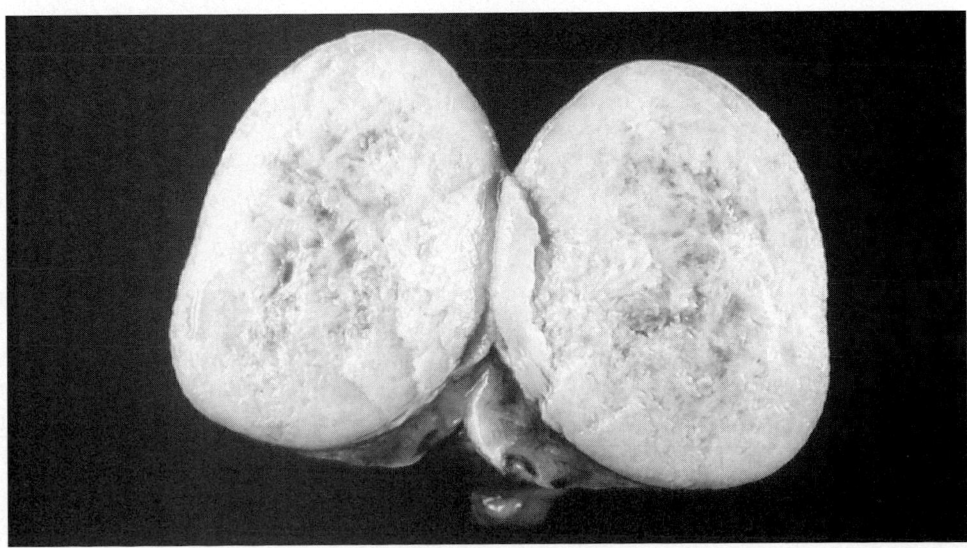

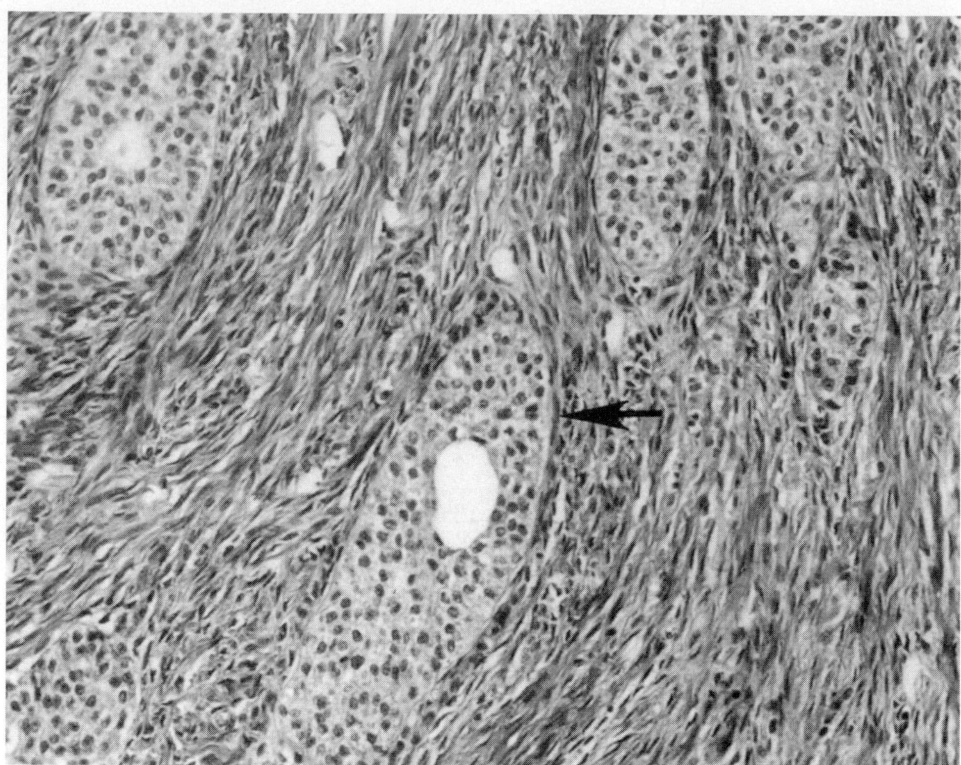

Figure 13.24 Benign Brenner tumor of the ovary. Note the nests of transitional metaplasia *(arrow)* found within the fibrotic stroma. (From **Berek JS, Hacker NF.** *Practical gynecologic oncology,* 2nd ed. Baltimore: Lippincott Williams & Wilkins, 1994:145.)

Diagnosis

A complete pelvic examination, including rectovaginal examination and Pap test, should be performed. Estimations of the size of a mass should be presented in centimeters rather than in comparison to common objects or fruit (e.g., orange, grapefruit, tennis ball, golf ball). After pregnancy has been excluded, one simple office technique that can help determine whether a mass is uterine or adnexal includes sounding and measuring the depth of the uterine cavity.

Other Studies **Endometrial sampling with an endometrial biopsy or D & C is mandatory when both a pelvic mass and abnormal bleeding are present.** An endometrial lesion—carcinoma or hyperplasia—may coexist with a benign mass such as a leiomyoma. In a woman with leiomyomas, abnormal bleeding cannot be assumed to be caused solely by the fibroids. Clinicians differ in recommendations about the need for endometrial biopsy when the diagnosis is leiomyomas with regular menses.

Studies of the urinary tract may be necessary if urinary symptoms are prominent, including cystometric measurements if incontinence or pressure is a prominent symptom. Cystoscopy may sometimes be necessary or appropriate to rule out intrinsic bladder lesions. Ultrasonography or an intravenous pyelogram may be appropriate to demonstrate ureteral deviation, compression, or dilation in the presence of moderately large and laterally located fibroids or other pelvic mass. Such findings rarely provide an indication for surgical intervention for otherwise asymptomatic leiomyomas.

Laboratory Studies Laboratory studies that are indicated for women of reproductive age with a pelvic mass include pregnancy test, cervical cytology, complete blood count, erythrocyte sedimentation rate, and testing of stool for occult blood. The value of tumor markers, such as CA125 in a premenopausal woman with a pelvic mass, has been widely debated. **A number of benign conditions, including uterine leiomyomas, PID, pregnancy, and endometriosis can cause elevated CA125 levels, and thus may lead to unnecessary surgical intervention.**

Imaging Studies Other studies may be necessary or appropriate. The most commonly indicated study is pelvic ultrasonography, which will help document the origin of the mass to determine whether it is uterine, adnexal, bowel, or gastrointestinal. The ultrasonographic examination also provides information about the size of the mass and its consistency—unilocular cyst, mixed echogenicity (Fig. 13.25), multiloculated cyst, solid cyst (Fig. 13.26)—which can help determine management.

The value of transvaginal and transabdominal ultrasonography in the diagnosis of pelvic masses has been compared. Transvaginal scanning has the advantage of providing additional information about the internal architecture or anatomy of the mass. Heterogeneous pelvic masses, described as tuboovarian abscesses on transabdominal ultrasonography, can be separated on transvaginal scans into pyosalpinx, hydrosalpinx, tuboovarian complex, and tuboovarian abscess (103) (Fig. 13.27).

The diagnostic accuracy of transvaginal ultrasonography in diagnosing endometrioma can be quite high (Fig. 13.28). Endometriomas can have a variety of ultrasonographic appearances, from purely cystic to varying degrees of complexity with septation or debris, to a solid appearance. A scoring system that can help predict benign versus malignant adnexal masses is presented in Table 13.9. Other ultrasonographic indices have been developed in an attempt to predict the risk of malignancy in ovarian masses (138,139). The indices have included not only characterizations of morphology such as septations, solid components, and ovarian size, but also demographic factors (i.e., age) as well as color flow imaging and Doppler waveform analysis (140,141). Although an analysis of such features may be helpful, histologic confirmation of surgically removed persistent masses remains the standard of care (142).

Figure 13.25 Transvaginal ultrasonogram of a unilocular ovarian cyst. This is characteristic of a benign process or corpus luteum cyst.

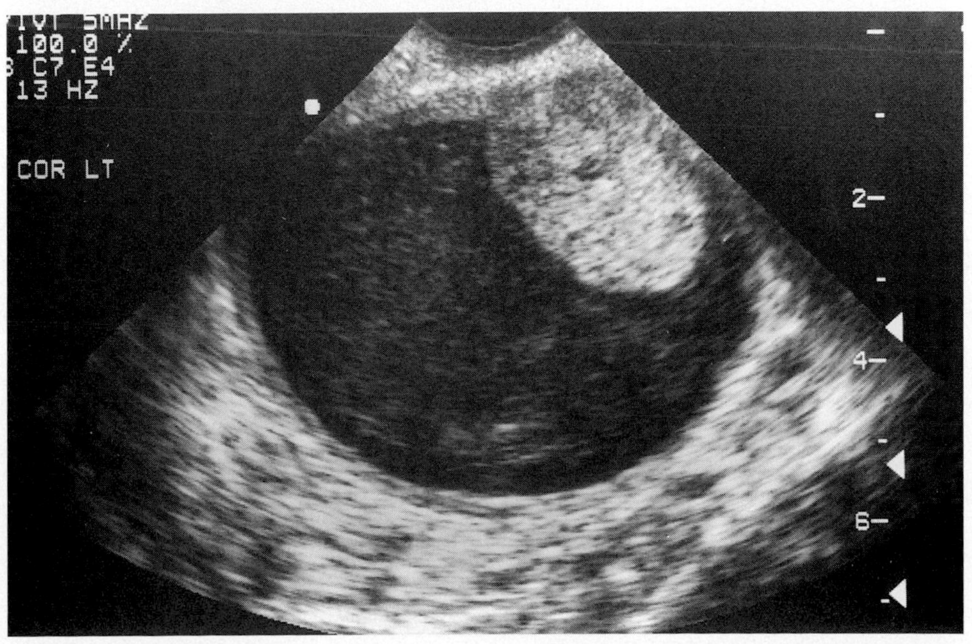

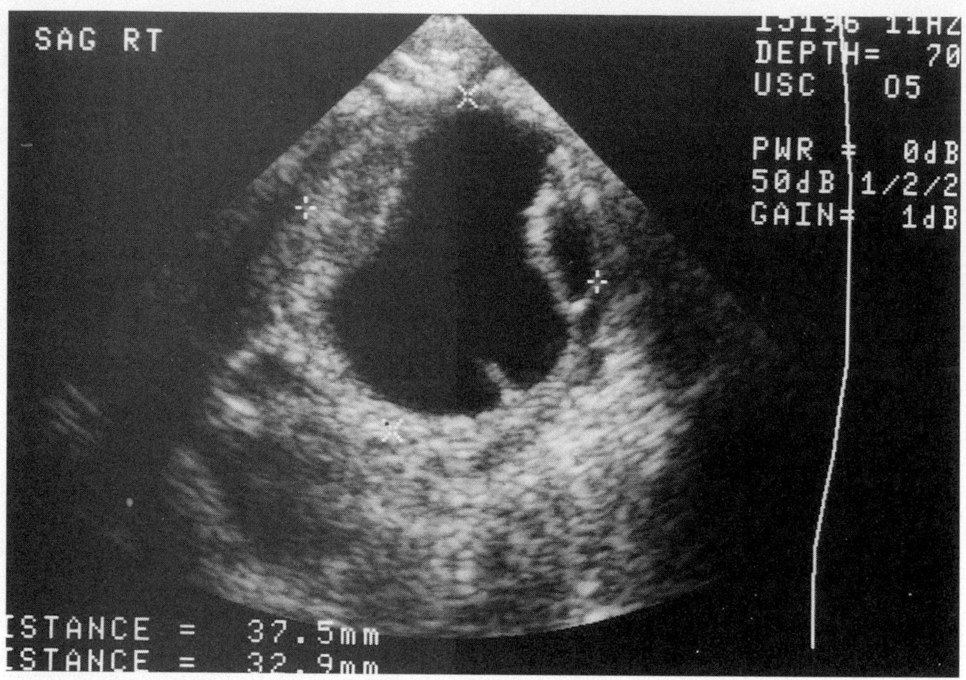

Figure 13.26 Transvaginal ultrasonogram of a complex, predominantly solid mass.

CT is seldom indicated as a primary diagnostic procedure, although it may be helpful in planning treatment when a malignancy is strongly suspected or when a nongynecologic disorder may be present. An abdominal flat plate radiograph is not a primary diagnostic procedure, although taken for other indications it may reveal calcifications that can assist in the discovery or diagnosis of a mass. Pelvic calcifications (teeth) consistent with a benign

Figure 13.27 Transvaginal ultrasonogram of bilateral tuboovarian abscesses.

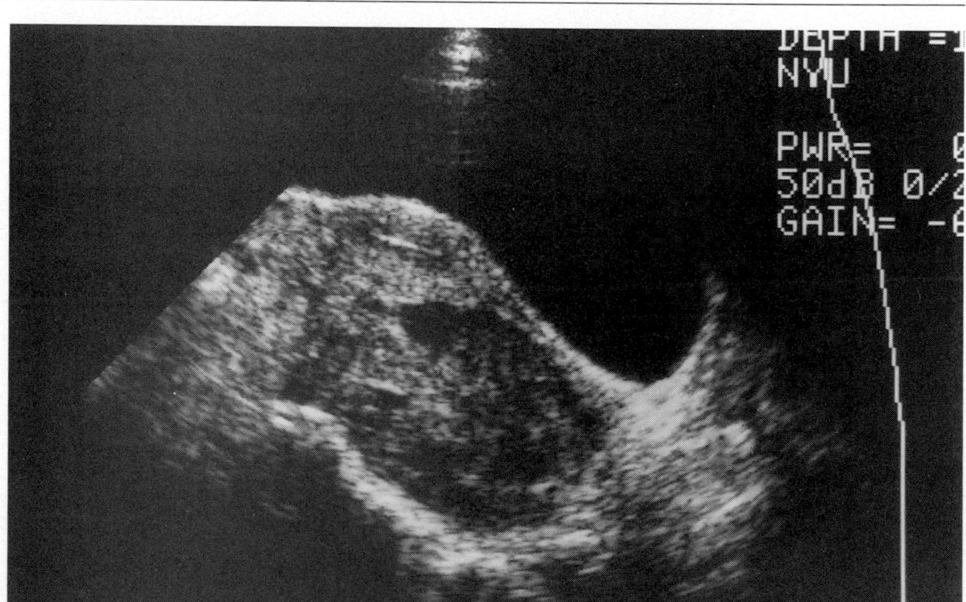

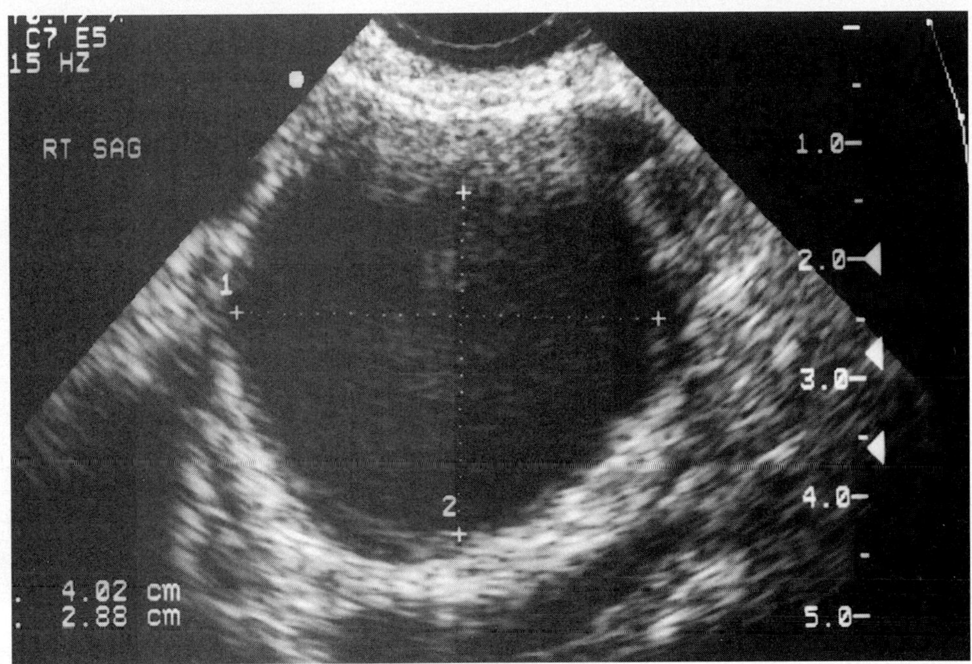

Figure 13.28 Transvaginal ultrasonogram of an endometrioma of the ovary.

cystic teratoma (Fig. 13.29), a calcified uterine fibroid, or scattered calcifications consistent with psammoma bodies of a papillary serous cystadenoma can be seen on abdominal radiograph.

Hysteroscopy provides direct evidence of intrauterine pathology or submucous leiomyomas that distort the uterine cavity (see Chapter 21). Hysterosalpingography will demonstrate indirectly the contour of the endometrial cavity and any distortion or obstruction of the uterotubal junction secondary to leiomyomas, an extrinsic mass, or peritubal adhesions. The techniques combining hysterosalpingography, in which fluid is instilled into the uterine cavity, with transvaginal ultrasonography have been helpful in the diagnosis of intrauterine pathology.

Table 13.9. Ultrasonographic Scoring System for Adnexal Masses[a]

Clear cyst and smooth borders	1
Clear cyst with slightly irregular border; cyst with smooth walls but low-level echoes (i.e., endometrioma)	2
Cyst with low-level echoes with slightly irregular border but no nodularity (i.e., endometrioma); clear cyst in postmenopausal patient	3
Equivocal, nonspecific ultrasonographic appearance: solid ovarian enlargement or small cyst with irregular borders and internal echoes (hemorrhagic cyst or benign ovarian tumor)	4–6
Multiseptate or irregular cystic mass consistent in appearance with ovarian tumor (7, 5 less nodularity; 8–9, 5 more nodularity)	7–9
Pelvic mass as above, with ascites	10

[a] 1, benign; 10, malignant.
From **Finkler NJ, Benacerraf B, Lavin PT, et al.** Comparison of CA 125, clinical impression, and ultrasound in the preoperative evaluation of ovarian masses. *Obstet Gynecol* 1988;72:659, with permission.

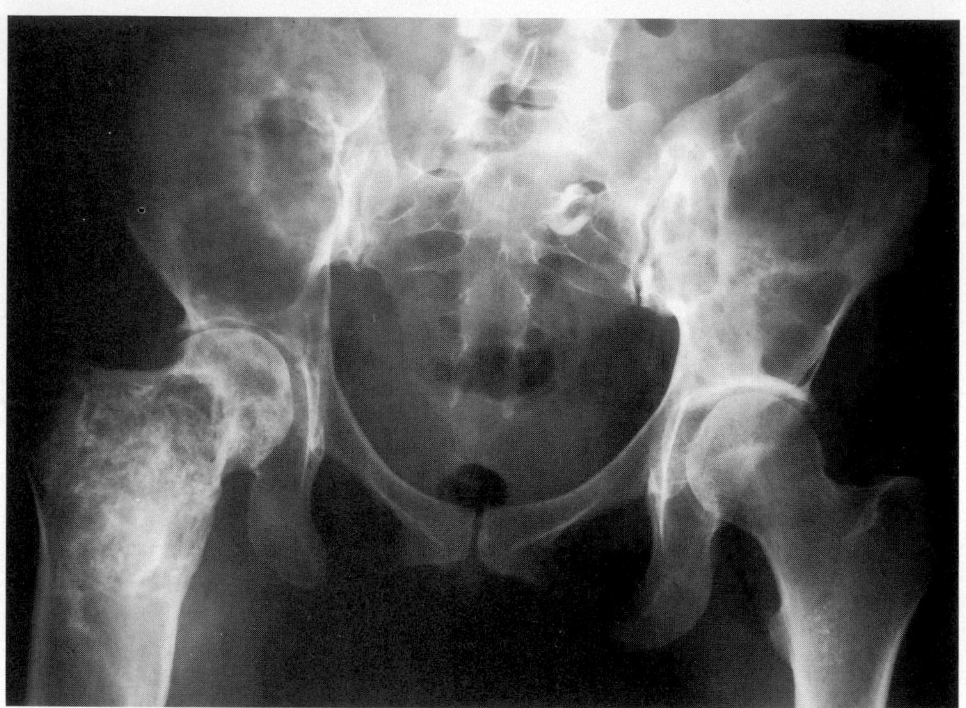

Figure 13.29 Benign cystic teratoma (dermoid cyst) of the ovary with teeth seen on abdominal radiograph.

MRI may be most useful in the diagnosis of uterine anomalies, although its value rarely justifies the increased cost of the procedure over ultrasonography for the diagnosis of other pelvic masses (143–145).

Management

The management of a pelvic mass is based on an accurate diagnosis. An explanation of this diagnosis should be conveyed to the patient, along with a discussion of the likely course of the disease (e.g., growth of uterine leiomyomas, regression of fibroids at menopause, regression of a follicular cyst, the uncertain malignant potential of an ovarian mass). All options for management should be presented and discussed, although it is appropriate for the physician to state a recommended approach with an explanation of the reasons for the recommendation. Management should be based on the primary symptoms and may include observation with close follow-up, temporizing surgical therapies, medical management, or definitive surgical procedures.

Management of Leiomyomas

Nonsurgical Management **Judicious patient observation and follow-up are indicated primarily for uterine leiomyomas; intervention is reserved for specific indications and symptoms** (146). Periodic examinations are indicated to ensure that the tumors are not growing rapidly. Uterine size should be recorded on the patient's chart, and the location of palpable and ultrasonographically localized leiomyomas should be described and diagrammed.

The use of GnRH agonists results in a 40% to 60% decrease in uterine volume and can be of value in some clinical situations. Treatment results in hypoestrogenism, which has been associated with reversible bone loss and symptoms such as hot flashes. Thus, treatment has been limited to short-term use, although low-dose hormonal replacement may be effective in minimizing the hypoestrogenic effects. Regrowth of leiomyomas is experienced within a few months after stopping therapy in about one-half of women treated. Some indications for the use of GnRH agonists in women with leiomyomas are as follows:

1. Preservation of fertility in women with large leiomyomas before attempting conception, or preoperative treatment before myomectomy
2. Treatment of anemia to allow recovery of normal hemoglobin levels before surgical management, minimizing the need for transfusion or allowing autologous blood donation
3. Treatment of women approaching menopause in an effort to avoid surgery
4. Preoperative treatment of large leiomyomas to make vaginal hysterectomy, hysteroscopic resection or ablation, or laparoscopic destruction more feasible
5. Treatment of women with medical contraindications to surgery
6. Treatment of women with personal or medical indications for delaying surgery.

Newer therapies combining GnRH agonists with estrogen add-back therapy have been promising in reducing side effects of agonist therapy alone, although this is a costly alternative (147). *Tibolone,* a synthetic steroid with estrogenic, progestational, and androgenic activity, has been widely used outside the United States for treatment of menopausal symptoms; its use with GnRH agonists as add-back therapy holds promise for longer-term therapy of leiomyoma (148). The use of GnRH antagonists holds promise, because it appears to be less likely than agonist therapy to result in bleeding early in therapy; it also causes rapid uterine shrinkage (149,150).

RU486, a progesterone antagonist, also has been shown to decrease the size of uterine leiomyoma (151). As the role of growth factors in leiomyoma-associated bleeding is better elucidated, treatment targeted at the growth factor or its receptor may prove useful. In addition, as the molecular biology and genetics of leiomyoma are better understood, newer nonsurgical therapies may be developed.

Surgical Therapy Determining potential indications for surgical treatment requires careful judgment and assessment of the degree of associated symptoms. **Asymptomatic leiomyomas do not usually require surgery.** Some indications for surgery include the following:

1. Abnormal uterine bleeding with resultant anemia, unresponsive to hormonal management
2. Chronic pain with severe dysmenorrhea, dyspareunia, or lower abdominal pressure or pain
3. Acute pain, as in torsion of a pedunculated leiomyoma, or prolapsing submucosal fibroid
4. Urinary symptoms or signs such as hydronephrosis after complete evaluation
5. Infertility, with leiomyomas as the only abnormal finding
6. Markedly enlarged uterine size with compression symptoms or discomfort.

Rapid enlargement of the uterus during the premenopausal years or any increase in uterine size in a postmenopausal woman have been suggested as indications for surgery because of the inability to exclude uterine sarcoma. Although the absolute risk of uterine sarcomas developing in a fibroid uterus has been reported to be less that 2 to 3 per 1,000, one study found sarcomas to be no more common in women with rapid uterine growth than those without such growth (152). However, rapid enlargement has not been well defined, and serial measurements may be hampered by variations in the interpretation of size by the examiner or series of examiners.

Hysterectomy has long been viewed as the definitive management of symptomatic uterine leiomyomas (Chapter 22). Myomectomy is an alternative to hysterectomy for patients who desire childbearing, who are young, or who prefer that the uterus be retained. Recent studies suggest that the morbidity of abdominal myomectomy and hysterectomy are similar, although previous reports had suggested higher risks for myomectomy, including the risks of hemorrhage and transfusion requirements (153,154). Blood loss and risk of transfusion are greater for women with larger uteri (155). Laparoscopic myomectomy minimizes the size of the abdominal incision, although several small incisions are required. The biggest concerns with laparoscopic myomectomy include the removal of large myomas through small incisions and the repair of the uterus (146). Instruments that efficiently morcellate the myomas have been developed, although skilled surgical techniques are required. There is controversy as to whether laparoscopic suturing provides strength and healing equivalent to that achieved with laparotomy. Risks include the need to convert to a laparotomy and the risk of uterine rupture with subsequent pregnancy (146). Vaginal myomectomy is indicated in the case of a prolapsed pedunculated submucous fibroid. Hysteroscopic resection of small submucous leiomyomas is a technique that may offer benefits for a selected group of patients (Chapter 21). **The recurrence risk for leiomyomas has been reported to be as high as 50% after myomectomy, with up to one-third requiring repeat surgery** (112,156). Endometrial ablation can decrease bleeding for women with primary intramural fibroids and can be performed using a variety of techniques, including laser ablation, thermal ablation, resection, or chemical destruction (146).

The preoperative use of GnRH agonists for both hysterectomy and myomectomy result in a decrease in uterine size. The expense, side effects, and time required to achieve a significant decrease in size are limitations to their use. The use of GnRH agonists may make surgical plans less distinct and thus myomectomy technically more difficult.

Nonextirpative approaches to the management of leiomyomas include myolysis and uterine artery embolization, although long-term safety and efficacy have not yet been demonstrated. Uterine artery embolization has been reported to have serious consequences, including infection, massive bleeding, and necrosis requiring emergency surgery (157). Pain is frequently a consequence. The procedure has been characterized as investigational (146). Myolysis involves the use of lasers to coagulate or needle electrodes to deliver an electrical current to individual leiomyomas (158).

Ovarian Masses

The now-routine application of ultrasound technology to gynecologic examinations has led to the more frequent detection of ovarian cysts. Ultrasonography is a relatively easy diagnostic study to perform, but this ease has led to the labeling of physiologic ovarian morphology, cystic follicles, as pathologic and the referral of patients for therapies, including surgery, without indications. **Treatment of ovarian masses that are suspected to be functional tumors is expectant.** A classic study popularized the use of oral contraceptives as suppressive therapy, although the results of this study have been misinterpreted (159). In this study, 286 patients (aged 16 to 48 years) with adnexal masses were treated with combination oral contraceptives. Eighty-one women had a persistent mass after this therapy; surgery was performed on these women, none of whom was found to have a physiologic cyst. This study has been interpreted to indicate that suspected functional cysts should be treated with oral contraceptives, although there are no data to indicate a more rapid resolution with oral contraceptives than with time alone. If a woman needs contraception and wishes to use oral contraceptives for birth control or for noncontraceptive indications, it is perfectly acceptable to prescribe them in this setting. However, **a number of randomized**

prospective studies have shown no acceleration of the resolution of functional ovarian cysts (which were associated with the use of clomiphene citrate or human menopausal gonadotropins) **with oral contraceptives compared with observation alone** (160–162). **However, oral contraceptives are effective in reducing the risk of subsequent ovarian cysts.**

Symptomatic cysts should be evaluated promptly, although mildly symptomatic masses suspected to be functional should be managed with analgesics rather than surgery to avoid the development of adhesions that may impair subsequent fertility. Surgical intervention is warranted in the presence of severe pain or the suspicion of malignancy or torsion. **On ultrasonography, large cysts and those that have multiloculations, septa, papillae, and increased blood flow should be suspected of neoplasia. If a malignant cyst is suspected at any age, exploratory laparotomy should be performed promptly.**

Ovarian or adnexal torsion is suspected on the basis of peritoneal signs and the acuity of onset. Doppler flow studies suggesting abnormal flow are highly predictive of torsion (163). The absence of internal ovarian flow is not specific to torsion, and may be seen with cystic lesions, although in these situations peripheral flow is typically visualized (164). Visualization of a twisted vascular pedicle has also been shown to be highly predictive (165). Normal flow does not exclude torsion, and in one study 60% of surgically confirmed cases of torsion had normal Doppler flow (163). **The management of suspected ovarian torsion, which can occur at any age, from prepubertal to postmenopausal, is surgical.** Previous studies have suggested that ovarian torsion requires oophorectomy on the basis that the untwisting (detorsion) of the ovarian pedicle would lead to emboli. Recent studies have suggested that the primary management should be detorsion with ovarian cystectomy, if a cyst is present; normal ovarian function frequently results even in ovaries that do not initially appear to be viable (166–168). This management is particularly important in prepubertal and young women (169). Oophoropexy may be helpful in preventing recurrent torsion (169,170).

Ultrasonographic or CT-directed aspiration procedures should not be used in women in whom there is a suspicion of malignancy. In the past, laparoscopic surgery for ovarian masses has been reserved for diagnostic or therapeutic purposes in patients at very low risk for malignancy. One survey of gynecologic oncologists' experiences with patients who had originally undergone laparoscopic management of malignant or borderline tumors suggested that so-called *benign* characteristics do not preclude malignancy and that laparoscopic management can be associated with partial or incomplete excision, delays in definitive surgery, or seeding and spread of disease (171–173). Even with frozen section, there is a possibility of a missed diagnosis of malignancy, which would necessitate reexploration. Whether this practice results in long-term compromise of outcome is unclear; thus, the laparoscopic management of complex masses that may be malignant remains controversial (171,174). More recently, the laparoscopic management of masses without selection for benign characteristics has been advocated provided the surgeon has expertise in operative laparoscopy, the capability for immediate and accurate pathologic examination is available, and appropriate further treatment can be instituted if indicated (including laparotomy for malignancy) (175).

The management of presumptive benign ovarian masses with operative laparoscopy has become increasingly common. The choice of surgical approach (laparotomy or laparoscopy) should be based on the surgical indications, the patient's condition, the surgeon's expertise and training, informed patient preference, and the most recent data supporting the chosen approach (176). The clear advantage of this technique is the shorter hospital stay, shorter recovery time, and lessened postoperative pain. Few controlled trials have been performed to compare the laparoscopic approach with laparotomy (128) (Chapter 21). Surgical complications include bowel injury, ureteral or other urinary tract injury, cannula site vessel injury, or incisional hernia (177). In one series the overall complication rate was 13.3% (177). Randomized clinical trials evaluating laparoscopy versus laparotomy in the treatment of ovarian masses have been performed and typically demonstrate a shorter hospitalization time with less postoperative pain and a shorter recovery period (135,178,179).

The role of laparoscopy has been even more controversial in the removal of dermoid cysts than with other benign masses. Concern centers around prevention of spill of the cyst contents. Randomized clinical trials have been reported with variable findings regarding spill; some studies suggest that cyst contents are more likely to spill with laparoscopy, whereas others do not find a difference or note no increase in morbidity when spillage occurred (180–182). Culdotomy and the use of an endoscopic specimen bag have been associated with lower rates of tumor spillage (182,183).

Postmenopausal Age Group

Differential Diagnosis

Ovarian Masses

During the postmenopausal years, the ovaries become smaller (129):

1. ***Before menopause,* the dimensions are approximately 3.5 × 2 × 1.5 cm.**
2. ***In early menopause,* the ovaries are approximately 2 × 1.5 × 0.5 cm.**
3. ***In late menopause,* they are even smaller: 1.5 × 0.75 × 0.5 cm.**

Barber has described the postmenopausal palpable ovary (PMPO) syndrome, suggesting that any ovary that is palpable on examination beyond the menopause is abnormal and deserves evaluation (184); however, this has not been shown to be a reliable predictor of malignancy (Chapter 32). Clearly, body habitus makes a difference in the ease of examination, but a postmenopausal ovary that, on palpation, is comparable in size to a premenopausal ovary is abnormally large. Ovarian cancer is predominantly a disease of postmenopausal women; the incidence increases with age, and the average patient age is about 56 to 60 years (Chapter 32).

With increased use of pelvic ultrasonographic evaluation, a new problem has arisen in postmenopausal women: the discovery of a small ovarian cyst. This is particularly troublesome in a woman who is entirely asymptomatic and whose ultrasonographic examination was performed for indications unrelated to pelvic pathology. It has been suggested that **when the cyst is asymptomatic, small (<5 cm in diameter), unilocular, and thin-walled, with a normal CA125 level, the risk of malignancy is extremely low and these masses can be followed conservatively, without surgery** (185–189). Surgery may be indicated in some women with a strong family history of ovarian, breast, endometrial, or colon cancer, or a mass that appears to be enlarging (see Chapter 32). The addition of color flow Doppler examination may be helpful in distinguishing benign from malignant masses (190,191).

Uterine and Other Masses

In women who have been receiving regular gynecologic care, the discovery of a new pelvic mass after menopause is worrisome because the likelihood of malignant neoplasm is high if it is an ovarian tumor. Many postmenopausal women have not had regular gynecologic care, however, so the discovery of a mass may reflect the persistence of uterine fibroids that had not previously been discovered. Some women may not remember having been told they had a pelvic mass. Thus, a review of medical records may be helpful in determining the preexistence of a benign pelvic mass. Other benign masses can occur in this age group, including paraovarian cysts and unusual tumors, such as benign retroperitoneal cysts of müllerian type (192).

Diagnosis

A personal and family medical history is helpful in detecting individuals at increased risk for the development of ovarian cancer. Several hereditary family cancer syndromes involve ovarian neoplasms (see Chapter 32). However, patients with hereditary forms of epithelial ovarian cancer account for only a small percentage of all cases; 90% to 95% of cases of ovarian cancer are sporadic and without identifiable heritable risk (193).

In one multicenter prospective study, the individual accuracy of pelvic examination, ultrasonography, and serum CA125 assessments in discriminating between benign and malignant pelvic masses was approximately the same (approximately 75%) (194). When the results of all three examinations were negative, no malignancy was found.

Management

The use of improved imaging techniques may allow the nonoperative management of ovarian masses that are probably benign (Table 13.9). When surgery is believed to be indicated, based on characteristics of the mass, a family or personal medical history, or the patient's desire for definitive diagnosis, selection of the appropriate surgical procedure is critical for effective therapy. The standard of care continues to be laparotomy, with appropriate staging procedures performed as necessary (Chapter 32), although laparoscopy has shown promise as a technique that offers the potential for lower morbidity. Ovarian cystectomy or oophorectomy may be indicated.

Vulvar Conditions

Vulvar and vaginal symptoms are a common initial complaint to gynecologists. The presence of vulvar symptoms may prompt a patient to seek care; however, this anatomic site is not one that is easily inspected by the patient. Thus, vulvar lesions may be noted on examination and may not have been noticed by the patient. Vulvar self-examination should be encouraged and could potentially result in the earlier diagnosis of vulvar lesions such as melanoma (195).

Neonatal

In the neonatal age group, various developmental and congenital abnormalities may be noted. Whereas an extensive discussion of these abnormalities is beyond the scope of this text, obstetricians will recognize that they must be prepared to deal with the parents and family when an infant is born with ambiguous genitalia. The etiology of these problems, as well as intersex disorders that may be discovered in an older child, can be complex. Chromosomal abnormalities, enzyme deficiencies (including 17- or 21-hydroxylase deficiency as causes of congenital adrenal hyperplasia), or prenatal masculinization of a female fetus resulting from maternal androgen-secreting ovarian tumors or, rarely, drug exposures can all result in genital abnormalities that are noted at birth. These abnormalities are addressed in Chapter 23.

Ambiguous genitalia represents a social and potential medical emergency that is best handled by a team of specialists, which may include urologists, neonatologists, endocrinologists, and pediatric gynecologists. The first questions parents ask after a baby is born include "Is it a boy or a girl?" In the case of ambiguous genitalia, the parents should be informed that the baby's genitals are not fully developed and, therefore, a simple examination of the external genitalia cannot determine the actual sex. The parents should be told that data will be collected but that it may take several days or longer to determine the baby's intended sex. In some situations, it may be best to state simply that the baby has some serious medical complications. The issues of gender assignment and timing of surgical therapy are controversial and should be managed by clinicians with extensive experience in the field (196,197).

Other genital abnormalities may be noted at birth, although few obstetricians or pediatricians carefully examine the external genitalia of female neonates. It has been argued that careful inspection of the external genitalia of all female infants should be performed, with gentle probing of the introitus and anus to determine the patency of the hymen or a possible imperforate anus. If patency is in doubt, a rectal thermometer may be used to gently test the patency. It has been suggested that this examination should be performed on all female infants in the delivery room (198). Various types of hymenal configurations in the newborn have been described, ranging from imperforate to microperforate, to cribriform, to hymenal bands, and hymens with central anterior, posterior, or eccentric orifices (199). An examination during the neonatal period would prevent the discovery of an imperforate hymen or vaginal septum only after a young woman experiences periodic pelvic and abdominal pain with the development of a large hematometra or hematocolpos.

Congenital vulvar tumors may include strawberry hemangiomas, which are relatively superficial vascular lesions, and large cavernous hemangiomas. Treatment is controversial; many lesions will spontaneously regress. Some clinicians have advocated cryotherapy, argon laser therapy, or sclerosing solutions (200).

Childhood

It may be difficult for a young child to describe vulvar sensations. Parents may notice the child crying during urination, scratching herself repeatedly, or complaining of vague symptoms. Often, the child's pediatrician will have evaluated the child for urinary tract infection. Evaluation for pinworms is also warranted, because pinworms can cause severe itching in the vulvar as well as perianal area. Vulvovaginitis is the most common gynecologic problem of childhood. Prepubertally, the vulva, vestibule, and vagina are anatomically and histologically vulnerable to infection with the bacteria typically present in the perianal area. The physical proximity of the vagina and vestibule to the anus can result in overgrowth of bacteria that can cause primary vulvitis and secondary vaginitis (see Chapter 15). Yeast infections are uncommon in prepubertal children who are toilet trained.

The clinician should be familiar with normal prepubertal genital anatomy and hymenal configuration (201,202). The unestrogenized vulvar vestibule is mildly erythematous and

Figure 13.30 **A:** Lichen sclerosus in a 7-year-old girl. (From **Novak ER, Woodruff JB,** eds. *Novak's gynecologic and obstetric pathology,* 7th ed. Philadelphia: WB Saunders, 1974:21, with permission.) **B:** Histologic appearance of lichen sclerosus.

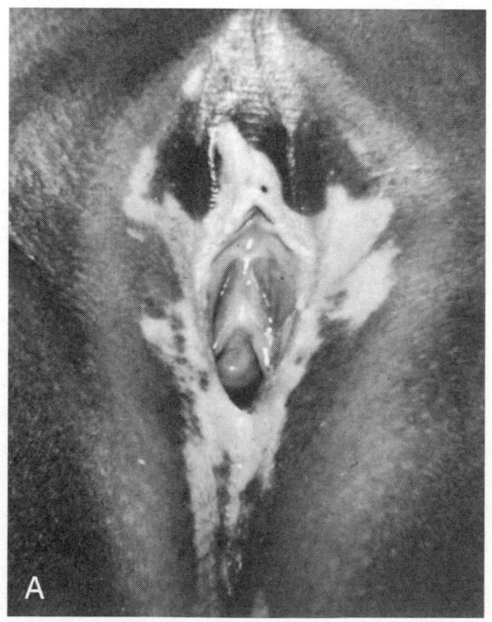

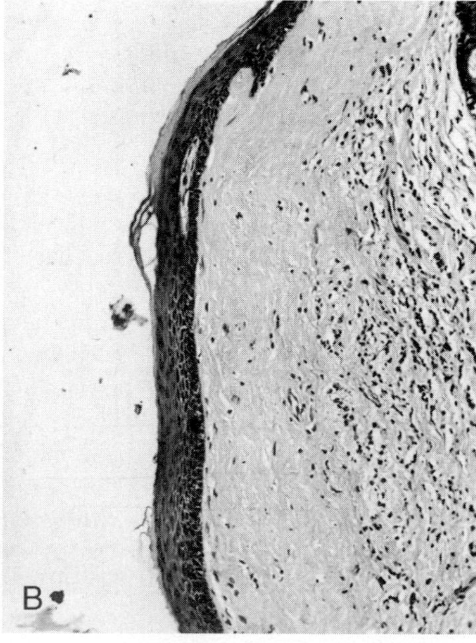

can be confused with infection. In addition, smegma around and beneath the prepuce may resemble patches of candida vulvitis. In prepubertal girls, the vulvar area is quite susceptible to chemical irritants.

Chronic skin conditions such as lichen sclerosus, psoriasis, seborrheic dermatitis, and atopic vulvitis may occur in children (203). Lichen sclerosus, the cause of which is not well established, has a characteristic "cigarette paper" appearance in a keyhole distribution (around the vulva and anus) (Fig. 13.30). Lichen sclerosus should be treated in pediatric patients as it is in adults; there is some suggestion that the condition may regress as the child progresses through adrenarche and menarche. The use of ultrapotent steroids topically has been successful in children as well as adults (204).

Labial agglutination may occur as a result of chronic vulvar inflammation from any cause (Fig. 13.31). The treatment of labial agglutination consists of a brief course (2 to 4 weeks) of externally applied estrogen cream. The area of agglutination (adhesion) will become thin as a result, and separation can often be performed in the office with the use of a topical anesthetic (e.g., lidocaine jelly) (Fig. 13.32). Urethral prolapse may cause acute pain or bleeding, or the presence of a mass may be noted.

Vulvovaginal complaints of any sort in a young child should prompt the consideration of possible sexual abuse. Sexually transmitted infections may occur in prepubertal children (205). Sensitive but direct questioning of the parent or caretaker and the child should be

Figure 13.31 Posterior labial agglutination in a 9-year-old girl.

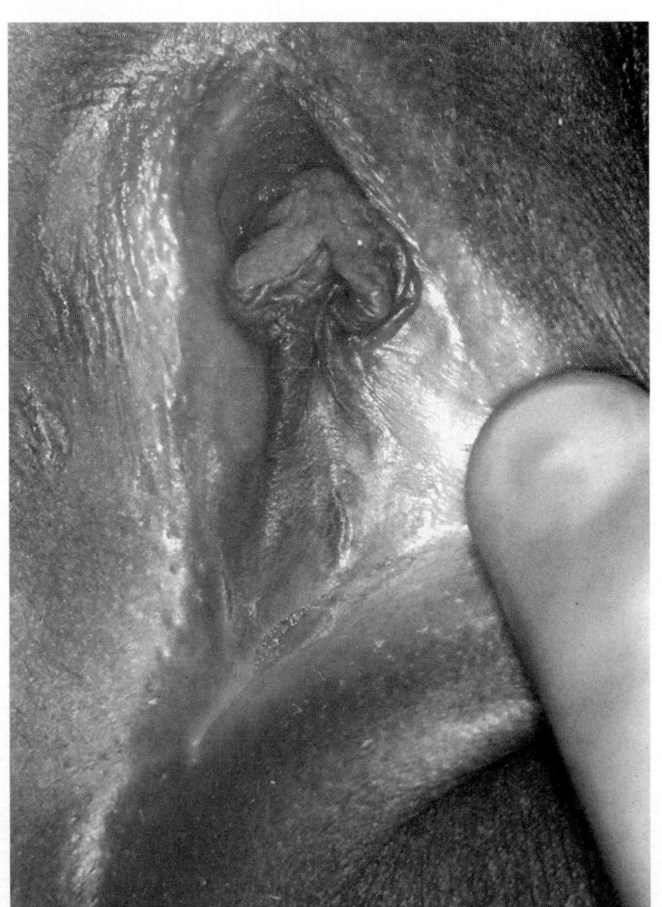

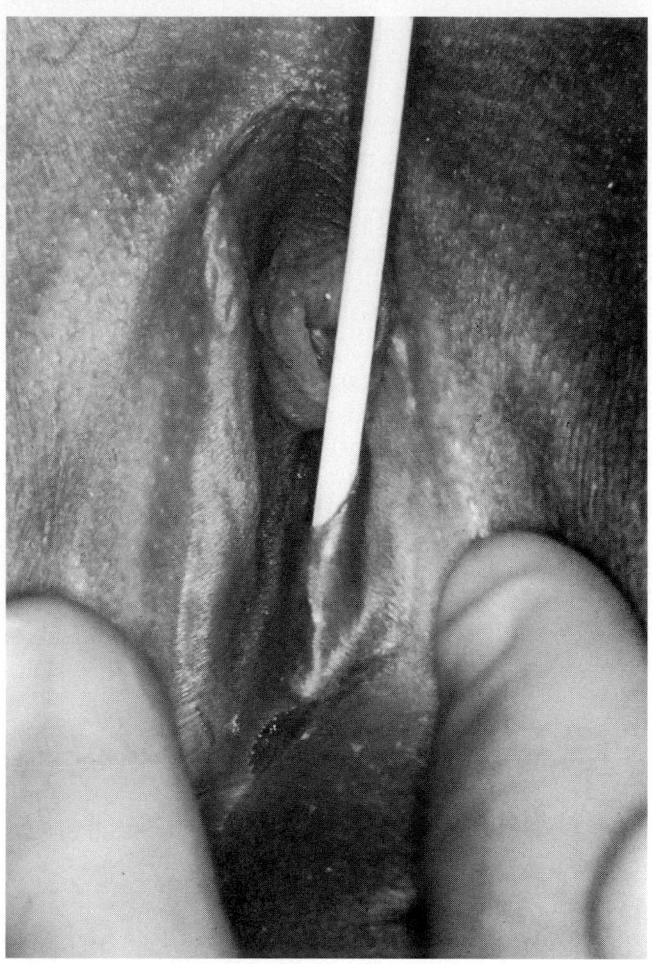

Figure 13.32 Cotton-tipped applicator placed inside the labial agglutination shown in Figure 13.31.

a part of the evaluation; if sexual abuse is suspected, reporting to the appropriate social services agency is required.

Adolescence

Adolescents with gonadal dysgenesis or androgen insensitivity may have abnormal pubertal development and primary amenorrhea (Chapter 23). Various developmental abnormalities—vaginal agenesis, imperforate hymen, transverse and longitudinal vaginal septa, vaginal and uterine duplications, hymenal bands, and septa—most commonly occur in early adolescence with amenorrhea (for the obstructing abnormalities) or with concerns such as inability to use tampons (for hymenal and vaginal bands and septa). These developmental abnormalities must be evaluated carefully to determine both external and internal anatomy.

A tight hymenal ring may be discovered because of concerns about the inability to use tampons or initiate intercourse. Manual dilation can be successful, as can small relaxing incisions at 6 o'clock and 8 o'clock in the hymenal ring. This can sometimes be done in the office using local anesthesia but may require conduction or general anesthesia in the operating room. Hymenal bands are not rare and also lead to difficulty in using tampons; they usually can be incised in the office using local anesthetic. The condition of hypertrophy of the labia minora has been described, along with surgical procedures to correct this developmental abnormality (206). This condition is more appropriately considered a variant of normal, with reassurance rather than a cosmetic surgical reduction as the primary therapy. Genital ulcerations may be noted in girls with leukemia or other cancers requiring chemotherapy

(207). The possibility of sexual abuse, incest, or involuntary intercourse should be considered for young adolescents with vulvovaginal complaints, STDs, or pregnancy.

Reproductive Age Women

In postmenarchal individuals, vulvar symptoms are most often related to a primary vaginitis and a secondary vulvitis. The presence of vaginal discharge can lead to vulvar irritative symptoms, or candidal vulvitis may be present. The causes of vaginitis and cervicitis are covered in Chapter 15. As noted, young children may have a difficult time describing vulvar symptoms; adult women describe vulvar symptoms using a variety of terms (itching, pain, discharge, discomfort, burning, external dysuria, soreness, pain with intercourse or sexual activity). Burning with urination from noninfectious causes may be difficult to distinguish from a urinary tract infection, although some women can distinguish pain when the urine hits the vulvar area (an external dysuria) from burning pain (often suprapubic in location) during urination. A urine culture may be necessary to help make the distinction. Itching is a very common vulvar symptom. A variety of vulvar conditions and lesions can present with pruritus.

A number of skin conditions that occur on other areas of the body may occur on the vulvar area. Table 13.10 contains a list of these conditions classified by either infectious or noninfectious causes. Whereas the diagnosis of some of these conditions is apparent from inspection alone (e.g., a skin tag) (Fig. 13.33), any lesions that appear atypical or in which the diagnosis is not clear should be analyzed by biopsy.

Pigmented vulvar lesions include benign nevi, lentigines, melanosis, seborrheic keratosis, and some vulvar intraepithelial neoplasias (VIN), especially multifocal VIN 3. Suspicious pigmented vulvar lesions, in particular, should warrant biopsy to rule out VIN or malignant melanoma (208). Approximately 10% of white women have a pigmented vulvar lesion; some of these lesions may be malignant (Chapter 33) or have the potential for progression (VIN) (Chapter 16). The behavior of some nevocellular lesions (representing about 2% of nevi)

Table 13.10. Subacute and Chronic Recurrent Conditions of the Vulva

Noninfectious	*Infectious*
Acanthosis nigricans	Cellulitis
Atopic dermatitis	Folliculitis
Behçets's disease	Furuncle/carbuncle
Contact dermatitis	Insect bites (e.g., chiggers, fleas)
Crohn's disease	Necrotizing fasciitis
Diabetic vulvitis[a]	Pubic lice
Hidradenitis suppurativa[a]	Scabies
Hyperplastic dystrophy	Tinea
Lichen sclerosus	
Mixed dystrophy	
Paget's disease	
Pseudo folliculitis	
Razor bumps	
Psoriasis	
Seborrheic dermatitis	
Vulvar intraepithelial neoplasia	

[a] Etiology unknown, often secondarily infected.

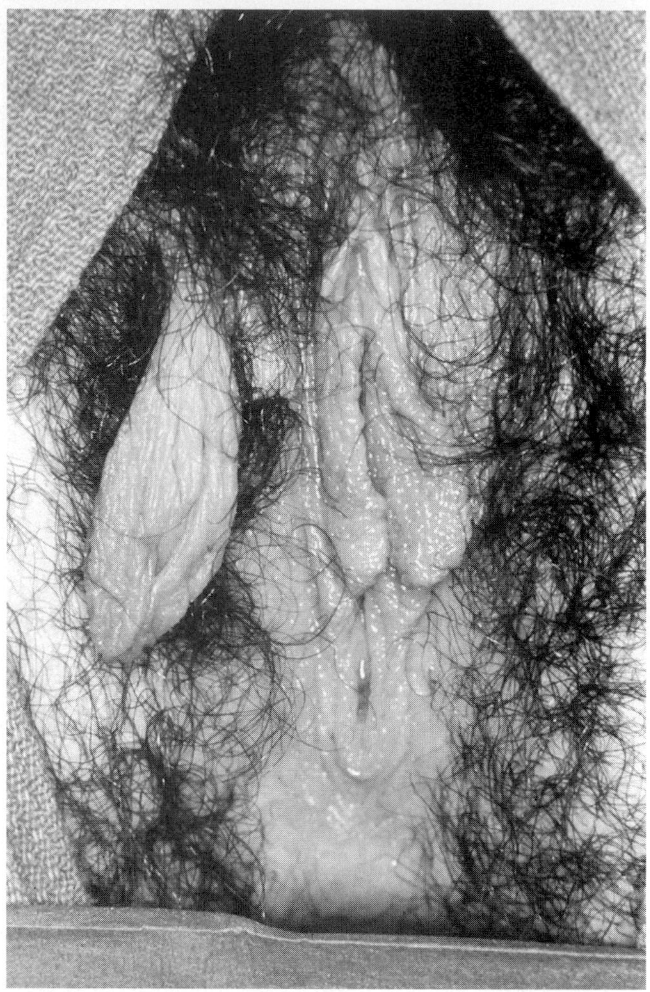

Figure 13.33 Large benign skin tag from left labium majus.

is not well established but has been linked to melanoma (209). Multiple hyperpigmented lesions of typical lentigo simplex and melanosis are common, and any areas with irregular borders should be evaluated by biopsy (Fig. 13.34).

Vulvar Biopsy

A vulvar biopsy is essential in distinguishing benign from premalignant or malignant vulvar lesions, especially because many types of lesions may have a somewhat similar appearance. Vulvar biopsies should be performed liberally to ensure that these lesions are diagnosed and treated appropriately. A prospective study of vulvar lesions evaluated by biopsy in a gynecologic clinic found lesions occurring in the following order of frequency: epidermal inclusion cyst (Fig. 13.35), lentigo, Bartholin duct obstruction, carcinoma in situ, melanocytic nevi, acrochordon, mucous cyst, hemangiomas, postinflammatory hyperpigmentation, seborrheic keratoses, varicosities, hidradenomas, verruca, basal cell carcinoma, and unusual tumors such as neurofibromas, ectopic tissue, syringomas, and abscesses (210). Clearly, the frequency with which a lesion would be reported after a tissue biopsy is related to the frequency with which all lesions of a given pathology are evaluated in this manner. Thus, this listing probably underrepresents such common lesions as condylomas.

Biopsy is easily performed in the office using a local anesthetic. Typically, 1% lidocaine is infiltrated beneath the lesion using a small (25- to 27-gauge) needle. Disposable punch biopsy instruments come in a variety of sizes from 2- to 6-mm in diameter. They have

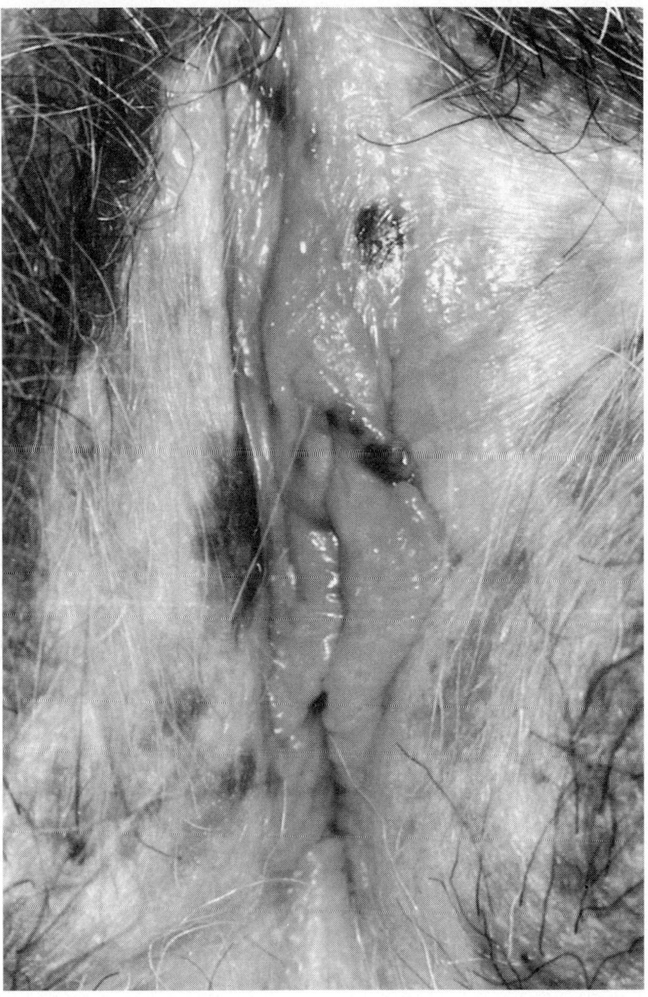

Figure 13.34 Lentigo simplex and melanosis of vulva. Note multiple hyperpigmented lesions. (From **Wilkinson EJ, Stone IK.** *Atlas of vulvar disease.* Baltimore: Lippincott Williams & Wilkins, 1995:41, with permission.)

the advantage of being sharp and thus facilitate obtaining a good specimen. Sterilizable instruments are also available and may be a more ecologically sound choice if they can be maintained and sharpened periodically. These skin biopsy instruments, along with fine forceps, scissors, and a scalpel, should be available in all outpatient gynecologic settings. For the smaller biopsies, it is usually unnecessary to place a suture. Topical silver nitrate can be used for hemostasis. Multiple tissue samples may be appropriate to obtain representative areas of a lesion if the lesion has a variable appearance or is multifocal. Although the vulvar biopsy procedure involves minimal discomfort, the biopsy sites will be painful for several days after the procedure. The prescription of a topical anesthetic such as 2% lidocaine jelly, to be applied periodically and before urinating, is appreciated by patients who require this procedure. Infection of the site can occur, and patients should be cautioned to report excessive erythema or purulent drainage.

Other Vulvar Conditions

Pseudofolliculitis, similar to what has been described as pseudofolliculitis barbae (razor bumps), may occur in women who follow the increasingly popular practice of shaving pubic hair to conform to a swimsuit (210). It consists of an inflammatory reaction surrounding an ingrown hair and occurs most commonly among individuals with curly hair, particularly African Americans.

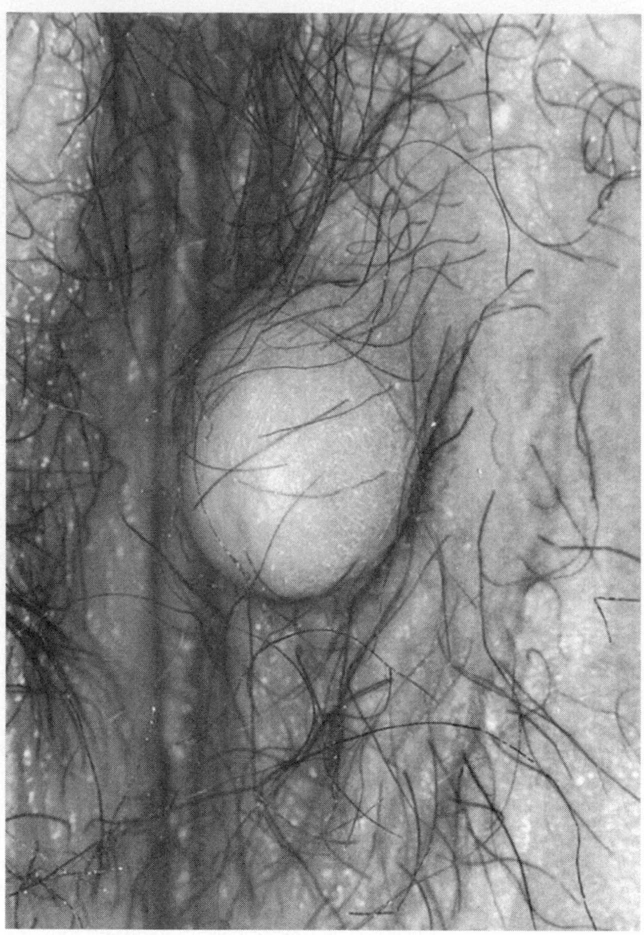

Figure 13.35 Inclusion cysts on right labium majus. (From **Wilkinson EJ, Stone IK.** *Atlas of vulvar disease.* Baltimore: Lippincott Williams & Wilkins, 1995:17, with permission.)

Fox-Fordyce disease is characterized by a chronic, pruritic eruption of small papules or cysts formed by keratin-plugged apocrine glands. It is commonly present over the lower abdomen, mons pubis, labia majora, and inner portions of the thighs. Hidradenitis suppurativa is a chronic condition involving the apocrine glands with the formation of multiple deep nodules, scars, pits, and sinuses that occur in the axilla, vulva, and perineum (Fig. 13.36). Hyperpigmentation and secondary infection are often seen. Hidradenitis suppurativa can be extremely painful and debilitating. It is often treated with antibiotics (with coverage of both aerobic and anaerobic bacteria). Estrogens or antiandrogen therapy has been attempted; surgical therapy with wide local excision may be necessary. Therapy with isotretinoin and steroids has been reported to be successful (211,212).

Acanthosis nigricans involves widespread velvety pigmentation in skin folds, particularly the axillae, neck, thighs, submammary area, and vulva and surrounding skin. It is of particular interest to gynecologists because of its association with hyperandrogenism and PCOS as such, it is associated with obesity, chronic anovulation, acne, glucose intolerance, and cardiovascular disease (37,213).

Intraepithelial Neoplasia

A classification of intraepithelial lesions of the vulva is presented in Table 16.13.

Extramammary Paget's disease of the vulva is an intraepithelial neoplasia containing vacuolated Paget's cells (Chapter 16). Clinically, it may have an appearance varying from moist,

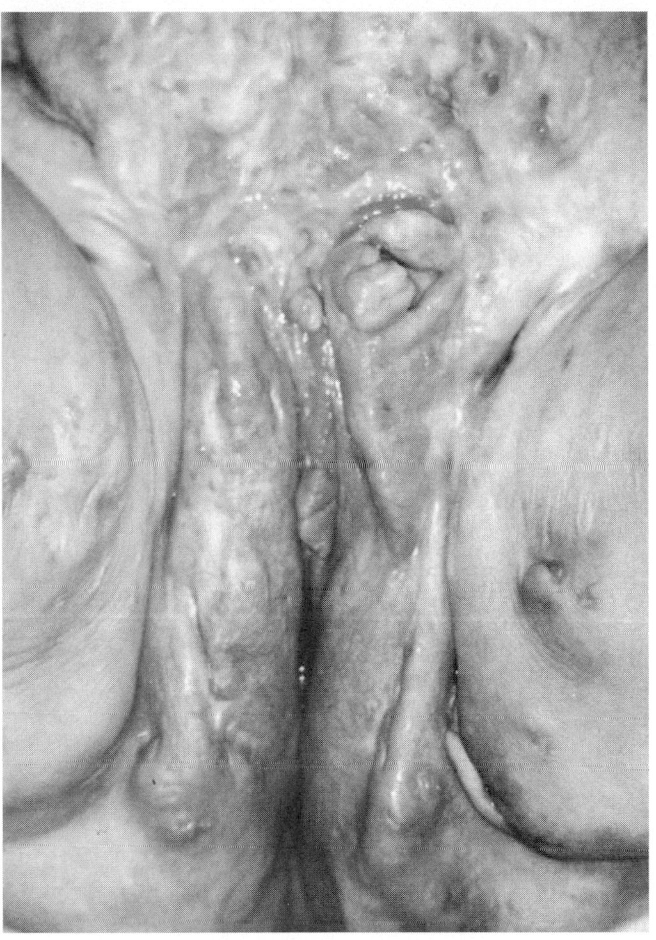

Figure 13.36 Hidradenitis suppurativa involving both labia majora and crease folds. (From **Wilkinson EJ, Stone IK.** *Atlas of vulvar disease.* Baltimore: Williams & Wilkins, 1995:150, with permission.)

oozing ulcerations to an eczematoid lesion with scaling and crusting, to a grayish lesion (200). A biopsy to confirm the diagnosis is mandatory.

Vulvar intraepithelial neoplasia is associated with human papillomavirus infection and is increasing in frequency, particularly among young women (Chapter 16) (214). Diagnosis requires biopsy of any suspicious vulvar lesions, particularly those that are pigmented or discolored. The increasing frequency of this entity makes a careful vulvar inspection mandatory during annual gynecologic examinations.

Vulvar Tumors, Cysts, and Masses

Condyloma acuminata are very common vulvar lesions and are usually easily recognized and treated with topical therapies such as tri- and bichloracetic acid. Other sexually transmitted organisms, such as the virus responsible for *molluscum contagiosum* and the lesions of *syphilis* and *condyloma lata,* may occasionally be mistaken for vulvar condyloma acuminata caused by the human papillomavirus (see Chapter 15). A summary of benign vulvar tumors is listed in Table 13.11. There is argument regarding whether sebaceous cysts exist on the vulva or whether these lesions are histopathologically epidermal or epidermal inclusion cysts (215). These cysts may result from the burial of fragments of skin after the trauma of childbirth or episiotomy.

It has been argued that the commonly cited concept of milk lines extending into the vulva and accounting for lesions of mammary-like anogenital glands (e.g., fibroadenoma, lactating

Table 13.11. Types of Vulvar Tumors

1. **Cystic Lesions**	3. **Anatomic**
Bartholin duct cyst	Hernia
Cyst in the canal of Nuck (hydrocele)	Urethral diverticulum
Epithelial inclusion cyst	Varicosities
Skene duct cyst	
	4. **Infections**
2. **Solid Tumors**	Abscess—Bartholin, Skene, periclitoral, other
Acrochordon (skin tag)	Condyloma lata
Angiokeratoma	Molluscum contagiosum
Bartholin gland adenoma	Pyogenic granuloma
Cherry angioma	
Fibroma	5. **Ectopic**
Hemangioma	Endometriosis
Hidradenoma	Ectopic breast tissue
Lipoma	
Granular cell myoblastoma	
Neurofibroma	
Papillomatosis	

glands) is not supported by observations in human embryos; such studies show that primordia of the mammary glands do not extend beyond the axillary-pectoral area (216). Eccrine or apocrine glands have been suggested as the probable source of these unusual lesions.

Bartholin duct cysts are common vulvar lesions. They result from occlusion of the duct with accumulation of mucus and are frequently asymptomatic. Infection of the gland may result in the accumulation of purulent material, with the formation of a rapidly enlarging, painful, inflammatory mass (a Bartholin abscess). An inflatable bulb-tipped catheter has been described by Word and is quite easy to use (217). The small catheter is inserted through a small stab wound into the abscess after infiltration of the skin with local anesthesia; the balloon of the catheter is inflated with 2 to 3 ml of saline and the catheter remains in place for 4 to 6 weeks, allowing epithelialization of a tract and the creation of a permanent gland opening.

Skene duct cysts are cystic dilations of the Skene glands, typically located adjacent to the urethral meatus within the vulvar vestibule (Fig. 13.37). Although most are small and often asymptomatic, they may enlarge and cause urinary obstruction, requiring excision.

The symptom of painful intercourse (dyspareunia) may be caused by many different vulvovaginal conditions, including common vaginal infections and vaginismus (Chapter 15). A careful sexual history is essential, as is a careful examination of the vulvar area and vagina. *Vulvodynia* is the term used to describe unexplained vulvar pain, sexual dysfunction, and the resultant psychological disability (218). The term *vulvar vestibulitis* has been used to describe a situation in which there is pain during intercourse, primarily during entry (219,220). The condition is characterized by tender areas surrounding the vulvar vestibule and hymenal ring (see Chapter 14). A number of recent studies have failed to demonstrate a consistent relationship with any genital infectious organism, including chlamydia, gonorrhea, *Trichomonas,* mycoplasma, *Ureaplasma, Gardnerella,* candida, or

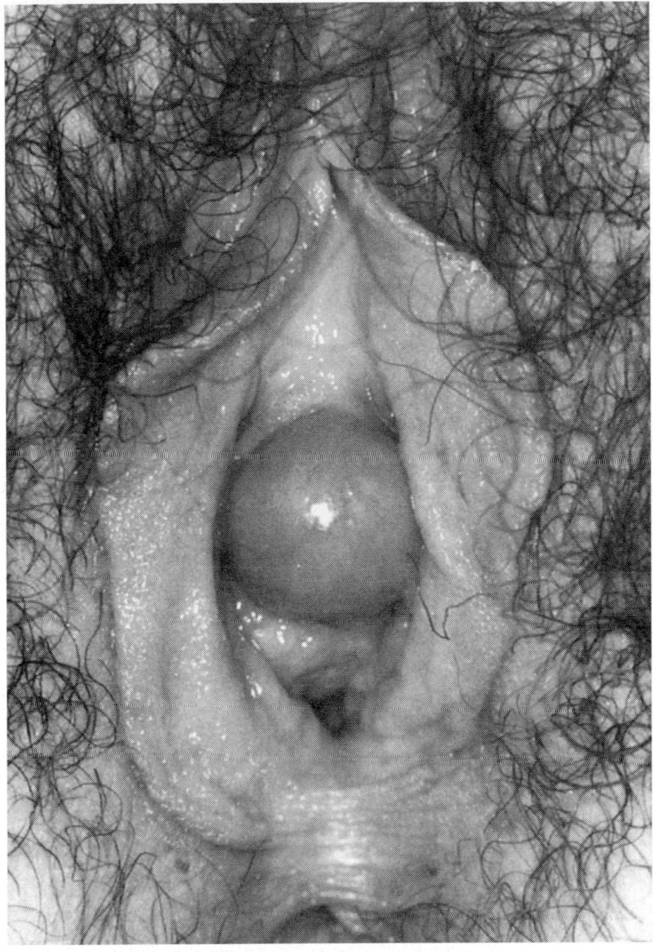

Figure 13.37 Skene duct cyst. (From **Wilkinson EJ, Stone IK.** *Atlas of vulvar disease.* Baltimore: Lippincott, Williams & Wilkins, 1995:21, with permission.)

human papillomavirus (221–223). Although the symptoms of dyspareunia with insertion can be disabling, no curative therapies have been found. Surgical therapies have been suggested, and both medical and behavioral therapies are of some benefit (224,225). The visible lesion of vestibular papillomatosis may be a nonspecific response to discharge or inflammation.

Vulvar Ulcers

A number of STDs can cause vulvar ulcers, including herpes simplex virus, syphilis, lymphogranuloma venereum, and granuloma inguinale (Chapter 15). *Crohn's disease* can include vulvar involvement with abscesses, fistulae, sinus tracts, fenestrations, and other scarring. Although medical treatment with systemic steroids and other systemic agents is the mainstay of therapy, surgical therapy of both intestinal and vulvar disease may be required.

Behçet's disease is characterized by genital and oral ulcerations with ocular inflammation. The cause and the most effective therapy are not well established.

Lichen planus also causes oral and genital ulcerations. Typically, there is desquamative vaginitis with erosion of the vestibule. Treatment is based on the use of both topical and systemic steroids. Plasma cell mucositis appears as erosions in the vulvar area, particularly the vestibule. Biopsy is essential in making the diagnosis.

Postmenopausal Women

Vulvar Dystrophies

Several vulvar conditions occur most commonly in postmenopausal women. Symptoms are primarily itching and vulvar soreness, in addition to dyspareunia.

In the past, numerous terms have been used to describe disorders of vulvar epithelial growth that produce a number of nonspecific gross changes. These terms have included leukoplakia, lichen sclerosus et atrophicus, atrophic and hyperplastic vulvitis, and kraurosis vulvae. The malignant potential of the vulvar dystrophies is less than 5%; at particular risk is the patient with cellular atypia on initial biopsy. The International Society for the Study of Vulvar Diseases (ISSVD) has recommended a classification of vulvar dystrophies, which is presented in Table 16.13.

Squamous Hyperplasia Squamous hyperplasia is seen most often in postmenopausal women but may occur during the reproductive years. Pruritus is the most common symptom. The lesion appears thickened and hyperkeratotic, and there may be excoriation. Squamous hyperplasia tends to be discrete but may be symmetric and multiple. Biopsies are necessary to make the diagnosis and to evaluate the presence of atypia and exclude malignancy.

The treatment is local application of a fluorinated corticosteroid ointment 2 times a day for 6 weeks. Typically, the lesion totally regresses. If a new lesion recurs, another biopsy should be performed and an additional 6 weeks of treatment with topical steroids should be given (224).

Lichen Sclerosus **Lichen sclerosus is the most common white lesion of the vulva** (Fig. 13.38). **Lichen sclerosus can occur at any age, although it is most common among postmenopausal women and prepubertal girls** (224). The symptoms are pruritus, dyspareunia, and burning. Lichen sclerosus characteristically is associated with decreased subcutaneous fat such that the vulva is atrophic, with small or absent labia minora, thin labia majora, and sometimes phimosis of the prepuce. The surface is pale with a shiny, crinkled pattern, often with fissures and excoriation. The lesion tends to be symmetric and often extends to the perineal and perianal areas. The diagnosis is confirmed by biopsy. Invasive cancer is only rarely associated with lichen sclerosus.

Treatment is with an ultrapotent topical steroid such as 0.05% clobetasol. Approximately 80% of patients have a satisfactory response (226). Maintenance therapy is important and may include the use of a lower potency steroid or the use of a topical emollient (227).

Urethral Lesions

Vulvar lesions that may be seen in other age groups, but that occur more commonly among older women, include urethral caruncles and prolapse of the urethral mucosa. Both conditions can be treated with topical or systemic estrogen preparations. Various vulvar skin lesions, including seborrheic keratoses and cherry hemangiomas (senile hemangiomas), occur more commonly on aging skin.

Vaginal Conditions

Vaginal discharge is one of the most common vaginal symptoms. Conditions ranging from vaginal candidiasis to chlamydia cervicitis to bacterial vaginosis to cervical carcinoma may cause vaginal discharge. Infectious vaginal conditions are addressed more completely in Chapter 15. Vaginal lesions may occasionally be palpable to a woman. More commonly, vaginal lesions are discovered on examination by a clinician. They may contribute to symptoms (such as bleeding or discharge) or they may be entirely asymptomatic. Vaginitis,

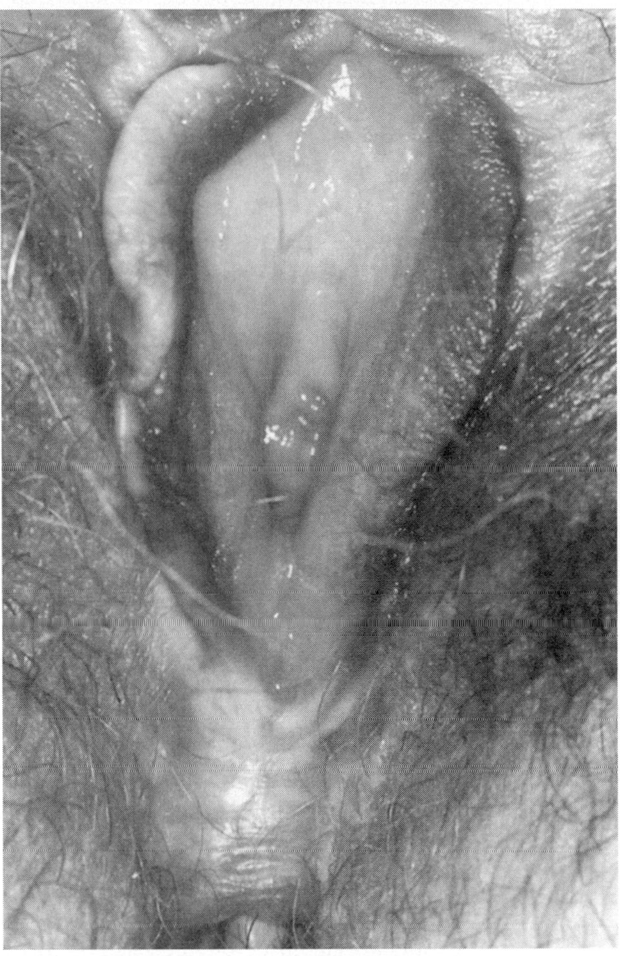

Figure 13.38 Lichen sclerosus of the vulva in a postmenopausal patient. (From **Wilkinson EJ, Stone IK.** *Atlas of vulvar disease.* Baltimore: Lippincott Williams & Wilkins, 1995:36, with permission.)

cervicitis, and vaginal or cervical lesions (including malignancies) can be causes of vaginal discharge. Other noninfectious causes of discharge are as follows:

1. Retained foreign body—tampon, pessary
2. Ulcerations—tampon-induced, lichen planus
3. Malignancy—cervical, vaginal
4. Postmenopausal atrophic vaginitis, postradiation vulvovaginitis

Pediatric

Sexual abuse should always be considered in prepubertal children with vaginal discharge. Although the use of routine STD cultures in girls with a history of sexual abuse has been questioned, vaginal culture for gonorrhea and chlamydia should be performed in girls with vaginal discharge (228). In prepubertal girls, vulvovaginitis is usually caused by multiple organisms that are present in the perineal area, although a single organism such as streptococcus or even, rarely, *Shigella* may be causative. Treatment should be initiated with a focus on hygienic and cleansing measures. A short-term (<4 weeks) course of topical estrogens and broad-spectrum antibiotics may be necessary. The problem can be recurrent.

A technique for obtaining vaginal cultures and for performing vaginal irrigation has been described by Pokorny (229). A catheter within a catheter can be fashioned using the tubing from an intravenous butterfly setup within a sterile urethral catheter. Nonbacteriostatic saline (1 ml) can be injected, aspirated, and sent for culture. Cultures taken in this manner are almost always better tolerated than cultures obtained using a cotton-tipped applicator. A larger quantity of saline can then be used to irrigate the vagina while the catheter is still within the vagina. Small foreign bodies can often be flushed from the vagina in this manner.

Adolescence and Older

Vaginal tampons have been associated with both microscopic and macroscopic ulcerations. Healing of the macroscopic ulcerations occurs within several weeks without specific therapy if tampon use is suspended. A follow-up examination to demonstrate healing is appropriate, with biopsy of any persistent ulcerations to rule out other lesions.

Toxic shock syndrome (TSS) has been associated with tampon use and vaginal *Staphylococcus aureus*–produced exotoxins. TSS consists of fever, hypotension, a diffuse erythroderma with desquamation of the palms and soles, plus involvement of at least three major organ systems (230). Vaginal involvement includes mucous membrane inflammation. TSS appears to be declining in frequency, and an increasing percentage of cases are not associated with menses (231).

Some vaginal lesions are asymptomatic and are noted incidentally on examination. *Fibroepithelial polyps* consist of polypoid folds of connective tissue, capillaries, and stroma covered by vaginal epithelium. Although they can be excised easily in the office, their vascularity can be troublesome, and excision is not necessary unless the diagnosis is in question. *Cysts of embryonic origin* can arise from mesonephric, paramesonephric, and urogenital sinus epithelium. *Gartner's duct cysts* are of mesonephric origin and are usually present on the lateral vaginal wall. They rarely cause symptoms and, therefore, do not require treatment. Other embryonic cysts can arise anterior to the vagina and beneath the bladder. Cysts that arise from the urogenital sinus epithelium are located in the area of the vulvar vestibule. *Vaginal adenosis,* the presence of epithelial-lined glands within the vagina, has been associated with *in utero* exposure to diethylstilbestrol. No therapy is necessary, other than close observation and periodic palpation to detect nodules that may need to be evaluated by biopsy to rule out vaginal clear cell adenocarcinoma (Chapter 31).

Women will sometimes describe a bulging lesion of the vagina and vulvar area, variably associated with symptoms of pressure or discomfort. The most common cause of such a lesion is one of the disorders of vaginal support: cystocele, rectocele, or urethrocele. Management of these conditions is discussed in Chapter 20. Other genital lesions, such as urethral diverticula or occasionally embryonic cysts, may cause similar symptoms.

References

1. **Biro FM, McMahon RP, Striegel-Moore R, et al.** Impact of timing of pubertal maturation on growth in black and white female adolescents: The National Heart, Lung, and Blood Institute Growth and Health Study. *J Pediatr* 2001;138:636–643.
2. **Herman–Giddens ME, Slora EJ, Wasserman RC, et al.** Secondary sexual characteristics and menses in young girls seen in office practice: a study from the Pediatric Research in Office Settings network. *Pediatrics* 1997;99:505–512.
3. **Marshall WA, Tanner JM.** Variations in pattern of pubertal changes in girls. *Arch Dis Child* 1969;44:291–303.
4. **Harlan WR, Harlan EA, Grillo GP.** Secondary sex characteristics of girls 12 to 17 years of age: the U.S. Health Examination Survey. *J Pediatr* 1980;96:1074–1078.
5. **Anveden-Hertzberg L, Gauderer MW, Elder JS.** Urethral prolapse: an often misdiagnosed cause of urogenital bleeding in girls. *Pediatr Emerg Care* 1995;11:212–214.
6. **Frasier LD.** Human papillomavirus infections in children. *Pediatr Ann* 1994;23:354–360.
7. **Neinstein LS, Goldenring J, Carpenter S.** Nonsexual transmission of sexually transmitted diseases: an infrequent occurrence. *Pediatrics* 1984;74:67–76.

8. **Pokorny SF.** Long-term intravaginal presence of foreign bodies in children. A preliminary study. *J Reprod Med* 1994;39:931–935.

9. **Herman-Giddens ME.** Vaginal foreign bodies and child sexual abuse. *Arch Pediatr Adolesc Med* 1994;148:195–200.

10. **American Medical Association.** Diagnostic and treatment guidelines on child sexual abuse. Chicago: American Medical Association, 1992.

11. **Dowd MD, Fitzmaurice L, Knapp JF, et al.** The interpretation of urogenital findings in children with straddle injuries. *J Pediatr Surg* 1994;29:7–10.

12. **Adams JA, Knudson S.** Genital findings in adolescent girls referred for suspected sexual abuse. *Arch Pediatr Adolesc Med* 1996;150:850–857.

13. **Emans SJ, Woods ER, Flagg NT, et al.** Genital findings in sexually abused, symptomatic and asymptomatic, girls. *Pediatrics* 1987;79:778–785.

14. **Muram D.** Child sexual abuse: relationship between sexual acts and genital findings. *Child Abuse Negl* 1989;13:211–216.

15. **Treloar A, Boynton R, Behn B, et al.** Variation of the human menstrual cycle through reproductive life. *Int J Fertil* 1970;12:77–126.

16. **Flug D, Largo RH, Prader A.** Menstrual patterns in adolescent Swiss girls: a longitudinal study. *Ann Hum Biol* 1984;11:495–508.

17. **World Health Organization Task Force on Adolescent Reproductive Health.** Longitudinal study of menstrual patterns in the early postmenarchal period, duration of bleeding episodes and menstrual cycles. *J Adolesc Health Care* 1986;7:236–244.

18. **Fraser IS, McCarron G, Markham R, et al.** Blood and total fluid content of menstrual discharge. *Obstet Gynecol* 1985;65:194–198.

19. **Fraser IS, McCarron G, Markham R.** A preliminary study of factors influencing perception of menstrual blood loss volume. *Am J Obstet Gynecol* 1984;149:788–793.

20. **Grimes DA.** Estimating vaginal blood loss. *J Reprod Med* 1979;22:190–192.

21. **Venturoli S, Porcu E, Fabbri R, et al.** Menstrual irregularities in adolescents: hormonal pattern and ovarian morphology. *Horm Res* 1986;24:269–279.

22. **Apter D, Vihko R.** Early menarche, a risk factor for breast cancer, indicates early onset of ovulatory cycles. *J Clin Endocrinol Metab* 1983;57:82–86.

23. **Abma JC, Sonenstein FL.** Sexual activity and contraceptive practices among teenagers in the United States, 1988 and 1995. *Vital Health Stat 2001.*

24. **Fraser IS, Hickey M, Song JY.** A comparison of mechanisms underlying disturbances of bleeding caused by spontaneous dysfunctional uterine bleeding or hormonal contraception. *Hum Reprod* 1996;11[Suppl 2]: 165–178.

25. **Rosenberg MJ, Long SC.** Oral contraceptives and cycle control: a critical review of the literature. *Adv Contracept* 1992;8[Suppl 1]:35–45.

26. **Rosenberg MJ, Burnhill MS, Waugh MS, et al.** Compliance and oral contraceptives: a review. *Contraception* 1995;52:137–141.

27. **Oakley D, Sereika S, Bogue EL.** Oral contraceptive pill use after an initial visit to a family planning clinic. *Fam Plann Perspect* 1991;23:150–154.

28. **Balassone ML.** Risk of contraceptive discontinuation among adolescents. *J Adolesc Health Care* 1989;10:527–533.

29. **Kaunitz AM.** Injectable depot medroxyprogesterone acetate contraception: an update for U.S. clinicians. *Int J Fertil Womens Med* 1998;43:73–83.

30. **Shoupe D, Mishell DR.** Norplant: subdermal implant system for long-term contraception. *Am J Obstet Gynecol* 1989;160:1286–1292.

31. **Kaunitz AM, Garceau RJ, Cromie MA.** Comparative safety, efficacy, and cycle control of Lunelle monthly contraceptive injection (medroxyprogesterone acetate and estradiol cypionate injectable suspension) and Ortho-Novum 7/7/7 oral contraceptive (norethindrone/ethinyl estradiol triphasic). Lunelle Study Group. *Contraception* 1999;60:179–187.

32. **Rockett H.** Bleeding patterns in Mirena users. *Br J Fam Plan* 1998;23:140.

33. **Krettek JE, Arkin SI, Chaisilwattana P, et al.** *Chlamydia trachomatis* in patients who used oral contraceptives and had intermenstrual spotting. *Obstet Gynecol* 1993;81:728–731.

34. **Claessens EA, Cowell CA.** Acute adolescent menorrhagia. *Am J Obstet Gynecol* 1981;139:277–280.

35. **Centers for Disease Control and Prevention.** 1998 guidelines for treatment of sexually transmitted diseases. *MMWR* 1998;47:1–111.

36. **Lawson MA, Blythe MJ.** Pelvic inflammatory disease in adolescents. *Pediatr Clin North Am* 1999;46:767–782.

37. **NICHD.** Androgens and women's health. *Clinician* 1994;12:1–30.

38. **Gordon CM.** Menstrual disorders in adolescents. Excess androgens and the polycystic ovary syndrome. *Pediatr Clin North Am* 1999;46:519–543.

39. **Dunaif A, Thomas A.** Current concepts in the polycystic ovary syndrome. *Annu Rev Med* 2001;52: 401–419.

40. **van Hooff MH, Voorhorst FJ, Kaptein MB, et al.** Polycystic ovaries in adolescents and the relationship with menstrual cycle patterns, luteinizing hormone, androgens, and insulin. *Fertil Steril* 2000;74:49–58.

41. **Imai A, Furui T, Matsunami K, et al.** Magnetic resonance evaluation of uterine malformation with corpus agenesis. *J Med* 1997;28:223–227.

42. **Henshaw SK.** Unintended pregnancy in the United States. *Fam Plann Perspect* 1998;30:24–29.

43. **The Alan Guttmacher Institute.** *Sex and America's teenagers.* New York: The Alan Guttmacher Institute, 1994:1–88.

44. **Isojarvi JI, Rattya J, Myllyla VV, et al.** Valproate, lamotrigine, and insulin-mediated risks in women with epilepsy. *Ann Neurol* 1998;43:446–451.

45. **Vainionpaa LK, Rattya J, Knip M, et al.** Valproate-induced hyperandrogenism during pubertal maturation in girls with epilepsy. *Ann Neurol* 1999;45:444–450.

46. **Rattya J, Vaininonpaa L, Knip M, et al.** The effects of valproate, carbamazepine, and oxcarbazepine on growth and sexual maturation in girls with epilepsy. *Pediatrics* 1999;103:588–593.

47. **Stubblefield PG.** Menstrual impact of contraception. *Am J Obstet Gynecol* 1994;170:1513–1522.

48. **Rosenberg MJ, Waugh MS, Burnhill MS.** Compliance, counseling and satisfaction with oral contraceptives: a prospective evaluation. *Fam Plann Perspect* 1998;30:89–92.

49. **Rosenberg MJ, Waugh MS, Meehan TE.** Use and misuse of oral contraceptives: risk indicators for poor pill taking and discontinuation. *Contraception* 1995;51:283–288.

50. **Archer DF, Philput CA, Weber ME.** Management of irregular uterine bleeding and spotting associated with Norplant. *Hum Reprod* 1996;11[Suppl 2]:24–30.

51. **Diaz S, Croxatto HB, Pavez M, et al.** Clinical assessment of treatments for prolonged bleeding in users of Norplant implants. *Contraception* 1990;42:97–109.

52. **Krassas GE.** Thyroid disease and female reproduction. *Fertil Steril* 2000;74:1063–1070.

53. **Nowak RA.** Fibroids: pathophysiology and current medical treatment. *Best Pract Res Clin Obstet Gynaecol* 1999;13:223–238.

54. **Okoronkwo MO.** Body weight and uterine leiomyomas among women in Nigeria. *West Afr J Med* 1999;18:52–54.

55. **Marshall LM, Spiegelman D, Barbieri RL, et al.** Variation in the incidence of uterine leiomyoma among premenopausal women by age and race. *Obstet Gynecol* 1997;90:967–973.

56. **Stewart EA, Nowak RA.** Leiomyoma-related bleeding: a classic hypothesis updated for the molecular era. *Hum Reprod Update* 1996;2:295–306.

57. **Kadir RA.** Frequency of inherited bleeding disorders in women with menorrhagia. *Lancet* 1998;351:485–489.

58. **Brenner PF.** Differential diagnosis of abnormal uterine bleeding. *Am J Obstet Gynecol* 1996;175:766–769.

59. **Rick ME.** Diagnosis and management of von Willebrand's syndrome. *Med Clin North Am* 1994;78:609–623.

60. **Soares SR, Barbosa dos Reis MM, Camargos AF.** Diagnostic accuracy of sonohysterography, transvaginal sonography, and hysterosalpingography in patients with uterine cavity diseases. *Fertil Steril* 2000;73:406–411.

61. **Dubinsky TJ, Stroehlein K, Abu-Ghazzeh Y, et al.** Prediction of benign and malignant endometrial disease: hysterosonographic-pathologic correlation. *Radiology* 1999;210:393–397.

62. **Kinkel K, Kaji Y, Yu KK, et al.** Radiologic staging in patients with endometrial cancer: a meta-analysis. *Radiology* 1999;212:711–718.

63. **Stock RJ, Kanbour A.** Prehysterectomy curettage. *Obstet Gynecol* 1975;45:537–541.

64. **Grimes DA.** Diagnostic dilation and curettage: a reappraisal. *Am J Obstet Gynecol* 1982;143:1–6.

65. **ACOG.** *Hysteroscopy.* Washington, DC: American College of Obstetricians and Gynecologists, 1994.

66. **ACOG Committee on Practice Bulletins—Gynecology.** *Management of anovulatory bleeding: clinical management guidelines for obstetrician-gynecologists.* Washington, DC: American College of Obstetricians and Gynecologists, 2000.

67. **Lethaby A, Augood C, Duckitt K.** Nonsteroidal anti-inflammatory drugs for heavy menstrual bleeding. [computer file] *Cochrane Database of Systematic Reviews* 2000;(2):CD000400.

68. **Cooke I, Lethaby A, Farquhar C.** Antifibrinolytics for heavy menstrual bleeding. [update in Cochrane Database Syst Rev. 2000;(4):CD000249]. [computer file] *Cochrane Database of Systematic Reviews* 2000;(2):CD000249.

69. **Lethaby A, Farquhar C, Cooke I.** Antifibrinolytics for heavy menstrual bleeding. [update of Cochrane Database Syst Rev. 2000;(2):CD000249]. [computer file] *Cochrane Database of Systematic Reviews* 2000;(4):CD000249.

70. **Lethaby A, Irvine G, Cameron I.** Cyclical progestogens for heavy menstrual bleeding. [computer file] *Cochrane Database of Systematic Reviews* 2000;(2):CD001016.

71. **Iyer V, Farquhar C, Jepson R.** Oral contraceptive pills for heavy menstrual bleeding. [computer file] *Cochrane Database of Systematic Reviews* 2000;(2):CD000154.

72. **Mishell DR.** Noncontraceptive health benefits of oral steroidal contraceptives. *Am J Obstet Gynecol* 1982;142:809–816.

73. **Larsson G, Milson I, Lindstedt G, et al.** The influence of a low-dose combined oral contraceptive on menstrual blood loss and iron status. *Contraception* 1992;46:327–334.

74. **Milsom I, Andersson K, Andersch B, et al.** A comparison of flurbiprofen, tranexamic acid, and a levonorgestrel-releasing intrauterine contraceptive device in the treatment of idiopathic menorrhagia. *Am J Obstet Gynecol* 1991;164:879–883.

75. **Hurskainen R, Teperi J, Rissanen P, et al.** Quality of life and cost-effectiveness of levonorgestrel-releasing intrauterine system versus hysterectomy for treatment of menorrhagia: a randomised trial. *Lancet* 2001;357:273–277.

76. **Haynes PJ, Hodgson J, Anderson AB, et al.** Measurement of menstrual blood loss in patients complaining of menorrhagia. *Br J Obstet Gynaecol* 1977;84:763–768.

77. **Nickelsen C.** Diagnostic and curative value of uterine curettage. *Acta Obstet Gynecol Scand* 1986;65:693–697.

78. **Alexander DA, Naji AA, Pinion SB, et al.** Randomised trial comparing hysterectomy with endometrial ablation for dysfunctional uterine bleeding: psychiatric and psychosocial aspects. *BMJ* 1996;312:280–284.

79. **Pinion SB, Parkin DE, Abramovich DR, et al.** Randomised trial of hysterectomy, endometrial laser ablation, and transcervical endometrial resection for dysfunctional uterine bleeding. *BMJ* 1994;309:979–983.

80. **Carlson KJ, Miller BA, Fowler FJ Jr.** The Maine Women's Health Study: I. Outcomes of hysterectomy. *Obstet Gynecol* 1994;83:556–565.

81. **Carlson KJ, Miller BA, Fowler FJ Jr.** The Maine Women's Health Study: II. Outcomes of nonsurgical management of leiomyomas, abnormal bleeding, and chronic pelvic pain. *Obstet Gynecol* 1994;83:566–572.

82. **Bachmann GA.** Psychosexual aspects of hysterectomy. *Womens Health Issues* 1990;3082:1284.

83. **Kenemans P, van Unnik GA, Mijatovic V, et al.** Perspectives in hormone replacement therapy. *Maturitas* 2001;38[Suppl 1]:S41–48.

84. **Shoupe D.** HRT dosing regimens: continuous versus cyclic-pros and cons. *Int J Fertil Womens Med* 2001;46:7–15.

85. **Feldman S, Berkowitz RS, Tosteson AN.** Cost-effectiveness of strategies to evaluate postmenopausal bleeding. *Obstet Gynecol* 1993;81:968–975.

86. **Kurman RJ, Kaminski PF, Norris HJ.** The behavior of endometrial hyperplasia. A long-term study of "untreated" hyperplasia in 170 patients. *Cancer* 1985;56:403–412.

87. **Breen JL, Maxson WS.** Ovarian tumors in children and adolescents. *Clin Obstet Gynecol* 1977;20:607–623.

88. **Lampkin BC, Wong KY, Kalinyak KA, et al.** Ovarian malignancies in children and adolescents. *Surg Clin North Am* 1985;65:1386.

89. **Norris HG, Jensen RD.** Relative frequency of ovarian neoplasms in children and adolescents. *Cancer* 1972;30:713–719.

90. **Diamond MP, Baxter JW, Peerman GCJ, et al.** Occurrence of ovarian masses in childhood and adolescence: a community-wide evaluation. *Obstet Gynecol* 1988;71:858–860.

91. **van Winter JT, Simmons PS, Podratz KC.** Surgically treated adnexal masses in infancy, childhood, and adolescence. *Am J Obstet Gynecol* 1994;170:1780–1789.

92. **Jabra AA, Fishman Ek, Taylor GA.** Primary ovarian tumors in the pediatric patient: CT evaluation. *Clin Imaging* 1993;17:199–203.

93. **Lazar EL, Stolar CJ.** Evaluation and management of pediatric solid ovarian tumors. *Semin Pediatr Surg* 1998;7:29–34.

94. **Kozlowski KJ.** Ovarian masses. *Adolesc Med* 1999;10:337–350.

95. **Schellhas HF.** Malignant potential of the dysgenetic gonad. Part 1. *Obstet Gynecol* 1974;44:289–309.

96. **Troche V, Hernandez E.** Neoplasia arising in dysgenetic gonads. *Obstet Gynecol Surv* 1986;41:74–79.

97. **Laufer MR, Goitein L, Bush M, et al.** Prevalence of endometriosis in adolescent girls with chronic pelvic pain not responding to conventional therapy. *J Pediatr Adolesc Gynecol* 1997;10:199–202.

98. **Hurd SJ, Adamson GD.** Pelvic pain: endometriosis as a differential diagnosis in adolescents. *Adolesc Pediatr Gynecol* 1992;5:3–7.

99. **Tolete-Velcek F, Hansbrough F, Kugaczewski J, et al.** Utero vaginal malformations: a trap for the unsuspecting surgeon. *J Pediatr Surg* 1989;24:736–740.

100. **Barnhart KT, Sondheimer SJ.** Contraception choice and sexually transmitted disease. *Curr Opin Obstet Gynecol* 1993;5:823–828.

101. **Farley TMM, Rosenberg MJ, Rowe PJ, et al.** Intrauterine devices and pelvic inflammatory disease: an international perspective. *Lancet* 1992;339:785–788.

102. **Mol BW, Ankum WM, Bossuyt PM, et al.** Contraception and the risk of ectopic pregnancy: a meta-analysis. *Contraception* 1995;2:337–341.

103. **Bulas DI, Ahlstrom PA, Sivit CJ, et al.** Pelvic inflammatory disease in the adolescent: comparison of transabdominal and transvaginal sonographic evaluation. *Radiology* 1992;83:435–439.

104. **Mitchell DG, Outwater EK.** Benign gynecologic disease: applications of magnetic resonance imaging. *Top Magn Reson Imaging* 1995;7:26–43.

105. **Schwartz LB, Seifer DB.** Diagnostic imaging of adnexal masses. A review. *J Reprod Med* 1992;37:63–71.

106. **Molander P, Cacciatore B, Sjoberg J, et al.** Laparoscopic management of suspected acute pelvic inflammatory disease. *J Am Assoc Gynecol Laparosc* 2000;7:107–110.

107. **Henry-Suchet J.** PID: clinical and laparoscopic aspects. *Ann N Y Acad Sci* 2000;900:301–308.

108. **Cibula D, Kuzel D, Fucikova Z, et al.** Acute exacerbation of recurrent pelvic inflammatory disease. Laparoscopic findings in 141 women with a clinical diagnosis. *J Reprod Med* 2001;46:49–53.

109. **Aboulghar MA, Mansour RT, Serour GI.** Ultrasonographically guided transvaginal aspiration of tuboovarian abscesses and pyosalpinges: an optional treatment for acute pelvic inflammatory disease. *Am J Obstet Gynecol* 1995;172:1501–1503.

110. **Buchweitz O, Malik E, Kressin P, et al.** Laparoscopic management of tubo-ovarian abscesses: retrospective analysis of 60 cases. *Surgical Endosc* 2000;14:948–950.

111. **Hernandez E, Miyazawa K.** The pelvic mass. Patients' ages and pathologic findings. *J Reprod Med* 1988;33:361–364.

112. **Buttram VC, Reiter RC.** Uterine leiomyomata: etiology, symptomatology, and management. *Fertil Steril* 1981;36:433–445.

113. **Townsend DE, Sparkes RS, Baluda MC, et al.** Unicellular histogenesis of uterine leiomyomas as determined by electrophoresis by glucose-6-phosphate dehydrogenase. *Am J Obstet Gynecol* 1970;107:1168–1173.

114. **Persaud V, Arjoon PD.** Uterine leiomyoma. Incidence of degenerative change and a correlation of associated symptoms. *Obstet Gynecol* 1970;35:432–436.

115. **Leibsohn S, d'Ablaing G, Mishell DR Jr, et al.** Leiomyosarcoma in a series of hysterectomies performed for presumed uterine leiomyomas. *Am J Obstet Gynecol* 1990;162:968–976.

116. **Lumsden MA, Wallace EM.** Clinical presentation of uterine fibroids. *Baillieres Clin Obstet Gynaecol* 1998;12:177–195.

117. **Katz VL, Dotters DJ, Droegemeuller W.** Complications of uterine leiomyomas in pregnancy. *Obstet Gynecol* 1989;73:593–596.

118. **Rosati P, Exacoustos C, Mancuso S.** Longitudinal evaluation of uterine myoma growth during pregnancy. A sonographic study. *J Ultrasound Med* 1992;11:511–515.

119. **Aharoni A, Reiter A, Golan D, et al.** Patterns of growth of uterine leiomyomas during pregnancy. A prospective longitudinal study. *Br J Obstet Gynaecol* 1988;95:510–513.

120. **Vergani P, Ghidini A, Strobelt N, et al.** Do uterine leiomyomas influence pregnancy outcome? *Am J Perinatol* 1994;11:356–358.

121. **Koonings PP, Campbell K, Mishell DR Jr, et al.** Relative frequency of primary ovarian neoplasms: a 10-year review. *Obstet Gynecol* 1989;74:921–926.

122. **Grimes DA, Hughes JM.** Use of multiphasic oral contraceptives and hospitalizations of women with functional ovarian cysts in the United States. *Obstet Gynecol* 1989;73:1037–1039.

123. **Hallatt JG, Steele CH Jr, Snyder M.** Ruptured corpus luteum with hemoperitoneum: a study of 173 surgical cases. *Am J Obstet Gynecol* 1984;149:5–9.

124. **Joshi R, Dunaif A.** Ovarian disorders of pregnancy. *Endocrinol Metab Clin North Am* 1995;24:153–169.

125. **Wajda KJ, Lucas JG, Marsh WL Jr.** Hyperreactio luteinalis. Benign disorder masquerading as an ovarian neoplasm. *Arch Path Lab Med* 1989;113:921–925.

126. **Vessey M, Metcalfe A, Wells C, et al.** Ovarian neoplasms, functional ovarian cysts, and oral contraceptives. *Br Med J Clin Res Ed* 1987;294:1518–1520.

127. **Holt VL, Daling JR, McKnight B, et al.** Functional ovarian cysts in relation to the use of monophasic and triphasic oral contraceptives. *Obstet Gynecol* 1992;79:529–533.

128. **Lanes SF, Birmann B, Walker AM, et al.** Oral contraceptive type and functional ovarian cysts. *Am J Obstet Gynecol* 1992;166:956–961.

129. **Grimes DA, Godwin AJ, Rubin A, et al.** Ovulation and follicular development associated with three low-dose oral contraceptives: a randomized controlled trial. *Obstet Gynecol* 1994;83:29–34.

130. **Holt VL, Kaling JR, McKnight B, et al.** Cigarette smoking and functional ovarian cysts. *Am J Epidemiol* 1994;139:781–786.

131. **Parazzini F, Moroni S, Negri E, et al.** Risk factors for functional ovarian cysts. *Epidemiology* 1996;7:547–549.

132. **Polson DW, Adams J, Wadsworth J, et al.** Polycystic ovaries—a common finding in normal women. *Lancet* 1988;1:870–872.

133. **Blaustein A, Kurman RJ.** *Blaustein's pathology of the female genital tract,* 4th ed. New York: Springer-Verlag, 1994:1280.

134. **Templeman CL, Fallat ME, Lam AM, et al.** Managing mature cystic teratomas of the ovary. *Obstet Gynecol Surv* 2000;55:738–745.

135. **Yuen PM, Yu MK, Yip SK, et al.** A randomized prospective study of laparoscopy and laparotomy in the management of benign ovarian masses. *Am J Obstet Gynecol* 1997;177:109–114.

136. **Mecke H, Savvas V.** Laparoscopic surgery of dermoid cysts—intraoperative spillage and complications. *Eur J Obstet Gynecol Reprod Biol* 2001;96:80–84.

137. **Stein AL, Koonings PP, Schlaerth JB, et al.** Relative frequency of malignant parovarian tumors: should parovarian tumors be aspirated? *Obstet Gynecol* 1990;75:1029–1031.

138. **Finkler NJ, Benacerraf B, Lavin PT, et al.** Comparison of serum CA 125, clinical impression, and ultrasound in the preoperative evaluation of ovarian masses. *Obstet Gynecol* 1988;72:659–664.

139. **Twickler DM, Forte TB, Santos-Ramos R, et al.** The Ovarian Tumor Index predicts risk for malignancy. *Cancer* 1999;86:2280–2290.

140. **Anandakumar C, Chew S, Wong YC, et al.** Role of transvaginal ultrasound color flow imaging and Doppler waveform analysis in differentiating between benign and malignant ovarian tumors. *Ultrasound Obstet Gynecol* 1996;7:280–284.

141. **Leeners B, Schild RL, Funk A, et al.** Colour Doppler sonography improves the pre-operative diagnosis of ovarian tumours made using conventional transvaginal sonography. *Eur J Obstet Gynecol Reprod Biol* 1996;64:79–85, 142.

142. **Jermy K, Luise C, Bourne T.** The characterization of common ovarian cysts in premenopausal women. *Ultrasound Obstet Gynecol* 2001;17:140–144.

143. **Patel VH, Somers S.** MR imaging of the female pelvis: current perspectives and review of genital tract congenital anomalies, and benign and malignant diseases. *Crit Rev Diagn Imaging* 1997;38:417–499.

144. **Woodward PJ, Gilfeather M.** Magnetic resonance imaging of the female pelvis. *Semin Ultrasound CT MR* 1998;19:90–103.

145. **Yamashita Y, Torashima M, Hatanaka Y, et al.** Adnexal masses: accuracy of characterization with transvaginal US and precontrast and postcontrast MR imaging. *Radiology* 1995;194:557–565.

146. **ACOG Committee on Practice Bulletins—Gynecology.** *Surgical alternatives to hysterectomy in the management of leiomyomas.* Washington, DC: American College of Obstetricians and Gynecologists, 2000.

147. **Broekmans FJ.** GnRH agonists and uterine leiomyomas. *Hum Reprod* 1996;11[Suppl 3]:3–25.

148. **Palomba S, Affinito P, Di Carlo C, et al.** Long-term administration of tibolone plus gonadotropin-releasing hormone agonist for the treatment of uterine leiomyomas: effectiveness and effects on vasomotor symptoms, bone mass, and lipid profiles. *Fertil Steril* 1999;72:889–895.

149. **Kettel LM, Murphy AA, Morales AJ, et al.** Rapid regression of uterine leiomyomas in response to daily administration of gonadotropin-releasing hormone antagonist. *Fertil Steril* 1993;60:642–646.

150. **Felberbaum RE, Ludwig M, Diedrich K.** Clinical application of GnRH-antagonists. *Mol Cell Endocrinol* 2000;166:9–14.

151. **Murphy AA, Kettel LM, Morales AJ, et al.** Regression of uterine leiomyomata in response to the antiprogesterone RU 486. *J Clin Endocrinol Metab* 1993;76:513–517.

152. **Parker WH, Fu YS, Berek JS.** Uterine sarcoma in patients operated on for presumed leiomyoma and rapidly growing leiomyoma. *Obstet Gynecol* 1994;83:414–418.

153. **Iverson RE, Chelmow D, Strohbehn K, et al.** Relative morbidity of abdominal hysterectomy and myomectomy for management of uterine leiomyomas. *Obstet Gynecol* 1996;88:415–419.

154. **Ecker JL, Foster TJ, Firiedman AJ.** Abdominal hysterectomy or abdominal myomectomy for symptomatic leiomyoma: a comparison of preoperative demography and postoperative morbidity. *J Gynecol Surg* 1995;11:11–18.

155. **Hillis SD, Marchbanks PA, Peterson HB.** Uterine size and risk of complications among women undergoing abdominal hysterectomy for leiomyomas. *Obstet Gynecol* 1996;87:539–543.

156. **Fedele L, Parazzini F, Luchini L, et al.** Recurrence of fibroids after myomectomy: a transvaginal ultrasonographic study. *Hum Reprod* 1995;10:1795–1796.

157. **Barbieri RL.** Ambulatory management of uterine leiomyomata. *Clin Obstet Gynecol* 1999;42: 196–205.

158. **Phillips DR, Milim SJ, Nathanson HG, et al.** Experience with laparoscopic leiomyoma coagulation and concomitant operative hysteroscopy. *J Am Assoc Gynecol Laparosc* 1997;4:425–433.

159. **Spanos WJ.** Preoperative hormonal therapy of cystic adnexal masses. *Am J Obstet Gynecol* 1973;116: 551–556.

160. **Steinkampf MP, Hammond KR, Blackwell RE.** Hormonal treatment of functional ovarian cysts: a randomized, prospective study. *Fertil Steril* 1990;54:775–777.

161. **MacKenna A, Fabres C, Alam V, et al.** Clinical management of functional ovarian cysts: a prospective and randomized study. *Hum Reprod* 2000;15:2567–2569.

162. **Turan C, Zorlu CG, Ugur M, et al.** Expectant management of functional ovarian cysts: an alternative to hormonal therapy. *Int J Gynaecol Obstet* 1994;47:257–260.

163. **Pena JE, Ufberg D, Cooney N, et al.** Usefulness of Doppler sonography in the diagnosis of ovarian torsion. *Fertil Steril* 2000;73:1047–1050.

164. **Quillin SP, Siegel MJ.** Transabdominal color Doppler ultrasonography of the painful adolescent ovary. *J Ultrasound Med* 1994;13:549–555.

165. **Lee EJ, Kwon JC, Joo HJ, et al.** Diagnosis of ovarian torsion with color Doppler sonography: depiction of twisted vascular pedicle. *J Ultrasound Med* 1998;17:83–89.

166. **Chapron C, Capella-Allouc S, Dubuisson JB.** Treatment of adnexal torsion using operative laparoscopy. *Hum Reprod* 1996;11:998–1003.

167. **Shalev E, Bustan M, Yarom I, et al.** Recovery of ovarian function after laparoscopic detorsion. *Hum Reprod* 1995;10:2965–2966.

168. **Oelsner G, Bider D, Goldenberg M, et al.** Long-term follow-up of the twisted ischemic adnexa managed by detorsion. *Fertil Steril* 1996;60:976–979.

169. **Righi RV, McComb PF, Fluker MR.** Laparoscopic oophoropexy for recurrent adnexal torsion. *Hum Reprod* 1995;10:3136–3138.

170. **Nagel TC, Sebastian J, Malo JW.** Oophoropexy to prevent sequential or recurrent torsion. *J Am Assoc Gynecol Laparosc* 1997;4:495–498.

171. **Canis M, Rabischong B, Botchorishvili R, et al.** Risk of spread of ovarian cancer after laparoscopic surgery. *Curr Opinion Obstet Gynecol* 2001;13:9–14.

172. **Hopkins MP, von Gruenigen V, Gaich S.** Laparoscopic port site implantation with ovarian cancer. *Am J Obstet Gynecol* 2000;182:735–736.

173. **Maiman M, Seltzer V, Boyce J.** Laparoscopic excision of ovarian neoplasms subsequently found to be malignant. *Obstet Gynecol* 1991;77:563–565.

174. **Ulrich U, Paulus W, Schneider A, et al.** Laparoscopic surgery for complex ovarian masses. *J Am Assoc Gynecol Laparosc* 2000;7:373–380.

175. **Dottino PR, Levine DA, Ripley DL, et al.** Laparoscopic management of adnexal masses in premenopausal and postmenopausal women. *Obstet Gynecol* 1999;93:223–228.

176. **ACOG Committee on Educational Bulletins.** *Operative laparoscopy.* Washington, DC: American College of Obstetricians and Gynecologists, 1997.

177. **Lok IH, Sahota DS, Rogers MS, et al.** Complications of laparoscopic surgery for benign ovarian cysts. *J Am Assoc Gynecologic Laparosc* 2000;7:529–534.

178. **Mais V, Ajossa S, Piras B, et al.** Treatment of nonendometriotic benign adnexal cysts: a randomized comparison of laparoscopy and laparotomy. *Obstet Gynecol* 1995;86:770–774.

179. **Deckardt R, Saks M, Graeff H.** Comparison of minimally invasive surgery and laparotomy in the treatment of adnexal masses. *J Am Assoc Gynecol Laparosc* 1994;1:333–338.

180. **Albini SM, Benadiva CA, Haverly K, et al.** Management of benign ovarian cystic teratomas: laparoscopy compared with laparotomy. *J Am Assoc Gynecol Laparosc* 1994;1:219–222.

181. **Nitke S, Goldman GA, Fisch B, et al.** The management of dermoid cysts—a comparative study of laparoscopy and laparotomy. *Isr J Med Sci* 1996;32:1177–1179.

182. **Campo S, Garcea N.** Laparoscopic conservative excision of ovarian dermoid cysts with and without an endobag. *J Am Assoc Gynecol Laparosc* 1998;5:165–170.

183. **Wang PH, Lee WL, Juang CM, et al.** Excision of mature teratoma using culdotomy, with and without laparoscopy: a prospective randomised trial. *Br J Obstet Gynaecol* 2001;108:91–94.

184. **Barber HR, Graber EA.** The PMPO syndrome (postmenopausal palpable ovary syndrome). *Obstet Gynecol* 1971;38:921–923.

185. **Kroon E, Andolf E.** Diagnosis and follow-up of simple ovarian cysts detected by ultrasound in postmenopausal women. *Obstet Gynecol* 1995;85:211–214.

186. **Ekerhovd E, Wienerroith H, Staudach A, et al.** Preoperative assessment of unilocular adnexal cysts by transvaginal ultrasonography: a comparison between ultrasonographic morphologic imaging and histopathologic diagnosis. *Am J Obstet Gynecol* 2001;184:48–54.

187. **Bailey CL, Ueland FR, Land GL, et al.** The malignant potential of small cystic ovarian tumors in women over 50 years of age. *Gynecol Oncol* 1998;69:3–7.

188. **Sasaki H, Oda M, Ohmura M, et al.** Follow-up of women with simple ovarian cysts detected by transvaginal sonography in the Tokyo metropolitan area. *Br J Obstet Gynaecol* 1999;106:415–420.

189. **Aubert JM, Rombaut C, Argacha P, et al.** Simple adnexal cysts in postmenopausal women: conservative management. *Maturitas* 1998;30:51–54.

190. **Kurjak A, Shalan H, Kupesic S, et al.** An attempt to screen asymptomatic women for ovarian and endometrial cancer with transvaginal color and pulsed Doppler sonography. *J Ultrasound Med* 1994;13:295–301.

191. **Bonilla-Musoles F, Ballester MJ, Simon C, et al.** Is avoidance of surgery possible in patients with perimenopausal ovarian tumors using transvaginal ultrasound and duplex color Doppler sonography? *J Ultrasound Med* 1993;12:33–39.

192. **de Peralta MN, Delahoussaye PM, Tornos CS, et al.** Benign retroperitoneal cysts of Müllerian type: a clinicopathologic study of three cases and review of the literature. *Int J Gynecol Pathol* 1994;13:273–278.

193. **ACOG Committee on Educational Bulletins.** *Ovarian cancer.* Washington, DC: American College of Obstetricians and Gynecologists, 1998.

194. **Schutter EM, Kenemans P, Sohn C, et al.** Diagnostic value of pelvic examination, ultrasound, and serum CA 125 in postmenopausal women with a pelvic mass. An international multicenter study. *Cancer* 1994;74:1398–1406.

195. **Panizzon RG.** Vulvar melanoma. *Semin Dermatol* 1996;15:67–70.

196. **Melton L.** New perspectives on the management of intersex. *Lancet* 2001;357:2110.

197. **Schober JM.** Sexual behaviors, sexual orientation and gender identity in adult intersexuals: a pilot study. *J Urol* 2001;165:2350–2353.

198. **Muram D, Buxton BH.** The importance of the gynecologic examination in the newborn. *J Tenn Med Assoc* 1983;76:239.

199. **Mor N, Merlob P, Reisner SH.** Types of hymen in the newborn infant. *Eur J Obstet Gynecol Reprod Biol* 1986;22:225–228.

200. **Kaufman RH, Friedrich EG, Gardner HL.** *Benign diseases of the vulva and vagina,* 3rd ed. Chicago: Year Book Medical Publishers, 1989:1–476.

201. **Pokorny SF, Kozinetz CA.** Configuration and other anatomic details of the prepubertal hymen. *Adolesc Pediatr Gynecol* 1988;1:97–103.

202. **Pokorny SF.** The genital examination of the infant through adolescence. *Curr Opin Obstet Gynecol* 1993;5:753–757.

203. **Pokorny SF.** Prepubertal vulvovaginopathies. *Obstet Gynecol Clin North Am* 1992;19:39–58.

204. **Garzon MC, Paller AS.** Ultrapotent topical corticosteroid treatment of childhood genital lichen sclerosus. *Arch Dermatol* 1999;135:525–528.

205. **Pokorny SF.** Child abuse and infections. *Obstet Gynecol Clin North Am* 1989;16:401–415.

206. **Rouzier R, Louis-Sylvestre C, Paniel BJ, et al.** Hypertrophy of labia minora: experience with 163 reductions. *Am J Obstet Gynecol* 2000;182:35–40.

207. **Muram D, Gold SS.** Vulvar ulcerations in girls with myelocytic leukemia. *South Med J* 1993;86:293–294.

208. **Ragnarsson-Olding BK, Kanter-Lewensohn LR, Lagerlof B, et al.** Malignant melanoma of the vulva in a nationwide, 25-year study of 219 Swedish females: clinical observations and histopathologic features. *Cancer* 1999;86:1273–1284.

209. **Rock B, Hood AF, Rock JA.** Prospective study of vulvar nevi. *J Am Acad Dermatol* 1990;22:104–106.

210. **Hood AF, Lumadue J.** Benign vulvar tumors. *Dermatol Clin* 1992;10:371–385.

211. **Fearfield LA, Staughton RC.** Severe vulval apocrine acne successfully treated with prednisolone and isotretinoin. *Clin Exp Dermatol* 1999;24:189–192.

212. **Brown CF, Gallup DG, Brown VM.** Hidradenitis suppurativa of the anogenital region: response to isotretinoin. *Am J Obstet Gynecol* 1988;158:12–15.

213. **Dunaif A.** Insulin action in the polycystic ovary syndrome. *Endocrinol Metab Clin North Am* 1999;28:341–359.

214. **Joura EA, Losch A, Haider-Angeler MG, et al.** Trends in vulvar neoplasia. Increasing incidence of vulvar intraepithelial neoplasia and squamous cell carcinoma of the vulva in young women. *J Reprod Med* 2000;45:613–615.

215. **Valdes CT, Malinak LR, Franklin RR.** *Benign diseases of the vulva and vagina.* **Kaufman RH, Friedrich EG, Gardner HL**, eds. Chicago: Year Book Medical Publishers, 1989:26–54.

216. **van der Putte SC.** Mammary-like glands of the vulva and their disorders. *Int J Gynecol Pathol* 1994;13:150–160.

217. **Word B.** A new instrument for office treatment of cysts and abscess of Bartholin's gland. *JAMA* 1964;190:777.

218. **Paavonen J.** Vulvodynia—a complex syndrome of vulvar pain. *Acta Obstet Gynecol Scand* 1995;74:243–247.

219. **Friedrich EG.** Vulvar vestibulitis syndrome. *J Reprod Med* 1987;32:110–114.

220. **Bazin S, Bouchard C, Brisson J, et al.** Vulvar vestibulitis syndrome: an exploratory case-control study. *Obstet Gynecol* 1994;83:47–50.

221. **Bergeron C, Moyal-Barracco M, Pelisse M, et al.** Vulvar vestibulitis. Lack of evidence for a human papillomavirus etiology. *J Reprod Med* 1994;39:936–938.

222. **Prayson RA, Stoler MH, Hart WR.** Vulvar vestibulitis. A histopathologic study of 36 cases, including human papillomavirus in situ hybridization analysis. *Am J Surg Pathol* 1995;19:154–160.

223. **Morin C, Bouchard C, Brisson J, et al.** Human papillomaviruses and vulvar vestibulitis. *Obstet Gynecol* 2000;95:683–687.

224. **ACOG Committee on Educational Bulletins.** *Vulvar nonneoplastic epithelial disorders.* Washington, DC: American Association of Obstetricians and Gynecologists, 1997.

225. **Bergeron S, Binik YM, Khalife S, et al.** A randomized comparison of group cognitive—behavioral therapy, surface electromyographic biofeedback, and vestibulectomy in the treatment of dyspareunia resulting from vulvar vestibulitis. *Pain* 2001;91:297–306.

226. **Bracco GL, Carli P, Sonni L, et al.** Clinical and histologic effects of topical treatments of vulval lichen sclerosus: a clinical evaluation; remission of symptoms in 75% of clobetasol, 10% in cream. *J Reprod Med* 1993;38:37–40.

227. **Cattaneo A, Carli P, De Marco A, et al.** Testosterone maintenance therapy: effects on vulvar lichen sclerosus treated with clobetasol propionate. *J Reprod Med* 1996;41:99–102.

228. **Siegel RM, Schubert CJ, Myers PA, et al.** The prevalence of sexually transmitted diseases in children and adolescents evaluated for sexual abuse in Cincinnati: rationale for limited STD testing in prepubertal girls. *Pediatrics* 1995;96:1090–1094.

229. **Pokorny SF, Stormer J.** Atraumatic removal of secretions from the prepubertal vagina. *Am J Obstet Gynecol* 1987;156:581–582.

230. **Schuchat A, Broome CV.** Toxic shock syndrome and tampons. *Epidemiol Rev* 1991;13:99–112.

231. **Hajjeh RA, Reingold A, Weil A, et al.** Toxic shock syndrome in the United States: surveillance update, 1979–1996. *Emerg Infect Dis* 1999;5:807–810.

Novak's Gynecology, 13th Edition. Edited by J.S. Berek. Lippincott Williams & Wilkins, Philadelphia © 2002.

14 Pelvic Pain and Dysmenorrhea

Julie A. Jolin
Andrea Rapkin

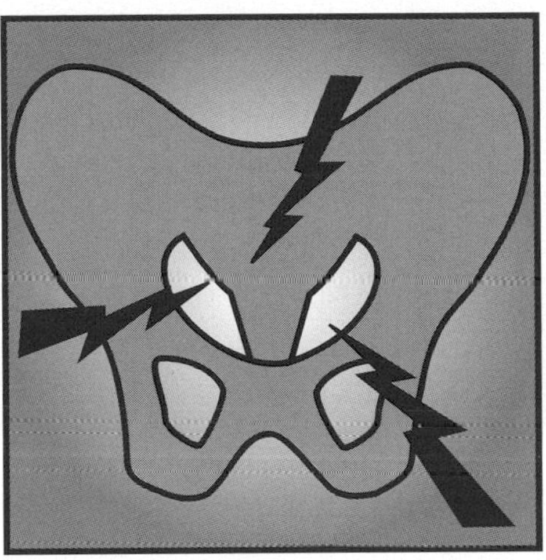

Pelvic pain is the most challenging symptom confronting the practitioner. The problems of acute, cyclic, and chronic pelvic pain encompass a large proportion of gynecologic complaints. The etiology of pelvic pain is diverse. Dysmenorrhea is one of the most common medical issues in gynecology.

***Acute pain* is intense and characterized by sudden onset, sharp rise, and short course. *Cyclic pain* refers to pain that occurs with a definite association to the menstrual cycle. *Dysmenorrhea,* or painful menstruation, is the most common cyclic pain phenomenon and is classified as *primary* or *secondary* on the basis of associated anatomic pathology** (1). ***Chronic pelvic pain* has been defined as pain of greater than 6 months' duration** (2). Whereas acute pain is often associated with profound autonomic reflex responses, such as nausea, emesis, diaphoresis, and apprehension, obvious autonomic reflex responses are not present in chronic pelvic pain. In addition, acute pelvic pain often is associated with signs of inflammation or infection, such as fever and leukocytosis, which are absent in chronic pain states. The pathophysiology of acute pelvic pain involves mediators of inflammation present in high concentration as a result of infection, ischemia, or chemical irritation (3,4). By contrast, the etiology of chronic pelvic pain often is obscure. Additionally, chronic pain is characterized by physiologic, affective, and behavioral responses that are quite different from those associated with acute pain (5).

Acute Pain

The differential diagnosis of acute pelvic pain is outlined in Table 14.1. Assessing the character of the pain is helpful in creating a differential diagnosis. **Rapid onset of pain is most consistent with perforation of a hollow viscus or ischemia. Colic or severe cramping pain is commonly associated with muscular contraction or obstruction of a hollow viscus, such as intestine or uterus, whereas pain perceived over the entire abdomen suggests a generalized reaction to an irritating fluid within the peritoneal cavity.**

Table 14.1. Differential Diagnosis of Acute Pelvic Pain

Gynecologic Disease or Dysfunction
Acute Pain
1. Complication of pregnancy a. Ruptured ectopic pregnancy b. Abortion, threatened or incomplete c. Degeneration of a leiomyoma 2. Acute infections a. Endometritis b. Pelvic inflammatory disease (acute PID) c. Tuboovarian abscess 3. Adnexal disorders a. Hemorrhagic functional ovarian cyst b. Torsion of adnexa c. Twisted paraovarian cyst d. Rupture of functional or neoplastic ovarian cyst
Recurrent Pelvic Pain
1. Mittelschmerz (midcycle pain) 2. Primary dysmenorrhea 3. Secondary dysmenorrhea
Gastrointestinal
1. Gastroenteritis 2. Appendicitis 3. Bowel obstruction 4. Diverticulitis 5. Inflammatory bowel disease 6. Irritable bowel syndrome
Genitourinary
1. Cystitis 2. Pylonephritis 3. Ureteral lithiasis
Musculoskeletal
1. Abdominal wall hematoma 2. Hernia
Other
1. Acute poryphyria 2. Pelvic thrombophlebitis 3. Aneurysm 4. Abdominal angina

The viscera are relatively insensitive to pain. The first perception of visceral pain is a vague, deep, poorly localizable sensation associated with autonomic reflex responses; however, once the pain becomes localized, the pain is called *referred pain*. Referred pain is well localized and superficial. It is appreciated within the nerve distribution or dermatome of the spinal cord segment innervating the involved viscus. The location of the referred pain provides insight into the location of the primary disease process. The innervation of the pelvic organs is outlined in Table 14.2 (3).

In the evaluation of acute pelvic pain, early diagnosis is critical because significant delay increases morbidity and mortality. Central to correct diagnosis is an accurate history (Fig. 14.1). The date and character of the last and previous menstrual periods and the presence of abnormal bleeding or discharge should be ascertained. Menstrual, sexual, and contraceptive history and the past history of sexually transmitted conditions and previous gynecologic disorders are important. The patient should be questioned about her medical history and any previous surgery. Pain history should be obtained, including how and when

Table 14.2. Nerves Carrying Painful Impulses from the Pelvic Organs

Organ	*Spinal Segments*	*Nerves*
Perineum, vulva, lower vagina	S2–S4	Pudendal, inguinal, genitofemoral, posterofemoral cutaneous
Upper vagina, cervix, lower uterine segment, posterior urethra, bladder trigone, uterosacral and cardinal ligaments, rectosigmoid, lower ureters	S2–S4	Sacral afferents traveling through the pelvic plexus
Uterine fundus, proximal fallopian tubes, broad ligaments, upper bladder, cecum appendix, terminal large bowel	T11–T12, L1	Thoracolumbar splanchnic nerves through uterine and hypogastric plexes
Outer two thirds of fallopian tubes, upper ureter	T9–T10	Thoracolumbar splanchnic nerves through mesenteric plexus
Ovaries	T9–T10	Thoracolumbar splanchnic nerves traveling with ovarian vessels through renal and aortic plexus and celiac and mesenteric ganglia

the pain started; the presence of gastrointestinal symptoms (e.g., anorexia, nausea, vomiting, constipation, obstipation, flatus pattern); urinary symptoms (e.g., urgency, frequency, hematuria, or dysuria); and signs of infection (e.g., fevers, chills).

Pathology

Abnormal Pregnancy

An ectopic pregnancy is defined as implantation of the fetus in the site other than the uterine cavity (see Chapter 17). Ninety-five percent of ectopic pregnancies develop in the fallopian tube. With the advent of sensitive pregnancy tests, misdiagnosis of ectopic pregnancy is less common. However, a substantial proportion of maternal mortality is still attributable to ectopic gestation.

Symptoms

Implantation of the fetus in the fallopian tube produces pain only with acute dilation of the tube. If tubal rupture occurs, localized abdominal pain tends to be temporarily relieved and is replaced by generalized pelvic and abdominal pain as the hemoperitoneum develops. Typically, there has been amenorrhea for 6 to 8 weeks and irregular bleeding or spotting related to fluctuating levels of human chorionic gonadotropin (hCG) and low progesterone concentrations. A mass in the cul-de-sac may produce an urge to defecate. Referred pain to the right shoulder often develops if the intraabdominal blood collection transverses the right colic gutter and irritates the diaphragm (C-3 to C-5 innervation). Dizziness or syncope can ensue if blood loss is significant.

Signs

Pulse and blood pressure taken in erect and supine positions (orthostatic vital signs) are especially helpful in documenting an early or small hemoperitoneum. In young women, there may be elevation of pulse or decrease in blood pressure only when altering position from supine to erect. Abdominal examination is usually notable for tenderness and guarding in one or both lower quadrants. With the development of hemoperitoneum, generalized abdominal distention and rebound tenderness are prominent, and bowel sounds are often

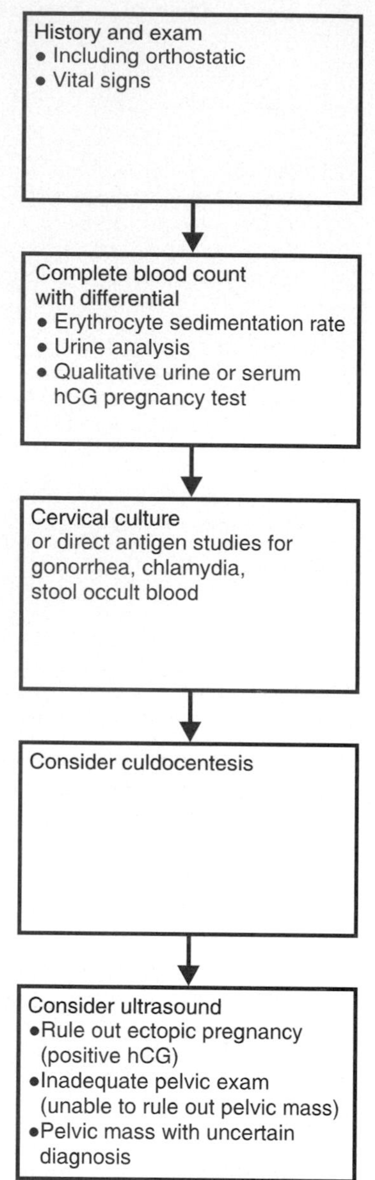

Figure 14.1 Diagnosis of acute pelvic pain.

decreased. Pelvic examination generally reveals mild tenderness on motion of the cervix. Adnexal tenderness is generally more pronounced on the side of the ectopic pregnancy. A mass consisting of a hematosalpinx or hematoma isolated by adhesions is sometimes present; however, a palpable mass is more often the corpus luteum of pregnancy. Low-grade fever and leukocytosis are uncommon but can be present if the tube has ruptured. The hematocrit often reveals progressive anemia indicating internal bleeding, although, because of vasoconstriction and subsequent hemoconcentration, low hematocrit is a late sign of blood loss in young women. The assessment of hematocrit must, therefore, be combined with evaluation of orthostatic vital signs.

Diagnosis

The diagnosis of ectopic pregnancy is discussed in Chapter 17. In women of reproductive age, serum or urine pregnancy test with sensitivity of greater than 20 IU/mL of hCG should be obtained; if positive, ectopic pregnancy must be excluded before the patient can be discharged or treated for another diagnosis. Acute pelvic pain during pregnancy can also result from other types of pathology. Once ultrasound has confirmed an intrauterine pregnancy, one must consider adnexal torsion, leakage or rupture of an ovarian cyst, degeneration of leiomyoma, or gastrointestinal or urinary pathology. Coexistent intrauterine and ectopic pregnancy is rare (1 in 30,000).

Leaking or Ruptured Ovarian Cyst

Functional cysts (e.g., follicle, corpus luteum) are the most common ovarian cysts and rupture more readily than do benign or malignant neoplasms. The pain associated with rupture of the ovarian follicle at the time of ovulation is called *mittleschmertz.* The small amount of blood leaking into the peritoneal cavity and high concentration of follicular fluid prostaglandins could cause this midcycle pelvic pain. However, the pain is mild or moderate and self-limited, and with an intact coagulation system, hemoperitoneum is unlikely. A hemorrhagic corpus luteum cyst can develop in luteal phase of the menstrual cycle. Rupture of this cyst can produce either a small amount of intraperitoneal bleeding or frank hemorrhage resulting in significant blood loss and hemoperitoneum.

Nonmalignant neoplasms, most commonly cystic teratomas (dermoid cysts) or cystadenomas, as well as inflammatory ovarian masses, such as endometriomas, can also leak or rupture. A history of a dermoid cyst or endometrioma that has not yet undergone surgical extirpation is not uncommon. Surgical exploration is indicated if rupture of the cyst leads to hemoperitoneum (corpus luteum) or chemical peritonitis (endometrioma, benign cyst teratoma), which could impair future fertility.

Symptoms

An ovarian cyst that is not torsing, rapidly expanding, infected, or leaking does not cause acute pain. A corpus luteum cyst is the most common cyst to rupture and lead to hemoperitoneum. Symptoms of a ruptured corpus luteum cyst are similar to those of a ruptured ectopic pregnancy. The onset of pain is usually sudden and is associated with increasing generalized abdominal pain and occasionally dizziness or syncope if a hemoperitoneum develops. A ruptured endometrioma or benign cystic teratoma (dermoid cyst) produces similar symptoms; however, dizziness and signs of hypovolemia are not present because blood loss is minimal.

Signs

Hypovolemia is present only when there is a hemoperitoneum. The most important sign is the presence of significant abdominal tenderness, often associated with rebound tenderness because of peritoneal irritation. The abdomen can be moderately distended with decreased bowel sounds. On pelvic examination, a mass is often present if the cyst is leaking and not completely ruptured. Fever and leukocytosis are rare. The hematocrit is decreased only if active bleeding is present.

Diagnosis

Pregnancy test, complete blood count, and ultrasound or culdocentesis confirm the diagnosis. Without orthostasis and with a relatively normal peripheral hematocrit, a hematocrit of 16% or less of the fluid obtained from the cul-de-sac is usually consistent with leakage of a small amount of blood into the peritoneal fluid and not a hemoperitoneum.

Management

Orthostasis, anemia, or hematocrit of the culdocentesis fluid of greater than 16% suggests hemoperitoneum and usually requires surgical treatment by laparoscopy or laparotomy. The culdocentesis is very helpful in determining the cause of peritonitis: fresh blood suggests a corpus luteum; chocolate "old" blood, an endometrioma; oily sebaceous fluid, a benign teratoma; purulent fluid, pelvic inflammatory disease (PID) or tuboovarian abscess. Patients who are not orthostatic or anemic and who have a small amount of blood in the cul-de-sac fluid (culdocentesis fluid hematocrit less than 16%) can often be observed in the hospital, without surgical intervention, or even discharged home from the emergency room after observation.

Torsion of Adnexa

Torsion (twisting) of the vascular pedicle of an ovary, fallopian tube, paratubal cyst, or rarely just a fallopian tube results in ischemia and rapid onset of acute pelvic pain. **A benign cystic teratoma is the most common neoplasm to undergo torsion.** Because of adhesions, ovarian carcinoma and inflammatory masses rarely are affected by torsion. It is also unusual for a normal tube and ovary to torse, although a polycystic ovary can undergo torsion.

Symptoms

The pain of torsion can be severe and constant or, if the torsion is partial and intermittently untwists, intermittent. The onset of the torsion and the symptoms of abdominal pain frequently coincide with lifting, exercise, or intercourse. Autonomic reflex responses are usually present (e.g., nausea, emesis, apprehension).

Signs

On examination, the abdomen is very tender, and localized rebound tenderness can be noted in the lower quadrants. The most important sign is the presence of a large pelvic mass on physical examination. Mild temperature elevation and leukocytosis may accompany the infarction. The diagnosis must be suspected in any woman with acute pain and unilateral adnexal mass.

Diagnosis

The process of torsion occludes the lymphatic and venous drainage of the involved adnexa; therefore, the mass rapidly increases in size and can be palpated on examination or visualized by ultrasound. Ultrasound confirms the presence of a mass but is not necessary if the examination reveals a large tender adnexal mass (at least 8 to 10 cm in diameter).

Management

Adnexal torsion must be treated surgically. If the tissue has not infarcted, the adnexa may be untwisted and a cystectomy performed if appropriate. If necrosis has occurred, an oophorectomy must be performed. Treatment may be accomplished by laparoscopy or laparotomy, depending on the size of the mass.

Acute Salpingo-oophoritis

The presentation and management of acute salpingo-oophoritis and PID are discussed in Chapter 15. PID is a polymicrobial infection consisting of the ascending spread of aerobic and anaerobic vaginal bacteria heralded by the acquisition of a sexually transmitted pathogen such as *Neisseria gonorrhea* or *Chlamydia trachomatis.* Transcervical instrumentation (endometrial biopsy) of the endometrial cavity (hysterosalpingogram, termination of pregnancy, or parturition) also can cause endometritis or salpingo-oophoritis.

Symptoms

Gonococcal PID is manifested by the acute onset of pelvic pain that increases with movement, fever, purulent vaginal discharge, and sometimes nausea and vomiting. The pain is often associated with a menstrual period, a time when pathogens have ready access to the upper genital tract. Chlamydial salpingo-oophoritis is associated with more insidious symptoms, which can be confused with the symptoms of irritable bowel.

Signs

Direct and rebound abdominal tenderness with palpation are usually notable on examination. The most important signs of acute salpingo-oophoritis are cervical motion tenderness and bilateral adnexal tenderness. Evaluation of the pelvis may be difficult because of acute pain, but lack of a discrete mass or masses differentiates acute salpingo-oophoritis from tuboovarian abscess or torsion. There is often leukocytosis, or at least an elevated erythrocyte sedimentation rate (ESR), a nonspecific, although more sensitive, sign of inflammation.

Diagnosis

For the clinical diagnosis of PID to be most accurate, lower abdominal tenderness with or without rebound, cervical motion tenderness and adnexal tenderness all must be present (6–8). The accuracy of the diagnosis is further increased in the presence of one or more of the following objective signs: fever, leukocytosis, inflammatory mass, culdocentesis revealing white cells or bacteria on Gram stain, gram-negative intracellular diplococci on Gram stain of the cervix, or positive chlamydia antigen test of the cervix. Appendicitis often is mistaken for PID.

Management

Salpingo-oophoritis may be treated on an outpatient basis with broad-spectrum oral antibiotics (7,9,10). Criteria for hospitalization include suspected tuboovarian abscess, pregnancy, presence of an intrauterine device, uncertain diagnosis, nausea and vomiting precluding administration of oral medication, upper peritoneal signs, and failure to respond to oral antibiotics within 48 hours. Hospitalization also should be considered for episodes of PID in young women who desire future childbearing. Outpatient antibiotic regimens are often successful for uncomplicated PID; however, the patient must be reassessed within 48 hours and, if not significantly improved, admitted to the hospital for intravenous antibiotic therapy. The treatment of acute PID is outlined in detail in Chapter 15.

Tuboovarian Abscess

Tuboovarian abscesses, a sequela of acute salpingitis, are usually bilateral, but unilateral abscess formation is not rare. The symptoms and signs are similar to those of acute salpingitis, although pain and fever have often been present for longer than 1 week before presentation to the emergency room. A ruptured tuboovarian abscess is a life-threatening surgical emergency because gram-negative endotoxic shock can develop rapidly.

Signs

Tuboovarian abscesses can be palpated on bimanual examination as very firm, exquisitely tender, bilateral fixed masses. The abscesses can be palpated or "point" in the pelvic cul-de-sac.

Diagnosis

The clinical diagnosis can be substantiated by ultrasonography. The differential diagnosis of a unilateral mass includes not only tuboovarian abscess but also adnexal torsion, endometrioma, leaking ovarian cyst, and periappendiceal abscess. If physical and ultrasound examination results are not definitive, laparoscopy or laparotomy must be performed.

Management

Unruptured tuboovarian abscesses may be treated medically with appropriate intravenous antibiotics and close monitoring to detect leakage or impending rupture. A ruptured tuboovarian abscess rapidly leads to diffuse peritonitis evidenced by tachycardia, rebound tenderness in all four quadrants of the abdomen, and, if progressive, hypotension and oliguria. Exploratory laparotomy with resection of infected tissue is mandatory.

Uterine Leiomyomas

Leiomyomas are uterine smooth muscle tumors. Discomfort may be present when myomas encroach on adjacent bladder, rectum, or supporting ligaments of the uterus, although acute pelvic pain attributable to uterine leiomyomas is rare. Acute pelvic pain can develop if the myoma undergoes degeneration or torsion. Degeneration of myomas occurs secondary to loss of blood supply, usually attributable to rapid growth associated with pregnancy. In a nonpregnant woman, degenerating uterine leiomyoma often is misdiagnosed, frequently being confused with subacute salpingo-oophoritis. A pedunculated subserosal leiomyoma can undergo torsion ischemic necrosis; when this situation occurs, it is associated with pain similar to that of adnexal torsion. When a submucous leiomyoma becomes pedunculated, the uterus contracts forcefully as if to expel a foreign body, and the resulting pain is similar to that of labor. The cramping pain is usually associated with hemorrhage.

Signs

Abdominal examination reveals an irregular solid mass or masses arising from the uterus. If degeneration occurs, the inflammation can cause abdominal tenderness in response to palpation and mild localized rebound tenderness. Elevation of temperature and leukocytosis also can occur.

Diagnosis and Management

Ultrasound is useful in distinguishing adnexal from uterine etiology of an eccentric mass. Degeneration of a leiomyoma is treated with observation and pain medication. A pedunculated, torsed, subserosal leiomyoma can easily be excised laparoscopically; however, surgery is not mandatory. A submucous leiomyoma with pain and hemorrhage should be excised transcervically, with hysteroscopic guidance if needed.

Endometriosis

A thorough discussion of endometriosis is presented in Chapter 26. Endometriosis is characterized by the presence and proliferation of endometrial tissue in sites outside the endometrial cavity. Women with endometriosis often experience dysmenorrhea (painful menses), dyspareunia (painful intercourse), and dyschezia (pain with bowel movements). There often is a history of luteal phase bleeding or infertility. Acute pain attributable to endometriosis is usually premenstrual and menstrual (dysmenorrhea); however, if nonmenstrual acute generalized pain occurs, a ruptured endometrioma (chocolate endometriotic cyst within the ovary) should be considered. In this situation, hemoperitoneum is absent, although the fluid from the chocolate cyst can cause chemical peritonitis.

Signs

The abdomen is often tender in the lower quadrants. Significant distention or rebound tenderness is usually not present. Pelvic examination often reveals a fixed, retroverted uterus with tender nodules in the uterosacral region or thickening of the cul-de-sac. An adnexal mass, if present, usually is fixed to the broad ligament and cul-de-sac.

Diagnosis

If a culdocentesis is performed, it will reveal the cyst contents of the ruptured endometrioma. If the diagnosis is unclear, ultrasound is helpful, and laparoscopy findings are definitive. In a patient who has an established diagnosis of endometriosis or who has recently been treated surgically for the disease, a trial of ovarian hormonal suppression (pseudomenopause) can be used to treat the condition and to confirm the correlation between the current pain and the underlying diagnosis of endometriosis.

Management

A ruptured endometrioma is an indication for laparoscopy or laparotomy with ovarian cystectomy or oophorectomy. If a small endometrioma (less than 3 cm) is suspected and there are no signs of rupture, medical management may proceed (see Chapter 26). Diagnostic laparoscopy can be performed if endometriosis or unruptured endometrioma is suspected but not confirmed.

Gastrointestinal Tract

Appendicitis is the most common intestinal source of acute pelvic pain in women. The symptoms and signs of appendicitis can be similar to those of PID. The first symptom of appendicitis is typically diffuse abdominal pain, especially epigastric pain, associated with anorexia and nausea. Within a matter of hours, the pain generally shifts to the right lower quadrant. Fever, chills, emesis, and obstipation may ensue. However, this classic symptom pattern is often lacking. Atypical abdominal pain can occur when the appendix is retrocecal or entirely within the true pelvis. In this setting, tenesmus and diffuse suprapubic pain may result. The patient with appendicitis is more likely to have pronounced and persistent gastrointestinal symptoms than the patient with salpingo-oophoritis.

Signs

Local tenderness is usually elicited on palpation of the right lower quadrant (McBurney point). The appearance of severe generalized muscle guarding; abdominal rigidity; rebound tenderness, right-sided mass, or tenderness on rectal examination; positive psoas sign (pain with forced hip flexion or passive extension of hip); and obturator signs (pain with passive internal rotation of flexed thigh) indicates appendicitis. A low-grade temperature is generally present, but the temperature may be normal. The pelvic examination is usually without cervical motion or bilateral adnexal tenderness, but right-sided unilateral adnexal tenderness can be present.

Diagnosis

Many patients with acute appendicitis have a normal total leukocyte count; however, the differential usually reveals a left shift. Ultrasound examination of the pelvic organs generally has normal findings, whereas the appendix may be abnormal on ultrasound or computed tomography scan. Gastrografin or barium enema with normal filling of the appendix rules out appendicitis. Diagnostic laparoscopy can be useful to rule out other sources of pelvic pathology, but it is occasionally difficult to visualize the appendix sufficiently to rule out early appendiceal inflammation.

Management

Laparotomy, with a false-positive rate of 20%, is an acceptable approach and is preferable to continued observation with rupture and peritonitis. Not only is a ruptured appendix life-threatening but it also may have profound sequelae for the fertility of a young woman of reproductive age.

Acute Diverticulitis

Acute diverticulitis is a condition in which there is inflammation of a diverticulum or outpouching of the wall of the colon, usually involving the sigmoid. Diverticulitis typically affects postmenopausal women but can occur in women in their 30s and 40s.

Symptoms

The severe, left lower quadrant pain of diverticulitis can follow a long history of symptoms of irritable bowel (bloating, constipation, and diarrhea), although diverticulosis usually is asymptomatic. Diverticulitis is less likely to lead to perforation and peritonitis than is appendicitis. Fever, chills, and constipation typically are present, but anorexia and vomiting are uncommon.

Signs

Abdominal examination reveals distention with left lower quadrant tenderness on direct palpation and localized rebound tenderness. Abdominal and pelvic examination may reveal a poorly mobile, doughy inflammatory mass in the left lower quadrant. Bowel sounds are hypoactive and, if peritonitis is present, absent. Leukocytosis frequently is observed.

Diagnosis and Management

Computed axial tomography scan is a useful adjunct to history and physical examination. A barium enema is contraindicated. Diverticulitis is initially managed medically with broad-spectrum intravenous antibiotics. A diverticular abscess often requires surgical intervention.

Intestinal Obstruction

The most common causes of intestinal obstruction in women are postsurgical adhesions, hernia formation, inflammatory bowel disease, and carcinoma of the bowel or ovary.

Symptoms

Intestinal obstruction is heralded by the onset of colicky abdominal pain, followed by abdominal distention, vomiting, constipation, and obstipation. Higher and more acute obstruction results in early vomiting, whereas colonic obstruction presents with a greater degree of abdominal distention and obstipation. Vomiting first consists of gastric contents, followed by bile, then material with feculent odor, depending on the level of obstruction.

Signs

Marked abdominal distention is present. At the onset of mechanical obstruction, bowel sounds are high pitched and maximal during an episode of colicky pain. As the obstruction progresses, bowel sounds decrease and, when absent, suggest ischemic bowel. Elevated white blood cell count and fever often are present in the late stages.

Diagnosis and Management

Abdominal x-ray series showing a characteristic gas pattern help to rule out ileus and to determine whether obstruction is partial or complete. Complete obstruction requires surgical management, whereas partial obstruction often can be managed with intravenous fluids and nasogastric suction. The cause of the obstruction should be determined and treated if possible.

Urinary Tract

Ureteral colic due to ureteral lithiasis is caused by a sudden increase in intraluminal pressure and associated inflammation. Urinary tract infections producing acute pain include cystitis and pyelonephritis.

Symptoms and Signs

The pain of lithiasis is typically severe and crampy; it can radiate from the costovertebral angle to the groin. Hematuria is often present. Cystitis is associated with dull suprapubic pain, urinary frequency, urgency, dysuria, and occasionally hematuria. Because urethritis can occur secondary to chlamydia or gonorrhea and has similar symptoms, these infections must be ruled out, if appropriate. Pyelonephritis is associated with flank and costovertebral angle pain, although lateralizing lower abdominal pain occasionally is present. There is pain with firm pressure over the costovertebral angle in the case of lithiasis or pyelonephritis. Peritoneal signs are absent. Suprapubic tenderness may accompany cystitis.

Diagnosis

Diagnosis of stone is afforded by urinalysis revealing red blood cells and ultrasound or CT urogram or intravenous pyelogram outlining the stone. In the case of urinary tract infection, the diagnosis is based on urinalysis revealing bacteria and leukocytes and subsequently confirmed by culture.

Management

Expectant medical and surgical management are both options for renal lithiasis. Nonpregnant women with pyelonephritis and all women with cystitis can be treated on an outpatient basis.

Diagnostic Tools

All women of reproductive age with acute pelvic pain should have a complete blood count with differential, ESR, urinalysis, and a sensitive qualitative urine or serum pregnancy test (Fig. 14.1). The sedimentation rate is nonspecific but often is the only abnormal laboratory finding in women with subacute PID. Other studies that may be helpful include culdocentesis with hematocrit, if bloody fluid is obtained, and Gram stain and culture, if the fluid is purulent. The presence of cul-de-sac mass precludes culdocentesis. Pelvic ultrasound is useful to rule out ectopic gestation or to assess the adnexae if the results of the examination are confusing or difficult to interpret because of obesity or guarding. Abdominal x-ray series or upper or lower Gastrografin studies are helpful to rule out gastrointestinal pathology when gastrointestinal symptoms predominate. Computed tomography scan is useful for evaluation of retroperitoneal masses or abscesses related to the gastrointestinal tract. Diagnostic laparoscopy is reserved for establishing the diagnosis in patients who have acute abdomen of uncertain cause, for elucidating the nature of an ambiguous adnexal mass, or for delineating whether a pregnancy is intrauterine or extrauterine (if ultrasound results are negative or equivocal). If there is a clinical evidence of salpingo-oophoritis, diagnostic laparoscopy can be used to confirm the diagnosis. Visualization is hampered if diagnostic laparoscopy is performed for a large pelvic mass (>12 cm) and is relatively contraindicated in patients with peritonitis, severe ileus, or bowel obstruction. In these settings, laparotomy is preferable.

Cyclic Pain: Primary and Secondary Dysmenorrhea

Dysmenorrhea is a common gynecologic disorder affecting up to 50% of menstruating women (11). ***Primary dysmenorrhea* refers to menstrual pain without pelvic pathology, whereas *secondary dysmenorrhea* is defined as painful menses associated with underlying pathology.** Primary dysmenorrhea usually appears within 1 to 2 years of menarche, when ovulatory cycles are established. The disorder affects younger women but may persist into the 40s. Secondary dysmenorrhea usually develops years after menarche and can occur with anovulatory cycles. The differential diagnosis of secondary dysmenorrhea is outlined in Table 14.3 (2).

Table 14.3. Peripheral Causes of Chronic Pelvic Pain

Gynecologic

Noncyclic

1. Adhesions
2. Endometriosis
3. Salpingo-oophoritis
   a. Acute
   b. Subacute
4. Ovarian remnant syndrome
5. Pelvic congestion syndrome (varicosities)
6. Ovarian neoplasms
7. Pelvic relaxation

Cyclic

1. Primary dysmenorrhea
2. Secondary dysmenorrhea
   a. Imperforate hymen
   b. Transverse vaginal septum
   c. Cervical stenosis
   d. Uterine anomalies (congenital malformation, bicornuate uterus, blind uterine horn)
   e. Intrauterine synechiae (Asherman's syndrome)
   f. Endometrial polyps
   g. Uterine leiomyoma
   h. Adenomyosis
   i. Pelvic congestion syndrome (varicosities)
   j. Endometriosis
3. Atypical cyclic
   a. Endometriosis
   b. Adenomyosis
   c. Ovarian remnant syndrome
   d. Chronic functional cyst formation

Gastrointestinal

1. Irritable bowel syndrome
2. Ulcerative colitis
3. Granulomatous colitis (Crohn's disease)
4. Carcinoma
5. Infectious diarrhea
6. Recurrent partial small bowel obstruction
7. Diverticulitis
8. Hernia
9. Abdominal angina
10. Recurrent appendiceal colic

Genitourinary

1. Recurrent or relapsing cystourethritis
2. Urethral syndrome
3. Interstitial cystitis
4. Ureteral diverticuli or polyps
5. Carcinoma of the bladder
6. Ureteral obstruction
7. Pelvic kidney

Neurologic

1. Nerve entrapment syndrome
2. Neuroma

Musculoskeletal

Low back pain syndrome

1. Congenital anomalies
2. Scoliosis and kyphosis
3. Spondylolysis

Table 14.3.—*continued*

4. Spondylolisthesis
5. Spinal injuries
6. Inflammation
7. Tumors
8. Osteoporosis
9. Degenerative changes
10. Coccydynia

Myofascial Syndrome

Systemic

1. Acute intermittent porphyria
2. Abdominal migraine
3. Systemic lupus erythematosus
4. Lymphoma
5. Neurofibromatosis

Primary Dysmenorrhea

The cause of primary dysmenorrhea is increased endometrial prostaglandin production (12–15). These compounds are found in higher concentration in secretory endometrium than in proliferative endometrium. The decline of progesterone levels in the late luteal phase triggers lytic enzymatic action, resulting in a release of phospholipids with the generation of arachidonic acid and activation of the cyclooxygenase pathway. The biosynthesis and metabolism of prostaglandins and thromboxane derived from arachidonic acid are depicted in Fig. 14.2 (14). Women with primary dysmenorrhea have higher uterine tone with high-amplitude contractions resulting in decreased uterine blood flow (16). Vasopressin concentrations are also higher in women with dysmenorrhea (17).

Symptoms

The pain of primary dysmenorrhea usually begins a few hours before or just after the onset of a menstrual period and may last up to 48 to 72 hours. The pain is similar to labor, with suprapubic cramping, and may be accompanied by lumbosacral backache, pain radiating down the anterior thigh, nausea, vomiting, diarrhea, and rarely syncopal episodes. The pain of dysmenorrhea is colicky in nature and is improved with abdominal massage, counterpressure, or movement of the body, unlike abdominal pain due to chemical or infectious peritonitis.

Signs

On examination, the vital signs are normal. The suprapubic region may be tender to palpation. Bowel sounds are normal, and there is no upper abdominal tenderness and no abdominal rebound tenderness. Bimanual examination at the time of the dysmenorrheic episode often reveals uterine tenderness; however, severe pain with movement of the cervix or palpation of the adnexal structures is absent. The pelvic organs are normal in primary dysmenorrhea.

Diagnosis

To diagnose primary dysmenorrhea, it is necessary to rule out underlying pelvic pathology and confirm the cyclic nature of the pain. The differential diagnosis of secondary dysmenorrhea includes primary dysmenorrhea and noncyclic pelvic pain. Whereas the diagnosis of primary dysmenorrhea is based on history and presence of a normal pelvic examination, the diagnosis of secondary dysmenorrhea may require review of a pain diary and an ultrasound examination or laparoscopy. During the pelvic examination, the size, shape, and mobility of the uterus, the size and tenderness of adnexal structures, and nodularity or fibrosis of uterosacral ligaments or rectovaginal septum should be assessed. Cervical studies for

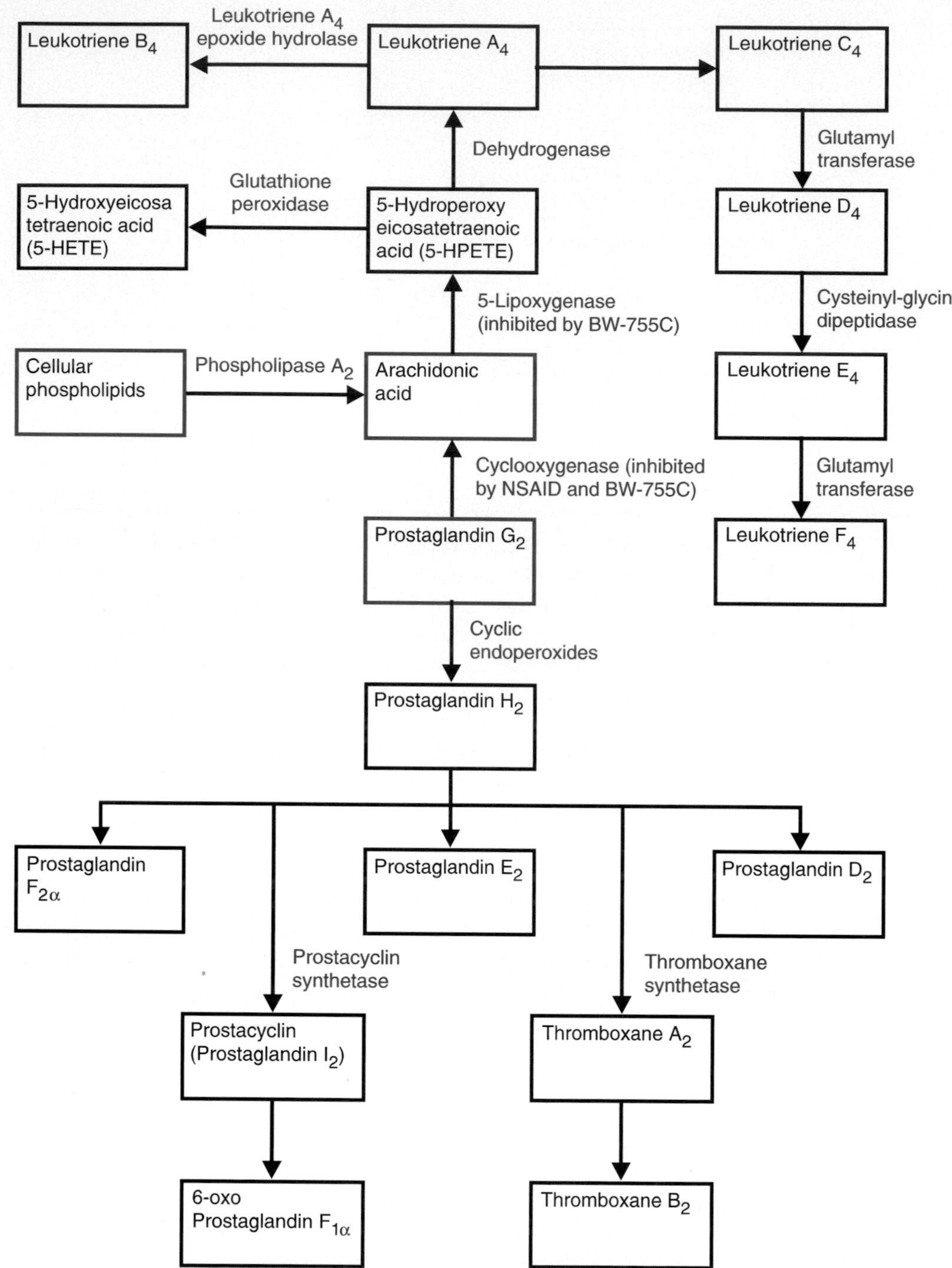

Figure 14.2 The biosynthesis and metabolism of prostaglandins and thromboxane derived from arachidonic acid. (From **Chaudhuri G.** Physiologic aspects of prostaglandins and leukotrienes. *Semin Reprod Endocrinol* 1985;3:219, with permission.)

gonorrhea and chlamydia and, if relevant, a complete blood count with an ESR are helpful to rule out subacute salpingo-oophoritis. If no abnormalities are found, a tentative diagnosis of primary dysmenorrhea can be established.

Treatment

Prostaglandin synthase inhibitors are effective for the treatment of primary dysmenorrhea in about 80% of women (18,19). **The inhibitors should be taken just before or**

at the onset of pain and then continuously every 6 to 8 hours to prevent reformation of prostaglandin by-products. The medication should be taken for the first few days of menstrual flow. A 4- to 6-month course of therapy is warranted before confirming treatment failure. Changes in dosages and types of inhibitors should be attempted if initial treatment is not successful. The medication may be contraindicated in patients with gastrointestinal ulcers or bronchospastic hypersensitivity to aspirin. Side effects are usually mild and include nausea, dyspepsia, diarrhea, and occasionally fatigue.

For the patient with primary dysmenorrhea who has no contraindications to oral contraceptive agents or who desires contraception, the oral contraceptives are the agent of choice. Oral contraceptives decrease endometrial proliferation and create an endocrine milieu similar to the early proliferative phase, when prostaglandin levels are lowest. **More than 90% of women with primary dysmenorrhea experience relief with oral contraception** (20). If the patient does not respond to this regimen, *hydrocodone* or *codeine* may be added for 2 to 3 days per month; however, before addition of the narcotic medication, psychological factors and other organic pathology should be ruled out with diagnostic laparoscopy. Pain management, in particular acupuncture or transcutaneous electrical nerve stimulation (TENS), may also be useful (21–23). In one study of women with primary dysmenorrhea undergoing TENS, 30% reported marked pain relief, 60% moderate pain relief, and 10% no relief (24). To evaluate more fully the evidence for treating primary dysmenorrhea with TENS and acupuncture, a forthcoming study by the Cochrane Library aims to analyze all prospective randomized controlled trials comparing these modalities with medical treatment or placebo (25). Methods used only rarely to treat primary dysmenorrhea include surgical laparoscopic uterine nerve ablation and presacral neurectomy.

Secondary Dysmenorrhea

Secondary dysmenorrhea usually occurs years after the onset of menarche. The definition does not reflect age of onset but rather is cyclic menstrual pain that occurs in association with underlying pelvic pathology. **The pain of secondary dysmenorrhea often begins 1 to 2 weeks before menstrual flow and persists until a few days after the cessation of bleeding.** The mechanisms underlying secondary dysmenorrhea are diverse and not fully elucidated, although most involve either excess prostaglandin production or hypertonic uterine contractions secondary to cervical obstruction, intrauterine mass, or the presence of a foreign body. However, nonsteroidal antiinflammatory agents and oral contraceptive pills are less likely to provide pain relief in women with secondary dysmenorrhea than in those with primary dysmenorrhea. The most common cause of secondary dysmenorrhea is endometriosis, followed by adenomyosis and intrauterine device (for a discussion of endometriosis, see diagnosis of acute and chronic pain, this chapter and Chapter 26). The differential diagnosis of secondary dysmenorrhea is outlined in Table 14.3. The management of secondary dysmenorrhea is treatment of the underlying disorder.

Adenomyosis

Dysmenorrhea associated with adenomyosis often begins up to a week before menses and may not resolve until after the cessation of menses. Associated dyspareunia, dyschezia, and metrorrhagia increase the probability of the diagnosis. Whereas endometriosis is characterized by ectopic endometrium appearing within the peritoneal cavity, adenomyosis is defined as presence of endometrial tissue within the myometrium, at least one high-power field from the basis of the endometrium. Adenomyosis, endometriosis, and uterine leiomyomas frequently coexist. Although occasionally noted in women in the younger reproductive years, the average age of symptomatic women is usually older than 40 years.

Symptoms

Adenomyosis often is asymptomatic. Symptoms typically associated with adenomyosis include excessively heavy or prolonged menstrual bleeding and dysmenorrhea, often beginning up to a week before the onset of a menstrual flow.

Signs

The uterus is diffusely enlarged, although usually less than 14 cm in size, and is often soft and tender, particularly at the time of menses. Mobility of the uterus is not restricted, and there is no associated adnexal pathology.

Diagnosis

Adenomyosis is a clinical diagnosis, and imaging studies, although helpful, are not definitive. Because of their cost and negligible improvement in diagnostic accuracy, these studies are not recommended routinely. In women with diffuse uterine enlargement and a negative pregnancy test, secondary dysmenorrhea may be attributed to adenomyosis; however, the pathologic confirmation of suspected adenomyosis can be made only at the time of hysterectomy. In one study to confirm preoperative diagnosis of adenomyosis before hysterectomy, the clinical diagnosis of adenomyosis was confirmed in only 48% of the cases (26).

Management

The management of adenomyosis clearly depends on the patient's age and desire for future fertility. Relief of secondary dysmenorrhea due to adenomyosis can be ensured after hysterectomy, but less invasive approaches can be tried initially. Nonsteroidal antiinflammatory agents, oral contraceptives, and menstrual suppression using progestins have all been found to be useful.

Chronic Pelvic Pain

Chronic pelvic pain remains an inclusive, general diagnosis that encompasses many more specific causes from endometriosis to nerve entrapment syndrome. Various forms of chronic pelvic pain affect 12% to 15% of women in the United States (27). The differential diagnosis of chronic pelvic pain is outlined in Table 14.3. Patients with chronic pelvic pain are frequently anxious and depressed. Their marital, social, and occupational lives have usually been disrupted. These patients have often had poor treatment outcomes after traditionally effective gynecologic and medical therapy and may have undergone multiple unsuccessful surgical procedures for pain. About 12% of hysterectomies are performed for pelvic pain, and 30% of patients who present to pain clinics have already had a hysterectomy (28,29). **Anywhere from 20% to 80% of patients undergoing laparoscopy for chronic pelvic pain have no intraperitoneal pathology or have tissue distortion that does not correlate with the pain** (2). **Additionally, the relationship can be inconsistent between the pain response and certain types of prevalent intraperitoneal pathology, such as endometriosis, adhesions, or venous congestion** (2). **Nongynecologic causes of pain, such as irritable bowel syndrome, interstitial cystitis, abdominal wall or pelvic floor myofascial syndrome, or nerve entrapment, are frequently overlooked but common causes of chronic pelvic pain.**

Recent investigations have suggested that "plasticity" of the nervous system or alterations in signal processing may be involved in the maintenance of painful states (2,4,30). Various neurohumoral modulators, such as prostaglandins, vasoactive intestinal peptide, substance P, and endorphins, can modulate peripheral neurotransmission and also affect neurotransmission at the level of the spinal cord (31). The spinal cord is not a simple conduit between the periphery and the brain. It is an important site of "gating" mechanisms, such as excitation, inhibition, convergence, and summation of neural stimuli (32). The pain sensation is also modified by neurotransmitters within the brain, such as norepinephrine, serotonin, and γ-aminobutyric acid (GABA), as well as by endogenous endorphin and nonendorphin algesic systems. Different regions of the brain are also important in altering the sensory and affective components of the pain response. **Evidence from animal studies indicates that**

supraspinal factors can interact at the level of the dorsal horn to modulate the sensory perception of pain from the pelvic viscera (33). The sensory and affective component of pain is affected by early experience, conditioning, fear, arousal, depression, and anxiety (30,34).

Evaluation of Chronic Pelvic Pain

Figure 14.3 outlines an approach to the patient with chronic pelvic pain. On the first visit, a thorough pain history should be performed, addressing the nature of each pain complaint: location, radiation, severity, aggravating and alleviating factors; effect of menstrual cycle, stress, work, exercise, intercourse, and orgasm; the context in which pain arose; and the social and occupational toll of the pain.

The patient should be questioned about symptoms specific to the types of pathology (see Table 14.3):

1. Genital (abnormal vaginal bleeding, discharge, dysmenorrhea, dyspareunia, infertility)
2. Enterocoelic (constipation, diarrhea, flatulence, hematochezia, and relationship of pain to bowel movements)
3. Musculoskeletal (trauma, exacerbation with exercise, or postural changes)
4. Urologic (urgency, frequency, nocturia, dysuria, incontinence, hematuria)

The history should include gynecologic, medical, and surgical factors; medication intake; prior evaluations for pain; and operative and pathology reports (2).

Symptoms of an acute process (fever, anorexia, nausea, emesis, significant diarrhea, obstipation, abdominal distention, undiagnosed uterine bleeding, pregnancy, or recent abortion) should alert the physician to the possibility of an acute condition requiring immediate medical or surgical intervention. This occurrence is especially important if symptoms are accompanied by elevated temperature, orthostasis, peritoneal signs, pelvic or abdominal mass, abnormal complete blood count, positive genital or urinary tract cultures, or a positive pregnancy test.

A complete physical examination should be performed, with particular attention directed to the abdominal, lumbosacral, external genital, vaginal, bimanual, and rectovaginal examination. The examination should include evaluation of the abdomen with muscles tensed (head raised off the table or with straight leg raising) to differentiate abdominal wall and visceral sources of pain. Abdominal wall pain is augmented and visceral pain is diminished with these maneuvers (35,36). The patient should be examined while standing for hernias, both abdominal (inguinal and femoral) and pelvic (cystocele and enterocele). An attempt should be made to locate by palpation the tissues that reproduce the patient's pain. If abdominal wall sources of pain are noted, it is useful to block these areas with local anesthetics and then perform the pelvic examination (35,36).

The Psychological Component

A pain history includes the current and past psychological history addressing psychosocial factors; history of past (or current) physical, sexual, or emotional abuse; history of psychiatric hospitalization; suicide attempts; and chemical dependency (2). The attitude of the patient and her family toward the pain, resultant behavior of the patient and her family, and current upheavals in the patient's life should be discussed. The part of the history addressing sensitive issues may have to be reobtained after establishing rapport with the patient.

It is vital to appreciate the various influences that can distort pain perception and expression. A distinction can be drawn between factors leading to a painful condition and those now

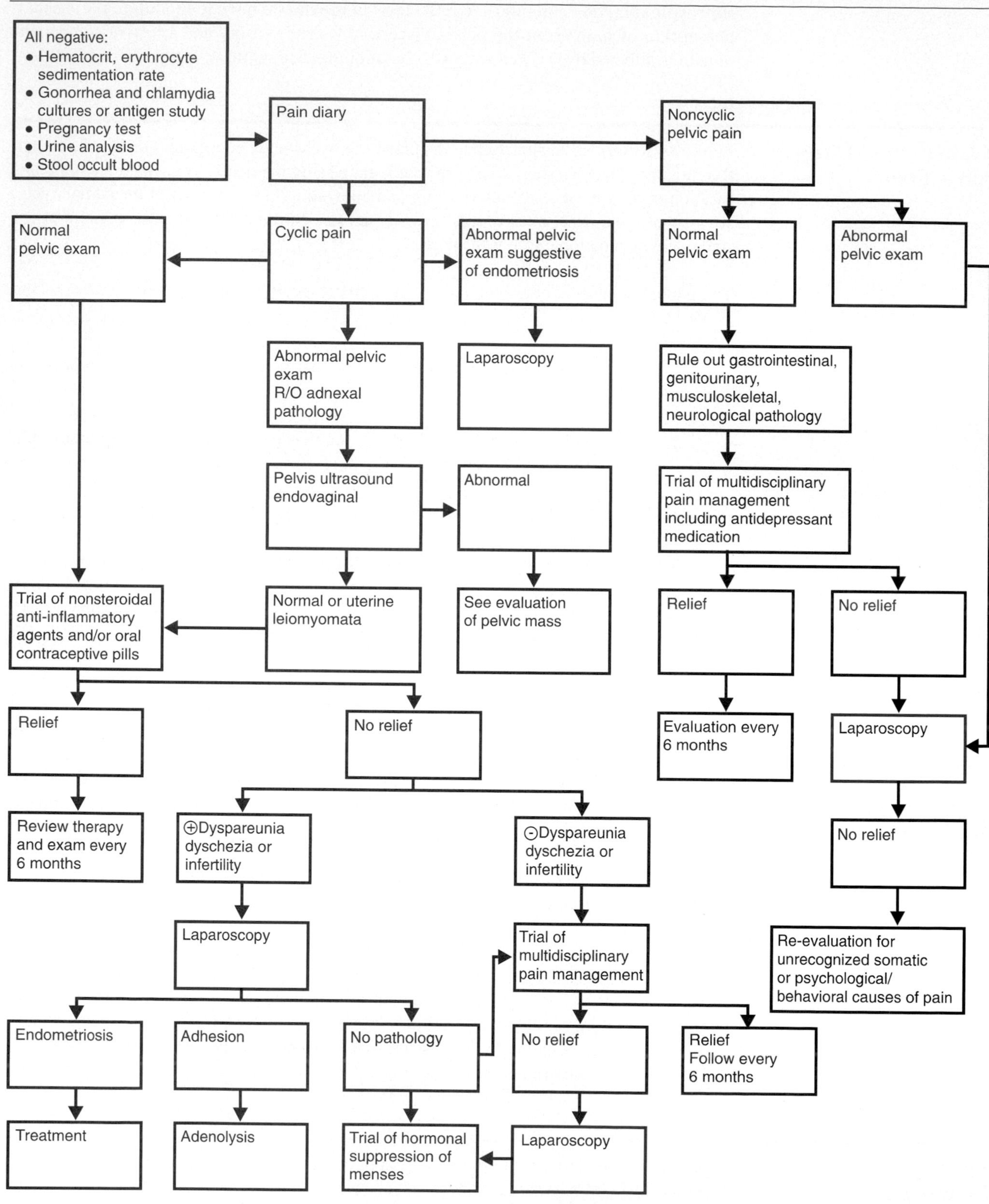

Figure 14.3 Evaluation of chronic pelvic pain.

maintaining it. Whatever the original cause of the pain, when pain has persisted for any length of time, it is likely that other facts are now maintaining or at least contributing to it. The full physical evaluation, outlined previously, should be accompanied by a review of psychosocial factors. Pain is commonly accompanied by anxiety and depression, and these conditions need to be carefully assessed and treated (2). In a typical gynecologic setting, referral to a psychologist for parallel evaluation can evoke resistance. The inference is drawn that the referring physician is ascribing the pain to psychological causes. The patient needs to understand the reason for this referral and to be reassured that it is a routine and necessary part of the evaluation.

Gynecologic Causes

The most common gynecologic pathologies noted at the time of laparoscopy performed for chronic pelvic pain are endometriosis and adhesions. For a thorough discussion of endometriosis and treatment, see Chapter 26.

Other Gynecologic Pathology: Leiomyomas, Ovarian Tumors, Pelvic Relaxation

Patients with obvious gynecologic pathology, such as benign or malignant ovarian cysts, uterine leiomyomas of sufficient size to encroach on supporting ligaments or other somatic structures, or significant pelvic relaxation should be evaluated and managed as is appropriate for the underlying condition (see Chapters 13 and 20). Pain associated with these conditions is generally not severe, and appropriate surgical management is therapeutic.

Endometriosis

Endometriosis can be demonstrated in 15% to 40% of patients undergoing laparoscopy for chronic pelvic pain (37). Endometriosis produces a low-grade inflammatory reaction (38). However, the cause of the pain is not well established. There is no correlation between the location of disease and pain symptoms (39,40). There also appears to be no relationship between the incidence or severity of pain and the stage of the endometriotic lesions, and as many as 30% to 50% of patients have no pain regardless of stage. Similarly, 40% to 60% of patients have no tenderness on examination regardless of stage (40). However, deeply infiltrating rectovaginal septum lesions are strongly associated with pain (41,42), and **vaginal and uterosacral endometrioses are associated with complaints of deep dyspareunia** (43). Prostaglandin E and $F_{2\alpha}$ production from explants of petechial lesions present in mild, low-stage disease was found to be significantly greater than from the explants of powder-burn or black lesions, which are more common in patients with higher-stage endometriosis (44). Therefore, prostaglandin production may account for severe pain in some patients with mild disease.

Clinically, it is possible to determine whether there is a relationship between pain and endometriosis because of the hormonal sensitivity of the disease. **It has been debated whether a laparoscopic diagnosis of chronic pelvic pain secondary to endometriosis is necessary to initiate treatment. Recent reports have suggested otherwise, including one study that showed significant efficacy of gonadotropin-releasing hormone (GnRH) agonist treatment based on empirical diagnosis** (45). After induction of a hypoestrogenic state with GnRH analogues, those patients with pelvic pain and dysmenorrhea related to endometriosis should experience relief. The pain relief usually occurs within 2 months of treatment, but pain often returns to the pretreatment level by 18 months after treatment (46). **During long-term (12 or more months) treatment with GnRH analogues, hormonal add-back therapy (i.e., *norethindrone acetate,* 5 mg daily, with or without estrogen) prevents the long-term hypoestrogenic side effects, such as bone loss, with continued pain relief** (47). Intermenstrual pain that is not as consistently associated with endometriosis as is dysmenorrhea is somewhat less responsive to hormonal manipulation. **Endometriosis may benefit from surgical intervention, such as electrodissection, laser vaporization, or excision. In fact, in one recent prospective, randomized, double-blinded study with 63 women, laparoscopic laser treatment benefited 90% of women who initially responded at 1-year follow-up** (48).

Adhesions

Adhesions noted at the time of laparoscopy are often in the same general region of the abdomen as the pelvic pain complaint (49); however, **neither the specific location (i.e., adnexa structures, parietal, visceral peritoneum, or bowel) nor density of the adhesions correlates consistently with the presence of pain symptoms** (50). Uncontrolled prospective studies of adenolysis have not consistently demonstrated a significant reduction in pain scores (51). In one study of lysis of adhesions, a subgroup of women with anxiety, depression, multiple somatic symptoms, and social and occupational disruption responded poorly to adhesiolysis. The group without these symptoms did have significant improvement in pain (51). A prospective study, however, noted a significant improvement in pain on two of three methods of assessment only if the adhesions were dense and involved the bowel (52).

Symptoms

Noncyclic abdominal pain, sometimes increased with intercourse or activity, is a common pain complaint in women with adhesions, but there is no symptom pattern specific for adhesions. **Chronic pelvic pain developing from adhesions likely results from restriction of bowel mobility and distention** (53). Furthermore, dense adhesions involving bowel can result in a partial or complete bowel obstruction.

Signs

The abdominal wall must be carefully elevated for myofascial or neurologic sources of pain. Most women with adhesions with have had a prior surgical procedure with possible injury to abdominal wall structures that may be the cause of pain. Decreased mobility of pelvic organs or adnexal enlargement can often be noted in patients with adhesions.

Diagnosis

Diagnostic laparoscopy is recommended if other somatic causes are ruled out and the results of the psychological evaluation are negative. **Recent advances in microlaparoscopy have enabled the development of a new technique known as "conscious pain mapping," whereby physicians may better locate the specific adhesions associated with pelvic pain using local anesthesia and conscious sedation** (54). **In an observational study of 50 women using local anesthesia, manipulation of appendiceal and pelvic adhesions contributed to observed pelvic pain** (55). **Further studies are needed to correlate the lysis of such painful adhesions with pain relief.**

Management

At this time, the causal role of adhesions in the genesis of pelvic pain is uncertain, and lysis is recommended only after thorough multidisciplinary evaluation and in the context of an integrated treatment approach that addresses stress, mood, and associated behavioral responses. Repeated surgical procedures for lysis are not recommended.

Pelvic Congestion

In 1954, Taylor suggested that emotional stress could lead to autonomic nervous system dysfunction manifested as smooth muscle spasm and congestion of the veins draining the ovaries and uterus (56). Transuterine venography in women with chronic pelvic pain often reveals delayed disappearance of contrast medium from the uterine and ovarian veins (57). Considering that pregnant and postpartum women have asymptomatic pelvic congestion, the role of congested veins in the causation of pelvic pain is uncertain. The specific neurotransmitters involved in mediating sympathetic efferent maintained pain syndrome are unknown.

Signs and Symptoms

Typical symptoms include lower abdominal and back pain, secondary dysmenorrhea, dyspareunia, abnormal uterine bleeding, chronic fatigue, and irritable bowel symptoms. Pain usually begins with ovulation and lasts until the end of menses. The uterus is often bulky, and the ovaries are enlarged with multiple functional cysts. The uterus, parametria, and uterosacral ligaments are tender.

Diagnosis

Transuterine venography has been the primary method for diagnosis, although other modalities, such as pelvic ultrasound, magnetic resonance imaging, and laparoscopy, may demonstrate varicosities (58). Because of the cost and possible side effects of treatment, further management should be based on related symptoms and not simply on the presence of varicosities.

Management

Treatment of suspected pelvic congestion ranges from the less invasive hormonal suppression and cognitive behavioral pain management to the more invasive ovarian vein embolization or hysterectomy. Low-estrogen, progestin-dominant continuous oral contraceptives, high-dose progestins, and GnRH analogues often provide pain relief. Hormonal suppression should be the initial mode of treatment for women with suspected pelvic congestion. *Medroxyprogesterone acetate,* 30 mg daily, has been found to be useful (59). Concurrently, a multidisciplinary approach incorporating psychotherapy, behavioral pain management, or both is important. A positive interaction between medroxyprogesterone acetate and pain management has been noted (59). **Technically more invasive, transcatheter embolotherapy selectively catheterizes the ovarian and internal iliac veins, followed by contrast venography and embolization** (60). **Several small, uncontrolled studies with limited follow-up have reported pain reduction with transcatheter embolization of pelvic veins** (61–63). For women who have completed their childbearing, hysterectomy with possible oophorectomy is a reasonable option.

Salpingo-oophoritis

Patients with salpingo-oophoritis usually present with symptoms and signs of acute infection. Atypical or partially treated infection may not be associated with fever or peritoneal signs. Subacute or atypical salpingo-oophoritis is often a sequela of chlamydia or mycoplasma infection. Alternatively, a patient with multiple partners may develop frequent recurrent infections (64). Patients with initial gonococcal PID are more likely to develop recurrent infections (65). The mechanism for this increased susceptibility to future infections has not been delineated, although it has been suggested that the fallopian tube and cervix may lose some of their natural protective mechanisms against microorganisms.

Abdominal tenderness, cervical motion, and bilateral adnexal tenderness are typical of pelvic infection. A complete blood count and ESR as well as cervical study for gonorrhea and chlamydia should be performed. In all situations, laparoscopy, with peritoneal fluid cultures, is usually diagnostic. Patients with either abnormal ESR or abnormal clinical examination should be treated empirically for salpingo-oophoritis before laparoscopy.

Ovarian Remnant Syndrome

Chronic pelvic pain in a patient who has had a hysterectomy and bilateral salpingo-oophorectomy for severe endometriosis or PID may be caused by the ovarian remnant syndrome. Ovarian remnant syndrome results from residual ovarian cortical tissue that is left *in situ* after a difficult dissection in an attempt to perform an oophorectomy. Often, the patient has had multiple pelvic operations with the uterus and adnexa removed sequentially.

Symptoms

The patient usually complains of lateralizing pelvic pain, often cycling with ovulation or the luteal phase, described as sharp and stabbing or as constant, dull, and nonradiating, possibly with associated genitourinary or gastrointestinal complaints (66). Symptoms tend to arise 2 to 5 years after initial oophorectomy. A tender mass in the lateral region of the pelvis is pathognomonic.

Diagnosis

Ultrasonography usually confirms a mass with the ultrasonographic characteristics of ovarian tissue. In a patient who has had bilateral salpingo-oophorectomy and is not taking hormonal replacement, estradiol and follicle-stimulating hormone (FSH) assays reveal a characteristic premenopausal picture, although on occasion the remaining ovarian tissue may not be active enough to suppress FSH levels (67,68).

Management

Initial medical treatment with either *danazol,* high-dose progestins, or oral contraceptives usually provides mixed results. Patients usually experience relief of pain with a GnRH agonist, although these medications are impractical for long-term therapy. **Those who achieve relief with GnRH agonists also were relieved by subsequent surgery** (69). Laparoscopic examination is usually nonproductive because the ovarian mass may be missed or adhesions may prevent accurate diagnosis. Laparotomy is necessary for treatment, and the corrective surgery tends to be arduous, often involving inadvertent cystotomy, enterotomy, postoperative small bowel obstructions, and hematoma formation. Surgical pathology usually reveals the presence of ovarian tissue, sometimes with endometriosis, corpus lutea or follicle cysts, and fibrous adhesions (67,68).

Gastroenterologic Causes

The uterus, cervix, and adnexa share with the lower ileum, sigmoid colon, and rectum the same visceral innervation, with pain signals traveling through sympathetic nerves to spinal cord segments T10 to L1 (70). It is often difficult, therefore, to determine whether lower abdominal pain is of gynecologic or enterocoelic origin. Skillful medical history and examination are necessary to distinguish gynecologic from gastrointestinal etiology of pain.

Irritable Bowel Syndrome

Irritable bowel syndrome (IBS) is one of the more common causes of lower abdominal pain and may account for up to 60% of referrals to the gynecologist for chronic pelvic pain (70). The exact etiology of IBS is unknown; however, patients with IBS have pain with smaller volume of distention of the bowel than those without IBS (71). These patients also have an abnormal pain referral pattern with colonic distention. Visceral hypersensitivity or hyperalgesia has been postulated as the cause of pain, although the cause of this hyperalgesia is not known (72).

Symptoms

The predominant symptom of IBS is abdominal pain. Other symptoms include abdominal distention, excessive flatulence, alternating diarrhea and constipation, increased pain before a bowel movement, decreased pain after a bowel movement, and pain exacerbated by events that increase gastrointestinal motility, such has high-fat diet, stress, anxiety, depression, and menses. The pain is usually intermittent, occasionally constant, cramplike, and more likely to occur in the left lower quadrant. The criteria for diagnosis include at least 12 weeks (not necessarily consecutive) in the preceding 12 months of abdominal discomfort or pain that has at least two of the following features: relief with defecation, onset associated with change in stool frequency, or onset associated with change in form (appearance) of stool.

Signs

On physical examination, the finding of a palpable tender sigmoid colon or discomfort during insertion of the finger into the rectum and finding hard feces in the rectum are suggestive of IBS (70).

Diagnosis

The diagnosis of IBS is usually based on history and physical examination, and although suggestive, especially in young women, the findings are not specific. In one study, 91% of patients with IBS had two or more IBS symptoms (abdominal distention, relief of pain with bowel movement, more frequent bowel movements with the onset of pain, looser bowel movements with the onset of pain), whereas 30% of patients with organic disease had two or more of these symptoms (73). Therefore, a complete blood count, stool sample to test for white cells and occult blood, and sigmoidoscopy or colonoscopy or barium enema are usually required, particularly in older individuals and in young individuals who have not responded to initial treatment. The results of these studies are all normal in patients with IBS.

Management

Current medical therapy for IBS is generally unsatisfactory, and placebo response rates are high (74). A multidisciplinary program consisting of medical and psychological approaches is recommended. The treatment consists of reassurance, education, stress reduction, bulk-forming agents, and low-dose tricyclic antidepressants. The multidisciplinary management approach addresses the cognitive, affective, and behavioral components of the pain. Therapy may decrease the intensity of nociceptor stimulation as well as change the interpretation of the meaning of pain.

Inflammatory bowel disease, such as Crohn's disease or ulcerative colitis, infectious enterocolitis, intestinal neoplasms, appendicitis, and hernia must be ruled out with appropriate history and physical examination, complete blood count, and stool cultures as well as visualization of colonic mucosa when appropriate.

Urologic Causes

Chronic pelvic pain of urologic origin may be related to recurrent cystourethritis, urethral syndrome, sensory urgency of uncertain cause, as well as interstitial cystitis. With an appropriate diagnostic workup, infiltrating bladder tumors, ureteral obstruction, renal lithiasis, and endometriosis can easily be ruled out as possible causes.

Urethral Syndrome

***Urethral syndrome* is defined as a symptom complex including dysuria, frequency and urgency of urination, suprapubic discomfort, and often dyspareunia in the absence of abnormality of urethra or bladder.** The cause of urethral syndrome is uncertain and has been attributed to a subclinical infection, urethral obstruction, and psychogenic and allergic factors (75).

Symptoms

Urinary urgency, frequency, suprapubic pressure, and other less frequent symptoms such as bladder or vaginal pain, urinary incontinence, postvoid fullness, dyspareunia, and suprapubic pain are commonly observed.

Signs

Physical and neurologic examinations should be performed. The anal reflex should document that S2 to S4 spinal segments have not been interrupted (75). Anatomic abnormalities, including pelvic relaxation, urethral caruncle, and hypoestrogenism, should be evaluated. The patient should also be evaluated for vaginitis. The urethra should be carefully palpated to detect purulent discharge.

Diagnosis

A clean catch or catheterized urine specimen for routine urinalysis and culture should be obtained to rule out urinary tract infection. As indicated, urethral and cervical cultures for chlamydia should be obtained, and a wet prep for vaginitis should be performed. Urethral syndrome should be considered if the results of urine and urethral cultures are negative, the evaluation does not disclose vulvovaginitis, and no allergic phenomenon causing contact dermatitis of the urethra can be detected. Ureoplasma, chlamydia, candida, trichomonas, gonorrhea, and herpes should be ruled out. Cystoscopic evaluation should be performed to rule out urethral diverticulum, interstitial cystitis, and cancer.

Management

Various forms of therapy have been suggested for urethral syndrome. Those patients in whom no infectious agent is present but who have sterile pyuria respond to a 2- to 3-week course of *doxycycline* or *erythromycin* (75). Long-term, low-dose antimicrobial prophylaxis is often used in women with urgency and frequency symptoms who have had a history of recurrent urinary tract infections. Some of these women may continue to have symptoms when their urine is not infected and then redeveloped bacteria over time (75). It is recommended that all postmenopausal women be given a trial of local estrogen therapy for about 2 months. If there is no improvement after antibiotic or estrogen therapy, urethral dilation can be considered. Positive results also have been noted with biofeedback techniques (75).

Interstitial Cystitis

Interstitial cystitis occurs more often in women than men. Most patients are between 40 and 60 years of age. The cause of interstitial cystitis is unknown, although an autoimmune etiology is generally accepted (75).

Symptoms

Symptoms include severe and disabling urinary frequency and urgency, nocturia, dysuria, and occasional hematuria. Suprapubic, pelvic, urethral, vaginal, or perineal pain is common and can be relieved partially by emptying of the bladder.

Signs

Pelvic examination usually reveals anterior vaginal wall and suprapubic tenderness. Urinalysis may reveal microhematuria without pyuria, although results may be normal.

Diagnosis

The diagnosis is based on symptoms and characteristic cystoscopic findings (75,76). Cystoscopy performed in the awake patient may reveal only bladder hypersensitivity; under anesthesia, however, with sufficient distention of the bladder, submucosal hemorrhages and cracking of the mucosa may be noted (70). Although the histologic features of the biopsy specimen are nonspecific, there is usually submucosal edema, vasodilation, and infiltration by macrophages, plasma cells, and eosinophils.

Management

Because the etiology is uncertain, management has been empirical. Various pharmaceutical approaches, including anticholinergic, antispasmodic, and antiinflammatory agents, have been used. **Response to treatment also has been noted with the use of tricyclic antidepressants or *pentosan polysulfate sodium,* which is approved for therapy** (77). Hydrostatic bladder distention may produce temporary relief by creating detrussor ischemia and decreased innervation of the bladder wall. Biofeedback and behavioral therapy has also been used with some success (75).

Neurologic and Musculoskeletal Causes

Nerve Entrapment

Abdominal cutaneous nerve injury or entrapment may occur spontaneously or within weeks to years after transverse suprapubic skin or laparoscopy incisions (35,78). The ilioinguinal or ileohypogastric nerves may become trapped between the transverse and internal oblique muscles, especially when the muscles contract. Alternatively, the nerve may be ligated or traumatized during the surgery. Symptoms of nerve entrapment include burning, aching pain in the dermatomal distribution of the involved nerve (79,80). Hip flexion and exercise exacerbate pain. The pain is usually judged as coming from the abdomen, not the skin.

Signs

On examination, the pain usually can be localized with the fingertip. The maximal point of tenderness in an iliohypogastric or ilioinguinal injury is usually at the rectus margin, medial and inferior to the anterior iliac spine. Tentative diagnosis is confirmed with the diagnostic nerve block with 0.25% *bupivacaine.* Patients usually report immediate relief of symptoms after injection, and at least 50% experience relief lasting longer than a few hours (35).

Management

Many patients may require no further intervention, although some patients require up to five biweekly injections. If injection is successful in producing only limited pain relief and there are no contributory visceral or psychological factors, cryoneurolysis or surgical removal of the involved nerve is recommended.

Myofascial Pain

Myofascial syndrome has been documented in about 15% of patients with chronic pelvic pain (81). These patients are noted to have trigger points if examined carefully (82). Trigger points are initiated by pathogenic autonomic reflex of visceral or muscular origin (82,83). The referred pain of the trigger point occurs in a dermatomal distribution, and it is thought to be due to nerves from the muscle or deeper structures sharing a common second-order neuron in the spinal cord. Painful trigger points characteristically can be abolished with the injection of local anesthetic into the painful points (82). Trigger points are often present in women with chronic pelvic pain irrespective of presence or type of underlying pathology. In one study, 89% of women with chronic pelvic pain had abdominal, vaginal, or lumbosacral trigger points (82). In the absence of the initial or continued organic pathology, various factors are theorized to predispose to the chronicity of the myofascial syndrome, including psychological, hormonal, and biomechanical factors (83,84).

Symptoms

Abdominal wall pain is often exacerbated during the premenstrual period or by stimuli to the dermatome of trigger points (e.g., full bladder, bowel, or any stimulation to organs that share the dermatome of the involved nerve) (36).

Signs

On examination, fingertip pressure on the trigger points evokes local and referred pain. Tensing of the rectus muscles by either straight leg lifting or raising the head off the table increases the pain. A specific jump sign can be elicited by palpation with fingertip or a cotton swab. An electric (tingling) sensation confirms correct needle placement (36,82).

Management

Injection of the trigger point with 3 mL of 0.25% bupivacaine provides relief that usually outlasts the duration of the anesthetic action. After four to five biweekly injections, the procedure should be abandoned if long-lasting relief is not obtained (82). Concomitant with injection of trigger points, multidisciplinary pain management should be undertaken, especially if anxiety, depression, history of physical or sexual abuse, sexual dysfunction, or social or occupational disruption are present.

Low Back Pain Syndrome

Women complaining of lower back pain without pelvic pain rarely have gynecologic pathology as the cause of their pain. However, low back pain may accompany gynecologic pathology. Back pain may be caused by gynecologic, vascular, neurologic, psychogenic, or respondologenic (related to the axial skeleton and its structure) pathology (2).

Symptoms

Women with low back pain syndrome often have pain occurring after trauma or physical exertion, in the morning on arising, or with fatigue. Nongynecologic low back pain can intensify with the menstrual cycle.

Signs

Examination consists of inspection, evaluation with movement, and palpation. Various anatomic structures in the spine should be considered as sources of pain. Muscles, vertebral joints, and disks (including lumbosacral junction, paravertebral sacrospinal muscles, and sacroiliac joints) are common sources of spondylogenic pain that must be examined carefully (2,85).

Diagnosis

Diagnostic imaging studies performed while the patient is standing, lying, and sitting with maximal flexion can be helpful. An elevated ESR suggests pain of inflammatory or neoplastic origin.

Management

Orthopedic or rheumatologic consultation should be sought before initiating management for back pain unless the source could be referred gynecologic pain.

Psychological Factors

From a psychological perspective, various factors may promote the chronicity of pain, including the meaning attached to the pain, anxiety, the ability to redirect attention, personality, mood state, past experience, and reinforcement contingencies that may amplify or attenuate pain (2). The Minnesota Multiphasic Personality Inventory (MMPI) studies of women with chronic pelvic pain reveal a high prevalence of a convergence "V" profile (elevated scores on the hypochondriasis, hysteria, and depression scales). Studies of MMPI profiles of women with chronic pain without obvious pathology compared with women with endometriosis-related pain or controls suggest that MMPI profiles are unable to distinguish patients with obvious organic findings. Both pain groups differ from controls (2). **Furthermore, treatment resulting in subjective improvement in pain severity and increased activity level produces a significant improvement in personality profile** (86).

There is also a close relationship between depression and pain (87). Both give rise to similar behavior, such as behavioral and social withdrawal and decreased activity, and may be mediated by the same neurotransmitters, including as norepinephrine, serotonin, and endorphins (2). Antidepressants appear to relieve both depression and pain. Childhood physical and sexual abuse has also been noted to be more prevalent in women with chronic pelvic pain than those with other types of pain and controls (52% versus 12%) (88). **In a comparison of women with chronic pelvic pain, women with nonpelvic chronic pain (headache), and pain-free women, a higher lifetime prevalence of major sexual abuse (56%) and physical abuse (50%) was found in the chronic pelvic pain group** (89). Individual differences in personality and habitual coping strategies may also influence response to pain and pain recurrence.

Management Approach

In patients with no obvious pathology and in those with pathology that has an equivocal role in pain production, multidisciplinary therapy is usually preferable. This approach incorporates the skills of the gynecologist, psychologist, and ideally anesthesiologist. A low dose of a tricyclic antidepressant is combined with behavioral therapy directed toward reducing reliance on pain medication, increasing activity, and relieving the impact the pain has on the women's overall lifestyle (2). Women with depression should be treated with an appropriate therapeutic dose of antidepressant medication (90). **Only one small, randomized, controlled trial has looked at the effect of selective serotonin reuptake inhibitors on pelvic pain. It failed to show a significant difference in pain or functional ability in a short follow-up period** (91). The approach to women with chronic pain must be therapeutic, supportive, and sympathetic. Offering regular follow-up appointments instead of asking the patient to return only if pain persists reinforces pain behavior. Specific skills can be taught to the patient using cognitive behavioral approaches. Women are offered ways to enhance opportunities for control of pain. Psychotherapy is indicated for women who have pronounced depression, sexual difficulties, or indications of past trauma. Various strategies, including relaxation techniques, stress management, sexual and marital counseling, hypnosis, and other psychotherapeutic approaches, have been found to be useful. Acupuncture may also be helpful (92). Diagnostic uterosacral, hypogastric, or epidural nerve blocks can be used (93).

Multidisciplinary Approach

Various studies of multidisciplinary pain management have been performed. Retrospective, uncontrolled studies revealed relief of pain in 85% of the subjects (92,94). One prospective randomized study revealed a similar response rate, which was significantly better than that of traditional therapy (95).

Surgical Therapy

Laparoscopy

Those women with disabling cyclic pain that does not respond to nonsteroidal antiinflammatory medication or oral contraceptives should undergo laparoscopic evaluation. Diagnostic laparoscopy has become a standard procedure in the evaluation of patients with chronic noncyclic pelvic pain; however, laparoscopy should be withheld until other nongynecologic somatic or visceral causes of pain have been eliminated. During diagnostic laparoscopy, endometriotic lesions should be excised for biopsy, and if infection is suspected, cultures should be performed. All visible endometriosis should be surgically excised or electrocoagulated. Patients with dysmenorrhea may benefit from transection of the uterosacral ligaments. The uterosacral ligaments carry the principal afferent nerve supply from the uterus to the hypogastric nerve. The original procedure was performed by a colpotomy and was noted to have a success rate of 70% (96). Laparoscopic nerve ablation was found to relieve dysmenorrhea in 85% of patients (97). **Nonrandomized retrospective and prospective studies have suggested that diagnostic laparoscopy provides a positive psychological effect on the treatment of chronic pelvic pain** (98).

Lysis of Adhesions

The role of pelvic adhesions in pain is unclear (2). Adhesiolysis, even by laparoscopy, is frequently complicated by adhesion reformation (99). However, other etiologies must be treated first. Psychological consultation and management should precede or accompany the lysis of adhesions.

Presacral Neurectomy

Presacral neurectomy or sympathectomy was first described for dysmenorrhea (100). The discovery of highly successful medical therapies has largely supplanted presacral neurectomy; however, presacral neurectomy may be indicated for primary or secondary dysmenorrhea unrelieved by traditional therapy and unresponsive to multidisciplinary pain management. The response rate to presacral neurectomy for secondary dysmenorrhea varies between 50% and 75% (2,99). The neurectomy only relieves pain deriving from the cervix, uterus, and proximal fallopian tubes (T11 to L2). The nerve supply to the adnexal structures (T9 to T10) bypasses the hypogastric nerve. Therefore, lateralizing visceral pain is unlikely to be relieved by presacral neurectomy. Intraoperative complications, such as hemorrhage or ureteral injury, can occur in a small percentage of cases. The sacral nerve supply is unaffected by division of the presacral nerve; thus, normal micturition, defecation, and parturition are preserved. A local anesthetic hypogastric block performed under fluoroscopic guidance can help to predict the response to this operation.

Hysterectomy

Hysterectomy has often been performed to cure pelvic pain; however, 30% of patients presenting to pain clinics have already undergone hysterectomy without experiencing pain relief (28). Hysterectomy is particularly useful for women who have completed childbearing and have secondary dysmenorrhea or chronic pain related to endometriosis, to uterine pathology, such as adenomyosis, or to pelvic congestion. Before recommending hysterectomy for pain or unilateral adnexectomy for unilateral pain, it is useful to apply the PREPARE pneumonic in discussions with the patient (101): the *P*rocedure that is being done, *R*eason or indication, *E*xpectation or desired outcome of the procedure, *P*robability that the outcome will be achieved, *A*lternatives and nonsurgical options, and *R*isks as well as *Expense* (see Chapter 3). Hysterectomy for central pelvic pain in women with dysmenorrhea, dyspareunia, and uterine tenderness provided relief of pain in 77% of women in one retrospective study (102) and in 74% of women in one prospective cohort study (103). Nevertheless, 25% of women in the retrospective study noted a persistence or worsening of pain at 1-year follow-up (104).

References

1. **Dawood MY.** Dysmenorrhea. *Clin Obstet Gynecol* 1990;3(2):168–178.
2. **Rapkin AJ, Reading AE.** *Curr Probl Obstet Gynecol Fertil* 1991;14(4):99–137.
3. **Bonica JJ.** General considerations of pain in the pelvis and perineum. In: **Bonica JJ, Loeser JD, Chapman CR, et al,** eds. *The management of pain II.* Philadelphia: Lea & Febiger, 1990:1283–1312.
4. **Rapkin AJ.** Gynecologic pain in the clinic: is there a link with the basic research? In: **Gebhart GF,** ed. *Visceral pain.* Seattle: IASP Press, 2002:469–480.
5. **Bonica JJ.** Neurophysiologic and pathologic aspects of acute and chronic pain. *Arch Surg* 1977;112:750–761.
6. **Kahn JG, Walker CK, Washington AE, et al.** Diagnosing pelvic inflammatory disease. *JAMA* 1991;266(18):2594–2604.

7. **Centers for Disease Control and Prevention.** 1993 Sexually transmitted diseases treatment guidelines. *MMWR Morb Mortal Wkly Rep* 1993;42(RR-14):1–13.

8. **Sellors J, Mahony J, Goldsmith C, et al.** The accuracy of clinical findings and laparoscopy in pelvic inflammatory disease. *Am J Obstet Gynecol* 1991;164:113–120.

9. **Centers for Disease Control and Prevention.** Recommendations for the prevention and control of Chlamydia trachomatis infections. *MMWR Morb Mortal Wkly Rep* 1993;42(RR-12):1–36.

10. **Holmes KK, Mårdh PA, Sparling PF, et al.** *Sexually transmitted diseases,* 2nd ed. New York: McGraw-Hill, 1990.

11. **The American College of Obstetricians and Gynecologists.** *Dysmenorrhea.* ACOG Technical Bulletin 1983;63.

12. **Wiqvist NE, Lindblom B, Wilhelmsson L.** The patho-physiology of primary dysmenorrhea. *Res Clin Forums* 1979;1:47–54.

13. **Lundstrom V, Green K.** Endogenous levels of prostaglandin in F_2-alpha and its main metabolites in plasma and endometrium of normal and dysmenorrheic women. *Am J Obstet Gynecol* 1978;130:640–646.

14. **Chaudhuri G.** Physiologic aspects of prostaglandins and leukotrienes. *Semin Reprod Endocrinol* 1985;3(3):219–230.

15. **Rapkin AJ, Berkley KJ, Rasgon NL.** Dysmenorrhea. In: **Yaksh TL,** ed. *Anesthesia: biologic foundation.* New York: Raven Press, 1995.

16. **Akerlund M, Stromberg P, Forsling ML.** Primary dysmenorrhea and vasopression. *Br J Obstet Gynecol* 1979;86:484–487.

17. **Akerlund M, Stromberg P, Forsling ML.** Primary dysmenorrhea and vasopressin. *Br J Obstet Gynecol* 1979;86:484–487.

18. **The Medical Letter: Drugs for Dysmenorrhea.** *The medical letter on drugs and therapeutics.* New Rochelle, NY: 1979;21:81–84.

19. **Filler WW, Hall WC.** Dysmenorrhea and its therapy. *Am J Obstet Gynecol* 1970;106:104–109.

20. **Chan WY, Dawood MY.** Prostaglandin levels in menstrual fluid of non-dysmenorrheic and dysmenorrheic subjects with and without oral contraceptive or ibuprofen therapy. *Adv Prostaglandin Thromboxane Res* 1980;8:1443–1447.

21. **Helms JM.** Acupuncture for the management of primary dysmenorrhea. *Obstet Gynecol* 1987;69:51–56.

22. **Lundberg T, Bondesson L, Lundstrom V.** Relief of primary dysmenorrhea by transcutaneous electrical nerve stimulation. *Acta Obstet Gynecol Scand* 1985;64:491.

23. **Mannheimer JS, Whalen EC.** The efficacy of transcutaneous electrical nerve stimulation in dysmenorrhea. *Clin J Pain* 1985;1:75.

24. **Kaplan B, Peled Y, Pardo J, et al.** Transcutaneous electrical nerve stimulation (TENS) as a relief for dysmenorrhea. *Clin Exp Obstet Gynecol* 1994;21:87–90.

25. **Wilson M, Farquhar C, Kennedy S, et al.** Trancutaneous electrical nerve stimulation and acupuncture for primary dysmenorrhoea [protocol]. *Cochrane Library* 2000;4.

26. **Lee NC, Dikcer RC, Rubin GL, et al.** Confirmation of the preoperative diagnoses for hysterectomy. *Am J Obstet Gynecol* 1984;150:283–287.

27. **Mathias SD, Kuppermann M, Liberman RF, et al.** Chronic pelvic pain: prevalence, health-related quality of life, and economic correlates. *Obstet Gynecol* 1996;87:321–327.

28. **Reiter RC.** A profile of women with chronic pelvic pain. *Clin Obstet Gynecol* 1990;33:130–136.

29. **Chamberlain A, La Ferla J.** The gynecologists approach to chronic pelvic pain. In: **Burroughs JD, et al,** ed. *Handbook of chronic pain management,* vol 33. Amsterdam: Elsevier, 1987:371–382.

30. **Wall PD.** The John J. Bonica distinguished lecture. Stability and instability of central pain mechanisms. In **Dubner R, et al,** ed. *Proceedings of the Fifth World Congress on Pain.* Amsterdam: Elsevier Science, 1988:13–24.

31. **Janig W, Morrison JFB.** Functional properties of spinal visceral afferents supplying abdominal and pelvic organs, with special emphasis on visceral nociception. In **Cervero F, et al,** eds. *Visceral sensation.* New York: Elsevier Science, 1986:87–114.

32. **Cervergo F, Tattersall JEH.** Somatic and visceral sensory integration in the thoracic spinal cord. In **Cervero F, et al,** eds. *Visceral sensation.* New York: Elsevier Science, 1986:189–205.

33. **Berkley KJ, Hubscher CH.** Visceral and somatic sensory tracks through the neuroaxis and their relation to pain: lessons from the rat female reproductive system. In: **Gebhart GF,** ed. *Visceral pain, progress in pain research and management,* vol 5. Seattle: IASP Press, 1995:195–216.

34. **Bonica JJ.** The management of pain: biochemistry and modulation of nociception and pain. In: **Loeser JD, Chapman CR, Fordyce WE,** eds. *The management of pain II.* Philadelphia: Lea & Febiger, 1990:95–121.

35. **Greenbaum DS, Greenbaum RB, Joseph JG, et al.** Chronic abdominal wall pain diagnostic validity and costs. *Dig Dis Sci* 1994;39(9):1935–1941.

36. **Slocumb JC.** Chronic somatic myofascial, and neurogenic abdominal pelvic pain. *Clin Obstet Gynecol* 1990;33:145–153.

37. **Vercellini P, Fedele L, Molteni P, et al.** Laparoscopy in the diagnosis of gynecologic chronic pelvic pain. *Int J Gynaecol Obstet* 1990;32:261–267.

38. **Hill JA, Anderson DJ.** Lymphocyte activity in the presence of peritoneal fluid from fertile women and infertile women with and without endometriosis. *Am J Obstet Gynecol* 1989;161:861–864.

39. **Fedele L, Parazzini F, Bianchi S, et al.** Stage and localization of pelvic endometriosis and pain. *Fertil Steril* 1990;53:155–158.

40. **Fukaya T, Hoshiai H, Yajima A.** Is pelvic endometriosis always associated with chronic pain? A retrospective study of 618 cases diagnosed by laparoscopy. *Am J Obstet Gynecol* 1993;169:719–722.

41. **Cornillie FJ, Oosterlynck D, Lauweryns JM.** Deeply infiltrating pelvic endometriosis: histology and clinical significance. *Fertil Steril* 1990;53:978–983.

42. **Konincky RP, Meuleman C, Demeyere S, et al.** Suggestive evidence that pelvic endometriosis is a progressive disease, whereas deeply infiltrating endometriosis is associated with pelvic pain. *Fertil Steril* 1991;55:759–765.

43. **Vercellini P, Trespedi L, De Giorgi O, et al.** Endometriosis and pelvic pain: relation to disease stage and localization. *Fertil Steril* 1996;65:299–304.

44. **Vernon MW, Beard JS, Graves K, et al.** Classification of endometriotic implants by morphologic appearance and capacity to synthesize prostaglandin F. *Fertil Steril* 1984;46:801–806.

45. **Ling FW.** Randomized controlled trial of depot leuprolide in patients with chronic pelvic pain and suspected endometriosis. Pelvic Pain Study Group. *Obstet Gynecol* 1999;93:51–58.

46. **Fedele L, Bianchi S, Baglione S, et al.** Stage and localization of pelvic endometriosis and pain. *Fertil Steril* 1989;73:1000–1004.

47. **Hornstein MD, Surrey ES, Weisberg GW, et al.** Leuprolide acetate depot and hormonal add-back in endometriosis: a 12-month study. *Obstet Gynecol* 1998;91:16–24.

48. **Sutton CJ, Pooley AS, Ewen SP, et al.** Follow-up report on a randomized controlled trial of laser laparoscopy in the treatment of pelvic pain associated with minimal to moderate endometriosis. *Fertil Steril* 1997;68:1070–1074.

49. **Stout AL, Steege JF, Dodson WC, et al.** Relationship of laparoscopic findings to self-report of pelvic pain. *Am J Obstet Gynecol* 1991;73–79.

50. **Rapkin AJ.** Adhesions and pelvic pain: a retrospective study. *Obstet Gynecol* 1986;68:13–15.

51. **Steege JF, Scott AL.** Resolution of chronic pelvic pain after laparoscopic lysis of adhesions. *Am J Obstet Gynecol* 1991;165:278–283.

52. **Peters AAW, Trimbos-Kemper GCM, Admiral C, et al.** A randomized clinical trial on the benefit of adhesiolysis in patients with intraperitoneal adhesions and chronic pelvic pain. *Br J Obstet Gynecol* 1992; 99:59–62.

53. **Duffy DM, diZerga GS.** Adhesion controversies: pelvic pain as a cause of adhesions, crystalloids on preventing them. *J Reprod Med* 1996;41:19–26.

54. **Palter SF.** Microlaparoscopy under local anesthesia and conscious pain mapping for the diagnosis and management of pelvic pain. *Curr Opin Obstet Gynecol* 1999;11:387–393.

55. **Almeida OD, Val-Gallas JM.** Conscious pain mapping. *J Am Assoc Gynecol Laparosc* 1997;4:587–590.

56. **Taylor HC Jr.** Pelvic pain based on a vascular and autonomic nervous system disorder. *Am J Obstet Gynecol* 1954;67:1177–1196.

57. **Beard RW, Highman JH, Pearce S, et al.** Diagnosis of pelvic varicosities in women with chronic pelvic pain. *Lancet* 1984;2:946–949.

58. **Gupta A, McCarthy S.** Pelvic varices as a cause for pelvic pain: MRI appearance. *Magn Reson Imaging* 1994;12:679–681.

59. **Farquhar CM, Rogers V, Franks S, et al.** A randomized controlled trial of medroxyprogesterone acetate and psychotherapy for the treatment of pelvic congestion. *Br J Obstet Gynecol* 1989;96:1153–1162.

60. **Venbrux AC, Lambert DL.** Embolization of the ovarian veins as a treatment for patients with chronic pelvic pain caused by pelvic venous incompetence (pelvic congestion syndrome). *Curr Opin Obstet Gynecol* 1999;11:387–393.

61. **Sichlau MJ, Yao JST, Vogelzang RL.** Transcatheter embolotherapy for the treatment of pelvic congestion syndrome. *Obstet Gynecol* 1994;83:892–896.

62. **Capasso P, Simons C, Trotteur G, et al.** Treatment of symptomatic pelvic varices by ovarian vein embolization. *Cardiovasc Intervent Radiol* 1997;20:107–111.

63. **Tarazov PG, Prozorovskij KV, Ryzhkov VK.** Pelvic pain syndrome caused by ovarian varices: treatment by transcatheter embolization. *Acta Radiol* 1997;38:1023–1025.

64. **Eschenbach DA, Holmes KK.** Acute pelvic inflammatory disease: current concepts of pathogenesis, etiology, and management. *Clin Obstet Gynecol* 1975;197(18):35–36.

65. **Sweet RL, Giggs RS.** Pelvic inflammatory disease. In: **Sweet R, Gibbs RS,** eds. *Infectious disease of the female genital tract: part 1.* Baltimore: Williams & Wilkins, 1985:53–77.

66. **Lafferty HW, Angioli R, Rudolph J, et al.** Ovarian remnant syndrome: experience at Jackson Memorial Hospital, University of Miami, 1985 through 1993. *Am J Obstet Gynecol* 1996;174:641–645.

67. **Steege JF.** Ovarian remnant syndrome. *Obstet Gynecol* 1987;70:64–67.

68. **Price FV, Edwards R, Buchsbaum HJ.** Ovarian remnant syndrome: Difficulties in diagnosis and management. *Obstet Gynecol Surv* 1990;45:151–156.

69. **Carey MP, Slack MC.** GnRH analogue in assessing chronic pelvic pain in women with residual ovaries. *Br J Obstet Gynaecol* 1996;103:150–153.

70. **Rapkin AJ, Mayer EA.** Gastroenterologic causes of chronic pelvic pain. In: **Ling FW,** ed. *Obstetrics and Gynecology Clinics of North America. Contemporary management of chronic pelvic pain.* Philadelphia: WB Saunders, 1993;4:663–682.

71. **Hightower NC, Roberts JW.** Acute and chronic lower abdominal pain of enterologic origin in chronic pelvic pain. In: **Ranaer,** ed. *Chronic pelvic pain in women.* New York: Springer–Verlag, 1981: 110–137.

72. **Mayer EA, Gebhart GF.** Functional bowel disorders and the visceral hyperalgesia hypothesis. In: **Mayer ER, Raybould HE,** eds. *Pain research and clinical management,* vol 9. Amsterdam: Elsevier, 1993; 1:3–28.

73. **Whitehead WE, Schustger MM.** *Gastrointestinal disorders.* San Diego: Academic Press, 1985.

74. **Klein KB.** Controlled treatment trials in the irritable bowel syndrome: a critique. *Gastroenterology* 1988;95:232.

75. **Karram MM.** Frequency, urgency, and painful bladder syndromes. In: **Walters MD, Karram MM,** eds. *Clinical urogynecology.* St. Louis: Mosby, 1993:285–298.

76. **Messing EM, Stamey TA.** Interstitial cystitis following colocystoplasty. *Urology* 1973;2:28.

77. **Sant GR.** Interstitial cystitis: a urogynecologic perspective. *Contemp Obstet Gynecol* 1998;840;119–130.

78. **Sippo WC, Burghardt A, Gomez AC.** Nerve entrapment after pfannansteil incision. *Am J Obstet Gynecol* 1987;157:420–421.

79. **Bonica JJ.** Pelvic and perineal pain caused by other disorders. In: **Loeser JD, Chapman CR, Fordyce WE,** eds. *The management of pain II.* Philadelphia: Lea & Febiger, 1990;69:1383–1394.

80. **Bonica JJ.** Applied anatomy relevant to pain. In: **Loeser JD, Chapman CR, Fordyce WE,** eds. *The management of pain II.* Philadelphia: Lea & Febiger, 1990:133–158.

81. **Reiter RC.** Occult somatic pathology in women with chronic pelvic pain. *Clin Obstet Gynecol* 1990;33:154–160.

82. **Slocumb JC.** Neurological factors in chronic pelvic pain: trigger points and the abdominal pelvic pain syndrome. *Am J Obstet Gynecol* 1984;149:536–543.

83. **Travell J.** Myofascial trigger points: clinical view. *Adv Pain Res Ther* 1976;1:919–926.

84. **Ling FW, Slocumb JC.** Use of trigger point injections in chronic pelvic pain. In: **Ling FW,** ed. *Obstetrics and Gynecology Clinics of North America: Contemporary management of chronic pelvic pain.* Philadelphia: WB Saunders, 1993;20(4):809–815.

85. **Nachemson AL.** Low back pain: its etiology and treatment. *Clin Med* 1971;78:18–24.

86. **Duleba AJ, Jubanyik KJ, Greenfield DA, et al.** Changes in personality profile associated with laparoscopic surgery for chronic pelvic pain. *J Am Assoc Gynecol Laparosc* 1998;5:389–395.

87. **Wood DP, Weisner MG, Reiter RC.** Psychogenic chronic pelvic pain. *Clin Obstet Gynecol* 1990;33:179–195.

88. **Rapkin AJ, Kames LD, Darke LL, et al.** History of physical and sexual abuse in women with chronic pelvic pain. *Obstet Gynecol* 1990;76:90–96.

89. **Walling MK, Reiter RC, O'Hara MW, et al.** Abuse history and chronic pain in women. I. Prevalence of sexual abuse and physical abuse. *Obstet Gynecol* 1994;84:193–199.

90. **Walker EA, Sullivan MD, Stenchever MA.** Use of antidepressants in the management of women with chronic pelvic pain. In: **Ling FW,** ed. *Obstetrics and Gynecology Clinics of North America: Contemporary management of chronic pelvic pain.* Philadelphia: WB Saunders, 1993;20(4):743–751.

91. **Engel CC Jr, Walker EA, Engel AL, et al.** A randomized, double–blind crossover trial of sertraline in women with chronic pelvic pain. *J Psychosom Res* 1998;44:203–207.

92. **Rapkin AJ, Kames LD.** The pain management approach to chronic pelvic pain. *J Reprod Med* 1987;32:323–327.

93. **McDonald JS.** Management of chronic pelvic pain. In: **Ling FW,** ed. *Obstetrics and Gynecology Clinics of North America: Contemporary management of chronic pelvic pain.* Philadelphia: WB Saunders, 1993;20(4):817–838.

94. **Milburn A, Reiter RC, Rhomberg AT.** Multidisciplinary approach of chronic pelvic pain. In: **Ling FW,** ed. *Obstetrics and Gynecology Clinics of North America: Contemporary management of chronic pelvic pain.* Philadelphia: WB Saunders, 1993;20(4):643–661.

95. **Peters AAW, van Dorst E, Jellis B, et al.** A randomized clinical trial to compare two different approaches in women with chronic pelvic pain. *Obstet Gynecol* 1991;77:740.

96. **Doyle IB.** Paracervical uterine denervation by transection of the cervical plexus for the relief of dysmenorrhea. *Am J Obstet Gynecol* 1955;70:1–16.

97. **Lichten EM, Bombard J.** Surgical treatment of primary dysmenorrhea with laparoscopic uterine nerve ablation. *J Reprod Med* 1987;32:37–41.

98. **Elcombe S, Gath D, Day A.** The psychological effects of laparoscopy on women with chronic pelvic pain. *Psychol Med* 1997;27:1041–1050.

99. **Parsons LH, Stovall TG.** Surgical management of chronic pelvic pain. In: **Ling FW,** ed. *Obstetrics and Gynecology Clinics of North America: Contemporary management of chronic pelvic pain.* Philadelphia: WB Saunders, 1993:765–778.

100. **Cotte G.** Resection of the presacral nerves in the treatment of obstinate dysmenorrhea. *Am J Obstet Gynecol* 1937;33:1034–1040.

101. **Reiter RC, Lench JB, Gambone JC.** Clinical commentary: consumer advocacy, elective surgery, and the "golden era of machine." *Obstet Gynecol* 1989;74:815–817.

102. **Stovall TG, Ling FW, Crawford DA.** Hysterectomy for chronic pelvic pain of presumed uterine etiology. *Obstet Gynecol* 1990;75:676–679.

103. **Hillis SD, Marchbanks PA, Peterson HB.** The effectiveness of hysterectomy for chronic pelvic pain. *Obset Gynecol* 1995;86:941–945.

104. **ACOG Criteria Set.** Hysterectomy, abdominal or vaginal for chronic pelvic pain. Number 29, November 1997. Committee on Quality Assessment. American College of Obstetricians and Gynecologists. *Int J Gynaecol Obstet* 1998;60:316–317.

15 Genitourinary Infections and Sexually Transmitted Diseases

David E. Soper

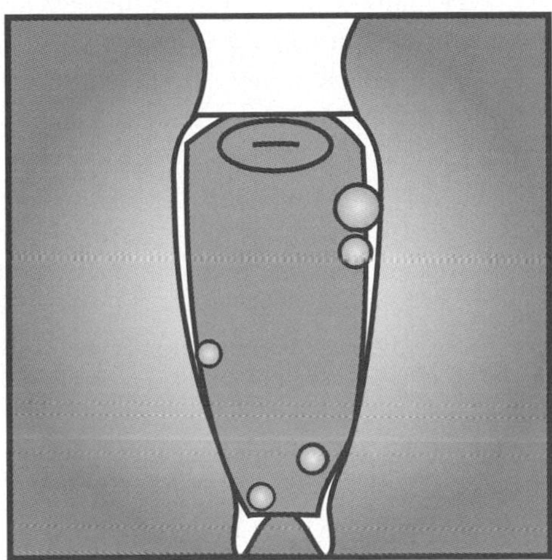

Genitourinary tract infections are among the most frequent disorders for which patients seek care from gynecologists. By understanding the pathophysiology of these diseases and having an effective approach to their diagnosis, physicians can institute appropriate antimicrobial therapy to treat these conditions and reduce long-term sequelae.

The Normal Vagina

Normal vaginal secretions are composed of vulvar secretions from sebaceous, sweat, Bartholin, and Skene glands; transudate from the vaginal wall; exfoliated vaginal and cervical cells; cervical mucous; endometrial and oviductal fluids; and microorganisms and their metabolic products. The type and amount of exfoliated cells, cervical mucus, and upper genital tract fluids are determined by biochemical processes that are influenced by hormone levels (1). Vaginal secretions may increase in the middle of the menstrual cycle because of an increase in the amount of cervical mucus. These cyclic variations do not occur when oral contraceptives are used and ovulation does not occur.

The vaginal desquamative tissue is made up of vaginal epithelial cells that are responsive to varying amounts of estrogen and progesterone. Superficial cells, the predominant cell type in women of reproductive age, predominate when estrogen stimulation is present. Intermediate cells predominate during the luteal phase because of progestogenic stimulation. Parabasal cells predominate in the absence of either hormone, a condition that may be found in postmenopausal women who are not receiving hormonal replacement therapy.

The normal vaginal flora is predominantly aerobic, with an average of six different species of bacteria, the most common of which is hydrogen peroxide–producing lactobacilli. The microbiology of the vagina is determined by factors that affect the ability of bacteria to survive (2). These factors include vaginal pH and the availability of glucose for bacterial metabolism. **The pH of the normal vagina is lower than 4.5, which is maintained by the production of lactic acid.** Estrogen-stimulated vaginal epithelial cells are rich in glycogen. Vaginal epithelial cells break down glycogen to monosaccharides, which can then be converted by the cells themselves and lactobacilli to lactic acid.

Normal vaginal secretions are floccular in consistency, white in color, and usually located in the dependent portion of the vagina (posterior fornix). Vaginal secretions can be analyzed by a wet-mount preparation. A sample of vaginal secretions is suspended in 0.5 mL of normal saline in a glass tube, transferred to a slide, covered with a slip, and assessed by microscopy. Some clinicians prefer to prepare slides by suspending secretions in saline placed directly on the slide. Secretions should not be placed on the slide without saline because this method causes drying of the vaginal secretions and does not result in a well-suspended preparation. Microscopy of normal vaginal secretions reveals many superficial epithelial cells, few white blood cells (less than 1 per epithelial cell), and few, if any, clue cells. **Clue cells are superficial vaginal epithelial cells with adherent bacteria, usually *Gardnerella vaginalis,* which obliterates the crisp cell border when visualized microscopically.** Potassium hydroxide 10% (KOH) may be added to the slide, or a separate preparation can be made, to examine the secretions for evidence of fungal elements. The results are negative in women with normal vaginal microbiology. Gram stain reveals normal superficial epithelial cells and a predominance of gram-positive rods (lactobacilli).

Vaginal Infections

Bacterial Vaginosis

Bacterial vaginosis (BV) has previously been referred to as nonspecific vaginitis or *Gardnella* vaginitis. It is an alteration of normal vaginal bacterial flora that results in the loss of hydrogen peroxide–producing lactobacilli and an overgrowth of predominantly anaerobic bacteria (3,4). **The most common form of vaginitis in the United States is BV** (5). Anaerobic bacteria can be found in less than 1% of the flora of normal women. In women with BV, however, the concentration of anaerobes, as well as *G. vaginalis* and *Mycoplasma hominis,* is 100 to 1,000 times higher than in normal women. Lactobacilli are usually absent.

It is not known what triggers the disturbance of normal vaginal flora. It has been postulated that repeated alkalinization of the vagina, which occurs with frequent sexual intercourse or use of douches, plays a role. After normal hydrogen peroxide–producing lactobacilli disappear, it is difficult to reestablish normal vaginal flora, and recurrence of BV is common.

Numerous studies have shown an association of BV with significant adverse sequelae. Women with BV are at increased risk for pelvic inflammatory disease (PID) (6), postabortal PID (7), postoperative cuff infections after hysterectomy (8), and abnormal cervical cytology (9). Pregnant women with BV are at risk for premature rupture of the membranes (10), preterm labor and delivery (10), chorioamnionitis, and postcesarean endometritis (11). It is not known whether screening for, and treatment of, BV will decrease the risk for these adverse sequelae.

Diagnosis

Bacterial vaginosis is diagnosed on the basis of the following findings (12):

1. A fishy vaginal odor, which is particularly noticeable following coitus, and vaginal discharge are present.
2. Vaginal secretions are gray and thinly coat the vaginal walls.
3. The pH of these secretions is higher than 4.5 (usually 4.7 to 5.7).

4. Microscopy of the vaginal secretions reveals an increased number of clue cells, and leukocytes are conspicuously absent. In advanced cases of BV, more than 20% of the epithelial cells are clue cells.

5. The addition of KOH to the vaginal secretions (the "whiff" test) releases a fishy, amine-like odor.

Culture of *G. vaginalis* is not recommended as a diagnostic tool because of its lack of specificity.

Treatment

Ideally, treatment of BV should inhibit anaerobes but not vaginal lactobacilli. The following treatments are effective (13):

1. *Metronidazole,* an antibiotic with excellent activity against anaerobes but poor activity against lactobacilli, is the drug of choice for the treatment of BV. A dose of 500 mg administered orally twice a day for 7 days should be used. Patients should be advised to avoid using alcohol during treatment with oral *metronidazole* and for 24 hours thereafter.

2. *Metronidazole* gel, 0.75%, one applicator (5 g) intravaginally once or twice daily for 5 days, may also be prescribed.

3. An alternative regimen uses a single, 2-g oral dose of *metronidazole.*

The overall cure rates range from 75% to 84% for the above regimens (13).

Clindamycin in the following regimens also is effective:

1. *Clindamycin* cream, 2%, one applicator full (5 g) intravaginally at bedtime for 7 days

2. *Clindamycin,* 300 mg, orally twice daily for 7 days

3. *Clindamycin* ovules, 100 mg, intravaginally once at bedtime for 3 days

Many clinicians prefer intravaginal treatment because of a lack of systemic side effects such as mild-to-moderate gastrointestinal upset and unpleasant taste. Treatment of the male sexual partner has not been shown to improve therapeutic response and therefore is not recommended.

Trichomonal Vaginitis

Trichomonal vaginitis is caused by the sexually transmitted, flagellated parasite, *Trichomonas vaginalis.* The transmission rate is high; 70% of males contract the disease after a single exposure to an infected female, which suggests that the rate of male-to-female transmission is even higher. The parasite is an anaerobe that has the ability to generate hydrogen to combine with oxygen to create an anaerobic environment. It exists only in trophozoite form. Trichomonal vaginitis often accompanies BV, which can be diagnosed in up to 60% of patients with trichomonal vaginitis.

Diagnosis

Local immune factors and inoculum size influence the appearance of symptoms. Symptoms and signs may be much milder in patients with a smaller inoculum of trichomonads, and trichomonal vaginitis often is asymptomatic (14,15).

1. Trichomonal vaginitis is associated with a profuse, purulent, malodorous vaginal discharge that may be accompanied by vulvar pruritus.

2. Vaginal secretions may exude from the vagina.

3. In patients with high concentrations of organisms, a patchy vaginal erythema and colpitis macularis ("strawberry" cervix) may be observed.

4. The pH of the vaginal secretions is usually higher than 5.0.

5. Microscopy of the secretions reveals motile trichomonads and increased numbers of leukocytes.

6. Clue cells may be present because of the common association with BV.

7. The whiff test may also be positive.

Morbidity associated with trichomonal vaginitis may be related to BV. Patients with trichomonal vaginitis are at increased risk for postoperative cuff cellulitis following hysterectomy (8). Pregnant women with trichomonal vaginitis are at increased risk for premature rupture of the membranes and preterm delivery. Because of the sexually transmitted nature of trichomonal vaginitis, women with this infection should be tested for other sexually transmitted diseases (STDs), particularly *Neisseria gonorrhoeae* and *Chlamydia trachomatis*. Serologic testing for syphilis and human immunodeficiency virus (HIV) infection should also be considered.

Treatment

The treatment of trichomonal vaginitis can be summarized as follows:

1. *Metronidazole* is the drug of choice for treatment of vaginal trichomoniasis. Both a single-dose (2 g orally) and a multidose (500 mg twice daily for 7 days) regimen are highly effective and have cure rates of about 95%.

2. The sexual partner should also be treated.

3. *Metronidazole* gel, although highly effective for the treatment of BV, should not be used for the treatment of vaginal trichomoniasis.

4. Women who do not respond to initial therapy should be treated again with *metronidazole,* 500 mg, twice daily for 7 days. If repeated treatment is not effective, the patient should be treated with a single 2-g dose of *metronidazole* once daily for 3 to 5 days.

5. Patients who do not respond to repeated treatment with *metronidazole* and for whom the possibility of reinfection has been excluded should be referred for expert consultation. In these uncommon refractory cases, an important part of management is to obtain cultures of the parasite to determine its susceptibility to *metronidazole.*

Vulvovaginal Candidiasis

It is estimated that as many as 75% of women experience at least one episode of vulvovaginal candidiasis (VVC) during their lifetimes (16). Almost 45% of women will experience two or more episodes (17). Fortunately, few are plagued with a chronic, recurrent infection. *Candida albicans* is responsible for 85% to 90% of vaginal yeast infections. Other species of *Candida,* such as *C. glabrata* and *C. tropicalis,* can cause vulvovaginal symptoms and tend to be resistant to therapy. Candida are dimorphic fungi existing as blastospores, which are responsible for transmission and asymptomatic colonization, and as mycelia, which result from blastospore germination and enhance colonization and facilitate tissue invasion. The extensive areas of pruritus and inflammation often associated with minimal invasion of the lower genital tract epithelial cells suggest that an extracellular toxin or enzyme may play a role in the pathogenesis of this disease. A hypersensitivity phenomenon also may be responsible for the irritative symptoms associated with VVC, especially for patients with chronic, recurrent disease. Patients with symptomatic disease usually have an increased concentration of these microorganisms ($>10^4$/mL) compared with asymptomatic patients ($<10^3$/mL) (18).

Factors that predispose women to the development of symptomatic VVC include antibiotic use (19,20), pregnancy (21), and diabetes (22). Through a mechanism referred to as *colonization resistance,* lactobacilli prevent the overgrowth of the opportunistic fungi. Antibiotic use disturbs the normal vaginal flora, decreasing the concentration of lactobacilli and other normal flora, and thus allowing an overgrowth of fungi. Pregnancy and diabetes are both associated with a qualitative decrease in cell-mediated immunity, leading to a higher incidence of candidiasis.

Diagnosis

The symptoms of VVC consist of vulvar pruritus associated with a vaginal discharge that typically resembles cottage cheese.

1. The discharge can vary from watery to homogeneously thick. Vaginal soreness, dyspareunia, vulvar burning, and irritation may be present. External dysuria ("splash" dysuria) may occur when micturition leads to exposure of the inflamed vulvar and vestibular epithelium to urine. Examination reveals erythema and edema of the labia and vulvar skin. There may be discrete pustulopapular peripheral lesions. The vagina may be erythematous with an adherent, whitish discharge. The cervix appears normal.

2. The pH of the vagina in patients with VVC is usually normal (4,5).

3. Fungal elements, either budding yeast forms or mycelia, appear within as many as 80% of cases. The results of saline preparation of the vaginal secretions usually are normal, although there may be a slight increase in the number of inflammatory cells in severe cases.

4. The whiff test is negative.

5. A presumptive diagnosis can be made in the absence of microscopy-proven fungal elements if the pH and the results of the saline preparation are normal. A fungal culture is recommended to confirm the diagnosis.

Treatment

1. Topically applied azole drugs are the most commonly available treatment for VVC and are more effective than *nystatin* (13) (Table 15.1). Treatment with azoles results in relief of symptoms and negative cultures among 80% to 90% of patients who have completed therapy. Symptoms usually take 2 to 3 days to resolve. There is a trend to shorten the duration of therapy to 1 to 3 days. Although the shorter period of therapy implies a shortened duration of treatment, because the short-course formulations have higher concentrations of the antifungal agent, they cause an inhibitory concentration in the vagina that persists for several days.

2. An oral antifungal agent, *fluconazole,* used in a single 150-mg dose, has been approved for the treatment of VVC. It appears to have equal efficacy when compared with topical azoles in the treatment of mild-to-moderate VVC (23). Patients should be advised that their symptoms will not disappear for 2 to 3 days so that

Table 15.1. Vulvovaginal Candidiasis—Topical Treatment Regimens

Butoconazole
2% cream, 5 g intravaginally for 3 days*†
2% cream, 5 g BI-BSR, single intravaginal application*
Clotrimazole
1% cream, 5 g intravaginally for 7–14 days*†
100-mg vaginal tablet for 7 days*†
100-mg vaginal tablet, two tablets for 3 days*
500-mg vaginal tablet, single dose*
Miconazole
2% cream, 5 g intravaginally for 7 days*†
200-mg vaginal suppository for 3 days*
100-mg vaginal suppository for 7 days*†
Nystatin
100,000-Units vaginal tablet, one tablet for 14 days
Ticonazole
6.5% ointment, 5 g intravaginally, single dose*
Terconazole
0.4% cream, 5 g intravaginally for 7 days*
0.8% cream, 5 g intravaginally for 3 days*
80-mg suppository for 3 days*

* Oil-based, may weaken latex condoms.
† Available as over-the-counter preparation.
From **Centers for Disease Control and Prevention.** *The sexually transmitted diseases treatment guidelines.* Washington, DC: Centers for Disease Control and Prevention. 2002, with permission.

they will not expect additional treatment. Patients with severe symptoms may benefit from an additional 150-mg dose given 72 hours after the first dose.

3. Adjunctive treatment with a weak topical steroid, such as 1% *hydrocortisone* cream, may be helpful in relieving some of the external irritative symptoms.

Chronic Vulvovaginal Candidiasis

A small number of women develop chronic recurrent VVC. These women experience persistent irritative symptoms of the vestibule and vulva. Burning replaces itching as the prominent symptom in patients with chronic VVC. The diagnosis should be confirmed by direct microscopy of the vaginal secretions and by fungal culture. **Many women with chronic vaginitis presume that they have a chronic yeast infection when this is not the case. Many of these patients have chronic atopic dermatitis or atrophic vulvovaginitis.**

The treatment of patients with chronic VVC consists of inducing a remission of chronic symptoms with *ketoconazole* (400 mg/day) or *fluconazole* (150 mg/3 days) until symptoms resolve. Patients should then be maintained on prophylactic doses of these agents (*ketoconazole,* 100 mg/d; *fluconazole,* 150 mg weekly) for 6 months (24).

Inflammatory Vaginitis

Desquamative inflammatory vaginitis is a clinical syndrome characterized by diffuse exudative vaginitis, epithelial cell exfoliation, and a profuse purulent vaginal discharge (25). The cause of inflammatory vaginitis is unknown, but Gram stain findings reveal a relative absence of normal long gram-positive bacilli (lactobacilli) and their replacement with gram-positive cocci, usually streptococci. Women with this disorder have a purulent vaginal discharge, vulvovaginal burning or irritation, and dyspareunia. A less frequent complaint is vulvar pruritus. Vaginal erythema is present, and there may be an associated vulvar erythema, vulvovaginal ecchymotic spots, and colpitis macularis. The pH of the vaginal secretions is uniformly higher than 4.5 in these patients.

Initial therapy is the use of 2% *clindamycin* cream, one applicator full (5 g) intravaginally once daily for 7 days. Relapse occurs in about 30% of patients, who should be retreated with intravaginal 2% *clindamycin* cream for 2 weeks. When relapse occurs in postmenopausal patients, supplementary hormonal replacement therapy should be considered.

Atrophic Vaginitis

Estrogen plays an important role in the maintenance of normal vaginal ecology. Women undergoing menopause, either occurring naturally or secondary to surgical removal of the ovaries, may develop inflammatory vaginitis, which may be accompanied by an increased, purulent vaginal discharge. In addition, they may note dyspareunia and postcoital bleeding resulting from atrophy of the vaginal and vulvar epithelium. Examination reveals atrophy of the external genitalia, along with a loss of the vaginal rugae. The vaginal mucosa may be somewhat friable in areas. Microscopy of the vaginal secretions shows a predominance of parabasal epithelial cells and an increased number of leukocytes.

Atropic vaginitis is treated with topical estrogen vaginal cream. Use of 1 g of *conjugated estrogen cream* intravaginally each day for 1 to 2 weeks generally provides relief. Systemic estrogen replacement therapy should be considered to prevent recurrence of this disorder.

Cervicitis

The cervix is made up of two different types of epithelial cells: squamous epithelium and glandular epithelium. The cause of cervical inflammation depends on the epithelium affected. The ectocervical epithelium can become inflamed by the same microorganisms that are responsible for vaginitis. In fact, the ectocervical squamous epithelium is an extension of and is continuous with the vaginal epithelium. Trichomonas, candida, and herpes simplex virus (HSV) can cause inflammation of the ectocervix. Conversely, *N. gonorrhoeae* and *C. trachomatis* infect only the glandular epithelium and are responsible for mucopurulent endocervicitis (MPC) (26).

Diagnosis

The diagnosis of MPC is based on the finding of a purulent endocervical discharge, generally yellow or green in color and referred to as "mucopus" (27).

1. After removal of ectocervical secretions with a large swab, a small cotton swab is placed into the endocervical canal and the cervical mucus is extracted. The cotton swab is inspected against a white or black background to detect the green or yellow color of the mucopus. In addition, edema, erythema, and friability of the zone of ectopy (glandular epithelium) are present. Although edema and erythema of the endocervix can be difficult to distinguish, friability or easily induced bleeding can be assessed by touching the ectropion with a cotton swab or spatulum.

2. Placement of the mucopus on a slide that can be Gram stained will reveal the presence of an increased number of neutrophils (>30 per high-power field). The presence of intracellular gram-negative diplococci, leading to the presumptive diagnosis of gonococcal endocervicitis, also may be detected. If the Gram stain results are negative for gonococci, the presumptive diagnosis is chlamydial MPC.

3. Tests for both gonorrhea (culture on Thayer-Martin media or polymerase chain reaction [PCR]) and chlamydia (cell culture, enzyme-linked immunosorbent assay [ELISA], chlamydiazyme, direct fluorescent antibody [MicroTrak], or PCR) should be performed. The microbial etiology of endocervicitis is unknown in about 50% of cases in which gonococci or chlamydia are not detected.

Table 15.2. Treatment Regimens for Gonococcal and Chlamydial Infections

***Neisseria gonorrhoeae* endocervicitis**
Cefixime, 400 mg orally (single dose), *or* *Ceftriaxone,* 125 mg intramuscularly (single dose), *or* *Ciprofloxacin,* 500 mg orally (single dose)*, *or* *Ofloxacin,* 400 mg orally (single dose)*, *or* levofloxacin 250 mg orally in a single dose (quinolones should not be used for infections acquired in Asia or the Pacific, including Hawaii)
***Chlamydia trachomatis* endocervicitis**
Azithromycin, 1 g orally (single dose), *or* *Doxycycline,* 100 mg orally twice daily for 7 days, *or* *Ofloxacin,* 300 mg orally twice daily for 7 days, *or* levofloxacin, 500 mg orally for 7 days *Erythromycin* base, 500 mg orally 4 times a day for 7 days, *or* *Erythromycin ethylsuccinate,* 800 mg orally 4 times a day for 7 days

From **Centers for Disease Control and Prevention.** *The sexually transmitted diseases treatment guidelines.* Washington, DC: Centers for Disease Control and Prevention, 2002, with permission.

Treatment of MPC consists of an antibiotic regimen recommended for the treatment of uncomplicated lower genital tract infection with both chlamydia and gonorrhea (13) (Table 15.2). It is imperative that all sexual partners be treated with a similar antibiotic regimen. MPC is commonly associated with BV, which, if not treated concurrently, leads to a significant persistence of the symptoms and signs of MPC.

Pelvic Inflammatory Disease

PID is caused by microorganisms colonizing the endocervix ascending to the endometrium and fallopian tubes. PID is a clinical diagnosis implying that the patient has upper genital tract infection and inflammation. The inflammation may be present at any point along a continuum that includes endometritis, salpingitis, and peritonitis (Fig. 15.1).

PID commonly is caused by the sexually transmitted microorganisms *N. gonorrhoeae* and *C. trachomatis* (28–30). Endogenous microorganisms found in the vagina, particularly the BV microorganisms, also often are isolated from the upper genital tract of women with PID. The BV microorganisms include anaerobic bacteria such as *Prevotella* and peptostreptococci as well as *G. vaginalis*. BV often occurs in women with PID, and the resultant complex alteration of vaginal flora may facilitate the ascending spread of pathogenic bacteria by enzymatically altering the cervical mucus barrier (31). Less frequently, respiratory pathogens such as *Haemophilus influenzae,* group A streptococci, and pneumococci can colonize the lower genital tract and cause PID.

Diagnosis

Traditionally, the diagnosis of PID has been based on a triad of symptoms and signs, including pelvic pain, cervical motion and adnexal tenderness, and the presence of fever. It is now recognized that there is wide variation in many symptoms and signs among women with this condition, which makes the diagnosis of acute PID difficult. Many women with PID exhibit subtle or mild symptoms that are not readily recognized as PID. Consequently, delay in diagnosis and therapy probably contributes to the inflammatory sequelae in the upper reproductive tract (32).

In the diagnosis of PID, the goal is to establish guidelines that are sufficiently sensitive to avoid missing mild cases but sufficiently specific to avoid giving antibiotic therapy to women who are not infected. Genitourinary tract symptoms may indicate PID; therefore, the diagnosis of PID should be considered in women with any genitourinary symptoms, including, but not limited to, lower abdominal pain, excessive vaginal discharge, menorrhagia,

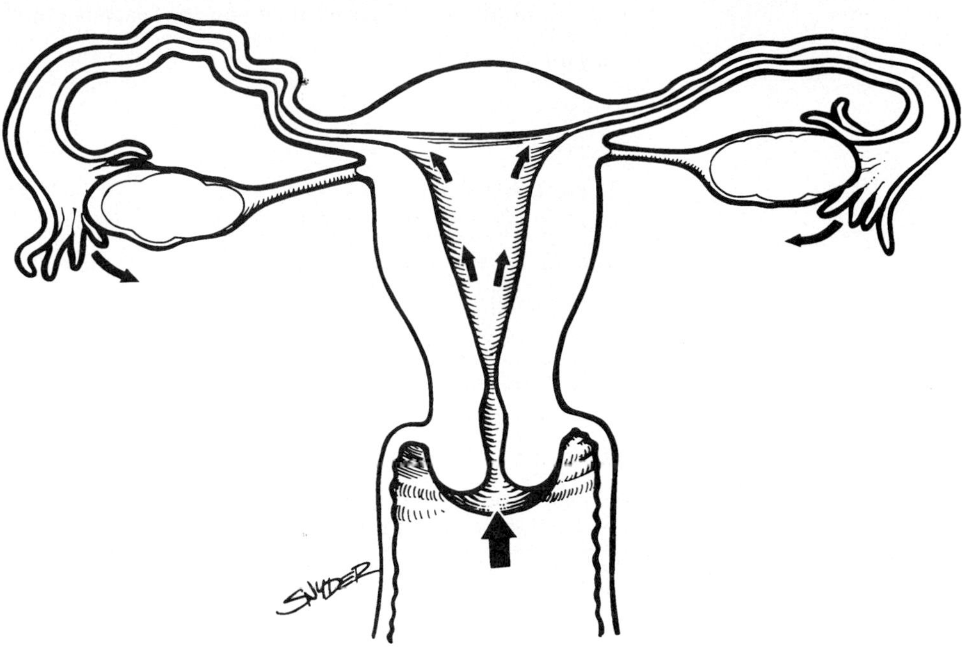

Figure 15.1 Microorganisms originating in the endocervix ascend into the endometrium, fallopian tubes, and peritoneum, causing pelvic inflammatory disease (endometritis, salpingitis, peritonitis). (From **Soper DE.** Upper genital tract infections. In: **Copeland LJ,** ed. *Textbook of gynecology.* Philadelphia: WB Saunders, 1993:521.)

metrorrhagia, fever, chills, and urinary symptoms (33). **Some women may develop PID without having any symptoms.**

Pelvic organ tenderness, either uterine tenderness alone or uterine tenderness with adnexal tenderness, is present in patients with PID. Cervical motion tenderness suggests the presence of peritoneal inflammation, which causes pain when the peritoneum is stretched by moving the cervix and causing traction of the adnexa on the pelvic peritoneum. Direct or rebound abdominal tenderness may be present.

Evaluation of lower genital tract secretions, both vaginal and endocervical, is a crucial part of the workup of a patient with PID (34). In women with PID, an increased number of polymorphonuclear leukocytes may be detected in a wet mount of the vaginal secretions or in the mucopurulent discharge.

More elaborate tests may be used in women with severe symptoms because an incorrect diagnosis may cause unnecessary morbidity (35) (Table 15.3). These tests include endometrial biopsy to confirm the presence of endometritis, ultrasound or radiologic tests to characterize a tuboovarian abscess (TOA), and laparoscopy to confirm salpingitis visually.

Treatment

Therapy regimens for PID must provide empirical, broad-spectrum coverage of likely pathogens (13,36), including *N. gonorrhoeae, C. trachomatis,* gram-negative facultative bacteria, anaerobes, and streptococci. Recommended regimens for the treatment of PID are listed in Table 15.4. Hospitalization is recommended, especially when the diagnosis is uncertain, pelvic abscess is suspected, clinical disease is severe, or compliance with an outpatient regimen is in question. Hospitalized patients can be considered for discharge when their fever has lysed (<99.5°F for more than 24 hours), the white blood cell count has become normal, rebound tenderness is absent, and repeat examination shows marked amelioration of pelvic organ tenderness (37).

Table 15.3. Clinical Criteria for the Diagnosis of Pelvic Inflammatory Disease

Symptoms
None necessary
Signs
Pelvic organ tenderness Leukorrhea and/or mucopurulent endocervicitis
Additional criteria to increase the specificity of the diagnosis
Endometrial biopsy showing endometritis Elevated C-reactive protein or erythrocyte sedimentation rate Temperature higher than 38°C Leukocytosis Positive test for gonorrhea or chlamydia
Elaborate criteria
Ultrasound documenting tuboovarian abscess Laparoscopy visually confirming salpingitis

Table 15.4. CDC Guidelines for Treatment of Pelvic Inflammatory Disease

Outpatient Treatment
Regimen A
Ofloxacin, 400 mg orally 2 times daily for 14 days, or *Levofloxacin,* 500 mg orally once daily for 14 days *With or Without:* *Metronidazole,* 500 mg orally 2 times daily for 14 days
Regimen B
Cefoxitin, 2 g intramuscularly, plus *probenecid,* 1 g orally concurrently, or *Ceftriaxone,* 250 mg intramuscularly, or Equivalent cephalosporin *Plus:* *Doxycycline,* 100 mg orally 2 times daily for 14 days *With or Without:* *Metronidazole,* 500 mg orally twice a day for 14 days
Inpatient Treatment
Regimen A
Cefoxitin, 2 g intravenously every 6 hours, *or* *Cefotetan,* 2 g intravenously every 12 hours, *Plus:* *Doxycycline,* 100 mg orally or intravenously every 12 hours
Regimen B
Clindamycin, 900 mg intravenously every 8 hours *Plus:* *Gentamicin,* loading dose intravenously or intramuscularly (2 mg/kg of body weight) followed by a maintenance dose (1.5 mg/kg) every 8 hours

From **Centers for Disease Control and Prevention.** *The sexually transmitted diseases treatment guidelines.* Washington, DC: Centers for Disease Control and Prevention, 2001, with permission.

Sexual partners of women with PID should be evaluated and treated for urethral infection with chlamydia or gonorrhea (Table 15.2). Urethral tests from male sexual partners of women with nongonococcal, nonchlamydial PID commonly reveals the presence of one of these STDs (38,39).

Tuboovarian Abscess

TOA is an end-stage process of acute PID. TOA is diagnosed when a patient with PID has a pelvic mass that is palpable during bimanual examination. The condition usually reflects an agglutination of pelvic organs (tube, ovary, bowel) forming a palpable complex. Occasionally, an ovarian abscess can result from the entrance of microorganisms through an ovulatory site. **Treatment of TOA involves the use of an antibiotic regimen administered in a hospital** (Table 15.4). **About 75% of women with TOA respond to antimicrobial therapy alone. Failure of medical therapy suggests the need for drainage of the abscess** (40). Although this may require surgical exploration, percutaneous drainage guided by imaging studies (ultrasound or computed tomography scan) has been used successfully.

Other Major Infections

Genital Ulcer Disease

In the United States, most patients with genital ulcers have genital HSV or syphilis (41–43). Chancroid is the next most common cause of sexually transmitted genital ulcers, followed by the rare occurrence of lymphogranuloma venereum (LGV) and granuloma inguinale (donovanosis). These diseases are associated with an increased risk for HIV infection. Other infrequent and noninfectious causes of genital ulcers include abrasions, fixed drug eruptions, carcinoma, and Behçet's disease.

Diagnosis

A diagnosis based on history and physical examination often is inaccurate. Therefore, evaluation of all women with genital ulcers should include a serologic test for syphilis (43). Because of the consequences of inappropriate therapy, such as tertiary disease and congenital syphilis in pregnant women, diagnostic efforts are directed at excluding syphilis. An optimal workup of the patient with a genital ulcer includes the performance of a dark-field examination or direct immunofluorescence test for *Treponema pallidum,* culture or antigen test for HSV, and culture for *Haemophilus ducreyi.* Dark-field or fluorescent microscopes and selective media to culture for *H. ducreyi* are often not available in most offices and clinics. Even after complete testing, the diagnosis remains unconfirmed in one fourth of patients with genital ulcers. For this reason, most clinicians base their initial diagnosis and treatment recommendations on their clinical impression of the appearance of the genital ulcer (Fig. 15.2) and knowledge of the most likely cause in their patient population (42).

Several clinical presentations are highly suggestive of specific diagnoses:

1. **A nonpainful and minimally tender ulcer, not accompanied by inguinal lymphadenopathy, is likely to be syphilis, especially if the ulcer is indurated.** A nontreponemal rapid plasma reagin (RPR) test, or venereal disease research laboratory (VDRL) test, and a confirmatory treponemal test—fluorescent treponemal antibody absorption (FTA ABS) or microhemagglutinin–*T. pallidum* (MHA TP), should be used to diagnose syphilis presumptively. The results of nontreponemal tests usually correlate with disease activity and should be reported quantitatively.

2. **Grouped vesicles mixed with small ulcers, particularly with a history of such lesions, are almost pathognomonic of genital herpes.** Nevertheless, laboratory confirmation of the diagnosis is recommended because the diagnosis of genital herpes is traumatic for many women, alters their self-image, and affects their perceived ability to enter new sexual relationships and bear children. Culture is the most sensitive and specific test; sensitivity approaches 100% in the vesicle stage and 89% in the pustular stage and drops to as low as 33% in patients with ulcers. Nonculture tests are about 80% as sensitive as culture.

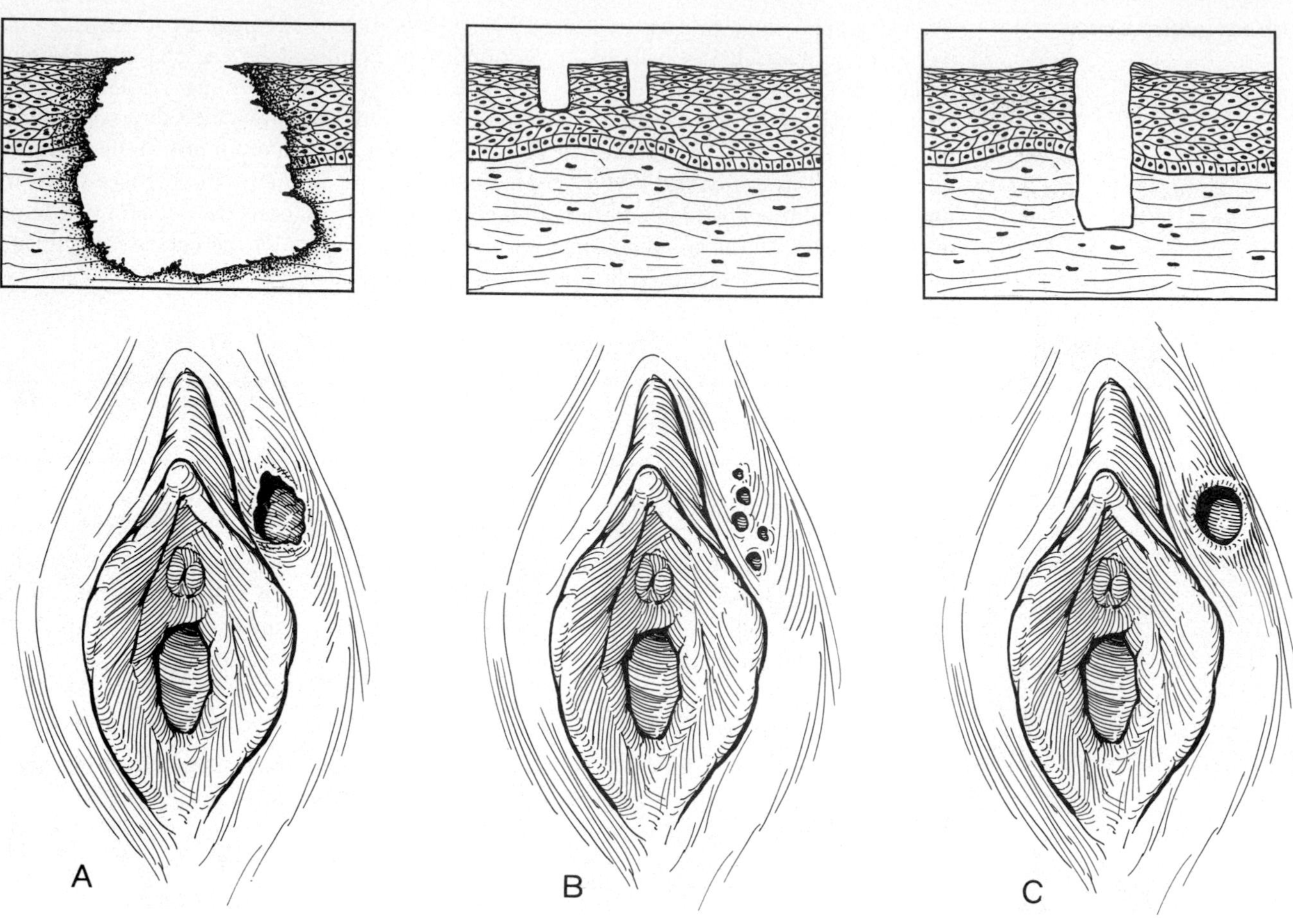

Figure 15.2 Showing the appearance of the ulcers of chancroid (A), herpes (B), and syphilis (C). The ulcer of chancroid has irregular margins and is deep with undermined edges. The syphilis ulcer has a smooth, indurated border and a smooth base. The genital herpes ulcer is superficial and inflamed. (Modified from **Schmid GP, Shcalla WO, DeWitt WE.** Chancroid. In: **Morse SA, Moreland AA, Thompson SE,** eds. *Atlas of sexually transmitted diseases.* Philadelphia: JB Lippincott, 1990.)

Because false-negative results are common with HSV cultures, especially in patients with recurrent infections, type-specific serologic tests (type-specific glycoprotein G-based antibody assay) are useful in confirming a clinical diagnosis of genital herpes.

3. **One to three extremely painful ulcers, accompanied by tender inguinal lymphadenopathy, are unlikely to be anything except chancroid.** This is especially true if the adenopathy is fluctuant.

4. **An inguinal bubo accompanied by one or several ulcers is most likely chancroid. If there is no ulcer, the most likely diagnosis is LGV.**

Treatment

Chancroid Recommended regimens for the treatment of chancroid include *azithromycin,* 1 g orally in a single dose; *ceftriaxone,* 250 mg intramuscularly in a single dose; *ciprofloxacin,* 500 mg orally twice a day for 3 days; or *erythromycin* base, 500 mg orally 4 times daily for 7 days. Patients should be reexamined 3 to 7 days after initiation of therapy to ensure the gradual resolution of the genital ulcer, which can be expected to heal within 2 weeks unless it is unusually large.

Herpes A first episode of genital herpes should be treated with acyclovir, 400 mg orally three times a day; or *famciclovir,* 250 mg orally three times a day; or *valacyclovir,* 1.0 orally twice a day for 7 to 10 days or until clinical resolution is attained. Although these agents provide partial control of the symptoms and signs of clinical herpes, it neither eradicates latent virus nor affects subsequent risk, frequency, or severity of recurrences after the drug is discontinued. Daily suppressive therapy (*acyclovir,* 400 mg orally twice daily; or *famciclovir,* 250 mg twice daily; or *valacyclovir,* 1.0 g orally once a day) reduces the frequency of HSV recurrences by at least 75% among patients with six or more recurrences of HSV per year. Suppressive treatment does not totally eliminate symptomatic or asymptomatic viral shedding or the potential for transmission.

Syphilis **Parenteral *penicillin G* administration is the preferred treatment of all stages of syphilis.** *Benzathine penicillin G,* 2.4 million units intramuscularly in a single dose, is the recommended treatment for adults with primary, secondary, or early latent syphilis. The Jarisch-Herxheimer reaction is an acute febrile reaction accompanied by headache, myalgia, and other symptoms—that may occur within the first 24 hours after any therapy for syphilis; patients should be advised of this possible adverse reaction.

Latent syphilis is defined as those periods after infection with *T. pallidum* when patients are seroreactive but show no other evidence of disease. Patients with latent syphilis of longer than 1 year's duration or of unknown duration should be treated with *benzathine penicillin G,* 7.2 million units total, administered as three doses of 2.4 million units intramuscularly each, at 1-week intervals. All patients with latent syphilis should be evaluated clinically for evidence of tertiary disease (e.g., aortitis, neurosyphilis, gumma, and iritis). Quantitative nontreponemal serologic tests should be repeated at 6 months and again at 12 months. An initially high titer (1:32) should decline at least fourfold (two dilutions) within 12 to 24 months.

Genital Warts

External genital warts (EGWs) are a manifestation of human papillomavirus (HPV) infection (44). The nononcogenic HPV types 6 and 11 are usually responsible for EGWs. The warts tend to occur in areas most directly affected by coitus, namely the posterior fourchette and lateral areas on the vulva. Less frequently, warts can be found throughout the vulva, in the vagina, and on the cervix. Minor trauma associated with coitus can cause breaks in the vulvar skin, allowing direct contact between the viral particles from an infected male and the basal layer of the epidermis of his susceptible sexual partner. Infection may be latent or may cause viral particles to replicate and produce a wart. EGWs are highly contagious; more than 75% of sexual partners develop this manifestation of HPV infection when exposed.

The goal of treatment is removal of the warts; it is not possible to eradicate the viral infection. Treatment is most successful in patients with small warts that have been present for less than 1 year. It has not been determined whether treatment of EGWs reduces transmission of HPV. Selection of a specific treatment regimen depends on the anatomic site, size, and number of warts, as well as expense, efficacy, convenience, and potential adverse effects (Table 15.5). Recurrences more often result from reactivation of subclinical infection than reinfection by a sex partner; therefore, examination of sex partners is not absolutely necessary. However, many of these sex partners may have EGWs and may benefit from therapy and counseling concerning transmission of warts.

Human Immunodeficiency Virus

It is estimated that almost 20% of individuals with HIV are women. Intravenous drug use and heterosexual transmission each are responsible for about 40% of acquired immunodeficiency syndrome (AIDS) cases in women in the United States (45). Infection with HIV produces a spectrum of disease that progresses from an asymptomatic state to

Table 15.5. Treatment Options for External Genital and Perianal Warts

Modality (%)	*Efficacy (%)*	*Recurrence Risk*
Cryotherapy	63–88	21–39
Imiquimod 5% cream*	33–72	13–19
Podophyllin 10%–25%	32–79	27–65
Podofilox 0.5%*	45–88	33–60
Triochloroacetic acid 80%–90%	81	36
Electrodesiccation or cautery	94	22
Laser†	43–93	29–95
Interferon	44–61	0–67

* May be self-applied by patients at home.
† Expensive; reserve for patients who have not responded to other regimens.

full-blown AIDS. The pace of disease progression in untreated adults is variable. The median time between infection with HIV and the development of AIDS is 10 years, with a range from a few months to more than 12 years. In a study of adults infected with HIV, symptoms developed in 70% to 85% of infected adults, and AIDS developed in 55% to 60% within 12 years after infection. The natural history of the disease can be significantly altered by antiretroviral therapy. Women with HIV-induced altered immune function are at increased risk for infections such as tuberculosis (TB), bacterial pneumonia, and *Pneumocystis carinii* pneumonia (PCP). Because of its impact on the immune system, HIV affects the diagnosis, evaluation, treatment, and follow-up of many other diseases and may decrease the efficacy of antimicrobial therapy for some STDs.

Diagnosis

Infection is most often diagnosed by HIV type 1 antibody tests. Antibody testing begins with a sensitive screening test such as ELISA or a rapid assay. If confirmed by Western blot or other supplemental testing, a positive antibody test result means a person is infected with HIV and is capable of transmitting the virus to others. HIV antibody is detectable in more than 95% of patients within 6 months of infection. Women diagnosed with any STD, particularly genital ulcer disease, should be offered HIV testing (42). Women at risk for STD, such as those with multiple sexual partners or whose partners have multiple sexual partners, should be offered HIV testing.

The initial evaluation of an HIV-positive woman includes screening for diseases associated with HIV such as TB and STDs, administration of recommended vaccinations (hepatitis B, pneumococcal, and influenza), and behavioral and psychosocial counseling. Intraepithelial neoplasia is strongly associated with HPV infection and has been found to occur in high frequency in women co-infected with HPV and HIV.

Treatment

Decisions regarding the initiation of antiretroviral therapy should be guided by monitoring the laboratory parameters of HIV RNA (viral load) and $CD4^+$ T–cell count, as well as the clinical condition of the patient. The primary goals of antiretroviral therapy are maximal and durable suppression of viral load, restoration or preservation of immunologic function, improvement of quality of life, and reduction of HIV-related morbidity and mortality. For the most part, women with acute retroviral syndrome, those within 6 months of HIV seroconversion, and all symptomatic patients should be offered treatment. In addition, treatment should be offered to those women with fewer than 350 $CD4^+$ T cells or plasma HIV RNA levels exceeding 30,000 copies/mL (bDNA assay). Patients must be willing to accept therapy to avoid the emergence of resistance due to poor compliance. It has been shown that dual nucleoside regimens plus a protease inhibitor provide a better durable clinical benefit than monotherapy.

In addition, patients with less than 200 $CD4^+$ T cells/μL should receive prophylaxis against opportunistic infections such as trimethoprim-sulfamethoxazole or aerosol pentamidine for the prevention of PCP pneumonia.

Urinary Tract Infection

Acute Cystitis

Women with acute cystitis generally have an abrupt onset of multiple, severe urinary tract symptoms including dysuria, frequency, and urgency associated with suprapubic or low back pain. Suprapubic tenderness may be noted on physical examination. Urinalysis reveals pyuria and sometimes hematuria. Several factors increase the risk for cystitis, including sexual intercourse, the use of a diaphragm and a spermicide, delayed postcoital micturition, and a history of a recent urinary tract infection (47–49).

Esherichia coli is the most common pathogen isolated from the urine of young women with acute cystitis, and it is present in 80% of cases (50). *Staphylococcus saprophyticus* is present in an additional 5% to 15% of patients with cystitis. The pathophysiology of cystitis in women involves the colonization of the vagina and urethra with coliform bacteria from the rectum. For this reason, the effects of an antimicrobial agent on the vaginal flora play a role in the eradication of bacteriuria.

Treatment

High concentrations of *trimethoprim* and the fluoroquinolones in vaginal secretions result in eradicating *E. coli* but minimally altering normal anaerobic and microaerophilic vaginal flora. An increasing linear trend in the prevalence of resistance among *E. coli* (9% to 18%) to *trimethoprim* and *trimethoprim-sulfamethoxazole* has been noted. In contrast, no such increase in resistance was noted with *nitrofurantoin* and *ciprofloxacin. Nitrofurantoin* (macrocrystals, 100 mg orally twice daily for 7 days) or a *fluoroquinolone* (*ciprofloxacin,* 250 mg orally twice daily for 3 days) are the optimal choices for empirical 3-day therapy for uncomplicated cystitis (51).

In patients with typical symptoms, an abbreviated laboratory workup followed by empirical therapy is suggested. The diagnosis can be presumed if pyuria is detected by microscopy or leukocyte esterase testing. Urine culture is not necessary, and a short course of antimicrobial therapy should be given. No follow-up visit or culture is necessary unless symptoms persist or recur.

Recurrent Cystitis

About 20% of premenopausal women with an initial episode of cystitis have recurrent infections. More than 90% of these recurrences are caused by exogenous reinfection. Recurrent cystitis should be documented by culture to rule out resistant microorganisms. Patients may be treated by one of three strategies: (a) continuous prophylaxis, (b) postcoital prophylaxis, or (c) therapy initiated by the patient when symptoms are first noted.

Postmenopausal women may also have frequent reinfections. Hormonal replacement therapy or topically applied estrogen cream, along with antimicrobial prophylaxis, is helpful in treating these patients.

Urethritis

Women with dysuria caused by urethritis have a more gradual onset of mild symptoms, which may be associated with abnormal vaginal discharge or bleeding related to concurrent cervicitis. Patients may also have a new sex partner or experience lower abdominal pain. Physical examination may reveal the presence of mucopurulent cervicitis or vulvovaginal herpetic lesions. *C. trachomatis, N. gonorrhoeae,* or genital herpes may cause acute urethritis. Pyuria is present on urinalysis, but hematuria is rarely seen. Treatment regimens for chlamydia and gonococcal infections are presented in Table 15.2.

Occasionally, vaginitis caused by *C. albicans* or trichomonas is associated with dysuria. On careful questioning, patients generally describe external dysuria, sometimes associated with vaginal discharge, and pruritus and dyspareunia. They usually do not experience urgency or frequency. Pyuria and hematuria are absent.

Acute Pyelonephritis

The clinical spectrum of acute, uncomplicated pyelonephritis in young women ranges from gram-negative septicemia to a cystitis-like illness with mild flank pain. *E. coli* accounts for more than 80% of these cases. Microscopy of unspun urine reveals pyuria and gram-negative bacteria. A urine culture should be obtained in all women with suspected pyelonephritis; blood cultures should be performed in those who are hospitalized because results are positive in 15% to 20% of cases. In the absence of nausea and vomiting and severe illness, outpatient oral therapy can be given safely. Patients who have nausea and vomiting, are moderately to severely ill, and are pregnant should be hospitalized. Outpatient treatment regimens include *trimethoprim-sulfamethoxazole* (160 to 800 mg every 12 hours) or a quinolone (e.g., *ofloxacin,* 200 to 300 mg every 12 hours) for 10 to 14 days. Inpatient treatment regimens include the use of parenteral *ceftriaxone* (1 to 2 g daily), *ampicillin* (1 g every 6 hours), and *gentamicin* (especially if *Enterococcus* species are suspected) or *aztreonam* (1 g every 8 to 12 hours). Symptoms should resolve after 48 to 72 hours. If fever and flank pain persist after 72 hours of therapy, ultrasound or computed tomography should be considered to rule out a perinephric or intrarenal abscess or ureteral obstruction. A follow-up culture should be obtained 2 weeks after the completion of therapy.

References

1. **Huggins GR, Preti G.** Vaginal odors and secretions. *Clin Obstet Gynecol* 1981;24:355–377.
2. **Larsen B.** Microbiology of the female genital tract. In: **Pastorek J,** ed. *Obstetric and gynecologic infectious disease.* New York: Raven Press, 1994:11–26.
3. **Eschenbach DA, Davick PR, Williams BL, et al.** Prevalence of hydrogen peroxide-producing Lactobacillus species in normal women and women with vaginal vaginosis. *J Clin Microbiol* 1989;27:251–256.
4. **Spiegel CA, Amsel R, Eschenbach DA, et al.** Anaerobic bacteria in nonspecific vaginitis. *N Engl J Med* 1980;303:601–607.
5. **Kent HL.** Epidemiology of vaginitis. *Am J Obstet Gynecol* 1991;165:1168–1176.
6. **Eschenbach DA, Hillier S, Critchlow C, et al.** Diagnosis and clinical manifestations of bacterial vaginosis. *Am J Obstet Gynecol* 1988;158:819–828.
7. **Larsson P, Platz-Christensen JJ, Thejls H, et al.** Incidence of pelvic inflammatory disease after first trimester legal abortion in women with bacterial vaginosis after treatment with metronidazole: a double-blind randomized study. *Am J Obstet Gynecol* 1992;166:100–103.
8. **Soper DE, Bump RC, Hurt WG.** Bacterial vaginosis and trichomoniasis vaginitis are risk factors for cuff cellulitis after abdominal hysterectomy. *Am J Obstet Gynecol* 1990;163:1016–1023.
9. **Platz-Christensen JJ, Sundstrom E, Larsson PG.** Bacterial vaginosis and cervical intraepithelial neoplasia. *Acta Obstet Gynecol Scand* 1994;73:586–588.
10. **Martius J, Eschenbach DA.** The role of bacterial vaginosis as a cause of amniotic fluid infection, chorioamnionitis and prematurity: a review. *Arch Gynecol Obstet* 1900;247:1–13.
11. **Watts DH, Krohn MA, Hillier SL, et al.** Bacterial vaginosis as a risk factor for postcesarean endometritis. *Obstet Gynecol* 1990;75:52–58.
12. **Amsel R, Totten PA, Spiegel CA, et al.** Nonspecific vaginitis: diagnostic criteria and microbial and epidemiologic associations. *Am J Med* 1983;74:14–22.
13. **Centers for Disease Control.** *The sexually transmitted diseases treatment guidelines.* Washington, DC: Centers for Disease Control, 2002.
14. **Wolner-Hanssen P, Krieger JN, Stevens CE, et al.** Clinical manifestations of vaginal trichomoniasis. *JAMA* 1989;261:571–576.
15. **Krieger JN, Tam MR, Stevens CE, et al.** Diagnosis of trichomoniasis: comparison of conventional wet-mount examination with cytologic studies, cultures, and monoclonal antibody staining of direct specimens. *JAMA* 1988;259:1223–1227.
16. **Hurley R, De Louvois J.** Candida vaginitis. *Postgrad Med J* 1979;55:645–647.
17. **Hurley R.** Recurrent Candida infection. *Clin Obstet Gynecol* 1981;8:208–213.

18. **Sobel JD, Faro S, Force RW, et al.** Vulvovaginal candidiasis: epidemiologic, diagnostic, and therapeutic considerations. *Am J Obstet Gynecol* 1998;178:203–211.

19. **Caruso LJ.** Vaginal moniliasisis after tetracycline therapy. *Am J Obstet Gynecol* 1964;90:374.

20. **Oriel JD, Waterworth PM.** Effect of minocycline and tetracycline on the vaginal yeast flora. *J Clin Pathol* 1975;28:403.

21. **Morton RS, Rashid S.** Candidal vaginitis: natural history, predisposing factors and prevention. *Proc R Soc Med* 1977;70(Suppl 4):3–12.

22. **Odds FC.** *Candida and candidiasis.* Baltimore: University Park Press, 1979:104–110.

23. **Brammer KW.** Treatment of vaginal candidiasis with a single oral dose of fluconazole. *Eur J Clin Microbiol Infect Dis* 1988;7:364–367.

24. **Sobel JD.** Management of recurrent vulvovaginal candidiasis with intermittent ketoconazole prophylaxis. *Obstet Gynecol* 1985;65:435–460.

25. **Sobel JD.** Desquamative inflammatory vaginitis: a new subgroup of purulent vaginitis responsive to topical 2% clindamycin therapy. *Am J Obstet Gynecol* 1994;171:1215–1220.

26. **Kiviat NB, Paavonen JA, Wolner-Hanssen P, et al.** Histopathology of endocervical infection caused by Chlamydia trachomatis, herpes simplex virus, Trichomonas vaginalis, and Neisseria gonorrhoeae. *Hum Pathol* 1990;21:831–837.

27. **Brunham RC, Paavonen J, Stevens CE, et al.** Mucopurulent cervicitis: the ignored counterpart in women of urethritis in men. *N Engl J Med* 1984;311:1–6.

28. **Soper DE, Brockwell NJ, Dalton HP.** Microbial etiology of urban emergency department acute salpingitis: treatment with ofloxacin. *Am J Obstet Gynecol* 1992;167:653–660.

29. **Sweet RL, Draper DL, Schachter J, et al.** Microbiology and pathogenesis of acute salpingitis as determined by laparoscopy: what is the appropriate site to sample? *Am J Obstet Gynecol* 1980;138:985–989.

30. **Wasserheit JN, Bell TA, Kiviat NB, et al.** Microbial causes of proven pelvic inflammatory disease and efficacy of clindamycin and tobramycin. *Ann Intern Med* 1986;104:187–193.

31. **Soper DE, Brockwell NJ, Dalton HP, et al.** Observations concerning the microbial etiology of acute salpingitis. *Am J Obstet Gynecol* 1994;170:1008–1017.

32. **Hillis SD, Joesoef R, Marchbanks PA, et al.** Delayed care of pelvic inflammatory disease as a risk factor for impaired fertility. *Am J Obstet Gynecol* 1993;168:1503–1509.

33. **Wolner-Hanssen P, Kiviat NB, Holmes KK.** Atypical pelvic inflammatory disease: subacute, chronic, or subclinical upper genital tract infection in women. In: **Holmes KK, March P-A, Sparking PF,** eds. *Sexually transmitted diseases,* 2nd ed. New York: McGraw-Hill, 1990:614–620.

34. **Westrom L.** Diagnosis and treatment of salpingitis. *J Reprod Med* 1983;28:703–708.

35. **Soper DE.** Diagnosis and laparoscopic grading of acute salpingitis. *Am J Obstet Gynecol* 1991;164:1370–1376.

36. **Peterson HB, Walker CK, Kahn JG, et al.** Pelvic inflammatory disease: key treatment issues and options. *JAMA* 1991;266:2605–2611.

37. **Soper DE.** Pelvic inflammatory disease. *Infect Dis Clin North Am* 1994;8:821–840.

38. **Gilstrap LC 3d, Herbert WN, Cunningham FG, et al.** Gonorrhea screening in the male consorts of women with pelvic infection. *JAMA* 1977;238:965–966.

39. **Potterat JJ, Phillips L, Rothenberg RB, et al.** Gonococcal pelvic inflammatory disease: case-finding observations. *Am J Obstet Gynecol* 1980;138:1101–1104.

40. **Reed SD, Landers DV, Sweet RL.** Antibiotic treatment of tuboovarian abscesses: comparison of broad-spectrum B-lactam agents versus clindamycin-containing regimens. *Am J Obstet Gynecol* 1991;164:1556–1562.

41. **Corey L, Adams HG, Brown ZA, et al.** Genital herpes simplex virus infection: clinical manifestations, course, and complications. *Ann Intern Med* 1983;98:958–972.

42. **Schmid GP.** Approach to the patient with genital ulcer disease. *Med Clin North Am* 1990;74:1559–1572.

43. **Hutchinson CM, Hook EW.** Syphilis in adults. *Med Clin North Am* 1990;74:1389–1416.

44. **Beutner KR, Richwald GA, Wiley DJ, et al.** External genital warts: report of the American Medical Association Consensus Conference. AMA Expert Panel on External Genital Warts. *Clin Infect Dis* 1998;27:796–806.

45. **Dinsmoor MJ.** HIV infection and pregnancy. *Clin Perinatol* 1994;21:85–94.

46. **Centers for Disease Control and Prevention.** Guidelines for the use of antiretroviral agents in HIV-infected adults and adolescents [On-line]. February 5, 2001. Available: http://www.hivatis.org.

47. **Remis RS, Gurwith MJ, Gurwith D, et al.** Risk factors for urinary tract infection. *Am J Epidemiol* 1987;126:685–694.

48. **Fihn SD, Latham RH, Roberts P, et al.** Association between diaphragm use and urinary tract infection. *JAMA* 1985;254:240–245.

49. **Strom BL, Collins M, West SL, et al.** Sexual activity, contraceptive use, and other risk factors for symptomatic and asymptomatic bacteriuria: a case-control study. *Ann Intern Med* 1987;107:816–823.

50. **Stamm WE, Counts GW, Running KR, et al.** Diagnosis of coliform infection in acutely dysuric women. *N Engl J Med* 1982;307:463–468.

51. **Gupta K, Scholes D, Stamm WE.** Increasing prevalence of antimicrobial resistance among uropathogens causing acute uncomplicated cystitis in women. *JAMA* 1999;281:736–738.

16 Intraepithelial Disease of the Cervix, Vagina, and Vulva

Kenneth D. Hatch
Jonathan S. Berek

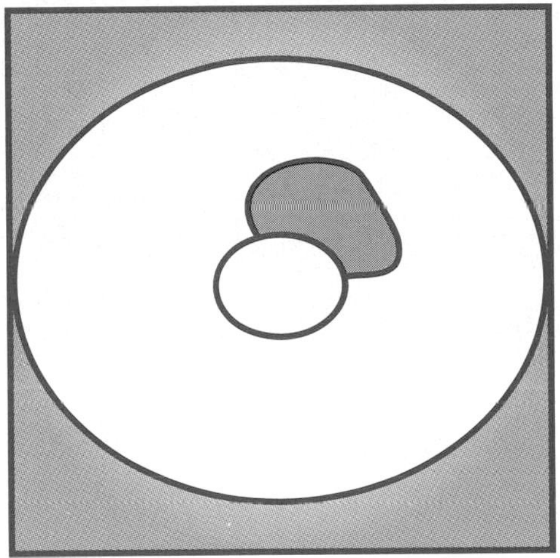

Intraepithelial disease frequently occurs and often coexists in the cervix, vagina, and vulva. The cause and epidemiologic basis are common in all three locations, and treatment typically is ablative and conservative. Early diagnosis and management are essential to prevent disease from progressing to invasive cancer.

Cervical Intraepithelial Neoplasia

The concept of *preinvasive disease* of the cervix was introduced in 1947, when it was recognized that epithelial changes could be identified that had the appearance of invasive cancer but were confined to the epithelium (1). Subsequent studies showed that if these lesions are not treated, they can progress to cervical cancer (2). Improvements in cytologic assessment led to the identification of early precursor lesions called *dysplasia,* which signaled possible development of future cancer. For a number of years, carcinoma *in situ* (CIS) was treated very aggressively (most often with hysterectomy), whereas dysplasias were believed to be less significant and were not treated or were treated by colposcopic biopsy and cryosurgery. The concept of *cervical intraepithelial neoplasia* (CIN) was introduced in 1968, when Richart indicated that all dysplasias have the potential for progression (3). It is now recognized that most CIN 1 lesions regress spontaneously if untreated (4); nevertheless, CIN refers to a lesion that may progress to invasive carcinoma. This term is equivalent to the term *dysplasia,* which means abnormal maturation; consequently, proliferating metaplasia without mitotic activity should not be called dysplasia. Squamous metaplasia should not be diagnosed as dysplasia (or CIN) because it does not progress to invasive cancer.

The criteria for the diagnosis of intraepithelial neoplasia may vary according to the pathologist, but the significant features are cellular immaturity, cellular disorganization, nuclear abnormalities, and increased mitotic activity. The extent of the mitotic activity, immature cellular proliferation, and nuclear atypicality identify the degree of neoplasia. If the mitoses and immature cells are present only in the lower one third of the epithelium, the lesion

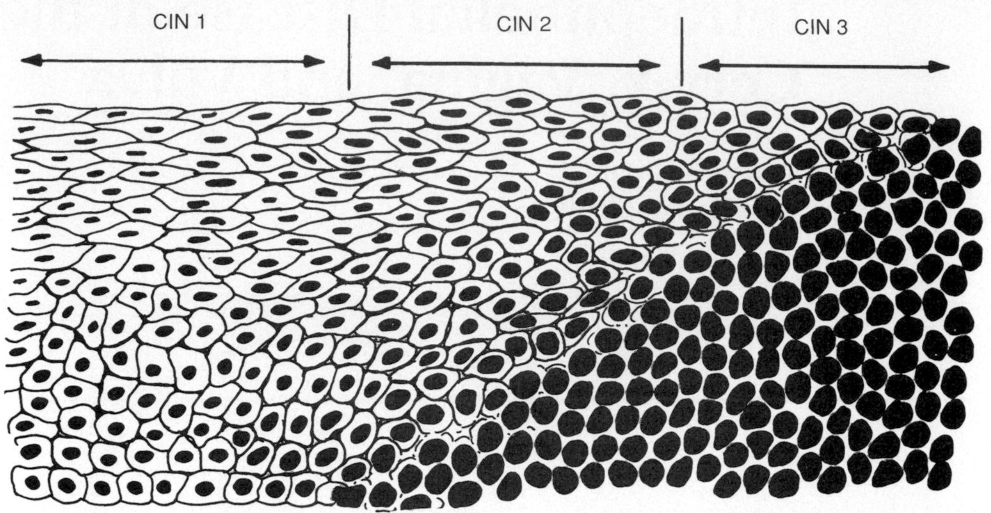

Figure 16.1 Diagram of the different grades of cervical intraepithelial neoplasia.

usually is designated as CIN 1. Involvement of the middle and upper thirds is diagnosed as CIN 2 and CIN 3, respectively (Fig. 16.1).

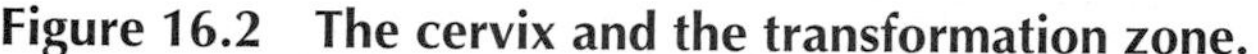

Cervical Anatomy

The cervix is composed of *columnar epithelium,* which lines the endocervical canal, and *squamous epithelium,* which covers the exocervix (5). The point at which they meet is called the *squamocolumnar junction* (SCJ) (Figs. 16.2 and 16.3).

The SCJ rarely remains restricted to the external os. Instead, it is a dynamic point that changes in response to puberty, pregnancy, menopause, and hormonal stimulation (Fig. 16.4). In

Figure 16.2 The cervix and the transformation zone.

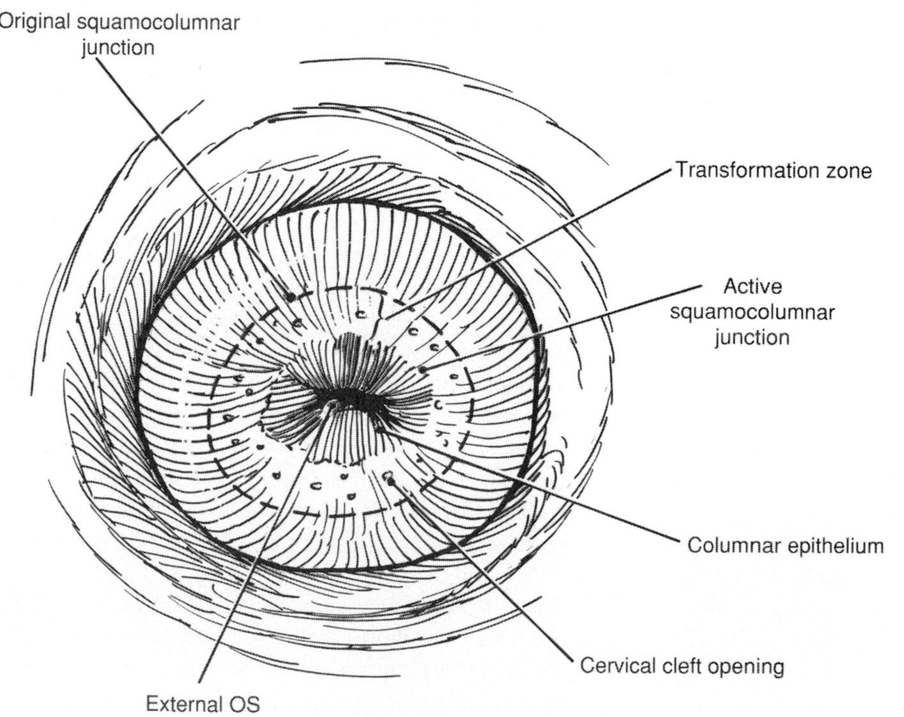

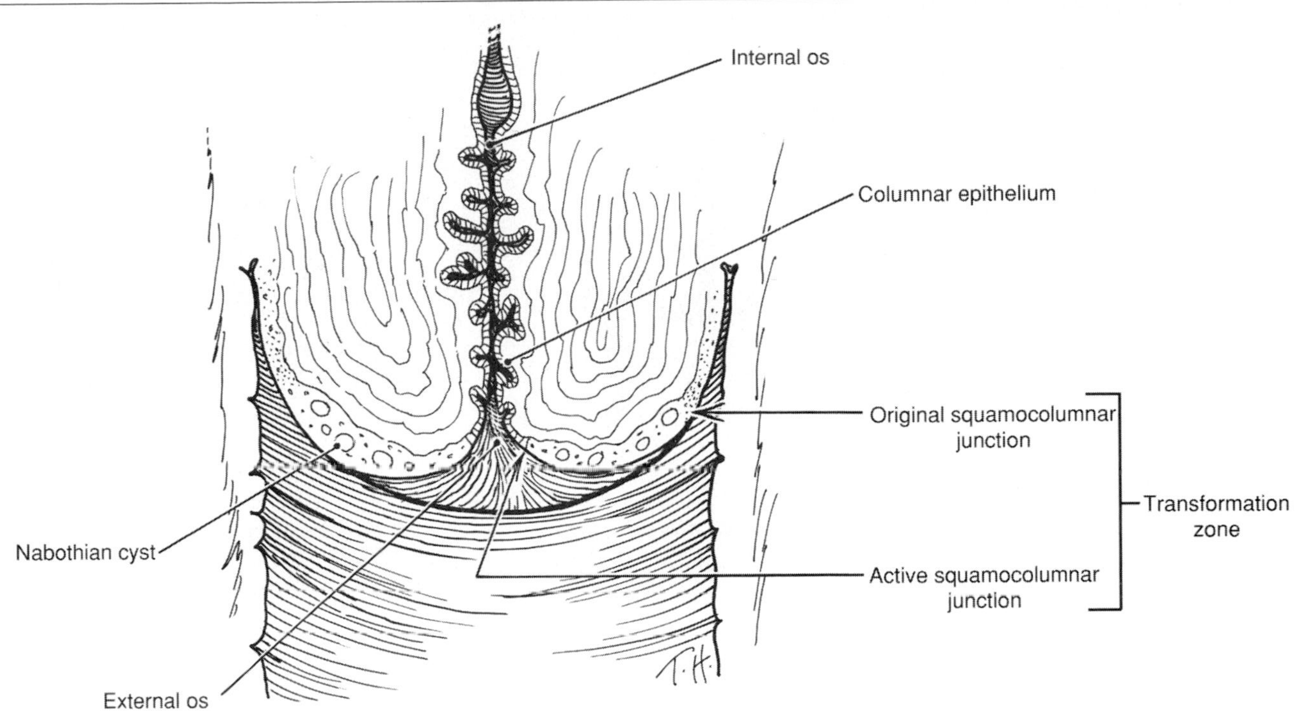

Figure 16.3 Cross-section of the cervix and the endocervix.

neonates, the SCJ is located on the exocervix. At menarche, the production of estrogen causes the vaginal epithelium to fill with glycogen. Lactobacilli act on the glycogen to the pH, stimulating the subcolumnar reserve cells to undergo *metaplasia* (5).

Metaplasia advances from the original SCJ inward, toward the external os, and over the columnar villi. This process establishes an area called the *transformation zone.* The transformation zone extends from the original SCJ to the physiologically active SCJ. As the metaplastic epithelium in the transformation zone matures, it begins to produce glycogen and eventually resembles the original squamous epithelium, colposcopically and histologically.

In most cases, CIN is believed to originate as a single focus in the transformation zone at the advancing SCJ. The anterior lip of the cervix is twice as likely to develop CIN as the posterior lip, and CIN rarely originates in the lateral angles. Once CIN occurs, it can progress horizontally to involve the entire transformation zone but usually does not replace the original squamous epithelium. This progression usually results in CIN with a sharp external border. Proximally, CIN involves the cervical clefts, and this area tends to have the most severe CIN lesions. The extent of involvement of these cervical glands has significant therapeutic implications because the entire gland must be destroyed to ensure elimination of the CIN (5).

The only way to determine where the original SCJ was located is to look for nabothian cysts or cervical cleft openings, which indicate the presence of columnar epithelium. Once the metaplastic epithelium matures and forms glycogen, it is called the *healed* transformation zone and is relatively resistant to oncogenic stimuli. However, the entire SCJ with early metaplastic cells is more susceptible to oncogenic factors, which may cause these cells to transform into CIN. Therefore, **CIN is most likely to begin either during menarche or after pregnancy, when metaplasia is most active. Conversely, a woman who has reached menopause without developing CIN has little metaplasia and is at a lower risk.** It has been established that oncogenic factors are introduced through sexual intercourse. Several agents, including sperm, seminal fluid histones, trichomonas, chlamydia, herpes simplex virus, and human papillomavirus (HPV), have been studied. It is now known that HPV plays an important role in the development of CIN.

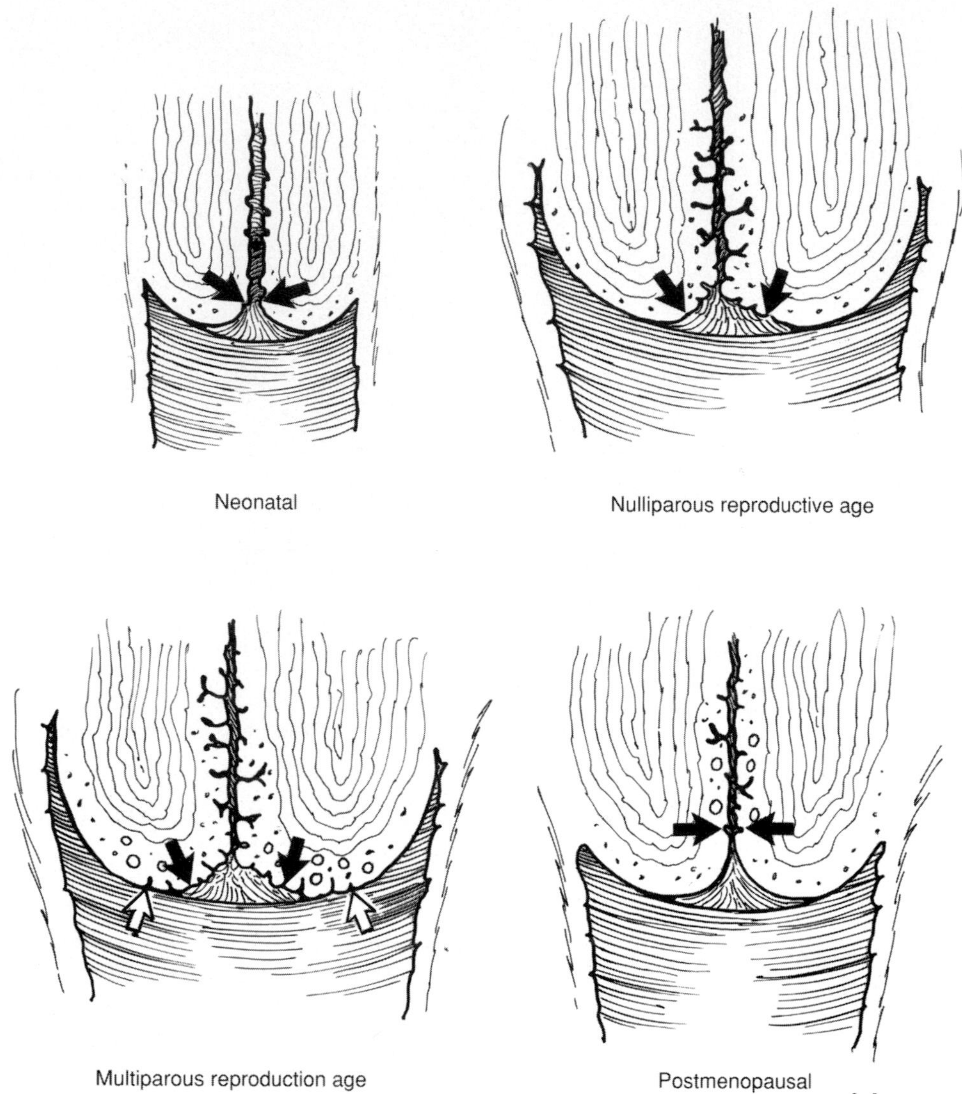

Figure 16.4 Different locations of the transformation zone and the squamocolumnar junction during a woman's lifetime. The *arrows* mark the active transformation zone.

Normal Transformation Zone

The original squamous epithelium of the vagina and exocervix is described as having four layers (5):

1. The *basal layer* is a single row of immature cells with large nuclei and a small amount of cytoplasm.

2. The *parabasal layer* includes two to four rows of immature cells that have normal mitotic figures and provide the replacement cells for the overlying epithelium.

3. The *intermediate layer* includes four to six rows of cells with larger amounts of cytoplasm in a polyhedral shape separated by an intercellular space. Intercellular bridges, where differentiation of glycogen production occurs, can be identified with light microscopy.

4. The *superficial layer* includes five to eight rows of flattened cells with small uniform nuclei and a cytoplasm filled with glycogen. The nucleus becomes pyknotic,

and the cells detach from the surface (exfoliation). These cells form the basis for Papanicolaou (Pap) testing.

Columnar Epithelium Columnar epithelium has a single layer of columnar cells with mucus at the top and a round nucleus at the base. The glandular epithelium is composed of numerous ridges, clefts, and infoldings and, when covered by squamous metaplasia, leads to the appearance of gland openings. Technically, the endocervix is not a gland, but the term *gland openings* is often used.

Metaplastic Epithelium Metaplastic epithelium, found at the SCJ, begins in the subcolumnar reserve cell (Fig. 16.4). Under stimulation of lower vaginal acidity, the reserve cells proliferate, lifting the columnar epithelium. The immature metaplastic cells have large nuclei and a small amount of cytoplasm without glycogen. As the cells mature normally, they produce glycogen, eventually forming the four layers of epithelium. The metaplastic process begins at the tips of the columnar villi, which are exposed first to the acid vaginal environment. As the metaplasia replaces the columnar epithelium, the central capillary of the villus regresses, and the epithelium flattens out, leaving the epithelium with its typical vascular network. As metaplasia proceeds into the cervical clefts, it replaces columnar epithelium and similarly flattens the epithelium. The deeper clefts, however, may not be completely replaced by the metaplastic epithelium, leaving mucus-secreting columnar epithelium trapped under the squamous epithelium. Some of these glands open onto the surface; others are completely encased, with mucus collecting in nabothian cysts. Gland openings and nabothian cysts mark the original SCJ and the outer edge of the original transformation zone (5).

Human Papillomavirus

The cytologic changes of HPV were first recognized by Koss and Durfee (6) in 1956 and given the term *koilocytosis.* Their significance was not recognized until 20 years later, when Meisels and colleagues (7) reported these changes in mild dysplasia (Fig. 16.5). Molecular biologic studies have demonstrated high levels of HPV DNA and capsid antigen, indicating productive viral infection in these koilocytic cells (8). The HPV genome has been demonstrated in all grades of cervical neoplasia (9). As the CIN lesions become more severe (Fig. 16.6), the koilocytes disappear, the HPV copy numbers decrease, and the capsid antigen disappears, indicating that the virus is not capable of reproducing in less differentiated cells (10). Instead, it appears that portions of the HPV DNA become integrated into the host cell. Integration of the transcriptionally active DNA into the host cell appears to be necessary for malignant growth (11). Malignant transformation appears to require the expression of E6 and E7 oncoproteins produced by HPV (12). Because HPV will not grow in cell culture, there is no direct evidence of the carcinogenesis of HPV. However, a cell culture system has been described for growing keratinocytes that allows for stratification and will produce differentiated specific keratinase (13). When normal cells are transfected with the plasmid-containing HPV-16, the transfected cells produced cystologic abnormalities identical to those seen in intraepithelial neoplasia. The E6 and E7 oncoproteins are identifiable in the transfected cell lines, providing the strongest laboratory evidence of a cause-and-effect relationship (14). Cervical cancer cell lines that contain active copies of HPV 16 or 18 (SiHa, HeLa, C 4-11, Ca Ski) demonstrate the presence of HPV-16 E6 and E7 oncoproteins (15).

HPV DNA can be detected in most women with cervical neoplasia (16,17). There is a 10-fold or greater risk for cervical neoplasia associated with the detection of HPV DNA. The relative risk for neoplasia associated with HPV is as high as 40, with a lower 95% confidence limit of 15 (16). **The percentage of intraepithelial neoplasia apparently attributed to HPV infection approaches 90%** (17).

Although the number of known genital HPV types now exceeds 20, only certain types count for about 90% of high-grade intraepithelial lesions and cancer (HPV-16, -18, -31, -33, -35, -39, -45, -51, -52, -56, and -58) (17). **Type 16 is the most common HPV**

Figure 16.5 Cervical intraepithelial neoplasia grade 1 with koilocytosis. The normal maturation process and differentiation from the basal and parabasal layers to the intermediate and superficial layers are maintained. In the upper layers, koilocytes are characterized by perinuclear halos, well-defined cell borders, and nuclear hyperchromasia, irregularity, and enlargement. (From **Fu YS, Woodruff JD.** Pathology. In: **Berek JS, Hacker NF,** eds. *Practical gynecologic oncology,* 2nd ed. Baltimore: Williams & Wilkins, 1994:118, with permission.)

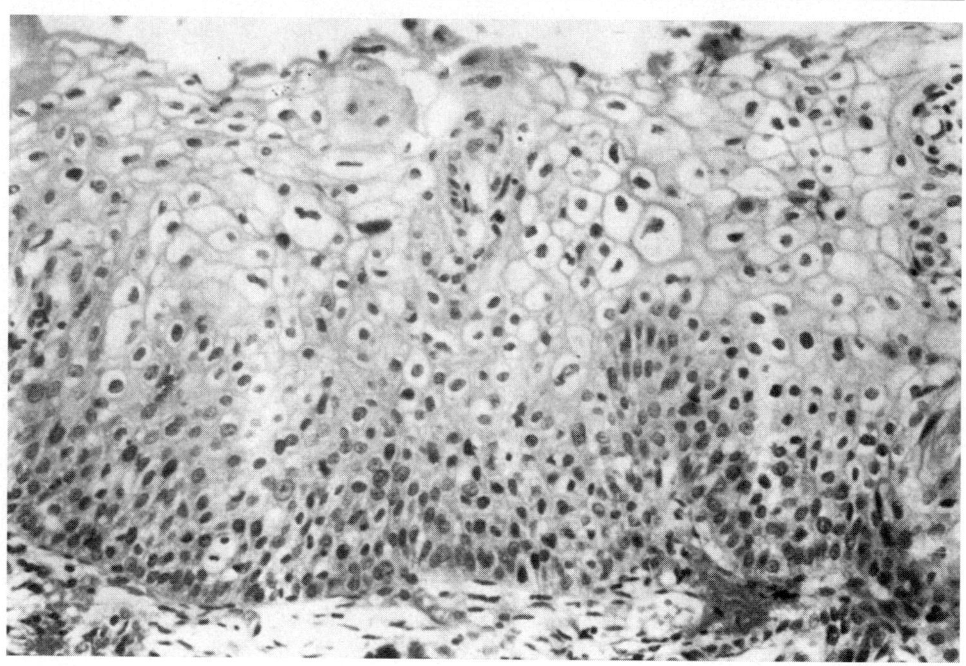

Figure 16.6 Cervical intraepithelial neoplasia grade 3 with the entire thickness of the epithelium replaced by abnormal cells that have large hyperchromatic, irregular nuclei. The normal maturation is lost. Mitotic figures are seen in the superficial layers *(left upper corner).* (From **Fu YS, Woodruff JD.** Pathology. In: **Berek JS, Hacker NF,** eds. *Practical gynecologic oncology,* 2nd ed. Baltimore: Williams & Wilkins, 1994:119, with permission.)

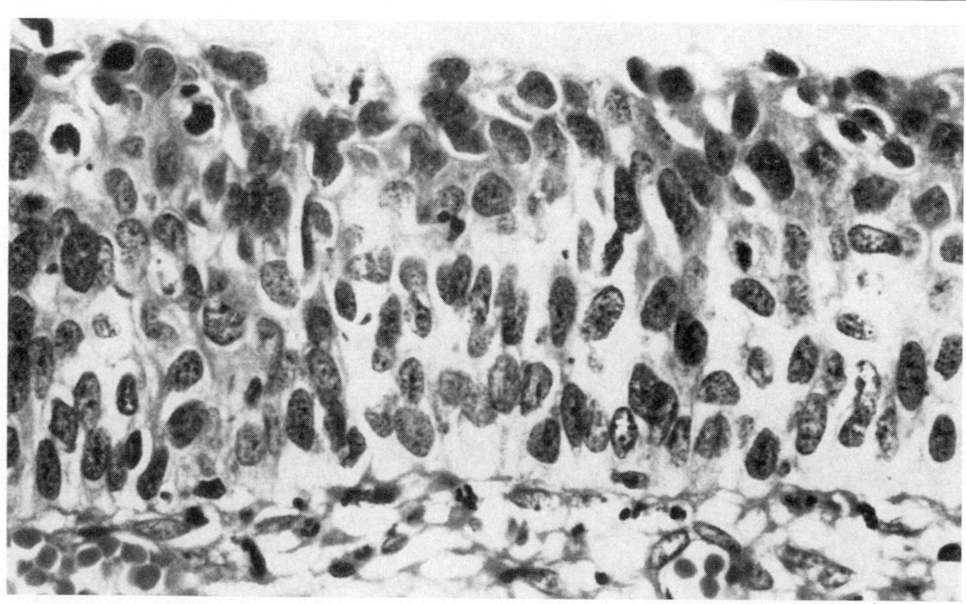

type in invasive cancer and in CIN 2 and CIN 3 and is found in 47% of women in both categories (18). It is also the most common HPV type in women with normal cytology.

Unfortunately, HPV-16 is not very specific; it can be found in 16% of women with low-grade lesions and in up to 14% of women with normal cytology. **HPV-18 is found in 23% of women with invasive cancers, 5% of women with CIN 2 and CIN 3, 5% of women with HPV and CIN 1, and fewer than 2% of patients with negative findings** (17). **Therefore, HPV-18 is more specific than HPV-16 for invasive tumors.**

Usually, HPV infections do not persist. Most women have no apparent clinical evidence of disease, and the infection is eventually suppressed or eliminated (16). Other women exhibit low-grade cervical lesions that may regress spontaneously. A minority of women exposed to HPV develop persistent infection that may progress to CIN (16,19). Factors that may have a role in this progression include smoking, contraceptive use, infection with other sexually transmitted diseases, or nutrition (16,18). Any factor that influences the integration of HPV DNA into the human genome may cause progression to invasive disease (20).

Papanicolaou Test Classification

In 1988, the first National Cancer Institute (NCI) workshop was held in Bethesda, Maryland, resulted in the development of the Bethesda System for cytologic reporting (21). A standardized method of reporting cytology findings was needed to facilitate peer review and quality assurance. **Recently, the terminology was refined in the Bethesda III System (2001) potentially premalignant squamous lesions fall into three categories: *atypical squamous cells* (ASC), *low-grade squamous intraepithelial lesions* (LSIL), and *high-grade squamous intraepithelial lesions* (HSIL)** (22). **The ASC category is subdivided into two categories: those of unknown significance (ASC-US), and those in which high-grade lesions must be excluded (ASC-H). Low-grade squamous intraepithelial lesions include CIN 1 (mild dysplasia) and the changes of HPV, termed *koilocytotic atypia.* The HSIL category includes CIN 2 and CIN 3 (moderate dysplasia, severe dysplasia, and carcinoma *in situ*).** A comparison of the various terms as they relate is shown in Table 16.1.

Table 16.1. Comparison of Cytology Classification Systems

Bethesda System	*Dysplasia/CIN System*		*Papanicolaou System*
Within normal limits	Normal		I
Infection (organism should be specified)	Inflammatory atypia (organism)		II
Reactive and reparative changes			
Squamous cell abnormalities			
Atypical squamous cells (1) of undetermined significance **(ASC-US)**	Squamous atypia HPV atypia, exclude **LSIL**		IIR
(2) exclude high-grade lesions **(ASC-H)**	Exclude **HSIL**		
Low-grade squamous intraepithelial lesion **(LSIL)**	HPV atypia Mild dysplasia	**CIN 1**	III
High-grade squamous intraepithelial lesion **(HSIL)**	Moderate dysplasia	**CIN 2**	III
	Severe dysplasia Carcinoma *in situ*	**CIN 3**	IV
Squamous cell carcinoma	Squamous cell carcinoma		V

CIN, cervical intraepithelial neoplasia.
Updated from **Berek JS, Hacker NF,** eds. *Practical gynecologic oncology,* 2nd ed. Baltimore: Williams & Wilkins, 1994:205, with permission.

Cellular changes associated with HPV (i.e., koilocytosis and CIN 1) are incorporated within the category of LSIL because the natural history, distribution of various HPV types, and cytologic features of both of these lesions are the same (20). **Long-term follow-up studies have shown that lesions properly classified as koilocytosis progress to high-grade intraepithelial neoplasia in 14% of cases** (22) **and that lesions classified as mild dysplasia progress to severe dysplasia or CIS in 16% of cases** (4). It was initially thought that lesions classified as koilocytosis would contain only low-risk HPV types, such as 6 and 11, whereas high-risk HPV types, such as 16 and 18, would be limited to true neoplasms, including CIN 1, thus justifying the distinction. Histopathologic and molecular virologic correlation, however, has demonstrated a similar heterogeneous distribution of low- and high-risk HPV types in both koilocytosis and CIN 1 (23). Studies evaluating the dysplasia, CIS, and CIN terminology have demonstrated a lack of interobserver and intraobserver reproducibility (24). The greatest lack of reproducibility is between koilocytosis and CIN 1 (25). Thus, on the basis of clinical behavior, molecular biologic findings, and morphologic features, HPV changes and CIN 1 appear to be the same disease. The rationale for combining CIN 2 and CIN 3 into the category of HSIL is similar. The biologic studies reveal the similar mix of high-risk HPV types in the two lesions, and the separation of the lesions has been shown to be irreproducible (24,25). In addition, the management of CIN 2 and CIN 3 is similar, so that separation serves no useful clinical purpose.

Diagnosis

The Papanicolaou Test

The Pap test has been successful in reducing the incidence of cervical cancer by 79% and the mortality by 70% since 1950 (26). Despite this, there will be 4,100 deaths in the United States in 2002 (27), and cases of cancer continue to occur in patients who have had regular Pap tests. The Agency for Health Care and Policy Research (AHCPR) undertook a literature review of conventional cervical cytology testing techniques and compared them to newer technologies designed to reduce the false-negative rate (28). The AHCPR project analyzed five reports and concluded that the sensitivity of conventional cytologic testing in detecting cervical cancer precursor lesions was 51%. This is a false-negative rate of 49%. Previously, it had been widely believed that sensitivity of the Pap test was in the 80% range (29). Recommendations for Pap test screening were based on this perceived 80% sensitivity. The recommendation that three annual Pap tests be performed is predicated on a false-negative rate that would reduce the risk for missed lesions to less than 1% after the first three tests. If the test sensitivity were 80%, then the sensitivity of three negative tests would be 99.2%, which achieves the screening goal. However, the 51% test sensitivity would have a sensitivity of only 86.8% after three tests.

It is obvious that improvement in the conventional Pap test technique is necessary. False-negative errors occur in sampling, preparation, and interpretation. Sampling errors occur because a lesion is too small to exfoliate cells or the device used did not pick up the cells and transfer them to the glass slide. Preparation errors may occur because of poor fixation on the glass slide, leading to air-drying and an inability to interpret the results. The slide may also be too thick and obscured by vaginal discharge, blood, or mucus. The thick slide also leads to poor fixation because the fixative does not penetrate the cell sample. Interpretive errors occur when the slide contains diagnostic cells that the screening technician did not identify.

Sampling and preparation errors can be alleviated by using a liquid-based media to collect the cytologic sample. The AHCPR reported that liquid-based cytology assessment improved the sensitivity of the Pap test to the stated goal of 80%. The cell sample is collected with an endocervical brush used in combination with a plastic spatula or with a plastic broom. The sample is then rinsed in a vial containing liquid preservative. This technique transfers 80% to 90% of the cells to the liquid media, as compared with the only 10% to 20%

transferred to the glass slide with conventional cytologic testing. In addition, using liquid-based media eliminates air-drying. The cells are retrieved from the vial by passing the liquid through a filter, which traps the larger epithelial cells, separating them from the small blood and inflammatory cells. This leads to a thin layer of diagnostic cells properly preserved and more easily interpreted by the cytologist. This technique reduces the rate of unsatisfactory smears encountered with conventional cytologic testing by 70% to 90% (32). Liquid-based cytology is now performed by more than 50% of the laboratories in the United States.

A second new technology of cervical cytologic assessment, the AutoPap Screening System, has been approved by the U.S. Food and Drug Administration for primary screening and rescreening of samples initially read as normal. This technique uses an automated microscope coupled to a special digital camera. The system scans the slide and uses computer imaging techniques to analyze each field of view on the slide. Computer algorithms are then used to rank each slide on the basis of the probability that the sample may contain an abnormality. The selected slides are then reviewed by a cytotechnologist or a cytopathologist. This technique has reduced the false-negative rate by 32% (33). The AutoPap Screening System is not in widespread use at the moment.

Atypical Squamous Cells

The ASC category is restricted to those test results disclosing abnormal cells that are truly of unknown significance. The ASC category does not include benign, reactive, and reparative changes that should be coded as normal in the Bethesda system. Because of the lack of diagnostic criteria and the fear of medical-legal action, the diagnosis has become quite common, ranging from 3% to 25% in some centers (34). When standardized diagnostic criteria are used, the rate of ASC results should be 3% to 5% (35). **The older term, ASCUS (Bethesda II classification) is now subdivided into ASC-US and ASC-H (Bethesda III classification).**

The cytologic diagnosis of ASCUS is associated with a 10% to 20% incidence of CIN 1 and a 3% to 5% risk for CIN 2 or 3 (36–39). It has become apparent that CIN 1 is most often a benign HPV infection and will regress spontaneously in more than 60% of the cases (40); therefore, the goals of triage of an ASCUS Pap test result is to identify more advanced CIN 2 and 3 lesions.

Triage options include the following: 1) Repeat Pap test every 4 to 6 months with referral for colposcopy if any subsequent abnormality is detected; 2) Immediate colposcopy; 3) HPV testing.

The option of repeat Pap testing is weakened by the 20% to 50% false-negative rate in identifying CIN lesions as well as the noncompliance of the patient. About 50% of patients will still undergo colposcopy because of subsequent abnormal Pap test results, making this option nearly as costly as immediate colposcopy (36). Immediate colposcopy is assumed to be the most sensitive method of detecting CIN 2 or 3 (36,39). Because 80% of patients will not have significant lesions, it is important to not overinterpret the colposcopic findings and to be conservative in performing biopsies. There is also the risk that pathologists will overinterpret the biopsy results and the patient will be diagnosed with CIN when metaplasia is the only finding. Several studies have documented the usefulness of HPV testing in the assessment of ASCUS Pap test results (41–43). These studies have shown that HPV testing can identify patients 90% of the patients with CIN 2 or 3 lesions.

To compare the aforementioned triage method in a prospective randomized fashion, the NCI funded an ASCUS/LSIL Triage Study (ALTS) whose results for ASCUS were recently published (44). Patients with ASCUS or LSIL were randomized to three triage arms: (a) immediate colposcopy, (b) HPV test, and (c) conservative management by repeat Pap test.

There were 1,163 women in the immediate colposcopy group, and 14 refused the examination. The results of colposcopy are assumed to reflect the prevalent disease rates, which were as follows: CIN 1, 14.3%; CIN 2, 16.1%; and CIN 3, 5%. Thus, 75% of the women with ASCUS had negative colposcopy results and did not have a biopsy (25%) or had a biopsy that had negative results. The HPV test results were positive in 56.1% of the patients, and 6.1% of the patients did not return for colposcopy. Of the 494 who underwent colposcopy, the results were as follows: CIN 1, 22.5%; CIN 2, 11.9%; and CIN 3, 15.6%. The sensitivity of HPV test was 95.9% for the detection of CIN 2 and 96.3% for the detection of CIN 3.

In the conservatively managed group, only one follow-up Pap test was reported. To be effective, it is recognized that Pap test must be done every 6 months. Despite this, the results of the single follow-up Pap test were included. Using a cutoff that includes any positive finding of ASCUS or greater, the sensitivity is 85% for CIN 2 and 85.3% for CIN 3, with 58.6% of patients being referred for colposcopy. If LSIL is used as a cutoff, 26.2% of the patients are referred, with sensitivity of 64.0% for both CIN 2 and 3. Using HSIL as the cutoff, 6.9% are referred, and the sensitivity falls to 44%.

The conclusion of the ALTS trial is that HPV triage is highly sensitive in identifying CIN 2 and 3 lesions, with an acceptable rate of referral for colposcopy. Cost-effective analysis of the findings will await the completion of the conservative arm of the study.

In 2001, the American Society for Colposcopy and Cervical Pathology (ASCCP) sponsored an NCI Consensus Conference to provide guidelines for the management of abnormal cervical cytology. They utilized information from the ALTS Trial and used Bethesda III terminology. Women with ASL-US should be managed with 1) a program of 2 repeat pap smears with referral of any abnormality to colposcopy 2) immediate colposcopy 3) testing for high risk type HPV. Testing for HPV DNA is the preferred method when liquid-based cytology is used. Women who are positive will be referred for colposcopy, and those who are negative will return to yearly cytology (41).

Low-grade Squamous Intraepithelial Lesions

The cytologic diagnosis of LSIL is reproducible and accounts for 1.6% of cytologic diagnoses (35). About 75% of the patients have CIN, with 20% being CIN 2 or 3 (36–38). These patients require additional evaluation. The ALTS trial closed the HPV test arm early because the HPV positivity rate was 82% and, therefore, was not a valid discriminator in determining the presence of disease. The immediate colposcopy arm and cytology follow-up have not been published. Until these data are available, **the standard practice is to perform colposcopy to evaluate a single LSIL result.**

High-grade Squamous Intraepithelial Lesions

Any woman with a cytologic specimen suggesting the presence of HSIL should undergo colposcopy and directed biopsy. After colposcopically directed biopsy and determination of the distribution of the lesion, ablative therapy and destruction of the entire T-zone should be performed.

Colposcopy Findings

Acetowhite Epithelium **Epithelium that turns white after application of acetic acid (3% to 5%) is called *acetowhite epithelium*** (28). **The application of acetic acid coagulates the proteins of the nucleus and cytoplasm and makes the proteins opaque and white** (5).

The acetic acid does not affect mature, glycogen-producing epithelium because the acid does not penetrate below the outer one third of the epithelium. The cells in this region have very small nuclei and a large amount of glycogen (not protein). These areas appear pink during colposcopy. Dysplastic cells are those most affected. They contain large nuclei with abnormally large amounts of chromatin (protein). The columnar villi become "plumper" after acetic acid is applied; these cells are then easier to see. They appear slightly white, particularly in the presence of the beginning signs of metaplasia. The immature metaplastic cells have larger nuclei and also show some effects of the acetic acid. Because the metaplastic epithelium is very thin, it is not as white or opaque as CIN but instead appears gray and filmy (5).

Leukoplakia Translated literally, *leukoplakia* is white plaque (5). In colposcopic terminology, this plaque is white epithelium visible before application of acetic acid. Leukoplakia is caused by a layer of keratin on the surface of the epithelium. Immature squamous epithelial cells have the potential to develop into keratin-producing cells or glycogen-producing cells. In the vagina and on the cervix, the normal differentiation is toward glycogen. Keratin production is abnormal in the cervicovaginal mucosa. Several things can cause leukoplakia, including HPV; keratinizing CIN; keratinizing carcinoma; chronic trauma from diaphragm, pessary, or tampon use; and radiotherapy.

Leukoplakia should not be confused with the white plaque of a monilial infection, which can be completely wiped off with a cotton-tipped applicator. Currently, the most common reason for leukoplakia is HPV infection (Fig. 16.7). Because it is not possible to see through the thick keratin layer to the underlying vasculature during colposcopy, such areas should undergo biopsy to rule out keratinizing carcinoma.

Punctation ***Punctation* refers to dilated capillaries terminating on the surface, which appear from the ends as a collection of dots** (Fig. 16.8). When these vessels occur in a

Figure 16.7 Cervical intraepithelial neoplasia type 1, mild dysplasia associated with human papillomavirus infection of the cervix. There is a shiny, snow-white color and a micropapillary surface contour. (From **Berek JS, Hacker NF,** eds. *Practical gynecologic oncology,* 2nd ed. Baltimore: Williams & Wilkins, 1994:207, with permission.)

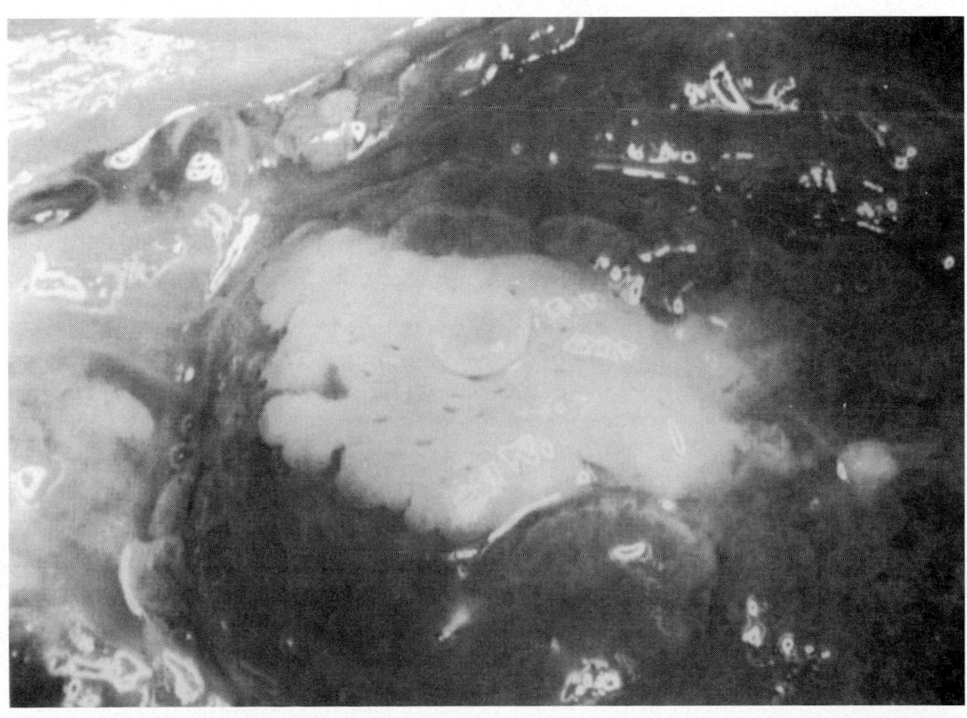

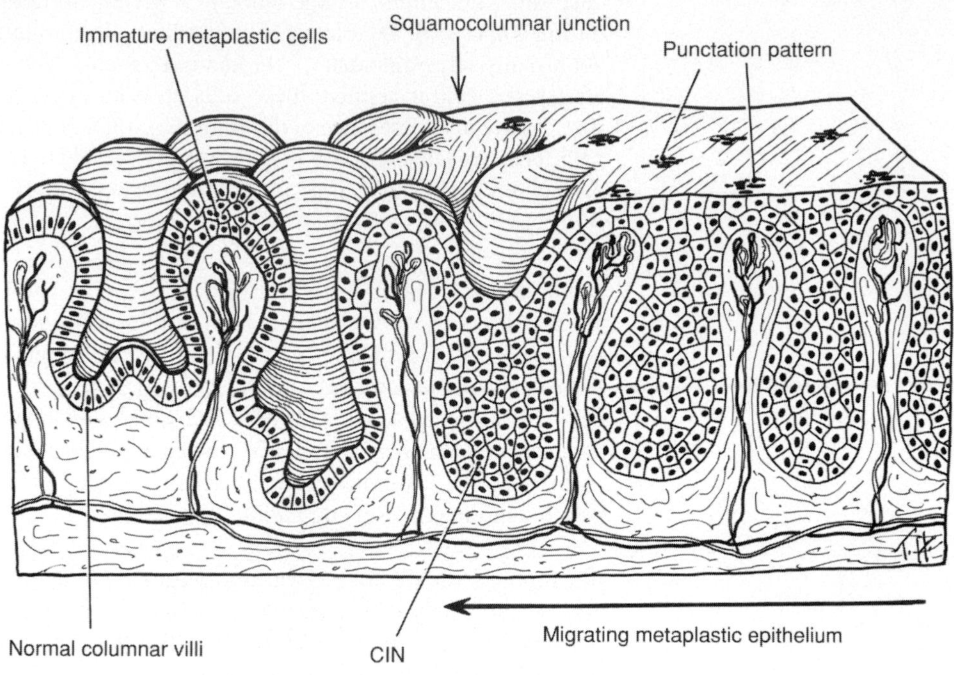

Figure 16.8 Diagram of punctation. The central capillaries of the columnar villi are preserved and produce the punctate vessels on the surface.

well-demarcated area of acetowhite epithelium, they indicate an abnormal epithelium—most often CIN (5) (Fig. 16.9). The punctate vessels are formed as the metaplastic epithelium migrates over the columnar villi. Normally, the capillary regresses; however, when CIN occurs, the capillary persists and appears more prominent.

Mosaic **Terminal capillaries surrounding roughly circular or polygonal-shaped blocks of acetowhite epithelium crowded together are called mosaic because their appearance is similar to mosaic tile** (Fig. 16.10). These vessels form a "basket" around the blocks of abnormal epithelium. They may arise from a coalescence of many terminal punctate vessels or from the vessels that surround the cervical gland openings (5). Mosaicism tends to be associated with higher-grade lesions and CIN 2 (Fig. 16.11) and CIN 3 (Fig. 16.12).

Atypical Vascular Pattern **Atypical vascular patterns are characteristic of invasive cervical cancer** and include looped vessels, branching vessels, and reticular vessels. These patterns are discussed in Chapter 31.

Endocervical Curettage The entire coagulant from the endocervical curettage (ECC), placed on a piece of filter paper or brown paper towel, is immersed in 10% buffered formalin or Bouin's solution. Absorbent paper towels should be avoided because they disintegrate when they become wet. The cheapest paper towels provide the best surface.

Cervical Biopsy The cervical biopsy sample is placed on a dry paper towel. The biopsy should be oriented on its side with the surface at right angles to the surface of the paper. It should be allowed to dry for a minute to ensure attachment to the piece of paper and then placed in the fixative with the specimen down. The specimen and paper will float, and the specimen will stay attached to the undersurface of the paper with its proper orientation. This allows the pathologist to orient the biopsy in the paraffin block and avoid tangential sectioning.

Figure 16.9 Human papillomavirus/cervical intraepithelial neoplasia type 1 presents as a white lesion with surface spicules.

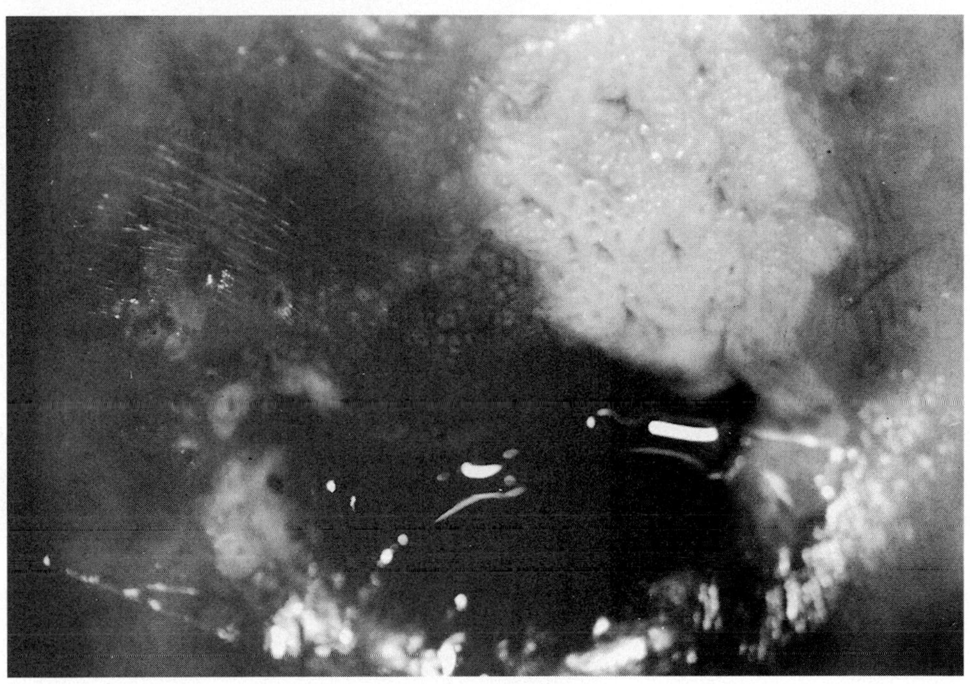

Figure 16.10 Mosaic pattern. This pattern develops as islands of dysplastic epithelium proliferate and push the ends of the superficial blood vessels away, creating a pattern that looks like mosaic tiles.

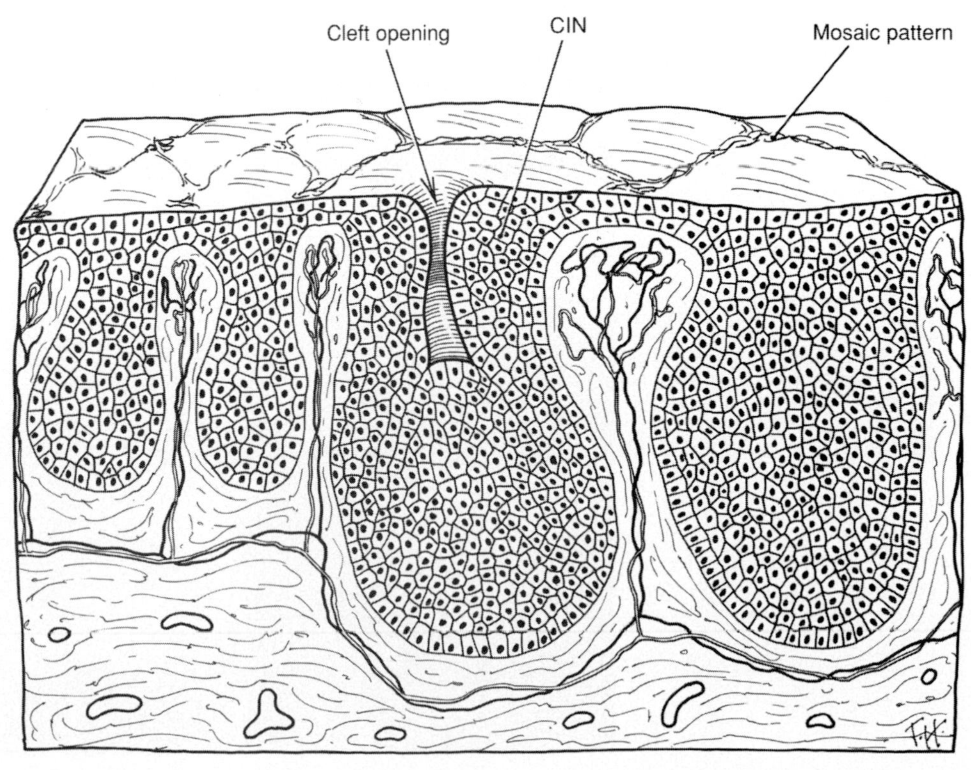

Figure 16.11 Human papillomavirus/cervical intraepithelial neoplasia grade 2. Cribriform pattern of HPV at periphery with mosaicism and punctation near the squamocolumnar junction.

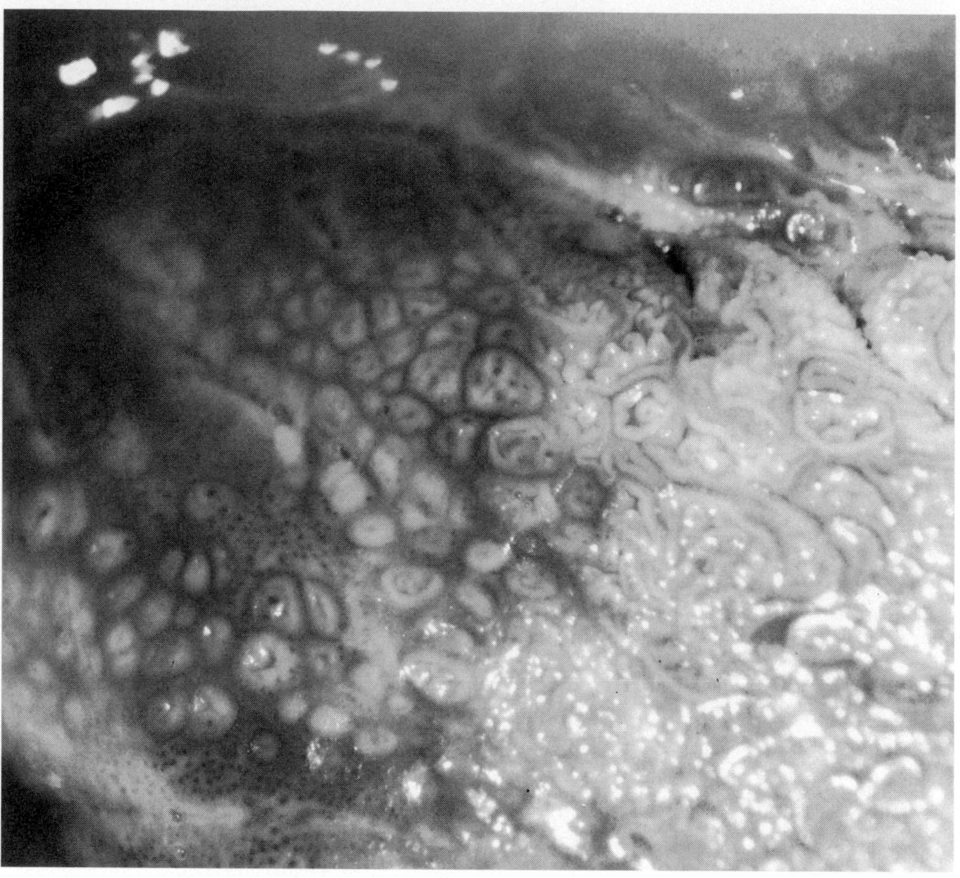

Figure 16.12 Cervical intraepithelial neoplasia grade 3, showing a white lesion with associated punctation and coarse mosaicism.

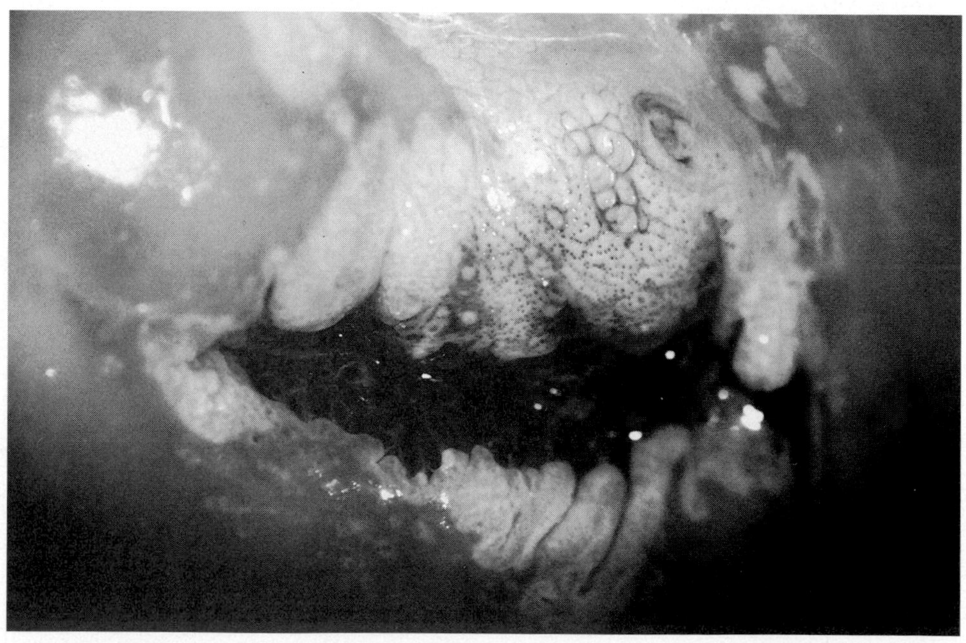

Correlation of Findings

Ideally, both the pathologist and colposcopist should review the colposcopic findings and the results of cytologic assessment, cervical biopsy, and ECC before deciding therapy (45–47). This is particularly true when operators are first learning the technique of colposcopy. The cytology results should not be sent to one laboratory and the histology results to another. The colposcopist should not treat the report but rather treat the disease. When the cytology and biopsy results correlate, the colposcopist can be reasonably certain that the worst lesion has been identified. If the cytology indicates a more significant lesion than the histology, the patient should undergo further evaluation and additional biopsies as necessary. An algorithm for the evaluation, treatment, and follow-up of an abnormal Pap test is presented in Fig. 16.13.

Figure 16.13 An algorithm for the evaluation, treatment, and follow-up of an abnormal Papanicolaou test.

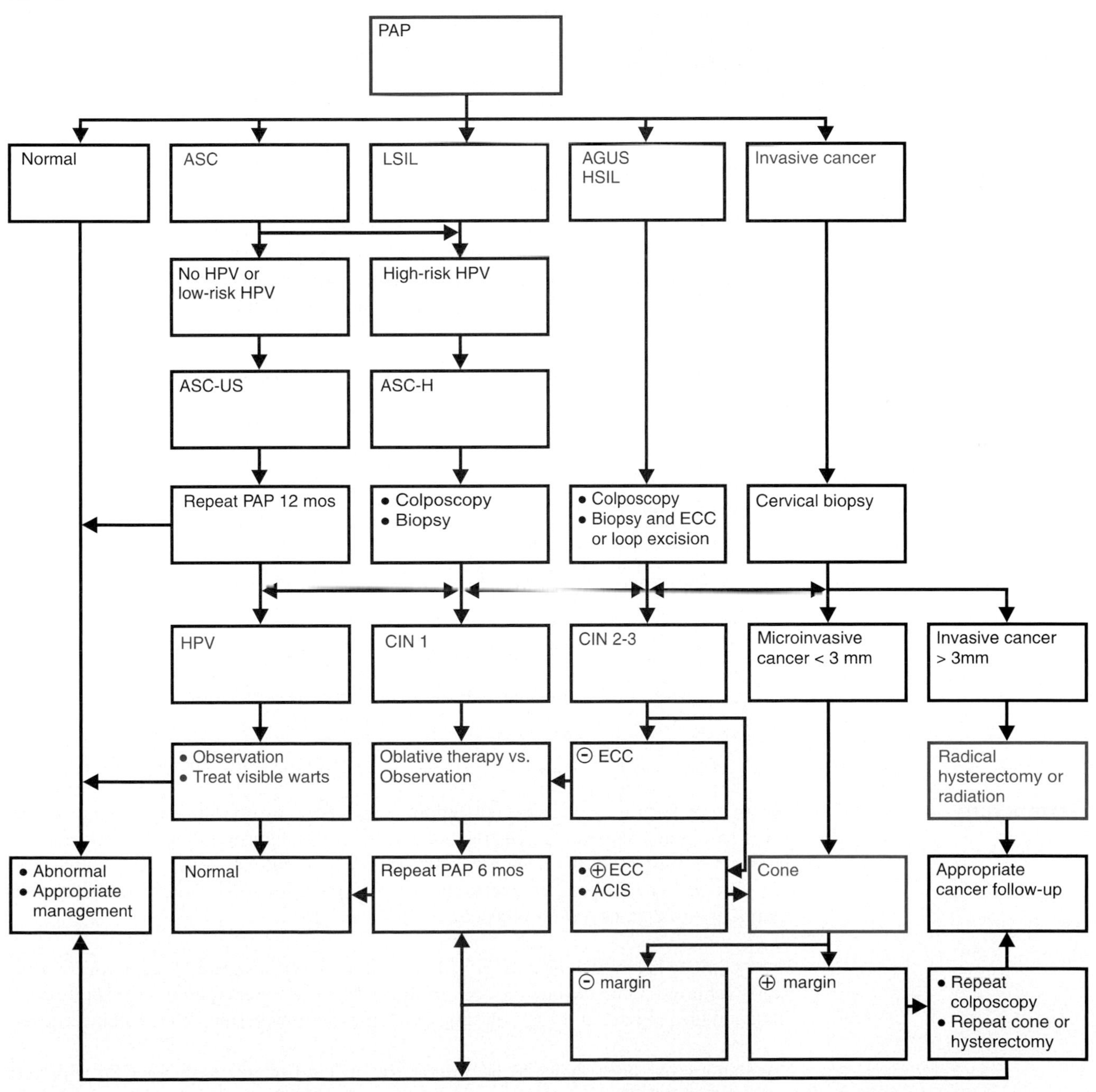

Colposcopic Terminology

CIN 1

The spontaneous regression rate of biopsy-proven CIN 1 is 60% to 85% in prospective studies (48–51). The regressions typically occur within a 2-year follow-up with cytology and colposcopy. This information has led to the recommendation that patients who have biopsy diagnoses of CIN 1 with satisfactory colposcopy and who agree to the evaluation every 6 months may be treated by observation. If the lesions progress during follow-up or persist at 2 years, ablative treatment should be performed.

For patients who prefer treatment and for those who progress or persist, the choice of treatment is optional. A randomized prospective trial comparing cryosurgery to laser and laser electrosurgical excision procedure (LEEP) showed no difference in persistent disease rate (4%) or recurrent disease rate (17%) (52). Cryosurgery has the advantage of low cost and ease of use. The disadvantages are lack of tissue specimen, inability to adapt to lesion size, and posttreatment vaginal discharge.

CIN 2 and 3

There is agreement that all CIN 2 and 3 lesions require treatment. This recommendation is based on a metaanalysis showing that CIN 2 progresses to CIS in 20% of cases and to invasion in 5%. Progression of CIS to invasion is 5% (49).

Although CIN can be treated with a variety of techniques, the preferred treatment for CIN 2 and 3 has become LEEP. These techniques allow a specimen to be sent for evaluation and enable the pathologist to identify occult microinvasive cancer or adenomatous lesions. This ensures that adequate treatment of these lesions is accomplished. The persistent and recurrent disease rates are 4% to 10% (52,53).

Treatment of CIN

Most of the ablative techniques used to treat CIN can be performed in an outpatient setting, which is one of the main objectives in the management of this disease. Because all therapeutic modalities carry an inherent recurrence rate of up to 10%, cytologic follow-up at about 3-month intervals for 1 year is necessary. Ablative therapy is appropriate when the following conditions exist:

1. There is no evidence of microinvasive or invasive cancer on cytology, colposcopy, ECC, or biopsy.
2. The lesion is located on the ectocervix and can be seen entirely.
3. There is no involvement of the endocervix as determined by colposcopy and ECC.

Cryotherapy

Cryotherapy destroys the surface epithelium of the cervix by crystallizing the intracellular water, resulting in the eventual destruction of the cell. The temperature needed for effective destruction must be in the range of (−20° to −30°C). Nitrous oxide (−89°C) and carbon dioxide (−65°C) produce temperatures below this range and, therefore, are the most commonly used gases for this procedure.

The technique believed to be most effective is a freeze-thaw-freeze method in which an ice ball is achieved 5 mm beyond the edge of the probe. The time required for this process is related to the pressure of the gas; the higher the pressure, the faster the ice ball is achieved.

Cryotherapy has been shown to be an effective method of treatment for CIN with very acceptable failure rates under certain conditions (54–57). It is a relatively safe procedure

Table 16.2. Results of Cryotherapy for Cervical Intraepithelial Neoplasia (CIN) Compared to Grade of CIN

	CIN 1		*CIN 2*		*CIN 3*	
Author (Ref. No.)	***No.***	***Failure (%)***	***No.***	***Failure (%)***	***No.***	***Failure (%)***
Ostergard (55)	13/205	6.3	7/93	7.5	9/46	19.6
Creasman (56)	15/276	5.4	17/235	7.2	46/259	17.8
Andersen (54)	—	—	9/123	7.3	17/74	23.0
Benedet (57)	7/143	4.9	19/448	4.2	65/1,003	6.5
TOTAL	35/624	5.6	50/899	5.6	137/1,382	9.9

with few complications. Cervical stenosis is rare but can occur. Posttreatment bleeding is uncommon and is usually related to infection.

Cure rates are related to the grade of the lesion; CIN 3 has a greater chance of failure (Table 16.2). Townsend has shown that cures are also related to the size of the lesion; those "covering most of the ectocervix" have failure rates as high as 42%, compared with a 7% failure rate for lesions less than 1 cm in diameter (58). Positive findings on ECC also can reduce the cure rate significantly. Endocervical gland involvement is important because the failure rate in women with gland involvement was 27%, compared with 9% in those who did not have such involvement (59).

Cryotherapy should be considered acceptable therapy when the following criteria are met:

1. Cervical intraepithelial neoplasia, grade 1 to 2
2. Small lesion
3. Ectocervical location only
4. Negative ECC findings
5. No endocervical gland involvement on biopsy

Laser

Laser vaporization therapy may be chosen for patients in whom the presence of invasive cancer has been ruled out, the entire lesion can be seen, and ECC results are negative (60–65). Laser vaporization is particularly applicable in the following situations:

1. Large lesions that the cryoprobe cannot adequately cover
2. Irregular cervix with a "fish mouth" appearance and deep clefts
3. Extension of disease to the vagina or satellite lesions on the vagina
4. Lesions with extensive glandular involvement in which the treatment must reach beyond the deepest gland cleft

The major advantage of laser vaporization therapy is the ability to control exactly the depth and width of destruction by direct vision through the colposcope. Several studies have demonstrated that CIN can be found at an average of 1.2 mm and up to a depth of 5.2 mm inside the cervical crypts, regardless of whether the lesion is located in the exocervix or endocervix (59). Wright has shown that destruction or resection of the tissue to a depth of 3.8 mm ablates all the involved glands in 99.7% of cases (62). Nevertheless, the tissue should be ablated to a depth of 7 mm, which is the location of the deepest endocervical gland. Both CIN 2 and CIN 3 with glandular involvement have deeper crypt involvement than CIN 1 lesions without endocervical gland involvement (61).

The other major advantage of laser therapy is the rapid posttreatment healing phase. This process takes about 3 to 4 weeks, after which time a new epithelium has formed completely and, in most cases, has a mature glycogen-containing epithelium. The healed cervix has a normal appearance with a small visible transformation zone at the cervical os.

Tissue Interaction When the laser beam contacts tissue, its energy is absorbed by the water in the cells, causing it to boil instantly. The cells explode into a puff of vapor (thus the term *laser vaporization*). The protein and mineral content is incinerated by the heat and leaves a charred appearance at the base of the exposed area. The depth of laser destruction is a function of the power of the beam (in watts), the area of the beam (in millimeters squared), and the length of time the laser remains in the tissue. The beam must be moved uniformly across the tissue surface to prevent deep destruction. The laser beam vaporizes a central area and leaves a narrow zone of heat necrosis surrounding the laser crater. The goal of laser vaporization is to minimize this area of tissue necrosis. This goal is accomplished by using high wattage (20 watts) with medium beam size (1.5 mm) and moving the beam uniformly but quickly over the surface. The zone of thermal necrosis will be 0.1 mm when the laser is used in this manner. Some lasers have a function called *super pulse,* in which the laser beam is electronically switched off and on thousands of times per second, thereby allowing the tissue to cool between pulses to create less thermal necrosis.

Results of Laser Therapy Laser therapy has extremely varied results (60–67). In general, the earlier reports showed a lower success rate; the improvement in success rate is attributed to the realization that the entire transformation zone needed to be treated, not just the individual identified lesions (Table 16.3). The therapeutic efficacy of laser conization versus knife conization is shown in Table 16.4, and a comparison of intraoperative and postoperative bleeding with the two procedures is listed in Table 16.5.

The carbon dioxide laser is an excellent tool for the treatment of CIN. In properly selected patients, the success rate with laser vaporization is higher than 95% (Table 16.4). For patients who need diagnostic conization, the cone can be obtained by laser excision performed on an outpatient basis with less blood loss and fewer complications than with a cold knife conization (67–72).

Table 16.3. Success Rate for Laser Vaporization

	CIN 1		*CIN 2*		*CIN 3*	
Author (Ref. No.)	***No.***	***NED (%)***	***No.***	***NED (%)***	***No.***	***NED (%)***
Burke (61)	49	41 (83.6)	42	36 (85.7)	40	31 (77.5)
Wright (62)	110	108 (98.2)	140	133 (95)	190	179 (94.2)
Rylander (63)	22	21 (95.5)	49	48 (97.9)	133	116 (87.2)
Jordan (64)	142	140 (98.6)	153	145 (94.7)	416	390 (93.8)
Baggish (65)	741	675 (91.1)	1,048	978 (93.3)	1,281	1,228 (96)
Benedet (66)	312	301 (96.5)	472	428 (90.7)	773	702 (90.8)
TOTAL	1,376	1,286 (93.5)	1,904	1,768 (92.9)	2,833	2,646 (93.4)

Table 16.4. Therapeutic Efficiency of Cervical Conization: Comparison Between Laser and Knife Techniques

	Percentage of patients who are "cured" by conization		
Author (Ref. No.)	***Laser (%)***	***Author (Ref. No.)***	***Knife (%)***
Larsson (67)	95.6	Larsson (67)	94.0
Bostofte (60)	93.2	Bostofte (60)	90.2
Wright (62)	96.2	Bjerre* (69)	94.8
Baggish (68)	97.5	Kolstad* (70)	97.6

*Patients had negative cone margins.

Loop Electrosurgical Excision

Loop electrosurgical excision is a valuable tool for the diagnosis and treatment of CIN (73–83). It has the advantage of being able to perform simultaneously a diagnostic and therapeutic operation during one outpatient visit (61–71).

The tissue effect of electricity depends on the concentration of electrons (size of the wire), the power (watts), and the water content of the tissue. If low power or a large-diameter wire is used, the effect will be electrocautery, and the thermal damage to tissue will be extensive. If the power is high (35 to 55 watts) and the wire loop is small (0.5 mm), the effect will be electrosurgical, and the tissue will have little thermal damage. The actual cutting is a result of a steam envelope developing at the interface between the wire loop and the water-laden tissue. This envelope is then pushed through the tissue, and the combination of electron flow and acoustical events separates the tissue. After the excision, a 5-mm diameter ball electrode is used, and the power is set at 50 watts. The ball is placed near the surface so that a spark occurs between the ball and the tissue. This process is called *electrofulguration,* and it results in some thermal damage that leads to hemostasis. If too much fulguration occurs, the patient will develop an eschar with more discharge, and the risk for infection and late bleeding will be higher.

Loop excision should not be used before identification of an intraepithelial lesion that requires treatment. The risk of the "see and treat" philosophy is that in women with only metaplasia, the entire transformation zone will be removed along with varying amounts of the cervical canal, thus potentially compromising fertility (81–83). **This is particularly true of young women, who may have large, immature transformation zones with extensive acetowhite areas.**

Complications following loop electrosurgical excision are fairly minimal and compare favorably with those following laser ablation and conization. Intraoperative hemorrhage,

Table 16.5. Perioperative and Postoperative Bleeding From Cervical Conization: Comparison between Laser and Knife Techniques

Percentage of patients undergoing conization who develop significant vaginal bleeding			
Author (Ref. No.)	***Laser (%)***	***Author (Ref. No.)***	***Knife (%)***
Larsson (67)	2.3	Larsson (67)	14.8
Bostofte (60)	5.0	Bostofte (60)	17.0
Wright (62)	12.2	Jones (71)	10.0
Baggish (68)	2.5	Luesley (72)	13.0

Table 16.6. Complications of Electrosurgical Excision

Complications	*No. of Patients*	*Operative Hemorrhage*	*Postoperative Hemorrhage*	*Cervical Stenosis*
Prendiville (73)	111	2	2	—
Whiteley (74)	80	0	3	—
Mor-Yosef (75)	50	1	3	—
Bigrigg (76)	1,000	0	6	—
Gunasekera (77)	98	0	0	—
Howe (78)	100	0	1	—
Minucci (79)	130	0	1	2
Wright (80)	432	0	8	2
Luesley (81)	616	0	24	7
TOTAL	2,617	3 (0.001%)	48 (1.8%)	11/6178 (1.0%)

postoperative hemorrhage, and cervical stenosis can occur but at acceptably low rates, as noted in Table 16.6. The SCJ is visible in more than 90% of patients after this procedure.

One advantage of loop excision over other ablative procedures is the ability to diagnose unsuspected invasive disease (Table 16.7). The loop has several advantages over the laser:

1. Treatment time is shorter.
2. It is easier to learn.
3. There is no hazard to eyesight.
4. Equipment breakdowns occur less often.
5. The cone sample is better.
6. There is less handling of the tissues.
7. Discomfort is reduced.

Table 16.7. Unsuspected Invasion in Electrosurgical Excision Specimens

Author (Ref. No.)	*Patients*	*Microinvasive*	*Invasive*
Prendiville (73)	102	1	—
Bigrigg (76)	1,000	5	—
Gunasekera (77)	98	—	1
Howe (78)	100	1	—
Chappatte (79)	100	3	—
Wright (80)	141	1	—
Luesley (81)	616	4	6 (Adenocarcinoma *in situ*)
TOTAL	2,157	15 (0.7%)	1 (0.04%)

Table 16.8. Grade of Discomfort of Large-loop Excision Versus Laser Conization

Side Effect	*Loop Excision (n = 98)*	*Laser (n = 101)*
Not unpleasant	80 (92%)	32 (32%)
Moderately unpleasant	16 (16%)	50 (50%)
Very unpleasant	2 (2%)	19 (18%)
Operative time	20–50 sec (mean, 16 sec)	4–15 min (mean, 6.5 min)

From **Gunasekera PC, Phipps JH, Lewis BV.** Large loop excision of the transformation zone (LLETZ) compared to carbon dioxide laser in the treatment of CIN: a superior mode of treatment. *Br J Obstet Gynecol* 1990;97:995–998, with permission.

One study of these two modes of therapy compared pain and operative time in a randomized fashion (77). Electrosurgical excision showed an advantage over laser therapy (Table 16.8).

The most important issue in selecting therapy is whether the loop is an effective means of eradicating CIN. A combined literature series indicated a recurrent rate of about 4% (Table 16.9). This rate compares favorably with the recurrence rate for other types of procedures used in the treatment of CIN.

Conization

Conization of the cervix plays an important role in the management of CIN. Before the availability of colposcopy, conization was the standard method of evaluating an abnormal Pap test result. Conization is both a diagnostic and therapeutic procedure and has the advantage over ablative therapies of providing tissue for further evaluation to rule out invasive cancer (67–72).

Conization is indicated for diagnosis in women with HSIL based on a Pap test under the following conditions:

1. Limits of the lesion cannot be visualized with colposcopy.
2. The SCJ is not seen at colposcopy.
3. ECC histologic findings are positive for CIN 2 or CIN 3.
4. There is a lack of correlation between cytology, biopsy, and colposcopy results.
5. Microinvasion is suspected based on biopsy, colposcopy, or cytology results.
6. The colposcopist is unable to rule out invasive cancer.

Table 16.9. Results of Loop Electrosurgical Excision

Author (Ref. No.)	*No. of Patients Treated*	*No. of Patients Recurred*
Prendiville (73)	102	2
Whiteley (74)	80	4
Bigrigg (76)	1,000	41
Gunasekera (77)	98	7
Luesley (81)	616	27
Murdoch (83)	600	16
TOTAL	2,496	97 (3.9%)

Table 16.10. Recurrence of Cervical Intraepithelial Neoplasia After Cone Biopsy

Author (Ref. No.)	*No. of Patients*	*Negative Margins*	*Positive Margins*
Larsson (67)	683	56	246
Bjerre (69)	1,226	64	429
Kolstad (70)	1,121	27	291
TOTAL	3,030	147 (4.9%)	966 (31.9%)

Lesions with positive margins are more likely to recur after conization (67–69) (Table 16.10). Dempoulos and associates (84) has shown that endocervical gland involvement also is predictive of recurrence (23.6% with gland involvement compared with 11.3% without gland involvement).

Hysterectomy

Hysterectomy is currently considered too radical for treatment of CIN. Coppleson (85) reported 38 cases of invasive cancer occurring after hysterectomy among 8,998 women (0.4%). The incidence of significant bleeding, infection, and other complications, including death, is higher with hysterectomy than with other means of treating CIN. There are some situations in which hysterectomy remains a valid and appropriate method of treatment for CIN:

1. Microinvasion
2. CIN 3 at limits of conization specimen
3. Poor compliance with follow-up
4. Other gynecologic problems requiring hysterectomy, such as fibroids, prolapse, endometriosis, and pelvic inflammatory disease

Glandular Cell Abnormalities

Atypical Glandular Cells of Undetermined Significance

The Bethesda system includes a category for glandular cell abnormalities (21). These cells may be classified as (a) adenocarcinoma or (b) atypical glandular cells of undetermined significance (AGUS). **Atypical endocervical cells are important because of their risk for significant disease.** In a series of 63 patients from whom subsequent cervical biopsy or hysterectomy specimens were evaluated, 17 women had CIN 2 or CIN 3, 5 women had adenocarcinoma *in situ,* and 2 women had invasive adenocarcinoma (86). An additional 8 patients had CIN 1, and 2 women had endometrial hyperplasia. Overall, 32 patients (50.8%) had significant cervical lesions. This is a much higher positive rate than that for ASCUS Pap test results.

In adenocarcinoma *in situ* (AIS), the endocervical glandular cells are replaced by tall columnar cells with nuclear stratification, hyperchromasia, irregularity, and increased mitotic activity (87). Cellular proliferation results in crowded, cribriform glands. However, the normal branching pattern of the endocervical glands is maintained. Most neoplastic cells resemble those of the endocervical mucinous epithelium. Endometrioid and intestinal cell types occur less often. About 50% of women with cervical AIS also have squamous CIN. Thus, some of the AIS lesions represent incidental findings in specimens removed for treatment of squamous neoplasia. Because AIS is located near or above the transformation zone, conventional cervical specimens may not be effective to sample AIS. Obtaining specimens by cytobrush may improve detection of AIS. If the focus of AIS is small, cervical biopsy and ECC may have negative findings. In such cases, a more comprehensive survey of the cervix in the form of conization is necessary. This type of specimen also allows exclusion of coexisting invasive adenocarcinoma. **The term *microinvasion* should not be used to describe adenocarcinomas.** Once the gland has been invaded, there is no definable technique for identifying the true "depth of invasion" because the invasion may have originated from the mucosal surface or the periphery of the underlying glands. The "breakthrough" of the basement membrane cannot truly be described; therefore, the tumor is either AIS or invasive adenocarcinoma.

With the recent apparent increase in invasive adenocarcinoma of the endocervix, more attention has been directed toward AIS. There is evidence that AIS may progress to invasive cancer (75). Boone and colleagues reported a series of 52 cases of adenocarcinoma of the uterine cervix in which the results of 18 endocervical biopsies were interpreted as negative 3 to 7 years before the presentation with cancer (87). In 5 of these cases, AIS was found.

Bertrand and associates studied the anatomic distribution of AIS in 23 women (88). All 23 patients had AIS involving both the surface and the glandular endocervical epithelium, often with the deepest glandular cleft also involved. The entire endocervical canal was at risk; nearly half of the patients had lesions between 1.5 and 3 cm from the external os. Fifteen patients had unifocal disease, 3 had multifocal disease, and 5 patients had AIS of undermined type. Eleven of the 23 patients had squamous intraepithelial lesions as well as AIS. Muntz reported 40 patients with AIS who had cervical conization (89). Twenty-three of 40 (58%) had coexisting squamous intraepithelial lesions, and 2 patients had invasive squamous cell carcinoma. Of the 22 patients who underwent hysterectomy, the margins on the cone specimen were positive in 10 patients, and 70% had residual AIS, including 2 patients with foci of invasive adenocarcinoma. One of the 12 patients with negative margins had focal residual adenocarcinoma in the hysterectomy specimen. Eighteen women had conization only with negative margins and had no relapse of disease after a medium interval of 3 years. Thus, positive margins on the conization specimen are significant findings in these patients.

Poyner and coauthors published the results of a more alarming study of 28 patients with AIS (90). Of the 8 patients with positive margins who underwent repeat conization or hysterectomy, 3 had residual AIS, and 1 patient had invasive adenocarcinoma. Four of 10 patients with negative margins who underwent hysterectomy or repeat conization had residual AIS. One patient in whom the cone margin could not be evaluated was found to have invasive adenocarcinoma. Of the 15 patients treated conservatively with repeat conization of the cervix and close follow-up, 7 (47%) had a recurrent glandular lesion detected after the conization, including invasive adenocarcinoma in two women. More disturbing is the finding that a glandular lesion was not suspected in 48% of the patients, based on Pap test and ECC results obtained before conization of the cervix.

AIS must be considered a serious cancer precursor of adenocarcinoma. The entire endocervical canal is at risk, and detection of the lesion with cytologic assessment or ECC may not be reliable. Any patient with a positive cone margin should undergo repeat conization. If fertility is not desired, a hysterectomy should be performed because of the risk for recurrence, even in the presence of negative margins.

Vaginal Intraepithelial Neoplasia

Vaginal intraepithelial neoplasia (VAIN) often accompanies CIN and is believed to have a similar cause (91). VAIN lesions may be extensions onto the vagina from the CIN, or they may be satellite lesions occurring mainly in the upper vagina. Because the vagina does not have a transformation zone with immature epithelial cells to be infected by HPV, the mechanism of entry of HPV is by way of skin abrasions from coitus or tampon use. As

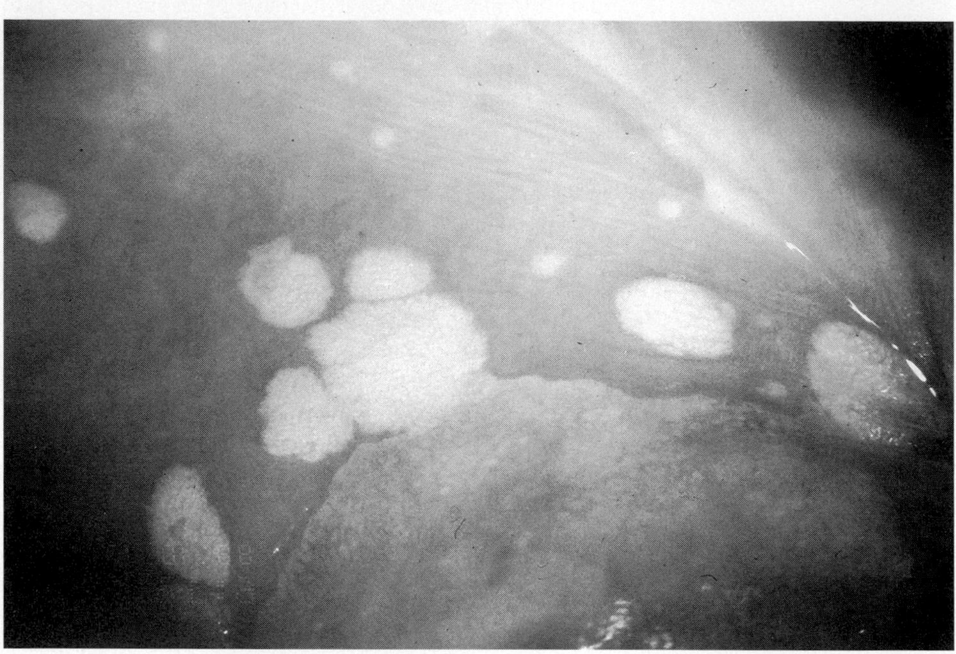

Figure 16.14 Vaginal condylomas in the posterior fornix.

these abrasions heal with metaplastic squamous cells, the HPV may begin its growth in a manner similar to that in the cervical transformation zone (Fig. 16.14).

Signs

VAIN lesions are asymptomatic. Because they often accompany active HPV infection, the patient may complain of vulvar warts or an odoriferous vaginal discharge from vaginal warts.

Screening

Women with an intact cervix should undergo routine cytologic screening. Because VAIN is nearly always accompanied by CIN, the Pap test result is likely to be positive when VAIN is present. The vagina should be carefully inspected by colposcopic examination at the time of colposcopy for any CIN lesion. Particular attention should be paid to the upper vagina. Women who have persistent positive Pap test results after treatment of CIN should be examined carefully for VAIN. For women in whom the cervix has been removed for cervical neoplasia, Pap testing should be performed at regular intervals initially, depending on the diagnosis and severity of lesion, and yearly thereafter.

Diagnosis

Colposcopic examination and directed biopsy are the mainstays of diagnosis of VAIN. Typically, the lesions are located along the vaginal ridges, are ovoid in shape and slightly raised, and often have surface spicules. VAIN 1 lesions usually are accompanied by a significant amount of koilocytosis, indicating their HPV origin (Fig. 16.15). As the lesions progress to VAIN 2, they have a thicker acetowhite epithelium, a more raised external border, and less iodine uptake (Fig. 16.16). When VAIN 3 occurs, the surface may become papillary, and the vascular patterns of punctation and mosaic may occur (Fig. 16.17). Early invasion is typified by vascular patterns similar to those of the cervix.

Treatment

Patients with VAIN 1 and HPV infection do not require treatment. These lesions often regress, are often multifocal, and recur quickly when treated with ablative therapy. VAIN 2 lesions are generally treated by laser ablation. VAIN 3 lesions are more likely

Figure 16.15 Human papillomavirus/vaginal intraepithelial neoplasia grade 1. Note the surface spicules with partial uptake of Lugol's stain.

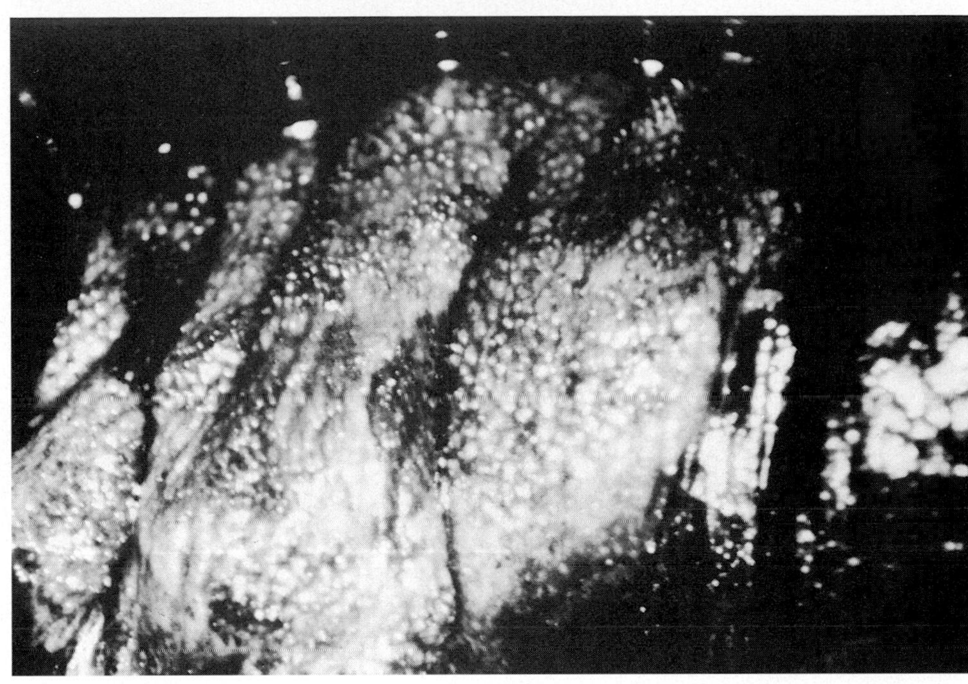

Figure 16.16 Vaginal intraepithelial neoplasia grade 2. There are multifocal raised, ovoid lesions on the vaginal rugae that are outlined by Lugol's stain.

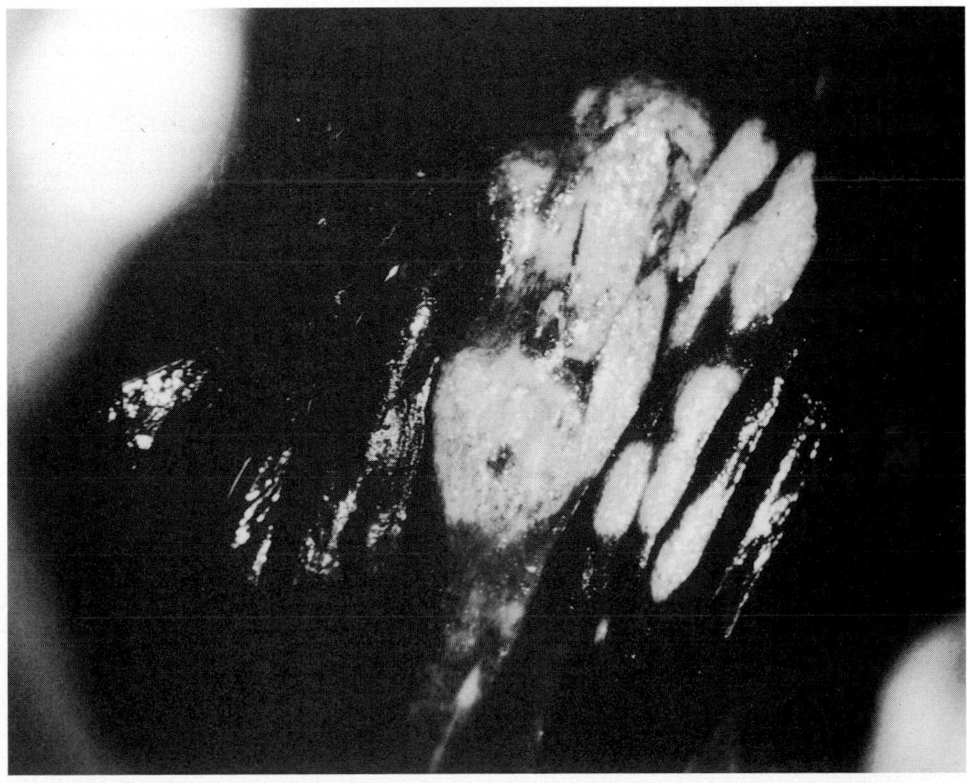

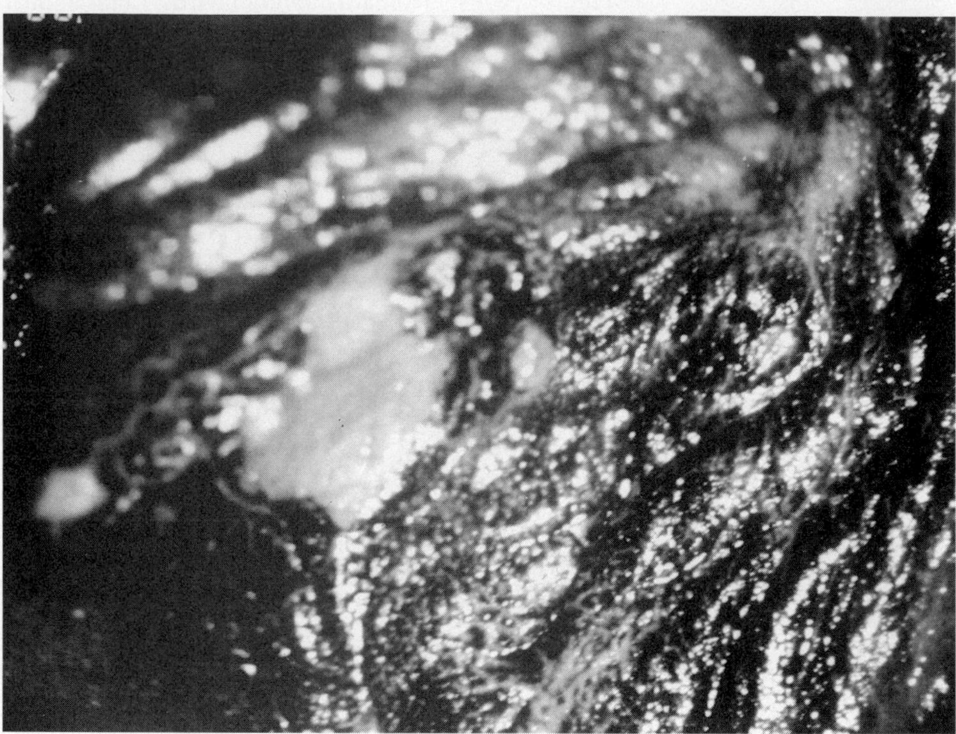

Figure 16.17 Vaginal intraepithelial neoplasia grade 3. The lesion is located in the center of human papillomavirus spicules with partial uptake of Lugol's stain.

to harbor an early invasive lesion. Hoffman and colleagues reported 32 patients who underwent upper vaginectomy for VAIN 3 (92). Occult invasive carcinoma was found in 9 patients (28%). It is recommended in older patients that VAIN 3 lesions located in the dimples of the vaginal cuff be excised to rule out occult invasive cancer. **VAIN 3 lesions that are adequately sampled to rule out invasive disease can be treated with laser therapy.**

Cryosurgery should not be used in the vagina because the depth of injury cannot be controlled and inadvertent injury to the bladder or rectum may occur. Superficial fulguration with electrosurgical ball cautery may be used under colposcopic control to observe the depth of destruction by wiping away the epithelial tissue as it is ablated. Excision is an excellent method for treatment of upper vaginal lesions in a small area. Occasionally, total vaginectomy will be required for a VAIN 3 lesion occupying the entire vagina. It should be accompanied by a split-thickness skin graft. This aggressive treatment for widespread vaginal lesions should not be used for VAIN 2.

The malignant potential of VAIN appears to be less than that of CIN. In a review of 136 cases of CIS of the vagina over a 30-year period (91), 4 cases (3%) progressed to invasive vaginal cancer despite the use of various treatment methods.

Vulvar Intraepithelial Disease

Vulvar Dystrophies

In the past, terms such as *leukoplakia, lichen sclerosis et atrophicus, primary atrophy, sclerotic dermatosis, atrophic and hyperplastic vulvitis,* and *kraurosis vulvae* have been used to denote disorders of epithelial growth and differentiation (93). In 1966, Jeffcoate (94) suggested that these terms did not refer to separate disease entities because their

Table 16.11. Classification of Epithelial Vulvar Diseases

Nonneoplastic epithelial disorders of skin and mucosa
Lichen sclerosus (lichen sclerosis et atrophicus)
Squamous hyperplasia (formerly hyperplastic dystrophy)
Other dermatoses
Mixed nonneoplastic and neoplastic epithelial disorders
Intraepithelial neoplasia
Squamous intraepithelial neoplasia
VIN 1
VIN 2
VIN 3 (severe dysplasia or carcinoma *in situ*)
Nonsquamous intraepithelial neoplasia
Paget's disease
Tumors of melanocytes, noninvasive
Invasive tumors

VIN, vulvar intraepithelial neoplasia.
From **Committee on Terminology, International Society for the Study of Vulvar Disease.** New nomenclature for vulvar disease. *Int J Gynecol Pathol* 1989;8:83, with permission.

macroscopic and microscopic appearances were variable and interchangeable. He assigned the generic term *chronic vulvar dystrophy* to the entire group of lesions.

The International Society for the Study of Vulvar Disease (ISSVD) recommended that the old "dystrophy" terminology be replaced by a new classification under the pathologic heading "nonneoplastic epithelial disorders of skin and mucosa." This classification is shown in Table 16.11. In all cases, diagnosis requires biopsy of suspicious-looking lesions, which are best detected by careful inspection of the vulva in a bright light aided, if necessary, by a magnifying glass (95).

The malignant potential of these nonneoplastic epithelial disorders is low, particularly now that the lesions with atypia are classified as vulvar intraepithelial neoplasia (VIN). However, patients with lichen sclerosis and concomitant hyperplasia may be at particular risk (96).

Vulvar Intraepithelial Neoplasms

As with the vulvar dystrophies, there has been confusion regarding the nomenclature for VIN. Four major terms have been used: *erythroplasia of Queyrat, Bowen's disease, carcinoma in situ simplex,* and *Paget's disease*. In 1976, the ISSVD decreed that the first three lesions were merely gross variants of the same disease process and that all of these entities should be included under the umbrella term *squamous cell carcinoma in situ* (stage 0) (81). In 1986, the ISSVD recommended the term *vulvar intraepithelial neoplasia* (Table 16.11).

VIN is graded as 1 (mild dysplasia), 2 (moderate dysplasia), or 3 (severe dysplasia or CIS) on the basis of cellular immaturity, nuclear abnormalities, maturation disturbance, and mitotic activity. In VIN 1, immature cells, cellular disorganization, and mitotic activity occur predominantly in the lower one third of the epithelium, whereas in VIN 3, immature cells with scanty cytoplasm and severe chromatinic alterations occupy most of the epithelium (Fig. 16.18). Dyskeratotic cells and mitotic figures occur in the superficial layer. The appearance of VIN 2 is intermediate between VIN 1 and VIN 3. Additional cytopathic changes of HPV infection, such as perinuclear halos with displacement of the nuclei by the intracytoplasmic viral protein, thickened cell borders, binucleation, and multinucleation, are common in the superficial layers of VIN, especially in VIN 1 and VIN 2. These viral changes are not definitive evidence of neoplasia but are indicative of viral exposure (97). Most vulvar condylomas are associated with HPV-6 and -11, whereas HPV-16 is detected in more than 80% of VIN cases by molecular techniques.

VIN 3 can be unifocal or multifocal. Typically, multifocal VIN 3 presents with small hyperpigmented lesions on the labia major (Fig. 16.19). Some cases of VIN 3 are more

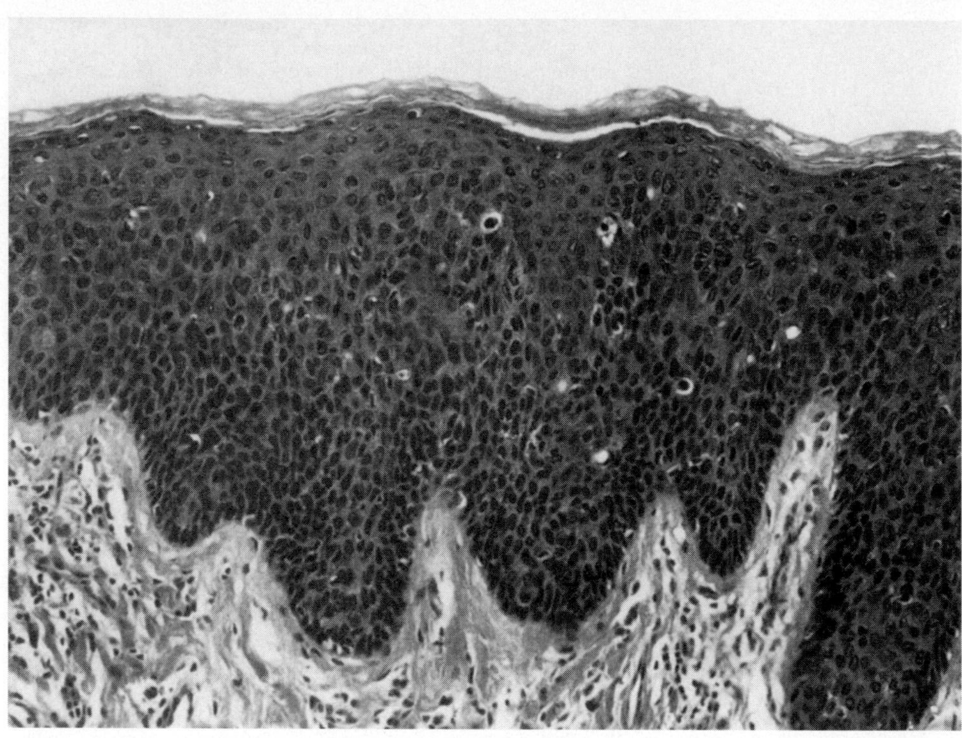

Figure 16.18 Carcinoma *in situ* of the vulva (vulvar intraepithelial neoplasia grade 3). Immature atypical cells are seen throughout epithelium. (From **Fu YS, Woodruff JD.** Pathology. In: **Berek JS, Hacker NF,** eds. *Practical gynecologic oncology,* 2nd ed. Baltimore: Williams & Wilkins, 1994:161, with permission.)

confluent, extending to the posterior fourchette and involving the perineal tissues. The term *bowenoid papulosis (bowenoid dysplasia)* has been used to describe multifocal VIN lesions ranging from grade 1 to 3. Clinically, patients with bowenoid papulosis present with multiple small pigmented papules (40% of cases) that are usually less than 5 mm in diameter. Most women with these lesions are in their 20s, and some are pregnant. After childbirth, the lesions may regress spontaneously. However, the term bowenoid papulosis is no longer recommended by the ISSVD.

Paget's Disease of the Vulva

Extramammary Paget's disease of the vulva (AIS) was described 27 years after the description by Sir James Paget of the mammary lesion that now bears his name (98). Some patients with vulvar Paget's disease have an underlying adenocarcinoma, although the precise frequency is difficult to ascertain.

Most cases of vulvar Paget's disease are intraepithelial. Because these lesions demonstrate apocrine differentiation, the malignant cells are believed to arise from undifferentiated basal cells, which convert into an appendage type of cell during carcinogenesis (Fig. 16.20). The "transformed cells" spread intraepithelially throughout the squamous epithelium and may extend into the appendages. In most patients with an underlying invasive carcinoma of the apocrine sweat gland, Bartholin gland, or anorectum, the malignant cells are believed to migrate through the dermal ductal structures and reach the epidermis. In such cases, metastasis to the regional lymph nodes and other sites can occur.

Paget's disease must be distinguished from superficial spreading melanoma. All sections should be studied thoroughly using differential staining, particularly periodic acid–Schiff (PAS) and mucicarmine stains. Mucicarmine has routinely positive results in the cells of Paget's disease and negative results in melanotic lesion.

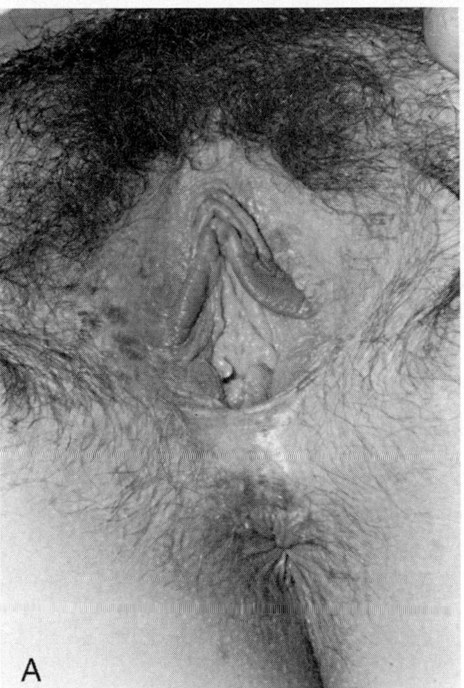

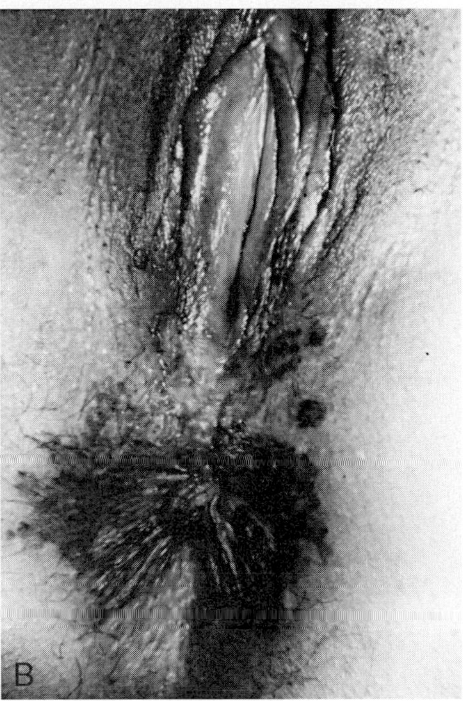

Figure 16.19 Vulvar intraepithelial neoplasia grade 3 (VIN 3). A: A multifocal VIN 3 lesion with multiple small hyperpigmented lesions on the labia major. **B:** VIN 3 with more confluent hyperpigmented areas on the posterior fourchette with extensive perianal involvement. (From **Berek JS, Hacker NF,** eds. *Practical gynecologic oncology,* 2nd ed. Baltimore: Williams & Wilkins, 1994:213, with permission.)

Clinical Features

Paget's disease of the vulva predominantly affects postmenopausal white women, and the presenting symptoms are usually pruritus and vulvar soreness. The lesion has an eczematoid appearance macroscopically and usually begins on the hair-bearing portions of the vulva (Fig. 16.21). It may extend to involve the mons pubis, thighs, and buttocks. Extension to involve the mucosa of the rectum, vagina, or urinary tract also has been described (99). The more extensive lesions are usually raised and velvety in appearance.

A second synchronous or metachronous primary neoplasm is associated with extramammary Paget's disease in about 30% of patients (100). Associated carcinomas have been reported in the cervix, colon, bladder, gallbladder, and breast. When the anal mucosa is involved, there usually is an underlying rectal adenocarcinoma (96).

Treatment

VIN The treatment of VIN has varied from wide excision to the performance of a superficial or "skinning" vulvectomy (101–104). Although the treatment originally recommended for CIS of the vulva was wide excision, fears that the disease frequently was preinvasive led to the widespread use of superficial vulvectomy (103). Because progression is relatively uncommon, typically occurring in 5% to 10% of cases (101), extensive surgery is not warranted. This is particularly true because many VIN lesions are found in premenopausal women.

The therapeutic alternatives for VIN are (a) simple excision, (b) laser ablation, and (c) superficial vulvectomy with or without split-thickness skin grafting.

Excision of small foci of disease produces excellent results and has the advantage of providing a histopathologic specimen. Although multifocal or extensive lesions may be difficult

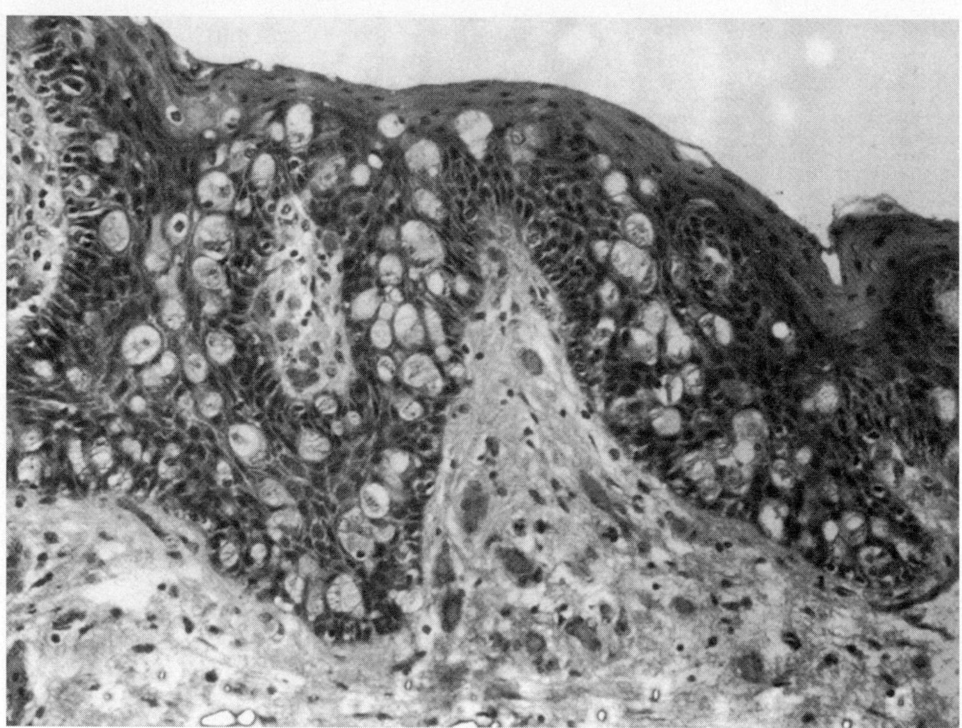

Figure 16.20 Paget's disease of vulva. The epidermis is permeated by abnormal cells with vacuolated cytoplasm and atypical nuclei. This heavy concentration of abnormal cells in the parabasal layers is typical of Paget's disease. (From **Fu YS, Woodruff JD.** Pathology. In: **Berek JS, Hacker NF,** eds. *Practical gynecologic oncology,* 2nd ed. Baltimore: Williams & Wilkins, 1994:162, with permission.)

to treat by this approach, it offers the potential for the most cosmetic result. Repeat excision is often necessary but can typically be accomplished without vulvectomy (102,104).

The carbon dioxide laser can be used for multifocal lesions but is unnecessary for unifocal disease. The disadvantages are that it can be painful and costly and does not provide a histopathologic specimen (105).

Superficial vulvectomy is appropriate for extensive and recurrent VIN (104). The goal of the surgery is to extirpate all of the disease while preserving as much of the normal vulvar anatomy as possible. The anterior vulva and the clitoris should be preserved if possible. In some patients, the disease extends up the anus, which also must be resected. An effort should be made to close the vulvar defect primarily, reserving the use of skin grafts for instances in which the vulvar defect cannot be closed because the resection is so extensive. Split-thickness skin grafts can be harvested from the thighs or buttocks, but the latter is more easily concealed (106).

Paget's Disease **Unlike squamous cell CIS, in which the histologic extent of disease usually correlates closely with the macroscopic lesion, Paget's disease usually extends well beyond the gross lesion** (107). This extension results in positive surgical margins and frequent local recurrence unless a wide local excision is performed (108). **Underlying adenocarcinomas are usually apparent clinically, but this finding does not occur invariably; therefore, the underlying dermis should be removed for adequate histologic evaluation.** For this reason, laser therapy is unsatisfactory in treating primary Paget's disease. If underlying invasive carcinoma is present, it should be treated in the same manner as a squamous vulvar cancer. This treatment usually requires radical vulvectomy and at least an ipsilateral inguinal-femoral lymphadenectomy.

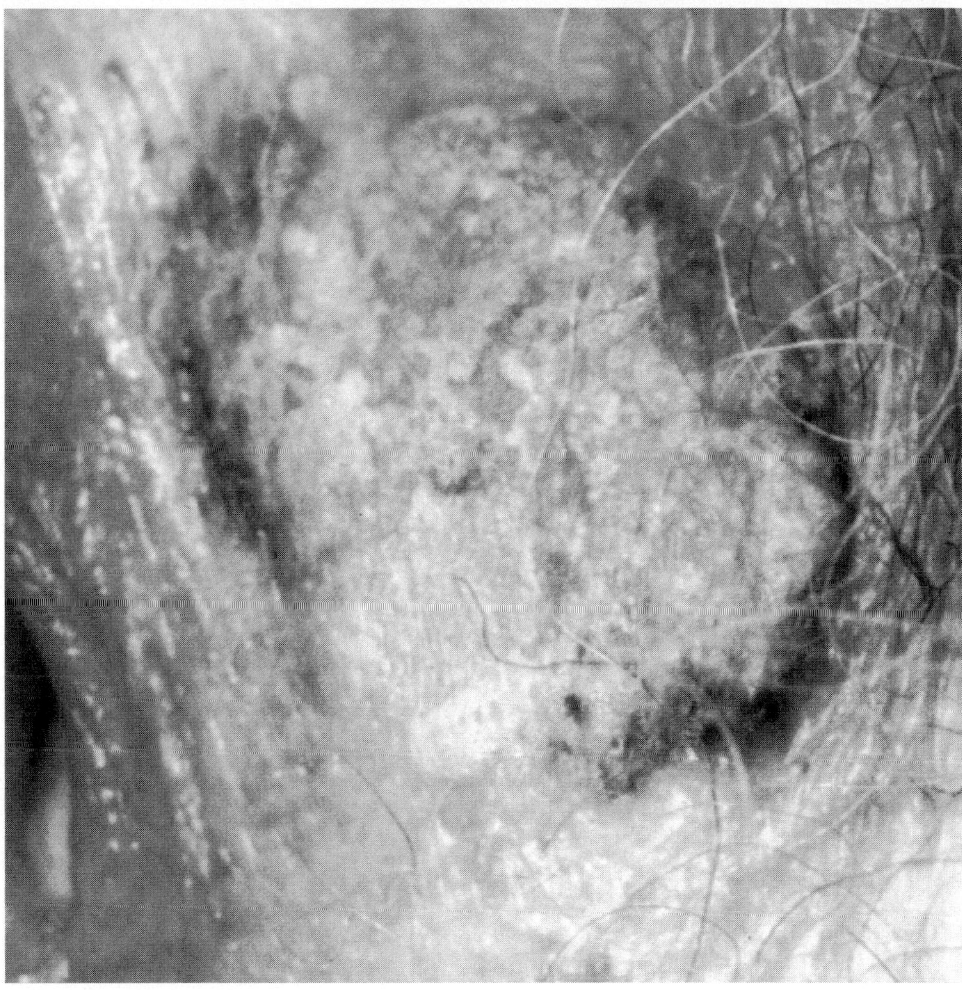

Figure 16.21 Paget's disease of the left labium majus treated by wide local excision. (From **Wilkinson EJ, Stone IK.** *Atlas of vulvar disease.* Baltimore: Williams & Wilkins, 1995:87, with permission.)

Recurrent lesions are almost always *in situ,* although there has been at least one report of an underlying adenocarcinoma in recurrent Paget's disease (100). In general, it is reasonable to treat recurrent lesions with surgical excision.

References

1. **Pund ER, Nieburgs H, Nettles JB, et al.** Preinvasive carcinoma of the cervix uteri: seven cases in which it was detected by examination of routine endocervical smears. *Arch Pathol Lab Med* 1947;44:571–577.
2. **Koss LG, Stewart FW, Foote FW, et al.** Some histological aspects of behavior of epidermoid carcinoma in situ and related lesions of the uterine cervix. *Cancer* 1963;16:1160–1211.
3. **Richart RM.** Natural history of cervical intraepithelial neoplasia. *Clin Obstet Gynecol* 1968;10:748.
4. **Nasiell K, Roger V, Nasiell M.** Behavior of mild cervical dysplasia during long-term follow-up. *Obstet Gynecol* 1986;5:665–669.
5. **Hatch KD.** *Handbook of colposcopy: diagnosis and treatment of lower genital tract neoplasia and HPV infections.* Boston: Little, Brown, 1989:7–19.
6. **Koss LG, Durfee GR.** Unusual patterns of squamous epithelium of the uterine cervix: cytologic and pathologic study of koilocytotic atypia. *Ann N Y Acad Sci* 1956;63:1235–1240.
7. **Meisels A, Fortin R, Roy M.** Condylomatous lesions of the cervix. II. Cytologic, colposcopic and histopathologic study. *Acta Cytol* 1977;21:379–390.
8. **Beckmann AM, Myerson D, Daling JR, et al.** Detection and localization of human papillomavirus DNA in human genital condylomas by in situ hybridization with biotinylated probes. *J Med Virol* 1985;16:265–273.

9. **Schneider A, Oltersdorf T, Schneider V, et al.** Distribution pattern of human papilloma virus 16 genome in cervical neoplasia by molecular in situ hybridization of tissue sections. *Int J Cancer* 1987;39:717–721.

10. **Crum CP, Mitao M, Levine RU, et al.** Cervical papilloma viruses segregate within morphologically distinct precancerous lesions. *J Virol* 1985;54:675–681.

11. **Durst M, Kleinheinz A, Hotz M, et al.** The physical state of human papillomavirus type 16 DNA in benign and malignant genital tumors. *J Gen Virol* 1985;66:1515–1522.

12. **Munger K, Phelps WC, Bubb V, et al.** The E6 and E7 genes of the human papillomavirus type 16 together are necessary and sufficient for transformation of primary human keratinocytes. *J Virol* 1989;63:4417–4421.

13. **McCance DJ, Kopan R, Fuchs E, et al.** Human papillomavirus type 16 alters human epithelial cell differentiation in vitro. *Proc Natl Acad Sci U S A* 1988;85:7169–7173.

14. **Dyson N, Howley PM, Munger K, et al.** The human papillomavirus-16E-oncoprotein is able to bind to the retinoblastoma gene produce. *Science* 1989;243:934–937.

15. **Yee CL, Krishnan-Hewiett I, Baker CC, et al.** Presences and expression of human papillomavirus sequences in human cervical carcinoma cell lines. *Am J Pathol* 1985;119:3261–3266.

16. **Koutsky LA, Holmes KK, Critchlow CW, et al.** A cohort study of the risk of cervical intraepithelial neoplasia grade 2 or 3 in relation to papillomavirus infection. *N Engl J Med* 1992;327:1272–1278.

17. **Lorincz AT, Reid R, Jenson AB, et al.** Human papillomavirus infection of the cervix: relative risk associations of 15 common anogenital types. *Obstet Gynecol* 1992;79:328–337.

18. **Bauer HM, Ting Y, Greer CE, et al.** Genital human papillomavirus infection in female university students as determined by a PCR-based method. *JAMA* 1991;265:472–477.

19. **Ley C, Bauer HM, Reingold A, et al.** Determinants of genital papillomavirus infection in young women. *J Natl Cancer Inst* 1991;83:997–1003.

20. **Shiffman MH.** Recent progress in defining the epidemiology of human papillomavirus infection and cervical cancer. *J Natl Cancer Inst* 1992;84:398–399.

21. **National Cancer Institute Workshop.** The 188 Bethesda system for reporting cervical/vaginal cytological diagnoses. *JAMA* 1989;262:931–934.

22. **Solomon D, Daveg D, Karman R, et al.** Terminology for reporting Results of Cervical Cytology. *JAMA* 2002;87:2114–2119.

23. **Willett GD, Kurman RJ, Reid R, et al.** Correlation of the histologic appearance of intraepithelial neoplasia of the cervix with human papillomavirus types: emphasis on the low grade lesions including so-called flat condyloma. *Int J Gynecol Pathol* 1989;8:18–25.

24. **Ismail SM, Colclough AB, Dinnen JS, et al.** Reporting cervical intraepithelial neoplasia (CIN): intra- and interpathologist variation and factors associated with disagreement. *Histopathology* 1990;16:371–376.

25. **Sherman ME, Schiffman MH, Erozan YS, et al.** The Bethesda system: a proposal for reporting abnormal cervical smears based on the reproducibility of cytopathologic diagnoses. *Arch Pathol Lab Med* 1992;116:1155–1158.

26. **Ries LAG, Kosary CL, Hankey BF, et al.** *SEER cancer statistics review 1973–1996*. Bethesda, MD: National Cancer Institute, 1999.

27. **Jemal A, Thomas A, Murray T, et al.** Cancer statistics, 2002. *CA Cancer J Clin* 2002;52:23–47.

28. ***Evidence report/technology assessment.*** Rockville, MD: Agency for Health Care Policy and Research, January 1999, No. 5.

29. **National Institutes of Health.** *Consensus statement* [On-line, April 1–3, 1996]. Cited November 15, 1999, 43(1):1–38.

30. **Linder J, Zahniser D.** ThinPrep pap testing to reduce false-negative cytology. *Arch Pathol Lab Med* 1998;122:139–144.

31. **Hutchinson ML, Isenstein LM, Goodman A, et al.** Homogeneous sampling accounts for the increased diagnostic accuracy using the ThinPrep processor. *Am J Clin Pathol* 1994;101:215–219.

32. **Bolick D, Hellman DJ.** Laboratory implementation and efficacy assessment of ThinPrep cervical cancer screening system. *Acta Cytol* 1998;42:209–213.

33. **McQuarrie HG, Ogden J, Costa M.** Understanding the financial impact of covering new screening technologies: the case of automated Pap smears. *J Reprod Med* 2000;45(11):898–906.

34. **Davey DD, Naryshkin S, Neilsen MI, et al.** Atypical squamous cells of undetermined significance: interlaboratory comparison and quality assurance monitors. *Diagn Cytopathol* 1994;11:390–396.

35. **Kurman RJ, Henson DE, Herbst AL, et al.** The National Cancer Institute Workshop. Interim guidelines for management of abnormal cervical cytology. *JAMA* 1994;271:1866–1869.

36. **Wright TC, Sun XW, Koulos J.** Comparison of management algorithms for the evaluation of women with low grade cytologic abnormalities. *Obstet Gynecol* 1995;85:202–210.

37. **Lonky NM, Navarre GL, Sanders S, et al.** Low grade Pap smears and the Bethesda system: a prospective cytopathologic analysis. *Obstet Gynecol* 1995;85:716–720.

38. **Kinney WK, Manos MM, Hurley LB, et al.** Where's the high-grade cervical neoplasia? The importance of the minimally abnormal pap smear. *Obstet Gynecol* 1998;91:973–976.

39. **Cox JJ, Lorincz AT, Schiffman MH.** HPV testing by hybrid capture appears to be useful in triaging women with a cytologic diagnosis of ASCUS. *Am J Obstet Gynecol* 1995;172:946–954.

40. **Melnikow J, Nuovo J, Willan AR, et al.** Natural history of cervical squamous intraepithelial lesions: a meta-analysis. *Obstet Gynecol* 1998;92(4, Part 2):727–735.

41. **Wright T, Lox J, Mossad L, et al.** 2001 Consensus Guidelines for the Management of Women with Cervical Cytological Abnormalities. *JAMA* 2002;287:2120–2129.

42. **Manos MM, Kinney WK, Hurley LH, et al.** Human papillomavirus DNA testing for equivocal pap results. *JAMA* 1999;281:1605–1610.

43. **Wright TC, Lorincz A, Ferris DG, et al.** Reflex human papillomavirus DNA testing in women with abnormal Pap smears. *Am J Obstet Gynecol* 1998;178:962–966.

44. **Solomon D, Schiffman M, Tarone R.** Comparison of three management strategies for patients with atypical squamous cells of undetermined significance: baseline results from a randomized trial. *J Natl Cancer Inst* 2001;93(4):293–318.

45. **Benedet JL, Anderson GH, Boyes DA.** Colposcopic accuracy in the diagnosis of microinvasive and occult invasive carcinoma of the cervix. *Obstet Gynecol* 1985;65:577–562.

46. **Townsend DE, Richart RM.** Diagnostic errors in colposcopy. *Gynecol Oncol* 1981;12:S259–S264.

47. **Urcuyo R, Rome RM, Nelson JH.** Some observations on the value of endocervical curettage performed as an integral part of colposcopic examination of patients with abnormal cervical cytology. *Am J Obstet Gynecol* 1977;128:787–792.

48. **Nasiell K, Roger V, Nasiell M.** Behavior of mild cervical dysplasia during long-term follow-up. *Obstet Gynecol* 1986;67(5):665–669.

49. **Oster AG.** Natural history of cervical intraepithelial neoplasia: a critical review. *Int J Gynecol Pathol* 1993;12:186–192.

50. **Lee SSN, Collins RJ, Pun TC, et al.** Conservative treatment of low grade squamous intraepithelial lesions (LSIL) of the cervix. *Int J Obstet Gynecol* 1998;60:35–40.

51. **Falls RK.** Spontaneous resolution rate of grade 1 cervical intraepithelial neoplasia in a private practice population. *Am J Obstet Gynecol* 1999;181:278–282.

52. **Mitchell MF, Tortolero-Luna G, Cook E, Whittaker L, et al.** A randomized clinical trial of cryotherapy, laser vaporization, and loop electrosurgical excision for treatment of squamous intraepithelial lesions of the cervix. *Obstet Gynecol* 1998;92:737–744.

53. **Alvarez RD, Helm CW, Edwards RP, et al.** Prospective randomized trial of LLETZ versus laser ablation in patients with cervical intraepithelial neoplasia. *Gynecol Oncol* 1994;52:175–179.

54. **Andersen ES, Thorup K, Larsen G.** Results of cryosurgery for cervical intraepithelial neoplasia. *Gynecol Oncol* 1988;30:21–25

55. **Ostergard DR.** Cryosurgical treatment of cervical intraepithelial neoplasia. *Obstet Gynecol* 1980;56:231–233.

56. **Creasman WT, Weed JC, Curry SL, et al.** Efficacy of cryosurgical treatment of severe cervical intraepithelial neoplasia. *Obstet Gynecol* 1973;41:501–505.

57. **Benedet JL, Miller DM, Nickerson KG, et al.** The results of cryosurgical treatment of cervical intraepithelial neoplasia at one, five, and ten years. *Am J Obstet Gynecol* 1987;157:268–273.

58. **Townsend DE.** Cryosurgery for CIN. *Obstet Gynecol Surv* 1979;34:828.

59. **Andersen MC, Hartley RB.** Cervical crypt involvement by intraepithelial neoplasia. *Am J Obstet Gynecol* 1980;55:546–550.

60. **Bostofte E, Berget A, Larsen JF, et al.** Conization by carbon dioxide laser or cold knife in the treatment of cervical intraepithelial neoplasia. *Acta Obstet Gynecol Scand* 1986;65:199–202.

61. **Burke L.** The use of the carbon dioxide laser in the therapy of cervical intraepithelial neoplasia. *Am J Obstet Gynecol* 1982;144:377–340.

62. **Wright VC.** Laser surgery for cervical intraepithelial neoplasia. *Acta Obstet Gynecol Scand* 1984;125(Suppl):17.

63. **Rylander E, Isberg A, Joelsson I.** Laser vaporization of cervical intraepithelial neoplasia: a five-year follow-up. *Acta Obstet Gynecol Scand Suppl* 1984;125:33–36.

64. **Jordan JA, Mylotte MJ, Williams DR.** The treatment of cervical intraepithelial neoplasia by laser vaporization. *Br J Obstet Gynecol* 1985;92:394–398.

65. **Baggish MS, Dorsey JH, Adelson M.** A ten-year experience treating cervical intraepithelial neoplasia with CO_2 laser. *Am J Obstet Gynecol* 1989;161:60–68.

66. **Benedet JL, Miller DM, Nickerson KG.** Results of conservative management of cervical intraepithelial neoplasia. *Obstet Gynecol* 1992;79:10–110.

67. **Larsson G, Gullberg BO, Grundsell H.** A comparison of complications of laser and cold knife conization. *Obstet Gynecol* 1983;62:213–217.

68. **Baggish MS.** A comparison between laser excisional conization and laser vaporization for the treatment of cervical intraepithelial neoplasia. *Am J Obstet Gynecol* 1986;155:39–44.

69. **Bjerre B, Eliasson G, Linell F, et al.** Conization as only treatment of carcinoma in situ of the uterine cervix. *Am J Obstet Gynecol* 1976;15:143–151.

70. **Kolstad P, Klem V.** Long-term follow-up of 1,121 cases of carcinoma in situ. *Obstet Gynecol* 1979;48:125–129.

71. **Jones III HW.** Treatment of cervical intraepithelial neoplasia. *Clin Obstet Gynecol* 1990;33:826–836.

72. **Luesley DM, McCann A, Terry PB, et al.** Complications of cone biopsy related to the dimensions of the cone and the influence of prior colposcopic assessment. *Br J Obstet Gynecol* 1985;92:158–162.

73. **Prendiville W, Cullimore J, Norman S.** Large loop excision of the transformation zone (LLETZ): a new method of management for women with cervical intraepithelial neoplasia. *Br J Obstet Gynecol* 1989;96:1054–1060.

74. **Whiteley PF, Olah KS.** Treatment of cervical intraepithelial neoplasia: experience with the low-voltage diathermy loop. *Am J Obstet Gynecol* 1990;162:1272–1277.

75. **Mor-Yosef S, Lopes A, Pearson S, et al.** Loop diathermy cone biopsy: instruments and methods. *Obstet Gynecol* 1990;75:884–886.

76. **Bigrigg MA, Codling BW, Pearson P, et al.** Colposcopic diagnosis and treatment of cervical dysplasia at a single clinic visit: experience of low-voltage diathermy loop in 1000 patients. *Lancet* 1990;336:229–231.

77. **Gunasekera PC, Phipps JH, Lewis BV.** Large loop excision of the transformation zone (LLETZ) compared to carbon dioxide laser in the treatment of CIN: a superior mode of treatment. *Br J Obstet Gynecol* 1990;97:995–998.

78. **Howe DT, Vincenti AC.** Is large loop excision of the transformation zone (LLETZ) more accurate than colposcopically directed biopsy in the diagnosis of cervical intraepithelial neoplasia? *Br J Obstet Gynecol* 1991;98:588–591.

79. **Minucci D, Cinel A, Insacco E.** Diathermic loop treatment for CIN and HPV lesions: a follow-up of 130 cases. *Eur J Gynecol Oncol* XII 1991;5:385–393.

80. **Wright TC, Gagnon S, Richart RM, et al.** Treatment of cervical intraepithelial neoplasia using the loop electrosurgical excision procedure. *Obstet Gynecol* 1991;79:173–178.

81. **Luesley DM, Cullimore J, Redman CWE, et al.** Loop diathermy excision of the cervical transformation zone in patients with abnormal cervical smears. *BMJ* 1990;300:1690–1693.

82. **Chappatte OA, Bryne DL, Raju KS, et al.** Histological differences between colposcopic-directed biopsy and loop excision of the transformation zone (LETZ): a cause for concern. *Gynecol Oncol* 1991;43:46–50.

83. **Murdoch JB, Grimshaw RN, Monaghan JM.** Loop diathermy excision of the abnormal cervical transformation zone. *Int J Gynecol Cancer* 1991;1:105–111.

84. **Demopoulos RI, Horowitz LF, Vamvakas EC.** Endocervical gland involvement by cervical intraepithelial neoplasia grade 3. *Cancer* 1991;68:1932–1936.

85. **Coppleson M.** Management of preclinical carcinoma of the cervix. In: **Jordan JA, Singer A,** eds. *The cervix uteri.* London: WB Saunders, 1976:453.

86. **Goff B, Atanasoff P, Brown E, et al.** Endocervical glandular atypia in Papanicolaou smears. *Obstet Gynecol* 1992;79:101–104.

87. **Boone ME, Baak JPA, Kurver JPH, et al.** Adenocarcinoma in situ of the cervix: an underdiagnosed lesion. *Cancer* 1981;48:768–773.

88. **Bertrand M, Lickrish MB, Colgan TJ.** The anatomic distribution of cervical adenocarcinoma in situ: implications for treatment. *Am J Obstet Gynecol* 1987;157:21–25.

89. **Muntz HG, Bell DA, Lage JM, et al.** Adenocarcinoma in situ of the uterine cervix. *Obstet Gynecol* 1992;80:935–939.

90. **Pyonor EA, Barakat RR, Hoskins WJ.** Management and follow-up of patients with adenocarcinoma in situ of the uterine cervix. *Gynecol Oncol* 1995;57:158–164.

91. **Benedet JL, Saunders BH.** Carcinoma in situ of the vagina. *Am J Obstet Gynecol* 1984;148:695–699.

92. **Hoffman MS, DeCesare SL, Roberts WS, et al.** Upper vaginectomy for in situ and occult superficially invasive carcinoma of the vagina. *Am J Obstet Gynecol* 1992;166:30–33.

93. **Gardner HL, Friedrich EG Jr, Kaufman RH, et al.** The vulvar dystrophies, atypias, and carcinoma in situ: an invitational symposium. *J Reprod Med* 1976;17:131–137.

94. **Jeffcoate TNA.** Chronic vulval dystrophies. *Am J Obstet Gynecol* 1966;95:61–74.

95. **Committee on Terminology, International Society for the Study of Vulvar Disease.** New nomenclature for vulvar disease. *Int J Gynecol Pathol* 1989;8:83.

96. **Rodke G, Friedrich EG, Wilkinson EJ.** Malignant potential of mixed vulvar dystrophy (lichen sclerosis associated with squamous cell hyperplasia). *J Reprod Med* 1988;33:545–550.

97. **Rusk D, Sutton GP, Look KY, et al.** Analysis of invasive squamous cell carcinoma of the vulva and vulvar intraepithelial neoplasia for the presence of human papillomaviral DNA. *Obstet Gynecol* 1991;77:918–922.

98. **Dubreuilh W.** Pigmentation of the skin due to demodex folliculorum. *Br J Dermatol* 1901;13:403.

99. **Lee RA, Dahlin DC.** Paget's disease of the vulva with extension into the urethra, bladder, and ureters: a case report. *Am J Obstet Gynecol* 1981;140:834–836.

100. **Hart WR, Millman JB.** Progression of intraepithelial Paget's disease of the vulva to invasive carcinoma. *Cancer* 1977;40:2333–2337.

101. **Buscema J, Woodruff JD, Parmley T, et al.** Carcinoma in situ of the vulva. *Obstet Gynecol* 1980;55:225 230.

102. **Friedrich EG, Wilkinson EJ, Fu YS.** Carcinoma in situ of the vulva: a continuing challenge. *Am J Obstet Gyncol* 1980;136:880–843.

103. **Rutledge F, Sinclair M.** Treatment of intraepithelial carcinoma of the vulva by skin excision and graft. *Am J Obstet Gynecol* 1968;102:806 812.

104. **Chafee W, Ferguson K, Wilkinson EJ.** Vulvar intraepithelial neoplasia (VIN): principles of surgical therapy. *Colpo Gynecol Surg* 1988;4:125–130.

105. **Reid R.** Superficial laser vulvectomy. III. A new surgical technique for appendage-conserving ablation of refractory condylomas and vulvar intraepithelial neoplasia. *Am J Obstet Gynecol* 1985;152:504–509.

106. **Berek JS, Hacker NF, Lagasse LD.** Reconstructive operations. In: **Knapp RC, Berkowitz RS,** eds. *Gynecologic oncology,* 2nd ed. Philadelphia: WB Saunders, 1994:420–432.

107. **Gunn RA, Gallager HS.** Vulvar Paget's disease: a topographic study. *Cancer* 1980;46:590–594.

108. **Stacy D, Burrell MO, Franklin EW III.** Extramammary Paget's disease of the vulva and anus: use of intraoperative frozen-section margins. *Am J Obstet Gynecol* 1986;155:519–523.

17 Early Pregnancy Loss and Ectopic Pregnancy

Thomas G. Stovall

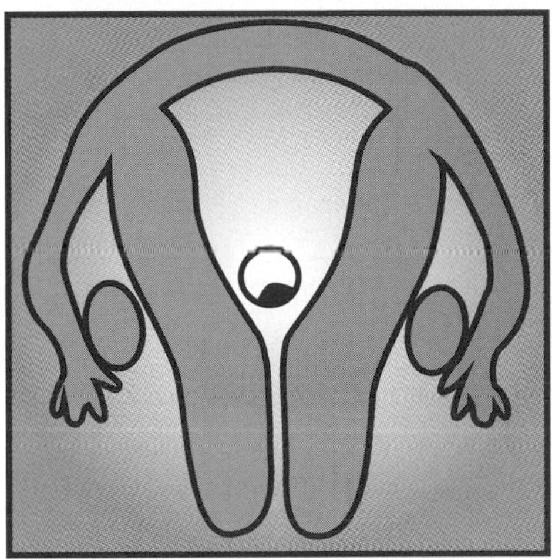

An abnormal gestation is either intrauterine or extrauterine. Extrauterine or ectopic pregnancy occurs when the fertilized ovum becomes implanted in tissue other than the endometrium. Although most ectopic gestations are located in the ampullary segment of the fallopian tube, such pregnancies may also occur in other sites (Table 17.1). Abnormal intrauterine pregnancy often results in pregnancy loss early in gestation. Such abnormalities can be related to a number of factors. With both abnormal intrauterine and extrauterine gestation, early recognition is key to diagnosis and management.

Abnormal Intrauterine Pregnancy

Spontaneous Abortion

Anembryonic gestation, inevitable abortion, incomplete abortion, and completed abortion are types of first-trimester abortions. **About 15% to 20% of known pregnancies terminate in spontaneous abortion. With the use of serial human chorionic gonadotropin (hCG) measurements to detect early subclinical pregnancy losses, the percentage increases to 30%. About 80% of spontaneous pregnancy losses occur in the first trimester; the incidence decreases with each gestational week.** In a study of 347 patients with a first-trimester pregnancy documented by ultrasound, the overall pregnancy loss was 6.1% to 4.2% in patients without bleeding and 12.4% in patients with bleeding (1). In women who have had one prior spontaneous abortion, the rate of spontaneous abortion in a subsequent pregnancy is about 20%; in women who have had three consecutive losses, the rate is 50%. The causes of this condition are varied and most often unknown (Table 17.2). Patients should be reassured that, in most cases, spontaneous abortion does not recur.

Threatened Abortion

***Threatened abortion* is defined as vaginal bleeding before 20 weeks of gestation. It occurs in about 30% to 40% of all pregnancies.** The bleeding is usually light and may be associated with mild lower abdominal or cramping pain. It is often not possible to differentiate clinically between threatened abortion, completed abortion, and ectopic pregnancy in an unruptured tube. The differential diagnosis in these patients includes consideration

Table 17.1. Definitions of Types of Abnormal Intrauterine and Extrauterine Pregnancies

Extrauterine Pregnancy	
Tubal pregnancy	A pregnancy occurring in the fallopian tube—most often these are located in the ampullary portion of the fallopian tube
Interstitial pregnancy	A pregnancy that implants within the interstitial portion of the fallopian tube
Abdominal pregnancy	Primary abdominal pregnancy—the first and only implantation occurs on a peritoneal surface Secondary abdominal pregnancy—implantation originally in the tubal ostia, subsequently aborted, and then reimplanted onto a peritoneal surface
Cervical pregnancy	Implantation of the developing conceptus in the cervical canal
Ligamentous pregnancy	A secondary form of ectopic pregnancy in which a primary tubal pregnancy erodes into the mesosalpinx and is located between the leaves of the broad ligament
Heterotopic pregnancy	A condition in which ectopic and intrauterine pregnancies coexist
Ovarian pregnancy	A condition in which an ectopic pregnancy implants within the ovarian cortex
Abnormal Intrauterine Pregnancy	
Incomplete abortion	Expulsion of some but not all of the products of conception before 20 completed weeks of gestation
Complete abortion	Spontaneous expulsion of all fetal and placental tissue from the uterine cavity before 20 weeks of gestation
Inevitable abortion	Uterine bleeding from a gestation of less than 20 weeks' gestation, accompanied by cervical dilation but without expulsion of placental or fetal tissue through the cervix
Anembryonic gestation	An intrauterine sac without fetal tissue present at more than 7.5 weeks of gestation
First-trimester fetal death	Death of the fetus in the first 12 weeks of gestation
Second-trimester fetal death	Death of the fetus between 13 and 24 weeks of gestation
Recurrent spontaneous abortion	The loss of more than three pregnancies before 20 weeks' gestation

Table 17.2. Potential Causes of Spontaneous Pregnancy Loss

Pathologic (blighted) ovum—anembryonic gestation
Embryonic anomalies
Chromosomal anomalies
Increased maternal age
Uterine anomalies
Intrauterine device
Teratogen
Mutagen
Maternal disease
Placental anomalies
Extensive maternal trauma

of possible cervical polyps, vaginitis, cervical carcinoma, gestational trophoblastic disease, ectopic pregnancy, trauma, and foreign body. On physical examination, the abdomen usually is not tender and the cervix is closed. Bleeding can be seen coming from the os, and there is no cervical motion or adnexal tenderness. Although most patients experience bleeding at 8 to 10 weeks of gestation, the actual loss usually occurs before 8 weeks of gestation. Only 3.2% of patients experience a pregnancy loss after 8 weeks of gestation (2).

Evaluation of a threatened abortion should include serial hCG measurements unless the patient has an intrauterine pregnancy documented by ultrasound, eliminating the possibility of an ectopic pregnancy. Endovaginal ultrasonography can detect a gestational sac at an hCG level of 1,000 to 2,000 mIU/mL. By 7 weeks of gestation, a fetal pole with fetal cardiac activity can be seen. When a gestational sac is visualized, subsequent loss of the pregnancy occurs in 11.5% of patients. If a yolk sac is present, the loss rate is 8.5%; with an embryo of 5 mm, the loss rate is 7.2%; with an embryo of 6 to 10 mm, the loss rate is 3.2%; and when the embryo is 10 mm, the loss rate is only 0.5%. The fetal loss rate after 14 weeks of gestation is about 2% (3). Transvaginal measurement of gestational sac size is useful in differentiating viable from nonviable intrauterine pregnancies. A mean sac diameter greater than 13 mm without a visible yolk sac or a mean sac diameter greater than 17 mm lacking an embryo predicts nonviability in all cases (4).

There is no effective therapy for a threatened intrauterine pregnancy. Bedrest, although advocated, is not effective. Progesterone or sedatives should not be used. All patients should be counseled and reassured so that they understand the situation. Treatment should be given for any vaginal infection.

Inevitable Abortion

With an *inevitable abortion,* the volume of bleeding is often greater, and the cervical os is open and effaced, but no tissue has been passed. Most patients have crampy lower abdominal pain, and some have cervical motion or adnexal tenderness. When it is certain that the pregnancy is not viable because the cervical os is dilated or excessive bleeding is present, suction curettage should be performed. Blood type and Rh determination and a complete blood count should be obtained if there is any concern about the amount of bleeding. **Rh_0(D) immune globulin (RhoGAM) should be given either before or after the uterus is evacuated if the patient's blood is Rh negative.**

Incomplete Abortion

An incomplete abortion is a partial expulsion of the pregnancy tissue. Before 6 weeks of gestation, the placenta and fetus are generally passed together, but after this time, they are often passed separately. Although most patients have vaginal bleeding, only some have passed tissue. Lower abdominal cramping is invariably present, and the pain may be described as resembling labor. On physical examination, the cervix is dilated and effaced, and bleeding is present. Often, clots are admixed with products of conception. If the bleeding is profuse, the patient should be examined promptly for tissue protruding from the cervical os; removal of this tissue with a ring forceps reduces the bleeding. A vasovagal bradycardia may occur and responds to removal of the tissue. All patients with an incomplete abortion should undergo suction curettage as quickly as possible. A complete blood count, maternal blood type, and Rh determination should be obtained; **Rh-negative patients should receive Rh_0(D) immune globulin.**

If the patient is febrile, broad-spectrum antibiotic therapy should be administered before suction curettage is performed to reduce the incidence of postabortal endometritis and pelvic inflammatory disease, thereby reducing potential deleterious effects on fertility. The antibiotic regimen chosen should be similar to the regimens used for treatment of pelvic inflammatory disease (PID). In patients who do not have clinical signs of infection, prophylactic antibiotic therapy should be instituted. Suggested regimens include *doxycycline* (100 mg orally twice daily), *tetracycline* (250 mg orally four times daily for 5 to 7 days) or another antibiotic of similar spectrum.

Ectopic Gestation

Incidence

The most comprehensive data available on ectopic pregnancy rates have been collected by the Centers for Disease Control and Prevention (5). They show a significant increase in the number of ectopic pregnancies in the United States during the past 20 years (Fig. 17.1). In 1989, the latest year for which statistics were published, there were an estimated 88,400 ectopic pregnancies, at a rate of 16 ectopic pregnancies per 1,000 reported pregnancies. These numbers represent a fivefold increase compared with the 1970 rates. The highest rates occurred in women aged 35 to 44 years (27.2 per 1,000 reported pregnancies). When the data are analyzed by race, the risk for ectopic pregnancy among African Americans and other minorities (20.8 per 1,000) is 1.6 times greater than the risk among whites (13.4 per 1,000). In 1988, 44 deaths were attributed to complications of ectopic pregnancy, which represents 15% of all maternal deaths. The risk for death is higher for African Americans and other minorities than for whites (6). For both races, teenagers have the highest mortality rates, but the rate for African American and other minority teenagers is almost five times that for white teenagers. **After an ectopic pregnancy, there is a 7- to 13-fold increase in the risk for a subsequent ectopic pregnancy. The chance that a subsequent pregnancy will be intrauterine is 50% to 80%, and the chance that the pregnancy will be tubal is 10% to 25%; the remaining patients will be infertile** (7–9). Many variables make accurate assessment of risk very difficult (e.g., size and location of the ectopic pregnancy, status of the contralateral adnexa, treatment method, and history of infertility).

Figure 17.1 Estimation of the number of ectopic pregnancies (United States, 1970–1989). *Dashed lines* represent the upper and lower limits of 95% confidence intervals.

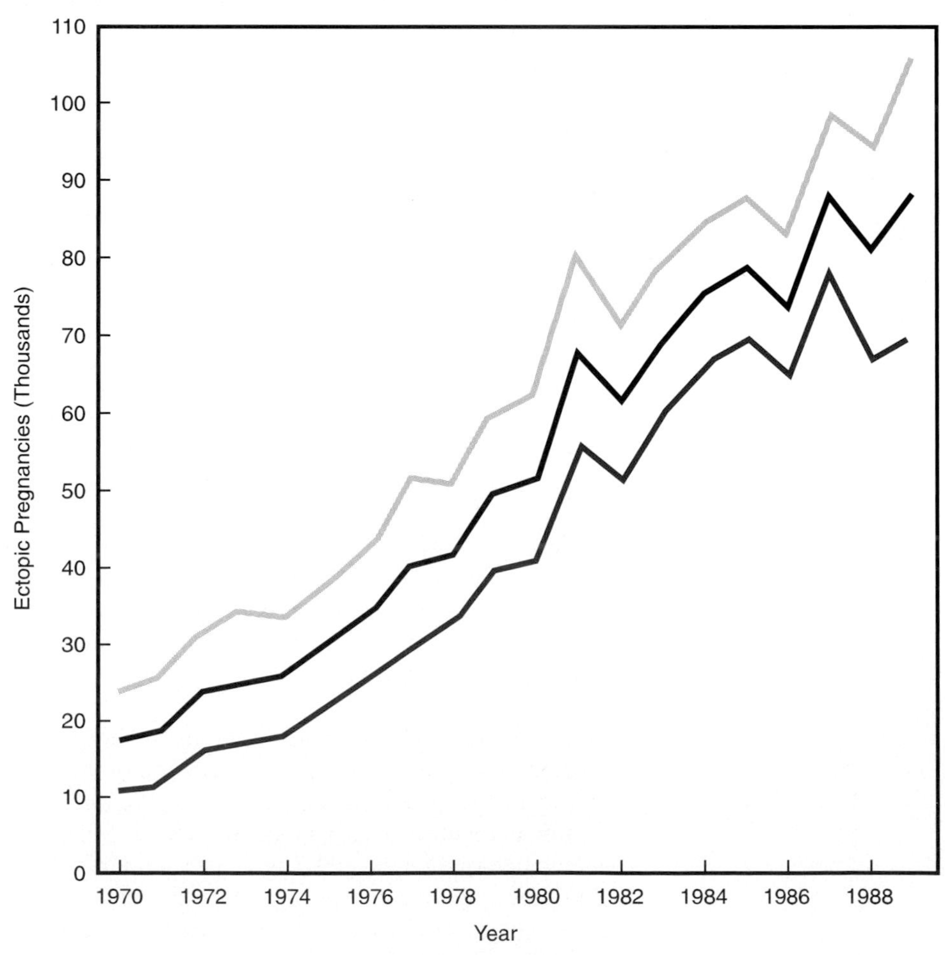

Etiology and Risk Factors

Tubal damage results from inflammation, infection, and surgery. Inflammation and infection may cause damage without complete tubal obstruction. Complete blockage may result from salpingitis, incomplete tubal ligation, tubal fertility surgery, partial salpingectomy, or congenital midsegment tubal atresia (10–14). Damage to the mucosal portion of the tube or fimbria accounts for about half of all tubal pregnancies (15). Tubal diverticula may result in abnormalities that entrap the blastocyst or impede transport (16,17). Tubal pregnancy may occur in a blocked tube with contralateral tubal patency, with the sperm migrating across the abdomen to fertilize an egg released from the blocked side.

Myoelectrical activity is responsible for propulsive activity in the fallopian tube (16). This activity facilitates movement of the sperm and ova toward each other and propels the zygote toward the uterine cavity. Estrogen increases smooth muscle activity, and progesterone decreases muscle tone. Aging results in progressive loss of myoelectrical activity along the fallopian tube, which may explain the increased incidence of tubal pregnancy in perimenopausal women (16). Hormonal control of the muscular activity in the fallopian tube may explain the increased incidence of tubal pregnancy associated with failures of the morning-after pill, minipill, progesterone-containing intrauterine devices (IUDs), and ovulation induction. Blighted ova occur more commonly in tubal conceptions than in intrauterine conceptions, although there is no increase in the incidence of chromosomal abnormalities in ectopic pregnancies (18).

Independent factors consistently shown to increase the risk for tubal pregnancy include the following:

1. Previous laparoscopically proven PID
2. Previous tubal pregnancy
3. Current IUD use
4. Previous tubal surgery for infertility

Many other factors, including contraceptive choice, prior surgery, previous pregnancies, and fertility status, also have been identified.

Pelvic Infection

The relationship of PID, tubal obstruction, and ectopic pregnancy is well documented (13,19). In a study of 415 women with laparoscopically proven PID, the incidence of tubal obstruction increased with successive episodes of PID: 13% after one episode, 35% after two, and 75% after three (19). Furthermore, after one episode of PID, the ratio of ectopic pregnancy to intrauterine pregnancy was 1 in 24, a sixfold increase over the incidence for women with laparoscopically negative results (1 in 147). In a prospective study of 1,204 patients followed until first pregnancy after infection, 47 of 746 (6%) women with laparoscopically documented PID had a tubal gestation, which is significantly higher than the 0.9% incidence in the control group (20).

Chlamydia is an important pathogen causing tubal damage and subsequent tubal pregnancy. Because many cases of chlamydia salpingitis are indolent, cases may not be recognized or, if recognized, may be treated on an outpatient basis. Chlamydia has been cultured from 7% to 30% of patients with tubal pregnancy (7,21). A strong association between chlamydia infection and tubal pregnancy has been shown with serologic tests for chlamydia (22–25). Conception is three times as likely to be tubal in women with anti–*Chlamydia trachomatis* titers higher than 1:64 than in those women whose titers were negative (7,26).

Contraceptive Use

Inert and copper-containing IUDs prevent both intrauterine and extrauterine pregnancies (27,28). **Women who conceive with an IUD in place, however, are 0.4 to 0.8 times more likely to have a tubal pregnancy than those not using contraceptives. However, because IUDs prevent implantation more effectively in the uterus than in the tube, a woman conceiving with an IUD is 6 to 10 times more likely to have a tubal pregnancy than if she conceives without using contraception** (27,28).

With copper IUDs, 4% of contraceptive failures are tubal pregnancies. Progesterone IUDs are less effective than copper IUDs in preventing tubal pregnancy; 17% of failures result in tubal pregnancy. Furthermore, the rate of ectopic pregnancy in women using progesterone IUDs is higher than in women not using contraceptives: 1.9 per 100 woman-years (versus 0.5 for copper IUDs) (29). This finding suggests that failures occur for different reasons. Although all IUDs prevent intrauterine implantation, copper IUDs prevent fertilization by cytotoxic and phagocytic effects on the sperm and oocytes. Progesterone-containing IUDs are probably less effective in preventing conception.

Duration of IUD use does not increase the absolute risk for tubal pregnancy (1.2 per 1,000 years of exposure), but with increasing use, there is an increase in the percentage of pregnancies that are tubal (30). It is unclear whether past use of IUDs increases the risk for tubal pregnancy. Only past use of the Dalkon shield is associated with a twofold increased risk (31). One study showed that previous use of an IUD for longer than 2 years was associated with a fourfold risk, but this risk was present for only the first year after discontinuation of IUD use (27). However, subsequent studies have found no increased risk for tubal pregnancy following IUD use (30,32).

The risk of the pregnancy being ectopic with combination oral contraceptive use has been calculated to be 0.5% to 4% (27,28,33). Past use of oral contraceptives does not increase the subsequent risk for ectopic pregnancy (8). Progesterone-only contraceptives, including oral contraceptives (minipill) and subdermal implants (*Norplant*), protect against both intrauterine and ectopic pregnancy when compared with no contraceptive use. If a pregnancy does occur, however, the chance of the pregnancy being ectopic is 4% to 10% for the minipill (34,35) and up to 30% if pregnancy occurs while implants are in place (36,37). Condom and diaphragm use protects against both intrauterine and ectopic pregnancy, and there is no increased incidence of ectopic pregnancy (30,33,38).

Sterilization

The greatest risk for pregnancy, including ectopic pregnancy, occurs in the first 2 years after sterilization (39). Despite a greater proportion of poststerilization failures resulting in ectopic pregnancy, the absolute rate of ectopic pregnancy is decreased. Calculating cumulative lifetime risk for ectopic pregnancy according to method of contraception, sterilized women have a lower cumulative risk for ectopic pregnancy than IUD users or nonusers of contraception, and women using barrier methods or oral contraceptives have the lowest risk (40).

The risk for tubal pregnancy after any sterilization procedure is 5% to 16% (10,39,40). The risk depends on the sterilization technique: about half of postelectrocautery failures are ectopic, compared with 12% after nonlaparoscopic, nonelectrocautery procedures (41). Laparoscopic coagulation has a reduced risk for pregnancy compared with mechanical devices, but the risk for ectopic pregnancy is increased ninefold when a failure does occur (10,42,43).

Tubal repair or reconstruction may be performed to correct an obstruction, lyse adhesions, or evacuate an unruptured ectopic pregnancy. Although it is clear that tubal surgery is associated with an increased risk for ectopic pregnancy, it is unclear whether the increased risk results from the surgical procedure or from the underlying problem. A fourfold to fivefold increased risk is associated with salpingostomy, neosalpingostomy, fimbroplasty, anastomosis, and lysis of complex peritubal and periovarian adhesions (7,11,43). After tubal surgery, the overall rate of ectopic pregnancy is 2% to 7%, and the viable intrauterine pregnancy rate is 50%.

There has been a concern that conservation of the tube at the time of removal of an ectopic pregnancy would increase the risk for recurrent ectopic pregnancy. However, after either tubal removal or conservation, the rates for intrauterine pregnancy (40%) and ectopic pregnancy (12%) have been found to be identical (44). In another study, the incidence of ectopic pregnancy could be predicted by the status of the contralateral tube: normal (7%), abnormal (18%), or absent (25%) (42). In a study of pregnancy outcomes of 1,152 patients treated for ectopic pregnancy, preservation of the tube did not increase the incidence of repeat ectopic pregnancy, but it did improve overall fertility rates (45).

Sterilization reversal also increases risk for ectopic pregnancy. The exact risk depends on the method of sterilization, site of tubal occlusion, residual tube length, coexisting disease, and surgical technique. In general, the risk for reanastomosing a cauterized tube is about 15%, and it is less than 3% for reversal of Pomeroy or Fallope ring procedures (46,47).

Prior Abdominal Surgery

Many patients with ectopic pregnancies have a history of previous abdominal surgery (7,8,48). The role of abdominal surgery in ectopic pregnancy is unclear. In one study, there appeared to be no increased risk for cesarean delivery, ovarian surgery, or removal of an unruptured appendix (49). Other studies have shown that ovarian cystectomy or wedge resection increases the risk for ectopic pregnancy, presumably as a result of peritubal scarring (50,51). Although there is general agreement that an increased risk for ectopic pregnancy is associated with a ruptured appendix (7,43), one study did not confirm this finding (49).

Other Causes

Abortion There is no established association between ectopic pregnancy and spontaneous abortion (7,9,52). With recurrent abortion (fewer than two consecutive abortions) the risk is increased 2 to 4 times. This may reflect a shared risk factor, such as with luteal phase defect. Uncomplicated elective abortion, regardless of the number of procedures or gestational age at which they were performed, is not associated with increased risk (7,8,53,54). In areas with a high incidence of illegal abortion, the risk is increased 10-fold. Presumably, this increased incidence is secondary to postoperative infection and improperly performed procedures (54).

Infertility Although the incidence of ectopic pregnancy increases with age and parity, there is also a significant increase in nulliparous women undergoing infertility treatment (7,8,44). For nulliparous women, conceptions after at least 1 year of unprotected intercourse are 2.6 times more likely to be tubal (55). Additional risks for infertile women are associated with specific treatments, including reversal of sterilization, tuboplasty, ovulation induction, and *in vitro* fertilization (IVF).

Hormonal alterations characteristic of *clomiphene citrate* and gonadotropin ovulation-induction cycles may predispose tubal implantation. About 1.1% to 4.6% of conceptions associated with ovulation induction are ectopic pregnancies (8,55). In many of these patients, the results of hysterosalpingography are normal, and there is no evidence of intraoperative tubal pathology. Hyperstimulation, with high estrogen levels, may play a role in tubal pregnancy (56,57); however, not all studies have shown this relationship (58).

The first pregnancy obtained with IVF was a tubal pregnancy (59). About 2% to 8% of IVF conceptions are tubal. Tubal factor infertility is associated with a further increased risk of 17% (60–62). Predisposing factors are unclear but may include placement of the embryo high in the uterine cavity, fluid reflux into the tube, and a predisposing tubal factor that prevents the refluxed embryo from returning to the uterine cavity.

Salpingitis Isthmica Nodosa Salpingitis isthmica nodosa (SIN) is a noninflammatory pathologic condition of the tube in which tubal epithelium extends into the myosalpinx and forms a true diverticulum. The reported prevalence ranges from 1 in 146 to 11 in 100. This condition is found more often in the tubes of women with an ectopic pregnancy than in nonpregnant women (17,63,64). Myometrial electrical activity over the diverticula has been found to be abnormal (16). Whether tubal pregnancy is caused by SIN or whether the association is coincidental is unknown.

Endometriosis or Leiomyomas Endometriosis or leiomyomas can cause tubal obstruction. However, neither is commonly associated with ectopic pregnancy.

Diethylstilbestrol Women exposed to diethylstilbestrol (DES) *in utero* who subsequently conceive are at increased risk for ectopic pregnancy. In several case-control studies, these women were more than twice as likely to have a tubal pregnancy (65,66). The Collaborative Diethylstilbestrol-Adenosis Project, which monitored 327 DES-exposed women, found that about 50% had uterine cavity abnormalities (65). In DES-exposed women, the risk for ectopic pregnancy was 13% in those who had uterine abnormalities compared with 4% in those who had a normal uterus. No specific type of defect was related to the risk for ectopic pregnancy.

Smoking Current cigarette smoking is associated with a more than twofold increased risk for tubal pregnancy (28,51,67–69). A case-control study showed a dose relationship: current smokers of more than 20 cigarettes a day had a relative risk of 2.5 compared with nonsmokers, whereas smokers of 1 to 10 cigarettes had a risk of 1.3 (68). Alterations of tubal motility, ciliary activity, and blastocyst implantation are associated with nicotine intake.

Histologic Characteristics

Chorionic villi, usually found in the lumen, are pathognomic findings of tubal pregnancy. Gross or microscopic evidence of an embryo is seen in two thirds of cases (70). An unruptured tubal pregnancy is characterized by irregular dilation of the tube, with a blue discoloration caused by hematosalpinx. The ectopic pregnancy may not be readily apparent. Bleeding associated with tubal pregnancies is mainly extraluminal but may be luminal (hematosalpinx) and may extrude from the fimbriated end. A hematoma is frequently seen surrounding the distal segment of the tube. Patients who have tubal pregnancies that spontaneously resolve and those treated with *methotrexate* frequently have an enlargement of the ectopic mass associated with blood clots and extrusion of tissue from the fimbriated end. Hemoperitoneum is nearly always present but is confined to the cul-de-sac unless tubal rupture has occurred. The natural progression of tubal pregnancy is either expulsion from the fimbriated end (tubal abortion), involution of the conceptus, or rupture, usually around the eighth gestational week. Some tubal pregnancies form a chronic inflammatory mass that is associated with involution and reestablishment of menses and thus is difficult to diagnose. Extensive histologic sampling may be required to disclose a few ghost villi.

Histologic findings associated with tubal gestation include evidence of chronic salpingitis and SIN. Inflammation associated with salpingitis causes adhesions as a result of fibrin deposition. Healing and cellular organization lead to permanent scarring between folds of tissue. This scarring may allow transport of sperm but not the passage of the larger blastocyst. About 45% of patients with tubal pregnancies have pathologic evidence of prior salpingitis (71).

The etiology of SIN is unknown but is speculated to be an adenomyosis-like process or, less likely, inflammation (72,73). This condition is rare before puberty, indicating a noncongenital origin. Tubal diverticula are identified in about half of patients who have ectopic pregnancies, as opposed to 5% of women who do not have ectopic pregnancies (17).

Histologic findings include the Arias-Sella reaction, which is characterized by localized hyperplasia of endometrial glands that are hypersecretory (74). The cells have enlarged

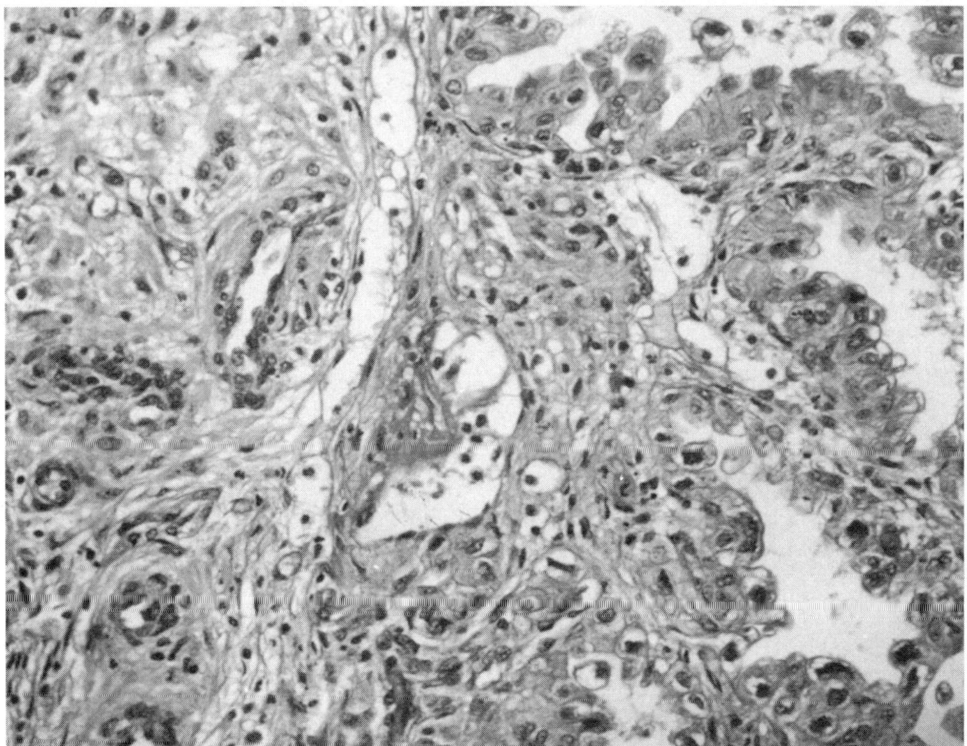

Figure 17.2 The Arias-Stella reaction of the endometrium. The glands are closely packed and hypersecretory with large, hyperchromatic nuclei suggesting malignancy. (From **Berek JS, Hacker NF.** *Practical gynecologic oncology,* 2nd ed. Baltimore: Williams & Wilkins, 1994:125, with permission.)

nuclei that are hyperchromatic and irregular. The Arias-Sella reaction is a nonspecific finding that can be seen in patients with intrauterine pregnancies (Fig. 17.2).

Diagnosis

The diagnosis of ectopic pregnancy is complicated by the wide spectrum of clinical presentations, from asymptomatic cases to acute abdomen and hemodynamic shock. The diagnosis and management of a ruptured ectopic pregnancy is straightforward; the primary goal is achieving hemostasis. If an ectopic pregnancy can be identified before rupture or irreparable tubal damage, consideration may be given to optimizing future fertility. With patients presenting earlier in the disease process, the number of those without symptoms or with minimal symptoms has increased. Therefore, there must be a high degree of suspicion of ectopic pregnancy, especially in areas of high prevalence. History and physical examination identify patients at risk, improving the probability of detection of ectopic pregnancy before rupture.

History

Patients who have an ectopic pregnancy generally have an abnormal menstrual pattern or the perception of a spontaneous pregnancy loss. Pertinent history includes the menstrual history, previous pregnancy, history of infertility, current contraceptive status, risk factor assessment, and current symptoms.

The classic symptom triad of ectopic pregnancy is pain, amenorrhea, and vaginal bleeding. This symptom group is present in only about 50% of patients, however, and is most typical in patients in whom an ectopic pregnancy has ruptured. Abdominal pain is the most common presenting complaint, but the severity and nature of the pain vary widely. There is no pathognomonic pain that is diagnostic of ectopic pregnancy.

Pain may be unilateral or bilateral and may occur in the upper or lower abdomen. The pain may be dull, sharp, or crampy and either continuous or intermittent. With rupture, the patient may experience transient relief of the pain, as stretching of the tubal serosa ceases. Shoulder and back pain, thought to result from hemoperitoneal irritation of the diaphragm, may indicate intraabdominal hemorrhage.

Physical Examination

The physical examination should include measurements of vital signs and examination of the abdomen and pelvis. Frequently, the findings before rupture and hemorrhage are nonspecific, and vital signs are normal. The abdomen may be nontender or mildly tender, with or without rebound. The uterus may be slightly enlarged, with findings similar to a normal pregnancy (75). Cervical motion tenderness may or may not be present. An adnexal mass may be palpable in up to 50% of cases, but the mass varies markedly in size, consistency, and tenderness. A palpable mass may be the corpus luteum and not the ectopic pregnancy. With rupture and intraabdominal hemorrhage, the patient develops tachycardia followed by hypotension. Bowel sounds are decreased or absent. The abdomen is distended, with marked tenderness and rebound tenderness. Cervical motion tenderness is present. Frequently, the pelvic examination is inadequate because of pain and guarding.

History and physical examination may or may not provide useful diagnostic information. The accuracy of the initial clinical evaluation is less than 50% (76). Additional tests are frequently required to differentiate early viable intrauterine pregnancy or suspected ectopic or abnormal intrauterine pregnancy.

Laboratory Assessment

Quantitative β-hCG measurements are the diagnostic cornerstone for ectopic pregnancy. The hCG enzyme immunoassay, with a sensitivity of 25 mIU/mL, is an accurate screening test for detection of ectopic pregnancy. The assay is positive in virtually all documented ectopic pregnancies.

Reference Standards There are three reference standards for β-hCG measurement. The World Health Organization introduced the First International Standard (1st IS) in the 1930s. Testing for hCG and its subunits have improved over the years. The Second International Standard (2nd IS), introduced in 1964, has varying amounts of hCG α and β subunits. A purified preparation of β-hCG is now available. Originally referred to as the First International Reference Preparation (1st IRP), the test standard is now referred to as the Third International Standard (3rd IS). Although each standard has its own scale, as a general rule, the 2nd IS is about half of the 3rd IS. For example, if a level is reported as 500 mIU/mL (2nd IS), it is equivalent to a level of 1,000 mIU/mL (3rd IS). The assay standard used must be known in order to interpret hCG results correctly (77). In several recent articles, attention has been drawn to a problem known as phantom hCG, in which the presence of heterophile antibodies or proteolytic enzymes causes a false-positive hCG result. Because the antibodies are large glycoproteins, significant quantities of the antibody are not excreted in the urine. Thus, in the patient with hCG levels less than 1,000 mIU/mL, a confirmatory positive urine pregnancy test should be obtained before instituting treatment (78,79).

Doubling Time The hCG level correlates with the gestational age (80). During the first 6 weeks of amenorrhea, the serum hCG level increases exponentially. Thus, during this time period, the doubling time of hCG is relatively constant, regardless of the initial level. After the sixth week of gestation, when the hCG levels are higher than 6,000 to 10,000 mIU/mL, the hCG rise is slower and not constant (81).

The hCG doubling time can differentiate an ectopic pregnancy from an intrauterine pregnancy—a 66% rise in the hCG level over 48 hours (85% confidence level) represents the lower limit of normal values for viable intrauterine pregnancies (82). **About 15% of patients with viable intrauterine pregnancies have less than a 66% rise in hCG**

level over 48 hours, and a similar percentage with an ectopic pregnancy have more than a 66% rise. If the sampling interval is reduced to 24 hours, the overlap between normal and abnormal pregnancies is even greater. Patients with a normal intrauterine pregnancy usually have more than a 50% rise in the hCG level over 48 hours when the starting level is less than 2,000 mIU/mL. **The hCG pattern that is most predictive of an ectopic pregnancy is one that has reached a plateau (a doubling time of more than 7 days). For falling levels, a half-life of less than 1.4 days is rarely associated with an ectopic pregnancy, whereas a half-life of more than 7 days is most predictive of ectopic pregnancy.**

Serial hCG levels are usually required when the initial ultrasound examination is indeterminate (i.e., when there is no evidence of an intrauterine gestation or extrauterine cardiac activity consistent with an ectopic pregnancy). When the hCG level is less than 2,000, doubling time predicts viable intrauterine gestation (normal rise) versus nonviability (subnormal rise). With normally rising levels, a second ultrasound is performed when the level is expected (by extrapolation) to reach 2,000 mIU/mL. Abnormally rising levels (less than 2,000 mIU/mL) indicate a nonviable pregnancy. The location (i.e., intrauterine versus extrauterine) must be determined surgically, either by laparoscopy or dilation and curettage. Indeterminate ultrasonography results, and an hCG level of less than 2,000 mIU/mL is diagnostic of nonviable gestation, either ectopic pregnancy or a complete abortion. As a general rule, a completed abortion has a rapidly falling hCG level (50% over 48 hours), whereas levels of an ectopic pregnancy rise or plateau.

Single hCG Level A single hCG measurement has limited usefulness because there is considerable overlap of values between normal and abnormal pregnancies at a given gestational age. The ectopic pregnancy site and hCG level do not correlate (83). Also, many patients in whom the diagnosis of ectopic pregnancy is being considered are uncertain about their menstrual dates. A single hCG level may be useful when measured by sensitive enzyme immunoassays that, if negative, exclude a diagnosis of ectopic pregnancy. Measurement of a single level may also be helpful in predicting pregnancy outcome after timed conceptions using advanced reproductive technology. If the hCG level is more than 300 mIU/mL on day 16 to 18 after artificial insemination, there is an 88% chance of a live birth (84). If the hCG level is less than 300 mIU/mL, the chance of a live birth is only 22%. Also, a single hCG level may facilitate the interpretation of ultrasonography when an intrauterine gestation is not visualized. An hCG level greater than the ultrasound discriminatory zone indicates a possible extrauterine pregnancy. However, determination of serial hCG levels may be needed to differentiate an ectopic pregnancy from a completed abortion. Further tests are required for patients in whom ultrasonography examinations are inconclusive and hCG levels are below the discriminatory zone.

Serum Progesterone

In general, the mean serum progesterone level in patients with ectopic pregnancies is lower than that in patients with normal intrauterine pregnancies (85,86). However, in studies of more than 5,000 patients with first-trimester pregnancies, a spectrum of progesterone levels in patients with both normal and abnormal pregnancies has been found (87–89). About 70% of patients with a viable intrauterine pregnancy have serum progesterone levels higher than 25 ng/mL, whereas only 1.5% of patients with ectopic pregnancies have serum progesterone levels higher than 25 ng/mL, and most of these pregnancies exhibit cardiac activity (87–89).

A serum progesterone level can be used as an ectopic pregnancy screening test for both normal and abnormal pregnancy, particularly in settings in which hCG levels and ultrasonography are not readily available. A serum progesterone level of less than 5 ng/mL is highly suggestive of an abnormal pregnancy, but it is not 100% predictive. The risk for a normal pregnancy with a serum progesterone level of less than 5 ng/mL is about 1 in 1,500 (90). Because of this, serum progesterone measurements alone cannot be used to predict pregnancy nonviability.

Other Endocrinologic Markers

In an effort to improve early ectopic pregnancy detection, various endocrinologic and protein markers have been studied. Estradiol levels increase slowly from conception until 6 weeks of gestation and then rise rapidly as placental production of estradiol increases (91). Estradiol levels are significantly lower in ectopic pregnancies when compared with viable pregnancies. However, there is considerable overlap between normal and abnormal pregnancies as well as between intrauterine and extrauterine pregnancies (92,93).

Maternal serum creatine kinase has been studied as a marker for ectopic pregnancy diagnosis (94). Maternal serum creatine kinase levels were significantly higher in all patients with tubal pregnancy when compared with those in patients who had missed abortions or normal intrauterine pregnancies, but no correlation was found between the creatine kinase level and the clinical presentation of the patient, and there was no correlation with the hCG levels.

Schwangerschafts protein 1 (SP_1), also known as pregnancy-associated plasma protein C (PAPP-C) or pregnancy-specific β glycoprotein (PSBS), is produced by the syncytiotrophoblast (92). The main advantage of SP_1 level assessment may be in the diagnosis of conception after recent hCG administration. A level of 2 ng/L might be used for the diagnosis of pregnancy; however, it is doubtful that a diagnosis can be established before delay of menses. Although the SP level increases late in all patients with a nonviable pregnancy, a single SP level does not have prognostic value (95).

Relaxin is a protein hormone produced solely by the corpus luteum of pregnancy. It appears in the maternal serum at 4 to 5 weeks of gestation, peaks at about 10 weeks of gestation, and decreases until term (96). Relaxin levels are significantly lower in ectopic pregnancies and spontaneous abortions than in normal intrauterine pregnancies. Prorenin and active renin levels are significantly higher in viable intrauterine pregnancies than in either ectopic pregnancies or spontaneous abortions, with a single level of more than 33 pg/mL excluding the diagnosis of ectopic pregnancy (97). However, the clinical utility of relaxin, prorenin, and renin levels in diagnosing ectopic pregnancy has not yet been determined.

CA125 is a glycoprotein, the origin of which is uncertain during pregnancy. Levels of CA125 rise during the first trimester and return to a nonpregnancy range during the second and third trimesters. After delivery, maternal serum concentrations increase again (98,99). CA125 levels have been studied in an effort to predict spontaneous abortion. Although a positive correlation has been found between elevated CA125 levels 18 to 22 days after conception and spontaneous abortion, repeat measurements at 6 weeks of gestation did not correlate with outcome (100). Conflicting results have been reported—one study showed a higher serum CA125 level in normal than in ectopic pregnancies 2 to 4 weeks after a missed menses, whereas another study found higher CA125 levels for ectopic pregnancies compared with normal pregnancies (101,102).

Maternal serum α-fetoprotein (AFP) levels are elevated in ectopic pregnancies (103,104); however, the use of AFP measurements as a screening technique for ectopic pregnancy has not been studied. A combination of AFP with three other markers—β-hCG, progesterone, and estradiol—has a 98.5% specificity and 94.5% accuracy for the prediction of ectopic pregnancy.

C-reactive protein is an acute-phase reactant that increases with trauma or infection. Levels of this protein are lower in patients with ectopic pregnancy than in patients with an acute infectious process. Thus, when an infectious process is part of the differential diagnosis, measurement of C-reactive protein may be beneficial (105).

Ultrasound

Improvements in ultrasonography have resulted in the earlier diagnosis of intrauterine and ectopic gestations (106). However, the sensitivity of the β-hCG assay usually allows the diagnosis of pregnancy before direct visualization by ultrasonography.

The complete examination should include both transvaginal and transabdominal ultrasonography. Transvaginal ultrasonography is superior to transabdominal ultrasonography in evaluating intrapelvic structures. The closeness of the vaginal probe to the pelvic organs allows use of higher frequencies (5 to 7 mHz), which improves resolution. The diagnosis of an intrauterine pregnancy can be made 1 week earlier with transvaginal than with transabdominal ultrasound. The demonstration of an empty uterus, detection of adnexal masses and free peritoneal fluid, and direct signs of ectopic pregnancy are more reliably established with a transvaginal procedure (107–111). Transabdominal ultrasonography permits visualization of both the pelvis and abdominal cavity and should be included as part of the complete ectopic pregnancy evaluation to detect adnexal masses and hemoperitoneum.

The earliest ultrasonographic finding of an intrauterine pregnancy is a small fluid space and the gestational sac, surrounded by a thick echogenic ring, located eccentrically within the endometrial cavity. The earliest normal gestational sac is seen at 5 weeks of gestation with transabdominal ultrasonography and at 4 weeks of gestation with transvaginal ultrasonography (112). **As the gestational sac grows, a yolk sac is seen within it, followed by an embryo with cardiac activity.**

The appearance of a normal gestational sac may be simulated by intrauterine fluid collection, the pseudogestational sac, which occurs in 8% to 29% of patients with ectopic pregnancy (113–115). This ultrasonographic lucency, centrally located, probably represents bleeding into the endometrial cavity by the decidual cast. Clots within this lucency may mimic a fetal pole.

Morphologically, identification of the double decidual sac sign (DDSS) is the best known method of ultrasonographically differentiating true sacs from pseudosacs (116). The double sac, believed to be the decidua capsularis and parietalis, is seen as two concentric echogenic rings separated by a hypoechogenic space. Although useful, there are some limitations of sensitivity and specificity—the DDSS sensitivity ranges from 64% to 95% (115). Pseudosacs may occasionally appear as the DDSS; intrauterine sacs of failed pregnancies may appear as pseudosacs.

The appearance of a yolk sac within the gestational sac is superior to the DDSS in proving an intrauterine pregnancy (117). The yolk sac is consistently visible on transabdominal ultrasonography with a gestational sac size of 2 cm, and on transvaginal ultrasonography at a gestational sac size of 0.6 to 0.8 cm (118,119). Intrauterine sacs smaller than 1 cm on transabdominal ultrasonography and smaller than 0.6 cm on transvaginal ultrasonography are considered indeterminate. Larger sacs without DDSS or yolk sac represent either a failed intrauterine or ectopic pregnancy.

The presence of cardiac activity within the uterine cavity is definitive evidence of an intrauterine pregnancy. This finding essentially eliminates the diagnosis of ectopic pregnancy because the incidence of combined intrauterine and extrauterine pregnancy is 1 in 30,000.

The demonstration of an adnexal gestational sac with a fetal pole and cardiac activity is the most specific but least sensitive sign of ectopic pregnancy, occurring in only 10% to 17% of cases (105,120,121). The recognition of other characteristics of ectopic pregnancy has improved ultrasonographic sensitivity. Adnexal rings (fluid sacs with thick echogenic rings) that have a yolk sac or nonliving embryo are accepted as specific ultrasonographic signs of ectopic pregnancy (122). Adnexal rings are visualized in 22% of ectopic pregnancies using transabdominal ultrasonography and in 38% using transvaginal ultrasonography (107). Other studies have identified adnexal rings in 33% to 50% of ectopic pregnancies (105,121). The adnexal ring may not always be apparent because bleeding around the sac results in the appearance of a nonspecific adnexal mass.

Complex or solid adnexal masses are frequently associated with ectopic pregnancy (1,3,19); however, the mass may represent a corpus luteum, endometrioma, hydrosalpinx, ovarian neoplasm (e.g., dermoid cyst), or pedunculated fibroid. Free cul-de-sac fluid is frequently associated with ectopic pregnancy and is no longer considered evidence of rupture. The presence of intraabdominal free fluid should raise concern about tubal rupture (123).

Accurate interpretation of ultrasonography findings requires correlation with the hCG level (discriminatory zone) (114,119,122,124). **All viable intrauterine pregnancies can be visualized by transabdominal ultrasonography for serum hCG levels higher than 6,500 mIU/mL; none are seen at 6,000 mIU/mL. Nonvisualization of an intrauterine gestation with serum hCG levels higher than 6,500 mIU/mL indicates an abnormal (failed intrauterine or ectopic) pregnancy. Intrauterine sacs seen at hCG levels below the discriminatory zone are abnormal and represent either failed intrauterine pregnancies or the pseudogestational sacs of ectopic pregnancy.** If there is no definite sign of an intrauterine gestation (the empty uterus sign) and the hCG level is below the discriminatory zone, the differential diagnosis includes the following considerations:

1. Normal intrauterine pregnancy too early for visualization
2. Abnormal intrauterine gestation
3. Recent abortion
4. Ectopic pregnancy
5. Nonpregnant

The discriminatory zone has been lowered progressively with improvements in ultrasonography resolution. Discriminatory zones for transvaginal ultrasonography have been reported at levels from 1,000 to 2,000 mIU/mL (114,119,122,124). Discriminatory zones vary according to the expertise of the examiner and capability of the equipment.

Although the discriminatory zone for intrauterine pregnancy is well established, there is no such zone for ectopic pregnancy. Levels of hCG have not been shown to correlate with the size of ectopic pregnancy. Regardless of how high the hCG level may be, nonvisualization does not exclude ectopic pregnancy. An ectopic pregnancy may be present anywhere in the abdominal cavity, making ultrasonographic visualization difficult.

Doppler Ultrasound

A Doppler shift occurs whenever the source of an ultrasound beam is moving. The usual sources of Doppler-shifted frequencies are red blood cells. The presence of intravascular blood flow, flow direction, and flow velocity can be determined (125). Pulsed Doppler provides ultrasonographic control over which vessels are sampled. The vascular information is provided both by the shape of the time-velocity waveform (high- or low-resistance flow) and by its systolic, diastolic, and mean velocities (or Doppler frequency shifts) (126). Color-flow Doppler ultrasonography analyzes very-low-amplitude signals from an entire ultrasound tomogram; the Doppler shift is then modulated into color. This information is used to gauge generalized tissue vascularity and to guide pulsed Doppler vascular sampling of specific vessels.

The waveform in the uterine arteries in the nongravid state and in the first trimester of pregnancy shows a high-resistance (little or no diastolic flow), low-velocity pattern. Conversely, a high-velocity, low-resistance signal is localized to the area of developing placentation (127–129). This pattern, seen near the endometrium, is associated with normal and abnormal intrauterine pregnancies and is termed *peritrophoblastic flow*. Whereas transvaginal ultrasonography requires a well-developed double decidual sac (or possibly cardiac activity) to localize an intrauterine gestation, the use of Doppler techniques allows detection of an intrauterine pregnancy at an earlier date. The combined use of Doppler and two-dimensional imaging allows the differentiation of pseudogestational sacs and true intrauterine gestational sacs (130) and the differentiation of the empty uterus sign as either the presence of an intrauterine pregnancy (normal and abnormal) or absence of an intrauterine pregnancy (with an increased risk for ectopic pregnancy) (123).

A similar high-velocity, low-impedence flow characterizes ectopic pregnancies. The addition of Doppler to the ultrasonographic evaluation of suspected ectopic pregnancy improves diagnostic sensitivity for individual diagnoses: from 71% to 87% for ectopic pregnancy, from 24% to 59% for failed intrauterine pregnancy, and from 90% to 99% for normal intrauterine pregnancy (122,123,130).

Dilation and Curettage

Uterine curettage is performed when the pregnancy has been confirmed to be nonviable and the location of the pregnancy cannot be determined by ultrasonography. The decision to evacuate the uterus in the presence of a positive pregnancy test must be made with caution to avoid the unintentional disruption of a viable intrauterine pregnancy. Although suction curettage traditionally has been performed in the operating room, it can now be accomplished under local anesthesia on an outpatient basis. Endometrial sampling methods (e.g., a Novak curettage or Pipelle endometrial sampling device) are accurate in diagnosing abnormal uterine bleeding, but their reliability for intrauterine pregnancy evacuation has not been studied. These devices might miss intrauterine villi and falsely suggest the diagnosis of ectopic pregnancy.

It is essential to confirm the presence of trophoblastic tissue as rapidly as possible so that therapy may be instituted. Once tissue is obtained by curettage, it can be added to saline, in which it will float (Fig. 17.3). Decidual tissue does not float. Chorionic villi are usually identified by their characteristic lacy frond appearance. The sensitivity and

Figure 17.3 When floated in saline, chorionic villi are often readily distinguishable as lacy fronds of tissue. (From **Stovall TG, Ling FW.** *Extrauterine pregnancy: clinical diagnosis and management.* New York: McGraw-Hill, 1993:186, with permission.)

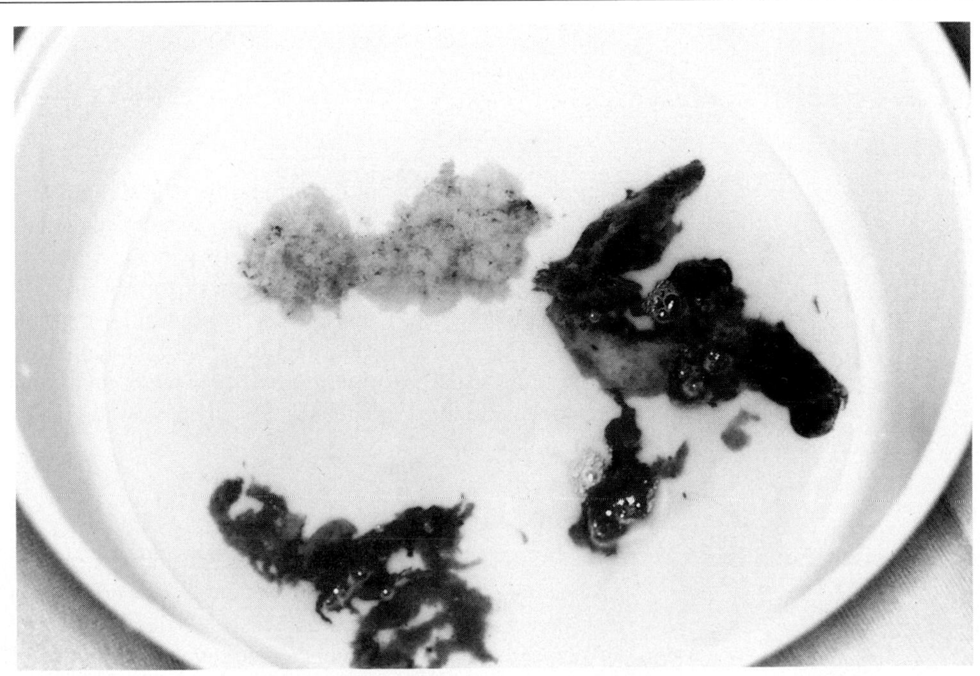

specificity of this technique are 95% when the tissue is examined with the aid of a dissecting microscope. Because flotation of curettings is not 100% accurate in differentiating an intrauterine from extrauterine gestation, histologic confirmation or serial β-hCG level measurement is required. A rapid assessment of the presence of chorionic villi may be obtained with frozen section, which avoids the at least 48-hour waiting period for permanent histologic evaluation. Immunocytochemical staining techniques have been used to identify intermediate trophoblasts that are not normally identified by light microscopy (74).

When frozen section is not available, serial hCG levels permit rapid diagnosis. After evacuation of an abnormal intrauterine pregnancy, the hCG level decreases by >15% within 12 to 24 hours. A borderline fall may represent interassay variability. A repeat level should be obtained in 24 to 48 hours to confirm the decline. If the uterus is evacuated and the pregnancy is extrauterine, the hCG level plateaus or continues to increase, indicating the presence of extrauterine trophoblastic tissue.

Culdocentesis

Culdocentesis has been used widely as a diagnostic technique for ectopic pregnancy. With the use of hCG testing and transvaginal ultrasound, however, culdocentesis is rarely indicated. The purpose of the procedure is to determine the presence of nonclotting blood, which increases the likelihood of ruptured ectopic pregnancy. After exposing the posterior vaginal fornix with a bivalve vaginal speculum, the posterior lip of the cervix is grasped with a tenaculum. The cul-de-sac is then entered through the posterior vaginal wall with an 18- to 20-gauge spinal needle with a syringe attached. As the cul-de-sac is entered, suction is applied, and the intraperitoneal contents are aspirated. If nonclotting blood is obtained, the results are positive. In the presence of serous fluid, results are negative. A lack of fluid return or clotted blood is nondiagnostic.

Historically, if the culdocentesis results were positive, laparotomy was performed for a presumed diagnosis of ruptured tubal pregnancy. However, **the results of culdocentesis do not always correlate with the status of the pregnancy.** Although about 70% to 90% of patients with ectopic pregnancy have a hemoperitoneum demonstrated by culdocentesis, only 50% of patients have a ruptured tube (131). Furthermore, about 6% of women with positive culdocentesis results do not have an ectopic gestation at the time of laparotomy. Nondiagnostic taps occur in 10% to 20% of patients with ectopic pregnancy and, therefore, are not definitive.

Laparoscopy

Laparoscopy is the gold standard for the diagnosis of ectopic pregnancy. Generally, the fallopian tubes are easily visualized and evaluated, although the diagnosis of ectopic pregnancy is missed in 3% to 4% of patients who have very small ectopic gestations. The ectopic gestation is usually seen distorting the normal tubal architecture. With earlier diagnosis, there is an increasing possibility that a small ectopic pregnancy may not be visualized. Pelvic adhesions or previous tubal damage may compromise assessment of the tube. False-positive results occur when tubal dilation or discoloration is misinterpreted as an ectopic pregnancy, in which case the tube can be incised unnecessarily and damaged.

Diagnostic Algorithm

The presenting symptoms and physical findings of patients with an unruptured ectopic pregnancy are similar to those of patients with a normal intrauterine pregnancy (89). History, risk factor assessment, and physical examination are the initial steps in the management of suspected ectopic pregnancy. Patients in a hemodynamically unstable condition should undergo immediate surgical intervention. Patients with a stable, relatively asymptomatic condition may be assessed as outpatients.

If the diagnosis of ectopic pregnancy can be confirmed without laparoscopy, several potential benefits result. First, both the anesthetic and surgical risks of laparoscopy are avoided; second, medical therapy becomes a treatment option. Because many ectopic pregnancies occur in histologically normal tubes, resolution without surgery may spare the tube from additional trauma and improve subsequent fertility. An algorithm for the diagnosis of ectopic pregnancy without laparoscopy proved to be 100% accurate in a randomized clinical trial (132,133) (Fig. 17.4). This screening algorithm combines the use of history and physical examination, serial hCG levels, serum progesterone levels, vaginal ultrasonography, and dilation and curettage. When hCG levels and transvaginal ultrasonography are available in a timely fashion, serum progesterone screening is not required. Serial hCG levels are used to assess pregnancy viability, correlated with transvaginal ultrasonography findings, and measured serially after a suction curettage.

In this algorithm, **transvaginal ultrasonography is used as follows:**

1. **The identification of an intrauterine gestational sac or pregnancy effectively excludes the presence of an extrauterine pregnancy.** If the patient has a rising hCG level of more than 2,000 mIU/mL, and no intrauterine gestational sac is identified, the patient is considered to have an extrauterine pregnancy and can be treated without further testing.

2. **Adnexal cardiac activity, when seen, definitively confirms the diagnosis of ectopic pregnancy.**

3. **A tubal mass as small as 1 cm can be identified and characterized.** Masses greater than 3.5 cm with cardiac activity or larger than 4 cm without cardiac activity should not be treated with medical therapy.

Suction curettage is used to differentiate nonviable intrauterine pregnancies from ectopic gestations (less than 50% rise in hCG level over 48 hours, an hCG level of less than 2,000 mIU/mL, and an indeterminate sonogram). Performance of this procedure avoids unnecessary use of methotrexate in patients with abnormal intrauterine pregnancy that can only be diagnosed by evacuating the uterus. An unlikely potential problem with suction curettage is missing either an early nonviable intrauterine pregnancy or combined intrauterine and extrauterine pregnancies.

Treatment

Ectopic pregnancy can be treated either medically or surgically. Both methods are effective, and the choice depends on the clinical circumstances, the site of the ectopic pregnancy, and the available resources.

Surgical Treatment

Operative management is the most widely used treatment for ectopic pregnancy. There has been debate about which surgical procedure is best. Salpingo-oophorectomy was once considered appropriate because it was theorized that this technique would eliminate transperitoneal migration of the ovum or zygote, which was thought to predispose to recurrent ectopic pregnancy (134). Ovarian removal results in all ovulations occurring on the side with the remaining normal fallopian tube. Subsequent studies have not confirmed that ipsilateral oophorectomy increases the likelihood of conceiving an intrauterine pregnancy; therefore, this practice is not recommended (135).

Salpingectomy Versus Salpingostomy

Linear salpingostomy is currently the procedure of choice when the patient has an unruptured ectopic pregnancy and wishes to retain her potential for future fertility. The products of conception are removed through an incision made into the tube on its antimesenteric border. The procedure can be accomplished with either a needle tip cautery,

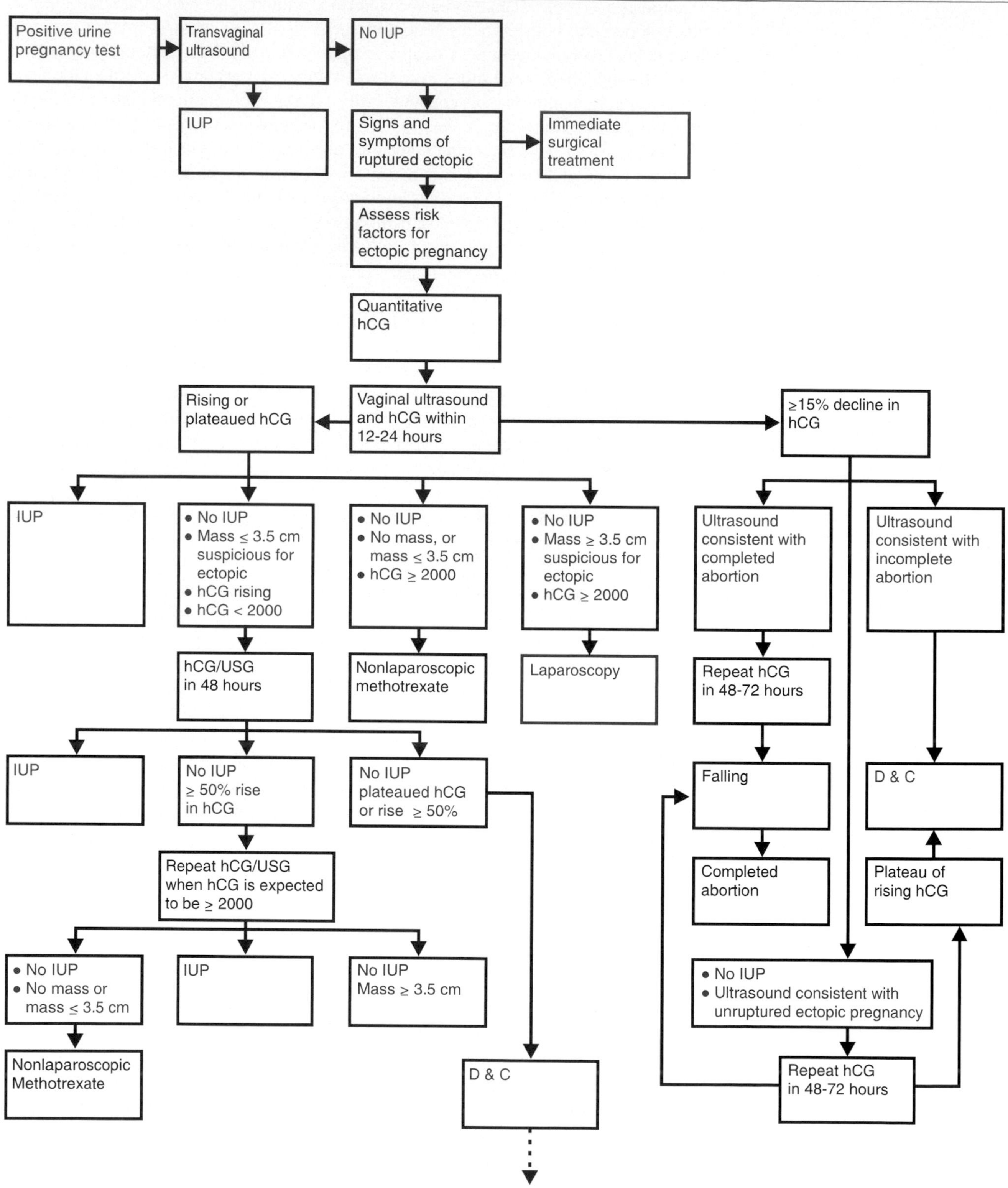

Figure 17.4 Nonlaparoscopic algorithm for diagnosis of ectopic pregnancy.

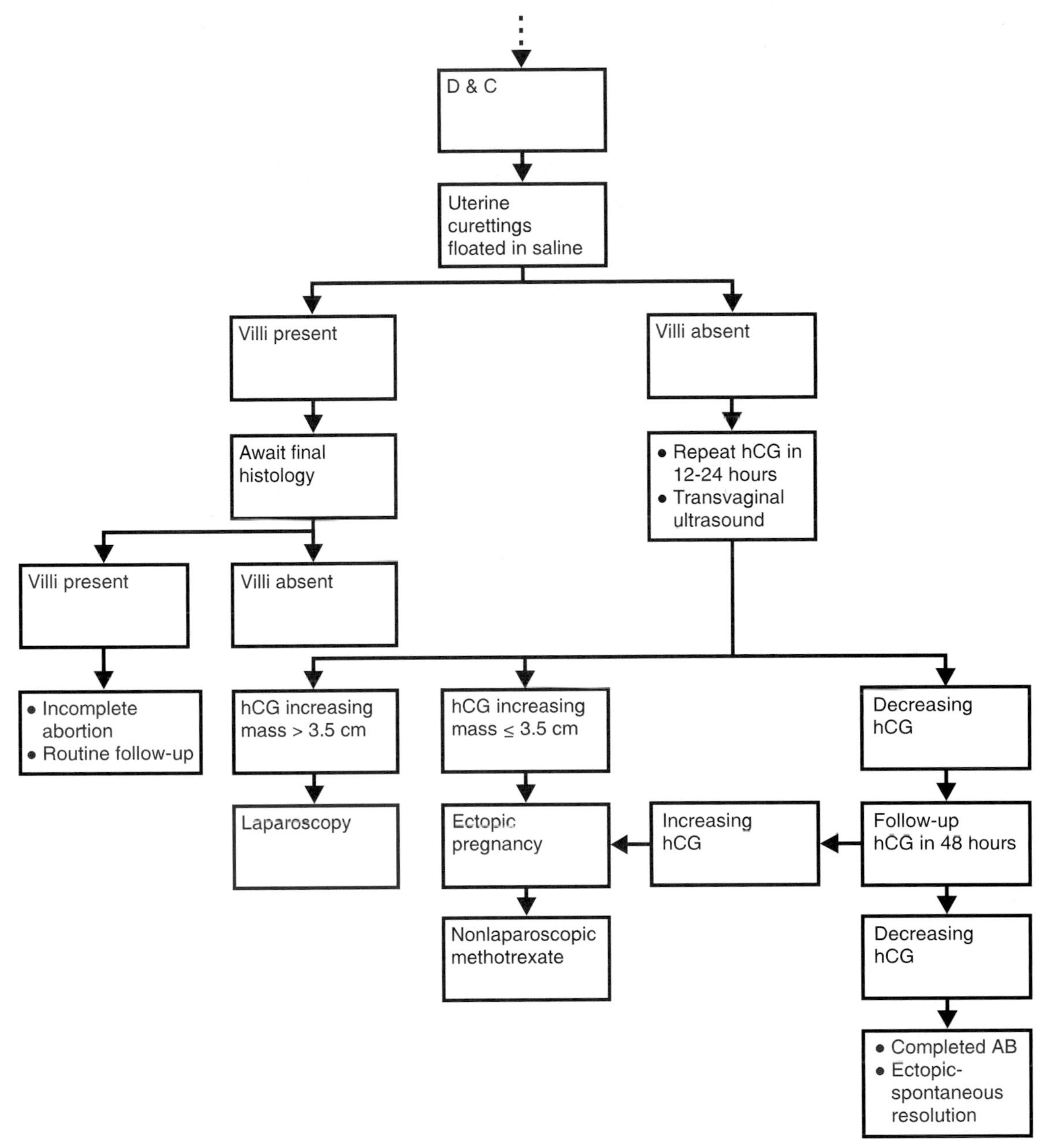

Figure 17.4—*continued*

laser, scalpel, or scissors. It can be done by operative laparoscopic techniques or laparotomy. In a study in which patients treated with either salpingectomy or salpingostomy were followed for a period of 3 years to about 12.5 years, there was no difference in pregnancy rates (136). A history of infertility is the most significant determinant of future fertility, and such patients are probably served better by salpingectomy to decrease their subsequent chance of a recurrent ectopic pregnancy. Linear salpingostomy is as effective as segmental resection with primary reanastomosis, even for ectopic pregnancies occurring in the isthmic tubal segment, and it is technically less difficult and has a shorter operative time (137).

Milking the tube to effect a tubal abortion has been advocated; if the pregnancy is fimbrial, this technique may be effective. However, when milking was compared with linear salpingostomy for ampullary ectopic pregnancies, milking was associated with a twofold increase in the recurrent ectopic pregnancy rate (138).

Laparotomy Versus Laparosocpy

Salpingostomy, salpingectomy, or segmental resection can be accomplished by laparoscopy or laparotomy. The approach used depends on the hemodynamic stability of the patient, the size and location of the ectopic mass, and the surgeon's expertise. **Laparotomy is indicated when the patient becomes hemodynamically unstable, whereas laparoscopy is reserved for patients who are hemodynamically stable. A ruptured ectopic pregnancy does not necessarily require laparotomy.** However, if large blood clots are present or the intraabdominal blood cannot be evacuated in a timely manner, laparotomy should be considered. Cornual or interstitial pregnancies often require laparotomy, although laparoscopic management has been described (139). Laparotomy is chosen for the management of most ovarian and abdominal pregnancies. In some cases, the patient may have extensive abdominal or pelvic adhesive disease, making laparoscopy difficult and laparotomy more feasible.

Laparoscopy has advantages over laparotomy for management of ectopic pregnancy. In a case-control study of 50 patients comparing the use of laparoscopy and laparotomy for ectopic pregnancy management, hospital stay was significantly shorter (1.3 ± 0.8 versus 3.0 ± 1.1 days), operative time was shorter (78 ± 26 versus 104 ± 27 minutes), and convalescence was shorter (9 ± 8 versus 26 ± 16 days) in the laparoscopy group (140). In a randomized study in which 30 patients in each group were compared, patients undergoing laparoscopic management had less estimated blood loss, shorter hospital stay, equivalent tubal pregnancy rates, and similar pregnancy and persistent trophoblast rates (141). In another study, patients were assigned during alternate months to undergo laparoscopic management (n = 26) or laparotomy (n = 37) (142). There were no differences in operative time, although patients undergoing laparoscopy had a significant decrease in blood loss, postoperative hospital stay, narcotic requirement, and time to return to normal activity. Laparoscopic management was associated with significant cost savings when compared with laparotomy (more than $5,528 ± $1,586 versus more than $6,793 ± $155). Using a prospective analysis, 105 patients with tubal pregnancy were stratified with regard to age and risk factors and then randomized to undergo either laparoscopic management or laparotomy (143). Subsequently, 73 patients underwent second-look laparoscopy to assess the degree of adhesion formation. Patients treated by laparotomy had significantly more adhesions at the surgical site than those treated by laparoscopy, but tubal patency rates were similar. Pregnancy rates were not analyzed.

Reproductive Outcome

Reproductive outcome after ectopic pregnancy is usually evaluated by determining tubal patency by hysterosalpingography, the subsequent intrauterine pregnancy rate, and the recurrent ectopic pregnancy rate. Pregnancy rates are similar in patients treated by either laparoscopy or laparotomy. Tubal patency on the ipsilateral side after conservative laparoscopic management is about 84%.

In a study of 143 patients followed after undergoing laparoscopic procedures for ectopic pregnancy, the overall intrauterine pregnancy rates for laparoscopic salpingostomy (60%) and laparoscopic salpingectomy (54%) were not significantly different (144). If the patient had evidence of tubal damage, pregnancy rates (42%) were significantly lower than in those women who did not have tubal damage (79%). In another study, the reproductive outcome of 188 patients followed for a mean of 7.2 years (range, 3 to 15 years) was reported after conservation by laparotomy for ectopic pregnancy (145). An intrauterine pregnancy occurred in 83 (70%) patients, with a recurrent ectopic pregnancy rate of 13%, suggesting that reproductive outcome after an ectopic pregnancy treated by laparotomy is similar to that of patients undergoing laparoscopic or medical management. Thus, when compared with medical therapy, surgical management appears to have equal reproductive outcome, although a prospective randomized trial has not been reported.

Medical Treatment

The drug most frequently used for medical management of ectopic pregnancy is *methotrexate,* although other agents have been studied, including potassium chloride (KCl), hyperosmolar glucose, prostaglandins, and *RU-486.* These agents may be given systemically (intravenously, intramuscularly, or orally) or locally (laparoscopic direct injection, transvaginal ultrasound–directed injection, or retrograde salpingography).

Methotrexate

Methotrexate is a folic acid analogue that inhibits dehydrofolate reductase and thereby prevents synthesis of DNA. It has been used extensively in the treatment of gestational trophoblastic disease (see Chapter 34). Commonly reported side effects include leukopenia, thrombocytopenia, bone marrow aplasia, ulcerative stomatitis, diarrhea, and hemorrhagic enteritis. Other reported side effects include alopecia, dermatitis, elevated liver enzyme levels, and pneumonitis (146). However, no significant side effects have been reported at the low doses used for ectopic pregnancy treatment. Minor side effects have been reported with multiple doses; *citrovorum factor* reduces the incidence of these side effects and is generally used when prolonged treatment is required. Importantly, long-term follow-up of women treated with *methotrexate* for gestational trophoblastic disease shows no increase in congenital malformations, spontaneous abortions, or tumors recurring after chemotherapy (147). A smaller total dose of *methotrexate* is required, and shorter treatment duration is used for treatment of ectopic pregnancy than for gestational trophoplastic disease.

Initially, *methotrexate* was used for the treatment of trophoblastic tissue left *in situ* after exploration for an abdominal pregnancy (148). In 1982, Tanaka and colleagues treated an unruptured interstitial gestation with a 15-day course of intramuscular *methotrexate* (149). The use of *methotrexate* for primary treatment of ectopic pregnancy has been reported in more than 300 patients (150–159).

A trial of intramuscular *methotrexate* (1 mg/kg/day) followed by *citrovorum* factor (0.1 mg/kg/day) on alternate days was given to 100 patients with a success rate of 96% (153,155). This outpatient treatment protocol used *methotrexate* plus *citrovorum factor* given only until the hCG level began to decline. Treatment was given until there was at least a 15% decline between two consecutive daily hCG levels. *Citrovorum* factor is given on the day after the *methotrexate* is administered, even if no further *methotrexate* is indicated. Once *methotrexate* is discontinued, hCG levels are measured weekly until the results are negative. A second course of *methotrexate* plus *citrovorum factor* is given only if there is a plateau or rise in the hCG level. Of the 96 patients successfully treated, 17 required only one *methotrexate* and *citrovorum* factor dose, and 19 required four doses. Four patients treated with *methotrexate* failed therapy and required surgical treatment for tubal rupture, and each of these cases differed with respect to ectopic pregnancy size, hCG level, and time of rupture. Of five ectopic pregnancies with cardiac activity, four were successfully treated. No conclusions can be drawn regarding risk factors or predictors of ectopic pregnancy rupture.

Single-dose intramuscular *methotrexate* for ectopic pregnancy treatment was administered to 31 patients with an injection of 50 mg/m^2 without *citrovorum factor.* Of 30 patients, 29 (96.7%) were successfully treated, and no patients experienced *methotrexate*-related side effects. Some 200 patients have now been treated using the single-dose protocol outlined in Table 17.3. Compared with the multidose protocol, single-dose *methotrexate* is less expensive, patient acceptance is greater because less monitoring is required during treatment, the incidence of side effects is decreased, and the treatment results and prospects for future fertility are comparable.

Initiating Methotrexate Table 17.4 outlines a checklist that should be followed by the physician before initiating *methotrexate.* It also lists instructions that are helpful to the patient.

Table 17.3. Single-dose Methotrexate Protocol for Ectopic Pregnancy

Day	Therapy *
0	D & C, hCG
1	CBC, SGOT, BUN, creatinine, blood type and Rh
4	*Methotrexate* 50 mg/m^2 IM
7	hCG

CBC, complete blood count; SGOT, serum glutamic-oxaloacetic transaminase; BUN, blood urea nitrogen; IM, intramuscularly.
* If less than a 15% decline in human chorionic gonadotropin (hCG) level between days 4 and 7, give second dose of *methotrexate,* 50 mg/m^2, on day 7.
If more than a 15% decline in hCG level between days 4 and 7, follow weekly until hCG is below 10 mIU/mL.
In patients not requiring dilation and curettage (D & C) (hCG > 2,000 mIU/mL and no gestational sac on transvaginal ultrasonography), days 0 and 1 are combined.

Patient Follow-up After intramuscular administration of *methotrexate,* patients are monitored on an outpatient basis. Patients who report severe pain or pain that is prolonged are evaluated by measuring hematocrit levels and performing transvaginal ultrasonography. The ultrasonography findings during follow-up, although not usually helpful, can be used to provide reassurance that the tube has not ruptured (160). Cul-de-sac fluid is very common, and the amount of fluid may increase if a tubal abortion occurs. However, it is usually not necessary to intervene surgically unless the patient has a precipitous drop in hematocrit levels or she becomes hemodynamically unstable.

Patients are asked not to become pregnant for at least 2 months after treatment. Hysterosalpingography can be performed, although the procedure is not mandatory.

Candidates for Methotrexate **In order to maximize the safety of treatment and to eliminate the possibility of treating in the presence of a nonviable or early viable intrauterine pregnancy, patients considered candidates for *methotrexate* treatment**

Table 17.4. Initiation of Methotrexate: Physician Checklist and Patient Instructions

Physician Checklist

Obtain hCG level.
Perform transvaginal ultrasound within 48 hours.
Perform endometrial curettage if hCG level is less than 2,000 mIU/mL.
Obtain normal liver function (SGOT), normal renal function (BUN, creatinine), and a normal CBC (WBC < 2,000/mL and platelet count > 100,000)
Administer *Rhogam* if patient is Rh-negative.
Identify unruptured ectopic pregnancy smaller than 3.5 cm.
Obtain informed consent.
Prescribe $FeSO_4$, 325 mg PO bid if hematocrit is less than 30%.
Schedule follow-up appointment on days 4, 6, and 7.

Patient Instructions

Refrain from alcohol use, multivitamins containing folic acid, and sexual intercourse until hCG level is negative.
Call your physician:
  If you experience prolonged or heavy vaginal bleeding.
  The pain is prolonged or severe (lower abdomen and pelvic pain is normal during the first 10–14 days of treatment).
  Use oral contraception or barrier contraceptive methods.

About 4%–5% of women experience unsuccessful *methotrexate* treatment and require surgery.
hCG, human chorionic gonadotropin; SGOT, serum glutamic-oxaloacetic transaminase; BUN, blood urea nitrogen; CBC, complete blood count; WBC, white blood cell.

should include those to whom the following factors apply:

1. **An hCG level is present after salpingostomy or salpingotomy.**
2. **A rising or plateaued hCG level is present at least 12 to 24 hours after suction curettage.**
3. **No intrauterine gestational sac or fluid collection is detected by transvaginal ultrasound, the hCG level is greater than 2,000 mIU/mL, and an ectopic pregnancy mass of at least 3.5 to 4 cm is demonstrated.**

Ultrasound findings should be interpreted with caution because most unruptured ectopic pregnancies will be accompanied by fluid in the cul-de-sac.

Side Effects Opponents of *methotrexate* therapy cite potential side effects as the reason not to use it. Most reported side effects have occurred in patients treated with intravenous *methotrexate* with higher doses and for more prolonged treatment courses than are now required. When using the single-dose intramuscular regimen, the incidence of side effects is less than 1%, and the failure rate is comparable to that of conservative laparoscopic surgery. One problem that remains puzzling is the inability to predict treatment failures with the use of *methotrexate.* However, the same is true with conservative surgical procedures; thus, the need to monitor hCG levels after either salpingostomy or *methotrexate* remains. In a review of more than 350 women treated with intramuscular *methotrexate,* Lipscomb and associates found that a high hCG concentration was the most important factor associated with failure of treatment with a single-dose *methotrexate* protocol (161). In patients with an hCG level of less than 10,000 mIU/mL, the overall success rate was 93.4%, as compared with 60.7% when the hCG level was greater than 10,000 mIU/mL. Although surgical management of ectopic pregnancy remains the mainstay of treatment worldwide, *methotrexate* treatment is appropriate in select patient populations.

Reproductive Function Although there are few data, reproductive function after *methotrexate* treatment can be assessed on the basis of tubal patency and pregnancy outcome. Tubal patency is reported to be 50% to 100%, with a mean of 71%, after systemic *methotrexate* treatment. In two separate reports of 23 and 62 patients, the tubal patency rates on the ipsilateral side were 81.4% and 82.3%, respectively (156,162).

Pregnancy outcome after *methotrexate* administration was reported in a group of 14 patients who attempted pregnancy after multiple intramuscular doses. Of these 14 women, 11 (78.6%) became pregnant; 10 of 11 (90.9%) were intrauterine pregnancies, and one (9%) was an extrauterine pregnancy (156). The mean time from first attempting to achieving pregnancy was 2.3 months (range, 1 to 4 months). In another study of 49 patients who were attempting pregnancy after completion of single-dose intramuscular *methotrexate* administration, 39 (80%) became pregnant; 34 (87%) were intrauterine pregnancies, and 5 (13%) were ectopic pregnancies (163). The mean time from attempting to achieving pregnancy was 3.2 ± 1.1 months. In 87 pregnancies after *methotrexate* therapy, the combined intrauterine pregnancy rate was 86%, and the ectopic pregnancy rate was 14%.

In a combined series of 527 patients treated by laparoscopic linear salpingostomy or salpingotomy, the intrauterine pregnancy rate was 54%, and the recurrent ectopic pregnancy rate was 13% (164). Comparison of laparoscopically treated patients with *methotrexate*-treated patients suggests that the two methods have similar reproductive outcomes.

Other Drugs and Techniques

Salpingocentesis is a technique in which agents such as KCl, *methotrexate,* prostaglandins, and hyperosmolar glucose are injected into the ectopic pregnancy transvaginally using ultrasound guidance, by transcervical tubal cannulization, or by laparoscopy. Agents injected under ultrasound guidance have included *methotrexate* (165–169), KCl (170), combined *methotrexate* and KCl (171), and *prostaglandin* E_2 (172). The potential advantages of salpingocentesis include a one-time injection with the potential avoidance of systemic side effects. Reproductive function after this form of treatment has not been reported. Because of the limited experience, this treatment cannot be recommended until there is further study.

Agents injected into the amniotic sac at laparoscopy have included *prostaglandin* F_{2a} (173), hyperosmolar glucose (174), and *methotrexate* (175). This method has the obvious disadvantage of requiring laparoscopy, but it can be used if laparoscopy has been performed. Other agents reported for the treatment of ectopic pregnancy include *RU-486* (176) and anti-hCG antibody (177).

Types of Ectopic Pregnancy

Spontaneous Resolution

Some ectopic pregnancies resolve by resorption or by tubal abortion, obviating the need for medical or surgical therapy (178–182). The proportion of ectopic pregnancies that resolve spontaneously and the reason they do so while others do not are unknown. There are no specific criteria for patient selection that predict successful outcome after spontaneous resolution. A falling hCG level is the most common indicator used, but ectopic pregnancy rupture can occur even with falling hCG levels.

Persistent Trophoblastic Tissue

Persistent ectopic pregnancy occurs when a patient has undergone conservative surgery (e.g., salpingostomy, fimbrial expression) and viable trophoblastic tissue remains. Histologically, there is no identifiable embryo, the implantation is usually medial to the previous tubal incision, and residual chorionic villi are usually confined to the tubal muscularis. Peritoneal trophoblastic tissue implants may also be responsible for persistence (183–188).

The incidence of persistent ectopic pregnancy has increased with the increased use of surgery that conserves the tubes. Persistence is diagnosed when the hCG levels plateau after conservative surgery. Persistent ectopic gestation is best diagnosed by an initial measurement of serum hCG or progesterone 6 days postoperatively and at 3-day intervals thereafter (186).

Risk factors for persistent ectopic pregnancy are based on the type of surgical procedure, the initial hCG level, the duration of amenorrhea, and the size of the ectopic pregnancy. A slower decline of serum hCG levels has been seen in patients treated by salpingostomy compared with patients treated by salpingectomy. The incidence of persistence after laparoscopic linear salpingostomy ranges from 3% to 20% (189,190). It is uncertain whether the incidence of persistent ectopic pregnancy is the same or greater when the procedure is performed by laparoscopy versus laparotomy. In a review of medical records from 157 patients who underwent salpingostomy for intact ampullary ectopic pregnancy, 16 of 103 patients (16%) undergoing laparoscopic salpingostomy were treated for persistent ectopic pregnancy, whereas 1 of 54 women (2%) who had salpingostomy by laparotomy was treated for persistent ectopic pregnancy (185). Lundorff and colleagues reported that 23% of women with a preoperative hCG level of less than 3,000 mIU/mL developed persistent ectopic pregnancy, whereas only 1 of 67 with a level of more than 3,000 mIU/mL persisted (187). They also noted that 36% of women with an hCG level of more than 1,000 mIU/mL on the second postoperative day and 64% of patients with an hCG level of more than 1,000 mIU/mL on the seventh postoperative day developed persistence. Amenorrhea of less than 7 weeks' duration and ectopic mass smaller than 2 cm have also been reported to increase the risk for persistent ectopic pregnancy (185,187).

Treatment of persistent ectopic pregnancy can be either surgical or medical; surgical therapy consists of either repeat salpingostomy or, more commonly, salpingectomy. *Methotrexate* offers an alternative to patients who are hemodynamically stable at the time of diagnosis. *Methotrexate* may be the treatment of choice because the persistent trophoblastic tissue may not be confined to the tube and, therefore, not readily identifiable during repeat surgical exploration (190–192).

Chronic Ectopic Pregnancy

Chronic ectopic pregnancy is a condition in which the pregnancy does not completely resorb during expectant management. The condition arises when there is persistence of the chorionic villi with bleeding into the tubal wall, which is distended slowly and does not rupture. It may also arise from chronic bleeding from the fimbriated end of the fallopian tube with subsequent tamponade. In a series of 50 patients with a chronic ectopic pregnancy, pain was present in 86%, vaginal bleeding was present in 68%, and both symptoms were present in 58% (193). Ninety percent of the patients had amenorrhea ranging from 5 to 16 weeks (mean, 9.6 weeks). Most patients develop a pelvic mass that is usually symptomatic. The hCG level is usually low but may be absent; ultrasound may be helpful in the diagnosis; and rarely, bowel involvement or ureteral compression or obstruction exists (193,194).

This condition is treated surgically with removal of the affected tube. Often, the ovary must be removed because there is inflammation with subsequent adhesion development. A hematoma may be present secondary to chronic bleeding.

Nontubal Ectopic Pregnancy

Cervical Pregnancy The incidence of cervical pregnancy in the United States ranges from 1 in 2,400 to 1 in 50,000 pregnancies (195). A variety of conditions are thought to predispose to the development of a cervical pregnancy, including previous therapeutic abortion, Asherman's syndrome, previous cesarean delivery, *diethylstilbestrol* exposure, leiomyomas, and IVF (195–197).

The diagnostic criteria for cervical pregnancy were established based on histologic analysis of a hysterectomy specimen (195). Clinical criteria include the following findings (197):

1. The uterus is smaller than the surrounding distended cervix.
2. The internal os is not dilated.
3. Curettage of the endometrial cavity is nonproductive of placental tissue.
4. The external os opens earlier than in spontaneous abortion.

Ultrasonographic diagnostic criteria have also been described that are helpful in differentiating a true cervical pregnancy from an ongoing spontaneous abortion (Table 17.5). Magnetic

Table 17.5. Ultrasound Criteria for Cervical Pregnancy

1. Echo-free uterine cavity or the presence of a false gestational sac only
2. Decidual transformation of the endometrium with dense echo structure
3. Diffuse uterine wall structure
4. Hourglass uterine shape
5. Ballooned cervical canal
6. Gestational sac in the endocervix
7. Placental tissue in the cervical canal
8. Closed internal os

From **Hofmann HMH, Urdl W, Hofler H, et al.** Cervical pregnancy: case reports and current concepts in diagnosis and treatment. *Arch Gynecol Obstet* 1987;241:63–69, with permission.

Table 17.6. Criteria for Ovarian Pregnancy Diagnosis

1. The fallopian tube on the affected side must be intact.
2. The fetal sac must occupy the position of the ovary.
3. The ovary must be connected to the uterus by the ovarian ligament.
4. Ovarian tissue must be located in the sac wall.

From **Spiegelberg O.** Casusistik der ovarialschwangerschaft. *Arch Gynaecol* 1878;13:73, with permission.

resonance imaging of the pelvis has also been used in this situation (198). Other potential diagnoses that must be differentiated from cervical pregnancy include cervical carcinoma, cervical or prolapsed submucous leiomyomas, trophoblastic tumor, placenta previa, and low-lying placenta.

When a cervical pregnancy is diagnosed before surgery, the preoperative preparation should include blood typing and cross-matching, establishment of intravenous access, and detailed informed consent. This consent should include the possibility of hemorrhage that may require transfusion or hysterectomy. Nonsurgical treatment, including intraamniotic and systemic methotrexate administration, has been used successfully (199,200).

The diagnosis may not be suspected until the patient is undergoing suction curettage for a presumed incomplete abortion and hemorrhage occurs. In some cases, bleeding is light, whereas in others, there is hemorrhage. Various techniques that can be used to control bleeding include uterine packing, lateral cervical suture placement to ligate the lateral cervical vessels, placement of a cerclage, and insertion of an intracervical 30-mL Foley catheter in an attempt to tamponade the bleeding. Alternatively, angiographic artery embolization can be used; or, if laparotomy is required, an attempt can be made to ligate the uterine or internal iliac arteries (201–203). When none of these methods is successful, hysterectomy is required.

Ovarian Pregnancy A pregnancy confined to the ovary represents 0.5% to 1% of all ectopic pregnancies and is the most common type of nontubal ectopic pregnancy. The incidence ranges from 1 in 40,000 to 1 in 7,000 deliveries (204,205). The diagnostic criteria were described in 1878 by Spiegelberg (Table 17.6). Unlike tubal gestation, ovarian pregnancy is associated with neither PID nor infertility. The only risk factor associated with the development of an ovarian pregnancy is the current use of an intrauterine device.

Patients have symptoms similar to those of ectopic pregnancies in other sites. Misdiagnosis is common because it is confused with a ruptured corpus luteum in up to 75% of cases (204). As with other types of ectopic pregnancy, an ovarian pregnancy has also been reported after hysterectomy (206). Ultrasonography has made preoperative diagnosis possible in some cases (207).

The treatment of ovarian pregnancy has changed. Whereas oophorectomy has been advocated in the past, ovarian cystectomy has become the preferred treatment (208). It is possible to perform cystectomy using laparoscopic techniques (209,210). Treatment with methotrexate or prostaglandin injection has also been reported (210).

Abdominal Pregnancy Abdominal pregnancies are classified as primary and secondary. Table 17.7 lists criteria for classifying a primary abdominal pregnancy. Secondary abdominal pregnancies are by far the most common and result from tubal abortion or rupture or, less often, from subsequent implantation within the abdomen after uterine rupture. The incidence of abdominal pregnancy varies from 1 in 372 to 1 in 9,714 live births (211). Abdominal pregnancy is associated with high morbidity and mortality, with the risk for death 7 to 8 times greater than from tubal ectopic pregnancy and 90 times greater than from intrauterine pregnancy. There are scattered reports of term abdominal pregnancies. When this occurs, perinatal morbidity and mortality are high, usually as a result of growth

Table 17.7. Studdiford's Criteria for Diagnosis of Primary Abdominal Pregnancy

1. Presence of normal tubes and ovaries with no evidence of recent or past pregnancy
2. No evidence of uteroplacental fistula
3. The presence of a pregnancy related exclusively to the peritoneal surface and early enough to eliminate the possibility of secondary implantation after primary tubal nidation

restriction and congenital anomalies such as fetal pulmonary hypoplasia, pressure deformities, and facial and limb asymmetry. The incidence of congenital anomalies ranges from 20% to 40% (212).

The presentation of patients with an abdominal pregnancy varies and depends on the gestational age. In the first and early second trimester, the symptoms may be the same as with tubal ectopic gestation; in advanced abdominal pregnancy, the clinical presentation is more variable. The patient may complain of painful fetal movement, fetal movements high in the abdomen, or sudden cessation of movements. Physical examination may disclose persistent abnormal fetal lies, abdominal tenderness, a displaced uterine cervix, easy palpation of fetal parts, and palpation of the uterus separate from the gestation. The diagnosis may be suspected when there are no uterine contractions after *oxytocin* infusion. Other diagnostic aids include abdominal x-ray, abdominal ultrasound, computed tomography scanning, and magnetic resonance imaging (213,214).

Because the pregnancy can continue to term, the potential maternal morbidity and mortality are very high. As a result, surgical intervention is recommended when an abdominal pregnancy is diagnosed. At surgery, the placenta can be removed if its vascular supply can be identified and ligated, but hemorrhage can occur, requiring abdominal packing that is left in place and removed after 24 to 48 hours. Angiographic arterial embolization has been described (215). If the vascular supply cannot be identified, the cord is ligated near the placental base, and the placenta is left in place. Placental involution can be monitored using serial ultrasonography and hCG levels. Potential complications of leaving the placenta in place include bowel obstruction, fistula formation, and sepsis as the tissue degenerates. Methotrexate treatment appears to be contraindicated because a high rate of complications has been reported, including sepsis and death, believed to be a result of rapid tissue necrosis (216).

Interstitial Pregnancy Interstitial pregnancies represent about 1% of ectopic pregnancies. These patients tend to present later in gestation than those with tubal pregnancies. Interstitial pregnancies often are associated with uterine rupture; therefore, they represent a disproportionately large percentage of fatalities from ectopic pregnancy. Treatment is cornual resection by laparotomy, although laparoscopic management has also been described (217).

Interligamentous Pregnancy Interligamentous pregnancy is a rare form of ectopic pregnancy that occurs in about 1 in every 300 ectopic pregnancies (218). An interligamentous pregnancy usually results from trophoblastic penetration of a tubal pregnancy through the tubal serosa and into the mesosalpinx, with secondary implantation between the leaves of the broad ligament. It can also occur if a uterine fistula develops between the endometrial cavity and the retroperitoneal space. As with an abdominal pregnancy, the placenta may be adherent to the uterus, bladder, and pelvic sidewalls. If possible, the placenta should be removed; when this is not possible, it can be left *in situ* and allowed to resorb. As in abdominal pregnancy, there are reported cases of live birth with this type ectopic gestation (218).

Heterotropic Pregnancy Heterotropic pregnancy occurs when there are coexisting intrauterine and ectopic pregnancies. The reported incidence varies widely from 1 in 100 to 1 in 30,000 pregnancies (219). Patients who have undergone ovulation induction have a much higher incidence of heterotropic pregnancy than those who have a spontaneous conception. An intrauterine pregnancy is seen during ultrasound examination, and an extrauterine pregnancy may be overlooked easily. Serial hCG levels are often not helpful because the intrauterine pregnancy causes the hCG level to rise appropriately.

The treatment of the ectopic pregnancy is operative; once the ectopic pregnancy has been removed, intrauterine pregnancy continues in most patients. It may be possible to use nonchemotherapeutic medical treatment such as KCl by transvaginal or laparoscopically directed injection for treatment of the ectopic pregnancy.

Multiple Ectopic Pregnancies Twin or multiple ectopic gestations occur less frequently than heterotropic gestations and may appear in a variety of locations and combinations. About 250 twin ectopic gestations have been reported (220). Although most reports are confined to twin tubal gestations, ovarian, interstitial, and abdominal twin pregnancies have been reported. Twin and triplet gestations have been reported following partial salpingectomy (221) and IVF (222). Management is similar to that for other types of ectopic pregnancy and is somewhat dependent on the location of the pregnancy.

Pregnancy After Hysterectomy The most unusual form of ectopic pregnancy is one that occurs after either vaginal or abdominal hysterectomy (223,224). Such a pregnancy may occur after supracervical hysterectomy because the patient has a cervical canal that may provide intraperitoneal access. Pregnancy may occur in the perioperative period with implantation of the fertilized ovum in the fallopian tube. Pregnancy after total hysterectomy probably occurs secondary to a vaginal mucosal defect that allows sperm into the abdominal cavity.

References

1. **Hill LM, Guzick D, Fries J, et al.** Fetal loss rate after ultrasonically documented cardiac activity between 6 and 14 weeks menstrual age. *J Clin Ultrasound* 1991;19:221–223.
2. **Simpson JL, Mills JL, Holmes LB, et al.** Low fetal loss rates after ultrasound-proved viability in early pregnancy. *JAMA* 1987;258:2555–2557.
3. **Goldstein SR.** Embryonic death in early pregnancy: a new look at the first trimester. *Obstet Gynecol* 1994;84:294–297.
4. **Tongsong T, Wanapirak C, Srisomboon J, et al.** Transvaginal ultrasound in threatened abortions with empty gestational sacs. *Int J Gynaecol Obstet* 1994;46:297–301.
5. **Goldner TE, Lawson HW, Xia Z, et al.** Surveillance for ectopic pregnancy—United States, 1970–1989. *MMWR Morb Mortal Wkly Rep* CDC Surveillance Summary 1993;42(SS-6):73–85.
6. **National Center for Health Statistics.** *Annual summary of births, marriages, divorces and deaths: United States, 1989.* Hyattsville, MD: US Department of Health and Human Services, Public Health Service, 1990;38(13):23.
7. **Diquelou JY, Pia P, Tesquier L, et al.** The role of Chlamydia trachomatis in the infectious etiology of extra-uterine pregnancy. *J Gynecol Obstet Biol Reprod* (Paris) 1988;17:325–332.
8. **Chow WH, Daling JR, Cates W Jr, et al.** Epidemiology of ectopic pregnancy. *Epidemiol Rev* 1987;9:70–94.
9. **Levin AA, Schoenbaum SC, Stubblefield PG, et al.** Ectopic pregnancy and prior induced abortion. *Am J Public Health* 1982;72:253–256.
10. **Chi IC, Potts M, Wilkens L.** Rare events associated with tubal sterilizations: an international experience. *Obstet Gynecol Surv* 1986;41:7–19.
11. **Lavy G, Diamond MP, DeCherney AH.** Ectopic pregnancy: its relationship to tubal reconstructive surgery. *Fertil Steril* 1987;47:543–556.
12. **Cartwright PS, Entman SS.** Repeat ipsilateral tubal pregnancy following partial salpingectomy: a case report. *Fertil Steril* 1984;42:647–648.
13. **Richardson DA, Evans MI, Talerman A, et al.** Segmental absence of the mid-portion of the fallopian tube. *Fertil Steril* 1982;37:577–579.
14. **Wanerman J, Wulwick R, Brenner S.** Segmental absence of the fallopian tube. *Fertil Steril* 1986;46:525–527.

15. **Weinstein L, Morris MB, Dotters D, et al.** Ectopic pregnancy—a new surgical epidemic. *Obstet Gynecol* 1983;61:698–701.

16. **Pulkkinen MO, Talo A.** Tubal physiologic consideration in ectopic pregnancy. *Clin Obstet Gynecol* 1987;30:164–172.

17. **Persaud V.** Etiology of tubal ectopic pregnancy: radiologic and pathologic studies. *Obstet Gynecol* 1970;36:257–263.

18. **Elias S, LeBeau M, Simpson JL, et al.** Chromosome analysis of ectopic human conceptuses. *Am J Obstet Gynecol* 1981;141:698–703.

19. **Westrom L, Bengtsson LPH, Mardh P-A.** Incidence, trends, and risks of ectopic pregnancy in a population of women. *BMJ* 1981;282:15–18.

20. **Westrom L.** Influence of sexually transmitted diseases on sterility and ectopic pregnancy. *Acta Eur Fertil* 1985;16:21–24.

21. **Berenson A, Hammill H, Martens M, et al.** Bacteriologic findings with ectopic pregnancy. *J Reprod Med* 1991;36:118–120.

22. **Coste J, Job-Spira N, Fernandez H, et al.** Risk factors for ectopic pregnancy: a case-control study in France, with special focus on infectious factors. *Am J Epidemiol* 1991;133:839–849.

23. **Svensson L, Mardh P-A, Ahlgren M, et al.** Ectopic pregnancy and antibodies to Chlamydia trachomatis. *Fertil Steril* 1985;44:313–317.

24. **Brunham RC, Binns B, McDowell J, et al.** Chlamydia trachomatis infection in women with ectopic pregnancy. *Obstet Gynecol* 1986;67:722–726.

25. **Miettinen A, Heinonen PK, Teisala K, et al.** Serologic evidence for the role of Chlamydia trachomatis, Neisseria gonorrhoeae, and Mycoplasma hominis in the etiology of tubal factor infertility and ectopic pregnancy. *Sex Transm Dis* 1990;17:10–14.

26. **Chow JM, Yonekura ML, Richwald GA, et al.** The association between Chlamydia trachomatis and ectopic pregnancy: a matched-pair, case-control study. *JAMA* 1990;263:3164–3167.

27. **Ory HW.** The Women's Health Study. Ectopic pregnancy and intrauterine contraceptive devices: new perspectives. *Obstet Gynecol* 1981;57:137–144.

28. **The World Health Organization's Programme of Research, Development and Research Training in Human Reproduction: Task Force on Intrauterine Devices for Fertility Regulation.** A multinational case-control study of ectopic pregnancy. *Clin Reprod Fertil* 1985;3(2):131–143.

29. **Sivin I.** Dose- and age-dependent ectopic pregnancy risks with intrauterine contraception. *Obstet Gynecol* 1991;78:291–298.

30. **Vessey M, Meisler L, Flavel R, et al.** Outcome of pregnancy in women using different methods of contraception. *Br J Obstet Gynaecol* 1979;86:548–556.

31. **Chow WH, Daling JR, Weiss NS, et al.** IUD use and subsequent tubal ectopic pregnancy. *Am J Public Health* 1986;76:536–539.

32. **Wilson JC.** A prospective New Zealand study of fertility after removal of copper intrauterine contraceptive devices for conception and because of complications: a four-year study. *Am J Obstet Gynecol* 1989;160:391–396.

33. **Franks AL, Beral V, Cates W Jr, et al.** Contraception and ectopic pregnancy risk. *Am J Obstet Gynecol* 1990;163:1120–1123.

34. **Rantakyla P, Ylostalo P, Jarvinen PA, et al.** Ectopic pregnancies and the use of intrauterine device and low dose progestogen contraception. *Acta Obstet Gynecol Scand* 1977;56:61–62.

35. **Liukko P, Erkkola R, Laakso L.** Ectopic pregnancies during use of low-dose progestogens for oral contraception. *Contraception* 1977;16:575–580.

36. **Sivin I.** International experience with NORPLANT and NORPLANT-2 contraceptives. *Stud Fam Plann* 1988;19:81–94.

37. **Shoupe D, Mishell DR Jr, Bopp BL, et al.** The significance of bleeding patterns in Norplant implant users. *Obstet Gynecol* 1991;77:256–260.

38. **Trussell J, Kost K.** Contraceptive failure in the United States: a critical review of the literature. *Stud Fam Plann* 1987;18:237–283.

39. **Cheng MC, Wong YM, Rochat RW, et al.** Sterilization failures in Singapore: an examination of ligation techniques and failure rates. *Stud Fam Plann* 1977;8:109–115.

40. **DeStefano F, Peterson HB, Layde PM, et al.** Risk of ectopic pregnancy following tubal sterilization. *Obstet Gynecol* 1982;60:326–330.

41. **McCausland A.** High rate of ectopic pregnancy following laparoscopic tubal coagulation failures: incidence and etiology. *Am J Obstet Gynecol* 1980;136:97–101.

42. **Langer R, Bukovsky I, Herman A, et al.** Conservative surgery for tubal pregnancy. *Fertil Steril* 1982;38: 427–430.

43. **Lavy G, DeCherney AH.** The hormonal basis of ectopic pregnancy. *Clin Obstet Gynecol* 1987;30:217–224.

44. **DeCherney AH, Cholst I, Naftolin F.** Structure and function of the fallopian tubes following exposure to diethylstilbestrol (DES) during gestation. *Fertil Steril* 1981;36:741–745.

45. **Hallatt JG.** Tubal conservation in ectopic pregnancy: a study of 200 cases. *Am J Obstet Gynecol* 1986;154:1216–1221.

46. **Lennox CE, Mills JA, James GB.** Reversal of female sterilization: a comparative study. *Contraception* 1987;35:19–27.

47. **Hulka JF, Halme J.** Sterilization reversal: results of 101 attempts. *Am J Obstet Gynecol* 1988;159:767–774.

48. **Marchbanks PA, Annegers JF, Coulam CB, et al.** Risk factors for ectopic pregnancy: a population-based study. *JAMA* 1988;259:1823–1827.

49. **Ni H, Daling JR, Chu J, et al.** Previous abdominal surgery and tubal pregnancy. *Obstet Gynecol* 1990;75:919–922.

50. **Trimbos-Kemper T, Trimbos B, van Hall E.** Etiological factors in tubal infertility. *Fertil Steril* 1982;37:384–388.

51. **Weinstein D, Polishuk WZ.** The role of wedge resection of the ovary as a cause for mechanical sterility. *Surg Gynecol Obstet* 1975;141:417–418.

52. **Shoupe D, Mishell DR.** Norplant: subdermal implant system for long-term contraception. *Am J Obstet Gynecol* 1989;160:1286–1292.

53. **Burkman RT, Mason KJ, Gold EB.** Ectopic pregnancy and prior induced abortion. *Contraception* 1988;37:21–27.

54. **Kalandidi A, Doulgerakis M, Tzonou A, et al.** Induced abortions, contraceptive practices, and tobacco smoking as risk factors for ectopic pregnancy in Athens, Greece. *Br J Obstet Gynaecol* 1991;98:207–213.

55. **Marchbanks PA, Coulam CB, Annegers JF.** An association between clomiphene citrate and ectopic pregnancy: a preliminary report. *Fertil Steril* 1985;44:268–270.

56. **McBain JC, Evans JH, Pepperell RJ, et al.** An unexpectedly high rate of ectopic pregnancy following the induction of ovulation with human pituitary and chorionic gonadotropin. *Br J Obstet Gynaecol* 1980;87:5–9.

57. **Gemzell C, Guillome J, Wang CF.** Ectopic pregnancy following treatment with human gonadotropins. *Am J Obstet Gynecol* 1982;143:761–765.

58. **Oelsner G, Blankstein J, Menashe Y, et al.** The role of gonadotropins in the etiology of ectopic pregnancy. *Fertil Steril* 1989;52:514–516.

59. **Steptoe PC, Edwards RG.** Reimplantation of a human embryo with subsequent tubal pregnancy. *Lancet* 1976;1:880–882.

60. **Carson SL, Dickey RP, Gocial B, et al.** Outcome in 242 in vitro fertilization: embryo replacement or gamete intrafallopian transfer-induced pregnancies. *Fertil Steril* 1989;51:644–650.

61. **Herman A, Ron-El R, Golan A, et al.** The role of tubal pathology and other parameters in ectopic pregnancies occurring in in vitro fertilization and embryo transfer. *Fertil Steril* 1990;54:864–868.

62. **Dor J, Seidman DS, Levron D, et al.** The incidence of combined intrauterine and extrauterine pregnancy after in vitro fertilization and embryo transfer. *Fertil Steril* 1991;55:833–834.

63. **Dubuisson JB, Aubriot FX, Cardone V, et al.** Tubal causes of ectopic pregnancy. *Fertil Steril* 1986;46:970–972.

64. **Homm RJ, Holtz G, Garvin AJ.** Isthmic ectopic pregnancy and salpingitis isthmica nodosa. *Fertil Steril* 1987;48:756–760.

65. **Barnes AB, Colton T, Gundersen J, et al.** Fertility and outcome of pregnancy in women exposed in utero to diethylstilbestrol. *N Engl J Med* 1980;302:609–613.

66. **Herbst AL, Hubby MM, Blough RR, et al.** A comparison of pregnancy experience in DES-exposed and DES-unexposed daughters. *J Reprod Med* 1980;24:62–69.

67. **Kullander S, Kaellen B.** A prospective study of smoking and pregnancy. *Acta Obstet Gynecol Scand* 1971;50:83–94.

68. **Coste J, Job-Spira N, Fernandez H.** Increased risk of ectopic pregnancy with maternal cigarette smoking. *Am J Public Health* 1991;81:199–201.

69. **Handler A, Davis F, Ferre C, et al.** The relationship of smoking and ectopic pregnancy. *Am J Public Health* 1989;79:1239–1242.

70. **Niles JH, Clark JFJ.** Pathogenesis of tubal pregnancy. *Am J Obstet Gynecol* 1969;105:1230–1234.

71. **Westrom L.** Effect of acute pelvic inflammatory disease on fertility. *Am J Obstet Gynecol* 1975;121:707–713.

72. **Benjamin CL, Beaver DC.** Pathogenesis of salpingitis isthmica nodosa. *Am J Clin Pathol* 1951;21:212–222.

73. **Wrork DH, Broders AC.** Adenomyosis of the fallopian tube. *Am J Obstet Gynecol* 1942;44:412–432.

74. **Kurman RJ, Main CS, Chen HC.** Intermediate trophoblast: a distinctive form of trophoblast with specific morphological, biochemical, and functional features. *Placenta* 1984;5:349–369.

75. **Stabile I, Grudzinskas JG.** Ectopic pregnancy: a review of incidence, etiology, and diagnostic aspects. *Obstet Gynecol Surv* 1990;45:335–347.

76. **Tuomivaara L, Kauppila A, Puolakka J.** Ectopic pregnancy—an analysis of the etiology, diagnosis and treatment in 552 cases. *Arch Gynecol* 1986;237:135–147.

77. **Storring PL, Gaines-Das RE, Bangham DR.** International reference preparation of human chorionic gonadotrophin for immunoassay: potency estimates in various bioassays and protein binding assay systems; and international reference preparations of the alpha and beta subunits of human chorionic gonadotrophin for immunoassay. *J Endocrinol* 1980;84:295–310.

78. **Cole LA.** Phantom hCG and phantom choriocarcinoma. *Gynecol Oncol* 1998;71:325–329.

79. **Rotmensch S, Cole LA.** False diagnosis and needless therapy of presumed malignant disease in women with false-positive human chorionic gonadotropic concentration. *Lancet* 2000;35:712–715.

80. **Marshall JR, Hammond CB, Ross GT, et al.** Plasma and urinary chorionic gonadotropin during early human pregnancy. *Obstet Gynecol* 1968;32:760–764.

81. **Daus K, Mundy D, Graves W, et al.** Ectopic pregnancy: what to do during the 20-day window. *J Reprod Med* 1989;34:162–166.

82. **Kadar N, Caldwell BV, Romero R.** A method of screening for ectopic pregnancy and its indications. *Obstet Gynecol* 1981;58:162–165.

83. **Cartwright PS, Moore RA, Dao AH, et al.** Serum beta-human chorionic gonadotropin levels relate poorly with the size of a tubal pregnancy. *Fertil Steril* 1987;48:679–680.

84. **Pearlstone AC, Oei ML, Wu TCJ.** The predictive value of a single, early human chorionic gonadotropin measurement and the influence of maternal age on pregnancy outcome in an infertile population. *Fertil Steril* 1992;57:302–304.

85. **Milwidsky A, Adoni A, Segal S, et al.** Chorionic gonadotropin and progesterone levels in ectopic pregnancy. *Obstet Gynecol* 1977;50:145–147.

86. **Radwanska E, Frankenberg J, Allen EI.** Plasma progesterone levels in normal and abnormal early human pregnancy. *Fertil Steril* 1978;30:398–402.

87. **Stovall TG, Ling FW, Andersen RN, et al.** Improved sensitivity and specificity of a single measurement of serum progesterone over serial quantitative beta-human chorionic gonadotrophin in screening for ectopic pregnancy. *Hum Reprod* 1992;7:723–725.

88. **Stovall TG, Ling FW, Cope BJ, et al.** Preventing ruptured ectopic pregnancy with a single serum progesterone. *Am J Obstet Gynecol* 1989;160:1425–1431.

89. **Stovall TG, Kellerman AL, Ling FW, et al.** Emergency department diagnosis of ectopic pregnancy. *Ann Emerg Med* 1990;19:1098–1103.

90. **Cowan BD, Vandermolen DT, Long CA, et al.** Receiver operator characteristics, efficiency analysis, and predictive value of serum progesterone concentration as a test for abnormal gestations. *Am J Obstet Gynecol* 1992;166:1729–1734.

91. **Barnes ER, Oelsner G, Benveniste R, et al.** Progesterone, estradiol, and alpha-human chorionic gonadotropin secretion in patients with ectopic pregnancy. *J Clin Endocrinol Metab* 1986;62:529–531.

92. **Witt BR, Wolf GC, Wainwright CJ, et al.** Relaxin, CA125, progesterone, estradiol, Schwangerschaft protein, and human chorionic gonadotropin as predictors of outcome in threatened and non-threatened pregnancies. *Fertil Steril* 1990;53:1029–1036.

93. **Guillaume J, Benjamin F, Sicuranza BJ, et al.** Serum estradiol as an aid in the diagnosis of ectopic pregnancy. *Obstet Gynecol* 1990;76:1126–1129.

94. **Lavie O, Beller U, Neuman M, et al.** Maternal serum creatine kinase: a possible predictor of tubal pregnancy. *Am J Obstet Gynecol* 1993;169:1149–1150.

95. **Ho PC, Chan SYW, Tang GWK.** Diagnosis of early pregnancy by enzyme immunoassay of Schwangerschafts-protein 1. *Fertil Steril* 1988;49:76–80.

96. **Bell RJ, Eddie LW, Lester AR, et al.** Relaxin in human pregnancy serum measured with an homologous radioimmunoassay. *Obstet Gynecol* 1987;69:585–589.

97. **Meunier K, Mignot TM, Maria B, et al.** Predictive value of the active renin assay for the diagnosis of ectopic pregnancy. *Fertil Steril* 1991;55:432–435.

98. **Niloff JM, Knapp RC, Schaetzl E, et al.** CA125 antigen levels in obstetric and gynecologic patients. *Obstet Gynecol* 1984;64:703–707.

99. **Kobayashi F, Sagawa N, Nakamura K, et al.** Mechanism and clinical significance of elevated CA125 levels in the sera of pregnant women. *Am J Obstet Gynecol* 1989;160:563–566.

100. **Check JH, Nowroozi K, Winkel CA, et al.** Serum CA125 levels in early pregnancy and subsequent spontaneous abortion. *Obstet Gynecol* 1990;75:742–744.

101. **Brumsted JR, Nakajima ST, Badger G, et al.** Serum concentration of CA125 during the first trimester of normal and abnormal pregnancies. *J Reprod Med* 1990;35:499–502.

102. **Sadovsky Y, Pineda J, Collins JL.** Serum CA125 levels in women with ectopic and intrauterine pregnancies. *J Reprod Med* 1991;36:875–878.

103. **Cederqvist LL, Killackey MA, Abdel-Latif N, et al.** Alpha-fetoprotein and ectopic pregnancy. *BMJ* 1983;286:1247–1248.

104. **Grosskinsky CM, Hage ML, Tyrey L, et al.** hCG, progesterone, alpha-fetoprotein, and estradiol in the identification of ectopic pregnancy. *Obstet Gynecol* 1993;81:705–709.

105. **Theron GB, Shepherd EGS, Strachan AF.** C-reactive protein levels in ectopic pregnancy, pelvic infection and carcinoma of the cervix. *S Afr Med J* 1986;69:681–682.

106. **Cacciatore B.** Can the status of tubal pregnancy be predicted with transvaginal sonography? A prospective comparison of sonographic, surgical, and serum hCG findings. *Radiology* 1990;177:481–484.

107. **Thorsen MK, Lawson TL, Aiman EJ, et al.** Diagnosis of ectopic pregnancy: endovaginal vs transabdominal sonography. *Am J Roentgenol* 1990;155:307–310.

108. **Bateman BG, Nunley WC Jr, Kolp LA, et al.** Vaginal sonography findings and hCG dynamics of early intrauterine and tubal pregnancies. *Obstet Gynecol* 1990;75:421–427.

109. **Cacciatore B, Stenman UH, Ylostalo P.** Comparison of abdominal and vaginal sonography in suspected ectopic pregnancy. *Obstet Gynecol* 1989;73:770–774.

110. **Fleischer AC, Pennell RG, McKee MS, et al.** Ectopic pregnancy: features at transvaginal sonography. *Radiology* 1990;174:375–378.

111. **Timor-Tritsch IE, Yeh MN, Peisner DB, et al.** The use of transvaginal ultrasonography in the diagnosis of ectopic pregnancy. *Am J Obstet Gynecol* 1989;161:157–161.

112. **Bree RL, Marn CS.** Transvaginal sonography in the first trimester: embryology, anatomy, and hCG correlation. *Semin Ultrasound CT MRI* 1990;11:12–21.

113. **Cacciatore B, Ylostalo P, Stenman UH, et al.** Suspected ectopic pregnancy: ultrasound findings and hCG levels assessed by an immunofluorometric assay. *Br J Obstet Gynaecol* 1988;95:497–502.

114. **Abramovici H, Auslender R, Lewin A, et al.** Gestational-pseudogestational sac: a new ultrasonic criterion for differential diagnosis. *Am J Obstet Gynecol* 1983;145:377–379.

115. **Nyberg DA, Filly RA, Laing FC, et al.** Ectopic pregnancy, diagnosis by sonography correlated with quantitative HCG levels. *J Ultrasound Med* 1987;6:145–150.

116. **Bradley WG, Fiske CE, Filly RA.** The double sac sign of early intrauterine pregnancy: use in exclusion of ectopic pregnancy. *Radiology* 1982;143:223–226.

117. **Nyberg DA, Mack LA, Harvey D, et al.** Value of the yolk sac in evaluating early pregnancies. *J Ultrasound Med* 1988;7:129–135.

118. **Jain KA, Hamper UM, Sanders RC.** Comparison of transvaginal and transabdominal sonography in the detection of early pregnancy and its complications. *AJR Am J Roentgenol* 1988;151:1139–1143.

119. **Bree RL, Edwards M, Bohm VM, et al.** Transvaginal sonography in the evaluation of normal early pregnancy: correlation with HCG level. *Am J Roentgenol* 1989;53:75–79.

120. **Nyberg DA, Hughes MP, Mack LA, et al.** Extrauterine findings of ectopic pregnancy at transvaginal US: importance of echogenic fluid. *Radiology* 1991;178:823–826.

121. **Rottem S, Thaler I, Levron J, et al.** Criteria for transvaginal sonographic diagnosis of ectopic pregnancy. *J Clin Ultrasound* 1990;18:274–279.

122. **Nyberg DA, Mack LA, Laing FC, et al.** Early pregnancy complications: endovaginal sonographic findings correlated with human chorionic gonadotropin levels. *Radiology* 1988;167:619–622.

123. **Emerson DS, Cartier MS, Altieri LA, et al.** Diagnostic efficacy of endovaginal color Doppler flow imaging in an ectopic pregnancy screening program. *Radiology* 1992;183:413–420.

124. **Bernaschek G, Rudelstorfer R, Csaicsich P.** Vaginal sonography versus serum human chorionic gonadotropin in early detection of pregnancy. *Am J Obstet Gynecol* 1988;158:608–612.

125. **Diamond MP, DeCherney AH.** *Ectopic pregnancy.* Philadelphia: WB Saunders, 1991:163.

126. **Menard A, Crequat J, Mandelbrot L, et al.** Treatment of unruptured tubal pregnancy by local injection of methotrexate under transvaginal sonographic control. *Fertil Steril* 1990;54:47–50.

127. **Campbell S, Pearce JM, Hackett G, et al.** Qualitative assessment of uteroplacental blood flow: early screening test for high-risk pregnancies. *Obstet Gynecol* 1986;68:649–653.

128. **McCowan LM, Ritchie K, Mo LY, et al.** Uterine artery flow velocity waveforms in normal and growth-retarded pregnancies. *Am J Obstet Gynecol* 1988;158:499–504.

129. **Taylor KJ, Ramos IM, Feyock AL, et al.** Ectopic pregnancy: duplex Doppler evaluation. *Radiology* 1989;173:93–97.

130. **Dillon EH, Feyock AL, Taylor KJW.** Pseudogestational sacs: Doppler US differentiation from normal or abnormal intrauterine pregnancies. *Radiology* 1990;176:359–364.

131. **Vermesh M, Graczykowski JW, Sauer MV.** Reevaluation of the role of culdocentesis in the management of ectopic pregnancy. *Am J Obstet Gynecol* 1990;162:411–413.

132. **Stovall TG, Ling FW, Carson SA, et al.** Serum progesterone and uterine curettage in the differential diagnosis of ectopic pregnancy. *Fertil Steril* 1992;57:456–458.

133. **Stovall TG, Ling FW.** Ectopic pregnancy: diagnostic and therapeutic algorithms minimizing surgical intervention. *J Reprod Med* 1993;38:807–812.

134. **Jeffcoate TN.** Salpingectomy or salpingo-oophorectomy. *J Obstet Gynaecol Br Emp* 1955;62:214–215.

135. **Schenker JG, Eyal F, Polishuk WZ.** Fertility after tubal surgery. *Surg Gynecol Obstet* 1972;135:74–76.

136. **Ory SJ, Nnadi E, Herrmann R, et al.** Fertility after ectopic pregnancy. *Fertil Steril* 1993;60:231–235.

137. **Timonen S, Nieminen U.** Tubal pregnancy: choice of operative methods of treatment. *Acta Obstet Gynecol Scand* 1967;46:327–339.

138. **Smith HO, Toledo AA, Thompson JD.** Conservative surgical management of isthmic ectopic pregnancies. *Am J Obstet Gynecol* 1987;157:604–610.

139. **Hill GA, Segars JH Jr, Herbert CM III.** Laparoscopic management of interstitial pregnancy. *J Gynecol Surg* 1989;5:209–212.

140. **Brumsted J, Kessler C, Gibson C, et al.** A comparison of laparoscopy and laparotomy for the treatment of ectopic pregnancy. *Obstet Gynecol* 1988;71:889–892.

141. **Vermesh M, Silva PD, Rosen GF, et al.** Management of unruptured ectopic gestation by linear salpingostomy: a prospective, randomized clinical trial of laparoscopy versus laparotomy. *Obstet Gynecol* 1989;73:400–404.

142. **Murphy AA, Nager CW, Wujek JJ, et al.** Operative laparoscopy versus laparotomy for the management of ectopic pregnancy: a prospective trial. *Fertil Steril* 1992;57:1180–1185.

143. **Lundorff P, Hahlin M, Kallfelt B, et al.** Adhesion formation after laparoscopic surgery in tubal pregnancy: a randomized trial versus laparotomy. *Fertil Steril* 1991;55:911–915.

144. **Silva PD, Schaper AM, Rooney B.** Reproductive outcome after 143 laparoscopic procedures for ectopic pregnancy. *Obstet Gynecol* 1993;81:710–715.

145. **Langer R, Raziel A, Ron-El R, et al.** Reproductive outcome after conservative surgery for unruptured tubal pregnancies—a 15-year experience. *Fertil Steril* 1990;53:227–231.

146. **Berkowitz RS, Goldstein DP, Jones MA, et al.** Methotrexate with citrovorum factor rescue: reduced chemotherapy toxicity in the management of gestational trophoblastic neoplasms. *Cancer* 1980;45:423–426.

147. **Rustin GJS, Rustin F, Dent J, et al.** No increase in second tumors after cytotoxic chemotherapy for gestational trophoblastic tumors. *N Engl J Med* 1983;308:473–476.

148. **St. Clair JT, Whealer DA, Fish SA.** Methotrexate in abdominal pregnancy. *JAMA* 1969;208:529–531.

149. **Tanaka T, Hayashi H, Kutsuzawa T, et al.** Treatment of interstitial ectopic pregnancy with methotrexate: report of a successful case. *Fertil Steril* 1982;37:851–852.

150. **Ory SJ, Villanueva AL, Sand PK, et al.** Conservative treatment of ectopic pregnancy with methotrexate. *Am J Obstet Gynecol* 1986;154:1299–1306.

151. **Ichinoe K, Wake N, Shinkai N, et al.** Nonsurgical therapy to preserve oviduct function in patients with tubal pregnancies. *Am J Obstet Gynecol* 1987;156:484–487.

152. **Sauer MV, Gorrill MJ, Rodi IA, et al.** Nonsurgical management of unruptured ectopic pregnancy: an extended clinical trial. *Fertil Steril* 1987;48:752–755.

153. **Stovall TG, Ling FW, Buster JE.** Outpatient chemotherapy of unruptured ectopic pregnancy. *Fertil Steril* 1989;51:435–438.

154. **Stovall TG, Ling FW, Gray LA, et al.** Methotrexate treatment of unruptured ectopic pregnancy: a report of 100 cases. *Obstet Gynecol* 1991;77:749–753.

155. **Stovall TG, Ling FW, Gray LA.** Single-dose methotrexate for treatment of ectopic pregnancy. *Obstet Gynecol* 1991;77:754–757.

156. **Stovall TG, Ling FW.** Single-dose methotrexate: an expanded clinical trial. *Am J Obstet Gynecol* 1993;170:1840–1841.

157. **Hoppe D, Bekkar BE, Nager CW.** Single-dose system methotrexate for the treatment of persistent ectopic pregnancy after conservative surgery. *Obstet Gynecol* 1994;83:51–54.

158. **Schafer D, Kryss J, Pfuhl JP, et al.** Systemic treatment of ectopic pregnancy with single-dose methotrexate. *J Am Assoc Gynecol Laparosc* 1994;1:213–218.

159. **Henry MA, Gentry WL.** Single injection of methotrexate for treatment of ectopic pregnancies. *Am J Obstet Gynecol* 1994;171:1584–1587.

160. **Brown DL, Felker RE, Stovall TG, et al.** Serial endovaginal sonography of ectopic pregnancies treated with methotrexate. *Obstet Gynecol* 1991;77:406–409.

161. **Lipscomb GH, McCord ML, Stovall TG, et al.** Predictors of success of methotrexate treatment in women with tubal ectopic pregnancies. *N Engl J Med* 1999;341:1974–1978.

162. **Kooi S, Kick HCLV.** Treatment of tubal pregnancy by local injection of methotrexate after adrenaline injection into the mesosalpinx: a report of 25 patients. *Fertil Steril* 1990;54:580–584.

163. **Stovall TG, Ling FW, Buster JE.** Reproductive performance after methotrexate treatment of ectopic pregnancy. *Am J Obstet Gynecol* 1990;162:1620–1624.

164. **Vermesh M.** Conservative management of ectopic gestation. *Fertil Steril* 1990;53:382–387.

165. **Menard A, Crequat J, Mandelbrot L, et al.** Treatment of unruptured tubal pregnancy by local injection of methotrexate under transvaginal sonographic control. *Fertil Steril* 1990;54:47–50.

166. **Shalev E, Peleg D, Bustan M, et al.** Limited role for intratubal methotrexate treatment of ectopic pregnancy. *Fertil Steril* 1995;63:20–24.

167. **Tulandi T, Atri M, Bret P, et al.** Transvaginal intratubal methotrexate treatment of ectopic pregnancy. *Fertil Steril* 1992;58:98–100.

168. **Fernandez H, Benifla JL, Lelaidier C, et al.** Methotrexate treatment of ectopic pregnancy: 100 cases treated by primary transvaginal injection under sonographic control. *Fertil Steril* 1993;59:773–777.

169. **Fernandez H, Pauthier S, Daimerc S, et al.** Ultrasound-guided injection of methotrexate versus laparoscopic salpingotomy in ectopic pregnancy. *Fertil Steril* 1995;63:25–29.

170. **Oelsner G, Admon D, Shalev E, et al.** A new approach for the treatment of interstitial pregnancy. *Fertil Steril* 1993;59:924–925.

171. **Aboulghar MA, Mansour RT, Serour GI.** Transvaginal injection of potassium chloride and methotrexate for the treatment of tubal pregnancy with a live fetus. *Hum Reprod* 1990;5:887–888.

172. **Feichtinger W, Kemeter P.** Treatment of unruptured ectopic pregnancy by needling of sac and injection of methotrexate or PGE_2 under transvaginal sonography control. *Arch Gynecol Obstet* 1989;246:85–89.

173. **Hagstrom HG, Hahlin M, Sjöblom P, et al.** Prediction of persistent trophoblastic activity after local prostaglandin F_{2a} injection for ectopic pregnancy. *Hum Reprod* 1994;9:1170–1174.

174. **Laatikainen T, Tuomivaara L, Kauppila K.** Comparison of a local injection of hyperosmolar glucose solution with salpingostomy for the conservative treatment of tubal pregnancy. *Fertil Steril* 1993;60:80–84.

175. **Kojima E, Abe Y, Morita M, et al.** The treatment of unruptured tubal pregnancy with intratubal methotrexate injection under laparoscopic control. *Obstet Gynecol* 1990;75:723–725.

176. **Kenigsberg D, Porte J, Hull M, et al.** Medical treatment of residual ectopic pregnancy: RU 486 and methotrexate. *Fertil Steril* 1987;47:702–703.

177. **Frydman R, Fernandez H, Troalen F, et al.** Phase I clinical trial of monoclonal anti-human chorionic gonadotropin antibody in women with an ectopic pregnancy. *Fertil Steril* 1989;52:734–738.

178. **Garcia AJ, Aubert JM, Sama J, et al.** Expectant management of presumed ectopic pregnancies. *Fertil Steril* 1987;48:395–400.

179. **Carson SA, Stovall TG, Ling FW, et al.** Low human chorionic somatomammotropin fails to predict spontaneous resolution of unruptured ectopic pregnancies. *Fertil Steril* 1991;55:629–630.

180. **Fernandez H, Rainhorn JD, Papiernik E, et al.** Spontaneous resolution of ectopic pregnancy. *Obstet Gynecol* 1988;71:171–174.

181. **Gretz E, Quagliarello J.** Declining serum concentrations of the beta-subunit of human chorionic gonadotropin and ruptured ectopic pregnancy. *Am J Obstet Gynecol* 1987;156:940–941.

182. **Makinen JI, Kivijarvi AK, Irjala KMA.** Success of non-surgical management of ectopic pregnancy. *Lancet* 1990;335:1099.

183. **Seifer DB, Gutmann JN, Doyle MB, et al.** Persistent ectopic pregnancy following laparoscopic linear salpingostomy. *Obstet Gynecol* 1990;76:1121–1125.

184. **Pouly JL, Mahnes H, Mage G, et al.** Conservative laparoscopic treatment of 321 ectopic pregnancies. *Fertil Steril* 1986;46:1093–1097.

185. **Seifer DB, Gutmann JN, Grant WD, et al.** Comparison of persistent ectopic pregnancy after laparoscopic salpingostomy versus salpingostomy at laparotomy for ectopic pregnancy. *Obstet Gynecol* 1993;81:378–382.

186. **Vermesh M, Silva PD, Sauer MV, et al.** Persistent tubal ectopic gestation: patterns of circulating beta-human chorionic gonadotropin and progesterone, and management options. *Fertil Steril* 1988;50:584–588.

187. **Lundorff P, Hahlin M, Sjoblom P, et al.** Persistent trophoblast after conservative treatment of tubal pregnancy: prediction and detection. *Obstet Gynecol* 1991;77:129–133.

188. **Cartwright PS.** Peritoneal trophoblastic implants after surgical management of tubal pregnancy. *J Reprod Med* 1991;36:523–524.

189. **Foulot H, Chapron C, Morice PH, et al.** Failure of laparoscopic treatment for peritoneal trophoblastic implants. *Hum Reprod* 1994;9:92–93.

190. **Higgins KA, Schwartz MB.** Treatment of persistent trophoblastic tissue after salpingostomy with methotrexate. *Fertil Steril* 1986;45:427–428.

191. **Rose PG, Cohen SM.** Methotrexate therapy for persistent ectopic pregnancy after conservative laparoscopic management. *Obstet Gynecol* 1990;76:947–949.

192. **Bengtsson G, Bryman I, Thorburn J, et al.** Low-dose oral methotrexate as second-line therapy for persistent trophoblast after conservative treatment of ectopic pregnancy. *Obstet Gynecol* 1992;79:589–591.

193. **Cole T, Corlett RC Jr.** Chronic ectopic pregnancy. *Obstet Gynecol* 1982;59:63–68.

194. **Rogers WF, Shaub M, Wilson R.** Chronic ectopic pregnancy: ultrasonic diagnosis. *J Clin Ultrasound* 1977;5:257–260.

195. **Parente JT, Ou CS, Levy J, et al.** Cervical pregnancy analysis: a review and report of five cases. *Obstet Gynecol* 1983;62:79–82.

196. **Weyerman PC, Verhoeven ATM, Alberda AT.** Cervical pregnancy after in vitro fertilization and embryo transfer. *Am J Obstet Gynecol* 1989;161:1145–1164.

197. **Hofmann HMH, Urdl W, Hofler H, et al.** Cervical pregnancy: case reports and current concepts in diagnosis and treatment. *Arch Gynecol Obstet* 1987;241:63–69.

198. **Bader-Armstrong B, Shah Y, Rubens D.** Use of ultrasound and magnetic resonance imaging in the diagnosis of cervical pregnancy. *J Clin Ultrasound* 1989;17:283–286.

199. **Stovall TG, Ling FW, Smith WC, et al.** Successful nonsurgical treatment of cervical pregnancy with methotrexate. *Fertil Steril* 1988;50:672–674.

200. **Oyer R, Tarakjian D, Lev-Toaff A, et al.** Treatment of cervical pregnancy with methotrexate. *Obstet Gynecol* 1988;71:469–471.

201. **Bernstein D, Holzinger M, Ovadia J, et al.** Conservative treatment of cervical pregnancy. *Obstet Gynecol* 1981;58:741–742.

202. **Wharton KR, Gore B.** Cervical pregnancy managed by placement of a Shirodkar cerclage before evacuation: a case report. *J Reprod Med* 1988;33:227–229.

203. **Nolan TE, Chandler PE, Hess LW, et al.** Cervical pregnancy managed without hysterectomy: a case report. *J Reprod Med* 1989;34:241–243.

204. **Hallatt JG.** Primary ovarian pregnancy: a report of twenty-five cases. *Am J Obstet Gynecol* 1982;143:55–60.

205. **Grimes HG, Nosal RA, Gallagher JC.** Ovarian pregnancy: a series of 24 cases. *Obstet Gynecol* 1983;61:174–180.

206. **Malinger G, Achiron R, Treschan O, et al.** Case report: ovarian pregnancy-ultrasonographic diagnosis. *Acta Obstet Gynecol Scand* 1988;67:561–563.

207. **DeVries K, Atad J, Arodi J, et al.** Primary ovarian pregnancy: a conservative surgical approach by wedge resection. *Int J Fertil* 1981;26:293–294.

208. **Van Coevering RJ, Fisher JE.** Laparoscopic management of ovarian pregnancy: a case report. *J Reprod Med* 1988;33:774–776.

209. **Russell JB, Cutler LR.** Transvaginal ultrasonographic detection of primary ovarian pregnancy with laparoscopic removal: a case report. *Fertil Steril* 1989;51:1055–1056.

210. **Koike H, Chuganji Y, Watanabe H, et al.** Conservative treatment of ovarian pregnancy by local prostaglandin F_{2a} injection [Letter]. *Am J Obstet Gynecol* 1990;163:696.

211. **Atrash HK, Friede A, Hogue CJR.** Abdominal pregnancy in the United States: frequency and maternal mortality. *Obstet Gynecol* 1987;69:333–337.

212. **Rahman MS, Al-Suleiman SA, Rahman J, et al.** Advanced abdominal pregnancy-observations in 10 cases. *Obstet Gynecol* 1982;59:366–372.

213. **Stanley JH, Horger EO III, Fagan CJ, et al.** Sonographic findings in abdominal pregnancy. *AJR Am J Roentgenol* 1986;147:1043–1046.

214. Harris MB, Angtuaco T, Frazer CN, et al. Diagnosis of a viable abdominal pregnancy by magnetic resonance imaging. *Am J Obstet Gynecol* 1988;159:150–151.

215. Martin JN Jr, Ridgway LE III, Connors JJ, et al. Angiographic arterial embolization and computed tomography-directed drainage for the management of hemorrhage and infection with abdominal pregnancy. *Obstet Gynecol* 1990;76:941–945.

216. Martin JN Jr, Sessums JK, Martin RW, et al. Abdominal pregnancy: current concepts of management. *Obstet Gynecol* 1988;71:549–557.

217. Pasic R, Wolfe WM. Laparoscopic diagnosis and treatment of interstitial ectopic pregnancy: a case report. *Am J Obstet Gynecol* 1990;163:587–588.

218. Vierhout ME, Wallenburg HCS. Intraligamentary pregnancy resulting in a live infant. *Am J Obstet Gynecol* 1985;152:878–879.

219. Reece EA, Petrie RH, Sirmans MF, et al. Combined intrauterine and extrauterine gestations: a review. *Am J Obstet Gynecol* 1983;146:323–330.

220. Olsen ME. Bilateral twin ectopic gestations with intraligamentous and interstitial components: a case report. *J Reprod Med* 1994;39:118–120.

221. Adair CD, Benrubi GI, Sanchez-Ramos L, et al. Bilateral tubal ectopic pregnancies after bilateral partial salpingectomy: a case report. *J Reprod Med* 1994;39:131–133.

222. Goffner L, Bluth MJ, Fruauff A, et al. Ectopic gestation associated with intrauterine triplet pregnancy after in vitro fertilization. *J Ultrasound Med* 1993;12:63–64.

223. Jackson P, Barrowclough IW, France JT, et al. A successful pregnancy following total hysterectomy. *Br J Obstet Gynaecol* 1980;87:353–355.

224. Nehra PC, Loginsky SJ. Pregnancy after vaginal hysterectomy. *Obstet Gynecol* 1984;64:735–737.

18 Benign Breast Disease

Baiba J. Grube
Armando E. Giuliano

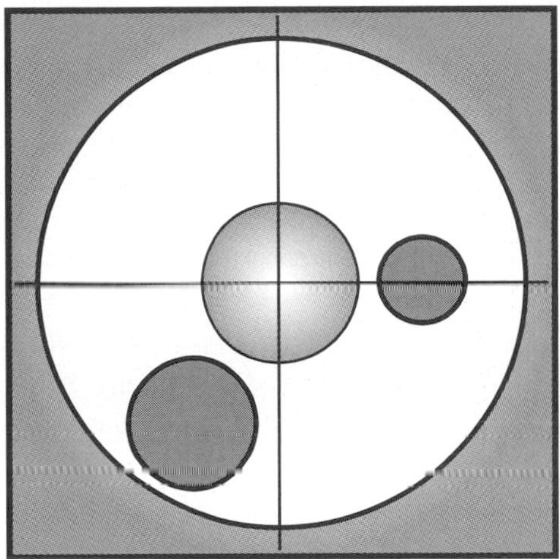

Diagnosis and management of common benign breast conditions, particularly those that mimic malignancy, and an appreciation of treatment options are essential for the practicing gynecologist (1). Benign breast disease is a complex entity of its own with a range of physiologic changes and clinical manifestations that have an impact on a woman's health independent of breast cancer risk (2).

Detection

History

Evaluation of a new breast complaint begins with symptom assessment by a thorough clinical history (3). The history should include questions regarding current symptoms, duration of the condition, fluctuation of the signs and symptoms, and factors that aggravate or relieve the complaint. Specific questions should address the following points:

Nipple discharge
Characteristics of discharge (appearance, spontaneous or nonspontaneous, unilateral or bilateral, single or multiple duct involvement)
Breast mass (size and change in size, density, or texture)
Breast pain (cyclic versus continuous)
Association of symptoms with menstrual cycle
Change in breast shape, size, or texture
Previous breast biopsies.

The patient should be questioned about risk factors:

Age of menarche
Age of first pregnancy
Age of menopause
Family history of breast cancer
Number of first-degree relatives with breast cancer and their ages when diagnosed
Other malignancies (ovary, colon, and prostate)
Pathology of previous breast biopsy.

It is important to obtain a thorough list of medications taken, including hormone therapy and herbal medications such as phytoestrogens. The gestational history should take into consideration the possibility of a current pregnancy. A personal history of exposure to radiation, especially in the treatment of childhood malignancies, is associated with a higher incidence of developing breast cancer (4). The goal of breast evaluation is to determine clearly if the complaint represents a benign breast condition or is suggestive of a neoplastic process.

Physical Examination

Breast tumors, particularly cancerous ones, usually are asymptomatic and are discovered only by physical examination or screening mammography. Typically, the breast changes slightly during the menstrual cycle. During the premenstrual phase, most women have increased innocuous nodularity and mild engorgement of the breast. Rarely, this can obscure an underlying lesion and make examination difficult. Findings should be carefully documented in the medical record to serve as a baseline for future reference.

Inspection

Inspection is done initially while the patient is seated comfortably with her arms relaxed at her sides. The breasts are compared for symmetry, contour, and skin appearance. Edema or erythema is identified easily, and skin dimpling or nipple retraction is shown by having the patient raise her arms above her head and then press her hands on her hips, thereby contracting the pectoralis muscles (Fig. 18.1). Palpable and even nonpalpable tumors that distort Cooper's ligaments may lead to skin dimpling with these maneuvers.

Palpation

While the patient is seated, each breast should be palpated methodically. Some physicians recommend palpating the breast in long strips, but the exact palpation technique used is probably not as important as the thoroughness of its application over the entire breast. One very effective method is to palpate the breast in enlarging concentric circles until the entire breast has been covered. A pendulous breast can be palpated by placing one hand between the breast and the chest wall and gently palpating the breast between both examining hands. The axillary and supraclavicular areas should be palpated for enlarged lymph nodes. The entire axilla, the upper outer quadrant of the breast, and the axillary tail of Spence are palpated for possible masses.

While the patient is supine with one arm over her head, the ipsilateral breast is again methodically palpated from the clavicle to the costal margin. If the breast is large, a pillow or towel should be placed beneath the scapula to elevate the side being examined; otherwise the breast tends to fall to the side, making palpation of the lateral hemisphere more difficult.

The major features to be identified on palpation of the breast are temperature, texture and thickness of skin, generalized or focal tenderness, nodularity, density, asymmetry, dominant masses, and nipple discharge. Most premenopausal patients have normally nodular breast parenchyma. The nodularity is diffuse but predominantly in the upper outer quadrants where there is more breast tissue. These benign parenchymal nodules are small, similar in size, and indistinct. By comparison, breast cancer is usually a nontender, firm mass with irregular margins. This mass feels distinctly different from the surrounding nodularity. A malignant mass may be fixed to the skin or to the underlying fascia. A suspicious mass is usually unilateral. Similar findings in both breasts are unlikely to represent malignant disease (5).

Breast Self-examination

Breast self-examination (BSE) increases early detection of cancer and may improve the survival of patients with breast carcinoma (6–8). In fact, most breast cancers are detected first by the patient rather than by the physician. Although young women have a low incidence of breast cancer, it is important to teach self-examination early so that it becomes habitual. Organizations such as the American Cancer Society sponsor courses in BSE. Reassurance,

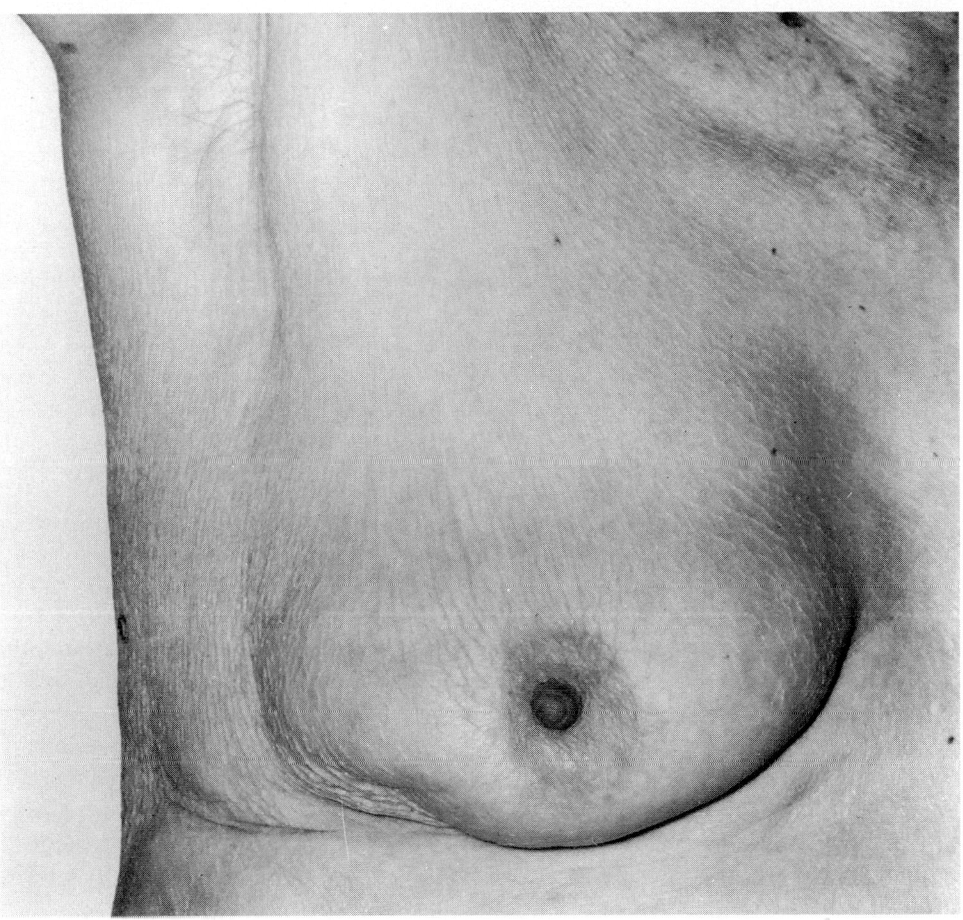

Figure 18.1 Raising the arm reveals retraction of the skin of the lower outer quadrant caused by a small palpable carcinoma. (From **Giuliano AE.** Breast disease. In: **Berek JS, Hacker NF,** eds. *Practical gynecologic oncology,* 3rd ed. Baltimore: Lippincott Williams & Wilkins, 2000:640, with permission.)

support, and patient education may encourage women to overcome psychological barriers to routine BSE (9). One study evaluated three different methods of instruction to determine compliance with BSE (10). The first arm evaluated the impact of physician message alone, the second arm assessed physician message in conjunction with a BSE class, and the third arm added follow-up reinforcement by phone or postcard to physician message and BSE class. The third produced the highest percentage of women doing BSE and is the ideal method of engaging patients to perform BSE.

The woman should inspect her breasts while standing or sitting before a mirror, looking for any asymmetry, skin dimpling, or nipple retraction. Elevating her arms over her head or pressing her hands against her hips to contract the pectoralis muscles will highlight any skin dimpling. While standing or sitting, she should carefully palpate her breasts with the fingers of the opposite hand. This may be performed while showering, because soap and water may increase the sensitivity of palpation. Finally, she should lie down and again palpate each quadrant of the breast, as well as the axilla.

Premenopausal women should examine their breasts monthly during the week after menses. It is helpful for all women to examine their breasts at the same time each month to develop a routine. All women should be instructed to report any abnormalities or changes to their physicians. If the physician cannot confirm the patient's findings, the examination should be repeated in 1 month or after her next menstrual period.

Breast Imaging

Mammography and ultrasonography are the most reliable and common imaging techniques for early detection of breast lesions (11,12). Full-field digital mammography is a modification of screen-film mammography, which records mammographic images on a computer (13). The U.S. Food and Drug Administration (FDA) approved a digital mammography system in March 2000 (14). This technology is still considered investigational and is not widely available (15). Some proposed advantages include lower radiation exposure, ability to manipulate a computerized image for optimal viewing, and distance consultations through telemammography (16). Magnetic resonance imaging (MRI) may be valuable for assessing breast lesions of an indeterminate nature detected by clinical and mammographic examination or occurring in patients who have implants (17). MRI and positron emission tomography (PET) have been used to identify occult lesions (18,19). Novel developments in breast imaging can be anticipated that will use functional imaging and molecular biology to create better methods to quantify the extent of disease as well as response to therapeutic interventions (20,21). A promising new approach uses technetium-99m (^{99m}Tc) sestamibi to detect breast cancer, especially in women with dense breast tissue (22).

Mammography

Slowly growing breast cancers can be identified by mammography at least 2 years before the mass reaches a size detectable by palpation (23). In fact, mammography is the only reproducible method of detecting nonpalpable breast cancer. However, its accurate use requires state-of-the-art equipment and a skilled radiologist. Vigorous compression of the breast is necessary to obtain good images, and patients should be forewarned that breast compression is uncomfortable. With a good technique and well-maintained modern equipment, the average mean glandular dose per mammographic image for all facilities in the United States inspected under the Mammography Quality Standards Act in the first one-half of 1997 was 1.6 mGy (160 mrad) (24).

Indications for Mammography

There are several indications for mammography:

1. To screen, at regular intervals, women who are at high risk for developing breast cancer. About one-third of the abnormalities detected on screening mammography prove malignant when biopsy is performed (25).
2. To evaluate a questionable or ill-defined breast mass or other suspicious change in the breast.
3. To establish a baseline breast mammogram and reevaluate patients at yearly intervals to diagnose a potentially curable breast cancer before it has been diagnosed clinically.
4. To search for occult breast cancer in a patient with metastatic disease in axillary nodes or elsewhere from an unknown primary origin.
5. To screen for unsuspected cancer prior to cosmetic operations or biopsy of a mass.
6. To monitor breast cancer patients who have been treated with a breast-conserving operation and radiation.

Screening

Approximately 35% to 50% of early breast cancers can be discovered only by mammography, and about 20% can be detected only by palpation. Mass screening programs to evaluate asymptomatic, healthy women combine physical examination with mammographic screening to identify breast abnormalities. During the past 25 years, there has been an increase in mammography, mammographic screening, and public awareness. The cancer detection rate for screening mammograms is 5 per 1,000 screening examinations (26). It is 11-fold higher for diagnostic mammograms at 55 per 1,000 diagnostic mammographic examinations (26). The mean diameter of breast cancers at diagnosis has decreased from 3 cm from 1979 to 1983 to 2 cm from 1989 to 1993, and this downward trend appears to be continuing (27,28). As the mean maximal diameter of breast cancers has decreased, there has been a simultaneous decrease in the number of positive axillary lymph nodes (28). Detecting breast cancer before it has spread to the axillary nodes greatly increases the chance of survival; about 85% of such women will survive at least 5 years (28).

Mammography's lack of sensitivity in dense breast tissue has led to questions concerning its screening value in women 40 to 50 years of age. In February 1993, the National Cancer Institute (NCI) held an international workshop on screening for breast cancer (23). The purpose of this workshop was to undertake a critical review of recent clinical screening trials. The participants examined only randomized studies and focused on clinical evidence related to the efficacy of breast cancer screening in various age groups. Of the eight randomized trials identified, only the Health Insurance Plan (HIP) project demonstrated a beneficial effect of screening for women between 40 and 49 years of age. This benefit was seen 10 to 18 years after entry into the study and resulted in a 25% decrease in deaths from breast cancer. Several Swedish trials showed a 13% decrease in breast cancer mortality for women in this age group after 12 years of follow-up; however, this decrease was not statistically significant (29,30). In a metaanalysis of five randomized trials, the breast cancer rates were independent of screening in women aged 40 to 49 years (31). The beneficial effect of screening in women aged 50 to 69 years was confirmed by all clinical trials. The efficacy of screening in women older than 70 years of age was inconclusive because of the small sample size.

This topic was once again revisited in 1997. The American Cancer Society (ACS) convened a workshop on breast cancer screening in 1997 to establish guidelines for early detection of breast cancer (32). The ACS recommends monthly BSE and clinical breast examination every 3 years between ages 18 and 39. They recommend a baseline mammogram at age 40 and annual mammography for women beginning at age 40 with no upper age limit (32). This recommendation has been adopted by the American Medical Association, American College of Radiology, American Society of Clinical Oncology, and the American College of Obstetricians and Gynecologists (33,34). In contrast, the NCI also met in 1997 to discuss, debate, and reach a consensus statement for breast cancer screening (35). They concluded that a beneficial effect was seen in women over 50 years of age, but a 17% reduction in breast cancer deaths in the 40- to 49-year age group with screening was not felt to be significant enough to mandate annual mammography examinations. The NCI recommendations for women with an average risk of breast cancer is screening mammography every 1 to 2 years for women between ages 40 and 49. Women with higher risk should seek the advice of a physician and have their individual risk assessed. In an overview of breast cancer screening, Kopans condemns the arbitrary categorization of women into two age groups ($<$50 and $\geq$50 years) (36). There is not an abrupt change in screening parameters at this age cutoff, and breast cancer in the younger woman is no less serious a problem, with potential years of life lost. He concludes that screening should begin at age 40 and continue on an annual basis to reduce breast cancer mortality by 24%.

There is a consensus that annual physical and mammographic examinations should be performed for women 50 years of age and older. Screening of women older than 70 years of age should be performed after consideration of the patient's comorbid conditions and her overall state of health. Recent reports evaluating the use of mammography in the older population revealed significantly smaller lesions and earlier stage of disease (37), with a 40% reduction in breast cancer mortality at 10 years (38) and a lower incidence of metastatic disease at time of breast cancer diagnosis (39).

Mammographic Abnormalities

A mammographic abnormality includes a mass (solid versus cystic), microcalcifications (benign, indeterminate, suspicious), asymmetric density, architectural distortion, and appearance of a new density. Mammographic abnormalities should be identified on two views and triangulate to the same location on those two views. Examples of mammographic abnormalities can be reviewed in several internet radiology libraries (40). Calcifications can be macrocalcifications, which are coarse and usually represent benign degenerative breast conditions. In breast cancer, the most common diagnostic mammographic abnormalities are clustered pleomorphic microcalcifications (41). Typically, five to eight or more calcifications are aggregated in one part of the breast. These calcifications may be associated with a mammographic mass density. A mass density may appear without evidence of calcifications. It can represent a cyst, benign tumor, or a malignancy. A malignant density usually has irregular or ill-defined borders and may lead to architectural distortion, which may be subtle and difficult to detect in a dense breast. Other mammographic findings suggesting breast cancer are architectural distortion, asymmetric density, skin thickening or retraction, or nipple retraction.

Mammographic Reports

The American College of Radiology has recommended the Breast Imaging Reporting and Data System (BI-RADS) as a standardized scheme for describing mammographic lesions (42). There are eight morphologic categories (42):

1. Calcification distribution
2. Number of calcification
3. Description of calcification
4. Mass margin
5. Shape of mass
6. Density of mass
7. Associated findings
8. Special cases.

In the BI-RADS system, there are six categories for mammographic findings (43):

1. 0 is incomplete, needs further imaging
2. 1 is negative
3. 2 is a benign finding
4. 3 is probably benign, short-interval follow-up recommended
5. 4 is a suspicious finding and biopsy should be considered
6. 5 is highly suggestive of malignancy and appropriate action should be undertaken.

The patient should be referred to a surgeon if the report identifies a lesion as a category 4 or 5 (44). A category 0 indicates incomplete evaluation and further diagnostic studies are

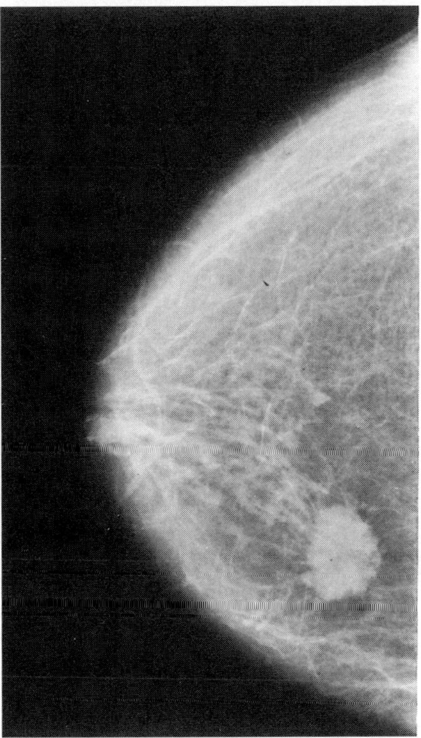
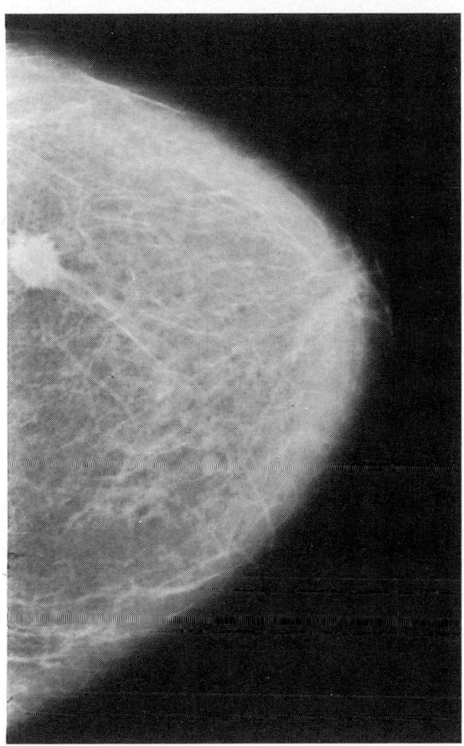

Figure 18.2 Bilateral mammography shows the extent of breast carcinoma, illustrating the importance of bilateral mammography in the workup of a clinically apparent mass. (From **Giuliano AE.** Breast disease. In: **Berek JS, Hacker NF,** eds. *Practical gynecologic oncology,* 3rd ed. Baltimore: Lippincott Williams & Wilkins, 2000:642, with permission.)

required. A category 3 is a finding which is most likely benign and a short-interval follow-up is recommended.

Biopsy must be performed on patients with a dominant or suspicious mass despite absence of mammographic findings (45). Mammography should be performed before biopsy so other suspicious areas can be noted and the contralateral breast can be checked (Fig. 18.2).

Correlation of Findings

Mammography is never a substitute for biopsy because it may not reveal clinical cancer, especially when it occurs in the dense breast tissue of young women with fibrocystic changes. In fact, the sensitivity of mammography varies from approximately 60% to 90%, depending on the patient's age (breast density) and the size, location, and mammographic appearance of the tumor.

Mammography is less sensitive in young women with dense breast tissue than in older women, who tend to have fatty breasts in which mammography can detect at least 90% of malignancies. Small tumors, particularly those without calcifications, are more difficult to detect, especially in women with dense breasts. The specificity of mammography is about 30% to 40% for nonpalpable mammographic abnormalities and 85% to 90% for clinically evident malignancies (46).

Ultrasonography

Reliable, portable computer-enhanced ultrasonography with high-frequency transducers and improved imaging is now available to evaluate and treat problems of the breast (47). It is a sensitive, minimally invasive technique that is being used more frequently in evaluating some breast symptoms, especially in younger women with dense breast tissue (48). There are some lesions that can be detected only with ultrasonography (49). It is the preferred modality to distinguish a solid from a cystic mass (47). Screening breast ultrasonography identifies many irregularities and hypoechoic areas; the significance of these findings must be validated in prospective randomized studies (50). Most experts advise against screening ultrasonography. However, the role of ultrasonography to identify breast cancer is continuing to undergo evaluation (51,52).

Ultrasonography may be especially useful if the patient feels a mass, but the physician cannot detect an abnormality and the mammogram does not disclose one. Ultrasonography cannot reliably detect microcalcifications, and it is not as useful as mammography for fatty breasts. Ultrasonography may be useful in identifying noncalcified cancers in the dense breast tissue of premenopausal women, but it is usually used to distinguish a benign cyst from a solid tumor.

Handheld or real-time ultrasonography is 95% to 100% accurate in differentiating solid masses from cysts (53). However, this is of limited clinical value because a dominant mass should be evaluated by biopsy, and a cystic mass can be studied by needle aspiration, which is far less expensive than ultrasonography. The primary role of handheld ultrasonography is in the evaluation of a benign-appearing, nonpalpable density identified by mammography. If such a lesion proves to be a simple cyst, no further workup is necessary. Rarely, ultrasonography may identify a small cancer within a cyst—an intracystic carcinoma. These complex cysts warrant surgical biopsy.

Magnetic Resonance Imaging

MRI is increasing in popularity as a means of imaging the breast (17,54). It tends to be highly sensitive but not very specific, leading to biopsies of many benign lesions. Image enhancement with gadolinium can discriminate between benign and malignant lesions with varying degrees of accuracy.

Several roles have been proposed for breast MRI. Its lack of radiation exposure makes MRI ideal for mass screening of healthy women, although such widespread use is probably too costly. There may be a role for MRI in evaluation of specific conditions such as (a) focal, asymmetric areas detected mammographically, (b) postoperative scar, and (c) exclusion of silicone leak with implants. Focal asymmetry is usually benign but can represent a malignancy, and MRI may help identify patients in whom focal asymmetric areas should undergo biopsy. Usually, a scar can easily be distinguished from recurrent tumor based on the evaluation and diminution of the scar over time. Some scars, however, do not diminish rapidly and are confused with cancer or, more commonly, with recurrent cancer after breast-conserving operation and radiation. Ideally, such cases are evaluated with MRI, sometimes obviating the need for biopsy. MRI is extremely useful in identifying silicone released by a ruptured breast implant in patients with augmented breasts (Fig. 18.3). In patients with implants, MRI with gadolinium may be performed to detect breast cancer, even if free silicone is not suspected.

The International Cooperative Magnetic Resonance Mammography Study that is currently under way will help identify the advantages and limitations of MRI. At present, MRI should be considered only after conventional imaging is performed; it should be used neither as a screening tool nor a substitute for mammography or biopsy.

Technetium-99m Sestamibi Scan

Technetium-99m sestamibi is an agent approved for coronary imaging. It is metabolized in the mitochondria. Evaluation of patients using physical examination, mammography, ultrasonography, and sestamibi scan indicate an 88% positive predictive value and a 93% negative predictive value with a sensitivity of 84% and a specificity of 95% (55). In a

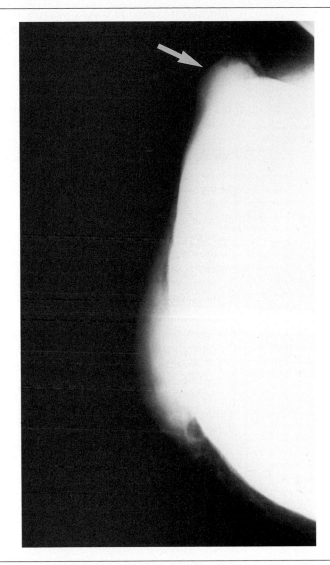

Figure 18.3 Mammography shows implant and extracapsular free silicone *(arrow).*

multicenter prospective cohort clinical trial comparing mammography to sestamibi, a positive scintimammogram increases the ability to predict the presence of malignant disease (56). This modality is still undergoing evaluation.

Positive Emission Tomography Scan

PET is a diagnostic modality that assesses the metabolic activity of tumors. Radioactive fluorodeoxyglucose (FDG) is an analog of glucose that is metabolized by tissues of high metabolic rates. In two prospective trials comparing PET to mammography, primary breast lesions were correctly identified and lymph nodes status was determined with a high degree of sensitivity using PET (57,58). PET has been used to identify occult breast lesions with positive axillary lymph nodes (59).

Breast Biopsy

The diagnosis of breast cancer depends ultimately on examination of tissue removed by biopsy. Because cancer is found in the minority of patients who require biopsy for diagnosis of a breast mass, treatment should never be undertaken without an unequivocal histologic diagnosis of cancer.

The safest course is biopsy examination of all dominant masses found on physical examination and, in the absence of a mass, of suspicious lesions shown by mammography. About 30% of lesions suspected to be cancer prove on biopsy to be benign, and about 15% of lesions believed to be benign prove to be malignant (25). Dominant masses or suspicious nonpalpable mammographic findings must be evaluated by biopsy (44,45). Histologic diagnosis should be obtained before conservation management to monitor breast mass. An exception may be a premenopausal woman with a nonsuspicious mass presumed to be fibrocystic disease. However, an apparently fibrocystic lesion that does not completely resolve within several menstrual cycles should be sampled for biopsy. Any mass in a postmenopausal woman who is not taking estrogen replacement should be presumed to be malignant. Figures 18.4 and 18.5 present algorithms for management of breast masses in premenopausal and postmenopausal patients. Simultaneous evaluation of a breast mass using clinical breast examination, radiography, and fine-needle aspiration biopsy can lower the risk of missing cancer to only 1%, effectively reducing the rate of diagnostic failure and increasing the quality of patient care (60). Ultrasonography is frequently used in addition to these techniques; although not studied, it most likely further reduces the risk of failure to diagnose cancer.

If the presence of breast cancer is strongly suggested by physical examination, the diagnosis can be confirmed by fine-needle cytologic assessment or core biopsy, and the patient may be counseled regarding treatment. Treatment should not be determined based on results of physical examination and mammography alone, in the absence of biopsy results. **The most reasonable approach to the diagnosis and treatment of breast cancer is outpatient biopsy (either needle or excision), followed by definitive surgery at a later date if needed.** This two-step approach allows patients to adjust to the diagnosis of cancer, carefully consider alternative forms of therapy, and seek a second opinion if they wish. Studies have shown no adverse effect from the 1- to 2-week delay associated with the two-step procedure (61). However, the two-step procedure should be reexamined in view of the increasing popularity of lumpectomy. Suspicious lesions may best be excised as the definitive lumpectomy specimen even if biopsy has not shown malignancy. The lumpectomy is, in essence, a biopsy that ensures a rim of normal tissue around the mass. It is better performed with the mass removed in its entirety than after a prior excisional biopsy.

Fine-needle Aspiration

Fine-needle aspiration cytology is a useful technique whereby cells from a breast tumor are aspirated with a small (usually 22-gauge) needle and examined by a pathologist. Precise guidelines for this technique are available (62). It can be performed easily, with no morbidity, and is much less expensive than excisional or open biopsy. However, it requires the availability of a pathologist skilled in the cytologic diagnosis of breast cancer to interpret the results, and it is subject to sampling problems, particularly when lesions are deep. Cytologic diagnoses must be correlated with clinical and imaging findings to achieve triple-test concordance and to decrease the false-negative rate (63). The triple test, comprising fine-needle aspiration, physical examination, and mammography, is the foundation of breast evaluation. The triple-test results are more powerful than each modality alone (64). The incidence of false-positive diagnoses was 0% to 0.3%, and the rate of false-negative diagnoses was 1.4% to 2.3% in several recent studies (64,65).

Most experienced clinicians will not leave a dominant mass in the breast even when fine-needle aspiration cytology results are negative. Some clinicians will monitor a mass when results of the clinical diagnosis, breast imaging studies, and cytologic studies are all in

Figure 18.4 Algorithm for management of breast masses in premenopausal women. (From **Giuliano AE.** Breast disease. In: **Berek JS, Hacker NF,** eds. *Practical gynecologic oncology,* 3rd ed. Baltimore: Lippincott Williams & Wilkins, 2000:652, with permission.)

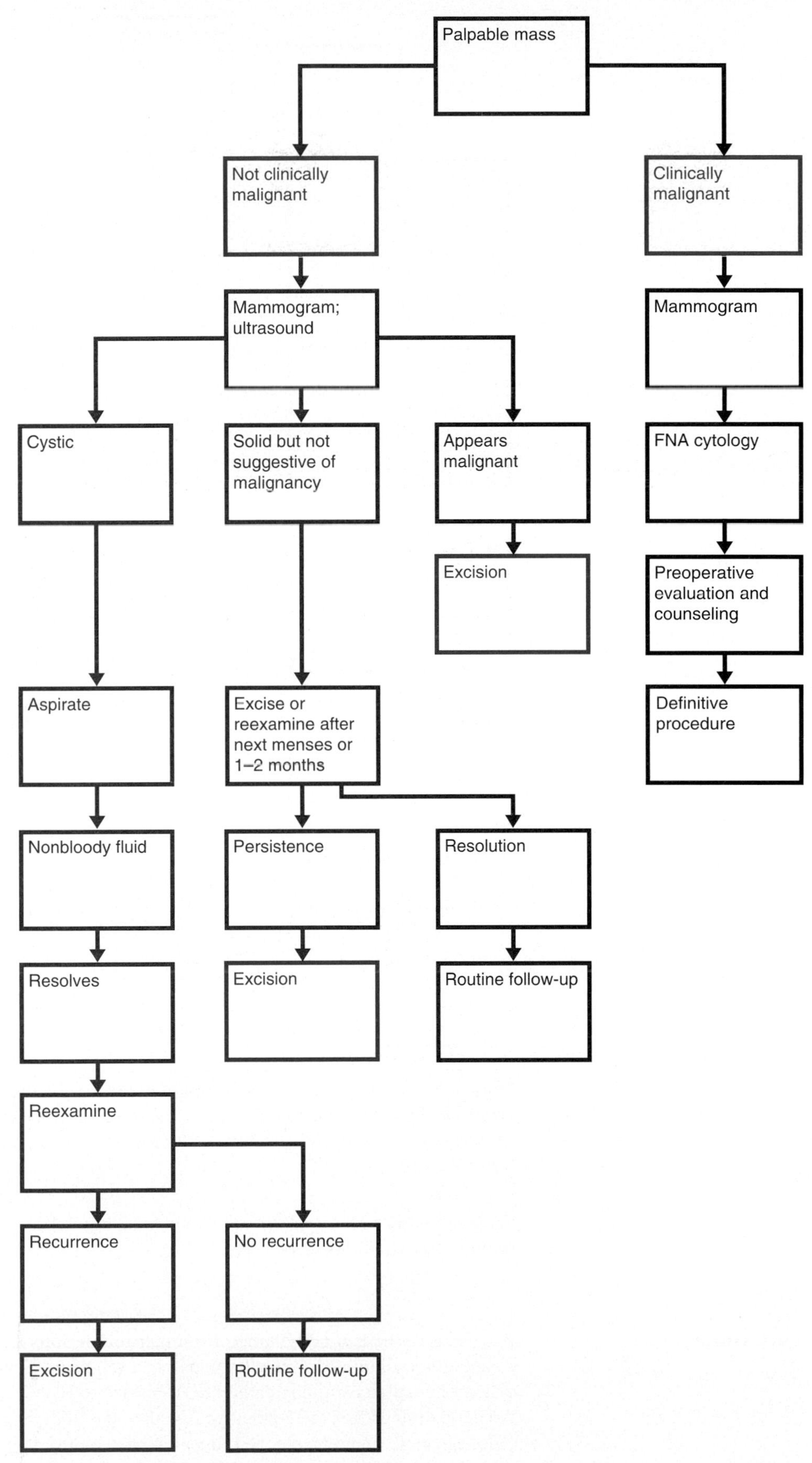
Palpable mass
Not clinically malignant
Clinically malignant
Mammogram; ultrasound
Mammogram
Cystic
Solid but not suggestive of malignancy
Appears malignant
FNA cytology
Excision
Preoperative evaluation and counseling
Aspirate
Excise or reexamine after next menses or 1–2 months
Definitive procedure
Nonbloody fluid
Persistence
Resolution
Resolves
Excision
Routine follow-up
Reexamine
Recurrence
No recurrence
Excision
Routine follow-up

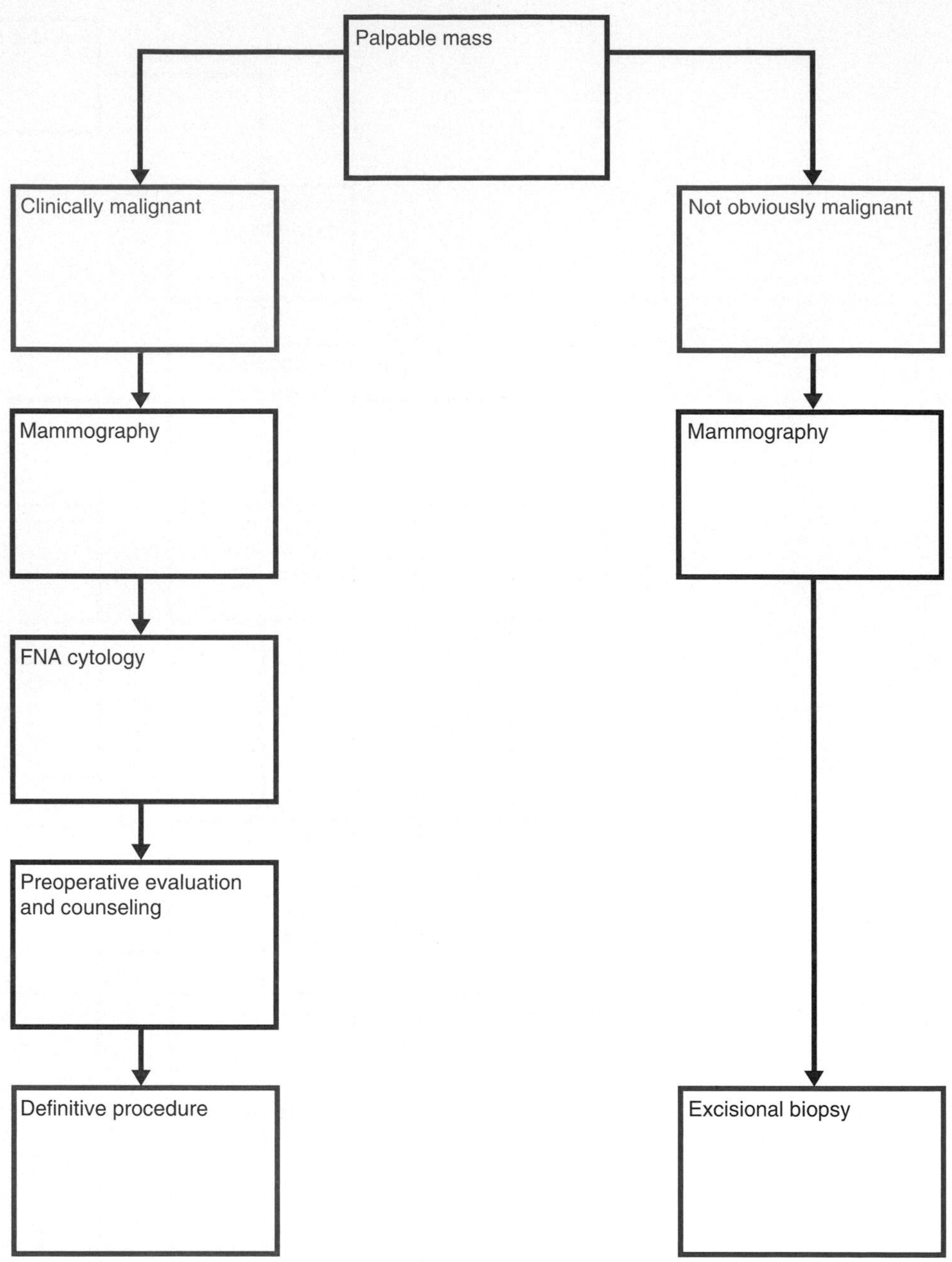

Figure 18.5 Algorithm for management of breast masses in postmenopausal women. (From **Giuliano AE.** Breast disease. In: **Berek JS, Hacker NF,** eds. *Practical gynecologic oncology,* 3rd ed. Baltimore: Lippincott Williams & Wilkins, 2000:653, with permission.

agreement. However, occasionally a malignancy will be diagnosed later, and such cases require periodic follow-up.

Core Biopsy

A core of tissue can be obtained from palpable lesions using a large cutting needle (66). Image-guided large-core needle biopsy is a reliable diagnostic alternative to surgical excision of suspicious nonpalpable breast lesions (67). As in the case of any needle biopsy, the main drawback is false-negative findings caused by improper positioning of the needle. False-negative findings may be reduced if core biopsy is performed with ultrasonographic direction.

Open Biopsy

Open biopsy with local anesthesia as a separate procedure prior to deciding on definitive treatment is the most reliable means of diagnosis. It is required when the results of needle biopsy are nondiagnostic or equivocal.

Histologic Analysis

Histologic evaluation with hematoxylin and eosin (H&E) staining confirms benign or malignant disease. Images of benign and malignant breast lesions can be viewed through the Internet Pathology Laboratory for Medical Education (68). The estrogen, progesterone, her-2/*neu* receptor status, and proliferative indices of the tumor should be determined during initial biopsy. This assessment is performed on paraffin-fixed tissue by immunohistochemistry (69). Her-2/*neu* assessment in breast cancer by immunohistochemistry (IHC) is appropriate for patients with tumors that score 3+. Fluorescence *in situ* hybridization (FISH) is recommended for 2+ IHC to more accurately assess her-2/*neu* amplification and provide better prognostic information (70).

Nipple Discharge and Nipple Lavage

Cytologic examination of nipple discharge or cyst fluid is rarely performed. Mammography (or ductography) and breast biopsy may be performed when nipple discharge or cyst fluid is bloody or cytologically questionable. However, excision and examination of the involved ductal system is the preferred method of diagnosis, and cytologic assessment should not be relied on for diagnosis.

Ductal lavage using a microcatheter is a new modality that has recently been investigated in high-risk women (71). Patients undergo gentle nipple suction to elicit nipple fluid. A duct that yields fluid is then cannulated with a microcatheter and 10 to 20 ml of saline are introduced in 2- to 4-ml increments. The cytologic assessment of a sample obtained by ductal lavage is more sensitive than that of nipple aspiration. Ductal lavage is a better modality to obtain a large number of cells for cytological evaluation. It is safe and well tolerated (71).

Benign Breast Conditions

Benign breast disorders account for a significant number of breast complaints. These conditions are frequently considered in relation to the possibility of excluding breast cancer and are often not recognized for their own associated morbidity (72). In order to provide appropriate management, it is important to consider benign breast disorders from four aspects, (a) clinical picture, (b) medical significance, (c) treatment intervention, (d) and pathologic etiology (73).

Hughes has described a conceptual framework to understanding benign breast problems that is called Aberrations of Normal Development and Involution (ANDI) (2,72,73). It includes symptomatology, histology, endocrine state, and pathogenesis in a progression from a normal to a disease state. Most benign breast conditions arise from normal changes in breast development, hormone cycling, and reproductive evolution (72).

There are three life cycles that reflect different reproductive phases in a woman's life and are associated with unique breast manifestations.

1. During the early reproductive period (15 to 25 years) there is lobule and stromal formation. The ANDI conditions associated with this period are fibroadenoma (mass) and juvenile hypertrophy (excessive breast development). In this first stage the progression from ANDI to a disease state results in the formation of giant fibroadenomas and multiple fibroadenomas.

2. During the mature reproductive period (25 to 40 years) cyclic hormonal changes affect glandular tissue and stroma. In this second period the ANDI is an exaggeration of these cyclic effects, such as cyclic mastalgia and generalized nodularity.

3. The third phase is involution of lobules and ducts or epithelia turnover, which occurs during ages 35 to 55 years. The ANDI associated with lobular involution are macrocysts (lumps) and sclerosing lesions (mammographic abnormalities). Those associated with ductal involution are duct dilation (nipple discharge) and periductal fibrosis (nipple retraction), and those with epithelial turnover are mild hyperplasia (pathologic description).

With ductal involution, progression to disease states during this period results in periductal mastitis with bacterial infections and abscess formation. Disease conditions with increased epithelial turnover are epithelial hyperplasias with atypia. Hughes feels that this framework allows the clinician to understand the pathogenesis of these conditions and to understand that these disorders are aberrations of a normal process that does not usually require any specific treatment (72).

Fibrocystic Change

Fibrocystic change, the most common lesion of the breast, is an imprecise term that covers a spectrum of clinical signs and symptoms and histologic changes (66). Macroscopic cysts occur in approximately 7% of women and microscopic, nonpalpable cysts in close to 40% of women (74). The term refers to a histologic picture of fibrosis, cyst formation, and epithelial hyperplasia (73). It is common in women 35 to 55 years of age but rare in postmenopausal women not taking hormone replacement therapy. The presence of estrogen seems necessary for the clinical symptoms to occur. This is supported by the observation that it is present bilaterally, increased in the perimenopausal age group, and responsive to endocrine therapy (75). In essence, a diagnosis of fibrocystic change is of little clinical significance as long as malignancy is excluded. These lesions are always associated with benign changes in the breast epithelium.

Cysts arise from the breast lobules and are an aberration of normal breast involution. The potassium-to-sodium ratio is a convenient marker to distinguish cyst subtypes (76). Cysts are either lined by apocrine epithelium with a high potassium-to-sodium ratio and a higher hormone or steroid concentration (type I); or by flattened lobule epithelium with a low potassium-to-sodium ratio and a higher concentration of albumin, CEA, CA125, and steroid hormone–binding globulin (type II) (75,77). A recent study has demonstrated that apocrine cysts produce and secrete large amounts of prostate-specific antigen (PSA) (78). The role of this serine protease in proliferative breast disease is not fully understood.

Clinical Findings

Fibrocystic changes may produce an asymptomatic mass but more often are accompanied by pain or tenderness and sometimes nipple discharge. In many cases, discomfort coincides with the premenstrual phase of the cycle, when the cysts tend to enlarge. Fluctuation in size and rapid appearance or disappearance of a breast mass are common. Multiple or bilateral masses appear frequently, and many patients have a history of a transient mass in the breast or cyclic breast pain. Cyclic breast pain is the most common symptom of fibrocystic changes.

Differential Diagnosis

Pain, fluctuation in size, and multiplicity of lesions are the features most helpful for differentiation from carcinoma. If a dominant mass is present, however, the diagnosis of cancer should be suspected until it is disproved by biopsy. Final diagnosis of the mass usually depends on biopsy.

Diagnostic Tests

Patients with cystic disease may have a discrete fibrocystic mass that is frequently indistinguishable from carcinoma on the basis of clinical findings. Mammography may be helpful, but there are no mammographic signs diagnostic of fibrocystic change. Ultrasonography is useful in differentiating a cystic from a solid mass. The finding of a simple cyst rules out carcinoma. **Any suspicious lesion should be biopsied.** Microscopic findings include cysts (gross and microscopic), papillomatosis, adenosis, fibrosis, and ductal epithelial hyperplasia (79).

When the diagnosis of fibrocystic change has been established by previous biopsy or is practically certain because the history is classic, aspiration of a discrete mass suggestive of a cyst is indicated. Aspiration may be performed with ultrasonographic guidance, but this usually is not necessary (80). Benign cyst fluid is straw colored to dark green to brownish and does not need to be submitted for cytologic evaluation (5). The patient is reexamined at intervals thereafter. Further cysts will occur in 30% of patients, cause anxiety, and require repeated evaluations (74). Biopsy should be performed if no cyst fluid is obtained, if the fluid is bloody, if a mass persists after aspiration, or if at any time during follow-up a persistent mass is noted. Even if a needle biopsy is performed and results are negative for malignancy, a suspicious mass that does not resolve over several months should be excised. Surgery should be conservative, because the primary objective is to exclude cancer. Simple mastectomy or extensive removal of breast tissue is rarely, if ever, indicated for fibrocystic disease. Most patients do not require treatment.

Mastalgia

Mastalgia is a recognized organic condition (81,82). Approximately 70% of women experience severe breast pain at some time in their lives (83). More than 30% of women seen in surgical breast clinics suffer from mastalgia (84). In 15% of the patients the mastalgia is so severe that it alters lifestyle and requires treatment (83). Mastalgia interferes with sexual (48%), physical (37%), social (12%), and work or school activities (8%) (85).

Cyclic mastalgia is related to exaggerated premenstrual symptoms associated with breast engorgement, pain, and tenderness (86). Noncyclic mastalgia is independent of menstrual cycles and more difficult to treat. Breast pain associated with generalized fibrocystic changes is best treated by avoiding trauma and by wearing (night and day) a brassiere that gives good support and protection (87). Hormone therapy is not advisable because it does not relieve symptoms and has undesirable side effects. Recognized treatments include bromocriptine, danazol, evening primrose oil, and tamoxifen, although tamoxifen is not approved for this use (88–91). A survey of surgeons in Great Britain revealed that 75% prescribed danazol as first-line therapy (81). Other treatments included analgesia (21%), diuretics (18%), local excision (18%), bromocriptine (15%), evening primrose oil (13%), tamoxifen (9%), a well-fitting bra (3%), and no treatment (10%) (81). In this study, breast specialists were more likely to initiate therapy with evening primrose oil, tamoxifen, vitamin B_6, and analgesia. In another study the first-line therapy was evening primrose oil containing essential fatty acids (γ-linolenic acid [GLA]), with danazol and bromocriptine reserved for second-line treatment (83). In a prospective mastalgia trial, women were given eight capsules of evening primrose oil daily for 4 months (320 mg GLA) (92). Those who responded had a lower level of essential fatty acids at the time of initiation when compared with poor responders, suggesting that evening primrose oil increases essential fatty acids and that this increase may be associated with the improvement in symptoms in the responders. Danazol (100 to 200 mg twice daily orally), a synthetic androgen, has been used for patients with severe pain (89). This treatment suppresses pituitary gonadotropins, and its androgenic effects (acne, edema, hirsutism) are usually intolerable; therefore, it probably should not be used. A recent study was conducted to evaluate the response to administration of danazol (200 mg daily) during the luteal phase (93). This approach to therapy reduces the premenstrual mastalgia with virtually no side effects. In one study, taking progesterone agents for birth control reduced cyclic breast pain to 2.3% of women compared with 4.9% who did not take such medication (84). Further studies may be warranted to see whether medroxyprogesterone acetate suppresses cyclic mastalgia in reproductive-age women. Bromocriptine (2.5 mg twice daily) given for 3 to 6 months was effective in women with an abnormal thyrotropin-releasing hormone (TRH) level (90). Patients who have normal TRH levels or are resistant to bromocriptine responded favorably to progesterone and systemic nonsteroidal antiinflammatory drugs.

The role of caffeine consumption in the aggravation of fibrocystic change is controversial (94–97). Results of some studies suggest that eliminating caffeine from the diet is associated with improvement of symptoms (96,97). Many patients are aware of these studies and report relief of symptoms after discontinuing intake of coffee, tea, and chocolate. Similarly, many women find vitamin E (150 to 600 IU daily) or B_6 (200 to 800 mg/day) helpful (98,99). However, observations about these effects have been difficult to confirm and are anecdotal (100–102). A recent review of nutritional interventions for fibrocystic breast conditions that evaluated evening primrose oil, vitamin E, or pyridoxine suggested that there are insufficient data to draw clear conclusions about their effectiveness (103). Exacerbations of pain, tenderness, and cyst formation may occur at any time until menopause, when symptoms usually subside unless patients are taking estrogen. A patient with fibrocystic changes should be advised to examine her own breasts each month just after menstruation and to inform her physician if a mass appears.

Fibrocystic Change and Cancer

Fibrocystic change is not associated with an increased risk of breast cancer unless there is histologic evidence of epithelial proliferative changes, with or without atypia (104–109). The common coincidence of fibrocystic disease and malignancy in the same breast reflects that one in every nine women will develop breast cancer, and as many as 80% of biopsies show fibrocystic changes. Page and Dupont (107) evaluated the relationship between fibrocystic change and breast cancer in 10,366 women who underwent biopsy from 1950 until 1968 and were followed for a median of 17 years. Approximately 70% of the biopsies showed nonproliferative breast disease, whereas 30% showed proliferative breast disease. Cytologic atypia were present in 3.6% of cases. Women with nonproliferative disease had no increased risk of breast cancer, whereas women with proliferative breast disease and no atypical hyperplasia had a twofold higher risk of breast cancer. **Patients whose biopsy results showed atypical ductal or lobular hyperplasia had an approximately fivefold higher risk than women with nonproliferative disease to develop invasive breast cancer in either breast.** Patients with carcinoma *in situ* have an 8- to 10-fold risk of developing breast cancer. This risk is bilateral for lobular lesions and local for ductal lesions. A family history of breast cancer added little risk for women with nonproliferative disease, but family history plus atypia increased breast cancer risk 11-fold. The presence of cysts alone did not increase the risk of breast cancer, but cysts combined with a family history of breast cancer increased the risk about threefold (66,104–109). Women with these risk factors (family history of breast cancer and proliferative breast disease) should be followed carefully with physical examination and mammography. For such women, age-specific probability of developing invasive breast carcinoma in the next 10 years is 1 in 2,000 (age 20), 1 in 256 (age 30), 1 in 67 (age 40), 1 in 39 (age 50) and 1 in 29 (age 60) (105). The relative risk changes with the type of proliferative lesion diagnosed.

Benign Tumors

Fibroadenoma

Fibroadenomas are the most common benign tumors of the breast. In one series, they account for 50% of all breast biopsies (110). They usually occur in young women (age 20 to 35 years) and may occur in teenagers (111). In women younger than 25 years, fibroadenomas are more common than cysts. They rarely occur after menopause, although occasionally they are found, often calcified, in postmenopausal women. For this reason, it is postulated that fibroadenomas are responsive to estrogen stimulation. A recent study reports the *de novo* occurrence of fibroadenoma in 51 women over age 35 years, who had no evidence of a palpable or mammographic visualized lesion in well-documented prior visits (112).

Although the presence of a fibroadenoma does not increase the risk of breast carcinoma, this subject still generates controversy (113). Because transformation of a fibroadenoma into cancer is rare and regression is frequent, current management recommendations are conservative (110).

On gross examination, fibroadenomas appear encapsulated and sharply delineated from the surrounding breast parenchyma. Microscopically, they have an epithelial and a stromal component. In longstanding lesions and in postmenopausal patients, calcifications may be observed within the stroma. Fibroadenomas may appear in multiples. Clinically, a young patient usually notices a mass while showering or dressing. Most masses are 2 to 3 cm in diameter when detected, but they can become extremely large (i.e., the giant fibroadenoma). On physical examination, they are firm, smooth, and rubbery. They do not elicit an inflammatory reaction, are freely mobile, and cause no dimpling of the skin or nipple retraction. They are often bilobed, and a groove can be palpated on examination. Mammographically, they have typical benign-appearing features with smooth, clearly defined margins.

A suspected fibroadenoma should be confirmed by either excisional biopsy or fine-needle aspiration cytology. Complete excision of a fibroadenoma with local anesthesia can be performed to treat the lesion and confirm the absence of malignancy. However, a young woman with a clinical fibroadenoma can undergo needle cytology and observation of the mass (114). Rarely will the fibroadenoma increase to more than 2 to 3 cm in size. Large or growing fibroadenomas must be excised.

Multiple Fibroadenomas

Multiple fibroadenomas have been reported in premenopausal women undergoing immunosuppression for transplant (115–118). It is an uncommon syndrome that raises issues regarding appropriate treatment. Excision of all lesions through separate incisions could leave significant scarring and deformity. Excision of these mobile lesions through a single periareolar incision has been suggested, but this approach can lead to significant ductal disruption (119). Alternatively, these lesions can be treated with observation based on triple-test concordance of a classic clinical examination with histologic corroboration with FNA and ultrasonographic diagnostic criteria consistent with a fibroadenoma (116).

Phyllodes Tumor

Cystosarcoma phyllodes, which is perhaps best referred to as a *phyllodes tumor,* may occur at any age but tends to be more common in women who are in their late thirties, forties, and fifties (120–123). These lesions are rarely bilateral and usually appear as isolated masses that are difficult to distinguish clinically from a fibroadenoma. Patients often relate a long history of a previously stable nodule that suddenly increases in size. Size is not a diagnostic criterion, although phyllodes tumors tend to be larger than fibroadenomas, probably because of their rapid growth. There are no good clinical criteria by which to distinguish a phyllodes tumor from a fibroadenoma.

The histologic distinction between fibroadenoma, benign phyllodes tumor, and malignant phyllodes tumor can be very difficult (124). Tumors judged by the pathologist to be benign tend to recur locally in up to 10% of patients (121–123). Malignant phyllodes tumors tend to recur locally and usually metastasize to the lung, although brain, pelvic, and bone metastases have also been reported (121,123). The stromal component of the tumor is malignant and metastasizes, behaving like a sarcoma. Axillary involvement is extremely unusual. Often, the appearance of metastasis is the first sign that a phyllodes tumor is malignant.

Treatment is wide local excision (120–123,125). Primary excision or reexcision with normal breast margins is recommended (122). Massive tumors, or large tumors in relatively small breasts, may require mastectomy; otherwise, mastectomy should be avoided and axillary lymph node dissection is not indicated. Typically, a patient will undergo excisional biopsy of a mass believed to be fibroadenoma, but histologic examination will reveal a phyllodes tumor. When the pathologic diagnosis is phyllodes tumor, complete reexcision of the area should be undertaken so that the prior biopsy site and any residual tumor are removed. Recurrence is associated with margin involvement, whereas death correlates with size and grade (126). Chemotherapy for metastatic phyllodes tumors should be based on regimens for sarcoma, not adenocarcinoma (122). Radiation therapy has generally not been used in the treatment of phyllodes tumors. When there is bulky tumor, positive margins, recurrence, or malignant histology radiation therapy may be of some benefit (127).

Breast Conditions Requiring Evaluation

Nipple Discharge

Nipple discharge is the breast symptom in 4.8% of patients seeking evaluation of a breast complaint, with 2.6% spontaneous and 2.2% provoked (128). Nipple discharge is infrequently found to be associated with carcinoma, with only 4 of 104 cases (3.8%) being due to malignancy (129). The most common causes of nipple discharge in nonlactating women are solitary intraductal papilloma, carcinoma, papillomatosis, and fibrocystic change with ectasia of the ducts (130). **Following are the important characteristics of the discharge and other factors to be evaluated by history and physical examination** (130):

1. Nature of discharge (serous, bloody, or milky)
2. Association with a mass
3. Unilateral or bilateral
4. Single or multiple ducts
5. Discharge that is spontaneous (persistent or intermittent) or expressed by pressure at a single site or on entire breast
6. Relation to menses
7. Premenopausal or postmenopausal
8. Hormonal medication (contraceptive pills or estrogen).

Unilateral, spontaneous, bloody, or serosanguinous discharge from a single duct is usually caused by an intraductal papilloma or, rarely, by an intraductal cancer. In either case, a mass may not be palpable. The involved duct may be identified by pressure at different sites around the nipple and at the margin of the areola. Bloody discharge is more suggestive of cancer but is usually caused by a benign papilloma in the duct. Cytologic examination is usually of no value but may identify malignant cells (129). Negative findings do not rule out cancer, which is more likely in women over 50 years of age. In any case, the involved duct—and a mass, if present—should be excised (129–131). Although ductography may identify a filling defect prior to excision of the duct system, this study is of little value (129). A new technology, fiberoptic ductoscopy, is emerging to evaluate patients with nipple discharge (132). In 259 patients with nipple discharge, it successfully detected intraductal papillary lesions in 92 patients (36%). Further experience and understanding of this technology may guide breast surgery for nipple discharge, and is being used for the assessment of margins in breast cancer value.

In premenopausal women, spontaneous multiple-duct discharge, unilateral or bilateral, is most marked just before menstruation. It often is caused by fibrocystic change. Discharge may be green or brownish. Papillomatosis and ductal ectasia are usually seen on biopsy. If a mass is present, it should be removed. Milky discharge from multiple ducts in nonlactating women presumably reflects increased secretion of pituitary prolactin; serum prolactin and thyroid-stimulating hormone levels should be evaluated to detect a pituitary tumor or hypothyroidism. Hypothyroidism may cause galactorrhea. Alternatively, phenothiazines may cause milky discharge that disappears when medication is discontinued. Oral contraceptive agents may cause clear, serous, or milky discharge from multiple ducts or, less often, from a single duct. The discharge is more evident just before menstruation and disappears when the medication is stopped. If discharge does not stop and is from a single duct, surgical exploration should be performed.

When localization is not possible and no mass is palpable, the patient should be reexamined every week for 1 month. When unilateral discharge persists, even without definite localization or tumor, surgical exploration must be considered. The alternative is careful follow-up at intervals of 1 to 3 months. Mammography should be performed. Chronic unilateral nipple discharge, especially if it is bloody, is an indication for resection of the involved ducts. Purulent discharge may originate in a subareolar abscess and requires excision of the abscess and related lactiferous sinus (133).

Erosive Adenomatosis of the Nipple

Erosive adenomatosis is a rare benign condition of the nipple that mimics Paget's disease (134). Patients seek treatment for pruritus, burning, and pain. On clinical examination the nipple can appear ulcerated, crusting, scaling, indurated, and erythematous. The nipple can be enlarged and more prominent during menstrual cycles (135). The differential diagnosis includes squamous cell carcinoma, psoriasis, contact dermatitis, seborrheic keratosis, adenocarcinoma metastatic to the skin, and unusual primary tumors of the nipple (134). Biopsy should be performed to diagnose the lesion. Local excision is curative (134).

Fat Necrosis

Fat necrosis of the breast is rare but clinically important because it produces a mass, often accompanied by skin or nipple retraction, which is indistinguishable from carcinoma. Trauma is presumed to be the cause, although only about one-half of patients have a history of injury to the breast. Ecchymosis is occasionally seen near the tumor. Tenderness may or may not be present. If untreated, the mass associated with fat necrosis gradually disappears. Fat necrosis often has a confusing clinical picture. Diagnostic imaging studies are usually insufficient (136). As a rule, the safest course is needle core or excisional biopsy of the entire mass to rule out carcinoma (136). Fat necrosis is common after segmental resection and radiation therapy or transverse rectus abdominis musculocutaneous (TRAM) flap (137).

Breast Abscess

Lactational Abscesses

Infection in the breast is rare unless the patient is lactating. During lactation, an area of redness, tenderness, and induration frequently develops in the breast. The organism most commonly found in these abscesses is *Staphylococcus aureus* (138). In its early stages, the infection can often be reversed while nursing is continued from that breast by administering an antibiotic such as *dicloxacillin* 250 mg 4 times daily, or *oxacillin,* 500 mg 4 times daily for 7 to 10 days. If the lesion progresses to a localized mass with local and systemic signs of infection, an abscess is present. It should be drained, and nursing should be discontinued.

Nonlactational Abscess

Rarely, infections or abscesses may develop in young or middle-aged women who are not lactating (139). The current approach to nonlactional abscess is conservative (140). A suspected abscess should be evaluated with preliminary ultrasonography to assess the presence of an inflammatory mass, frank pus, solitary cavity, or a multiloculated abscess (141). Aspiration of pus, if present, and antibiotic therapy is instituted with reaspiration if necessary (140). Bacteriologic analysis of 22 abscesses in nonlactating women shows a preponderance of gram-positive cocci including *Staphylococcus epidermidis* (11 women), *Staphylococcus aureus* (3 women), *Proteus mirabilis* (3 women), *Pseudomonas aeruginosa* (1 woman), and sterile abscess (4 women) (141). If these infections recur after multiple aspirations, incision and drainage followed by excision of the involved lactiferous duct(s) at the base of the nipple may be necessary during a quiescent interval. In virtually all cases, mammillary sinus can be demonstrated as the cause of reinfection or persistent infection (142). Because inflammatory carcinoma must always be considered in the presence of erythema of the breast, findings suggestive of abscesses are an indication for incision and biopsy of any indurated tissue. Patients should not undergo prolonged treatment for an apparent infection unless biopsy has eliminated the possibility of inflammatory carcinoma.

Disorders of Breast Augmentation

Estimates indicate that nearly 4 million women in the United States have undergone augmentation mammoplasty. Breast implants are usually placed under the pectoralis muscle or, less desirably, in the subcutaneous tissue of the breast. Most implants are made of an outer silicone shell filled with a silicone gel or saline.

The complications of breast implantation are significant. About 15% to 25% of patients develop capsule contraction or scarring around the implant, leading to a firmness and distortion of the breast that can be painful and sometimes requires removal of the implant and capsule. Implant rupture may occur in as many as 5% to 10% of women, and bleeding of gel through the capsule is even more common (143). In April 1992, the FDA concluded that the safety and effectiveness of silicone gel breast implants had not been established and called for additional preclinical and clinical studies (144). The FDA advised symptomatic women with ruptured implants to discuss the need for surgical removal with their physicians. When there is no evidence of associated symptoms or rupture, implant removal is generally not indicated because the risks of removal are probably greater than those of retention. If screening ultrasonography shows no rupture, the probability of rupture is 2.2% (145). If ultrasonography shows rupture, true rupture is present in 37.8%. In this setting a large number of women would have normal implants removed. When MRI is used in addition to ultrasonography, the probability of rupture increases to 86%.

A suggested association between silicone gel and autoimmune disease has been poorly documented (146,147). A retrospective cohort study from the Mayo Clinic showed no increased incidence of autoimmune disorders among women with silicone implants (148). Subsequent studies have demonstrated no clinical data proving an increased incidence of connective tissue disorders in patients with silicone gel breast implants (149–151). Even so, patients who have symptoms suggestive of an autoimmune disorder should discuss with their physician the risks and benefits of implant removal.

Any association between implants and an increased incidence of breast cancer is unlikely (152). However, breast cancer may develop in any patient with a silicone gel prosthesis.

References

1. **Marchant DJ.** Controversies in benign breast disease. *Surg Oncol Clin North Am* 1998;7:285–298.
2. **Hughes LE, Mansel RE, Webster DJT.** *Benign disorders and diseases of the breast,* 2nd ed. Barcelona, Spain: WB Saunders, 2000.
3. **Kelsey JL.** Breast cancer epidemiology: summary and future directions. *Epidemiol Rev* 1993;15:256–263.
4. **Wolden SL, Lamborn KR, Cleary SF, et al.** Second cancers following pediatric Hodgkin's disease. *J Clin Oncol* 1998;16:536–544.
5. **Cady B, Steele GD, Morrow M, et al.** Evaluation of common breast problems: guidance for primary care providers. *CA Cancer J Clin* 1998;48:49–63.
6. **Solomon LJ, Mickey RM, Rairikar CJ, et al.** Three-year prospective adherence to three breast cancer screening modalities. *Prev Med* 1998;27:781–786.
7. **Harvey BJ, Miller AB, Baines CJ, et al.** Effect of breast self-examination techniques on the risk of death from breast cancer. *CMAJ* 1997;157:1205–1212.

8. **Baines CJ, To T.** Changes in breast self-examination behavior achieved by 89,835 participants in the Canadian National Breast Screening Study. *Cancer* 1990;66:570–576.

9. **Vietri V, Poskitt S, Slaninka SC.** Enhancing breast cancer screening in the university setting. *Cancer Nursing* 1997;20:323–329.

10. **Strickland CJ, Feigl P, Upchurch C, et al.** Improving breast self-examination compliance: a Southwest Oncology Group randomized trial of three interventions. *Prev Med* 1997;26:320–332.

11. **Watson L.** The role of ultrasound in breast imaging. *Radiol Technol* 2000;71:441–459.

12. **Simonetti G, Cossu E, Montanaro M, et al.** What's new in mammography. *Eur J Radiol* 1998;27[Suppl 2]:S234–241.

13. **Lewin JM, Hendrick RE, D'Orsi CJ, et al.** Comparison of full-field digital mammography with screen-film mammography for cancer detection: results of 4,945 paired examinations. *Radiology* 2001;218:873–880.

14. **White J.** FDA approves system for digital mammography. *J Natl Cancer Inst* 2000;92:442.

15. **Pisano ED, Yaffe MJ, Hemminger BM, et al.** Current status of full-field digital mammography. *Acad Radiol* 2000;7:266–280.

16. **Lou SL, Sickles EA, Huang HK, et al.** Full-field direct digital telemammography: technical components, study protocols, and preliminary results. *IEEE Trans Inform Tech Biomed* 1997;1:270–278.

17. **Harms SE.** Breast magnetic resonance imaging. *Semin Ultrasound CT MR* 1998;19:104–120.

18. **Block EF, Meyer MA.** Positron emission tomography in diagnosis of occult adenocarcinoma of the breast. *Am Surgeon* 1998;64:906–908.

19. **Olson JA, Morris EA, Van Zee KJ, et al.** Magnetic resonance imaging facilitates breast conservation for occult breast cancer. *Ann Surg Oncol* 2000;7:411–415.

20. **Williams MB, Pisano ED, Schnall MD, et al.** Future directions in imaging of breast diseases. *Radiology* 1998;206:297–300.

21. **Reynolds HE.** Advances in breast imaging. *Hematol Oncol Clin North Am* 2000;13:333–348.

22. **Khalkhali I, Villanueva-Meyer J, Edell SL, et al.** Diagnostic accuracy of ^{99m}Tc-sestamibi breast imaging: multicenter trial results. *J Nucl Med* 2000;41:1973–1979.

23. **Fletcher SW, Black W, Harris R, et al.** Report of the International Workshop on Screening for Breast Cancer. *J Natl Cancer Inst* 1993;85:1644–1656.

24. **Haus AG, Yaffe MJ.** Breast imaging: screen-film and digital mammography, image quality and radiation dose considerations. *Radiol Clin North Am* 2000;38:871–898.

25. **Bassett LW, Liu TH, Giuliano AE, et al.** The prevalence of carcinoma in palpable vs. impalpable, mammographically detected lesions. *AJR Am J Roentgenol* 1991;157:21–24.

26. **Dee KE, Sickles EA.** Medical audit of diagnostic mammography examinations: comparison with screening outcomes obtained concurrently. *AJR Am J Roentgenol* 2001;176:729–733.

27. **Cady B, Stone MD, Schuler JG, et al.** The new era in breast cancer: invasion, size, and nodal involvement dramatically decreasing as a result of mammographic screening. *Arch Surg* 1996;131:301–308.

28. **Tabar L, Fagerberg G, Day NE, et al.** Breast cancer treatment and natural history: new insights from results of screening. *Lancet* 1992;339:412–414.

29. **Parker SH.** Percutaneous large core breast biopsy. *Cancer* 1994;74:256–262.

30. **Leis HJ.** Concepts regarding breast biopsies. *Breast Dis* 1991;4:223.

31. **Kopans DB.** Screening for breast cancer and mortality reduction among women 40 to 49 years of age. *Cancer* 1994;74:311–322.

32. **Leitch AM, Dodd GD, Costanza M, et al.** American Cancer Society guidelines for the early detection of breast cancer: update 1997. *CA Cancer J Clin* 1997;47:150–153.

33. **Alexander W.** ASCO and ACOG update: breast cancer screening and prevention. *Oncol Issues* 1999;14:27–28.

34. **Dershaw DD.** Mammographic screening of the high-risk woman. *Am J Surg* 2000;180:288–289.

35. **NCI.** Statement from the National Cancer Institute on the National Cancer Advisory Board recommendations on mammography. Bethesda, MD: National Cancer Institute, 1997.

36. **Kopans DB.** An overview of the breast cancer screening controversy. *J Natl Cancer Inst Monogr* 1997;22:1–3.

37. **Gabriel H, Wilson TE, Helvie MA.** Breast cancer in women 65 to 74 years old: earlier detection by mammographic screening. *AJR Am J Roentgenol* 1997;168:23–27.

38. **Van Dijck JA, Verbeek AL, Beex LV, et al.** Breast-cancer mortality in a non-randomized trial on mammographic screening in women over age 65. *Int J Cancer* 1997;70:164–168.

39. **Smith-Bindman R, Kerlikowski K, Gebretsadik T, et al.** Is screening mammography effective in elderly women? *Am J Med* 2000;108:112–119.

40. **Smith JK.** UNC Radiology Teaching File. Available at: http://www.ibiblio.org/jksmith/UNC-Radiology-Webserver/Mammography.html. University of North Carolina Department of Radiology, 2001. Accessed

41. **Sickles EA.** Mammographic features of 300 consecutive nonpalpable breast cancers. *AJR Am J Roentgenol* 1986;146:661–663.

42. **Baker JA, Kornguth PJ, Floyd CE Jr.** Breast imaging reporting and data system standardized mammography lexicon: observer variability in lesion description. *AJR Am J Roentgenol* 1996;166:773–778.

43. **American College of Radiology.** *Breast imaging reporting and data system (BI-RADS),* 3rd ed. Reston, VA: American College of Radiology, 1998.

44. **D'Orsi C, Mendelson E, Bassett L, et al.** Work-up of nonpalpable breast masses: American College of Radiology, ACR appropriateness criteria. *Radiology* 2000;215:965–972.

45. **Evans WP III, Mendelson E, Bassett L, et al.** Appropriate imaging work-up of palpable breast masses: American College of Radiology, ACR appropriateness criteria. *Radiology* 2000;215:961–964.

46. **Sickles EA, Ominsky SH, Sollitto RA, et al.** Medical audit of a rapid-throughput mammography screening practice: methodology and results of 27,114 examinations. *Radiology* 1990;175:323–327.

47. **Velez N, Earnest DE, Staren ED.** Diagnostic and interventional ultrasound for breast disease. *Am J Surg* 2000;180:284–287.

48. **Buchberger W, DeKoekkoek-Doll P, Springer P, et al.** Incidental findings on sonography of the breast: clinical significance and diagnostic workup. *AJR Am J Roentgenol* 1999;173:921–927.

49. **Kolb TM, Lichy J, Newhouse JH.** Occult cancer in women with dense breast: detection with screening US—diagnostic yield and tumor characteristics. *Radiology* 1998;196:123–134.

50. **Kopans DB.** Breast-cancer screening with ultrasonography. *Lancet* 1999;354:2096–2097.

51. **Malich A, Boehm T, Facius M, et al.** Differentiation of mammographically suspicious lesions: evaluation of breast ultrasound, MRI mammography and electrical impedance scanning as adjunctive technologies in breast cancer detection. *Clin Radiol* 2001;56:278–283.

52. **Blohmer JU, Oellinger H, Schmidt C, et al.** Comparison of various imaging methods with particular evaluation of color Doppler sonography for planning surgery for breast tumors. *Arch Gynecol Obstet* 1999;262:159–171.

53. **Sickles EA, Filly RA, Callen PW.** Benign breast lesions: ultrasound detection and diagnosis. *Radiology* 1984;151:467–470.

54. **Brenner RJ.** Breast MR imaging. *Magn Reson Imaging Clin N Am* 1994;2:705–723.

55. **Clifford EJ, Lugo-Zamudio C.** Scintimammography in the diagnosis of breast cancer. *Am J Surg* 1996;172:483–486.

56. **Sampalis FS, Reid T, Martin G, et al.** International prospective evaluation of scintimammography with teenetium-99m sestamibi: interim results. *Am J Surg* 2001;182:399–403.

57. **Adler LP, Crowe JP, al-Kaisi NK, et al.** Evaluation of breast masses and axillary lymph nodes with F-18 2-deoxy-1-fluoro-D-glucose PET. *Radiology* 1993;187:743–750.

58. **Tse NY, Hoh CK, Hawkins MJ, et al.** The application of positron emission tomographic imaging with fluorodeoxyglucose to the evaluation of breast disease. *Ann Surg* 1992;216:27–34.

59. **Block EFJ, Meyer MA.** Positron emission tomography in diagnosis of occult adenocarcinoma of the breast. *Am Surgeon* 1998;64:906–908.

60. **Osuch JR, Bonham VL, Morris LL.** Primary care guide to managing a breast mass: step-by-step workup. *Medscape Womens Health* 1998;3:4.

61. **King TA, Cederbom GJ, Champaign JL, et al.** A core breast biopsy diagnosis of invasive carcinoma allows for definitive surgical treatment planning. *Am J Surg* 1998;176:497–501.

62. **Abati A, Subcommittee Members.** The uniform approach to breast fine needle aspiration biopsy: a synopsis. *Acta Cytol* 1996;40:1120–1126.

63. **Boerner S, Sneige N.** Specimen adequacy and false-negative diagnosis rate in fine-needle aspirates of palpable breast masses. *Cancer* 1998;84:344–348.

64. **Schmidt WA, Wachtel MS, Jones MK, et al.** The triple test: A cost-effective diagnostic tool. *Lab Med* 1994;25:715–719.

65. **Arisio R, Cuccorses C, Accinelli G, et al.** Role of fine-needle aspiration biopsy in breast lesions: analysis of a series of 4,110 cases. *Diagn Cytopathol* 1998;18:462–467.

66. **McDivitt RW, Stevens JA, Lee NC, et al.** Histologic types of benign breast disease and the risk for breast cancer. The Cancer and Steroid Hormone Study Group. *Cancer* 1992;69:1408–1414.

67. **Meyer JE, Smith DN, Lester SC, et al.** Large-core needle biopsy of nonpalpable breast lesions. *JAMA* 1999;281:1638–1641.

68. **Bingham M, Blaylock RC, Byrne JLB, et al.** The internet pathology laboratory for medical education. Available at: http://www-medlib.med.utah.edu/WebPath/breshtml/brestidx.html

69. **Vetrani A, Fulciniti F, Di Benedetto G, et al.** Fine-needle aspiration biopsies of breast masses: an additional experience with 1153 cases (1985–1988) and a metaanalysis. *Cancer* 1992;69:736–740.

70. **Kakar S, Puangsuvan N, Stevens JM, et al.** Her-2/*neu* assessment in breast cancer by immunohistochemistry and fluorescence in situ hybridization comparison of results and correlation with survival. *Mol Diagn* 2000;5:191–192.

71. **Dooley WC, Ljung M-B, Veronesi V, et al.** Ductal lavage for detection of cellular atypia in women at high risk for breast cancer. *J Natl Cancer Inst* 2001;93:1624–1632.

72. **Hughes LE.** Classification of benign breast disorders: the ANDI classification based on physiologic processes with the normal breast. *Br Med Bull* 1991;47:251–257.

73. **Hughes LE.** Benign breast disorders: the clinician's view. *Cancer Detect Prev* 1992;16:1–5.

74. **Mansel RE, Harrison BJ, Melhuish J, et al.** A randomized trial of dietary intervention with essential fatty acids in patients with categorized cysts. *Ann N Y Acad Sci* 1990;586:288–294.

75. **Dixon JM.** Cystic disease and fibroadenoma of the breast: natural history and relation to breast cancer risk. *Br Med Bull* 1991;47:258–271.

76. **Bradlow HL, Fleisher M, Breed CN, et al.** Biochemical classification of patients with gross cystic breast disease. *Ann N Y Acad Sci* 1990;586:12–16.

77. **Dogliotti L, Orlandi F, Caraci P, et al.** Biochemistry of breast cyst fluid: an approach to understanding intercellular communication in the terminal duct lobular units. *Ann N Y Acad Sci* 1990;586:17–28.

78. **Mannello F, Bocchiotti GD, Bianchi G, et al.** Quantification of prostate-specific antigen immunoreactivity in human breast cyst fluids. *Breast Cancer Res Treat* 1996;38:247–252.

79. **Azzopardi JG.** Terminology of benign diseases and the benign epithelial hyperplasias. In: **Azzopardi JG,** ed. *Problems in breast pathology.* Philadelphia: WB Saunders, 1979:23.

80. **Meyer JE, Christian RL, Frenna TH, et al.** I. Image-guided aspiration of solitary occult breast cysts. *Arch Surg* 1992;127:435.

81. **BeLieu RM.** Mastodynia. *Obstet Gynecol Clin North Am* 1994;24:461–477.

82. **Tavaf-Motamen H, Ader DN, Browne MW, et al.** Clinical evaluation of mastalgia. *Arch Surg* 1998;133:211–214.

83. **Holland PA, Gateley CA.** Drug therapy of mastalgia. What are the options? *Drugs* 1994;48:709–716.

84. **Euhus DM, Uyehara C.** Influence of parenteral progesterones on the prevalence and severity of mastalgia in premenstrual women: a multi-institutional cross-sectional study. *J Am Coll Surg* 1997;184:596–604.

85. **Browne MW.** Prevalence and impact of cyclic mastalgia in a United States clinic-based sample. *Am J Obstet Gynecol* 1997;177:126–132.

86. **Goodwin PJ, Miller A, Del Giudice ME, et al.** Breast health and associated premenstrual symptoms in women with severe cyclic mastopathy. *Am J Obstet Gynecol* 1997;176:998–1005.

87. **Maddox PR, Mansel RE.** Management of breast pain and nodularity. *World J Surg* 1989;13:699–705.

88. **Faiz O, Fentiman IS.** Management of breast pain. *Int J Clin Pract* 2000;54:228–232.

89. **Gateley CA, Miers M, Mansell RE, et al.** Drug treatments for mastalgia: 17 years experience in the Cardiff Mastalgia Clinic. *J R Soc Med* 1992;85:12–15.

90. **Rea N, Bove F, Gentile A, et al.** Prolactin response to thyrotropin-releasing hormone as a guideline for cyclical mastalgia treatment. *Minerva Med* 1997;88:479–487.

91. **Kontostolis E, Stefanidis K, Navrozoglou I, et al.** Comparison of tamoxifen with danazol for treatment of cyclical mastalgia. *Gynecol Endocrinol* 1997;11:393–397.

92. **Gateley CA, Maddox PR, Pritchard GA, et al.** Plasma fatty acid profiles in benign breast disorders. *Br J Surg* 1992;79:407–409.

93. **O'Brien PMS, Abukhalil IEH.** Randomized controlled trial of the management of premenstrual syndrome and premenstrual mastalgia using luteal phase–only danazol. *Am J Obstet Gynecol* 1999;180:18–23.

94. **Allen SS, Froberg DG.** The effect of decreased caffeine consumption on benign proliferative breast disease: a randomized clinical trial. *Surgery* 1987;101:720–730.

95. **Heyden S, Muhlbaier LH.** Prospective study of "fibrocystic breast disease" and caffeine consumption. *Surgery* 1984;96:479–484.

96. **Russell LC.** Caffeine restriction as initial treatment for breast pain. *Nurse Pract* 1989;14:36–37.

97. **Lawson DH, Jick H, Rothman KJ.** Coffee and tea consumption and breast disease. *Surgery* 1981;90:801–803.

98. **London RS, Sundaram GS, Murphy L, et al.** The effect of α-tocopherol on premenstrual symptomatology: a double-blind study. *J Am Coll Nutr* 1983;2:115–122.

99. **Abraham GE.** Nutritional factors in the etiology of the premenstrual tension syndromes. *J Reprod Med* 1983;28:446–464.

100. **Meyer EE, Sommers DK, Reitz CJ, et al.** Vitamin E and benign breast disease. *Surgery* 1990;107:549–551.

101. **Smallwood J, Ah-Kye D, Taylor I.** Vitamin B_6 in the treatment of premenstrual mastalgia. *Br J Clin Pract* 1986;40:532–533.

102. **Ernster VL, Goodson WH III, Hunt TK, et al.** Vitamin E and benign breast "disease." A double-blind, randomized clinical trial. *Surgery* 1985;97:490–494.

103. **Horner NK, Lampe JW.** Potential mechanisms of diet therapy for fibrocystic breast conditions show inadequate evidence of effectiveness. *J Am Diet Assoc* 2000;100:1368–1380.

104. **Hutter RVP.** Is fibrocystic disease of the breast precancerous? [Consensus Meeting]. *Arch Pathol Lab Med* 1986;110:171–173.

105. **Fitzgibbons PL, Henson DE, Hutter RV, et al.** Benign breast changes and the risk of subsequent breast cancer: an update of the 1985 consensus statement. *Arch Pathol Lab Med* 1998;122:1053–1055.

106. **London SJ, Connolly JL, Schnitt SJ, et al.** A prospective study of benign breast disease and the risk of breast cancer. *JAMA* 1992;267:941–944.

107. **Page DL, Dupont WD.** Anatomic markers of human premalignancy and risk of breast cancer. *Cancer* 1990;66:1326–1335.

108. **Page DL.** The woman at high risk for breast cancer: importance of hyperplasia. *Surg Clin North Am* 1996;76:223–230.

109. **Simpson JF, Page DL.** Pathology of preinvasive and excellent-prognosis breast cancer. *Curr Opin Oncol* 1997;9:512–519.

110. **Greenberg R, Skornick Y, Kaplan O.** Management of breast fibroadenomas. *J Gen Intern Med* 1998;13:640–645.

111. **Dent DM, Cant PJ.** Fibroadenoma. *World J Surg* 1989;13:701–710.

112. **Foxcroft L, Evans E, Hirst C.** Newly arising fibroadenomas in women aged 35 and over. *Aust N Z J Surg* 1998;68:419–422.

113. **Dupont WD, Page DL, Parl FF, et al.** Long-term risk of breast cancer in women with fibroadenoma. *N Engl J Med* 1994;331:10–15.

114. **Hindle WH, Alonzo LJ.** Conservative management of breast fibroadenomas. *Am J Obstet Gynecol* 1991;164:1647–1650.

115. **Baxi M, Agarwal A, Mishra A, et al.** Multiple bilateral giant juvenile fibroadenomas of breast. *Eur J Surg* 2000;166:828–830.

116. **Williamson MER, Lyons K, Hughes LE.** Multiple fibroadenomas of the breast: a problem of uncertain incidence and management. *Ann R Coll Surg Engl* 1993;75:161–163.

117. **Foster ME, Garrahan N, Williams S.** Fibroadenoma of the breast: a clinical and pathological study. *J R Coll Surg Edinb* 1988;33:16–19.

118. **Campbell A, Moazami N, Ditkoff BA, et al.** Short-term outcome of chromic immunosuppression on the development of breast lesions in premenopausal heart and lung transplant patients. *J Surg Res* 1998;78:27–30.

119. **Naraynsingh V, Rajy GC.** Familial bilateral fibroadenomas of the breast. *Postgrad Med J* 1985;64:439–440.

120. **Reinfuss M, Mitus J, Duda K, et al.** The treatment and prognosis of patients with phyllodes tumor of the breast: an analysis of 170 cases. *Cancer* 1996;77:910–916.

121. **Chaney AW, Pollack A, McNeese MD, et al.** Primary treatment of cystosarcoma phyllodes of the breast. *Cancer* 2000;89:1502–1511.

122. **Mangi AA, Smith BL, Gadd MA, et al.** Surgical management of phyllodes tumors. *Arch Surg* 1999;134:487–492.

123. **Zissis C, Apostolikas N, Konstantinidou A, et al.** The extent of surgery and prognosis of patients with phyllodes tumor of the breast. *Breast Cancer Res Treat* 1998;48:205–210.

124. **Krishnamurthy S, Ashfaq R, Shin HJ, et al.** Distinction of phyllodes tumor from fibroadenoma: a reappraisal of an old problem. *Cancer* 2000;90:342–349.

125. **Zurrida S, Bartoli C, Galimberti V, et al.** Which therapy for unexpected phyllode tumour of the breast? *Eur J Cancer* 1992;28:654–657.

126. **de Roos WK, Kaye P, Dent DM.** Factors leading to local recurrence or death after surgical resection of phyllodes tumours of the breast. *Br J Surg* 1999;86:396–399.

127. **Chaney AW, Pollack A, McNeese MD, et al.** Adjuvant radiotherapy for phyllodes tumor of breast. *Radiat Oncol Investig* 1998;6:264–267.

128. **Gulay H, Bora S, Kilicturgay S, et al.** Management of nipple discharge. *J Am Coll Surg* 1994;178:471–474.

129. **King TA, Carter KM, Bolton JS, et al.** A simple approach to nipple discharge. *Am Surgeon* 2000;66:960–966.

130. **Florio MG, Manganaro T, Pollicino A, et al.** Surgical approach to nipple discharge: a ten-year experience. *J Surg Oncol* 1999;71:235–238.

131. **Gulay H, Bora S, Kilicturgay S, et al.** Management of nipple discharge. *J Am Coll Surg* 1994;178:471–474.

132. **Shen KW, Wu J, Lu JS, et al.** Fiberoptic ductoscopy for patients with nipple discharge. *Cancer* 2000;89:1512–1519.

133. **Dixon JM.** Outpatient treatment of non-lactational breast abscesses. *Br J Surg* 1992;79:56–57.

134. **Miller L, Tyler W, Marron M, et al.** Erosive adenomatosis of the nipple: a benign imitator of malignant breast disease. *Cutis* 1997;59:91–92.

135. **Bourlond J, Bourlond-Reinert L.** Erosive adenomatosis of the nipple. *Dermatology* 1992;185:319–324.

136. **Harrison RL, Britton P, Warren R, et al.** Can we be sure about a radiological diagnosis of fat necrosis of the breast. *Clin Radiol* 2000;55:119–123.

137. **Kroll SS, Gherardini G, Martin JE, et al.** Fat necrosis in free and pedicled TRAM flaps. *Plast Reconstr Surg* 1998;102:1502–1507.

138. **Dixon JM.** Repeated aspiration of breast abscess in lactating women. *BMJ* 1988;297:1517–1518.

139. **Edmiston CJ, Walker AP, Krepel CJ, et al.** The nonpuerperal breast infection: aerobic and anaerobic microbial recovery from acute and chronic disease. *J Infect Dis* 1990;162:695–699.

140. **O'Hara RJ, Dexter SPL, Fox JN.** Conservative management of infective mastitis and breast abscesses after ultrasonographic assessment. *Br J Surg* 1996;83:1413–1414.

141. **Ferrara JJ, Leveque J, Dyess DL, et al.** Nonsurgical management of breast infections in nonlactating women: a word of caution. *Am Surgeon* 1990;56:668–671.

142. **Maier WP, Au FC, Tang CK.** Nonlactational breast infection. *Am Surgeon* 1994;60:247–250.

143. **Nemecek JA, Young VL.** How safe are silicone breast implants? *South Med J* 1993;86:932–944.

144. **Kessler DA.** The basis of the FDA's decision on breast implants. *N Engl J Med* 1992;326:1713–1715.

145. **Chung KC, Greenfield ML, Walters M.** Decision-analysis methodology in the work-up of women with suspected silicone breast implant rupture. *Plast Reconstr Surg* 1998;102:689–695.

146. **Duffy MJ, Woods JE.** Health risks of failed silicone gel breast implants: a 30-year clinical experience. *Plast Reconstr Surg* 1994;94:295–299.

147. **Sanchez-Guerrero J, Schur PH, Sergent JS, et al.** Silicone breast implants and rheumatic disease. Clinical, immunologic, and epidemiologic studies. *Arthritis Rheum* 1994;37:158–168.

148. **Gabriel SE, O'Fallon WM, Kurland LT, et al.** Risk of connective tissue diseases and other disorders after breast implantation. *N Engl J Med* 1994;330:1697–1702.

149. **Karlson EW, Hankinson SE, Liang MH, et al.** Association of silicone breast implants with immunologic abnormalities: a prospective study. *Am J Med* 1999;106:11–19.

150. **Blackburn WD Jr, Grotting JC, Everson MP.** Lack of evidence of systemic inflammatory rheumatic disorders in symptomatic women with breast implants. *Plastic Reconstr Surg* 1997;99:1054–1060.

151. **Contant CM, Swaak AJ, Wiggers T, et al.** First evaluation of the Dutch Working Party on silicone breast implants (SBI) and the silicone-related symptom complex (SRSC). *Clin Rheumatol* 2000;19:458–463.

152. **Bryant H, Brasher P.** Breast implants and breast cancer–reanalysis of a linkage study. *N Engl J Med* 1995;332:1535–1539.

Novak's Gynecology, 13th Edition. Edited by J.S. Berek. Lippincott Williams & Wilkins, Philadelphia © 2002.

19 Preoperative Evaluation and Postoperative Management

Daniel L. Clarke-Pearson
Angeles Alvarez
Laura Havrilesky
Johnathan Lancaster

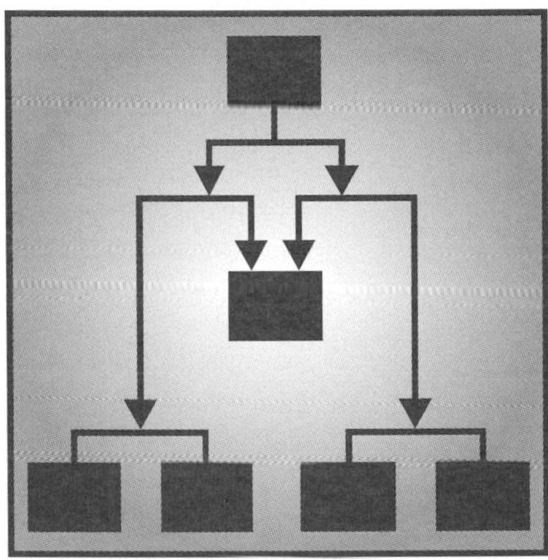

The successful outcome of gynecologic surgery is based on thorough evaluation, careful preoperative preparation, and attentive postoperative care. Approaches to the general perioperative management of patients undergoing major gynecologic surgery who have specific medical problems that could complicate the surgical outcome are presented in this chapter.

Medical History and Physical Examination

The hazards of undertaking surgery without a thorough understanding of a patient's medical history and performing a complete physical examination cannot be overstated. The preoperative medical history should include any significant medical illnesses that might be aggravated by surgery or anesthesia.

1. **Inquiry should be made regarding medications currently being taken as well as those discontinued within the months prior to surgery.** This inquiry should include notation of nonprescription drugs being taken and the use of oral contraceptives, which many patients consider a routine part of their lives rather than a medication. In addition, information on the use of alternative therapies, herbs, and vitamins should be elicited. Specific instructions must be given to the patient regarding the need to discontinue any medications prior to surgery (e.g., *aspirin* or oral contraceptives) as well as those medications that should be continued (e.g., cardiac or antihypertensive medications).

2. **The patient should be questioned regarding known allergies to medications (e.g., sulfa and *penicillin*), foods, or environmental agents.** A history of sensitivity to shellfish may be the only clue to an iodine sensitivity, which may

be significant because iodinated intravenous contrast material is used for intravenous pyelography (IVP), enhanced computed tomography (CT) scanning, and venography and arteriography. A history of hypersensitivity to intravenously administered iodine-containing compounds or shellfish should be clearly noted, and the patient should not be exposed to iodine-containing compounds unless such exposure is absolutely mandatory. When intravenous contrast material must be used, administration of a glucocorticoid preparation may prevent life-threatening anaphylactic reactions.

3. **Previous surgical procedures, and the patient's course following those surgical procedures, should be reviewed to identify complications of previous operations that might be avoided.** Pertinent medical records from prior surgery should be obtained and reviewed. Reactions and response to anesthetic techniques should be evaluated with the anesthesiologist in charge. The patient should be asked about specific complications, such as excessive bleeding, wound infection, deep vein thrombosis, peritonitis, or bowel obstruction. A history of pelvic surgery should alert the gynecologist to the possibility of distorted surgical anatomy and possible preexisting injury to adjacent organ systems, such as small bowel adhesions in the pelvis or ureteral stenosis from previous periureteral scarring. Intravenous pyelography may be helpful in such cases to establish ureteral anatomy and patency and to identify any preexisting abnormality. Many patients may not be entirely clear about the extent of the previous surgical procedure or the details of intraoperative findings. Therefore, operative notes from previous pelvic operations should be obtained and reviewed to determine the details of the procedure and findings. This is particularly important in patients who have had surgery for pelvic inflammatory disease, pelvic abscess, endometriosis, or pelvic malignancy.

4. **Family history may identify familial traits that might complicate planned surgery.** A family history of excessive intraoperative or postoperative bleeding, malignant hyperthermia, and other potentially inherited conditions should be sought. A general review of systems should also be included in the questioning in an effort to identify any coexisting medical or surgical conditions. Inquiry about gastrointestinal and urologic function is particularly important before undertaking pelvic surgery, and many gynecologic diseases also involve adjacent nongynecologic viscera.

5. **Although many women undergoing gynecologic surgical procedures are otherwise healthy, with pathology identified only on pelvic examination, other major organ systems should not be neglected in the physical examination.** Identification of abnormalities such as a heart murmur or pulmonary compromise should lead the surgeon to obtain additional testing and consultation in order to minimize intraoperative and postoperative complications. Decisions regarding additional testing or consultation should be made in conjunction with the anesthesiologist.

Laboratory Evaluation

The selection of appropriate preoperative laboratory studies will depend on the extent of the anticipated surgical procedure and the patient's medical status.

1. For patients undergoing general anesthesia, a blood count, including hematocrit, white blood cell count, and platelet count, should be obtained routinely.

2. The results of serum chemistry and liver function tests are rarely abnormal in asymptomatic patients who have no significant factors in their medical history and who are not taking medications.

3. Coagulation studies are of little value unless the patient has a significant risk factor in her medical history (1).

4. In women under 40 years of age, a chest radiograph and electrocardiography are of very low yield in identifying asymptomatic cardiopulmonary disease and thus may not be necessary (2,3). However, women over 40 years of age and those undergoing major gynecologic surgical procedures should have a chest radiograph, electrocardiography, and serum electrolyte analysis preoperatively. If the results of these studies are normal, they will serve as baseline data for comparison to other studies that may be required in the evaluation of a postoperative complication.

Radiographic evaluation of adjacent organ systems should be undertaken based on patients' needs.

1. Intravenous pyelography is helpful to delineate ureteral patency and course, especially in the presence of a pelvic mass, gynecologic cancer, or congenital müllerian anomaly. **However, an IVP is not of significant value in the evaluation of most patients undergoing pelvic surgery (4).**

2. A barium enema or upper gastrointestinal studies with small bowel assessment may be of significant value in evaluating some patients before pelvic surgery. Because of the proximity of the female genital tract to the lower gastrointestinal tract, the rectum and sigmoid colon may be involved with benign (endometriosis or pelvic inflammatory disease) or malignant gynecologic conditions. Conversely, a pelvic mass could have a gastrointestinal origin such as a diverticular abscess or a mass of inflamed small intestines (Crohn's disease). Clearly, any patient with gastrointestinal symptoms should be further evaluated.

3. Other imaging studies, including ultrasonography, CT scanning, or magnetic resonance imaging (MRI), are useful only in selected patients.

Preoperative Discussion and Informed Consent

The verbal and nonverbal rapport and trust that exist between the patient and her gynecologist begin on the initial office visit and should be built on during each subsequent visit. During the initial discussion, the physician should explain in sufficient detail to the patient the findings of the examination, the results of testing, the natural history of the disease process, and the goals of the surgical procedure. Because most gynecologic surgery is elective, the gynecologist has the opportunity to evaluate the patient from a medical point of view, as well as to allow the patient to develop psychological coping mechanisms and to answer questions that may not have been discussed initially. The surgeon should be available to discuss in person or by phone any questions that arise before actual hospital admission.

The goals of the preoperative discussion are to allay the patient's anxiety and fears and to answer any questions. The discussion should serve as the basis to expand further on issues relative to the surgery, its expected outcome, and risks as well as to obtain signed informed consent (5). Informed consent is an educational process for the patient and her family and fulfills the physician's need to convey information in understandable terms. The following items should be discussed and, after each item, the patient and family should be invited to ask questions:

1. The nature and extent of the disease process

2. The extent of the actual operation proposed and the potential modifications of the operation, depending on intraoperative findings

3. The anticipated benefits of the operation, with a conservative estimate of successful outcome

4. The risks and potential complications of the surgery

5. Alternative methods of therapy and the risks and results of those alternative methods of therapy

6. The results likely if the patient is not treated.

A discussion of the nature and the extent of the disease process should include an explanation in lay terms of the significance of the disease. Is it life-threatening, or will it likely result in significant disability or dysfunction? To what extent does the disease process alter the patient's daily living? If untreated, could the disease resolve spontaneously, or could it potentially worsen? What is the time course and natural history of the disease?

The goals of surgery should be discussed in detail. Some gynecologic surgical procedures are performed purely for diagnostic purposes (e.g., dilation and curettage, cold knife conization, a diagnostic laparoscopy, or staging laparotomy), while most are clearly aimed at correcting an anatomic defect or a specific disease process. The extent of the surgery should be outlined, including which organs will be removed. Most patients like to be informed regarding the type of surgical incision and the estimated duration of anesthesia.

The expected outcome of the surgical procedure should be explained. If the procedure is being performed for diagnostic purposes, the outcome will depend on surgical or pathologic findings that are not known before surgery. When treating anatomic deformity or disease, the expected success of the operation should be discussed, as well as the potential for failure of the operation. This discussion should include the probability of failure (i.e., failure of tubal sterilization or the possibility that stress urinary incontinence may not be alleviated). When treating cancer, the possibility of finding more advanced disease and the potential need for adjunctive therapy (e.g., postoperative radiation therapy or chemotherapy) should be mentioned. Other issues of importance to the patient include discussion of loss of fertility or loss of ovarian function. These issues should be raised by the physician to ensure that the patient adequately understands the pathophysiology that may result from the surgery and to allow her to express her feelings regarding these emotionally charged issues.

The risks and potential complications of the surgical procedure should be discussed with the patient, including the most frequent complications of the particular procedure. For most major gynecologic surgery, the risks include intraoperative and postoperative hemorrhage, postoperative infection, venous thrombosis, and injury to adjacent viscera. If the patient has a preexisting medical problem, what additional risks might be encountered? Unanticipated findings at the time of surgery should also be mentioned. For example, if the ovaries are found unexpectedly to be diseased, it may be the best surgical judgment that they should be removed.

The usual postoperative course should be discussed in enough detail to allow the patient to understand what to expect in the days following surgery. Information regarding the need for a suprapubic catheter or prolonged central venous monitoring helps the patient accept her postoperative course and avoids surprises to the patient that may be very disconcerting. The expected duration of the recovery period, both in and out of the hospital, should be noted.

Alternative methods of therapy should be mentioned as part of the preoperative discussion. Other medical management or surgical approaches should be discussed, along with their potential benefits and complications. Finally, the patient should have an understanding of the outcome of the disease if nothing is done. Following this discussion, it should be clear to the patient why the proposed surgery is the appropriate next step in her care. The preoperative discussion and signing of the consent form should include witnesses—a family member and another member of the health care team. The informed consent discussion detailing the information given to the patient should be documented in the patient's chart.

The anesthesiologist responsible for the surgical procedure should also have the opportunity to examine the patient, review her laboratory findings, and discuss the proposed anesthetic method with the patient. In many institutions, the consent to the administration of anesthetic is included in the surgical consent form, whereas in other institutions it is a separate form that should be obtained by the anesthesiologist after appropriate preoperative discussion.

General Considerations

Nutrition

In general, patients undergoing elective gynecologic surgery have adequate nutritional stores and, for the most part, do not require nutritional support. However, **all patients should have a nutritional assessment, especially those undergoing surgery for gynecologic cancer and other major gynecologic procedures in which a prolonged postoperative recovery is expected.** Reassessment of nutritional status should also be performed at regular intervals postoperatively until the patient has successfully returned to a regular diet.

A nutritional assessment includes a careful history and physical examination, which are the most useful, reliable, and cost-effective methods of assessing a patient's nutritional status. In particular, information about recent weight loss as well as the patient's dietary history should be noted. Evidence of malnutrition that can be detected on physical examination includes temporal wasting, muscle wasting, ascites, and edema. Accurate height and weight measurements should be obtained and an ideal body weight, percent ideal body weight, and percent usual body weight may be calculated. Patients who have lost less than 6% of their ideal body weight do not need preoperative nutritional intervention. However, **patients who have lost more than 12% of their ideal body weight should be considered for preoperative intervention.** Patients who have lost between 6% and 12% of their body weight should undergo further studies to determine if preoperative intervention is needed. In addition to routine preoperative laboratory tests, data on albumin, transferrin, zinc, lipids, and liver function may be obtained. In selected patients, additional laboratory assessments such as vitamin B_{12}, folate, copper, manganese, prothrombin time, and creatinine values may be useful in the nutritional assessment.

A variety of techniques have been developed to determine nutritional state, including isotope dilution, γ neutron activation, and anthropometric measurements. Anthropometric measurements of skin-fold thickness and arm-muscle circumference provide an estimate of total body fat and lean muscle mass. Isotope dilution techniques have been used to determine the ratios of exchangeable sodium and potassium, which can determine body cell mass and thus give another parameter for chronic malnutrition. Whole body counters that can measure radioactive intracellular calcium can also be used to determine skeletal muscle mass. More recently, γ neutron activation has been used to measure total body nitrogen, which is currently considered the state-of-the-art method for the determination of total body protein (6,7). Unfortunately, these measurements have not been reproducible and traditionally have been poor predictors of nutritional status and clinical outcome (8,9).

The degree of malnutrition can in part be determined by serum concentrations of albumin, transferrin, prealbumin, and retinal binding protein (RBP). The levels of these serum proteins are greatly influenced by the patient's level of hydration. Prealbumin and RBP have the shortest half-lives, and levels are depressed very early in comparison with serum transferrin and albumin, which have half-lives of 8 and 20 days, respectively (10). A quick assessment of malnutrition can be performed based on the patient's weight, appetite, and serum albumin levels. **An unintentional weight loss of $\geq$5 pounds over 3 weeks, anorexia, or**

a serum albumin level <3.5 g/dl are indicative of malnutrition. Serum albumin was determined to be a decent substitute for the Prognostic Nutritional Index (PNI), which is a time-consuming calculation, in assessing malnutrition in women with gynecologic malignancies (11).

No single test accurately predicts the outcome in malnourished surgical patients. A number of formulas incorporating a variety of nutritional indices have been proposed to assess the perioperative risk secondary to malnutrition. Mullen and co-workers have prospectively evaluated a model that incorporates albumin (ALB), triceps skin-fold thickness (TSF), transferrin (TFN), and delayed hypersensitivity (DH). By a step-wise regression analysis, a linear predictive model called the PNI was developed to relate these factors. It is calculated as follows:

$$\mathbf{PNI\ (\%) = 158 - 16.6\,(ALB) - 0.78\,(TSF) - 0.20\,(TFN) - 5.8\,(DH).}$$

This model was tested on 100 patients undergoing elective surgery and was shown to be valid (12).

Despite the variety of tests and calculations, the decisions regarding the need for nutritional support should be based on several individualized factors. These factors include the patient's prior nutritional state, the anticipated length of time in which the patient will not be able to eat, the severity of surgery, and the likelihood of complications. The nutritional assessment should also determine whether the cause of the malnutrition is increased enteral loss (malabsorption, intestinal fistula), decreased oral intake, increased nutritional requirements as a result of hypermetabolism (sepsis, malignancy), or a combination of these factors. Moderate to severe malnutrition occurs either as a consequence of the patient's diagnosis or possibly from the therapeutic modality used to treat her disease (13,14). Severe malnutrition, if not corrected, can contribute to further postoperative complications by causing altered immune function, chronic anemia, impaired wound healing and, eventually, multiple organ system failure and death.

The patient's nutritional requirements are also increased by surgery. Indices of nutrition were abnormal in 50% of patients who were hospitalized for more than 1 week after surgery (14). Surgery increases the nutritional requirements for several reasons. First, there is a period following surgery during which oral intake is not allowed or is very limited. In addition, the operation itself causes increased protein catabolism, increased energy requirements, and a negative nitrogen balance. If the surgery is uncomplicated and the patient is without food for less than 7 days, this response is limited and patients usually recover without the need for nutritional support. An adequate diet is defined as providing 75% of estimated caloric and protein needs. Therefore, if an adequate oral diet is not expected for 7 to 10 days, perioperative nutritional support may be required to avoid progressive malnutrition and its associated complications. Perioperative nutritional support can reduce operative morbidity and decrease hospitalization when it is commenced early in the postoperative course. Therefore, in patients with either normal nutritional indices or mild or moderate malnutrition who will be undergoing surgical procedures likely to require a prolonged catabolic period of more than 7 to 10 days, total parenteral nutrition (TPN) should be instituted in the early postoperative period as soon as the patient is hemodynamically stable. This type of management should be strongly considered in patients undergoing pelvic exenterations, urinary diversions, or multiple enterectomies (15).

Preoperative nutritional support is indicated for patients who have significant preexisting malnutrition or who require major elective surgery. Preoperative nutritional support is recommended for at least 5 to 7 days prior to surgery to correct electrolyte imbalances and nutritional deficits. Starker and others recommended the following markers to determine adequate nutritional support: weight, fluid status, and serum albumin. In this study patients who exhibited weight loss, diuresis, and a rise in serum albumin after initiation of TPN had an extremely low risk of postoperative morbidity. In contrast, patients who exhibited additional fluid retention, weight gain, and a decline in serum albumin had a significantly higher risk of postoperative complications. In this group of patients, an additional 5 to 7 days of TPN was recommended before proceeding with surgical interventions (16). Nutritional support should be tapered and stopped at midnight prior to surgery and then restarted 24 to 72 hours after the procedure and continued until the patient is able to meet nutritional requirements.

Calculation of Caloric Requirements

The most precise method for calculating a patient's daily caloric requirements is indirect calorimetry. This method is very costly, however, and is not used routinely in clinical practice. Caloric requirements can be calculated based on Long's modification of the Harrison-Benedict formula for actual energy expenditure (AEE) (17). This is the most accurate available method to calculate an individual's AEE.

$$\textbf{AEE (women)} = (\textbf{655.10} + \textbf{9.56 weight [kg]} + \textbf{4.85 height [cm]} - \textbf{4.68 age [yr]}) \times \textbf{activity factor} \times \textbf{injury factor}$$

- Activity factor: confined to bed (1.2), out of bed (1.3)
- Injury factory: minor surgery (1.2), skeletal trauma (1.3), major sepsis (1.6), severe burn (2.1)

1. **The daily caloric requirements can be met by providing 1,000 calories more than the patient's basal energy expenditure.** Alternatively, daily caloric requirements can be met by giving the patient 35 kcal/kg per day for maintenance and 45 kcal/kg per day for anabolic states. Daily nitrogen requirements may be met by providing 1 g of nitrogen (6.25 g of protein) for every 125 to 150 calories.

2. **The maximal rate of glucose oxygenation in adults is approximately 7 g/kg per day.** Patients with very high caloric requirements or diabetes mellitus should receive calories in excess of this in the form of lipids. *Insulin* should be used to maintain serum glucose concentration between 150 and 250 mg/dl, and it may be added directly to the TPN solution. Glucose administration in excess of the caloric requirements can lead to fatty infiltration of the liver and other metabolic complications.

3. **Lipid in a 10% to 20% emulsion can be given as further caloric supplement.** More calories can be given in the form of free fatty acids, which are the major source of energy for most peripheral tissues. When lipids are used as a major source of calories, a minimum of 50 to 150 g/day of glucose should also be given to provide a substrate for the central nervous system. Most patients can tolerate up to 2 g of fat/kg per day, and daily dosages should not exceed 4 g of fat/kg per day. These lipid emulsions are isotonic and can be delivered simultaneously with the protein and carbohydrate mixture in a 3-liter bag for infusion over 24 hours. In general, 30% to 50% of nonprotein calories should be supplied in lipid form. Serum triglyceride levels should be monitored to ensure that the patient can metabolize the fat.

4. **In addition to calories and protein, nutritional support should be maintained in terms of electrolytes, vitamins, and trace elements.** Daily maintenance requirements for electrolytes are as follows: sodium, 60 to 120 mEq; potassium, 30 to 40 mEq; chloride, 60 to 120 mEq; magnesium, 8 to 10 mEq; calcium, 200 to 400 mg; and phosphorous, 300 to 400 mg. A number of vitamins and trace elements must also be supplied to ensure that the patient is eumetabolic.

Route of Administration

After the decision has been made that nutritional support is required, the appropriate route of administration must be determined. Enteral nutrition should be considered primarily because it is easy to deliver, associated with the fewest complications, linked to enhanced wound healing, and relatively inexpensive (18). Contraindications to this route of delivery include intestinal obstruction, gastrointestinal bleeding, and diarrhea. Many different types are commercially available and can be chosen based on their caloric content, fat content, protein content, osmolality, viscosity, and price. Depending on the patient's problem, the route of delivery may be through a Dobhoff feeding tube, a gastrostomy tube, or a feeding jejunostomy tube. If the gastrointestinal tract is unusable for more than 7 days postoperatively, TPN should be implemented.

Total parenteral nutrition must be delivered through a central vein and has gained wide acceptance as a means of providing nutritional support for surgically ill patients. It must be delivered through a subclavian or internal jugular vein, and the catheter must be placed using meticulous sterile surgical technique. Proper daily care is required to avoid infectious complications, and a eumetabolic state may be obtained if multivitamins (including folate and B_{12}) and trace metals (cobalt, iodine, manganese, and zinc) are used to supplement the 2 to 3 L/day of TPN solution. Essential fatty acids are supplied weekly, and iron may be added if hyperalimentation is prolonged and bone marrow stores have become depleted. Appropriate adjustments in the contents of the TPN are required for patients with liver, renal, or cardiac dysfunction. When managed by an experienced team, the most frequent complication, infection, can be reduced to a very reasonable level (5% to 10%) (19).

Postoperative Outcome

A number of retrospective clinical studies, mostly from the general surgical literature, have demonstrated that nutritional support improves postoperative outcome in a variety of categories, including surgical complications, sepsis, wound infections, and mortality. A number of prospective randomized trials, however, have failed to demonstrate that the widespread use of preoperative TPN improves clinical outcome (20–24). The largest, most carefully executed, prospective, randomized trial evaluating perioperative TPN use was reported by the Veterans Affairs Total Parenteral Nutrition Cooperative Study Group (24). The study evaluated a series of 395 malnourished patients who were randomly assigned to receive TPN for 7 to 15 days before surgery and 3 days postoperatively (treatment arm) or no perioperative TPN (control arm). The patients were then followed for 90 days after the surgery and were evaluated in terms of morbidity and mortality. Major complications during the first 30 days, as well as the overall 90-day mortality rates, were then analyzed and were similar in both the treated and control arms. However, in a small group of patients with extremely severe malnutrition, the incidence of noninfectious complications was significantly less common in the group given TPN. In this study, severe malnutrition was defined as a nutritional risk index score of less than 83. The authors of that study concluded that preoperative TPN should be limited to patients who were severely malnourished unless there were other specific indications.

The effect of postoperative TPN on outcome was evaluated in patients undergoing major surgery, regardless of their nutritional status. Three hundred patients were randomized to either TPN or prolonged glucose administration for up to 15 days. There were no significant differences among the two groups with respect to mortality rate or complications. Sixty percent of patients were tolerating enteral intake by 8 to 9 days after surgery, signifying that the majority of patients do not require nutritional support. However, 20% of patients in the glucose-only arm were unable to tolerate oral intake within 15 days of their operations. For these patients, institution of TPN represented a life-saving therapy. Unfortunately, a method of preoperative identification of this group has not been established. Interestingly 20% of the TPN-only arm could not tolerate the nutritional therapy and required treatment modifications. This group had a higher mortality rate than the glucose arm that subsequently required parenteral nutrition (36% versus 21%, $P < 0.10$). Therefore, suboptimal nutrition includes not only too little nutrition, but also too much nutritional support (25).

In summary, clinical trials have demonstrated that TPN can improve nutritional status as measured by biochemical assays, immune function, and nitrogen balance. The effect of TPN on clinical outcome, however, is less well established. Despite what would seem reasonable based on common sense as well as preoperative nutritional parameters, the data do not support TPN for mild to moderately malnourished patients. With severe malnutrition, preoperative TPN would seem to be beneficial and should be instituted.

Fluid and Electrolytes

Water constitutes approximately 50% to 55% of the body weight of the average woman. Two-thirds of this water is contained in the intracellular compartment. One-third is contained in the extracellular compartment, of which one-fourth is contained in plasma, and the remaining three-fourths is in the interstitium.

Osmolarity, or tonicity, is a property derived from the number of particles in a solution. Sodium and chloride are the primary electrolytes contributing to the osmolarity of the extracellular compartment. Potassium and, to a lesser extent, magnesium and phosphate are the major intracellular electrolytes. Water flows freely between the intracellular and the extracellular spaces to maintain osmotic neutrality throughout the body. Any shifts in osmolarity in any fluid spaces within the body are accompanied by corresponding shifts in free water from spaces of lower to higher osmolarity, thus maintaining equilibrium.

The average adult daily fluid maintenance requirement is approximately 30 ml/kg per day, or 2,000 to 3,000 ml/day (26). **This is offset partially by insensible losses of 1,200 ml/day, which includes losses from the lungs (600 ml), skin (400 ml), and gastrointestinal tract (200 ml).** Urinary output from the kidney will provide the remainder of the fluid loss, and this output will vary depending on total body intake of water and sodium. Approximately 600 to 800 mOsm of solute are excreted by the kidney per day. Healthy kidneys can concentrate urine up to approximately 1,200 mOsm and, therefore, the minimum output can range between 500 and 700 ml/day. The maximal urine output of the kidney can be as high as 20 L/day, as seen in patients with diabetes insipidus. In healthy individuals, the kidney adjusts output commensurate with daily fluid intake.

The major extracellular buffer used in the acid-base balance is the bicarbonate-carbonic acid system: $CO_2 + H_2O - H_2CO_3 - H^+ + HCO_3^-$ (27). Typically, the body will maintain a bicarbonate-to-carbonic acid ratio of 20.1 in order to maintain an extracellular pH of 7.4. Both the lung and the kidney play integral roles in the maintenance of normal extracellular pH via retention or excretion of carbon dioxide and bicarbonate. Under conditions of alkalosis, minute ventilation decreases and renal excretion of bicarbonate increases to restore the normal ratio of bicarbonate to carbonic acid. The opposite occurs with acidosis.

Ultimately, the kidney plays the most important role in fluid and electrolyte balance through excretion and retention of water and solute. Circulating antidiuretic hormone and aldosterone help modulate the process. Serum osmolarity affects hypothalamic release of antidiuretic hormone and aldosterone secretion in response to renal perfusion. Under states of dehydration or hypovolemia, serum antidiuretic hormone levels increase, leading to increased resorption of water in the distal tubule of the kidney. In addition, increased aldosterone release promotes increased sodium and water retention. The opposite occurs in states of fluid excess. As a result, individuals with normal renal function and circulating antidiuretic hormone and aldosterone levels maintain normal serum osmolarity and electrolyte composition, despite daily fluctuations of fluid and electrolyte intake.

Various disease states can alter the normal fluid and electrolyte homeostatic mechanisms, making perioperative fluid and electrolyte management more difficult. Patients with intrinsic renal disease are unable to excrete solute and to maintain acid-base balance. In patients undergoing the stress of chronic starvation or severe illness, there may be an inappropriately high level of circulating antidiuretic hormone and aldosterone, resulting in fluid and sodium retention. With severe cardiac disease, secondary renal hypoperfusion can lead to increased aldosterone synthesis and, therefore, increased sodium and water retention by the kidney. Finally, patients with severe diabetes can have significant osmotic diuresis as well as acid-base dysfunction secondary to circulating ketoacids. Correction and optimization of renal, cardiac, or endocrine disorders preoperatively are imperative and will often rectify fluid and electrolyte abnormalities.

Fluid and electrolyte management in the preoperative and perioperative periods requires knowledge of the daily fluid and electrolyte requirements for maintenance, replacement of ongoing fluid and electrolyte losses, as well as correction of any existing abnormalities.

Fluid and Electrolyte Maintenance Requirements

The body adjusts to higher and lower volumes of intake by changes in plasma tonicity. Alterations in plasma tonicity induce adjustments in circulating antidiuretic hormone levels, which ultimately regulate the amount of water retained in the distal tubule of the kidney. In the preoperative and the early postoperative periods, it is usually only necessary to replace sodium and potassium. Chloride is automatically replaced, concomitant with sodium and potassium, because chloride is the usual anion used to balance sodium and potassium in electrolyte solutions. There are various commercially available solutions containing 40 mmol of sodium chloride, with smaller amounts of potassium, calcium, and magnesium designed to meet the requirements of a patient who is receiving 3 L of intravenous fluids per day. The daily requirement, however, can be met by any combination of intravenous fluids. For example, 2 liters of D5 (5% dextrose)/0.45 normal saline (7 mEq sodium chloride each), supplemented with 20 mEq of potassium chloride, followed by 1 liter of D5W (5% dextrose in water) with 20 mEq of potassium chloride, would suffice.

Fluid and Electrolyte Replacement

Fluid and electrolyte losses beyond the daily average must be replaced by appropriate solutions. The choice of solutions for replacement depends on the composition of the fluids lost. Often, it is difficult to measure free water loss, particularly in patients who have high losses from the lungs, skin, or the gastrointestinal tract. Weighing these patients daily can be very useful. Up to 300 g of weight loss daily can be attributable to weight loss from catabolism of protein and fat in the patient who is taking nothing by mouth (26). Anything beyond this, however, would be due to fluid loss and should be replaced accordingly.

Patients with a high fever can have increased pulmonary and skin loss of free water, sometimes in excess of 2 to 3 L/day. These losses should be replaced with free water in the form of D5W. Perspiration typically has one-third the osmolarity of plasma and can be replaced with D5W or, if excessive, with D5/0.25 normal saline.

The patient with acute blood loss needs replacement with appropriate isotonic fluid or blood or both. There are a wide range of plasma volume expanders, including albumin, dextran, and hetastarch solutions, which contain large-molecular-weight particles (>50,000 molecular weight). These particles are slow to exit the intravascular space, and about one-half of the particles remain after 24 hours. These solutions are expensive, however, and for most cases, simple replacement with 0.9 normal saline or lactated Ringer's solution will suffice. One-third of the volume of lactated Ringer's solution or normal saline typically will remain in the intravascular space, and the remainder goes to the interstitium.

Appropriate replacement of gastrointestinal fluid loss depends on the source of fluid loss in the gastrointestinal tract. Gastrointestinal secretions beyond the stomach and up to the colon are typically isotonic with plasma, with similar amounts of sodium, slightly lower amounts of chloride, slightly alkaline pH, and more potassium (in the range of

10 to 20 mEq/L). Under normal conditions, stool is hypotonic. However, under conditions of increased flow (i.e., severe diarrhea), stool contents are isotonic with a composition similar to that of the small bowel contents. Gastric contents are typically hypotonic, with one-third the sodium of plasma, increased amounts of hydrogen ion, and low pH.

In patients who have gastric outlet obstruction, nausea, and vomiting, or who undergo nasogastric suction, appropriate replacement of gastric secretions can be provided with a solution such as D5/0.45 normal saline with 20 mEq/L of potassium. Potassium supplementation is particularly important to prevent hypokalemia in these patients, whose kidneys attempt to conserve hydrogen ions in the distal tubule of the kidney in exchange for potassium ions.

In patients with bowel obstruction, 1 to 3 liters of fluid can be sequestered daily in the gastrointestinal tract. This fluid should be replaced with isotonic saline or lactated Ringer's solution. Similarly, patients with enterocutaneous fistulas or new ileostomies should receive replacement with isotonic fluids.

Correction of Existing Fluid and Electrolyte Abnormalities

Patients who have fluid or electrolyte abnormalities preoperatively can pose a diagnostic challenge. The correct diagnosis and therapy is contingent on a correct assessment of total body fluid and electrolyte status. The management of hyponatremia, for example, may be either fluid restriction or fluid replacement. The choice of treatment depends on whether there is overall extracellular fluid excess and normal body sodium stores or decreased overall total body sodium stores and extracellular fluid. A detailed history is necessary to disclose any underlying medical illness and to assess the amount and duration of any abnormal fluid losses or intake. Initial evaluation should include an assessment of hemodynamic, clinical, and urinary parameters in order to determine the overall level of hydration as well as the fluid status of the extracellular fluid compartment. The patient who has good skin turgor, moist mucosa, stable vital signs, and good urinary output is well hydrated. Nonpitting edema is indicative of extracellular fluid excess, whereas patients with orthostasis, sunken eyes, parched mouth, and decreased skin turgor clearly have extracellular volume contraction. A patient's overall extracellular fluid status does not always reflect the hydration status of the intravascular compartment, however. A patient can have increased interstitial fluid and yet be intravascularly dry, requiring replacement with isotonic fluid.

The laboratory workup for patients who may have preexisting fluid problems should include assessment of blood hematocrit, serum chemistry, glucose, blood urea nitrogen (BUN) and creatinine, urine osmolarity, and urine electrolyte levels. Serum osmolarity is mainly a function of the concentration of sodium and is given by the following equation:

$$\mathbf{2 \times Na^{+} + glucose\ (mg/dl)/18 + BUN\ (mg/dl)/2.8.}$$

Normal serum osmolarity is typically 290 to 300 mOsm. Blood hematocrit will rise or fall inversely at a rate of 1% per 500-ml alteration of extracellular fluid volume. The BUN-to-creatinine ratio is typically 10:1 but will rise to a ratio of greater than 20:1 under conditions of extracellular fluid contraction. Under conditions of extracellular fluid deficit, urine osmolarity will typically be high (>400 mOsm), whereas urine sodium concentration is low (<15 mEq/L) indicative of an attempt by the kidney to conserve sodium. Under conditions of extracellular fluid excess or in cases of renal disease in which the kidney has impaired ability to retain sodium and water, urine osmolarity will be low and urine sodium will be high (>30 mEq/L). Finally, changes in sodium can give insight into the degree of extracellular fluid excess or deficit. In the average person, the serum sodium rises by 3 mmol/L for every liter of water deficit and falls by 3 mmol/L for each liter of water excess. One must be careful in making these estimates, however, because patients with prolonged water and electrolyte loss can have low serum sodium levels and marked water deficits.

Specific Electrolyte Disorders

Hyponatremia

Because sodium is the major extracellular cation, shifts in serum sodium levels are usually inversely correlated with the hydration state of the extracellular fluid compartment. The pathophysiology of hyponatremia, then, is usually expansion of body fluids leading to excess total body water (27,28). Symptomatic hyponatremia usually does not occur until the serum sodium is below 120 to 125 mEq/L. The severity of the symptoms (nausea, vomiting, lethargy, seizures) is related more to the rate of change of serum sodium than to the actual serum sodium level.

Hyponatremia in the form of extracellular fluid excess can be seen in patients with renal or cardiac failure as well as in conditions such as nephrotic syndrome, in which total body salt and water are increased, with a relatively greater increase in the latter. Administration of hypertonic saline to correct the hyponatremia would be inappropriate in this setting. The treatment should include, in addition to correcting the underlying disease process, water restriction with diuretic therapy. Inappropriate secretion of antidiuretic hormone (ADH) can occur with head trauma, pulmonary or cerebral tumors, and states of stress. The abnormally elevated ADH results in excess water retention. Treatment includes water restriction and, if possible, correction of the underlying cause. *Demeclocycline* has been shown to be effective in this disorder via its action in the kidney.

Inappropriate replacement of body salt losses with water alone will result in hyponatremia. This will typically occur in patients losing large amounts of electrolytes secondary to vomiting, nasogastric suction, diarrhea, or gastrointestinal fistulas, and who received replacement with hypotonic solutions. Simple replacement with isotonic fluids and potassium will usually correct the abnormality. Rarely, rapid correction of the hyponatremia is necessary, in which case hypertonic saline (3%) can be administered. Hypertonic saline should be administered very cautiously in order to avoid a rapid shift in serum sodium, which will induce central nervous system dysfunction.

Hypernatremia

Hypernatremia is an uncommon condition that can be life-threatening if severe (serum sodium >160 mEq/L). The pathophysiology is extracellular fluid deficit. The resultant hyperosmolar state leads to decreased water volume in cells in the central nervous system, which, if severe, can cause disorientation, seizures, intracranial bleeding, and death. The causes include excessive extrarenal water loss, which can occur in patients who have a high fever, have undergone tracheostomy in a dry environment, or have extensive thermal injuries; who have diabetes insipidus, either central or nephrogenic; and who have iatrogenic salt loading. The treatment involves correction of the underlying cause (correction of fever, humidification of the tracheostomy, administration of pitressin for control of central diabetes insipidus) and replacement with free water either by the oral route or intravenously with D5W. As with severe hyponatremia, marked hypernatremia should be corrected slowly.

Hypokalemia

Hypokalemia may be encountered preoperatively in patients with significant gastrointestinal fluid loss (prolonged emesis, diarrhea, nasogastric suction, intestinal fistulas) and marked urinary potassium loss secondary to renal tubular disorders (renal tubular acidosis, acute tubular necrosis, hyperaldosteronism, prolonged diuretic use). It can also arise from prolonged administration of potassium-free parenteral fluids in patients who are restricted from ingesting anything by mouth. The symptoms associated with hypokalemia include neuromuscular disturbances, ranging from muscle weakness to flaccid paralysis, and cardiovascular abnormalities, including hypotension, bradycardia, arrhythmias, and enhancement of digitalis toxicity. These symptoms rarely occur unless the serum potassium is <3 mEq/L. The treatment is potassium replacement. Oral therapy is preferable in patients who are on an oral diet. If necessary, potassium replacement can be given intravenously in doses that should not exceed 10 mEq/hr.

Hyperkalemia

Hyperkalemia is encountered infrequently in preoperative patients. It is usually associated with renal impairment but can also be seen in patients who have adrenal insufficiency, are taking potassium-sparing diuretics, and have marked tissue breakdown such as that occurring with crush injuries, massive gastrointestinal bleeding, or hemolysis. The clinical manifestations are mainly cardiovascular. Marked hyperkalemia (potassium >7 mEq/L) can result in bradycardia, ventricular fibrillation, and cardiac arrest. The treatment chosen depends on the severity of the hyperkalemia and whether there are associated cardiac abnormalities detected with electrocardiography. *Calcium gluconate* (10 ml of a 10% solution), given intravenously, can offset the toxic effects of hyperkalemia on the heart. One ampule each of sodium bicarbonate and D50, with or without insulin, will cause a rapid shift of potassium into cells. Over the longer term, cation exchange resins such as *sodium polystyrene sulfate* (*Kayexalate*), taken orally or by enema, will bind and decrease total body potassium. Hemodialysis is reserved for emergent conditions in which other measures are not sufficient or have failed.

Postoperative Fluid and Electrolyte Management

Several hormonal and physiologic alterations in the postoperative period may complicate fluid and electrolyte management. The stress of surgery induces an inappropriately high level of circulating ADH. Circulating aldosterone levels also are increased, especially if sustained episodes of hypotension have occurred either intraoperatively or postoperatively. The elevated levels of circulating ADH and aldosterone make patients prone to sodium and water retention postoperatively.

Total body fluid volume may be altered significantly postoperatively. First, 1 ml of free water is released for each gram of fat or tissue that is catabolized and, in the postoperative period, several hundred milliliters of free water is released daily from tissue breakdown, particularly in the patient who has undergone extensive intraabdominal dissection and who is restricted from ingesting food and fluids by mouth. This free water is often retained in response to the altered levels of ADH and aldosterone. Second, fluid retention is further enhanced by third spacing, or sequestration of fluid in the surgical field. **The development of an ileus may result in an additional 1 to 3 liters of fluid per day being sequestered in the bowel lumen, bowel wall, and peritoneal cavity.**

In contrast to renal sodium homeostasis, the kidney lacks the capacity for retention of potassium. In the postoperative period, the kidneys will continue to excrete a minimum of 30 to 60 mEq/L of potassium daily, irrespective of the serum potassium level and total body potassium stores (27). If this potassium loss is not replaced, hypokalemia may develop. Tissue damage and catabolism during the first postoperative day usually result in the release of sufficient intracellular potassium to meet the daily requirements. However, beyond the first postoperative day, potassium supplementation is necessary.

Correct maintenance of fluid and electrolyte balance in the postoperative period starts with the preoperative assessment, with emphasis on establishing normal fluid and electrolyte parameters prior to surgery. Postoperatively, close monitoring of daily weight, urine output, serum hematocrit, serum electrolytes, and hemodynamic parameters will yield the necessary information to make correct adjustments in crystalloid replacement. The normal daily fluid and electrolyte requirements must be met, and any unusual fluid and electrolyte losses, such as from the gastrointestinal tract, lungs, or skin, must be replaced. After the first few postoperative days, third-space fluid begins to mobilize back into the intravascular space, and ADH and aldosterone levels revert to normal. The excess fluid retained perioperatively is thus mobilized and excreted through the kidneys, and exogenous fluid requirements decrease. The patient with inadequate cardiovascular or renal reserve is prone to fluid overload during this time of third-space reabsorption, especially if intravenous fluids are not appropriately reduced.

The most common fluid and electrolyte disorder in the postoperative period is fluid overload. The fluid excess can occur concomitant with normal or decreased serum sodium. Large amounts of isotonic fluids are usually infused intraoperatively and postoperatively to maintain blood pressure and urine output. Because the infused fluid is often isotonic with plasma, it will remain in the extracellular space. Under such conditions, serum sodium will remain within normal levels. Fluid excess with hypotonicity (decreased serum sodium) can occur if large amounts of isotonic fluid losses (e.g., blood and gastrointestinal tract) are inappropriately replaced with hypotonic fluids. Again, the predisposition toward retention of free water in the immediate postoperative period compounds the problem. An increase in body weight occurs concomitant with the fluid expansion. In the patient who is not allowed anything by mouth, catabolism should induce a daily weight loss as great as 300 g/day. Clearly, the patient who is gaining weight in excess of 150 g/day is in a state of fluid expansion. Simple fluid restriction will correct the abnormality. When necessary, diuretics can be used to increase urinary water excretion.

States of fluid dehydration are uncommon but will occur in patients who have large daily fluid losses that are not replaced. Gastrointestinal losses should be replaced with the appropriate fluids. Patients with high fevers should be given appropriate free water replacement, because up to 2 L/day of free water can be lost through perspiration and hyperventilation. Although these increased losses are difficult to monitor, a reliable estimate can be obtained by monitoring body weight.

Postoperative Acid-base Disorders

A variety of metabolic, respiratory, and electrolyte abnormalities in the postoperative period can result in an imbalance in normal acid-base homeostasis, leading to alkalosis or acidosis. Changes in the respiratory rate will directly affect the amount of carbon dioxide that is exhaled. *Respiratory acidosis* will result from carbon dioxide retention in patients who have hypoventilation from central nervous system depression. This condition can result from oversedation with narcotics, particularly in the presence of concurrent severe chronic obstructive pulmonary disease. *Respiratory alkalosis* can result from hyperventilation caused by excitation of the central nervous system by drugs, pain, or excess ventilator support. Numerous metabolic derangements can result in *alkalosis* or *acidosis.* Proper fluid and electrolyte replacement as well as maintenance of adequate tissue perfusion will help prevent most acid-base disorders that occur during the postoperative period.

Alkalosis

The most common acid-base disorder encountered in the postoperative period is alkalosis (27). Alkalosis is usually of no clinical significance and resolves spontaneously. Several etiologic factors may include hyperventilation associated with pain; posttraumatic transient hyperaldosteronism, which results in decreased renal bicarbonate excretion; nasogastric suction, which removes hydrogen ions; infusion of bicarbonate during blood transfusions in the form of citrate, which is converted to bicarbonates; administration of exogenous alkali; and use of diuretics. Alkalosis can usually be corrected easily with removal of the inciting cause, as well as with correction of extracellular fluid and potassium deficits (Table 19.1). Full correction can usually be safely achieved over 1 to 2 days.

Marked alkalosis, with serum pH higher than 7.55, can result in serious cardiac arrhythmias or central nervous system seizures. Myocardial excitability is particularly pronounced with concurrent hypokalemia. Under such conditions, fluid and electrolyte replacement may not be sufficient to correct the alkalosis rapidly. *Acetazolamide* (250 to 500 mg), orally

Table 19.1. Causes of Metabolic Alkalosis

Disorder	*Source of Alkali*	*Cause of Renal HCO Retention*
Gastric alkalosis	Gastric mucosa	↓ECF, ↓K
Nasogastric suction		
Vomiting		
Renal alkalosis		
Diuretics	Renal epithelium	↓ECF, ↓K
Respiratory acidosis and diuretics		↓ECF, ↓K, ↑P_{CO_2}
Exogenous base	$NaHCO_3$, Na citrate, Na lactate	Coexisting disorder of ECF, K, Pa_{CO_2}

↓ECF, extracellular fluid depletion; ↓K, potassium depletion; ↑P_{CO_2}, carbon dioxide retention; $NaHCO_3$, sodium bicarbonate; Pa_{CO_2}, partial pressure of carbon dioxide, arterial.

or intravenously, can be given 2 to 4 times daily to induce renal bicarbonate diuresis. Treatment with an acidifying agent is rarely necessary and should be reserved for acutely symptomatic patients (i.e., those with cardiac or central nervous system dysfunction) or for patients with advanced renal disease. Under such conditions, HCl (5 to 10 mEq/hr of a 100-mmol solution) can be given via a central intravenous line. Ammonium chloride can also be given orally or intravenously but should not be given to patients with hepatic disease.

Acidosis

***Metabolic acidosis* is less common than alkalosis during the postoperative period, but acidosis can potentially be serious because of its effect on the cardiovascular system.** Under conditions of acidosis, there are decreased myocardial contractility, a propensity for vasodilation of the peripheral vasculature leading to hypotension, and refractoriness of the fibrillating heart to defibrillation (27). These effects promote decompensation of the cardiovascular system and can hinder attempts at resuscitation.

Metabolic acidosis results from a decrease in serum bicarbonate levels caused by the consumption and replacement of bicarbonate by circulating acids or the replacement by other anions such as chloride. The proper workup includes a measurement of the anion gap:

$$\textbf{Anion gap} = (\mathbf{Na^+ + K^+}) - (\mathbf{Cl^- + HCO_3^-}) = \textbf{10 to 14 mEq/L (normal)}.$$

The anion gap is also composed of circulating protein, sulfate, phosphate, citrate, and lactate (29).

With metabolic acidosis, the anion gap can be increased or normal. An increase in circulating acids will consume and replace bicarbonate ion, thus increasing the anion gap. The causes include an increase in circulating lactic acid secondary to anaerobic glycolysis, such as that seen under conditions of poor tissue perfusion; increased ketoacids, as with cases of severe diabetes or starvation; exogenous toxins; and renal dysfunction, which leads to increased circulating sulfates and phosphates (30). The diagnosis can be established via a thorough history and measurement of serum lactate (normal <2 mmol/L), serum glucose, and renal function parameters. Metabolic acidosis in the face of a normal anion gap is usually the result of an imbalance of the ions chloride and bicarbonate, which occurs under conditions leading to excess chloride and decreased bicarbonate. Hyperchloremic acidosis can be seen in patients who have undergone saline loading. Bicarbonate loss will be seen in patients with small bowel fistulas, new ileostomies, severe diarrhea, or renal tubular acidosis. Finally, in patients with marked extracellular volume expansion, which often occurs postoperatively, the relative decrease in serum sodium and bicarbonate will result in a mild acidosis. A summary of the various causes of metabolic acidosis is shown in Table 19.2.

Table 19.2. Causes of Metabolic Acidosis

	Normal Anion Gap	
High Anion Gap	***Hyperkalemic***	***Hypokalemic***
Uremia	Hyporeninism	Diarrhea
Ketoacidosis	Primary adrenal failure	Renal tubular acidosis
Lactic acidosis	NH_2Cl	Ileal and sigmoid bladders
Aspirin	Sulfur poisoning	Hyperalimentation
Paraldehyde	Early chronic renal failure	
Methanol	Obstructive uropathy	
Ethylene glycol		
Methyl malonic aciduria		

NH_2Cl, chloramine.
From **Narins RG, Lazarus MJ.** Renal system. In: **Vandam LD,** ed. *To make the patient ready for anesthesia: medical care of the surgical patient,* 2nd ed. Menlo Park, CA: Addison Wesley, 1984:67–114.

The treatment of metabolic acidosis depends on the cause. In patients with lactic acidosis, restoration of tissue perfusion is imperative. This can be accomplished through cardiovascular and pulmonary support as needed, oxygen therapy, and aggressive treatment of systemic infection wherever appropriate. Ketosis from diabetes can be corrected gradually with *insulin* therapy. Ketosis resulting from chronic starvation or from lack of caloric support postoperatively can be corrected with nutrition. In patients with normal anion gap acidosis, bicarbonate losses from the gastrointestinal tract should be replaced, excess chloride administration can be curtailed and, where necessary, a loop diuretic can be used to induce renal clearance of chloride. Dilutional acidosis can be corrected with mild fluid restriction.

Bicarbonates should not be given unless serum pH is lower than 7.2 or severe cardiac complications secondary to acidosis are present. Furthermore, close monitoring of serum potassium levels is mandatory. Under states of acidosis, potassium will exit the cell and enter the circulation. The patient with a normal potassium concentration and metabolic acidosis is actually depleted of intracellular potassium. Treatment of the acidosis without potassium replacement will result in severe hypokalemia with its associated risks. A summary of the various acid-base abnormalities and associated therapies is shown in Table 19.3.

Perioperative Pain Management

Although satisfactory analgesia is easily achievable with currently available methods, patients continue to suffer unnecessarily from postoperative pain. Studies have consistently shown that 30% to 40% of patients suffer moderate to severe pain in the postoperative period (31). There are several reasons for the existing inadequacies in pain management. First, patient expectations of pain relief are low and they are not aware of the extent of analgesia that they should expect. In a study of the perception of pain relief after surgery, 86% of patients had moderate to severe pain after surgery, but 70% felt that the pain was as severe as they had expected (32). Second, there is a lack of formal physician training in pain management. This lack is epitomized by the commonly written order prescribing a range of narcotic to be given intramuscularly every 3 to 4 hours as needed, leaving pain management decisions to the nursing staff, with no attempt made to titrate the dose of the prescribed narcotic commensurate with individual patient requirements. Third, attitudes continue to be influenced by the common misconception that the use of narcotics in the postoperative period can result in opioid dependance. In one review, 20% of nurses responding to a staff questionnaire expressed concern that the use of opioid analgesics during the postoperative period could cause addiction (32). Studies have confirmed that nurses will administer less than one-fourth of the total dose of narcotic that is prescribed on an as-needed basis. In order to facilitate acute pain management and reduce the number of adverse outcomes, the American Society of Anesthesiologists has established practice guidelines for acute pain management (33).

Table 19.3. Acid-Base Disorders and Their Treatment

Primary Disorder	Defect	Common Causes	Compensation	Treatment
Respiratory acidosis	Carbon dioxide (hypoventilation)	Central nervous system depression Airway and lung impairment	Renal excretion of acid salts Bicarbonate retention Chloride shift into red blood cells	Restoration ventilation Control of excess dioxide production
Respiratory alkalosis	Hyperventilation	Central nervous excitation system Excess ventilator support	Renal excretion of sodium, potassium bicarbonate Absorption of hydrogen and chloride ions Lactate release from red blood cells	Correction hyperventilation
Metabolic acidosis	Excess loss of base Increased nonvolatile acids	Excess chloride versus sodium Increased bicarbonate loss Lactic, ketoacidosis Uremia Dilutation acidosis	Respiratory alkalosis Renal excretion of hydrogen and chloride ions Resorption of potassium bicarbonate	Increase sodium load give bicarbonate for pH <7.2 Restore buffers, protein, hemoglobin
Metabolic acidosis	Excess loss of chloride and potassium Increased bicarbonate	Gastrointestinal losses of chloride Excess intake of bicarbonate Diuretics Hypokalemia Extracellular fluid volume contraction	Respiratory acidosis May be hypoxia Renal excretion of bicarbonate and potassium Absorption of hydrogen and chloride ions	Increased chloride content Potassium replacement Acetazolamide (Diamox) to waste bicarbonate Vigorous volume replacement Occasional 0.1 NaHCl as needed

NaHCl, sodium hydrochloride.

The *minimal effective analgesic concentration* (MEAC) refers to the serum concentration of a drug below which very little analgesia is achieved. At the MEAC, receptor and plasma concentrations of a drug are in equilibrium. Steady-state drug concentrations above the MEAC are difficult to achieve with intramuscular depot injection (34). In one study, patients receiving intramuscular injections with *meperidine hydrochloride* (*Demerol*) every 4 hours experienced marked intra- and interpatient variations in narcotic drug peak concentrations as well as in the time required to reach these peaks. As a result, serum concentrations of drug were above the MEAC an average of only 35% of each 4-hour dosing interval (35). Variable pain control following intermittent intramuscular injections is the result of inadequate, highly variable, and unpredictable blood concentrations (36). Adequate analgesia can be achieved through intramuscular or subcutaneous modes of administration, but unpredictable absorption can make titration difficult. Small intravenous boluses can be more easily titrated but may be shorter acting, requiring more frequent injections and thus intensive nursing care, whereas larger intravenous boluses may be associated with a higher incidence of central nervous system and respiratory depression. **The *patient-controlled analgesia (PCA) technique,* which allows patients to self-administer small doses of narcotic on demand, allows titration of measured boluses of narcotic as needed to relieve pain and can provide a more thorough analgesia with maintenance of steady-state drug concentrations above the MEAC.**

Irrespective of the route of administration, analgesics must be front loaded in order to provide prompt analgesia from the start. Without front loading, attainment of the MEAC will not occur for at least three elimination half-lives of the narcotic agent that is used. After front loading, additional small boluses of narcotic can be administered until analgesia is achieved. From the total dose of drug required to achieve analgesia, maintenance drug

Table 19.4. Guidelines for Front-Loading IV Analgesics for Relief of Postoperative Pain

Drug	Total Front-Loaded Dose	Increments	Cautions
Morphine	0.08–0.12 mg/kg	0.03 mg/kg q 10 min	Histaminergic effects; nausea; biliary colic; reduce dose for elderly
Meperidine	1.0–1.5 mg/kg	0.30 mg/kg q 10 min	Reduce dose or change drug for impaired renal function
Codeine	0.5–1.0 mg/kg	1/3 of total q 15 min	Nausea
Fentanyl	0.4–1.0 μg/kg	0.2–0.5 μg/kg q 6 min	Bradycardia; minimal hemodynamic alterations

dosages can then be determined and administered either as a continuous infusion or on a scheduled basis, so that the dose of drug administered offsets the amount that is cleared (Table 19.4). Thereafter, prescribed doses of narcotic can be adjusted as needed.

Patient-controlled Analgesia

PCA devices are electronically controlled infusion pumps that deliver a preset dose of narcotic into a patient's indwelling intravenous catheter upon patient request. The devices all contain delay intervals or lockout times during which patient demands for more narcotic are not met. These devices eliminate the delay between the onset of pain and the administration of analgesic agents, a common problem inherent with on-demand analgesic orders in busy hospital wards. Patient-controlled analgesia has enjoyed excellent patient acceptance. Compared with conventional intramuscular injections, serum narcotic levels have significantly lower variability in patients using PCA (34). Patients using PCA have been shown to have improved analgesia, a lower incidence of postoperative pulmonary complications, and less confusion than those given intramuscular narcotics (37). Furthermore, the total dose of narcotic used has been lower with PCA than with conventional intramuscular depot injection.

The use of PCA does not by any means eliminate the adverse side effects of narcotics. Potentially life-threatening respiratory depression is seen in as many as 0.5% of patients using PCA. The use of a continuous narcotic infusion in addition to demand dosing has been associated with a fourfold increase in respiratory depression. Elderly patients and those with preexisting respiratory compromise also are at risk for respiratory depression (34).

Carefully supervised regimens using continuous infusions, on-demand intramuscular therapy, or fixed dosage schedules (every-4-hour dosing) with on-demand supplementation can have analgesic efficacy comparable with PCA. Nonetheless, the type of close supervision required to achieve adequate on-demand analgesia without PCA is difficult to maintain. Use of PCA shortens the time between the onset of pain and the administration of pain medication, provides more continuous access to analgesics, and allows for an overall steadier state of pain control.

Epidural and Spinal Analgesia

Anesthetics and narcotics administered either in the epidural space or intrathecally are among the most potent analgesic agents available; the efficacy of these agents is greater than that provided by intravenous PCA techniques. These drugs can be administered in one of several ways, including a single-shot dose given by epidural or intrathecal injection, intermittent injection given either on schedule or on demand, and continuous infusion.

Because of the risk of central nervous system infections and headaches, intrathecal administration is usually limited to a single dose of narcotic, local anesthetic, or both. In comparison with epidural administration, duration of action for a single dose is increased via the intrathecal route as a result of the high concentrations of drug attained in the cerebrospinal fluid. However, the risk of central nervous system and respiratory depression, as well as systemic hypotension, also is increased. Even the low doses of opioids required for intrathecal analgesia have been associated with an increased risk of respiratory depression (38). Therefore, some investigators have warned against the use of intrathecal spinal analgesia outside the intensive care setting.

Epidural administration is the preferred approach and provides extended (>24 hours) pain control during the postoperative period. Relative contraindications are the presence of coagulopathy, sepsis, and hypotension. Both anesthetic and narcotic agents have been used with excellent efficacy. Among the anesthetic agents, *bupivacaine* has been the most popular, providing excellent analgesia with minimal toxicity. Epidural analgesia is most suited for pain control in the lower abdomen and extremities. Potential adverse effects of epidural anesthetic agents include urinary retention, motor weakness, hypotension, and central nervous system and cardiac depression. In contrast to anesthetic agents, opioids offer excellent analgesia without accompanying sympathetic blockade. Epidural opioids tend to have a much longer duration of action, and hypotension is a rare complication. Compared with epidural anesthetics, however, there is a higher incidence of nausea and vomiting, respiratory depression, and pruritus (39).

Compared with analgesics administered intramuscularly or intravenously, epidural analgesia has been shown to be associated with improved pulmonary function postoperatively, a lower incidence of pulmonary complications, a decrease in postoperative venous thromboembolic complications (most likely secondary to earlier ambulation), fewer gastrointestinal side effects, a lower incidence of central nervous system depression, and shorter convalescence (39). Severe respiratory depression is the most serious potential complication, seen in fewer than 1% of patients. A lower incidence of respiratory depression is seen with the more lipophilic drugs such as *fentanyl,* which is quickly absorbed within the spinal cord and is therefore less likely to diffuse to the central nervous system respiratory control centers. Pruritus, nausea, and urinary retention are common but can be easily managed and are usually of little clinical significance. Cost is perhaps the main and most limiting drawback of epidural analgesia.

Close monitoring by nursing staff is required for safe administration of epidural analgesia. However, an intensive care setting is not necessary. Epidural analgesics can be administered safely in a hospital ward setting under close nursing supervision, using respiratory monitoring with hourly ventilatory checks during the first 8 hours of epidural analgesia.

Nonsteroidal Antiinflammatory Drugs

Nonsteroidal antiinflammatory drugs (NSAIDs) are becoming increasingly popular for the postoperative treatment of pain in patients undergoing major and minor surgical procedures. The NSAID *ketorolac* is a potent drug that can be given intravenously or intramuscularly. *Ketorolac* has a slightly slower onset of activity than *fentanyl* but has an analgesic potency comparable to *morphine.* The theoretical advantages of NSAIDs over opioids include absence of respiratory depression, lack of abuse potential, decreased sedative effects, decreased nausea, early return of bowel function, and faster recovery. In clinical studies, *ketorolac* has been found to have analgesic effects similar to those of morphine in postoperative orthopedic patients and, when used in conjunction with PCA, significantly reduced opioid requirements (40,41). Studies in gynecologic populations have been less positive. One study found no differences in pain scores, *morphine* consumption, or side effects between patients given *ketorolac* intravenously compared with placebo following hysterectomy (42). Because of the potential advantages, many advocate the addition of NSAIDs to opioid therapy for perioperative pain management.

Potential adverse effects associated with the use of NSAIDs include an increased risk of renal compromise (particularly in patients suffering from acute hypovolemia), gastrointestinal side effects, hypersensitivity reactions, and bleeding. Although NSAIDs cause a modest increase in bleeding time, this does not appear to be clinically significant. Controlled prospective studies have not demonstrated a significant increase in blood loss in patients who receive NSAIDs perioperatively. These agents should be used with extreme care, if at all, in patients with asthma, because 5% to 10% of adult patients with asthma are sensitive to *aspirin* and other NSAID preparations. *Ketorolac* is active when administered both intravenously and orally, making it easy to administer in the perioperative setting for patients undergoing minor procedures.

Antibiotic Prophylaxis

Infection at the operative site is a common cause of morbidity in patients undergoing gynecologic surgery. Procedures such as vaginal hysterectomy, abdominal hysterectomy, surgical drainage of pelvic abscess, selected cases of pregnancy termination, and radical surgery for gynecologic malignancy carry a significant risk of postoperative infection. Other risk factors for the development of wound infection include prolonged operative time, prolonged preoperative admission, concurrent infection, and presence of malignancy. Such infections result in considerable morbidity as well as prolonged hospitalization, increased rates of readmission, and substantial cost. Prophylactic antibiotics have been used in an effort to reduce these problems.

Pathogens that can cause contamination during gynecologic surgery are organisms indigenous to the vaginal tract, including gram-positive and gram-negative aerobes and anaerobes (Table 19.5). The primary pathogenic bacteria include coliforms, streptococci, fusobacteria, and *Bacteroides*.

Prophylactic antibiotic use in patients undergoing vaginal hysterectomy is highly effective and widely accepted as the standard of care. A review of the placebo-controlled trials in the literature regarding antibiotic prophylaxis in vaginal and abdominal hysterectomy included 48 studies of 5,524 patients who underwent vaginal hysterectomy and 30 studies of 3,752 patients who underwent abdominal hysterectomy (43). In vaginal hysterectomy, prophylactic antibiotics decreased febrile morbidity from 40% in control patients to 15% in treated patients and lowered pelvic infection rates from 25% in control patients to 5% in treated patients. In this analysis the benefits of prophylaxis were less pronounced with abdominal hysterectomy; prophylactic antibiotics reduced febrile morbidity from 28% in control patients to 16% in treated patients, pelvic infections from 10% to 5%, and wound infections from 8% to 3%. More recently, a metaanalysis of 25 randomized controlled trials revealed that use of antibiotic prophylaxis reduced the incidence of serious infections after abdominal hysterectomy from 21.1% (373 of 1,768) to 9% (166 of 1,836) (44). The authors concluded that because preoperative antibiotics are highly effective in prevention of serious infections associated with total abdominal hysterectomy, they should be used routinely.

The antibiotic chosen for prophylaxis for gynecologic surgery should have activity against the broad range of vaginal organisms. The first- and second-generation cephalosporins are

Table 19.5. Bacteria Indigenous to the Lower Genital Tract

Lactobacillus	*Enterobacter agglomerans*
Diphtheroids	*Klebsiella pneumoniae*
Staphylococcus aureus	*Proteus mirabilis*
Staphylococcus epidermidis	*Proteus vulgaris*
Streptococcus agalactiae	*Morganella morganii*
Streptococcus faecalis	*Citrobacter diversus*
α-Hemolytic streptococci	
Group D streptococci	*Bacteroides* species
Peptostreptococci	*B. bivius*
Peptococcus	*B. disiens*
Clostridium	*B. fragilis*
Gaffky anaerobia	*B. melaninogenicus*
Escherichia coli	
Fusobacterium	
Enterobacter cloacae	

well suited for this purpose because of their activity against gram-positive, gram-negative, and anaerobic organisms. Most classes of antibiotics (including *penicillin, tetracycline, sulfonamide,* broad-spectrum *penicillin,* and cephalosporins) and anaerobic drugs (clindamycin, *metronidazole*) have been shown to be effective prophylactically, but none has been shown to be consistently more effective than first-generation cephalosporins (45–48).

The timing of administration of the prophylactic antibiotic agent is important. Antibiotics given for prophylaxis are most active if present in tissues prior to contamination with an inoculum of bacteria (49). **For patients who undergo hysterectomy, the antibiotic should be present in the tissues prior to opening of the vaginal cuff, at which time vaginal organisms enter the pelvic cavity. Infusion of an antibiotic within 30 minutes of surgery is ideal for this purpose.** For long surgical procedures, particularly when there is a large blood loss or when an antibiotic agent with a short half-life is used, a second antibiotic dose should be given intraoperatively.

Many prospective studies have shown that short courses of prophylactic antibiotics (24 hours or shorter) are as efficacious as longer ones (49). Moreover, several clinical trials have found that one perioperative dose of prophylactic antibiotics is sufficient (50–52). The use of one dose of a prophylactic antibiotic has many advantages, including decreased cost, decreased toxicity, minimal alteration of host flora, and decreased induction of pathogen resistance.

Despite the advantages of using prophylactic antibiotics, the importance of good surgical technique must be emphasized. Delicate handling of tissues, good hemostasis, adequate drainage, and avoidance of unnecessarily large pedicles in ligatures promote healing and lower the risk of complications.

Postoperative Infections

Infections are a major source of morbidity in the postoperative period. Risk factors for infectious morbidity include the absence of perioperative antibiotic prophylaxis, contamination of the surgical field from infected tissues or from spillage of large bowel contents, an immunocompromised host, poor nutrition, chronic and debilitating severe illness, poor surgical technique, and preexisting focal or systemic infection. Sources of postoperative infection can include the lung, urinary tract, surgical site, pelvic side wall, vaginal cuff, abdominal wound, and sites of indwelling intravenous catheters. Early identification and treatment of infection will result in the best outcome from these potentially serious complications.

Although infectious morbidity is an inevitable complication of surgery, the incidence of infections can be decreased by the appropriate use of simple preventive measures. In cases that involve transection of the large bowel, spillage of fecal contents inevitably occurs. A thorough preoperative mechanical and antibiotic bowel preparation in combination with systemic antibiotic prophylaxis will help decrease the incidence of postoperative pelvic and abdominal infections in these patients. The surgeon can further decrease the risk of postoperative infections by using meticulous surgical technique. Blood and necrotic tissue are excellent media for the growth of aerobic and anaerobic organisms. In cases in which there is higher-than-usual potential for serum and blood to collect in spaces that have been contaminated by bacterial spill, closed-suction drainage may reduce the risk of infection. Antibiotic therapy, rather than prophylaxis, should be initiated during surgery in patients who have frank intraabdominal infection or pus.

Elective surgical procedures should be postponed in patients who have infections preoperatively. In an epidemiologic study conducted by the Centers for Disease Control and Prevention, the incidence of nosocomial surgical infections ranged from 4.3% in community hospitals to 7% in municipal hospitals (53). Urinary tract infections accounted for approximately 40% of these nosocomial infections. Infections of the skin and wound accounted for approximately one-third of the infections, and respiratory tract infections accounted for approximately 16%. In patients who had any type of infection prior to surgery, the risk of infection at the surgical wound site was increased fourfold. Rates of infection were higher in older patients, in patients with increased length of surgery, and in those with increased length of hospital stay prior to surgery. The relative risk was 3 times higher in patients with a community-acquired infection prior to surgery. These community-acquired infections included infections of the urinary and respiratory tracts.

Historically, the standard definition of febrile morbidity for surgical patients has been the presence of a temperature higher than or equal to 100.4°F (38°C) on two occasions at least 4 hours apart during the postoperative period, excluding the first 24 hours. However, other **sources have defined fever as two consecutive temperature elevations greater than 101.0°F (38.3°C)** (54,55). Febrile morbidity has been estimated to occur in as many as one-half of patients; however, it is often self-limited, resolving without therapy, and is usually noninfectious in origin (56). Overzealous evaluations of postoperative fever, especially during the early postoperative period, are time consuming, expensive, and sometimes uncomfortable for the patient (55). **The value of 101.0°F is more useful than 100.4°F to distinguish an infectious cause from an inconsequential postoperative fever.**

The assessment of a febrile surgical patient should include a review of the patient's history with regard to risk factors. Both the history and the physical examination should focus on the potential sites of infection (Table 19.6). The examination should include inspection of the pharynx, a thorough pulmonary examination, percussion of the kidneys to assess for costovertebral angle tenderness, inspection and palpation of the abdominal incision, examination of sites of intravenous catheters, and an examination of the extremities for evidence of deep venous thrombosis or thrombophlebitis. In gynecologic patients, an appropriate workup may also include inspection and palpation of the vaginal cuff for signs of induration, tenderness, or purulent drainage. A pelvic examination should also be performed in order to identify a mass consistent with a pelvic hematoma or abscess and to look for signs of pelvic cellulitis.

Patients with fever in the early postoperative period should have an aggressive pulmonary toilet, including incentive spirometry (55). If the fever persists beyond 72 hours postoperatively, additional laboratory and radiologic data may be obtained. The evaluation may include complete and differential white blood cell counts and a urinalysis. In one study, a routine urine culture had a yield of only 9%; therefore, culture should not be analyzed unless indicated by the urinalysis results or symptoms (54). Routine chest radiographs have a yield of 12.5% and should be obtained in asymptomatic patients as well as those with signs and symptoms localizing to the lung (54). Blood cultures can also be obtained but will most likely be of little yield unless the patient has a high fever (102°F). In patients with costovertebral angle tenderness, IVP may be indicated to rule out the presence of ureteral damage or obstruction from surgery, particularly in the absence of laboratory evidence of

Table 19.6. Posthysterectomy Infections

Operative Site	*Nonoperative Site*
Vaginal cuff	Urinary tract
Pelvic cellulitis	Asymptomatic bacteriuria
Pelvic abscess	Cystitis
Supervaginal, extraperitoneal	Pyelonephritis
Intraperitoneal	Respiratory
Adnexa	Atelectasis
Cellulitis	Pneumonia
Abscess	Vascular
Abdominal incision	Phlebitis
Cellulitis	Septic pelvic thrombophlebitis
Simple	
Progressive bacterial synergistic	
Necrotizing fascitis	
Myonecrosis	

urinary tract infection. Patients who have persistent fevers without a clear localizing source should undergo CT scanning of the abdomen and pelvis to rule out the presence of an intraabdominal abscess. Finally, if fever persists in patients who have had gastrointestinal surgery, a barium enema or upper gastrointestinal series with small bowel assessment may be indicated late in the course of the first postoperative week to rule out an anastomotic leak or fistula.

Urinary Tract Infections

Historically, the urinary tract has been the most common site of infection in surgical patients (53). However, the incidence reported in the more recent gynecologic literature has been less than 4% (56,57). This decrease in urinary tract infections is most likely the result of increased perioperative use of prophylactic antibiotics. The incidence of postoperative urinary tract infection in gynecologic surgical patients not receiving prophylactic antibiotics has been confirmed to be as high as 40% (58), and **even a single dose of perioperative prophylactic antibiotic has been shown to decrease the incidence of postoperative urinary tract infection from 35% to 4%** (59).

Symptoms of a urinary tract infection may include urinary frequency, urgency, and dysuria. In patients with pyelonephritis, other symptoms include headache, malaise, nausea, and vomiting. A urinary tract infection is diagnosed on the basis of microbiology and has been defined as the growth of 10^5 organisms/ml of urine cultured. Most infections are caused by coliform bacteria, with *Escherichia coli* being the most frequent pathogen. Other pathogens include *Klebsiella, Proteus,* and *Enterobacter* species. *Staphylococcus* organisms are the causative bacteria in fewer than 10% of cases.

Despite the high incidence of urinary tract infections in the postoperative period, few of these infections are serious. Most are confined to the lower urinary tract, and pyelonephritis is a rare complication (60). Catheterization of the urinary tract, either intermittently or continuously with the use of an indwelling catheter, has been implicated as a main cause of urinary tract contamination (61). In fact, more than 1 million catheter-associated urinary tract infections occur yearly in the United States, and **catheter-associated bacteria remains the most common etiology of gram-negative bacteremia in hospitalized patients.** Bacteria adhere to the surface of urinary catheters and grow within bile films, which appear to protect embedded bacteria from antibiotics, making treatment less effective. Therefore, the use of urinary tract catheters should be minimized. An indwelling catheter should be removed or replaced in a patient undergoing treatment for catheter-related infections.

The treatment of urinary tract infection includes hydration and antibiotic therapy. Commonly prescribed and effective antibiotics include penicillin, sulfonamides, cephalosporins, fluoroquinolones, and nitrofurantoin. The choice of antibiotic should be based on knowledge of the susceptibility of organisms cultured at a particular institution. In some institutions, for example, more than 40% of *E. coli* strains are resistant to *ampicillin.* For uncomplicated urinary tract infections, an antibiotic that has good activity against *E. coli* should be given in the interim while awaiting results of the urine culture and sensitivity data.

Patients who have a history of recurrent urinary tract infections, those with chronic indwelling catheters (Foley catheters or ureteral stents), and those who have urinary conduits should be treated with antibiotics that will be effective against the less common urinary pathogens such as *Klebsiella* and *Pseudomonas.* Chronic use of the fluoroquinolones for prophylaxis is not advised, because these agents are notorious for inducing antibiotic-resistant strains of bacteria.

The respiratory tract is an uncommon site for infectious complications in gynecologic surgical patients. Hemsell noted only six cases of pneumonia in more than 4,000 women who underwent elective hysterectomy (56). This low incidence is probably a reflection of the young age and good health status of gynecologic patients in general. In acute care facilities, pneumonia is a frequent hospital-acquired infection, particularly in elderly patients

(62). Risk factors include extensive or prolonged atelectasis, preexistent chronic obstructive pulmonary disease, severe or debilitating illness, central neurologic disease causing an inability to clear oropharyngeal secretions effectively, and nasogastric suction (62). In surgical patients, early ambulation and aggressive management of atelectasis are the most important preventive measures. The role of prophylactic antibiotics remains unclear.

A significant proportion (40% to 50%) of hospital-acquired pneumonias are caused by gram-negative organisms. These organisms gain access to the respiratory tract from the oral pharynx. Gram-negative colonization of the oral pharynx has been shown to be increased in patients in acute care facilities and has been associated with the presence of nasogastric tubes, preexisting respiratory disease, mechanical ventilation, tracheal intubation, and paralytic ileus, as a result of microbial overgrowth in the stomach (63). Interestingly, the use of antimicrobial drugs seems to significantly increase the frequency of colonization of the oral pharynx with gram-negative bacteria.

A thorough lung examination should be included in the assessment of all febrile surgical patients. In the absence of significant lung findings, a chest radiograph is probably of little benefit in patients at low risk for postoperative pulmonary complications. In patients with pulmonary findings or with risk factors for pulmonary complications, a chest radiograph should be obtained. A sputum sample should also be obtained for Gram stain and culture. The treatment should include postural drainage, aggressive pulmonary toilet, and antibiotics. The antibiotic chosen should be effective against both gram-positive and gram-negative organisms, and in patients who are receiving assisted ventilation, the antibiotic spectrum should include drugs that are active against *Pseudomonas* organisms.

Phlebitis

Intravenous catheter–related infections are common; the reported incidence is from 25% to 35% (64). The intravenous site should be inspected daily, and the catheter should be removed if there is any associated pain, redness, or induration. Unfortunately, phlebitis can occur even with close surveillance of the intravenous site. In one study, more than 50% of the cases of phlebitis became evident more than 12 hours after discontinuation of intravenous catheters (65). In addition, fewer than one-third of patients had symptoms related to the intravenous catheter site 24 hours prior to the diagnosis of phlebitis.

Intravenous catheters should be inserted using sterile technique, and they should be changed frequently. The institution of intravenous therapy teams has decreased the incidence of phlebitis by as much as 50% (64). This decrease is related not so much to surveillance of the intravenous catheter site as it is to frequent changing of intravenous catheters. The incidence of catheter-related phlebitis increases significantly after 72 hours. Therefore, intravenous catheters should be changed at least every 3 days.

Phlebitis can be diagnosed based on the presence of fever, pain, redness, induration, or a palpable venous cord. Occasionally, suppuration will be present. Phlebitis is usually self-limited and resolves within 3 to 4 days. The treatment includes application of warm, moist compresses and prompt removal of any catheters from the infected vein. Antibiotic therapy with antistaphylococcal agents should be instituted for catheter-related sepsis. Excision or drainage of an infected vein is rarely necessary.

Wound Infections

The results of a prospective study of more than 62,000 wounds were revealing in regard to the epidemiology of wound infections (66). The wound infection rate varied markedly, depending on the extent of contamination of the surgical field. The wound infection rate for clean surgical cases (infection not present in the surgical field, no break in aseptic technique, no viscus entered) was lower than 2%, whereas the incidence of wound infections with dirty, infected cases was 40% or higher. Preoperative showers with *hexachlorophene* slightly lowered the infection rate for clean wounds, whereas preoperative shaving of the wound site with a razor increased the infection rate. A 5-minute wound preparation immediately before surgery was as effective as preparation for 10 minutes. The wound infection rate increased with the duration of preoperative hospital stay as well as with the duration of surgery. In addition, incidental appendectomy increased the risk of wound infection in patients undergoing clean surgical procedures. The study concluded that the incidence of wound infections could be decreased by short preoperative hospital stays, hexachlorophene showers prior to surgery, minimizing shaving of the wound site, use of meticulous surgical technique, decreasing operative time as much as possible, bringing drains out through sites other than the wound, and dissemination of information to surgeons regarding their wound infection rates. A program instituting these conclusions led to a fall in the clean wound infection rate from 2.5% to 0.6% over an 8-year period. The wound infection rate in most gynecologic services has been lower than 5%, reflective of the clean nature of most gynecologic operations.

The symptoms of wound infection often occur late in the postoperative period, usually after the fourth postoperative day, and may include fever, erythema, tenderness, induration, and purulent drainage. Wound infections which occur on postoperative days 1 through 3 are generally caused by streptococcal and *Clostridia* infections. The management of wound infections is mostly mechanical and involves opening the infected portion of the wound above the fascia, with cleansing and debridement of the wound edges as necessary. Wound care, consisting of debridement and dressing changes 2 to 3 times daily with mesh gauze, will promote growth of granulation tissue, with gradual filling in of the wound defect by secondary intention. Clean, granulating wounds can often be secondarily closed with good success, shortening the time required for complete wound healing.

The technique of delayed primary wound closure can be used in contaminated surgical cases to lower the incidence of wound infection. Briefly, this technique involves leaving the wound open above the fascia at the time of the initial surgical procedure. Vertical interrupted mattress sutures through the skin and subcutaneous layers are placed 3 cm apart but are not tied. Wound care is instituted immediately after surgery and continued until the wound is noted to be granulating well. Sutures may then be tied and the skin edges further approximated using sutures or staples. **Using this technique of delayed primary wound closure, the overall wound infection rate has been shown to be decreased from 23% to 2.1% in high-risk patients** (67).

Pelvic Cellulitis

Vaginal cuff cellulitis is present to some extent in most patients who have undergone hysterectomy. It is characterized by erythema, induration, and tenderness at the vaginal cuff. Occasionally, a purulent discharge from the apex of the vagina may also be present. The cellulitis is often self-limited and does not require any treatment. Fever, leukocytosis, and pain localized to the pelvis may accompany severe cuff cellulitis and most often signifies extension of the cellulitis to adjacent pelvic tissues. In such cases, broad-spectrum antibiotic therapy should be instituted with coverage for gram-negative, gram-positive, and anaerobic organisms. If purulence at the vaginal cuff is excessive or if there is a fluctuant mass noted at the vaginal cuff, the vaginal cuff should be gently probed and opened with a blunt instrument. The cuff can then be left open for dependent drainage or, alternatively, a drain can be placed into the lower pelvis through the cuff and removed when drainage, fever, and symptoms in the lower pelvic region have resolved.

Intraabdominal and Pelvic Abscess

The development of an abscess in the surgical field or elsewhere in the abdominal cavity is an uncommon complication after a gynecologic surgery. It is most likely to occur in contaminated cases in which the surgical site is not adequately drained or as a secondary complication of hematomas. The causative pathogens in patients who have intraabdominal abscesses are usually polymicrobial in nature. The aerobes most commonly identified include *E. coli, Klebsiella, Streptococcus, Proteus,* and *Enterobacter.* Anaerobic isolates are also common, usually from the *Bacteroides* group. These pathogens arise mainly from the vaginal tract but also can be derived from the gastrointestinal tract, particularly when the colon has been entered at the time of surgery.

Intraabdominal abscess is sometimes difficult to diagnose. The evolving clinical picture is often one of persistent febrile episodes with a rising white blood cell count. Findings on abdominal examination may be equivocal. If an abscess is located deep in the pelvis, it may be palpable by pelvic or rectal examination. For abscesses above the pelvis, the diagnosis will depend on radiologic confirmation.

Ultrasonography can occasionally delineate fluid collections in the upper abdomen as well as in the pelvis. However, bowel gas interference makes visualization of fluid collections or abscesses in the midabdomen difficult to distinguish. **CT scanning is therefore much more sensitive and specific for diagnosing intraabdominal abscesses and often is the radiologic procedure of choice.** Occasionally, if conventional radiologic methods fail to identify an abscess and the index of suspicion for an abscess remains high, labeled leukocyte scanning may be useful for locating the infected focus.

Standard therapy for intraabdominal abscess is evacuation and drainage combined with appropriate parenteral administration of antibiotics. Abscesses located low in the pelvis, particularly in the area of the vaginal cuff, can often be reached through a vaginal approach. In many patients, the ability to drain an abscess by placement of a drain percutaneously under CT guidance has obviated the need for surgical exploration. With CT guidance, a pigtail catheter is placed into an abscess cavity via either transperineal, transrectal, or transvaginal approaches. The catheter is left in place until drainage decreases. Transperineal and transrectal drainage of deep pelvic abscesses has been successful in 90% to 93% of patients, obviating the need for surgical management (68,69). **For those patients in whom radiologic drainage is not successful, however, surgical exploration and evacuation are indicated.** The gold standard of initial antibiotic therapy has been the combination of *ampicillin, gentamicin,* and *clindamycin.* Adequate treatment can also be achieved with currently available broad-spectrum single agents (including the broad-spectrum *penicillin*), second- and third-generation cephalosporins, *levofloxacin* and *metronidazole,* and the *sulbactam-clavulanic acid*–containing preparations (70–73).

Necrotizing Fasciitis

Necrotizing fasciitis is an uncommon infectious disorder; approximately 1,000 cases occur annually in the United States (74). The disorder is characterized by a rapidly progressive bacterial infection that involves the subcutaneous tissues and fascia while characteristically sparing underlying muscle. Systemic toxicity is a frequent feature of this disease, as manifested by the presence of dehydration, septic shock, DIC, and multiple organ system failure.

The pathogenesis of necrotizing fasciitis involves a polymicrobial infection of the dermis and subcutaneous tissue. Hemolytic streptococcus was initially believed to be the primary pathogen responsible for the infection in necrotizing fasciitis (75). However, it is now evident that numerous other organisms are often cultured in addition to streptococcus, including other gram-positive organisms, coliforms, and anaerobes (75–79). Bacterial enzymes such as hyaluronidase and lipase released in the subcutaneous space destroy the fascia and adipose tissue and induce a liquefactive necrosis. In addition, noninflammatory intravascular coagulation or thrombosis subsequently occurs. Intravascular coagulation results in ischemia and necrosis of the subcutaneous tissues and skin (76,77). Late in the course of the infection, destruction of the superficial nerves produces anesthesia in the involved skin. The release of bacteria and bacterial toxins into the systemic circulation can cause septic shock, acid-base disturbances, and multiple organ impairment.

The diagnostic criteria for necrotizing fasciitis include extensive necrosis of the superficial fascia and subcutaneous tissue with peripheral undermining of the normal skin, a moderate to severe systemic toxic reaction, the absence of muscle involvement, *Clostridia* in wound and blood culture and major vascular occlusion, intensive leukocytic infiltration, and necrosis of subcutaneous tissue (80).

Most patients with necrotizing fasciitis suffer pain, which in the early stages of the disease is often disproportionately greater than that expected from the degree of cellulitis present. Late in the course of the infection, the involved skin may actually be anesthetized secondary to necrosis of superficial nerves. Temperature abnormalities, both hyperthermia and hypothermia, are common concomitant with the release of bacterial toxins as well as with bacterial sepsis, which is present in up to 40% of patients (81). The involved skin is initially tender, erythematous, and warm. Edema develops and the erythema spreads diffusely, fading into normal skin, characteristically without distinct margins or induration. Subcutaneous microvascular thrombosis induces ischemia in the skin, which becomes cyanotic and blistered. Eventually, as necrosis develops, the skin becomes gangrenous and may slough spontaneously. Most patients will have leukocytosis and acid-base abnormalities. Finally, subcutaneous gas may develop, which can be identified by palpation and by radiograph. The finding of subcutaneous gas by radiograph is often indicative of clostridial infection, although it is not a specific finding and may be caused by other organisms. These organisms include *Enterobacter, Pseudomonas,* anaerobic streptococci, and *Bacteroides* (82) which, unlike clostridial infections, spare the muscles underlying the affected area. A tissue biopsy specimen for Gram stain and aerobic and anaerobic culture should be obtained from the necrotic center of the lesion in order to identify the etiologic organisms (77). Although necrotizing fasciitis is often diagnosed during surgery, a high index of suspicion as well as liberal use of frozen-section biopsy can often provide an early life-saving diagnosis and minimize morbidity (83).

Predisposing risk factors for necrotizing fasciitis include diabetes mellitus, alcoholism, an immunocompromised state, hypertension, peripheral vascular disease, intravenous drug abuse, and obesity (74,76,79,82,84). The most frequent site of infection has been in the extremities (77), but the infection can occur anywhere in the subcutaneous tissues, including the head and neck, trunk, and perineum. Necrotizing fasciitis has been known to occur after trauma, surgery, burns, and lacerations; as a secondary complication in perirectal infections or Bartholin duct abscesses; and *de novo* (74–77,83). Increased age, delay in diagnosis, inadequate debridement during initial surgery, extensive disease at the time of diagnosis, and the presence of diabetes mellitus are all factors that have been associated with an increased likelihood of mortality from necrotizing fasciitis (74,81). Clearly, early diagnosis and aggressive management of this lethal disease have led to improved survival. In an earlier series, the mortality rate was consistently higher than 30%; in more recent series, the mortality rate has decreased to less than 10% (82,85,86).

Successful management of necrotizing fasciitis involves early recognition, immediate initiation of resuscitative measures (including correction of fluid, acid-base, electrolyte, and hematologic abnormalities), aggressive surgical debridement and redebridement as necessary, and broad-spectrum antibiotic therapy. Many patients will benefit from central venous monitoring, as well as from high-caloric nutritional support.

During surgery, the incision should be made through the infected tissue down to the fascia. An ability to undermine the skin and subcutaneous tissues with digital palpation often will confirm the diagnosis. Multiple incisions can be made sequentially toward the periphery of the affected tissue until well-vascularized, healthy, resistant tissue is reached at all margins. The remaining affected tissue must be excised. The wound can then be packed and sequentially debrided on a daily basis as necessary until healthy tissue is displayed at all margins.

Hyperbaric oxygen therapy may be of some benefit, particularly in patients for whom culture results are positive for anaerobic organisms. Retrospective nonrandomized studies (74,87) have demonstrated that the addition of hyperbaric oxygen therapy to surgical debridement and antimicrobial therapy appear to significantly decrease both wound morbidity and overall mortality in patients with necrotizing fasciitis. The demonstrated benefit of hyperbaric therapy in one study (74) was remarkable, given that patients receiving hyperbaric oxygen were sicker and had a higher incidence of diabetes mellitus, leukocytosis, and shock.

After the initial resuscitative efforts and surgical debridement, the primary concern is the management of the open wound. Allograft and xenograft skin can be used to cover open wounds, thus decreasing heat and evaporative water loss. Interestingly, temporary biologic closure of open wounds also seems to decrease bacterial growth (88). Amniotic membranes have also been shown to be an effective wound covering in patients with necrotizing fasciitis (84). Recently a new technology has been developed to expedite wound healing. The vacuum-assisted closure (VAC) method is a subatmospheric pressure technique that has been demonstrated in laboratory and clinical studies to significantly improve wound healing. The VAC device as a method for wound control has demonstrated significant promotion of wound healing in laboratory and clinical studies (89,90). In situations in which spontaneous closure is not likely, the VAC device may allow for the development of a suitable granulation bed and prepare the tissue for graft placement, thereby increasing the probability of graft survival. Finally, skin flaps can be mobilized to help cover open wounds once the infections have resolved and granulation has begun.

Gastrointestinal Preparation

Preparation of the lower gastrointestinal tract prior to elective gynecologic surgery has several goals. In most gynecologic surgery, when the gastrointestinal tract is not entered, mechanical preparation of the bowel reduces gastrointestinal contents and thus allows more room in the abdomen and pelvis, facilitating the surgical procedure. If a rectosigmoid colon enterotomy occurs, the mechanical bowel preparation eliminates formed stool and reduces the risk of bacterial contamination, thus reducing infectious complications. Mechanical bowel preparation may be accomplished by several methods (Table 19.7). The traditional use of laxatives and enemas requires at least 12 to 24 hours and generally causes moderate abdominal distention and crampy pain. In addition, nursing supervision of enema administration and the need for intravenous fluid replacement makes this regimen relatively

Table 19.7. Bowel Preparation Regimens to Begin Day Prior to Surgery

Time	*Mechanical Prep*	*Antibiotic Prep*
Preoperative day 2		
PM	Clear liquid diet	
Preoperative day 1		
Noon	Clear liquid diet *Magnesium citrate* (240 cc PO), or *GoLYTELY* (4 L PO over 3 hr)	
1 PM		*Erythromycin* base 500 mg PO, plus *Neomycin* 1 gm PO *Metronidazole* 500 mg PO may be substituted
2 PM		Repeat PO antibiotics
8 PM	Enemas until clear IV D5/0.5 NS + 20 mEq KCl at 125 cc/hr (optional)	
11 PM		Repeat PO antibiotics
Operative day		
12 midnight	Nothing by mouth	
AM	Surgery	Prophylactic IV antibiotics

IV, intravenous; D5, 5% dextrose; NS, normal saline; PO, per os.

expensive. Randomized trials comparing traditional mechanical bowel preparation with oral gut lavage (*PEG electrolyte solution [GoLYTELY]*) have found that the use of approximately 4 liters of *GoLYTELY* (administered until the rectal effluent is clear) provides more complete, faster, and more comfortable bowel preparation (91). Furthermore, the fluid loss following gut lavage with *GoLYTELY* appears to be clinically insignificant. Gut lavage can usually be performed at home the day prior to scheduled surgery. If the patient cannot drink the 4 liters, the *GoLYTELY* may be administered through a small-caliber nasogastric tube. The ingestion of 4 liters of fluid is problematic for many patients. An alternative mechanical preparation method is the use of oral *sodium phosphate* (*Phospho-Soda*). When evaluated in a randomized trial comparing the 4 liters of *GoLYTELY* with oral *sodium phosphate*, colonoscopic examination disclosed that both methods were equally effective in colonic cleansing and more patients preferred the sodium phosphate method (92).

High infection rates after colonic surgery have led to investigation of methods aimed at reducing these significant complications. Although mechanical bowel preparation is an essential part of all colonic surgery preparation regimens, it does not reduce the infection rate satisfactorily. Reduction of the number of pathogenic flora in the colon is the primary strategy to reduce infection after colonic surgery. The colon has the greatest concentration of bacteria in the body, including both aerobes and anaerobes. Anaerobes outnumber aerobes by 1,000:1. After reducing the bacterial load by mechanical preparation, the administration of antibiotics can further reduce the bacterial count in the colon. Of the many trials reported, the most widely accepted regimen combines *erythromycin* base and *neomycin* administered orally (Table 19.7) (93–95). Many surgeons substitute *metronidazole* for the *erythromycin;* there is no significant difference in infection rates, but patients tolerate *metronidazole* better than *erythromycin.* **The use of oral antibiotics 24 hours prior to colonic resection has reduced the infection rate from approximately 40%, to 5% to 10%, in randomized trials.** Because these oral antibiotics are poorly absorbed and many do little to reduce infection from vaginal contamination, an intravenous antibiotic (first-generation cephalosporin) can be added to the preoperative regimen. **Antibiotic bowel prophylaxis should be used for patients who are likely to undergo colorectal surgery (pelvic exenteration, ovarian cancer debulking) and those who are at high risk for rectal injury (such as severe cases of endometriosis or pelvic inflammatory disease).**

Postoperative Gastrointestinal Complications

Ileus

Following abdominal or pelvic surgery, most patients will experience some degree of intestinal ileus. The exact mechanism by which this arrest and disorganization of gastrointestinal motility occurs is unknown, but it appears to be associated with the opening of the peritoneal cavity and is aggravated by manipulation of the intestinal tract and prolonged surgical procedures. Infection, peritonitis, and electrolyte disturbances may also result in ileus. For most patients undergoing common gynecologic operations, the degree of ileus is minimal and gastrointestinal function returns relatively rapidly, allowing the resumption of oral intake within a few days of surgery. Patients who have persistently diminished bowel sounds, abdominal distention, and nausea and vomiting require further evaluation and more aggressive management.

Ileus is usually manifested by abdominal distention and should be evaluated initially by physical examination. Pertinent points of the abdominal examination include assessment of the quality of bowel sounds and palpation in search of tenderness or rebound. The possibility that the patient's signs and symptoms may be associated with a more serious intestinal obstruction or other intestinal complication must be considered. Pelvic examination should be performed to evaluate the possibility of a pelvic abscess or hematoma that may contribute to the ileus. **Abdominal radiograph to evaluate the abdomen in the flat (supine) position as well as in the upright position usually will aid in the diagnosis of an ileus. The**

most common radiographic findings include dilated loops of small and large bowel as well as air-fluid levels while the patient is in the upright position. Sometimes, massive dilation of the colon or stomach may be noted. The remote possibility of distal colonic obstruction suggested by a dilated cecum should be excluded by rectal examination, proctosigmoidoscopy, or barium enema. In the postoperative gynecology patient, especially in the upright position, the flat plate of the abdomen may also show evidence of free air. This is a common finding following surgery, which lasts 7 to 10 days in some instances and is not indicative of a perforated viscus in most patients.

The initial management of a postoperative ileus is aimed at gastrointestinal tract decompression and maintenance of appropriate intravenous replacement fluids and electrolytes.

1. **A nasogastric tube should evacuate the stomach of its fluid and gaseous contents.** Prolonged nasogastric suction continues to remove swallowed air, which is the most common source of air in the small bowel. Some clinicians prefer to use a longer small intestinal tube (Cantor or Miller-Abbott tube) (96). This tube, which usually has a mercury-filled bag on its distal tip, may be propelled by peristalsis through the pylorus and into the small bowel, thus allowing a better evacuation of the small bowel. The disadvantage of long tubes is that they take a longer time to become positioned and may not enter the small bowel as a result of the decreased intestinal motility associated with ileus.

2. **Fluid and electrolyte replacement must be adequate to keep the patient well perfused.** Significant amounts of third-space fluid loss occur in the bowel wall, the bowel lumen, and the peritoneal cavity during the acute episode. Gastrointestinal fluid losses from the stomach may lead to a metabolic alkalosis and depletion of other electrolytes as well. Careful monitoring of serum chemistry levels and appropriate replacement are necessary.

3. **Most cases of severe ileus will begin to improve over a period of several days.** In general, this is recognized by reduction in the abdominal distention, return of normal bowel sounds, and passage of flatus or stool. Follow-up abdominal radiographs should be obtained as necessary for further monitoring.

4. **When the gastrointestinal tract function appears to have returned to normal, the nasogastric tube may be removed and a liquid diet may be instituted.**

5. **If a patient shows no evidence of improvement during the first 48 to 72 hours of medical management, other causes of ileus should be sought.** Such cases may include ureteral injury, peritonitis from pelvic infection, unrecognized gastrointestinal tract injury with peritoneal spill, or fluid and electrolyte abnormalities such as hypokalemia. With persistent ileus, the use of water-soluble upper gastrointestinal contrast studies may assist in the resolution, but prospective randomized data regarding this maneuver are lacking.

Small Bowel Obstruction

Obstruction of the small bowel following major gynecologic surgery occurs in approximately 1% to 2% of patients (97). The most common cause of small bowel obstruction is adhesions to the operative site. If the small bowel becomes adherent in a twisted position, partial or complete obstruction may result from distention, ileus, or bowel wall edema. Less common causes of postoperative small bowel obstruction include entrapment of the small bowel into an incisional hernia and an unrecognized defect in the small bowel or large bowel mesentery. **Early in its clinical course, a postoperative small bowel obstruction may exhibit signs and symptoms identical to those of ileus. Initial conservative management as outlined for the treatment of ileus is appropriate.** Because of the potential for mesenteric vascular occlusion and resulting ischemia or perforation, worsening symptoms of abdominal pain, progressive distention, fever, leukocytosis, or acidosis should be evaluated carefully because immediate surgery may be required.

In most cases of small bowel obstruction following gynecologic surgery, the obstruction is only partial and the symptoms usually resolve with conservative management.

1. **Further evaluation after several days of conservative management may be necessary.** Evaluation of the gastrointestinal tract with barium enema and an upper gastrointestinal study with small bowel assessment are appropriate. In most cases, complete obstruction is not documented, although a narrowing or tethering of the segment of small bowel may indicate the site of the problem.

2. **Further conservative management with nasogastric decompression and intravenous fluid replacement may allow time for bowel wall edema or torsion of the mesentery to resolve.**

3. **If resolution is prolonged and the patient's nutritional status is marginal, the use of total parenteral nutrition may be necessary.**

4. **Conservative medical management of postoperative small bowel obstruction usually results in complete resolution.** However, if persistent evidence of small bowel obstruction remains after full evaluation and an adequate trial of medical management, exploratory laparotomy may be necessary to surgically evaluate and manage the obstruction. In most cases, lysis of adhesions is all that is required, although a segment of small bowel that is badly damaged or extensively sclerosed from adhesions may require resection and reanastomosis.

Colonic Obstruction

Postoperative colonic obstruction following surgery for most gynecologic conditions is exceedingly rare. It is almost always associated with a pelvic malignancy, which in most cases will have been known at the time of the initial operation. Advanced ovarian carcinoma is the most common cause of colonic obstruction in postoperative gynecologic surgery patients, and it is caused by extrinsic impingement on the colon by the pelvic malignancy. Intrinsic colonic lesions may be undetected, especially in a patient with some other benign gynecologic condition. When colonic obstruction is manifested by abdominal distention and abdominal radiographs reveal a dilated colon and enlarging cecum, further evaluation of the large bowel is required by barium enema or colonoscopy. **Dilation of the cecum to more than 10 to 12 cm in diameter as viewed by abdominal radiograph requires immediate evaluation and surgical decompression by performing colectomy or colostomy.** Surgery should be performed as soon as the obstruction is documented. Conservative management of colonic obstruction is not appropriate because the complication of colonic perforation has an exceedingly high mortality rate.

Diarrhea

Episodes of diarrhea often occur following abdominal and pelvic surgery as the gastrointestinal tract returns to its normal function and motility. However, prolonged and multiple episodes may represent a pathologic process such as impending small bowel obstruction, colonic obstruction, or pseudomembranous colitis. Excessive amounts of diarrhea should be evaluated by abdominal radiographs and stool samples tested for the presence of ova and parasites, bacterial culture, and *Clostridium difficile* toxin. Proctoscopy and colonoscopy may also be advisable in severe cases. Evidence of intestinal obstruction should be managed as outlined previously. Infectious causes of diarrhea should be managed with the appropriate antibiotics as well as fluid and electrolyte replacement. *C. difficile*–associated pseudomembranous colitis may result from exposure to any antibiotic. Discontinuation of these antibiotics (unless they are needed for another severe infection) is advisable, along with the institution of appropriate therapy. Oral *metronidazole* is a suitable agent for instituting therapy and is less expensive than vancomycin. Therapy should be continued until the diarrhea abates, and several weeks of oral therapy may be required in order to obtain complete resolution of the pseudomembranous colitis.

Fistula

Gastrointestinal fistulas are relatively rare following gynecologic surgery. They are most often associated with malignancy, prior radiation therapy, or surgical injury to the large or small bowel that was improperly repaired or unrecognized. Signs and symptoms of gastrointestinal fistula are often similar to those of small bowel obstruction or ileus, except that a fever is usually a more prominent component of the patient's symptoms. When fever is associated with gastrointestinal dysfunction postoperatively, evaluation should include early assessment of the gastrointestinal tract to confirm its continuity. **When fistula is suspected, the use of water-soluble gastrointestinal contrast material is advised to avoid the complication of barium peritonitis.** Evaluation with abdominal pelvic CT scan may also assist in identification of a fistula and associated abscess. **Recognition of an intraperitoneal gastrointestinal leak or fistula formation usually requires immediate surgery, unless the fistula has drained spontaneously through the abdominal wall or vaginal cuff.**

An *enterocutaneous fistula* arising from the small bowel and draining spontaneously through the abdominal incision may be managed successfully with medical therapy. Therapy should include nasogastric decompression, replacement of intravenous fluids as well as TPN, and appropriate antibiotics to treat an associated mixed bacterial infection. If the infection is under control and there are no other signs of peritonitis, the surgeon may consider allowing potential resolution of the fistula over a period of up to 2 weeks. Some authors have suggested the use of somatostatin to decrease intestinal tract secretion and allow earlier healing of the fistula. In some cases, the fistula will close spontaneously with this mode of management. If the enterocutaneous fistula does not close with conservative medical management, surgical correction with resection, bypass, or reanastomosis will be necessary.

A *rectovaginal fistula* that occurs following gynecologic surgery is usually the result of surgical trauma that may have been aggravated by the presence of extensive adhesions in the rectovaginal septum associated with endometriosis, pelvic inflammatory disease, or pelvic malignancy. **A small rectovaginal fistula may be managed with a conservative medical approach, in the hope that decreasing the fecal stream will allow closure of the fistula.** A small fistula that allows continence except for an occasional leak of flatus may be managed conservatively until the inflammatory process in the pelvis resolves. At that point, usually several months later, correction of the fistula is appropriate. Large rectovaginal fistulas for which there no hope of spontaneous closure are best managed by performing an initial diverting colostomy followed by repair of the fistula after inflammation has resolved. After the fistula closure is healed and deemed successful, the colostomy can be closed.

Thromboembolism Prophylaxis

Risk Factors

Deep venous thrombosis and pulmonary embolism, although largely preventable, are significant complications in postoperative patients. The magnitude of this problem is relevant to the gynecologist, because 40% of all deaths following gynecologic surgery are directly attributed to pulmonary emboli (98). Pulmonary embolism is also the second leading cause of death in women who undergo a legally induced abortion (99) and the most frequent cause of postoperative death in patients with uterine (100) or cervical carcinoma (101).

The causal factors of venous thrombosis were first proposed by Virchow in 1858 and include the following: a hypercoagulable state, venous stasis, and vessel intima injury. Two prospective studies have evaluated risk factors associated with the postoperative occurrence of deep venous thrombosis in patients undergoing gynecologic surgery. In one study, the risk factors of 124 patients undergoing vaginal and abdominal surgery for benign gynecologic disease were studied (102). Five factors were identified to be associated with postoperative deep venous thrombosis: (a) increasing age, (b) presence of varicose veins, (c) being overweight, (d) prolonged euglobulin lysis time, and (e) presence of serum fibrin-related antigen. In another prospective study, the risk factors associated with venous thromboembolic complications were also assessed in 411 patients undergoing major abdominal and pelvic surgery (103). Preoperative risk factors identified in this study include advanced age; nonwhite race; increasing stage of malignancy; history of deep venous thrombosis, lower extremity edema, or venous stasis changes; presence of varicose veins; being overweight; and a history of radiation therapy. Intraoperative factors associated with postoperative deep venous thrombosis included increased anesthesia time, increased blood loss, and the need for transfusion in the operating room. It is important to recognize these risk factors in order to provide the appropriate level of venous thrombosis prophylaxis.

Prophylactic Methods

During the past 2 decades, a number of prophylactic methods have undergone clinical trials that showed significant reduction in the incidence of deep venous thrombosis, and a few studies have demonstrated a reduction in fatal pulmonary emboli (100–133). The ideal prophylactic method would be effective, free of significant side effects, well accepted by the patient and nursing staff, widely applicable to most patient groups, and inexpensive.

Low-dose *Heparin*

The use of small doses of subcutaneously administered *heparin* for the prevention of deep venous thrombosis and pulmonary embolism is the most widely studied of all prophylactic methods. More than 25 controlled trials have demonstrated that *heparin,* given subcutaneously 2 hours preoperatively and every 8 to 12 hours postoperatively, is effective in reducing the incidence of deep venous thrombosis. The value of low-dose *heparin* in preventing fatal pulmonary emboli was established by a randomized, controlled, multicenter international trial that showed a significant reduction in fatal postoperative pulmonary emboli in general surgery patients receiving low-dose *heparin* every 8 hours postoperatively (104). Trials of low-dose *heparin* use in gynecologic surgery patients are limited, and a clear consensus regarding the value of low-dose *heparin* in all groups of patients has not been established because of differences in patient selection and length of follow-up. Three randomized controlled studies used the same regimen of low-dose *heparin* administration: 5,000 units subcutaneously 2 hours preoperatively and every 12 hours for 7 days postoperatively. Two trials were conducted in patients with benign gynecologic conditions (98%); all patients were older than 40 years of age, and follow-up was discontinued at the time of discharge from hospital (105,106). One trial showed a 23% incidence of deep venous thrombosis in the control group, compared with a 6% incidence of deep venous thrombosis in the patients treated with low-dose *heparin* (106). This difference was statistically significant ($P = 0.05$). Although this was a randomized trial, the control group contained a larger number of patients with malignancy and, when the cancer patients were excluded from the trial analysis, there was no significant value to the use of low-dose *heparin* in patients with benign conditions. In the other study, the nontreated control group had a 29% incidence of deep venous thrombosis compared with a 3.6% incidence in the group treated with low-dose *heparin* ($P = 0.001$) (105). A third trial evaluated a larger group of patients receiving treatment in gynecologic oncology unit, only 16% of whom had benign gynecologic conditions; follow-up included the first 6 weeks postoperatively (107). In this trial, there was no difference in the incidence of thromboembolic complications between the control group (12.4%) and the group treated with low-dose *heparin* (14.8%) (107).

In a subsequent trial (108), two more intense *heparin* regimens were evaluated in high-risk gynecologic oncology patients. *Heparin* was given either in a regimen of 5,000 units subcutaneously 2 hours preoperatively and every 8 hours postoperatively, or 5,000 units subcutaneously every 8 hours preoperatively (a minimum of three preoperative doses) and every 8 hours postoperatively. Both of these prophylaxis regimens were effective in significantly reducing the incidence of postoperative deep venous thrombosis in patients with gynecologic cancers.

Although low-dose *heparin* is considered to have no measurable effect on coagulation, most large series have noted an increase in the bleeding complication rate, especially a higher incidence of wound hematoma. Up to 10% to 15% of otherwise healthy patients develop a transiently prolonged activated partial thromboplastin time (APTT) after 5,000 units of *heparin* is given subcutaneously (109). Retrospective studies have suggested that low-dose *heparin* contributed to an increased occurrence of lymphocysts (110,111). A prospective study demonstrated an increase in retroperitoneal lymph drainage volume in patients treated with low-dose *heparin,* but there was no increase in the incidence of lymphocysts (109). Although relatively rare, thrombocytopenia is associated with low-dose *heparin* use and has been found in 6% of patients after gynecologic surgery (109). If patients remain on low-dose *heparin* therapy for greater than 4 days, it is reasonable to perform a platelet count to assess the possibility of heparin-induced thrombocytopenia.

Low-molecular-weight Heparin

Low-molecular-weight heparin (*LMWH*) consists of fragments of unfractionated *heparin* that vary in size from 4,500 to 6,500 daltons. When compared with unfractionated *heparin, LMWH* has more anti-Xa and less antithrombin activity, leading to less effect on partial thromboplastin time. Decreased platelet inhibition and microvascular bleeding has been noted with *LMWH* use, which may also lead to fewer bleeding complications (112). An increased half-life of 4 hours (in both intravenous and subcutaneous administrations) leads to increased bioavailability when compared with unfractionated *heparin.* The increase in half-life of *LMWH* allows the convenience of once-a-day dosing. Several commercially available *LMWH* preparations are internationally available but only two (i.e., *enoxaparin* and *dalteparin*) have been approved by the Food and Drug Administration for deep venous thrombosis prophylaxis in the United States.

Four randomized controlled trials have compared *LMWH* with unfractionated *heparin* in patients undergoing gynecologic surgery. All studies showed a similar incidence of deep venous thrombosis. Bleeding complications (113–115) were also similar between the unfractionated *heparin* and *LMWH* groups. In a trial evaluating *LMWH* (*dalteparin*) in a gynecologic cancer population, the *LMWH* was associated with fewer bleeding complications than would have been expected. The rate of thromboembolism was approximately 2% in this collective group of 521 operative patients, with deep venous thrombosis diagnosed in 7 patients receiving unfractionated *heparin* and 3 patients receiving *LMWH* prophylaxis. A recent metaanalysis of patients undergoing general surgery and gynecologic surgery from 32 trials likewise indicated that daily *LMWH* administration is as effective as unfractionated *heparin* in deep venous thrombosis prophylaxis without any difference in hemorrhagic complications (116). Caution should be maintained in interpretation of assimilated data involving *LMWH,* because different anti-Xa activities are associated with the different preparations (117). In a comparison of prophylactic methods of deep venous thrombosis treatment, *LMWH* has been suggested by some investigators to be more cost effective than unfractionated *heparin* because of the convenience of once-daily dosing (118,119).

Mechanical Methods

Stasis in the veins of the legs while the patient is undergoing surgery has been clearly demonstrated and continues postoperatively for varying lengths of time. Stasis occurring in the capacitance veins of the calf during surgery, in addition to the hypercoagulable state induced by surgery, are the prime factors contributing to the development of acute postoperative deep venous thrombosis. Prospective studies of the natural history of postoperative venous thrombosis have shown that the calf veins are the predominant site of thrombi and that most thrombi develop within 24 hours of surgery (120). Reduction of venous stasis in the perioperative period by various mechanical methods has been less extensively investigated than pharmacologic methods such as low-dose *heparin*. However, mechanical prophylactic methods may play an important role in the prevention of postoperative deep vein thrombosis.

Although probably of only modest benefit, reduction of stasis by short preoperative hospital stays and early postoperative ambulation should be encouraged for all patients. Elevation of the foot of the bed, raising the calf above heart level, allows gravity to drain the calf veins and should further reduce stasis. More active forms of mechanical prophylaxis include elastic gradient compression stockings and external pneumatic leg compression.

Elastic Stockings In a survey of general surgeons in the United States, gradient elastic stockings were second only to low-dose *heparin* as the prophylactic method of choice in high-risk and moderately high-risk surgical patients (121). The simplicity of elastic stockings and the absence of significant side effects are probably the two most important reasons that they are often included in routine postoperative care. Controlled studies of graduated pressure stockings are limited but do suggest modest benefit when they are carefully fitted (122). Poorly fitted stockings may be hazardous to some patients who develop a tourniquet effect at the knee or midthigh (99). Variations in human anatomy do not allow perfect fit of all patients to available stocking sizes.

External Pneumatic Compression The largest body of literature dealing with the reduction of postoperative venous stasis deals with intermittent external compression of the leg by pneumatically inflated sleeves placed around the calf or leg during intraoperative and postoperative periods. Various pneumatic compression devices and leg sleeve designs are available, and currently one method has not been shown to be superior to others. Single-chambered calf compression devices have been studied most extensively in gynecologic surgery and appear to significantly reduce the incidence of deep venous thrombosis on a level similar to that of low-dose *heparin*. In addition to increasing venous flow and pulsatile emptying of the calf veins, external pneumatic compression also appears to augment endogenous fibrinolysis, which may result in lysis of very early thrombi before they become clinically significant (123).

The duration of postoperative external pneumatic compression has differed in various trials. External pneumatic compression may be effective only when used in the operating room or for the first 24 hours postoperatively (124,125), although they should remain in use in patients who are not ambulatory.

Used in patients undergoing major surgery for gynecologic malignancy, external pneumatic compression has been found to reduce nearly threefold the incidence of postoperative venous thromboembolic complications (126). To determine the effectiveness of this approach, calf compression was applied intraoperatively and continued for the first 5 postoperative days. In a subsequent trial of similar patients that was designed to evaluate whether external pneumatic compression might achieve similar benefits when used only intraoperatively and for the first 24 hours postoperatively, there was no reduction of deep venous thrombosis when compared with the control group (127). Because of stasis and their hypercoagulable states, patients with gynecologic malignancies may remain at risk for a longer period than general surgical patients and therefore appear to benefit from longer use of external pneumatic compression.

External pneumatic leg compression has no significant side effects or risks. Although patient intolerance has been cited as a drawback to its use, anecdotal experience does not support this perception. However, we have had only 5 patients of nearly 900 treated with external pneumatic compression request removal because of discomfort. The equipment is easily managed by the nursing staff, and although the initial capital outlay for external pneumatic compressors may seem large, the cost per patient is slightly less than that of low-dose *heparin* given for 7 days postoperatively (128).

The risk factors associated with the failure of external compression to prevent deep venous thrombosis has been investigated in a retrospective analysis of 1,862 consecutive gynecologic surgery patients who received postoperative intermittent pneumatic compression at Duke University between 1992 and 1997. A history of prior deep venous thrombosis, diagnosis of cancer, and age greater than 60 years were factors independently associated with the development of deep venous thrombosis despite external pneumatic compression prophylaxis ($P < 0.05$). Patients having two or more of these factors had a 16-fold increased risk of postoperative deep vein thrombosis despite prophylaxis ($P < 0.05$) (129). In these extremely high-risk patients, combined methods of prophylaxis ought to be considered.

Combination Prophylaxis

Combination therapy using *heparin* and compression stockings has been utilized in other high-risk surgical patients in an attempt to diminish both the hypercoagulability and venous stasis that can be found in postoperative patients at high risk for thromboembolism. The prophylactic use of low-dose *heparin* has been compared with low-dose *heparin* combined with graduated compression stockings in deep vein thrombosis prophylaxis among general surgery patients. Willie-Jorgensen and associates (130), in an investigation involving 245 patients undergoing acute extensive abdominal operations, demonstrated that the rate of postoperative deep vein thrombosis was significantly lower among 79 patients receiving a combination regimen of graduated compression stockings and low-dose *heparin* (i.e., 5,000 units subcutaneously 1 hour preoperatively and 12 hours postoperatively) than patients receiving only the low-dose *heparin* regimen ($P = 0.013$). A statistically significant improvement ($P < 0.05$) in postoperative deep vein thrombosis was similarly noted by the same investigators in the evaluation of 176 patients undergoing elective abdominal surgery (131). A metaanalysis of six studies involving 898 general surgery patients has shown that combination therapy with low-dose *heparin* and graduated compression stockings provides significantly better deep vein thrombosis prophylaxis postoperatively than either single modality (odds ratio 0.40; 95% CI 0.27 to 0.59) (132). Recently, a multicenter prospective randomized clinical trial demonstrated that combination prophylaxis consisting of graduated compression stockings and *LMWH* was more effective in deep vein thrombosis prevention than graduated compression stockings alone (relative risk 0.52; 95% CI 0.17 to 0.95, $P = 0.04$) (133). Such combination prophylaxis might be considered in the highest risk gynecologic oncology patients, although the efficacy, risks, and costs have not been studied.

Management of Postoperative Deep Venous Thrombosis and Pulmonary Embolism

Because pulmonary embolism is the leading cause of deaths following gynecologic surgical procedures, identification of high-risk patients and the use of prophylactic venous thromboembolism regimens is an essential part of management (98,100,101). In addition, the early recognition of deep vein thrombosis and pulmonary embolism and immediate treatment are critical. Although pulmonary emboli arise from the deep venous system of the leg, following gynecologic surgery the pelvic veins are a known source of fatal pulmonary emboli as well.

The signs and symptoms of deep vein thrombosis of the lower extremities include pain, edema, erythema, and prominent vascular pattern of the superficial veins. These signs and symptoms are relatively nonspecific; 50% to 80% of patients with these symptoms will not actually have deep vein thrombosis (134). Conversely, approximately 80% of patients with symptomatic pulmonary emboli have no signs or symptoms of thrombosis in the lower extremities (135). Because of the lack of specificity when signs and symptoms are recognized, additional diagnostic tests should be performed to establish the diagnosis of deep vein thrombosis.

Venography Although venography has been the gold standard for diagnosis of deep vein thrombosis, other diagnostic studies are accurate when performed by a skilled technologist and, in most patients, may replace the need for routine contrast venography. Venography is moderately uncomfortable, requires the injection of a contrast material that may cause allergic reaction or renal injury, and may result in phlebitis in approximately 5% of patients (136). Fortunately, newer diagnostic tests have been developed that are less invasive yet have a high accuracy rate in most patients.

Doppler Ultrasound B-mode duplex Doppler imaging is currently the most common technique used in the diagnosis of symptomatic venous thrombosis, especially when it arises in the proximal lower extremity. With duplex Doppler imaging, the femoral vein can be visualized and clots may be seen directly (137). Compression of the vein with the ultrasonographic probe tip allows assessment of venous collapsibility; the presence of a thrombus diminishes vein wall collapsibility. Doppler imaging is less accurate when evaluating the calf venous system and the pelvic veins.

Impedance Plethysmography Impedance plethysmography is a noninvasive study that measures the change in electrical impedance of the lower extremities when venous blood flow and volume are altered by an occlusive cuff on the thigh. This study may be performed at the patient's bedside and repeated as often as necessary without any risk to the patient. Correlation with venography in symptomatic patients approaches 95% (138,139). The test is effective in the identification of deep venous thrombi in the popliteal, femoral, and external iliac segments. It is less accurate (30%) in identifying calf vein thrombosis and does not identify thrombi occurring in the internal iliac venous system. False-positive results are primarily due to extrinsic venous compression. In gynecology, this might include a large pelvic mass compressing the external iliac or common iliac vein.

Magnetic Resonance Imaging MRI has a sensitivity and specificity comparable to venography. In addition, MRI may detect thrombi in pelvic veins which are not imaged by venography (140). The primary drawback to MRI is the time involved in examining the lower extremity and pelvis as well as the expense of this technology.

Deep Venous Thrombosis

The treatment of postoperative deep venous thrombosis requires the immediate institution of anticoagulant therapy. Treatment may be with either unfractionated *heparin* or LMWHs, followed by 3 to 6 months of oral anticoagulant therapy with *warfarin.*

Unfractionated Heparin After venous thromboembolism is diagnosed, unfractionated *heparin* should be initiated to prevent proximal propagation of the thrombus and allow physiologic thrombolytic pathways to dissolve the clot. After an initial bolus of 5,000 units intravenously, a continuous infusion of 30,000 units per day should be implemented and dosage adjusted to maintain APTT levels at a therapeutic range of 1.5 to 2.5 times the control value. Patients having subtherapeutic APTT levels in the first 24 hours have a risk of recurrent thromboembolism 15 times the risk of patients with appropriate levels. Administration of subcutaneous *heparin* also results in a higher likelihood of subtherapeutic prophylaxis when compared with continuous intravenous infusion. Thus management should entail aggressive use of intravenous *heparin* to achieve prompt anticoagulation. Oral anticoagulant (*warfarin*) should be started on the first day of *heparin* infusion. International normalized ration (INR) should be monitored daily until a therapeutic level is achieved. The change in the INR resulting from *warfarin* administration often precedes the anticoagulant effect by approximately 2 days, during which time low protein C levels are associated with a transient hypercoagulable state. Therefore, *heparin* should be administered until the INR has been maintained in a therapeutic range for at least 2 days, confirming the proper *warfarin* dose. Intravenous *heparin* may be discontinued in 5 days if an adequate INR level has been established. Patients experiencing a thromboembolic event for the first time should take *warfarin* for approximately 3 to 6 months to prevent recurrent thromboembolism. Longer periods of anticoagulation should be considered in patients experiencing a recurrence. Indefinite anticoagulation has not been shown to decrease the risk of deep venous thrombosis recurrence, and the risks of bleeding are increased in patients who maintain prolonged therapy.

Low-molecular-weight Heparin *LMWH* has been shown to be effective in the treatment of venous thromboembolism and has a cost-effective advantage over intravenous *heparin* in that it may be administered in the outpatient setting. The dosages used in treatment of thromboembolism are unique and weight adjusted according to each *LMWH* preparation. Because *LMWH* has a minimal effect on APTT, serial laboratory monitoring of APTT levels is not necessary. Similarly, monitoring of anti-Xa activity has not been shown to be of benefit in a dose adjustment of *LMWH*. The increased bioavailability associated with *LMWH* allows for once- or twice-daily dosing, potentially making outpatient management for a subset of patients an option. A metaanalysis involving more than 1,000 patients from 19 trials suggests that *LMWH* is more effective in preventing recurrent thromboembolism, safer, and less costly when compared with unfractionated *heparin*.

Pulmonary Embolism

Many of the signs and symptoms of pulmonary embolism are associated with other, more commonly occurring pulmonary complications following surgery. The classic findings of pleuritic chest pain, hemoptysis, shortness of breath, tachycardia, and tachypnea should alert the physician to the possibility of a pulmonary embolism. Many times, however, the signs are much more subtle and may be suggested only by a persistent tachycardia or a slight elevation in the respiratory rate. Patients suspected of pulmonary embolism should be evaluated initially by chest radiography, electrocardiography, and arterial blood gas assessment. Any evidence of abnormality should be further evaluated by ventilation–perfusion lung scan, searching for evidence of decreased perfusions in areas of adequate ventilation. Unfortunately, a high percentage of lung scans may be interpreted as indeterminate. In this setting, careful clinical evaluation and judgment are required to decide whether pulmonary arteriography should be obtained to document or exclude the presence of a pulmonary embolism.

The treatment of pulmonary embolism is as follows:

1. Immediate anticoagulant therapy, identical to that outlined for the treatment of deep vein thrombosis, should be initiated.

2. Respiratory support, including oxygen and bronchodilators and an intensive care setting, may be necessary.

3. Although massive pulmonary emboli are usually quickly fatal, pulmonary embolectomy has been performed successfully on rare occasions.

4. Pulmonary artery catheterization with the administration of thrombolytic agents bears further evaluation and may be important in patients with massive pulmonary embolism.

5. A vena cava interruption may be necessary in situations in which anticoagulant therapy is ineffective in the prevention of rethrombosis and repeated embolization from the lower extremities or pelvis. A vena cava umbrella or filter may be situated percutaneously or a large clip can be used to obstruct the vena cava above the level of the thrombosis. In most cases, however, anticoagulant therapy is sufficient to prevent repeat thrombosis and embolism and to allow the patient's own endogenous thrombolytic mechanisms to lyse the pulmonary embolus.

Management of Medical Problems

Endocrine Disease

The three most frequent endocrine disorders that occur in patients undergoing gynecologic surgery are diabetes mellitus, thyroid disease, and adrenal abnormalities. The pathophysiology of these disorders aids in understanding the effects of surgery on patients with these problems.

Diabetes Mellitus

It is estimated that approximately six million people in the United States (2.5% of the population) have diabetes mellitus (DM) and that about one-half of these individuals will undergo surgery at some point in their lives. Approximately 75% of individuals with DM will have surgery after they are 50 years of age. Many of these procedures are a direct result of the complications of DM: retinopathy, nephropathy, large- and small-vessel occlusive disease, and coronary artery disease. It is the direct effect of DM on the end organs that determines the risk of surgery rather than the type or duration or the control of the condition itself.

Diabetes mellitus is a complicated medical disorder of glucose metabolism that is related to a lack of production of or resistance to *insulin.* Patients with DM experience exaggerated hyperglycemia during surgery. This hyperglycemia is multifactorial in origin and is secondary to increased catecholamine production, which inhibits pancreatic release of insulin and causes increased *insulin* resistance at the end organs. Elevations in instrumental hormones such as cortisol, growth hormone, and glucagon also enhance gluconeogenesis and glycogenolysis. Goals of the preoperative assessment and perioperative management are to ensure metabolic homeostasis and to anticipate problems arising from preexisting complications.

Preoperative Risk Assessment

Large- and small-vessel arterial occlusive disease is the single most important risk factor in the preoperative setting. A careful history and physical examination should be performed to determine the presence or absence of coronary artery or cerebral vascular disease. Assessment of end-organ disease in the retina, kidney, and carotid arteries, or evidence of peripheral vascular disease by the presence of foot ulcers, should alert the clinician to the possibility of small- or large-vessel disease. When extended surgery is possible, as with surgery for gynecologic cancer, exercise stress testing or *dipyridamole-thallium imaging* should be considered to rule out occult coronary artery disease. Diabetic nephropathy should be documented carefully preoperatively. Imaging studies using contrast dye should be avoided, and alternative testing should be performed to reduce the incidence of acute tubular necrosis. If a contrast study must be performed, adequate hydration both before and after the procedure is essential.

Preoperative evaluation should include examination of the skin and urine sediment to detect asymptomatic infection. There is a known predisposition for patients with DM to have gram-negative and staphylococcal pneumonia as well as an increased incidence of gram-negative and group B streptococcal sepsis (141). Seven percent of individuals with diabetes will have postoperative gram-negative sepsis, a rate approximately 7 times higher than in the nondiabetic population. These complications occur more often in patients with poor glucose control, probably due to impaired leukocyte function in the presence of hyperglycemia (142,143). Patients with DM have an increased risk of wound dehiscence and wound infection as well as decreased amounts of collagen formation, fibroblast growth, and capillary growth, presumably secondary to the pathophysiology of small-vessel disease (144–146).

Autonomic neuropathy has been documented in patients with DM, and these autonomic impairments can lead to intraoperative hypotension, cardiac arrhythmias, and sudden death as well as abnormal motility of the esophagus, stomach, and small intestine (147). Peripheral sensory and motor neuropathies may or may not be present. The presence of any manifestations of autonomic neuropathy intraoperatively should prompt close monitoring of the affected organ system during the postoperative period (148).

Perioperative Management

The general goal for glucose control during surgery is to maintain the glucose level between 150 and 200 mg/dl. Perioperative hyperglycemia (>250 mg/dl) is associated with increased susceptibility to infection and poor wound healing. Extreme hyperglycemia predisposes patients to metabolic acidosis, and surgery should be canceled until normal acid-base balance has been documented. Hyperosmolar hyperglycemic nonketotic states must be recognized before surgery. Electrolyte disturbances, especially those related to sodium and potassium, should be corrected preoperatively. Hypoglycemia should be avoided at all costs during the perioperative period.

The history and type of DM are important factors to consider when devising a perioperative management plan. Patients with non–*insulin*-dependent diabetes (type II) whose condition is controlled with oral hypoglycemic agents or diet are best treated with intravenous fluids containing no dextrose and generally should not be given insulin intraoperatively. Oral administration of hypoglycemic agents should be discontinued approximately 24 hours prior to the surgery. Hyperglycemic episodes in the perioperative period are treated with regular *insulin* only for blood sugar levels in excess of 250 mg/dl.

Insulin-dependent or type I diabetes poses a more difficult problem. Preoperatively, the goals include avoiding ketoacidosis and hypoglycemia as well as, but to a lesser extent, hyperglycemia. Traditionally, approximately one-third to one-half of the patient's usual daily dose of *NPH insulin* (intermediate acting) is given subcutaneously the morning of surgery. An infusion of 5% dextrose is then given intraoperatively, and additional regular *insulin* can be administered in the operating room and every 6 hours afterward if necessary (141). Alternatively, the continuous infusion of *insulin* and glucose in a fixed ratio has been advocated (149,150). The patient is much more prone to significant hypoglycemia, however, when a continuous infusion of *insulin* is given. Because of the severe implications associated with intraoperative hypoglycemia, this method may pose risks and has not been shown to improve the surgical outcome or lessen morbidity. There is no single regimen that is clearly superior for the intraoperative management of type I diabetics. However, a continuous intravenous *insulin* infusion is indicated for patients with unstable type I diabetes, those who require emergency surgery while in ketoacidosis, and those undergoing long, complex procedures (142).

Postoperative monitoring of patients with DM includes careful monitoring of serum glucose levels approximately every 6 hours until the patient is eating and her condition is stable on preoperative regimens. The serum glucose level should be maintained at less than 250 mg/dl, and regular *insulin* should be given on a sliding scale in carefully defined increments of the glucose level. It is essential to prevent the development of severe hypoglycemia or hyperglycemia and the associated complications of diabetic ketoacidosis or a hyperosmolar state. Compulsive perioperative management may obviate some of the infectious and wound healing complications that are more common in these patients (144).

Hyperthyroidism

Thyroid dysfunction should be suspected in any patient who has a history of hyperthyroidism, uses thyroid replacement medication or antithyroid medication, has had prior thyroid surgery, or is undergoing radioactive iodine therapy. Diffuse toxic goiter (Graves' disease), is the most common cause of hyperthyroidism. Any physical findings suggestive of weight loss, tachycardia, proptosis, or myxedema should initiate a more extensive laboratory evaluation of thyroid function. Total thyroxin, free T_3, free thyroxin (T_4), and thyroid-stimulating hormone (TSH) tests are useful in diagnosis.

Because of the risk of thyroid storm, a new diagnosis of hyperthyroidism necessitates postponement of elective surgery until adequate treatment with antithyroid medication can be initiated. Ideally, a euthyroid state should be maintained for 3 months prior to elective surgery. In emergent situations, β-blockers can be used to counter sympathomimetic drive such as palpitations, diaphoresis, and anxiety. Antithyroid medications such as *propylthiouracil*

(PTU) or radioactive iodine do not render patients euthyroid quickly enough for urgent surgery. At best, *PTU* (100 to 200 mg every 6 hours) and a β-blocker can be implemented for 2 weeks prior to surgery; with careful monitoring, optimal results can be achieved (151).

When thyroid dysfunction is corrected and maintained for several months, surgery can proceed without additional perioperative monitoring. Antithyroid medications should be resumed with return of bowel function. In the emergent setting however, close monitoring of the patient for tachycardia, arrhythmias, and hypertension is necessary. β-Blockade can control these symptoms until definitive therapy can be initiated after recovery from surgery. Any signs suggestive of the development of thyroid storm, including hemodynamic instability, tachycardia, arrhythmias, hyperreflexia, diarrhea, or congestive heart failure, mandate transfer to an intensive care setting for optimal monitoring and management in consultation with a medical endocrinologist. Such thyroid instability can be triggered by underlying infection, which requires prompt diagnosis and treatment to facilitate management of this medical emergency.

Hypothyroidism

The prevalence of subclinical hypothyroidism is approximately 1% in the adult population (152). Many such cases are secondary to previous antithyroid therapy (radioactive iodine or thyroidectomy) for hyperthyroidism. A history of lethargy, cold intolerance, lassitude, weight gain, fluid retention, constipation, dry skin, hoarseness, periorbital edema, and brittle hair can be indicative of inadequate thyroid function. In this setting, physical findings of increased relaxation phase of deep tendon reflexes, cardiomegaly, pleural or pericardial effusions, or peripheral edema should stimulate further investigation of thyroid function by assessment of TSH levels. Temporal elevation of TSH can occur in the postoperative setting.

When elective surgery is planned for patients with hypothyroidism, it should be postponed until thyroid replacement therapy has been initiated (153). *Thyroxin* dosage (0.025 mg/day) should be doubled every 2 weeks until the patient is taking a dose of 0.15 mg daily. Dosage levels can ultimately be titrated against TSH levels. In the urgent surgical setting, thyroid replacement should be initiated postoperatively with return of bowel function. Close postoperative monitoring is essential. In severely myxedematous patients in whom surgery cannot be avoided, *thyroxin* (0.3 to 0.5 mg) given intravenously will saturate the carrier protein–binding sites. Standard replacement therapy can then be given until the thyroid function tests and TSH levels determine the optimal dose. In these patients, additional measures are usually necessary because of the severe hypothyroid state. With major abdominal surgery, free water restriction, ventilatory support, diuretics, and nasogastric suction are usually necessary until the patient's condition is stabilized after surgery. Additionally, *hydrocortisone* should be given intravenously (100 to 300 mg every 8 hours) to avoid the possibility of decreased adrenal reserve.

Adrenal Insufficiency

Adrenal insufficiency may result in catastrophic postoperative complications, including death. In patients undergoing surgery, insufficiency most often occurs secondary to the exogenous use of glucocorticoids. Therefore, the physician should ascertain whether a patient has used exogenous steroids for asthma, malignant conditions, arthritis, or irritable bowel syndrome. The type of steroid use, the route, the dose, the duration, and the temporal relationship to the timing of the surgical procedure must be determined. The classification of the surgical procedure and its associated stress should also be taken into consideration. High doses of exogenous steroids for prolonged periods can cause circulatory collapse, and they have adverse effects on wound healing and immunocompetence.

The daily replacement dose of cortisol is approximately 5 to 7.5 mg of *prednisone*. Suppression of the hypothalamic–pituitary–adrenal axis for more than a few weeks may produce relative adrenal insufficiency. When systemic steroids are used for longer periods, adrenal insufficiency may persist for up to 1 year (154). A number of biochemical tests have been recommended to preoperatively evaluate the function of the adrenal gland. The easiest and safest test to assess hypothalamic–pituitary–adrenal function is the *cosyntropin* stimulation test. *Cosyntropin,* a synthetic analog of adrenocorticotropic hormone, is given in a dose of 250 μg, intravenously, and a blood sample is collected 30 minutes after the injection and assayed for plasma cortisol. A plasma cortisol value of >500 nmol/L (18 to 20 μg/dl) indicates adequate adrenal function (155). If the history regarding exogenous steroid use is unclear, then the *cosyntropin* stimulation test should be performed preoperatively to determine if the patient will need perioperative glucocorticoid coverage.

Guidelines for perioperative steroid coverage have been recommended by Salem and co-workers based on clinical and research findings (155). The amount of glucocorticoid replacement should be equivalent to the normal physiologic response to surgical stress. In response to major surgical procedures, adults secrete 75 to 150 mg glucocorticoid a day. In contrast, during minor procedures only 50 mg of glucocorticoid is released (156). For minor surgical stress, the glucocorticoid target is approximately 25 mg of *hydrocortisone* equivalent. Therefore, the patient should receive 25 mg of *hydrocortisone* preoperatively and then resume the normal glucocorticoid dose the next day. For moderate surgical stress (i.e., as with abdominal hysterectomy) the glucocorticoid target is 50 to 75 mg of *hydrocortisone* equivalent per day for 1 to 2 days. The patient should receive her normal daily dose preoperatively, followed by 50 mg of *hydrocortisone* intravenously administered during surgery. Salem and co-workers recommended that patients should receive 60 mg *hydrocortisone* (20 mg every 8 hours) intravenously on postoperative day 1 and then return to their preoperative dose, given either enterally or parenterally on postoperative day 2. For major surgical stress, the glucocorticoid target range is 100 to 150 mg *hydrocortisone* equivalent per day for 2 to 3 days. The patient should receive her normal daily dose within 2 hours preoperatively, followed by 50 mg of *hydrocortisone* intravenously every 8 hours after the initial dose for the first 2 to 3 days after surgery (155).

Whether patients need even this amount of perioperative steroids is unknown. A randomized blinded trial evaluating perioperative steroid use in patients with secondary adrenal insufficiency was performed at the Veterans Affairs Medical Center. Patients who had been taking at least 7.5 mg of *prednisone* daily and had secondary adrenal insufficiency were randomized to two groups. The subjects underwent major surgical procedures; one group received perioperative saline injections and the other received cortisol. All patients received their usual daily steroid dose. Two patients had hypotension, one from each group, which was reversible with fluid replacement. When given their daily dose of steroids for surgical procedures, patients with secondary adrenal insufficiency do not experience serious hypotension secondary to insufficient glucocorticoid levels (157). Therefore, perioperative glucocorticoid coverage should be individualized, based on the patient's preoperative dosage requirements and the type of surgical procedure (155).

Administration of high-dose steroids should be stopped as soon as possible postoperatively because it can inhibit wound healing and promote infection. Hypertension and glucose intolerance also can develop. It is safe to abruptly discontinue steroid use after a few days of therapy. Addison's disease is uncommon but should be considered in the differential diagnosis if the patient develops perioperative hypotension. In addition to blood and isotonic fluid replacement, a "stress" dose of steroids should be given if adrenal insufficiency is suspected and sepsis and hypovolemia have been excluded.

When a prolonged or involved procedure is performed and longer steroid use is necessary, careful tapering will be required. The recommended approach is to halve the dose of *hydrocortisone* on a daily basis until a dose of 25 mg is reached. Eliminating one dose each day until the drug has been stopped is the safest method of withdrawal.

Cardiovascular Diseases

The incidence of perioperative cardiovascular complications has decreased markedly as a result of improvements in preoperative detection of high-risk patients, preoperative preparation, and surgical and anesthetic techniques (158).

Preoperative Evaluation

The goal of a preoperative cardiac evaluation is to determine the presence of heart disease, its severity, and the potential risk to the patient during the perioperative period. Every patient should be questioned about symptoms of cardiac disease including chest pain, dyspnea on exertion, peripheral edema, wheezing, syncope, claudication, or palpitations. Patients with a history of cardiac disease should be evaluated for worsening of symptoms, which indicates progressive or poorly controlled disease. Records of previous treatment should be obtained. Prescriptions for antihypertensive, anticoagulant, antiarrhythmic, antilipid, or antianginal medications may be the only indication of cardiac problems. In patients without known heart disease, the presence of DM, hyperlipidemia, hypertension, tobacco use, or a family history of heart disease identifies a group of patients at higher risk for heart disease who should be more carefully screened.

On physical examination, the presence of findings such as hypertension, jugular venous distention, laterally displaced point of maximum impulse, irregular pulse, third heart sound, pulmonary rales, heart murmurs, peripheral edema, or vascular bruits should prompt a more complete evaluation. Laboratory evaluation of patients with known or suspected heart disease should include a blood count and serum chemistry analysis. Patients with heart disease tolerate anemia poorly. Serum sodium and potassium levels are particularly important in patients taking diuretics and digitalis. Blood urea nitrogen and creatinine values provide information on renal function and hydration status. Assessment of blood glucose levels may detect undiagnosed DM. Chest radiograph and electrocardiography are mandatory as part of the preoperative evaluation, and the results may be particularly helpful when compared with those of previous studies.

Coronary Artery Disease

Coronary artery disease is a major risk factor for patients undergoing abdominal surgery. In an adult population without a prior history of myocardial infarction, the incidence of myocardial infarction following surgery is 0.1% to 0.7% (159). In **patients who have had a prior myocardial infarction, however, the reinfarction rate is 2.8% to 7%** (160). The risk of reinfarction is inversely proportional to the length of time between infarction and surgery. At 3 months or less, the risk of reinfarction is 5.7%, and from 3 to 6 months, the rate falls to 2.3%. Six months after myocardial infarction, the reinfarction rate is 1.5% (159). Fortunately, careful perioperative management can lower the reinfarction rate even in patients who have had recent infarctions. Perioperative myocardial infarction is associated with a mortality rate of 26% to 70% (160).

Because of the high mortality and morbidity associated with perioperative myocardial infarction, much effort has been made to predict perioperative cardiac risk. **A prospective evaluation of preoperative cardiac risk factors using a multivariate analysis identified independent cardiac risk factors for patients undergoing noncardiac surgery** (161). Using these factors, a cardiac risk index was created that placed a patient in one of four risk classes. High-risk clinical factors included age over 70 years, myocardial infarction within 6 months prior to surgery, congestive heart failure, and atrial and ventricular arrhythmias. More recent studies have added to and modified the commonly accepted list of risk factors, which are listed in Table 19.8 (160). Additional risk factors include unstable angina, DM, uncontrolled hypertension, history of stroke, and abnormal electrocardiogram.

In addition to clinical predictors, cardiac risk is also determined by the risk level of the proposed operation and the functional capacity of the patient. High-risk procedures include

Table 19.8. Risk Factors for Perioperative Cardiovascular Risk (160)

Major
Unstable or severe angina
Recent myocardial infarction (>7 days but <30 days)
Decompensated congestive heart failure
Symptomatic arrhythmias
Intermediate
Mild angina
Prior myocardial infarction by history or ECG
Compensated or prior congestive heart failure
Diabetes mellitus
Minor
Advanced age
Abnormal ECG (LVH, LBBB, ST-T abnormalities)
Rhythm other than sinus
Low functional capacity
History of stroke
Uncontrolled systemic hypertension

ECG, electrocardiogram; LVH, left ventricular hypertrophy; BBB, bundle branch block.

emergent major operations, aortic and vascular procedures, and prolonged surgical procedures associated with large fluid shifts or blood loss. Intermediate-risk procedures include other intraperitoneal operations, whereas low-risk procedures include endoscopic surgery, breast surgery, and superficial procedures. The patient's functional status is assessed by a thorough history; risk classification is summarized in Table 19.9. Patients with poor functional capacity have higher perioperative cardiac risk and should be considered for preoperative cardiac function testing (160).

In an effort to quantitate preoperative cardiac risk, several tests have been used to assess cardiovascular function. *Exercise stress testing* prior to surgery can identify patients who have ischemic heart disease not apparent at rest. These patients have been shown to be at increased risk of developing cardiac complications in the perioperative period. In a study of patients undergoing peripheral vascular surgery, a high-risk group of patients was identified who had ischemic electrocardiographic changes when they exercised to less than 75% of their maximal predicted heart rate. In this group, the incidence of perioperative myocardial infarction was 25% and the overall cardiac mortality rate was 18.5%. Conversely,

Table 19.9. Functional Capacity Assessment from Clinical History (160)

Excellent
Carry 24 lb up eight steps
Carry objects that weigh 80 lb
Outdoor work (shovel snow, spade soil)
Recreation (ski, basketball, squash, handball, jog or walk 5 mph)
Moderate
Have sexual intercourse without stopping
Walk at 4 mph on ground level
Outdoor work (garden, rake, weed)
Recreation (roller skate, dance)
Poor
Shower and dress without stopping
Basic housework
Walk 2.5 mph on level ground
Recreation (golf, bowl)

no perioperative infarctions occurred in patients who were able to exercise to more than 75% of their maximal predicted heart rate and who had no electrocardiographic evidence of ischemia (162). However, the prognostic value of stress testing was not supported in another prospective study that found that only an abnormal preoperative resting electrocardiogram was an independent risk factor (163). The exercise stress test must be selectively applied to a high-risk population because its predictive value is dependent upon the prevalence of the disease. Therefore, it is not prudent to screen all patients preoperatively; it is preferable to rely on a careful history to identify patients with symptoms of cardiac disease for whom the test would be most predictive.

Exercise stress testing is limited in some patients who cannot exercise because of musculoskeletal disease, pulmonary disease, or severe cardiac disease. *Dipyridamole-thallium scanning* may be used to overcome the limitations of exercise stress testing. This study has a high degree of sensitivity and specificity, and it relies on the ability of dipyridamole to dilate normal coronary arteries but not stenotic vessels. Normally perfused myocardium readily takes up thallium when it is given intravenously. Conversely, hypoperfused myocardium does not demonstrate good uptake of thallium when scanned 5 minutes after injection. Reperfusion and uptake of thallium 3 hours after injection identify viable but high-risk myocardium. Old infarctions are identified as areas without uptake. Several studies have shown a risk of perioperative myocardial infarction in patients with areas of reperfusion of thallium uptake ranging from 20% to 33% (164,165). The dipyridamole-thallium scan is applicable for patients who are unable to exercise because it uses a medically induced "stress."

Dobutamine stress echocardiography is another test to evaluate cardiac risk in patients who are unable to exercise. This method identifies regional cardiac wall motion abnormalities after dobutamine infusion to identify patients at high risk for cardiac events. Positive and negative predictive values are similar to those of dipyridamole-thallium testing (166,167).

It is rare for patients who are younger than 50 years and who do not have diabetes, hypertension, hypercholesterolemia, or coronary artery disease to suffer a perioperative myocardial infarction. However, patients with coronary artery disease are at increased risk of myocardial infarction in the postoperative period. Prevention, early recognition, and treatment are important, because myocardial infarctions that occur in the postoperative period have mortality rates of approximately 50% and are more lethal than those that are not associated with surgery.

Nearly two-thirds of postoperative myocardial infarctions occur during the first 3 days postoperatively. Although the pathophysiologic factors are complex, the causes of postoperative myocardial ischemia and infarction are related to decreased myocardial oxygen supply coupled with increased myocardial oxygen requirements. In postoperative patients, conditions that decrease oxygen supply to the myocardium include tachycardia, increased preload, hypotension, anemia, and hypoxia (168). Conditions that increase myocardial oxygen consumption are tachycardia, increased preload, increased afterload, and increased contractility. Tachycardia and increased preload are the most important causes of ischemia, because both conditions decrease oxygen supply to the myocardium while simultaneously increasing myocardial oxygen demand. Tachycardia decreases the diastolic time which, when the coronary arteries are perfused, decreases the volume of oxygen available to the myocardium. Increased preload increases the pressure exerted by the myocardial wall on the arterioles within it, thus decreasing myocardial blood flow.

Other factors associated with perioperative myocardial ischemia include physiologic responses to the stress of intubation, intravenous or intraarterial line placement, emergence from anesthesia, pain, and anxiety. This stress results in catecholamine stimulation of the cardiovascular system, resulting in increased heart rate, blood pressure, and contractility, which may induce or worsen myocardial ischemia. Loss of intravascular volume because of third spacing of fluids or postoperative hemorrhage can also induce ischemia.

Postoperative myocardial infarction is often difficult to diagnose. Chest pain, which is present in 90% of nonsurgical patients with myocardial infarction, may be present in only 50% of patients with postoperative infarction, because of the masking of myocardial pain by coexisting surgical pain and the use of analgesia (159). Thus, it is important to maintain a high level of suspicion for postoperative infarction in patients with coronary artery disease. The presence of arrhythmia, congestive heart failure, hypotension, dyspnea, or elevations of pulmonary artery pressure may indicate infarction and should prompt a thorough cardiac investigation and electrocardiographic monitoring. **Measurement of creatinine phosphokinase myocardial band (CPK-MB) isoenzyme and troponin T levels are the most sensitive and specific indicators of myocardial infarction, and assessments should be obtained for all patients suspected of myocardial infarction.**

Despite the high incidence of silent myocardial infarction, routine use of postoperative electrocardiography (ECG) for all patients with cardiovascular disease is controversial. Many patients will exhibit P-wave changes that spontaneously resolve and do not represent ischemia or infarction. Conversely, patients with proven myocardial infarctions may show few, if any, ECG abnormalities. If routine screening of asymptomatic patients is desired, ECGs should be obtained 24 hours following surgery, because it has been shown that significant ECG changes that occur immediately postoperatively will persist for 24 hours. It is prudent to continue serial ECG assessments for at least 3 days postoperatively.

Postoperative management of patients with coronary artery disease is based on maximizing delivery of oxygen to the myocardium as well as decreasing myocardial oxygen utilization. Most patients benefit from supplemental oxygen in the postoperative period, although special care should be exercised in patients with chronic obstructive pulmonary disease. Oxygenation can be easily monitored by pulse oximetry. Anemia is detrimental because of loss of oxygen-carrying capacity as well as resultant tachycardia and should, therefore, be carefully corrected in high-risk patients.

Patents with coronary artery disease may benefit from pharmacologic control of hyperadrenergic states that result from increased postoperative catecholamine production. β-Blockers decrease heart rate, myocardial contractility, and systemic blood pressure, all of which are increased by adrenergic stimulation. Perioperative β-blockade with atenolol has been shown to significantly reduce perioperative ischemia, myocardial infarction, and overall mortality caused by cardiac death and congestive heart failure in the perioperative period (169,170). For patients receiving β-blockade therapy prior to surgery, that therapy should be continued in the perioperative period because abrupt withdrawal results in a rebound hyperadrenergic state.

Although prophylactic nitrates have been used in the perioperative period for many years, this practice remains controversial. *Nitroglycerin* enhances blood flow to ischemic areas, increases collateral flow, increases myocardial oxygenation, and reduces angina (171–174). The route of administration, dosage, and duration of therapy are controversial; thus, perioperative treatment with nitrates should be initiated in consultation with a cardiologist. Likewise, calcium-channel blockers have not proved useful in the prophylaxis of perioperative myocardial ischemia (175).

Congestive Heart Failure

Patients with congestive heart failure (CHF) face a substantially increased risk of myocardial infarction during and after surgery (161). The postoperative development of pulmonary edema is a grave prognostic sign and results in death in a high percentage of patients (176). Because patients with heart failure at the time of surgery are significantly more likely to develop pulmonary edema perioperatively, every effort should be made to diagnose and treat CHF before surgery (177). The signs and symptoms of CHF are listed in Table 19.10 and should be assessed based on preoperative history and physical examination.

Table 19.10. Signs and Symptoms of Congestive Heart Failure

1. Presence of an S_3 gallop
2. Jugular venous distention
3. Lateral shift of the point of maximal impulse
4. Lower extremity edema
5. Basilar rales
6. Increased voltage on electrocardiogram
7. Evidence of pulmonary edema or cardiac enlargement on chest radiograph
8. Tachycardia

Patients who are able to perform usual daily activities without developing CHF are at limited risk of perioperative heart failure.

To prevent severe postoperative complications, congestive heart failure must be corrected preoperatively. Treatment usually relies on aggressive diuretic therapy, although care must be taken to avoid dehydration, which may result in hypotension during the induction of anesthesia. Hypokalemia can result from diuretic therapy and is especially deleterious to patients who are also taking digitalis. In addition to diuretics and digitalis, treatment often includes the use of preload- and afterload-reducing agents. Optimal use of these drugs and correction of CHF may be aided by consultation with a cardiologist. In general, it is preferable to continue the usual regimen of cardioactive drugs throughout the perioperative period. In patients with severe or intractable CHF, the perioperative measurement of left ventricular filling (wedge) pressure with a pulmonary artery catheter (Swan-Ganz) may be extremely helpful to guide perioperative fluid management.

Postoperative CHF results most frequently from excessive administration of intravenous fluids and blood products. Other common postoperative causes are myocardial infarction, systemic infection, pulmonary embolism, and cardiac arrhythmias. The cause of postoperative heart failure must be diagnosed because, to be successful, treatment should be directed simultaneously to the underlying cause.

Postoperative diagnosis of CHF is often more difficult than preoperative diagnosis because the signs and symptoms of CHF are not specific and may result from other causes (Table 19.10). The most reliable method of detecting CHF is chest radiography, in which the presence of cardiomegaly or evidence of pulmonary edema is a helpful diagnostic feature.

Acute postoperative CHF frequently manifests as pulmonary edema. Treatment of pulmonary edema may include the use of intravenous furosemide, supplemental oxygen, including morphine sulfate, and elevation of the head of the bed. Intravenous aminophylline may be useful if cardiogenic asthma is present. Electrocardiography, in addition to laboratory evaluation, including arterial blood gas, serum electrolyte, and renal function chemistry measurements, should be obtained expediently. If the patient's condition does not improve rapidly, she should be transferred to an intensive care unit.

Arrhythmias

Nearly all arrhythmias found in otherwise healthy patients are asymptomatic and of limited consequence. In patients with underlying cardiac disease, however, even brief episodes of arrhythmias may result in significant cardiac morbidity and mortality.

Preoperative evaluation of arrhythmias by a cardiologist and anesthesiologist is important because many anesthetic agents as well as surgical stress contribute to the development or worsening of arrhythmias. In patients undergoing continuous electrocardiographic monitoring during surgery, a 60% incidence of arrhythmias, excluding sinus tachycardia, has been reported (178). Patients with heart disease have an increased risk of arrhythmias, most commonly ventricular arrhythmias (178). Conversely, patients without cardiac disease are more likely to develop supraventricular arrhythmias during surgery. Patients taking antiarrhythmic medications prior to surgery should continue taking those drugs during the perioperative period. Initiation of antiarrhythmic medications is rarely indicated preoperatively, but consultation with a cardiologist is recommended for patients in whom arrhythmias are detected prior to surgery.

Patients with first-degree atrioventricular (AV) block or asymptomatic Mobitz I (Wenckebach) second-degree AV block require no preoperative therapy. Conversely, a pacemaker is appropriate in patients with symptomatic Mobitz II second- or third-degree AV block before elective surgery (179). In emergency situations, a pacing pulmonary artery catheter can be used. Prior to performing surgery on patients with a permanent pacemaker, the type and location of the pacemaker should be determined because electrocautery units may interfere with demand-type pacemakers (180). When performing gynecologic surgery on patients with pacemakers, it is preferable to place the electrocautery unit ground plate on the leg to minimize interference. In patients with a demand pacemaker in place, the pacemaker should be converted preoperatively to the fixed-rate mode.

Surgery is not contraindicated in patients with bundle branch blocks or hemiblocks. Complete heart block rarely develops during noncardiac surgical procedures in patients with conduction system disease (181–183). However, the presence of a left bundle branch block may indicate the presence of aortic stenosis, which can increase surgical mortality if it is severe.

Valvular Heart Disease

Although there are many forms of valvular heart disease, primarily two types—aortic and mitral stenosis—are associated with significantly increased operative risk (184). Patients with significant aortic stenosis appear to be at greatest risk, which is further increased if atrial fibrillation, congestive heart failure, or coronary artery disease is also present. Significant stenosis of aortic or mitral valves should be repaired prior to elective gynecologic surgery (160).

Severe valvular heart disease is usually evident during physical exertion. Common findings in such patients are listed in Table 19.11. The classic history presented by patients with severe aortic stenosis includes exercise dyspnea, angina, and syncope, whereas symptoms of mitral stenosis are paroxysmal and effort dyspnea, hemoptysis, and orthopnea. Most patients have a remote history of rheumatic fever. Severe stenosis of either valve is considered to be a

Table 19.11. Signs and Symptoms of Valvular Heart Disease

Aortic stenosis
1. Systolic murmur at right sternal border, which radiates into carotids
2. Decreased systolic blood pressure
3. Apical heave
4. Chest radiograph with calcified aortic ring, left ventricular enlargement
5. Electrocardiogram with high R waves, depressed T waves in lead I and precordial leads
Mitral stenosis
1. Precordial heave
2. Diastolic murmur at apex
3. Mitral opening snap
4. Suffused face and lips
5. Chest radiograph with left atrial dilation
6. Electrocardiogram with large P waves and right axis deviation

Table 19.12. Recommendations for Prophylaxis of Bacterial Endocarditis for Genitourinary and Gastrointestinal Procedures (185)

High-Risk Patients	***Agents***	***Regimen***
Standard regimen	*Ampicillin* and	2.0 g IM or IV within 30 min of starting procedure; 1.0 g IM or IV 6 hr later
	Gentamicin	1.5 mg/kg (not to exceed 120 mg) within 30 min of starting procedure
Penicillin-allergic	*Vancomycin* and	1.0 g IV over 1–2 hr completed within 30 min of starting procedure
	Gentamicin	1.5 mg/kg (not to exceed 120 mg) within 30 min of starting procedure
Moderate-Risk Patients	***Agents***	***Regimen***
Standard regimen	*Ampicillin* or *Amoxicillin*	2.0 g IM or IV within 30 min of starting procedure 2.0 g orally 1 hr before procedure
Penicillin-allergic	*Vancomycin*	1.0 g IV over 1–2 hr completed within 30 min of starting procedure

valvular area of less than 1 cm^2, and diagnosis can be confirmed by echocardiography or cardiac catheterization.

Patients with valvular abnormalities have been subdivided by the American Heart Association into risk groups for the development of subacute bacterial endocarditis following surgery (185). Patients with prosthetic valves are classified as high risk, whereas patients with mitral valve prolapse with regurgitation, history of rheumatic heart disease, or bicuspid aortic valve are considered at moderate risk. **Patients in both high- and moderate-risk groups should receive prophylactic antibiotics immediately preoperatively to prevent subacute bacterial endocarditis.** Table 19.12 outlines the American Heart Association recommendations for antibiotic prophylaxis (185).

Patients with aortic and mitral stenosis tolerate sinus tachycardia and other *tachyarrhythmias* poorly. In patients with aortic stenosis, sufficient digitalization should be provided to correct preoperative tachyarrhythmias, and *propranolol* may be used to control sinus tachycardia. Patients with mitral valve stenosis often have atrial fibrillation and, if present, digitalis should be used to reduce rapid ventricular response.

Patients with mechanical heart valves usually tolerate surgery well (186). Management of these patients requires antibiotic prophylaxis (Table 19.12) and discontinuation of anticoagulant therapy during the perioperative period. Usually, *warfarin* (*Coumadin*) is withheld several days prior of surgery and anticoagulation is obtained by intravenous administration of *heparin* (187). The *heparin* is discontinued 6 to 8 hours prior to surgery and resumed a few days postoperatively (188). The patient is returned to oral *warfarin* maintenance therapy. Alternatively, *warfarin* can be stopped 1 to 3 days perioperatively and restarted several days postoperatively. Perioperative heparinization is indicated in patients who have more thrombogenic valves, such as the Starr-Edwards valve, and valves in the tricuspid position (179). Both methods of management have essentially no risk of thromboembolic complications and bleeding complication rates of approximately 15%.

In the postoperative period, patients with mitral stenosis should be carefully monitored for pulmonary edema because they may not be able to compensate for the amount of intravenous fluid administered during surgery. Patients with mitral stenosis also frequently have pulmonary hypertension and decreased airway compliance. Therefore, they may require more pulmonary support and therapy postoperatively, including prolonged mechanical ventilation.

Table 19.13. Common Parenteral Antihypertensives

Drug	Route	Initial Dose	Onset	Duration	Side Effects
Nitroprusside	IV infusion	0.5 μg/min	Immediate	2–5 minutes	Tachycardia, nausea
Labetalol	IV infusion	20 mg	5–10 minutes	4 hours	Bronchospasm, dizziness, nausea
Esmolol	IV infusion	50 μg/min	2 hours	9 minutes	Headache, somnolence, dizziness, hypotension
Nifedipine	Sublingual	10 mg	5 minutes	2 minutes	Hypotension, headache, dizziness, nausea, peripheral edema
Verapamil	IV infusion	5–10 mg	3–5 minutes	2–5 hours	Nausea, headache, hypotension, dizziness, pulmonary edema

IV, intravenous.

For patients with significant aortic stenosis, it is imperative that a sinus rhythm be maintained during the postoperative period. Even sinus tachycardia can be deleterious because it shortens the diastolic time. Bradycardia less than 45 beats per minute should be treated with atropine. Supraventricular dysrhythmias may be controlled with *verapamil* or direct-current cardioversion. Particular attention should be provided to the maintenance of proper fluid status, digoxin levels, electrolyte levels, and blood replacement.

Hypertension

Patients with controlled essential hypertension have no increased risk of perioperative cardiac morbidity or mortality (177). However, patients with concomitant heart disease are at elevated risk and should be completely evaluated by a cardiologist preoperatively. Laboratory studies should include an ECG, chest radiograph, blood count, urinalysis, and serum electrolytes and creatinine measurement. Antihypertensive medications should be continued perioperatively. Of note, β-blockers should be continued, parenterally if necessary, to avoid rebound tachycardia, hypercontractility, and hypertension.

Patients with diastolic pressures higher than 110 mmHg or systolic pressures higher than 180 mmHg should receive medication to control their hypertension prior to surgery. Chronically hypertensive patients are very susceptible to intraoperative hypotension because of impaired autoregulation of blood flow to the brain and, therefore, require a higher mean arterial pressure to maintain adequate perfusion (189). Conversely, during induction of anesthesia episodes of hypertension occur, and such episodes are seen more frequently in patients with baseline hypertension.

Postoperative hypertension is usually treated parenterally because gastrointestinal absorption may be diminished, and transdermal absorption can be erratic in patients who are cold and rewarming. Commonly used parenteral antihypertensives are listed in Table 19.13.

Hemodynamic Monitoring

Hemodynamic monitoring has become integral to the perioperative management of patients with cardiovascular and pulmonary disease. The major impetus for this advancement resides in the need for the quantitative estimate of cardiac function, resulting in the development of bedside pulmonary artery catheterization. The impact of monitoring of cardiac function is demonstrated by the significant reduction of myocardial infarctions in high-risk patients who are aggressively monitored for 72 to 96 hours postoperatively (190).

Before the development of the pulmonary artery catheter, central venous pressure (CVP) measurement was used to assess intravascular volume status and cardiac function. To measure the CVP, a catheter is placed in the central venous system, most frequently the superior vena cava. A water manometer or a calibrated pressure transducer is connected to the CVP line, thus allowing an estimation of right atrial pressure to be obtained. Right atrial pressure is determined by the balance between cardiac output and venous return. Cardiac output is determined by heart rate, myocardial contractility, preload, and afterload. Thus, if the pulmonary vascularity and left ventricular function are normal, the CVP accurately reflects the left ventricular end-diastolic pressure (LVEDP). The LVEDP reflects cardiac output or systemic perfusion and has been considered the standard estimator of left ventricular pump function. Venous return is determined primarily by the mean systemic pressure, which propels blood toward the heart, balanced against resistance to venous return, which acts in the opposite direction. Thus, if right ventricular function is normal, the CVP accurately reflects intravascular volume.

Left and right ventricular function is frequently abnormal or discordant; therefore, the relationship of CVP to cardiac function and to intravascular volume is not maintained. When this occurs, measurement of pulmonary artery occlusion pressure is required to accurately assess volume status and cardiovascular function. The use of a pulmonary artery catheter also allows detection of changes in cardiovascular function with more sensitivity and rapidity than clinical observation.

The balloon-tipped pulmonary artery catheter (Swan-Ganz catheter) can provide measurement of pulmonary artery and pulmonary artery occlusion pressures (191). The catheter can measure cardiac output, be used to perform intracavitary electrocardiography, and provide temporary cardiac pacing. The standard pulmonary artery occlusion catheter is a 7-French, radiopaque, flexible, polyvinyl chloride, 4-lumen catheter with a 1.5-ml latex balloon at its distal tip. Most often, a right internal jugular cannulation is used for placement of the catheter, because this site provides the most direct access into the right atrium and has fewer complications when compared with a subclavian route of placement. After the catheter is placed into the right atrium, the balloon is inflated and the catheter is pulled by blood flow through the right ventricle into the pulmonary artery. The position of the catheter can be identified and followed by the various pressure waveforms generated by the right atrium, right ventricle, and pulmonary artery. As the catheter passes through increasingly smaller branches of the pulmonary artery, the inflated balloon eventually occludes the pulmonary artery. **The distal lumen of the catheter, which is beyond the balloon, measures left atrial pressure (LAP) and, in the absence of mitral valvular disease, LAP approximates LVEDP. Thus, pulmonary–capillary wedge pressure (PCWP) equals the LAP, which equals LVEDP and is normal at 8 to 12 mm Hg.** Additionally, because the standard pulmonary artery catheter has an incorporated thermistor, thermodilution studies can be performed to determine cardiac output. This thermodilution method is performed by injecting cold 5% dextrose in water through the proximal port of the catheter, which cools the blood entering the right atrium. The change in temperature measured at the more distal thermistor (4 cm from the catheter tip) generates a curve proportional to cardiac output. Knowledge of the cardiac output is helpful in establishing cardiovascular diagnoses. For example, a patient with hypotension, low-to-normal wedge pressure, and a cardiac output of 3 L/min is most likely hypovolemic. Conversely, the same patient with a cardiac output of 8 L/min is probably septic with resultant low systemic vascular resistance.

Pulmonary artery catheters are associated with a small but significant complication rate. The complications can be grouped into those occurring during venous cannulation and those resulting from the catheter or its placement. The most common problems encountered during venous access are cannulation of the carotid or subclavian artery and introduction of a pneumothorax. Problems resulting from the catheter itself include dysrhythmias, sepsis, and disruption of the pulmonary artery. Pulmonary artery catheters should be placed under the supervision of experienced personnel in a setting in which complications can be rapidly diagnosed and treated.

The effect of pulmonary artery catheter use on patient outcome has become controversial. In 1996 Dalen and Bone recommended a reevaluation of pulmonary artery catheters and initiation of randomized clinical trials to assess their benefit (192). At that time, Connors and others published a large study demonstrating a higher mortality rate in patients who received a pulmonary artery catheter than those that did not have a pulmonary artery catheter (193). The design of this study was questionable, however, and it was retrospective and not randomized. A recent metaanalysis evaluating 12 randomized clinical trials demonstrated a statistically significant reduction in morbidity (63% versus 74%, $P < 0.01$) in the pulmonary artery catheter group, but no significant difference in mortality (194). Future large randomized clinical trials comparing pulmonary artery catheters to central venous catheters for the treatment of critical care patients are currently under way, and it is hoped a consensus regarding who will benefit from pulmonary artery catheters will eventually be established.

Hematologic Disorders

The presence of hematologic disorders, although uncommon in gynecologic patients, significantly affects operative morbidity and mortality and therefore should be considered routinely in preoperative evaluation. Preoperative assessment should include consideration of anemia, platelet and coagulation disorders, white blood cell function, and immunity.

Anemia

Moderate anemia is not in itself a contraindication to surgery because it can be corrected by transfusion. If possible, surgery should be postponed until the cause of the anemia can be identified and the anemia corrected without resorting to transfusion. **Current anesthetic and surgical practice ideally recommend a hemoglobin level of >10 g/dl or a hematocrit of >30%. Such numbers are only guidelines, and should be applied on an individual basis.** Oxygen-carrying capacity and tissue oxygenation is provided by the circulating blood volume. Usually this capacity is reflected by the hemoglobin level and hematocrit. Under certain circumstances, however, this is not the case. After an acute blood loss or before plasma expansion by extracellular fluid has occurred, hematocrit measurements may be normal despite a low circulating blood volume. Conversely, overhydration may result in low hematocrit and hemoglobin levels despite adequate red blood cell mass.

Individual tolerance of anemia depends on overall physical fitness and cardiovascular reserve. The effects of anemia depend on its magnitude, the rate at which it occurs, the oxygen requirement of the patient, and the ability of physiologic mechanisms to compensate (195). Maintenance of adequate tissue perfusion requires an increase in cardiac output as hemoglobin concentration falls (196). A patient with ischemic heart disease will not tolerate anemia as well as a healthy young patient. Therefore, the presence of cardiac, pulmonary, or other serious illness justifies a more conservative approach to the management of anemia. Conversely, patients with longstanding anemia may have normal blood volume levels and tolerate surgical procedures well. There is no evidence that mild to moderate anemia increases perioperative morbidity or mortality (197).

Patients with normal hematocrit levels may store three or more units of autologous blood preoperatively to reduce the need for allogenic blood transfusion and minimize the risk of infections and immunologic problems (198). *Recombinant human erythropoietin* may increase collection and reduce preoperative anemia in these patients (199). Further, intraoperative blood collection and homologous transfusion can be employed to limit need for allogenic blood transfusion.

Platelet and Coagulation Disorders

Surgical hemostasis is provided by platelet adhesion to injured vessels, which plugs the opening as the coagulation cascade is activated, resulting in the formation of fibrin clots. Thus, functional platelets and coagulation pathways are necessary to prevent excessive surgical bleeding. Platelet dysfunction is encountered more frequently preoperatively than coagulation disorders.

Platelets may be deficient in both number and function. The normal peripheral blood count is 150,000 to 400,000 per mm^3, and the normal lifespan of a platelet is approximately 10 days. Although there is no clear-cut correlation between the degree of thrombocytopenia and the presence or amount of bleeding, several generalizations can be made. If the platelet count is higher than 100,000/mm^3 and the platelets are functioning normally, there is little chance of bleeding during surgical procedures. Patients with a platelet count higher than 75,000/mm^3 almost always have normal bleeding times, and a platelet count higher than 50,000/mm^3 is probably adequate. **A platelet count lower than 20,000/mm^3 will often be associated with severe and spontaneous bleeding.** Platelet counts higher than 1,000,000/mm^3 are often, paradoxically, associated with bleeding.

If the patient's platelet count is lower than 100,000/mm^3, an assessment of bleeding time should be obtained. If the bleeding time is abnormal and surgery must be performed, an attempt should be made to raise the platelet count by administering platelet transfusions immediately before surgery. In patients with immune destruction of platelets, human leukocyte antigen (HLA)–matched donor-specific platelets may be required to prevent rapid destruction of transfused platelets. If surgery can be postponed, a hematology consultation should be obtained to identify and treat the cause of the platelet abnormality.

Abnormally low platelet counts result from either decreased production or increased consumption of platelets. Although there are numerous causes of thrombocytopenia, most are exceedingly uncommon. Decreased platelet production may be drug induced and has been associated with the use of *sulfonamides, cinchona alkaloids, thiazide diuretics, nonsteroidal antiinflammatory drugs (NSAIDs)*, gold salts, *penicillamine, anticonvulsants,* and *heparins* (200). Decreased platelet count is a feature of several diseases, including vitamin B_{12} and folate deficiency, aplastic anemia, myeloproliferative disorders, renal failure, and viral infections. Inherited congenital thrombocytopenia is extremely rare. More commonly, thrombocytopenia results from immune destruction of platelets by diseases such as idiopathic thrombocytopenia purpura and collagen vascular disorders. Consumptive thrombocytopenia is a feature of disseminated intravascular coagulation (DIC), which is encountered most frequently in conjunction with sepsis or malignancy in the preoperative population.

Platelet dysfunction is most often acquired, but may be inherited. Occasionally, a patient with von Willebrand's disease, the second most common inherited disorder of coagulation, may be encountered in the preoperative setting. More commonly, however, platelet dysfunction results from the use of drugs (e.g., *aspirin* and *amitriptyline*), and patients with resulting prolonged bleeding times should have the drug withheld for 7 to 10 days before surgery. Uremia and hepatic diseases can also affect platelet function.

Platelet dysfunction is more difficult to diagnose than abnormalities of platelet count. A history of easy bruising, petechiae, bleeding from mucous membranes, or prolonged bleeding from minor wounds may signify an underlying abnormality of platelet function. Such dysfunction can be identified with the help of a bleeding time, but full characterization of the underlying etiology should be carried out with hematologic consultation. If at all possible, surgery should be postponed until therapy has been instituted.

Similarly, disorders of the coagulation cascade are often diagnosed through a personal or family history of excessive bleeding during minor surgery, childbirth, or menses. Deficiency of factor VIII (hemophilia) and factor IX (Christmas disease) are the most commonly encountered inherited disorders of coagulation. There are few commonly prescribed drugs that affect coagulation factors, the exceptions being *warfarin* and *heparin.* Disease states that may be associated with decreased coagulation factor levels are primarily liver disease, vitamin K deficiency (secondary to obstructive biliary disease, intestinal malabsorption, or antibiotic reduction of bowel flora), and DIC.

Preoperative laboratory screening for coagulation deficiencies is controversial. Routine screening in patients without historical evidence of a bleeding problem is not warranted

(201). However, patients who are seriously ill or who will be undergoing extensive surgical procedures should undergo testing preoperatively to determine prothrombin time, partial thromboplastin time, fibrinogen level, and platelet count.

White Blood Cells and Immune Function

Abnormally high or low white blood cell counts are not an absolute contraindication to surgery; however, they should be considered relative to the need for surgery. Evaluation of an elevated or decreased white blood cell count should be undertaken prior to elective surgery. Clearly, **patients with absolute granulocyte counts lower than 1,000/mm^3 are at increased risk of severe infection and perioperative morbidity and mortality, and should undergo surgery only for life-threatening indications** (202).

Blood Component Replacement

Most hematologic problems observed in the postoperative period are related to perioperative bleeding and blood component replacement. Although the primary cause of the bleeding is usually lack of surgical hemostasis, other factors, including deranged coagulation, may compound the problem. Such coagulopathy can result from massive transfusion (less than one blood volume) and is thought to be due to dilution of platelets and labile coagulation factors by platelet- and factor-poor packed red blood cells (PRBCs), fibrinolysis, and DIC.

Reports of massive transfusions in soldiers reveal that for those in whom thrombocytopenia developed following red blood cell replacement, bleeding diatheses that responded to infusion of fresh blood but not fresh-frozen plasma (FFP) also developed (203). The investigators concluded that dilutional thrombocytopenia is a major cause of posttransfusion bleeding. However, more recently, in a prospective, randomized, double-blind study, prophylactic platelet administration during massive transfusion was not helpful (204). Although it seems that these studies are contradictory, they demonstrate the need for obtaining platelet counts during transfusion of large amounts of blood. If clinical evidence of excessive bleeding exists and the platelet count is lower than 100,000/mm^3, platelets should be transfused, because they are consumed during surgery and higher levels are required to maintain hemostasis following surgery.

Packed red blood cells, which may be stored for several weeks, are used for most postoperative transfusions. Most clotting factors are stable for long periods. The exceptions are factors V and VIII, which decrease to 15% and 50% of normal, respectively. Despite this loss, these factors rarely decrease below levels required for hemostasis. In 1985, a National Institutes of Health consensus conference concluded that there was little or no scientific evidence to support the use of FFP for bleeding diatheses following multiple blood transfusions except in the presence of clinical bleeding, platelet count higher than 100,000/mm^3, and a partial thromboplastin time greater than 1.5 times control. A task force of the American Society of Anesthesiologists (205) recently **recommended critical values for replacement in patients with massive transfusion and microvascular bleeding:**

1. Platelet counts $<$50,000/mm^3 (with intermediate platelet counts, i.e., 50,000/mm^3 to 100,000/mm^3 the transfusion of platelet concentrates should be based on the risk for more significant bleeding)
2. Elevated ($>$1.5 times normal) prothrombin or activated partial thromboplastin time values
3. Coagulation factor concentrations less than 30%
4. Fibrinogen concentrations less than 80 to 100 mg/dl.

Donor blood is stored in the presence of citrate, which chelates calcium to prevent clotting, raising the theoretical risk of hypocalcemia following massive transfusion. However, citrate is metabolized at a rate equivalent to 20 units of blood transfused per hour; thus, routine supplementation of calcium is unnecessary. Close monitoring of calcium levels is required in patients with hypothermia, liver disease, or hyperventilation, because citrate metabolism may be slowed. Hepatic metabolism of citrate to bicarbonate can result in metabolic alkalosis following transfusion, resulting in subsequent hypokalemia, despite the high level of extracellular potassium in stored blood.

Pulmonary Disease

In patients undergoing abdominal surgery, several pulmonary physiologic changes occur secondary to immobilization, anesthetic irritation of the airways, and the splinting of breathing that inevitably occurs with incisional pain. Pulmonary physiologic changes include a decrease in the functional residual capacity (FRC) and vital capacity (VC), an increase in ventilation–perfusion mismatching, and impaired mucociliary clearance of secretions from the tracheobronchial tree. These changes result in transient hypoxemia and atelectasis that, untreated, can progress to pneumonia in the postoperative period (206,207). Postoperative pulmonary dysfunction is more pronounced in patients with advanced age, preexisting lung disease, obesity, a significant history of smoking, and upper abdominal surgery (206).

Most postoperative pulmonary complications occur in patients who have preexisting pulmonary disease. In these patients, the incidence of pulmonary complications is higher than 70%, as compared with the low incidence (2% to 5%) that occurs in individuals with healthy lungs (206,208). The risk of postoperative pulmonary complications is lower in patients undergoing lower abdominal surgery as compared with upper abdominal surgery and in those undergoing nonthoracic, nonabdominal surgery as compared with abdominal operations. The presence of chronic obstructive pulmonary disease markedly increases the risk (206,209).

Preoperative spirometry is of unproved value in patients undergoing abdominal surgery in whom the risk of postoperative pulmonary complications is low (210–213). In high-risk patients, preoperative spirometry should be performed with and without bronchodilators in order to identify patients who may benefit from preoperative treatment with inhaled β_2 agonists and steroids. These patients include those with a history of chronic cough or dyspnea, evidence of pulmonary abnormalities by either physical examination or chest radiograph, and a history of chronic obstructive pulmonary disease, as well as patients with a significant history of smoking. In addition to the preoperative spirometric evaluation, an arterial blood gas assessment should be performed. The spirometric abnormalities most often associated with postoperative atelectasis and pneumonia are shown in Table 19.14.

Young, healthy patients rarely have abnormal chest radiographic examination results. Therefore, chest radiographs should not be performed routinely in these patients. Most patients with abnormal chest radiographs have history or physical examination findings suggestive

Table 19.14. Predictors of Postoperative Pulmonary Complications[a]

Parameter	*Value*
Maximal breathing capacity	<50% predicted
FEV_1	<1 L
FVC	<70% predicted
FEV_1/FVC	<65% predicted
$Pa{O_2}$	<60 mm Hg
$Pa{CO_2}$	>45 mm Hg

FEV, forced expiration volume; FVC, forced vital capacity; $Pa{O_2}$, partial pressure of oxygen, arterial; $Pa{CO_2}$, partial pressure of carbon dioxide, arterial.
[a]Complication defined as atelectasis or pneumonia.
From **Blosser SA, Rock P.** Asthma and chronic obstructive lung disease. In: **Breslow MJ, Miller CJ, Rogers MC,** eds. *Perioperative management.* St Louis: Mosby, 1990:259–280.

of pulmonary disease (214). Chest radiographs should be limited to patients older than 40 years, patients with a history of smoking, patients with a history of pulmonary disease, and patients who have evidence of cardiopulmonary disease.

Asthma

The prevalence of bronchial asthma is increasing worldwide, and approximately 10% of people have suffered an asthma attack (215). Asthma is a disease that is characterized by a history of episodic wheezing, physiologic evidence of reversible obstruction of the airways, either spontaneously or following bronchodilator therapy, and pathologic evidence of chronic inflammatory changes in the bronchial submucosa. Asthma is not a disease of airway physiology in which hypertrophy and increased contractility of bronchial smooth muscle is the dominant lesion; rather, it is an inflammatory disease affecting the airways that secondarily results in epithelial damage, leukocytic infiltration, and increased sensitivity of the airways to a number of different stimuli. The treatment of asthma is directed toward relaxing the airways and alleviating inflammation with glucocorticoids.

Despite advances in pharmacologic management, morbidity and mortality from asthma have been increasing in recent years (216). This most likely cause has been the result of underdiagnosis and undertreatment of this disease (217). Multiple stimuli have been noted to precipitate or exacerbate asthma, including environmental allergens or pollutants, respiratory tract infections, exercise, cold air, emotional stress, use of β-adrenergic blockers, and aspirin (218). Management of asthma includes removal of the inciting stimuli as well as use of appropriate pharmacologic therapy.

The severity of clinical asthma correlates with measurements of the severity of the inflammatory response in the lung (219). Some investigators have referred to asthma as a chronic eosinophilic bronchitis (217). Numerous mediators, including interleukin-3, interleukin-5, granulocyte-macrophage colony-stimulating factors, tumor necrosis factor-α, and interferon-γ, are released in the lungs by eosinophils, macrophages, and T cells. The mediators induce microvascular leakage, bronchoconstriction, and epithelial damage, which block the distal airways. The optimal therapy for asthma involves not only managing the acute symptoms but also long-term management of the inflammatory component of the disease.

Pharmacotherapy of Asthma

The recognition of asthma as an inflammatory condition that should be treated with anti-inflammatory agents has led to the use of glucocorticoids for treatment. Glucocorticoids have become the first-line therapy for chronic asthma because they inhibit mediator release from eosinophils and macrophages, inhibit the late response to allergens, and reduce hyperresponsiveness of the bronchioles (217). Inhaled steroids have greatly reduced the steroid dose required to achieve optimal results. The steroid effect is dose related, but many patients with asthma can achieve control using low-dose inhaled steroids (1,000 g/day). Onset of action is slow (several hours), and up to 3 months of steroid therapy may be required for optimal improvement of bronchial hyperresponsiveness. Even with acute exacerbation of asthma, steroid treatment can enhance the beneficial effect of β-adrenergic treatment.

During acute exacerbations of asthma, a short course of oral steroids may be necessary in addition to inhaled steroids. For adults with chronic asthma, however, only a minority will require chronic oral steroid therapy. Patients taking oral steroids should receive intravenous steroid support perioperatively.

Until recently, β_2-adrenergic agonists were considered the first-line drugs for asthma. These drugs, inhaled 4 to 6 times daily, rapidly relax smooth muscle in the airways and are effective for up to 6 hours. Studies of β_2 agonists in chronic asthma, however, have failed to show any influence of these agents on the inflammatory component of asthma. Furthermore, it has been suggested that the long-term use of this class of drugs can lead to a worsening of asthma (217). Thus β_2 agonists are now recommended for use for short-term relief of bronchospasm or as first-line treatment for patients with very infrequent symptoms or symptoms provoked solely by exercise (220).

Methylxanthines, such as *theophylline,* have been relegated to third-line status in the management of asthma. It is doubtful whether these drugs have any additional benefit in patients who are using maximal inhaler therapy. The xanthines are limited by their narrow therapeutic window. It is necessary to achieve a serum concentration of at least 10 g/ml; at levels higher than 20 g/ml significant toxicity develops, including nausea, tremor, and central nervous system excitation. Xanthines have a limited antiinflammatory effect and no effect on bronchial hyperresponsiveness or eosinophilic degranulation. In addition, plasma concentrations can be altered by drugs or environmental factors, requiring an adjustment in the *theophylline* dose. Smoking and *phenobarbital* use, for example, increase clearance of theophylline by the liver, whereas clearance of *theophylline* is decreased with hepatic disease and cardiac failure or with the concomitant use of certain drugs, including *ciprofloxacin, cimetidine, erythromycin,* and *troleandomycin.*

Anticholinergic agents are weak bronchodilators that work via inhibition of muscarinic receptors in the smooth muscle of the airways. The quaternary derivatives such as *ipratropium bromide (Atrovent)* are available in an inhaled form that is not absorbed systemically. Anticholinergic drugs may provide additional benefit in conjunction with standard steroid and bronchodilator therapy but should not be used as single-agent therapy because they do not inhibit mast cell degranulation, do not have any effect on the late response to allergens, and do not have an antiinflammatory effect.

Cromolyn sodium is highly active in the treatment of seasonal allergic asthma in children and young adults. It is usually not as effective in older patients or in patients in whom asthma is not caused by allergy (220). The drug is taken by inhalation but has a relatively short duration of action (3 to 4 hours). It has a mild antiinflammatory effect but is less effective than inhaled cortical steroids, and its role as a single agent is limited.

Perioperative Management of Asthma

In patients with asthma, elective surgery should be postponed whenever possible until pulmonary function and pharmacotherapeutic management are optimized. The preoperative evaluation may include pulmonary function testing and arterial blood gas assessment, depending on the severity of the symptoms and concern regarding ventilation and oxygenation. Preoperative chest physiotherapy, bronchodilator therapy, systemic hydration, and appropriate antibiotics will improve the reversible components of asthma (221). For mild asthma, the use of inhaled β-adrenergic agonists preoperatively may be all that is required. For chronic asthma, optimization of steroid therapy will greatly decrease alveolar inflammation and bronchiolar hyperresponsiveness. Inhaled β_2 agonists should be added to therapy as needed for further control of asthma. Each drug prescribed should be used in maximal dosage before adding an additional agent. For patients undergoing emergent surgery who have significant bronchoconstriction, a multimodal approach should be instituted, including aggressive bronchodilator inhalation therapy, intravenous *aminophylline,* as well as steroid therapy. Ideally, steroid therapy can be instituted 3 to 6 days preoperatively. In all patients with asthma, pharmacotherapeutic response can be demonstrated by an improvement in the peak expiratory flow rate based on pulmonary function testing (220).

Chronic Obstructive Pulmonary Disease

Chronic obstructive pulmonary disease (COPD) is the greatest risk factor for the development of postoperative pulmonary complications. The term *COPD* has been used to encompass both chronic bronchitis and emphysema, disease entities that often occur in tandem. Cigarette smoke is implicated in the pathogenesis of both, and any treatment plan must include cessation of smoking (222). *Chronic bronchitis* is defined as the presence of productive cough on most days for at least 3 months per year and for at least 2 successive years (223). It is characterized by chronic airway inflammation and excessive mucus production. The histologic changes of emphysema include destruction of alveolar septa and distension of airspaces distal to terminal alveoli. The destruction of alveolar septa is most likely caused by serine elastase, released by neutrophils exposed to cigarette smoke (222). The destruction of alveoli results in air trapping, loss of pulmonary elastic recoil, collapse of the airways in expiration, increased work of breathing, significant ventilation–perfusion mismatching, and an ineffective cough (219). The impaired ability to cough effectively and clear secretions predisposes patients with COPD to atelectasis and pneumonia in the postoperative period.

COPD and a history of heavy smoking account for the majority of postoperative pulmonary complications in gynecologic surgical patients. The severity of COPD can be determined preoperatively via a thorough history, physical examination, pulmonary function tests, and arterial blood gas assessments. Preoperative evaluation should be performed to assess reversible components of COPD, such as bronchospasm or infection. Several studies have suggested that preoperative pulmonary preparation of patients with preexisting lung disease can decrease the incidence of postoperative pulmonary complications by 50% to 70% (224–227).

The severity of COPD can be quantitated with pulmonary function testing (206,208,228). Typically, patients with COPD demonstrate impaired expiratory air flow, manifested by diminished forced expiratory volume (FEV_1), forced vital capacity (FVC), FEV_1/FVC, and maximal expiratory flow rate (MEFR). In one study, patients with abnormal pulmonary function test results had a 70% incidence of postoperative pulmonary complications, as compared with a 3% incidence of complications in patients who had normal spirography results (208). In patients considered to be at high risk, the incidence of complications was highest in those undergoing abdominal surgery (92%) or thoracic surgery (78%) and lowest in those undergoing surgery outside the abdomen (26%). Guidelines for preoperative spirometry include the following: lung resection; coronary artery bypass or upper abdominal surgery in a patient with a positive smoking history or dyspnea; lower abdominal surgery in a patient with uncharacterized pulmonary symptoms or history of pulmonary disease without recent spirometry within 60 days, especially if the surgery will be extensive, prolonged, or require strenuous postoperative rehabilitation (229).

Arterial blood gas measurement may show varying degrees of hypoxemia and hypercapnia and can be used for prognostic purposes; PaO_2 levels lower than 70 mm Hg and $PaCO_2$ levels higher than 45 mm Hg are associated with an increase in the risk of postoperative pulmonary complications and the need for mechanical ventilation postoperatively (230). $PaCO_2$ levels higher than 50 mm Hg are associated with increased postoperative respiratory failure and should caution against elective surgery (221).

The preoperative preparation of the patient at risk for postoperative pulmonary complications should include cessation of smoking for as long as possible preoperatively. Whereas 2 to 3 days of smoking abstinence are sufficient for carboxyhemoglobin levels to return to normal (231), 2 months of smoking abstinence is required to significantly lower the risk of postoperative pulmonary complications (232). Longer periods of abstinence can thus be considered in patients undergoing elective surgery.

In patients with severe COPD, maximal improvement in airflow limitation can be achieved with a therapeutic trial of high-dose oral glucocorticoids followed by a 2-week trial of high-dose inhaled steroid (*beclomethasone* 1.5 mg/day or the equivalent) in addition to inhaled bronchodilator therapy. Ideally, oral and inhaled steroid therapy should be initiated 1 to 2 weeks preoperatively. Inhaled steroids, in particular, address the inflammatory component of COPD. Oral steroid therapy initiated preoperatively should be maintained throughout the perioperative period and then tapered postoperatively. β-Adrenergic agonist therapy can be initiated at least 72 hours preoperatively and is beneficial in patients who have demonstrated either clinical or spirometric improvement with bronchodilator therapy.

Patients with COPD and an active bacterial infection, as suggested by purulent sputum, should undergo a full course of antibiotic therapy prior to surgery. The antibiotic used should cover the most likely etiologic organisms, *Streptococcus pneumoniae* and *Haemophilus influenzae*. In any patient with acute upper respiratory infection, surgery should be delayed if possible. In the absence of evidence of an acute infection, the use of antibiotics to sterilize the sputum should be avoided because this practice may lead to bacterial resistance.

Instruction in deep breathing maneuvers and chest physical therapy are easily instituted, and these measures can be started the evening before surgery (232). Steps to improve skeletal muscle strength include good nutrition and treatment of hypokalemia (221). Prophylactic measures, such as smoking cessation, pharmacotherapy administration, and aggressive pulmonary toilet, should be instituted preoperatively and continued postoperatively to minimize the incidence of atelectasis and pneumonia.

Postoperative Pulmonary Management

Atelectasis

Atelectasis accounts for more than 90% of all postoperative pulmonary complications. The pathophysiology involves a collapse of the alveoli resulting in ventilation–perfusion mismatching, intrapulmonary venous shunting, and a subsequent drop in the PaO_2. Collapsed alveoli are susceptible to superimposed infection, and if managed improperly atelectasis will progress to pneumonia. Patients with atelectasis have a decreased FRC as well as decreased lung compliance, resulting in increased work during breathing. Despite the decrease in PaO_2, the PCO_2 remains unaffected unless atelectatic changes progress to large volumes of the lung or there is preexisting lung disease.

Physical findings associated with atelectasis may include a low-grade fever. Auscultation of the chest may reveal decreased breath sounds at the bases or dry rales upon inspiration. Percussion of the posterior thorax may suggest elevation of the diaphragm. Radiologic findings include the presence of horizontal lines or plates noted on the posteroanterior chest radiographs, occasionally with adjacent areas containing hyperinflation. These changes are most pronounced during the first 3 postoperative days.

Therapy for atelectasis should be aimed at expanding the alveoli and increasing the functional residual capacity. The most important maneuvers are those that promote maximal inspiratory pressure, which is maintained for as long as possible. This exercise promotes not only an expansion of the alveoli but also secretion of surfactant, which stabilizes alveoli. It can be achieved with aggressive supervised use of incentive spirometry, deep breathing exercises, coughing and, in some cases, the use of positive expiratory pressure with a mask (continuous positive airway pressure). Oversedation should be avoided, and patients should be encouraged to ambulate and change positions frequently. Fiberoptic bronchoscopy for removal of mucopurulent plugs should be reserved for patients who fail to improve with the usual measures.

Cardiogenic (High-pressure) Pulmonary Edema

Cardiogenic pulmonary edema can result from myocardial ischemia, myocardial infarction, or from intravascular volume overload, particularly in patients who have low cardiac reserve or renal failure. The process usually begins with an increase in the fluid in the alveolar septa and bronchial vascular cuffs, ultimately seeping into the alveoli. Complete filling of the alveoli impairs secretion and production of surfactant. Concomitant with alveolar flooding, there is a decrease in lung compliance, impairment of the oxygen diffusion capacity, and an increase in the arteriolar–alveolar oxygen gradient. Ventilation–perfusion mismatching in the lung results in a decrease in the PaO_2, resulting eventually in decreased oxygenation of the tissues and impairment of cardiac contractility.

Symptoms may include tachypnea, dyspnea, wheezing, and use of the accessory muscles of respiration. Clinical signs may include distention of the jugular veins, peripheral edema, rales upon auscultation of the lungs, and an enlarged heart. Radiographic findings may include the presence of bronchiolar cuffing as well as increased interstitial fluid markings extending to the periphery of the lung. The diagnosis can be further confirmed with the use of central hemodynamic monitoring, which will denote an elevated central venous pressure and, more specifically, an elevation in the pulmonary–capillary wedge pressure.

The patient's volume status should be evaluated thoroughly. In addition, myocardial ischemia or infarction should be ruled out by performing ECG and analyzing cardiac enzyme levels. The management of cardiogenic pulmonary edema includes oxygen support, aggressive diuresis, and afterload reduction to increase the cardiac output. In the absence of myocardial infarction, an inotropic agent may be used. Mechanical ventilation should be reserved for cases of acute respiratory failure.

Noncardiogenic Pulmonary Edema (Adult Respiratory Distress Syndrome)

In contrast to cardiogenic pulmonary edema, in which alveolar flooding is a result of an increase in the hydrostatic pressure of the pulmonary capillaries, alveolar flooding in patients with adult respiratory distress syndrome (ARDS) is the result of an increase in pulmonary capillary permeability. The primary pathophysiologic process is one of damage to the capillary side of the alveolar–capillary membrane. This damage results in rapid movement of fluid containing high concentrations of protein from the capillaries to the pulmonary parenchyma and alveoli. Lung compliance decreases and oxygen diffusion capacity is impaired, resulting in hypoxemia. If not managed aggressively, respiratory failure may result. Even if managed aggressively, the mortality rate associated with ARDS is 60% to 70% (221). There are a number of causes as well as several distinct states of ARDS. The causes of ARDS include shock, sepsis, massive nonlung trauma (as from fractures or burns), multiple red blood cell transfusions, aspiration injury, inhalation injury, pneumonia, pancreatitis, DIC, and fat emboli (221). Irrespective of the cause, which should be identified and treated if possible, the evolving clinical findings and management are very similar.

Clinically, ARDS passes through several stages. Initially, patients develop tachypnea and dyspnea with no remarkable findings on clinical evaluation or on chest radiograph. Chest radiographs will eventually reveal bilateral diffuse pulmonary infiltrates. As lung compliance becomes impaired, functional residual capacity, tidal volume, and vital capacity decrease. The PaO_2 decreases and, characteristically, increases only marginally with oxygen supplementation. An attempt should be made to maintain the arterial oxygen level above 90%. This may be achievable initially by administering oxygen by mask. For patients with severe hypoxemia, endotracheal intubation with positive-pressure ventilation should be instituted. Guidelines for initial ventilatory support are changing, and new lung-protective ventilation strategies are being advocated. One strategy advocates the use of high positive end-expiratory pressure (PEEP), low tidal volume, permissive hypercapnia, and pressure-limited ventilatory modes. The low-tidal-volume strategy may confer a survival advantage, and available data support its use in patients with ARDS (233). Multicenter trials are currently under way to assess differences in PEEP and FIO_2 levels, and the use of glucocorticoids.

Attempts to manage and treat the cause of ARDS also must include aggressive efforts toward hemodynamic and circulatory resuscitation in patients with shock. Nosocomial pneumonia is present in 50% of patients with ARDS, and broad-spectrum antibiotic therapy should be administered as appropriate for patients with suspected pneumonia or sepsis. Patients who have DIC may require replacement with cryoprecipitate or FFP. Other measures for general care should include the placement of a nasogastric tube, gastric acid suppression with H^2 blockers, and administration of steroids in patients with the fat emboli syndrome.

Hemodynamic monitoring is invaluable and should be initiated early in the course of the disease process. Patients with any evidence of fluid overload should receive aggressive diuresis, whereas others may require fluid resuscitation for maintenance of tissue perfusion while the pulmonary–capillary wedge pressure is maintained below 15 mm Hg. Pulmonary wedge pressure may be falsely elevated when PEEP is being applied. The goal of management is to maintain the lowest pulmonary–capillary wedge pressure, with acceptable cardiac output and blood pressure. In the presence of hypotension and oliguria, inotropic support with *dopamine* or *dobutamine* is helpful.

With aggressive management, particularly if the inciting cause is identified and treated, ARDS can be reversed during the first 48 hours with few sequelae. After the first 48 hours, however, progression of the ARDS will cause lung damage that may leave residual pulmonary fibrosis. With progression beyond 10 days, multiple organ system failure occurs and the mortality rate is higher than 80% (234).

Renal Disease

The need for surgical intervention in patients with renal impairment has resulted in the development of a very specialized medical approach to their care. Special precautions are necessary to compensate for the kidney's impaired ability to regulate fluids and electrolytes and excrete metabolic waste products. Equally important are the unique problems that develop in patients with chronic renal impairment, including an increased risk of sepsis, coagulation defects, impaired immune function and wound healing, and a propensity to develop specific acid-base abnormalities. Special consideration must be given to a variety of different medications, anesthetic agents, and numerous hematologic and nutritional factors that are important in the successful surgical care of patients with renal insufficiency.

Management of fluid levels and cardiovascular hemodynamics in patients with acute or chronic renal impairment is paramount. Intravascular fluid volume changes that lead to hypertension or hypotension are very common in these patients and are often difficult to manage secondary to autonomic dysfunction, acidosis, and other problems that are inherent to the underlying kidney disease. Patients undergoing dialysis for whom major abdominal or pelvic surgery is contemplated should be treated using a Swan-Ganz catheter intraoperatively and postoperatively. The results of physical examination and central venous pressure monitoring correlate poorly with left cardiac filling pressures. Swan-Ganz catheter measurements will help guide fluid replacement and avoid volume overload. Invasive hemodynamic monitoring should be continued as needed throughout the first postoperative week because third spacing will occur during this period.

Postoperative dialysis is usually necessary to avoid problems associated with fluid overload and hyperkalemia. Dialysis-dependent patients should undergo dialysis approximately 24 hours following surgery. A short-lived but rather significant fall in the number of platelets occurs during dialysis, and *heparin* is used in hemodialysis equipment to prevent clotting. Because of these factors and concerns about postoperative bleeding, dialysis is usually avoided during the first 12 to 24 hours following surgery. Although ischemic heart disease is the most common cause of death in patients with renal insufficiency, it is not a major cause of perioperative mortality (235). A large percentage of perioperative deaths of patients with renal insufficiency are associated with hyperkalemia that is controlled most effectively by dialysis (236).

Patients with chronic renal failure are at an increased risk for postoperative infections resulting from abnormalities in neutrophil and monocyte function (237). Appropriate preoperative antibiotic prophylaxis and an accurate assessment of nutritional status will lower the incidence of postoperative infectious complications.

The major hematologic concern in patients with chronic renal insufficiency is the increased incidence of bleeding. These bleeding problems are secondary to abnormal bleeding times and, in particular, disorders of platelet function related to a decreased amount of factor VIII and von Willebrand antigen in the serum of uremic patients. Anemia, which is common in patients with renal insufficiency, can contribute to prolonged bleeding times (238).

Abnormalities in arachidonic acid metabolism, acquired platelet storage pool deficiency, and disturbed regulation of platelet calcium content all account for an increased tendency for uremic patients to have significant bleeding during surgery (239). Therefore, the bleeding time should be routinely checked preoperatively in these patients and abnormalities should be corrected before surgery. Options for the correction of bleeding time in uremic patients include infusion of *desmopressin* or *cryoprecipitate,* both of which act to increase plasma levels of factor VIII and von Willebrand antigen (240,241).

Normal renal function is essential for maintenance of acid-base balance in the body. Patients with renal insufficiency can have a normal anion gap or an elevated anion gap acidosis. When mild renal insufficiency develops, a normal anion gap can be seen, whereas in more significant and severe renal dysfunction, an elevated anion gap acidosis occurs. Hemodialysis corrects metabolic acidosis. If a patient is severely acidotic (pH less than 7.15) and emergency surgery is planned, correction of the blood pH to 7.25 using intravenous sodium bicarbonate is indicated. Correction of metabolic acidosis should be carried out slowly, however, because in patients with hypocalcemia seizures may be precipitated (241). It is also important to exclude other causes of elevated anion gap acidosis, such as ketoacidosis secondary to diabetes, lactic acidosis secondary to infection or, in rare instances, poisoning with *ethylene glycol, methanol,* or *aspirin.*

Impaired kidney function causes phosphate retention by the kidney and impaired vitamin D metabolism. Therefore, hypocalcemia is common in patients with renal insufficiency, but tetany and other signs of hypocalcemia are relatively uncommon because metabolic acidosis raises the level of ionized calcium. Oral phosphate binders such as *aluminum hydroxide* (1 to 2 g per meal) and dietary phosphate restriction (1 g per day) is the usual treatment for hypocalcemia-hyperphosphatemia in patients with renal insufficiency. In chronic situations, because of central nervous system toxicity associated with elevated aluminum levels, it is preferable to treat hypocalcemia-hyperphosphatemia with large doses of *calcium carbonate* (6 to 12 g per day) rather than with the standard aluminum-containing antacids (242).

Approximately 20% of patients with renal insufficiency will exhibit clinical evidence of protein calorie malnutrition. Vitamin deficiencies, most notably with water-soluble vitamins, also occur with dialysis. Nutritional disturbances in patients with chronic renal insufficiency arise secondary to deficiencies in protein intake, and studies have shown that, in patients with chronic renal insufficiency, their kidneys are hyperfiltrating (243). Postoperatively, both protein and caloric intake may need to be increased dramatically to meet catabolic demands in surgical patients. As much as 1.5 g/kg of protein and 45 kcal/kg of calories may be needed (243).

Wound healing is impaired in patients with chronic renal failure, and wound dehiscence and evisceration are potential problems. Wound healing is most appropriately aided by nutritional assessment preoperatively and maintenance of adequate caloric and protein intake in the perioperative setting. Antibiotic prophylaxis should be used in these patients, and uremia should be treated with dialysis as indicated. A running mass-closure of the midline vertical incision with continuous monofilament sutures should be used to further decrease the risk of wound dehiscence and evisceration (244).

Patients with chronic renal disease have an altered ability to excrete drugs and are prone to significant metabolic derangements secondary to the altered bioavailability of many commonly used medications. Because of this, as well as the effect of dialysis on drug pharmacokinetics, the gynecologic surgeon and nephrologist must be aware of the lowered metabolism and bioavailability of narcotics, barbiturates, muscle relaxants, antibiotics, and other drugs that require renal clearance. Of particular note is the inability of patients with renal insufficiency to clear the neuromuscular blockade caused by *pancuronium* (245). Care must be taken with *D-tubocurarine,* especially if repeated doses are given (246). *Midazolam, propofol, vecuronium,* and *atracurium* have been safely used in patients with renal failure (241). *Succinylcholine* has been reported to cause significant hyperkalemic responses in patients with renal failure (247). *Succinylcholine* can be used safely in patients with chronic renal insufficiency. Careful monitoring of the serum potassium level is necessary (248).

Perioperative acute renal failure in previously normal patients may be caused by decreased renal perfusion, nephrotoxins, or both. Patients with impaired cardiac function, intravascular volume depletion, sepsis, or hypotension fall under the first category. Nephrotoxic medications such as *aminoglycosides,* chemotherapeutic agents such as *cisplatin,* or iodinated contrast agents fall under the second category (249–251). The risk of renal impairment becomes cumulative if more than one of these factors exist at the same time, and especially if a variety of factors are associated with intervascular volume depletion (252). Several measurements should be used to avoid acute renal failure. All nephrotoxic drugs should be discontinued when possible; when it is not practical to withdraw medication, strict attention should be paid to the pharmacokinetic characteristics of each drug as well as to the regular measurements of the serum creatinine. Patients with diabetes should be given reduced doses of radiocontrast agents and should be well hydrated because they are particularly susceptible to renal injury from these materials (253). Volume repletion is essential to lower the incidence of renal impairment (254).

Liver Disease

Management of perioperative problems in gynecologic patients with liver disease requires a comprehensive understanding of normal liver physiology and the pathophysiology underlying diseases of the liver that may complicate surgery or recovery. Patients with liver disease often have numerous complicated problems involving nutrition, coagulation, wound healing, encephalopathy, and infection.

History and Physical Examination

Patients with a history of alcohol abuse, drug use, hepatitis, jaundice, blood product exposure, or a family member with liver disease should undergo biochemical evaluation. During the physical examination, note should be made of any jaundice, signs of muscle wastage, ascites, right upper quadrant tenderness, or hepatomegaly.

Laboratory Testing

The biochemical profile (alkaline phosphatase, calcium, lactic acid dehydrogenase, bilirubin, serum glutamic-oxaloacetic transaminase, cholesterol, uric acid, phosphorous, albumin, total protein, and glucose) has not been shown to be useful for routine preoperative evaluation (255). Mild abnormalities lead to further extensive testing that require consultation, delays in surgery, and increased cost without net benefit. A possible exception is selected use of biochemical testing when the history or physical examination reveals abnormalities. Patients with known liver disease should undergo albumin and bilirubin testing using the Child's risk classification (Table 19.15). This system was originally designed to predict mortality following portosystemic shunt surgery. It divides patients into three classes of severity based on five easily assessed clinical parameters. Measurement of prothrombin time may also be helpful in patients with significant histories of liver disease. If a history of hepatitis is ascertained, the patient should be tested for serum aminotransferase, alkaline phosphatase, bilirubin, and albumin levels. Serologic documentation of hepatitis is also important. If a

Table 19.15. Child's Classification of Liver Dysfunction

	Child Classification		
Parameter	***A***	***B***	***C***
Bilirubin	<2.0	2.0–3.0	>3.0
Albumin	>3.5	3.0–3.5	<3.0
Ascites	None	Easily controlled	Poor controlled
Encephalopathy	None	Mild	Advanced
Nutritional status	Excellent	Good	Poor

patient has a known malignancy, there may be some benefit from biochemical testing of the liver as a screen for metastatic disease, although this has not been proved conclusively.

Anesthesia

With few exceptions, most anesthetic agents, including those administered by epidural or spinal routes, reduce hepatic blood flow and decrease oxygenation of the liver. Other perioperative factors—hemorrhage, intraoperative hypotension, hypercarbia, congestive heart failure, and intermittent positive pressure ventilation, especially in critically ill patients—lead to decreased hepatic perfusion and hypoxia (256).

Drug Metabolism

Patients with altered liver function should be carefully monitored because of the prolonged action of many medications used during surgery. In addition to impaired metabolism, hypoalbuminemia decreases drug binding, which alters serum levels and biliary clearance rates. The degree of hepatic metabolism varies greatly, depending on the type of medication being considered. For inhalation anesthetics, *isoflurane* is preferred because it undergoes minimal hepatic metabolism in comparison with *halothane* or *enflurane.* Narcotics, induction agents, sedatives, and neuromuscular blocking agents all undergo abnormal metabolism in patients with decompensated liver disease. *Diazepam, meperidine,* and *phenobarbital* cause prolonged depression of consciousness and may precipitate hepatic encephalopathy because of their altered rates of clearance. *Sufentanil* and *oxazepam* are the preferred narcotics, and *benzodiazepine* should be used for patients with altered liver function. Muscle relaxants, such as *D-tubocurarine, pancuronium,* and *vecuronium,* cause prolonged neuromuscular blockade in patients with impaired liver function and are not ideal drugs to use in this situation. *Atracurium* is not metabolized by the liver and, therefore, is the preferred muscle relaxant for patients with abnormal hepatic function. *Succinylcholine* metabolism is greatly prolonged in patients with hepatic dysfunction and must be used with great caution (257).

Determination of Operative Risk

Although it is well known that acute hepatobiliary damage results in increased morbidity and mortality in the surgical patient, estimating the operative risk in patients with hepatic dysfunction is troublesome, because it is often difficult to determine which patients are at risk based on the history and physical examination. The most accurate method for risk assessment of surgery in patients with hepatic dysfunction is Child's classification (Table 19.15). Using this system, accurate assessment of morbidity and mortality can be directly related to the degree of liver dysfunction (258). The Child's classification has been shown to be useful for patients undergoing a variety of different types of abdominal surgery. Operative mortalities of 10%, 31%, and 76% have been reported for each of the three Child's classifications, respectively (259). The major cause of perioperative death was sepsis. This classification correlated significantly with postoperative complications such as bleeding, renal failure, wound dehiscence, and sepsis.

Acute Viral Hepatitis

Acute viral hepatitis poses an increased risk of operative complications and perioperative mortality and, therefore, elective surgery is contraindicated (260). Elective surgery should be delayed for approximately 1 month after the results of all biochemical tests have returned to normal (261). In patients with ectopic pregnancy, hemorrhage, or bowel obstruction secondary to malignancy, however, surgical intervention must take place before normalization of serum transaminase (260). In these situations, the perioperative morbidity (12%) and mortality (9.5%) rates are much higher than when they are performed under ideal situations (257).

Chronic Hepatitis

Chronic hepatitis is a group of disorders characterized by inflammation of the liver for at least 6 months. The disease is divided by morphologic and clinical criteria into chronic persistent hepatitis and chronic active hepatitis. A liver biopsy is usually required to establish the extent and type of injury. The surgical risk in these patients correlates most closely with the disease severity. The risk of surgery in patients with asymptomatic or mild disease is minimal, in contrast to a significant risk for those patients who have symptomatic chronic active hepatitis (262). Elective surgery is contraindicated in symptomatic patients, and nonelective surgery is associated with significant morbidity (261). In the nonelective situation, patients taking long-term glucocorticoid therapy should be given appropriate stress coverage with a higher dose of glucocorticoids during the perioperative period. Preoperatively, patients who are not taking steroids should receive *prednisone* and *azathioprine,* which have been shown to reduce the perioperative risk of complications and may result in remission in up to 80% of patients (263). More recently, a controlled randomized trial of prednisone and *interferon-α* has documented regression of the hepatitis B core antigen and hepatitis B viral DNA replication in approximately 30% of patients (264). *Interferon-α* has also been used in the treatment of hepatitis C. Consideration should be given to using these medications for patients in whom surgery cannot be avoided but is not emergent.

Asymptomatic carriers of the hepatitis B virus (individuals who test positive for the hepatitis B surface antigen) are not at increased risk for postoperative complications in the absence of elevated aminotransferase levels and liver inflammation. There is, however, a significant risk to the health care professional when operating on these individuals. In cases of needle stick in which the patient's hepatitis status is unknown, both the health care worker and the patient should be tested for HCV antibody and HBV serologic markers. If markers for HBV infection are present, hepatitis B immune globulin should be administered to unvaccinated medical personnel. A vaccination series should then be initiated during the early postoperative period. If the health care worker is immune (surface antibody positive), no treatment is necessary (257). All medical personnel, and especially those in the surgical subspecialties, should receive a full course of recombinant hepatitis B vaccine as recommended by the Centers for Disease Control and Prevention (265).

Alcoholic Liver Disease

Alcoholic liver disease encompasses a spectrum of diseases including fatty liver, acute alcoholic hepatitis, and cirrhosis. Elective surgery is not contraindicated in patients with fatty liver because liver function is preserved. If nutritional deficiencies are discovered, they should be corrected prior to elective surgery. Acute alcoholic hepatitis is characterized on biopsy by hepatocyte edema, polymorphonuclear leukocyte infiltration, necrosis, and the presence of Mallory bodies. Elective surgery in these patients is contraindicated (266). Abstinence from alcohol for approximately 6 to 12 weeks along with clinical resolution of the biochemical abnormalities are recommended before surgery is considered. Severe alcoholic hepatitis may persist for several months despite abstinence and, if any question of continued activity exists, a liver biopsy should be repeated (267). In cases of urgent or emergent surgery on patients with alcohol dependence, a benzodiazepine taper is appropriate as prophylaxis against alcohol withdrawal.

Cirrhosis

Cirrhosis is an irreversible liver lesion characterized histologically by parenchymal necrosis, nodular degeneration, fibrosis, and a disorganization of hepatic lobular architecture. The most serious complication of cirrhosis is portal venous hypertension that ultimately leads to bleeding from esophageal varices, ascites, and hepatic encephalopathy. Conventional liver biochemical test results correlate poorly with the degree of liver impairment in patients with cirrhosis. Hepatic dysfunction, however, may be somewhat quantitated by low albumin levels and prolonged prothrombin times.

Surgical risk is clearly increased in patients with cirrhosis, although it is substantially greater in emergency surgery than in elective surgery. Perioperative mortality correlates with the severity of cirrhosis and can be estimated through the use of the Child's classification (Table 19.15). Surgery in patients with Child's class A cirrhosis can usually be performed without significant risk, whereas surgery in patients with Child's class B or C poses a major risk and requires careful preoperative consideration. Meticulous preoperative preparation may improve the surgical outcome (268).

References

1. **Rohrer MJ, Michelotti MC, Nahrwold DL.** A prospective evaluation of the efficacy of preoperative coagulation testing. *Ann Surg* 1989;208:554–557.
2. **Lamers RJ, van Engelshoven JM, Pfaff A.** Once again, the routine preoperative thorax photo. *Ned Tijdschr Geneeskd* 1989;133:2288–2291.
3. **Loder RE.** Routine preoperative chest radiography. *Anesthesiology* 1987;66:195–198.
4. **Piscitelli JT, Simel DL, Addison WA.** Who should have intravenous pyelograms before hysterectomy for benign disease? *Obstet Gynecol* 1987;69:541–545.
5. **Easley HA, Hammond CB.** Informed consent in obstetrics and gynecology. *Postgrad Obstet Gynecol* 1986;10:1–12.
6. **Shizgal HM, Spanier AH, Kurtz RS.** Effect of parenteral nutrition on body composition in the critically ill patient. *Am J Surg* 1976;131:156–161.
7. **Hill GL, Beddoe AH.** In vivo neutron activation in metabolic and nutritional studies. *J Clin Surg* 1982;1:270.
8. **Bozzetti F, Migliavacca S, Gallus G, et al.** "Nutritional" markers as prognostic indicators of postoperative sepsis in cancer patients. *JPEN J Parenter Enteral Nutr* 1985;9:464–470.
9. **Blackburn GL, Bistrian BR, Maini BS, et al.** Nutritional and metabolic assessment of the hospitalized patient. *JPEN J Parenter Enteral Nutr* 1977;1:11–22.
10. **Bistrian BR.** Nutritional assessment of the hospitalized patient: a practical approach. In: **Wright RA, Heymsfield SN,** eds. *Nutritional assessment.* Boston: Blackwell Science, 1984.
11. **Santoso JT, Canada T, Latson B, et al.** Prognostic nutritional index in relation to hospital stay in women with gynecologic cancer. *Obstet Gynecol* 2000;95:844–846.
12. **Mullen JL, Buzby GP, Matthews DC, et al.** Reduction of operative morbidity and mortality by combined preoperative and postoperative nutritional support. *Ann Surg* 1980;192:604–613.
13. **Bistrian BR, Blackburn GL, Hallowell E, et al.** Protein status of general surgical patients. *JAMA* 1974;230:858–860.
14. **Hill GL, Blackett RL, Pickford I, et al.** Malnutrition in surgical patients. An unrecognised problem. *Lancet* 1977;1:689–692.
15. **Soper JT, Berchuck A, Creasman WT, et al.** Pelvic exenteration. Factors associated with major surgical morbidity. *Gynecol Oncol* 1989;35:93–98.
16. **Starker PM, Lasala PA, Askanazi J, et al.** The response to TPN. A form of nutritional assessment. *Ann Surg* 1983;198:720–724.
17. **Long CL, Schaffel N, Geiger JW, et al.** Metabolic response to injury and illness. Estimation of energy and protein needs from indirect calorimetry and nitrogen balance. *JPEN J Parenter Enteral Nutr* 1979;3:452–456.
18. **Barbul A, Purtill WA.** Nutrition in wound healing. *Clin Dermatol* 1994;12:133–140.
19. **Heymsfield SB, Horowitz J, Lawson DH.** Enteral hyperalimentation. In: **Berk JE,** ed. *Developments in digestive diseases,* vol 3. Philadelphia: Lea & Febiger, 1980:59–83.
20. **Holter AR, Rosen HM, Fischer JE.** The effects of hyperalimentation on major surgery in patients with malignant disease: a prospective study. *Acta Chir Scand Suppl* 1976;466:86–87.
21. **Sako K, Lore JM, Kaufman S, et al.** Parenteral hyperalimentation in surgical patients with head and neck cancer. A randomized study. *J Surg Oncol* 1981;16:391–402.
22. **Thompson BR, Julian TB, Stremple JF.** Perioperative total parenteral nutrition in patients with gastrointestinal cancer. *J Surg Res* 1981;30:497–500.
23. **Bellantone R, Doglietto G, Bossola M, et al.** Preoperative parenteral nutrition of malnourished surgical patients. *Acta Chir Scand* 1988;154:249–251.
24. **Anonymous.** Perioperative total parenteral nutrition in surgical patients. The Veterans Affairs Total Parenteral Nutrition Cooperative Study Group. *N Engl J Med* 1991;325:525–532.
25. **Sandstrom R, Drott C, Hyltander A, et al.** The effect of postoperative intravenous feeding (TPN) on outcome following major surgery evaluated in a randomized study. *Ann Surg* 1993;217:185–195.
26. **Pestana C.** *Fluids and electrolytes in the surgical patient,* 5th ed. Baltimore: Williams & Wilkins, 2000.
27. **Miller TA, Duke JH.** Fluid and electrolyte management. In: **Dudrick SJ, Baue AE, Eiseman B, et al.,** eds. *Manual of preoperative and postoperative care.* Philadelphia: WB Saunders, 1983:38–67.

28. **Cogan MG.** *Fluid and electrolytes.* Connecticut: Appleton & Lange, 1991.

29. **Narins RG, Lazarus MJ.** Renal systems. In: **Vandam LD,** ed. *To make the patient ready for anesthesia: medical care of the surgical patient,* 2nd ed. Stoneham, MA: Butterworth, 1984:67–114.

30. **Wish JB, Cacho CP.** Acid/base and electrolyte disorders. In: **Sivak ED, Higgins TL, Seiver A,** eds. *The high risk patient: management of the critically ill.* Baltimore: Williams & Wilkins, 1995:755–782.

31. **Edwards WT.** Optimizing opioid treatment of postoperative pain. *J Pain Symptom Manage* 1990;5[Suppl 1]: S24–36.

32. **Kuhn S, Cooke K, Collins M, et al.** Perceptions of pain relief after surgery. *BMJ* 1990;300:1687–1690.

33. **American Society of Anesthesiologists Task Force on Pain Management, Acute Pain Section.** Practice guidelines for acute pain management in the perioperative setting. A report by the American Society of Anesthesiologists Task Force on Pain Management, Acute Pain Section. *Anesthesiology* 1995;82:1071–1081.

34. **Etches RC.** Patient-controlled analgesia. *Surg Clin North Am* 1999;79:297–312.

35. **Austin KL, Stapleton JV, Mather LE.** Multiple intramuscular injections: a major source of variability in analgesic response to meperidine. *Pain* 1980;8:47–62.

36. **Jain S, Datta S.** Postoperative pain management. *Chest Surg Clin N Am* 1997;7:773–799.

37. **Egbert AM, Parks LH, Short LM, et al.** Randomized trial of postoperative patient-controlled analgesia vs intramuscular narcotics in frail elderly men. *Arch Intern Med* 1990;150:1897–1903.

38. **Rawal N, Arner S, Gustafsson LL, et al.** Present state of extradural and intrathecal opioid analgesia in Sweden. A nationwide follow-up survey. *Br J Anaesth* 1987;59:791–799

39. **Rawal N.** Epidural and spinal agents for postoperative analgesia. *Surg Clin North Am* 1999;79:313–344.

40. **DeAndrade JR, Maslanka M, Maneatis T, et al.** The use of ketorolac in the management of postoperative pain. *Orthopedics* 1994;17:157–166.

41. **Etches RC, Warriner CB, Badner N, et al.** Continuous intravenous administration of ketorolac reduces pain and morphine consumption after total hip or knee arthroplasty. *Anesth Analg* 1995;81:1175–1180.

42. **Parker RK, Holtmann B, Smith I, et al.** Use of ketorolac after lower abdominal surgery. Effect on analgesic requirement and surgical outcome. *Anesthesiology* 1994;80:6–12.

43. **Hirsch HA.** Prophylactic antibiotics in obstetrics and gynecology. *Am J Med* 1985;78:170–176.

44. **Mittendorf R, Aronson MP, Berry RE, et al.** Avoiding serious infections associated with abdominal hysterectomy. A meta-analysis of antibiotic prophylaxis. *Am J Obstet Gynecol* 1993;169:1119–1124.

45. **Munck JM, Jensen HK.** Preoperative clindamycin treatment and vaginal drainage in hysterectomy. *Acta Obstet Gynecol Scand* 1989;68:241–245.

46. **Gerber B, Wilken H.** Effectiveness of perioperative preventive use of antibiotics with metronidazole or doxycycline in vaginal hysterectomy. *Zentralbl Gynakol* 1989;111:1542–1548.

47. **Friese S, Willems FT, Loriaux SM, et al.** Prophylaxis in gynaecological surgery: a prospective randomized comparison between single dose prophylaxis with amoxicillin/clavulanate and the combination of cefuroxime and metronidazole. *J Antimicrob Chemother* 1989;24:213–216.

48. **Chodak GW.** Use of systemic antibiotics for prophylaxis in surgery. *Arch Surg* 1977;112:326–234.

49. **Hemsell DL.** Prophylactic antibiotics in gynecologic and obstetric surgery. *Rev Infect Dis* 1991;13[Suppl 10]:S821–S841.

50. **Hemsell DL, Johnson EF, Heard MC, et al.** Single-dose piperacillin versus triple-dose cefoxitin prophylaxis at vaginal and abdominal hysterectomy. *South Med J* 1989;82:438–442.

51. **Orr JW Jr, Sisson PF, Patsner B, et al.** Single-dose antibiotic prophylaxis for patients undergoing extended pelvic surgery for gynecologic malignancy. *Am J Obstet Gynecol* 1990;162:718–721.

52. **Mayer HO, Petru E, Haas J, et al.** Perioperative antibiotic prophylaxis in patients undergoing radical surgery for gynecologic cancer: single dose versus multiple dose administration. *Eur J Gynaecol Oncol* 1993;14:177–181.

53. **Brachman PS, Dan BB, Haley RW, et al.** Nosocomial surgical infections: incidence and cost. *Surg Clin North Am* 1980;60:15–25.

54. **Lyon DS, Jones JL, Sanchez A.** Postoperative febrile morbidity in the benign gynecologic patient. Identification and management. *J Reprod Med* 2000;45:305–309.

55. **O'Grady NP, Barie PS, Bartlett J, et al.** Practice parameters for evaluating new fever in critically ill adult patients. Task Force of the American College of Critical Care Medicine of the Society of Critical Care Medicine in collaboration with the Infectious Disease Society of America. *Crit Care Med* 1998;26:392–408.

56. **Hemsell DL.** Infections after gynecologic surgery. *Obstet Gynecol Clin North Am* 1989;16:381–400.

57. **Bartzen PJ, Hafferty FW.** Pelvic laparotomy without an indwelling catheter. A retrospective review of 949 cases. *Am J Obstet Gynecol* 1987;156:1426–1432.

58. **Kingdom JC, Kitchener HC, MacLean AB.** Postoperative urinary tract infection in gynecology: implications for an antibiotic prophylaxis policy. *Obstet Gynecol* 1990;76:636–638.

59. **Ireland D, Tacchi D, Bint AJ.** Effect of single-dose prophylactic co-trimoxazole on the incidence of gynaecological postoperative urinary tract infection. *Br J Obstet Gynaecol* 1982;89:578–580.

60. **Boyd ME.** Postoperative gynecologic infections. *Can J Surg* 1987;30:7–9.

61. **Kunin CM.** Urinary tract infections. *Surg Clin North Am* 1980;60:223–231.

62. **Harkness GA, Bentley DW, Roghmann KJ.** Risk factors for nosocomial pneumonia in the elderly. *Am J Med* 1990;89:457–463.

63. **Eickhoff TC.** Pulmonary infections in surgical patients. *Surg Clin North Am* 1980;60:175–183.

64. **Tomford JW, Hershey CO, McLaren CE, et al.** Intravenous therapy team and peripheral venous catheter-associated complications. A prospective controlled study. *Arch Intern Med* 1984;144:1191–1194.

65. **Hershey CO, Tomford JW, McLaren CE, et al.** The natural history of intravenous catheter–associated phlebitis. *Arch Intern Med* 1984;144:1373–1375.

66. **Cruse PJ, Foord R.** The epidemiology of wound infection. A 10-year prospective study of 62,939 wounds. *Surg Clin North Am* 1980;60:27–40.

67. **Brown SE, Allen HH, Robins RN.** The use of delayed primary wound closure in preventing wound infections. *Am J Obstet Gynecol* 1977;127:713–717.

68. **Sperling DC, Needleman L, Eschelman DJ, et al.** Deep pelvic abscesses. Transperineal US-guided drainage. *Radiology* 1998;208:111–115.

69. **Nelson AL, Sinow RM, Oliak D.** Transrectal ultrasonographically guided drainage of gynecologic pelvic abscesses. *Am J Obstet Gynecol* 2000;182:1382–1388.

70. **Crombleholme WR, Ohm-Smith M, Robbie MO, et al.** Ampicillin/sulbactam versus metronidazole-gentamicin in the treatment of soft tissue pelvic infections. *Am J Obstet Gynecol* 1987;156:507–512.

71. **Cunningham FG.** Treatment and prevention of female pelvic infection: the quest for single-agent therapy. *Am J Obstet Gynecol* 1987;157:485–488.

72. **Hemsell DL, Heard MC, Nobles BJ, et al.** Single-agent therapy for women with acute polymicrobial pelvic infections. *Am J Obstet Gynecol* 1987;157:488–490.

73. **Goldstein EJ.** Possible role for the new fluoroquinolones (levofloxacin, grepafloxacin, trovafloxacin, clinafloxacin, sparfloxacin, and DU-6859a) in the treatment of anaerobic infections: review of current information on efficacy and safety. *Clin Infect Dis* 1996;23[Suppl 1]:S25–S30.

74. **Riseman JA, Zamboni WA, Curtis A, et al.** Hyperbaric oxygen therapy for necrotizing fasciitis reduces mortality and the need for debridements. *Surgery* 1990;108:847–850.

75. **Meleney RL.** Hemolytic streptococcus gangrene. *Arch Surg* 1925;9:317–321.

76. **Umbert IJ, Winkelmann RK, Oliver GF, et al.** Necrotizing fasciitis: a clinical, microbiologic, and histopathologic study of 14 patients. *J Am Acad Dermatol* 1989;20:774–781.

77. **Wilkerson R, Paull W, Coville FV.** Necrotizing fasciitis. Review of the literature and case report. *Clin Orthop* 1987;187–192.

78. **Marrie TJ, Costerton JW.** In vivo ultrastructural study of microbes in necrotizing fascitis. *Eur J Clin Microbiol Infect Dis* 1988;7:51–53.

79. **Sudarsky LA, Laschinger JC, Coppa GF, et al.** Improved results from a standardized approach in treating patients with necrotizing fasciitis. *Ann Surg* 1989;206:661–665.

80. **Fisher JR, Conway MJ, Takeshita RT, et al.** Necrotizing fasciitis. Importance of roentgenographic studies for soft-tissue gas. *JAMA* 1979;241:803–806.

81. **Clayton MD, Fowler JE, Sharifi R, et al.** Causes, presentation and survival of fifty-seven patients with necrotizing fasciitis of the male genitalia. *Surg Gynecol Obstet* 1990;170:49–55.

82. **Hirn M, Niinikoski J.** Management of perineal necrotizing fasciitis (Fournier's gangrene). *Ann Chir Gynaecol* 1989;78:277–281.

83. **Stamenkovic I, Lew PD.** Early recognition of potentially fatal necrotizing fasciitis. The use of frozen-section biopsy. *N Engl J Med* 1984;310:1689–1693.

84. **Rothman PA, Wiskind AK, Dudley AG.** Amniotic membranes in the treatment of necrotizing fasciitis complicating vulvar herpes virus infection. *Obstet Gynecol* 1989;76:534–536.

85. **Eltorai IM, Hart GB, Strauss MB, et al.** The role of hyperbaric oxygen in the management of Fournier's gangrene. *Int Surg* 1986;71:53–58.

86. **Kaiser RE, Cerra FB.** Progressive necrotizing surgical infections—a unified approach. *J Trauma* 1981;21:349–355.

87. **Korhonen K, Klossner J, Hirn M, et al.** Management of clostridial gas gangrene and the role of hyperbaric oxygen. *Ann Chir Gynaecol* 1999;88:139–142.

88. **Robson MC, Krizek TJ, Koss N, et al.** Amniotic membranes as a temporary wound dressing. *Surg Gynecol Obstet* 1973;136:904–906.

89. **Argenta LC, Morykwas MJ.** Vacuum-assisted closure: a new method for wound control and treatment. Clinical experience. *Ann Plast Surg* 1977;38:563–577.

90. **Morykwas MJ, Argenta LC, Shelton-Brown EI, et al.** Vacuum-assisted closure: a new method for wound control and treatment. Animal studies and basic foundation. *Ann Plast Surg* 1997;38:553–562.

91. **Beck DE, Harford FJ, DiPalma JA.** Comparison of cleansing methods in preparation for colonic surgery. *Dis Colon Rectum* 1985;28:491–495.

92. **Cohen SM, Wexner SD, Binderow SR, et al.** Prospective, randomized, endoscopic-blinded trial comparing precolonoscopy bowel cleansing methods. *Dis Colon Rectum* 1994;37:689–696.

93. **Clarke JS, Condon RE, Bartlett JG, et al.** Preoperative oral antibiotics reduce septic complications of colon operations: results of prospective, randomized, double-blind clinical study. *Ann Surg* 1977;186:251–259.

94. **Fry DE.** Antibiotics in surgery, an overview. *Ann Surg* 1988;155:11–15.

95. **Menaker GJ.** The use of antibiotics in surgical treatment of the colon. *Gynecol Obstet* 1987;164:581–586.

96. **Wolfson PJ, Bauer JJ, Gelernt IM, et al.** Use of the long tube in the management of patients with small intestinal obstruction due to adhesions. *Arch Surg* 1985;120:1001–1006.

97. **Ratcliff JB, Kapernick P, Brooks GG, et al.** Small bowel obstruction and previous gynecologic surgery. *South Med J* 1983;76:1349–1350, 1360.

98. **Jeffcoate TNA, Tindall VR.** Venous thrombosis and embolism in obstetrics and gynecology. *Aust N Z J Obstet Gynaecol* 1965;5:119–130.

99. **Kimball AM, Hallum VA, Cates W.** Deaths caused by pulmonary thromboembolism after legally induced abortion. *Am J Obstet Gynecol* 1978;132:169–174.

100. **Clarke-Pearson DL, Jelovsek FR, Creasman WT.** Thromboembolism complicating surgery for cervical and uterine malignancy; incidence, risk factors, and prophylaxis. *Obstet Gynecol* 1983;61:87–94.

101. **Creasman WT, Weed JC Jr.** Radical hysterectomy. In: **Schaefer G, Grager EA,** eds. *Complications in obstetrics and gynecology surgery.* Hagerstown, MD: Harper & Row, 1981:389–398.

102. **Clayton JK, Anderson JA, McNicol GP.** Preoperative prediction of postoperative deep vein thrombosis. *BMJ* 1976;2:910–912.

103. **Clarke-Pearson DL, DeLong E, Synan IS, et al.** Variables associated with postoperative deep venous thrombosis: a prospective study of 411 gynecology patients and creation of a prognostic model. *Obstet Gynecol* 1987;69:146–150.

104. **Kakkar VV.** Prevention of fatal postoperative pulmonary embolism by low-dose heparin. An international multicenter trial. *Lancet* 1975;2:145–151.

105. **Ballard RM, Bradley-Watson PJ, Johnstone FD, et al.** Low doses of subcutaneous heparin in the prevention of deep venous thrombosis after gynecologic surgery. *J Obstet Gynaecol Br Commonw* 1973;80:469–472.

106. **Taberner DA, Poller L, Burslem RW, et al.** Oral anticoagulants controlled by British comparative thromboplastin versus dose heparin prophylaxis of deep venous thrombosis. *BMJ* 1978;1:272–274.

107. **Clarke-Pearson DL, Coleman RE, Synan IS, et al.** Venous thromboembolism prophylaxis in gynecologic oncology: a prospective controlled trial of low-dose heparin. *Am J Obstet Gynecol* 1983;145:606–613.

108. **Clarke-Pearson DL, DeLong E, Synan IS, et al.** A controlled trial of two low-dose heparin regimens for the prevention of postoperative deep vein thrombosis. *Obstet Gynecol* 1990;75:684–689.

109. **Clarke-Pearson DL, DeLong E, Synan IS, et al.** Complications of low-dose heparin prophylaxis in gynecologic oncology surgery. *Obstet Gynecol* 1984;64:689–694.

110. **Catalona WJ, Kadmon D, Crane DB.** Effect of mini-dose heparin on lymphocele formation following extraperitoneal pelvic lymphadenectomy. *J Urol* 1979;123:890–895.

111. **Piver MS, Malfetano JH, Lele SB, et al.** Prophylactic anticoagulation as a possible cause of inguinal lymphocyst after radical vulvectomy and inguinal lymphadenectomy. *Obstet Gynecol* 1983;62:17–21.

112. **Tapson VF, Hull RD.** Management of venous thromboembolic disease. The impact of low-molecular weight heparin. *Chest* 1995;16:281–294.

113. **Borstad E, Urdal K, Handeland G, et al.** Comparison of low molecular weight heparin vs unfractionated heparin in gynecological surgery II. Reduced dose of low molecular weight heparin. *Acta Obstet Gynecol Scand* 1992;71:471–475.

114. **Heilmann L, Kruck M, Schindler AE.** Prevention of thrombosis in gynecology. Double-blind comparison of LMW heparin and unfractionated heparin. *Geburtshilfe Frauenheilkd* 1989;49:803–807.

115. **Kaaja R, Lehtovirta P, Venesmaa P, et al.** Comparison of enoxaparin, a low-molecular weight heparin and unfractionated heparin, with or without dihydroergotamine, in abdominal hysterectomy. *Eur J Obstet Gynecol Reprod Bio* 1992;47:141–145.

116. **Jorgensen LN, Willie-Jorgensen P, Hauch O.** Prophylaxis of postoperative thromboembolism with low molecular weight heparins. *Br J Surg* 1993;80:689–704.

117. **Haas S, Haas P.** Efficacy of low molecular weight heparins. An overview. *Semin Thromb Hemost* 1993;19:101–106.

118. **Bergovst D, Lindgren B, Matzsch T.** Comparison of the cost of preventing postoperative deep vein thrombosis with either unfractionated or low molecular weight heparin. *Br J Surg* 1996;83:1548–1552.

119. **Anderson DR, O'Brien BJ, Levine MN, et al.** Efficacy and cost of low-molecular weight heparin compared with standard heparin for the prevention of deep vein thrombosis after total hip arthroplasty. *Ann Intern Med* 1993;119:1105–1112.

120. **Clarke-Pearson DL, Synan IS, Coleman RE, et al.** The natural history of postoperative venous thromboembolism in gynecologic oncology: a prospective study of 283 patients. *Am J Obstet Gynecol* 1984;148:1051–1054.

121. **Conti S, Daschbach M.** Venous thromboembolism prophylaxis: a survey of its use in the United States. *Arch Surg* 1982;117:1036–1040.

122. **Scurr JH, Ibrahim SZ, Faber RG, et al.** The efficacy of graduated compression stocking in the prevention of deep vein thrombosis. *Br J Surg* 1977;64:371–373.

123. **Allenby F, Boardman L, Pflug JJ, et al.** Effects of external pneumatic intermittent compression on fibrinolysis in man. *Lancet* 1973;2:1412–1414.

124. **Salzman EW, Ploet J, Bettlemann M, et al.** Intraoperative external pneumatic calf compression to afford long-term prophylaxis against deep vein thrombosis in urological patients. *Surgery* 1980;87:239–242.

125. **Nicolaides AN, Fernandes e Fernandes J, Pollock AV.** Intermittent sequential pneumatic compression of the legs in the prevention of venous stasis and postoperative deep venous thrombosis. *Surgery* 1980;87:69–76.

126. **Clarke-Pearson DL, Synan IS, Hinshaw W, et al.** Prevention of postoperative venous thromboembolism by external pneumatic calf compression in patients with gynecologic malignancy. *Obstet Gynecol* 1984;63:92–98.

127. **Clarke-Pearson DL, Creasman WT, Coleman RE, et al.** Perioperative external pneumatic calf compression as thromboembolism prophylaxis in gynecologic oncology: report of a randomized controlled trial. *Gynecol Oncol* 1984;18:226–232.

128. **Slazman EW, Davies GC.** Prophylaxis of venous thromboembolism: analysis of cost effectiveness. *Ann Surg* 1980;191:207–218.

129. **Maxwell GL, Dodge R, Synan I, et al.** Risk factors which predispose patients to thromboembolism despite prophylaxis with external pneumatic compression. *Gynecol Oncol* 1999;72:455(abst).

130. **Willie-Jorgensen P, Hauch O, Dimo B, et al.** Prophylaxis of deep venous thrombosis after acute abdominal operation. *Surg Gynecol Obstet* 1991;172:44–48.

131. **Willie-Jorgensen P, Thorup J, Fischer A, et al.** Heparin with and without graded compression stockings in the prevention of thromboembolic complications of major abdominal surgery. A randomized trial. *Br J Surg* 1985;72:579–581.

132. **Willie-Jorgensen P.** Prophylaxis of postoperative thromboembolism with combined modalities. *Semin Thromb Hemost* 1991;17:272–279.

133. **Agnelli G, Piovella F, Buoncristiani P, et al.** Enoxaparin plus compression stockings alone in the prevention of venous thromboembolism after elective neurosurgery. *N Engl J Med* 1998;339:80–85.

134. **Haegger K.** Problems of acute deep vein thrombosis. *Angiology* 1969;20:219–222.

135. **Palko PA, Namson EM, Fedonik SO.** The early detection of deep venous thrombosis using ^{135}I-tagged fibrinogen. *Can J Surg* 1964;7:215–220.

136. **Athanasoulis CA.** Phlebography for the diagnosis of deep leg vein thrombosis, prophylactic therapy of deep venous thrombosis and pulmonary embolism. DHEW Publication No. 76–886. Washington, DC: National Institutes of Health, 1975:62–76.

137. **Lensing AWA, Pradoni P, Bandjes D, et al.** Detection of deep-vein thrombosis by real-time B-mode ultrasonography. *N Engl J Med* 1989;320:342–348.

138. **Wheeler HB, O'Donnel JA, Anderson FA.** Occlusive cuff impedance phlebography. a diagnostic procedure for venous thrombosis and pulmonary embolism. *Prog Cardiovasc Dis* 1974;17:199–204.

139. **Clarke-Pearson DL, Creasman WT.** Diagnosis of deep vein thrombosis in obstetrics and gynecology in impedance phlebography. *Obstet Gynecol* 1981;58:52–59.

140. **Montgomery KD, Potter HG, Helfet DL.** Magnetic resonance venography to evaluate the deep venous system of the pelvis in patients who have acetabular fracture. *J Bone Joint Surg* 1995;77:1639–1649.

141. **Reynolds C.** Management of the diabetic surgical patient. *Postgrad Med* 1985;77:266–279.

142. **Jacober SJ, Sowers JR.** An update on perioperative management of diabetes. *Arch Intern Med* 1999;159:2405–2411.

143. **Hirsch IB, McGill JB.** Role of insulin in management of surgical patients with diabetes mellitus. *Diabetes Care* 1990;13:980–991.

144. **Galloway JA, Shuman CR.** Diabetes and surgery. A study of 667 cases. *Am J Med* 1963;34:177–191.

145. **Zonszein J, Santangele RP, Mackin JF, et al.** Propanol therapy in thyrotoxicosis: a review of 84 patients undergoing surgery. *Am J Med* 1979;66:411–416.

146. **Goldman DR.** Surgery in patients with endocrine dysfunction. Preoperative consultation. *Med Clin North Am* 1987;71:499–506.

147. **James ML.** Endocrine disease and anesthesia. *Anesth Analg* 1970;25:232–252.

148. **Hirsch IB, McGill JB, Cryer PE, et al.** Perioperative management of surgical patients with diabetes mellitus. *Anesthesiology* 1991;74:346–359.

149. **Alberti KG, Thomas DJ.** The management of diabetes during surgery. *Br J Anaesth* 1979;51:693–710.

150. **Walts LF.** Perioperative management of diabetes mellitus. *Anesthesiology* 1981;55:104–108.

151. **Goldman DR.** Surgery in patients with endocrine dysfunction. Preoperative consultation. *Med Clin North Am* 1987;71:499–506.

152. **Pirich C, Mullner M, Sinzinger H.** Prevalence and relevance of thyroid dysfunction in 1922 cholesterol screening participants. *J Clin Epidemiol* 2000;53:623–629.

153. **Pronovost PH, Parris KH.** Perioperative management of thyroid disease. Prevention of complications related to hyperthyroidism and hypothyroidism. *Postgrad Med* 1995;98:83–86.

154. **Grader AL, Neg KL, Nicholson WE, et al.** Natural history of pituitary-adrenal recovery following long-term suppression with corticosteroids. *J Clin Endocrinol Metab* 1965;25:11.

155. **Salem M, Tainsh REJ, Bromberg J, et al.** Perioperative glucocorticoid coverage. A reassessment 42 years after emergence of a problem. *Ann Surg* 1994;219:416–425.

156. **Kehlet, H.** *Clinical course and hypothalamic-pituitary-adrenocortical function in glucocorticoid-treated surgical patients.* Copenhagen: FADL's Forlag, 1976.

157. **Glowniak JV, Loriaux DL.** A double-blind study of perioperative steroid requirements in secondary adrenal insufficiency. *Surgery* 1997;121:123–129.

158. **Becker RC, Underwood DA.** Myocardial infarction in patients undergoing noncardiac surgery. *Cleve Clin J Med* 1987;54:25–28.

159. **Rao TL, Jacobs KH, El-Etr AA.** Reinfarction following anesthesia in patients with myocardial infarction. *Anesthesiology* 1983;59:499–505.

160. **Mehta RH, Bossone E, Eagle KA.** Perioperative cardiac risk assessment for noncardiac surgery. *Cardiologia* 1999;44:409–418.

161. **Goldman L, Caldera DL, Nussbaum SR, et al.** Multifactorial index of cardiac risk in noncardiac surgical procedures. *N Engl J Med* 1977;297:845–850.

162. **Cutler BS, Wheeler HB, Paraskos JA, et al.** Applicability and interpretation of electrocardiographic stress testing in patients with peripheral vascular disease. *Am J Surg* 198;141:501–506.

163. **Carliner NH, Fisher ML, Plotnick GD, et al.** Routine preoperative exercise testing in patients undergoing major noncardiac surgery. *Am J Cardiol* 1985;56:51–58.

164. **Coley CM, Field TS, Abraham SA, et al.** Usefulness of dipyridamole-thallium scanning for preoperative evaluation of cardiac risk for nonvascular surgery. *Am J Cardiol* 1992;69:1280–1285.

165. **Baron JF, Mundler O, Bertrand M, et al.** Dipyridamole-thallium scintigraphy and gated radionuclide angiography to assess cardiac risk before abdominal aortic surgery. *N Engl J Med* 1994;330:663–669.

166. **Lane RT, Sawada SG, Segar DS, et al.** Dobutamine stress echocardiography for assessment of cardiac risk before noncardiac surgery. *Am J Cardiol* 1991;68:976–977.

167. **Davila-Roman VG, Waggoner AD, Sicard GA, et al.** Dobutamine stress echocardiography predicts surgical outcome in patients with an aortic aneurysm and peripheral vascular disease. *J Am Coll Cardiol* 1993;21:957–963.

168. **Kaplan J.** Hemodynamic monitoring. In: **Kaplan J,** ed. *Cardiac anesthesia.* New York: Grune & Stratton, 1987:179–226.

169. **Mangano DT, Layug EL, Wallace A, et al.** Effect of atenolol on mortality and cardiovascular morbidity after noncardiac surgery. Multicenter Study of Perioperative Ischemia Research Group. *N Engl J Med* 1996;335:1713–1720.

170. **Wallace A, Layug B, Tateo I, et al.** Prophylactic atenolol reduces postoperative myocardial ischemia. *Anesthesiology* 1998;88:7–17.

171. **McGregor M.** The nitrates and myocardial ischemia. *Circulation* 1982;66:689–691.

172. **Coriat P, Daloz M, Bousseau D, et al.** Prevention of intraoperative myocardial ischemia during noncardiac surgery with intravenous nitroglycerin. *Anesthesiology* 1984;61:193–198.

173. **Gallagher J, Moore RA, Jose AB, et al.** Prophylactic nitroglycerin infusions during coronary artery bypass surgery. *Anesthesiology* 1986;64:785–789.

174. **Thomson I, Mutch W, Culligan J.** Failure of intravenous nitroglycerin to prevent intraoperative myocardial ischemia during fentanyl-pancuronium anesthesia. *Anesthesiology* 1984;61:385–390.

175. **Warltier DC, Pagel PS, Kersten JR.** Approaches to the prevention of perioperative myocardial ischemia. *Anesthesiology* 2000;92:253–259.

176. **Cooperman LH, Price HL.** Pulmonary edema in the operative and postoperative period. a review of 40 cases. *Ann Surg* 1970;172:883–891.

177. **Goldman L.** Cardiac risk factors and complications in non-cardiac surgery. *Medicine* 1978;57:357–370.

178. **Kuner J, Enescu V, Utsu F, et al.** Cardiac arrhythmias during anesthesia. *Dis Chest* 1967;52:580–587.

179. **Blaustein AS.** Preoperative and perioperative management of cardiac patients undergoing noncardiac surgery. *Cardiol Clin* 1995;13:149–161.

180. **Lerner SM.** Suppression of a demand pacemaker by transurethral electrocautery. *Anesth Analg* 1973; 52:703–706.

181. **Rooney SM, Goldner PL, Muss E.** Relationship of right bundle branch block and marked left axis deviation to complete heart block during general anesthesia. *Anesthesiology* 1976;44:64–66.

182. **Bellocci F, Santarelli P, DiGennaro M, et al.** The risk of cardiac complications in surgical patients with bifascicular block. A clinical and electrophysiologic study in 98 patients. *Chest* 1980;77:343–348.

183. **Berg GR, Kofler MN.** The significance of bilateral bundle branch block in the preoperative patient. A retrospective electrocardiographic and clinical study in 30 patients. *Chest* 1971;59:62–67.

184. **Skinner JF, Pearce ML.** Surgical risk in the cardiac patient. *J Chronic Dis* 1964;17:57–72.

185. **Dajani AS, Taubert KA, Wilson W, et al.** Prevention of bacterial endocarditis. Recommendations by the American Heart Association. *JAMA* 1997;277:1794–1801.

186. **Maille JG, Dyrda I, Paiement B, et al.** Patients with cardiac valve prosthesis: subsequent anesthetic management for noncardiac surgical procedures. *Can Anaesth Soc J* 1973;20:207–216.

187. **Katholi RE, Nolan SP, McGuire LB.** The management of anticoagulation during noncardiac operations in patients with prosthetic heart valves. A prospective study. *Am Heart J* 1978;96:163–165.

188. **Tinker JH, Tarhan S.** Discontinuing anticoagulant therapy in surgical patients with cardiac valve prostheses. Observations in 180 operations. *JAMA* 1978;239:738–739.

189. **Strandgaard S, Olesen J, Skinhoj E, et al.** Autoregulation of brain circulation in severe arterial hypertension. *BMJ* 1973;1:507–510.

190. **Rao TL, Jacobs KH, El-Etr AA.** Reinfarction following anesthesia in patients with myocardial infarction. *Anesthesiology* 1983;59:499–505.

191. **Swan HJ, Ganz W, Forrester J, et al.** Catheterization of the heart in man with use of a flow-directed balloon-tipped catheter. *N Engl J Med* 1970;283:447–451.

192. **Dalen JE, Bone RC.** Is it time to pull the pulmonary artery catheter? *JAMA* 1996;276:916–918.

193. **Connors AFJ, Speroff T, Dawson NV, et al.** The effectiveness of right heart catheterization in the initial care of critically ill patients. *JAMA* 1996;276:889–897.

194. **Ivanov R, Allen J, Calvin JE.** The incidence of major morbidity in critically ill patients managed with pulmonary artery catheters: a meta-analysis. *Crit Care Med* 2000;28:615–619.

195. **Greenburg AG.** Benefits and risks of blood transfusion in surgical patients. *World J Surgery* 1996;20:1189–1193.

196. **Renzi RM, Kaye W, Greenburg AG.** Oxygen utilization in the critically ill patient. In: **Barrie PS, Shires GT,** eds. *Surgical intensive care.* Boston: Little, Brown and Company, 1993:211–226.

197. **National Institutes of Health.** Summary of NIH consensus development conference on perioperative red cell transfusion. *Am J Hematol* 1989;31:144–150.

198. **D'Ambra MN, Kaplan DK.** Alternatives to allogenic blood use in surgery. acute normovolemic hemodilution and preoperative autologous donation. *Am J Surg* 1995;[Suppl 6A]:170.

199. **Goodnough LT.** Increased preoperative collection of autologous blood with recombinant human erythropoietin therapy. *N Engl J Med* 1989;321:1163–1168.

200. **Pedersen-Bjergaard U, Andersen M, Hansen PB.** Drug-specific characteristics of thrombocytopenia caused by non-cytotoxic drugs. *Eur J Clin Pharmacol* 1998;54:701–706.

201. **Myers ER, Clarke-Pearson DL, Olt GJ, et al.** Preoperative coagulation testing on a gynecologic oncology service. *Obstet Gynecol* 1994;83:438–444.

202. **Bodey GP, Buckley M, Sathe YS, et al.** Quantitative relationships between circulating leukocytes and infection in patients with acute leukemia. *Ann Intern Med* 1966;64:328–340.

203. **Miller RD, Robins TO, Tong MJ, et al.** Coagulation defects associated with massive blood transfusions. *Ann Surg* 1971;174:794–799.

204. **Reed RL II, Ciavarella D, Heimbach DM, et al.** Prophylactic platelet administration during massive transfusion: a prospective, randomized, double-blind clinical study. *Ann Surg* 1986;203:40–46.

205. **American Society of Anesthesiologists Task Force on Blood Component Therapy.** Practice guidelines for blood component therapy. *Anesthesiology* 1996;84:732–747.

206. **Mohr DN, Jett JR.** Preoperative evaluation of pulmonary risk factors. *J Gen Intern Med* 1988;3:277–287.

207. **Hotchkiss RS.** Perioperative management of patient with chronic obstructive pulmonary disease. *Int Anesthesiol Clin* 1988;26:134–142.

208. **Stein M, Cassara EL.** Preoperative pulmonary evaluation and therapy for surgery patients. *JAMA* 1970;211:787–790.

209. **Forthman HJ, Shepard A.** Postoperative pulmonary complications. *South Med J* 1969;62:1198–1200.

210. **De Nino LA, Lawrence VA, Averyt EC, et al.** Preoperative spirometry and laparotomy: blowing away dollars. *Chest* 1997;111:1536–1541.

211. **Lawrence VA, Dhanda R, Hilsenbeck SG, et al.** Risk of pulmonary complications after elective abdominal surgery. *Chest* 1996;110:744–750.

212. **Zibrak JD, O'Donnell CR.** Indications for preoperative pulmonary function testing. *Clin Chest Med* 1993;14:227–236.

213. **Zibrak JD, O'Donnell CR, Marton K.** Indications for pulmonary function testing. *Ann Intern Med* 1990;112:763–771.

214. **Sagel SS, Evens RG, Forrest JV, et al.** Efficacy of routine screening and lateral chest radiographs in a hospital-based population. *N Engl J Med* 1974;291:1001–1004.

215. **Woolcock AJ, Peat JK.** Evidence for the increase in asthma worldwide. *Ciba Found Symp* 1997;206:122–134.

216. **Galant SP.** Treatment of asthma. New and time-tested strategies. *Postgrad Med* 1990;87:229–236.

217. **Barnes PJ.** A new approach to the treatment of asthma. *N Engl J Med* 1989;321:1517–1527.

218. **Drazen JM, Israel E, O'Byrne PM.** Treatment of asthma with drugs modifying the leukotriene pathway. *N Engl J Med* 1999;340:197–206.

219. **Blosser SA, Rock P.** Asthma and chronic obstructive lung disease, perioperative management. In: **Breslow MJ, Miller CJ, Rogers MC,** eds. St Louis: Mosby, 1990:259–280.

220. **Hargreave FE, Dolovich J, Newhouse MT.** The assessment and treatment of asthma. A conference report. *J Allergy Clin Immunol* 1990;85:1098–1111.

221. **Stoelting RK, Dierdorf SF.** *Anesthesia and co-existing disease.* New York, Churchill Livingstone, 1993.

222. **Flenley DC.** Chronic obstructive pulmonary disease. *Dis Mon* 1988;34:537–599.

223. **Barnes PJ.** Chronic obstructive pulmonary disease. *N Engl J Med* 2000;343:269–280.

224. **Tarhan S, Moffitt EA, Sessler AD, et al.** Risk of anesthesia and surgery in patients with chronic bronchitis and chronic obstructive pulmonary disease. *Surgery* 1973;74:720–726.

225. **Gracey DR, Divertie MB, Didier EP.** Preoperative pulmonary preparation of patients with chronic obstructive pulmonary disease: a prospective study. *Chest* 1979;76:123–129.

226. **Castillo R, Haas A.** Chest physical therapy. Comparative efficacy of preoperative and postoperative in the elderly. *Arch Phys Med Rehabil* 1985;66:376–379.

227. **Marienau ME, Buck CF.** Preoperative evaluation of the pulmonary patient undergoing nonpulmonary surgery. *J Perianesth Nurs* 1998;13:340–348.

228. **Schwaber JR.** Evaluation of respiratory status in surgical patients. *Surg Clin North Am* 1970;50:637–644.

229. **Hnatiuk OW, Dillard TA, Torrington KG.** Adherence to established guidelines for preoperative pulmonary function testing. *Chest* 1995;107:1294–1297.

230. **Nunn JF, Milledge JS, Chen D, et al.** Respiratory criteria of fitness for surgery and anaesthesia. *Anaesthesia* 1988;43:543–551.

231. **Anderson ME, Belani KG.** Short-term preoperative smoking abstinence. *Am Fam Physician* 1990;41:1191–1194.

232. **Warner MA, Offord KP, Warner ME, et al.** Role of preoperative cessation of smoking and other factors in postoperative pulmonary complications: a blinded prospective study of coronary artery bypass patients. *Mayo Clin Proc* 1989;64:609–616.

233. **Weinacker AB, Vaszar LT.** Acute respiratory distress syndrome: physiology and new management strategies. *Annu Rev Med* 2001;52:221–237.

234. **Smith G.** Management of post-operative pain. *Can J Anaesth* 1989;36:S1–S4.

235. **Broyer M, Brunner FP, Brynger H, et al.** Demography of dialysis and transplantation in Europe, 1984. *Nephrol Dial Transplant* 1986;1:1–8.

236. **Blumberg A, Weidman P, Shaw S, et al.** Effect of various therapeutic approaches on plasma potassium and major regulating factors in terminal renal failure. *Am J Med* 1988;85:507–512.

237. **Lewis SL, Van Epps DE.** Neutrophil and monocyte alterations in chronic dialysis patients. *Am J Kidney Dis* 1987;9:381–395.

238. **Hellem A, Borchgrevink C, Ames S.** The role of red cells in hemostasis. The relationship between hematocrit, bleeding time, and platelet adhesiveness. *Br J Haematol* 1961;7:42–50.

239. **Remuzzi G.** Bleeding disorders in uremia: pathophysiology and treatment. *Adv Nephrol Necker Hosp* 1989;18:171–186.

240. **Mannucci PM, Remuzzi G, Pusineri F, et al.** Deamino-8-D-arginine vasopressin shortens the bleeding time in uremia. *N Engl J Med* 1983;308:8–12.

241. **Stoelting RK, Dierdoff SF.** Renal disease. In: **Stoelting RK, Dierdoff SF,** eds. *Anesthesia and co-existing disease,* 3rd ed. New York: Churchill Livingstone, 1993:289–312.

242. **Sherrard DJ.** Aluminum toxicity. In: **Ferris TF**, ed. *The kidney.* Washington, DC: National Kidney Foundation, 1988:31–36.

243. **Hostetter TH, Olson JL, Rennke HG, et al.** Hyperfiltration in remnant nephrons: a potentially adverse response to renal ablation. *Am J Physiol* 1981;241:85–93.

244. **Gallup DG, Nolan TE, Smith RP.** Primary mass closure of midline incisions with a continuous polyglyconate monofilament absorbable suture. *Obstet Gynecol* 1990;76:872–875.

245. **Miller RD.** Pharmacology of muscle relaxants and their antagonists. In: **Miller RD,** ed. *Anesthesia,*2nd ed. New York: Churchill Livingstone, 1986:920.

246. **Mazze RI.** Anesthesia for patients with abnormal renal function and genitourinary problems. In: **Miller RD,** ed. *Anesthesia,* 2nd ed. New York: Churchill Livingstone, 1986:1648.

247. **Roth F, Wuthrich H.** The clinical importance of hyperkalemia following suxamethonium administration. *Br J Anaesth* 1969;41:311–315.

248. **Silberman H.** Renal failure and the surgeon. *Surg Gynecol Obstet* 1977;144:775–784.

249. **Hou SH.** Hospital-acquired renal insufficiency: a prospective study. *Am J Med* 1983;74:243–248.

250. **Bullock ML, Umen AJ, Finkelstein MS.** The assessment of risk factors in 462 patients with acute renal failure. *Am J Kidney Dis* 1985;5:97–103.

251. **Meyer RD.** Risk factors and comparison of clinical nephrotoxicity of aminoglyosides. *Am J Med* 1986;80:119–125.

252. **Shusterman N, Strom BL, Murray TG, et al.** Risk factors and outcome of hospital-acquired acute renal failure: clinical epidemiologic study. *Am J Med* 1987;83:65–71.

253. **Harkonen S, Kjellstrand CM.** Contrast nephropathy. *Am J Nephrol* 1981;1:69–72.

254. **Bush HL, Huse JB, Johnson WC, et al.** Prevention of renal insufficiency after abdominal aortic aneurysm resection by optimal volume loading. *Arch Surg* 1981;116:1517–1524.

255. **Cebul RD, Beck JR.** Biochemical profiles. Applications in ambulatory screening and preadmission testing of adults. *Ann Intern Med* 1987;106:403–413.

256. **Batchelder BM, Cooperman LH.** Effects of anesthetics on splanchnic circulation and metabolism. *Surg Clin North Am* 1975;55:787–794.

257. **Maze M, Bass NM.** Anesthesia and the hepatobiliary system. In: **Miller RD**, ed. *Anesthesia.* New York: Churchill Livingstone, 2000:1960–1972.

258. **Child CG, Turcotte JG.** Surgery and portal hypertension. In: **Child CG,** ed. *The liver and portal hypertension,* 3rd ed. Philadelphia: WB Saunders, 1964:1–85.

259. **Garrison RN, Cryer HM, Howard DA, et al.** Clarification of risk factors for abdominal operations in patients with hepatic cirrhosis. *Ann Surg* 1984;199:648–655.

260. **Terblanche J.** Sclerotherapy for prophylaxis of variceal bleeding. *Lancet* 1986;1:961–963.

261. **LaMont JT.** The liver. In: **Vandam LD,** ed. *To make the patient ready for anesthesia: medical care of the surgical patient.* Menlo Park, CA: Addison Wesley, 1984:47–66.

262. **Blamey SL, Fearon KCH, Gilmour WH, et al.** Prediction of risk in biliary surgery. *Br J Surg* 1983;70:535–538.

263. **Czaja Aj, Summerskill WH.** Chronic hepatitis. To treat or not to treat? *Med Clin North Am* 1978;62:71–85.

264. **Perrillo RP, Schiff ER, Davis GL, et al.** A randomized controlled trial of interferon α-IIB alone and after prednisone withdrawal for the treatment of chronic hepatitis B. *N Engl J Med* 1990;323:295–301.

265. **Immunization Practices Advisory Committee.** Recommendations for protection against viral hepatitis. *Ann Intern Med* 1985;103:391–402.

266. **Chiang PP.** Perioperative management of the alcohol-dependent patient. *Am Fam Physician* 1995;52:2267–2273.

267. **Matloff DS, Kapkan MM.** Gastroenterology. In: **Molitch ME,** ed. *Management of medical problems in surgical patients.* Philadelphia: FA Davis Co, 1982:219–252.

268. **Sirinek KR, Burk RR, Brown M, et al.** Improving survival in patients with cirrhosis undergoing major abdominal operations. *Arch Surg* 1987;122:271–273.

20 Incontinence, Prolapse, and Disorders of the Pelvic Floor

Shawn A. Menefee
L. Lewis Wall

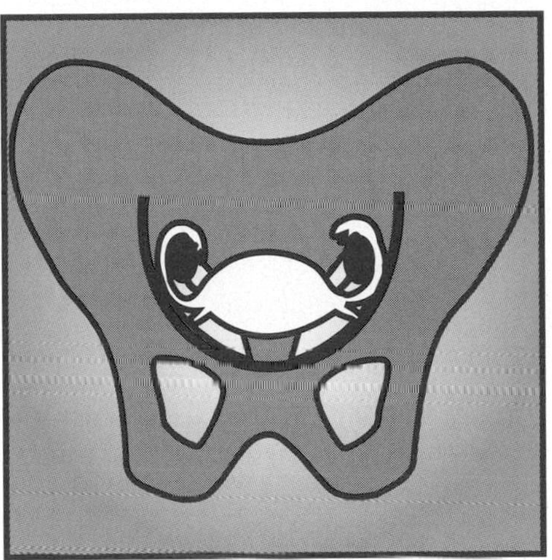

The genital and urinary tracts are intimately associated anatomically and embryologically from the earliest stages of their development. The bladder is located directly above the anterior vaginal wall, and the urethra is fused to it. Both of these structures, as well as other structures of the pelvic floor, are placed at risk during pregnancy and childbirth. Each organ system in the pelvic floor—urinary, genital, intestinal—traverses the pelvis and exits through its own orifice. Thus, these systems are intricately related in function and anatomic support (1). Disorders of each of these components should be evaluated in light of their impact on the function of the surrounding structures and the functional anatomy of the pelvic floor. The term *urogynecology* has been coined to describe the area of gynecology that deals with disorders of the female lower urinary tract; however, it has become apparent that urinary tract disorders are only one facet of a wide range of pelvic floor disorders that afflict women. As part of this growing recognition, the American Board of Obstetrics and Gynecology and the American Board of Urology have recently agreed to begin the process of jointly accrediting fellowship programs in Female Pelvic Medicine and Reconstructive Surgery. This effort to train both urologists and gynecologists in the treatment of all aspects of pelvic floor dysfunction is a positive step toward improving the care of patients afflicted with these common conditions.

Pelvic Floor Anatomy

The striated muscles of the pelvic floor, in combination with their fascial attachments, work together across the entire pelvis to prevent pelvic organ displacement, to maintain continence, and to control expulsive activities. An appreciation of the fact that these organ systems have complex interrelationships should help clinicians realize that patients' problems are not necessarily limited to a single organ; rather, each disturbance of pelvic support or continence exists within a complex pelvic "ecosystem" and, as a result, may be linked to problems in other organ systems.

Pelvic Support

The bony pelvis surrounds and protects its contents but, by itself, actually provides them with little support. The pelvic organs are supported primarily by the muscular activity of the pelvic floor, aided by ligamentous attachments. Rather than functioning as a rigid structure, the pelvic floor muscles provide dynamic support through constant activity, functioning more like a self-regulating trampoline that continually adjusts its tension in response to changing circumstances (2,3).

The functional anatomy of the muscles of the pelvic floor (the levator ani) has been studied for many years but remains poorly understood (4). The pelvic floor muscles contract to maintain urinary and fecal incontinence and relax to permit bowel and bladder emptying. The pelvic floor plays a role in normal female sexual responsiveness (5). It must distend tremendously to allow the delivery of a term infant but must contract again during the postpartum period to allow its varied functions to continue. Because the urethra, bladder, rectum, and supporting structures of the pelvis are all part of the pelvic floor, the functions of these organs cannot really be understood without an understanding of the pelvic musculature (see Chapter 5) (6,7).

Levator Ani Muscle

The nomenclature of the pelvic muscles has long been subject to debate. The levator ani muscle (the broad general term for most of the muscles of the pelvic floor) has been described as consisting of a diaphragmatic portion (iliococcygeus) and the more important pubovisceral portion (8). The iliococcygeus portion of the levator ani consists of a thin muscular sheet that arises from the pelvic sidewall on either side of the arcus tendineus and ischial spine and inserts into a midline raphe behind the rectum. The pubovisceral (pubococcygeus) portion of the levator ani muscle consists of a thick U-shaped band of muscle arising from the pubic bone and attaching to the lateral walls of the vagina and rectum (Fig. 20.1). Therefore, the rectum is supported by a muscular sling that pulls it toward the pubic bones when these muscles contract. This muscular band is often called the *puborectalis* or the *pubococcygeus* muscle, but a more accurate term is the *pubovisceral* muscle because these muscles arise from the pubic bone and insert directly onto pelvic viscera or provide a supporting sling for them.

When the pubovisceral muscle contracts, it pulls the rectum, vagina, and urethra anteriorly toward the pubic bone and constricts the lumens of these pelvic organs (Fig. 20.2). It is this contractile property that is so important in maintaining urinary and fecal continence and in providing support for the genital organs (vagina, cervix, uterus) that lie upon and are supported by the levator plate. The medial portions of the pubovisceral muscle (levator ani) pass laterally to the arcus tendineus fasciae of the pelvis and attach to the endopelvic fascia surrounding the vaginal wall at a point opposite the upper half of the urethra (9–11) (Fig. 20.3). The pubovisceral muscle attaches to a web of endopelvic fascia rather than directly to the urethra in this area. This portion of the muscle (puborectalis) contains large quantities of type I ("slow-twitch") muscle fibers that are tonically contracted. This baseline level of muscular activity provides constant resilient support for the urethra. At the same time, type II ("fast-twitch") fibers allow the pubovisceral muscle to respond quickly to rapid changes in intraabdominal pressure (coughing, sneezing) and to maintain urethral closure under such conditions (12). Reflex contraction of both types of muscle fibers helps support all of the contents of the pelvis.

As with the external anal sphincter, the levator ani muscles exhibit constant baseline tone in addition to their ability to contract and offset increases in intraabdominal pressure that would force pelvic contents downward. The phenomenon of constant baseline tone is separate from the ability of these muscles to contract forcefully. This aspect of pelvic muscle function is poorly understood, but it is critical for proper pelvic support because closure of the pelvic floor allows the pelvic viscera to rest on a muscular shelf. The constant adjustments in muscle activity maintain pelvic floor closure in response to changing circumstances and keep the pelvic ligaments from stretching.

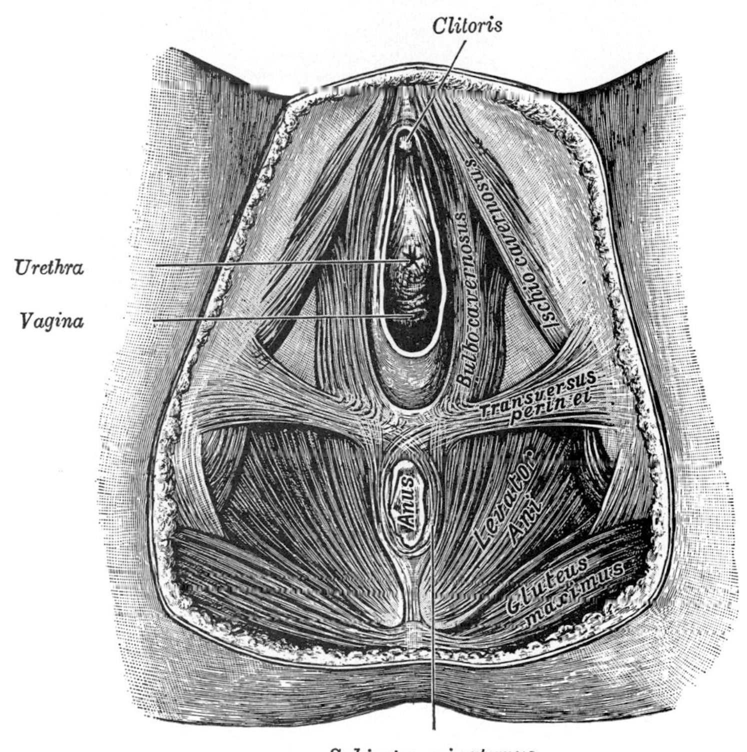

Figure 20.1 The levator ani muscles, as seen from below. (From **Goss CM,** ed. *Gray's anatomy of the human body.* 28th ed. Philadelphia, Lee & Febiger, 1966:447, with permission.)

Pelvic Ligaments

It is often erroneously believed that the various pelvic ligaments are the most important factors in pelvic support. Ligaments are poorly suited to maintaining support over time because fibrous tissues elongate when subjected to constant tension. The pelvic ligaments serve mainly to keep structures in positions where they can be supported by muscular activity rather than acting as weight-bearing structures themselves. The loss of normal muscular

Figure 20.2 A: The "pubovisceral" muscle at rest. **B:** Contraction of the pubovisceral muscle constricts the lumens of the urethra, vagina, and rectum, augmenting closure of all three organs.

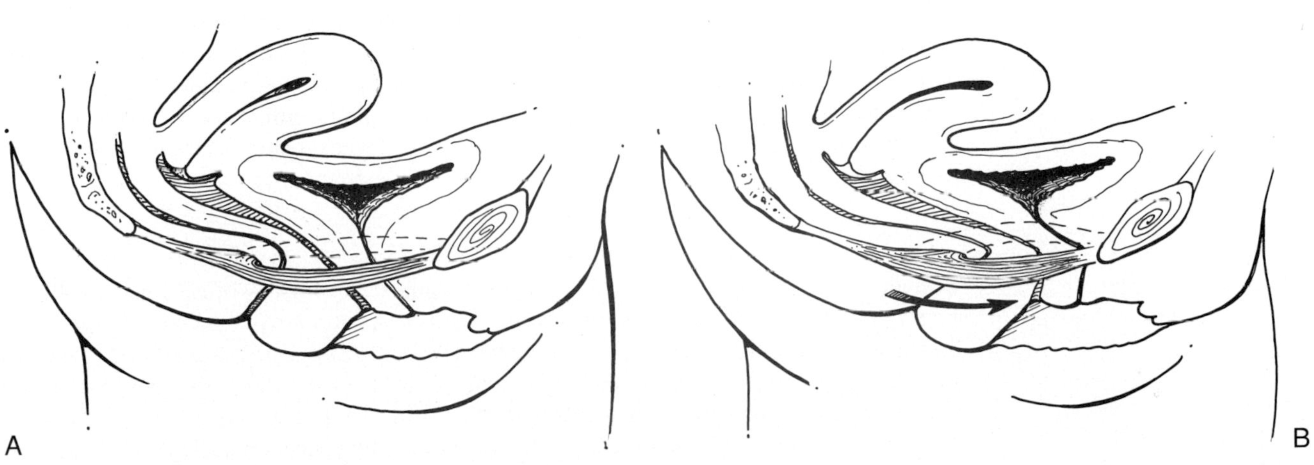

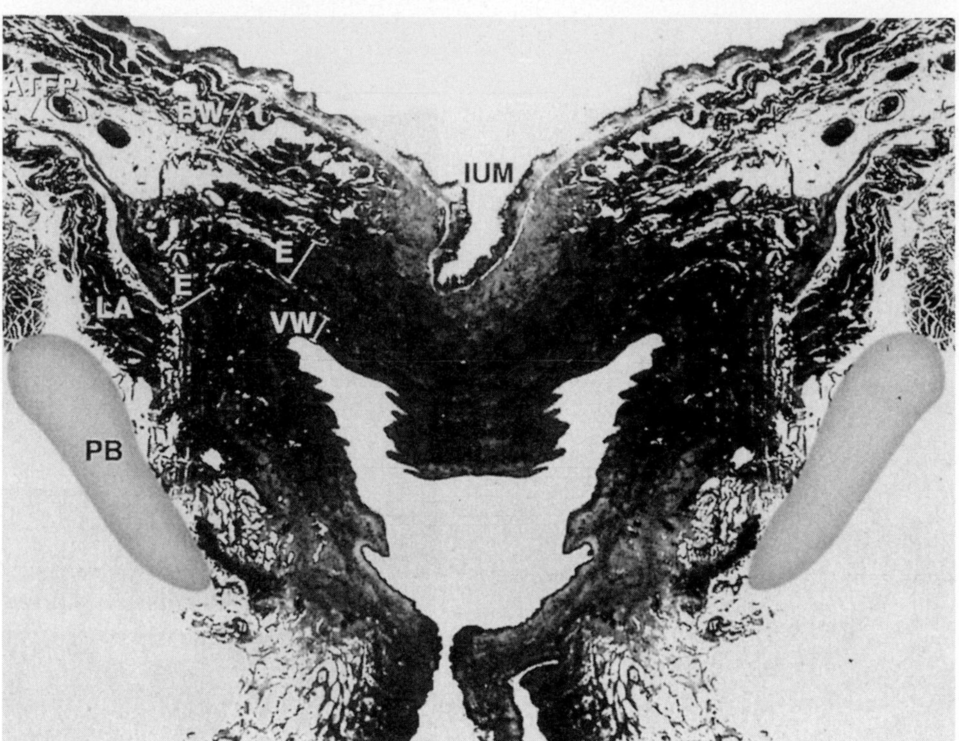

Figure 20.3 Frontal section of the cadaver of a 21-year-old woman at the vesical neck showing the supportive layer formed by the vaginal wall *(VW)* and the endopelvic fascia *(E)* attached to the pelvic wall at the arcus tendineus fasciae pelvis *(ATFP)* on the inner surface of the levator ani *(LA)* at the level of the proximal urethral and internal urinary meatus *(IUM)*. The area where the pubic bones were removed is shaded *(PB)*. The image is reconstructed from a specimen made from the left side of the body by reflecting it across the midline. (From **Delancey J.** Structural support of the urethra as it relates to stress urinary incontinence: the hammock hypothesis. *Am J Obstet Gynecol* 1994;170:1715, with permission.)

support leads to sagging and widening of the urogenital hiatus and predisposes patients to the development of pelvic organ prolapse (13) (Fig. 20.4).

Although fascia and ligaments are believed to be essential for support of the pelvic organs, this belief comes more from the amount of attention given to these structures in the performance of gynecologic surgery than from any empiric evidence regarding their role in pelvic support. However, the pelvic ligaments (i.e., the round, infundibulopelvic, and cardinal) are loose condensations of areolar tissue, blood vessels, and muscle fibers. By themselves, they have little supportive strength; rather, they function as "moorings" to hold the uterus and vagina in place. The pelvic ligaments and the endopelvic fascia attach the uterus and vagina to the pelvic sidewalls so that these structures can be supported by the muscles of the pelvic floor. The entire complex then rests on the levator plate, where it can be closed by increases in intraabdominal pressure by a flap-valve effect (14).

Connective Tissue

Connective tissue is the "glue" of the body. It is composed primarily of elastin and collagen fibers in a polysaccharide ground substance. The composition of connective tissue is not constant but varies in different sites throughout the body. Connective tissue forms capsules to help maintain the structural integrity of organs. It forms the fascia that covers muscles and the tendons and allows them to attach to other structures in the body. If connective tissue fails, muscular support is weak because the attachments that permit muscles to exercise their functions are unreliable (15). Connective tissue is not static; instead, it is a dynamic tissue

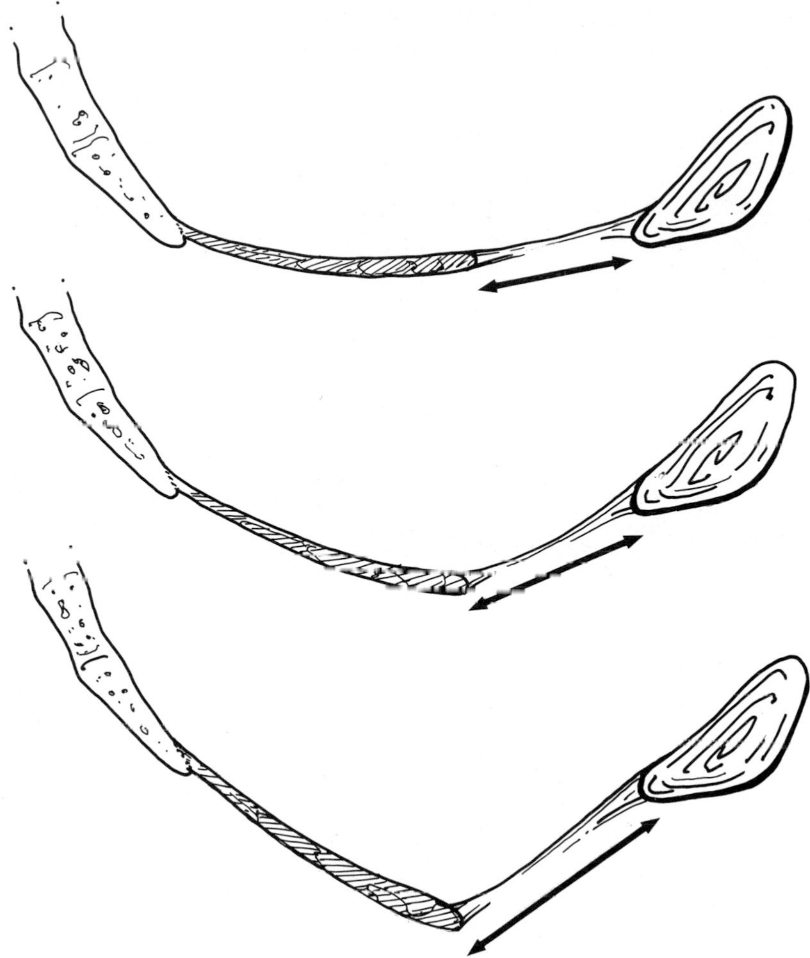

Figure 20.4 Supportive role of the levator plate. Note how muscle tone in the levator muscle complex keeps the urogenital hiatus constricted and relatively closed (*top*). As muscle tone is lost, the levator plate sags, gradually widening the levator hiatus and predisposing the patient to the development of prolapse (*bottom*).

that undergoes constant turnover and remodeling in response to stress. Connective tissue turnover and repair are especially important in relation to wound healing and recovery from surgery. Hormonal changes appear to have significant effects on collagen, and these effects are probably of great importance during pregnancy and parturition, as well as in aging (16–18). Exercise appears to increase collagen turnover, as measured by increased proline hydroxylase activity in 69-year-old women who exercised for 8 weeks (19). Nutrition has an important role in the maintenance of connective tissue integrity. Vitamin C deficiency (scurvy) produces defects in collagen synthesis and repair that can result in the breakdown of seemingly normal connective tissue, even including the reopening of old, previously healed wounds (20).

Studies suggest that connective tissue abnormalities are a significant factor contributing to prolapse and related conditions. For example, joint hypermobility is a common clinical marker for abnormal collagen levels. Several studies have now shown an association between joint hypermobility and pelvic floor prolapse (21,22). Studies evaluating patients with a history of Ehlers-Danlos syndrome, a disorder of collagen synthesis, have revealed an increased incidence of urinary incontinence associated with this disorder (23,24). Fibroblasts grown in tissue culture from the fascia of women with recurrent genital prolapse have an imbalance of collagen types, with excessive synthesis of weaker type III collagen (25). Both collagen content and collagen strength appear to be decreased in the fascia of women with stress incontinence (26,27). However, pelvic support defects are affected by many different factors, and the ultimate clinical presentation (and perhaps the surgical solution) may be different for each patient (28).

Lower Urinary Tract Function

The bladder is a complex organ that has a relatively simple function: to store urine effortlessly, painlessly, and without leakage and to discharge urine voluntarily, effortlessly, completely, and painlessly. To meet these demands, the bladder must have normal anatomic support as well as normal neurophysiologic function.

Normal Urethral Closure

Normal urethral closure is maintained by a combination of intrinsic and extrinsic factors. The extrinsic factors include the levator ani muscles, the endopelvic fascia, and their attachments to the pelvic sidewalls and the urethra. This forms a hammock beneath the urethra that responds to increases in intraabdominal pressure by remaining tense, allowing the urethra to be closed against the posterior supporting shelf (Fig. 20.5). When this supportive mechanism becomes faulty for some reason—the endopelvic fascia has detached from its normal points of fixation, muscular support has weakened, or a combination of these two processes—normal support is lost, and anatomic hypermobility of the urethra and bladder neck develops. For many women, this loss of support is severe enough to cause loss of closure during periods of increased intraabdominal pressure, and stress incontinence results. However, many women remain continent in spite of loss of urethral support (11).

The intrinsic factors contributing to urethral closure include the striated muscle of the urethral wall, vascular congestion of the submucosal venous plexus, the smooth muscle of the urethral wall and associated blood vessels, the epithelial coaptation of the folds of the

Figure 20.5 Lateral view of the pelvic floor drawn from a three-dimensional reconstruction with the urethra, vagina, and fascial tissues transected at the level of the vesical neck. Note how the urethra is compressed against the underlying supportive tissues by the downward force *(arrow)* generated by a cough or sneeze. (From **Delancey J.** Structural support of the urethra as it relates to stress urinary incontinence: the hammock hypothesis. *Am J Obstet Gynecol* 1994;170:1718, with permission.)

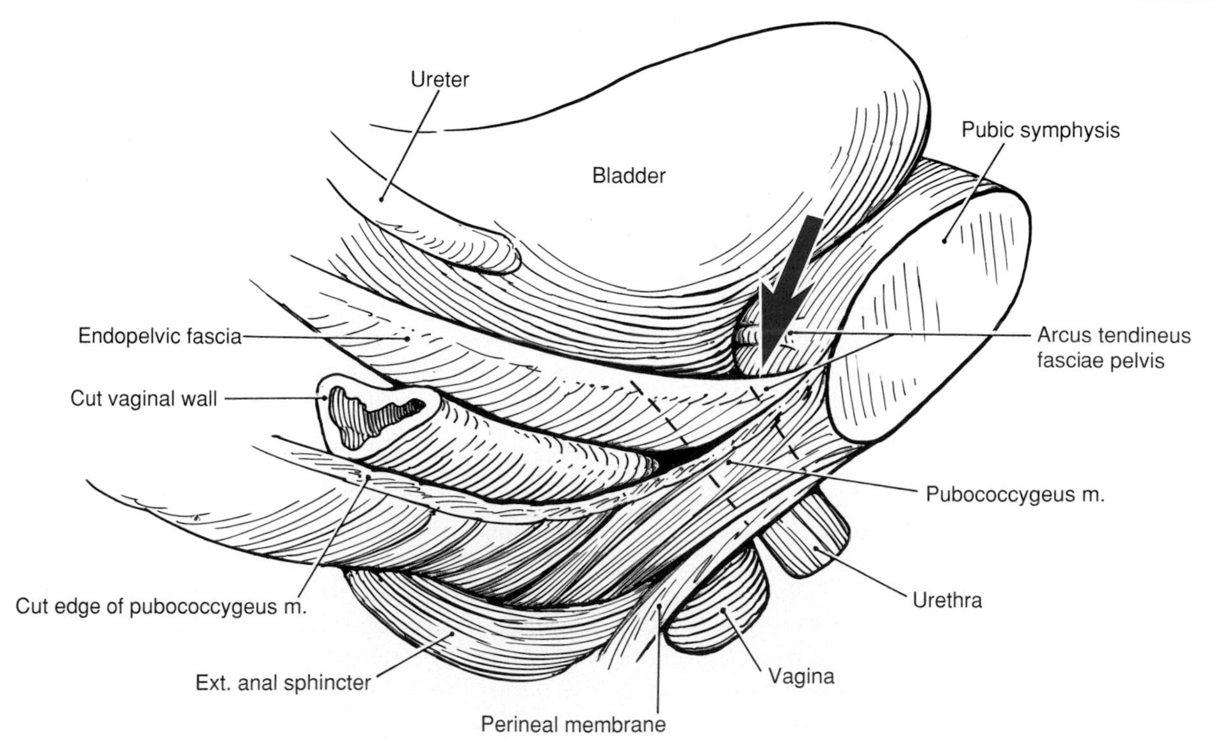

urethral lining, urethral elasticity, and the tone of the urethra as mediated by α-adrenergic receptors of the sympathetic nervous system. The intrinsic competence of the urethral closure mechanism can be affected by congenital developmental defects, scarring from trauma or multiple unsuccessful surgical procedures, estrogen deficiency, and neurologic injury. Stress incontinence resulting from intrinsic sphincteric deficiency is more difficult to correct than that occurring from loss of proper anatomic support. Urethral support alone, however, is not responsible for ensuring the integrity of the closure mechanism. The bladder is an autonomic organ under voluntary control, and neurophysiology plays a role in its function, although our understanding of these complex processes is limited (29).

The Bladder

The bladder is a bag of smooth muscle that stores urine and contracts to expel urine under voluntary control. It is a low-pressure system that expands to accommodate increasing volumes of urine without an appreciable rise in pressure. This function appears to be mediated primarily by the sympathetic nervous system. During bladder filling, there is an accompanying increase in outlet resistance. This action is manifest as increasing muscle fiber recruitment, as seen with electromyography of the pelvic floor and urethra while performing filling cystometry. The bladder muscle (the detrusor) should remain inactive during bladder filling, without involuntary contractions. When the bladder has filled to a certain volume, fullness is registered by tension-stretch receptors, which signal the brain to initiate a micturition reflex. This reflex is permitted or not permitted by cortical control mechanisms, depending on the social circumstances and the state of the patient's nervous system. Normal voiding is accomplished by voluntary relaxation of the pelvic floor and urethra, accompanied by sustained contraction of the detrusor muscle, leading to complete bladder emptying.

Innervation

The lower urinary tract receives its innervation from three sources: (a) the sympathetic and (b) parasympathetic divisions of the autonomic nervous system and (c) the neurons of the somatic nervous system (external urethral sphincter). The *autonomic nervous system* consists of all efferent pathways with ganglionic synapses that lie outside the central nervous system. Although knowledge of the norepinephrine of the autonomic nervous system is incomplete, it appears that the sympathetic system primarily controls bladder storage and that the parasympathetic nervous system controls bladder emptying. The somatic nervous system plays only a peripheral role in neurologic control of the lower urinary tract through its innervation of the pelvic floor and external urethral sphincter.

The sympathetic nervous system originates in the thoracolumbar spinal cord, principally T11 through L2 or L3. The ganglia of the sympathetic nervous system are located close to the spinal cord and use acetylcholine as the preganglionic neurotransmitter. The postganglionic neurotransmitter in the sympathetic nervous system is norepinephrine, and it acts on two types of receptors: α receptors, located principally in the urethra and bladder neck, and β receptors, located principally in the bladder body. Stimulation of α receptors increases urethral tone and thus promotes closure. α-Adrenergic receptor blockers have the opposite effect. Stimulation of β receptors decreases tone in the bladder body.

The *parasympathetic nervous system* controls bladder motor function—bladder contraction and bladder emptying. The parasympathetic nervous system originates in the sacral spinal cord, primarily in S2 to S4, as does the somatic innervation of the pelvic floor, urethra, and external anal sphincter. Sensation in the perineum is also controlled by sensory fibers that connect with the spinal cord at this level. For this reason, examination of perineal sensation, pelvic muscle reflexes, and pelvic muscle or anal sphincter tone is relevant to clinical evaluation of the lower urinary tract. The parasympathetic neurons have long preganglionic neurons and short postganglionic neurons, which are located in the end organ. Both the preganglionic and postganglionic synapses use acetylcholine as their neurotransmitter, acting on muscarinic receptors. Because acetylcholine is the main neurotransmitter used in bladder muscle contraction, virtually all drugs used to control detrusor muscle overactivity have anticholinergic properties. Unfortunately, cholinergic stimulants appear to be ineffective in promoting bladder emptying, even though they cause bladder muscle strips to contract in a laboratory setting, thus making medical treatment of voiding dysfunction unsuccessful in most cases.

Bladder storage and bladder emptying involve the interplay of the sympathetic and parasympathetic nervous systems. The modulation of these activities appears to be influenced by a variety of nonadrenergic, noncholinergic neurotransmitters and neuropeptides, which fine-tune the system at various facilitative and inhibitory levels in the spinal cord and higher areas of the central nervous system (30–32). Thus, neuropathology at almost any level of the neurourologic axis can have an adverse effect on lower urinary tract function.

Micturition

Micturition is triggered by the peripheral nervous system controlled by the central nervous system. It is useful to consider this event as occurring at a micturition threshold, a bladder volume at which reflex detrusor contractions occur. The threshold volume is not fixed but instead is variable, and it can be altered depending on the contributions made by sensory afferents from the perineum, bladder, colon, and rectum as well as input from the higher centers of the nervous system. The micturition threshold is, therefore, a floating threshold that can be altered or reset by various influences.

The spinal cord and higher centers of the nervous system have complex patterns of inhibition and facilitation. The most important facilitative center above the spinal cord is the pontine-mesencephalic gray matter of the brain stem, often called the *pontine micturition center,* which serves as the final common pathway for all bladder motor neurons. Transection of the tracts below this level leads to disturbed bladder emptying, whereas destruction of tracts above this level leads to detrusor hyperreflexia. The cerebellum serves as a major center for coordinating pelvic floor relaxation and the rate, force, and range of detrusor contractions, and there are multiple interconnections between the cerebellum and the brain-stem reflex centers. Above this level, the cerebral cortex and related structures exert inhibitory influences on the micturition reflex. Thus, the upper cortex exerts facilitative influences that release inhibition, permitting the anterior pontine micturition center to send efferent impulses down the complex pathways of the spinal cord, where a reflex contraction in the sacral micturition center generates a detrusor contraction that causes bladder emptying.

Colorectal Function

The sigmoid (S-shaped) colon begins at the pelvic brim and straightens as it enters the pelvis to become the rectum. Below the cul-de-sac, it expands into the rectal ampulla, filling the posterior pelvis from the left side. An anorectal angle of 90 degrees is formed at this point by the action of the puborectalis portion of the levator ani muscle complex, separating the anal canal below from the rectum above. **The anorectal angle is believed to be one factor among several that are important in the maintenance of normal anal continence. The puborectalis muscle maintains this angle through its normal tone, and during normal defecation, it relaxes to depress the pelvic floor and then contracts to elevate the pelvic floor during and after bowel emptying.**

The anorectal continence mechanism consists of an *internal sphincter* composed of smooth muscle and an *external sphincter* composed of striated muscle. The internal sphincter is a visceral muscle under autonomic control and normally has a high resting tone. The external sphincter is a striated muscle under voluntary control. In addition, there are sensory nerves in the rectum and pelvic floor. Continence is maintained at the level of the internal anal sphincter by gradual increases in the level of tonic contraction of the internal anal sphincter. This seal works only if the anal lining is sufficiently bulky to permit closure, and it is maintained by a combination of vascularity and infolding of the anal lining. The contractile efficiency of the internal sphincter is aided by contraction of the external anal sphincter. Rapid rectal distention causes a reflex relaxation of the internal anal sphincter. Under these circumstances, continence is maintained by contraction of the external sphincter. The efficiency of this process is closely linked to rectal sensation. Afferent sensation from the rectum appears to travel with the parasympathetic nerves to sacral segments S2 to S4. Sensation from the anal canal also travels to these sacral segments through the inferior hemorrhoidal branches of the pudendal nerve. The sensory apparatus of the rectum allows patients to distinguish between solid feces, liquid stool, and flatus. Impairment of this ability can have serious social consequences.

Innervation

The innervation of the gut is similarly complex. There are two ganglionic complexes in the bowel wall: (a) a *myenteric plexus* between the longitudinal and circular muscle coats, and (b) a *submucosal plexus.* The innervation of the smooth muscle of the bowel involves excitatory and inhibitory nonadrenergic, noncholinergic neurotransmitters and cotransmitters, primarily acetylcholine, substance P, and vasoactive intestinal polypeptide. The sphincters appear to be under separate neuronal control from nonsphincteric smooth muscle of the bowel. Sympathetic stimulation (norepinephrine) appears to cause contraction of the internal anal sphincter, whereas parasympathetic stimulation causes relaxation of the internal anal sphincter. The internal anal sphincter receives sympathetic innervation by the hypogastric nerves from L5, and the parasympathetic innervation comes from sacral segments S1 to S3. The external anal sphincter is innervated by branches of the pudendal nerve, originating in the sacral segments S2 to S4, with some branches from the coccygeal nerve plexus (S4 to S5).

Like the bladder, the colon and rectum undergo a filling and emptying cycle; unlike the bladder, the lower end of the gastrointestinal tract is not a closed viscus but rather a one-way conduit through which waste matter passes (33). Like the bladder, colorectal function can be categorized into storage (continence) and emptying (defecation) components.

Anal Continence

Anal continence is maintained by a combination of colonic compliance and mechanisms for retention in the rectosigmoid that keep the distal rectum collapsed and empty. The forces of retention are both mechanical and physiologic. The mechanical forces promoting retention of stool involve the S-shaped anteroposterior angulations of the sigmoid colon and the spiral folds in the lumen formed by the valves of Houston. Also, the puborectalis muscle creates a sharp angulation of the anorectum, which is accentuated by contraction of this muscle. Increases in intraabdominal pressure accentuate these angulations. These pressure increases have been postulated to create a flap-valve effect, which helps occlude the upper anal canal during periods of increased intraabdominal pressure (34); however, the principal mechanism of action may actually be a sphincter-like function exerted by puborectalis contraction (35). A flutter-valve effect may also be created in the collapsed anorectum (33,36). Retention of stool is further helped by a reverse pressure gradient between the rectum and the rectosigmoid colon. Waves of muscle contraction are both more frequent and of higher amplitude in the rectum than they are in the sigmoid.

The most important factors in maintaining fecal continence are sphincteric factors. The anus has both internal and external sphincters. Both of these sphincters are tonically contracted in the resting state, with the internal sphincter more so than the external sphincter. The external sphincter contains both slow-twitch and fast-twitch fibers. It remains tonically contracted even during sleep. In addition to its tonic baseline contractility, the external anal sphincter can respond with a quick, forceful contraction during periods of stress to maintain anal control, and its degree of contraction varies with posture and activity. The internal sphincter is at or near its state of maximal contraction all of the time. It relaxes only to allow the passage of stool when the rectum reaches a threshold of distention. When this occurs, relaxation of the internal sphincter allows the passage of matter into the distal anal canal. This stimulates multiple nerve endings to give warning of an impending movement of matter, which is detected as solid, liquid, or gaseous in nature. Continence is maintained by a reflex contraction of the external anal sphincter, which occurs concurrently with internal sphincter relaxation.

Voluntary contraction of the anal sphincter, in conjunction with rectal compliance, allows the individual to withhold a bowel movement until it is appropriate to release it.

Defecation

Defecation is the emptying phase of the colonic cycle. This may occur involuntarily in certain pathologic states or as a response to prolonged overdistention of the rectum, but defecation usually is a voluntary process. Voluntary defecation begins with closure of the glottis, which helps increase intraabdominal pressure, and by closure of the muscles of the pelvic floor. The diaphragm descends, and the muscles of the abdominal wall are contracted, raising intraabdominal pressure. The anal sphincter also contracts, further increasing intraabdominal pressure. Segmental contractions in the colon are inhibited. When the bolus of feces reaches the upper rectum, the muscles of the pelvic floor relax, the pelvic floor descends, and the acute rectal angle that existed at rest is straightened. Constriction of the distal muscles allows pressure to build up in the rectum, and when the internal sphincter relaxes, the bolus of stool is expelled. As the bolus passes, there is complete inhibition of electrical activity in the external sphincter, which contracts again only after the stool has been passed. The act of defecation represents the only known condition in which the external sphincter responds to increased intraabdominal pressure by relaxation rather than by contraction. At the end of defecation, the pelvic floor is elevated to its normal position, and the sphincters return to their tonically contracted resting state ("the closing reflex").

The complex intricate mechanisms involved in maintenance of continence and defecation are poorly understood, grossly undervalued, and generally taken for granted until impairment occurs (34). The same is undoubtedly true for all aspects of pelvic floor function.

Lower Urinary Tract Dysfunction

Symptoms arising in the lower urinary tract account for a significant number of patient visits to gynecologists. Disturbances in bladder function produce a wide variety of urinary tract symptoms. To help the clinician organize an initial patient evaluation, these symptoms can be classified according to whether they are disturbances of storage, emptying, sensation, or bladder contents (Table 20.1).

Urinary Incontinence

Urinary incontinence is defined as involuntary loss of urine that is a social or hygienic problem and that is objectively demonstrable (37). Urinary incontinence is a symptom, not a diagnosis. It is not a normal part of aging, although the prevalence of the problem increases with age, and it is not a trivial complaint. Urinary incontinence affects 13 million Americans, with an estimated 1 million new cases diagnosed each year. The total annual cost to care for patients with incontinence in the United States is estimated at $11.2 billion in the community and $5.2 billion in nursing homes (38). The differential diagnosis of urinary incontinence is extensive (Table 20.2); however, urinary incontinence is almost always treatable. It can almost always be improved and frequently can be cured, often using relatively simple, nonsurgical interventions.

Principles of Investigation

The initial evaluation of most patients with incontinence is not difficult, but it requires a systematic approach to consider all possible causes. The following items should be part of the basic evaluation:

1. History
2. Physical examination
3. Urinalysis, with urine culture and cytology as appropriate

Table 20.1. Classification and Definition of Lower Urinary Symptoms in Women

I. Abnormal Storage

Incontinence: Involuntary urine loss that is a social or hygienic problem
Stress incontinence: Incontinence occurring under conditions of increase intraabdominal pressure
Urge incontinence: Incontinence accompanied by a strong desire to void
Mixed incontinence: Stress and urge incontinence occurring together
Unconscious incontinence: Incontinence occurring without urgency and without conscious recognition of leakage
Frequency: The number of voids per day, from waking in the morning until falling asleep at night
Nocturia: The number of times the patient is awakened from sleep to void at night
Nocturnal enuresis: Urinary incontinence during sleep

II. Abnormal Emptying

Hesitancy: Trouble initiating voiding
Straining to void: Voiding accompanied by abdominal straining
Poor stream: Decreased force of flow of the urinary stream
Intermittent stream: A stop and start pattern of urination
Incomplete emptying: A persistent feeling of bladder fullness after voiding
Postmicturition dribble: Urine loss occurring just after normal voiding has been completed
Acute urinary retention: Sudden inability to void, resulting in painful bladder overdistention and the need for catheterization to obtain relief

III. Abnormal Sensation

Urgency: A strong desire to void
Dysuria: Burning pain with urination
Bladder pain: Conscious, hurting, suprapubic pain in the bladder
Flank pain: Pain between the lower rib cage and the ilial crest
Pressure: A feeling of heaviness or constant force being exerted in the bladder or lower pelvis
Loss of bladder sensation: Decreased sensation in the bladder

IV. Abnormal Bladder Contents

Abnormal color
Abnormal smell
Hematuria
Pneumaturia
Stones
Foreign bodies

4. Measurement of postvoid residual urine

5. Frequency/volume bladder chart

When these steps have been completed, some patients benefit from urodynamic studies to create a more comprehensive bladder biophysical profile before treatment.

History

Every incontinent patient should undergo a thorough history, including a review of symptoms, general medical history, review of past surgery, and current medications. It is helpful to write down the patient's chief complaint in her own words and expand the history from this point. The patient's most troubling symptoms must be ascertained—how often she leaks urine, how much urine she leaks, what provokes urine loss, what helps the problem or makes it worse, and what treatment (if any) she has had in the past.

The general medical history often reveals systemic illnesses that have a direct bearing on urinary incontinence, such as diabetes mellitus (which produces osmotic diuresis if glucose

Table 20.2. Differential Diagnosis of Urinary Incontinence

I. Extraurethral incontinence

A. Congenital
   1. Ectopic ureter
   2. Bladder exstrophy
   3. Other
B. Acquired (fistulas)
   1. Ureteric
   2. Vesical
   3. Urethral
   4. Complex combinations

II. Transurethral incontinence

A. Genuine stress incontinence
   1. Bladder neck displacement (anatomic hypermobility)
   2. Instrinsic sphincteric dysfunction
   3. Combined
B. Detrusor overactivity
   1. Idiopathic detrusor instability
   2. Neuropathic detrusor hyperreflexia
C. Mixed incontinence
D. Urinary retention with bladder distention and overflow
   1. Genuine stress incontinence
   2. Detrusor hyperactivity with impaired contractility
   3. Combinations
E. Urtheral diverticulum
F. Congenital urethral abnormalities (e.g., epispadias)
G. Uninhibited urethral relaxation (urethral instability)
H. Functional and transient incontinence

control is poor), vascular insufficiency (which can lead to incontinence at night when peripheral edema is mobilized into the vascular system, resulting in increased diuresis), chronic pulmonary disease (which can lead to stress incontinence from chronic coughing), or a wide variety of neurologic conditions that can affect the neurourologic axis at any point from the cerebral cortex to the peripheral nervous system.

Many medications affect the lower urinary tract (39,40).

1. Sedatives such as the benzodiazepines may accumulate in the patient's system and cause confusion and secondary incontinence, particularly for elderly patients.

2. Alcohol may have similar effects to benzodiazepines and also impairs mobility as well as produces diuresis.

3. Anticholinergic drugs may impair detrusor contractility and may lead to voiding difficulty and overflow incontinence. Drugs with anticholinergic properties are widespread and include antihistamines, antidepressants, antipsychotics, opiates, antispasmodics, and drugs used to treat Parkinson's disease.

4. α-Adrenergic agents may have a profound effect on the lower urinary tract. α-Agonists, which are often found in over-the-counter cold remedies, increase outlet resistance and may lead to voiding difficulty.

5. α-Blockers, which are often used in the treatment of hypertension (e.g., prazosin, terazosin), may decrease urethral closure and lead to stress incontinence (41).

6. Calcium-channel blockers may reduce bladder smooth muscle contractility and lead to voiding problems or incontinence; they may also cause peripheral edema, which may lead to nocturia or nighttime urine loss.

7. Angiotensin-converting enzyme inhibitors may result in a chronic and bothersome cough that can result in increasing stress urinary incontinence in an otherwise asymptomatic patient (42).

Physical Examination

The physical examination of the patient with incontinence should include detection of general medical conditions that may affect the lower urinary tract. Such conditions include cardiovascular insufficiency, pulmonary disease, occult neurologic processes (e.g., multiple sclerosis, stroke, Parkinson's disease, and anomalies of the spine and lower back), as well as abnormalities of genitourinary development. The pelvic examination, including an evaluation of urethral support, is of crucial importance.

1. Patients with urinary incontinence should be examined with a full bladder, particularly if stress incontinence is a complaint.

2. The patient should stand with her feet separated to shoulder width and cough several times to see if the physical sign of stress incontinence can be demonstrated. If urine loss occurs, confirm with the patient that this is the problem that has been bothering her. Many multiparous women may lose a small amount of urine during such an examination but not be bothered by it.

3. Many women with urge incontinence caused by detrusor overactivity may demonstrate urine loss during a cough stress test, but this finding may not be relevant to their real complaint. The physical findings must be set within the context of the patient's history to be relevant.

4. The patient's complaint should be reproduced by the physician and confirmed with the patient, particularly if surgery is contemplated.

Urinalysis

Examination of the urine by dipstick testing and microscopy is necessary to exclude infection, metabolic abnormalities, and kidney disease.

1. Urine culture will help rule out infection, which can be associated with incontinence.

2. Urine cytology is useful as a screening test for urinary tract malignancy, but the utility of the test depends greatly on the accuracy of the laboratory performing the cytology. Routine urinary cytology is not helpful, but testing should be performed in women older than 50 years of age with irritative urinary tract symptoms, particularly if those symptoms are of sudden onset.

3. Hematuria should be evaluated with cytology, intravenous urography, and cystoscopy. Bladder biopsy should be performed by the surgeon who will treat the patient in the event that a malignancy is discovered.

Measurement of Postvoid Residual Urine

Incomplete bladder emptying is a frequent cause of incontinence. Patients with a large postvoid residual urine have a diminished functional bladder capacity because of the dead space occupied in the bladder by retained urine. This stagnant pool of urine is also a frequent source of urinary tract infections, because the major defense of the bladder against infection is frequent, complete emptying.

A large postvoid residual can contribute to urinary incontinence in two ways. If the bladder is overdistended, increases in intraabdominal pressure can force urine past the urethral sphincter, causing stress incontinence. In some cases, bladder overdistention may provoke an uninhibited contraction of the detrusor muscle, leading to incontinence. Both conditions may exist together, further complicating the problem.

Patients with an elevated postvoid residual urine should begin a regimen of clean, intermittent self-catheterization to improve bladder emptying. In many cases, this technique may be the only therapy needed to correct the incontinence and eliminate recurrent urinary tract infections. The recent development of sacral nerve root neuromodulation for nonobstructive voiding dysfunction now offers an additional treatment option for some of these women (43).

Frequency/Volume Bladder Chart

A frequency/volume bladder chart is an invaluable aid in the evaluation of patients with urinary incontinence, but use of this tool often is neglected (44,45). A frequency/volume chart is a voiding record kept by the patient for several days. Use of a plastic measuring "hat" that fits over the patient's toilet bowl is very helpful in keeping accurate records. Patients should be instructed to write down the time of every void on the chart and measure the amount of urine voided. The time of any incontinent episodes should be recorded, and it is also helpful to maintain an annotated record of symptoms or activities associated with urine loss. If desired, the patient can also be instructed to keep a record of fluid intake, although in most cases intake can be estimated with some accuracy from the amount of urine produced.

A frequency/volume bladder chart gives an accurate record of 24-hour urinary output, the total number of daily voids, the average voided volume, and the functional bladder capacity (largest volume voided in normal daily life). This information allows the clinician to confirm complaints of urinary frequency with objective data and to determine whether part of the patient's problem is an abnormally high (or low) urinary output. For example, incontinence is a common complaint of many patients with diabetes, and the first step in the management of such patients is to control their blood glucose levels and decrease their urinary output rather than using medications or surgery, which often is ineffective. Conversely, many patients with incontinence decrease their fluid intake dramatically in an attempt to control their urine loss, not realizing that the resulting highly concentrated urine is often much more irritating to their bladders than a higher volume of a more diluted urine. **As a rule, daily urine output should be 1,500 to 2,500 mL, with an average voided volume of about 250 mL, a functional bladder capacity (largest voided volume) of 400 to 600 mL, and seven or eight voids per day.** The frequency/volume chart is the foundation for conservative management of urinary incontinence based on fluid manipulation and behavioral management of voiding habits.

Urodynamic Studies

At its most basic level, a urodynamic study is anything that provides objective evidence about lower urinary tract function (46). In this sense, measurement of a patient's voided urine volume and catheterization to determine her postvoid residual urine are urodynamic studies. A frequency/volume chart is also a valuable urodynamic study. Obtaining clinically useful information does not always require the use of expensive, complex technology.

Bladder Filling Test If a patient with a complaint of urinary incontinence comes for her examination without a full bladder, a great deal of information can be obtained by a simple bladder filling test (47). The patient should urinate and measure the volume she voids. The residual urine can be measured by draining it through a 10- or 12-Fr. red rubber catheter placed into the bladder. Once the residual urine has been drained out, a bag of sterile water or saline attached to the catheter can be used to fill the patient's bladder at a rate of 60 to 75 mL/min until her functional bladder capacity is reached.

If the patient experiences urgency with accompanying urine loss during bladder filling, it is highly likely that she has motor urge incontinence caused by detrusor overactivity. If the patient leaks an isolated spurt of urine each time she coughs, and this leakage is demonstrated repetitively and confirmed as the problem for which she is seeking help, she has stress incontinence. Further evaluation is required for patients who exhibit mixed incontinence (the presence of both stress and urge incontinence), who exhibit prolonged leakage with coughing (suggestive of a cough-induced detrusor contraction), who have marked incontinence with a nearly empty bladder or with minimal effort, who develop incontinence after their prolapse is treated, or who report incontinence that cannot be verified by simple testing.

Multichannel Urodynamic Studies Multichannel urodynamic studies produce a biophysical profile of a patient's bladder and urethral function, but such studies are helpful only if they are interpreted with reference to the patient's history and the results of her physical examination. Clinicians who recommend that patients undergo urodynamic studies without first taking a careful history and performing a thorough physical examination are likely to obtain useless or irrelevant information from these expensive investigations. A detailed history and a thorough physical examination often can predict reliably the type of incontinence when these findings are combined with those derived from some simple urodynamic tests (48–50).

A wide variety of sophisticated studies of bladder and urethral function have been developed to measure various aspects of bladder storage and bladder emptying. These studies include uroflowmetry, filling cystometry, pressure-flow voiding studies (with and without simultaneous electromyography of the pelvic floor), urethral pressure profilometry, and determination of leak-point pressure.

The bladder is affected by neural impulses running along afferent and efferent sensory pathways and generates a pressure–volume relationship in the cycle of micturition (Fig. 20.6). As bladder volume increases, tension-stretch receptors in the bladder wall are activated, and the afferent sensory impulses gradually lead to a desire to void. Normally, this occurs between 150 and 250 mL. Normally, a patient is able to suppress a micturition reflex until an appropriate time. She should then be able to relax the pelvic floor and generate a sustained contraction of the bladder detrusor muscle until emptying is complete, after which the detrusor relaxes and the cycle begins again.

Cystometry Cystometry is the technique by which the pressure–volume relationship of the bladder is measured. It can be divided into two phases: (a) filling cystometry and (b) voiding cystometry (also called a ***pressure-flow study***). Simple cystometry is carried out when bladder pressure only is measured during filling. Because the bladder is an intraabdominal organ, however, the pressure recorded in the bladder is a combination of several other pressures, most notably the pressure created by the activity of the detrusor muscle itself and the pressure exerted on the bladder by the weight of the surrounding intraabdominal contents (e.g., uterus, intestines, straining, or exertion). For this reason, the technique of subtracted cystometry is used.

Subtracted cystometry is an attempt to measure the pressure exerted in the bladder by the activity of the detrusor muscle. Subtracted cystometry is carried out by measuring *total intravesical pressure* (P_{ves}) with a bladder pressure catheter, approximating *intraabdominal pressure* (P_{abd}) by measuring either rectal or vaginal pressure, and using an electronic instrument to subtract the latter from the former to give the *true detrusor* pressure (P_{det}) or the subtracted pressure:

$$\mathbf{P_{det} = P_{ves} - P_{abd}}$$

Measurements can be made using either expensive electronic microtip transducer pressure catheters or inexpensive fluid-filled pressure lines. The technique for such a study is shown in Figure 20.7.

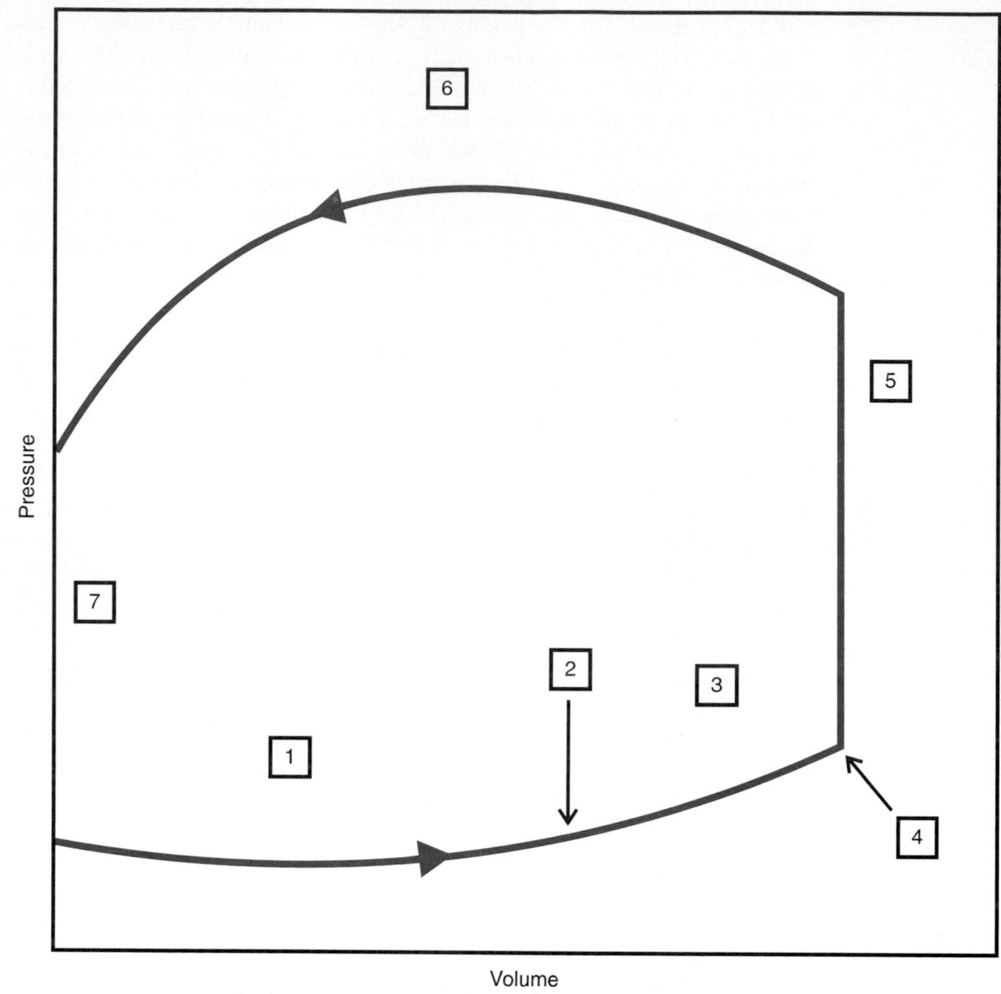

Figure 20.6 Pressure–volume relationship of the micturition cycle. (1) The normal bladder accommodates increasing urine volumes without a significant increase in pressure. (2) At about 200 mL, the first sensation of bladder fullness is appreciated. (3) The micturition reflex can be suppressed until a socially acceptable time and place for urination presents itself. (4) At this time, a voluntary detrusor contraction is initiated, in conjunction with pelvic floor relaxation. (5) There is a brief isometric pressure rise before the bladder neck is open and flow starts. (6) Normal voiding is accomplished by a sustained detrusor contraction until bladder emptying is complete. (7) The detrusor muscle then relaxes and the process of filling begins anew. (From **Wall LL, Addison WA.** Basic cystometry in gynecologic practice. *Postgrad Obstet Gynecol* 1988;26[2]:2, with permission.)

1. Fluid (usually sterile water or saline, sometimes radiographic contrast dye) is infused at a rate of 50 to 100 mL/min. The volume infused and the pressure measurements are recorded continuously. The patient's bladder may be filled with her lying supine, in a modified lithotomy position, sitting, or standing. When possible, standing cystometry is usually preferable because most patients with incontinence complain of this problem when they are erect.

2. The point at which any leakage occurs should be noted carefully.

3. During filling, the point at which the first desire to void is experienced should be noted, along with the point at which the patient experiences a strong desire to void, urgency, and her cystometric capacity.

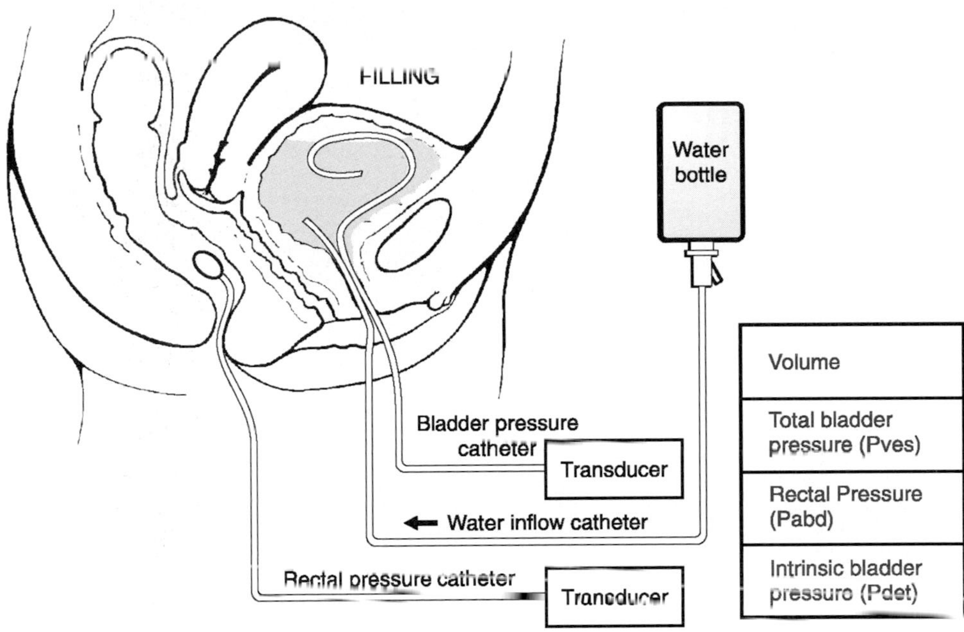

Figure 20.7 Subtracted filling cystometry. Pressure catheters are in place in the bladder and rectum. An additional filling catheter has been placed in the bladder. Volume infused, total bladder pressure, rectal (abdominal) pressure, and subtracted detrusor pressure (intrinsic bladder pressure) are recorded. (From **Wall LL, Addison WA.** Basic cystometry in gynecologic practice. *Postgrad Obstet Gynecol* 1988;26(2):3).

4. Provocative maneuvers are performed, such as coughing, heel bouncing, and listening to the sound of running water in an attempt to produce urinary incontinence and to provoke any uninhibited detrusor contractions, which may be the cause of the patient's symptoms.

Normal cystometric values for women are shown in Table 20.3.

At *cystometric capacity* (ideally, the same as the patient's functional bladder capacity), the filling catheter should be removed, leaving only the pressure measurement lines in place (Fig. 20.8). If the pressures are allowed to equilibrate for 1 minute, bladder compliance can be calculated by dividing the bladder volume in milliliters by the pressure of water in centimeters. The patient should then void. The urine flow rate can be measured and

Table 20.3. Approximate Normal Values of Female Bladder Function

- Residual urine <50 mL
- First desire to void occurs between 150 and 250 mL infused
- Strong desire to void does not occur until after 250 mL
- Cystometric capacity between 400 and 600 mL
- Bladder compliance between 20 and 100 mL/cm H_2O measured 60 sec after reaching cystometric capacity
- No uninhibited detrusor contractions during filling, despite provocation
- No stress or urge incontinence demonstrated, despite provocation
- Voiding occurs due to a voluntarily initiated and sustained detrusor contraction
- Flow rate during voiding is >15 mL/sec with a detrusor pressure of less than 50 cm H_2O

(From **Wall LL, Norton P, Delancey J.** *Practical urogynecology.* Baltimore: Williams & Wilkins, 1993, with permission.)

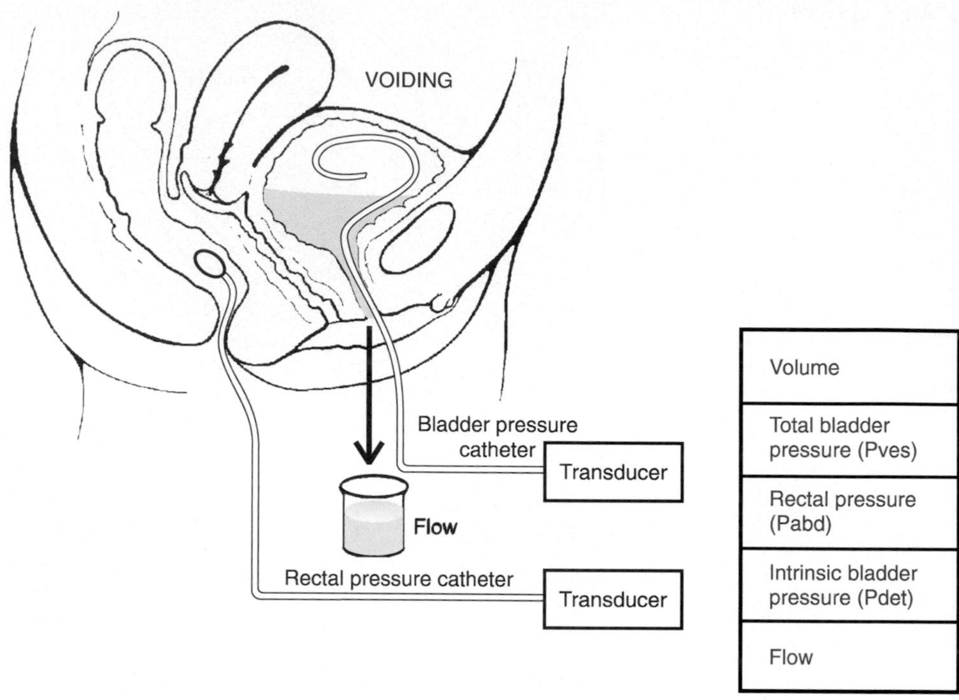

Figure 20.8 Pressure–flow voiding study. The filling catheter has been removed. Volume voided, urine flow rate, total bladder pressure, rectal (abdominal) pressure, and subtracted detrusor pressure are recorded. (From **Wall LL, Addison WA.** Basic cystometry in gynecologic practice. *Postgrad Obstet Gynecol* 1988;26[2]:3, with permission).

correlated with the detrusor pressure. This technique allows a better assessment of voiding function than measurement of urine flow rate alone.

Urethral Pressure Profile

In addition to an assessment of filling and emptying, specific urodynamic tests allow some quantitative assessment of sphincteric integrity. The urethral pressure profile is a test designed to measure urethral closure. Because continence requires the pressure in the urethra to be higher than the pressure in the bladder, it was believed that measuring the pressure differential between the two would provide useful clinical information. The urethral pressure profile is generated by slowly pulling a pressure-sensitive catheter through the urethra from the bladder, which is usually filled with a standardized volume of fluid (Fig. 20.9). The urethral closure pressure (P_{close}) is the difference between the urethral pressure (P_{ure}) and the bladder pressure (P_{ves}):

$$\mathbf{P_{close} = P_{ure} - P_{ves}}$$

Although this pressure can be used to differentiate groups of normal women from groups of those with stress incontinence (women with stress incontinence tend to have higher urethral pressure levels than those who do not), there is considerable overlap between the two groups. It has also been suggested that women with stress incontinence with low urethral closure pressure (<20 cm H_2O) have a poorer prognosis for surgical outcome than women who do not have this condition; however, there is considerable debate about this (51–53). Because stress incontinence, by definition, occurs during increases in intraabdominal pressure that are generated by some kind of physical activity, it is not obvious why measurement of resting urethral pressure should be relevant to stress-related leakage, which is a dynamic event. In general, the urethral pressure profile has been a disappointing test with questionable clinical utility.

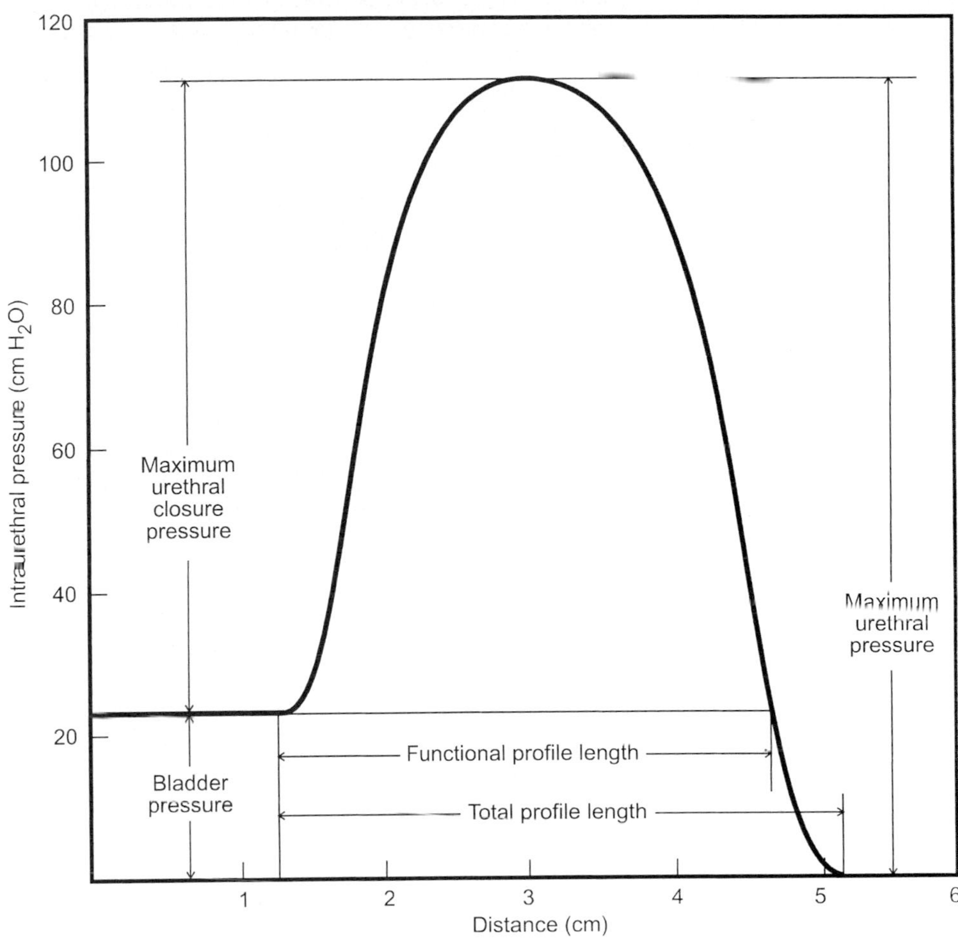

Figure 20.9 Parameters normally measured during urethral pressure profile studies (International Continence Society).

Leak-Point Pressure Test

A more promising test appears to be the leak-point pressure test (54). The idea behind this test is quite simple: the amount of force that it takes to produce stress incontinence should be related to the severity of the stress incontinence and to the strength of the sphincteric unit. **The leak-point pressure is the intravesical (or sometimes intraabdominal) pressure measured at the moment that stress incontinence occurs.** It is usually determined at a bladder volume of 200 mL, but the technique has not been completely standardized. When the appropriate bladder volume has been reached, patients are asked to cough with gradually increasing force (cough leak-point pressure), and finally to strain slowly (Valsalva) to increase intravesical pressure gradually. The lowest pressure at which leakage occurs is recorded as the cough or the Valsalva leak-point pressure. If leakage is not demonstrated, the highest pressure that has been obtained can be recorded with the notation "no leakage" to the specified pressure as measured in cm H_2O. This figure appears to give a reasonable estimation of sphincteric strength. Standardization and interpretation of these tests are in early stages, and further research is required.

Extraurethral Causes of Incontinence

Involuntary urine loss can occur through two basic routes. Most urinary incontinence represents unwanted urine loss through the urethra (transurethral incontinence); however, urine loss can also occur through abnormal openings. These openings can be created by congenital causes or some form of trauma. The congenital causes of urinary incontinence are not common and usually are easy to diagnose. The most extreme cases are caused by bladder exstrophy, in which there is a congenital absence of the lower anterior abdominal wall and anterior portion of the bladder, resulting in the entire bladder opening directly to the outside (55). Such cases are diagnosed at birth, and before the advent of modern reconstructive surgery, these infants usually died very early in life from sepsis.

Ectopic Ureter

The most common and most subtle congenital anomaly causing extraurethral urine loss is an ectopic ureter (56). Generally, ectopic ureters are detected early in life, but occasionally one may escape detection until adolescence or early adulthood. In infancy, an ectopic ureter should be suspected when a mother seeks care for her baby whom she says is never dry. Normally, infants have periods of dryness interspersed with periods of wetness. If a parent notes that every time the baby is checked her diaper is wet, this is the first clue that an ectopic ureter may exist because this ureter will most likely drain outside the bladder, causing continuous urinary leakage. Most commonly, the ectopic ureter drains into the vagina, but occasionally, it may drain into the urethra distal to the point of continence. Ectopic ureter has been reported as an uncommon cause of suburethral mass (57). This condition can be diagnosed easily by excretory urography.

Urinary Fistula

A traumatic opening between the urinary tract and the outside is called a *fistula*. Worldwide, the most common cause of fistulas is obstructed labor. This was also true in the Western world 150 years ago, but advances in the provision of basic obstetric services and advanced obstetric intervention have virtually eliminated this problem in developed countries. The rest of the world is not so fortunate.

Obstructed labor often occurs in rural areas where girls are married young (sometimes as early as 9 or 10 years of age) and where transportation is poor and access to medical services is limited. In such circumstances, pregnancy often occurs shortly after menstruation begins and before maternal skeletal growth is complete. When labor begins, cephalopelvic disproportion is common, and little can be done to correct fetal malpresentations. Women may be in labor as long as 5 to 6 days without intervention, and if they survive, they usually give birth to a stillborn infant. In such cases, the soft tissues of the pelvis have been crushed by constant pressure from the fetal head, leading to an ischemic vascular injury and subsequent tissue necrosis. When this tissue sloughs, a genitourinary or rectovaginal fistula develops. Many of these patients have complex or multiple fistulas, involving total destruction of the urethra and sloughing of the entire bladder base. Obstetric fistulas are frequently as large as 5 to 6 cm in diameter.

After such fistulas develop, the lives of these young women (most of whom are younger than 20 years of age) are ruined unless they can gain access to curative surgical services. The constant, uncontrolled dribble of urine makes them offensive to their husbands and family members. They can no longer live with their families. Most of them eventually become destitute social outcasts—and yet these are otherwise healthy functional young women. The social and economic costs of this problem are enormous, but the problem has largely been neglected by the world medical community. The morbidity associated with obstetric fistulas remains, along with the related problem of maternal mortality, one of the single most neglected issues in international women's health care (58).

In the industrialized world, the most common causes of genitourinary fistulas are surgery, malignancy, and radiation therapy or the interrelation of all three factors. Most often, a vesicovaginal fistula develops after an otherwise uncomplicated vaginal or abdominal hysterectomy in which a small portion of the bladder was inadvertently trapped in a surgical clamp or was transfixed by a suture. These fistulas most often occur at the vaginal apex and are no larger than 1 to 2 mm. The amount of urine that can leak through a fistula of any size, however, is enormous.

A wide variety of techniques are available for fistula repair (59,60). **Traditionally, fistula repair is has been performed after a waiting period to allow the resolution of inflammation and formation of scar tissue.** This is particularly important in the case of obstetric fistulas, in which the extent of the vascular injury to the soft tissues of the pelvis may not be apparent for many weeks. However, there has been a recent trend toward early closure of small gynecologic fistulas (61). The keys to closure of a vesicovaginal fistula include wide mobilization of tissue planes so that the fistula edges can be approximated without any tension, close approximation of tissue edges, closure of the fistula in several layers, and meticulous attention to postoperative bladder drainage for 10 to 14 days. The closure of large fistulas will be enhanced by the use of tissue grafts (e.g., Martius labial fat-pad grafts, gracilis muscle flaps) that bring an additional blood supply to nourish an area that has sustained vascular injury.

Stress Urinary Incontinence

Stress incontinence occurs during periods of increased intraabdominal pressure (e.g., sneezing, coughing, or exercise) when the intravesical pressure rises higher than the pressure that the urethral closure mechanism can withstand, and urine loss results. Stress urinary incontinence is the most common form of transurethral urinary incontinence in women. A community survey of 1,060 randomly selected women older than 18 years of age in South Wales, for example, revealed that 22% of women had this complaint (62). In a survey of 144 collegiate female varsity athletes, 27% complained of stress incontinence while participating in their sport (63). The activities most likely to produce urinary loss were jumping, high-impact landings, and running. Even in otherwise fit and vigorous women, the continence mechanism is particularly susceptible to stress incontinence.

The term *stress incontinence* refers to three distinct entities: a symptom, a sign, and a condition (37). Confusion can occur if the differences between these three entities are not appreciated.

Symptoms and Signs

The *symptom* of stress incontinence refers to the patient's complaint that she leaks urine when intraabdominal pressure is increased. Such urine leakage may result from a variety of conditions: genuine stress incontinence, a detrusor contraction provoked by coughing or change of position, incomplete bladder emptying, or a urethral diverticulum. The patient's complaint of stress incontinence makes it likely, but not certain, that she has this problem, but the complaint must be confirmed by some objective means. A patient should never undergo surgery for stress incontinence on the basis of symptoms alone.

The *sign* of stress incontinence refers to the physical demonstration of urine loss during conditions of increased intraabdominal pressure (e.g., coughing) while the patient is being examined. Mere demonstration of stress urinary leakage during a physical examination does not mean that the patient has a clinical problem with stress incontinence. According to the International Continence Society's definition, incontinence exists when urine loss becomes a social or hygienic problem (37). Many women experience occasional stress urinary leakage that is merely annoying or inconvenient. These women do not consider themselves incontinent, nor do they need surgery; however, studies have also shown that there is little relationship between the volume of urine lost and the distress that it causes a patient with incontinence (64).

Genuine Stress Incontinence

A specific technical term, *genuine stress incontinence,* is used to refer to the urodynamic diagnosis of stress incontinence (37). **Genuine stress incontinence is said to exist when a patient has demonstrable urinary leakage when intravesical pressure exceeds**

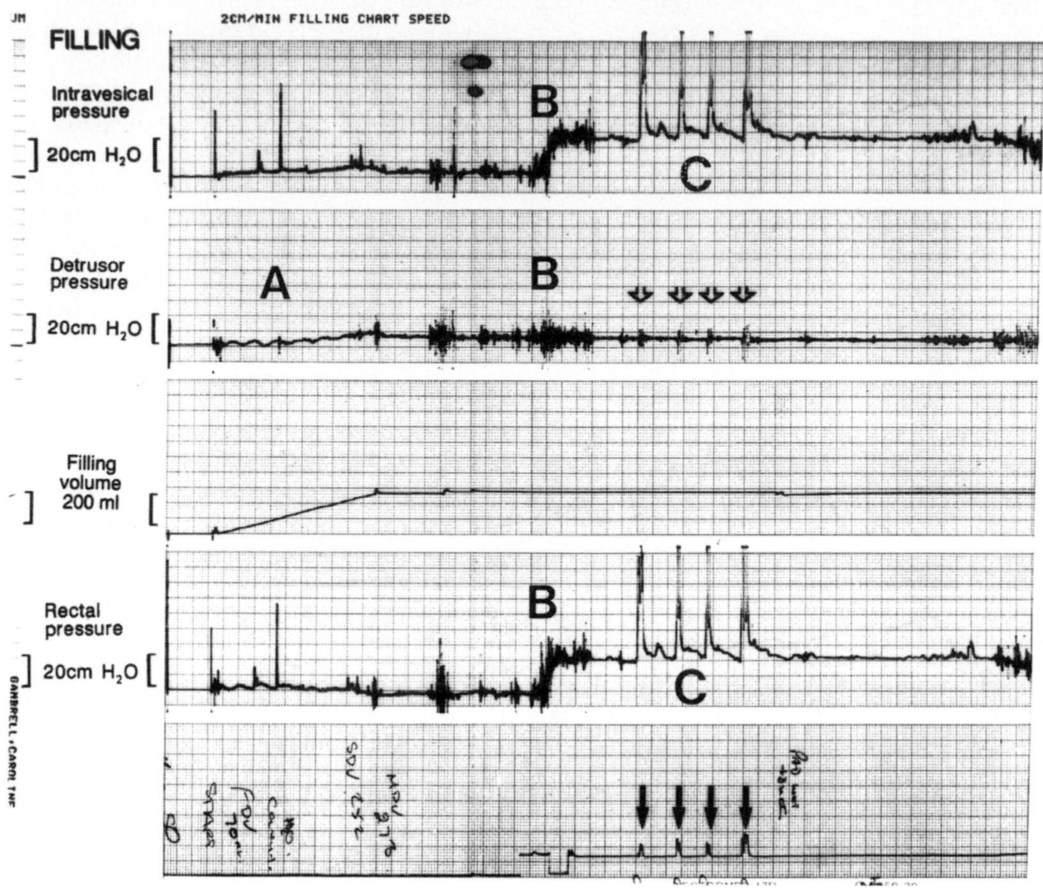

Figure 20.10 Subtracted cystometrogram showing a stable bladder with genuine stress incontinence. During the filling phase **(A)**, there is no rise in detrusor pressure. When the patient stands **(B)**, there is a rise in intravesical and rectal pressure as the position of the intraabdominal contents changes, but the subtracted detrusor pressure remains stable. When the patient coughs in the erect position **(C)**, the detrusor remains stable. Coughs appear as sharp, isolated pressure spikes. The presence of leakage confirms that the patient has genuine stress incontinence owing to ineffective urethral closure rather than detrusor overactivity.

the maximum urethral closure pressure in the absence of a detrusor contraction. This term can only be used for a patient who has undergone urodynamic testing and who has met these test criteria, which prove that her urine loss is caused by ineffective urethral closure during periods of increased intraabdominal pressure (Fig. 20.10). This urodynamic diagnosis must be analyzed with reference to the patient's complaint; one may have genuine stress incontinence that is nonetheless not a clinical problem or is a less severe problem than urge incontinence caused by detrusor muscle overactivity.

The clinical condition of stress incontinence includes a spectrum of symptoms ranging in severity. At one end of the spectrum is the female athlete who leaks only a tiny amount during vigorous physical activity; at the other end of the spectrum is the frail elderly woman who leaks large amounts of urine during minimal physical effort. The degree to which either woman is bothered by her leakage is influenced by her cultural values and expectations regarding urinary continence and incontinence.

Biobehavioral Model **A biobehavioral model of stress incontinence can be created by examining the interaction of three variables: the biologic strength of the sphincteric mechanism, the level of physical stress placed on the closure mechanism, and the woman's expectations about urinary control** (Fig. 20.11). This model explains the enormous variation that exists among the symptoms, the degree of demonstrable leakage, and a

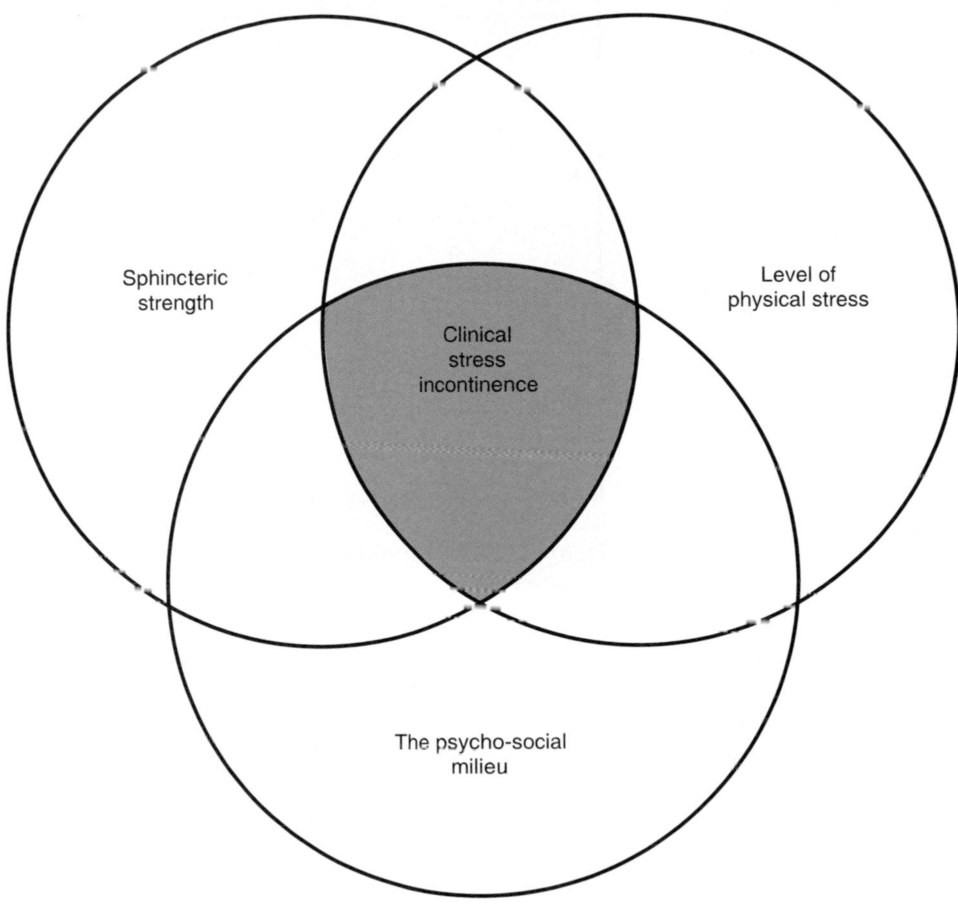

Figure 20.11 A biobehavioral model of stress incontinence. Clinical stress urinary incontinence results from the interaction of three distinct components: the inherent biologic strength of the urinary sphincter, the level of physical stress placed on the sphincter, and the psychosocial milieu in which the patient lives (i.e., her personal and cultural expectations concerning urinary control and urinary incontinence).

patient's response to her stress incontinence. Modification of any one of these factors may influence the patient's clinical status. For example, many patients give up certain physical activities (e.g., running, dancing, aerobics) when they experience stress incontinence. Limiting their activities may eliminate the incontinence problem, but it does so at a certain cost to their quality of life. Other women learn to cope with stress incontinence by adopting new body postures during physical activities that prevent them from leaking or by strengthening their pelvic muscles to compensate for increased exertion. Other women may be profoundly relieved to find out that the small amount of leakage they experience from time to time is not abnormal. In any case, the interaction of these three biopsychosocial factors opens up a variety of strategies for the management of stress incontinence. Surgical intervention is only one strategy, and it addresses only the biologic competence of the sphincteric mechanism rather than either of the other factors that interact to produce the clinical problem.

Interaction of Extrinsic and Intrinsic Urethral Support Effective urethral closure is maintained by the interaction of extrinsic urethral support and intrinsic urethral integrity, each of which is influenced by several factors (i.e., muscle tone and strength, innervation, fascial integrity, urethral elasticity, coaptation of urothelial folds, urethral vascularity). In the clinical setting, damaged urethral support is manifest clinically by urethral hypermobility, which often results in incompetent urethral closure during physical activity and presents as stress urinary incontinence. Intrinsic urethral functioning is more complicated and is not nearly as well understood as urethral support (65).

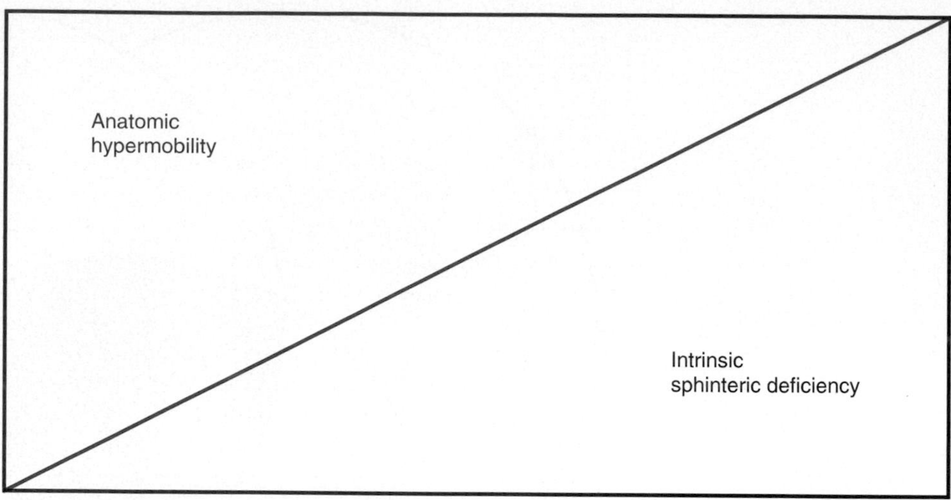

Figure 20.12 Interaction of anatomic urethral hypermobility with intrinsic sphincteric deficiency in patients with stress incontinence. The problem is not an "either-or" dichotomy, but rather one of degree.

Clinical appreciation of the importance of extrinsic support and intrinsic urethral function have led surgeons to separate stress incontinence into two broad types:

1. That caused by anatomic hypermobility of the urethra, which produces faulty urethral closure under stress

2. That caused by intrinsic sphincteric weakness or deficiency

The former type is more prevalent, probably accounting for somewhere between 80% and 90% of stress urinary incontinence.

The latter type is less common and more challenging to treat. Although this concept is useful, in most cases, patients cannot be distinguished easily as belonging to one category or another but instead are affected to some degree by both factors that interact to produce the clinical condition of stress incontinence (Fig. 20.12). The challenge is deciding which factor predominates because this decision will have a direct bearing on the type of treatment chosen.

Nonsurgical Treatment

Many extrinsic, as well as intrinsic, factors influence urethral closure, and surgery is not the only option, nor is it always the best choice, for this condition. **Nonsurgical approaches to stress incontinence are based on manipulation of the factors that contribute to the condition. These approaches may involve reducing factors that worsen the problem (e.g., obesity, smoking, or excessive fluid intake) or by intervening actively to enhance the ability of the patient's pelvic floor to compensate for increased intraabdominal pressure** (e.g., making adaptive changes in posture, rehabilitating pelvic muscles, improving estrogen status, using α-adrenergic stimulants, or wearing a device to improve urethral support).

Muscle Strengthening By its connection with the endopelvic fascia, the musculature of the levator ani complex provides substantial support for the urethra, vagina, and rectum as they descend through the pelvic floor (66). The periurethral levator ani muscles contain both type I (slow-twitch) and type II (fast-twitch) muscle fibers, which allows them to maintain tone over a long period and to increase tone suddenly to compensate for the increased abdominal pressure that occurs with coughing, sneezing, and straining. These muscle groups can be rehabilitated through exercise and physical therapy (67). There are two possible ways in which this therapy improves stress urinary incontinence. First, strengthening the striated urogenital sphincter could enhance its ability to constrict the urethral lumen, yielding a stronger closure force in the urethra at rest or increasing the forces of urethral closure generated during a cough or other stressful situations. Second, because the levator ani muscles play an important role in pelvic and urethral support, exercise could improve the support of the proximal urethra, generating improved continence during a cough, when the muscles are active, without producing a noticeable rise in resting urethral pressure measurements.

Kegel was the first person to investigate pelvic floor muscle strengthening. He developed the patient's awareness of the pubococcygeus muscle and instructed her in exercises to strengthen this muscle with a crude pneumatic biofeedback device called a perineometer. He stressed the importance of supervised instruction and encouragement in the performance of these exercises and reported good success rates in relieving symptomatic stress incontinence by his program. Although nearly all gynecologists are familiar with these exercises, they rarely are taught and used as Kegel did originally, and this form of therapy has often degenerated into a few brief words of oral instruction in which the patient is told to stop and start her urine stream a few times each day while voiding. Programs based on this approach are not only disappointing in their results but also can train women to become dysfunctional voiders.

For muscular rehabilitation of the pelvic floor to be effective, exercises must be supervised, performed regularly, and aided by some form of feedback so that the patient can judge her progress. Careful supervision makes a dramatic difference in the degree of success that can be obtained (67,68). Using an intensive program of physical therapy over 3 months with pretherapy and posttherapy urodynamic and radiographic evaluations, Benvenuti and colleagues cured 32% of their patients with genuine stress incontinence and brought about marked improvement in symptoms in the remaining 68%. Both tonic and phasic contractility of the pubococcygeus muscle were improved, and there was clear-cut improvement of bladder neck support, as seen on radiographic evaluation in 13 of 15 patients who underwent repeat studies. After 12 to 36 months of follow-up, 77% reported that they had maintained the functional level they had attained at the end of treatment (69).

Similarly, Peattie and co-workers trained 30 premenopausal women with genuine stress incontinence in pelvic muscle rehabilitation with an ingenious form of resistive therapy using a set of weighted vaginal cones (70). These cones are of the same size but of increasing weight (from 20 to 100 g). After inserting a cone into the vagina, it can only be retained in place by contracting the pelvic floor. As one cone is successfully retained for 15 minutes, the next heaviest cone is used, thus progressively increasing the retained weight. The feeling that the cone is slipping out of the vagina results in a form of sensory biofeedback that causes an increased contraction in the pelvic floor in an attempt to retain it. At the end of 1 month of therapy, 19 patients (70%) reported cure or significant improvement of symptoms, and only 11 (37%) opted for subsequent surgical intervention.

Physical therapy will not cure or improve all cases of stress incontinence; however, properly supervised and rigorously performed techniques for pelvic muscular rehabilitation can play a significant role in the treatment of genuine stress incontinence (69). Patients can expect improvement in their symptoms by tensing the musculature of the pelvic floor and holding these contractions for 5 seconds each, 15 to 20 times per session, three sessions per day. This will strengthen slow-twitch muscle fibers. Patients should also practice a similar number of rapid contractions to strengthen the fast-twitch muscle fibers. Pelvic muscle exercises should be taught to patients one-on-one during a pelvic examination because many patients contract the wrong muscles; teaching Kegel exercises to large groups in classrooms is not worthwhile. Because pelvic muscle rehabilitation is virtually without side effects, involves the patient in her own care, and may prevent the development of subsequent pelvic organ prolapse if used regularly, physicians should be encouraged to incorporate pelvic muscle exercises into routine health maintenance programs for women.

Drug Therapy The tone of the urethra and bladder neck is maintained in large part by α-adrenergic activity from the sympathetic nervous system. For this reason, many pharmacologic agents have been used with varying degrees of success to treat stress incontinence. These drugs include *imipramine* (which has a concomitant relaxing effect on the detrusor), *ephedrine, pseudoephedrine, phenylpropanolamine,* and *norepinephrine.* Unfortunately, many of these compounds also increase vascular tone and may, therefore, lead to problems with hypertension, a condition that afflicts many postmenopausal women with stress incontinence. These effects may preclude the use of α-agonists in such patients. A recent U.S. Food and Drug Administration (FDA) statement urged caution in the use of *phenylpropanolamine,* an α-agonist, in women because of an apparent increased epidemiologic risk for hemorrhagic cerebral vascular accidents. Although the risk remains very low, it is not possible to predict who is at risk for this complication (71). The use of these agents in the treatment of stress urinary incontinence appears to be more limited than originally thought. Of equal importance, however, is the role of α-blockers such as *prazosin* in causing stress incontinence. These drugs are commonly used in treating hypertension because of their relaxing effects on vascular smooth muscle; however, they may also relax the bladder neck and urethra to the point at which incontinence develops. For patients who have symptoms of stress incontinence while taking this or a related drug, their antihypertensive medication should be changed before surgery is considered because their incontinence may resolve spontaneously with a change of medication (41).

Postmenopausal women with urogenital atrophy resulting from estrogen deprivation and concurrent urinary incontinence should receive hormone replacement therapy as part of their therapeutic regimen unless such therapy is contraindicated. Not only will many complaints of urgency, frequency, and irritation often disappear, but evidence suggests that estrogen replacement enhances the effectiveness of α-adrenergic receptors in the urethra (72,73).

Electrical Stimulation In addition to physical therapy and selected pharmacologic agents, electrical stimulation therapy has been used to treat stress incontinence. This treatment may offer advantages to women with moderate to severe weakness of the pelvic floor muscles who have difficulty performing pelvic muscle exercises themselves. Electrical stimulation, particularly when used in conjunction with individual instruction by a pelvic floor physical therapist, also is useful in teaching the patient which muscles to exercise. Passage of an electrical current through the muscles of the pelvic floor causes them to contract and simultaneously causes a reflex inhibition of detrusor activity. The stimulus can be applied transvaginally or transrectally in either continuous or intermittent fashion. When compared with sham devices and pelvic floor exercises, electrostimulation has produced mixed results in the treatment of stress urinary incontinence (74,75). Although many authors have reported good success rates using these devices, patient acceptance of the technique is often poor, and the device may fail because of mechanical problems. Although this mode of therapy remains an option for patients with stress incontinence, it is unlikely to be used extensively at present outside a research setting. Recently, a new device using pulsed magnetic technology has been developed for strengthening the pelvic floor in the treatment of urinary incontinence. This device produces a rapidly pulsing magnetic field that passes through air, skin, fat, and bone with minimal attenuation. *Extracorporeal magnetic innervation* has been used to treat women with both stress and urge incontinence in a noninvasive treatment session (it does not require internal probes or electrodes). A typical treatment session lasts 20 minutes and includes both high- and low-frequency stimulation with the patient sitting fully clothed on the treatment chair. The recommended treatment course consists of twice weekly sessions for 6 to 8 weeks. The research is currently limited by short duration of follow-up and small numbers of patients, but the concept is attractive, and this therapy may offer a more acceptable form of treatment for many women with pelvic floor dysfunction (76,77).

Surgical Management

Operations for stress incontinence can be classified into four broad categories (78–80):

1. Traditional anterior vaginal colporrhaphy
2. Operations to correct stress incontinence resulting from anatomic hypermobility (retropubic bladder neck suspension operations, needle suspension procedures, tension-free vaginal tape, and some sling procedures)
3. Operations for stress incontinence resulting from intrinsic sphincteric weakness or dysfunction (sling operations and periurethral injections)
4. Salvage operations (intentionally obstructive sling operations, implantation of an artificial urinary sphincter, urinary diversion)

Anterior Colporrhaphy Anterior vaginal repair is the oldest operation for stress incontinence in gynecology. It was described by Howard Kelly in 1914 (81). He believed that stress incontinence was caused by an open vesical neck rather than from loss of urethral support, and he designed an operation to cure this condition by pulling the bladder neck closed using periurethral Kelly plication sutures. This operation remained the standard first approach to stress incontinence until the middle of the twentieth century and still is popular among many practitioners.

Many different operations have been lumped together under the term *anterior colporrhaphy*, including simple plication of the bladder neck, elevation of the bladder neck by plicating the fascia under the urethra, and elevation and fixation of the bladder neck by passing sutures lateral to the urethra and driving the needles anteriorly into the back of the pubic symphysis for fixation.

The mechanism of action of this operation, when it works, is preventing excessive displacement of endopelvic fascia beneath the urethra so that the urethra can be closed during coughing or sneezing. The main advantage of this operation is that it avoids an abdominal incision, which may not be well tolerated by older women. It also allows the operation to be performed in conjunction with other vaginal surgery, such as vaginal hysterectomy for uterine prolapse.

The problem with most techniques of anterior colporrhaphy is that they do not hold up well over time (82–84). In essence, this operation attempts to take weak support from below and to push it back up from below, with hope that these structures will maintain their strength and position over time. Although there have been excellent long-term results shown with anterior colporrhaphy, most of these reports use specific techniques requiring skillful dissection of the endopelvic fascia, deep bold bites of suture, and fixation of permanent sutures to the pubic bone from below: in essence, a transvaginal retropubic bladder neck suspension (85,86). Most surgical series that have evaluated techniques of anterior colporrhaphy for stress incontinence show long-term success rates of only 35% to 65%, a figure that most would regard as unacceptably low. Anterior colporrhaphy should be reserved primarily for patients requiring cystocele repair who do not have significant stress incontinence.

Surgery to Correct Urethral Hypermobility

Retropubic Urethropexy The modern era of retropubic surgery for stress incontinence began in 1949, when Marshall, Marchetti, and Krantz described their technique for urethral suspension in a male with postprostatectomy incontinence (87). Since that time, a variety of modifications of this operation have been described, all of which share at least

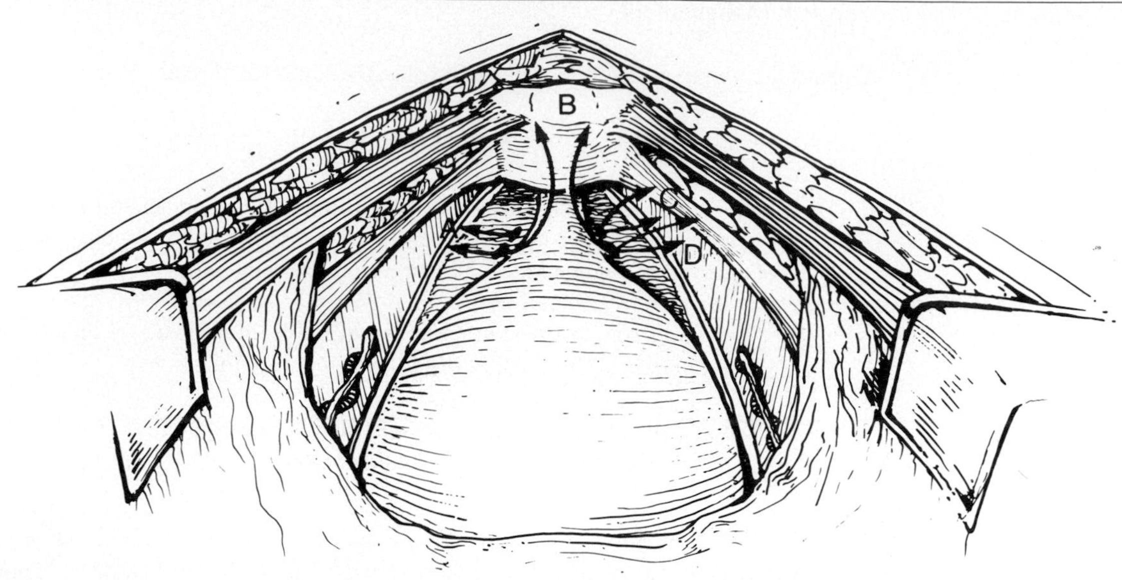

Figure 20.13 Points of reattachment of the endopelvic fascia during retropubic bladder neck suspension operations. A: Arcus tendineus fascia pelvis. **B:** Periosteum of the pubic symphysis. **C:** Ileopectineal ligament (Cooper's ligament). **D:** Obturator internus fascia. (From **Wall LL.** Stress urinary incontinence. In **Rock JA, Thompson JD,** eds. *TeLinde's operative gynecology.* 8th ed. Philadelphia: JB Lippincott, 1997, with permission.)

two characteristics: they are performed through an open low abdominal incision or with laparoscopically assisted exposure of the space of Retzius, and they all involve attachment of the periurethral or perivesical endopelvic fascia to some other supporting structure in the anterior pelvis (Fig. 20.13). In the Marshall-Marchetti-Krantz operation, the periurethral fascia is attached to the back of the pubic symphysis. Another approach, the Burch colposuspension, involves the attachment of the fascia at the level of the bladder neck to the iliopectineal ligament (Cooper's ligament) (88,89). With the paravaginal repair, the lateral endopelvic fascia along the urethra and bladder is reattached to the arcus tendinous fascia pelvis (90,91). In the Turner-Warwick vaginoobturator shelf procedure, the endopelvic fascia, vagina, or both are attached to the fascia of the obturator internus muscle (92,93). All of these operations cure stress incontinence by correcting anatomic hypermobility of the urethra and bladder neck. The long-term success rate for patients undergoing these operations as primary procedures for stress incontinence is in the range of 70% to 90% (94–98).

Retropubic urethropexy has had high success rates; however, the traditional route, which requires an abdominal incision, results in increased morbidity when compared with transvaginal corrective procedures. Presumably, laparoscopically assisted retropubic urethropexy would have a decreased recovery time when compared with the traditional open approach; however, the learning curve is prolonged with this technique, and the published results of the success rate of this operation to date are mixed (99–101). Many surgeons have made substantial modifications to the operation in an attempt to perform it laparoscopically, and these modifications may be a factor explaining these differences in outcome.

No operation is perfect, however (102,103). Depending on how high and tight the suspending sutures are tied, these operations may introduce an element of urethral kinking or obstruction, with subsequent voiding difficulty (104–106). This can be a significant long-term complication for patients undergoing this type of surgery. Operations that put sutures directly into the pubic symphysis may cause debilitating osteitis pubis, which can disable an otherwise healthy woman for several months. The normal vaginal axis is almost horizontal, with the vagina resting on top of the levator plate (Fig. 20.14). Because the vagina is a tubular structure, pulling up on the anterior vagina also elevates the posterior vagina. This

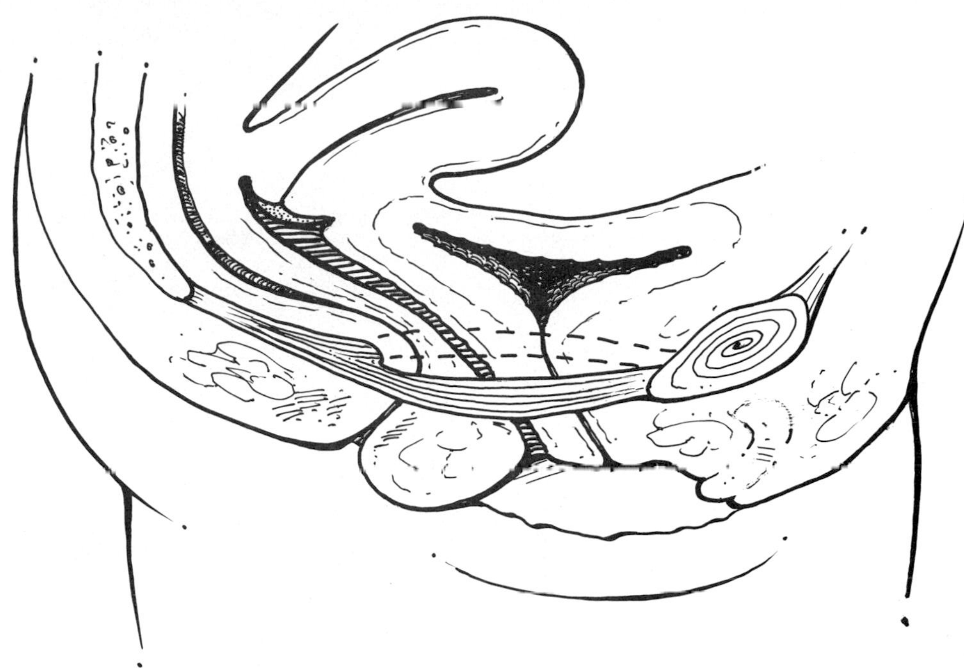

Figure 20.14 Normal location of structures over the pelvic floor. Note that the normal vagina is almost horizontal, lying over the levator plate. Any operation that pulls the vagina forward, away from its normal location, increases the risk of enterocele formation and the development of rapidly progressive prolapse.

can pull the posterior vagina up out of its normal position, opening the rectouterine pouch of Douglas and thereby predisposing patients to enterocele formation, uterine prolapse, and vaginal vault eversion. For this reason, culdoplasty can be performed at the time of bladder neck suspension to reduce the incidence of future prolapse (107).

Transvaginal Urethropexy Needle suspension procedures are so named because they suspend the urethra and bladder neck through a technique that involves passage of sutures between the vagina and anterior abdominal wall using a specially designed long needle carrier. To perform these operations, a vaginal incision is typically made at the level of the bladder neck, the endopelvic fascia is perforated, the space of Retzius is entered from below, and a permanent suture is passed down through a low abdominal incision through the retropubic space, where it is fixed to the endopelvic fascia at the level of the bladder neck. The long needle is then passed back up through the retropubic space to the abdominal incision, where it is tied in place (Fig. 20.15). The first needle suspensions were performed by a gynecologist, Dr. Armand Pereyra, in the 1950s, but many urologic surgeons have since made modifications to the technique (108–113).

These operations are designed to correct stress incontinence resulting primarily from anatomic hypermobility of the bladder neck and urethra. If the suspending sutures are pulled too tight, an element of obstruction can be created. They are relatively simple and take less time to perform than open procedures, but this advantage is often offset by the fact that they are not as effective in curing stress incontinence. Initial cure rates are between 70% and 90%, but these rates appear to decrease significantly over time in many series, with 5-year success rates of 50% or less (95,114–118). In addition to a lower success rate, other complications include perforation of the bladder or urethra by the long needles, infections, formation of granulation tissue around sutures and the synthetic bolsters often used in fixing the sutures to the fascia at the bladder neck or abdominal wall, development of prolapse as a result of changes created in the vaginal axis, chronic pulling pelvic pain created by the suspension sutures, and nerve entrapment syndromes (119–122). Because the long-term

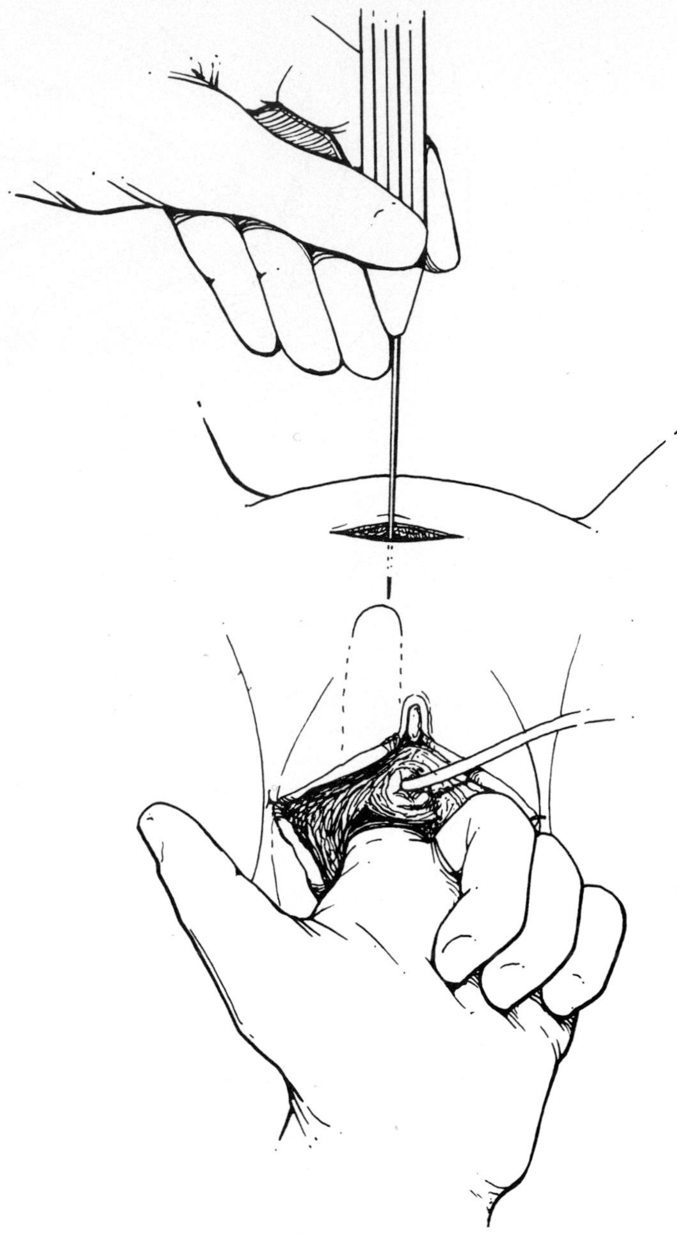

Figure 20.15 Guidance of the long needle through the space of Retzius using the surgeon's index finger. (From **Wall LL.** Stress urinary incontinence. In **Rock JA, Thompson JD,** eds. *TeLinde's operative gynecology.* 8th ed. Philadelphia: JB Lippincott, 1997, with permission.)

success rate of needle urethropexy is poor, this operation is falling out of favor. Surgeons performing needle urethropexy should know their long-term continence rates to make sure that they are offering their patients an appropriate treatment option.

Tension-free Vaginal Tape The poor success rates of needle urethropexy operations have led many surgeons to search for a similarly attractive, low-morbidity operation with better long-term success. Ulmson described a new technique for correcting stress urinary incontinence in 1996 (123). This technique involves the use of polypropylene mesh placed under the midurethra with minimal tension. To perform this operation, a small midurethral incision is made in the vaginal epithelium mucosa. A 40- × 1-cm mesh tape covered by a plastic sheath and attached to two 5 mm-curved trocars is passed lateral to the urethra and through the endopelvic fascia into the retropubic space. The trocar is then passed along the back of the pubic bone, through the rectus fascia, into two small suprapubic skin incisions. The tension on the tape is adjusted, the sheath is removed, and the remaining tape is cut off at the level of the skin. This technique has the advantage of being performed quickly using limited anesthesia (less than 30 minutes in experienced hands). The procedure requires the use of a catheter guide to deviate the urethra and cystoscopy to ensure that bladder or urethral perforations are recognized immediately because the trocar is passed blindly.

The short-term results reported to date by various authors are encouraging, but long-term data must be evaluated before the role of this operation in the treatment of stress incontinence can be determined (124,125). The complications reported appear to be similar to those occurring with needle urethropexies. Concern about the use of synthetic materials placed through a vaginal incision remain; reports of transvaginal sling operations performed using other types of synthetic materials have documented complications with this approach in the past (126–128).

Sling Procedures and Periurethral Injections

Sling Operations After reviewing reports that included patient follow-up for more than 48 months, the American Urological Association and the Female Stress Urinary Incontinence Guidelines Panel concluded that the two most effective surgical treatments for stress incontinence are retropubic bladder neck suspensions and sling procedures (130). This panel confirmed that the use of sling operations in women with complex or recurrent stress urinary incontinence is a safe and effective treatment. Given the high success rates with complex incontinence, many surgeons are now performing sling procedures as a primary procedure, rather than reserving such operations for patients who have failed previous operations. Traditionally, sling operations have been used principally for patients with complicated stress incontinence, usually resulting from intrinsic sphincteric damage or weakness. Probably no more than 15% to 20% of women with stress incontinence need a sling procedure to be cured. Patients requiring a sling typically have demonstrable stress incontinence with normal urethral support or stress incontinence with a low leak-point pressure. Other candidates might be women with stress incontinence who engage in very heavy occupational lifting, who have severe chronic obstructive lung disease, and who have posthysterectomy vaginal vault eversion. Such patients appear to have an increased risk for surgical failure if their stress incontinence is treated with an anterior colporrhaphy, retropubic operation, or needle suspension. Although sling operations do provide urethral support, they work primarily by compressing the urethral lumen at the level of the bladder neck to compensate for a faulty urethral closure mechanism; that is, they work by creating some degree of outlet obstruction (Fig. 20.16).

Sling operations have traditionally been performed using a combined vaginal and abdominal approach. The anterior vagina is opened, the space of Retzius is dissected on each side of the bladder neck, and a sling is passed around the bladder neck and urethra and is then attached to the anterior rectus fascia or some other structure to cradle the urethra in a supporting hammock. This both supports the urethra and allows it to be compressed during periods of increased intraabdominal pressure (130–140). The sling can be made of organic or inorganic materials. Organic materials can be autologous tissues harvested from the patient (e.g., fascia lata, rectus fascia, tendon, round ligament, rectus muscle, vagina), processed allografts from human donors (e.g., fascia lata, dermis), or heterologous tissues harvested from another species and processed for surgical use (e.g., ox dura mater, porcine dermis). Synthetic materials (e.g., Silastic, Gore-Tex, Marlex) are popular because of their consistent strength and easy availability, but these substances are often plagued by problems with erosion and infection when they are used around the urethra (127–129).

Technologic advances have made it possible to perform sling procedures completely through the vaginal approach using bone anchors, bone screws, and suture capturing devices. These devices decrease the morbidity resulting from an abdominal incision and may

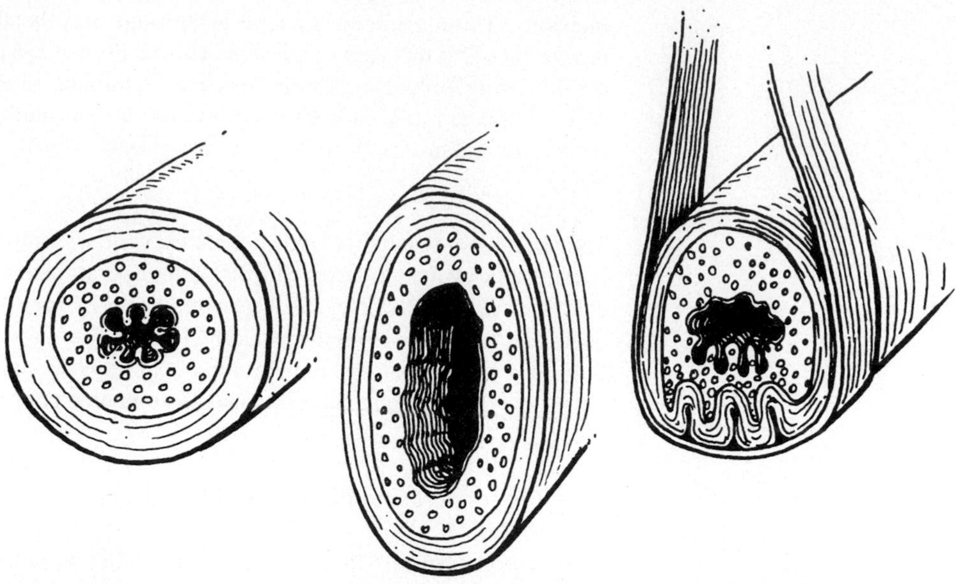

Figure 20.16 Mechanism of action of sling procedures for stress incontinence. A: Normal urethra. **B:** Incompetent urethra with intrinsic sphincteric deficiency. The lumen is gaping, scarred, and has lost its normal coaptation and pliability. **C:** Correction of intrinsic sphincteric deficiency using a sling operation. The urethra is supported and the urethral lumen is partially compressed by the sling. (From **Wall LL.** Stress urinary incontinence. In **Rock JA, Thompson JD,** eds. *TeLinde's operative gynecology.* 8th ed. Philadelphia: JB Lippincott, 1997, with permission.

allow for earlier discharge and resumption of normal activity. The safety and efficacy of these modifications to the traditional sling procedure must be confirmed with comparative long-term outcome studies.

The most common problem encountered by patients for whom a sling procedure has been performed is obstructed voiding after surgery. The sling does not have to be pulled tight to work, but the common temptation of less experienced surgeons is to make the sling too tight in hopes of ensuring that the patient is cured. Not infrequently, patients with a sling require long-term bladder drainage using either a suprapubic catheter or clean intermittent self-catheterization. The symptoms of obstructed voiding—urgency, frequency, urge incontinence, incomplete emptying, low flow, intermittent stream, hesitancy, and increased residual urine—typically improve over time and often resolve. Some patients, however, require long-term self-catheterization. This possibility should be discussed with patients before surgery.

The number of sling procedures performed for stress urinary incontinence has increased markedly over the past several years. The use of donor allograft tissue for implantation has resulted in decreased morbidity and ease of performing these surgical procedures. The short-term results of surgery with these allografts have been promising; however, the concern over long-term results and reports of early failures necessitates additional research before human allografts can be recommended for most sling procedures (139–141). Sling procedures for simple and complex stress urinary incontinence continue to be an important treatment option with low morbidity when performed by experienced surgeons.

Periurethral Injections A less invasive treatment of intrinsic urethral failure is attempting to restore urethral closure by injecting a material around the periurethral tissues to facilitate their coaptation under conditions of increased intraabdominal pressure (142–147). This approach has been tried for years with limited success, but advances in chemistry have allowed the development of materials better suited to the injection procedure, namely *polytetrafluoroethylene paste* (*Polytef*), *glutaraldehyde cross-linked bovine collagen* (*Contigen*), and *pyrolytic carbon-coated zirconium beads* (*Durasphere*). A small-gauge needle is inserted into the periurethral tissues, and the material is injected along the urethra at the level of the bladder neck. This seems to work by bulking up the bladder neck, allowing enhanced urethral closure under stress, rather than by changing the resting urethral pressure. *Teflon* is harder to work with and requires the use of a power-injector. It also has been shown to migrate to other areas of the body under some circumstances. *Contigen* can be passed easily through small-bore needles under local anesthesia but requires preoperative skin testing to check for possible allergic reactions (3%). *Durasphere* is nonantigenic (thus no skin testing is required) and does not migrate. *Durasphere* appears to have similar reduction in leakage episodes as compared with collagen and is more likely to require only a single injection (147). This bulking agent does require a larger-gauge needle for injection and is somewhat more difficult to inject than collagen. These techniques may require several injections to achieve continence, and the long-term success of these operations remains poorly studied. The development of a bulking agent that is easy to inject, is nonantigenic, has a minimal inflammatory response, and does not degrade or migrate should result in increased efficacy in properly selected patients.

Salvage Operations

The best opportunity to cure stress incontinence occurs at the time of the initial operation. Subsequent surgeries have a lower success rate, and the chances of success seem to diminish with each subsequent operation (65). In some cases, the surgeon is faced with a scarred, fibrotic nonfunctional urethra in a hopelessly incontinent patient. This type of patient requires what can best be called "salvage" operations—a last ditch effort for cure. Such patients may benefit from periurethral collagen injections. Others may benefit from the placement of a deliberately obstructive sling, with the plan that the patient will drain her bladder by self-catheterization for the rest of her life. Still others may benefit from the implantation of an artificial urinary sphincter, a high-technology approach to incontinence that appears to work better for males than females (148,149). Finally, others may require urinary diversion. Only a small percentage of women with stress incontinence require such measures.

Urinary Incontinence Caused by Detrusor Overactivity

Although stress incontinence is the most common type of urinary continence in women, urge incontinence caused by detrusor overactivity is the most common form of incontinence in older women and the second most common form of urinary incontinence overall (150). In this condition, urine loss is caused not by failure of urethral support or closure but rather by uninhibited contractions of the detrusor muscle. Patients with this condition typically experience sudden, unexpected loss of large volumes of urine or leakage associated with a sudden urge to urinate that cannot be controlled. In both cases, urine loss occurs from an unsuppressed contraction of the bladder muscle, a failure to inhibit the micturition reflex. **When this occurs as the result of a known neuropathologic process relevant to bladder disorders (e.g., stroke, Parkinson's disease, multiple sclerosis), it is referred to as *detrusor hyperreflexia*. In cases in which there is no evidence of neuropathology (most cases), the condition is referred to as *detrusor instability*.** Both conditions can be called *detrusor overactivity* (65). Detrusor overactivity should be suspected in all cases in which the patient has symptoms of urgency, frequency, and urge incontinence. For patients who have frequency and urgency without incontinence, detrusor overactivity rarely is the cause of their problem. For most such cases, the cause of the symptoms is a disorder of bladder sensation (151,152).

Diagnosis

The diagnosis of incontinence caused by detrusor overactivity can be confirmed by cystometry. A rule for all incontinence evaluations is to demonstrate incontinence and confirm

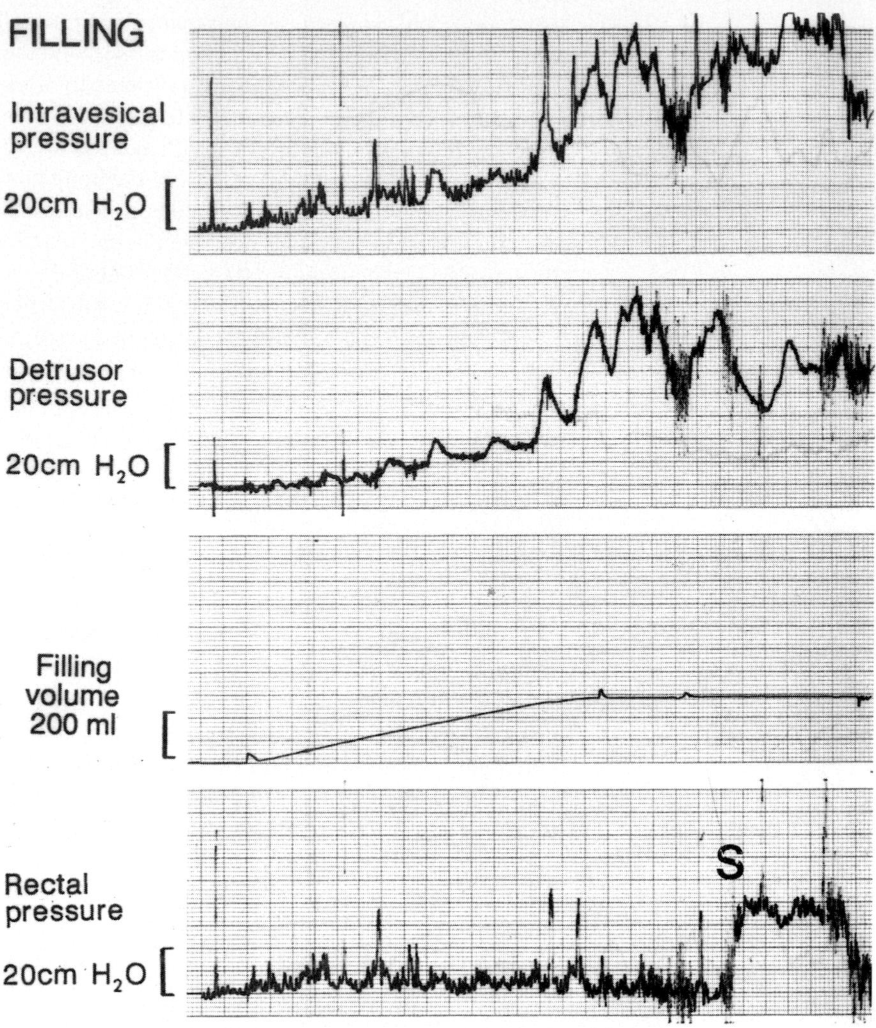

Figure 20.17 Subtracted cystometrogram showing detrusor overactivity. Notice that the rectal pressure stays relatively constant throughout bladder filling in the supine position, whereas there are phasic changes in intravesical pressure and subtracted detrusor pressure. These changes are diagnostic of uninhibited contractions of the detrusor muscle. In this patient, these contractions produced a large amount of urine loss. Note that the rise in rectal pressure that occurs when the patient stands *(S)* provokes an additional detrusor contraction.

with the patient that what has been demonstrated reproduces her complaint. Subtracted filling cystometrography for patients with an overactive detrusor should show phasic pressure waves that produce urgency and urge incontinence (Fig. 20.17). False-negative and false-positive results can occur. False-positive results occur for patients with asymptomatic detrusor activity, detrusor activity that is irrelevant to the complaint, or detrusor activity that is situational (e.g., caused by test anxiety). The false-negative results occur because 20-minute cystometrography is not always an accurate measure of daily bladder activity. Looking for detrusor instability with such a test is like looking for an episodic cardiac arrhythmia using 12-lead electrocardiography, as opposed to looking for the arrhythmia using a 24-hour Holter monitor. The sensitivity of the latter test is far greater than that of the former. The same principles apply to stationary subtracted cystometry when compared with long-term ambulatory urodynamic studies (153–155). In most patients with a strong history of urge incontinence, a detrusor problem is the cause of leakage.

Treatment

Detrusor overactivity can be treated using drugs or behavioral modification (150). The best initial choice is probably a combination of the two therapies. If possible, long-term management of this condition should be based on behavioral therapy for two main reasons. The first is that the drugs used in treating detrusor instability have unpleasant anticholinergic side effects. Most patients tire of these problems over time and discontinue medications. Second, the cure rates with behavioral treatment are comparable to those with drug therapy, and any drug therapy for this condition will be enhanced by modifying the behavior that contributes to detrusor overactivity.

Drug Therapy

The drugs used in treating detrusor muscle overactivity can be grouped into different categories according to their pharmacologic characteristics; however, for all practical purposes, these drugs are anticholinergic agents that exert their effects on the bladder by blocking the activity of acetylcholine at muscarinic receptor sites. Most of these drugs have a short half-life, which means that they must be taken frequently. All of these drugs have side effects, the most common of which are dry mouth resulting from decreased saliva production, increased heart rate because of vagal blockade, feelings of constipation resulting from decreased gastrointestinal motility, and occasionally, blurred vision caused by blockade of the sphincter of the iris and the ciliary muscle of the lens of the eye. Other drugs, such as *imipramine,* may produce orthostatic hypotension and cardiac arrhythmias. Patients should be encouraged to titrate their medication to their symptoms and to vary the dosage (within acceptable limits) according to their needs.

The introduction of two new medications for the treatment of detrusor overactivity has resulted in significant attention being given to urinary incontinence in the media—*tolterodine* and long-acting *oxybutynin. Tolterodine* (*Detrol*) is a muscarinic receptor antagonist with a long half life, which means it can be taken once or twice daily. *Tolterodine* has demonstrated similar efficacy to immediate-release *oxybutynin* in the reduction of urinary frequency and episodes of urge-related urinary leakage. Significant reduction in the common complaint of a bothersome dry mouth was found in the *tolterodine* group compared with the group taking immediate-release *oxybutynin* and the placebo group (156,157). Long-acting *oxybutynin* (*Ditropan XL*) relies on a slow-release mechanism known as oral osmotic (OROS) technology to deliver a constant dose of *oxybutynin* throughout the day. By reducing fluctuations in serum levels through this constant-release mechanism, the new delivery system attempts to reduce the side-effect profile associated with traditional formulations. Long-acting *oxybutynin* appears to have better patient compliance and reduced side-effects while maintaining efficacy similar to that of immediate-release *oxybutynin* (158,159).

A list of medications and the usual dosage ranges are given in Table 20.4. In general, it is best to start with a lower dose (particularly for elderly patients) and to increase it as needed to a higher, more frequent dosage. Patients with neuropathic detrusor hyperreflexia generally need more medication than patients with idiopathic detrusor instability. Patients should be warned of the anticholinergic side effects. Patients should be particularly advised about the symptom of a dry mouth and told that this is not due to thirst. Some patients increase their

Table 20.4. Drugs Useful in Treating Detrusor Overactivity

Drug	Dose
Tolterodine	1–2 mg PO b.i.d.
Tolterodine, long-acting	4 mg PO q.d.
Hyoscyamine sulfate	0.125–0.25 mg PO q. 4–6 hr
Hyoscyamine sulfate, extended release	0.375 mg PO b.i.d.
Oxybutynin chloride	5–10 mg PO t.i.d./q.i.d.
Oxybutynin chloride XL	5–15 mg PO q.d.
Dicyclomine hydrochloride	20 mg PO q.i.d.

fluid intake to combat this problem, with a subsequent worsening of their incontinence. If dry mouth is a problem, patients should relieve it by chewing gum, sucking on a piece of hard candy, or eating a piece of moist fruit.

Behavioral Therapy

Behavioral therapy for detrusor instability is based on the assumption that the underlying pathophysiology is the escape of the detrusor from the cortical control over micturition that had previously been established during childhood toilet-training. The object of bladder retraining (or *bladder drill,* as it is sometimes called) is to reestablish the authority of the cerebral cortex over bladder function. This is performed through a regimen of timed voiding, gradually increasing the intervals between voids until the cycle of urgency, frequency, and urge incontinence is broken.

Behavioral therapy is carried out as follows:

1. The patient is instructed to void on a timed schedule, starting with a relatively frequent interval of every hour while she is awake.

2. When she wakes up in the morning, she voids at 6:00 AM, 7:00 AM, 8:00 AM, and so forth throughout the day. If it is 7:00 AM, and she does not feel the need to void, she must do so anyway. The object is to make her bladder do what she wants it to do, instead of responding to the whims of her bladder. If it is 7:55 AM and she is desperate to urinate, she cannot do so. She must wait until 8:00 AM, even if this means that she leaks some urine onto a pad. When the appropriate time arrives, she can empty her bladder.

3. At night, the patient is allowed to void only when she is awakened from sleep by the need to do so.

4. When she can maintain this schedule for 1 week, the voiding interval is increased by 15 minutes. It is increased gradually by 15 minutes every week until a normal voiding interval of 2.5 to 3 hours has been established.

This program works very well for patients with detrusor instability. The secret of success is gradual increases in the interval between voids. The best predictor of success is patient compliance; those who follow this program get excellent results. **Unfortunately, patients who have suffered a neurologic insult that has resulted in detrusor hyperreflexia do not respond very well to bladder retraining because the problem is actually one of neural pathway destruction rather than the need to reestablish cortical control mechanisms.** Frequently, these patients have a trigger volume of urine that sets off a contraction that they cannot control voluntarily. Such patients may benefit from a timed voiding schedule in which they void at regular intervals (such as every 2 hours) to keep their bladder volume below the trigger point. Attempting to lengthen the interval between voids often does not work well.

Functional Electrical Stimulation

Functional electrical stimulation similar to that used with stress urinary incontinence has also been used in treating overactive bladders that have not responded to other medical and behavioral therapy. Several prospective, double-blind studies have demonstrated cure or improvement in 50% of patients with overactive bladders (160,161) using this technology. Economic and reimbursement issues, as well as issues related to access, patient compliance, and acceptability of the therapy, have limited the use of electrical stimulation for the treatment of detrusor overactivity in the past, but many of these questions are being answered, opening up a whole new range of exciting treatment possibilities in the future.

Sacral Nerve Root Neuromodulation

Even with the development of newer anticholinergic medications with fewer side effects, there continues to be a select group of patients with overactive bladders who remain refractory to standard medical and behavioral treatment. Surgical treatment of this condition has traditionally involved substantial morbidity and major urinary denervation, reconstruction, or both in order to achieve therapeutic benefits. For example, augmentation cystoplasty for refractory urge incontinence has significant short-term operative morbidity and often results in long-term voiding dysfunction that requires clean intermittent catheterization to achieve bladder emptying. The development of implantable sacral nerve root stimulators has led to FDA approval of sacral root neuromodulation in patients with refractory urinary urgency and frequency, urge incontinence, and voiding dysfunction. This therapy offers patients with severe symptoms an alternative to urinary augmentation or diversion. Sacral nerve stimulation therapy is performed in two phases. In the first phase, a percutaneous nerve evaluation test (PNE) is performed to determine which patients respond to this type of therapy. This phase is followed by surgical implantation of a permanent electrode lead adjacent to the third sacral nerve root connected to a pulse generator in those patients who are identified as appropriate candidates after a successful test stimulation (this technique results in more than 50% improvement in symptoms).

A multicenter prospective study demonstrated that 63% of test patients responded to the initial procedure. After implantation, 47% of patients became completely dry, and 77% were successful in eliminating "heavy" leakage episodes. Despite substantial success in nearly 80% of patients who received implants, 30% of patients required further surgical revision because of pain or other complications at the generator or implant site. There were no permanent injuries or nerve damage in the initial trials (162,163). This therapy offers an alternative to radical surgery for many patients in whom other treatment options have been unsuccessful.

Mixed Incontinence

Patients are said to have mixed incontinence when they have motor urge incontinence as a result of detrusor overactivity along with stress incontinence. Because most patients have mixed symptoms, every effort should be made to confirm the diagnosis and to demonstrate stress and urge incontinence objectively before establishing such a diagnosis. Patients with mixed incontinence often pose complicated management problems, and controversy exists regarding the best method of treating them. In the confirmed presence of both types of urinary incontinence, one reasonable approach is to try to determine which symptom is more bothersome to the patient—stress incontinence or urge incontinence—and to proceed from that point (164). Others advocate using conservative therapy to treat urge incontinence first, proceeding with surgery only if stress incontinence persists. Because patients with mixed incontinence have a lower continence rate after surgery than patients with genuine stress incontinence alone, this approach is reasonable. However, some patients experience the *de novo* onset of detrusor overactivity after stress incontinence surgery, and detrusor instability resolves in some patients with mixed incontinence after surgery for stress incontinence. **Bladder neck suspension surgery is contraindicated for patients with detrusor instability alone as the cause of their incontinence. Patients with mixed incontinence, a small functional bladder capacity, and high-pressure detrusor contractions on filling cystometry should undergo operations for stress incontinence only after careful consideration of their individual circumstances and a comprehensive clinical and urodynamic evaluation.**

Functional or Transient Incontinence

In addition to stress incontinence and incontinence caused by detrusor overactivity, a variety of other conditions may cause involuntary urine loss that is a social or hygienic problem (Table 20.2). Among the most important of these causes are those that are loosely categorized as functional or transient. The factors leading to urinary incontinence of this type are medically reversible conditions. This gives them heightened importance (particularly for

Table 20.5. Reversible Causes of Incontinence

Delirium
Infection
Atrophic urethritis and vaginitis
Pharmacologic causes
Psychological causes
Excessive urine production
Restricted mobility
Stool impaction

(Modified from **Resnik N, Yalla S.** Management of urinary incontinence in the elderly. *N Engl J Med* 1985;313:800–805, with permission.)

older women) because appropriate medical intervention can cure or improve the continence problem without resorting to other forms of treatment.

Resnick has invented the useful mnemonic DIAPPERS to help remember these factors (165,166) (Table 20.5). *Delirium* is an acute confusional state that may result in incontinence caused by disorientation. It is often associated with serious underlying pathology. *Infection* may lead to detrusor overactivity, which can be reversed by appropriate antimicrobial therapy. *Atrophic urethritis* and *vaginitis* can be a significant cause of urgency and frequency in older women. *Pharmacologic agents* of many types can have an adverse impact on urinary tract function. *Psychiatric diagnoses* may also be accompanied by incontinence. *Excessive urine production*, such as that found in diabetes, hypercalcemia, or excessive fluid intake, often leads to incontinence by overwhelming a bladder's capabilities to deal with large volumes of fluid. *Restricted mobility* often is associated with incontinence, particularly for elderly patients who, because of arthritis or unsteady gait, cannot reach toilet facilities or undress themselves quickly enough when the urge to urinate arises. Bowel disorders are often found in association with urinary tract problems, partly because of the shared innervation of these organ systems. *Stool impaction* is often found in elderly patients with urinary incontinence; relief of the impaction by prescribing a good bowel regimen to prevent the problem from recurring is often associated with improvement in the function of both organ systems. All of these factors argue strongly for the inclusion of a good medical evaluation as part of the workup of any patient with urinary incontinence.

Disorders of Bladder Emptying, Storage, and Contents

Voiding Difficulty

For women, disorders of urine storage (incontinence) are more common than disorders of bladder emptying (voiding difficulty), which tend to be the predominant problems in men because of the longer urethra and the presence of a potentially enlarged and obstructing prostate gland. Nonetheless, **women do suffer from voiding difficulties, which may be defined as emptying dysfunction resulting from a failure of pelvic floor relaxation or failure of the detrusor muscle to contract appropriately.** True outflow obstruction (defined as a detrusor pressure of more than 50 cm H_2O in association with a urine flow rate of less than 15 mL/sec) is rare in women and, when seen, is usually found in patients who have undergone obstructive bladder neck surgery for stress incontinence (106,167).

For normal voiding to occur, the pelvic floor and urethral sphincter must relax, which should occur in conjunction with a coordinated contraction of the detrusor muscle that leads to complete bladder emptying. Of course, the bladder may be emptied by other mechanisms, such as by abdominal straining in the absence of a detrusor contraction, or simply by relaxation of the pelvic floor if the closure mechanism is exceptionally weak; however, complete bladder emptying is not the same as normal voiding. Some women may empty their bladders completely, but only by expending great effort over several minutes. In such cases, voiding is clearly abnormal, even though the bladder is empty when voiding ceases. In the worst cases, voiding is both difficult and incomplete.

An example of voiding difficulty is the *detrusor-sphincter dyssynergia* that occurs in some patients with multiple sclerosis and other neuropathic conditions (168,169). With this condition, there is a lack of coordination between detrusor contraction and urethral relaxation, and the urethral sphincter contracts at the same time as the detrusor. This means that outlet resistance to voiding increases at the same time that intravesical pressure is increasing; hence, voiding becomes difficult if not impossible. Great effort is required to overcome urethral resistance; the patient voids with an interrupted stop-and-start stream and usually leaves a significant amount of residual urine.

Treatment

Voiding difficulty can be managed in several different ways, depending on the cause of the condition. Patients with pelvic floor spasticity (in the absence of a neurologic insult) can often be trained to relax the pelvic floor through biofeedback therapy and to void normally.

Drug Therapy

Mild sedatives are sometimes helpful in this process, as are α-blockers (e.g., prazosin, phenoxybenzamine), which reduce urethral tone. For patients who are unable to generate a detrusor contraction, attempts have been made to enhance detrusor contractility using a cholinergic agonist such as bethanechol chloride. Although cholinergic medications are successful in making strips of bladder muscle contract in a laboratory, there is little evidence that such drugs are helpful clinically (170).

Self-Catheterization

The mainstay in the treatment of voiding difficulty, therefore, is clean intermittent self-catheterization (171). The implementation of self-catheterization programs revolutionized the treatment of voiding difficulties and urinary retention by eliminating the use of chronic indwelling catheters for many patients. **The most important protection against urinary tract infection is frequent and complete bladder emptying rather than avoidance of the introduction of a foreign body into the bladder.** Self-catheterization allows the patient to accomplish this task using a small (14-Fr.) plastic catheter that she inserts through the urethra into the bladder, draining its contents. The catheter is then removed, washed with soap and water, dried, and stored in a clean, dry place. Elaborate sterile procedures are not necessary. Although bacteria are introduced into the bladder in this process, frequent emptying through self-catheterization greatly reduces the risk for urinary tract infection for these patients. The urine of women after self-catheterization regimens will always be colonized with bacteria; however, this condition should not be treated unless symptomatic infection occurs.

Sacral Nerve Root Neuromodulation

Even though self-catheterization can be used to treat women who have all types of voiding dysfunction, some women find this difficult or cumbersome to perform. Neuromodulation of the sacral nerve roots (S3 or S4) has proved to be an effective treatment option for some patients with nonobstructive urinary retention as well as for some patients with refractory urge incontinence. If test stimulation results in successful voiding, the implanted pulse generator results in clinical improvement in voiding symptoms in 70% of patients (163). Although this technology requires a major surgical procedure, many women favor this therapy over lifelong self-catheterization.

Suppressive Antibiotics

Voiding difficulty and stress incontinence pose special surgical problems, and many women with these conditions do not void normally after surgery, particularly if an obstructive operation is performed. After surgery, voiding difficulty can be managed with self-catheterization and reassurance. If outflow obstruction is diagnosed on a pressure-flow voiding study (low flow in the presence of high pressure), however, it may be beneficial to take down the obstructive operative procedure and resuspend the bladder neck at a lower, less obstructed, level (106).

Chronic suppressive antibiotic therapy should not be used; instead, acute infections should be treated with an appropriate antibiotic for 3 days. This treatment prevents the selection of potentially dangerous drug-resistant bacteria, which pose a risk for these patients.

Acute Urinary Retention

Acute urinary retention exists when there is a sudden inability to void (172). The condition is painful, and, upon catheterization, a large volume of urine is released. Sometimes, the explanation is found readily, as in the case of a woman who develops urinary retention after the administration of an epidural anesthetic. A careful search should always be performed to determine the cause of the retention, particularly if any neurologic signs are present. The patient should be catheterized to decompress her bladder and prevent overdistention. Most patients should be taught self-catheterization. This procedure not only gives patients a better method of long-term bladder emptying than an indwelling catheter but also provides them with a "safety valve" in the event that the problem recurs unexpectedly in the future.

Disorders of Bladder Sensation

Most patients with disorders of bladder sensation experience pain rather than lack of bladder sensation. The cause of most painful bladder conditions is unknown, and the therapies currently used in treatment are only partially successful, similar to the treatment of most chronic pain syndromes. As a result, disorders of bladder sensation are among the most frustrating urogynecologic conditions.

Diagnosis

A careful history should be obtained, along with a sterile urine specimen for analysis and culture. Many women treated repetitively for chronic cystitis have taken multiple courses of antibiotics on the basis of symptoms without ever having had a culture-proven infection. Detrusor instability may be the cause of frequency, urgency, and urge incontinence but is not usually a factor in dysuria or painful urination. **Women older than 50 years of age (particularly smokers and workers exposed to chemicals) are at risk for bladder cancer, and this possibility must be considered, especially if hematuria is present. Urinary cytology is sometimes helpful in detecting early tumors of the urinary tract, and cystoscopy and intravenous urography are mandatory in the evaluation of patients with hematuria.**

Interstitial cystitis is a syndrome that presents as urgency, frequency, and bladder pain in the presence of a small bladder capacity, with bladder pain experienced on filling and relieved by voiding. Many different pathophysiologic processes factor into this condition, which complicates treatment (173). A number of possible causes must be considered in the differential diagnosis of painful voiding, including urethral diverticula; vulvar disease; endometriosis; chemical irritation from soaps, bubble bath, or feminine hygiene products; urinary stones; urogenital atrophy from estrogen deprivation; and sexually transmitted diseases (174).

The diagnosis of interstitial cystitis is largely one of exclusion; strict diagnostic guidelines have been developed for research protocols, but the criteria used to diagnose this condition in clinical practice are vague, shifting, and confusing. Hydrodistention of the bladder is believed to be of diagnostic value if Hunner's ulcers are seen; but this finding occurs infrequently in patients with irritative bladder symptoms. The cystoscopic findings of terminal hematuria and diffuse petechial hemorrhage or glomerulations are often seen on reinspection after filling to capacity. Bladder biopsies rarely assist in the diagnosis but may rule out other causes of the patient's symptoms. The use of a potassium chloride infusion test has been described in the evaluation of patients with painful bladder symptoms and is believed to be suggestive of interstitial cystitis in those patients with a positive response (175). The ideal diagnostic test for interstitial cystitis has not been determined.

Treatment

Typically, the clinician has no definitive diagnosis at the end of the evaluation and must rely on symptomatic treatment.

1. Frequency-urgency syndromes should be managed with a careful voiding regimen (similar to that used in the treatment of detrusor instability) and local care.
2. The use of urinary tract analgesics such as Urised is often helpful in reducing urethral irritation. Urised is a polypharmaceutical agent containing a mixture of *methenamine, methylene blue, phenyl salicylate, benzoic acid, atropine sulfate,* and *hyoscyamine,* which has a soothing effect on many irritative urethral symptoms.
3. Restricting the patient's intake of alcohol, caffeine, fruit juice, spices, artificial sweeteners, and food colorings often is helpful.
4. Instruction in the basics of vulvar and perineal hygiene is important (thorough drying; avoidance of most body powders, perfumes, or colored irritating soaps; avoidance of tight-fitting undergarments).
5. Hydrodistention of the bladder has been recommended as a treatment option and can result in clinical improvement in some patients.
6. *Pentosan polysulfate* (*Elmiron*) is an oral agent with *heparin*-like activity. This medication is designed to attempt to replacement of the glycoaminoglycan sulfate layer that is believed deficient in these patients.
7. Some patients benefit from the instillation of 50 mL of a 50% solution of *dimethylsulfoxide* (*DMSO*) for 20 to 30 minutes every other week for four or five sessions.
8. Because it has been theorized that bladder pain may result from increased histamine release, some patients benefit from medications that block these inflammatory mediators, such as *diphenhydramine hydrochloride,* 25 to 50 mg orally three times per day, in combination with 300 mg of *cimetidine* three times per day.

Pelvic Organ Prolapse

Pelvic support problems account for thousands of gynecologic surgical procedures each year, and yet our understanding of these conditions has advanced remarkably slowly over the past century. An increased appreciation of the various contributions of muscle, nerve, and connective tissue to pelvic organ support will probably change this situation within the next decade. Many basic questions have not yet been asked, and many basic clinical issues remain unresolved.

Definition and Classification

A prolapse is a downward or forward displacement of one of the pelvic organs from its normal location. Traditionally, prolapse has referred to displacement of the bladder, the uterus, or the rectum. These displacements have usually been graded on a scale of 0 to 3 (or 0 to 4); the grade increases with increasing severity of the prolapse, with 0 referring to no prolapse and 3 (or 4) referring to total prolapse ("procidentia") (176–179). All forms of female genital prolapse are described with reference to the vagina. True rectal prolapse (as contrasted to a rectocele) is discussed separately.

A variety of terms are used to describe female genital prolapse. Although these terms are generally unsatisfactory and somewhat inaccurate, they are so fixed in the literature that it is impossible to avoid discussing these terms.

- A *cystocele* is a downward displacement of the bladder.
- A *cystourethrocele* is a cystocele that includes the urethra as part of the prolapsing organ complex.
- A *uterine prolapse* is a descent of the uterus and cervix down the vaginal canal toward the vaginal introitus.
- A *rectocele* is a protrusion of the rectum into the posterior vaginal lumen.
- An *enterocele* is a herniation of the small bowel into the vaginal lumen.

Unfortunately, these descriptive terms are inaccurate and misleading. They prejudge the true nature of any prolapse by focusing attention on the bladder, rectum, or uterus rather than on the specific defects that are responsible for alterations in vaginal support. Furthermore, these terms are used in combination with an imprecise (and usually unspecified) system of grading, and they do not convey useful comparative information. The lack of an accurate system of classification of pelvic support defects has hampered progress in the clinical evaluation and treatment of patients with prolapse.

What is observed during a pelvic examination of patients with these conditions is an alteration in vaginal anatomy: anterior vaginal wall descent, posterior vaginal wall descent, a lateral vaginal support defect, cervical descent, or descent of the vaginal apex (in patients who have had a hysterectomy). To name these areas of vaginal descent after the organs that are presumed to be responsible for them prejudges many clinical issues and can lead the surgeon into problems for which he or she may not be prepared; for example, when an "occult" enterocele is discovered during a rectocele repair or when vaginal eversion occurs after surgery because its apex was not believed to be involved in the support defect. Similarly, lumping defects of vaginal support into organ compartments or broad categories such as "cystocele" or "rectocele" draws attention from the precise nature and location of the defects of pelvic support that are present.

As a result of the deficiencies in the traditional classification, the International Continence Society standardization of terminology of female pelvic organ prolapse was developed and published in 1996 (180). The International Continence Society, the American Urogynecologic Society, and the Society of Gynecologic Surgeons have all adopted this standard system for the classification of female pelvic organ prolapse. In this system, anatomic descriptions of specific sites in the vagina replace the traditional terms (i.e., cystocele, rectocele, enterocele). This descriptive system contains a series of nine site-specific measurements. The classification uses six points along the vagina (two points on the anterior, middle, and posterior compartments) measured in relation to the hymen. The anatomic position of the six defined points should be measured in centimeters proximal to the hymen (negative number) or distal to the hymen (positive number), with the plane of the hymen representing zero. Three other measurements in the pelvic organ prolapse quantitative examination (POPQ) include the genital hiatus, perineal body, and the total vaginal length.

The genital hiatus is measured from the middle of the external urethral meatus to the posterior midline hymen. The perineal body is measured from the posterior margin of

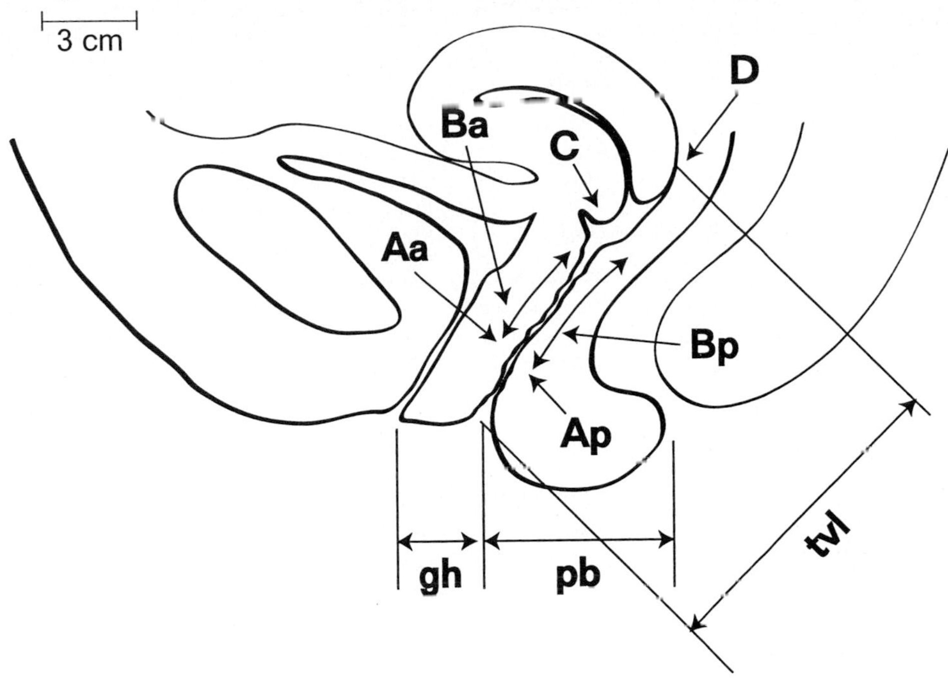

Figure 20.18 Standardization of terminology for female pelvic organ prolapse (POP-Q classification). This diagram demonstrates the anatomic position of the POP-Q sites including six sites involving the anterior *(Aa, Ba)*, middle *(C, D)*, and posterior *(Ap, Bp)* compartments with the genital hiatus *(gh)*, perineal body *(pb)*, and total vaginal length *(tvl)*. (From **Bump RC, Mattiasson A, Bo K, et al.** The standardization of terminology of female pelvic organ prolapse and pelvic floor dysfunction. *Am J Obstet Gynecol* 1996;175:12, with permission.)

the genital hiatus to the midanal opening. The total vaginal length is the greatest depth of the vagina in centimeters when the vaginal apex is reduced to its full normal position (Fig. 20.18). All measurements except the total vaginal length are measured at maximal straining.

The anterior vaginal wall measurements are termed Aa and Ba, with the Ba point moving depending on the amount of anterior compartment prolapse. Point Aa represents a point on the anterior vagina 3 cm proximal to the external urethral meatus, which corresponds to the bladder neck. By definition, the range of position of this point is −3 to +3. Point Ba represents the most distal or dependent point of any portion of the anterior vaginal wall from point Aa to just anterior to the vaginal cuff or anterior lip of the cervix. This point can vary depending on the nature of the patient's support defect. For example, point Ba is −3 in the absence of any prolapse (it is never less than −3) to a positive value equal to the total vaginal length in a patient with total eversion of the vagina.

The middle compartment consists of points C and D. Point C represents the most depend edge of the cervix or vaginal cuff after hysterectomy.

Point D is the location of the posterior fornix; it is omitted if the cervix is absent. This point represents the level of the uterosacral ligament attachment to the posterior cervix. It is meant to differentiate suspensory failure from cervical elongation.

The posterior compartment is measured similarly to the anterior compartment; the corresponding terms are Ap and Bp. The nine measurements can be recorded as a simple line of numbers (i.e., −3, −3, −8, −10, −3, −3, 11, 4, 3 for points Aa, Ba, C, D, Ap, Bp, total vaginal length, genital hiatus, and perineal body). The six vaginal sites have possible

Table 20.6. Possible Ranges of the Six Site-specific Pelvic Organ Prolapse Quantitative Examination Measurements

Points	*Description*	*Range*
Aa	Anterior wall 3 cm from hymen	−3 cm to +3 cm
Ba	Most dependent portion of rest of anterior wall	−3 cm to + TVL
C	Cervix or vaginal cuff	± TVL
D	Posterior fornix (if no prior hysterectomy)	± TVL or omitted
Ap	Posterior wall 3 cm from hymen	−3 cm to +3 cm
Bp	Most dependent portion of rest of posterior wall	−3 to + TVL

TVL, total vaginal length.
(Adapted from **Bump RC, Mattiasson A, Bo K, et al.** The standardization of terminology of female pelvic organ prolapse and pelvic floor dysfunction. *Am J Obstet Gynecol* 1996;175:11–12, with permission.)

ranges, which are dependent on the total vaginal length (Table 20.6). After collection of the site-specific measurements, stages are assigned according to the most dependent portion of the prolapse (Table 20.7). The POPQ examination often appears confusing on initial review; however, a measuring device (i.e., a marked ring forceps or marked cotton-tip applicator) can assist in instructing those unfamiliar with this staging system. The POPQ examination provides a standardized measurement system to allow for more accurate postoperative outcome assessments and to ensure uniform, reliable, and site-specific descriptions of pelvic organ prolapse. An inexpensive demonstration videotape describing the system and showing its use in several patients is available from the American Urogynecology Society.

Symptoms of Prolapse

Asymptomatic pelvic prolapse generally does not require treatment, but the patient should be informed that she is losing some aspects of pelvic support, which may require treatment in the future. Symptomatic prolapse may manifest in several different ways. The most common symptom is a feeling of pressure or that something is protruding from the vagina. Patients often say they feel like they are sitting on an egg or they may complain of a dragging discomfort, which is described as a low backache or feeling of heaviness. Generally, this feeling is relieved by lying down, is less noticeable in the morning, and worsens as the day progresses, particularly if patients are on their feet for long periods. Specific types of prolapse may be associated with specific symptoms. Loss of anterior vaginal support often leads to urethral hypermobility, which in turn often (but not necessarily) results in stress urinary incontinence. A large anterior vaginal prolapse (or vaginal vault eversion) can produce symptoms of voiding difficulty. In such cases, the large prolapse comes out below the urethra, either compressing it from below or kinking it so that bladder emptying is incomplete or intermittent. An anterior protrusion of the rectum into the vaginal canal (rectocele) can cause symptoms of inefficient rectal emptying, often described by the patient as constipation. In severe cases, the patient may have to splint the posterior vagina with a finger during defecation, thereby reducing the pocket that is trapping stool back into its normal position. In most cases, however, constipation in women has causes other than a

Table 20.7. Stages of Pelvic Organ Prolapse

Stage 0	No prolapse is demonstrated. Points Aa, Ap, Ba, Bp are all at −3 cm, and point C is between total vaginal length (TVL) and −(TVL − 2 cm).
Stage I	The most distal portion of the prolapse is >1 cm above the level of the hymen.
Stage II	The most distal portion of the prolapse is <1 cm proximal or distal to the plane of the hymen.
Stage III	The most distal portion of the prolapse is >1 cm below the plane of the hymen but no further than 2 cm less than the total vaginal length
Stage IV	Complete to nearly complete eversion of the vagina. The most distal portion of the prolapse protrudes to at ≥ + (TVL − 2) cm

(From **Bump RC, Mattiasson A, Bo K, et al.** The standardization of terminology of female pelvic organ prolapse and pelvic floor dysfunction. *Am J Obstet Gynecol* 1996;175:13, with permission.)

rectocele. The symptoms that result from a massive prolapse in which the entire uterus or vagina protrudes below the pelvic floor are self-explanatory.

Examination

In examining a patient with pelvic organ prolapse, all aspects of vaginal support should be carefully surveyed. Each area of vaginal anatomy should be described separately, and because **prolapse is almost invariably worse when the patient is upright, the clinician should become accustomed to examining patients in the standing position as well as in the standard dorsal lithotomy position.** The patient should stand on the floor with one foot elevated on a well-supported footstool. The examining gown can be lifted slightly to expose the genital region (Fig. 20.19). A standing pelvic examination allows the prolapse to be assessed when it is at its worst. A rectovaginal examination performed in this position is the best way of detecting an occult enterocele because the small bowel can be palpated easily in the cul-de-sac between the thumb and forefinger. A standing pelvic examination can be conducted quickly and efficiently.

For a patient with prolapse, the traditional speculum examination of the vagina should be supplemented with a site-specific examination of the vagina using either a single-bladed speculum (such as a Sims speculum) or by taking a traditional Graves speculum apart and using the posterior blade as a single-sided retractor. This technique allows the clinician to perform the POPQ measurements by obtaining an adequate view of the anterior, posterior, and lateral vagina, looking for specific defects of vaginal support (Fig. 20.20A–C). This is important because a large prolapse of one side of the vagina may hold a smaller prolapse from the other side in place. This can result in misdiagnosis, such as when a large cystocele obscures the presence of a large rectocele, or when eversion of the vaginal apex is mistaken for a large cystocele.

Figure 20.19 Standing examination of the patient to detect the extent of pelvic organ prolapse. An enterocele is detected during a standing rectovaginal examination by palpating the small bowel between the thumb and index finger.

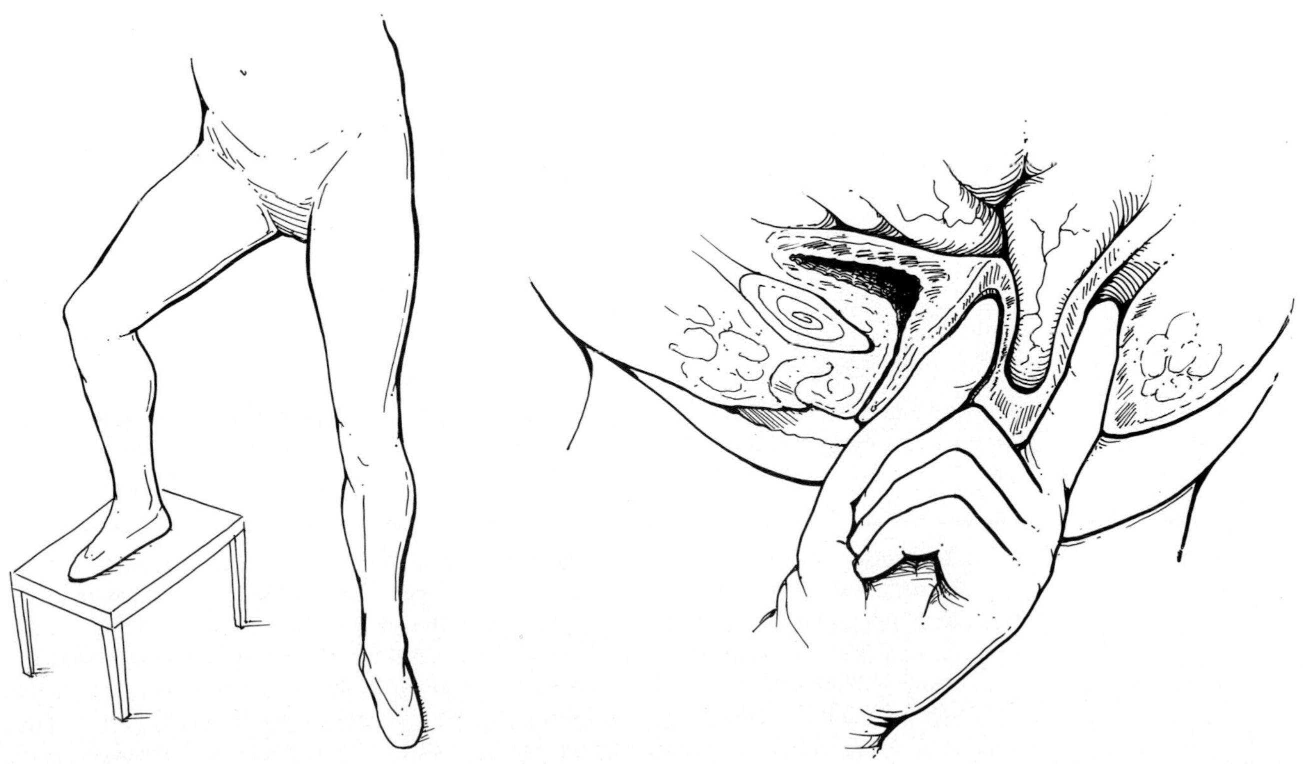

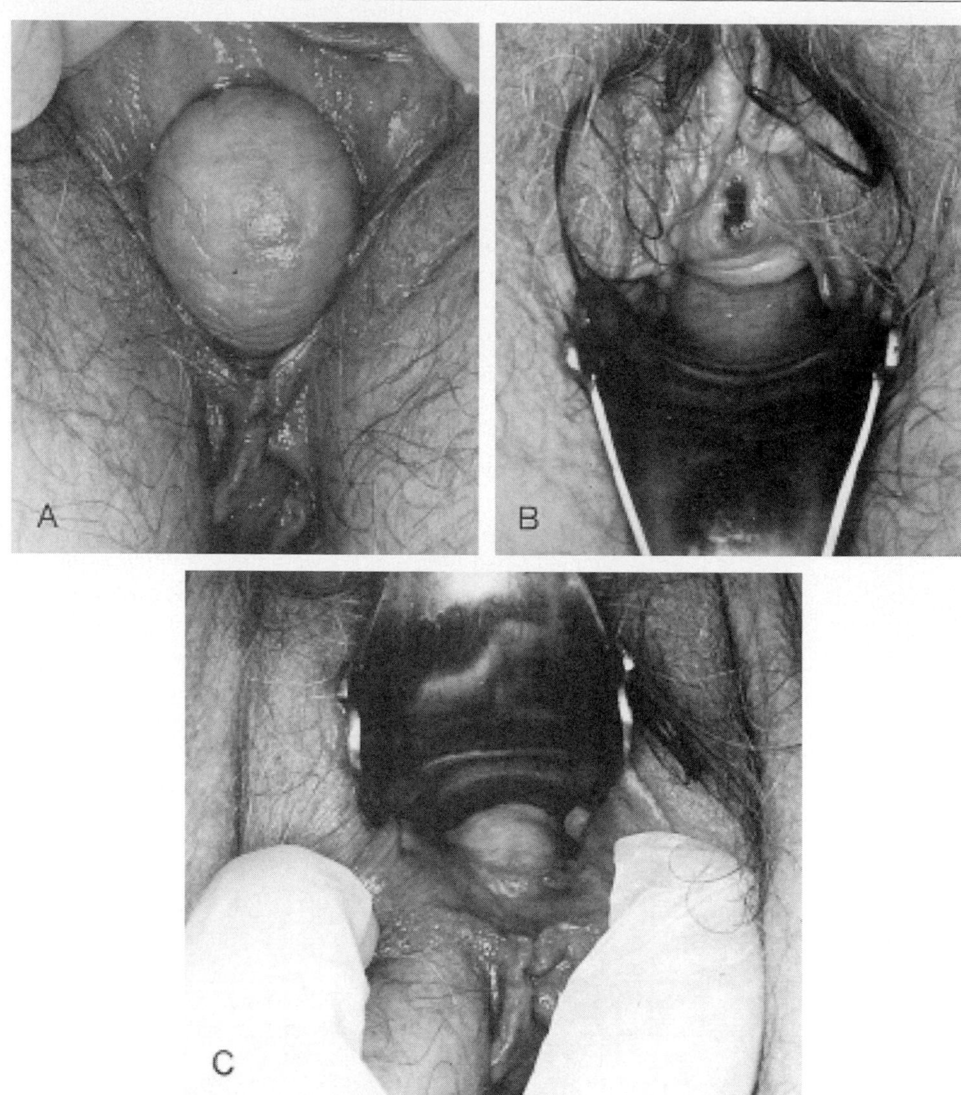

Figure 20.20 Examination of a prolapse whose nature is unclear. A: Without more careful examination, the components of this prolapse are uncertain. When a speculum is place posteriorly **(B)** and anteriorly **(C)** to inspect each vaginal wall separately, the prolapse goes away. This indicates that the patient has a prolapse of the vaginal apex, which has been elevated by the speculum in each instance. (From **Wall LL, Norton PA, DeLancey JOL.** Practical urodynamics. In: *Practical urogynecology.* Baltimore: Williams & Wilkins, 1993:307, with permission.)

As a general rule, any prolapse that lies within the vaginal lumen above the plane of the hymenal ring is of limited significance, particularly if the patient does not have symptoms.

Treatment

Asymptomatic prolapse does not need treatment. An exception is a woman with stress incontinence and prolapse who is about to undergo surgical bladder neck suspension. Most operations for stress incontinence elevate the anterior vagina and, in doing so, pull the posterior vagina forward. This opens the cul-de-sac, pulling it off the levator plate and thereby creating an opening for enterocele formation, the development of uterine prolapse, vaginal vault eversion, or worsening of an asymptomatic rectocele (108). Under these conditions, additional surgery in the form of a culdoplasty, rectocele or enterocele repair, or in some cases, hysterectomy, may be advisable.

Symptomatic prolapse can be treated conservatively or surgically, depending on the individual. Although pelvic muscle exercises may be of benefit to women with stress incontinence by strengthening urethral support, they have not proved beneficial for patients with significant prolapse. The pelvic muscles provide most of the support for the pelvic organs, after this support has become inefficient, increasing stress is placed on the connective tissue involved in pelvic support. When fascial attachments have been disrupted in the presence of poor muscular tone and clinically significant prolapse has developed, attempts to correct the problem by restoring muscular tone are not efficient. Pelvic muscle exercises are virtually never harmful, but under these circumstances, they are not likely to correct the problem.

Pessary

Conservative management of prolapse usually involves fitting the patient with a pessary. A wide variety of shapes and sizes of pessaries are available. The use of pessaries is an important part of gynecologic practice that has been neglected in contemporary gynecologic residency training programs (181). Each patient should be fitted individually with her pessary, much as each individual is fitted for a contraceptive diaphragm. The patient who is using a pessary should have a well-estrogenized vagina. Postmenopausal women should be given hormone replacement therapy, or alternatively, they should use intravaginal estrogen cream on a regular basis. **For women who are past menopause, it is preferable to use intravaginal estrogen cream 4 to 6 weeks before the pessary is inserted because this makes the pessary more comfortable to wear, dramatically increases compliance, and promotes long-term use.**

Complications of pessary use include chronic irritation and erosion of a pessary into the bladder, creating a vesicovaginal fistula (182,183). All such cases are caused by neglect rather than the pessary itself. Patients who are using pessaries, particularly older women, should be examined on a regular basis. Some pessaries, such as the silicone doughnut pessary, can be left in place for months at a time without removal or inspection. Other pessaries, such as the cube pessary, which provides vaginal support through a gentle suction effect, ideally should be removed by the patient at bedtime each night and replaced in the morning to avoid erosions. The exact schedule of care should be based on individual circumstances. At the initial fitting, the patient should be encouraged to insert and remove the pessary herself. If the pessary fits and the patient is comfortable, it is helpful to reexamine her within 1 week and at least every 4 to 6 months thereafter.

Surgery

Traditionally, prolapse has been treated by surgery, the nature of which depends on the type of prolapse. The goal of surgery should be to relieve the patient of her symptoms by repairing each aspect of abnormal pelvic support in a durable and long-lasting manner. A detailed description of the various operations for managing pelvic support defects is beyond the scope of this chapter and can be obtained elsewhere (184,185); however, a few general remarks are in order.

Most patients with prolapse have defects in more than one location; thus, attention should be paid to correcting all defects during the same operation. Operations for prolapse are generally, but not always, carried out through the vaginal route rather than through the abdominal surgical route. Some conditions, such as stress urinary incontinence, are more reliably handled by an abdominal operation.

Operations for Vaginal Prolapse

Vaginal Hysterectomy **Uterine prolapse is generally treated with vaginal hysterectomy, which may be accomplished by several different techniques.** The advantage of vaginal hysterectomy is that it allows other vaginal surgery (e.g., anterior and posterior colporrhaphy or enterocele repair) to be performed at the same time, without the need for a separate incision or for repositioning the patient. At the time of hysterectomy for prolapse, special attention should be paid to closing the cul-de-sac using a McCall culdoplasty and to reattaching the endopelvic fascia and the uterosacral ligaments to the vaginal cuff to provide additional support (186). These same steps should be performed with abdominal hysterectomy (187). This reattachment to the uterosacral ligaments can be used both as a prophylactic procedure to prevent future posthysterectomy vaginal vault prolapse and as treatment for uterine prolapse. A modification to the standard plication, the high lateral fixation of the vaginal apex bilaterally without midline plication of the uterosacral ligaments, recreates normal anatomy with durable results (188,189). With any reconstructive procedure that requires plication or suspension to the uterosacral complex, care must be taken to avoid the ureters and ensure their postoperative patency (190).

Manchester/Fothergill Operation An alternative to hysterectomy for patients with uterine prolapse is the Manchester operation, originally described in 1888 by Donald and subsequently modified by Fothergill. In this operation, the bladder is dissected off the cervix, which is then amputated. The cardinal ligaments are sewn to the anterior cervical stump, and the posterior vagina is closed over the rest of the opening. This operation is usually performed in conjunction with an anteroposterior colporrhaphy, and it is usually done for the sake of expediency in patients who are poor surgical risks and who do not desire future fertility.

Uteropexy Occasionally, marked uterine prolapse may develop in a young nulliparous patient who desires to retain her fertility. If prolapse cannot be managed successfully with a pessary, such patients present a surgical challenge. The older abdominal uterine suspension operations (Baldy-Webster, Gilliam, ventrofixation, or hysteropexy) do not work for patients with significant uterine prolapse. There is anecdotal evidence of success in such patients using sacrospinous ligament fixation or retroperitoneal abdominal uterosacropexy, suturing mesh or fascia to the uterosacral ligaments and then to the anterior longitudinal ligament of the sacrum. There is little information available regarding long-term follow-up of such patients.

Paravaginal Defect Repair Operation Anterior vaginal prolapse has been treated with anterior colporrhaphy, plicating the endopelvic fascia in the midline under the bladder neck. If the anterior vaginal prolapse results from a lateral detachment of the endopelvic fascia from the lateral pelvic sidewall, however, better results will be obtained by performing a lateral repair. In this technique, the endopelvic fascia is reattached to the arcus tendineus fasciae pelvis through what is referred to as a *paravaginal defect repair* operation (91,92,177,178). Although generally this procedure is performed through an abdominal incision, operating in the space of Retzius, some surgeons are now performing it through a vaginal incision. In patients with severe or recurrent anterior defects, the traditional repair is now being reinforced with fascia lata or another graft material (191,192).

Posterior Colporrhaphy Repair of posterior vaginal prolapse for rectocele and enterocele is also performed vaginally using posterior colporrhaphy. In a rectocele repair, the posterior vagina is opened, the rectum is dissected away from the pararectal fascia, and the levator ani muscles are plicated over the rectum in the midline, after which the vaginal epithelium is closed. Because of concern over postoperative dyspareunia, recent modifications of posterior colporrhaphy have included site-specific repair. In this technique, the posterior vaginal epithelium is opened in the traditional fashion, and breaks in vaginal muscularis or Denonvillier's fascia are identified by using a finger in the rectum to demonstrate the defect. The traumatic separations may occur in various directions and be of varying magnitude; however, it is usually possible to identify and repair these defects (193,194). The site-specific repair technique for posterior compartment relaxation offers a more logical correction than the standard plication procedure and appears to have success rates similar to those of traditional approaches but with less vaginal narrowing.

An enterocele is a peritoneal hernia, usually seen over the rectum, often appearing as a second bump higher up in the vaginal canal on examination. The peritoneal sac should be carefully identified, opened, and closed with several pursestring sutures of permanent material; the sac should be excised, and the vagina should be closed once more over the defect. If the perineal body is noted to be deficient and the patient has a gaping introitus, this deficit may be repaired by a perineorrhaphy or perineoplasty, in which the vaginal fourchette is opened and the base of the levator ani muscle is pulled together in the midline, providing renewed support for the lateral vagina at its outlet.

Operations for Complete Eversion of the Vagina

Among the most challenging cases are those involving complete eversion of the vagina in patients who have had a previous hysterectomy. This condition virtually always requires surgical correction because of the large size of the prolapse, its propensity to enlarge over time because of increases in intraabdominal pressure, and the rare danger of vaginal evisceration if it is not treated.

Colpectomy and Colpocleisis For some patients, particularly elderly women who are not sexually active and who lead a sedentary lifestyle, the condition can be managed by surgically removing the vagina and closing off the space (colpectomy and colpocleisis). The correction of a significant and bothersome pelvic prolapse in elderly patients can often be completed using this technique with local anesthesia. These operations have proved very successful in preventing recurrent prolapse if patients are selected properly (195). The surgeon must consider both the patient's future coital activity as well as underlying issues relating to self-image if consideration is given to an obliterative procedure.

Colpopexy A different procedure is required for younger women and for women who wish to retain sexual function. For these women, the condition can be managed transvaginally or transabdominally. With the transvaginal approach, vaginal eversion is corrected by suturing one or both sides of the vaginal apex (usually the right side) to the sacrospinous ligament with one or two sutures—a transvaginal sacrospinous colpopexy. Other transvaginal reconstructive procedures for the management of advanced posthysterectomy vaginal vault prolapse (stage 3 to 4) include enterocele ligation and uterosacral ligament suspension or vaginal vault suspension using the iliococcygeal fascia on the pelvic sidewall. These procedures are performed transvaginally and have demonstrated effectiveness in restoring normal vaginal anatomy (197,198). In the transabdominal approach, the vaginal apex is suspended from the anterior longitudinal ligament along the sacrum using a graft of fascia or artificial mesh that is sutured to the vagina and to the sacrum in a retroperitoneal position—a transabdominal sacral colpopexy. The vaginal suspension should always be combined with a meticulous culdoplasty to repair the enterocele that coexists with vaginal eversion. All these operations are highly successful in resuspending the vaginal apex (196–199). Because the lines of force produced by increases in intraabdominal pressure are directed across the vagina differently after the two operations, patients who have recurrent prolapse postoperatively tend to have different problems. As a rule, recurrent anterior vaginal prolapse is more common in patients with vaginal eversion if they have had a sacrospinous ligament fixation, whereas recurrent posterior vaginal prolapse is more common if they have undergone an abdominal sacral colpopexy. Some authors have suggested that recurrent posterior relaxation can be prevented by a colpoperineopexy in which mesh is attached all the way down to the perineal body during the suspension operation (200). It is unclear which is the best route for correcting posthysterectomy vaginal vault prolapse, and there are few clinical data comparing the vaginal or abdominal approaches (201,202). The most appropriate procedure must be individualized to each patient's clinical findings and the operating surgeon's expertise in reconstructive pelvic surgery.

Colorectal Dysfunction

Pelvic floor disorders span all three anatomic compartments of the pelvis: urinary, genital, and colorectal. Any approach to pelvic floor dysfunction that ignores colonic and rectal problems will not meet the needs of these women. Disorders of colonic and rectal function are disproportionately prevalent among women and represent a major area of continuing clinical neglect in women's health care (1). Although gynecologists and urologists have made great strides in jointly evaluating and treating urinary incontinence, to date neither specialty has done a creditable job of incorporating the treatment of posterior compartment problems into patient care. Because they are often the first physicians that women see for pelvic floor disorders, gynecologists have an obligation to become knowledgeable about common colorectal complaints. Not only can many of these problems be evaluated and treated initially by gynecologists, but a familiarity with colorectal conditions and a good working relationship with a colon and rectal surgeon or an interested gastroenterologist will also help educate practitioners of these specialties about the genitourinary complaints that frequently accompany disorders of the posterior pelvis. Among the more common conditions with which gynecologists should be familiar are anal incontinence, rectal prolapse, constipation, fecal impaction, and irritable bowel syndrome (see Chapter 14).

Anal Incontinence

Anal incontinence refers to involuntary passage of flatus or feces (either liquid or formed stool) through the anal canal. The term *anal incontinence* is therefore a more comprehensive term than *fecal incontinence,* which refers only to the involuntary passage of stool (203,204). Many women have disabling loss of gas, even though they are able to control feces. Although it is becoming more acceptable socially to talk about urinary incontinence, discussion of fecal loss still remains a taboo subject. Even patients with severe anal incontinence often will refuse to bring this problem to the attention of their doctor because of the extreme embarrassment involved. Physicians must ask patients directly (but sensitively) about loss of bowel control in order to elicit this complaint. The problem is more prevalent than most people realize: in one large household survey, 7.1% of the general population reported some degree of anal incontinence (205).

Diagnosis

Normal anal continence depends on the harmonious integration of many factors, including anal sphincter function, anorectal sensation and reflexes, colonic transit, rectal distensibility (compliance), stool consistency, stool volume, and the patient's level of mental functioning. As in the case of urinary incontinence, there are multiple potential causes of anal incontinence (203–209) (Table 20.8).

History

A thorough history regarding bowel function should delineate the nature and frequency of anal loss. Loss of flatus alone is usually (but not necessarily) less troublesome than frequent loss of formed stool. The presence of liquid stool or diarrhea often represents a challenge that a decompensated sphincter cannot withstand, and this condition may respond favorably to bulking agents. If the history is uncertain, administration of a normal saline enema often is helpful in determining the diagnosis. The patient who can retain 1,000 to 1,500 mL of normal saline without leakage is unlikely to have a significant problem with anal incontinence (207). Important pieces of information include changes in stool frequency or consistency, history of blood in the stool, associated medical conditions (especially diabetes and related neurologic problems), medication use, obstetric history, and any history of pelvic or perianal surgery. It is also important to determine whether the patient ever notices anything protruding from the anus because rectal prolapse often is associated with anal incontinence.

Examination

The perineum should be carefully inspected to determine the state of hygiene, the presence of fissures, and the status of the anal sphincter. Pelvic muscle reflexes should be checked in all patients with anal incontinence, and a vaginal and bimanual examination should

Table 20.8. Causes of Fecal Incontinence

Normal Pelvic Floor
Diarrheal states
Infectious diarrhea
Inflammatory bowel disease
Short gut syndrome
Laxative abuse
Radiation enteritis
Overflow
Impaction
Encopresis
Rectal neoplasms
Neurologic conditions
Congenital anomalies (e.g., myelomeningocele)
Multiple sclerosis
Dementia, strokes, tabes dorsalis
Neuropathy (e.g., diabetes)
Neoplasms of brain, spinal cord, cauda equina
Injuries to brain, spinal cord, cauda equina
Abnormal Pelvic Floor
Congenital anorectal malformation
Trauma
Accidental injury (e.g., impalement, pelvic fracture)
Anorectal surgery
Obstetrical injury
Aging
Pelvic floor denervation (idiopathic neurogenic incontinence)
Vaginal delivery
Chronic straining at stool
Rectal prolapse
Descending perineum syndrome

(From **Madoof RD, Williams JG, Caushaj PF.** Fecal incontinence. *N Engl J Med* 1992;326:1002–1007, with permission.)

be performed. The possibility of a disrupted sphincter or a rectovaginal fistula must be considered. The patient should be examined while straining to check for the presence of rectal prolapse. All patients should undergo a digital rectal examination with testing of the stool for occult blood: at least 50% of rectal carcinomas lie within reach of the examiner's finger. Many patients with fecal incontinence have a fecal impaction, which should be removed (210,211). The puborectalis muscle should be palpated through the posterior rectum. When the patient contracts this muscle, the examiner's finger should move anteriorly. Poor sphincter tone is indicated by gaping of the rectum when the puborectalis muscle is depressed. Direct inspection of the large intestine through the use of flexible sigmoidoscopy or colonoscopy should be considered in all patients.

Tests

The American Gastroenterological Association has recently reviewed the major tests currently available for the evaluation of anorectal function (212). Anorectal manometry, endoanal ultrasonography, and evacuation proctography (defecography) are the most useful diagnostic tests; there are others, but they are less useful in clinical decision making.

Anorectal Manometry Anorectal manometry is a test performed to evaluate anorectal sensation, resting and squeeze pressures, compliance (distensibility), and reflexes. The test may be performed with solid-state transducers or water-perfusion techniques. In anorectal manometry, the pressure-measuring device is slowly withdrawn through the rectum and anal canal at rest and during intermittent squeeze maneuvers. Pressure gradients are calculated, and the response of the anus and rectum to distention with an air-filled balloon is evaluated. Specific resting and squeeze values cannot distinguish continent from incontinent patients, but patients with low squeeze pressures are more likely, as a group, to be incontinent than those who have higher values. Patients with low anal compliance (often due to radiation fibrosis or proctitis) tend to have urgency symptoms; when these patients undergo anorectal surgery, they tend to have less successful operative outcomes. Measurement of sensory thresholds is important in patients with anal incontinence because one of the most effective interventions is biofeedback training to improve anorectal sensation (213).

Endoanal Ultrasonography Endoanal ultrasonography is performed using a rotating ultrasound probe inserted into the anal canal that produces a circumferential view of the anatomy of the internal and external anal sphincters. It is currently the procedure of choice for evaluating sphincter damage, particularly from obstetric causes. Endoanal ultrasonography performed after vaginal childbirth has revealed a very high rate of occult sphincter injury in women who did not have a known perineal laceration at delivery (214). Although many of these women do not have symptoms in the immediate postpartum period, the long-term consequences of occult sphincter injury are unclear. Such an injury may play an important role in the development of anal incontinence in later life. Endoanal ultrasonography is important in helping the clinician decide whether surgical repair will aid patients who have anal incontinence.

Evacuation Proctography Evacuation proctography is a radiographic test in which stool-like contrast material (usually a barium paste) is instilled into the rectum. The utility of the test can be enhanced by putting additional contrast in the bladder and vagina and by having the patient ingest contrast material before the study to opacify the small bowel. Cinefluoroscopic images are then taken with the patient sitting on a radiolucent commode so that the mechanism of rectal evacuation can be studied. The test is useful for evaluating puborectalis muscle function, detecting the presence of occult enteroceles, and evaluating patients for the presence of rectal prolapse and intussusception. These studies are most useful if done collaboratively by a pelvic floor physician and radiologist with special interest in this area (215).

Because the external anal sphincter is innervated by the pudendal nerve, assessment of pudendal nerve function would appear to have a role in the evaluation of patients with anal incontinence. Unfortunately, the pudendal nerve is hidden in the pelvis and traverses a tortuous pathway from the sacral spinal cord to the perineum, which varies significantly among different individuals. To date, it has not been possible to measure the length of the pudendal nerve accurately in individual patients; therefore, precise measurement of pudendal nerve conduction velocity (time of impulse transmission/length of pudendal nerve) is not possible. Numerous attempts have been made to correlate the time (latency) between a stimulus applied to the pudendal nerve at the ischial spine and its appearance at the anal sphincter, but the studies that correlate these results with clinical findings and surgical outcome are conflicting and their utility is questionable. The American Gastroenterology Association does not recommend this test in the evaluation of patients with fecal incontinence (212).

Treatment

Effective treatment of anal incontinence depends on its cause (204). The first step in treating fecal incontinence is usually bowel management, especially in patients with fecal impaction and resulting "overflow" incontinence. These patients respond well to disimpaction and the subsequent regular use of stool softeners and laxatives. Diarrhea can be evaluated and treated with bulking agents, often with surprisingly successful results. Antiflatulence preparations such as *Beano* (AK Pharma, Pleasantville, NJ) are often very helpful. High-fiber diets and stool-bulking agents will help the patient develop a more consistent stool that can be controlled more easily by the sphincter muscles. Antidiarrheal agents, such as loperamide or diphenoxylate with atropine, are also helpful. Daily tap water enemas can be used to help keep the rectum empty and to schedule predictable daily bowel movements. Biofeedback training is useful in helping patients regain control of sphincteric activity, especially when they have impaired rectal sensation. This technique allows patients to strengthen the muscles of the pelvic floor, to sense smaller volumes of stool in the rectum, and to improve their control over the anal sphincter mechanism, often with surprisingly good results (216).

Surgical repair should be considered in patients who have a demonstrable sphincter defect. The best results appear to be obtained using an overlapping sphincteroplasty rather than an end-to-end reapproximation of the torn sphincter (217). Although restoration of complete continence in most patients with an old sphincter injury is unlikely, the chance for substantial improvement is great enough that all patients should be offered the option of surgical repair if they are otherwise suitable candidates, irrespective of age (204). Patients with a rectovaginal fistula will obviously benefit from fistula closure. For some patients, construction of an anal neosphincter using transplanted gracilis muscle driven by an implanted pacemaker may be of benefit (218). Patients who have severe persistent incontinence after biofeedback therapy, medical management, and surgical treatment may be candidates for colostomy. An algorithm for the evaluation and treatment of fecal incontinence is given in Fig. 20.21 (204).

Rectal Prolapse

Rectal prolapse is relatively uncommon but nonetheless is a significant clinical problem for those unfortunate enough to experience it. About 90% of patients with rectal prolapse are women (219). Normally, the rectum is attached firmly to the levator ani muscle complex through an extensive interweaving of longitudinal muscle fibers. This attachment is important because the rectum undergoes multiple changes in position and location during the normal act of defecation. Without this attachment, the rectum would slip down through the levator muscle hiatus during defecation. In rectal prolapse, this actually occurs. An intussusception of the rectum develops (for reasons not totally clear). Gradually, over time, the intussusception pulls the rectum away from its sacral attachments, ultimately allowing it to appear at or beyond the anal verge. Predisposing factors associated with rectal prolapse are summarized in Table 20.9 (219).

Diagnosis

Most patients with rectal prolapse consider the presence of the prolapse itself as the major problem. Many patients have constipation; however, fecal incontinence also is commonly associated with rectal prolapse. Stretch injury of the pudendal and pelvic nerves may cause denervation injury to the rectum and resultant incontinence, but this finding is not always present. As the prolapse worsens, patients must replace the rectum manually to defecate. Occasionally, a rectal prolapse may become incarcerated; rarely, there is a transanal evisceration of small bowel from a ruptured rectal prolapse.

Patients with rectal prolapse should be examined while straining. If their sphincter tone is poor and the anus is patulous, subsequent surgical repair may not be satisfactory. If the tone of the pelvic muscles is good, however, the prognosis is more favorable. An important point is whether the prolapse is a full-thickness prolapse of the rectum or whether it is only a prolapse of the rectal mucosa. Examination of patients with rectal prolapse should include both digital examination and a thorough proctosigmoidoscopic or colonoscopic examination because a colonic cancer or sigmoidal polyp may form at the point at which an intussusception develops. Changes associated with the solitary rectal ulcer syndrome are frequently seen in patients with early rectal prolapse. The value of evacuation proctography in the evaluation of rectal prolapse is well established (215,220,221).

Treatment

Partial or incomplete rectal mucosal prolapse generally can be treated with anal surgery, often involving only excision of the affected area. Complete rectal prolapse is a more complicated problem, with more than 200 operations having been described for the treatment

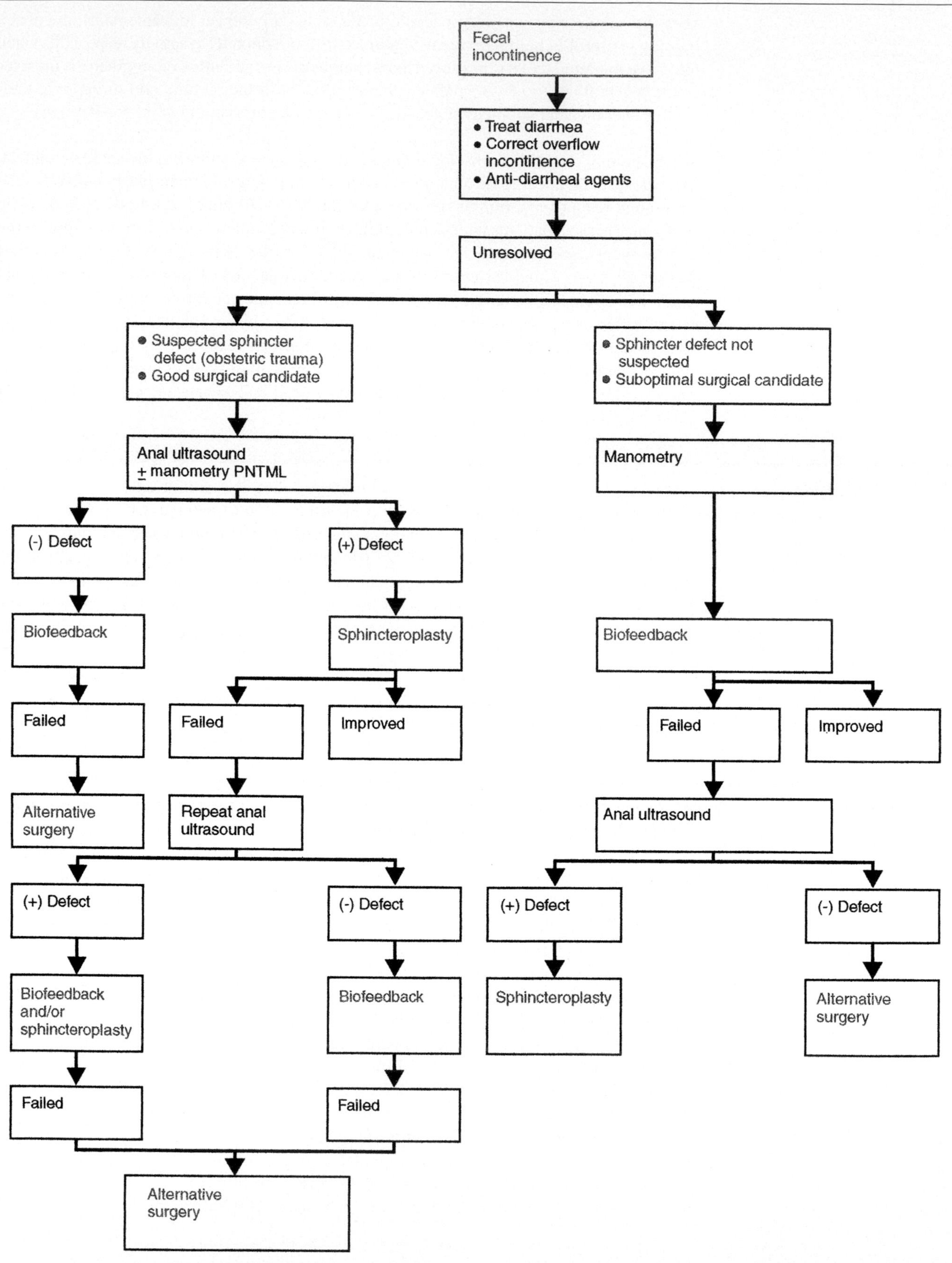

Figure 20.21 Treatment algorithm for fecal incontinence. (From **Soffer EE, Hull T.** Fecal incontinence: a practical approach to evaluation and treatment. *Am J Gastroentererol* 2000;95:1879, with permission.)
PNTML, pudendal nerve terminal motor latency

Table 20.9. Factors Associated with or Predisposing to Rectal Prolapse

Poor bowel habits (especially constipation)
Neurologic disease (e.g., congenital anomaly, cauda equina lesion, spinal cord injury, senility)
Female sex
Nulliparity
Redundant rectosigmoid
Deep pouch of Douglas
Patulous anus (weak internal sphincter)
Diastasis of levator ani muscle (defect in pelvic floor)
Lack of fixation of rectum to sacrum
Intussusception (also, secondary to colonic lesions)
Operative procedure (e.g., hemorrhoidectomy, fistulectomy, abdominoanal pull-through)

(From **Corman ML.** Rectal prolapse. In: *Colon and rectal surgery.* 2nd ed. Philadelphia: JB Lippincott, 1989:209–247, with permission.)

of this condition. The proposed operations include or combine several modes of therapy, such as narrowing the anal orifice, obliteration of the cul-de-sac, restoration of the pelvic floor, resection of bowel, and suspension or fixation of the rectum. In general, some form of rectopexy appears to have the highest success rate, the lowest recurrence rate, and an acceptable level of complications. Several concise but comprehensive reviews of this subject have recently been prepared (222–224).

Constipation

Constipation is a common patient concern, yet there is no generally accepted definition of the term (225). Commonly used definitions include frequent straining at stool (more than 25% of the time) or fewer than three bowel movements per week. Nearly 95% of normal individuals have between three bowel movements per day and three bowel movements per week. In surveys of patients not seeking medical care for gastrointestinal disorders, between 10% to 20% appear to have symptoms of constipation; most of these individuals are female (226,227). Constipation is less frequent among the young and increases to its highest prevalence in old age. Because there is no generally accepted definition of constipation, the physician must generally take the patient's reports of this problem at face value and then attempt to understand what she means by this term. Constipation is a symptom, rather than a disease, produced by many different factors (228) (Table 20.10). Most patients who describe themselves as constipated can be treated with laxatives, increased fiber intake, and the development of regular dietary habits. Only a small percentage of patients have "intractable" constipation, but these patients should undergo an appropriate evaluation.

Diagnosis

Because of its high prevalence among women, physicians should be well versed in the treatment of constipation. The goal of treatment for patients with chronic constipation is restoration of normal frequency and consistency of stools without the need to strain during defecation (229). Restoration should be accomplished with as little artificial intervention as possible, and it should result in the diminution of any associated symptoms such as crampy abdominal pain or bloating. Because stool of normal consistency is about 70% water, the mainstays in the treatment of constipation are water and fiber. The fiber serves as a bulking agent that can trap water and promote an increased mass of stool. The normal dietary fiber intake should be 14 g/d. Unprocessed bran is the most readily available fiber supplement. If it is not available, *psyllium* can also be used. The type of fiber is not nearly as important as adequate fiber intake. One inexpensive and highly useful dietary recipe for use

Table 20.10. Causes of Constipation

Anorectal Disorders	Anal fissure; anal stenosis; anterior mucosal prolapse; descending perineum syndrome; hemorrhoids; perineal abscess; rectocele; tumors
Colonic Disorders	Irritable bowel syndrome; diverticular disease, tumors; strictures; carcinoma; Crohn's disease; diverticulitis; ulcerative colitis; ischemic colitis; tuberculosis; amebiasis; syphilis; lymphogranuloma venereum; hernias; volvulus; intussusception; ulcerative colitis with right-sdied fecal stasis; pneumatosis cystoides intestinalis; idiopathic slow transit constipation
Pelvic Causes	Pregnancy and the puerperium; ovarian and uterine tumors; endometriosis
Neuromuscular Causes	*Peripheral causes:* Hirschprung's disease; autonomic neuropathy; Chaga's disease; intestinal pseudoobstruction *Central causes:* cerebrovascular accident; cerebral tumors; Parkinson's disease; meningocele; disseminated sclerosis; tabes dorsalis; paraplegia; cauda equina tumor; trauma to the lumbosacral cord or cauda equina; Shy-Drager syndrome *Muscular causes:* dermatomyositis; dystrophia myotonica; progressive systemic sclerosis
Psychiatric Disorders	Depression; anorexia nervosa; denied bowel action
Endocrine Causes	Diabetes mellitus; hypercalcemia; hypothyroidism; hypopituitarism; pheochromocytoma
Metabolic Causes	Hypokalemia; lead poisoning; porphyria; uremia
Environmental Causes	Debility; dehydration; immobilization; use of a bed pan
Drug-induced	Anesthetics; analgesics; antacids containing aluminum and calcium; anticholinergics; anticonvulsants; antidepressives; antihypertensives; antiparkinsonian drugs; diuretics; ganglion-blocking drugs; iron; habitual laxatives abuse; monoamine oxidase inhibitors; oral contraceptives; psychotherapeutic agents.

(From **Moriatry KJ, Irving MH.** Constipation. *BMJ* 1992;304:1237–1240, with permission.)

by constipated patients involves mixing about 1 cup of Miller's bran, $^1/_2$ cup of applesauce, and $^1/_4$ cup of prune juice to desired consistency, storing it under refrigeration, and taking 1 to 2 tablespoons per day. This can be taken straight, or mixed with fruit or cereal, and titrated to the desired results.

Treatment

Laxatives are an important adjunct to fiber and water in the treatment of constipation. Literally hundreds of laxative preparations are available. They can be divided into two main groups: stimulant laxatives and mechanical laxatives. Stimulant laxatives (e.g., *cascara, senna,* castor oil, *bisacodyl,* and *diphenylmethane*) cause increased peristaltic activity in the colon. Stimulant laxatives may be used occasionally, but chronic use should be avoided because the bowel may become dependent on them. Side effects of stimulant laxatives can include cramps and urgent, explosive defecation. The mechanical laxatives include salts such as sodium phosphate or magnesium sulfate, mineral oil, and surfactants such as *docusate sodium.* These agents increase peristalsis by changing stool consistency or increasing stool bulk. Agents such as lactulose produce an osmotic catharsis. Oral agents such as mineral oil work by decreasing water absorption from the stool, thereby keeping it soft. If taken orally, mineral oil should be used with caution because inhalation can lead to serious aspiration pneumonia, particularly in elderly or debilitated patients.

Enemas and suppositories are also useful. An enema is particularly helpful in removing an acute fecal impaction. The best enemas are usually the simplest: warm tap water or equal parts of water, glycerin, and mineral oil. The use of these agents is preferable to soap enemas or hypertonic phosphate enemas, which are particularly irritating. Injudicious use of enemas can cause electrolyte imbalances or colonic perforation. Suppositories are helpful in the periodic evacuation of the lower bowel. Insertion of a simple glycerin suppository will usually initiate defecation within 1 hour without chemical stimulation of the colon.

Attention should always be paid to other factors influencing the normal action of the gut. Patients should be taught not to suppress defecation but to make use of the normal gastrocolic reflex that promotes a call to stool about 30 minutes after a meal (usually breakfast). Regular meals help promote regular bowel movements. Regular exercise, even exercise as simple as a brisk walk, has an important influence on regular defecation, as well as on general fitness and well-being.

Attention to good bowel habits, adequate fiber intake, and occasional laxative use should help prevent fecal impaction. Although this condition can occur at any age, elderly and institutionalized patients are at particular risk for impaction (210). Continued passage of stool does not rule out impaction. Many impacted patients develop diarrhea and anal incontinence, as well as nausea, anorexia, vomiting, and abdominal pain, as loose bowel contents bypass the point of impaction. The diagnosis of fecal impaction can usually be established by rectal examination, although a fecal impaction is sometimes located high in the colon. The impacted stool may be hard or soft and may be a single mass or multiple pellets. If the patient's presentation suggests an impaction but one cannot be detected on rectal examination, it may be useful to obtain an x-ray of the abdomen. Fecal masses or unusual air-fluid levels may be detected with this technique. Once diagnosed, the impaction should be removed by fragmenting the fecal mass manually and removing it piecemeal. This usually can be accomplished using local anesthesia (*lidocaine* jelly) and liberal amounts of lubricant, combined with pressure on the posterior vagina. After the mass has been broken up, tap water enemas and *bisacodyl* suppositories will help finish expelling it. The patient should then be placed on a bowel regimen thereafter to prevent the recurrence of future impactions.

Conservative measures, including adequate fluid intake, a high-fiber diet, and occasional laxative use, should allow most women with constipation to regain normal bowel habits of at least three movements per week. If a trial of 3 to 6 months of conservative therapy in a compliant patient is unsuccessful in relieving the constipation, further evaluation should be undertaken. Constipation is not a diagnosis but rather is a symptom that may be associated with many different pathologic states. The major concerns in the evaluation of intractable constipation are ruling out an underlying colonic pathology (i.e., carcinoma, intussusception) and picking up those patients with altered colonic motility ("slow-transit" constipation) or a nonrelaxing puborectalis muscle ("spastic pelvic floor syndrome").

Gynecologists in particular should be on guard against the common assumption that all women with constipation and a rectocele have a condition that is correctable by surgery. Concomitant pathology often is present. The further examination of patients with constipation should include endoscopic examination of the colon and rectum and referral to a colorectal physiology laboratory for more sophisticated studies, including segmental colonic transit studies, anorectal manometry, pelvic floor electromyography, and defecography (225). If blood is present in the stool, if the constipation is painful, if constipation is the result of a sudden change in bowel habits, or if the clinician is otherwise suspicious of a more serious disease process, these studies should be performed earlier in the course of treatment. When the usual sets of studies reveal no cause, constipation is considered functional or nonorganic (226). Most patients with severe functional constipation are young women (227–229). Many of these women appear to have disordered colonic motility of unknown etiology, and many of them exhibit paradoxical contraction (rather than relaxation) of the pelvic floor during defecation, resulting in fecal outflow obstruction. This condition has been termed the spastic pelvic floor syndrome. Although they are refractory to treatment by fiber supplementation and laxatives, some of these patients appear to benefit from biofeedback therapy that enables them to learn normal patterns of defecation and to relax the pelvic floor during a bowel movement (230). The possibility that they may have been victims of sexual abuse should always be considered in the differential diagnosis of such patients.

References

1. **Wall LL, DeLancey JOL.** The politics of prolapse: a revisionist approach to disorders of the pelvic floor in women. *Perspect Biol Med* 1991;34:486–496.
2. **Parks AG, Porter NH, Melzack J.** Experimental study of the reflex mechanism controlling the muscles of the pelvic floor. *Dis Colon Rectum* 1962;5:407–414.
3. **Zacharin RF.** Pulsion enterocele: review of functional anatomy of the pelvic floor. *Obstet Gynecol* 1980;55:135–140.
4. **Dickinson RL.** Studies of the levator ani muscle. *Am J Obstet Dis Women* 1889;22:897–917.
5. **Kegel AJ.** Sexual functions of the pubococcygeus muscle. *West J Obstet Gynecol* 1952;60:521–524.
6. **Gillan P, Brindley GS.** Vaginal and pelvic floor responses to sexual stimulation. *Psychophysiology* 1979;16:471–481.
7. **Wall LL.** The muscles of the pelvic floor. *Clin Obstet Gynecol* 1993;36:910–925.
8. **Lawson JO.** Pelvic anatomy I: pelvic floor muscles. *Ann R Coll Surg Engl* 1974;54:244–252.
9. **DeLancey JOL.** Structural aspects of the extrinsic continence mechanism. *Obstet Gynecol* 1988;72:296–301.
10. **DeLancey JOL.** Correlative study of paraurethral anatomy. *Obstet Gynecol* 1986;68:91–97.
11. **DeLancey JOL.** Structural support of the urethra as it relates to stress urinary incontinence: the hammock hypothesis. *Am J Obstet Gynecol* 1994;170:1713–1723.
12. **Gosling JA, Dixson JS, Critchley HOD, et al.** A comparative study of the human external sphincter and periurethral levator ani muscles. *Br J Urol* 1981;53:35–41.
13. **Berglas B, Rubin IC.** Study of the supportive structures of the uterus by levator myography. *Surg Gynecol Obstet* 1953;97:677–692.
14. **DeLancey JOL.** Anatomy and biomechanics of genital prolapse. *Clin Obstet Gynecol* 1993;36:897–909.
15. **Norton PA.** Pelvic floor disorders: the role of fascia and ligaments. *Clin Obstet Gynecol* 1993;36:926–938.
16. **Bird J.** The effects of pregnancy on joint mobility. *J Orthop Res* 1984;41:345–349.
17. **Brincat M, Versi E, Moniz C, et al.** Skin collagen changes in postmenopausal women receiving different regimens of estrogen. *Obstet Gynecol* 1987;70:123–127.
18. **Castelo-Branco C, Duran M, Gonzalez-Merlo J.** Skin collagen changes related to age and hormone replacement therapy. *Maturitas* 1992;15:113–119.
19. **Suominen H, Heikken E, Parkatti T.** Effects of eight weeks physical training on muscle and connective tissue of the m. vastus lateralis in 69-year-old-men and women. *J Gerontol* 1977;32:33–37.
20. **Lind J.** *A treatise on the scurvy.* 3rd ed. S. Crowder London: 1772:113.
21. **Al-Rawi R, Al-Rawi L.** Joint hypermobility in multiparous Iraqi women with genital prolapse. *Lancet* 1982;1:439–441.
22. **Norton P, Baker J, Sharp H, et al.** Genitourinary prolapse: its relationship with joint mobility. *Neurourol Urodyn* 1990;9:321–322.
23. **McIntosh LJ, Stantiski DF, Mallett VT, et al.** Ehlers-Danlos syndrome: a relationship between joint hypermobility, urinary incontinence, and pelvic floor prolapse. *Gynecol Obstet Invest* 1996;41:135–139.
24. **Carley ME, Schaffer J.** Urinary incontinence and pelvic organ prolapse in women with Marfan or Ehlers syndrome. *Am J Obstet Gynecol* 2000;182:1021–1023.
25. **Norton P, Boyd C, Deak S.** Abnormal collagen ratios in women with genitourinary prolapse. *Neurourol Urodyn* 1992;11:2–4.
26. **Ulmsten U, Ekman G, Giertz G, et al.** Different biochemical composition of connective tissue in continent and stress incontinent women. *Acta Obstet Gynecol Scand* 1987;66:455–457.
27. **Kondo A, Narushima M, Yoshikawa Y, et al.** Pelvic fascia strength in women with stress urinary incontinence in comparison with those who are continent. *Neurourol Urodyn* 1994;13:507–513.

28. **Ball T.** Anterior and posterior cystocele: cystocele revisited—an account of the twilight hours of some antifascialists and fascialists as I knew them. *Clin Obstet Gynecol* 1964;9:1062–1064.

29. **Torrens M, Morrison JFB.** *The physiology of the lower urinary tract.* New York: Springer-Verlag, 1987.

30. **Burnstock G.** Nervous control of smooth muscle by transmitters, co-transmitters, and modulators. *Experientia* 1985;41:869–874.

31. **Burnstock G.** The changing face of autonomic neurotransmission. *Acta Physiol Scand* 1986;126:67–91.

32. **Daniel EE, Cowan W, Daniel VP.** Structural bases of neural and myogenic control of human detrusor muscle. *Can J Physiol Pharmacol* 1983;61:1247–1273.

33. **Schuster MM.** The riddle of the sphincters. *Gastroenterology* 1975;69:249–262.

34. **Parks AG.** Anorectal incontinence. *Proc R Soc Med* 1975;68:681–690.

35. **Bartolo DCC, Roe AM, Locke-Edmunds JC, et al.** Flap-valve theory of anorectal continence. *Br J Surg* 1986;73:1012–1014.

36. **Phillips SF, Edwards DAW.** Some aspects of anal continence and defecation. *Gut* 1965;6:396–406.

37. **Abrams P, Blaivas JG, Stanton SL, et al.** The standardisation of terminology of lower urinary tract function. *Scand J Urol Nephrol* 1988;114:5–18.

38. **United States Department of Health and Human Services.** Urinary incontinence in adults: acute and chronic management. Public Health Service. *Agency for Health Care Policy and Research: AHCPR Publications* No. 96-0682, March 1996.

39. **Bissada NK, Finkbeiner AE.** Urologic manifestations of drug therapy. *Urol Clin North Am* 1988;15:725–736.

40. **Ostergard DR.** The effect of drugs on the lower urinary tract. *Obstet Gynecol Surv* 1979;34:424–432.

41. **Wall LL, Addison WA.** Prazosin-induced stress incontinence. *Obstet Gynecol* 1990;75:558–560.

42. **Menefee SA, Chesson R, Wall LL.** Stress urinary incontinence due to prescription medication: alpha-blockers and angiotensin converting enzyme inhibitors. *Obstet Gynecol* 1998;91:853–854.

43. **Shaker HS, Hassouna M.** Sacral nerve root neuromodulation in idiopathetic nonobstructive chronic urinary retention. *J Urol* 1998;159:1516–1519.

44. **Siltberg H, Larsson G, Victor A.** Frequency/volume chart: the basic tool for investigating urinary symptoms. *Acta Obstet Scand* 1997;76:24–27.

45. **Wyman JF, Choi SC, Harkins SW, et al.** The urinary diary in the evaluation of incontinent women: a test-retest analysis. *Obstet Gynecol* 1988;71:812–817.

46. **Wall LL, Norton PA, DeLancey JOL.** Practical urodynamics. In: *Practical urogynecology.* Baltimore: Williams & Wilkins, 1993:83–124.

47. **Wall LL, Wisking AK, Taylor PA.** Simple bladder filling with a cough stress test compared to subtracted cystometry in the diagnosis of urinary incontinence. *Am J Obstet Gynecol* 1994;171:1472–1479.

48. **Videla FL, Wall LL.** Stress incontinence diagnosed without multichannel urodynamics studies. *Obstet Gynecol* 1998;91:965–968.

49. **Weber AM, Walters MD.** Cost-effectiveness of urodynamic testing before surgery for women with pelvic organ prolapse and stress urinary incontinence. *Am J Obstet Gynecol* 2000;183:1338–1347.

50. **Thompson PK, Duff DS, Thayer PS.** Stress incontinence in women under 50: does urodynamics improve surgical outcome? *Int Urogynecol J* 2000;11:285–289.

51. **Hilton P, Stanton SL.** Urethral pressure measurement by microtransducer: the results in symptom-free women and in those with genuine stress incontinence. *Br J Obstet Gynecol* 1983;90:919–933.

52. **Sand PK, Bowen LD, Panganiban R, et al.** The low pressure urethra as a factor in failed retropubic urethropexy. *Obstet Gynecol* 1987;69:399–402.

53. **Richardson DA, Ramahi A, Chalas E.** Surgical management of stress incontinence in patients with low urethral pressure. *Obstet Gynecol Invest* 1991;31:106–109.

54. **McGuire EJ, Fitzpatrick CC, Wan J, et al.** Clinical assessment of urethral sphincter function. *J Urol* 1993;150:1452–1454.

55. **Stanton SL.** Gynecologic complications of epispadias and bladder exstrophy. *Am J Obstet Gynecol* 1974;119:749–754.

56. **Mitchell RJ.** An ectopic vaginal ureter. *J Obstet Gynaecol Br Commw* 1961;68:299–302.

57. **Boyd SD, Raz S.** Ectopic ureter presenting in midline urethral diverticulum. *Urology* 1993;41:571–574.

58. **Tahzib F.** Epidemiological determinants of vesicovaginal fistulas. *Br J Obstet Gynaecol* 1983;90:387–391.

59. **Fitzpatrick C, Elkins TE.** Plastic surgical techniques in the repair of vesicovaginal fistulas: a review. *Int Urogynecol J* 1993;4:287–295.

60. **Arrowsmith SD.** Genitourinary reconstruction in obstetric fistulas. *J Urol* 1994;152:403–406.

61. **Menefee SA, Elkins TE.** Urinary fistula. *Curr Opin Obstet Gynecol* 1996;8:380–385.

62. **Yarnell JW, Voyle GJ, Richards CJ, et al.** The prevalence and severity of urinary incontinence in women. *J Epidemiol Comm Health* 1981;35:71–74.

63. **Nygaard I, DeLancey JO, Arnsdorf L, et al.** Exercise and incontinence. *Obstet Gynecol* 1990;75:848–851.

64. **Frazer MI, Haylen BT, Sutherst JR.** The severity of urinary incontinence in women: comparison of subjective and objective tests. *Br J Urol* 1989;63:14–15.

65. **Wall LL, Helms M, Peattie AB, et al.** Bladder neck mobility and the outcome of surgery for genuine stress incontinence: a logistic regression analysis of lateral bead-chain cystourethrograms. *J Reprod Med* 1994;39:429–435.

66. **Wall LL.** The muscles of the pelvic floor. *Clin Obstet Gynecol* 1993;36:910–925.

67. **Wall LL, Davidson TG.** The role of muscular re-education by physical therapy in the treatment of genuine stress incontinence. *Obstet Gynecol Surv* 1992;47:322–331.

68. **Bo K, Larsen S.** Pelvic floor muscle exercise for the treatment of stress urinary incontinence: classification and characterization of responders. *Neurourol Urodyn* 1992;11:497–508.

69. **Benvenuti F, Caputo GM, Bandinelli S, et al.** Reeducative treatment of female genuine stress incontinence. *Am J Phys Med* 1987;66:155–168.

70. **Peattie AB, Plevnik S, Stanton SL.** Vaginal cones: a conservative method of treating genuine stress incontinence. *Br J Obstet Gynaecol* 1988;95:1049–1053.

71. **Kernan WN, Viscoli CM, Brass LM, et al.** Phenylpropanolamine and risk of hemorrhagic stroke. *N Engl J Med* 2000;343:1826–1832.

72. **Fantl JA, Wyman JF, Anderson RL, et al.** Postmenopausal urinary incontinence: comparison between non-estrogen supplemented and estrogen-supplemented women. *Obstet Gynecol* 1988;71:823–828.

73. **Schrieter F, Fuchs P, Stockamp K.** Estrogenic sensitivity of alpha-receptors in the urethra musculature. *Urol Int* 1976;31:13–19.

74. **Luber KM, Wolde-Tsadik G.** Efficacy of functional electrical stimulation in treating genuine stress urinary incontinence: a randomized clinical trial. *Neurourol Urodyn* 1997;16:543–551.

75. **Sand PK, Richardson DA, Staskin DR, et al.** Pelvic floor electrical stimulation in the treatment of genuine stress urinary incontinence: a multicenter, placebo-controlled trial. *Am J Obstet Gynecol* 1995;173:72–79.

76. **Galloway NTM, El-Galley RES, Sand PK, et al.** Update on extracorporeal magnetic innervation therapy for stress urinary incontinence. *Urology* 2000;56[Suppl 6A]:82–86.

77. **Galloway NTM, El-Galley RES, Sand PK, et al.** Extracorporeal magnetic innervation therapy for stress urinary incontinence. *Urology* 1999;53:1108–1111.

78. **Hurt G.** *Urogynecologic surgery.* Philadelphia: Lippincott Williams & Wilkins, 2000.

79. **Stanton SL, Tanagho EA.** *Surgery of female incontinence.* 2nd ed. London: Springer-Verlag, 1986.

80. **Wall LL.** Stress urinary incontinence. In: **Rock JA, Thompson JD,** eds. *TeLinde's operative gynecology.* 8th ed. Philadelphia: JB Lippincott, 1997.

81. **Kelly HA, Dumm WM.** Urinary incontinence in women without manifest injury to the bladder. *Surg Gynecol Obstet* 1914;18:444–450.

82. **Bailey KV.** A clinical investigation into uterine prolapse with stress incontinence: treatment by modified Manchester colporrhaphy. *J Obstet Gynaecol Br Emp* 1954;61:291–301.

83. **Colombo M, Vitobello D, Proietti F, et al.** Randomised comparison of Burch colposuspension versus anterior colporrhaphy in women with stress urinary incontinence and anterior vaginal wall prolapse. *Br J Obstet Gynaecol* 2000;107:544–551.

84. **Stanton SL, Cardozo LD.** A comparison of vaginal and suprapubic surgery in the correction of incontinence due to urethral sphincter incompetence. *Br J Urol* 1979;51:497–499.

85. **Beck RP, McCormick S.** Treatment of urinary stress incontinence with anterior colporrhaphy. *Obstet Gynecol* 1982;59:269–274.

86. **Beck RP, McCormick S, Nordstrom L.** A 25-year experience with 519 anterior colporrhaphy procedures. *Obstet Gynecol* 1991;78:1011–1018.

87. **Marshall VF, Marchetti AA, Krantz KE.** The correction of stress incontinence by simple vesicourethral suspension. *Surg Gynecol Obstet* 1949;88:509–518.

88. **Burch JC.** Urethrovaginal fixation to Cooper's ligament for correction of stress incontinence, cystocele and prolapse. *Am J Obstet Gynecol* 1961;81:281–290.

89. **Burch JC.** Cooper's ligament urethrovesical suspension for stress incontinence: nine years experience—results, complications, technique. *Am J Obstet Gynecol* 1968;100:764–774.

90. **Richardson AC, Lyon JB, Williams NL.** Treatment of stress urinary incontinence due to paravaginal fascial defect. *Obstet Gynecol* 1981;57:357–362.

91. **Shull BL, Baden WFA.** A six-year experience with paravaginal defect repair for stress urinary incontinence. *Am J Obstet Gynecol* 1989;160:1432–1440.

92. **Turner-Warwick R.** Turner-Warwick vagino-obturator shelf urethral repositioning procedure. In: **Gingell C, Abrams P,** eds. *Controversies and innovations in urologic surgery.* New York: Springer-Verlag, 1988:195–200.

93. **German KA, Kynaston H, Weight S, et al.** A prospective randomized trial comparing a modified needle suspension procedure with the vagina/obturator shelf procedure for genuine stress incontinence. *Br J Urol* 1994;74:188–190.

94. **Bergman A, Ballard CA, Kooning PP.** Comparison of three different surgical procedures for genuine stress incontinence: prospective randomized study. *Am J Obstet Gynecol* 1989;160:1102–1106.

95. **Bergman A, Elia G.** Three surgical procedures for genuine stress incontinence: five year follow-up of a prospective randomized study. *Am J Obstet Gynecol* 1995;173:66–71.

96. **Van Geelen JM, Theeuwes AG, Eskes TK, et al.** The clinical and urodynamics effects of anterior vaginal repair and Burch colposuspension. *Am J Obstet Gynecol* 1988;159:137–144.

97. **Alcalay M, Monga A, Stanton SL.** Burch colposuspension: a 10–20 year follow up. *Br J Obstet Gynecol* 1995;102:740–745.

98. **Herbertsson G, Iosif C.** Surgical results and urodynamic studies 10 years after retropubic colpocystourethropexy. *Acta Obstet Gynecol Scand* 1993;72:298–301.

99. **Lui CY.** Laparoscopic treatment of genuine urinary stress incontinence. *Clin Obstet Gynecol* 1994;8:789–798.

100. **Saida MH, Gallagher MS, Skop IP, et al.** Extraperitoneal laparoscopic colposuspension: short-term cure rate, complications and duration of hospital stay comparison with Burch colposuspension. *Obstet Gynecol* 1998;92:619–625.

101. **Das S.** Comparative outcome analysis of laparoscopic colposuspension, abdominal colposuspension and vaginal needle suspension for female urinary incontinence. *J Urol* 1998;160:368–371.

102. **Persky L, Guerriere K.** Complications of Marshall-Marchetti-Krantz urethropexy. *Urology* 1976;8:469–471.

103. **Galloway NTM, Davies N, Stephenson TP.** The complications of colposuspension. *Br J Urol* 1987;60:122–124.

104. **Zimmern PE, Hadley HR, Leach GE, et al.** Female urethral obstruction after Marshall-Marchetti-Krantz operation. *J Urol* 1987;138:517–520.

105. **Webster GD, Kreder KJ.** Voiding dysfunction following cystourethropexy: its evaluation and management. *J Urol* 1990;144:670–673.

106. **Lose G, Jorgensen L, Mortensen SO, et al.** Voiding difficulties after colposuspension. *Obstet Gynecol* 1987;69:33–38.

107. **Wiskind AK, Creighton SM, Stanton SL.** The incidence of prolapse after the Burch colposuspension. *Am J Obstet Gynecol* 1992;167:399–405.

108. **Pereyra AJ.** A simplified surgical procedure for the correction of stress incontinence in women. *West J Surg* 1959;67:223–256.

109. **Pereyra AJ, Lebherz TB.** Combined urethral vesical suspension vaginal urethroplasty for correction of urinary stress incontinence. *Obstet Gynecol* 1967;30:537–546.

110. **Pereyra AJ, Lebherz TB.** The revised Pereyra procedure. In: **Buchsbaum H, Schmidt JD,** eds. *Gynecologic and obstetric urology.* Philadelphia: WB Saunders, 1978:208–222.

111. **Stamey TA.** Endoscopic suspension of vesical neck for urinary incontinence in females. *Ann Surg* 1980;192:465–471.

112. **Hadley HR, Zimmern PE, Staskin DR, et al.** Transvaginal needle bladder neck suspension. *Urol Clin North Am* 1985;12:291–303.

113. **Gittes RF, Loughlin KR.** No-incision pubovaginal suspension for stress incontinence. *J Urol* 1987;138:568–570.

114. **O'Sullivan DC, Chilton CP, Munson KW.** Should Stamey colposuspension be our primary surgery for stress incontinence? *Br J Urol* 1995;75:457–460.

115. **Hilton P, Mayne C.** The Stamey endoscopic bladder neck suspension: a clinical and urodynamic investigation including actuarial follow-up over four years. *Br J Obstet Gynaecol* 1991;98:1141–1149.

116. Peattie A, Stanton S. The Stamey operation for correction of genuine stress incontinence in the elderly woman. *Br J Obstet Gynaecol* 1989;96:983–986.

117. Trockman BA, Leach GE, Hamilton J, et al. Modified Pereyra bladder neck suspension: 10-year mean followup using outcomes analysis in 125 patients. *J Urol* 1995;154:1841.

118. Tebyani N, Patel H, Yamaguchi R, et al. Percutaneous needle bladder neck suspension for the treatment of stress urinary incontinence in women: long-term results. *J Urol* 2000;163:1510–1512.

119. Birhle W, Tarantino AF. Complications of retropubic bladder neck suspension. *Urology* 1990;35:213–214.

120. Miyazaki F, Shook G. Ilioinguinal nerve entrapment during needle suspension for stress incontinence. *Obstet Gynecol* 1992;80:246–248.

121. Weiss RE, Cohen E. Erosion of buttress following bladder neck suspension. *Br J Urol* 1992;69:656–657.

122. Zedric SA, Burros HM, Hanno PM, et al. Bladder calculi in women after urethrovesical suspension. *J Urol* 1988;139:1047–1048.

123. Falconer C, Ekman-Ordeberg G, Malstrom A, et al. Clinical outcome and changes in connective tissue metabolism after intravaginal slingoplasty in stress incontinence women. *Int Urogynecol J* 1996;7:133–137.

124. Ulmsten U, Johnson P, Rezapour M. A three-year follow up of tension free vaginal tape for surgical treatment of female stress urinary incontinence. *Br J Obstet Gynaecol* 1999;106:345–350.

125. Ulmsten U, Falconer C, Johnson P, et al. A multicenter study of tension-free vaginal tape for surgical treatment of stress urinary incontinence. *Int Urogynecol J* 1998;9:210–213.

126. Weinberger MW, Ostergard DR. Long term clinical and urodynamic evaluation of the polytetrafluoroethylene suburethral sling for treatment of genuine stress incontinence. *Obstet Gynecol* 1995;86:92–96.

127. Kobashi KC, Dmochowski R, Mee S, et al. Erosion of polyester pubovaginal sling. *J Urol* 1999;162:2070–2072.

128. Clemens JQ, Delancey JO, Faerber GJ, et al. Urinary tract erosions after synthetic pubovaginal slings: diagnosis and management strategy. *Urology* 2000;56:589–595.

129. Leach GE, Dmochowski RR, Appell RA, et al. Female stress urinary incontinence clinical guidelines panel summary report on surgical management of female stress incontinence. *J Urol* 1997;158:875–880.

130. Parker RT, Addison WA, Wilson CJ. Fascia lata urethrovesical suspension for recurrent stress urinary incontinence. *Am J Obstet Gynecol* 1979;135:843–852.

131. Beck RP, Lai AR. Results in treating 88 cases of recurrent urinary stress incontinence with the Oxford fascia lata sling procedure. *Am J Obstet Gynecol* 1982;142:649–651.

132. Beck RP, McCormick S, Nordstrom L. The fascia lata sling procedure for treating recurrent genuine stress incontinence. *Obstet Gynecol* 1988;72:699–703.

133. Chaikin DC, Rosenthal J, Blaivas JG. Pubovaginal fascial sling for all types of stress urinary incontinence: long-term analysis. *J Urol* 1998;160:1312–1316.

134. Cross CA, Cespedes RD, McGuire EJ. Our experience with pubovaginal slings in patients with stress urinary incontinence. *J Urol* 1998;159:1195–1198.

135. Breen JM, Geer BE, May GE. The fascia lata suburethral sling for treating recurrent urinary stress incontinence. *Am J Obstet Gynecol* 1997;177:1363–1366.

136. Stanton SL, Brindley GS, Holmes DM. Silastic sling for urethral sphincter incompetence. *Br J Obstet Gynaecol* 1985;92:747–750.

137. Horbach NS, Blanco JS, Ostergard DR, et al. A suburethral sling procedure with polytetrafluoroethylene for the treatment of genuine stress incontinence with low urethral closure pressure. *Obstet Gynecol* 1988;71:648–652.

138. Rottenberg RD, Weil A, Brioschi PA, et al. Urodynamic and clinical assessment of the Lyodura sling operation for urinary stress incontinence. *Br J Obstet Gynaecol* 1985;92:829–834.

139. Wright EJ, Iselin CE, Carr LK, et al. Pubovaginal sling using cadaveric allograft for the treatment of intrinsic deficiency. *J Urol* 1998;160:759–762.

140. Amundsen CL, Visco AG, Ruiz H, et al. Outcome in 104 pubovaginal slings using freez-dried allograft fascia lata from a single tissue bank. *Urology* 2000;56(6A):2–8.

141. FitzGerald MP, Mollenhauer J, Bitterman P, et al. Functional failure of fascia lata allografts. *Am J Obstet Gynecol* 1999;181:1339–1346.

142. Murless BC. The injection treatment of stress incontinence. *J Obstet Gynaecol Br Emp* 1938;45:67–73.

143. Beckingham IJ, Wemyss-Holden G, Lawrence WT. Long-term follow-up of women treated with periurethral Teflon injections for stress incontinence. *Br J Urol* 1992;69:580–583.

144. Swami S, Batista JE, Abrams P. Collagen for female stress urinary incontinence after a minimum 2-year follow-up. *Br J Urol* 1997;80:757–761.

145. **Dmochowski RR, Appell RA.** Injectable agents in the treatment of stress urinary incontinence in women: where are we now? *Urology* 2000;56(6A):32–40.

146. **Appell RA.** Injectables for urethral incompetence. *World J Urol* 1990;8:208–211.

147. **Lightner D, Diokno A, Synder J.** Study of Durasphere in the treatment of stress urinary incontinence: a multicenter, double blind randomized, comparative study. *J Urol* 2000;163:166.

148. **Webster GD, Perez LM, Khoury JM, et al.** Management of type III stress incontinence using artificial urinary sphincter. *Urology* 1992;39:499–503.

149. **Diokno AC, Hollander JB, Alderson TP.** Artificial urinary sphincter for recurrent female urinary incontinence: indications and results. *J Urol* 1987;138:778–780.

150. **Wall LL.** Diagnosis and management of urinary incontinence due to detrusor instability. *Obstet Gynecol Surv* 1990;45:1S–47S.

151. **Koefoot RB, Webster GD.** Urodynamic evaluation in women with frequency, urgency symptoms. *Urology* 1983;6:648–651.

152. **Coolsaet BLRA, Blok C, van Venrouji GEFM, Tan B.** Subthreshold detrusor instability. *Neurourol Urodyn* 1985;4:309–311.

153. **Van Waalwijk Van Doorn ESC, Remmers A, Janknegt RA.** Conventional and extramural ambulatory urodynamic testing of the lower urinary tract in female volunteers. *J Urol* 1992;147:1319–1326.

154. **Griffiths CJ, Assi MS, Styles RA, et al.** Ambulatory monitoring of bladder and detrusor pressure during natural filling. *J Urol* 1989;142:780–784.

155. **Gorton E, Stanton S.** Ambulatory urodynamics: do they help clinical management. *Br J Obstet Gynecol* 2000;107:316–319.

156. **Appell R.** Clinical efficacy and safety of tolterodine in the treatment of overactive bladder: a pooled analysis. *Urology* 1997;50:90–96.

157. **Abrams P, Freeman R, Anderstrom C, et al.** Tolterodine, a new antimuscarinic agent: as effective but better tolerated than oxybutynin in patients with an overactive bladder. *Br J Urol* 1998;81:801–810.

158. **Gleason DG, Susset J, White C, et al.** Evaluation of a new once daily formulation of oxybutynin for the treatment of urinary urge incontinence. *Urology* 1999;54:420–423.

159. **Anderson RU, Mobley D, Blank B, et al.** Once daily controlled versus immediate release oxybutynin chloride for urge urinary incontinence. *J Urol* 1999;161:1809–1812.

160. **Brubaker L, Benson JT, Bent A, et al.** Transvaginal electrical stimulation for female urinary incontinence. *Am J Obstet Gynecol* 1997;177:536–540.

161. **Yamanishi T, Yasuda K, Sakakibara R, et al.** Randomized, double-blind study of electrical stimulation for urinary incontinence due to detrusor overactivity. *Urology* 2000;55:353–357.

162. **Schmidt RA, Jonas U, Oleson KA, et al.** Sacral nerve stimulation for treatment of refractory urinary urge incontinence. *J Urol* 1999;162:352–357.

163. **Siegel SW, Catanzaro F, Dijkema HE, et al.** Long-term results of a multicenter study on sacral nerve stimulation for treatment of urinary urge incontinence, urgency-frequency, and retention. *Urology* 2000;56(6A):87–91.

164. **Wall LL, Norton PA, DeLancey JOL.** Mixed incontinence. In: *Practical urogynecology.* Baltimore: Williams & Wilkins, 1993:215–220.

165. **Resnick N, Yalla S.** Management of urinary incontinence in the elderly. *N Engl J Med* 1985;313:800–805.

166. **Resnick N, Yalla S, Laurino E.** An algorithmic approach to urinary incontinence in the elderly. *Clin Res* 1986;34:832–837.

167. **Carlson KV, Rome S, Nitti.** Dysfunctional voiding in women. *J Urol* 2001;165:143–148.

168. **Rackley RR, Appell RA.** Evaluation and management of lower urinary tract disorders in women with multiple sclerosis. *Int Urogynecol J Pelvic Floor Dysfunct* 1999;10:139–143.

169. **McGuire EJ, Savastano JA.** Urodynamic findings and long term outcome management of patients with multiple sclerosis induced lower urinary tract dysfunction. *J Urol* 1984;132:713–715.

170. **Finkbeiner A.** Is bethanechol chloride clinically effective in promoting bladder emptying. *J Urol* 1985;134:443–449.

171. **Lapides J, Diokno A, Silber S, et al.** Clean intermittent self-catheterization in the treatment of urinary tract disease. *J Urol* 1972;107:458–461.

172. **Preminger GM.** Acute urinary retention in female patients: diagnosis and treatment. *J Urol* 1983;130: 112–113.

173. **Batra AK, Hanno DM, Wein AJ.** Interstitial cystitis. *Am Urol Assoc Update Series* 1999;18.

174. **Wall LL, Norton PA, DeLancey JOL.** Sensory disorders of the bladder and urethra: frequency/urgency/dysuria/bladder pain. In: *Practical urogynecology.* Baltimore: Williams & Wilkins, 1993:255–273.

175. **Parson CL, Stein DC, Bidair M, et al.** Abnormal sensitivity to intravesical potassium in interstitial cystitis and radiation cystitis. *Neurourol Urodyn* 1994;113:515–520.

176. **Baden WF, Walker T.** Genesis of the vaginal profile. *Clin Obstet Gynecol* 1972;15:1048–1054.

177. **Richardson AC, Lyon JB, Williams NL.** A new look at pelvic relaxation. *Am J Obstet Gynecol* 1976;126:568–573.

178. **Shull BL, Capen CV, Riggs MW, et al.** Preoperative and postoperative analysis of site-specific pelvic support defects in 81 women treated with sacrospinous ligament suspension and pelvic reconstruction. *Am J Obstet Gynecol* 1992;166:1764–1771.

179. **Baden WF, Walker T.** *Surgical repair of vaginal defects.* Philadelphia: JB Lippincott, 1992.

180. **Bump RC, Mattiasson A, Bo K, Brubaker LP, et al.** The standardization of terminology of female pelvic organ prolapse and pelvic floor dysfunction. *Am J Obstet Gynecol* 1996;175:10–17.

181. **Zeitlin MP, Lebherz TB.** Pessaries in the geriatric patient. *J Am Geriatr Soc* 1992;40:635–639.

182. **Russell JK.** The dangerous vaginal pessary. *BMJ* 1961;1:1595–1597.

183. **Goldstein I, Wise GJ, Tancer ML.** A vesicovaginal fistula and intravesical foreign body: a rare case of the neglected pessary. *Am J Obstet Gynecol* 1990;163:589–591.

184. **Nichols DH.** *Gynecology, obstetric, and related surgery.* 2nd ed. St. Louis: Mosby-Yearbook, 1999:462–503.

185. **Thompson JD, Rock JA.** *TeLinde's operative gynecology.* 8th ed. Philadelphia: JB Lippincott, 1996: 969–1086.

186. **McCall M.** Posterior culdoplasty: surgical correction of enterocele during vaginal hysterectomy: a preliminary report. *Obstet Gynecol* 1957;10:595–602.

187. **Wall LL.** A technique for modified McCall culdoplasty at the time of abdominal hysterectomy. *J Am Coll Surg* 1994;178:507–509.

188. **Shull BL, Bachofen C, Coates KW, et al.** A transvaginal approach to repair of apical and other associated sites of pelvic organ prolapse with uterosacral ligaments. *Am J Obstet Gynecol* 2000;183:1365–1374.

189. **Barber MD, Visco AG, Weidner AC, et al.** Bilateral uterosacral vaginal vault suspension with site-specific endopelvic fascia defect repair for treatment of pelvic organ prolapse. *Am J Obstet Gynecol* 2000;183:1402–1411.

190. **Harris RL, Cundiff GW, Theofrastous JP, et al.** The value of intraoperative cystoscopy in urogynecologic and reconstructive pelvic surgery. *Am J Obstet Gynecol* 1997;177:1367–1369.

191. **Hale DS.** Surgical management of pelvic organ prolapse. In: **Stenchever MA, Benson JT,** eds. *Atlas of clinical gynecology: urogynecology and reconstructive pelvic surgery.* 1st ed. New York: McGraw-Hill, 2000:9.7–9.8.

192. **Chesson RR, Schlossberg SM, Elkins TE, et al.** The use of fascia lata graft for correction of severe or recurrent anterior vaginal wall defects. *J Pelv Surg* 1999;5:96–103.

193. **Cundiff GW, Weidner AC, Visco AG, et al.** An anatomic and functional assessment of the discrete defect rectocele repair. *Am J Obstet Gynecol* 1998;179:1451–1456.

194. **Glavind K, Madsen H.** A prospective study of the discrete fascial defect rectocele repair. *Acta Obstet Gynecol Scand* 2000;79:145–147.

195. **DeLancey JO, Morley GW.** Total colpocleisis for vaginal eversion. *Am J Obstet Gynecol* 1997;176:1228–1235.

196. **Morley GW, DeLancey JOL.** Sacrospinous ligament fixation for eversion of the vagina. *Am J Obstet Gynecol* 1988;158:872–881.

197. **Shull BL, Capen CV, Riggs MW, et al.** Bilateral attachment of the vaginal cuff to the iliococcygeus fascia: an effective method of cuff suspension. *Am J Obstet Gynecol* 1993;168:1669–1677.

198. **Webb MJ, Aronson MP, Ferguson LK, et al.** Posthysterectomy vaginal vault prolapse: primary repair in 693 patients. *Obstet Gynecol* 1998;92:281–285.

199. **Addison WA, Livengood CH, Sutton GP, et al.** Abdominal sacral colpopexy with Mersilene mesh in the retroperitoneal position in the management of posthysterectomy vaginal vault prolapse and enterocele. *Am J Obstet Gynecol* 1985;153:140–146.

200. **Fox SD, Stanton SL.** Vault prolapse and rectocele: assessment of repair using sacrocolpopexy with mesh interposition. *Br J Obstet Gynec* 2000;107:1371–1375.

201. **Sze EH, Kohni N, Miklos JR, et al.** A retrospective comparison of abdominal sacrocolpopexy with Burch colposuspension versus sacrospinous fixation with transvaginal needle suspension for management of

vaginal vault prolapse and coexisting stress incontinence. *Int Urogynecol J Pelvic Floor Dysfunct* 1999;10: 390–393.

202. **Benson JT, Lucente V, McClellean E.** Vaginal versus abdominal reconstructive surgery for the treatment of pelvic support defects: a randomized study with long-term outcome evaluation. *Am J Obstet Gynecol* 1996;175:1418–1422.

203. **Madoof RD, Williams JG, Caushaj PF.** Fecal incontinence. *N Engl J Med* 1992;326:1002–1007.

204. **Soffer EE, Hull T.** Fecal incontinence: a practical approach to evaluation and treatment. *Am J Gastroenterol* 2000;95:1873–1880.

205. **Drossman DA, Zhming L, Andruzzi E, et al.** U.S. householder survey of functional gastrointestinal disorders. *Dig Dis Sci* 1993;38:1569–1580.

206. **Toglia MR, DeLancey JOL.** Anal incontinence and the obstetrician-gynecologist. *Obstet Gynecol* 1994;84:731–740.

207. **Jorge JMN, Wexner SD.** Etiology and management of fecal incontinence. *Dis Colon Rectum* 1993;36:77–97.

208. **Kiff ES.** Faecal incontinence. *BMJ* 1992;305:702–704.

209. **Read NW, Harford WV, Schmulen AC, et al.** A clinical study of patients with fecal incontinence and diarrhea. *Gastroenterology* 1979;76:747–756.

210. **Wrenn K. Fecal impaction.** *N Engl J Med* 1989;321:658–662.

211. **Read NW, Abouzekry L.** Why do patients with faecal impaction have faecal incontinence? *Gut* 1986;27:283–287.

212. **Diamant NE, Kamm MA, Wald A, et al.** AGA position paper on anorectal testing techniques. *Gastroenterology* 1999;116:735–760.

213. **Sun WM, Read NW, Miner PB.** Relationship between rectal sensation and anal function in normal subjects and patients with faecal incontinence. *Gut* 1990;31:1056–1061.

214. **Sultan AH, Kamm MA, Hudson CN, et al.** Anal-sphincter disruption during vaginal delivery. *N Engl J Med* 1993;329:1905–1911.

215. **Kelvin FM, Maglinte DDT, Benson JT.** Evacuation proctography (defecography): an aid to the investigation of pelvic floor disorders. *Obstet Gynecol* 1994;83:307–314.

216. **Enck P.** Biofeedback training in disordered defecation: a critical review. *Dig Dis Sci* 1993;38:1953–1960.

217. **Parks AG, McPartlin JF.** Later repair of injuries of the anal sphincter. *J R Soc Med* 1971;64:1187–1189.

218. **Seccia M.** Study protocols and functional results in 86 electrostimulated gracilosphincters. *Dis Colon Rectum* 1994;37:897–904.

219. **Corman ML.** Rectal prolapse. In: *Colon and rectal surgery.* 2nd ed. Philadelphia: JB Lippincott, 1989: 209–247.

220. **Kuijpers JHC, De Morree H.** Toward a selection of the most appropriate procedure in the treatment of complete rectal prolapse. *Dis Colon Rectum* 1988;31:355–357

221. **Broden B, Snellman B.** Procidentia of the rectum studied with cineradiography: a contribution to the discussion of causative mechanism. *Dis Colon Rectum* 1968;11:330–347.

222. **Eu KW, Seow-Choen F.** Functional problems in adult rectal prolapse and controversies in surgical treatment. *Br J Surg* 1997;84:904–911.

223. **Kuijpers HC.** Treatment of complete rectal prolapse: to narrow, to wrap, to suspend, to fix, to encircle, to plicate or to resect? *World J Surg* 1992;16:826–830.

224. **Duthie GS, Bartolo DCC.** Abdominal rectopexy for rectal prolapse: a comparison of techniques. *Br J Surg* 1992;79:107–113.

225. **Mollen RMHG, Claassen ATPN, Kuijpers JHC.** The evaluation and treatment of functional constipation. *Scand J Gastroenterol* 1997;32;[Suppl 223]:8–17.

226. **Thompson WG, Heaton KW.** Functional bowel disorders in apparently healthy people. *Gastroenterology* 1980;79:283–288.

227. **Drossman DA, Sandler RS, McKee DC, et al.** Bowel patterns among subjects not seeking health care: use of a questionnaire to identify a population with bowel dysfunction. *Gastroenterology* 1982;83:529–534.

228. **Moriarty KJ, Irving MH.** ABC or colorectal disease. Constipation. *BMJ* 1992;304:1237–1240.

229. **Shafik A.** Constipation: pathogenesis and management. *Drugs* 1993;45:528–540.

230. **Kamm MA.** Idiopathic constipation: any movement? *Scand J Gastroenterol Suppl* 1992;192:106–109.

231. **Read NW, Timms JM, Barfield LJ, et al.** Impairment of defecation in young women with severe constipation. *Gastroenterology* 1986;90:53–60.

232. **Preston DM, Lennard-Jones JE.** Severe chronic constipation of young women: idiopathic slow transit constipation. *Gut* 1986;27:41–48.

233. **Preston DM, Lennard-Jones JE.** Anismus in chronic constipation. *Dig Dis Sci* 1985;30:413–418.

234. **Bleijenberg G, Juijpers HC.** Treatment of spastic pelvic floor syndrome with biofeedback. *Dis Colon Rectum* 1987;30:108–111.

21 Gynecologic Endoscopy

Malcom G. Munro
Andrew I. Brill

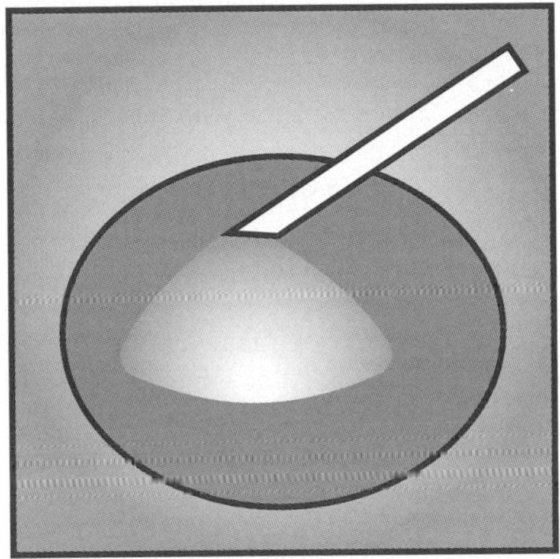

Endoscopy is a procedure that uses a narrow telescope to view the interior of a viscus space. Although the first medical endoscopic procedures were performed more than 100 years ago, the potential of this method has only recently been realized. Endoscopes are currently used to perform a variety of operations. In gynecology, endoscopes are used most often to diagnose conditions by direct visualization of the peritoneal cavity (laparoscopy) or the inside of the uterus (hysteroscopy).

When used appropriately, endoscopic surgery offers the benefits of reduced pain, improved cosmesis, lower cost, and faster recovery. The indications for endoscopic surgery are outlined here and detailed in the appropriate chapters. The technology, potential uses, and complications of laparoscopy and hysteroscopy are summarized here.

Laparoscopy

The past three decades have witnessed rapid progress and technologic advances in laparoscopy (1–12). Operative laparoscopy was developed in the 1970s; and in the early 1980s, laparoscopy was first used to direct the application of electrical or laser energy for the treatment of advanced stages of endometriosis (6–7). The use of high-resolution, lightweight video cameras in operative laparoscopy has made it easier to view the pelvis during the performance of complex procedures (7–10). Subsequently, many other procedures that were previously performed using traditional techniques, such as hysterectomy, became feasible with the laparoscope (11). However, the endoscopic approach may have drawbacks in some patients. Although some laparoscopic procedures appear to reduce the cost and morbidity associated with surgery, others have not been shown to be effective replacements for more traditional operations. The techniques and indications for operative endoscopy are evolving.

Diagnosis

The objective lens of a laparoscope can be positioned to allow wide-angle or magnified views of the peritoneal cavity. Laparoscopy is the standard method for the diagnosis of endometriosis and adhesions because no other imaging technique provides the same degree of sensitivity and specificity.

There are limitations to laparoscopy, however. The view is restricted, and if tissue or fluid becomes attached to the lens, vision may be obscured. Also, soft tissues or the inside of a hollow viscus cannot be palpated. For assessment of soft tissue, an imaging modality, such as ultrasonography, computed tomography (CT), or magnetic resonance imaging (MRI) scans, is superior. Because of its ability to view soft tissue, ultrasonography is more accurate than laparoscopy for the evaluation of the inside of adnexal masses. The intraluminal contour of the uterus can be demonstrated only by hysteroscopy or contrast imaging. Ultrasonography, in combination with serum assays of β-human chorionic gonadotropin (β-hCG) and progesterone, can be used to diagnose ectopic pregnancy, usually allowing medical therapy to be given without laparoscopic confirmation (12). As a result of the advances in blood tests and imaging technology, laparoscopy is more often used to confirm a clinical impression than for initial diagnosis.

Laparoscopy may disclose abnormalities that are not necessarily related to the patient's problem. Although endometriosis, adhesions, leiomyomas, and small cysts in the ovaries are common, they are frequently asymptomatic. Thus, diagnostic laparoscopy must be performed prudently, interpreting findings in the context of the clinical problem and other diagnoses.

Therapy

The role of laparoscopy in the operative management of gynecologic conditions is still being defined. Many procedures previously in the domain of traditional abdominal and vaginal operations are feasible with laparoscopy. In addition to the benefits of endoscopic procedures in general, laparoscopic surgery is less likely than laparotomy to form adhesions. Because sponges are not used, the amount of direct peritoneal trauma is reduced substantially, and contamination of the peritoneal cavity is minimized. The lack of exposure to air allows the peritoneal surface to remain more moist and, therefore, less susceptible to injury and adhesion formation.

Despite these advantages, there are potential limitations: exposure of the operative field can be reduced, manipulation of the pelvic viscera is limited, and the caliber of the suture required may be larger than otherwise desired. In many cases, the cost of hospitalization increases, despite a shortened stay, because of prolonged operating room time and the use of more expensive surgical equipment and supplies. Efficacy may be reduced because surgeons may not adequately replicate the abdominal operation. In some patients, there is an increased risk for complications, which can be attributed to the innate limitations of laparoscopy, the level of surgical expertise, or both. With an adequate combination of ability, training, and experience, however, operative time and complications are comparable to those of traditional abdominal surgery.

Tubal Surgery

Sterilization Laparoscopic sterilization has been extensively used since the late 1960s and can be performed under local or general anesthesia. The tubes may be occluded by suture, clips, or Silastic rings, but electrosurgical desiccation with bipolar energy is the technique used most often (see Chapter 10). If an operative laparoscope is used, only one incision is required. Otherwise, a second port is needed for the introduction of the occluding instrument. Patients remain in the hospital for several hours, even when general anesthesia is used. Postoperative pain is usually minor and related to the effects of the anesthesia, gas that remains in the peritoneal cavity (shoulder pain, dyspnea), and in the case of occlusive devices, pain at the surgical site. These effects normally disappear within a few days. The failure rate is about 5.4 per 1,000 woman-years (13,14).

Ectopic Gestation Ectopic gestation can be managed using laparoscopy to perform the same procedures done with laparotomy, including salpingostomy, salpingectomy, and segmental resection of a portion of the oviduct (see Chapter 17) (15). Salpingostomy is performed with scissors, a laser, or an electrosurgical electrode after carefully injecting the mesosalpinx with a dilute *vasopressin*-containing solution (20 units per 100 mL of normal saline). For salpingectomy, the vascular pedicles are usually secured with electrosurgical desiccation, ligatures, clips, or a combination thereof. Tissue is removed from the peritoneal cavity through one of the laparoscopic ports.

When salpingostomy is performed by any route, there is about a 5% chance that trophoblastic tissue remains. In such instances, medical treatment with *methotrexate* is considered appropriate (see Chapter 17). Consequently, β-hCG levels should be measured weekly until there is confidence that complete excision has occurred (16,17).

Ovarian Surgery

Ovarian Masses Laparoscopic removal of selected ovarian masses is a well-established procedure (18,19). However, controversy exists regarding the selection of tumors that can be removed by laparoscopy, because of concerns about an adverse effect on prognosis with malignant tumors (20). Preoperative ultrasonography is mandatory. Sonolucent lesions with thin walls and no solid components are at very low risk for malignancy and, therefore, are suitable for laparoscopic removal. For postmenopausal women, the measurement of CA125 may be useful in identifying candidates for laparoscopic management (21,22). Lesions with ultrasonographic findings suggestive of mature teratoma (dermoid) may also be suitable for endoscopic management (23). The ovarian tumors should be assessed by frozen histologic section, and any malignancy should be managed expeditiously by laparotomy (22,24).

Oophorectomy and cystectomy are performed similar to those for laparotomy (16). For cystectomy, scissors are used to separate the cyst from the ovary; if oophorectomy is performed, the vascular pedicles are ligated with sutures, clips, linear cutting staplers, electrosurgical desiccation, or a combination thereof. Most cysts are drained before extraction, through either a laparoscopic cannula or a posterior colpotomy. If there is concern about the impact of spilled cyst contents, the specimen can be removed in a retrieval bag inserted into the peritoneal cavity.

Although in the past the ovary has routinely been closed after cystectomy, this practice may be unnecessary and could contribute to the formation of adhesions (25). However, complete disruption of the ovarian cortex may make closure necessary. If so, the edges of the ovarian incision can be sutured.

Other Ovarian Surgery

Many cases of ovarian torsion previously treated by laparotomy and oophorectomy can be managed laparoscopically (26,27). If there is no apparent necrosis, the adnexa should be untwisted. Otherwise, adnexectomy is indicated.

Polycystic ovarian syndrome can be treated laparoscopically using electrosurgery and laser vaporization (28–30). Although such procedures have been shown to be successful, the occurrence of postoperative adhesions in 15% to 20% of patients underscores the need first to exhaust medical treatment (31,32).

Uterine Surgery

Myomectomy

Laparoscopic myomectomy, although feasible, is rarely performed, in part because its efficacy is yet to be established, especially as it relates to the treatment of infertility and menorrhagia (33,34). Also, laparoscopic myomectomy requires more technical skills than many other endoscopic procedures.

Unless the myoma involves the endometrial cavity, it is unlikely to contribute to heavy menstrual bleeding. Leiomyomas that cause pressure are often large and located in or near vital vascular structures. Myomectomy should be performed only when indicated (as opposed to expectant or medical management), and laparotomy should be used if there are technical limitations (35). **The only leiomyomas that are clearly appropriate candidates for laparoscopic excision are those pedunculated or subserosal lesions that cause pain in association with torsion** (16,36).

Hysterectomy

In many patients, hysterectomy can be performed under laparoscopic direction. **Laparoscopic hysterectomy encompasses a variety of procedures, including the facilitation of vaginal hysterectomy with variable extents of endoscopic dissection, supracervical hysterectomy by dissection, amputation and mechanical removal of the fundus, and the removal of the entire uterus with the assistance of the laparoscope** (37). The procedure is performed with scissors, sutures, electricity, clips, and, in some instances, linear cutting and stapling devices to dissect or ligate pedicles. Laparoscopic hysterectomy offers no advantage for women in whom vaginal hysterectomy is possible because the endoscopic approach is more expensive and has a higher risk for postoperative morbidity (38,39).

Infertility Operations

Laparoscopic treatment of infertility includes operations used to reconstruct the normal anatomic relationships altered by an inflammatory process: fimbrioplasty, adhesiolysis, and salpingostomy for distal obstruction (40). Fimbrioplasty is distinguished from salpingostomy because it is performed in the absence of preexisting complete distal obstruction. Endometriosis associated with adnexal distortion can be treated by laparoscopic adhesiolysis. There is no known additional benefit of laparoscopic (or medical) treatment to coexistent active endometriosis. Laparoscopy has been superseded by ultrasound for the retrieval of oocytes for *in vitro* fertilization but is still used for procedures in which gametes (gamete intrafallopian transfer) or zygotes (zygote intrafallopian transfer) are placed into the fallopian tube.

Adhesiolysis may be accomplished by blunt or sharp dissection with scissors, laser, or an electrosurgical electrode. These instruments are usually passed through an ancillary port; those who use laser energy frequently use the channel of the operating laparoscope. Although there has been controversy regarding the most appropriate modality, both methods are probably equally effective in appropriately trained hands.

Laparoscopic operations for the treatment of mechanical infertility are probably equally effective to similar procedures performed by laparotomy. In patients with extensive adhesions, however, the effectiveness of all procedures is limited. Assisted reproductive technologies such as *in vitro* fertilization and embryo transfer are necessary in these situations (16,41).

Endometriosis

The laparoscopic management of endometriomas parallels that of adnexal masses, although the ultrasonographic complexity of endometriomas may make it difficult to distinguish them preoperatively from a neoplasm. The relationship of the endometrioma to the ovarian cortex and stroma makes it difficult to find surgical dissection planes. There is a tendency either to compromise the function of the remaining ovary by attempting complete removal or to leave part of the endometrioma in place. Therefore, for women who want to retain their fertility, electrosurgical or laser ablative techniques may be used to treat endometriotic tissue that is adherent to the remaining ovary.

Multifocal endometriosis may be treated by mechanical excision or ablation, the latter using coagulation or vaporization with either electrical or laser energy. With proper use, each energy source creates about the same amount of thermal injury (42,43). Endometriosis is frequently deeper than appreciated, making excisional techniques valuable in many instances (16,41).

Pelvic Floor Disorders

Laparoscopy can be used to guide procedures to treat pelvic floor prolapse, including enterocele repair, vaginal vault suspension, paravaginal repair, and retropubic cystourethropexy for urinary stress incontinence. Although these conditions can be treated vaginally, the abdominal approach may offer benefits, particularly with retropubic urethropexy. There is some evidence that this procedure is effective when compared with the traditional approaches (44,45). The laparoscopic treatment of enterocele and vault prolapse may be useful in patients who require abdominal approaches after failure of a previous vaginal procedure.

Gynecologic Malignancies

The role of laparoscopy in the management of gynecologic malignancy has not been clearly established (24,46,47). However, a number of ongoing research protocols relating to cervical, endometrial, and ovarian cancer should help document this role. Lymph node biopsies performed by laparoscopy can be coupled with vaginal hysterectomy for the management of early-stage endometrial cancer. The potential for laparoscopic lymphadenectomy has fostered a resurgence of interest in vaginal radical hysterectomy for stage I carcinoma of the cervix. Laparoscopy is also being investigated for the staging of early ovarian malignancy and for second-look surgery.

Patient Preparation and Communication

The prospective patient must understand the rationale, alternatives, risks, and potential benefits of the selected approach. She should know what would probably happen if the procedure were not done and expectant management were used.

The expectations and risks of diagnostic laparoscopy, as well as those of any other procedures that may be needed, must be explained. The risks of laparoscopy include those associated with anesthesia, infection, bleeding, and injury to the abdominal and pelvic viscera. Infection is uncommon with laparoscopic surgery. For procedures involving extensive dissection, there is a higher risk for visceral injury. The potential for these risks should be clearly presented. The patient should be given realistic expectations regarding postoperative disability. **Because pain and visceral dysfunction normally continue to improve after uncomplicated laparoscopy, the patient should be instructed to communicate immediately any regression in her recovery.** After diagnostic or brief operative procedures, patients can be discharged on the day of surgery and usually require 24 to 72 hours away from work or school. If extensive dissection is performed or the surgery lasts longer than 2 hours, hospital admission may be necessary, and the period of disability may be longer.

If the colon may be involved, mechanical bowel preparation should be performed to help improve visualization and minimize the need for a colostomy if the colon is entered. The patient should arrange for a friend or family member to discuss the results of the procedure and to drive her home if she is discharged the same day. Mild analgesia is often necessary.

Technique

Laser and electrical sources of energy manifest their effect by conversion to thermal energy. Highly focused energy produces vaporization or cutting, whereas less focused energy causes desiccation and tissue coagulation. Animal studies fail to demonstrate differences in injury characteristics (41–43). Randomized controlled studies have shown no differences in fertility outcomes in women undergoing CO_2 laser surgery and electrosurgery (48). Therefore, differences in results are more likely to be caused by other factors, such as patient selection, extent of disease, and degree of surgical expertise. With proper education, modern equipment, and adherence to safety protocols, these techniques can be used safely. To facilitate the discussion of laparoscopic equipment, supplies, and techniques, it is useful to divide procedures into "core competencies," which are as follows:

1. Patient positioning
2. Operating room organization
3. Peritoneal access
4. Visualization
5. Manipulation of tissue and fluid
6. Cutting, hemostasis, and tissue fastening
7. Tissue extraction
8. Incision management

Patient Positioning

Proper positioning of the patient is essential for safety, comfort of the operator, and optimal visualization of the pelvic organs. Laparoscopy is performed on an operating table that can be rotated around the patient's long axis and tipped to create a steep, head-down (Trendelenburg) position. The footrest can be dropped to allow access to the perineum. The patient is placed in the low lithotomy position, with the legs supported in stirrups and the buttocks protruding slightly from the lower edge of the table (Fig. 21.1). The thighs are usually kept in the neutral position to preserve the sacroiliac angle, reducing the tendency of bowel to slide into the peritoneal cavity. **The feet should rest flat, and the lateral aspect of the knee should be protected with padding or a special stirrup to avoid peroneal nerve injury.** The knees should be kept in at least slight flexion to minimize stretching of the sciatic nerve and to provide more stability in the Trendelenburg position. **The arms are positioned at the patient's side by adduction and pronation to allow freedom of movement for the surgeon and to lower the risk for brachial plexus injury** (Fig. 21.2). Care must be exercised to protect the patient's fingers and hands from injury when the foot of the table is raised or lowered. After the patient is properly positioned, the bladder should be emptied with a catheter and a uterine manipulator attached to the cervix.

Operating Room Organization

The arrangement of instruments and equipment is important for safety and efficiency. The orientation depends on the operation, the instruments used, and whether the surgeon is right- or left-handed. An orientation for a right-handed operator is shown in Fig. 21.2.

For pelvic surgery, the monitor should be placed at the foot of the table within the angle formed by the patient's legs. If a second monitor is used, one should be positioned at each foot of the patient. If upper abdominal surgery is also to be performed, the additional monitor should be moved to the head of the operating table.

The surgeon stands by the patient's left side, at an angle facing the patient's contralateral foot. The nurse or technician and instrument table are positioned near the foot of the operating table to avoid obscuring the video monitor. The insufflator is placed on the patient's right side, in front of the surgeon, to allow continuous monitoring of the inflation rate and intraabdominal pressure. The electrosurgical generator is also positioned on the patient's right side to permit visualization of the power output. When a laser is used through a second puncture site, it is also placed to the patient's right. When the laser is passed through the channel of an operating laparoscope, however, it is situated on the patient's left side, beside the surgeon.

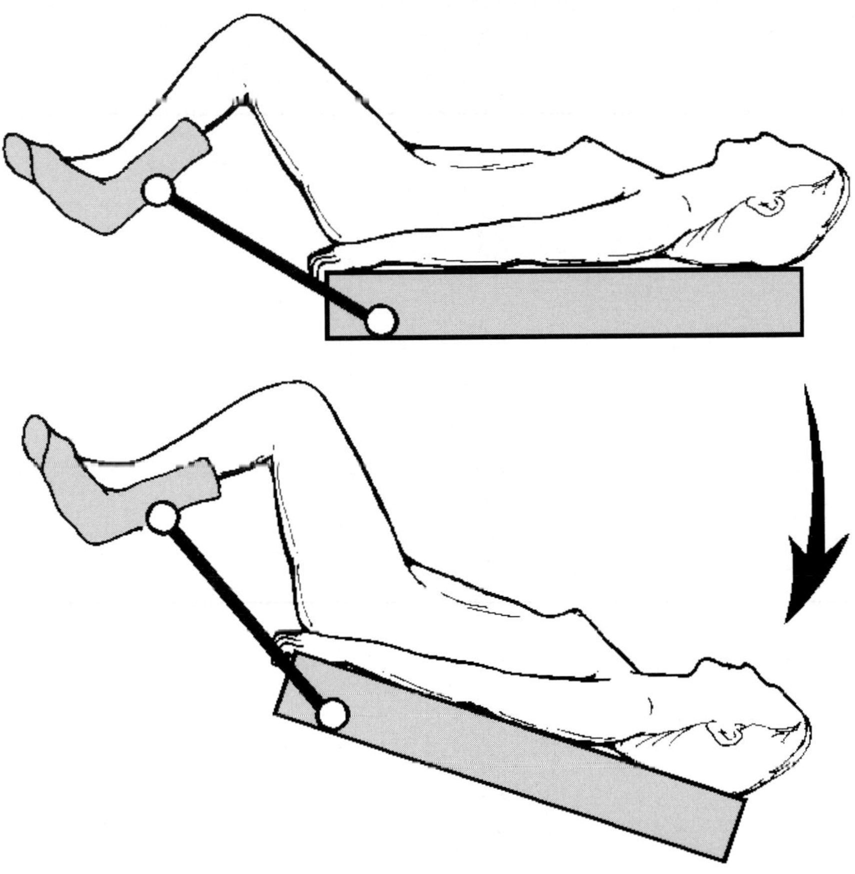

Figure 21.1 Patient positioning: the low lithotomy position. The patient's buttocks are positioned so that the perineum is at the edge of the table. The legs are well supported with stirrups, with the thighs in slight flexion. Too much flexion may impede the manipulation of laparoscopic instruments while in the Trendelenburg (head-down) position.

Peritoneal Access

Before inserting the laparoscope, a cannula or port must be positioned in the abdominal wall to establish access to the peritoneal cavity. The *closed technique* is a blind approach in which the cannula is introduced with a sharp trocar used to penetrate the abdominal layers. In *open laparoscopy,* entry into the peritoneal cavity is achieved by a minilaparotomy, with the cannula fixed into position with sutures or other suitable techniques. Gynecologists have generally favored a closed technique, preinflating the peritoneal cavity with CO_2 through a hollow needle. In either case, additional cannulas are inserted by sharp trocars under direct vision to allow the use of laparoscopic hand instruments such as scissors, probes, and other manipulating devices.

Cannula insertion is aided by an understanding of the normal anatomy, especially the location of vessels (Fig. 21.3). A "safety zone" exists inferior to the sacral promontory in the area bounded cephalad by the bifurcation of the aorta, posteriorly by the sacrum, and laterally by the iliac vessels (49). In women placed in the Trendelenburg position, the great vessels are situated more cephalad and anterior, making them more vulnerable to injury unless appropriate adjustments are made in the angle of insertion (Fig. 21.4). Therefore, positioning of the insufflation needle, the initial trocar, and the cannula is best accomplished with the patient in a horizontal position. This approach also facilitates the evaluation of the upper abdomen, which is limited if the intraperitoneal contents are shifted cephalad by the head-down position.

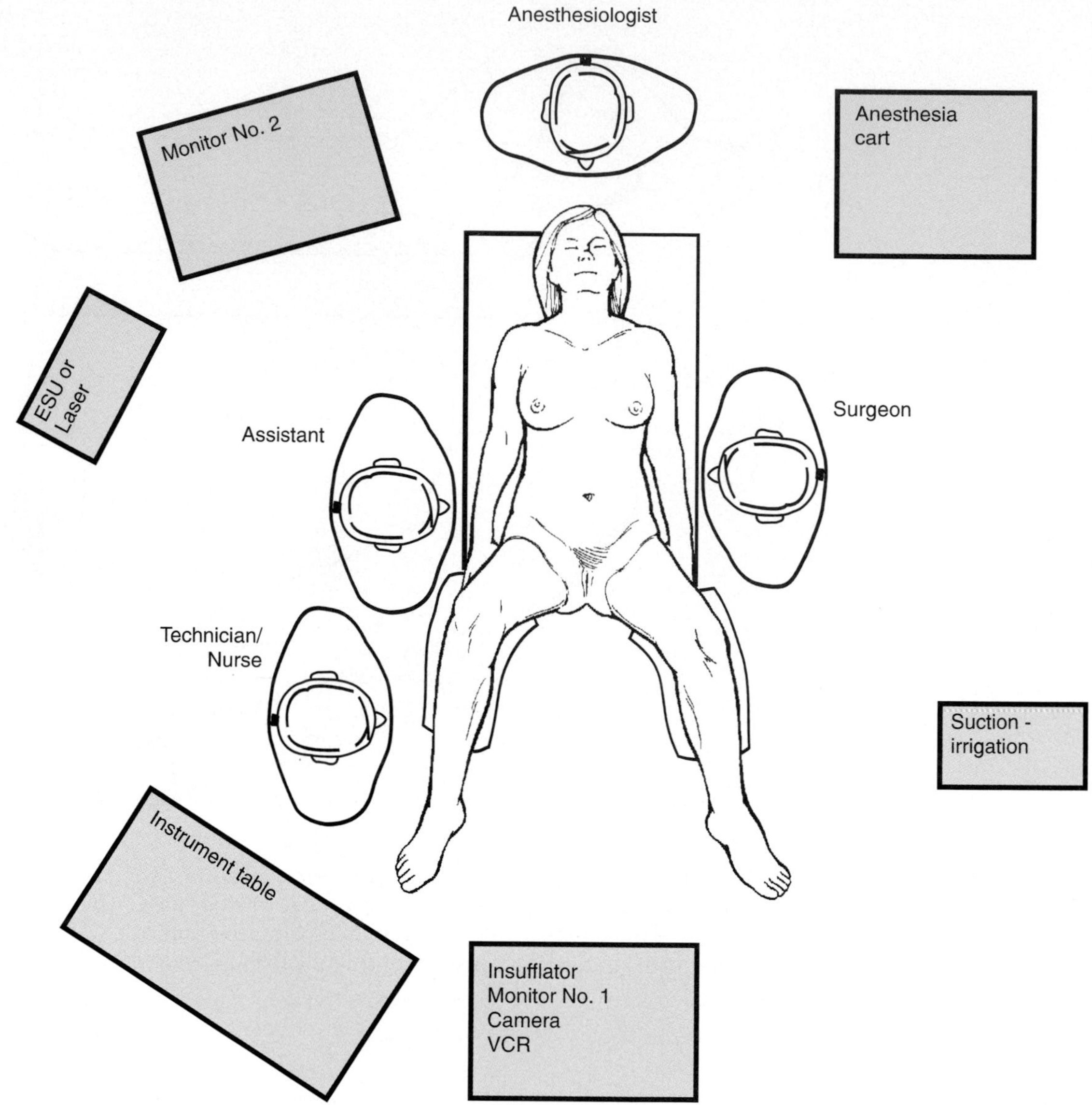

Figure 21.2 Operating room organization. The patient's arms are at the sides. The right-handed surgeon stands on the patient's left. Instruments and equipment are distributed around the patient within view of the surgeon. For pelvic surgery, the monitor should be located between the patient's legs. For upper abdominal surgery, or when operating from below, a monitor should be placed near the patient's head.

Insufflation Needles

Virtually all insufflation needles are modifications of the hollow needle designed by Verres (Fig. 21.5). In cases uncomplicated by previous pelvic surgery, the preferred site for insertion is as close as possible to (or within) the umbilicus, where the abdominal wall is the thinnest.

1. **A 3-mm incision adequate for the needle is made with a small scalpel, and the abdominal wall is elevated by gripping it in the midline below the umbilicus.** Safe insertion of the insufflation needle mandates that the instrument be maintained in a midline, sagittal plane while the operator directs the tip between the iliac vessels, anterior to the sacrum but inferior to the bifurcation of the aorta and the proximal aspect of the vena cava. Therefore, in women of average weight, the insufflation needle is directed at a 45-degree angle to the patient's spine. In heavy to obese individuals, this angle may be increased incrementally to nearly 90 degrees, accounting for the increasing thickness of the abdominal wall and the

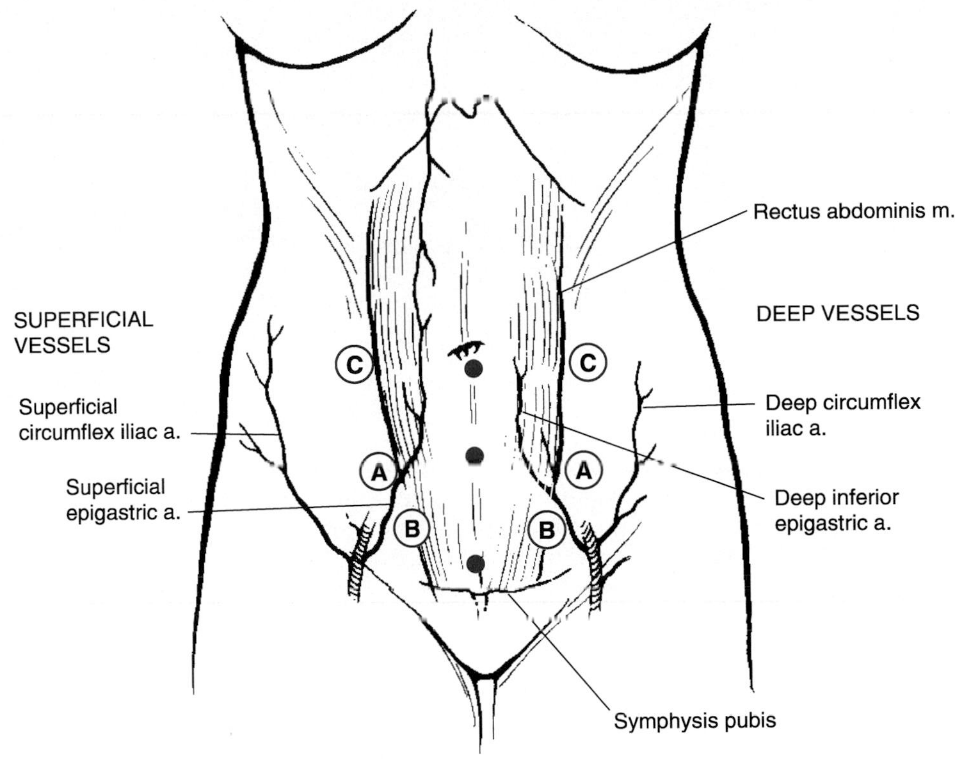

Figure 21.3 Vascular anatomy of the anterior abdominal wall. Location of the vessels that can be traumatized when inserting trocars into the anterior abdominal wall.

tendency of the umbilicus to gravitate caudad with increasing abdominal girth (49). The needle's shaft is held by the tips of the fingers and steadily but purposefully guided into position only far enough to allow the tip's entry into the peritoneal cavity. The tactile and visual feedback created when the needle passes through the facial and peritoneal layers of the abdominal wall may provide guidance and help prevent overaggressive insertion attempts. This proprioceptive feedback is less apparent with disposable needles than with the classic Verres needle. With

Figure 21.4 Vascular anatomy. Location of the great vessels and their changing relationship to the umbilicus with increasing patient weight (*from left to right*).

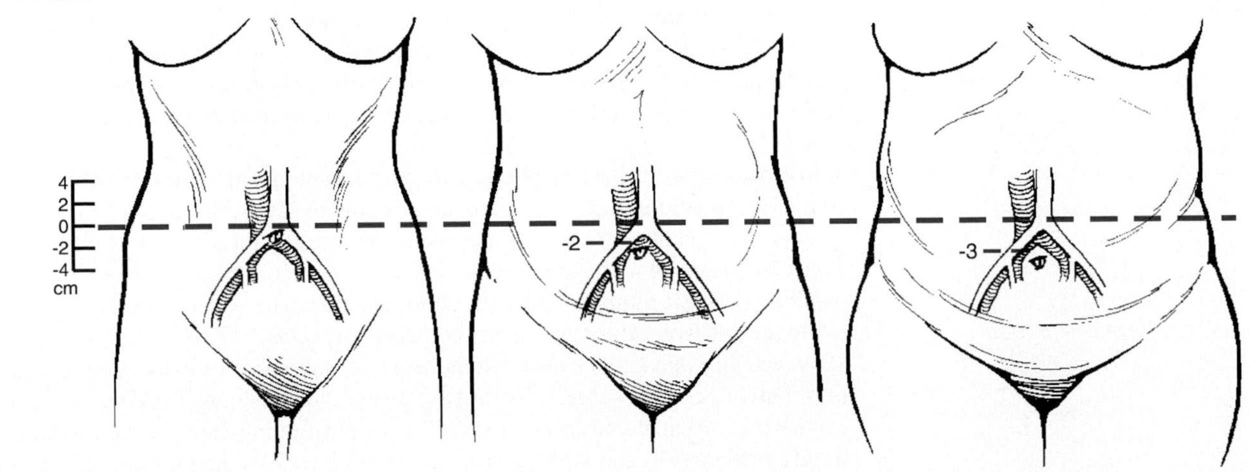

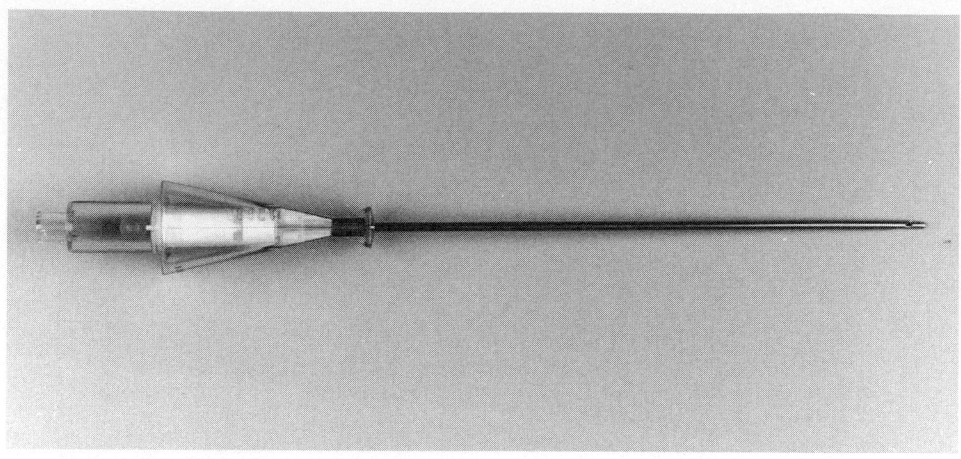

Figure 21.5 Insufflation needle (Ethicon Endosurgery, Inc., Cincinnati, OH). When pressed against tissue such as fascia or peritoneum, the spring-loaded blunt obturator is pushed back into the hollow needle, revealing its sharpened end. When the needle enters the peritoneal cavity, the obturator springs back into position, protecting the intraabdominal contents from injury. The handle of the hollow needle allows the attachment of a syringe or tubing for insufflation of the distention gas.

the former, the surgeon must listen to the "clicks" as the needle obturator retracts when it passes through the rectus fascia and the peritoneum. The needle should never be forced.

2. **In instances in which known or suspected intraabdominal adhesions surround the umbilicus, alternative sites for insufflation needle insertion should be used.** These include the pouch of Douglas, the fundus of the uterus, and the left upper quadrant, most often at the left costal margin (Fig. 21.6). The left upper quadrant is preferred if there has been no previous surgery in this area. In such patients, the stomach must be decompressed with a nasogastric or orogastric tube before the puncture.

3. **Before insufflation, the operator should try to detect whether the insufflation needle has been malpositioned in the omentum, mesentery, blood vessels, or hollow organs such as the stomach or bowel.** Using a syringe attached to the insufflation needle, blood or gastrointestinal contents may be aspirated. This examination may be facilitated by injecting a small amount of saline into the syringe. If the needle is appropriately positioned, negative intraabdominal pressure is created by lifting the abdominal wall. This negative pressure may be demonstrated by aspiration of a drop of saline placed over the open, proximal end of the needle or, preferably, by using the digital pressure gauge on the insufflator.

4. **Additional signs of proper placement may be sought after starting insufflation.** The intraabdominal pressure reading should be low, reflecting only systemic resistance to the flow of CO_2. Consequently, there should be little deviation from a baseline measurement, generally less than 10 mm Hg. The pressure varies with respiration and is slightly higher in obese patients. The earliest reassuring sign is the loss of liver "dullness" over the lateral aspect of the right costal margin. However, this sign may be absent if there are dense adhesions in the area, usually the result of previous surgery. Symmetric distention is unlikely to occur when the needle is positioned extraperitoneally. Proper positioning can also be shown by lightly compressing the xiphoid process, which increases the pressure measured by the insufflator.

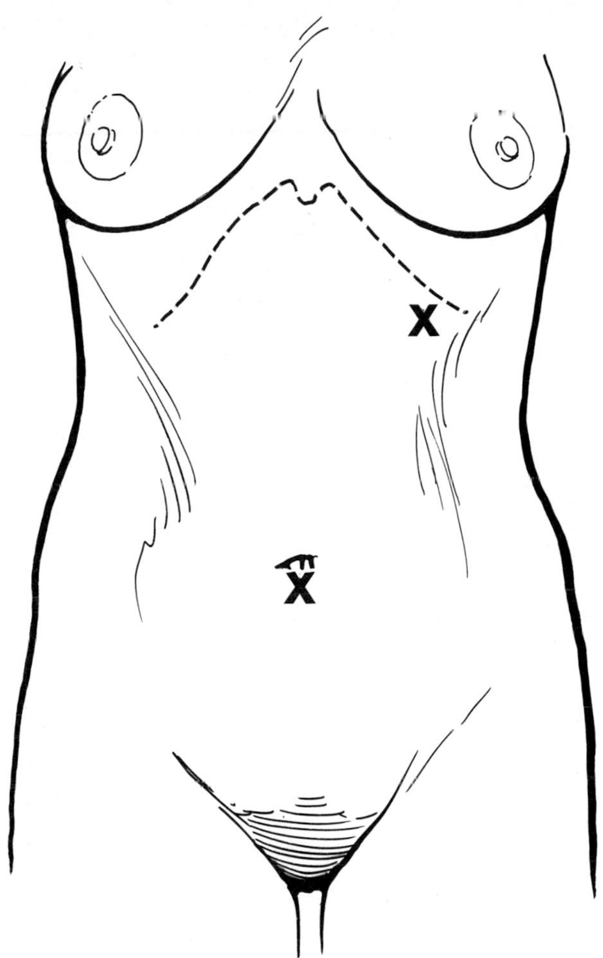

Figure 21.6 Insufflation needle and cannula insertion sites. In most instances, both the insufflation needle, if used, and the primary cannula are inserted through the umbilicus. When subumbilical adhesions are known or suspected, the insufflation needle may be placed through the pouch of Douglas or in the left upper quadrant after evacuation of the gastric contents with an orogastric tube.

5. **The amount of gas transmitted into the peritoneal cavity should depend on the measured intraperitoneal pressure, not the volume of gas inflated.** Intraperitoneal volume capacity varies significantly between individuals. Many surgeons prefer to insufflate to 20 mm Hg for positioning of the cannulas. This level usually provides enough counterpressure against the peritoneum, facilitating trocar introduction and potentially reducing the chance of bowel or posterior abdominal wall and vessel trauma. After placement of the cannulas, the pressure should be dropped to 10 to 12 mm Hg, which essentially eliminates hypercarbia or decreased venous return of blood to the heart.

Laparoscopic Cannulas

Laparoscopic cannulas are necessary to allow the insertion of laparoscopic instruments into the peritoneal cavity while maintaining the pressure created by the distending gas (Figs. 21.7 and 21.8). Cannulas are hollow tubes with a valve or sealing mechanism at or near the proximal end. The cannula may be fitted with a Luer-type port that allows attachment to tubing connected with the CO_2 insufflator. Larger-diameter cannulas (8 to 12 mm) may be fitted with adapters or specialized valves that allow the insertion of smaller-diameter instruments without loss of intraperitoneal pressure.

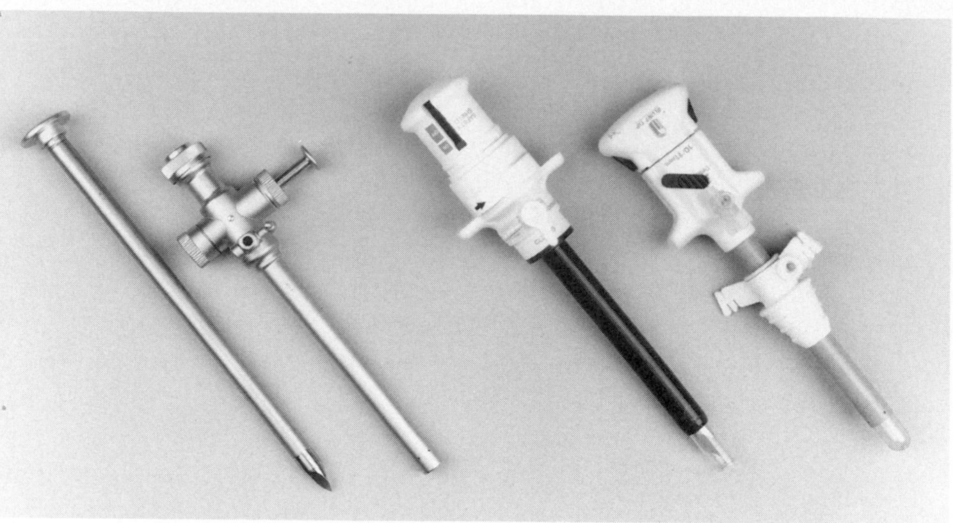

Figure 21.7 Primary laparoscopic cannulas. *Left to right:* a nondisposable 10-mm cannula with the obturator removed (Olympus America, Inc., Woodbury, NY), a disposable 5- to 12-mm cannula with a "safety" sheath (Autosuture, Inc, Norwalk, CT), and a Hasson cannula used in open laparoscopy (Ethicon Endosurgery, Inc., Cincinnati, OH).

The trocar is a longer instrument of slightly smaller diameter that is passed through the cannula, exposing its tip. Most trocars have sharp tips, allowing penetration of the abdominal wall after a small skin incision. Many disposable trocar-cannula systems are designed with a safety mechanism—usually a pressure-sensitive spring that either retracts the trocar or deploys a protective sheath around its tip after passage through the abdominal wall. None

Figure 21.8 Ancillary laparoscopic cannulas: 5-mm laparoscopic cannulas for ancillary instruments. *Top:* Apple Medical, Boston, MA (disposable). *Middle:* Wolf, Laguna Niguel, CA (nondisposable). These cannulas neither have nor require ports or safety sheaths and are therefore less expensive than other cannulas. *Bottom:* Core Surgical Inc. (Jacksonville, FL).

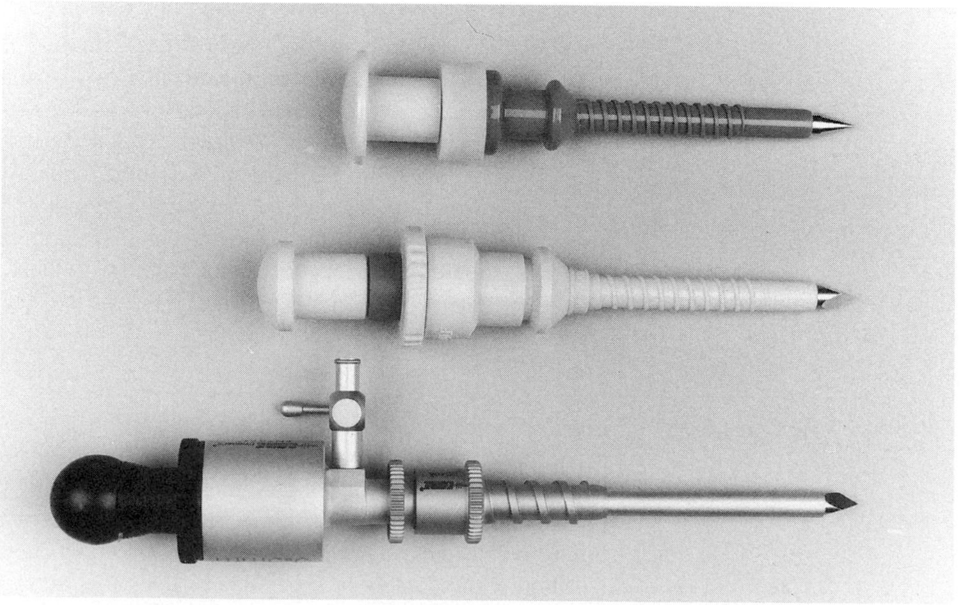

of these protective devices has been shown to make the procedure safer; however, they all increase the cost.

Cannulas can be inserted following minilaparotomy (open laparoscopy), after the successful creation of a pneumoperitoneum (secondary puncture), or without previously instilling intraperitoneal gas (primary puncture). With open laparoscopy, there is less risk for injury to blood vessels and abdominal viscera. However, open laparoscopy cannot prevent all insertion accidents because intestine can be entered inadvertently no matter how small the laparotomy. There is little evidence that secondary puncture is necessary, at least when there are no preexisting abdominal wall adhesions. Therefore, in women with no previous surgery, the primary puncture can be performed with a sharp-tipped trocar-cannula system, which lowers the cost by eliminating the need for the insufflation needle and by reducing operating time. The first, or primary, cannula must be of sufficient caliber to permit passage of the laparoscope and is usually inserted in or at the lower border of the umbilicus. The incision should be extended only enough to allow insertion of the cannula; otherwise, leakage of gas may occur around the sheath. For the primary puncture, an assistant should elevate the abdominal wall. For the secondary puncture, it is unnecessary to lift the abdominal wall during insertion. Both hands can be positioned on the device, using one to provide counterpressure and control to prevent "overshoot" and resultant injury to bowel or vessels. The angle of insertion is the same as for the insufflation needle; adjustments are made according to the patient's weight and body habitus. The laparoscope should be inserted to confirm proper intraperitoneal placement before the insufflation gas is allowed to flow. Laparoscope cannulas can become dislodged and slip out of the incision during a procedure. There are a variety of cannula attachments designed to prevent slippage.

Previous abdominal surgery increases the incidence of adhesions of the bowel to the anterior abdominal wall, frequently near the umbilicus and in the path of the primary trocar. In such patients, another primary insertion site should be selected, even if it is used solely for conveying a narrow "scout" laparoscope, some types of which can be inserted through an insufflation needle (Fig. 21.9). Using such a laparoscope, the presence of adhesions under the incision can be confirmed or excluded, and the umbilical cannula can be inserted under direct vision. Alternate insertion sites for primary cannulas are shown in Fig. 21.6. Of these

Figure 21.9 Scout laparoscopes. *Top:* the 2.7-mm-diameter Olympus/Ethicon Endosurgery system. The Imagyn outer sheath is introduced with a standard diameter 15-cm insufflation needle, and the Olympus/Ethicon system is inserted with a 3-mm needle. *Bottom:* the 2-mm-diameter Imagyn laparoscope (Imagyn, Inc., Laguna Niguel, CA).

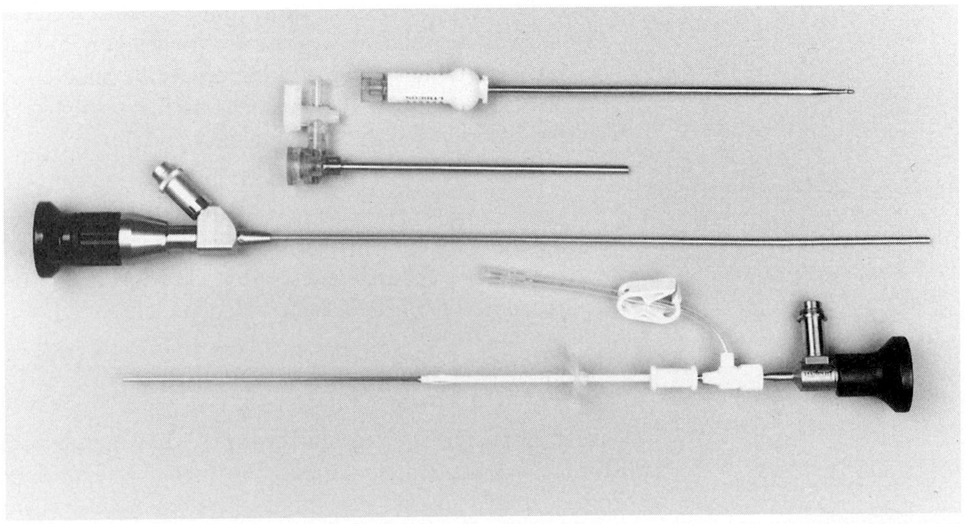

locations, the left upper quadrant is the most useful because adhesions are rarely present. Nasogastric or orogastric suction must be applied preceding insertion to improve vision and reduce the risk for gastric injury.

Ancillary Cannulas

Ancillary cannulas are necessary to perform most diagnostic and operative laparoscopic procedures. Most of the currently available disposable ancillary cannulas are identical to those designed for insertion of the primary cannula. However, many of the integrated design features of the primary cannula are unnecessary for ancillary cannulas. Consequently, simple cannulas without safety sheaths and insufflation ports are sufficient (Fig. 21.8).

Proper positioning of these cannulas depends on a sound knowledge of the abdominal wall vascular anatomy. They should always be inserted under direct vision because injury to bowel or major vessels can occur. Before insertion, the bladder should be drained with a urethral catheter. The insertion sites depend on the procedure, the disease, the patient's body habitus, and the surgeon's preference. The most useful and cosmetically acceptable site for an ancillary cannula is usually in the midline of the lower abdomen, about 2 to 4 cm above the symphysis. The ancillary cannula should not be inserted too close to the symphysis because it limits the mobility of the ancillary instruments and access to the cul-de-sac.

Lower-quadrant cannulas are useful for operative laparoscopy, but the inferior epigastric vessels must be located in order to avoid injury (Fig. 21.3). Transillumination of the abdominal wall from within permits the identification of the superficial inferior epigastric vessels in most thin women. However, the deep inferior epigastric vessels cannot be identified by this mechanism because of their location deep to the rectus sheath. **The most consistent landmarks are the medial umbilical ligaments (obliterated umbilical arteries) and the exit point of the round ligament into the inguinal canal.** At the pubic crest, the deep inferior epigastric vessels begin their cephalad course between the medially located umbilical ligament and the laterally positioned exit point of the round ligament. The trocar should be inserted medial or lateral to the vessels if they are visualized. **If the vessels cannot be seen and it is necessary to position the cannula laterally, the cannula should be placed 3 to 4 cm lateral to the medial umbilical ligament or lateral to the lateral margin of the rectus abdominis muscle.** If the insertion is placed too far laterally, it will endanger the deep circumflex epigastric artery. The risk for injury can be minimized by placing a 22-gauge spinal needle through the skin at the desired location, directly observing the entry through the laparoscope. This provides reassurance that a safe location has been identified and allows visualization of the peritoneal needle hole, which provides a precise target for inserting the trocar.

Even after a proper incision, the abdominal wall vessels can be injured if the trocar is directed medially. Large-diameter trocars are more likely to cause injury; therefore, the smallest cannulas necessary to perform the procedure should be used. Ancillary cannulas should not be placed too close together because this results in "knitting" of the hand instruments, which compromises access and maneuverability.

Visualization

During endoscopy, the image must be transferred through an optical system. Although direct optical viewing is feasible and often used for diagnostic purposes, virtually all operative laparoscopy is performed using video guidance.

Operative versus Diagnostic Equipment

Laparoscopes used for operative purposes have a straight channel, parallel to the optical axis, for the introduction of operating instruments. An advantage of such an endoscope is that it provides an additional port for the insertion of instruments and the tangential application of laser energy. However, operative endoscopes are of relatively larger caliber than diagnostic

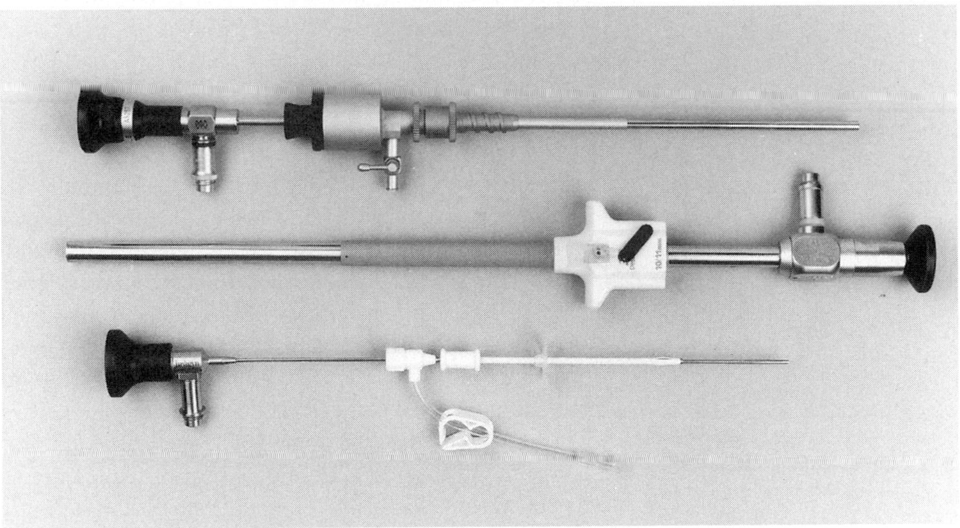

Figure 21.10 Laparoscopes. *Top to bottom:* 5-mm diameter (Olympus, Inc., Woodbury, NY), 10 mm diameter (Karl Storz, Agoura Hills, CA), and 2-mm diameter (Imagyn, Inc., Laguna Niguel, CA) laparoscopes. The 2-mm laparoscope can be inserted by a very narrow cannula passed through an insufflation needle.

laparoscopes and have smaller fields of view and increased electrosurgical risks. Diagnostic laparoscopes permit better visualization at a given diameter and are associated with fewer electrosurgical risks.

Diameter

Narrow-diameter laparoscopes allow limited transfer of light both into and out of the peritoneal cavity; therefore, they require a more sensitive camera or a more powerful light source for adequate illumination. Ideal illumination is provided by 10-mm diagnostic laparoscopes, but improvements in optics are making more procedures feasible with smaller-caliber devices (Fig. 21.10).

Lenses

Most laparoscope lenses are made of optical-quality glass. The use of fibers is necessary for very-small-caliber laparoscopes (<3 mm in diameter) because lens integrity is not well protected by the flexible sheath. Relatively large-caliber fibers tend to "pixellate" the image, although the use of densely packed, fine-caliber fibers reduces this tendency, and with an adequate number and quality of fibers, it is eliminated altogether.

Viewing Angle

The viewing angle depicts the relationship of the visual field to the axis of the endoscope and is usually either zero or 30 degrees to the horizontal. The zero-degree scope is the standard for gynecologic surgery. However, the 30-degree angle provides some advantage in difficult situations such as the performance of retropubic urethropexy.

Imaging Systems

Video Cameras

The video camera captures the image transmitted by the endoscope with one or three light-sensitive, charged-coupled device (CCD) chips located in the camera head and coupled with the endoscope. Generally, the camera is attached to the eyepiece of the laparoscope, but with newer instruments, the chip will be affixed to the end of the device ("chip-on-a-stick"), obviating the need for an optical channel. In either case, the image is transmitted to the body of the camera located outside the operative field, where it is processed and sent to a recording device or monitor.

The key functional features of a camera are its light sensitivity and its horizontal resolution. Light sensitivity is measured in lux (1 lux = 1 lumen/m^2); lower minimum lux ratings reflect increased sensitivity of the chips in the camera. The most sensitive cameras are rated at 1 lux, but for adequate imaging, the rating should be no higher than 5 lux when used with a 10-mm laparoscope and a 250- to 300-watt light source. Horizontal resolution is measured in lines; the best single-chip and triple-chip resolutions are about 500 and 700 lines, respectively. The images with the highest resolution are provided by cameras that separate chrominance from luminance (sometimes referred to as Y/C or S-Video) or by those that separate the three components of color (RGB—red, green, blue). These cameras are to be distinguished from the lower-resolution composite signals that are provided with standard coaxial cable television. However, the additional cost of triple-chip technology at this time is justified only for the creation of teaching videos or still images for publication.

Monitors

The resolution capability of the monitor should be at least equal to that provided by the camera. The best available monitors have the potential to display about 800 horizontal lines of resolution. This degree of resolution is not produced by S-Video or RGB systems; therefore, expensive Y/C- or RGB-capable cameras are unnecessary.

Light Sources

The more light transmitted through the endoscope, the better the visualization. The best currently available output is achieved from 250 to 300 watts, usually using xenon or metal halide bulbs. Most camera systems are integrated with the light source to vary light output automatically, depending on the amount of exposure required.

Light Cables

Light guides or cables transmit light from the source to the endoscope. They may be constructed of densely packed fibers (fiberoptic) or can be fluid filled. Fiberoptic cables lose function over time, particularly if they are bent at sharp angles, which breaks the fibers. Fluid-filled guides may initially supply more light but are less convenient than fiberoptic cables because they are heavier and less flexible.

Camera–Endoscope Couplers

These instruments connect the video camera to the laparoscope. Couplers with a beam splitter allow direct visualization by the surgeon with simultaneous video monitoring for the assistants. By sending the image through two optical channels, however, the brightness of each is reduced. Couplers also vary in focal length, which affects both the amount of screen occupied by the circular image and the depth of field in focus. For example, a coupler with a wide-angled 28-degree lens will fill all of the screen but will have less depth of field in focus than the smaller image of a 32-degree lens.

Some laparoscopes attach directly to the camera, making a coupler unnecessary. This feature further enhances light transmission and reduces problems with fogging of the lens.

Intraperitoneal Distention

Insufflation Machines

The insufflator delivers CO_2 from a gas cylinder to the patient through tubing connected to one of the ports on the laparoscope. Most insufflators can be set to maintain a predetermined intraabdominal pressure. High flow rates (9 to 20 L/min) are especially useful for maintaining exposure when suction of smoke or fluid depletes the volume of intraperitoneal gas.

Laparoscopic Lifting Systems

Intraperitoneal retractors attached to a pneumatic or mechanical lifting system can be used to create an intraperitoneal space much like a tent. This "gasless" or "apneumic" technique may have some advantages over pneumoperitoneum, particularly in patients with cardiopulmonary disease. Also, airtight cannulas are not necessary, and instruments do not need to have a uniform, narrow, cylindrical shape. Consequently, some conventional instruments may be used directly through the incisions.

Manipulation of Fluid and Tissue

Fluid Management

Fluid may be instilled into the peritoneal cavity through wide-caliber arthroscopy or cystoscopy tubing using pressure provided by gravity, an infusion cuff, or a high-pressure mechanical pump. The pumps deliver fluid faster than the other techniques, and the highly pressurized stream of fluid may facilitate blunt dissection (hydro- or aqua-dissection). Removal of small volumes of fluid can be performed with a syringe attached to a cannula, but for large volumes, it is necessary to use suction generated by a machine or a wall source.

The cannulas used for suction and irrigation depend on the irrigation fluid used and the fluid being removed. For ruptured ectopic gestations or other procedures in which there is a large amount of blood and clots, large-diameter cannulas (7 to 10 mm) are preferred. Cannulas with narrow tips are more effective in generating the high pressure needed for hydrodissection.

If large volumes of fluid are required, isotonic fluids should be used to avoid fluid overload and electrolyte imbalance. If electrosurgery is to be performed, however, small volumes of a nonelectrolyte-containing solution such as glycine or sorbitol can be used for hemostasis and irrigation. *Heparin* (1,000 to 5,000 U/L) can be added to irrigating solution to prevent blood from clotting, thus allowing it to be removed more easily.

Tissue Manipulation

Uterine Manipulators

A properly designed uterine manipulator should have an intrauterine component, or obturator, and a method for fixation of the device to the uterus. A hollow obturator attached to a port allows intraoperative instillation of liquid dye to demonstrate tubal patency. Articulation of the probe permits acute anteversion or retroversion, both of which are extremely useful maneuvers. If the uterus is large, longer and wider obturators are used so that the manipulations can be performed more effectively. An articulated uterine manipulator is shown in Fig. 21.11.

Grasping Forceps

The forceps used during laparoscopy should replicate those used in open surgery. Disposable instruments generally do not have the quality, strength, and precision of nondisposable forceps. Instruments with teeth (toothed forceps) are necessary to grasp the peritoneum

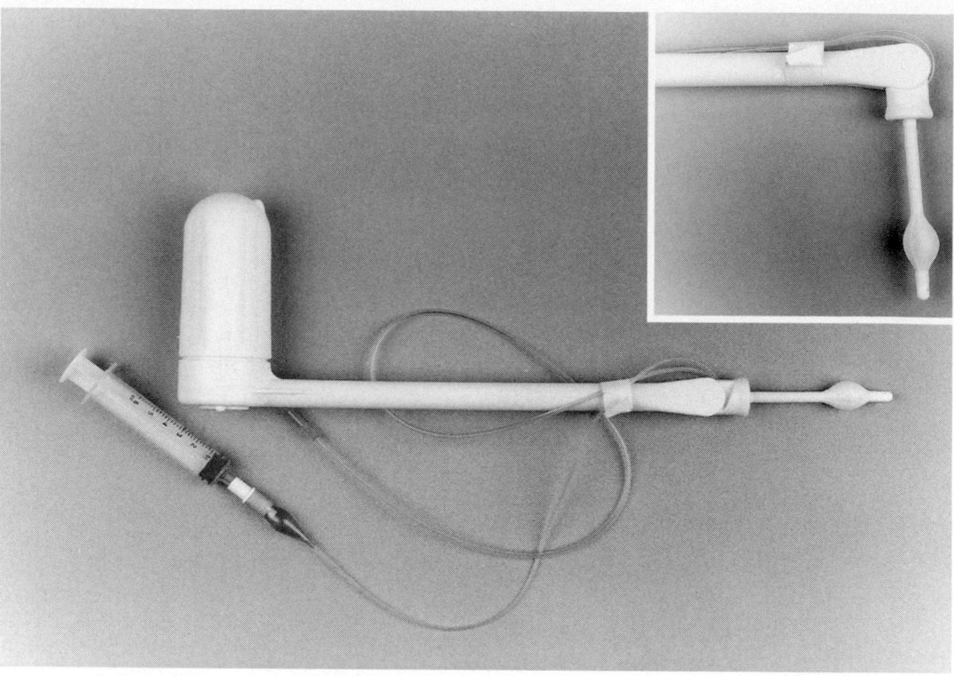

Figure 21.11 Uterine manipulators. The disposable Clearview (Ethicon Endo-surgery, Cincinnati, OH) manipulator is demonstrated. *Inset* is a demonstration of the ability of the obturator to articulate, allowing the uterus to be anteverted or retroverted more easily and completely.

or the edge of ovary securely in order to remove an ovarian cyst. Minimally traumatic instruments designed like Babcock clamps are needed to retract the fallopian tube safely. Tenaculum-like instruments are desirable to retract leiomyomas or the uterus. A ratchet is useful to hold tissue in the absence of hand pressure. The instrument should be insulated and capable of transmitting unipolar or bipolar electrical energy for hemostasis.

Cutting, Hemostasis, and Tissue Fixation

Cutting can be achieved by mechanical means, electricity, laser energy, and ultrasonic energy (Fig. 21.12). The methods for maintaining or securing hemostasis include sutures, clips, linear staplers, energy sources, and topical or injectable substances (Fig. 21.13). Secure apposition or tissue fixation may be accomplished with sutures, clips, or staples. Because of the visual, tactile, and mechanical limitations of laparoscopy, prevention of bleeding is important.

Cutting

The most useful cutting instruments are scissors. Because it is difficult to sharpen laparoscopic scissors, most surgeons prefer disposable instruments that may be used until dull and then discarded. Another mechanical cutting tool is the linear stapler-cutter that can simultaneously cut and hemostatically staple the edges of the incision. The cost and large dimensions of the instruments limit their practical use to only a few highly selected situations, such as separation of the uterus from the ovary and fallopian tube during laparoscopic hysterectomy.

Electrosurgical electrodes that are narrow or pointed are capable of generating the high-power densities necessary to vaporize or cut tissue. Continuous or modulated, usually unipolar, sine-wave outputs are used. For optimal results, they should be used in a noncontact fashion, following (not leading) the energy. Specially designed bipolar cutting probes are available that have one integrated electrode shaped as a needle and the other band-shaped

Figure 21.12 Laparoscopic cutting devices. *Top to bottom:* pointed microscissors (Ethicon Endosurgery, Cincinnati, OH), curved dissecting scissors (Microsurge, Needham, MA), a narrow-angled electrode (Ethicon, Cincinnati, OH), a GIA-30 linear cutter stapler (Autosuture, U.S. Surgical, Norwalk, CT).

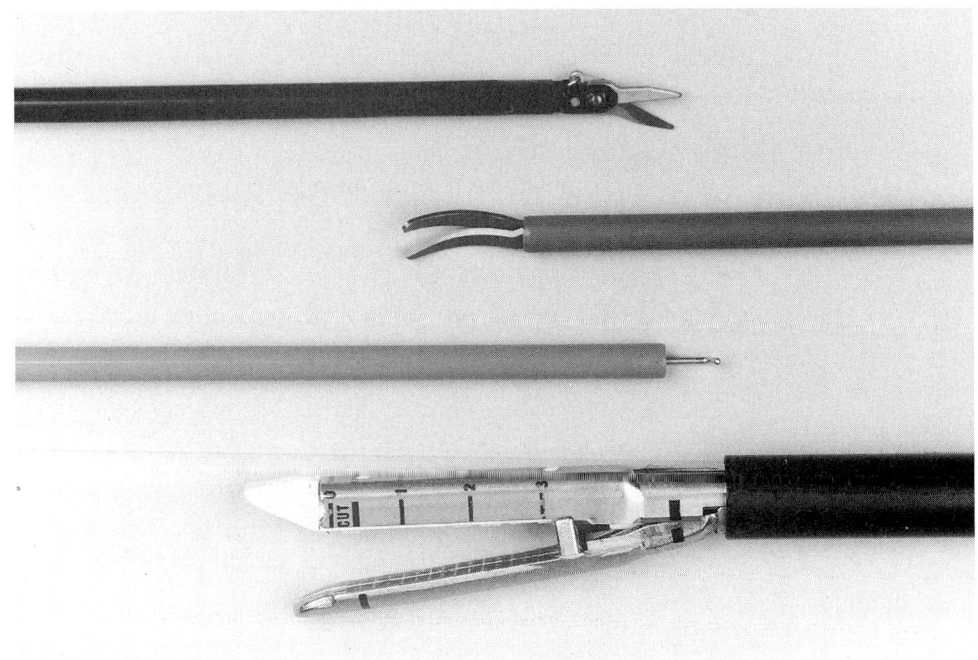

Figure 21.13 Hemostatic devices. *Left to right:* preloaded microfibrillar collagen (MedChem Products Inc., Woburn, MA), 1-cm clip applier (U.S. Surgical, Norwalk, CT), monopolar grasping forceps (Ethicon Endosurgery, Cincinnati, OH), GIA-30 linear with stapler (Autosuture, U.S. Surgical, Norwalk, CT), Clarke knot manipulator (Marlow, Inc., Willoughby, OH), Endoloop pretied ligature (Autosuture, U.S. Surgical, Norwalk, CT).

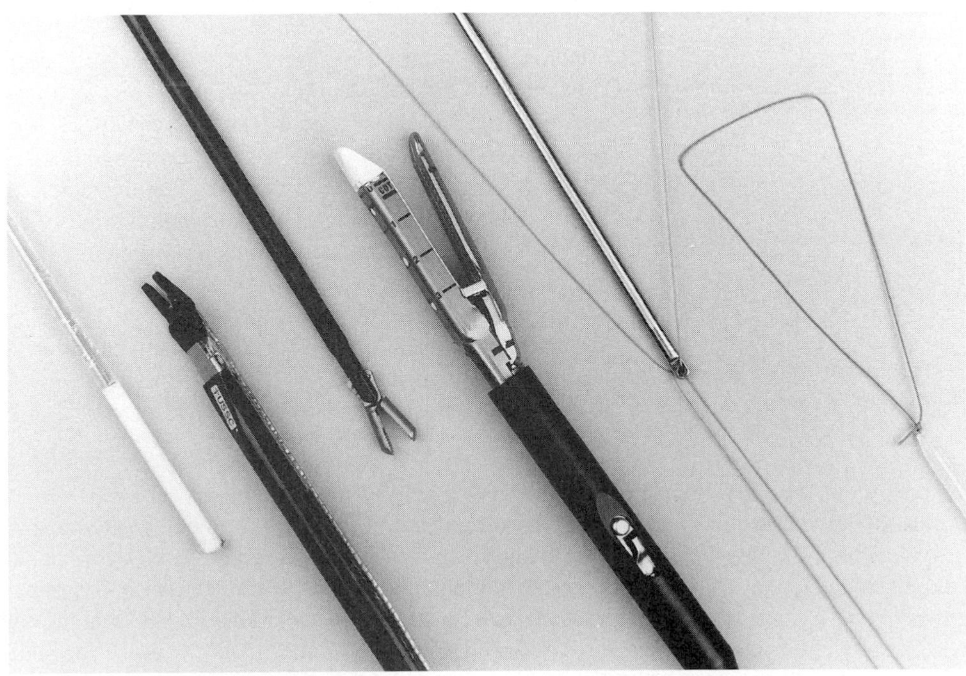

electrode designed to be dispersive. Laparoscopic scissors with unipolar or bipolar electrosurgical attachments are designed to cut mechanically with energy used simultaneously for desiccation and hemostasis when cutting tissue that has small blood vessels.

Laser energy can be focused to vaporize and cut tissue. The most efficient cutting instrument is the CO_2 laser, which has the drawback of requiring linear transmission because light cannot be effectively conducted along bendable fibers. The potassium-titanyl-phosphate (KTP) and neodymium:yttrium, aluminum, garnet (Nd:YAG) lasers are also effective cutting tools. They are capable of propagating energy along bendable quartz fibers but result in slightly greater thermal injury than electrical or CO_2 laser energy. Because of such limitations and the additional expense, these lasers are of limited value.

A laparoscopic instrument has been developed that uses ultrasonic energy for cutting. The device consists of a vibrating pizo electrode located in a handle that causes linear oscillation of a probe tipped with a blade, hook, or clamp. The rapid oscillation (55 kHz) of the probe allows the tip to cut mechanically or create hemostasis by tissue coagulation. In low-density tissue, cutting is augmented by the process of cavitation, in which reduction of local atmospheric pressure allows vaporization of intracellular water at body temperature.

Hemostasis and Tissue Fixation

Electricity is the least expensive and most versatile method for achieving hemostasis during laparoscopy. The process of electrical desiccation (coagulation) is achieved by contacting the tissue, activating the electrode using continuous "cutting" current of adequate power to heat and coagulate the tissue. For large-caliber vessels, the tissue should be compressed before the electrode is activated, allowing the edges of the vessel to seal or coapt. Either unipolar or bipolar grasping devices may be used. Fulguration is near-contact spraying of tissue with unipolar, high-voltage energy from the "coagulation" side of the electrosurgical generator. This technique is useful for control of superficial bleeding.

Clips may be placed with specially designed laparoscopic instruments. Nonabsorbable clips made of titanium are useful for relatively narrow vessels, and longer, self-retaining clips are generally preferred for larger vessels. Clips may be of particular value when securing relatively large vessels near an important structure such as the ureter.

Laparoscopic suturing has only recently become accepted as a method of maintaining hemostasis (50). The cost of materials is far less than that of clips or linear staplers, although operating time may be longer. The two basic methods for securing a ligature around a blood vessel are with intracorporeal and extracorporeal knots, depending on where the suture is tied. Intracorporeal knots are derived from the standard instrument knot and are formed within the peritoneal cavity. Extracorporeal knots are created outside the abdomen under direct vision and then transferred into the peritoneal cavity by knot manipulators (Fig. 21.13) (51).

Topical agents such as microfibrillar collagen are available in 5- and 10-mm diameter laparoscopic applicators (Fig. 21.13). Local injection of diluted vasopressin may be used to maintain hemostasis for myomectomy or removal of ectopic pregnancy.

Removal of Tissue

After excising tissue, it is usually necessary to remove it from the peritoneal cavity. Small samples can be pulled through an appropriate-sized cannula with grasping forceps; however, larger specimens may not fit. If the specimen is cystic, it may be drained by a needle or incised, shrinking it to a size suitable for removal through the cannula or one of the small laparoscopic incisions. Because of the concern for malignancy, an alternative is to place the specimen in an endoscopic retrieval bag before drainage to prevent spillage. More solid tissue may be morcellated with scissors, ultrasonic equipment, or electrosurgery.

Electrosurgical morcellation requires special bipolar needles or, if the monopolar technique is used, that the specimen remain attached to the patient to preserve the integrity of the electrical circuit.

Larger specimens may be removed by inserting a larger cannula through an incision in the cul-de-sac (posterior culdotomy) or by extending one of the laparoscopy incisions. With the exception of colpotomy, extension of the umbilical incision may be the most cosmetic approach because removal of the tissue can be directed from an endoscope positioned in one of the ancillary ports.

Incision Management

Dehiscence and hernia risk increase when the fascial incision is made by a trocar that is larger than 10 mm in diameter (52). Closure of the fascia should take place under direct laparoscopic vision to prevent the accidental incorporation of bowel into the incisions. A small-caliber laparoscope passed through one of the narrow cannulas can be used to direct the fascial closure using curved needles or a ligature carrier especially designed for this purpose.

Complications

Laparoscopic procedures can be complicated by infections, trauma, or hemorrhage, as well as by problems associated with anesthetic use. The incidence of infection is lower than with procedures performed by laparotomy. Conversely, problems associated with visualization in conjunction with the change in anatomic perspective may increase the risk for damage to blood vessels or vital structures such as the bowel, ureter, or bladder.

Some complications are more common with laparoscopy than with procedures performed by laparotomy or the vagina. The instillation of large amounts of fluid into the peritoneal cavity may contribute to electrolyte disturbances or fluid overload. The prolonged use of intraperitoneal gas under pressure may cause metabolic abnormalities or may adversely affect cardiorespiratory function. The intraperitoneal use of electrical or laser energy creates the potential for a variety of complications that can be minimized by knowledge of the energy source, meticulous technique, and maintenance of the instruments.

Anesthetic and Cardiopulmonary Complications

One third of the deaths associated with minor laparoscopic procedures such as sterilization are secondary to complications of anesthesia (52). The potential complications of general anesthesia include hypoventilation, esophageal intubation, gastroesophageal reflux, bronchospasm, hypotension, narcotic overdose, cardiac arrhythmias, and cardiac arrest. These risks can be enhanced by some of the inherent features of gynecologic laparoscopy. For example, the Trendelenburg position, in combination with the increased intraperitoneal pressure provided by pneumoperitoneum, places greater pressure on the diaphragm, increasing the risk for hypoventilation, hypercarbia, and metabolic acidosis. This position, combined with anesthetic agents that relax the esophageal sphincter, promotes regurgitation of gastric content, which in turn can lead to aspiration, bronchospasm, pneumonitis, and pneumonia.

Parameters of cardiopulmonary function associated with both CO_2 and N_2O insufflation include reduced PO_2, O_2 saturation, tidal volume, and minute ventilation and increased respiratory rate. The use of intraperitoneal CO_2 as a distention medium is associated with an increase in PCO_2 and a decrease in pH. Elevation of the diaphragm may be associated with basilar atelectasis, resulting in right-to-left shunt and a ventilation–perfusion mismatch (53).

Carbon Dioxide Embolus

Carbon dioxide is the most widely used peritoneal distention medium, largely because of the rapid absorption of CO_2 in blood. However, if large amounts of CO_2 gain access to the central venous circulation, if there is peripheral vasoconstriction, or if the splanchnic blood flow is decreased by excessively high intraperitoneal pressure, severe cardiorespiratory compromise may result.

The signs of CO_2 embolus include sudden and otherwise unexplained hypotension, cardiac arrhythmia, cyanosis, and heart murmurs. The end-tidal CO_2 may increase, and findings consistent with pulmonary edema may occur. Accelerating pulmonary hypertension may occur, resulting in right-sided heart failure.

Because gas embolism may result from direct intravascular injection through an insufflation needle, the proper placement of the needle must be ensured. The intraperitoneal pressure should be maintained at less than 20 mm Hg and, except for the initial placement of trocars, at 8 to 12 mm Hg. The risk for CO_2 embolus is also reduced by careful hemostasis because open venous channels are the portal of entry for gas into the systemic circulation. The anesthesiologist should continuously monitor the patient's color, blood pressure, heart sounds, heartbeat, and end-tidal CO_2 to allow early recognition of the signs of CO_2 embolus.

If CO_2 embolus is suspected or diagnosed, the surgeon must evacuate the CO_2 from the peritoneal cavity and place the patient in the left lateral decubitus position, with the head below the level of the right atrium. A large-bore central venous line should be inserted immediately to allow aspiration of gas from the heart. Because the findings are nonspecific, other causes of cardiovascular collapse should be excluded.

Cardiovascular Complications

Cardiac arrhythmias occur relatively frequently during laparoscopic surgery and are related to a number of factors, the most significant of which are hypercarbia and acidemia. Early reports of laparoscopy-associated arrhythmia were associated with spontaneous respiration; therefore, most anesthesiologists have adopted the practice of mechanical ventilation during laparoscopic surgery. The incidence of hypercarbia is reduced by operating with intraperitoneal pressures less than 12 mm Hg (54).

The risk for cardiac arrhythmia also may be reduced by using NO_2 as a distending medium. However, although NO_2 is associated with a decreased incidence of arrhythmia, it is insoluble in blood. External lifting systems avoid the complication of hypercarbia and can also provide protection against cardiac arrhythmia.

Hypotension can occur because of decreased venous return secondary to very high intraperitoneal pressure, and this condition may be potentiated by volume depletion. Vagal discharge may occur in response to increased intraperitoneal pressure, which can cause hypotension secondary to cardiac arrhythmias (55). All of these side effects are more dangerous for patients with preexisting cardiovascular disease.

Gastric Reflux

Gastric regurgitation and aspiration can occur during laparoscopic surgery, especially in patients with obesity, gastroparesis, hiatal hernia, or gastric outlet obstruction. In these patients, the airway must be maintained with a cuffed endotracheal tube, and the stomach must be decompressed (e.g., with a nasogastric tube). The lowest necessary intraperitoneal pressure should be used to minimize the risk for aspiration. Patients should be moved out of the Trendelenburg position before being extubated. Routine preoperative administration of metoclopramide, H_2-blocking agents, and nonparticulate antacids also reduces the risk.

Extraperitoneal Insufflation

The most common causes of extraperitoneal insufflation are preperitoneal placement of the insufflating needle and leakage of CO_2 around the cannula sites. Although this condition is usually mild and limited to the abdominal wall, subcutaneous emphysema can become extensive, involving the extremities, the neck, and the mediastinum. Another relatively common site for emphysema is the omentum or mesentery, a circumstance that may be mistaken for preperitoneal insufflation.

Subcutaneous emphysema may be identified by the palpation of crepitus, usually in the abdominal wall. Emphysema can extend along contiguous fascial plains to the neck, where it can be visualized directly. Such a finding may reflect mediastinal emphysema, which may indicate impending cardiovascular collapse (56–58).

The risk for subcutaneous emphysema is reduced by the proper positioning of the insufflation needle and by maintaining a low intraperitoneal pressure after placement of the desired cannulas. Other approaches that reduce the chance of subcutaneous emphysema include open laparoscopy and the use of abdominal wall lifting systems that make gas unnecessary.

If the insufflation has occurred extraperitoneally, the laparoscope can be removed, and the procedure can be repeated. However, difficulty may ensue because of the altered anterior peritoneum. Open laparoscopy or the use of an alternate site, such as the left upper quadrant, should be considered. One approach is to leave the laparoscope in the expanded preperitoneal space while the insufflation needle is reinserted under direct vision through the peritoneal membrane caudad to the tip of the laparoscope (59).

In mild cases of subcutaneous emphysema, the findings quickly resolve after evacuation of the pneumoperitoneum, and no specific intraoperative or postoperative therapy is required. When the extravasation extends to the neck, it is usually preferable to terminate the procedure because pneumomediastinum, pneumothorax, hypercarbia, and cardiovascular collapse may result.

At the end of the procedure, it is prudent to obtain a chest x-ray. The patient's condition should be managed expectantly unless a tension pneumothorax results, in which case immediate evacuation must be performed using a chest tube or a wide-bore needle (14 to 16 gauge) inserted in the second intercostal space in the midclavicular line.

Electrosurgical Complications

Complications of electrosurgery occur secondary to thermal injury from unintended or inappropriate use of the active electrode, current diversion to an undesirable path, and injury at the site of the dispersive electrode. Active electrode injury can occur with either unipolar or bipolar instruments, whereas trauma secondary to current diversion or dispersive electrode accidents occurs only with unipolar technique. Complications of electrosurgery are reduced by adherence to safety protocols coupled with a sound understanding of the principles of electrosurgery and the circumstances that can lead to injury (16).

Active Electrode Trauma

If the foot pedal is accidentally depressed, tissue adjacent to the electrode will be traumatized. Commonly, the bowel or ureter is involved, or, if the electrode lies on the abdomen, the skin is burned. Direct extension injuries occur when the zone of vaporization or coagulation extends to large blood vessels or vital structures such as the bladder, ureter, or bowel. Bipolar technique may reduce but does not eliminate the risk for thermal injury to adjacent tissue (60). Therefore, blood vessels should be isolated before desiccation, especially when they are near vital structures, and appropriate amounts of energy must be applied to allow an adequate margin of noninjured tissue.

The diagnosis of direct thermal visceral injury may be difficult. If unintended activation of the electrode occurs, nearby intraperitoneal structures should be evaluated carefully. The appearance can be affected by several factors, including the output of the generator, the type of electrode, its proximity to tissue, and the duration of its activation. The diagnosis of visceral thermal injury is often delayed until signs and symptoms of fistula or peritonitis appear. Because these complications may not manifest until 2 to 10 days after surgery, patients should be advised to report any postoperative fever or increasing abdominal pain.

Unintended activation injuries can be prevented if the surgeon is always in direct control of electrode activation and if all electrosurgical hand instruments are removed from the peritoneal cavity when not in use. When removed from the peritoneal cavity, the instruments should be detached from the electrosurgical generator, or they should be stored in an insulated pouch near the operative field. These measures prevent damage to the patient's skin if the electrode is accidentally activated.

Thermal injury to the bowel, bladder, or ureter that is recognized at the time of laparoscopy should be managed immediately with laparotomy, taking into consideration the potential extent of the zone of coagulative necrosis (61). Incisions made with the focused energy from a pointed electrode are associated with a minimal amount of surrounding thermal injury. Prolonged or even transient contact with a relatively large-caliber electrode may produce thermal necrosis that extends several centimeters. In such cases, wide excision or resection will be necessary.

Current Diversion

Current diversion can occur when electrons find a direct path out of the patient's body through grounded sites other than the dispersive electrode. Alternatively, the current can be diverted directly to other tissues before it reaches the tip of the active electrode. In either case, if the power density becomes high enough, unintended and severe thermal injury can result.

Alternate Ground Site Burns

These injuries can occur only with ground-referenced electrosurgical generators (ESUs) because they lack an isolated circuit. In such generators, when the dispersive electrode becomes detached, unplugged, or otherwise ineffective, the current seeks any grounded conductor. If the conductor has a small surface area, the current or power density may become high enough to cause thermal injury (Fig. 21.14). Examples include electrocardiograph patch electrodes or the conductive metal components of the operating table.

Modern ESUs are designed with isolated circuits and impedance monitoring systems that shut down the machine if dispersive electrode detachment occurs. Because ground-referenced machines without such safeguards are still in use, it is important to know the type of ESU used in the operating room.

Insulation Defects

If the insulation coating the shaft of an electrosurgical electrode becomes defective, it can allow current diversion to adjacent tissue, often bowel, potentially resulting in significant injury (Fig 21.15A). Therefore, the instruments should be examined before each procedure to detect worn or obviously defective insulation. When applying unipolar electrical energy, the shaft of the instrument should be kept away from vital structures and, if possible, totally visible in the operative field.

Direct Coupling

Direct coupling occurs when an activated electrode touches and energizes another metal conductor such as a laparoscope, cannula, or other instrument, especially one that is not insulated. If the conductor is near or in contact with other tissue, a thermal injury can result (Fig 21.15B). Direct coupling can be prevented by removing the electrode when it is not in

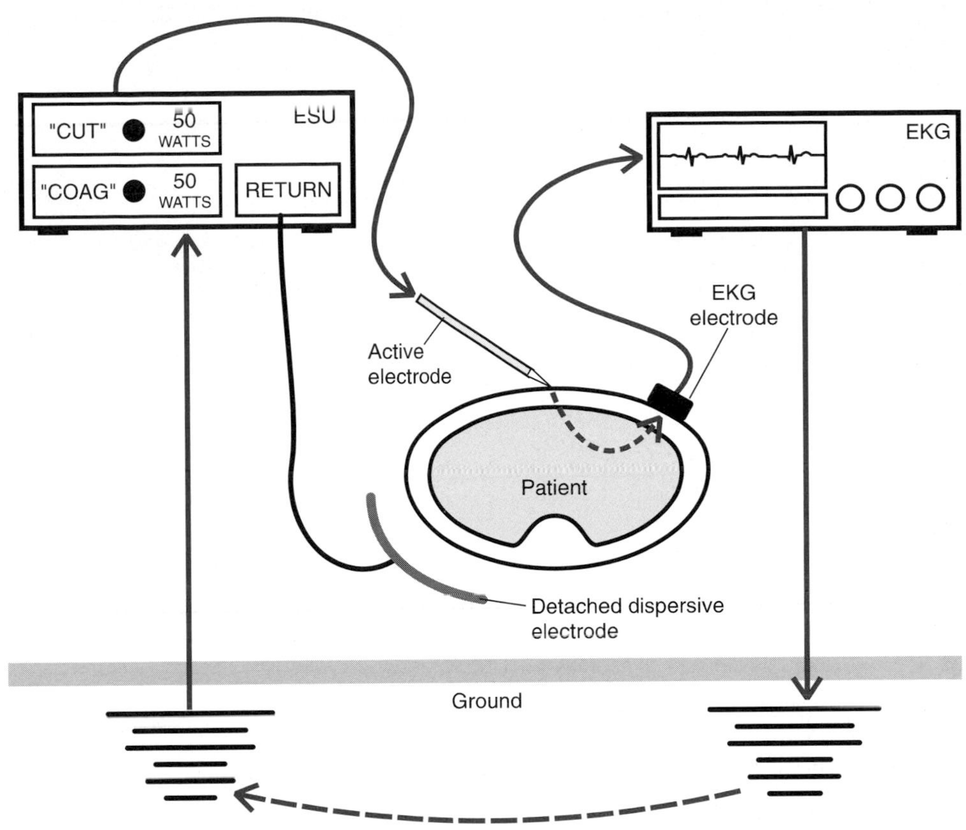

Figure 21.14 Risk of ground-referenced generators. Current diversion along alternate pathways is a risk associated with ground referenced electrosurgical generators, particularly if the dispersive electrode is detached. In the example depicted, the relatively high current density at the electrocardiogram electrode site may result in a skin burn.

use and by visually confirming that there is no contact with other conductive instruments before activation.

Capacitive Coupling

Capacitance is the ability of a conductor to establish an electrical current in an unconnected but nearby circuit. An electrical field is established around the shaft of any activated laparoscopic unipolar electrode, a circumstance that makes the electrode a capacitor. This field is harmless if the circuit is completed through a dispersive, low-power density pathway (Fig. 21.16). For example, if capacitative coupling occurs between the laparoscopic electrode and a metal cannula positioned in the abdominal wall, the current harmlessly "returns" to the abdominal wall, where it traverses to the dispersive electrode (Fig. 21.16A). However, if the metal cannula is anchored to the skin by a nonconductive plastic retaining sleeve or anchor (a hybrid system), the current will not return to the abdominal wall because the sleeve acts as an insulator (Fig. 21.16B). Instead, the capacitor will have to "look" elsewhere to complete the circuit. Therefore, bowel or any other nearby conductor can become the target of a relatively high-power density discharge (Fig. 21.16C). This mechanism can also occur when a unipolar electrode is inserted through an operating laparoscope that, in turn, is passed through a nonconductive plastic laparoscopic cannula. In this configuration, the plastic port acts as the insulator. If the electrode capacitively couples with the metal laparoscope, nearby bowel will be at risk for significant thermal injury (61,62).

Capacitative coupling can be prevented by avoiding the use of hybrid laparoscope-cannula systems that contain a mixture of conductive and nonconductive elements. Instead, it is

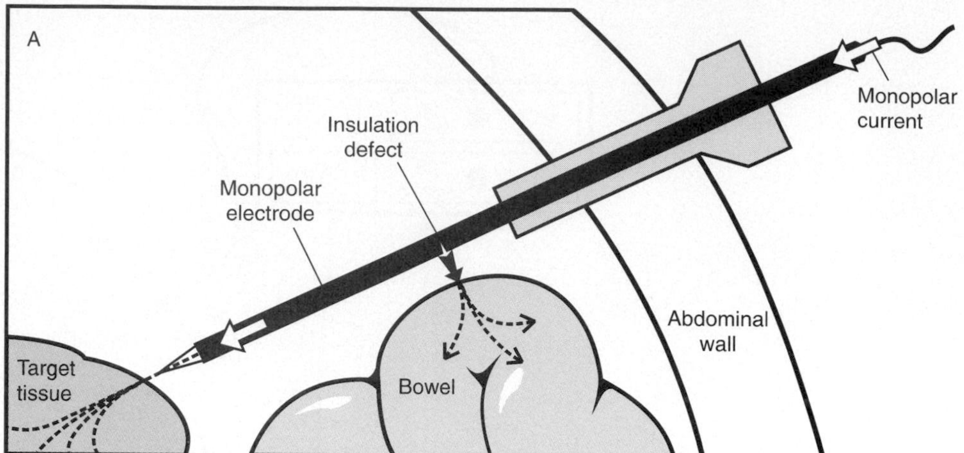

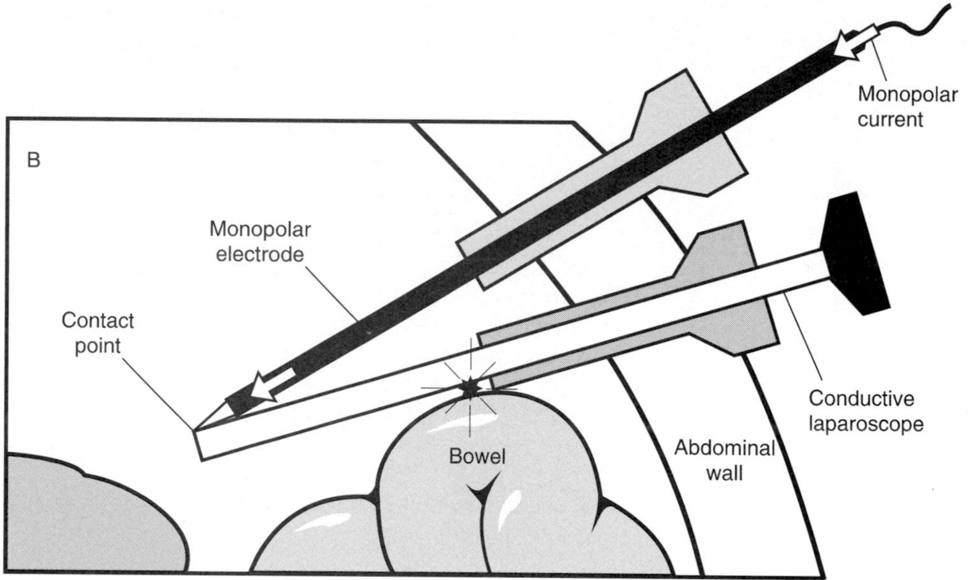

Figure 21.15 Direct coupling. Direct coupling is a potential complication of monopolar electrosurgery and may occur secondary to defects in the insulation (**A**) or, classically, to contract with a conductive instrument that in turn touches other intraperitoneal structures. In the example depicted (**B**), the active electrode is touching the laparoscope, and current is transferred to bowel through a small enough contact point that thermal injury results. Another common target of such coupling is to noninsulated hand instruments.

preferred that all-plastic or all-metal cannula systems be used. When operating laparoscopes are used, all-metal cannula systems should be the rule unless there is no intent to perform unipolar electrosurgical procedures through the operating channel.

Dispersive Electrode Burns

The use of isolated-circuit electrosurgical generators with return electrode monitors has virtually eliminated dispersive electrode–related thermal injury. Return electrode monitoring is actually accomplished by measuring the impedance in the dispersive electrode (patient pad), which should always be low because of the large surface area. Without such devices, partial detachment of the "patient pad" could result in a thermal injury because reducing the surface area of the electrode raises the current density (Fig. 21.17).

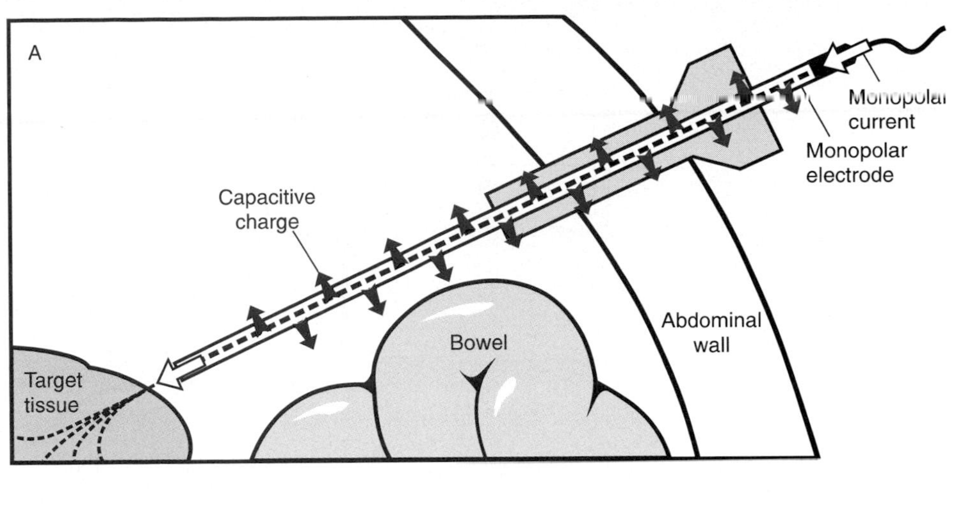

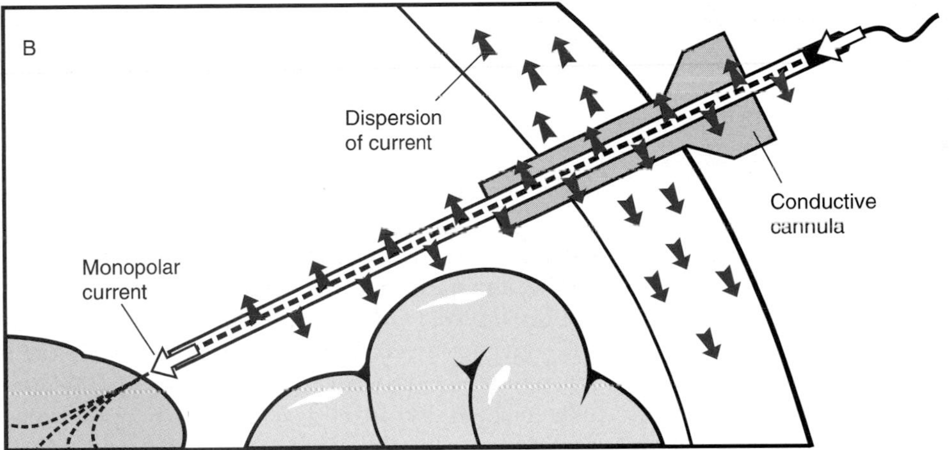

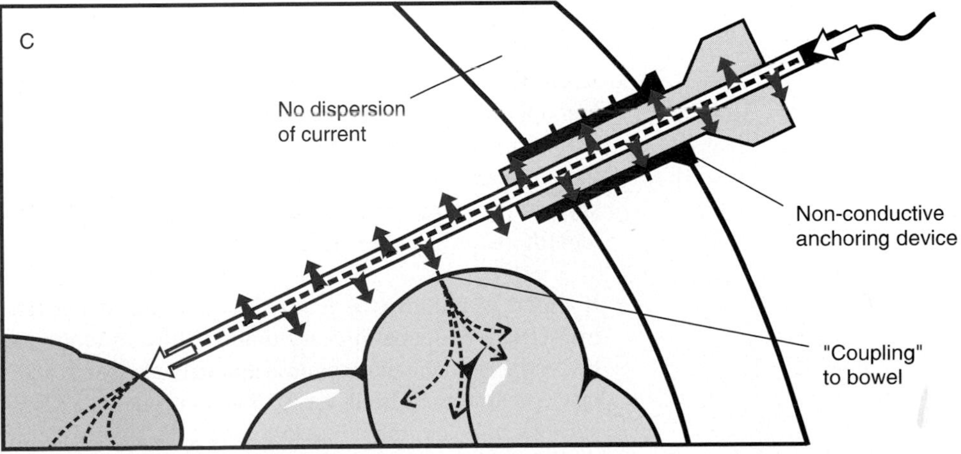

Figure 21.16 Capacitative coupling. A: All activated monopolar electrodes emit a surrounding charge, proportional to the voltage of the current. This makes the electrode a potential capacitor. **B:** Generally, as long as the charge is allowed to disperse through the abdominal wall, no sequelae result. However, if the "return" to the dispersive electrode is blocked by insulation, such as a plastic anchor (**C**), the current can couple to a conductive cannula or directly to bowel.

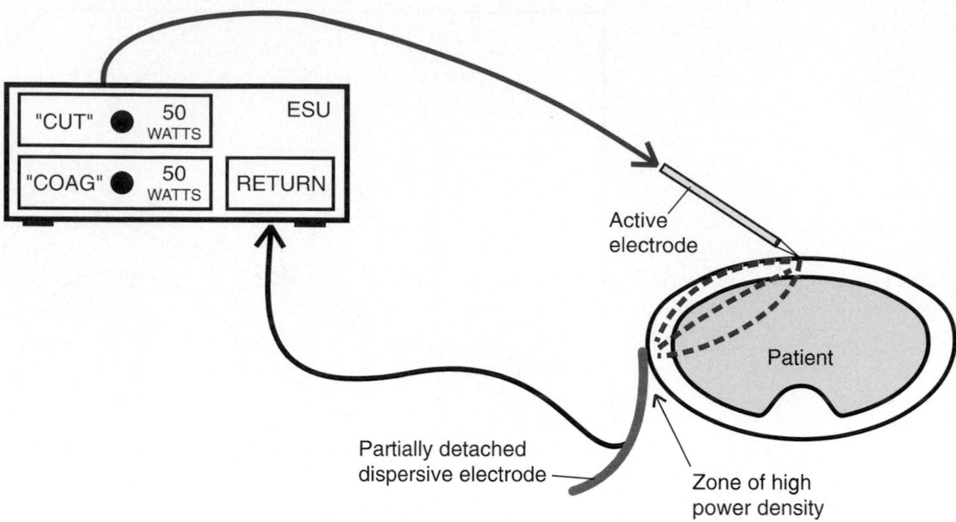

Figure 21.17 Dispersive electrode burns. If the dispersive electrode becomes partially detached, the current density may increase to the point that a skin burn results.

Hemorrhagic Complications

Great Vessel Injury

The most dangerous hemorrhagic complications are injuries to the great vessels, including the aorta and the vena cava, the common iliac vessels and their branches, and the internal and external iliac arteries and veins. The injuries most often occur secondary to insertion of an insufflation needle but may be created by the tip of the primary or ancillary trocars. The vessels most frequently damaged are the aorta and the right common iliac artery as it branches from the aorta in the midline. The anatomically more posterior location of the vena cava and the iliac veins provides relative protection, but not immunity, from injury (63). Although most of these injuries are small and amenable to repair with suture, some are larger and require ligation with or without the insertion of a vascular graft. Deaths have been reported.

After vascular injury, patients usually develop profound hypotension with or without hemoperitoneum. In some instances, blood is aspirated through the insufflation needle before the introduction of the distending gas. Frequently, the bleeding may be contained in the retroperitoneal space, which usually delays the diagnosis; consequently, hypovolemic shock may develop. To avoid late recognition, the course of each great vessel must be identified before completing the procedure.

If blood is withdrawn from the insufflation needle, it should be left in place while immediate preparations are made to obtain blood products and perform laparotomy. If hemoperitoneum is diagnosed upon initial visualization of the peritoneal cavity, a grasping instrument may be used, if possible, to occlude the vessel temporarily. Upon entry into the peritoneal cavity, the aorta and vena cava should immediately be compressed just below the level of the renal vessels to gain at least temporary control of blood loss. The most appropriate course of action depends on the site and extent of injury.

Abdominal Wall Vessel Injury

The abdominal wall vessels most commonly injured during laparoscopy are the superficial inferior epigastric vessels as they branch from the femoral artery and vein and course cephalad in each lower quadrant. They are invariably damaged by the initial passage of an ancillary trocar or by the introduction of a wider device later in the procedure. The problem may be recognized immediately by the observation of blood dripping along the cannula or out through the incision. However, the bleeding may be obstructed by the cannula until it is withdrawn at the end of the operation.

The more serious injuries are those to the deep inferior epigastric vessels, which are branches of the external iliac artery and vein that course cephalad but are deep to the rectus fascia and often deep to the muscles (Fig. 21.3). More laterally located are the deep circumflex iliac vessels, which are not often encountered in laparoscopic surgery. Laceration of these vessels may cause profound blood loss, particularly when the trauma is unrecognized and causes extraperitoneal bleeding.

Signs of injury, in addition to blood dripping down the cannula, include the postoperative appearance of shock and abdominal wall discolorization or hematoma located near the incision. In some instances, the blood may track to a more distant site, presenting as a pararectal or vulvar mass. Delayed diagnosis may be prevented by laparoscopic evaluation of each peritoneal incision after removal of the cannula.

Superficial inferior epigastric vessel trauma usually stops spontaneously; therefore, expectant management is appropriate. A straight ligature carrier can be used to repair lacerated deep inferior epigastric vessels. If a postoperative hematoma develops, local compression should be used initially. Open removal or aspiration of the hematoma should not be undertaken because it may inhibit the tamponade effect and increase the risk for abscess. However, if the mass continues to enlarge or if signs of hypovolemia develop, the wound must be explored.

Intraperitoneal Vessel Injury

Hemorrhage may result from inadvertent entry into a vessel or failure of a specific occlusive technique. In addition to delayed hemorrhage, there may be a further delay in diagnosis at laparoscopy as a result of the restricted visual field and the temporary occlusive pressure exerted by CO_2 in the peritoneal cavity.

Inadvertent division of an artery or vein is usually evident immediately. Transected arteries may go into spasm and bleed minutes to hours later, going unnoticed temporarily because of the limited visual field of the laparoscope. Therefore, at the end of the procedure, all areas of dissection must be carefully examined. CO_2 should be vented, which decreases the intraperitoneal pressure so that blood vessels temporarily occluded by higher pressure can be recognized.

Gastrointestinal Complications

The stomach, the small bowel, and the colon can be injured during laparoscopy. Mechanical entry into the large or small bowel can occur 10 times more often when laparoscopy is performed in patients who have had prior intraperitoneal inflammation or abdominal surgery. Loops of intestine can adhere to the abdominal wall under the insertion site and be injured (64–66).

Insufflation Needle Injuries

Needle entry into the gastrointestinal tract may be more common than reported because it often occurs unnoticed and without further complication. Gastric entry may be identified by the increased filling pressure, asymmetric distention of the peritoneal cavity, or aspiration of gastric particulate matter through the lumen of the needle. Initially, the hollow, capacious stomach may allow the insufflation pressure to remain normal. Signs of bowel entry are the same as those for gastric injury, with the addition of feculent odor.

If particulate debris is identified, the needle should be left in place, and an alternate insertion site should be identified, such as the left upper quadrant. Immediately after successful entry into the peritoneal cavity, the site of injury is identified. Defects must be repaired immediately.

Trocar Injuries

Damage caused by a sharp trocar is usually more serious than needle injury. Inadvertent gastric entry usually results from stomach distention because of aerophagia, difficult or improper intubation, or mask induction with inhalation anesthetic. Most often, the injury is created by the primary trocar, although ancillary cannulas may also result in visceral injury.

The risk for gastric perforation can be minimized with the selective use of preoperative nasogastric or oral gastric suction when left upper-quadrant entries are used or when the intubation was difficult. Open laparoscopy can reduce but not eliminate the risk for gastrointestinal complications. For high-risk patients, left upper quadrant needle insertion with a properly decompressed stomach may be preferable (67–69).

If the trocar of a primary cannula penetrates the bowel, the condition is usually diagnosed when the mucosal lining of the gastrointestinal tract is visualized. If the large bowel is entered, a feculent odor may be noted. However, the injury may not be immediately recognized because the cannula may not stay within the bowel or may pass through the lumen. Such injuries usually occur when a single loop of bowel is adherent to the anterior abdominal wall. The injury may not be recognized until peritonitis, abscess, enterocutaneous fistula, or death occurs (70,71). Therefore, at the end of the procedure, the removal of the primary cannula must be viewed either through the cannula or an ancillary port, a process facilitated by routine direct visualization of closure of the incision of the primary port.

Trocar injuries to the stomach and bowel require repair as soon as they are recognized. If the injury is small, a trained operator can repair the defect by laparoscopy using a double layer of running 2-0 or 3-0 absorbable suture. Extensive lesions may require resection and reanastomosis, which in most instances requires laparotomy. The preoperative use of mechanical bowel preparation in selected high-risk cases minimizes the need for laparotomy or colostomy.

Dissection and Thermal Injury

It is often easier to recognize intestinal injury that occurs during dissection than thermal injury to the bowel, particularly if the latter was created with electrical or laser energy. Even if thermal injury is recognized, it is difficult to estimate by visual inspection the extent of the damage because the zone of desiccation may exceed the area of visual damage. In some patients, the diagnosis is delayed until the development of peritonitis and fever, usually a few days later but occasionally not for several weeks (72). When mechanical bowel trauma is recognized during the dissection, treatment is the same as that described for trocar injury. If the diagnosis is delayed until the postoperative recognition of peritonitis, laparotomy must be performed immediately.

Thermal injury may be handled expectantly if the lesion seems superficial and confined. In a study of 33 women with such injuries who were managed expectantly in the hospital, only 2 required laparotomy for perforation (72).

Urologic Injury

Laparoscopy-associated damage to the bladder or ureter may occur secondary to mechanical or thermal trauma. Ideally, such injury should be prevented; otherwise, it is essential that the lesion be identified intraoperatively.

Bladder Injury

Bladder injury can occur from a trocar perforation of the undrained bladder but may also occur while dissecting the bladder from adherent structures or from the anterior uterus (73,74). The injury may be readily apparent by direct visualization. If an indwelling catheter is in place, hematuria or pneumaturia (CO_2 in the catheter drainage system) may be noticed. A bladder laceration can be confirmed by injecting sterile milk or a diluted methylene blue solution through a transurethral catheter. Thermal injury to the bladder, however, may not be initially apparent and, if missed, can present as peritonitis or a fistula.

Routine preoperative bladder drainage usually prevents trocar-related cystotomies. Separation of the bladder from the uterus or other adherent structures requires good visualization, appropriate retraction, and excellent surgical technique. Sharp mechanical dissection is preferred, particularly when relatively dense adhesions are present.

Very-small-caliber injuries to the bladder (1 to 2 mm) may be treated with bladder catheterization for 5 to 7 days. If repair is undertaken immediately, catheterization is unnecessary. When a larger injury is identified, it can be repaired laparoscopically (73–75). However, if the laceration is near the trigone or involves the trigone, an open procedure should be used. The mechanism of injury should be taken into consideration in making this evaluation because electrical injuries often extend beyond the visible limits of the apparent defect.

For small lesions, closure may be performed with layers of absorbable 2-0 to 3-0 sutures. If there is thermal injury, the coagulated portion should be excised. Postoperative catheterization with either a transurethral or suprapubic catheter should be maintained for 2 to 5 days for small fundal lacerations and for 10 to 14 days for injuries to the trigone. **Cystography should be performed before removal of the urinary catheter.**

Ureteral Injury

The most common cause of ureteral injury during laparoscopy is electrosurgical trauma (76,77). However, ureteral injury can occur after mechanical dissection and the use of linear cutting and stapling devices (78–80). Although intraoperative recognition of ureteral injury is possible, the diagnosis is usually delayed (76). Ureteral lacerations may be confirmed intraoperatively visually or with the intravenous injection of indigo carmine. Thermal injury presents up to 14 days after surgery with fever, abdominal or flank pain, and peritonitis. Leukocytosis may be present, and intravenous pyelography shows extravasation of urine or a urinoma. Mechanical obstruction from staples or a suture can be recognized intraoperatively only by direct visualization. Ureteral obstruction presents a few days to 1 week after surgery with flank pain and often fever (80). Abdominal ultrasound may be helpful, but intravenous pyelography can more precisely identify the site and degree of the obstruction.

Discharge or continuous incontinence is a delayed sign of ureterovaginal or vesicovaginal fistulas. A bladder fistula can be confirmed by detecting dye on a tampon previously placed in the vagina after filling the bladder with methylene blue. With a ureterovaginal fistula, the methylene blue will not pass into the vagina, but it can be detected with the intravenous injection of indigo carmine.

Knowledge of the course of the ureter through the pelvis is a prerequisite to reducing the risk for injury. The ureter can usually be seen through the peritoneum of the pelvic sidewall between the pelvic brim and the attachment of the broad ligament. However, because of variation from one patient to another or the presence of disease, the location of the ureter can become obscured, making it necessary to enter the retroperitoneal space. The techniques used for retroperitoneal dissection are also important factors in reducing the risk for ureteric injury. Blunt and sharp dissection with scissors is preferred, although hydrodissection can be used (81). The selective placement of ureteral stents may also be helpful.

Ureteral injury can be treated immediately if it is diagnosed intraoperatively. Although very limited damage may heal over a ureteral stent left in place for 10 to 21 days, repair is indicated in most patients. Although laparoscopic repair of ureteric lacerations and transections has been performed, most injuries require laparotomy (76,82).

When the diagnosis of ureteral injury is delayed, the bladder should be drained with a catheter. Incomplete or small obstructions or lacerations may be treated successfully with either a retrograde or anterograde ureteral stent. Urinomas may be drained percutaneously. If a stent cannot be placed successfully, a percutaneous nephrostomy should be performed before operative repair is undertaken.

Neurologic Injury

Peripheral nerve injury is usually related either to poor positioning of the patient or to excessive pressure exerted by the surgeons. Nerve injury may also occur as a result of the surgical dissection.

In the extremities, the trauma may be direct, such as when the common peroneal nerve is compressed against the stirrups. The femoral nerve or the sciatic nerve or its branches may be overstretched and damaged by inappropriate positioning of the hip or the knee joint (83,84). Brachial plexus injuries may occur secondary to the surgeon or assistants leaning against the abducted arm during the procedure. If the patient is placed in a steep Trendelenburg position, the brachial plexus may be damaged because of the pressure exerted on the shoulder joint (85). In most cases, sensory or motor deficits are found as the patient emerges from anesthesia. The likelihood of brachial plexus injury can be reduced with adequate padding and support of the arms and shoulders or by placing the patient's arms in an adducted position.

Most injuries to peripheral nerves resolve spontaneously. The time to recovery depends on the site and severity of the lesion. For most peripheral injuries, full sensory nerve recovery occurs in 3 to 6 months. Recovery may be facilitated by physical therapy, appropriate braces, and electrical stimulation of the affected muscles. Open microsurgery should be performed for transection of major intrapelvic nerves.

Incisional Hernia and Wound Dehiscence

Incisional hernia after laparoscopy has been reported in more than 900 cases (51). Although no incision is immune to the risk, defects that are larger than 10 mm in diameter are particularly vulnerable (86,87). In most cases, these defects can be prevented by proper technique and closure of large defects. All ancillary cannulas should be removed under direct vision to ensure that bowel is not drawn into the incision. For incisions larger than 10 mm in diameter, the fascia should be closed while viewing the defect with the laparoscope to minimize the risk for intestinal injury. A small-diameter laparoscope should be used through a narrow cannula to facilitate incisional closure.

The most common defect is when intestinal hernia develops in the immediate postoperative period. The hernia may be asymptomatic or, within the first postoperative week, may cause pain, fever, periumbilical mass, obvious evisceration, and the symptoms and signs of mechanical bowel obstruction.

Because Richter's hernias contain only a portion of the intestine in the defect, the diagnosis is often delayed. Hernias most often occur in incisions lateral to the midline. The initial symptom is usually pain because the incomplete obstruction still allows the passage of intestinal contents. Fever can be present if incarceration occurs, and peritonitis may result from subsequent perforation. The condition is difficult to diagnose, requires a high index of suspicion, and may be confirmed with an ultrasound or a CT scan (88).

The management of laparoscopic incisional defects depends on the time of presentation and the presence and condition of entrapped bowel. Evisceration always requires surgical intervention. If the condition is diagnosed immediately, the intestine is replaced into the peritoneal cavity (if there is no evidence of necrosis or intestinal defect), and the incision is repaired, usually with laparoscopic guidance. If the diagnosis is delayed or the bowel is incarcerated or at risk for perforation, laparotomy is necessary to repair or resect the intestine.

Infection

Wound infections after laparoscopy are uncommon; most are minor skin infections that can be treated successfully with expectant management, drainage, or antibiotics (89). Severe necrotizing fasciitis can occur rarely (90). Bladder infection, pelvic cellulitis, and pelvic abscess have been reported (91).

The risk for infection associated with laparoscopy is much lower than that for infection associated with open abdominal or vaginal surgery. Prophylactic antibiotics should be offered to selected patients (e.g., those with enhanced risk for bacterial endocarditis and those for whom hysterectomy is planned). Patients should be instructed to monitor their body temperature after discharge and to report immediately a temperature higher than 38°C.

Hysteroscopy

The hysteroscopic lysis of intrauterine adhesions was first described in 1973 (92). The technique of endoscopically guided electrosurgical resection was adapted from urology to gynecology for the removal of uterine leiomyomas (93). Hysteroscopic division of uterine septa was developed using a technique in which scissors are passed along the outside of the endoscope (94). Hysteroscopic destruction of the endometrium has been reported using Nd:YAG laser vaporization, electrosurgical resection, and electrosurgical coagulation (95–97).

The use of diagnostic and operative hysteroscopy has been limited by the difficulties in obtaining a consistently acceptable image (as a result of inadequate distention, bleeding) and the perception that its therapeutic potential is low. Although hysteroscopic technology and techniques are still being developed, the current quality of the images is excellent because smaller-diameter endoscopes have been made possible by improvements in fiber technology. The concomitant use of ultrasound imaging can provide a view of the myometrial wall during resectoscopic procedures.

Because diagnostic hysteroscopy can be performed in an office or clinic setting without anesthetic, its widespread use has been advocated to investigate abnormal uterine bleeding. Hysteroscopic surgical procedures include removal of polyps, excision of leiomyomas, endometrial ablation, and division of adhesions and uterine septa. Some of these procedures are well established; others, although promising, require more clinical investigation. Hysteroscopy has been suggested as a method to replace blind sampling of the uterine cavity because it may provide better results at a lower cost (98,99).

Diagnostic Hysteroscopy

Diagnostic hysteroscopy can provide information that cannot be obtained by blind endometrial sampling (98–104). In most cases, the additional findings visible with hysteroscopy are endometrial polyps or submucous leiomyomas (101,102,104,105). Malignant or hyperplastic processes can be identified with hysteroscopy and directed biopsy (103). Hysteroscopic examination is probably superior to hysterography in the evaluation of the endometrial cavity (106,107). However, in some situations (e.g., endometritis, hyperplasia), curettage provides information not otherwise available by hysteroscopic evaluation, even when it is combined with directed biopsy (101,102,104,108). The principal advantage of diagnostic hysteroscopy is that structural anomalies (congenital or acquired) are more easily detected and defined. Potential indications for diagnostic hysteroscopy are as follows.

1. Unexplained abnormal uterine bleeding
   - Premenopausal
   - Postmenopausal

2. Selected infertility cases
   - Abnormal hysterography
   - Unexplained infertility

3. Recurrent spontaneous abortion

In most patients, diagnostic hysteroscopy can be performed in an office or clinic with minimal discomfort and at a much lower cost than in an operating room. For some patients, concerns about patient comfort or a preexisting medical condition may preclude office hysteroscopy.

Although hysteroscopy can, in many patients, provide more information than blind curettage, it should still be used prudently. For most patients, other investigative or therapeutic measures can be undertaken before, or instead of, diagnostic hysteroscopy. For women with perimenopausal and postmenopausal bleeding, office endometrial biopsy or curettage should be performed before diagnostic hysteroscopy. If a satisfactory diagnosis cannot be established, or if bleeding continues without explanation, office hysteroscopy and directed biopsy or repeat curettage is appropriate. For women in their reproductive years, medical or expectant management may be used initially, depending on the severity and inconvenience of the bleeding. For those who do not respond to medical regimens such as oral contraceptives, office hysteroscopy with biopsy or curettage can be performed for diagnosis (109).

For women with infertility, hysterosalpingography is the best initial imaging step because it provides information about the patency of the oviducts. In the presence of a suspicious or identified abnormality in the endometrial cavity, hysteroscopy can be performed to confirm the diagnoses, to define the abnormality, and perhaps to direct the removal of the lesion. Some consider hysteroscopy mandatory for these patients because of the high occurrence of false-negative radiologic images in those with intrauterine anomalies. However, there has been no evidence that identification and treatment of these "missed" anomalies improves pregnancy rates. Confirmation of patency of the oviduct is unnecessary in women who have recurrent abortions; therefore, these patients can be evaluated primarily with hysteroscopy.

Operative Hysteroscopy

Adhesiolysis, division of a uterine septum, resection of myomas, and endometrial destruction through resection, electrosurgical desiccation, or vaporization with the Nd:YAG laser can be performed hysteroscopically. Hysteroscopy may also be used to remove foreign bodies or to position instruments in the fallopian tube.

Foreign Body

If the string of an intrauterine device is absent, the device usually can be removed with a specially designed hook or a toothed curette (e.g., Novak). When removal is difficult or impossible, the location of the device may be confirmed by hysteroscopy, allowing removal with a grasping forceps.

Septum

When a single uterus with a divided cavity is present, hysteroscopic division of uterine septa improves reproductive outcome at a rate comparable to abdominal metroplasty, with reduced morbidity and cost (110–113). The procedure may be performed mechanically with scissors or with energy-based techniques such as the Nd:YAG laser or an electrosurgical knife or loop. Because most septa have few vessels, scissors can be used easily, and the minimal risk for thermal damage is avoided.

Endometrial Polyps

Although endometrial polyps can be removed with blind curettage, many are missed (101,102,104,105). Therefore, known or suspected endometrial polyps are more successfully treated with hysteroscopic guidance, which can often be performed in a clinic or office using local anesthesia. Hysteroscopy may be used either to evaluate the result of blind curettage, or preferably, to guide a grasping forceps. Alternatively, for larger polyps, a uterine resectoscope may be used to sever the stalk or morcellate the lesion.

Leiomyomas

Hysteroscopy may be used to remove intracavitary leiomyomas in women with menorrhagia or infertility (114–121). However, this approach is limited by the location and size of the leiomyomas. In some patients, excision is relatively easy, whereas in others, laparotomy is necessary.

Pedunculated leiomyomas may be removed by transecting the stalk with scissors or a resectoscope. For larger lesions, electrosurgical morcellation with a resectoscope may be necessary before removal. In some patients, hysteroscopy can be used to direct the attachment of a tenaculum so that the lesion can be twisted off. Although preferable, it is not absolutely necessary to remove the leiomyoma because it will be expelled spontaneously.

Selected submucous leiomyomas that extend into the uterine wall may be resected using a loop electrode. The extent of intramural involvement may be evaluated by performing abdominal ultrasound with saline instilled into the endometrial cavity (i.e., sonohysterography) (121). If the leiomyoma is too deeply imbedded in the myometrium, it may not be resectable, or the uterus might be perforated if overzealous attempts are made to remove the tumor. Selected intramural leiomyomas may be removed completely during a second procedure performed after a suitable interval (119). Instead of a second procedure, the Nd:YAG laser or bipolar electrosurgery can be used to desiccate the remaining portion of the leiomyomas, although the efficacy of this approach is unclear (115). Preoperative gonadotropin-releasing hormone (GnRH) agonists may help shrink submucous myomas, facilitating their complete removal (122–124).

Menorrhagia

Menorrhagia that does not respond to medications may be managed by endometrial ablation or resection (95–97, 117, 124–132). Ablation may be performed with the laser (95,125,126), by electrosurgical desiccation using a uterine resectoscope equipped with a blunt ball- or barrel-shaped electrode (97,132), or by thermal balloon ablation. Resection is performed with an electrosurgical loop electrode that can shave the endometrium (96,127,128). Complications of the procedure include fluid overload, electrolyte imbalances, bleeding, perforation, and intestinal injury (130). The risk for uterine perforation can be reduced by using a combination of resection and electrosurgical ablation; the latter is most suitable for the thinner areas of the myometrium in the cornu and on the lateral walls of the endometrial cavity (117). The preoperative use of GnRH analogues or *danazol* may reduce operating time, bleeding, and the amount of fluid required (134,135).

For many women, these procedures are successful in reducing or eliminating menses without hysterectomy or long-term medical therapy (136). Success rates vary and depend on the duration of follow-up and the definition of success. For many patients, amenorrhea is the goal, whereas for others, it is normalization of menses. About 75% to 95% of patients are satisfied with the surgical procedure after 1 year, and 30% to 90% of patients have amenorrhea. In comparative studies, there is no advantage of laser over electrosurgical techniques (125,130).

The long-term efficacy and impact of ablation or resection on women with adenomyosis is unknown. Because some endometrium inevitably cannot be ablated, there is the potential for endometrial cancer; therefore, postmenopausal women who have undergone ablation or resection should take progestin as a part of hormonal replacement therapy (136).

Sterilization

Hysteroscopic sterilization can be performed without entering the peritoneal cavity. Because the tubal ostia are usually visible during hysteroscopy, there are several potential options for sterilization: insertion of a plug, injection of a sclerosing agent, or destruction of the intramural portion of the oviduct. These procedures are being developed and should be performed only as part of an approved clinical trial (36).

Synechiae

Asherman's syndrome is the presence of adhesions in the endometrial cavity resulting in infertility or recurrent spontaneous abortion with or without amenorrhea.

These synechiae may be detected on a hysterogram but are best shown with diagnostic hysteroscopy. Relatively thin, fragile synechiae may be divided with the tip of a rigid diagnostic hysteroscope (137). Thicker lesions may require division by semirigid or rigid scissors or energy-based instruments such as a resectoscope or an operative hysteroscope with an Nd:YAG laser. Reproductive outcome depends on the extent of the preoperative endometrial damage (138–140).

Patient Preparation

Most diagnostic hysteroscopy procedures are performed in the office or clinic, whereas operative hysteroscopy is performed in an operating room or hospital surgicenter. The patient should understand the rationale for either procedure as well as the anticipated discomfort, the potential risks, and the expectant medical and surgical alternatives. The patient must understand the nature of the procedure and the chance of therapeutic success. A realistic estimate of success based on the operator's experience must be presented to the patient.

Diagnostic Hysteroscopy

Diagnostic hysteroscopy is designed to identify or exclude the presence of anatomic or structural abnormalities in the endometrial cavity that may contribute to bleeding, infertility, or recurrent pregnancy loss. The risks of diagnostic hysteroscopy are few, and they rarely have severe consequences. However, those related to anesthesia, perforation, bleeding, and the distention media should be discussed. After diagnostic hysteroscopy, most patients have slight vaginal bleeding and lower abdominal cramps. Severe cramps, dyspnea, and upper abdominal and right shoulder pain can develop if CO_2 passes into the peritoneal cavity. Consequently, the patient should be accompanied by a friend or relative who will escort her home.

Operative Hysteroscopy

Counseling before operative hysteroscopy varies depending on the planned procedure and the type of anesthesia used. The risks of operative hysteroscopy are higher and are potentially more dangerous than those of diagnostic hysteroscopy. **Failure to purge air sufficiently from inflow lines or cervical dilation and insertion of operative instruments into the uterine cavity may be sufficient to cause a clinically significant air embolus. The risk for emboli as room air or gas from electrosurgical combustibles increases with higher intrauterine pressures, longer procedures, and invasion into the deeper myometrial vasculature.** The use of large volumes of hypotonic distention media may not be tolerated in some patients if there is significant intravascular absorption, especially in patients with underlying cardiovascular disease. The patient must be aware of the risk for damage to the intestines or to the urinary tract. If damage occurs during the procedure, it may not be possible to complete the surgery, and laparotomy may be necessary to repair the problem.

Equipment and Technique

The equipment required depends on the reason for the procedure. The surgeon must be knowledgeable about the equipment, its mechanisms, and the technical specifications to facilitate efficiency, optimal clinical outcome, and a decreased probability of complications (Fig. 21.18). A typical hysteroscopy setup for diagnostic and minor operative procedures is shown in Fig. 21.19. Core competencies required for hysteroscopy are as follows:

1. Patient positioning and cervical exposure
2. Anesthesia
3. Cervical dilation
4. Uterine distention
5. Imaging
6. Intrauterine manipulation

Patient Positioning and Exposure

Hysteroscopy is performed in a modified dorsal lithotomy position; the patient is supine, and the legs are held in stirrups. For hysteroscopic procedures performed while the patient is conscious, comfort must be considered in conjunction with the need to gain good exposure of the perineum. Stirrups that hold and support the knees, calves, and ankles permit prolonged procedures. "Candy cane" stirrups should be avoided for hysteroscopic surgery on conscious patients.

Figure 21.18 Office hysteroscopy equipment. A typical diagnostic hysteroscopy setup. On the table are a hysteroscope, a video camera mount, and diagnostic instruments. On the cart is (*from top*) a super VHS 1/2-inch videotape recorder, a Sony high-resolution monitor, an Olympus hysteroscopic insufflator, and the Olympus video camera base and light source.

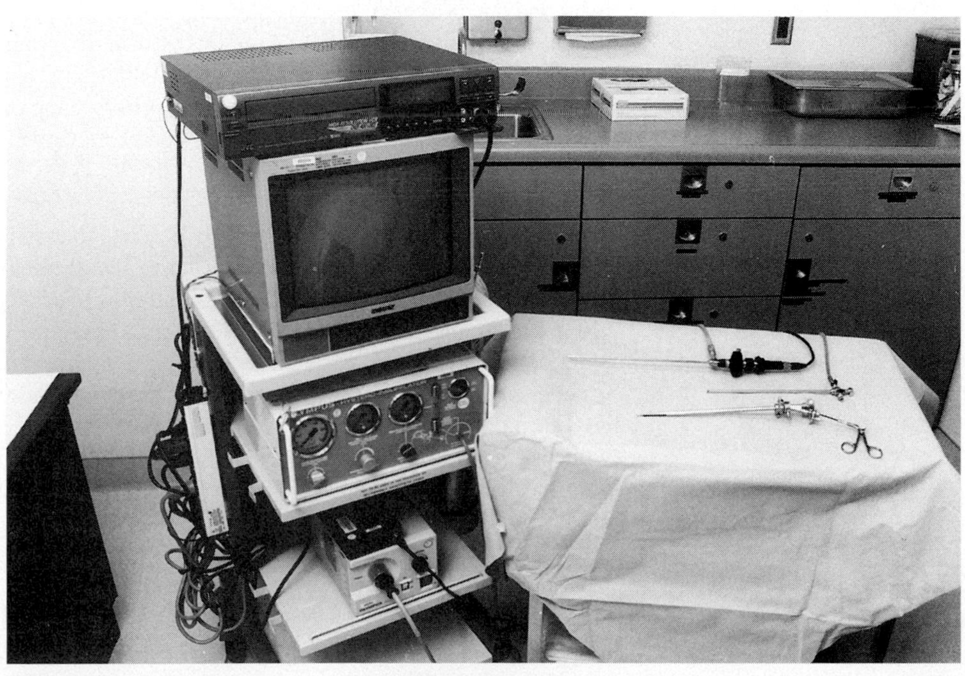

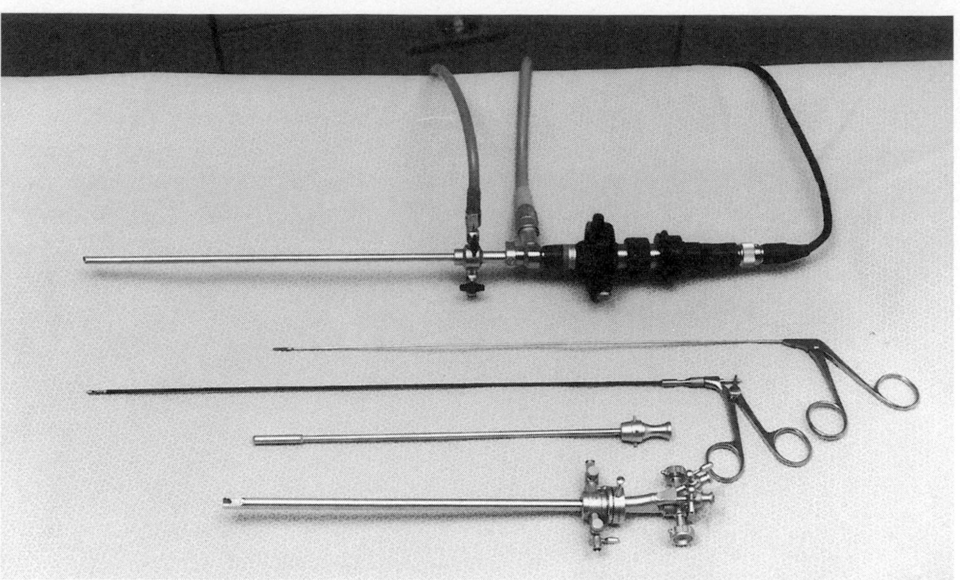

Figure 21.19 Diagnostic and minor operative hysteroscopic instruments. *Top to bottom:* a 4-mm-diameter hysteroscope in a 5-mm diagnostic sheath with attached CCD video camera, light cable and insufflation tubing; two semirigid hysteroscopic instruments—scissors and a biopsy forceps; the obturator for the operative sheath; the 7-mm operative sheath with two ports on the right side, allowing the introduction of the semirigid instruments.

The smallest speculum possible should be used to expose the cervix. A bivalve speculum hinged on only one side allows its removal without disturbing the other instruments needed. The use of weighted specula should be avoided in conscious patients.

Anesthesia

The anesthetic requirements for hysteroscopy vary greatly, depending on the patient's level of anxiety, the status of her cervical canal, the procedure, and the outside diameter of the hysteroscope or sheath. In some patients, diagnostic hysteroscopy is possible without anesthesia, especially if the patient is parous or if narrow-caliber (<3 mm in outside diameter) hysteroscopes are used. The pain of cervical dilation also is avoided or minimized by inserting a laminaria tent in the cervix 3 to 8 hours before the procedure. However, if left in place too long (e.g., longer than 24 hours), the cervix may overdilate, which is counterproductive for CO_2 insufflation.

For most diagnostic procedures, effective cervical anesthesia is obtained with an intracervical block. A spinal needle can be used to instill about 3 mL of 0.5% to 1% lidocaine into the anterior lip of the cervix. A tenaculum is used to grasp the cervix. An intracervical block is administered evenly around the circumference of the internal os. A paracervical block may also be injected into the uterosacral ligaments at the 4- and 8-o'clock positions, if necessary (141). Care must be taken to avoid intravascular injection. Additional topical anesthesia may be given by injecting 5 mL of 2% *mepivacaine* into the endometrial cavity with a syringe. Many operative procedures can be performed with this technique combined with intravenous anxiolytics or analgesics, as necessary. Alternatively, regional or general anesthesia may be used.

Cervical Dilation

Dilation of the cervix, although apparently simple, can be incorrectly performed in a way that compromises the whole procedure. If the objective lens of the hysteroscope cannot be placed in the endometrial cavity, the hysteroscopy cannot be done. The cervix should be dilated as atraumatically as possible. A uterine sound should not be used because it can traumatize the canal or the endometrium, causing unnecessary bleeding and uterine perforation.

Uterine Distention

Distention of the endometrial cavity is necessary to create a viewing space. The choices include CO_2 gas, high-viscosity 32% *dextran* 70, and a number of low-viscosity fluids, including glycine, sorbitol, saline, and dextrose in water. **A pressure of 45 mm Hg or higher is required for adequate distention of the uterine cavity. To minimize extravasation, this pressure should not exceed the mean arterial pressure.** For each of the fluids, there are several methods used to create this pressure by infusion into the endometrial cavity.

Sheaths

A rigid hysteroscope is passed into the endometrial cavity through an external sheath. The design and diameter of the sheath reflect both the dimensions of the endoscope and the purpose of the instrument. Diagnostic hysteroscopes have a sheath slightly wider than the telescope, allowing infusion of the distention media. Sheaths for operative hysteroscopes have one or two additional channels that permit the passage or efflux of distention media or the insertion of semirigid instruments or laser fibers. These sheaths are usually 7 to 8 mm in diameter, and some allow continuous flow of distention media in and out of the endometrial cavity (Fig. 21.16).

Media

CO_2 provides an excellent view for diagnostic purposes, but it is unsuitable for operative hysteroscopy and for diagnostic procedures when the patient is bleeding because there is no effective way to remove blood and other debris from the endometrial cavity. To prevent CO_2 embolus, the gas must be instilled by an insufflator that is specially designed for the procedure—the intrauterine pressure is kept below 100 mm Hg, and the flow rate is maintained at less than 100 mL/min.

Normal saline is a useful and safe medium for procedures that do not require electricity. Even if there is absorption of a significant volume of solution, saline does not cause electrolyte imbalance. Therefore, saline is a good fluid for minor procedures performed in the office.

Dextran 70 is useful for patients who are bleeding, because it does not mix with blood. However, it is expensive and tends to "caramelize" on instruments, which must be disassembled and thoroughly cleaned in warm water immediately after each use. Anaphylactic reactions, fluid overload, and electrolyte disturbances can occur.

For operative hysteroscopy, low-viscosity, nonconductive fluids such as 1.5% glycine and 3% sorbitol are used most often. These solutions can be used with electricity because there are no electrolytes to disperse the current and impede the electrosurgical effect. Both 1.5% glycine and 3% sorbitol are inexpensive and are readily available in 3-L bags suitable for continuous-flow hysteroscopy. Because each fluid is hypotonic, extravasation into the systemic circulation can be associated with fluid and electrolyte disturbances. Therefore, uterine "absorption" must be monitored continuously by collecting outflow from the sheath and subtracting it from the total infused volume. Absorbed volumes greater than 1 L mandate the measurement of electrolyte levels. If there is more than 2 L of extravasated fluid, the procedure should be stopped. Excessive circulating sorbitol may cause hyperglycemia, and large volumes of glycine may elevate levels of ammonia in the blood (142).

Delivery Systems

Syringes can be used for office diagnostic procedures and are especially good for infusing dextran solution. The syringe can be operated by the surgeon and is either connected directly to the sheath or attached by connecting tubing. Because this technique is so tedious, it is suited only for simple operations.

Continuous hydrostatic pressure is effectively achieved by elevating the vehicle containing the distention media above the level of the patient's uterus. The achieved pressure is the product of the width of the connecting tubing and the elevation—for operative hysteroscopy with 10-mm tubing, intrauterine pressure ranges from 70 to 100 mm Hg when the bag is between 1 and 1.5 m above the uterine cavity.

A pressure cuff may be placed around the infusion bag to elevate the pressure in the system. Caution must be exercised, however, because this technique causes extravasation if intrauterine pressure rises above the mean arterial pressure.

A variety of infusion pumps are available, ranging from simple devices to instruments that maintain a preset intrauterine pressure. Simple pump devices continue to press fluid into the uterine cavity regardless of resistance, whereas the pressure-sensitive pumps reduce the flow rate when the preset level is reached, thereby impeding the efflux of blood and debris and compromising the view.

Imaging

Endoscopes

Hysteroscopes are available in two basic types—flexible and rigid. Flexible hysteroscopes have lower resolution than rigid instruments of a similar diameter and are most useful for cannulation of the fallopian tube. For other uses, rigid hysteroscopes are more durable and provide a superior image. The most commonly used hysteroscopes are 4 mm in diameter, although those smaller than 3 mm in diameter are available. Small-diameter endoscopes have a somewhat lower resolution but are easier to pass through the cervix.

Oblique endoscopes are more useful for hysteroscopy than laparoscopy and are available in zero-degree, 12- to 15-degree, and 25- to 30-degree models (Fig. 21.20). The zero-degree telescope provides a panoramic view and is best for diagnostic procedures. Hysteroscopes with 25- to 30-degree angles are most often used for both diagnosis and therapy, although the 12- to 15-degree types are a suitable compromise useful for diagnosis, ablation, and resection.

Figure 21.20 Hysteroscope optics. Panoramic (08) and oblique (158 and 308) viewing angles.

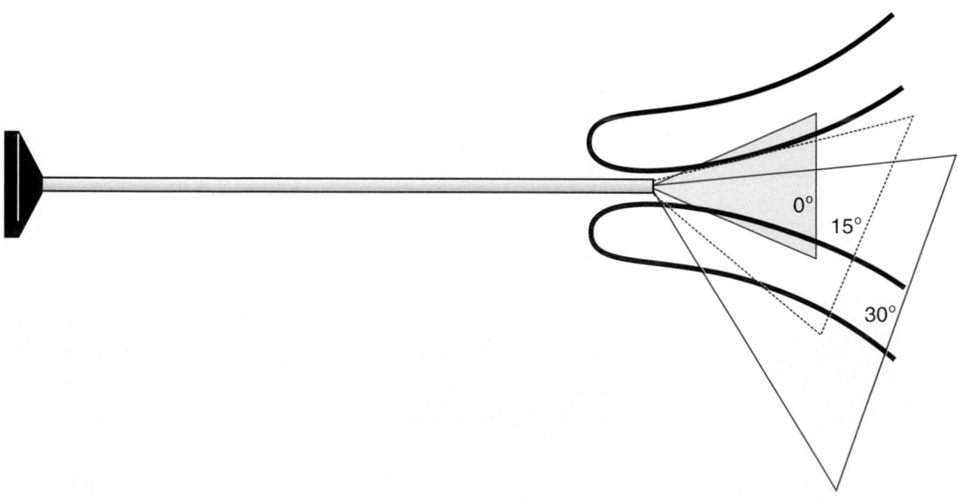

Light Sources and Cables

Adequate illumination of the endometrial cavity is essential. Because it runs from a standard 110- or 220-volt wall outlet, the light source requires no special electrical connections. For most cameras and endoscopes, the element must have at least 150 watts of power for direct viewing and preferably 250 watts or more for video and operative procedures (143).

Video Imaging

Although diagnostic hysteroscopy may be performed with direct visualization, it is best to use video guidance for prolonged operations. Video imaging is important for teaching and recording pathology and procedures. The cameras used for operative hysteroscopy often have greater technical requirements than those used for laparoscopy. The camera must be more sensitive because of the narrow diameter of the endoscope and the frequently dark background of the endometrial cavity, particularly when it is enlarged (Fig. 21.18).

Intrauterine Manipulation

The instruments available for use through operative hysteroscopes include grasping, cutting, and punch-biopsy devices. These tools are narrow and flexible enough to navigate the 1- to 2-mm diameter operating channel (Fig. 21.21). Their value is limited by their small size and flimsy construction. However, the scissors can be used to divide adhesions, the biopsy forceps can be used to sample targeted lesions, and the grasping forceps can be used to remove small polyps or intrauterine devices. Some operative hysteroscopes are designed to allow passage of fibers for the conduction of Nd:YAG laser.

The uterine resectoscope is similar to the one used in urology and is designed to apply electrical energy in the endometrial cavity (Fig. 21.22). An understanding of the principles of electrosurgery is mandatory for safe and effective use of this instrument. By sliding the "working element," one of a variety of electrode tips can be manipulated back and forth within the cavity. Tissue can be divided with a pointed electrode, excised with a loop, or desiccated with a rolling ball or bar. A clear operative field is maintained by the continuous flow of nonconductive distending media in and out of the cavity. Although basic

Figure 21.21 Hysteroscopy hand instruments. *From top:* biopsy forceps, grasping forceps, and scissors, each of which passes through the instrument channel of an operating hysteroscope. *Bottom:* a rigid sheath with integrated scissors.

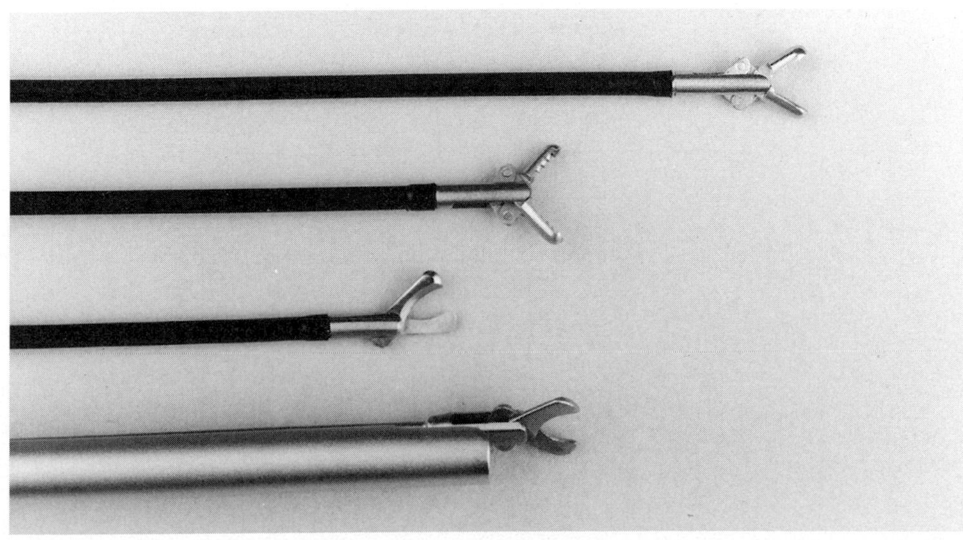

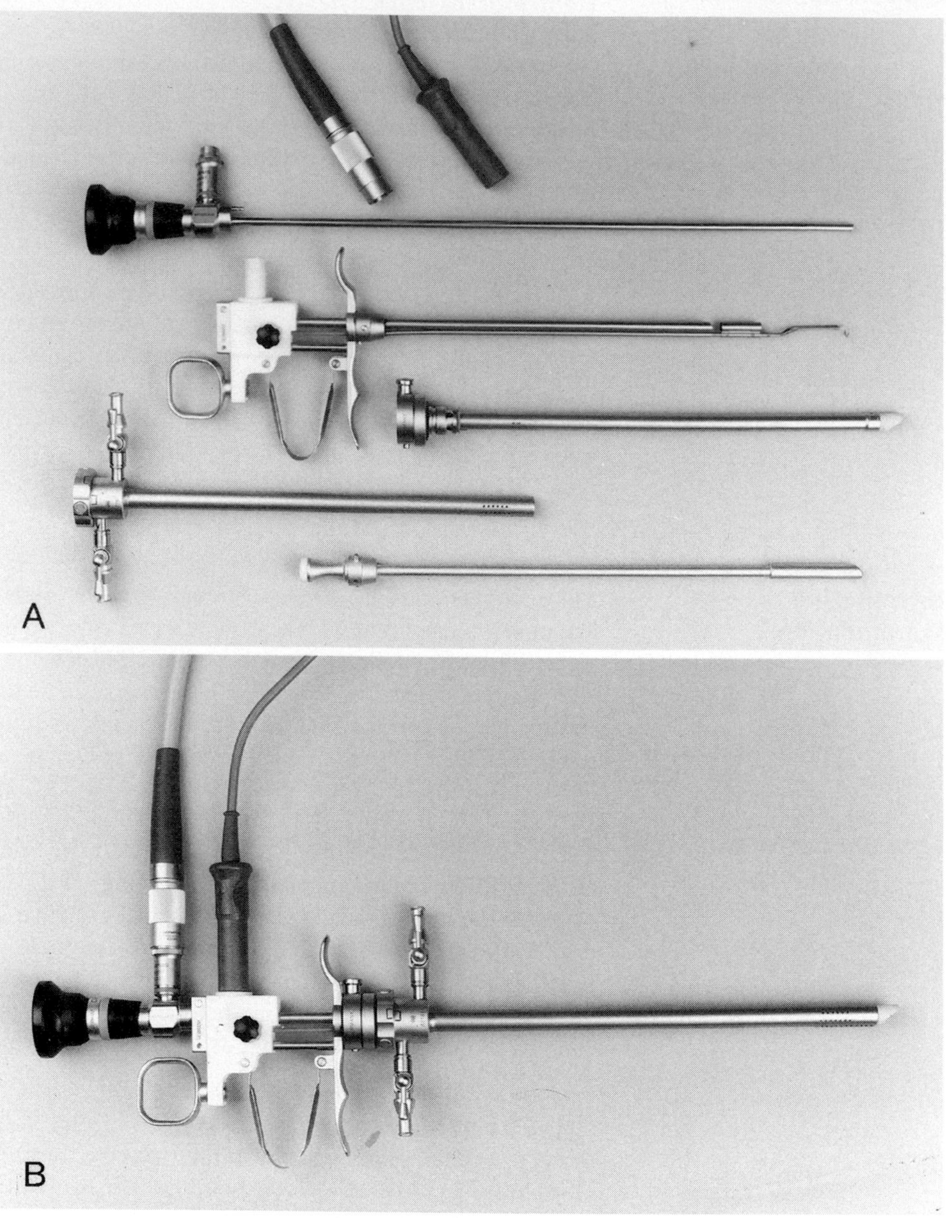

Figure 21.22 Uterine resectoscope (Olympus America, Inc., Woodbury, NY). **A** (*from top*): light guide (*left*) and monopolar electrosurgical cord (*right*); a 4-mm 128 endoscope; the Iglesas working element; an inner sheath; an outer sheath; the obturator. **B,** Fully assembled resectoscope.

design modifications have made the resectoscope more useful in gynecology, extraction of resected fragments is time consuming. The most effective approach is the periodic use of a uterine curette or polyp forceps inserted after removal of the hysteroscope.

Other Instruments

For any hysteroscopic procedure, it is necessary to have a cervical tenaculum, dilators, uterine curette, and appropriate-sized vaginal specula. When using the resectoscope, it is helpful to have a modern, solid-state, isolated circuit electrosurgical generator capable of delivering both modulated and nonmodulated radiofrequency current. Laparoscopy or laparotomy may be necessary for emergencies secondary to uterine perforation.

Complications

The potential risks of diagnostic hysteroscopy include uterine perforation, infection, excessive bleeding, and complications related to the distention media (144). The latter include CO_2 embolus and pulmonary edema secondary to overinfusion of 32% *dextran 70* (*Hyskon*) or low-viscosity fluids. Diagnostic hysteroscopy performed in the office has a low rate of complications (0% to 1%) (98–100). The risks of operative hysteroscopy are related to one of five aspects of the procedure performed: (a) anesthesia, (b) perforation, (c) bleeding, (d) the use of energy, and (e) the distention media.

Anesthesia

Local anesthesia is provided by the intracervical or paracervical injection of 0.5% to 2% lidocaine or mepivacaine solution, with or without a local vasoconstrictor such as adrenaline. Overdosage is prevented by ensuring that intravascular injection is avoided and by not exceeding the maximum recommended doses (*lidocaine,* 4 mg/kg; *mepivacaine,* 3 mg/kg). The use of a vasoconstrictor reduces the amount of systemic absorption of the agent, doubling the maximum dose that can be used.

Complications of intravascular injection or anesthetic overdose include allergy, neurologic effects, and impaired myocardial conduction. Allergy is characterized by the typical symptoms of agitation, palpitations, pruritus, coughing, shortness of breath, urticaria, bronchospasm, shock, and convulsions. Treatment measures include administration of oxygen, isotonic intravenous fluids, intramuscular or subcutaneous adrenaline, and intravenous prednisolone and aminophylline. Cardiac effects related to impaired myocardial conduction include bradycardia, cardiac arrest, shock, and convulsions. Emergency treatment measures include the administration of oxygen, intravenous *atropine* (0.5 mg), and intravenous *adrenaline* and the initiation of appropriate cardiac resuscitation. The most common central nervous system manifestations are paresthesia of the tongue, drowsiness, tremor, and convulsions. Options for therapy include intravenous diazepam and respiratory support.

Perforation

Perforation may occur during dilation of the cervix or during the hysteroscopic procedure. With perforation, the endometrial cavity does not distend, and the visual field is lost. When perforation occurs during dilation of the cervix, the procedure must be terminated, but usually there are no other injuries. If the uterus is perforated by a hysteroscopic instrument, the tip of a laser, or an activated electrode, there is a risk for bleeding or injury to the adjacent viscera. Therefore, the operation must be stopped and the instruments withdrawn under hysteroscopic guidance.

If there is evidence of bleeding or presumed visceral injury, laparoscopy or laparotomy should be performed. Injury to the uterus is relatively easy to detect with a laparoscope. However, mechanical or thermal injury to the bowel, ureter, or bladder is more difficult and may require laparotomy. If the patient's condition is managed expectantly, she should be advised of the situation and asked to report any symptoms of bleeding or visceral trauma.

Bleeding

Bleeding that occurs during or after hysteroscopy results from trauma to the vessels in the myometrium or injury to other vessels in the pelvis. Myometrial vessels can be lacerated during the resectoscopic procedures.

In planning operations that involve deep resection, autologous blood can be obtained before surgery. The risk for bleeding may be reduced by the preoperative injection of diluted vasopressin into the cervical stroma (145). The risk for injury to branches of the uterine artery can be lowered by minimizing the depth of resection in the lateral endometrial cavity near the uterine isthmus, where ablative techniques should be used. When bleeding is encountered during resectoscopic procedures, the ball electrode can be used to desiccate the vessel electrosurgically. Intractable bleeding may respond to the injection of diluted vasopressin or to the inflation of a 30-mL Foley catheter balloon in the endometrial cavity (117).

Thermal Trauma

The temperature of the uterine serosa does not rise significantly during electrosurgical coagulation of the endometrium, even at the cornu, which is the thinnest area of the myometrium (146). However, if an activated electrode or laser fiber penetrates the uterus, surrounding structures such as bowel, urinary tract, and blood vessels are at risk. An activated electrode or fiber should never be advanced, but if an activated electrode has penetrated the uterine wall, direct examination of the pelvic viscera is mandatory. Laparoscopy is the appropriate first step. The site of the perforation should be examined to exclude the presence of significant bleeding. Most perforations do not need to be repaired. However, the pelvic sidewalls, the bladder, and the small and large bowel should be carefully inspected. If the intestines are damaged, laparotomy is indicated to repair the damage (147).

Thermal injury to the intestine or ureter may be difficult to diagnose, and symptoms may not occur for several days to 2 weeks. Therefore, the patient should be advised of the symptoms that could indicate peritonitis.

Distention Media

Carbon Dioxide

CO_2 can cause emboli and result in serious intraoperative morbidity and death (148–150). These risks can be eliminated by not using CO_2 with operative procedures and by ensuring that the insufflation pressure is always lower than 100 mm Hg and that the flow rate is lower than 100 mL/min. The insufflator used must be especially designed for hysteroscopy; it is difficult to set laparoscopic insufflator flow rates below 1,000 mL/min.

Dextran 70

Dextran 70 is a hyperosmolar medium that can induce an allergic response, coagulopathy, and, if sufficient volumes are infused, vascular overload and heart failure (151,152). Because dextran is hydrophilic, it can draw 6 times its own volume into the systemic circulation. Consequently, the volume of this agent should be limited to less than 300 mL, particularly for office use.

Low-Viscosity Fluids

The low-viscosity fluids 1.5% glycine and 3% sorbitol are most often used, largely because of their low cost, compatibility with electrosurgery, and availability in large-volume bags. However, the use of a continuous-flow system with hypotonic media can create fluid and electrolyte disturbances.

1. Before undertaking a procedure using the resectoscope, baseline serum electrolyte levels should be measured. Women with cardiopulmonary disease should be evaluated carefully. The selective preoperative use of agents such as GnRH agonists may reduce operating time and media absorption.

2. In the operating room, media infusion and collection should take place in a closed system to allow accurate measurement of the "absorbed" volume. The volume should be calculated every 5 minutes or at least every 15 minutes.

3. The lowest intrauterine pressure necessary for adequate distention should be used to complete the operation, usually at a level that is below the mean arterial pressure. A good range is 70 to 80 mm Hg, which can be achieved with a specially designed pump or by maintaining the meniscus of the infusion bag 1 m above the level of the patient's uterus.

4. Deficits of more than 1 L require measurement of electrolyte levels. The procedure should be completed expeditiously. If the deficit is more than 2 L, the procedure should be terminated, and a diuretic such as mannitol or furosemide should be used as needed. In patients with cardiovascular compromise, deficits must be avoided (36).

Image Documentation

A small video camera can be used to teach and to coordinate the procedure better with the operating room team. It also allows the operation to be recorded for future reference. A video recorder may be attached to a video camera system. For optimal recording, the camera should be attached directly to the recorder so that the image is transmitted to the monitor for viewing during the operation. A number of video recording formats are available, each with inherent advantages and disadvantages. The best quality still images are obtained with a 35-mm single-lens reflex still camera and coupler. The use of a camera is often cumbersome, but the images taken from a standard still camera are of higher resolution than those obtained from videotape. Some video printers provide images suitable for a medical record. Newer digital cameras provide video still images, slides, or prints that are suitable for publication or teaching.

References

1. **Shapiro HI, Adler DH.** Excision of an ectopic pregnancy through the laparoscope. *Am J Obstet Gynecol* 1973;117:290–291.
2. **Gomel V.** Laparoscopic tubal surgery in infertility. *Obstet Gynecol* 1975;46:47–48.
3. **Gomel V.** Salpingostomy by laparoscopy. *J Reprod Med* 1977;18:265–267.
4. **Mettler L, Giesel H, Semm K.** Treatment of female infertility due to tubal obstruction by operative laparoscopy. *Fertil Steril* 1979;32:384–388.
5. **Steptoe PC, Edwards RG.** Birth after the reimplantation of a human embryo. *Lancet* 1978;2:366.
6. **Daniell JF.** Operative laparoscopy for endometriosis. *Semin Reprod Endocrinol* 1985;3:353.
7. **Howard FM, El-Minawi AM, Sanchez RA.** Conscious pain mapping by laparoscopy in women with chronic pelvic pain. *Obstet Gynecol* 2000:96(6);934–939.
8. **Brill AI, Nezhat F, Nezhat CH, et al.** The incidence of adhesions after prior laparotomy: a laparoscopic appraisal. *Obstet Gynecol* 1995;85(2):269–272.
9. **Fatum M, Rojansky N.** Laparoscopic surgery during pregnancy. *Obstet Gynecol Surv* 2001;56(1):50–59.
10. **Keye WR Jr.** Laparoscopy in the 1990s: "deja vu all over again." *Fertil Steril* 1996;66:511–512.
11. **Reich H, DeCaprio J, McGlynn F.** Laparoscopic hysterectomy. *J Gynecol Surg* 1989;5:213–216.
12. **Stovall G, Ling FW, Gray LA.** Single dose methotrexate for treatment of ectopic pregnancy. *Obstet Gynecol* 1991;77:754–757.
13. **Bhiwandiwala PP, Mumbord SD, Feldblum PJ.** A comparison of different laparoscopic sterilization occlusion techniques in 24,939 procedures. *Am J Obstet Gynecol* 1982;144:319–331.
14. **Ryder RM, Vaughan MC.** Laparoscopic tubal sterilization. Methods, effectiveness, and sequelae. *Obstet Gynecol Clin North Am* 1999;26:83–97.
15. **Maruri F, Azziz R.** Laparoscopic surgery for ectopic pregnancies: technology assessment and public health implications. *Fertil Steril* 1993;59:487–498.
16. **Gomel V, Taylor PJ.** *Diagnostic and operative laparoscopy.* St. Louis: CV Mosby, 1995.
17. **Gomel V.** Management of ectopic gestation: surgical treatment is usually best. *Clin Obstet Gynecol* 1995;38:353–361.
18. **Mecke H, Lehmann-Willenbrock E, Ibrahim M, et al.** Pelviscopic treatment of ovarian cysts in premenopausal women. *Gynecol Obstet Invest* 1992;34:36–42.
19. **Canis M, Mage G, Pouly J, et al.** Laparoscopic diagnosis of adnexal cystic masses: a twelve year experience with long-term followup. *Obstet Gynecol* 1994;83:707–712.
20. **Lehner R, Wenzl R, Heinzl H, et al.** Influence of delayed staging laparotomy after laparoscopic removal of ovarian masses later found malignant. *Obstet Gynecol* 1998;92:967–971.
21. **Parker WH, Berek JS.** Management of selected cystic adnexal masses in postmenopausal women by operative laparoscopy: a pilot study. *Am J Obstet Gynecol* 1990;163:1574–1577.

22. **Parker WH, Levine R, Howard F, et al.** A multicenter study of laparoscopic management of selected cystic adnexal masses in postmenopausal women. *J Am Coll Surg* 1994;179:733–737.

23. **Howard FM.** Surgical management of benign cystic teratoma: laparoscopy vs. laparotomy. *J Reprod Med* 1995;40:495–499.

24. **Canis M, Pouly JL, Wattiez A, et al.** Laparoscopic management of adnexal masses suspicious at ultrasound. *Obstet Gynecol* 1997;89:679–683.

25. **Operative Laparoscopy Study Group.** Postoperative adhesion development after operative laparoscopy: evaluation at early second-look laparoscopy. *Fertil Steril* 1991;55:700–704.

26. **Mage G, Canis M, Manhes H, et al.** Laparoscopic management of adnexal torsion. *J Reprod Med* 1989;34:520–524.

27. **Vancaillie T, Schmidt EH.** Recovery of ovarian function after laparoscopic treatment of adnexal torsion. *J Reprod Med* 1987;32:561–562.

28. **Gjönnaess H.** Polycystic ovarian syndrome treated by ovarian electrocautery through the laparoscope. *Fertil Steril* 1984;41:20–25.

29. **Kovacs G, Buckler H, Bangah M, et al.** Treatment of anovulation due to polycystic ovarian syndrome by laparoscopic ovarian cautery. *Br J Obstet Gynaecol* 1991;98:30–35.

30. **Huber J, Hosmann J, Spona J.** Polycystic ovarian syndrome treated by laser through the laparoscope. *Lancet* 1988;2(8604):215.

31. **Gürgan T, Kisnisci H, Yarali H, et al.** Evaluation of adhesion formation after laparoscopic treatment of polycystic ovarian disease. *Fertil Steril* 1991;56:1176–1178.

32. **Naether OGJ, Fischer R.** Adhesion formation after laparoscopic electrocoagulation of the ovarian surface in polycystic ovary patients. *Fertil Steril* 1993;60:95–98.

33. **Hasson H, Rotman C, Rana N, et al.** Laparoscopic myomectomy. *Obstet Gynecol* 1993;82:897–900.

34. **Dubuisso JB, Fauconnier A, Babaki-Fard K, et al.** Laparoscopic myomectomy: a current view. *Hum Reprod Update* 2000;6:588–594.

35. **Parker WH, Rodi I.** Patient selection for laparoscopic myomectomy. *J Am Assoc Gynecol Laparosc* 1994;2:23–26.

36. **Sutton C, Diamond MP.** *Endoscopic surgery for gynecologists.* St. Louis: CV Mosby, 1993:169–171.

37. **Munro MG, Parker WH.** A classification system for laparoscopic hysterectomy. *Obstet Gynecol* 1993;82:624–629.

38. **Summitt RL, Stovall TG, Lipscomb GH, et al.** Randomized comparison of laparoscopy-assisted vaginal hysterectomy with standard vaginal hysterectomy with standard vaginal hysterectomy in and outpatient setting. *Obstet Gynecol* 1992;80:895–901.

39. **Munro MG, Deprest JA.** Laparoscopic hysterectomy, does it work? Bicontinental review of the literature and clinical commentary. *Clin Obstet Gynecol* 1995;38(2):401–424.

40. **Raiga J, Canis M, Le Bouedec G, et al.** Laparoscopic management of adnexal abscesses: consequences for fertility. *Fertil Steril* 1996;66:712–717.

41. **Munro MG, Gomel V.** Fertility-promoting laparoscopically-directed procedures. *Reprod Med Rev* 1994;3:29–42.

42. **Filmar S, Jetha N, McComb P, et al.** A comparative histologic study on the healing process after tissue transection. I. Carbon dioxide laser and electromicrosurgery. *Am J Obstet Gynecol* 1991;77:563–565.

43. **Munro MG, Fu YS.** A randomized comparison of thermal injury characteristics of an electrosurgical laparoscopic loop electrode and the CO_2 laser in the rat uterine horn. *Am J Obstet Gynecol* 1995;172(4):1257–1262.

44. **Ross JW.** Multichannel urodynamic evaluation of laparoscopic Burch colposuspension for genuine stress incontinence. *Obstet Gynecol* 1998;91:55–59.

45. **Miklos JR, Kohli N.** Laparoscopic paravaginal repair plus Burch colposuspension: review and descriptive technique. *Urology* 2000;56[Suppl 1]:64–69.

46. **Fowler JM, Carter JR.** Laparoscopic management of the adnexal mass in postmenopausal women. *J Gynecol Tech* 1995;1:7–10.

47. **Possover M, Krause N, Plaul K, et al.** Laparoscopic para-aortic and pelvic lymphadenectomy: experience with 150 patients and review of the literature. *Gynecol Oncol* 1998;71:19–28.

48. **Tulandi T.** Salpingo-ovariolysis: a comparison between laser surgery and electrosurgery. *Fertil Steril* 1986;45:489–491.

49. **Nezhat F, Brill AI, Nezhat CH, et al.** Laparoscopic appraisal of the anatomic relationship of the umbilicus to the aortic bifurcation. *J Am Assoc Gynecol Laparosc* 1998;5:135–140.

50. **Munro MG.** Laparoscopic suturing techniques. In: Stovall T, Sammarco M, Steege J, eds. *Gynecologic endoscopy: principles in practice.* Baltimore: Williams & Wilkins, 1996:193–246.

51. **Boike GM, Miller CE, Spirtos NM, et al.** Incisional bowel herniations after operative laparoscopy: a series of nineteen cases and review of the literature. *Am J Obstet Gynecol* 1995;172:1726–1733.

52. **Peterson HB, DeStefano F, Rubin GL, et al.** Deaths attributable to tubal sterilization in the United States, 1977 to 1981. *Am J Obstet Gynecol* 1982;146:131–136.

53. **Hirvonen EA, Nuutinen LS, Kauko M.** Ventilatory effects, blood gas changes, and oxygen consumption during laparascopic hysterectomy. *Anesth Analg* 1995;80:961–966.

54. **Ishizaki Y, Bandai Y, Shimomura K, et al.** Safe intra-abdominal pressure of carbon dioxide pneumoperitoneum during laparoscopic surgery. *Surgery* 1993;114:549–554.

55. **Myles PS.** Brady arrhythmias and laparoscopy: a prospective study of heart rate changes with laparoscopy. *Aust N Z J Obstet Gynecol* 1991;31:171–173.

56. **Kent RB.** Subcutaneous emphysema and hypercarbia associated with laparoscopy. *Arch Surg* 1991;126: 1154–1156.

57. **Bard PA, Chen L.** Subcutaneous emphysema associated with laparoscopy. *Anesth Analg* 1990;71:101–102.

58. **Kalhan SB, Reaney JA, Collins RL.** Pneumomediastinum and subcutaneous emphysema during laparoscopy. *Cleve Clin J Med* 1990;57:639–642.

59. **Kabukoba JJ, Skillern LH.** Coping with extraperitoneal insufflation during laparoscopy: a new technique. *Obstet Gynecol* 1992;80:144–145.

60. **Grainger DA, Soderstrom RM, Schiff SF, et al.** Ureteral injuries at laparoscopy: insights into diagnosis, management, and prevention. *Obstet Gynecol* 1990;75:839–843.

61. **Corson SL.** Electrosurgical hazards in laparoscopy. *JAMA* 1974;227:1261.

62. **Engel T.** The electrical dynamics of laparoscopic sterilization. *J Reprod Med* 1975;15:33–42.

63. **Baadsgarrd SE, Bille S, Egeblad K.** Major vascular injury during gynecologic laparoscopy. *Acta Obstet Gynecol Scand* 1989;68:283–285.

64. **Chi IC, Feldblum PJ.** Laparoscopic sterilization requiring laparotomy. *Am J Obstet Gynecol* 1982;142: 712–713.

65. **Chi IC, Feldblum PJ, Baloh SA.** Previous abdominal surgery as a risk factor in interval laparoscopic sterilization. *Am J Obstet Gynecol* 1983;145:841–846.

66. **Franks AL, Kendrick JS, Peterson HB.** Unintended laparotomy associated with laparoscopic tubal sterilization. *Am J Obstet Gynecol* 1987;157:1102–1105.

67. **Penfield AJ.** How to prevent complications of open laparoscopy. *J Reprod Med* 1985;30:660–663.

68. **Reich H.** Laparoscopic bowel injury. *Surg Laparosc Endosc* 1992;2:74–78.

69. **Childers JM, Brzechfta PR, Surwit EA.** Laparoscopy using the left upper quadrant as the primary trocar site. *Gynecol Oncol* 1993;50:221–225.

70. **Deziel DJ, Millikan KW, Economou SG, et al.** Complications of laparoscopic cholecystectomy: a national survey of 4292 hospitals and an analysis of 77,614 cases. *Am J Surg* 1993;165:9–14.

71. **Wolfe BM, Gardiner BN, Leary BF, et al.** Endoscopic cholecystectomy: an analysis of complications. *Arch Surg* 1991;126:1192–1198.

72. **Mirhashemi R, Harlow BL, Ginsburg ES, et al.** Predicting risk of complications with gynecologic laparoscopic surgery. *Obstet Gynecol* 1998;92:327–331.

73. **Ostrzenski A, Ostrzenska KM.** Bladder injury during laparoscopic surgery. *Obstet Gynecol Surv* 1998;53: 175–180.

74. **Font GE, Brill AI, Stuhldreher PV, et al.** Endoscopic management of incidental cystotomy during operative laparoscopy. *J Urol* 1993;149:1130–1131.

75. **Reich H, McGlynn F.** Laparoscopic repair of bladder injury. *Obstet Gynecol* 1990;75:909–910.

76. **Gomel V, James C.** Intraoperative management of ureteral injury during operative laparoscopy. *Fertil Steril* 1991;55:416–419.

77. **Grainger DA, Soderstrom RM, Schiff SF, et al.** Ureteral injuries at laparoscopy: insights into diagnosis, management, and prevention. *Obstet Gynecol* 1990;75:839–843.

78. **Steckel J, Badillo F, Waldbaum RS.** Uretero-fallopian tube fistula secondary to laparoscopic fulguration of pelvic endometriosis. *J Urol* 1993;149:1128–1129.

79. **Kadar N, Lemmerling L.** Urinary fistulas during laparoscopic hysterectomy: causes and prevention. *Am J Obstet Gynecol* 1994;170:47–48.

80. **Woodland MB.** Ureter injury during laparoscopy-assisted hysterectomy with the endoscopic linear stapler. *Am J Obstet Gynecol* 1992;167:756–757.

81. **Nezhat C, Nezhat FR.** Safe laser endoscopic excision or vaporization of peritoneal endometriosis. *Fertil Steril* 1989;52:149–151.

82. **Nezhat C, Nezhat F.** Laparoscopic repair of ureter resected during operative laparoscopy. *Obstet Gynecol* 1992;80:543–544.

83. **Loffler FD, Dent D, Goodkin R.** Sciatic nerve injury in a patient undergoing laparoscopy. *J Reprod Med* 1978;21:371–372.

84. **al Hakin M, Katirjic B.** Femoral neuropathy induced by the lithotomy position: a report of 5 cases with a review of the literature. *Muscle Nerve* 1993;16:891–895.

85. **Reich H.** Laparoscopic treatment of extensive pelvic adhesions, including hydrosalpinx. *J Reprod Med* 1987;32:736–742.

86. **Bloom DA, Ehrlich RM.** Omental evisceration through small laparoscopy port sites. *J Endourol* 1993;7: 31–33.

87. **Plaus WJ.** Laparoscopic trocar site hernias. *J Laparoendosc Surg* 1993;3:567–570.

88. **Maco A, Ruchman RB.** CT diagnosis of post laparoscopic hernia. *J Comput Assist Tomogr* 1991;15:1054–1055.

89. **Chamberlain GVP, Carron-Brown J.** *Gynaecological laparoscopy.* London: Royal College of Obstetricians & Gynecologists, 1978.

90. **Sotrel G, Hirsch E, Edelin KC.** Necrotizing fascitis following diagnostic laparoscopy. *Obstet Gynecol* 1982;62(Suppl 3):675–695.

91. **Glew RH, Pokoly TB.** Tubovarian abscess following laparoscopic sterilization with silicone rubber bands. *Obstet Gynecol* 1980;50:760–762.

92. **Levine RU, Neuwirth RS.** Simultaneous laparoscopy and hysteroscopy for intrauterine adhesions. *Obstet Gynecol* 1973;42:441–445.

93. **Neuwirth RS, Amin JH.** Excision of submucous fibroids with hysteroscopic control. *Am J Obstet Gynecol* 1976;126:95–99.

94. **Chervenak FA, Neuwirth RS.** Hysteroscopic resection of uterine septa. *Am J Obstet Gynecol* 1981;141: 351–353.

95. **Goldrath MH, Fuller TA, Segal S.** Laser photovaporization of endometrium for the treatment of menorrhagia. *Am J Obstet Gynecol* 1983;147:869–872.

96. **DeCherney AH, Polan ML.** Hysteroscopic management if intrauterine adhesions and intractable uterine bleeding. *Obstet Gynecol* 1983;61:392–397.

97. **Townsend DE, Richart RM, Paskowitz RA, et al.** "Rollerball" coagulation of the endometrium. *Obstet Gynecol* 1987;679:679–682.

98. **Goldrath MH, Sherman AI.** Office hysteroscopy and suction curettage: can we eliminate the hospital diagnostic dilatation and curettage? *Am J Obstet Gynecol* 1985;152:220–229.

99. **Gimpelson RJ.** Office hysteroscopy. *Clin Obstet Gynecol* 1992;35:270–281.

100. **Itzkowic DJ, Laverty CR.** Office hysteroscopy and curettage: a safe diagnostic procedure. *Aust N Z J Obstet Gynecol* 1990;30:150–153.

101. **Gimpelson R, Rappold H.** A comparative study between panoramic hysteroscopy with directed biopsies and curettage: a review of 276 cases. *Am J Obstet Gynecol* 1988;158:489–492.

102. **Loffer FD.** Hysteroscopy with selective endometrial sampling compared with D&D for abnormal uterine bleeding: the value of a negative hysteroscopic view. *Obstet Gynecol* 1989;73:16–20.

103. **Iossa A, Cianferoni L, Ciatto S, et al.** Hysteroscopy and endometrial cancer diagnosis: a review of 2007 consecutive examinations in self-referred patients. *Tumori* 1991;77:479–483.

104. **Crescini C, Artuso A, Repetti F, et al.** Hysteroscopic diagnosis in patients with abnormal uterine hemorrhage and previous endometrial curettage. *Minerva Ginecol* 1992;44:233–235.

105. **Brooks PG, Serden SP.** Hysteroscopic findings after unsuccessful dilatation and curettage for abnormal uterine bleeding. *Am J Obstet Gynecol* 1988;158:1354–1357.

106. **Valle RF.** Hysteroscopy in the evaluation of female infertility. *Am J Obstet Gynecol* 1980;317:425–431.

107. **Golan A, Ron-El R, Herman A, et al.** Diagnostic hysteroscopy: its value in an in vitro fertilization transfer unit. *Hum Reprod* 1992;7:1433–1434.

108. **Marty R, Amouroux J, Haouet S, et al.** The reliability of endometrial biopsy performed during hysteroscopy. *Int J Gynaecol Obstet* 1991;34:151–155.

109. **Chambers JT, Chambers SK.** Endometrial sampling: When? Where? Why? With what? *Clin Obstet Gynecol* 1992;35:28–39.

110. **DeCherney AH, Russell JB, Graebe RA, et al.** Resectoscopic management of müllerian fusion defects. *Fertil Steril* 1986;45:726–728.

111. **Valle RF, Sciarra JJ.** Hysteroscopic treatment of the septate uterus. *Obstet Gynecol* 1986;67:253–257.

112. **March CM, Israel R.** Hysteroscopic management of recurrent abortion caused by the septate uterus. *Am J Obstet Gynecol* 1987;156:834–842.

113. **Daly DC, Maier D, Soto-Albers C.** Hysteroscopic metroplasty: six years' experience. *Obstet Gynecol* 1989;61:392–397

114. **Hart R, Molnar BG, Margos A.** Long term follow up of hysteroscopic myomectomy assessed by survival analysis. *Br J Obstet Gynaecol* 1999;106;700–705.

115. **Emanuel MH, Wamsteker K, Hart AA, et al.** Long-term results of hysteroscopic myomectomy for abnormal uterine bleeding. *Obstet Gynecol* 1999;93:743–748.

116. **Vercellini P, Zaina B, Yaylayan L, et al.** Hysteroscopic myomectomy: long-term effects on menstrual pattern and fertility. *Obstet Gynecol* 1999;94:341–347.

117. **Brill AL.** What is the role of hysteroscopy in the management of abnormal uterine bleeding? *Clin Obstet Gynecol* 1995;38:319–345.

118. **O'Connor H, Magos A.** Endometrial resection for the treatment of menorrhagia. *N Engl J Med* 1996;335: 151–156.

119. **Wamsteker K, Emanuel MH, de Kruif JH.** Transcervical hysteroscopic resection of submucous fibroids for abnormal uterine bleeding: results regarding the degree of intramural extension. *Obstet Gynecol* 1993; 82:736–740.

120. **Indman PD.** Hysteroscopic treatment of menorrhagia associated with uterine leiomyomas. *Obstet Gynecol* 1993;81:716–720.

121. **Cicinelli E, Romano F, Anastasio PS, et al.** Transabdominal sonohysterography, transvaginal sonography and hysteroscopy in the evaluation of submucous myomas. *Obstet Gynecol* 1995;85:42–47.

122. **Brooks PG.** Hysteroscopic surgery using the resectoscope: myomas, ablation, septa, synechiae. Does preoperative medication help? *Clin Obstet Gynecol* 1992;35:249–255.

123. **Sowter MC, Singla AA, Lethaby A.** Pre-operative endometrial thinning agents before hysteroscopic surgery for heavy menstrual bleeding. *Cochrane Database Syst Rev* 2000;2:CD001124.

124. **Scottish Hysteroscopy Audit Group.** A Scottish audit of hysteroscopic surgery for menorrhagia: complications and follow up. *Br J Obstet Gynecol* 1995;102:249–254.

125. **Overton C, Hargreaves J, Maresh M.** A national survey of the complications of endometrial destruction for menstrual disorders: the MISTLETOE study. Minimally Invasive Surgical Techniques—Laser, Endo Thermal or Endoresection. *Br J Obstet Gynecol* 1997;104:1351–1359.

126. **Lomano J.** Endometrial ablation for the treatment of menorrhagia: a comparison of patients with normal, enlarged and fibroid uteri. *Lasers Surg Med* 1991;11:8–12.

127. **Magos AL, Baumann R, Lockwood GM, et al.** Experience with the first 250 endometrial resections for menorrhagia. *Lancet* 1991;337:1074–1078.

128. **Wortman M, Daggett A.** Hysteroscopic endomyometrial resection: a new technique for the treatment of menorrhagia. *Obstet Gynecol* 1994;83:295–298.

129. **Garry R.** Endometrial ablation and resection: validation of a new surgical concept. *Br J Obstet Gynaecol* 1997;104:1329–1331.

130. **Pinion SB, Parkin DE, Abramovich DR, et al.** Randomised trial of hysterectomy, endometrial laser ablation and transcervical endometrial resection for dysfunctional uterine bleeding. *BMJ* 1994;309:979–983.

131. **Lethaby A, Shepperd S, Cooke I, et al.** Endometrial resection and ablation versus hysterectomy for heavy menstrual bleeding. *Cochrane Database Syst Rev* 2000;2:CD000329.

132. **Daniell JF, Kurtz BR, Ke RW.** Hysteroscopic endometrial ablation using the rollerball electrode. *Obstet Gynecol* 1992;80:329–332.

133. **Milad MP, Buckley AP, Keh PC.** Residual endometrium after uterine ballon ablation. *Obstet Gynecol* 1999; 93:838.

134. **Perino A, Chianchiano N, Petronio M, et al.** Role of leuprolide acetate depot in hysteroscopic surgery: a controlled study. *Fertil Steril* 1993;59:507–510.

135. **Goldrath MH.** Use of danazol in hysteroscopic surgery for menorrhagia. *J Reprod Med* 1990;35:91–96.

136. **Alexander DA, Naji AA, Pinion SB, et al.** Randomised trial comparing hysterectomy with endometrial ablation for dysfunctional uterine bleeding: psychiatric and psychological aspects. *BMJ* 1996;312:280–284.

137. **Sugimoto O.** Diagnostic and therapeutic hysteroscopy for traumatic intrauterine adhesions. *Am J Obstet Gynecol* 1978;131:539–547.

138. **March CM, Israel R.** Gestational outcome following hysteroscopic lysis of adhesions. *Fertil Steril* 1981;36:455–459.

139. **Valle RF, Schiarra JJ.** Intrauterine adhesions: classification, treatment and reproductive outcome. *Am J Obstet Gynecol* 1988;158:1459–1470.

140. **Schlaff WD, Hurst BS.** Preoperative sonographic measurement of endometrial pattern predicts outcome of surgical repair in patients with severe Asherman's syndrome. *Fertil Steril* 1995;63:410–413.

141. **Zupi E, Luciano AA, Valli E, et al.** The use of topical anesthesia in diagnostic hysteroscopy and endometrial biopsy. *Fertil Steril* 1995;63:414–416.

142. **Hoekstra PT, Kahnoski R, McCamish MA, et al.** Transurethral resection syndrome—a new perspective: encephalopathy with associated hyperammonemia. *J Urol* 1983;130:704–707.

143. **Brill AI.** Energy systems for operative hysteroscopy. *Obstet Gynecol Clin North Am* 2000;27:317–326.

144. **Jansen FW, Vredevogd CD, van Ulzen K, et al.** Complications of hysteroscopy: a prospective, multicenter study. *Obstet Gynecol* 2000;96:266–270.

145. **Phillips DR, Nathanson HG, Milim SJ, et al.** The effect of dilute vasopressin solution on blood loss during operative hysteroscopy: a randomized controlled trial. *Obstet Gynecol* 1996;88:761–766.

146. **Indman PD, Brown WW 3rd.** Uterine surface temperature changes caused by electrosurgical endometrial coagulation. *J Reprod Med* 1992;37:667–670.

147. **Sullivan B, Kenney P, Seibel M.** Hysteroscopic resection of fibroid with thermal injury to sigmoid. *Obstet Gynecol* 1992;80:546–547.

148. **Obenhaus T, Maurer W.** CO_2 embolism during hysteroscopy. *Anaesthetist* 1990;39:243–246.

149. **Vo Van JM, Nguyen NQ, Le Bervet JY.** A fatal gas embolism during a hysteroscopy-curettage. *Cah Anesthesiol* 1992;40:617–618.

150. **Stoloff DR, Isenberg RA, Brill AL.** Venous air and gas emboli in operative hysteroscopy. *J Am Assoc Gynecol Laparosc* 2001:8:181–192.

151. **Cholban MJ, Kalhan SB, Anderson RJ, et al.** Pulmonary edema and coagulopathy following intrauterine instillation of 32% dextran-70 (Hyskon). *J Clin Anesth* 1991;3:317–319.

152. **Golan A, Siedner M, Bahar M, et al.** High-output left ventricular failure after dextran use in an operative hysteroscopy. *Fertil Steril* 1990;54:939–941.

22 Hysterectomy

Thomas G. Stovall

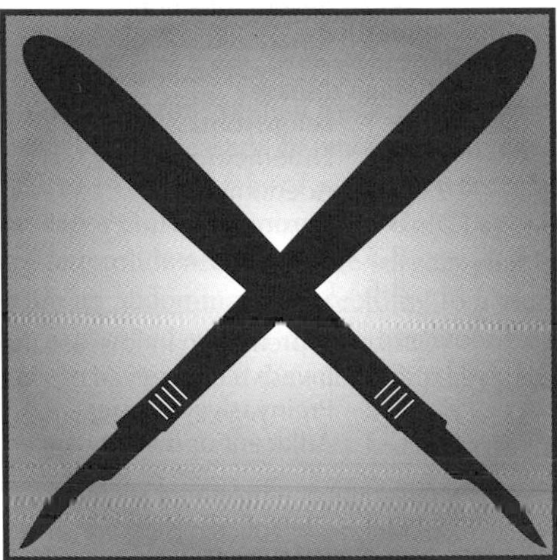

Hysterectomy is one of the most common surgical procedures performed. After cesarean delivery, it is the second most frequently performed major surgical procedure in the United States (1). In 1965, there were 426,000 hysterectomies performed in the United States, with an average length of hospital stay of 12.2 days. This number reached its peak in 1985, when 724,000 procedures were reported, with the length of stay decreasing to 9.4 days. The number of hysterectomies performed in the United States declined to 544,000 in 1991, with an average length of stay of 4.5 days. Of these 544,000 hysterectomies, 408,000 (75%) were performed abdominally, and 136,000 (25%) were performed vaginally (2,3). However, by 1998, the number of hysterectomies performed had increased to more than 600,000 (4). Using 1987 age-specific hysterectomy rates and the population projections supplied by the U.S. Census Bureau, it has been projected that there will be 824,000 hysterectomies in the year 2005 (5).

The rate of hysterectomy has varied between 6.1 and 8.6 per 1,000 women of all ages. A woman's chance of having a hysterectomy is dependent on a variety of factors, including her age, race, and where she lives, and the sex of her physician. Women between the ages of 20 and 49 years constituted the largest segment of women undergoing the procedure. The average age of a woman undergoing hysterectomy is 42.7 years and the median age is 40.9 years, which has remained constant since the 1980s. About 75% of all hysterectomies are performed in women between the ages of 20 and 49 years. The rates of hysterectomy vary by region of the country. The highest overall rate is in the southern states, where the rate tends to be higher for women aged 15 to 44 years. The lowest rates have consistently been in the northeastern portion of the United States. Hysterectomy is more often performed in African American than in white women and is performed more frequently by male gynecologists than by female gynecologists (6–9).

Indications

The indications for hysterectomy are listed in Table 22.1. In virtually all studies, uterine leiomyomas are consistently the leading indication for hysterectomy. As expected, the indications differ with the patient's age (10). For instance, whereas pelvic relaxation accounts for 16% of hysterectomies, this diagnosis is responsible for more than 33% of hysterectomies

Cholecystectomy

Gallbladder disease is about four times more common in women than men, and its highest incidence occurs between 50 and 70 years of age, when hysterectomy is most often performed. Thus, women may require both procedures. A combined procedure does not appear to result in increased febrile morbidity or length of hospital stay (72,73).

Abdominoplasty

Abdominoplasty performed at the time of hysterectomy is associated with a shorter hospital stay, a shorter operating time, and a lower intraoperative blood loss than when the two operations are performed separately (74,75). Liposuction also can be performed safely at the time of vaginal hysterectomy (76).

Technique

Negative results of a Pap test performed within the year should be obtained before performing a hysterectomy for benign disease. If the patient is 40 years of age or older and has not recently had a mammography, this examination should be performed. Endometrial sampling is recommended if the patient has reported abnormal uterine bleeding. In patients older than 40 years of age, a stool guaiac test should be performed.

Other preoperative testing should be dictated by the patient's specific medical conditions.

Abdominal Hysterectomy

Preoperative Preparation

Although not mandatory, a cleansing tap water or soap enema given on the evening before or the morning of the scheduled hysterectomy is preferred by some surgeons. To reduce the colony count of skin bacteria, the patient is asked to shower. Hair surrounding the incision area may be removed at the time of surgery or before surgery using a depilatory agent. Hair clipping is preferable to shaving because it decreases the incidence of incisional infection (77).

Patient Positioning The patient is placed in the dorsal supine position for the procedure. After the patient is anesthetized adequately, her legs are placed in the stirrups and a pelvic examination is performed to validate the in-office pelvic examination findings. A Foley catheter is placed in the bladder, and the vagina is cleansed with an iodine solution. The patient's legs are then straightened.

Skin Preparation Several methods for skin cleaning can be recommended, including a 5-minute iodine solution scrub followed by application of iodine solution, iodine solution scrub followed by alcohol with application of an iodine-impregnated occlusive drape, or an iodine-alcohol combination with or without application of an iodine-impregnated occlusive drape.

Surgical Technique

Incision The choice of incision should be determined by the following considerations:

1. Simplicity of the incision
2. The need for exposure
3. The potential need for enlarging the incision
4. The strength of the healed wound

5. Cosmesis of the healed incision

6. The location of previous surgical scars

The skin is opened with a scalpel, and the incision is carried down through the subcutaneous tissue and fascia. With traction applied to the lateral edges of the incision, the fascia is divided. The peritoneum is opened similarly. This technique minimizes the possibility of inadvertent enterotomy, entering the abdominal cavity.

Abdominal Exploration After entering the peritoneal cavity, the upper abdomen and the pelvis are explored systematically. The liver, gallbladder, stomach, kidneys, paraaortic lymph nodes, and large and small bowel should be examined and palpated. Cytologic sampling of the peritoneal cavity, if needed, should be performed before abdominal exploration.

Retractor Choice and Placement A variety of retractors have been designed for pelvic surgery. The Balfour and the O'Connor-O'Sullivan retractors are used most often. The Bookwalter retractor has a variety of adjustable blades that can be helpful, particularly in obese patients.

Elevation of the Uterus The uterus is elevated by placing broad ligament clamps at each cornu so that it crosses the round ligament. The clamp tip may be placed close to the internal os. This placement provides uterine traction and prevents backbleeding (Fig. 22.1).

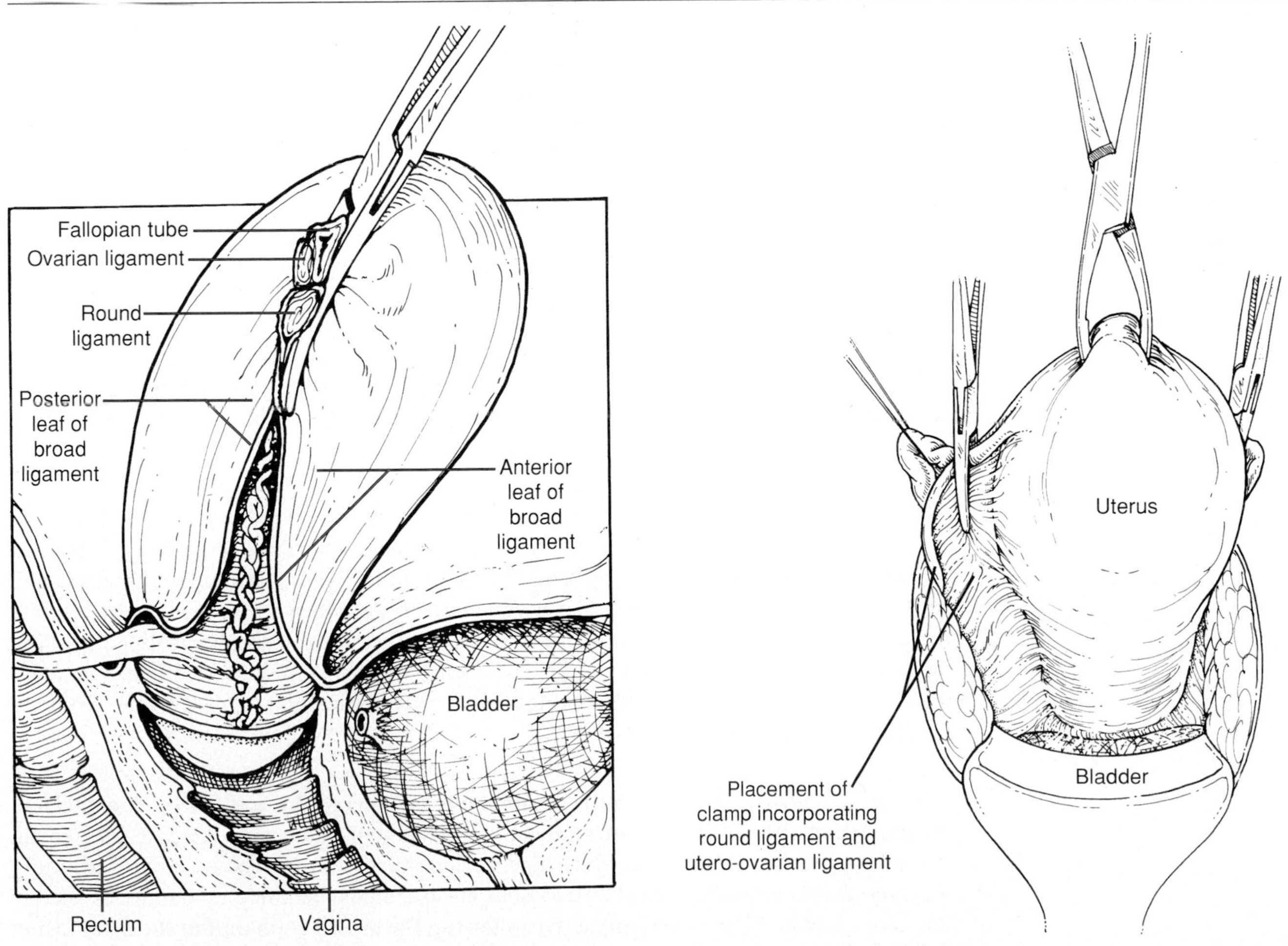

Figure 22.1 The uterus is elevated by placement of clamps across the broad ligament. (From **Mann WA, Stovall TG.** *Gynecologic surgery.* New York: Churchill Livingstone, 1996, with permission.)

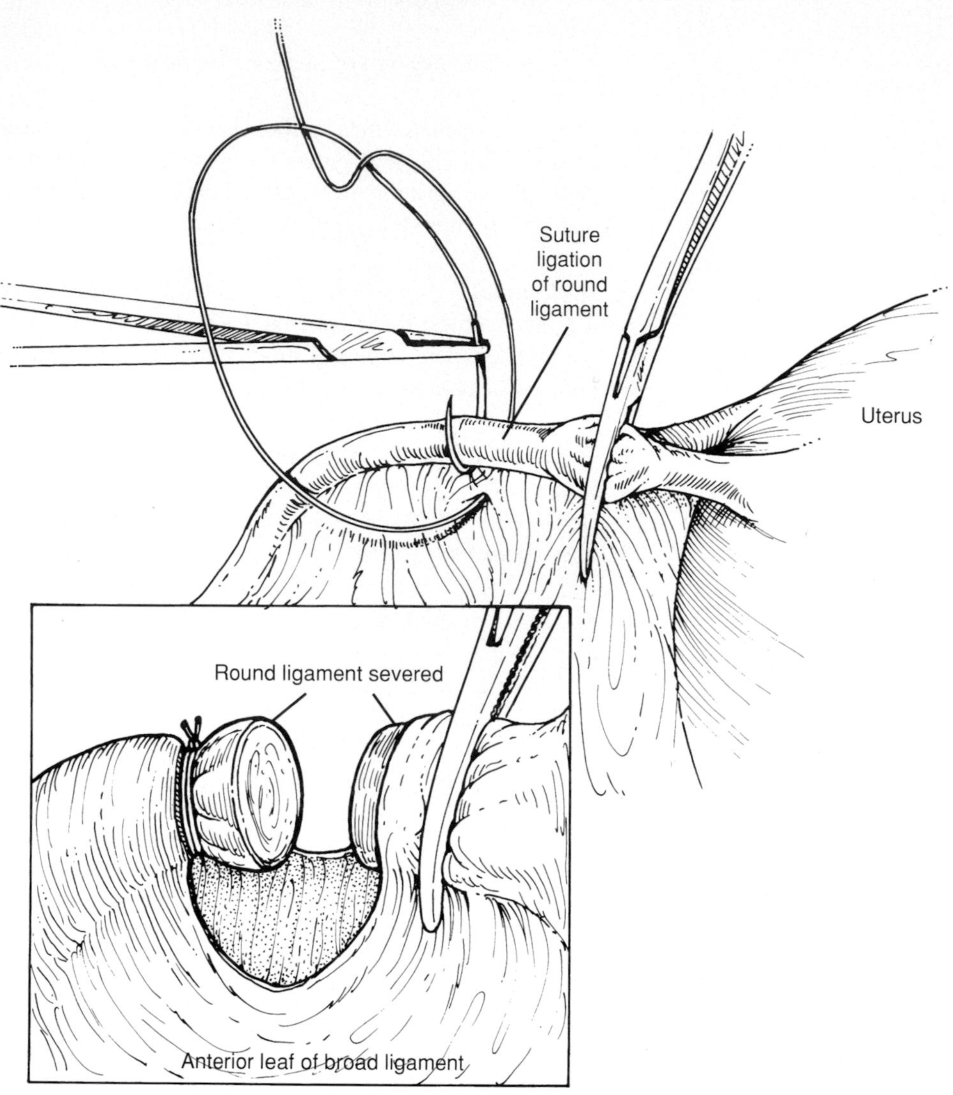

Figure 22.2 The round ligament is transected and the broad ligament is incised and opened. (From **Mann WA, Stovall TG.** *Gynecologic surgery.* New York: Churchill Livingstone, 1996.)

Round Ligament Ligation The uterus is deviated to the patient's left side, stretching the right round ligament. With the proximal portion held by the broad ligament clamp, the distal portion of the round ligament is ligated with a suture ligature or simply transected with Bovie cautery (Fig. 22.2). The distal portion can be grasped with forceps, and the round ligament is cut to separate the anterior and posterior leaves of the broad ligament. The anterior leaf of the broad ligament is incised with Metzenbaum scissors or electrocautery along the vesicouterine fold, separating the peritoneal reflection of the bladder from the lower uterine segment (Fig. 22.3).

Ureter Identification **The retroperitoneum is entered by extending the incision cephalad on the posterior leaf of the broad ligament.** Care must be taken to remain lateral to both the infundibulopelvic ligament and iliac vessels. The external iliac artery courses along the medial aspect of the psoas muscle and is identified by bluntly dissecting the loose alveolar tissue overlying it. **By following the artery cephalad to the bifurcation of the common iliac artery, the ureter is identified crossing the common iliac artery. The ureter should be left attached to the medial leaf of the broad ligament to protect its blood supply** (Fig. 22.4).

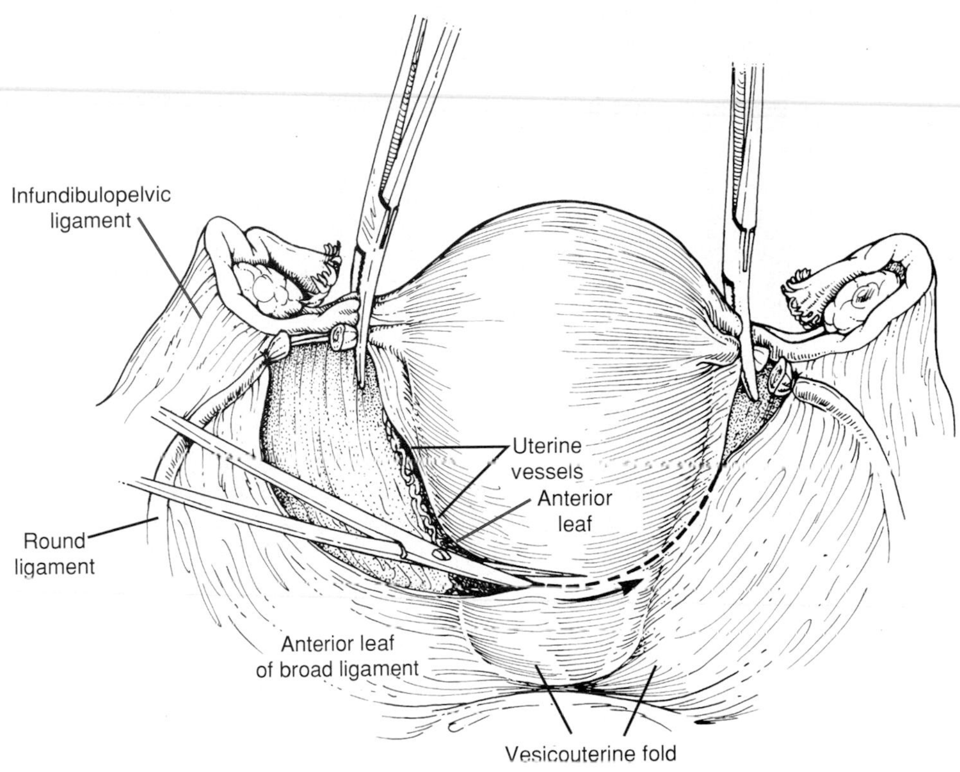

Figure 22.3 The incision in the anterior broad ligament is extended along the vesicouterine fold. (From **Mann WA, Stovall TG.** *Gynecologic surgery.* New York: Churchill Livingstone, 1996, with permission.)

Uteroovarian or Infundibulopelvic Ligament Ligation If the ovaries are to be preserved, the uterus is retracted toward the pubic symphysis and deviated to one side, placing tension on the contralateral infundibulopelvic ligament, the tube, and the ovary. **With the ureter under direct visualization, a window is created in the peritoneum of the posterior leaf of the broad ligament under the uteroovarian ligament and fallopian tube.** The tube and uteroovarian ligament are clamped on each side with a curved Heaney or Ballentine clamp, cut, and ligated with both a free-tie and a suture ligature. The medial clamp at the uterine cornu should control backbleeding; if it does not, the clamp should be repositioned to do so (Fig. 22.5).

If the ovaries are to be removed, the peritoneal opening is enlarged and extended cephalad to the infundibulopelvic ligament and caudad to the uterine artery. This opening allows proper exposure of the uterine artery, the infundibulopelvic ligament, and the ureter. In this manner, the ureter is released from its proximity to the uterine vessels and the infundibulopelvic ligament.

A curved Heaney or Ballentine clamp is placed lateral to the ovary (Fig. 22.6); care is taken to ensure that the entire ovary is included in the surgical specimen. The infundibulopelvic ligament on each side is cut and doubly ligated (Fig. 22.7). Alternatively, free ties can be passed around the infundibulopelvic ligament, two cephalad and one caudad, before the ligament is cut.

Bladder Mobilization Using Metzenbaum scissors, with the tips pointed toward the uterus, the bladder is sharply dissected from the lower uterine segment and cervix. Alternatively, Bovie electrocautery can be used. An avascular plane, which exists between the lower uterine segment and the bladder, allows for this mobilization. Tonsil clamps may be placed on the bladder edge to provide countertraction and easier dissection (Fig. 22.8).

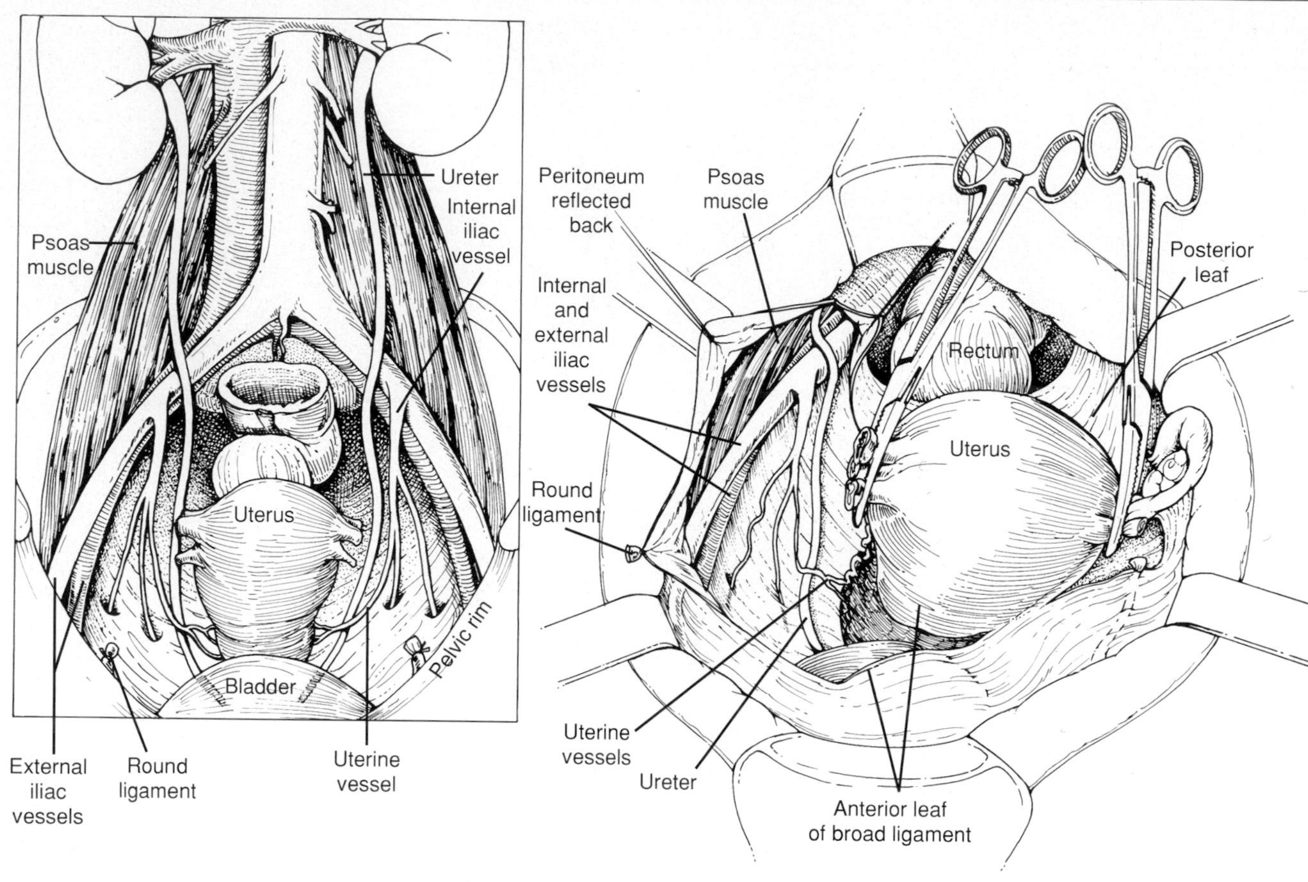

Figure 22.4 Identification of the ureter in the retroperitoneal space on the medial leaf of the broad ligament. (From **Mann WA, Stovall TG.** *Gynecologic surgery.* New York: Churchill Livingstone, 1996, with permission.)

Uterine Vessel Ligation The uterus is retracted cephalad and deviated to one side of the pelvis, stretching the lower ligaments. The uterine vasculature is dissected or "skeletonized" from any remaining areolar tissue, and a curved Heaney clamp is placed perpendicular to the uterine artery at the junction of the cervix and body of the uterus. Care is taken to place the tip of the clamp adjacent to the uterus at this anatomic narrowing. The vessels are cut, and the suture is ligated. The same procedure is repeated on the opposite side (Fig. 22.9).

Incision of Posterior Peritoneum If the rectum is to be mobilized from the posterior cervix, the posterior peritoneum between the uterosacral ligaments just beneath the cervix and rectum may be incised (Fig. 22.10). A relatively avascular tissue plane exists in this area, allowing mobilization of the rectum inferiorly out of the operative field. A sponge may be placed to control the venous oozing that often occurs.

Cardinal Ligament Ligation The cardinal ligament is divided by placing a straight Heaney clamp medial to the uterine vessel pedicle for a distance of 2 to 3 cm parallel to the uterus. The ligament is then cut, and the pedicle suture is ligated. This step is repeated on each side until the junction of the cervix and vagina is reached (Fig. 22.11).

Removal of the Uterus The uterus is placed on traction cephalad and the tip of the cervix is palpated. Curved Heaney clamps are placed bilaterally, incorporating the uterosacral ligament and upper vagina just below the cervix. **Care should be taken to avoid foreshortening the vagina.** The uterus is then removed with heavy curved scissors (Fig. 22.12).

Figure 22.5 Ligation of the uteroovarian ligament. (From **Mann WA, Stovall TG.** *Gynecologic surgery.* New York: Churchill Livingstone, 1996, with permission.)

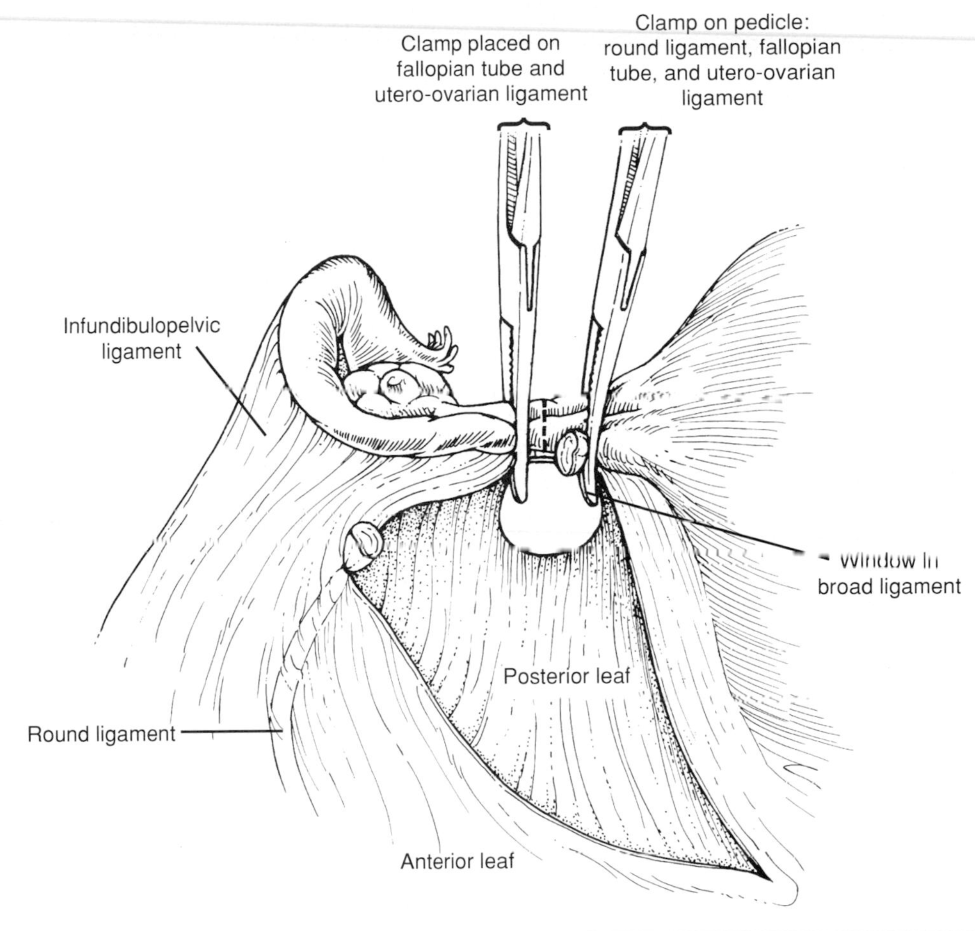

Figure 22.6 Ligation of the infundibulopelvic ligament. (From **Mann WA, Stovall TG.** *Gynecologic surgery.* New York: Churchill Livingstone, 1996, with permission.)

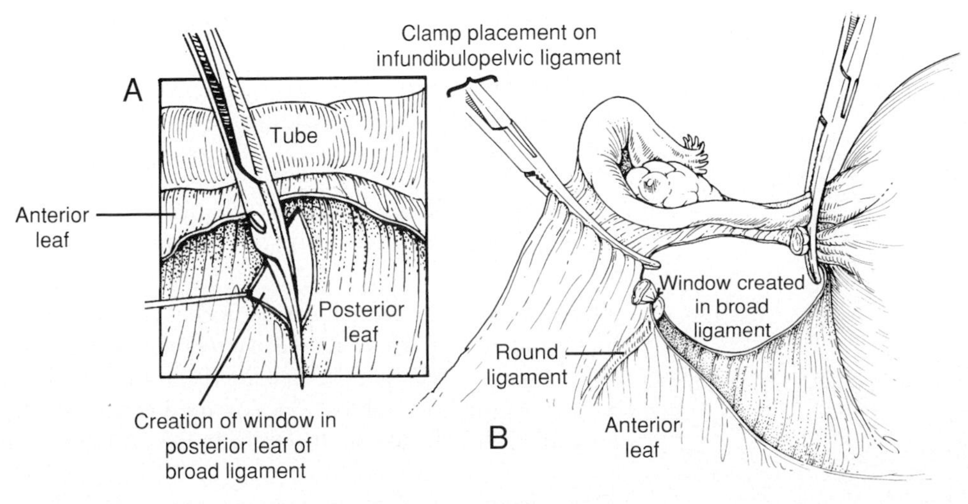

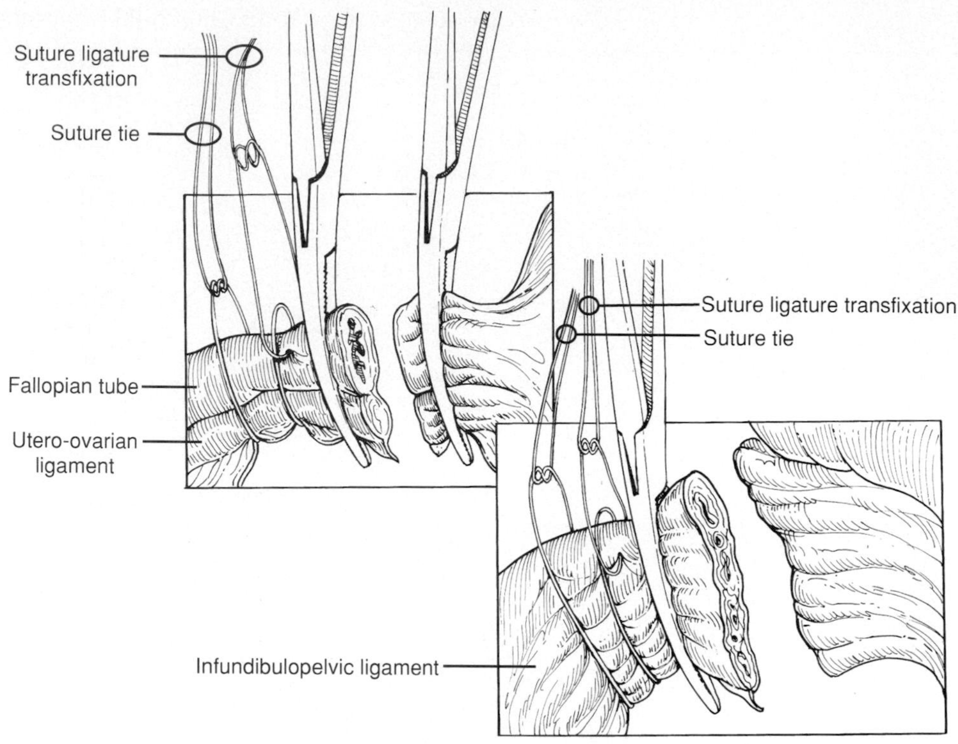

Figure 22.7 Transection of the infundibulopelvic ligament. (From **Mann WA, Stovall TG.** *Gynecologic surgery.* New York: Churchill Livingstone, 1996, with permission.)

Vaginal Cuff Closure Several techniques of vaginal cuff closure have been described. A figure-of-eight suture of 0-0 braided absorbable material is placed between the tips of the two clamps. The suture is used for both traction and hemostasis. Sutures are also placed at the tip of each clamp, and the pedicles are sutured with a Heaney stitch, thereby incorporating the uterosacral and cardinal ligament at the angle of the vagina (Fig. 22.13). Alternatively, the vaginal cuff can be left open to heal secondarily. If this method is used, a running-locked suture is used for hemostasis along the cuff edge (Fig. 22.14).

Irrigation and Hemostasis The pelvis is thoroughly irrigated with saline or lactated Ringer's solution. Meticulous care is taken to ensure hemostasis throughout the pelvis, particularly of the vascular pedicles. Ureteral position and integrity are checked again to ensure that they are intact and do not appear dilated.

Peritoneal Closure The pelvic peritoneum is not reapproximated. Research using animal models suggests that reapproximation may increase tissue trauma and promote adhesion formation (77).

If the ovaries have been retained, they may be suspended to the pelvic sidewall to minimize the risk of becoming retroperitoneal or adherent to the vaginal cuff.

Incision Closure The parietal peritoneum is not reapproximated as a separate layer. Fascia can be closed with an interrupted or a continuous 0-0 or 1-0 monofilament absorbable suture. A continuous suture may reduce the risk for necrosis, which may occur when interrupted sutures are tied too tightly (77). As with interrupted sutures, bites should be taken about 1 cm from the cut edge of the fascia and about 1 cm apart to prevent wound dehiscence.

Skin Closure The subcutaneous tissue should be irrigated, with careful attention given to maintaining hemostasis. Subcutaneous sutures are not used because they may increase

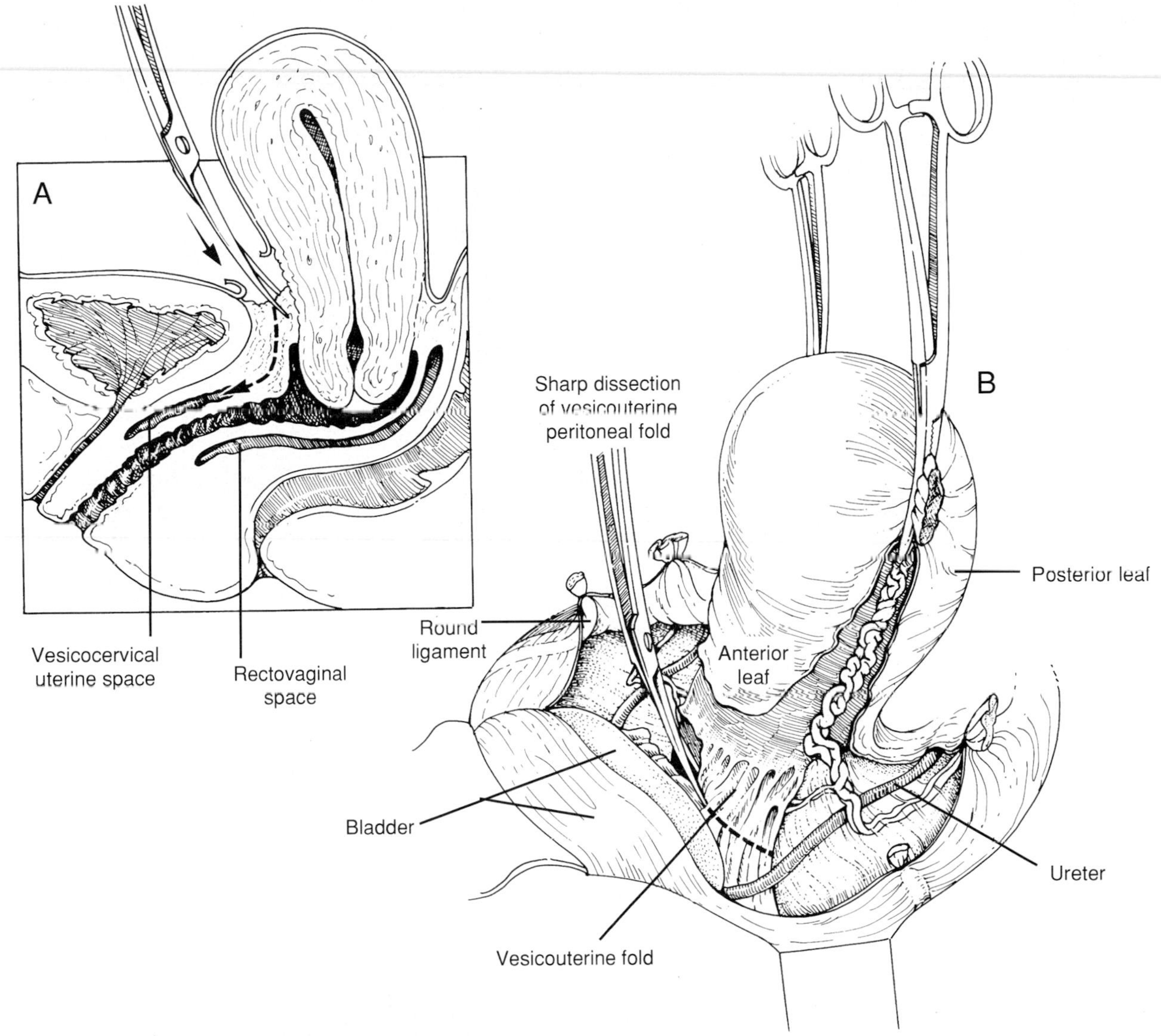

Figure 22.8 Dissection of the vesicouterine plane to mobilize the bladder. (From **Mann WA, Stovall TG.** *Gynecologic surgery.* New York: Churchill Livingstone, 1996, with permission.)

the incidence of wound infection (77). Skin staples or subcuticular sutures are used to reapproximate the skin edges. A bandage is applied and left in place for about 24 hours.

Intraoperative Complications

Most intraoperative injuries during abdominal hysterectomy can be traced to poor lighting, unsatisfactory assistance, undue haste, anatomic variants, or involvement of the injured organ in the disease process (78). Some of these factors can be eliminated with careful attention to detail and use of proper surgical technique. However, some operative injuries cannot be avoided by even the most skilled surgeons. The surgeon, therefore, must be prepared to recognize and repair these injuries. Even with a high level of attention to detail, injuries and complications, recognized and unrecognized, can still occur.

Ureteral Injuries

Injury to the pelvic ureter is one of the most formidable complications of hysterectomy (79–81). Because of the risk for subsequent renal impairment, injury to the ureter is far more serious than injury to the bladder or bowel (82,83).

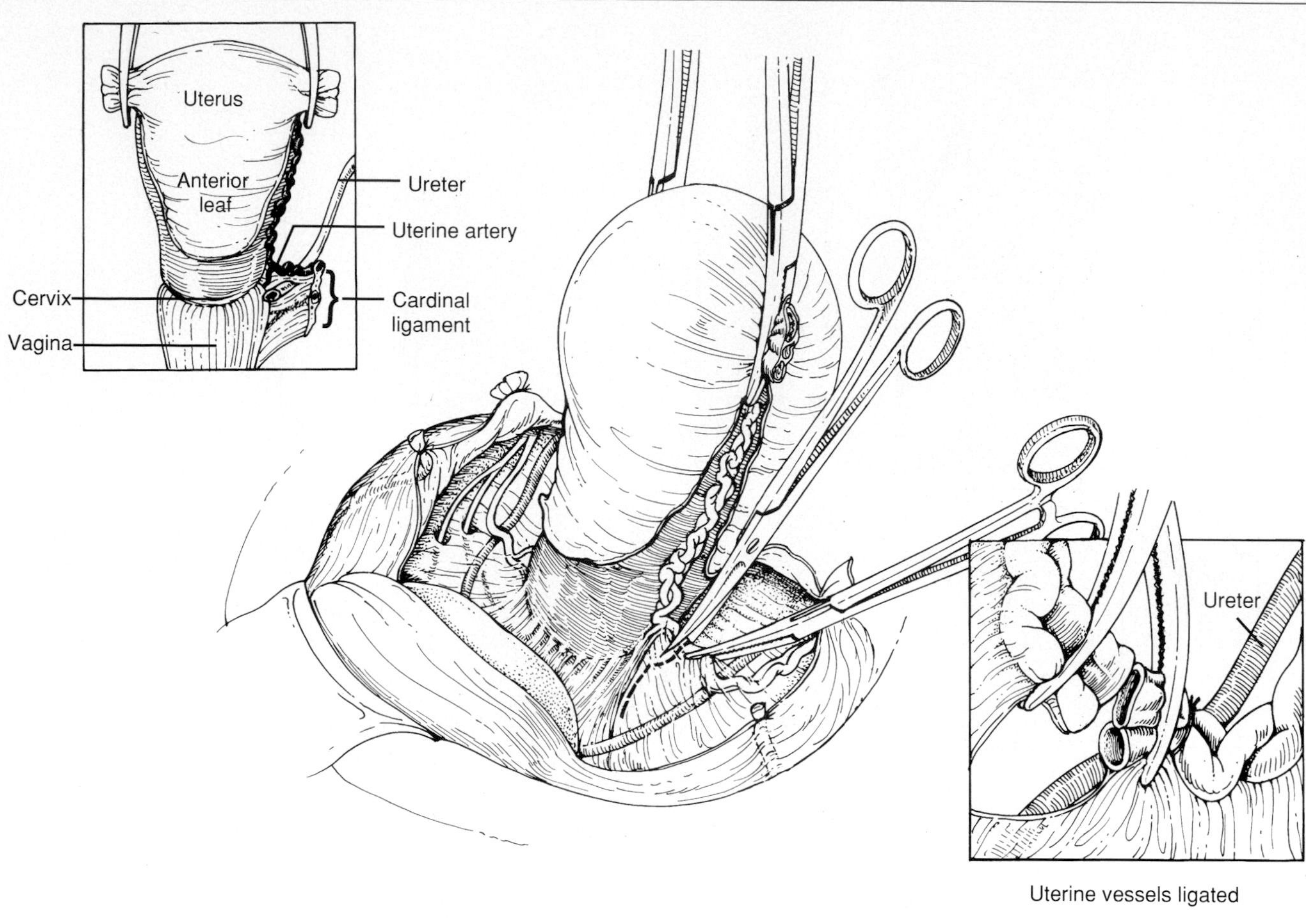

Figure 22.9 Ligation of the uterine blood vessels. (From **Mann WA, Stovall TG.** *Gynecologic surgery.* New York: Churchill Livingstone, 1996, with permission.)

It is essential to be aware of the proximity of the ureter to the other pelvic structures at all times. **Most ureteral injuries can be avoided by opening the retroperitoneum and directly identifying the ureter.** The use of ureteral catheters as a substitute for direct visualization is often of little help in patients with extensive fibrosis or scarring resulting from endometriosis, pelvic inflammatory disease, or ovarian cancer. In these instances, a false sense of security may actually increase an already high risk for ureteral injury (84). The use of ureteral catheters can also be associated with hematuria and acute urinary retention. Their complications are usually transitory in nature.

Direct visualization is accomplished by opening the retroperitoneum lateral to the external iliac artery. Blunt dissection of the loose areolar tissue is performed to visualize the artery directly. The artery may then be traced cephalad to the bifurcation of the internal and external iliac arteries. The ureter crosses the common iliac artery at its bifurcation and may be followed throughout its course in the pelvis.

Despite these precautions, ureteral injuries may occur. Prompt consultation is necessary if the surgeon has not been trained in ureteral repair. If a ureteral obstruction is suspected, confirmation may be obtained by intravenous injection of 1 ampule of indigo carmine dye, opening the dome of the bladder, and observing the presence or absence of bilateral spill of tinted urine. Alternatively, ureteral patency may be established by opening the dome of the bladder and positioning retrograde ureteral stents. Cystoscopic evaluation may replace opening the bladder to evaluate the spill of tinted urine (79–84).

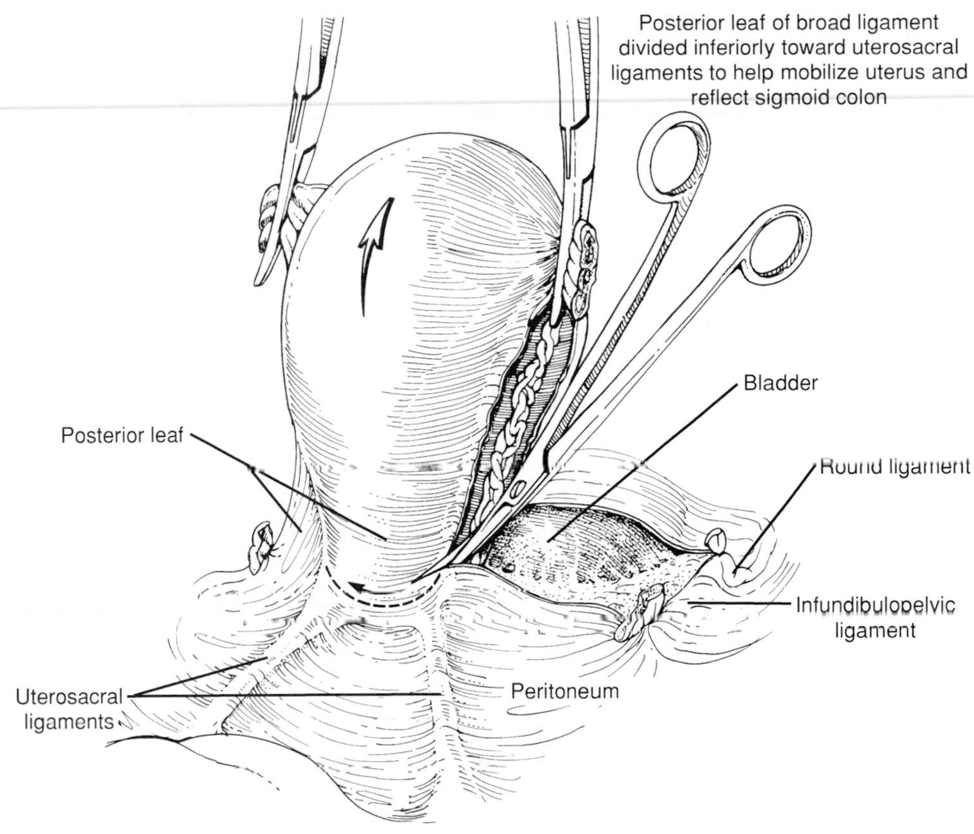

Figure 22.10 Incision of the rectouterine peritoneum and mobilization of the rectum from the posterior cervix. (From **Mann WA, Stovall TG.** *Gynecologic surgery.* New York: Churchill Livingstone, 1996, with permission.)

Bladder Injury

Because of the close anatomic relationship of the bladder, uterus, and upper vagina, the bladder is the segment of the lower urinary tract that is most vulnerable to injury (82,84). Bladder injury may occur on opening the peritoneum or, more frequently, during the dissection of the bladder off the cervix and upper vagina (85). Unless there is involvement of the bladder trigone, a bladder laceration is easily repaired. In the nonirradiated bladder, a one- or two-layer closure with a small-caliber braided absorbable suture such as a 3-0 polyglycolic acid is adequate. The bladder should be drained postoperatively. The length of time that drainage is required is controversial. If the bladder is not compromised, drainage should be continued at least until gross hematuria clears, which may occur as soon as 48 hours postoperatively. A more conservative practice is to continue drainage until the patient is ready for discharge, usually a total of 3 to 4 days. Elective incision into the dome of the bladder is performed similarly (85). If the trigone is involved, a surgeon trained in complicated urologic repair should be consulted.

Bowel Injury

Small bowel injuries are the most common intestinal injuries in gynecologic surgery (86). Small defects of the serosa or muscularis may be repaired using a single layer of continuous or interrupted 3-0 braided absorbable suture. Although single-layer closure of the small bowel has proved adequate, it is safer to close defects involving the lumen in two layers using a 3-0 braided absorbable suture. **The defect should be closed in a direction perpendicular**

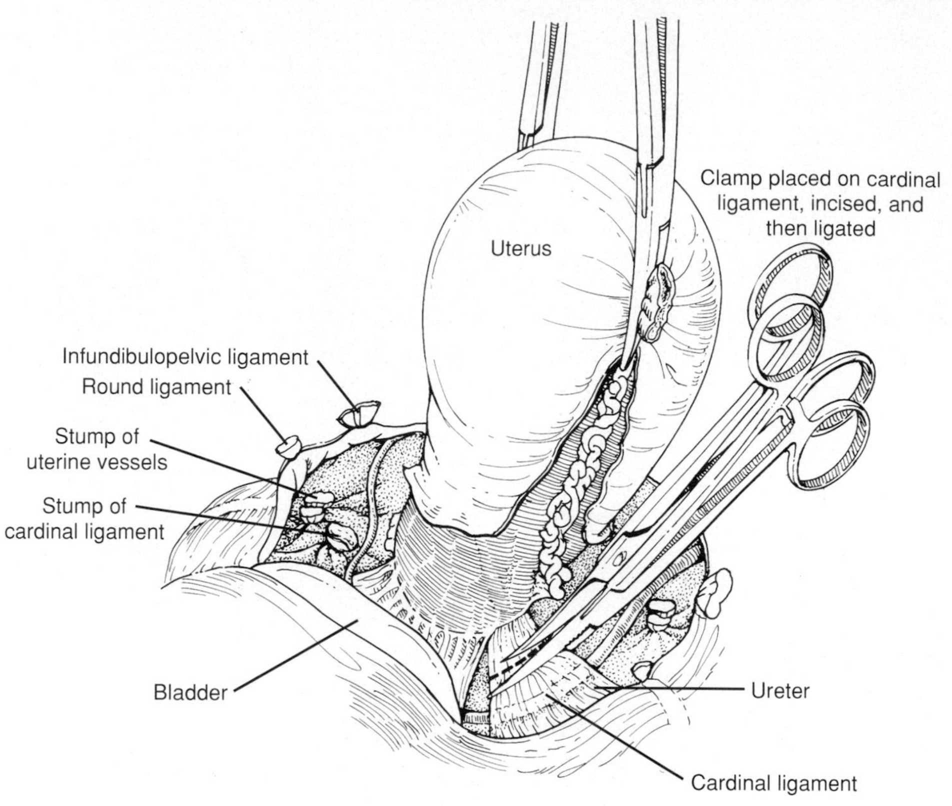

Figure 22.11 Ligation of the cardinal ligament. (From **Mann WA, Stovall TG.** *Gynecologic surgery.* New York: Churchill Livingstone, 1996, with permission.)

to the intestinal lumen. If a large area has been injured, resection with reanastomosis may be necessary (85,87).

Because the bacterial flora of the ascending colon is similar to that of the small bowel, injuries can be repaired in a similar manner. The transverse colon rarely is injured in normal gynecologic procedures because it is well outside the operative field. However, the descending colon and the rectosigmoid colon are intimately involved with the pelvic structures and are at significant risk for injury during gynecologic surgery. Injuries not involving the mucosa may be repaired with a single running layer of 2-0 or 3-0 braided absorbable suture. If the laceration involves the mucosa, it may be closed as with small bowel injuries if the colon has been prepared adequately. Otherwise, diverting colostomy may be necessary in some patients to protect the repair site from fecal contamination, especially if the defect is larger than 5 cm or if there is spillage of the bowel contents (85,87).

Hemorrhage

Significant arterial bleeding usually arises from the uterine arteries or the ovarian vessels near the insertion of the infundibulopelvic ligaments (88). Blind clamping of these vessels presents a risk for ureteral injury; therefore, the ureters should be identified in the retroperitoneal space and traced to the area of bleeding to avoid inadvertent ligation. It is best to apply a pressure pack to tamponade the bleeding and then slowly remove the pack in an effort to visualize, isolate, and individually clamp the bleeding vessels. Mass ligatures should be avoided. The use of surgical clips may be helpful. Venous bleeding, while less dramatic, is often more difficult to manage, particularly in the presence of extensive adhesions and fibroids. This type of bleeding can be controlled with pressure alone or with suture ligation. Bleeding from peritoneal edges or denuded surfaces may be controlled with pressure,

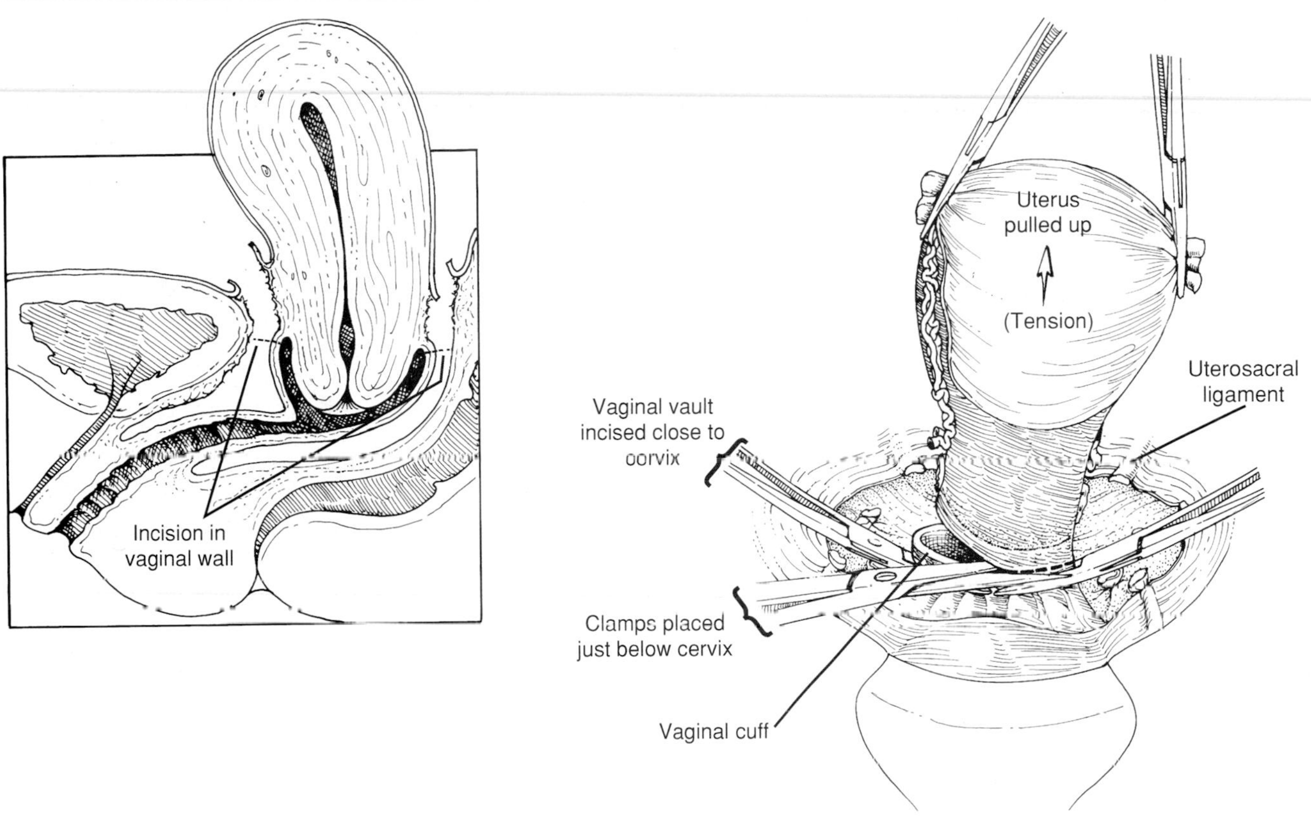

Figure 22.12 Removal of the uterus by transection of the vagina. (From **Mann WA, Stovall TG.** *Gynecologic surgery.* New York: Churchill Livingstone, 1996.)

application of topical agents such as thrombin or collagen, or cautery with the Bovie. A variety of laser techniques have been used to control bleeding.

Postoperative Management

Bladder Drainage Overdistention of the female bladder resulting from bladder trauma or the patient's reluctance to initiate the voluntary phase of voiding is one of the most common complications after abdominal hysterectomy (89). For this reason, an indwelling bladder catheter should be used for the first few postoperative hours until the patient is able to ambulate and urinate.

If retropubic urethropexy has been performed, consideration should be given to using a suprapubic catheter, which allows postvoid residual levels to be checked without repetitive catheterizations. This catheter may be removed when satisfactory postvoid residual levels of less than 100 mL have been obtained.

Diet In anticipation of the rare case in which the patient must be returned to the operating room, the patient is allowed only ice chips and liquids on the day of surgery. On the first postoperative day, assuming bowel sounds are present, diet is resumed, beginning with a soft diet and advancing to solid foods as tolerated. This dietary regimen assumes minimal intraoperative bowel manipulation and dissection. Early postoperative feeding has been shown not only to be safe but also to speed return of bowel function and recovery. In patients who have undergone pelvic and paraaortic lymph node dissection, bowel surgery, or other extensive dissections, clear liquids should not be given until flatus has been passed. The diet should be advanced only as tolerated.

Activity Early ambulation decreases the incidence of thrombophlebitis and pneumonia. Patients are encouraged to begin ambulation on their first postoperative day if possible

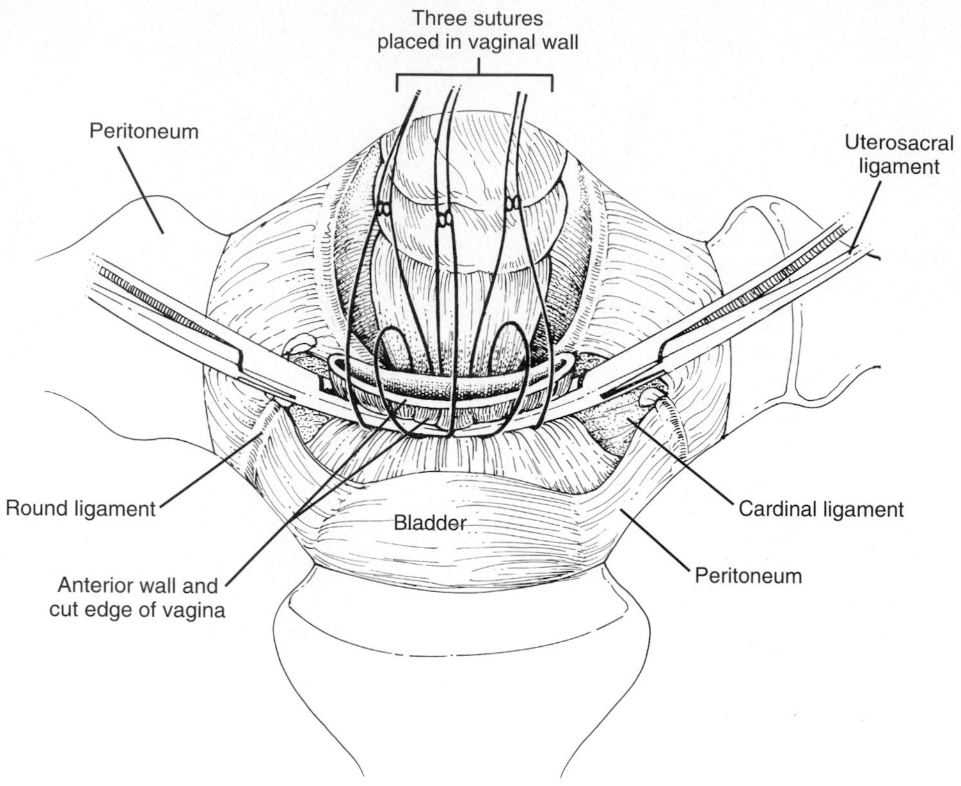

Figure 22.13 Vaginal cuff closure incorporating the uterosacral and cardinal ligaments. (From **Mann WA, Stovall TG.** *Gynecologic surgery.* New York: Churchill Livingstone, 1996, with permission.)

and to increase progressively their time out of bed as their strength improves. On discharge, the patient is instructed to avoid lifting more than 20 pounds for 6 weeks, thereby minimizing stress on fascia to allow full healing. Sexual intercourse is not recommended until 6 weeks after surgery, when the vaginal cuff is fully healed. Patients are instructed to avoid driving until full mobility returns because postoperative pain and tenderness may hinder sudden braking or steering maneuvers in emergency situations. With these exceptions,

Figure 22.14 A: Vaginal cuff left open with a running suture along the cuff. B: Peritoneum closed. (From **Mann WA, Stovall TG.** *Gynecologic surgery.* New York: Churchill Livingstone, 1996, with permission.)

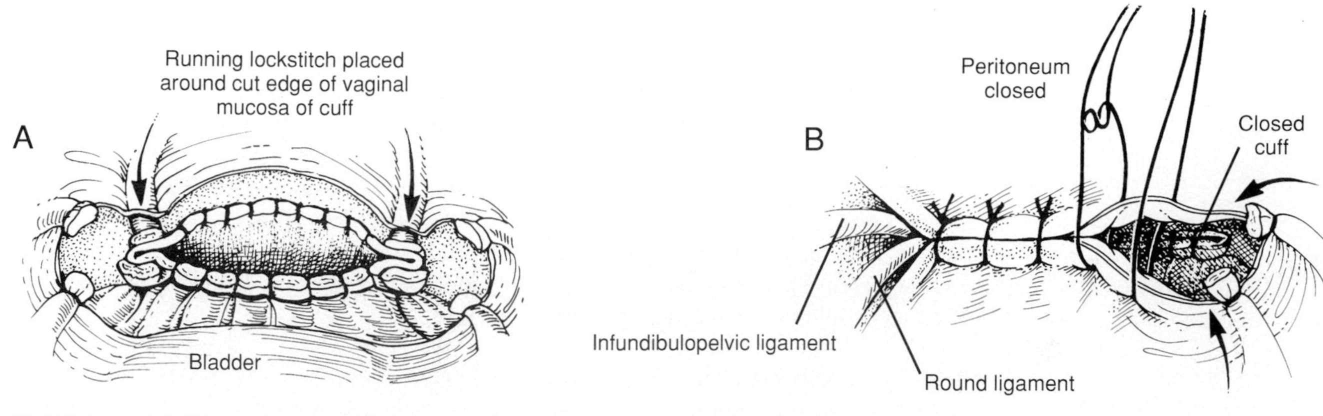

the patient is encouraged to return to normal activities as soon as she feels comfortable doing so.

Wound Care The abdominal incision normally requires little attention, except for ordinary hygienic measures. The wound is kept covered with a sterile bandage for the first 24 hours after surgery, by which time the incision has sealed itself. After the bandage has been removed, the incision should be cleaned daily with mild soap and water and kept dry.

Vaginal Hysterectomy

Preoperative Evaluation

Evaluation of Pelvic Support The most important observation in determining the feasibility of a vaginal hysterectomy is the demonstration of uterine mobility (89,90). A vaginal approach should not be chosen if the uterus is not freely mobile. Pelvic support structures are elevated at the initial pelvic examination. In patients with no apparent prolapse, poor pelvic support can often be demonstrated by observing descent of the uterus with a series of Valsalva maneuvers. Although vaginal hysterectomy is easier to perform when the uterine supporting ligaments are lax, it is not an absolute requirement. Some gynecologists advocate the application of a tenaculum to the anterior cervical lip, with subsequent traction applied as the patient bears down. Although this exercise may give some indication of uterine mobility, it is uncomfortable and not necessarily predictive of the success of vaginal hysterectomy. Therefore, **the practice of applying traction to the cervix with a tenaculum to demonstrate descent of an apparently well-supported uterus is not recommended.**

Evaluation of the Pelvis After assessment of pelvic support, the bony pelvis should be evaluated. Ideally, the angle of the pubic arch should be 90 degrees or greater, the vaginal canal should be ample, and the posterior vaginal fornix should be wide and deep. The surgeon may use a closed fist to approximate the bituberous diameter, which should exceed 10 cm. The size and shape of the female pelvis contributes to increased exposure.

Surgical Considerations

Patient Positioning Once the patient is in the dorsal lithotomy position, the buttocks should be positioned just over the table's edge. Several stirrup types are available, including those that support the entire leg and those that suspend the legs in straps. To avoid nerve injury, adequate padding should be used; marked flexion of the thigh and pressure points should be avoided. Trendelenburg (10- to 15-degree) positioning aids in the intravaginal visualization needed during surgery.

Vaginal Preparation A povidone-iodine solution is applied to the vagina, the bladder is drained, and the catheter is removed. Several methods for draping have been proposed, including individual or single-piece drapes; the method chosen is at the surgeon's discretion. There is usually no need to shave or clip the pubic hair. Individual drapes with an adhesive barrier should be used to hold the drapes in place and prevent the pubic hair from compromising the field.

Instruments Instruments specific to and useful in performing a vaginal hysterectomy include right-angled retractors, narrow Deaver retractors, weighted specula, Heaney needle holders, and an assortment of Briesky-Navratil vaginal retractors. Heaney and Heaney-Ballentine hysterectomy clamps are preferable. Several other clamps also are commonly used, including the Masterson clamp.

Lighting Overhead high-intensity lamps should be used and positioned to direct light over the operator's shoulder. In addition, the surgeon may prefer a headlight, which can be worn to provide direct horizontal lighting. Although not routinely used, a fiberoptic-lighted irrigating suction system can provide additional light and transilluminate tissue planes.

Suture Material Various suture materials have been advocated for gynecologic surgery. The type of suture material chosen should be based on the surgeon's preference. A synthetic delayed absorbable polyglactin or polyglycolic acid suture and atraumatic needles are generally preferable.

Procedure

The patient is examined while anesthetized to confirm prior findings and to assess uterine mobility and descent. The decision is then made whether to proceed vaginally or abdominally.

Grasping and Circumscribing the Cervix The anterior and posterior lips of the cervix are grasped with a single- or double-toothed tenaculum. With downward traction applied on the cervix, a circumferential incision is made in the vaginal epithelium at the junction of the cervix (Fig. 22.15).

Dissection of Vaginal Mucosa After the initial incision is made, the vaginal epithelium may be dissected sharply from the underlying tissue or pushed bluntly with an open sponge (Fig. 22.16). If the initial incision is made too close to the external cervical os, there is a greater amount of dissection required and associated bleeding. Therefore, this circumscribing incision should be made just below the bladder reflection. It is important to continue the dissection in the correct cleavage plane because dissection in the wrong plane will increase blood loss.

Posterior Cul-de-Sac Entry The peritoneal reflection of the posterior cul-de-sac (cul-de-sac of Douglas) can be identified by stretching the vaginal mucosa and underlying connective

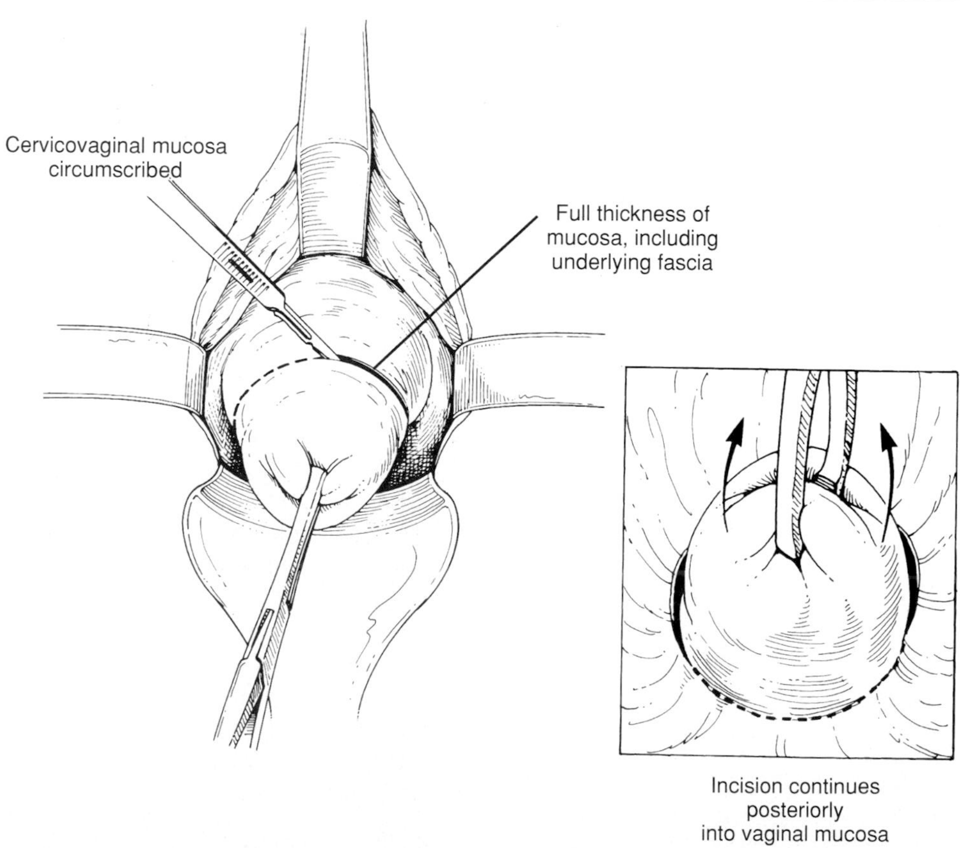

Figure 22.15 Circumferential incision in the vagina to infiltrate a vaginal hysterectomy. (From **Mann WA, Stovall TG.** *Gynecologic surgery.* New York: Churchill Livingstone, 1996, with permission.)

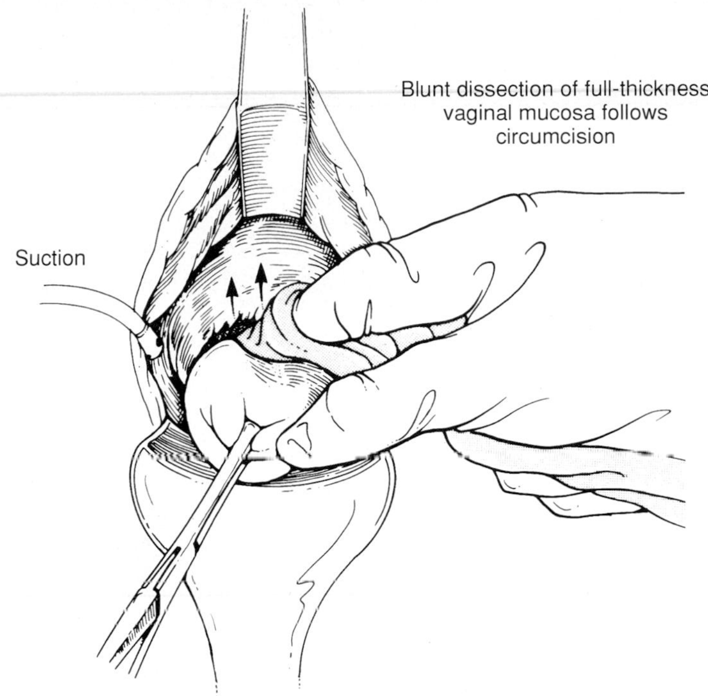
Blunt dissection of full-thickness vaginal mucosa follows circumcision
Suction

Figure 22.16 Dissection of the vaginal mucosa. (From **Mann WA, Stovall TG.** *Gynecologic surgery.* New York: Churchill Livingstone, 1996, with permission.)

tissue with forceps (Fig. 22.17). If difficulty is encountered (e.g., if the cervix is elongated and the peritoneum is not evident), the vaginal mucosa may be incised vertically to the point at which the cul-de-sac becomes more apparent.

If the vaginal mucosa has been dissected in the wrong plane, the hysterectomy may be begun extraperitoneally by clamping and cutting the uterosacral and cardinal ligaments close to the cervix. The posterior cul-de-sac will then become readily identifiable.

If the peritoneal reflection of the posterior cul-de-sac still cannot be identified, entry into the anterior peritoneum is attempted, and a finger is hooked into the posterior cul-de-sac to place tension on the peritoneum. The peritoneum is opened with Mayo scissors. An interrupted suture is placed to approximate the peritoneum and vaginal cuff and thus provide hemostasis (Fig. 22.18).

The posterior pelvic cavity is examined for pathologic alterations of the uterus or adhesive disease of the cul-de-sac. The weighted speculum is placed into the posterior cul-de-sac.

Uterosacral Ligament Ligation With retraction of the lateral vaginal wall and countertraction on the cervix, the uterosacral ligaments are clamped, with the tip of the clamp incorporating the lower portion of the cardinal ligaments (Fig. 22.19). The clamp is placed perpendicular to the uterine axis, and the pedicle is cut close to the clamp and sutured. A small pedicle (0.5 cm) distal to the clamp is optimal because a larger pedicle becomes necrotic and the tissue sloughs, which may present culture medium for microorganisms. The pedicle should be incised no more than one half to three fourths of the way around the tip of the clamp. Limiting the incision prevents the next pedicle, which may be vascular, from being cut.

When suturing any pedicle, the needle point is placed at the tip of the clamp, and the needle is passed through the tissue by a rolling motion of the operator's wrist. Once ligated, the uterosacral ligaments may be transfixed to the posterolateral vaginal mucosa (Fig. 22.20).

Figure 22.17 Entry into the posterior cul-de-sac. (From **Mann WA, Stovall TG.** *Gynecologic surgery.* New York: Churchill Livingstone, 1996, with permission.)

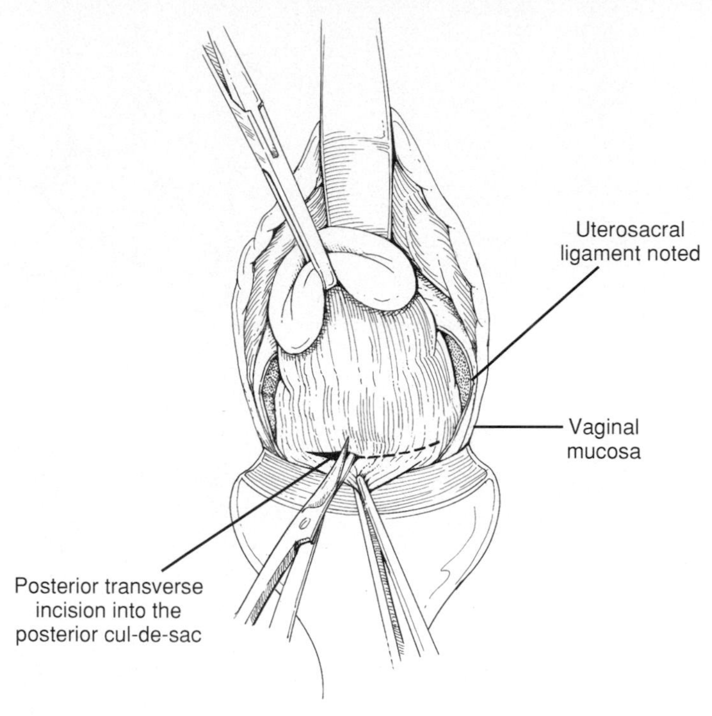

Figure 22.18 Interrupted suture is placed on posterior vaginal cuff and peritoneum for hemostasis. (From **Mann WA, Stovall TG.** *Gynecologic surgery.* New York: Churchill Livingstone, 1996, with permission.)

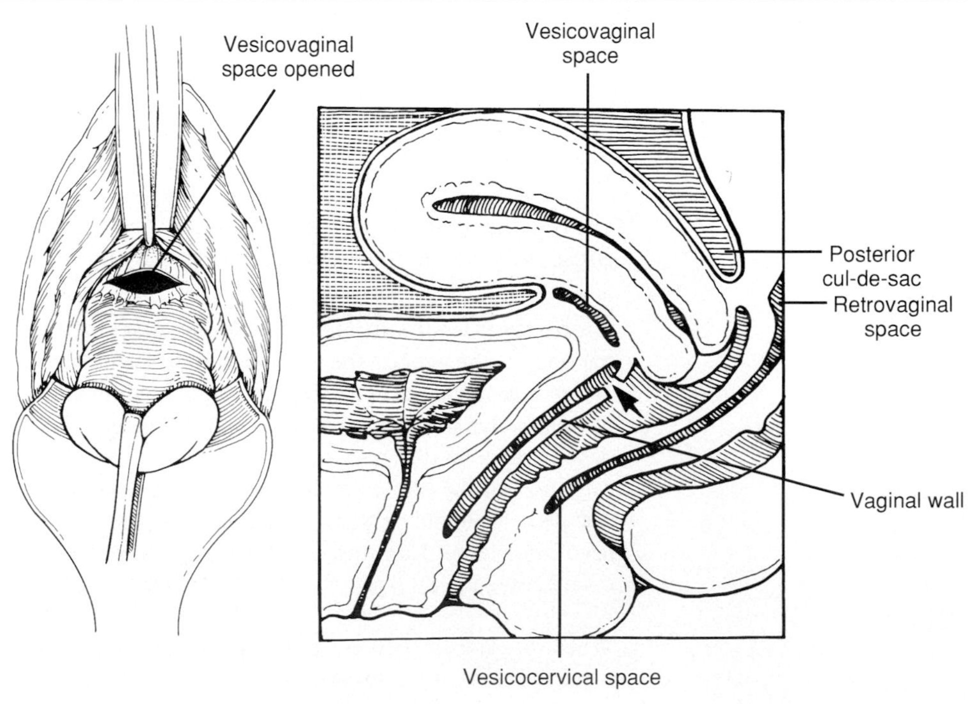

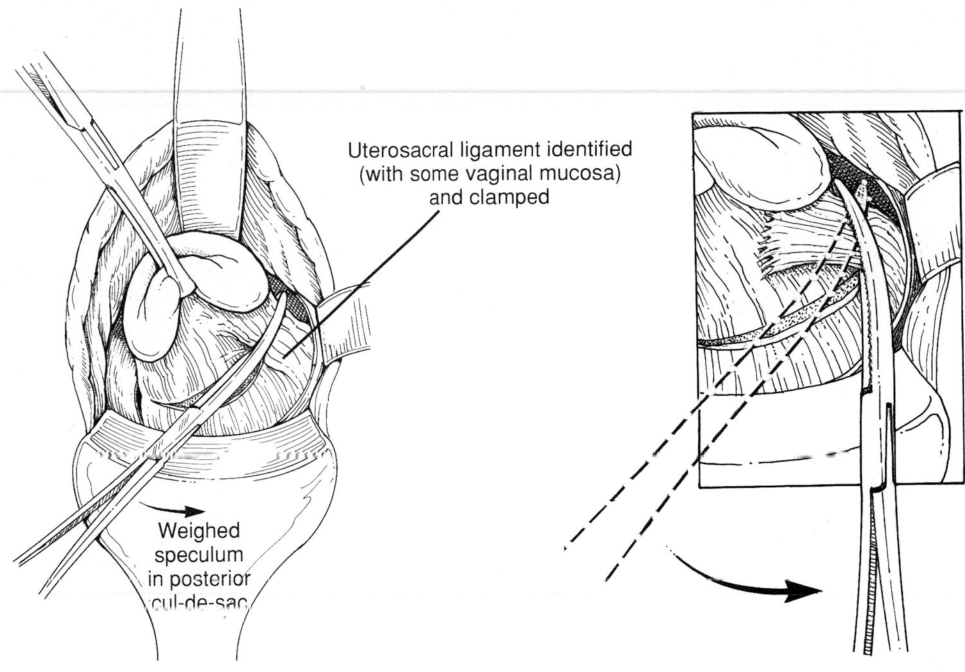

Figure 22.19 Ligation of the uterosacral ligaments. (From **Mann WA, Stovall TG.** *Gynecologic surgery.* New York: Churchill Livingstone, 1996, with permission.)

This suture may lend additional support to the vagina and provides hemostasis at this point on the vaginal mucosa. This suture is held with a hemostat to facilitate location of any bleeding at the completion of the procedure and to aid in the closure of vaginal mucosa.

Entry versus Nonentry into the Vesicovaginal Space (Cul-de-Sac) Downward traction is placed on the cervix. Using either Mayo scissors, with the points directed toward the uterus, or an open moistened 4 × 4 gauze sponge, the bladder is advanced. If the vesicovaginal peritoneal reflection is easily identified at this point, the vesicovaginal space may be entered. Otherwise, it may be preferable to delay entry. There is no danger in delaying entry so long as the operator has ascertained that the bladder has been advanced.

After the bladder has been advanced, a curved Deaver or Heaney retractor is placed in the midline, holding the bladder out of the operative field. This process precedes each step of the vaginal hysterectomy until the vesicovaginal space is entered.

Cardinal Ligament Ligation With traction on the cervix continued, the cardinal ligaments are identified, clamped, and cut. The suture is ligated (Fig. 22.21).

Advancement of Bladder The bladder again is advanced out of the operative field. A blunt dissection technique may be used; however, sharp dissection may be helpful if the patient has had previous surgery such as cesarean delivery, which may have scarred the bladder reflection.

Uterine Artery Ligation Contralateral and downward traction is placed on the cervix. With an effort to incorporate the anterior and posterior leaves of the visceral peritoneum, the uterine vessels are identified, clamped, and cut, and the suture is ligated (Fig. 22.22). A single suture and single clamp technique is adequate and decreases the potential risk for ureteral injury. When the uterus is large or when a fibroid distorts the anatomic relationships, a second suture may be required to ligate any remaining branches of the uterine artery.

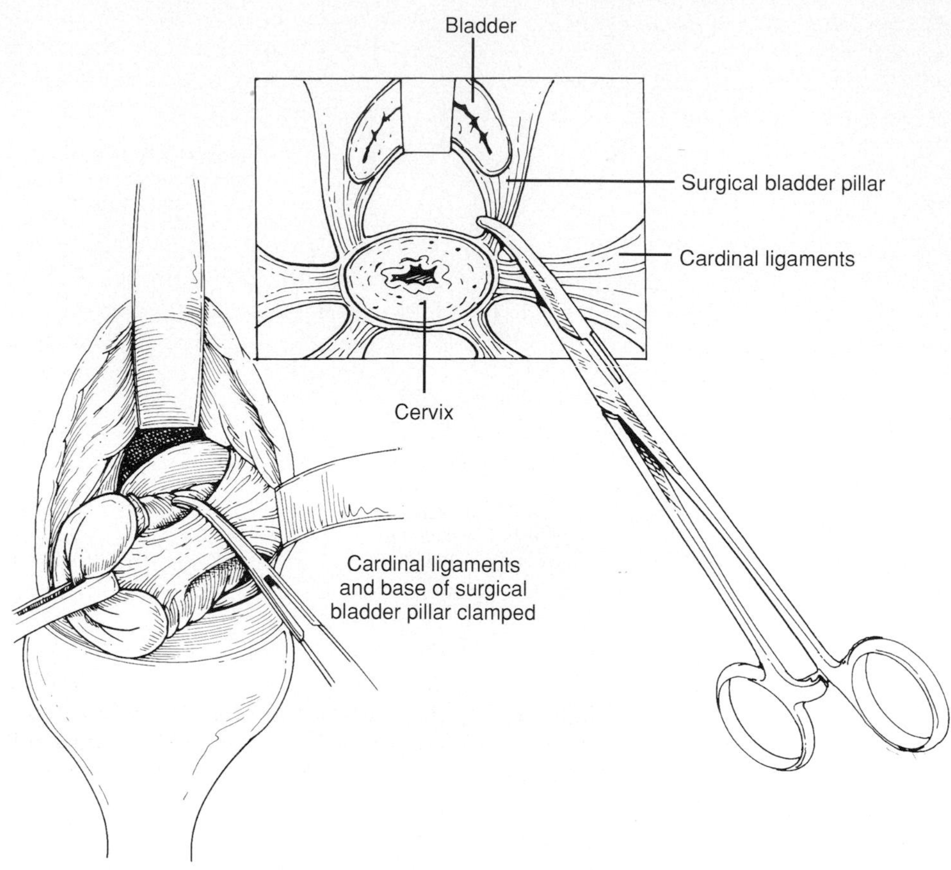

Figure 22.20 Transfixion of the uterosacral ligament to the posterolateral vaginal mucosa. (From **Mann WA, Stovall TG.** *Gynecologic surgery.* New York: Churchill Livingstone, 1996, with permission.)

Entry into the Vesicovaginal Space The anterior peritoneal fold usually can be identified readily just before or after clamping and suture ligation of the uterine arteries. The anterior peritoneal cavity should not be opened blindly because of the increased risk for bladder injury (Fig. 22.23). The peritoneum is grasped with forceps, tented, and opened with scissors with the tips pointed toward the uterus. A Heaney or Deaver retractor is then placed, and the peritoneal contents are identified. This retractor serves to keep the bladder out of the operative field.

Delivery of the Uterus A tenaculum is placed onto the uterine fundus in a successive fashion to deliver the fundus posteriorly (Fig. 22.24). The operator's index finger is used to identify the uteroovarian ligament and aid in clamp placement.

Uteroovarian and Round Ligament Ligation With the posterior and anterior peritoneum opened, the remainder of the broad ligament and uteroovarian ligaments are clamped, cut, and ligated (Fig. 22.25). The uteroovarian and round ligament complexes are double ligated with a suture tie followed by a ligature medial to the first suture. A hemostat is placed on the second suture to aid in the identification of any bleeding and to assist with peritoneal closure. A hemostat should not be placed on the first suture or any other vascular pedicle in order to avoid the risk for loosening the tie.

Removal of the Ovaries When the adnexa are removed, the round ligaments should be removed separately from the adnexal pedicles. Traction is placed on the uteroovarian pedicle. The ovary is drawn into the operative field by grasping it with a Babcock clamp. A Heaney clamp is placed across the infundibulopelvic ligament, and the ovary and tube are excised (Fig. 22.26). A transfixion tie and suture ligature are placed on the infundibulopelvic

Figure 22.21 Ligation of the cardinal ligament. (From **Mann WA, Stovall TG.** *Gynecologic surgery.* New York: Churchill Livingstone, 1996, with permission.)

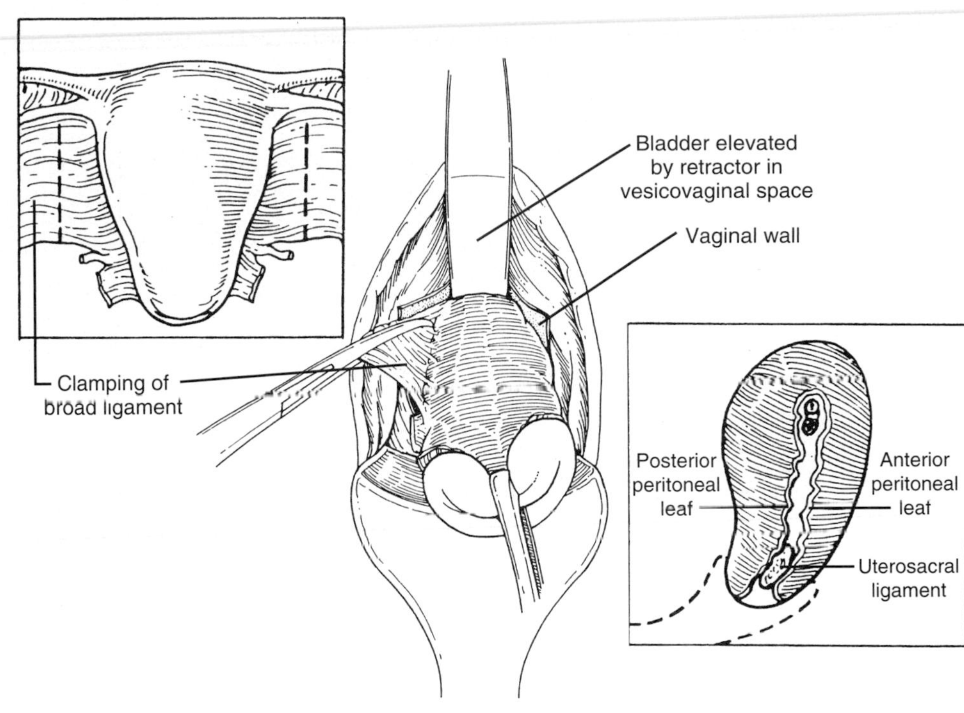

Figure 22.22 Ligation of the uterine artery. (From **Mann WA, Stovall TG.** *Gynecologic surgery.* New York: Churchill Livingstone, 1996.)

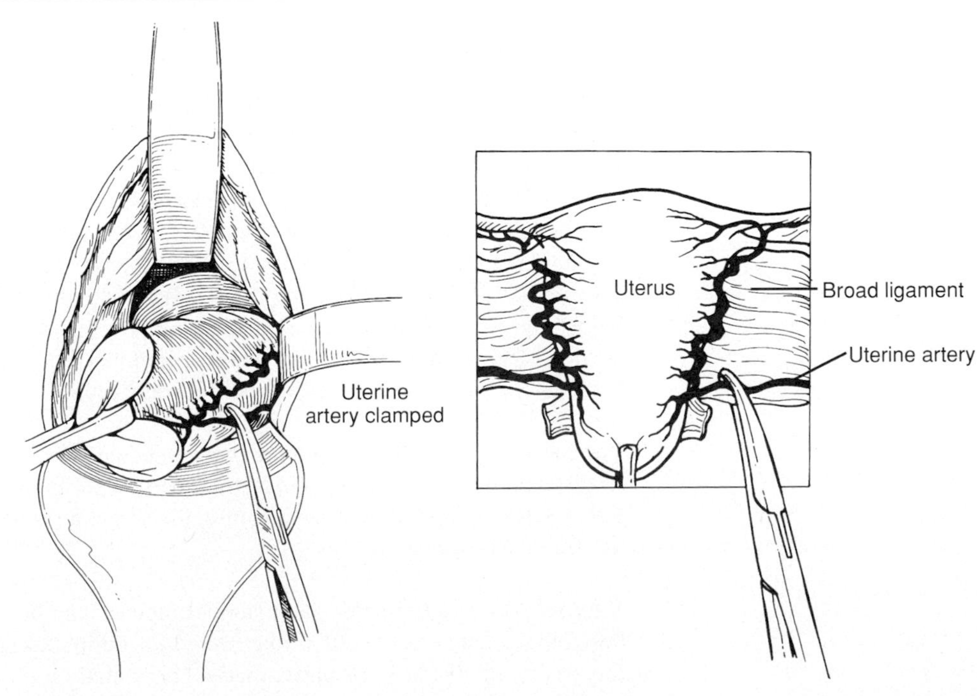

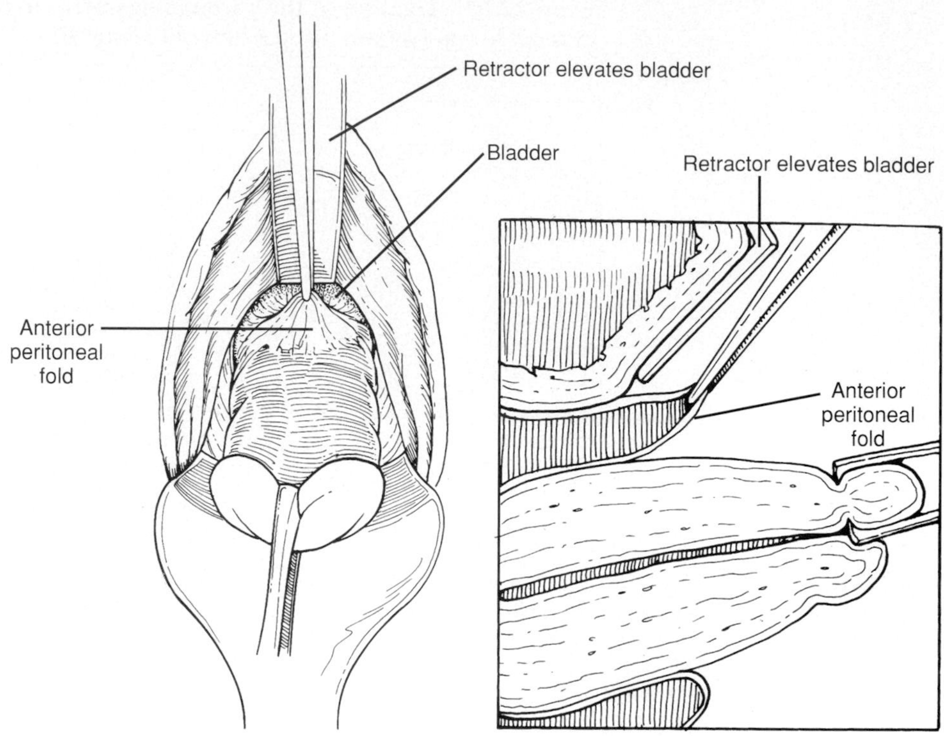

Figure 22.23 Entry into the vesicovaginal space. (From **Mann WA, Stovall TG.** *Gynecologic surgery.* New York: Churchill Livingstone, 1996, with permission.)

ligament. The surgeon should not be reluctant to remove the fallopian tube separately from the ovary if taking them together risks loss of the tissue pedicle or injury to the ureter or nearby blood vessels.

Hemostasis A retractor or tagged sponge is placed into the peritoneal cavity, and each of the pedicles is visualized and inspected for hemostasis. If additional sutures are required, they should be placed precisely with care to avoid the ureter or bladder.

Peritoneal Closure Because the pelvic peritoneum does not provide support and reforms in 24 hours after surgery, the peritoneum need not be reapproximated routinely. If it is believed to be important, the anterior peritoneal edge is identified and grasped with forceps. A continuous absorbable 0-0 suture is begun at the 12-o'clock position. The suture is continued in a pursestring fashion and incorporates the distal portion of the left upper pedicle and the left uterosacral ligament (Fig. 22.27). Tension is applied to the suture placed at the beginning of the procedure that incorporates the posterior peritoneum and vaginal mucosa. This allows for high posterior reperitonealization, which shortens the cul-de-sac and thus helps to prevent future enterocele formation. The right uterosacral ligament and the distal portion of the right upper pedicle are incorporated, and this continuous suture ends at the point on the anterior peritoneum where it was begun.

The intraabdominal tagged sponge is removed and inspected for the presence of blood at its distal end. The slack of the pursestring peritoneal suture is taken up by pulling the suture tight. Before tying the peritoneal suture, the surgeon should make certain that no prolapse of viscera has occurred.

Vaginal Mucosa Closure The vaginal mucosa can be reapproximated in a vertical or horizontal manner, using either interrupted or continuous sutures (Fig. 22.28). The vaginal mucosa is, in this case, reapproximated horizontally with interrupted absorbable sutures.

Figure 22.24 Delivery of the uterine fundus posteriorly. (From **Mann WA, Stovall TG.** *Gynecologic surgery.* New York: Churchill Livingstone, 1996, with permission.)

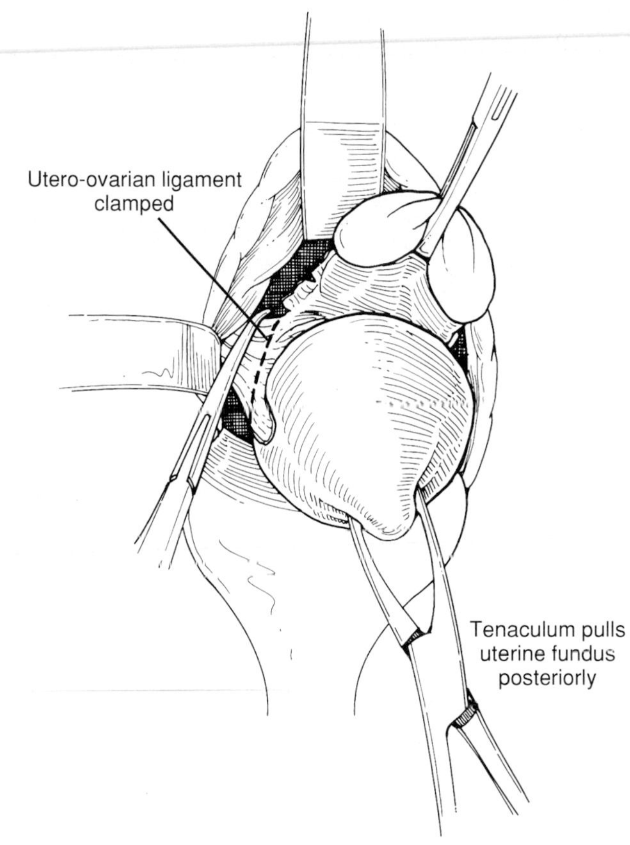

Figure 22.25 Ligation of the uteroovarian and round ligaments. (From **Mann WA, Stovall TG.** *Gynecologic Surgery.* New York: Churchill Livingstone, 1996, with permission.)

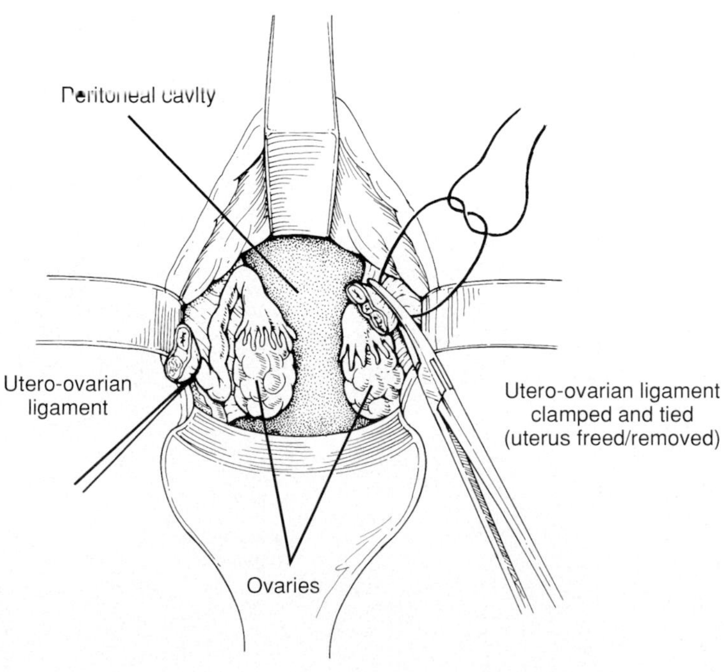

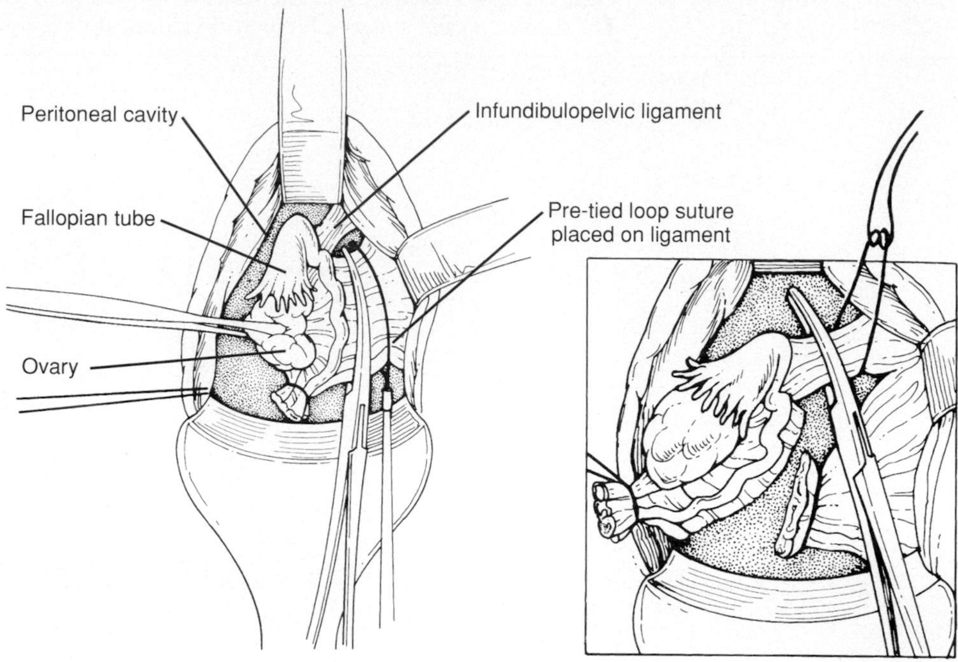

Figure 22.26 Removal of the ovaries and fallopian tubes by clamping across the infundibulopelvic ligament. (From **Mann WA, Stovall TG.** *Gynecologic surgery.* New York: Churchill Livingstone, 1996, with permission.)

The sutures are placed through the entire thickness of the vaginal epithelium, with care taken to avoid entering the bladder anteriorly. These sutures will obliterate the underlying dead space and produce an anatomic approximation of the vaginal epithelium, thereby decreasing the postoperative formation of granulation tissue.

Figure 22.27 Closure of the peritoneum. (From **Mann WA, Stovall TG.** *Gynecologic surgery.* New York: Churchill Livingstone, 1996, with permission.)

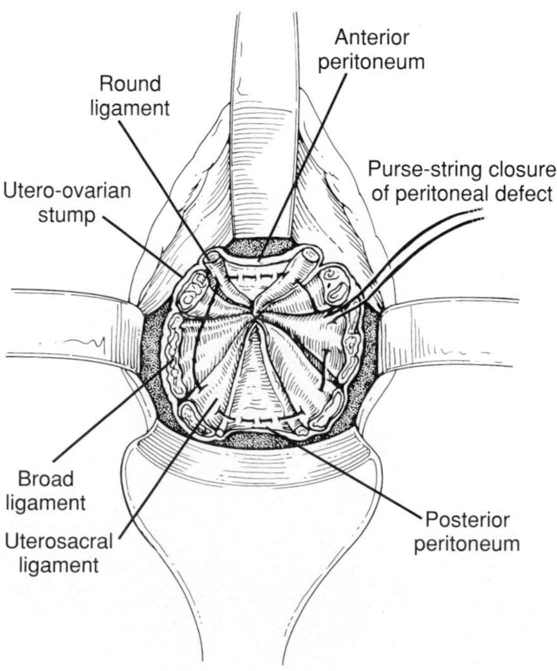

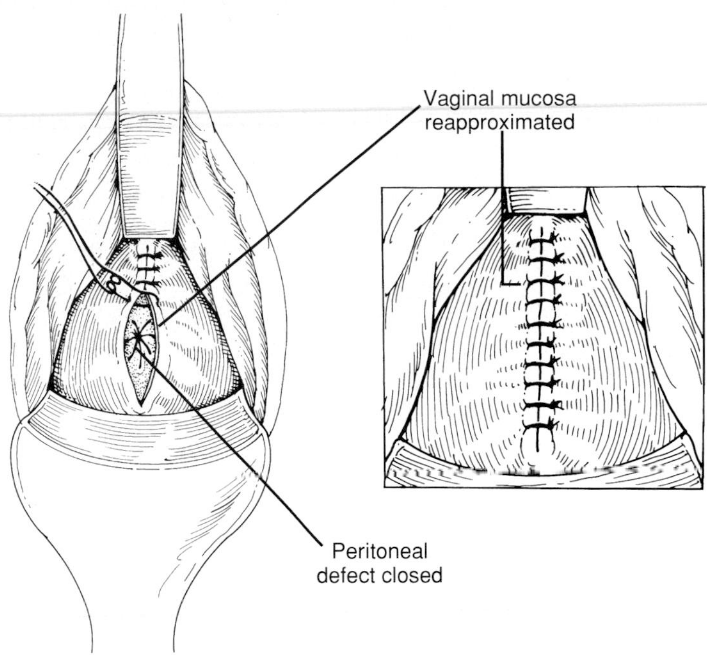

Figure 22.28 Closure of the vaginal mucosa. (From **Mann WA, Stovall TG.** *Gynecologic surgery.* New York: Churchill Livingstone, 1996, with permission.)

Bladder Drainage After completion of the procedure, the bladder is drained. Unless an anterior or posterior colporrhaphy or other reconstructive procedure is performed, a bladder catheter or vaginal packing is not mandatory.

Surgical Techniques for Selected Patients

Injection of Vaginal Mucosa The use of paracervical and submucosal injection of 20 to 30 mL of 0.5% *lidocaine* with 1:200,000 epinephrine before incision of the vaginal mucosa is believed by some to decrease postoperative pain and facilitate identification of surgical planes. There is no need to inject the cervix. Areas to be injected include the bladder pillars, lower portion of the cardinal ligament, uterosacral ligaments, and paracervical tissue. However, it has been shown that the incidence of cuff cellulitis and cuff abscess formation is increased when *epinephrine* is injected into the cervicovaginal mucosa.

Morcellation of the Large Uterus

Uterine morcellation is a well-known but often underutilized surgical procedure whereby the uterus is removed piecemeal. Several methods of uterine morcellation have been described (91), including hemisection or bivalving, wedge or "V" incisions, and intramyometrial coring. Before beginning any morcellation procedure, the uterine vessels must be ligated, and the peritoneal cavity must be entered.

When uterine hemisection or bivalving is performed, the cervix is split at the midline, and the uterus is cut into halves, which are removed separately (92,93). This method seems best suited for fundal, midline leiomyomas.

Wedge morcellation is best suited for anterior or posterior fibroids or for fibroids in the other broad ligaments (i.e., when the fibroids are away from the midline) (93–97). The cervix is amputated, and the myometrium is grasped with clamps. Wedge-shaped portions of myometrium are removed from the anterior or posterior uterine wall. The apex of the wedge is kept in the midline, thereby reducing the bulk of the myometrium. This process is repeated until the uterus can be removed or until a pseudocapsule of a fibroid can be grasped with a Leahy clamp or towel clip. Traction is then applied, and a "myomectomy" is performed.

When the intramyometrial coring technique is used, the myometrium above the site of the ligated vessels is incised parallel to the axis of the uterine cavity and serosa of the uterus. This incision is continued around the full circumference of the myometrium in a symmetric fashion beneath the uterine serosa. Traction is maintained on the cervix, and the avascular myometrium is cut to allow the undisturbed endometrial cavity, with a thick layer of myometrium, to be delivered with the cervix. As a result, the inside of the uterus with its unopened endometrial cavity is brought closer to the operator. Incision of the lateral portions of the myometrium medial to the remaining attachment of the broad ligament results in considerable additional descent of the uterus and greatly increases the mobility of the uterine fundus. The uterus is converted from a globular to an elongated tissue mass. The cored uterus is removed by clamping the uteroovarian pedicle and fallopian tubes.

McCall Culdoplasty

A McCall culdoplasty has been thought by some surgeons to help decrease future enterocele formation (96). Whether this is accurate remains open to debate. An absorbable suture is placed through the full thickness of the posterior vaginal wall at the point of the highest portion of the vaginal vault. The patient's left uterosacral ligament pedicle is grasped and sutured. The suture then incorporates the posterior peritoneum, between the uterosacral ligaments and the right uterosacral ligament. The suture is completed by passing the needle from the inside to the outside at the same point at which it was begun. The suture is tied, thereby approximating the uterosacral ligaments and the posterior peritoneum.

Schuchardt Incision

When vaginal exposure is difficult, the Schuchardt incision may be used (96). If the surgeon is right-handed, the incision is made on the patient's left side. To decrease blood loss, the area can be infiltrated with lidocaine-containing epinephrine. The incision follows a curved line from the 4-o'clock position at the hymenal margin to a point halfway between the anus and the ischial tuberosity. The incision may be continued as high as necessary in the vaginal vault to gain exposure. The depth of the incision is the medial portion of the pubococcygeus muscle, which may be divided in extreme cases. The incision must be closed in layers at the completion of the procedure.

Intraoperative Complications

Bladder Injury

Injury to the urinary bladder is one of the most common intraoperative complications associated with hysterectomy. **If the bladder is inadvertently entered, repair generally should be performed when the injury is discovered and not delayed until completion of surgery** (84). When bladder injury is recognized, the edges of the wound should be mobilized to assess the full extent of the injury and to allow repair without tension. This assessment should include visualization of the trigone to exclude injury to that area. The bladder may then be repaired with a single- or double-layered closure with a small-caliber absorbable suture. Methylene blue or a dye of sterile milk formula can be instilled into the bladder to ensure that the repair is adequate.

Bowel Injury

Because patients with suspected pelvic adhesions or obvious pelvic disease are excluded as candidates for vaginal hysterectomy, bowel injuries do not often occur. Bowel injuries more often are associated with the performance of a posterior colporrhaphy and are usually confined to the rectum (84,96).

If the rectum is entered, the injury is repaired with a single- or double-layer closure using a small-caliber absorbable suture, followed by copious irrigation. Postoperatively, the patient should be given a stool softener and a low-residue diet.

Hemorrhage

Intraoperative hemorrhage invariably is the result of failure to ligate securely a significant blood vessel, bleeding from the vaginal cuff, slippage of a previously placed ligature, or avulsion of tissue before clamping (96). Most intraoperative bleeding can be avoided with adequate exposure and good surgical technique. Using square knots with attention to proper knot-tying mechanisms will prevent bleeding in most cases. Likewise, the use of Heaney-type sutures minimizes ligature slippage and subsequent bleeding. When bleeding does occur, blind clamping, which may endanger the ureter, should be avoided. The bleeding vessel should be identified and precisely ligated with visualization of the ureter if necessary. If the location of the ureter is in question, it should be visualized before suturing a bleeding vessel. Although excessive blood loss occasionally occurs despite these precautions, it should be infrequent.

Perioperative Care

Bladder Drainage Postoperative bladder drainage should be employed after any procedure in which spontaneous, complete voiding is not anticipated. Reasons to consider closed bladder drainage include significant local pain, additional vaginal reparative procedures, surgery for stress incontinence, the use of a vaginal pack, and patient anxiety.

After vaginal hysterectomy without additional repair, most patients can void spontaneously, and therefore, catheter drainage is not required. The relative amount of pain after a vaginal hysterectomy is less than with abdominal hysterectomy and, in the absence of additional repairs or a pack, no obstructive effect should be present.

If the patient does not tolerate pain well postoperatively or is extremely anxious, the transurethral insertion of a 16-Fr. catheter after completing surgery is warranted. This catheter may also be inserted postoperatively if the patient is unable to void spontaneously on two attempts. Closed-catheter drainage after vaginal hysterectomy usually is not necessary for longer than 24 hours. The catheter is removed without clamping, and there is no need to obtain a urine specimen for culture and sensitivity.

Diet Although little manipulation of the bowel occurs during vaginal hysterectomy, there is some slowing of gastrointestinal motility. This slowing rarely occurs to a degree that limits some form of oral intake soon after surgery. Most patients experience some degree of nausea after surgery, which, combined with drowsiness from analgesics, usually makes them disinterested in food on the evening after surgery. A clear liquid diet is suitable during the first 24 hours after surgery. On the first full postoperative day, a regular diet can usually be consumed. The patient is often the best judge of what she can tolerate.

Perioperative Complications of Hysterectomy

A comprehensive discussion of postoperative complications after gynecologic surgery is presented in Chapter 19.

Wound Infections

Wound infections occur after 4% to 6% of abdominal hysterectomies (29). Measures believed to reduce the incidence of wound infections include a preoperative shower, no removal of hair, or if hair removal is necessary, removal of hair with clippers in the operating room, use of adhesive drapes and prophylactic antibiotics, and delayed primary closure (see Chapter 19).

Hemorrhage

Immediately after hysterectomy, hemorrhage may become apparent in one of two ways (88). First, bleeding from the vagina may be noted by the nursing staff or physician within the first few hours after surgery. Second, and less commonly, the patient may be noted to have little bleeding from the vagina but deteriorating vital signs manifested by low blood pressure and rapid pulse, falling hematocrit level, and flank or abdominal pain. The first presentation usually is in the form of bleeding from the vaginal cuff or one of the pedicles. The second presentation may be a retroperitoneal hemorrhage. Each situation is approached differently in its evaluation and treatment, but both involve the same general principles of rapid diagnosis, stabilization of vital signs, appropriate fluid and blood replacement, and constant surveillance of the patient's overall condition (98).

After vital signs are assessed, attention should be directed to the amount of bleeding. A small amount of bleeding is expected after any vaginal hysterectomy. However, steady bleeding 2 to 3 hours after surgery suggests lack of hemostasis. The patient should be taken promptly to the examining room, where the operative site is viewed using a large speculum and good lighting. If bleeding is not excessive, the vaginal cuff can be inspected, and in many instances, bleeding from the cuff edge will be found. Hemostasis can easily be achieved with one or two sutures placed through the mucosa.

If bleeding is excessive or appears to be coming from above the cuff, or if the patient is too uncomfortable to tolerate adequate examination, she should be taken to the operating room. General anesthesia should be administered and the vaginal operative site should be thoroughly explored. Any bleeding point may be sutured or ligated. However, bleeding that is coming from above the cuff or is extremely brisk usually cannot be controlled through the vaginal route. An exploratory laparotomy is necessary to examine the pelvic floor, identify and isolate the bleeding vessel, and achieve hemostasis. The ovarian vessels and uterine arteries should be thoroughly inspected because they often are the source of excessive vaginal bleeding. If it is difficult to localize bleeding to a specific pelvic vessel, ligation of the hypogastric artery may be necessary.

In the patient with little vaginal bleeding in whom vital signs have deteriorated, retroperitoneal hemorrhage should be suspected. Input and output should be monitored. Hematocrit assessment, along with cross-matching, should be performed immediately. Examination may reveal tenderness and dullness in the flank. In cases of intraperitoneal bleeding, abdominal distention may occur. Diagnostic radiologic studies can be used to confirm the presence of retroperitoneal or intraabdominal bleeding. Ultrasonography is one option for viewing low pelvic hematomas. CT provides better visualization of retroperitoneal spaces, however, and can delineate a hematoma.

If the patient's condition stabilizes rapidly with intravenous fluids, one of two approaches may be used for continued care. The first is to give the patient a transfusion and follow serial hematocrit assessments and vital signs. In many instances, retroperitoneal bleeding will tamponade and stop, forming a hematoma that may eventually be resorbed. The risk with this approach is that the hematoma will later become infected, necessitating surgical drainage. In some instances when the patient's condition is stable, radiologic embolization may be considered.

Another option is to perform abdominal exploratory surgery while the patient's condition is stable. This approach adds the morbidity of a second procedure but avoids the possibility of the patient's condition deteriorating with continued delay or the formation of a pelvic abscess. Once adequate exposure is obtained, the peritoneum over the hematoma should be opened, and the blood should be evacuated. All bleeding vessels should be identified and ligated. Again, if control of bleeding is difficult, consideration should be given to unilateral or bilateral ligation of the anterior division of the internal iliac artery. Once hemostasis is achieved, the pelvis should be drained using a closed system.

Urinary Tract Complications

Urinary Retention

Urinary retention after hysterectomy is an uncommon occurrence (32). If the urethra is unobstructed and retention occurs, it is usually the result of either pain or bladder atony resulting from anesthesia. Both are temporary effects.

If a catheter was not placed after surgery, retention can be relieved initially with the insertion of a Foley catheter for 12 to 24 hours. Most patients are able to void after the catheter is removed 1 day later. If the patient still has trouble voiding and urethral spasm is suspected, success often can be achieved with a skeletal muscle relaxant such as *diazepam* (2 mg twice a day). In most cases, waiting is the best course, and voiding usually occurs spontaneously.

Ureteral Injury

In patients who develop flank pain soon after vaginal hysterectomy, ureteral obstruction should be suspected. The incidence of ureteral injury is lower with vaginal hysterectomy than with abdominal hysterectomy (83). One risk factor for its occurrence is total uterine prolapse, in which the ureters are drawn outside the bony pelvis.

In a patient with flank pain in whom ureteral obstruction is suspected, intravenous pyelography and urinalysis should be performed (80). If obstruction is noted on intravenous pyelography, it is usually present near the ureterovesical junction. The first immediate step should be attempted passage of a catheter through the ureter under cystoscopic guidance. If a catheter can be passed through the ureter, it should be left in place for at least 4 to 6 weeks, allowing sutures to absorb and the obstruction or kinking to release. If the catheter cannot be passed through the ureter, the best course is to perform abdominal exploratory surgery and repair the ureter at the site of obstruction (79–84).

Vesicovaginal Fistula

Vesicovaginal fistulas occur most often after total abdominal hysterectomy for benign gynecologic disease (83). Intraoperative steps to avoid the formation of a vesicovaginal fistula include correct identification of the proper plane between the bladder and cervix, sharp rather than blunt dissection of the bladder, and care in clamping and suturing the vaginal cuff. The development of a postoperative vesicovaginal fistula after hysterectomy is rare; the incidence is as low as 0.2% (82,83).

Patients who have a postoperative vesicovaginal fistula develop a watery vaginal discharge 10 to 14 days after surgery. Some fistulas resulting from surgery are noted as early as the first 48 to 72 hours after surgery (84). After vaginal examination with a speculum, the diagnosis can usually be confirmed with the insertion of a cotton tampon into the vagina followed by the instillation of *methylene blue* or *indigo carmine* dye through a transurethral catheter. If the tampon stains blue, a vesicovaginal fistula is present. If no staining occurs, however, the presence of a ureterovaginal fistula must be ruled out by the intravenous injection of 5 mL of *indigo carmine* dye. Within 20 minutes, the tampon should stain blue if a ureterovaginal fistula is present. Intravenous pyelography should also be performed to rule out ureteral obstruction.

If a vesicovaginal fistula is diagnosed, a Foley catheter should be inserted for prolonged drainage. As many as 15% of fistulas spontaneously close with 4 to 6 weeks of continuous bladder drainage. If closure has not occurred by 6 weeks, operative correction is necessary. Waiting 3 to 4 months from the time of diagnosis before operative repair is recommended to allow reduction of inflammation and to improve vascular supply. After vaginal hysterectomy, the fistula site is above the bladder trigone and away from the ureters. Vaginal repair can be anticipated in most patients. The surgical correction is generally undertaken in a four-layered closure: the bladder mucosa, the seromuscular layer, the endopelvic fascia, and the vaginal epithelium.

Incidental cystotomy at the time of hysterectomy is more common than vesicovaginal fistula. When repaired correctly, cystotomy rarely results in the development of a fistula (82).

Prolapse of the Fallopian Tube

Posthysterectomy prolapse of the fallopian tube is a rare event and is often confused with granulation tissue at the vaginal apex (32). Predisposing factors for the development of fallopian tube prolapse include development of a hematoma and an abscess at the vaginal apex. As many as half of patients undergoing vaginal hysterectomy form some granulation tissue at the vaginal vault. In patients in whom granulation tissue persists after attempts to cauterize it or pain is experienced with attempts to remove it, fallopian tube prolapse should be suspected. A biopsy of the area is warranted and usually reveals tubal epithelium if a fallopian tube is present.

If fallopian tube prolapse is diagnosed, it should be repaired with surgery. In general, the surrounding vaginal mucosa should be opened and undermined widely. The tube is then ligated high and removed, followed by closure of the vaginal mucosa.

Discharge Instructions

Before discharging the patient, instructions should be reviewed. Printed postoperative instructions are helpful to the patient and should include the following information:

1. Avoid strenuous activity for the first 2 weeks and increase activity level gradually.
2. Avoid heavy lifting, douching, or sexual intercourse until instructed by the physician.
3. Bathe as needed using shower or tub baths.
4. Follow a regular diet.
5. Avoid straining for a bowel movement or urination. For constipation, use *Milk of Magnesia* or *Metamucil* (1 tsp in juice).
6. Call the physician if excessive vaginal bleeding or fever occurs.
7. Schedule a return appointment at the time specified by the physician.

The physician should provide telephone numbers for emergencies both during and after office hours. Typically, the first postoperative visit is scheduled about 4 weeks after discharge from the hospital. At the time of that visit, the patient should be ambulating well, and vaginal discharge or bleeding should be minimal. Speculum examination of the cuff should be gentle and cursory, but the patient should be assured that the healing process is proceeding normally. Finally, the patient's questions should be answered, and advice should be given on increasing her activity level, including sexual activity, work, and normal household activity.

Psychosomatic Aspects

The decision to proceed with hysterectomy should be made jointly by the patient and her physician. Factors leading a patient or her physician to choose hysterectomy and reasons that patients with similar conditions choose different treatments are uncertain. For many patients, the decision to undergo hysterectomy may be sudden. They face the potential risks of anesthesia and surgery, and, if premenopausal, they must also cope with the loss of menstruation and the ability to procreate. Many women are concerned that the procedure will result in a loss of femininity, a decrease in sexual satisfaction, or an increase in interpersonal problems with their spouses. The concern over the loss of the reproductive tract is greater than that related to the loss of other intraabdominal organs (99). To minimize the possibility that the patient has a poor outcome, preoperative counseling and preparation are essential.

Drellich and Bieber studied 23 women after hysterectomy. Most of these women regretted the loss of menstruation, which was true even for women who had experienced dysmenorrhea (100). Several of these women viewed the menstrual cycle as a way for the body to "rid itself of waste," and they felt better after the menstrual phase of their cycle.

Depression

There is wide variation in women's responses to hysterectomy. Most studies suggest that there is little evidence that hysterectomy increases the risk for depression. Some investigators have reported depression and an increased incidence of psychiatric symptoms after hysterectomy (101,102). Hollender reported that almost twice as many women were admitted to a psychiatric hospital after pelvic operations compared with other types of surgery (103). However, other authors have not found such an association (104), and some report a decrease in symptoms after hysterectomy (105–109). The impact of hysterectomy on the development of depression is unknown because most studies are retrospective and not well controlled for preoperative depression (see Chapter 12).

Patients who had a moderate amount of preoperative anxiety do much better postoperatively than patients with little or no anxiety or patients who had an exaggerated response (110). Both long delays before surgery and a very short time before surgery increase patients' anxiety. Thus, women should be scheduled for surgery several weeks in advance to avoid this problem (110). Women who planned to have children in the future had more problems during the immediate postoperative period. The patient's response to previous loss (e.g., death of family members) predicted her response after hysterectomy (111).

Sexuality

The incidence of sexual dysfunction after hysterectomy ranges from 10% to 40%. Estimates vary based on study variations, cultural variations, and the definitions used to determine the diagnosis. Some report a decrease in libido after hysterectomy, whereas others suggest that libido is increased because of the reduced fear of unwanted pregnancy (102,112). Humphries found that most patients do not have a change in their sexual practices after hysterectomy (113), whereas others report a deterioration of sexual relations (114). Preoperative anxiety about sexual functioning is often associated with an overall deterioration of sexual relations (115).

The literature supports that hysterectomy does not cause psychiatric sequelae or diminished sexual functioning in most patients. The best predictor of satisfaction after hysterectomy is the patient's preoperative understanding of the procedure. **The best predictor of postoperative sexual functioning is the patient's preoperative sexual satisfaction.** Preoperatively, these issues should be discussed with the patient, and her questions and concerns should be addressed to decrease the fear and anxiety associated with surgery.

References

1. **Benrubi GI.** History of hysterectomy. *J Fla Med Assoc* 1988;75:533–538.
2. **U.S. Department of Health and Human Services, Public Health Services, Center for Disease Control.** *National Hospital Discharge Survey, Annual Summary.* (Vital and Health Statistics. Series 13, Data from the National Health Survey). Hyattsville, MD: U.S. Department of Health and Human Services, 1991.
3. **Pokras R.** Hysterectomy: past, present and future. *Stat Bull Metrop Insur Co* 1989;70:12.
4. **Keshavarz H, Hillis S, Kieke B.** Hysterectomy surveillance—United States, 1994–1998. *Proceedings of the Fiftieth Annual Conference of the Epidemic Intelligence Service.* Center for Disease Control and Prevention. Atlanta, GA: April, 2001.
5. **Spencer G.** *Projections of the population of the United States, by age, sex, and race, 1983 to 2080.* (Current Population Reports. Population estimates and projections. Series P-25; no. 952). Washington, DC: U.S. Dept. of Commerce, Bureau of the Census, 1984.

6. **Roos NP.** Hysterectomy: variations in rates across small areas and across physicians' practices. *Am J Public Health* 1984;74:327–335.

7. **Dicker RC, Scally MJ, Greenspan JR, et al.** Hysterectomy among women of reproductive age: trends in the United States, 1970–1978. *JAMA* 1982;248:323–327.

8. **Domenighetti G, Luraschi P, Marazzi A.** Hysterectomy and sex of the gynecologist. *N Engl J Med* 1985;313:1482.

9. **Kjerulff KH, Guzinski GM, Langenberg PW, et al.** Hysterectomy and race. *Obstet Gynecol* 1993;82:757–764.

10. **Gambone JC, Reifer RC.** Hysterectomy. *Clin Obstet Gynecol* 1990;33:205–211.

11. **Parker WH, Fu YS, Berek JS.** Uterine sarcoma in patients operated for presumed leiomyomata and presumed rapidly growing leiomyoma. *Obstet Gynecol* 1994;83:814–878.

12. **Friedman AJ, Haas ST.** Should uterine size be an indication for surgical intervention in women with myomas? *Am J Obstet Gynecol* 1993;168:751–755.

13. **Coddington CC, Collins RL, Shawker THE.** Long-acting gonadotropin hormone-releasing analog used to treat uteri. *Fertil Steril* 1986;45:624–629.

14. **West CP, Lumsden MA, Lawson S.** Shrinkage of uterine fibroids during therapy with goserelin (Zoladex): a leutinizing hormone-releasing hormone agonist administered as a monthly subcutaneous depot. *Fertil Steril* 1987;48:45–51.

15. **Stovall TG, Ling FW, Henry LC.** A randomized trial evaluating leuprolide acetate prior to hysterectomy for leiomyomata. *Am J Obstet Gynecol* 1991;164:1420–1425.

16. **Nilsson L, Rybo G.** Treatment of menorrhagia. *Am J Obstet Gynecol* 1971;110:713–720.

17. **Dawood MY.** Current concepts in the etiology and treatment of primary dysmenorrhea. *Acta Obstet Gynecol Scan Suppl* 1986;138:7–10.

18. **Halbert DR, Demers LM, Fontana J, et al.** Prostaglandin levels in endometrial jet wash specimens in patients with dysmenorrhea before and after indomethacin therapy. *Prostaglandins* 1975;10:1047–1056.

19. **Chan WY, Dawood MY, Fuchs F.** Prostaglandins in primary dysmenorrhea: comparison of prophylactic and nonprophylactic treatment with ibuprofen and use of oral contraceptives. *Am J Med* 1981;70:535–541.

20. **Gambone JC, Reiter RC.** Nonsurgical management of chronic pelvic pain: a multidisciplinary approach. *Clin Obstet Gynecol* 1990;33:205–211.

21. **Reiter RC, Gambone JC.** Demographic and historic variables in women with idiopathic chronic pelvic pain. *Obstet Gynecol* 1990;75:428–432.

22. **Rapkin AJ, Kames LD.** The pain management approach to chronic pelvic pain. *J Reprod Med* 1987;32:323–327.

23. **Carlson KJ, Miller BA, Fowler FJ.** The Maine women's health study. I. Outcomes of hysterectomy. *Obstet Gynecol* 1994;83:556–565.

24. **Stovall TG, Ling FW, Crawford DA.** Hysterectomy for chronic pelvic pain of presumed uterine etiology. *Obstet Gynecol* 1990;75:676–679.

25. **Anderson MC, Hartley RB.** Cervical crypt involvement by intraepithelial neoplasia. *Obstet Gynecol* 1980;55:546–550.

26. **Enblad P, Adami HO, Glimelius B, et al.** The risk of subsequent primary malignant diseases after cancers of the colon and rectum: a nationwide cohort study. *Cancer* 1990;65:2091–2100.

27. **Stearns MW Jr.** Benign and malignant neoplasms of colon and rectum: diagnosis and management. *Surg Clin North Am* 1978;58:605–618.

28. **Gambone JC, Reiter RC, Lench JB.** Short-term outcome of incidental hysterectomy at the time of adnexectomy for benign disease. *J Womens Health* 1992;1:197–200.

29. **Easterday CL, Grimes DA, Riggs JA.** Hysterectomy in the United States. *Obstet Gynecol* 1983;62:203–212.

30. **Copenhaver EH.** Hysterectomy: vaginal versus abdominal. *Surg Clin North Am* 1965;45:751–763.

31. **White SC, Wartel LJ, Wade ME.** Comparison of abdominal and vaginal hysterectomies: a review of 600 operations. *Obstet Gynecol* 1971;37:530–537.

32. **Dicker RC, Greenspan JR, Strauss LT, et al.** Complications of abdominal and vaginal hysterectomy among women of reproductive age in the United States: the collaborative review of sterilization. *Am J Obstet Gynecol* 1982;144:841–848.

33. **Kovac SR.** Guidelines to determine the route of hysterectomy. *Obstet Gynecol* 1995;85:18–23.

34. **Hasson HM.** Cervical removal at hysterectomy for benign disease: risks and benefits. *J Reprod Med* 1993;38:781–790.

35. **Drife J.** Conserving the cervix at hysterectomy. *Br J Obstet Gynaecol* 1994;101:563–564.

36. **Kilkku P, Lehtinen V, Hirvonen T, et al.** Abdominal hysterectomy versus supravaginal uterine amputation: psychic factors. *Ann Chir Gynaecol Suppl* 1987;76:62–67.

37. **Kilkku P, Hirvonen T, Gronroos M.** Supra-vaginal uterine amputation vs. abdominal hysterectomy: the effects on urinary symptoms with special reference to pollakisuria, nocturia and dysuria. *Maturitas* 1981;3:197–204.

38. **Kilkku P, Gronroos M, Hirvonen T, et al.** Supravaginal uterine amputation vs. hysterectomy. *Acta Obstet Gynecol Scand* 1983;62:147–152.

39. **Kilkku P.** Supravaginal uterine amputation vs. hysterectomy: effects on coital frequency and dyspareunia. *Acta Obstet Gynecol Scand* 1983;62:141–145.

40. **Cartwright DS.** Diagnostic laparoscopy immediately preceding elective hysterectomy. *Proc Am Assoc Gynecol Laparosc* 1992;18:88–89.

41. **Stovall TG, Elder RE, Ling FW.** Predictors of pelvic adhesions. *J Reprod Med* 1989;34:345–348.

42. **Howard FM, Sanchez R.** A comparison of laparoscopically assisted vaginal hysterectomy and abdominal hysterectomy. *J Gynecol Surg* 1993;9:83–90.

43. **Jones RA.** Laparoscopic hysterectomy: a series of 100 cases. *Med J Aust* 1993;159:447–449.

44. **Kovac SR, Cruikshank SH, Retto HF.** Laparoscopic-assisted vaginal hysterectomy. *J Gynecol Surg* 1990;6:185–193.

45. **Saye WB, Espy GB III, Bishop MR, et al.** Laparoscopic Doderlein hysterectomy: a rational alternative to traditional abdominal hysterectomy. *Surg Laparosc Endosc* 1993;3:88–94.

46. **Summitt RL Jr, Stovall TG, Lipscomb GH, et al.** Randomized comparison of laparoscopic-assisted vaginal hysterectomy with standard vaginal hysterectomy in an outpatient setting. *Obstet Gynecol* 1992;80:895–901.

47. **Johns DA, Diamond MP.** Laparoscopically assisted vaginal hysterectomy. *J Reprod Med* 1994;39:424–428.

48. **Liu CY.** Laparoscopic hysterectomy: report of 215 cases. *Gynaecol Endosc* 1992;1:73–77.

49. **Nezhat F, Nezhat CH, Admon D, et al.** Complications and results of 361 hysterectomies performed at laparoscopy. *J Am Coll Surg* 1995;180:307–316.

50. **Raju KS, Auld BJ.** A randomized prospective study of laparoscopic vaginal hysterectomy versus abdominal hysterectomy each with bilateral salpingo-oophorectomy. *Br J Obstet Gynaecol* 1994;101:1068–1071.

51. **Nezhat F, Nezhat C, Gordon S, et al.** Laparoscopic versus abdominal hysterectomy. *J Reprod Med* 1992;37:247–250.

52. **Daniell JF, Kurtz BR, McTavish G, et al.** Laparoscopically assisted vaginal hysterectomy: the initial Nashville, Tennessee, experience. *J Reprod Med* 1993;38:537–542.

53. **Davis GD, Wolgamott G, Moon J.** Laparoscopically assisted vaginal hysterectomy as definitive therapy for stage III and IV endometriosis. *J Reprod Med* 1993;38:577–581.

54. **Coulam CB, Pratt JH.** Vaginal hysterectomy: is previous pelvic operation a contraindication? *Am J Obstet Gynecol* 1973;116:252–260.

55. **Mengert WF.** Mechanisms of uterine support and position. I. Factors influencing uterine support (an experimental study). *Am J Obstet Gynecol* 1936;31:775–782.

56. **Photopulos GJ, Stovall TG, Summitt RL Jr.** Laparoscopic-assisted vaginal hysterectomy, bilateral salpingo-oophorectomy, and pelvic lymph node sampling for endometrial cancer. *J Gynecol Surg* 1992;8:91–94.

57. **Sheth SS.** The place of oophorectomy at vaginal hysterectomy. *Br J Obstet Gynaecol* 1991;98:662–666.

58. **Schweppe KW, Beller FK.** Prophylactic oophorectomy. *Geburtshilfe Frauenheilkd* 1979;39(12):1024–1032.

59. **Randall CL, Hall DW, Armenia CS.** Pathology in the preserved ovary after unilateral oophorectomy. *Am J Obstet Gynecol* 1962;84(9):1233–1241.

60. **Lynch HT, Guirgis HA, Albert S, et al.** Familial association of carcinoma of the breast and ovary. *Surg Gynecol Obstet* 1974;138(5):717–724.

61. **American College of Obstetricians and Gynecologists.** *Familiar ovarian cancer.* ACOG Technical Bulletin. Washington, DC: American College of Obstetricians and Gynecologists, 1993.

62. **Ryan PJ, Harrison R, Blake GM, et al.** Compliance with hormone replacement therapy (HRT) after screening for postmenopausal osteoporosis. *Br J Obstet Gynaecol* 1992;99:1325–1328.

63. **Storer EH.** Appendix. In: **Schwartz SI,** ed. *Principles of surgery.* 3rd ed. New York: McGraw-Hill, 1979:1257–1267.

64. **Melcher DH.** Appendectomy with abdominal hysterectomy. *Lancet* 1971;1:810–811.

65. **Waters EG.** Elective appendectomy with abdominal and pelvic surgery. *Obstet Gynecol* 1977;50:511–517.

66. **Loeffler F, Stearn R.** Abdominal hysterectomy with appendicectomy. *Acta Obstet Gynecol Scand* 1967;46:435–443.

67. **Voitk AJ, Lowry JB.** Is incidental appendectomy a safe practice? *Can J Surg* 1988;31:448–451.

68. **Massoudnia N.** Incidental appendectomy in vaginal surgery. *Int Surg* 1975;60:89–90.

69. **Reiner IJ.** Incidental appendectomy at the time of vaginal surgery. *Tex Med* 1980;76:46–50.

70. **McGowan L.** Incidental appendectomy during vaginal surgery. *Am J Obstet Gynecol* 1966;95:588.

71. **Kovac SR, Cruikshank SH.** Incidental appendectomy during vaginal hysterectomy. *Int J Gynecol Obstet* 1993;43:62–63.

72. **Pratt JH, O'Leary JA, Symmonds RE.** Combined cholecystectomy and hysterectomy: a study of 95 cases. *Mayo Clin Proc* 1967;42:529–535.

73. **Murray JM, Gilstrap LC, Massey FM.** Cholecystectomy and abdominal hysterectomy. *JAMA* 1980;244:2305–2306.

74. **Hester TR, Baird W, Bostwick J, et al.** Abdominoplasty combined with other major surgical procedures: safe or sorry? *Plast Reconstr Surg* 1989;83:997–1004.

75. **Voss SC, Sharp HC, Scott JR.** Abdominoplasty combined with gynecologic surgical procedures. *Obstet Gynecol* 1986;67:181–186.

76. **Kovac SR.** Vaginal hysterectomy combined with liposuction. *Mo Med* 1989;86:165–168.

77. **Sanz L, Smith S.** Mechanisms of wound healing, suture material, and wound closure. In: **Buchsbaum HJ, Walton LA,** eds. *Strategies in gynecologic surgery.* New York: Springer-Verlag, 1986:53–76.

78. **Richardson AC, Lyon JB, Geraham EE.** Abdominal hysterectomy: relationship between morbidity and surgical technique. *Am J Obstet Gynecol* 1973;115:953–961.

79. **Masterson BJ.** Total abdominal hysterectomy. In: *Manual of gynecologic surgery.* 2nd ed. New York: Springer-Verlag, 1986:187–218.

80. **Masterson BJ.** Ureteral injuries. In: *Manual of gynecologic survey.* 2nd ed. New York: Springer-Verlag, 1986:339–349.

81. **Mattingly RF, Thompson JD.** Operative injuries of the ureter. In: *TeLinde's operative gynecology.* 6th ed. Philadelphia: JB Lippincott, 1985:325–344.

82. **Symmonds RE.** Ureteral injuries associated with gynecologic surgery: prevention and management. *Clin Obstet Gynecol* 1976;19:623–644.

83. **Symonds RE.** Incontinence: vesical and ureteral fistulas. *Clin Obstet Gynecol* 1984;27:499–514.

84. **Buchsbaum HJ, Walton LA.** *Strategies in gynecological surgery.* New York: Springer-Verlag, 1986:77–104.

85. **Berek JS.** Surgical techniques. In: **Berek JS, Hacker NF,** eds. *Practical gynecologic oncology*. 2nd ed. Baltimore: Williams & Wilkins, 1994:519–560.

86. **Walker FW.** Small intestine operative procedures. In: **Shackerford RT, Zuideema GE.** *Surgery for the alimentary tract.* 2nd ed. Philadelphia: WB Saunders, 1986:46–56.

87. **Shakerford RT, Zuideema GE.** *Surgery in the alimentary tract.* 2nd ed. Philadelphia: WB Saunders, 1986:312–335.

88. **Mitchell GW, Massey FM.** Bleeding 3 hours following vaginal hysterectomy. In: **Nichols DH,** ed. *Clinical problems, injuries and complications of gynecologic surgery.* Baltimore: Williams & Wilkins, 1988:151–153.

89. **Buchsbaum HJ.** Avoiding urinary tract injuries. In: **Buchsbaum HJ, Walton LA,** eds. *Strategies in gynecological surgery.* New York: Springer-Verlag, 1986:77–85.

90. **Copenhaver EH.** Vaginal hysterectomy: an analysis of indications and complications among 1,000 operations. *Am J Obstet Gynecol* 1962;84:123–128.

91. **Grody MHT.** Vaginal hysterectomy: the large uterus. *J Gynecol Surg* 1989;5:301–312.

92. **Kaser SR, Ikle FA, Hirsch HA.** *Atlas of gynecologic surgery.* 2nd ed. Philadelphia: WB Saunders, 1985.

93. **Kovac SR.** Intramyometrial coring as an adjunct to vaginal hysterectomy. *Obstet Gynecol* 1986;67:131–136.

94. **Lash AF.** A method for reducing the size of the uterus in vaginal hysterectomy. *Am J Obstet Gynecol* 1941;42:452–459.

95. **Lash AF.** Technique for removal of abnormally large uteri without entering the cavities. *Clin Obstet Gynecol* 1961;4:210–219.

96. **Nichols DH, Randall CL.** *Vaginal surgery.* 3rd ed. Baltimore: Williams & Wilkins, 1989:206–209.

97. **Pratt JH, Gunnar H.** Vaginal hysterectomy by morcellation. *Mayo Clin Proc* 1970;45:374–387.

98. **Shires GT, Canzaro PC, Lowry SF.** Fluid, electrolyte, and nutritional management of the surgical patient. In: **Schartz SL,** ed. *Principles of surgery.* 4th ed. New York: McGraw-Hill, 1984:45–80.

99. **Massler DJ, Devanesan MM.** Sexual consequences of gynecologic operations. In: **Comfort A,** ed. *Sexual consequences of disability.* Philadelphia: George F. Stickley, 1978:153–181.

100. **Drellich MG, Bieber I.** The psychological importance of the uterus and its function. *J Nerv Ment Dis* 1958;126:322–336.

101. **Lindemann E.** Observations on psychiatric sequelae to surgical operations in women. *Am J Psychiatry* 1941;98:132–137.

102. **Richards DH.** Depression after hysterectomy. *Lancet* 1973;2:430–432.

103. **Hollender MH.** A study of patients admitted to a psychiatric hospital after pelvic operations. *Am J Obstet Gynecol* 1960;79:498–503.

104. **Bragg RL.** Risk of admission to mental hospital following hysterectomy or cholecystectomy. *Am J Public Health* 1965;55:1403–1410.

105. **Martin RL, Roberts WV, Clayton PJ.** Psychiatric status after hysterectomy: a one year prospective follow-up. *JAMA* 1980;244:350–353.

106. **Moore JT, Tolley DH.** Depression following hysterectomy. *Psychosomatics* 1976;17:86–89.

107. **Hamptom PT, Tarnasky WG.** Hysterectomy and tubal ligation: a comparison of the psychological aftermath. *Am J Obstet Gynecol* 1974;119:949–952.

108. **Gath D, Cooper P, Day A.** Hysterectomy and psychiatric disorder. I. Levels of psychiatric morbidity before and after hysterectomy. *Br J Psychiatry* 1982;140:335–342.

109. **Lalinec-Michaud M, Engelsmann F, Marino J.** Depression after hysterectomy: a comparative study. *Psychosomatics* 1988;29:307–313.

110. **Janis IL.** *Psychological stress.* Psychoanalytical behavioral studies of surgical patients. New York: John Wiley & Sons, 1958.

111. **Menzer D, Morris T, Gates P, et al.** Patterns of emotional recovery from hysterectomy. *Psychosom Med* 1957;19:379–388.

112. **Huffman JW.** The effect of gynecologic surgery on sexual relations. *Am J Obstet Gynecol* 1950;59:915–917.

113. **Humphries PT.** Sexual adjustment after a hysterectomy. *Issues Health Care Women* 1980;2:1–14.

114. **Dennerstein L, Wood C, Burrows GD.** Sexual response following hysterectomy and oophorectomy. *Obstet Gynecol* 1977;49:92–96.

115. **Lindgren HC.** *Personality as a social phenomenon.* 2nd ed. New York: John Wiley & Sons, 1973:225–299.

SECTION

V

REPRODUCTIVE ENDOCRINOLOGY

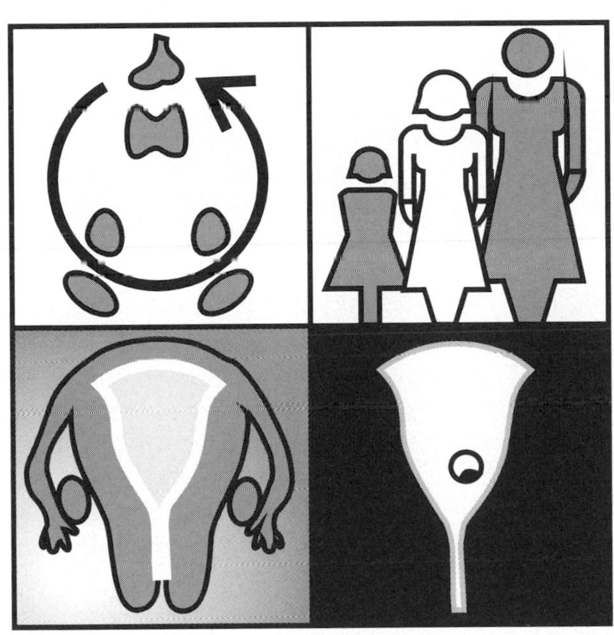

23 Puberty

Robert W. Rebar

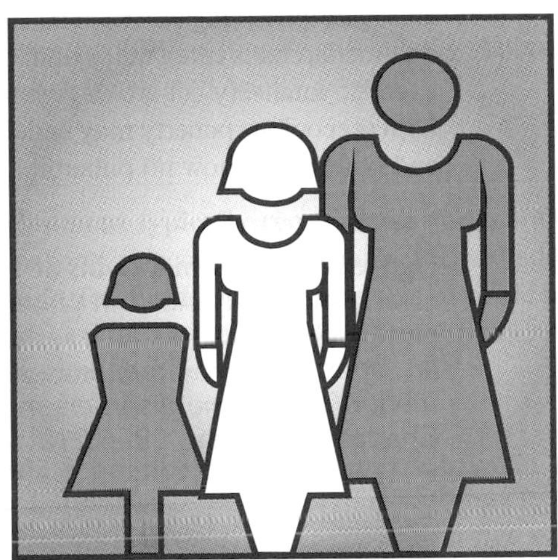

***Puberty* is defined as the period during which secondary sexual characteristics begin to develop and the capability of sexual reproduction is attained.** The physical changes accompanying pubertal development result directly or indirectly from maturation of the hypothalamus, stimulation of the sex organs, and secretion of sex steroids. Hormonally, puberty in humans is characterized by the resetting of the classic negative gonadal steroid feedback loop, alterations in circadian and ultradian (frequent) gonadotropin rhythms, and the acquisition in the woman of a positive estrogen feedback loop, which controls the monthly rhythm as an interdependent expression of gonadotropins and ovarian steroids.

The ability to evaluate and treat aberrations of pubertal development requires an understanding of the normal hormonal and physical changes that occur at puberty. An understanding of these changes is also important in evaluating young women with amenorrhea.

Normal Pubertal Development

Factors Affecting Time of Onset

The major determinant of the timing of the onset of puberty is no doubt genetic, but a number of other factors appear to influence both the age at onset and the progression of pubertal development. Among these influences are nutritional state, general health, geographic location, exposure to light, and psychological state (1). The concordance of the age of menarche in mother–daughter pairs and between sisters and in ethnic populations illustrates the importance of genetic factors (1). Typically, the age of menarche is earlier than average in children with moderate obesity (up to 30% above normal weight for age), whereas delayed menarche is common in those with severe malnutrition. Children who live in urban settings, closer to the equator, and at lower altitudes typically begin puberty earlier than those who live in rural areas, farther from the equator, and at higher elevations. Blind girls apparently undergo menarche earlier than sighted girls, suggesting some influence of light (2).

In western Europe, the age of menarche declined 4 months each decade between 1850 and 1960 (1). Recent data suggest that the trend toward earlier pubertal development is continuing among girls (but not boys) who live in the United States (3). It has been presumed that these changes represent improved nutritional status and healthier living conditions.

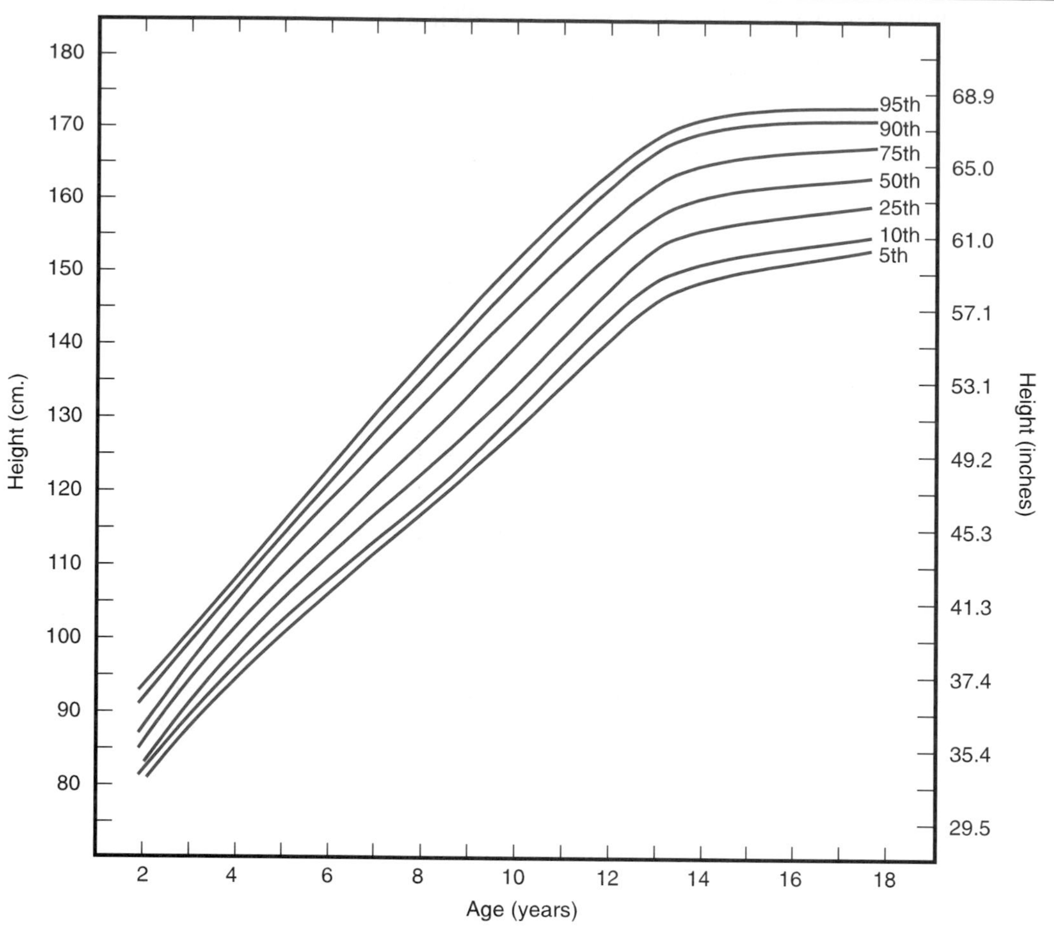

Figure 23.7 Growth chart showing stature by age percentiles for girls aged 2 to 18 years. Weight can be plotted in a similar fashion. Several excellent growth charts are available to clinicians, including those from Ross Laboratories (Columbus, OH), Serono Laboratories (Randolph, MA), and Genentech, Inc. (South San Francisco, CA). (From **Hamill PVV, Drizd TA, Johnson CL, et al.** Physical growth: National Center for Health Statistics percentiles. *Am J Clin Nutr* 1979;32:607–629, with permission; based on data from the National Center for Health Statistics.)

that has been proposed is shown in Table 23.2 (23). The incidence of these anomalies was estimated to be 0.02% of the female population several years ago (24), but the incidence may have increased as a result of the maternal ingestion of diethylstilbestrol (DES) and the resultant increase in anomalies of the lumen of the uterus (class VI) (25). Of the disorders unrelated to drugs, the septate uterus (class V) is most common.

Disorders of the outflow tract and uterus often occur as a part of a syndrome of malformations that include abnormalities of the skeletal and renal systems (Rokitansky-Küster-Hauser syndrome). Familial aggregates of the most common disorders of müllerian differentiation in females—müllerian aplasia and incomplete müllerian fusion—are best explained on the basis of polygenic and multifactorial inheritance (26). It is clear that the *HOX* genes, a family of regulatory genes that encode for transcription factors, are essential for proper development of the müllerian tract in the embryonic period (27), and *HOXA 13* has been found to be altered in hand–foot–genital syndrome.

The most common single anatomic disorder of puberty is the imperforate hymen, which prevents the passage of endometrial tissue and blood. These products can accumulate in the vagina (*hydrocolpos*) or uterus (*hydrometrocolpos*) and result in a bulging hymen that is often bluish in color. The affected individual often has a history of vague abdominal pain with approximately monthly exacerbations. It is sometimes difficult to distinguish an

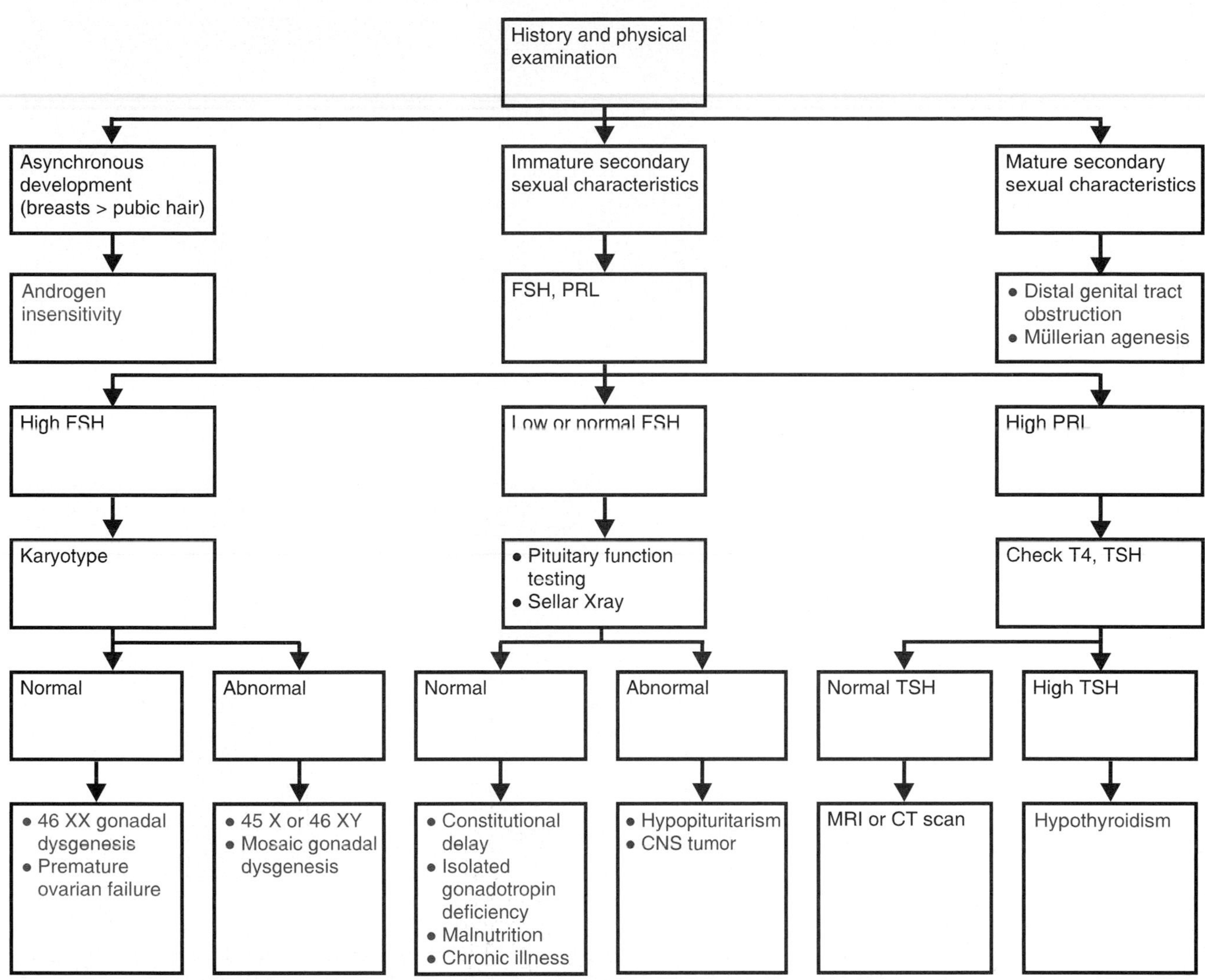

Figure 23.8 Flow diagram for the evaluation of delayed or interrupted pubertal development, including primary amenorrhea, in phenotypic girls. Girls with asynchronous development often present because of failure to menstruate. (From **Rebar RW.** Normal and abnormal sexual differentiation and pubertal development. In: **Moore TR, Reiter RC, Rebar RW, et al,** eds. *Gynecology and obstetrics: a longitudinal approach.* New York: Churchill Livingstone, 1993: 97–133.)

imperforate hymen from a transverse vaginal septum, and in most situations, examination under anesthesia is required.

Regardless of the cause, uterine anomalies not involving segmental müllerian agenesis or hypoplasia (class I) are compatible with normal pregnancy. However, increased fetal wastage has been reported (28). Uterine malformations have been associated with spontaneous abortion, premature labor, abnormal presentations, and complications of labor (i.e., retained placenta). Many of these uterine anomalies can be identified with hysterosalpingography (Fig. 23.9). Hysterosalpingography, laparoscopy, and hysteroscopy have been used to differentiate a septate uterus (class V) from a bicornuate uterus (class IV). It is now clear that magnetic resonance imaging (MRI) and endovaginal ultrasonography (sometimes with sonohysterography) are as accurate as these invasive techniques in identifying the abnormality (29).

Obstruction or malformation of the distal genital tract must be distinguished from androgen insensitivity. Individuals with androgen insensitivity have breast development

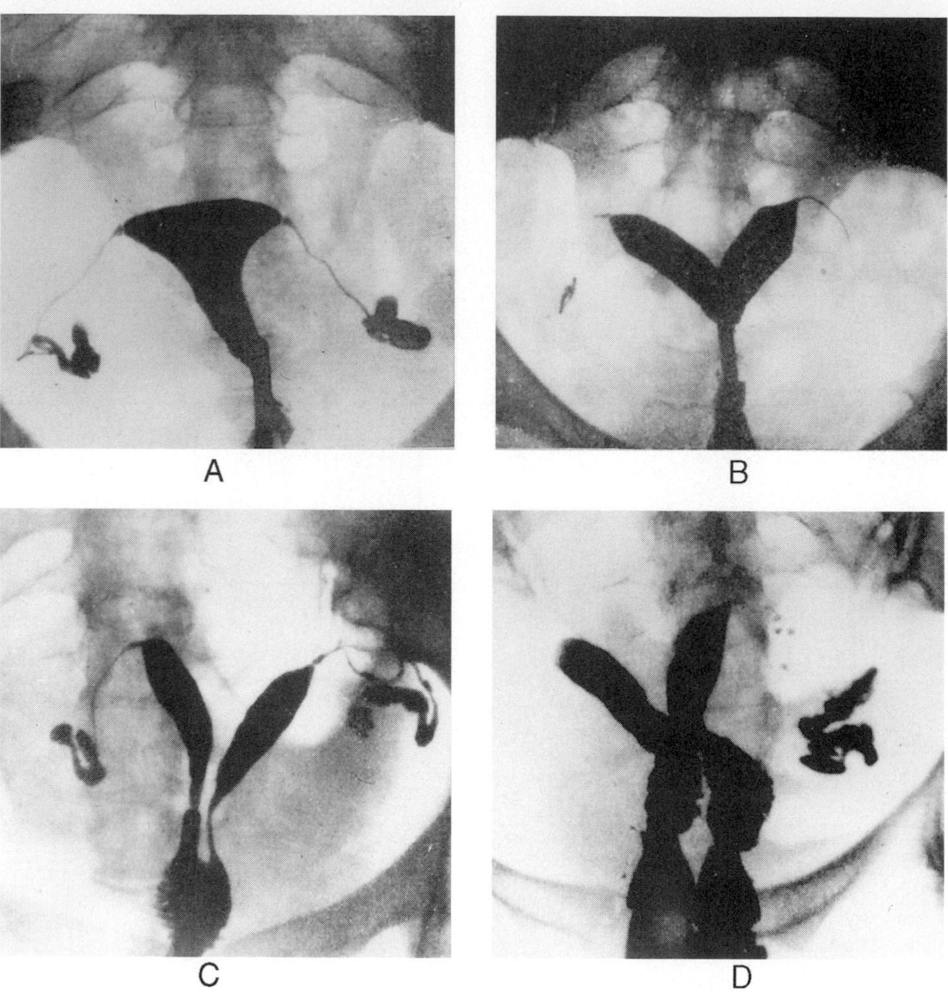

Figure 23.9 Hysterosalpingograms of normal and abnormal female genital tracts. The radiographic photographs have been reversed to accentuate the uterine cavities. **A:** Normal study with bilateral spill. **B:** Bicornuate uterus. **C:** Uterus didelphis. **D:** Uterus didelphis with double vagina. (Courtesy of Dr. A. Gerbie; from **Spitzer IB, Rebar RW.** Counselling for women with medical problems: ovary and reproductive organs. In: **Hollingsworth D, Resnik R,** eds. *Medical counselling before pregnancy.* New York: Churchill Livingstone, 1988:213–248, with permission.)

in the absence of significant pubic and axillary hair development; the vagina may be absent or foreshortened in these women.

Hypergonadotropic and Hypogonadotropic Hypogonadism

Basal levels of FSH and prolactin should be determined in individuals in whom secondary sex characteristics have not developed to maturity (Fig. 23.8). Bone age should be estimated from x-rays of the nondominant hand. If prolactin levels are elevated, thyroid function should be assessed to determine whether the individual has primary hypothyroidism. Paradoxically, primary hypothyroidism can result in precocious puberty as well. If thyroid function is normal, a hypothalamic or pituitary neoplasm is possible, and careful evaluation of the hypothalamic and pituitary area by MRI or computed tomography (CT) is indicated.

The karyotype should be determined in any individual with delayed puberty and increased basal FSH concentrations. Regardless of the karyotype, the individual with hypergonadotropic hypogonadism has some form of ovarian "failure."

Table 23.2. Classification of Müllerian Anomalies

Class I. Segmented müllerian agenesis or hypoplasia
A. Vaginal
B. Cervical
C. Fundal
D. Tubal
E. Combined
Class II. Unicornuate uterus
A. With a rudimentary horn
1. With a communicating endometrial cavity
2. With a noncommunicating cavity
3. With no cavity
B. Without any rudimentary horn
Class III. Uterus didelphis
Class IV. Bicornuate uterus
A. Complete to the internal os
B. Partial
C. Arcuate
Class V. Septate uterus
A. With a complete septum
B. With an incomplete septum
Class VI. Uterus with internal luminal changes

Adapted from **Buttrarm VC Jr, Gibbons WE.** Müllerian anomalies: a proposed classification (an analysis of 144 cases). *Fertil Steril* 1979;32:40, with permission.

Forms of Gonadal Failure

Turner's Syndrome **Most affected individuals have a 45X karyotype and Turner's syndrome; still others have mosaic karyotypes (i.e., 45X/46XX; 45X/46XY) and may present with the Turner's phenotype as well.** Intrauterine growth restriction is common in infants with a 45X karyotype. After birth, these patients generally grow slowly, beginning in the second or third year of life. They typically have many of the associated stigmata, including lymphedema at birth; a webbed neck; multiple pigmented nevi; disorders of the heart, kidneys (most commonly horseshoe), and great vessels (most commonly coarctation of the aorta); and small hyperconvex fingernails (30) (Fig. 23.10). Diabetes mellitus, thyroid disorders, essential hypertension, and other autoimmune disorders are often present in individuals with 45X karyotypes. Most 45X patients have normal intelligence, but many affected individuals have an unusual cognitive defect characterized by an inability to appreciate the shapes and relations of objects with respect to one another (i.e., space-form blindness). As they grow older, affected children typically are shorter than normal. Although they do not develop breasts at puberty, some pubic or axillary hair may develop because appropriate adrenarche can occur with failure of thelarche (i.e., breast development). **Although less severe short stature and some adolescent development may occur with chromosomal mosaicism, it is reasonable to assume that any short, slowly growing, sexually infantile girl has Turner's syndrome until proved otherwise because this disorder is so prevalent (about 1 in 2,500 newborn phenotypic females). In fact, the 45X karyotype is the single most frequent chromosomal disorder in humans, but most affected fetuses are aborted spontaneously early in pregnancy. However, trisomy is the most common chromosomal type or category of abnormality in first-trimester losses.**

Even in the presence of typical Turner stigmata, a karyotype is indicated to eliminate the possibility of any portion of a Y chromosome. If a Y chromosome is identified, surgical extirpation of the gonads is warranted to eliminate any possibility of a germ cell neoplasm (estimated 20% to 30% prevalence) (31,32). In individuals in whom there is no evidence of neoplastic dissemination, the uterus may be left *in situ* for donor *in vitro* fertilization

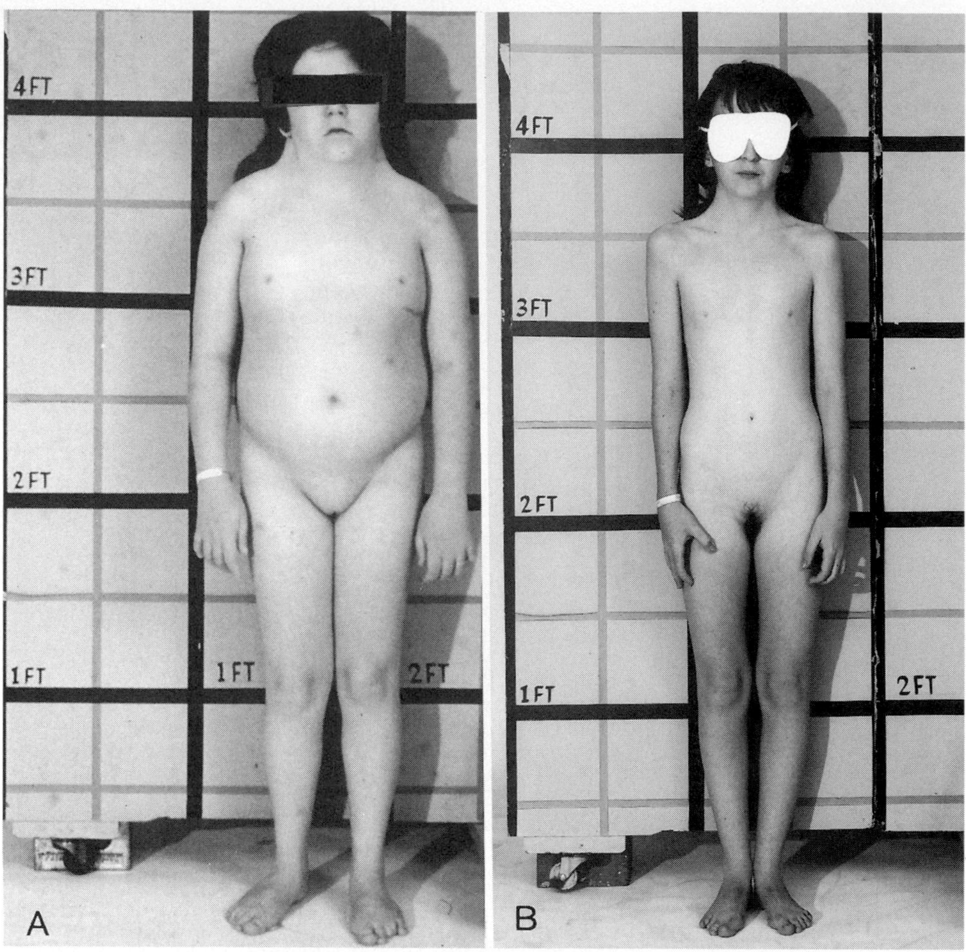

Figure 23.10 Typical appearance of two individuals with 45X gonadal dysgenesis. A: This 16-year-old individual has obvious short stature, a webbed neck, shortened fourth metatarsals, and a thoracotomy scar from the repair of the coarctation of the aorta that was performed at 13 years of age. **B:** This 13-year-old individual had evidence of adrenarche with some pubic and axillary hair development. She is quite short, but the stigmata of Turner's syndrome are less obvious than in the patient in **A.**

and embryo transfer. The evaluation of other commonly involved organ systems should include a careful physical examination, with special attention to the cardiovascular system, and thyroid function tests (including antibody assessment), fasting blood glucose, renal function tests, and intravenous pyelography or a renal ultrasonography.

Treatment of Turner's Syndrome To increase final adult height, treatment strategies using exogenous growth hormone (GH) are commonly accepted (33). It is not yet known what dose of GH is optimal or if an anabolic steroid such as oxandrolone will provide additional growth. However, GH in doses 25% greater than those recommended for GH deficiency are proving safe and effective, with a net increase in height of 8.1 cm over the average height of about 146 cm in untreated individuals.

The treatment of patients with Turner's syndrome is as follows:

1. **To promote sexual maturation, therapy with exogenous *estrogen* should be initiated when the patient is psychologically ready, at about 12 to 13 years of age, and after GH therapy is completed.**

2. Because the intent is to mimic normal pubertal development, therapy with low-dose *estrogen* alone (such as 0.3 to 0.625 mg *conjugated estrogens* orally each day) should be initiated.

3. Progestins (5 to 10 mg *medroxyprogesterone acetate* or 200 mg *micronized progesterone* orally for 12 to 14 days every 1 to 2 months) can be added to prevent endometrial hyperplasia after the patient first experiences vaginal bleeding or after 6 months of unopposed *estrogen* use if the patient has not yet had any bleeding.

4. The dose of *estrogen* is increased slowly over 1 to 2 years until the patient is taking about twice as much *estrogen* as is administered to postmenopausal women.

5. Girls with gonadal dysgenesis must be monitored carefully for the development of hypertension with estrogen therapy.

6. The patients and their parents should be counseled regarding the emotional and physical changes that will occur with therapy.

Mosaic Forms of Gonadal Dysgenesis Individuals with rare mosaic forms of gonadal dysgenesis may develop normally at puberty. The decision to initiate therapy with exogenous estrogen should be based mainly on circulating FSH levels because FSH levels in the normal range for the patient's age imply the presence of functional gonads.

Pregnancies can be achieved in these individuals, with success rates of more than 50%, by using donor oocytes (34).

Pure Gonadal Dysgenesis **The term *pure gonadal dysgenesis* refers to 46XX or 46XY phenotypic females who have streak gonads. This condition may occur sporadically or may be inherited as an autosomal recessive trait or as an X-linked trait in XY gonadal dysgenesis** (Fig. 23.11). Affected girls are typically of average height and have none of the stigmata of Turner's syndrome, but they have elevated levels of FSH because the streak gonads produce neither steroid hormones nor inhibin. When gonadal dysgenesis occurs in 46XY individuals, it is sometimes termed *Swyer's syndrome.* Surgical extirpation is warranted in individuals with a 46XY karyotype to prevent development of germ cell neoplasms. Both 46XX and 46XY forms of gonadal dysgenesis benefit from exogenous estrogen and are potential candidates for donor oocytes.

In early gonadal failure, the ovaries apparently develop normally but contain no oocytes by the expected age of puberty. These disorders are considered further in the discussion delineating the evaluation of amenorrhea (see Chapter 24).

Hypogonadotropic Hypogonadism

Hypothalamic–pituitary disturbances are usually associated with low levels of circulating gonadotropins (with both LH and FSH $\leq$10 mIU/mL) (35). There are both sporadic and familial causes of hypogonadotropic hypogonadism, and the differential diagnosis is extensive. Mutations in several genes have been shown to cause hypogonadotropic hypogonadism in humans (36). This condition can arise from abnormalities in hypothalamic GnRH secretion, impaired release of gonadotropins from the pituitary gland, or both. At least four genes have been identified as causes of hypogonadotropic hypogonadism: (a) *KAL,* (b) *DAX 1* (the gene for X-linked congenital adrenal hypoplasia), (c) *GNRHR* (the gene for the GnRH receptor), and (d) *PC1* (the gene for prohormone convertase 1) (37). Because defects in these four genes account for less than 20% of all cases of isolated hypogonadotropic hypogonadism, additional mutations probably exist but have yet to be identified. It is important to remember, however, that low levels of LH and FSH are normally present in the prepubertal years; thus, girls with constitutionally delayed puberty may mistakenly be presumed to have hypogonadotropic hypogonadism. **In fact, constitutional delay is the most**

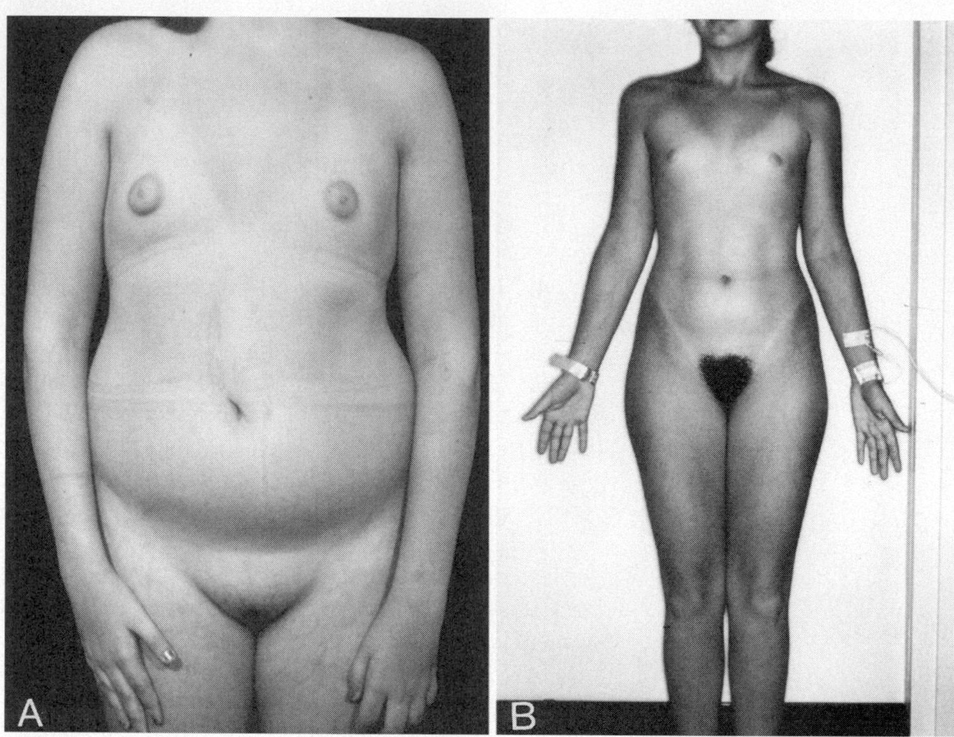

Figure 23.11 A: A 16-year-old individual with 46XX gonadal dysgenesis and primary amenorrhea. Circulating follicle-stimulating hormone (FSH) levels were markedly elevated. The small amount of breast development (Tanner stage 2) is unusual, but some pubertal development may occur in such patients. **B: A 16-year-old individual with 46XY gonadal dysgenesis who presented with primary amenorrhea and markedly elevated FSH levels.** Most affected individuals do not present with as much pubic and axillary hair development. The right gonad contained a dysgerminoma, but there was no evidence of metastases. (From **Rebar RW.** Normal and abnormal sexual differentiation and pubertal development. In: **Moore TR, Reiter RC, Rebar RW, et al,** eds. *Gynecology and obstetrics: a longitudinal approach.* New York: Churchill Livingstone, 1993:97–133, with permission.)

common cause of delayed puberty. Constitutional delayed growth and adolescence can be diagnosed only after careful evaluation excludes other causes of delayed puberty and longitudinal follow-up documents normal sexual development. The farther below the third percentile for height that the young girl is, the less likely it is that the cause is constitutional.

Kallmann's Syndrome As originally described in 1944 (38), Kallmann's syndrome consisted of the triad of anosmia, hypogonadism, and color blindness in men. Women may be affected as well, and other associated defects may include cleft lip and palate, cerebellar ataxia, nerve deafness, and abnormalities of thirst and vasopressin release. Because autopsy studies have shown partial or complete agenesis of the olfactory bulb, the term *olfactogenital dysplasia* has also been used to describe the disorder. These anatomic findings coincide with embryologic studies documenting that GnRH neurons originally develop in the epithelium of the olfactory placode and normally migrate into the hypothalamus (39). In some affected individuals, gene defects have been found in one protein, anosmin, that facilitates this neuronal migration, thus leading to an absence of GnRH neurons in the hypothalamus and olfactory bulbs and consequent hypogonadotropic hypogonadism and anosmia (Kallmann's syndrome) (40). The gene defect resulting in loss of this facilatory adhesion protein has been localized to the X chromosome in an X-linked form of the syndrome, and this locus has been designated *KAL1*. Because confirmed mutations in the coding sequence of the *KAL* gene occur only in a minority of individuals with Kallmann's syndrome (41), other mutations no doubt will be identified in the future. Moreover, the disorder is so heterogeneous that it appears likely that this disorder forms a structural continuum with other midline defects. Septooptic dysplasia represents the most severe disorder.

Clinically, affected individuals typically present with sexual infantilism and an eunuchoid habitus, but some degree of breast development may occur (Fig. 23.12). Primary amenorrhea is the rule. The ovaries are usually small, with follicles seldom developing beyond the primordial stage. Circulating gonadotropin levels are usually very low but almost invariably measurable. Affected individuals respond readily to pulsatile administration of exogenous GnRH, and clearly this is the most physiologic approach to ovulation induction (34). For women not seeking pregnancy, replacement therapy with exogenous estrogen and progestin is indicated.

Isolated gonadotropin deficiency can also occur in association with the Prader-Labhardt-Willi syndrome, which is characterized by obesity, short stature, hypogonadism, small hands and feet (acromicria), mental retardation, and infantile hypotonia; and in association with the Laurence-Moon-Bardet-Biedl syndrome, which is characterized by retinitis pigmentosa, postaxial polydactyly, obesity, and hypogonadism. Prader-Labhardt-Willi syndrome apparently results from rearrangements of chromosome 15q11 to q13, an imprinted region of the human genome (42). Laurence-Moon-Bardet-Biedl syndrome, inherited in an autosomal recessive manner, is apparently heterogeneous, with at least four involved gene loci having been mapped to date (43).

Multiple pituitary hormone deficiencies, which are usually hypothalamic in origin, may be congenital and either part of an inherited constellation of findings or sporadic. If growth hormone (GH) or thyroid-stimulating hormone (TSH) concentrations are subnormal, growth and pubertal development will be affected. Thus, the condition should be diagnosed before the age of puberty. Because individuals with hypopituitarism have a high mortality rate, predominantly caused by vascular and respiratory disease (44), it is important to identify affected individuals. Later age at diagnosis, female sex, and above all craniopharyngioma have been identified as significant independent risk factors. Untreated gonadotropin deficiency also is an important risk factor for early mortality.

Tumors of the Hypothalamus and Pituitary Several different tumors of the hypothalamic and pituitary regions may also lead to hypogonadotropic hypogonadism (45) (Fig. 23.13A). Except for craniopharyngiomas, these tumors are relatively uncommon in children. Craniopharyngiomas are usually suprasellar in location and may be asymptomatic well into the second decade of life. Such tumors may present as headache, visual disturbances, short stature or growth failure, delayed puberty, or diabetes insipidus. Visual field defects (including bilateral temporal hemianopsia), optic atrophy, or papilledema may be seen on physical examination. Laboratory evaluation should document hypogonadotropinism and may also reveal hyperprolactinemia as a result of interruption of hypothalamic dopamine inhibition of prolactin release. Radiographically, the tumor may be either cystic or solid and may show areas of calcification. Appropriate therapy for hypothalamic–pituitary tumors may involve surgical excision or radiotherapy (with adequate pituitary hormone replacement therapy) and is best decided by a team of physicians that includes an endocrinologist, a neurosurgeon, and a radiotherapist.

Other Central Nervous System Disorders Other central nervous system disorders that may lead to delayed puberty include infiltrative diseases, such as Langerhans-type histiocytosis, particularly the form known previously as Hand-Schüller-Christian disease (Fig. 23.13B). Diabetes insipidus is the most common endocrinopathy (because of infiltration of the supraoptic nucleus in the hypothalamus), but short stature resulting from GH deficiency, and delayed puberty caused by gonadotropin deficiency are not uncommon in this disorder (46).

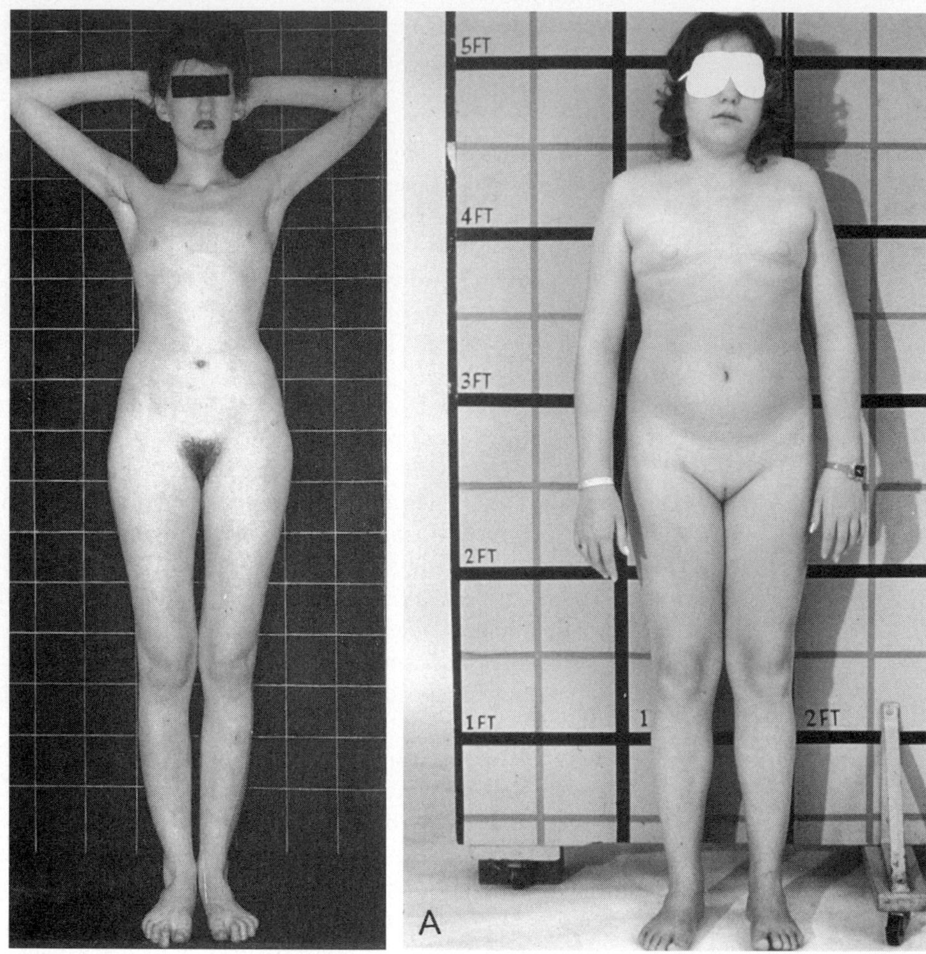

Fig. 23.12 Fig. 23.13A

Figure 23.12 A $21\frac{1}{2}$-year-old woman with Kallmann's syndrome. Note that the patient has some pubic and axillary hair. Bone age was 16 years. It is rare to see affected individuals today who were not given oral contraceptive agents to induce menses (with some consequent breast development). (From **Wilkins L.** *The diagnosis and treatment of endocrine disorders in childhood and adolescence.* 3rd ed. Springfield, IL: Charles C. Thomas, 1965, with permission.)

Figure 23.13 A: A 16-year-old girl with delayed puberty. Breast budding began at 11 years of age, but there was no further development. During the year before presentation, her scholastic performance in school deteriorated, she gained 25 lb, she became increasingly lethargic, and nocturia and polydypsia were noted. Initial evaluation documented low follicle-stimulating hormone, elevated prolactin, and a bone age of 10.5 years. Computed tomography scanning documented a large hypothalamic neoplasm that proved to be an ectopic germinoma. The patient was also documented to be hypothyroid and hypoadrenal and to have diabetes insipidus. Despite the elevated prolactin, she had no galactorrhea because of the minimal breast development. (From **Rebar RW.** Normal and abnormal sexual differentiation and pubertal development. In: **Moore TR, Reiter RC, Rebar RW, et al,** eds. *Gynecology and obstetrics: a longitudinal approach.* New York: Churchill Livingstone, 1993:97–133, with permission.)

Irradiation of the central nervous system for treatment of any neoplasm or leukemia may result in hypothalamic dysfunction. Although GH deficiency occurs most often, partial or complete gonadotropin deficiency may develop in some patients.

Severe chronic illnesses, often accompanied by malnutrition, may also lead to slowed growth in childhood and delayed adolescence. Regardless of the cause, weight loss to less than 80%

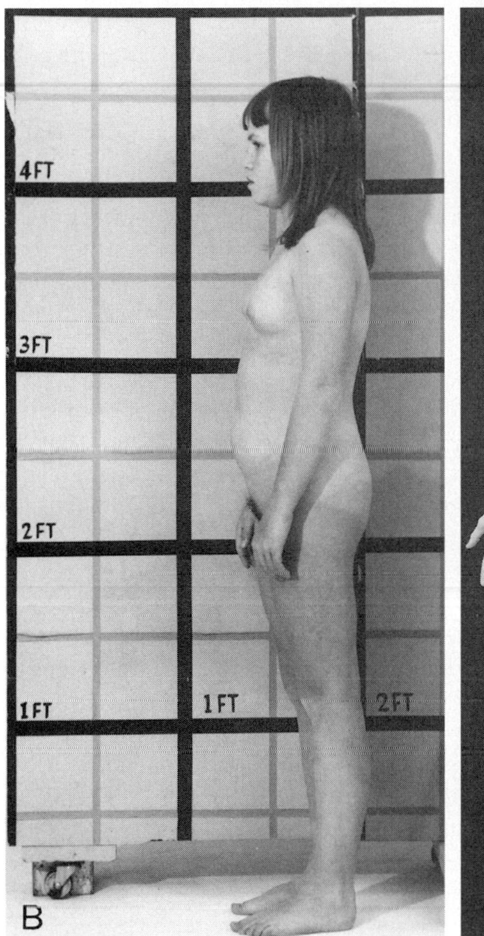

Fig. 23.13B

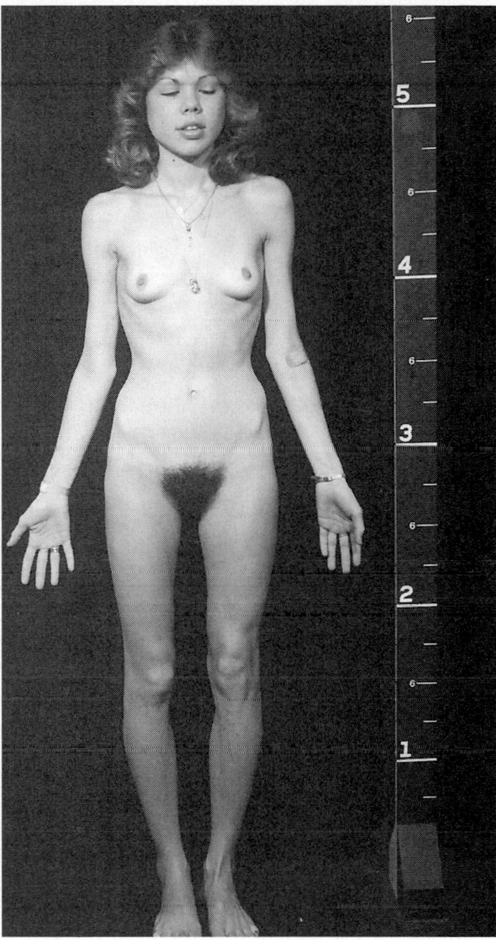

Fig. 23.14

Figure 23.13 B: A 16-year-old girl with primary amenorrhea who progressed in puberty until about 12 years of age. Breast budding occurred at about 10 years of age. The patient's short stature is obvious. She proved to have hypopituitarism. Classic radiographic findings established the diagnosis of Langerhans cell–type histiocytosis (Hand-Schüller-Christian disease).

Figure 23.14 An 18-year-old girl with anorexia nervosa. As is true of most such patients, pubertal development had been completed and menses initiated before anorexia led to marked weight loss.

to 85% of ideal body weight often results in hypothalamic GnRH deficiency. If adequate body weight and nutrition are maintained in chronic illnesses such as Crohn's disease or chronic pulmonary or renal disease, sufficient gonadotropin secretion usually is present to initiate and maintain pubertal development.

Anorexia Nervosa and Bulimia *Significant* weight loss and psychological dysfunction occur simultaneously with anorexia nervosa (47,48). Although many anorectic girls experience amenorrhea after pubertal development has begun, if the disorder begins sufficiently early, pubertal development may be delayed or interrupted (Fig. 23.14). The following constellation of associated findings confirms anorexia nervosa in most individuals:

1. Relentless pursuit of thinness
2. Amenorrhea, sometimes preceding the weight loss
3. Extreme inanition

4. Obsessive-compulsive personality often characterized by overachievement

5. Distorted and bizarre attitude toward eating, food, or weight

6. Distorted body image

Because normal body weight is commonly maintained in bulimia, it is unusual for bulimic patients to experience either delayed development or amenorrhea. Girls with anorexia nervosa may have, in addition to hypogonadotropic hypogonadism, partial diabetes insipidus, abnormal temperature regulation, chemical hypothyroidism with low serum triiodothyronine (T_3) and high reverse T_3 levels, and elevated circulating cortisol levels in the absence of evidence of hypercortisolism (49).

Fear of obesity, a syndrome of self-induced malnutrition common among teenage gymnasts and ballet dancers, also may slow growth and delay pubertal development (50). These children voluntarily reduce their caloric intake as much as 40%, leading to nutritional growth retardation. Any additive role for endurance training in the delayed development is possible, but the mechanisms are unclear at this point. These conditions are essentially severe forms of hypothalamic amenorrhea. It is clear, however, that delayed puberty will occur inevitably unless adequate caloric intake is provided.

Hyperprolactinemia Low levels of LH and FSH may be associated with hyperprolactinemia. As noted, galactorrhea cannot occur in the absence of complete breast development. Pituitary prolactinomas are rare during adolescence but must be considered when certain signs and symptoms are present. Many individuals with prolactinomas have a history of delayed menarche. The association between the ingestion of certain drugs (most often psychotropic agents and opiates in this age group) is well established. Primary hypothyroidism also is associated with hyperprolactinemia because increased levels of thyrotropin-releasing hormone (TRH) stimulate secretion of prolactin. The empty sella syndrome, in which the sella turcica is enlarged but has been replaced by cerebrospinal fluid, may also be associated with hyperprolactinemia.

Asynchronous Puberty

Asynchronous pubertal development is characteristic of androgen insensitivity (i.e., testicular feminization). Affected individuals typically present with breast development (usually only to Tanner stage 3) out of proportion with the amount of pubic and axillary hair (Fig. 23.15). In this disorder, 46XY individuals have bilateral testes, female external genitalia, a blindly ending vagina (often foreshortened and sometimes absent), and no müllerian derivatives (i.e., uterus and fallopian tubes) (51). Infrequently, patients may have clitoral enlargement and labioscrotal fusion at puberty, which is referred to as *incomplete androgen insensitivity.*

Asynchronous puberty is heterogeneous but is always related to some abnormality of the androgen receptor or of androgen action (52). In perhaps 60% to 70% of cases, androgen receptors cannot be detected (i.e., the patient is receptor negative). In the remaining cases, androgen receptors are present (i.e., receptor positive), but mutations in the androgen receptor have been detected or there is a defect at a more distal step in androgen action (i.e., a postreceptor defect). Receptor-positive individuals are indistinguishable clinically from receptor-negative individuals. Several different mutations in the androgen receptor gene, most of which occur within the androgen-binding domain of the receptor, have been identified in affected individuals who are receptor positive. Severe X-linked androgen receptor gene mutations cause complete androgen insensitivity, mild mutations impair virilization with or without infertility, and moderate mutations result in a wide phenotypic spectrum of expression among siblings (53).

Because the Sertoli cells of the testis make antimüllerian hormone (AMH), müllerian derivatives are absent in this disorder; thus, müllerian regression occurs normally. The testes are

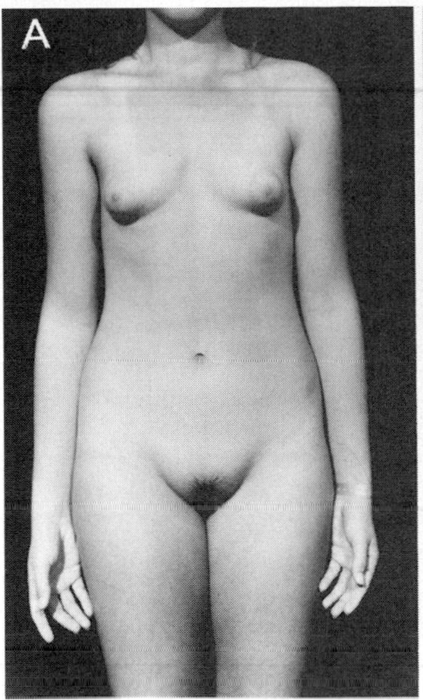

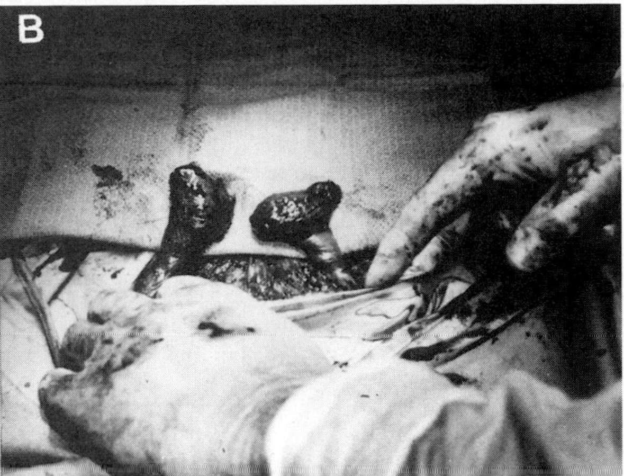

Figure 23.15 A: This 17-year-old individual presented with primary amenorrhea and was found to have a blind-ending vagina and bilateral inguinal masses. Circulating levels of testosterone were at the upper limits of the normal range for men and the karyotype was 46XY, confirming androgen insensitivity. **B: Two inguinal testes were found at surgery.** (From **Simpson JL, Rebar RW.** Normal and abnormal sexual differentiation and development. In: **Becker KL,** ed. *Principles and practice of endocrinology and metabolism.* 2nd ed. Philadelphia: JB Lippincott, 1995:788–822, with permission.)

often normal in size and may be located anywhere along the path of embryonic testicular descent—in the abdomen, inguinal canal, or labia. Half of all individuals with androgen insensitivity develop inguinal hernias. Recognizing that most such girls will be 46XX, it is important to determine the karyotype in prepubertal girls with inguinal hernias, especially if a uterus cannot be detected with certainty by ultrasound.

The frequency of gonadal neoplasia is increased with this condition, but the extent is uncertain (31). Most clinicians believe the risk for neoplasia is low before 25 years of age; thus, the testes should be left in place until after pubertal feminization, especially because the risk for neoplasia appears to increase with age. Exogenous estrogen should be provided after gonadectomy.

The diagnosis is often suspected by the typical physical findings and strongly suggested by normal (or even somewhat elevated) male levels of testosterone, normal or somewhat elevated levels of LH, and normal levels of FSH. The diagnosis is confirmed by a 46XY karyotype.

Interacting with the patient and family requires sensitivity and care. It may be inadvisable to begin by informing the patient of the karyotype; the psychological implications may be devastating because the patient has been reared as a female. Family members should be informed initially that müllerian aplasia occurred and that the risk for neoplasia mandates gonadectomy after puberty. Because the disorder can be inherited in an X-linked recessive fashion, families should undergo appropriate genetic counseling and screening to identify the possible existence of other affected family members.

Precocious Puberty

Although precocious pubertal development may be classified in several ways, it is perhaps simplest to think of the development as gonadotropin dependent (in which case it is

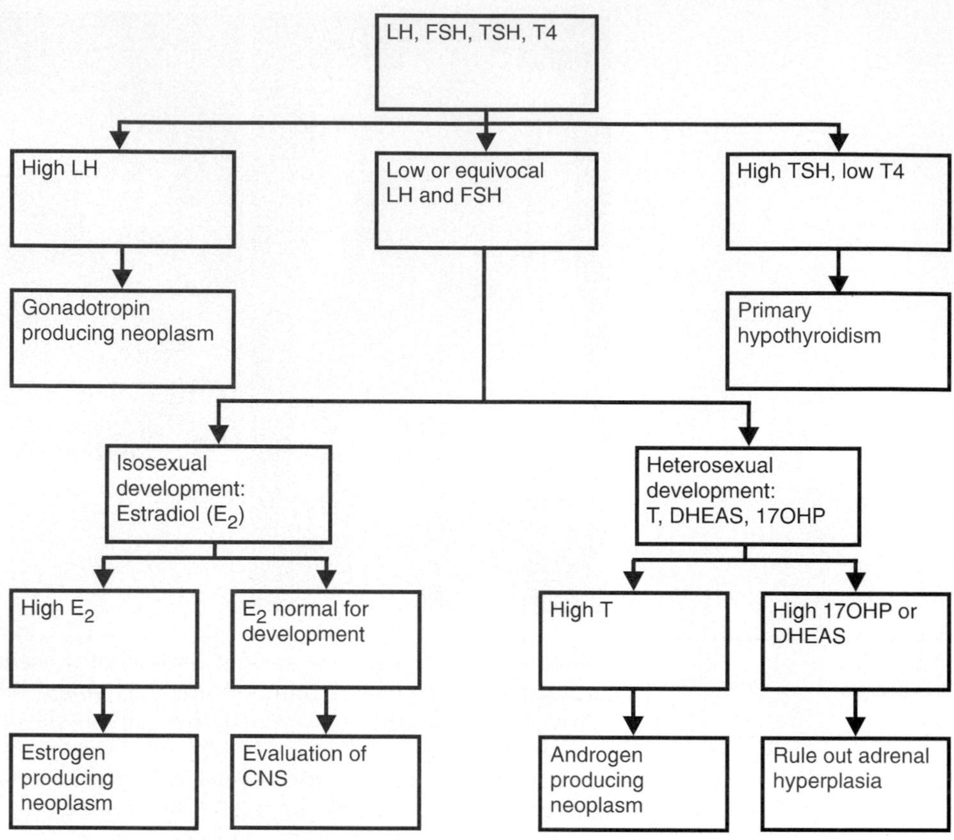

Figure 23.16 Flow diagram for the evaluation of precocious puberty in phenotypic females. (From **Rebar RW.** Normal and abnormal sexual differentiation and pubertal development. In: **Moore TR, Reiter RC, Rebar RW, et al,** eds. *Gynecology and obstetrics: a longitudinal approach.* New York: Churchill Livingstone, 1993:97–133, with permission.)

almost invariably of central origin) or gonadotropin independent (of peripheral origin). The evaluation of precocious puberty is as follows:

1. **Measurement of basal gonadotropin levels is the first step in the evaluation of a child with sexual precocity** (Fig. 23.16).

2. Thyroid function should also be evaluated to rule out primary hypothyroidism as the cause of precocious development.

3. High levels of LH (which really may be human chorionic gonadotropin detected because of cross-reactivity with LH in immunoassays) suggest a gonadotropin-producing neoplasm, most often a pinealoma (ectopic germinoma) or choriocarcinoma or, less often, a hepatoblastoma. (Gonadotropin-producing neoplasms are the only causes of precocious puberty in which the gonadotropin dependence does not equate with central precocious puberty.)

4. Low or pubertal levels of gonadotropins indicate the need to determine circulating estradiol concentrations in girls with isosexual development and to assess androgen levels, specifically testosterone, dehydroepiandrosterone sulfate, and 17α-hydroxyprogesterone in girls with heterosexual development.

5. Increased estradiol levels suggest an estrogen-secreting neoplasm, probably of ovarian origin.

6. Increased testosterone levels suggest an androgen-producing neoplasm of the ovary or the adrenal gland. Such neoplasms may be palpable on abdominal or rectal examination. Increased 17α-hydroxyprogesterone levels are diagnostic of 21-hydroxylase deficiency (i.e., congenital adrenal hyperplasia [CAH]). Dehydroepiandrosterone sulfate levels are elevated in various forms of CAH as well.

7. If the estradiol levels are compatible with the degree of pubertal development observed, evaluation of the central nervous system by MRI or CT scanning is warranted.

8. Bone age should always be assessed in evaluating an individual with sexual precocity.

Perhaps the most difficult decision for the gynecologist is determining how much evaluation is warranted for the young girl brought in by her mother for precocious breast budding only (*precocious thelarche*) or the appearance of pubic or axillary hair alone (*precocious pubarche* or *adrenarche*). In such cases, it is acceptable to many clinicians to follow the patient at frequent intervals and to proceed with evaluation if there is evidence of pubertal progression. The feasibility of this approach may depend on the concerns of the parents. Premature thelarche may be caused by increased sensitivity of the breasts to low levels of estrogen or to increased estradiol secretion by follicular cysts. Premature adrenarche or pubarche may be due to increased sensitivity to low levels of androgens and must be distinguished from late-onset (nonclassic) CAH. If there is no evidence of breast development and the appearance of sexually stimulated hair (i.e., precocious puberty) or of progression, these conditions are virtually always benign.

Constitutional sexual precocity is the most common cause of precocious puberty. It is often familial and represents the so-called "tail" of the gaussian curve (i.e., the early 2.5% for the age distribution for the onset of puberty).

Central (True) Precocious Puberty

In central precocious puberty, GnRH prematurely stimulates increased gonadotropin secretion. Central precocious puberty may occur in children in whom there is no structural abnormality, in which case it is termed *constitutional* or *idiopathic.* Alternatively, central precocious puberty may result from a tumor, infection, congenital abnormality, or traumatic injury affecting the hypothalamus. Tumors of the hypothalamus include hamartomas and, less frequently, neurogliomas and pinealomas. It appears that hamartomas produce GnRH in a pulsatile manner and thus stimulate gonadotropin secretion (54) (Fig. 23.17). A number of congenital malformations, including hydrocephalus, craniostenosis, arachnoid cysts, and septooptic dysplasia, also can be associated with precocious puberty (as well as with sexual infantilism).

Precocious Puberty of Peripheral Origin

In gonadotropin-independent precocious puberty, production of estrogens or androgens from the ovaries, adrenals, or rare steroid-secreting neoplasms leads to early pubertal development. Small functional ovarian cysts, typically asymptomatic, are common in children and may cause transient sexual precocity (55). Simple cysts (with a benign ultrasonographic appearance) can be observed and usually resolve over time. Of the various ovarian neoplasms that can secrete estrogens, granulosa-theca cell tumors occur most frequently but are still rare (56). Although such tumors may grow rapidly, more than two thirds are benign.

The McCune-Albright syndrome is characterized by polyostotic fibrous dysplasia of bone, irregular café-au-lait spots on the skin, and hyperfunctioning endocrinopathies. Girls develop sexual precocity as a result of functioning ovarian cysts. Other endocrinopathies may include hyperthyroidism, hypercortisolism, hyperprolactinemia, and acromegaly. It is now known that mutations of the GS_{α} subunit of the G protein, which couples extracellular hormonal signals to the activation of adenylate cyclase, are responsible

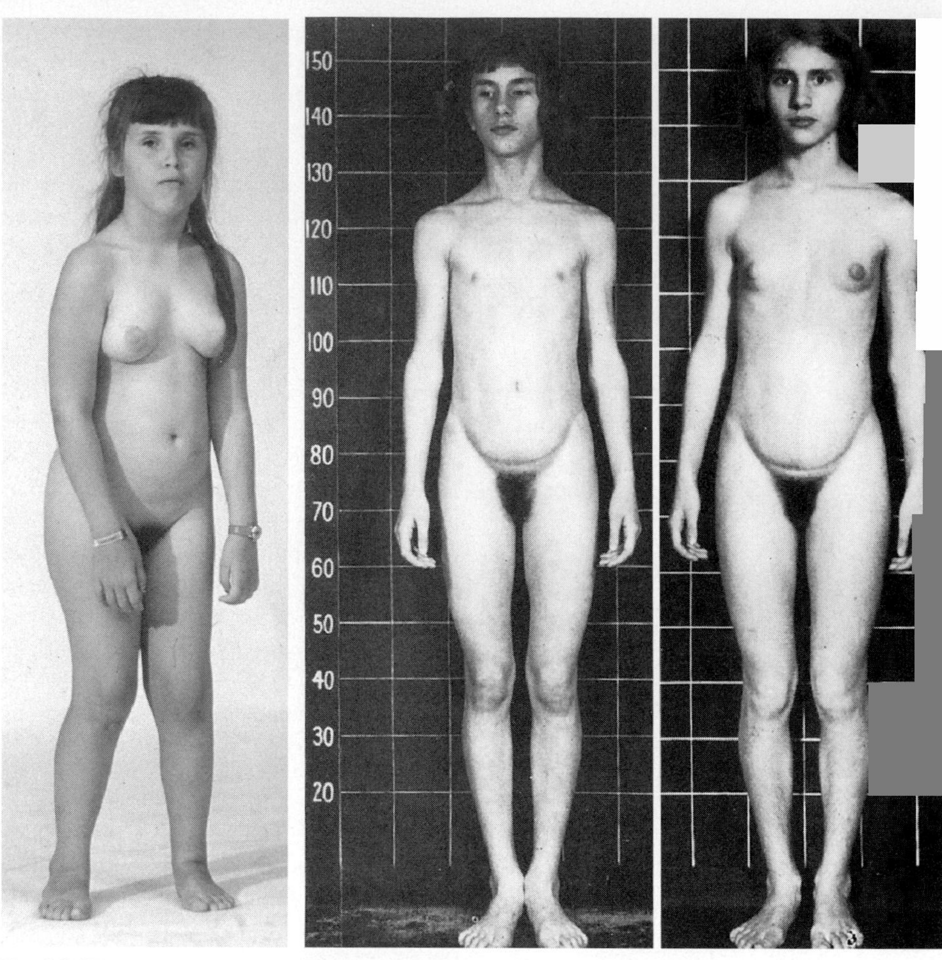

Fig. 23.17 Fig. 23.18 Left Fig. 23.18 Right

Figure 23.17 A $7\frac{1}{2}$-year-old girl with Tanner stage 4 pubertal development who began menstruating 1 month earlier. She was 57 inches tall (above the ninety-fifth percentile). Luteinizing hormone and follicle-stimulating hormone levels were consistent with her development. A large neoplasm that proved to be a hypothalamic hamartoma was present on computed tomography scan. Pubertal development began at about 5 years of age.

Figure 23.18 Left: A $10\frac{1}{2}$-year-old girl with 21-hydroxylase deficiency before treatment. 17-Ketosteroid (KS) excretion was 34 mg/day. **Right: The same patient after 9 months of therapy with cortisone** (17-KS excretion: 4.6 mg/day). (From **Wilkins L.** *The diagnosis and treatment of endocrine disorders in childhood and adolescence.* 3rd ed. Springfield, IL: Charles C. Thomas, 1965:439, with permission.)

for the autonomous hyperfunction of the endocrine glands and, presumably, for the other defects present in this disorder (57). Exposure to exogenous estrogens can mimic gonadotropin-independent precocious puberty. Ingestion of oral contraceptives, other estrogen-containing pharmaceutical agents, and estrogen-contaminated foods and the topical use of estrogens have been implicated in cases of precocious development in infants and children. Severe primary hypothyroidism has also been associated with sexual precocity; associated hyperprolactinemia may result in galactorrhea in affected individuals.

Congenital Adrenal Hyperplasia

Heterosexual precocious puberty is always of peripheral origin and is most often caused by CAH. Three adrenal enzyme defects—21-hydroxylase deficiency, 11β-

hydroxylase deficiency, and 3β-hydroxysteroid dehydrogenase deficiency—can lead not only to heterosexual precocity but also to virilization of the external genitalia because of increased androgen production beginning *in utero* (58). The clinical presentation of the various forms of CAH depend on (a) the affected enzyme, (b) the extent of residual enzymatic activity, and (c) the physiologic consequences of deficiencies in the end products and excesses of precursor steroids.

21-Hydroxylase Deficiency **Most patients with classic CAH have 21-hydroxylase deficiency** (Fig. 23.18). Neonatal screening suggests an incidence of about 1 in 15,000 births. This disorder is inherited as an autosomal recessive trait closely linked to the human leukocyte antigen (HLA) major histocompatibility complex on the short arm of chromosome 6. Thus, siblings with 21-hydroxylase deficiency usually have identical HLA types. There are various forms of 21-hydroxylase deficiency, including simple virilizing or classic (typically identified at birth because of genital ambiguity), salt-wasting (in which there is impairment of mineralocorticoid as well as glucocorticoid secretion), and late-onset or nonclassic (in which heterosexual development occurs at the expected age of puberty). All types involve alleles at the same locus. The nonclassic form is discussed in the following section on heterosexual pubertal development.

Deficiency of 21-hydroxylase results in the impairment of the conversion of 17α-hydroxyprogesterone to 11-deoxycortisol and of progesterone to deoxycorticosterone (Fig. 23.19). As a consequence, precursors accumulate, and there is increased conversion to adrenal androgens. Because the development of the external genitalia is controlled by androgens, in the classic form of this disorder, girls are born with ambiguous genitalia, including an enlarged clitoris, fusion of the labioscrotal folds, and the urogenital sinus. The internal female organs (including the uterus, fallopian tubes, and ovaries) develop normally because they are not affected by the increased androgen levels. Almost two thirds of affected newborns rapidly develop salt-wasting 21-hydroxylase deficiency, hyponatremia, hyperkalemia, and hypotension. During childhood, untreated girls with either the classic or salt-wasting form grow rapidly but have advanced bone ages, enter puberty early, experience early closure of their epiphyses, and ultimately are short in stature as adults. CAH, with appropriate therapy, is the only inherited disorder of sexual differentiation in which normal pregnancy and childbearing are possible. The classic and salt-wasting forms of 21-hydroxylase deficiency are easily diagnosed based on the presence of genital ambiguity and markedly elevated levels of 17α-hydroxyprogesterone. Some states have initiated neonatal screening programs to detect 21-hydroxylase deficiency at birth.

3β-Hydroxysteroid Dehydrogenase Deficiency of 3β-hydroxysteroid dehydrogenase (3β-HSD) affects the synthesis of glucocorticoids, mineralocorticoids, and sex steroids. Typically, levels of 17-hydroxypregnenolone and DHEA are elevated (Fig. 23.19). The classic form of the disorder, detectable at birth, is quite rare, and affected girls may be masculinized only slightly. In severe cases, salt-wasting may also be present.

A nonclassic form of this disorder may be associated with heterosexual precocious pubertal development (as is the classic form if untreated), but postpubertal hyperandrogenism occurs more often. The androgen excess in individuals with nonclassic 3β-HSD deficiency appears to result from androgens derived from the peripheral conversion of increased serum concentrations of DHEA. This disorder is inherited in autosomal recessive fashion, with allelism at the *3β-HSD* gene on chromosome 1 believed to be responsible for the varying degrees of enzyme deficiency.

11-Hydroxylase Deficiency The classic form of 11-hydroxylase deficiency is believed to constitute 5% to 8% of all cases of CAH. Deficiency in 11-hydroxylase results in the ability to convert 11-deoxycortisol to cortisol, resulting in the accumulation of androgen precursors (Fig. 23.19). Markedly elevated levels of 11-deoxycortisol and deoxycorticosterone are present in the disorder. Because deoxycorticosterone acts as a mineralocorticoid,

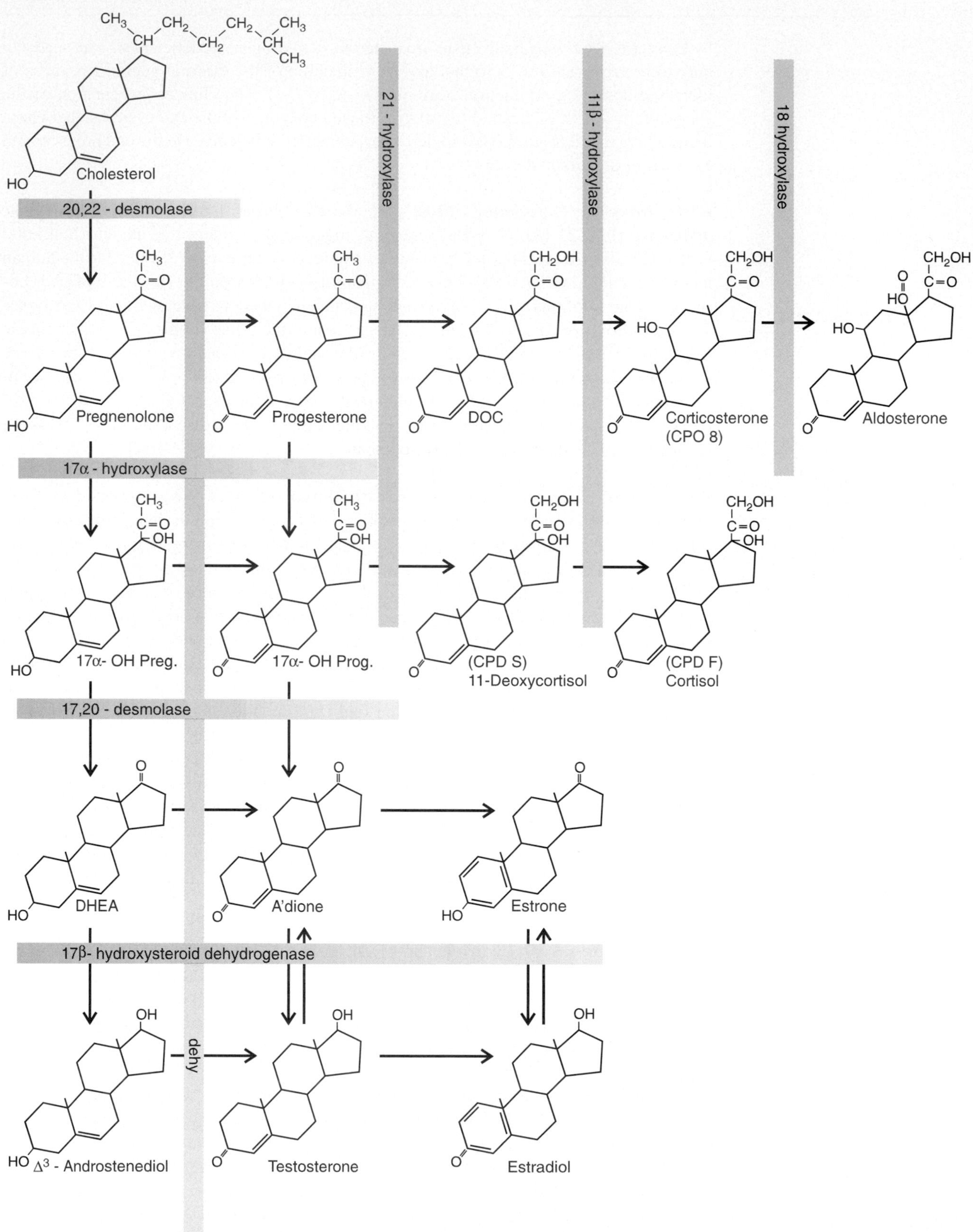

Figure 23.19 Gonadal and adrenal steroid pathways and the enzymes required for steroid conversion. (From **Rebar RW, Kenigsberg D, Hodgen GD.** The normal menstrual cycle and the control of ovulation. In: **Becker KL,** ed. *Principles and practice of endocrinology and metabolism.* 2nd ed. Philadelphia: JB Lippincott, 1995:868–880, with permission.)

many individuals with this disorder become hypertensive. A mild nonclassic form of 11-hydroxylase deficiency has been reported but apparently is very uncommon.

Treatment of Congenital Adrenal Hyperplasia **The treatment of CAH involves providing replacement doses of the deficient steroid hormones.** *Hydrocortisone* (10 to 20 mg/m^2 body surface area) or its equivalent is given daily in divided doses to suppress the elevated levels of pituitary corticotropin present and thus suppress the elevated androgen levels. With such treatment, signs of androgen excess should regress. In children, growth velocity and bone age should be monitored carefully because both overreplacement and underreplacement can result in premature closure of the epiphyses and short stature. Data now indicate that early diagnosis and compliance with therapy lead to adult height within 1 standard deviation of the anticipated target height in girls with 21-hydroxylase deficiency (59).

Mineralocorticoid replacement is generally required in individuals with 21-hydroxylase deficiency whether or not they are salt-losing. The intent of glucocorticoid therapy should be to suppress morning 17α-hydroxyprogesterone levels to between 300 and 900 ng/dL. Sufficient *fluorocortisone* should be given daily to suppress plasma renin activity to less than 5 mg/mL per hour. Girls with ambiguous genitalia may require reconstructive surgery, including clitoral recession and vaginoplasty. Timing of such surgery is debated, but the girl must be of appropriate size to permit the surgery to be as simple as possible.

Heterosexual Pubertal Development

The most common cause of heterosexual development at the expected age of puberty is polycystic ovarian syndrome (PCO) (Fig. 23.20). Because the syndrome is heterogeneous and poorly defined, clinical difficulties result in diagnosis and management (60). For the sake of simplicity, **PCO may be defined as LH-dependent hyperandrogenism** (61). Most clinical manifestations arise as a consequence of the hyperandrogenism and often include hirsutism beginning at or near puberty and irregular menses from the age of menarche because of oligoovulation or anovulation. Clinical manifestations are as follows:

1. Affected girls may be but are not necessarily somewhat overweight.
2. In rare instances, menarche may be delayed, and primary amenorrhea also may occur.
3. Basal levels of LH tend to be elevated in most affected individuals, and androgen production is invariably increased, even though circulating levels of androgens may be near the upper limits of the normal range in many affected women.
4. In anovulatory women, estrone levels are typically greater than estradiol levels.
5. Because circulating levels of estrogens are not diminished in PCO and androgen levels are only mildly elevated, affected girls become both feminized and masculinized at puberty. This is an important feature because girls with classic forms of CAH who do not experience precocious puberty (and even those who do) only become masculinized at puberty (i.e., they do not develop breasts).
6. Some degree of insulin resistance may be present, even in the absence of overt glucose intolerance (62).

Differential Diagnosis and Evaluation

Distinguishing PCO from the nonclassic forms of CAH is problematic and controversial (63,64). The evaluation is as follows:

1. Some clinicians advocate measurement of 17α-hydroxyprogesterone in all women who develop hirsutism. Although values of 17α-hydroxyprogesterone are

commonly elevated more than 100-fold in individuals with classic 21-hydroxylase deficiency, they may or may not be elevated in nonclassic late-onset forms of the disorder.

2. Measurement of 17α-hydroxyprogesterone also can identify women with various forms of 11-hydroxylase deficiency.

3. Basal levels of DHEAS as well as 17α-hydroxyprogesterone may be moderately elevated in patients with PCO, making the diagnosis even more difficult.

4. To screen for CAH, 17α-hydroxyprogesterone should be measured in early morning.

5. In women with regular cyclic menses, it is important to measure 17α-hydroxyprogesterone only in the follicular phase because basal levels increase at midcycle and in the luteal phase.

Measurements of 17α-hydroxyprogesterone appear to be of value in populations at high risk for nonclassic late-onset 21-hydroxylase deficiency. In the white population, the gene occurs in only about 1 in 1,000 individuals, but it occurs in 1 in 27 Ashkenazi Jews, 1 in 40 Hispanics, 1 in 50 Yugoslavs, and 1 in 300 Italians (58). The incidence is also increased among Eskimos and French Canadians. Alternatively, screening might be restricted to hirsute teenagers presenting with the more "typical" features of nonclassic 21-hydroxylase deficiency, including severe hirsutism beginning at puberty, "flattening" of the breasts (i.e., defeminization), shorter stature than other family members, and increased DHEAS levels (between 5,000 and 7,000 ng/mL). Women with a strong family history of hirsutism or hypertension might be screened as well (35) (Fig. 23.21).

Figure 23.20 Typical appearance of a young 21-year-old woman with polycystic ovarian syndrome. The patient is well feminized but has apparent hirsutism on her face **(A)** and on her torso **(B)**.

Figure 23.21 A 19-year-old girl with secondary amenorrhea and severe acne and hirsutism beginning at the normal age of puberty. Stimulatory testing with corticotropin documented nonclassic 21-hydroxylase deficiency. Flattening of the breasts is apparent. She was shorter than her one sister and her mother.

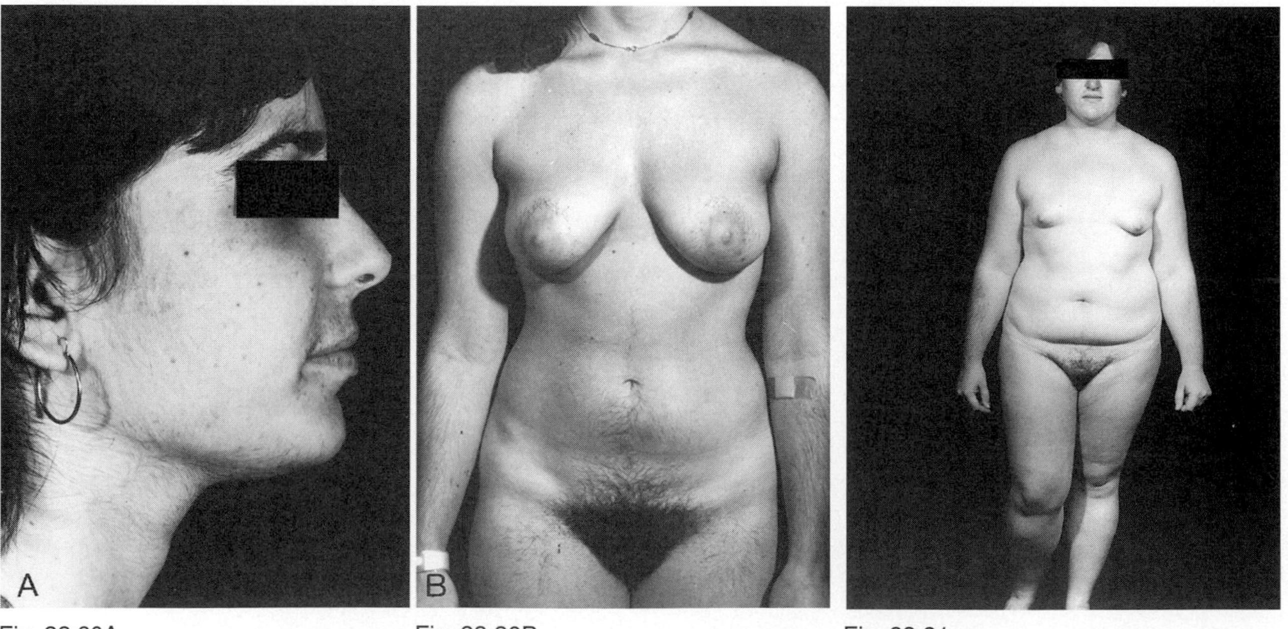

Fig. 23.20A Fig. 23.20B Fig. 23.21

Basal Levels of 17-Hydroxyprogesterone **Basal levels of 17α-hydroxyprogesterone higher than 800 ng/dL are virtually diagnostic of CAH. Levels between 300 and 800 ng/dL require stimulatory testing with corticotropin to distinguish between PCO and CAH. To complicate the situation even further, nonclassic 21-hydroxylase deficiency may occur even when basal levels of 17α-hydroxyprogesterone are below 300 ng/dL, thus requiring stimulatory testing in those cases as well.**

Cosyntropin Stimulation Test The most commonly used stimulatory test involves measurement of 17α-hydroxyprogesterone 30 minutes after administration of a bolus of 250 mg of synthetic cosyntropin (Cortrosyn) (65). In normal women, this value seldom exceeds 400 ng/dL. Patients with classic 21-hydroxylase deficiency achieve peak levels of 3,000 ng/dL or higher. Patients with nonclassic 21-hydroxylase deficiency commonly achieve levels of 1,500 ng/dL or more. Heterozygous carriers achieve peak levels up to about 1,000 ng/dL. In hirsute women with hypertension, 11-deoxycortisol levels can be determined during the test. If both 11-deoxycortisol and 17α-hydroxyprogesterone levels are increased, the rare 11-hydroxylase deficiency is present. Only measurements of several steroid precursors after corticotropin stimulation can identify individuals with nonclassic forms of 3β-HSD deficiency.

The elevated levels of 17α-hydroxyprogesterone present in all forms of 21-hydroxylase deficiency are rapidly suppressed by administration of exogenous corticoids. Even a single dose of a glucocorticoid such as dexamethasone will suppress 17α-hydroxyprogesterone in CAH but not in virilizing ovarian and adrenal neoplasms.

Hirsutism It has been suggested that androgen-receptor blockade may be preferable to glucocorticoids as primary treatment of nonclassic 21-hydroxylase deficiency (66). Although menses usually (but not always) become regular shortly after beginning therapy with glucocorticoids, the hirsutism in this disorder has proved to be remarkably refractory to glucocorticoids.

Distinguishing nonclassic forms of CAH from idiopathic hirsutism also may be problematic. Individuals with idiopathic hirsutism have regular ovulatory menses, thus effectively eliminating PCO from consideration. Confusion can be created by the fact that some women with nonclassic CAH may continue to ovulate. Basal levels of 17α-hydroxyprogesterone are normal in idiopathic hirsutism, as is the response to ACTH stimulation. Idiopathic hirsutism represents enhanced androgen action at the hair follicle (67).

Mixed Gonadal Dysgenesis

The term *mixed gonadal dysgenesis* is used to designate those individuals with asymmetric gonadal development, with a germ cell tumor or a testis on one side and an undifferentiated streak, rudimentary gonad, or no gonad on the other side. Most individuals with this rare disorder have a mosaic karyotype of 45X/46XY and are raised as females who then virilize at puberty. Gonadectomy is indicated to remove the source of androgens and eliminate any risk for neoplasia.

Reifenstein's Syndrome

Individuals who have rare forms of male pseudohermaphroditism, especially 5α-reductase deficiency (the so-called "penis at 12" syndrome) and the Reifenstein's syndrome, generally have ambiguous female genitalia with variable virilization at puberty. Cushing syndrome, too, may occur rarely during the pubertal years, as may adrenal or ovarian androgen-secreting neoplasms.

Genital Ambiguity at Birth

Because of the concerns of the parents and the need to prevent life-threatening complications, the infant with genital ambiguity should be evaluated promptly. Evaluation and treatment is best conducted by a team of physicians. The initial evaluation is as follows:

1. Cytogenetic and endocrine studies should be initiated promptly. Use of specific probes for the Y chromosome and fluorescent *in situ* hybridization can assist in obtaining a karyotype within 48 hours. Probes for many specific inherited disorders are now available.

2. To exclude CAH, the most common cause of genital ambiguity, serum levels of sodium, potassium, and 17α-hydroxyprogesterone and urinary excretion of 17-ketosteroids, pregnanetriol, and tetrahydrodeoxycortisol should be measured. Infants should be monitored closely to prevent development of dehydration, hyponatremia, and hyperkalemia.

3. It has been suggested that antimüllerian hormone be measured in infants with genital ambiguity because it is elevated in males and undetectable in females in the first several years of life (68).

Physical Signs

During the 3 to 4 days required for evaluation, it is important to be supportive of the parents. Many clinicians believe that it is important not to attach any unusual significance to the genital ambiguity and to treat the abnormality as just another "birth defect." Physicians should emphasize that the child should undergo normal psychosexual development regardless of the sex-of-rearing selected. Either a name compatible with either sex should be chosen or the naming of the infant should be delayed until the studies have been completed.

Although the diagnosis is not usually obvious on examination, there are some helpful distinguishing features (Fig. 23.22). In normal males, there is only a single midline frenulum on the ventral side of the phallus; in normal females, there are two frenula lateral to the midline. A female with clitoral enlargement still has two frenula, and a male with hypospadias has a single midline frenulum or several irregular fibrous bands (chordee).

It is important to determine whether any müllerian derivatives are present. Recent studies suggest that MRI may be the most effective way of evaluating the infant for the presence of müllerian tissue (69).

The location or consistency of the gonad may be helpful in deducing its composition. A gonad located in the labial or inguinal regions almost always contains testicular tissue. A testis is generally softer than an ovary or a streak gonad and is more apt to be surrounded by blood vessels imparting a reddish cast. An ovary is more often white, fibrous, and convoluted. A gonad that varies in consistency may be an ovotestis or a testis or a streak gonad that has undergone neoplastic transformation. If a well-differentiated fallopian tube is absent on only one side, the side without the tube probably contains a testis or ovotestis.

Diagnosis and Management

Although genital ambiguity is usually identified at birth, it may not be recognized for several years. Questions about changing the sex-of-rearing may arise. It has been believed that sex-of-rearing may be changed before 2 years of age without psychologically damaging the child, but experience with individuals with 5α-reductase deficiency suggests that gender changes may be made after 2 years of age in certain instances (70). In any case, surgery for genital ambiguity to make the external genitalia (and development) as compatible with the sex-of-rearing of the child is warranted but has not always been proved successful. Clitoral recession and clitorectomy are the most frequently performed surgical procedures.

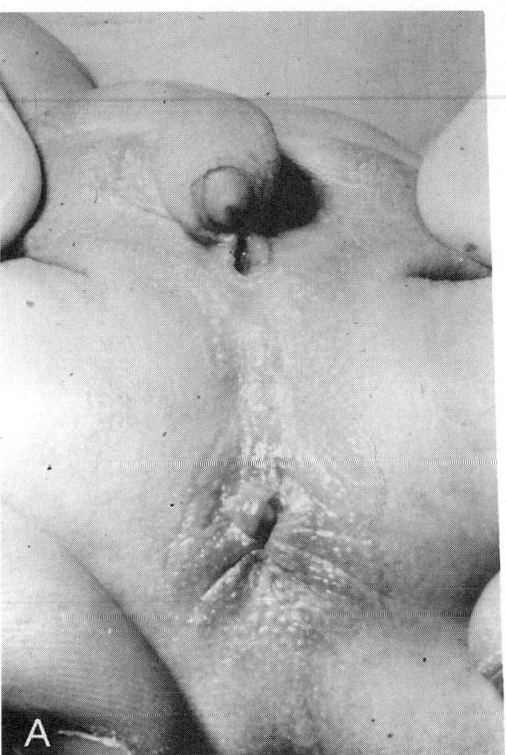

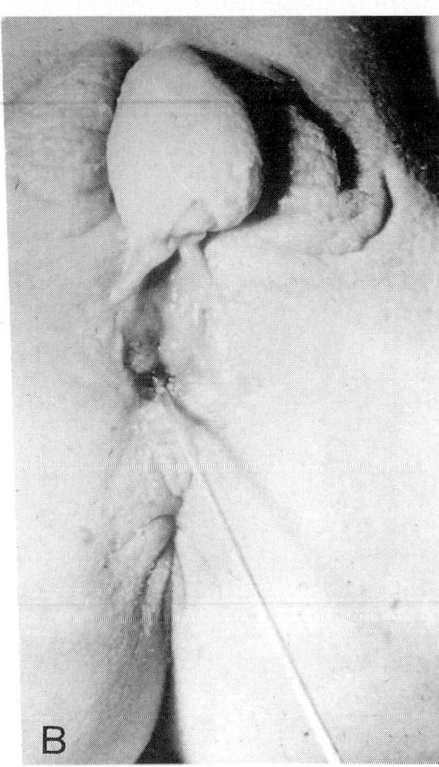

Figure 23.22 Two newborn girls with 46XX karyotypes and genital ambiguity. Both had clitoral hypertrophy, paired frenula, so-called scrotalization of the labia, and a common urogenital sinus (shown by the probe in **B**). Both were shown to have 21-hydroxylase deficiency. (From **Rebar RW.** Normal and abnormal sexual differentiation and pubertal development. In: **Moore TR, Reiter RC, Rebar RW, et al,** eds. *Gynecology and obstetrics: a longitudinal approach.* New York: Churchill Livingstone, 1993:97–133, with permission.)

It is possible to diagnose prenatally 21-hydroxylase deficiency in patients known to be at risk (58). The diagnosis is established by documenting elevated levels of 17α-hydroxyprogesterone or 21-deoxycortisol in amniotic fluid. Genetic diagnosis using specific probes and cells obtained by chorionic villus sampling or amniocentesis is also possible. Unfortunately, prenatal treatment of the fetus by administering dexamethasone to the mother is usually but not always successful in preventing genital ambiguity (71). Moreover, maternal complications, including hypertension, massive weight gain, and overt Cushing's syndrome, have been noted in about 1% of pregnancies in which the mothers are given low doses of dexamethasone. Despite the risks and the nonuniformity of beneficial outcome to affected female fetuses, many parents may choose prenatal medical treatment because of the psychological impact of ambiguous genitalia.

Teratogens

It is important to recognize that ambiguous genitalia can result from the maternal ingestion of various teratogens, most of which are synthetic steroids (Table 23.3). Exposure to the teratogen must occur early in pregnancy, during genital organogenesis. Moreover, not all exposed fetuses manifest the same anomalies or even the presence of any anomalies. In principle, most synthetic steroids with androgenic properties, including weakly androgenic progestins, can affect female genital differentiation. However, the doses required to produce genital ambiguity are generally so great that the concern is only theoretical. The one agent that clearly can lead to genital ambiguity when ingested in clinically used quantities is danazol. There is no evidence that inadvertent ingestion of oral contraceptives, which contain relatively low doses of either mestranol or ethinyl estradiol and a 19-nor-steroid, results in virilization (72,73).

Table 23.3. Androgens and Progestogens Potentially Capable of Producing Genital Ambiguity[a]

Proved	No Effect	Insufficient Data
Testosterone enanthate	Progesterone	Ethynodiol diacetate
Testosterone propionate	17α-Hydroxyprogesterone	Dimethisterone
Methylandrostenediol	Medroxyprogesterone	Norgestrel
6α-Methyltestosterone	Norethynodrel	Desogestrel
Ethisterone		Gestodene
Norethindrone		Norgestimate
Danazol		

[a] Those agents proved to cause genital ambiguity do so only when administered in relatively high doses. Insufficient data exist regarding effects of dimethisterone and norgestrel. In low doses (e.g., as in oral contraceptives), progestins, even including norethindrone, seem unlikely to virilize a female fetus.

References

1. **Tanner JM.** *Growth at adolescence.* 2nd ed. Oxford, UK: Blackwell Scientific Publications, 1962.
2. **Zacharias L, Wurtman RJ.** Blindness: its relation to age of menarche. *Science* 1964;144:1154–1155.
3. **Kaplowitz PB, Oberfield SE,** for the Drug and Therapeutics and Executive Committees of the Lawson Wilkins Pediatric Endocrine Society. Reexamination of the age limit for defining when puberty is precocious in girls in the United States: implications for evaluation and treatment. *Pediatrics* 1999;104:936–941.
4. **Frisch RE.** Body fat, menarche, and reproductive ability. *Semin Reprod Endocrinol* 1985;3:45–49.
5. **Maclure M, Travis LB, Willett W, et al.** A prospective cohort study of nutrient intake and age at menarche. *Am J Clin Nutr* 1991;54:649–656.
6. **deRidder CM, Thijssen JHH, Bruning PF, et al.** Body fat mass, body fat distribution, and pubertal development: a longitudinal study of physical and hormonal sexual maturation of girls. *J Clin Endocrinol Metab* 1992;75:442–446.
7. **Marshall WA, Tanner JM.** Variations in patterns of pubertal changes in girls. *Arch Dis Child* 1969;44: 291–303.
8. **Greulich WW, Pyle SI.** *Radiographic atlas of skeletal development of the hand and wrist.* 2nd ed. London: Oxford University Press, 1959.
9. **Bayley N, Pinneau SR.** Tables for predicting adult height from skeletal age: revised for use with the Greulich-Pyle hand standards. *J Pediatr* 1952;40:423–441.
10. **Kaplan SL, Grumbach MM, Aubert ML.** The ontogeny of pituitary hormones and hypothalamic factors in the human fetus: maturation of central nervous system regulation of anterior pituitary function. *Recent Prog Horm Res* 1976;32:161–243.
11. **Conte FA, Grumbach MM, Kaplan SL.** A diphasic pattern of gonadotropin secretion in patients with the syndrome of gonadal dysgenesis. *J Clin Endocrinol Metab* 1975;40:670–674.
12. **Boyar RM, Finkelstein JW, Roffwarg HP, et al.** Synchronization of augmented luteinizing hormone secretion with sleep during puberty. *N Engl J Med* 1972;287:582–586.
13. **Boyar RM, Rosenfeld RS, Kapen S, et al.** Simultaneous augmented secretion of luteinizing hormone and testosterone during sleep. *J Clin Invest* 1974;54:609–618.
14. **Boyar RM, Wu RHK, Roffwarg H, et al.** Human puberty: 24-hour estradiol patterns in pubertal girls. *J Clin Endocrinol Metab* 1976;43:1418–1421.
15. **Grumbach MM.** The neuroendocrinology of puberty. In: **Krieger DT, Hughes JC,** eds. Neuroendocrinology. Sunderland, MA: Sinauer Associates, 1980:249–258.
16. **Penny R, Olambiwonnu NO, Frasier SD.** Episodic fluctuations of serum gonadotropins in pre- and postpubertal girls and boys. *J Clin Endocrinol Metab* 1977;45:307–311.
17. **Korth-Schutz S, Levine LS, New MI.** Serum androgens in normal prepubertal and pubertal children and in children with precocious adrenarche. *J Clin Endocrinol Metab* 1976;42:117–124.
18. **Ducharme J-R, Forest MG, DePeretti E, et al.** Plasma adrenal and gonadal sex steroids in human pubertal development. *J Clin Endocrinol Metab* 1976;42:468–476.
19. **Lee PA, Xenakis T, Winer J, et al.** Puberty in girls: correlation of serum levels of gonadotropins, prolactin, androgens, estrogens and progestin with physical changes. *J Clin Endocrinol Metab* 1976;43:775–784.

20. **Judd HL, Parker DC, Siler TM, et al.** The nocturnal rise of plasma testosterone in pubertal boys. *J Clin Endocrinol Metab* 1974;38:710–713.

21. **Grumbach MM, Kaplan SL.** The neuroendocrinology of human puberty: an ontogenetic perspective. In: **Grumbach MM, Sizonenko PC, Aubert ML,** eds. *Control of the onset of puberty.* Baltimore: Williams & Wilkins, 1990:1–62.

22. **Rosenfield RL.** Current age of onset of puberty. *Pediatrics* 2000;105:622.

23. **Buttram VC Jr, Gibbons WE.** Müllerian anomalies: a proposed classification (an analysis of 144 cases). *Fertil Steril* 1979;32:40–46.

24. **Smith FR.** The significance of incomplete fusion of the müllerian ducts in pregnancy and parturition with a report on 35 cases. *Am J Obstet Gynecol* 1931;22:714–728.

25. **Herbst AL, Hubby MM, Azizi F, et al.** Reproductive and gynecological surgical experience in diethylstilbestrol-exposed daughters. *Am J Obstet Gynecol* 1981;141:1019–1028.

26. **Simpson JL.** Genetics of the female reproductive ducts. *Am J Med Genet* 1999;89:224–239.

27. **Taylor HS.** The role of HOX genes in the development and function of the female reproductive tract. *Semin Reprod Med* 2000;18:81–89.

28. **Buttram VC Jr, Reiter RC.** *Surgical treatment of the infertile female.* Baltimore: Williams & Wilkins, 1985:89.

29. **Pellerito JS, McCarthy SM, Doyle MB, et al.** Diagnosis of uterine anomalies: relative accuracy of MR imaging, endovaginal sonography, and hysterosalpingography. *Radiology* 1992;183:795–800.

30. **Simpson JL.** Localizing ovarian determinants through phenotypic-karyotypic deductions: progress and pitfalls. In: **Rosenfield R, Grumbach M,** eds. *Turner syndrome.* New York: Marcel Dekker, 1990:65–77.

31. **Simpson JL, Photopulos G.** The relationship of neoplasia to disorders of abnormal sexual differentiation. *Birth Defects* 1976;12:15–60.

32. **Manuel M, Katayama KP, Jones HW Jr.** The age of occurrence of gonadal tumors in intersex patients with a Y chromosome. *Am J Obstet Gynecol* 1976;124:293–300.

33. **Rosenfeld RG, Frane J, Attie KM, et al.** Six-year results of a randomized prospective trial of human growth hormone and oxandrolone in Turner syndrome. *J Pediatr* 1992;121:49–55.

34. **Rebar RW, Cedars MI.** Hypergonadotropic amenorrhea. In: **Filicori M, Flamigni C,** eds. *Ovulation induction: basic science and clinical advances.* Amsterdam: Elsevier Science B.V., 1994:115–121.

35. **Kustin J, Rebar RW.** Hirsutism in young adolescent girls. *Pediatr Ann* 1986;15:522.

36. **Achermann JC, Jameson JL.** Advances in the molecular genetics of hypogonadotropic hypogonadism. *J Pediatr Endocrinol Metab* 2001;14:3–15.

37. **Seminara SB, Oliveira LM, Beranova M, et al.** Genetics of hypogonadotropic hypogonadism. *J Endocrinol Invest* 2000;23:560–565.

38. **Kallmann FJ, Schoenfeld WA, Barrera SE.** The genetic aspects of primary eunuchoidism. *Am J Ment Defic* 1944;48:203–236.

39. **Schwanzel-Fukuda M, Jorgenson KL, Bergen HT, et al.** Biology of normal luteinizing hormone-releasing hormone neurons during and after their migration from olfactory placode. *Endocr Rev* 1992;13:623–634.

40. **Crowley WF Jr, Jameson JL.** Clinical counterpoint: gonadotropin-releasing hormone deficiency: perspectives from clinical investigation. *Endocr Rev* 1992;13:635–640.

41. **Oliveira LMB, Seminara SB, Beranova M, et al.** The importance of autosomal genes in Kallmann syndrome: genotype-phenotype correlations and neuroendocrine characteristics. *J Clin Endocrinol Metab* 2001;86: 1532–1538.

42. **Henek M, Wevrick R.** The role of genomic imprinting in human developmental disorders: lessons from Prader-Willi syndrome. *Clin Genet* 2001;59:156–164.

43. **Beales PL, Warner AM, Hitman GA, et al.** Bardet-Biedl syndrome: a molecular and phenotypic study of 18 families. *J Med Genet* 1997;34:92–98.

44. **Tomlinson JN, Holden N, Hills RK, et al.** Association between premature mortality and hypopituitarism. West Midlands Prospective Hypopituitary Study Group. *Lancet* 2001;357:425–431.

45. **Vance ML.** Hypopituitarism. *N Engl J Med* 1994;330:1651–1662.

46. **Braunstein GD, Whitaker JN, Kohler PO.** Cerebellar dysfunction in Hand-Schüller-Christian disease. *Arch Intern Med* 1973;132:387–390.

47. **Spitzer R.** *Diagnostic and statistical manual of mental disorders.* 4th ed. Washington, DC: American Psychiatric Association, 1994:53.

48. **Vigersky RA, Loriaux DL, Andersen AE, et al.** Anorexia nervosa: behavioral and hypothalamic aspects. *Clin Endocrinol Metab* 1976;5:517–535.

49. **Gold PW, Gwirtsman H, Avgerinos PC, et al.** Abnormal hypothalamic-pituitary-adrenal function in anorexia nervosa: pathophysiologic mechanisms in underweight and weight-corrected patients. *N Engl J Med* 1986;314:1335–1342.

50. **Vigersky RA, Andersen AE, Thompson RH, et al.** Hypothalamic dysfunction in secondary amenorrhea associated with simple weight loss. *N Engl J Med* 1977;297:1141–1145.

51. **Morris JM.** The syndrome of testicular feminization in male pseudohermaphrodites. *Am J Obstet Gynecol* 1953;65:1192.

52. **Griffin JE.** Androgen resistance the clinical and molecular spectrum. *N Engl J Med* 1992;326:611–618.

53. **Gottlieb B, Pinsky L, Beitel LK, et al.** Androgen insensitivity. *Am J Med Genet* 1999;89:210–217.

54. **Mahachoklertwattana P, Kaplan SL, Grumbach MM.** The luteinizing hormone-releasing hormone-secreting hypothalamic hamartoma is a congenital malformation: natural history. *J Clin Endocrinol Metab* 1993;77:118–124.

55. **Lyon AJ, DeBruyn R, Grant DB.** Transient sexual precocity and ovarian cysts. *Arch Dis Child* 1985;60: 819–822.

56. **Ein SH, Darte JM, Stephens CA.** Cystic and solid ovarian tumors in children: a 44-year review. *J Pediatr Surg* 1970;5:148–156.

57. **Weinstein LS, Shenker A, Gejman PV, et al.** Activating mutations of the stimulatory G protein in the McCune-Albright syndrome. *N Engl J Med* 1991;325:1688–1695.

58. **Speiser PW.** Congenital adrenal hyperplasia. In: **Becker KL,** ed. *Principles and practice of endocrinology and metabolism.* 2nd ed. Philadelphia: JB Lippincott, 1995:686–695.

59. **Engster EA, Dimeglio LA, Wright JC, et al.** Height outcome in congenital adrenal hyperplasia caused by 21-hydroxylase deficiency: a meta-analysis. *J Pediatr* 2001;138:3–5.

60. **Futterweit W.** Pathophysiology of polycystic ovarian syndrome. In: **Redmond GP,** ed. *Androgenic disorders.* New York: Raven Press, 1995:77–166.

61. **Rebar RW.** Disorders of menstruation, ovulation, and sexual response. In: **Becker KL,** ed. *Principles and practice of endocrinology and metabolism.* 2nd ed. Philadelphia: JB Lippincott, 1995:880–899.

62. **Lewy, VD, Danadian K, Witchel SF, et al.** Early metabolic abnormalities in adolescent girls with polycystic ovarian syndrome. *J Pediatr* 2001;138:38–44.

63. **Lobo RA, Goebelsmann U.** Adult manifestation of congenital hyperplasia due to incomplete 21-hydroxylase deficiency mimicking polycystic ovarian disease. *Am J Obstet Gynecol* 1980;138:720–726.

64. **Chrousos GP, Loriaux DL, Mann DL, et al.** Late-onset 21-hydroxylase deficiency mimicking idiopathic hirsutism or polycystic ovarian disease. *Ann Intern Med* 1982;96:143–148.

65. **New MI, Lorenzen F, Lerner AJ, et al.** Genotyping steroid 21-hydroxylase deficiency: hormonal reference data. *J Clin Endocrinol Metab* 1983;57:320–326.

66. **Spritzer P, Billaud L, Thalabard J-C, et al.** Cyproterone acetate versus hydrocortisone treatment in late-onset adrenal hyperplasia. *J Clin Endocrinol Metab* 1990;70:642–646.

67. **Horton R, Hawks D, Lobo R.** 3a, 17b-Androstanediol glucuronide in plasma: a marker of androgen action in idiopathic hirsutism. *J Clin Invest* 1982;69:1203–1206.

68. **Gustafson ML, Lee MM, Asmundson L, et al.** Müllerian inhibiting substance in the diagnosis and management of intersex and gonadal abnormalities. *J Pediatr Surg* 1993;28:439–444.

69. **Hricak H, Chang YCF, Thurner S.** Vagina: evaluation with MR imaging. I. Normal anatomy and congenital anomalies. *Radiology* 1991;179:593.

70. **Imperato-McGinley J, Guerrero L, Gautier T, et al.** Steroid 5a-reductase deficiency: an inherited form of male pseudohermaphroditism. *Science* 1974;186:1213–1215.

71. **Pang SY, Pollack MS, Marshall RN, et al.** Prenatal treatment of congenital adrenal hyperplasia due to 21-hydroxylase deficiency. *N Engl J Med* 1990;322:111–115.

72. **Schardein JL.** Congenital abnormalities and hormones during pregnancy: a clinical review. *Teratology* 1980;22:251–270.

73. **Bracken MB.** Oral contraception and congenital malformations in offspring: a review and meta-analysis of the prospective studies. *Obstet Gynecol* 1990;76:552–557.

74. **Wilkins L.** *The diagnosis and treatment of endocrine disorders in childhood and adolescence.* 3rd ed. Springfield, IL: Charles C. Thomas, 1965.

75. **Rebar RW.** Practical evaluation of hormonal status. In: **Yen SSC, Jaffe RB,** eds. *Reproductive endocrinology: physiology, pathophysiology and clinical management.* 3rd ed. Philadelphia: WB Saunders, 1991: 830.

76. **Marshall WA, Tanner JM.** Variation in the pattern of pubertal changes in boys. *Arch Dis Child* 1970;45: 13–23.

77. **Ross GT, VandeWiele RL, Frantz AG.** The ovaries and the breasts. In: **Williams RH,** ed. *Textbook of endocrinology.* 6th ed. Philadelphia: WB Saunders, 1981:355.

78. **Emans SJH, Goldstein DP.** The physiology of puberty. In: **Emans SJH, Goldstein DP,** eds. *Pediatric and adolescent gynecology.* 3rd ed. Boston: Little, Brown, 1990:95.

79. **Hamill PVV, Drizd TA, Johnson CL, et al.** Physical growth: National Center for Health Statistics percentiles. *Am J Clin Nutr* 1979;32:607–629.

80. **Rebar RW.** Normal and abnormal sexual differentiation and pubertal development. In: **Moore TR, Reiter RC, Rebar RW, et al,** eds. *Gynecology and obstetrics: a longitudinal approach.* New York: Churchill Livingstone, 1993:97–133.

81. **Spitzer IB, Rebar RW.** Counselling for women with medical problems. Ovary and reproductive organs. In: **Hollingsworth D, Resnik R,** eds. *Medical counselling before pregnancy.* New York: Churchill Livingstone, 1988:213–248.

82. **Simpson JL, Rebar RW.** Normal and abnormal sexual differentiation and development. In: **Becker KL,** ed. *Principles and practice of endocrinology and metabolism.* 2nd ed. Philadelphia: JB Lippincott, 1995:788–822.

83. **Rebar RW, Kenigsberg D, Hodgen GD.** The normal menstrual cycle and the control of ovulation. In: **Becker KL,** ed. *Principles and practice of endocrinology and metabolism.* 2nd ed. Philadelphia: JB Lippincott, 1995:868–880.

84. **Buttram VC Jr, Gibbons WE.** Müllerian anomalies: a proposed classification (an analysis of 144 cases). *Fertil Steril* 1979;32:40–46.

Novak's Gynecology, 13th Edition. Edited by J.S. Berek. Lippincott Williams & Wilkins, Philadelphia © 2002

24 Amenorrhea

Wendy J. Schillings
Howard McClamrock

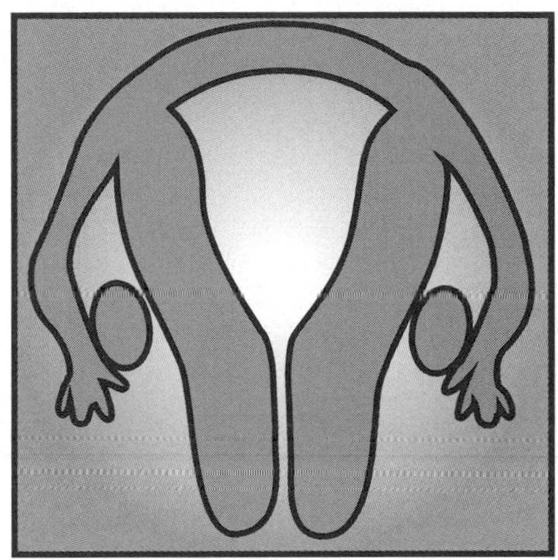

A complex hormonal interaction must take place in order for normal menstruation to occur. The hypothalamus must secrete gonadotropin-releasing hormone (GnRH) in a pulsatile fashion, which is modulated by neurotransmitters and hormones. The GnRH stimulates secretion of follicle-stimulating hormone (FSH) and luteinizing hormone (LH) from the pituitary, which promotes ovarian follicular development and ovulation. A normally functioning ovarian follicle secretes estrogen; after ovulation, the follicle is converted to a corpus luteum and progesterone is secreted in addition to estrogen. These hormones stimulate endometrial development. If pregnancy does not occur, estrogen and progesterone secretion decrease, and withdrawal bleeding begins. If any of the components (hypothalamus, pituitary, ovary, outflow tract, and feedback mechanism) are nonfunctional, bleeding cannot occur.

***Primary amenorrhea* is defined as the absence of menses by 16 years of age in the presence of normal secondary sexual characteristics, or by 14 years of age when there is no visible secondary sexual characteristic development.** The definition represents approximately two standard deviations from the mean age when secondary sexual characteristic development and menstruation should occur. **A woman who has previously menstruated can develop *secondary amenorrhea,* which is defined as absence of menstruation for three normal menstrual cycles or 6 months.**

Patients may develop slight alterations in the hypothalamic–pituitary–ovarian axis that are not severe enough to cause amenorrhea but instead cause anovulation. Anovulatory patients usually have irregular menses and may bleed excessively during menstruation because estrogen is unopposed. This often occurs at the beginning and end of the reproductive years. Luteal phase defect is caused by minimal alterations in the hypothalamic–pituitary–ovarian axis, and patients have regular menses along with infertility or recurrent pregnancy loss. Except for amenorrhea from anatomic and chromosomal etiologies, luteal phase defects and anovulation have causes similar to those of amenorrhea, but the hypothalamic, pituitary, or ovarian hormonal dysfunction is less severe or of shorter duration than with amenorrhea.

In order to detect the cause of amenorrhea, it is useful to determine whether secondary sexual characteristics are present (Fig. 24.1). The absence of secondary sexual characteristics indicates that a woman has never been exposed to estrogen stimulation.

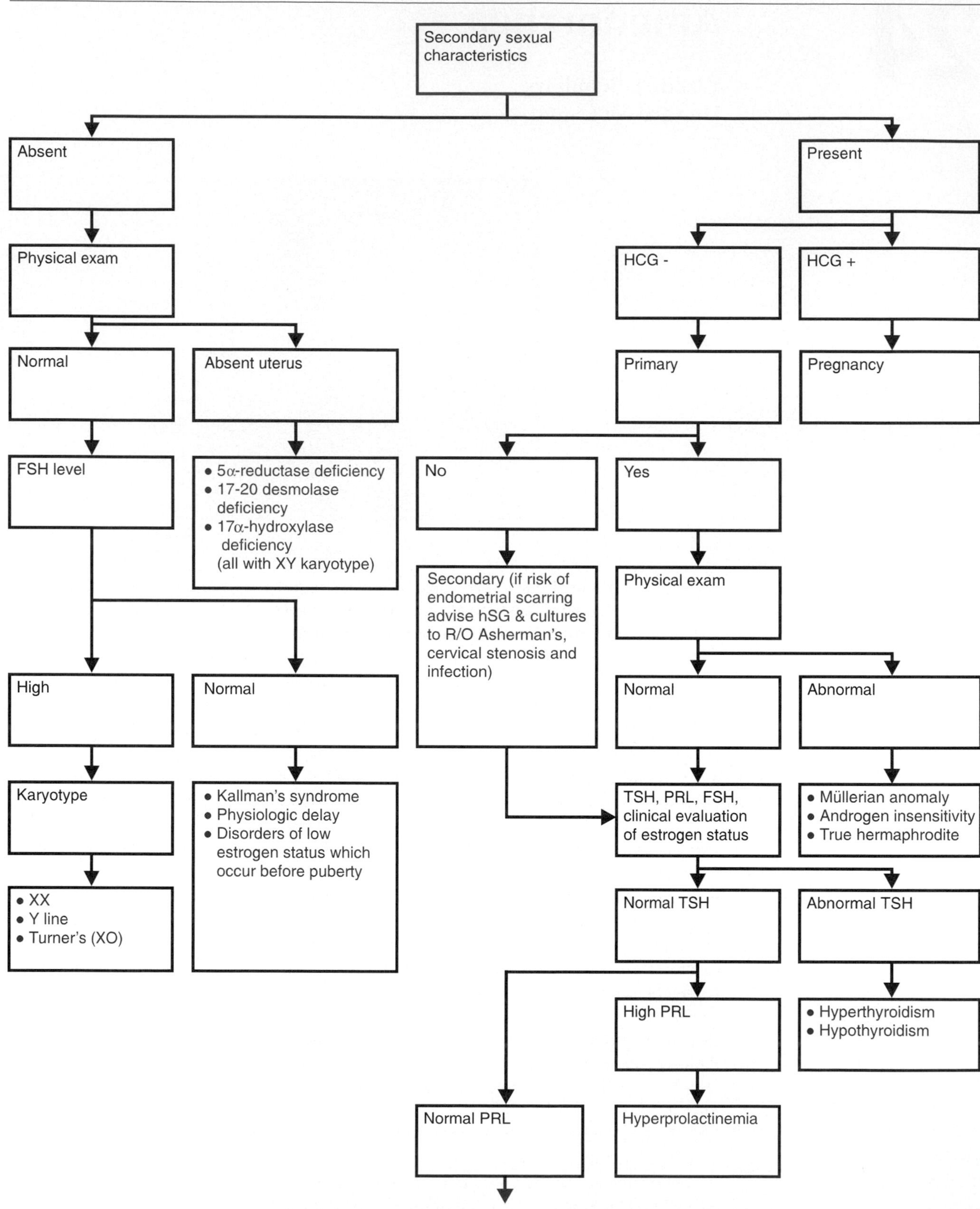

Figure 24.1 Decision tree for evaluation of amenorrhea.

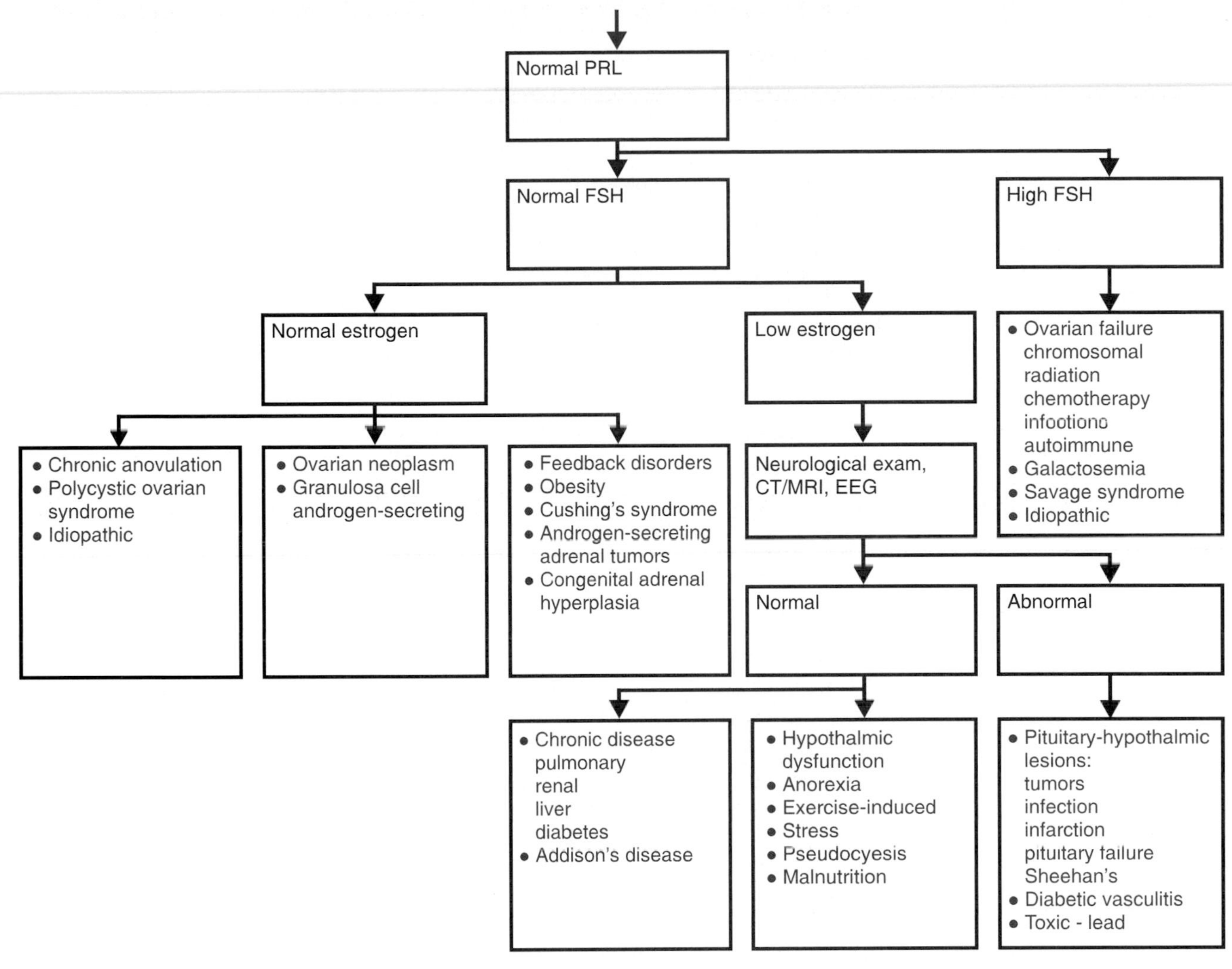

Figure 24.1—*continued*

Amenorrhea without Secondary Sexual Characteristics

Although the diagnosis and treatment of disorders associated with hypogonadism have been discussed in Chapter 23, they will also be mentioned here because these conditions may cause primary amenorrhea. Abnormal findings on physical examination may suggest certain enzyme deficiencies (Fig. 24.1). Because these conditions are very rare, however, it is more clinically relevant to discuss the causes of amenorrhea on the basis of gonadotropin status.

Causes of Primary Amenorrhea

Hypergonadotropic Hypogonadism

Primary gonadal failure and the resulting impaired secretion of gonadal steroids is manifested by elevated levels of LH and FSH that result from decreased negative feedback. Gonadal failure as well as primary amenorrhea are most often associated with genetic abnormalities (Table 24.1). **Approximately 30% of patients with primary amenorrhea have an associated genetic abnormality** (1). **The syndrome of gonadal dysgenesis, or Turner's syndrome, and its variants represent the most common form of hypogonadism**

Table 24.1. Amenorrhea Associated with a Lack of Secondary Sexual Characteristics

Abnormal physical examination
5α-reductase deficiency in XY individual
17, 20-desmolase deficiency in XY individual
17α-hydroxylase deficiency in XY individual
Hypergonadotropic hypogonadism
Gonadal dysgenesis
Pure gonadal dysgenesis
Partial deletion of X chromosome
Sex chromosome mosaicism
Environmental and therapeutic ovarian toxins
17α-hydroxylase deficiency in XX individual
Galactosemia
Other
Hypogonadotropic hypogonadism
Physiologic delay
Kallmann's syndrome
Central nervous system tumors
Hypothalamic/pituitary dysfunction

in women (see Chapter 23). Other disorders associated with primary amenorrhea include structurally abnormal X chromosomes, mosaicism, pure gonadal dysgenesis (46,XX and 46,XY with gonadal streaks), and 17α-hydroxylase deficiency. Individuals with these conditions have gonadal failure and cannot synthesize ovarian steroids. Therefore, gonadotropin levels are elevated because of the lack of negative estrogen feedback on the hypothalamic–pituitary axis. Patients with 17α-hydroxylase deficiency have primordial follicles, but gonadotropin levels are elevated because the enzyme deficiency prevents synthesis of sex steroids. Most patients with these conditions have primary amenorrhea and lack secondary sexual characteristics. Occasionally patients with a partial deletion of the X chromosome, mosaicism, or pure gonadal dysgenesis (46,XX) may synthesize enough estrogen in early puberty to induce breast development and a few episodes of uterine bleeding. Ovulation and, occasionally, pregnancy are possible.

Genetic Disorders

Gonadal Dysgenesis **Turner's syndrome (45,X) is the most common chromosomal abnormality causing gonadal failure and primary amenorrhea** (1,2). Turner's syndrome is discussed in Chapter 23.

Partial Deletions of the X Chromosome Individuals with partial deletions of the X chromosome have the karyotype 46,XX with part of one of the X chromosomes missing. The phenotype is variable, depending on the amount and location of the missing genetic material. Patients with a deletion of part of the long arm of the X chromosome (Xq−) often exhibit sexual infantilism, normal stature, no somatic abnormalities, and streak gonads (3,4). Some patients may be eunuchoid in appearance and have delayed epiphyseal closure. Patients with a deletion of the short arm of the X chromosome (Xp) and patients with isochrome of the long arm of the X chromosome, with or without mosaicism, usually are phenotypically similar to individuals with Turner's syndrome (5).

Mosaicism **Primary amenorrhea is associated with various mosaic states, the most common of which is 45,X/46,XX** (6). As discussed in Chapter 23, the clinical findings in patients with 45,X/47,XXX and 45,X/46,XX/47,XXX are similar to those in 45,X/46,XX and vary in estrogen and gonadotropin production, depending on the number of follicles in the gonads. When compared with the pure 45,X cell line, individuals with 45,X/46,XX are taller and have fewer abnormalities, although 80% of those with 45,X/46,XX mosaics are shorter than their peers and 66% have some somatic abnormalities. **Spontaneous menstruation occurs in approximately 20% of these patients** (6).

Pure Gonadal Dysgenesis **Pure gonadal dysgenesis refers to phenotypically female individuals who have sexual infantilism, primary amenorrhea with normal stature, and no chromosomal abnormalities (46,XX or 46,XY). The gonads are usually streaks, but there may be some development of secondary sexual characteristics as well as a few episodes of uterine bleeding. Mutations in the SRY (sex-determining region gene on the Y chromosome) have been identified in some XY females with gonadal dysgenesis** (7).

Enzyme Deficiencies

Congenital Lipoid Adrenal Hyperplasia **Patients with this autosomal recessive disorder have an inability to convert cholesterol to pregnenolone, which is the first step in steroid hormone biosynthesis.** A defect has not been found in the *P450scc* gene, which is the conversion enzyme responsible for this step in the pathway. Instead, 15 different mutations have been identified in the steroidogenic acute regulatory protein that facilitates the transport of cholesterol from the outer to the inner mitochondrial membrane. This protein appears to be the rate-limiting step for steroid hormone biosynthesis stimulated by tropic hormones. These patients in infancy suffer from hyponatremia, hyperkalemia, and acidosis. Both XX and XY individuals are phenotypically female. With appropriate mineralocorticoid and glucocorticoid replacement, these patients can survive into adulthood. Patients who are XY do not have a uterus and remain sexually infantile without hormone replacement, whereas XX patients may acquire some secondary sexual characteristics at puberty but develop early ovarian failure as a result of accumulation of cholesterol in the ovaries (8).

17α-Hydroxylase Deficiency **17α-Hydroxylase deficiency may be associated with either 46,XX or 46,XY karyotypes. The uterus is absent in individuals with 46,XY karyotype, a feature distinguishing them from individuals with 46,XX karyotype. Individuals with 17α-hydroxylase deficiency have primary amenorrhea, no secondary sexual characteristics, hypertension, and hypokalemia** (9). The diminished levels of 17α-hydroxylase that characterize this disorder lead to a reduction in cortisol production, which in turn causes an increase in adrenocorticotropic hormone (ACTH). 17α-Hydroxylase is not required for production of mineralocorticoids; thus, excessive amounts of mineralocorticoid are produced, resulting in sodium retention, loss of potassium, and hypertension. Over 20 mutations, which alter the reading frame of the gene, have been identified even though fewer than 200 people in the world have the disorder (10).

17,20-Desmolase Deficiency **Complete block in the δ-4 pathway of 17,20-desmolase leads to a female phenotype in individuals with an XY karyotype. The uterus is absent, and sexual development does not occur at puberty.** Although cortisol levels respond normally to ACTH stimulation, testosterone levels are low and do not respond to human chorionic gonadotropin (hCG) stimulation (11).

Aromatase Deficiency This rare autosomal recessive abnormality, which has been reported in only six cases, prevents the affected individual from aromatizing androgens to estrogen. This syndrome may be suspected even before birth because most mothers of affected children develop virilization during pregnancy. The placenta cannot convert the fetal androgens to estrogen, leading to androgen diffusion into the maternal circulation. The female child is born with clitoromegaly and posterior labioscrotal fusion. At puberty breasts do not develop, primary amenorrhea occurs, virilization worsens, growth spurt is absent, bone growth is delayed, and multicystic ovaries are present. The diagnostic hormonal pattern consists of an elevation of FSH, LH, testosterone, and dehydroepiandrosterone sulfate (DHEAS) levels and undetectable levels of estradiol.

Estrogen therapy has been shown to improve the ovarian and skeletal abnormalities, but it must be titrated to mimic normal estrogen levels. Therefore, only minimal amounts need to be given during childhood and then should be increased at puberty (12,13).

Gonadotropin Receptor Mutations

Luteinizing Hormone Receptor Mutation LH receptor inactivation caused by a homozygous premature stop codon was identified in a Brazilian family with 3,XY pseudohermaphroditism with primary amenorrhea in the absence of development of secondary sexual characteristics. The Leydig cells are unable to respond to LH; as a result, Leydig cell hypoplasia occurs, leading to early testicular failure and preventing masculinization. An XX sibling with the same mutation developed normal secondary sexual characteristics but was amenorrheic with elevated LH levels, normal FSH levels, and cystic ovaries (14).

Follicule-stimulating Receptor Mutation In six Finnish families, an autosomal recessive single amino acid substitution in the extracellular domain of the FSH receptor has been identified that prevents FSH binding. This leads to primary or early secondary amenorrhea, variable development of secondary sexual characteristics, and high levels of FSH and LH (15).

Other Causes of Primary Ovarian Failure

Amenorrhea and premature ovarian failure can occur in association with irradiation of the ovaries (16), chemotherapy with alkylating agents (e.g., *cyclophosphamide*) (17), or combinations of radiation and other chemotherapeutic agents. In girls, galactosemia often is associated with premature ovarian failure, but usually it is detected by newborn screening programs. Gonadotropin resistance, autoimmune ovarian failure, and ovarian failure resulting from infectious and infiltrative processes also have been described.

Hypogonadotropic Hypogonadism

Primary amenorrhea resulting from hypogonadotropic hypogonadism occurs when the hypothalamus fails to secrete adequate amounts of GnRH or when a pituitary disorder associated with inadequate production or release of pituitary gonadotropins is present.

Physiologic Delay **Physiologic or constitutional delay of puberty is the most common manifestation of hypogonadotropic hypogonadism. Amenorrhea may result from the delay of physical development caused by delayed reactivation of the GnRH pulse generator.** Levels of GnRH are functionally deficient in relation to chronologic age but normal in terms of physiologic development.

Kallmann's Syndrome **The second most common hypothalamic cause of primary amenorrhea associated with hypogonadotropic hypogonadism is insufficient pulsatile secretion of GnRH (Kallmann's syndrome), which has varied modes of genetic transmission,** as discussed in Chapter 23. Insufficient pulsatile secretion of GnRH leads to deficiencies in FSH and LH. Deficiencies in GnRH may also be caused by developmental or genetic defects, inflammatory processes, tumors, vascular lesions, or trauma. Patients with isolated deficiencies of LH and FSH usually are a normal height for their age, whereas patients with physiologic delay of puberty are usually short for their chronologic age but normal for their bone age (18).

Central Nervous System Tumors Central nervous system tumors that lead to primary amenorrhea, the most common of which is craniopharyngioma, are usually extracellular masses that interfere with synthesis and secretion of GnRH or stimulation of pituitary gonadotropins. Virtually all patients with these tumors have disorders in the production of other pituitary hormones as well as LH and FSH (19,20). Prolactin-secreting pituitary adenomas are rare in childhood and more commonly occur after development of secondary sexual characteristics.

Genetic Disorders

5α-Reductase Deficiency 5α-Reductase deficiency should also be considered as a cause of amenorrhea (21). Patients with this disorder are genotypically XY, frequently experience virilization at puberty, have testes (because of functioning Y chromosomes), and have no müllerian structures due to functioning müllerian-inhibiting factor (MIF). 5α-Reductase converts testosterone to its more potent form, dihydrotestosterone. **Patients with 5α-reductase deficiency differ from patients with androgen insensitivity, because they do not develop breasts at puberty and have low gonadotropin levels as a result of testosterone levels sufficient to suppress breast development and to allow normal feedback mechanisms to remain intact.** Normal male differentiation of the urogenital sinus and external genitalia do not occur, because dihydrotestosterone is required for this development. However, normal internal male genitalia derived from the Wolffian ducts are present because this development requires only testosterone.

Gonadotropin-releasing Hormone Receptor Mutations In two families with hypogonadotropic hypogonadism, compound heterozygous mutations (autosomal recessive inheritance) have been identified in the GnRH receptor gene. The GnRH receptor is a G-protein–coupled receptor. Functional studies show that the mutations either cause marked decrease in binding of GnRH to its receptor or prevent second-messenger signal transduction. Without a functional signal transduction, FSH and LH are not stimulated and are unable to promote follicular growth (22,23).

Follicle-stimulating Hormone Deficiency These patients usually seek treatment for delayed puberty and primary amenorrhea due to hypoestrogenism. They are distinguished from other hypoestrogenic patients by having decreased FSH levels and increased LH levels. These patients have low serum androgen levels despite the abnormal LH-to-FSH ratio, indicating that FSH-stimulated follicular development is a prerequisite for thecal cell androgen production. In some of these patients autosomal recessive mutations in the FSH β subunit, which impair dimerization of α and β subunits and prevent binding to the FSH receptor, have been identified (24). Pregnancy was achieved in one patient after induction of ovulation with injectable gonadotropins (25).

Other Hypothalamic and Pituitary Dysfunctions

Functional gonadotropin deficiency results from malnutrition, malabsorption, weight loss or anorexia nervosa, stress, excessive exercise, chronic disease, neoplasias, and marijuana use (26–30). Hypothyroidism, Cushing's syndrome, hyperprolactinemia, and infiltrative disorders of the central nervous system are rare causes of primary amenorrhea (31,32).

Diagnosis

A careful history and physical examination are necessary to appropriately diagnose and manage primary amenorrhea associated with hypogonadism. The physical examination may be particularly helpful in patients with Turner's syndrome. A history of short stature but consistent growth rate, a family history of delayed puberty, and normal physical findings (including assessment of smell, optical discs, and visual fields) may suggest physiologic delay. Headaches, visual disturbances, short stature, symptoms of diabetes insipidus, and weakness of one or more limbs suggest central nervous system lesions (20). Galactorrhea may be seen with prolactinomas, and the history of galactorrhea is also helpful when diagnosing postinfectious, inflammatory, or vascular lesions of the central nervous system; trauma; anorexia nervosa; stress-related amenorrhea; or other systemic disease processes.

The diagnostic workup is summarized as follows:

1. Assessment of the serum FSH level should be performed as the initial laboratory test unless the history and physical examination suggest otherwise. The FSH level differentiates hypergonadotropic and hypogonadotropic forms of hypogonadism.

If the FSH level is elevated, a karyotype is obtained. An elevated FSH level in combination with a 45,X karyotype confirms the diagnosis of Turner's syndrome. Partial deletion of the X chromosome, mosaicism, pure gonadal dysgenesis, and mixed gonadal dysgenesis are diagnosed by obtaining a karyotype.

2. Because of the association of coarctation of the aorta and thyroid dysfunction, patients with Turner's syndrome should undergo echocardiography and thyroid function studies.

3. If the karyotype is normal and the FSH is elevated, it is important to consider the diagnosis of 17α-hydroxylase deficiency because it may be a life-threatening disease if untreated. This diagnosis should be considered when testing indicates elevated serum progesterone levels (>3 ng/ml), a low 17α-hydroxyprogesterone level (<0.2 ng/ml), and an elevated serum deoxycorticosterone (DOS) level (33). The diagnosis is confirmed with an ACTH stimulation test. After ACTH bolus administration, affected individuals have markedly increased levels of serum progesterone compared with baseline levels and no change in serum 17α-hydroxyprogesterone levels.

4. If the screening FSH level is low, the diagnosis of hypogonadotropic hypogonadism is established.

5. If the history suggests the presence of a central nervous system lesion or galactorrhea, imaging of the head using computed tomography (CT) or magnetic resonance imaging (MRI) is helpful in the diagnosis. Suprasellar or intrasellar calcification in an abnormal sella is found in approximately 70% of patients with craniopharyngioma (20).

Physiologic delay is a diagnosis of exclusion that is difficult to distinguish from insufficient GnRH secretion. The diagnosis can be supported by a history suggesting physiologic delay, a radiograph showing delayed bone age, and the absence of a central nervous system lesion on CT or MRI scanning. Gonadotropin-deficient patients can usually be distinguished from patients with physiologic delay by their response to GnRH stimulation. Patients with physiologic delay have a normal LH response to GnRH stimulation for their bone age, in contrast with gonadotropin-deficient patients, in whom the LH and FSH responses are low (34).

Treatment of Amenorrhea

Individuals with primary amenorrhea associated with all forms of gonadal failure and hypergonadotropic hypogonadism need cyclic estrogen and progestin therapy to initiate, mature, and maintain secondary sexual characteristics. Prevention of osteoporosis is an additional benefit of estrogen therapy:

1. Therapy is usually initiated with 0.625 mg/day of conjugated estrogens or 1 mg/day of estradiol.

2. If the patient is short in stature, higher doses should not be used in an attempt to prevent premature closure of the epiphyses. Most of these patients are of normal height, however, and higher estrogen doses may be used initially and then reduced to the maintenance doses after several months.

3. Estrogens can be given daily in combination with progestin (medroxyprogesterone acetate) or progesterone to prevent unopposed estrogen stimulation of the endometrium in patients with a uterus. Medroxyprogesterone acetate may be administered daily at a dose of 2.5 mg or for 12 to 14 days every 1 to 2 months at a dose of 5 to 10 mg. Oral micronized progesterone may be administered at a dose

of 100 mg daily or 200 mg for 12 to 14 days every 1 to 2 months. Likewise, progesterone suppositories may be administered at a dose of 50 mg daily or 100 mg for 12 to 14 days every 1 to 2 months.

4. Occasionally, individuals with mosaicism and gonadal streaks may ovulate and be able to conceive either spontaneously or after the institution of estrogen replacement therapy (5).

5. If 17α-hydroxylase deficiency is confirmed, treatment is instituted with corticosteroid replacement as well as estrogen. Progestin is added if a uterus is present.

If possible, therapeutic measures are aimed at correcting the primary cause of amenorrhea:

1. Craniopharyngiomas may be resected with a transphenoidal approach or during craniotomy, depending on the size of the tumor. Some studies have shown improved prognosis with radiation therapy used in combination with limited tumor removal (20,35).

2. Germinomas are highly radiosensitive, and surgery is rarely indicated (36).

3. Prolactinomas and hyperprolactinemia often may respond to dopamine agonists (37).

4. Specific therapies are directed toward malnutrition, malabsorption, weight loss, anorexia nervosa, exercise amenorrhea, neoplasia, and chronic diseases.

5. Logically, it would appear that patients with hypogonadotropic hypogonadism of hypothalamic origin should be treated with long-term administration of pulsatile GnRH. This form of therapy is impractical, however, because of the necessity for the use of an indwelling catheter and a portable pump for prolonged periods. Therefore, these patients should be treated with cyclic estrogen and progestin therapy.

6. Patients with Kallmann's syndrome, as well as patients with exercise or stress amenorrhea and anorexia and weight loss, are treated with hormone replacement.

7. If the patient has physiologic delay of puberty, the only management required is reassurance that the anticipated development will occur eventually (38).

Individuals whose karyotypes contain a Y cell line (45,X/46,XY mosaicism, or pure gonadal dysgenesis 46,XY) are predisposed to gonadal ridge tumors such as gonadoblastomas, dysgerminomas, and yolk sac tumors. The gonads of these individuals should be removed when the condition is diagnosed to prevent malignant transformation (18,33). There is some evidence that hirsute individuals without Y chromosomes should also undergo gonad removal. One patient with hirsutism and the karyotype 45,X was noted to have a streak gonad; the contralateral gonad was dysgenic and contained developing follicles, well-differentiated seminiferous tubules, and Leydig cells. This patient was found to be H-Y antigen–positive (39).

Clomiphene citrate is ineffective in inducing ovulation in patients with hypogonadism who desire pregnancy, because such patients are hypoestrogenic. In patients with hypogonadism, ovulation induction with injectable gonadotropins is generally successful, and pulsatile treatment with GnRH may be used in patients who have normal pituitary function. In patients without ovarian function, oocyte donation may be appropriate. Because most patients with hypogonadism and lack of sexual development are young, pregnancy is not desired.

Amenorrhea with Secondary Sexual Characteristics and Anatomic Abnormalities

Causes

Anatomic Abnormalities

Amenorrhea occurs if there is blockage of the outflow tract or if the outflow tract is missing (Table 24.2). An intact outflow tract includes a patent vagina as well as a functioning cervix and uterus. Any transverse blockage of the müllerian system (Buttram and Gibbons classification I) will cause amenorrhea (40). Such outflow obstructions include imperforate hymen, transverse vaginal septum, and hypoplasia or absence of the uterus, cervix, and vagina (Mayer-Rokitansky-Küster-Hauser syndrome). Mayer-Rokitansky-Küster-Hauser syndrome has been associated with abnormal galactose metabolism (41). Of the patients with this syndrome 15% have an absent kidney, 40% have a double urinary collecting system (42), and 5% to 12% have skeletal abnormalities (43). Transverse blockage of the outflow tract with an intact endometrium frequently causes cyclic pain without menstrual bleeding in adolescents. The blockage of blood flow can cause hematocolpos, hematometra, or hemoperitoneum. Endometriosis may develop.

When the findings of the physical examination are normal, anatomic abnormalities may still be considered. A congenitally absent endometrium is a rare finding in patients with primary amenorrhea. Asherman's syndrome, which is more common with secondary amenorrhea or hypomenorrhea, may occur in patients with risk factors for endometrial or cervical scarring, such as a history of uterine or cervical surgery, infections related to use of an intrauterine device, and severe pelvic inflammatory disease. It is found in 39% of patients undergoing hysterosalpingography who have previously undergone postpartum curettage (44). Infections such as tuberculosis and schistosomiasis may cause Asherman's syndrome but are rare in the United States. Cervical stenosis resulting from surgical removal of dysplasia (cone biopsy, loop electroexcision procedure) may also lead to amenorrhea.

Androgen Insensitivity

Phenotypic females with complete congenital androgen insensitivity (previously called testicular feminization) develop secondary sexual characteristics but do not have menses. These patients are male pseudohermaphrodites. Genotypically, they are male (XY) but have a defect that prevents normal androgen receptor function, leading to

Table 24.2. Anatomic Causes of Amenorrhea

Secondary sexual characteristics present
Müllerian anomalies
Imperforate hymen
Transverse vaginal septum
Mayer-Rokitansky-Küster-Hauser syndrome
Androgen insensitivity
True hermaphrodites
Absent endometrium
Asherman's syndrome
Secondary to prior uterine or cervical surgery
Currettage, especially postpartum
Cone biopsy
Loop electroexcision procedure
Secondary to infections
Pelvic inflammatory disease
IUD-related
Tuberculosis
Schistosomiasis

IUD, intrauterine device.

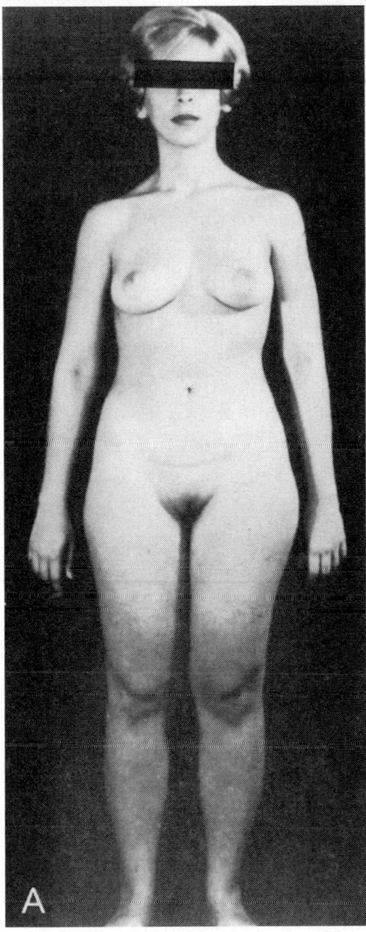

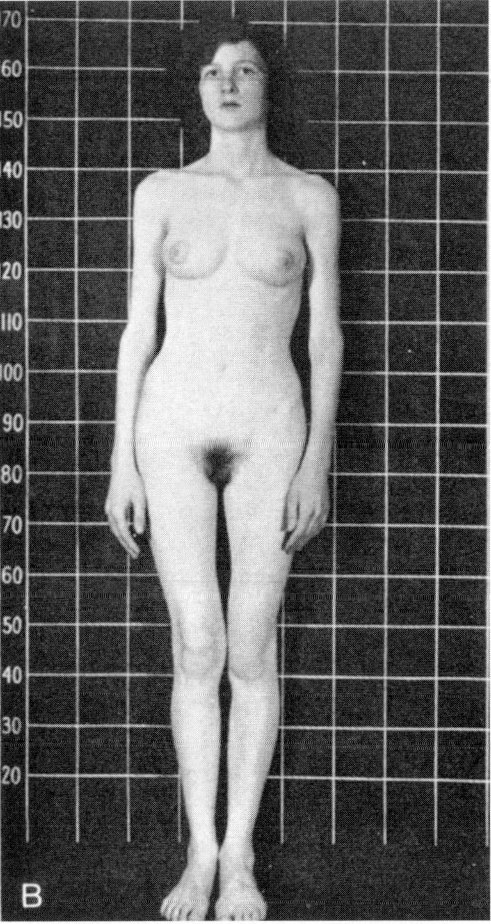

Figure 24.2 A: A well-developed patient with complete androgen insensitivity. Note the characteristic paucity of pubic hair and well-developed breasts. (From **Yen SSC, Jaffe RB.** *Reproductive endocrinology,* 3rd ed. Philadelphia: WB Saunders, 1991:497, with permission.) **B:** Another patient with androgen insensitivity syndrome with a contrasting thin body habitus. This is a 17-year-old twin 46,XY. (From **Jones HW Jr, Scott WW.** *Hermaphrodism, genital anomalies, and related endocrine disorders,* 2nd ed. Baltimore: Williams & Wilkins, 1971, with permission.)

the development of the female phenotype. Defects in the androgen receptor gene located on the X chromosome include absence of the gene that encodes for the androgen receptor and abnormalities in the androgen-binding domain of the receptor. Postreceptor defects also exist (45). Total serum testosterone concentration is in the range of normal males. Because anti–müllerian hormone is present and functions normally in these patients, internal female (müllerian) structures such as a uterus, vagina, and fallopian tubes are absent. Testes rather than ovaries are present in the abdomen or in inguinal hernias because of the presence of normally functioning genes on the Y chromosome. Patients have a blind vaginal pouch, and scant or absent axillary and pubic hair. These patients experience abundant breast development at puberty; however, the nipples are immature and the areolae are pale. Testosterone is not present during development to suppress the formation of breast tissues; at puberty, the conversion of testosterone to estrogen stimulates breast growth. Patients are unusually tall with eunuchoidal tendency (long arms with big hands and feet) (Fig. 24.2).

True Hermaphroditism

True hermaphroditism is a rare condition that should be considered as a possible cause of amenorrhea. Both male and female gonadal tissue is present in these patients, in

whom XX, XY, and mosaic genotypes have been found. Two-thirds of the patients menstruate, but menstruation has never been reported in XY genotypes. The external genitalia is usually ambiguous, and breast development frequently occurs in these individuals.

Diagnosis

Most congenital abnormalities can be diagnosed by physical examination:

1. An imperforate hymen is diagnosed by the presence of a bulging membrane that distends during Valsalva maneuver. Ultrasonography or MRI is useful to identify the müllerian anomaly when the abnormality cannot be identified by physical examination. The patient should also be examined for skeletal malformations and assessed with intravenous pyelography to detect concomitant renal abnormalities.

2. It is difficult to differentiate a transverse septum or complete absence of the cervix and uterus in a female from a blind vaginal pouch in a male pseudohermaphrodite. Androgen insensitivity is diagnosed when pubic and axillary hair is absent. To confirm the diagnosis, a karyotype determination should be performed to see whether a Y chromosome is present. In some patients, the defect in the androgen receptor is not complete and virilization occurs.

3. An absent endometrium is an outflow tract abnormality that cannot be diagnosed by physical examination in a patient with primary amenorrhea. This abnormality is so rare that, in a patient with normal physical findings, it may be advisable to proceed with evaluation of endocrine abnormalities. Absence of the endometrium should be suspected in patients with primary amenorrhea and normal secondary sexual characteristics when the results of hormonal studies are normal and the patients do not bleed after withdrawal of combined estrogen and progesterone replacement.

4. *Asherman's syndrome* also cannot be diagnosed by physical examination. It is diagnosed by performing hysterosalpingography, saline infusion, ultrasonography, or hysteroscopy. These tests will show either complete obliteration or multiple filling defects caused by synechiae (Fig. 24.3). If tuberculosis or schistosomiasis is suspected, endometrial cultures should be performed.

Figure 24.3 A: Intrauterine adhesion seen on hysterosalpingogram in a patient with Asherman's syndrome. B: Hysteroscopic view of intrauterine adhesion in a patient with Asherman's syndrome. (From **Donnez J, Nisolle M.** *The encyclopedia of visual medicine series—an atlas of laser operative laparoscopy and hysteroscopy.* New York: Parthenon Publishing Group, 1994:306, with permission.)

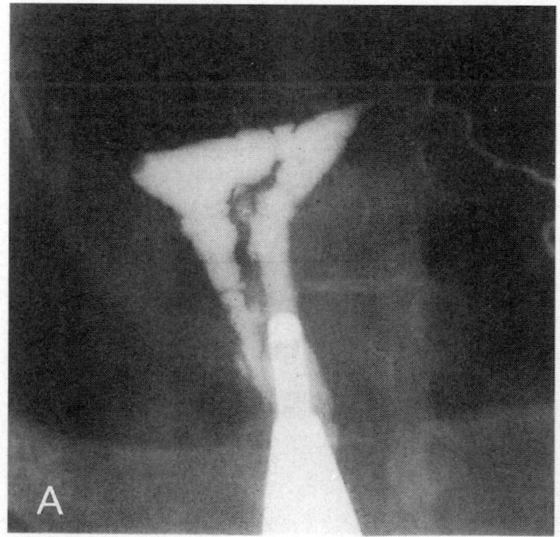

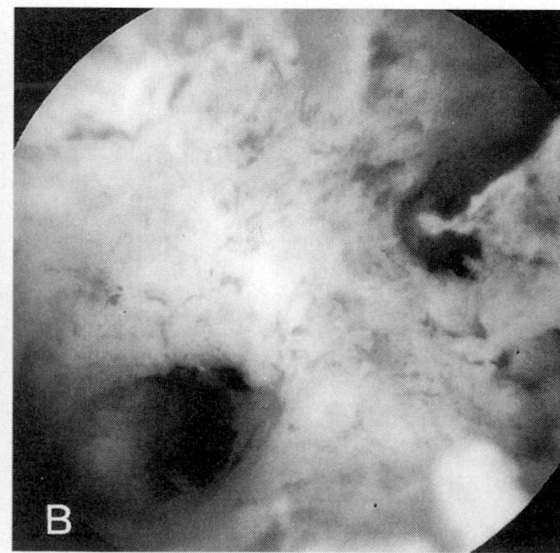

Treatment

The treatment of congenital anomalies can be summarized as follows:

1. **Treatment of an imperforate hymen involves making a cruciate incision to open the vaginal orifice.** Most imperforate hymens are not diagnosed until after a hematocolpos forms. It is unwise to place a needle into the hematocolpos without completely removing the obstruction because a pyocolpos may occur.

2. **If a transverse septum is present, surgical removal is required.** Forty-six percent of transverse septa occur in the upper one-third of the vagina, and 40% occur in the middle one-third of the vagina (46). Frank dilators should be used to distend the vagina until it is healed to prevent vaginal adhesions (47). Patients have a fully functional reproductive system after surgery; however, patients with repaired high transverse septa have lower pregnancy rates (48).

3. **Hypoplasia or absence of the cervix in the presence of a functioning uterus is more difficult to treat than other outflow obstructions.** Surgery to repair the cervix has not been successful, and hysterectomy is required (49). Endometriosis is a common finding, and it is questionable whether this condition should be treated with initial surgery or if it will resolve spontaneously after surgical repair of the obstruction. The ovaries should be retained to provide the benefits of estrogen and to allow for the possibility of future childbearing by removing mature oocytes for *in vitro* fertilization and using a surrogate mother for implantation.

4. **If the vagina is absent or short, progressive dilation is usually successful in making it functional** (47,50). If dilation fails or the patient is unable to perform dilation, the *McIndoe split thickness graft* technique may be performed (51,52). The initial use of vaginal dilators is required to maintain a functional vagina.

5. **In patients with complete androgen insensitivity, the testes should be removed after pubertal development is complete to prevent malignant degeneration** (53). In patients with testes, 52% develop a neoplasia, most often a gonadoblastoma. Almost one-half of the testicular neoplasms are malignant (dysgerminomas), but transformation usually does not occur until after puberty (54). In patients who develop virilization and have an XY karyotype, the testes should be removed immediately to preserve the female phenotype and to promote female gender identity. Bilateral laparoscopic gonadectomy is the preferred procedure for removal of intraabdominal testes.

6. **Adhesions in the cervix and uterus (Asherman's syndrome) can be removed using hysteroscopic resection with scissors or electrocautery.** A pediatric Foley catheter should be placed in the uterine cavity for 7 to 10 days postoperatively (along with systemic administration of broad-spectrum antibiotic therapy), and a 2-month course of high-dose estrogen therapy with monthly progesterone withdrawal is used to prevent reformation of adhesions. Eighty percent of patients thus treated achieve pregnancy, but complications including miscarriage, premature labor, placenta previa, and placenta accreta are common (55). Cervical stenosis can be treated by cervical dilation.

Amenorrhea with Secondary Sexual Characteristics and Nonanatomic Causes

Pregnancy must be considered in all women of reproductive age with amenorrhea. Thyroid dysfunction and hyperprolactinemia are also frequent causes of amenorrhea and are discussed further in Chapter 25. The three major causes of amenorrhea with secondary sexual characteristics are ovarian failure, pituitary and hypothalamic lesions, and abnormal hypothalamic GnRH secretion.

Causes

Ovarian Failure

Ovarian failure is a normal occurrence during menopause. The age of menopause is determined by genetic inheritance. Once a patient is exposed to estrogen, estrogen withdrawal causes hot flashes and vaginal dryness. This occurs in approximately 50% of patients, whether ovarian failure is premature or occurs at the normal age (56). Physical examination reveals vaginal mucosal atrophy and no cervical mucus. When ovarian failure occurs before 40 years of age, it is pathologic. Earlier failure may be caused by decreased follicular endowment or accelerated follicular atresia. If ovarian failure occurs before puberty, the patient's breasts will not develop (i.e., Turner's syndrome), and gonadal agenesis results (Tables 24.1 and 24.3).

Despite the numerous causes of ovarian failure, in most cases the etiology cannot be determined. In some patients, ovarian failure resolves spontaneously. Pregnancies have been reported to occur after the diagnosis of ovarian failure in <0.09% to 8.2% (56,57).

Cigarette smoking has been shown to have a clear inverse dose-response relationship with age of menopause (58). Other studies have confirmed this association, some eliminating potential confounding factors such as body weight that could affect the age of menopause (59). Cigarette smoking alters both gametogenesis and hormonogenesis, suggesting an effect on the follicle. Smoking has also been shown to increase the risk of diminished ovarian reserve (60).

Sex Chromosome Disorders **Deletion of the X chromosome (Turner's Syndrome) is associated with premature ovarian failure despite normal development of the ovaries due to accelerated atresia of the follicles** (61). Mosaicism of an XO or XY cell line may cause ovarian failure in patients younger than 30 years of age. A deletion of a portion of the X chromosome may be present in patients with premature ovarian failure. The Xq26–28 region is critical (62). Individuals with a 47,XXX karyotype also may develop ovarian failure. Familial ovarian failure is inherited by dominant mendelian inheritance in some cases (63).

Iatrogenic Causes Radiation, chemotherapy (especially alkylating agents such as cyclophosphamide) (64), surgical interference with ovarian blood supply, and infections can cause ovarian failure from early loss of follicles. At a radiation dose of 800 cGy, all patients

Table 24.3. Causes of Ovarian Failure After Development of Secondary Sexual Characteristics

Chromosomal etiology
Iatrogenic causes
  Radiation
  Chemotherapy
  Surgical alteration of ovarian blood supply

Infections
Autoimmune disorders
Galactosemia (mild form or heterozygote)
Savage syndrome
Cigarette smoking
Idiopathic

become sterile. Ovarian failure can be caused by as little as 150 cGy in some patients, especially if they are older than 40 years with limited follicle reserves.

Autoimmune Disorders Premature ovarian failure may be part of a polyglandular autoimmune syndrome. Antibodies are present in a variable number of patients with premature ovarian failure, depending on the autoimmune studies performed. One study showed that 92% of patients with premature ovarian failure had autoantibodies (65). However, only 20% of these patients exhibited signs of immunologic dysfunction, most frequently a thyroid disorder (57). Rarely, premature ovarian failure is associated with myasthenia gravis, idiopathic thrombocytopenic purpura, rheumatoid arthritis, vitiligo, autoimmune hemolytic anemia, diabetes mellitus, and other autoimmune disorders (66–68).

Galactosemia Galactosemia is caused by a lack of functional galactose-1-phosphate uridyl transferase. Galactose metabolites appear to have toxic effects on ovarian follicles, causing their premature destruction (69). There is also evidence that heterozygote carriers of this disorder may have suboptimal ovarian function (70). Early dietary modification may delay the ovarian failure.

Savage Syndrome In some patients follicles are present, but they do not mature in response to FSH because FSH receptors are absent or a postreceptor defect exists (67,71). In six Finnish families an autosomal recessive single amino acid substitution has been identified in the FSH receptor, which prevents binding of FSH (15). These patients experience ovarian resistance (Savage syndrome) as opposed to ovarian failure, in which no follicles are present. Except in the rare cases in which a genetic defect has been identified, ovarian biopsy is the only way to distinguish these disorders. Biopsy is not advised, however, because diagnosing resistant ovarian failure will not affect management. Although the use of GnRH agonists, estrogen therapy, and ovarian stimulation have been attempted in patients desiring pregnancy, studies have shown little success.

Pituitary and Hypothalamic Lesions

Hypothalamic Tumors In order for normal menstruation to occur, the hypothalamus must be able to secrete GnRH, and the pituitary must be able to respond with production and release of FSH and LH. Tumors of the hypothalamus or pituitary such as craniopharyngiomas, germinomas, tubercular or sarcoid granulomas, or dermoid cysts may prevent appropriate hormonal secretion. Patients with these disorders may exhibit neurologic abnormalities and abnormal secretion of other hypothalamic and pituitary hormones. Craniopharyngiomas are the most common tumors. They are located in the suprasellar region and frequently cause headaches and visual changes. The surgical and radiologic treatment of tumors may in itself cause further abnormalities in hormone secretion (Table 24.4).

Pituitary Lesions Hypopituitarism is rare because a large portion of the gland must be destroyed before decreased hormonal secretion affects the patient clinically. The pituitary gland may be destroyed by tumors (nonfunctioning or hormone secreting), infarction, infiltrating lesions such as lymphocytic hypophysitis, granulomatous lesions, and surgical or radiologic ablations.

Sheehan's syndrome is associated with postpartum necrosis of the pituitary resulting from a hypotensive episode that, in its severe form (pituitary apoplexy), causes shock. The patient may develop a localized severe retroorbital headache or abnormalities in visual fields and visual acuity. Patients with a mild form of postpartum pituitary necrosis experience failure to lactate, loss of pubic and axillary hair, and failure to resume menses after delivery.

Diabetic vasculitis and sickle cell anemia rarely manifest as pituitary failure. Hypopituitarism is associated with hyposecretion of ACTH and thyroid-stimulating hormone (TSH) as well as gonadotropins; therefore, thyroid and adrenal function also must be evaluated. If

Table 24.4. Pituitary and Hypothalamic Lesions

Pituitary and hypothalamic
Craniopharyngioma
Germinoma
Tubercular granuloma
Sarcoid granuloma
Dermoid cyst
Pituitary
Nonfunctioning adenomas
Hormone-secreting adenomas
Prolactinoma
Cushing's disease
Acromegaly
Primary hyperthyroidism
Infarction
Lymphocytic hypophysitis
Surgical or radiologic ablations
Sheehan's syndrome
Diabetic vasculitis

hypopituitarism occurs prior to puberty, menses and secondary sexual characteristics will not develop.

Growth hormone (GH), TSH, ACTH, and prolactin also are secreted by the pituitary, and the excess production of each by pituitary tumors causes menstrual abnormalities. The menstrual abnormalities are caused by adverse effects of these hormones on the GnRH pulse generator and not by directly effecting the ovary. **Prolactinomas are the most common hormone-secreting tumors in the pituitary** (see Chapter 25).

Altered Hypothalamic GnRH Secretion

The pulsatile secretion of GnRH is modulated by interactions with neurotransmitters and peripheral gonadal steroids. Endogenous opioids, corticotropin-releasing hormones (CRH), melatonin, and γ-aminobutyric acid (GABA) inhibit the release of GnRH, whereas catecholamines, acetylcholine, and vasoactive intestinal peptide (VIP) stimulate GnRH pulses. Dopamine and serotonin have variable affects (72). Chronic disease, malnutrition, stress, psychiatric disorders, and exercise inhibit GnRH pulses, thus altering the menstrual cycle (Table 24.5). Other hormonal systems that produce excess or insufficient hormones can cause abnormal feedback and adversely affect GnRH secretion. In hyperprolactinemia, Cushing's disease (excess ACTH), and acromegaly (excess GH) excess pituitary hormones are secreted that inhibit GnRH secretion. When the decrease in GnRH pulsatility is severe, amenorrhea results. With less severe alterations in GnRH pulsatility, anovulation can occur. Even slight defects in the pulsatility may result in luteal phase defect.

Anorexia Nervosa

Anorexia nervosa is an eating disorder that affects 5% to 10% of adolescent women in the United States. The criteria for anorexia nervosa as stated in the psychiatric diagnostic manual (DSM-IV) are refusal to maintain body weight above 15% below normal, an intense fear of becoming fat, altered perception of one's body image (i.e., patients see themselves as fat despite being underweight), and amenorrhea. Patients attempt to maintain their low body weight by food restriction, induced vomiting, laxative abuse, and intense exercise. **This is a life-threatening disorder with a mortality rate as high as 9%.** Amenorrhea may precede, coincide with, or follow the weight loss. Multiple hormonal patterns are altered. The 24-hour patterns of FSH and LH may show constantly low levels as seen in childhood or increased LH pulsatility during sleep consistent with the

Table 24.5. Abnormalities Affecting Release of Gonadotropin-Releasing Hormone

Variable estrogen status[a]
Anorexia nervosa
Exercise-induced
Stress-induced
Pseudocyesis
Malnutrition
Chronic diseases
Diabetes mellitus
Renal disorders
Pulmonary disorders
Liver disease
Chronic infections
Addison's disease
Hyperprolactinemia
Thyroid dysfunction
Euestrogenic states
Obesity
Hyperandrogenism
Polycystic ovary syndrome
Cushing's syndrome
Congenital adrenal hyperplasia
Androgen-secreting adrenal tumors
Androgen-secreting ovarian tumors
Granulosa cell tumor
Idiopathic

[a]Severity of the condition determines estrogen status—the more severe, the more likely to manifest as hypoestrogenism.

pattern seen in early puberty. Hypercortisolism is present despite normal ACTH levels, and the ACTH response to CRH administration is blunted. Circulating triiodothyronine (T_3) is low, yet circulating inactive reverse T_3 concentrations are high (73). Patients may develop cold and heat intolerance, lanugo hair, hypotension, bradycardia, and diabetes insipidus. They may have yellowish discoloration of the skin resulting from elevated levels of serum carotene caused by altered vitamin A metabolism.

Exercise and Stress-induced Disorders

In patients with exercise-induced amenorrhea, there is a decrease in the frequency of GnRH pulses, which is assessed by measuring a decreased frequency of LH pulses. These patients are usually hypoestrogenic, but less severe alterations may cause minimal menstrual dysfunction (anovulation or luteal phase defect). The decrease in LH pulsatility can be caused by hormonal alterations such as elevations in endogenous opioids, ACTH, prolactin, adrenal androgens, cortisol, and melatonin (74). Rates of amenorrhea by sport have been attributed to differences in body fat content. Runners and ballet dancers are at higher risk for amenorrhea than swimmers (75). Frisch and McArthur suggest that a minimum of 17% body fat is required for the initiation of menses and 22% body fat for the maintenance of menses (76). However, newer studies suggest that inappropriately low caloric intake during strenuous exercise is more important than body fat content (77). Higher intensity training, poor nutrition, stress of competition, and associated eating disorders increase an athlete's risk for menstrual dysfunction (78).

Stress-related amenorrhea can be caused by abnormalities in neuromodulation in hypothalamic GnRH secretion, similar to those that occur with exercise and anorexia nervosa. Excess endogenous opioids and elevations in CRH secretion inhibit the secretion of GnRH (72). These mechanisms are not fully understood but appear to be the common link between amenorrhea and chronic diseases, pseudocyesis, and malnutrition.

Obesity

Most obese patients have normal menstrual cycles, but the percentage of women with menstrual disorders increases from 2.6% in normal-weight patients to more than 8.4% in women 75% above ideal body weight. The menstrual disorder is more often irregular uterine bleeding with anovulation than amenorrhea. **Obese women have an excess number of fat cells in which extraglandular aromatization of androgens to estrogen occurs. They also have lower circulating levels of sex hormone–binding globulin, which allows a larger proportion of free androgens to be converted to estrone. Excess estrogen creates a higher risk for endometrial cancer for these women.** The decrease in sex hormone–binding globulin also allows an increase in free androgen levels, which initially are removed by an increased rate of metabolic clearance. This compensatory mechanism diminishes over time, and hirsutism can develop. Frequently, these patients are classified as having polycystic ovary (PCO) syndrome. Alterations in the secretion of endorphins, cortisol, insulin, growth hormone, and insulin-like growth factor-1 (IGF-1) may interact with the abnormal estrogen and androgen feedback to the GnRH pulse generator to cause menstrual abnormalities.

Other Hormonal Dysfunctions

The secretion of hypothalamic neuromodulators can be altered by feedback from abnormal levels of peripheral hormones. Excesses or deficiencies of thyroid hormone, corticosteroids, androgens, and estrogens can cause menstrual dysfunction. PCO syndrome usually causes irregular bleeding but may cause amenorrhea. It is likely that PCO syndrome is the result of peripheral alteration in IGF-1, androgen, and estrogen levels, which leads to hypothalamic dysfunction. Elevations in androgens (e.g., Sertoli-Leydig, hilus, and lipoid cell tumors) and estrogens (e.g., granulosa cell tumors) by ovarian tumors may lead to abnormal menstrual patterns, including amenorrhea. In patients who are hirsute and amenorrheic, androgen-secreting adrenal tumors and congenital adrenal hyperplasia should be considered.

Excess secretion of GH, TSH, ACTH, and prolactin from the pituitary gland can cause abnormal feedback inhibition of GnRH secretion, leading to amenorrhea. GH excess causes acromegaly, which may be associated with anovulation, hirsutism, and polycystic ovaries as a result of stimulation of the ovary by IGF-1. More commonly, GH excess is accompanied by amenorrhea, low gonadotropin levels, and elevated prolactin levels. Acromegaly is characterized by enlargement of facial features, hands, and feet, hyperhidrosis, visceral organ enlargement, and multiple skin tags. Cushing's disease is caused by an ACTH-secreting pituitary tumor manifested by truncal obesity, moon facies, hirsutism, proximal weakness, depression, and menstrual dysfunction.

Diagnosis

A pregnancy test (urine or serum hCG) should be performed in a reproductive-age woman with normal secondary sexual characteristics and normal pelvic examination findings who has amenorrhea. If the results of the pregnancy test are negative, amenorrhea should be evaluated using the following assessments:

1. Serum TSH level
2. Serum prolactin level
3. FSH levels
4. Estrogen status
5. Pituitary and hypothalamic function.

Thyroid-stimulating Hormone and Prolactin Levels

1. Sensitive TSH assays can be used to evaluate hypothyroidism and hyperthyroidism. Further evaluation of a thyroid disorder is required if abnormalities in TSH levels are found.

2. Hyperprolactinemia is a common cause of anovulation in women. If elevated TSH and prolactin levels are found, the hypothyroidism should be treated before hyperprolactinemia is treated. Often, the prolactin level will normalize with treatment of hypothyroidism because thyroid-releasing hormone, which is elevated in hypothyroidism, stimulates prolactin secretion.

Follicle-stimulating Hormone Levels

Serum FSH levels are required to determine whether the patient has hypergonadotropic, hypogonadotropic, or eugonadotropic amenorrhea. **A circulating FSH level of >40 mIU/ml indicated on at least two blood samples is indicative of hypergonadotropic amenorrhea.** Hypergonadotropism signifies that the cause of amenorrhea is at the level of the ovary. The history should reveal whether chemotherapy or radiation therapy are the cause for ovarian failure. Galactose-1-phosphate uridyl transferase level should be measured to assess whether the patient has galactosemia disease or is a carrier.

In patients less than 30 years of age with hypergonadotropic amenorrhea, a karyotype is required to rule out the presence of a Y cell line. *In situ* hybridization studies may prove the existence of Y chromosomal material with a Y-specific probe when the karyotype is normal (79). It is important to identify Y chromosomal material so it may be removed to prevent malignant degeneration.

There is much debate regarding the extent of an autoimmune workup required for a patient with ovarian failure.

1. It is reasonable to screen patients with nonspecific tests, such as those for antinuclear antibodies (ANA), rheumatoid factor (RF), and erythrocytic sedimentation rate (ESR).

2. A normal partial thromboplastin time (PTT) is sufficient to exclude lupus anticoagulant.

3. Assessments of serum electrolytes, calcium, and phosphorus concentrations can be used to evaluate the possibility that parathyroid autoantibodies are active.

4. Other assessments that should be performed include TSH, antithyroglobulin antibodies, and antimicrosomal antibodies to evaluate thyroid status, and 24-hour urinary free cortisol to evaluate the presence of antiadrenal antibodies.

5. A more extensive workup may include assessment of parietal cell antibodies, islets of Langerhans antibodies, and antiadrenal antibodies; it is unclear, however, if these tests will alter clinical management.

Tests should be repeated yearly because of the transient nature of autoimmune disorders.

In a patient with hypergonadotropic amenorrhea, it is not advisable to perform ovarian biopsy to determine whether follicles are present. Even if oocytes are found, no good method exists to stimulate those oocytes to ovulate. Some patients with negative biopsy results later ovulated spontaneously. This phenomenon can be explained by considering that the biopsy samples only a small portion of the ovary (57).

Assessment of Estrogen Status

Traditionally, estrogen status has been determined by giving *medroxyprogesterone acetate,* either 5 or 10 mg for 10 days, to determine whether the patient bleeds after withdrawal of the medication (usually 2 to 10 days after the last dose). There is a debate as to how much bleeding constitutes withdrawal bleeding. If vaginal bleeding does not occur after oral administration of *progesterone,* frequently 100 to 200 mg *progesterone* in oil is given intramuscularly. Other ways of testing for estrogen status may be quicker and easier. The development of vaginal dryness and hot flashes increase the likelihood of a diagnosis of hypoestrogenism. A sample of vaginal secretions can be obtained during the physical examination, and mucosal estrogen response can be demonstrated by the presence of superficial cells. A serum estradiol level higher than 40 pg/ml is considered adequate, but interassay discrepancies often exist.

The finding of vaginal bleeding after progesterone challenge is important when Asherman's syndrome is suspected. In a patient with primary amenorrhea and an apparently normal estrogen status, a progesterone challenge will diagnose the rare finding of congenitally absent endometrium. If estrogen status is questioned, 2.5 mg *conjugated estrogen* or 2 mg *micronized estradiol* can be given for 25 days with 5 to 10 mg of *medroxyprogesterone acetate* added for the last 10 days of therapy. Congenital absence of the endometrium is confirmed if no bleeding occurs with this regimen in a patient with primary amenorrhea and no physical abnormalities. Transvaginal ultrasonography to assess endometrial thickness may also be helpful. If similar findings occur in patients with secondary amenorrhea, Asherman's syndrome is diagnosed. **Asherman's syndrome must be confirmed by showing filling defects on hysterosalpingography or by visualizing adhesions with hysteroscopy.**

Assessment of the Pituitary and Hypothalamus

If the patient is hypoestrogenic and the FSH level is not high, pituitary and hypothalamic lesions should be excluded.

1. A complete neurologic examination, including electroencephalography (EEG), may help localize a lesion.

2. Either CT or MRI scanning should be performed to confirm the presence of a tumor. MRI can identify smaller lesions than can CT; if a lesion is too small for identification by MRI, it may be clinically insignificant.

3. After anatomic lesions have been excluded, the patient's history of weight changes, exercise, eating habits, body image, and career or school achievements are important factors in identifying anorexia nervosa, malnutrition, obesity, or exercise-induced or stress-induced menstrual disorders.

Amenorrheic patients who have hypothalamic dysfunction and are hypoestrogenic may have disorders similar to those who are well estrogenized. The hypothalamic dysfunction caused by chronic disease, anorexia nervosa, stress, and malnutrition may be more severe or may exist for a more prolonged time in hypoestrogenic patients than in euestrogenic patients.

Patients with appropriate clinical findings should undergo screening for other hormonal alterations as follows:

1. Androgen levels should be assessed in any hirsute patient to ensure that adrenal and ovarian tumors are not present as well as to diagnose PCO syndrome (Chapter 25).

2. Acromegaly is suggested by coarse facial features, large doughy hands, and hyperhidrosis and may be confirmed by measuring IGF-1 levels.

3. Cushing's syndrome should be ruled out by assessing 24-hour urinary cortisol levels or a 1-mg overnight *dexamethasone* suppression test in patients with truncal obesity, hirsutism, hypertension, and erythematous striae.

Treatment

The treatment of nonanatomic causes of amenorrhea associated with secondary sexual characteristics varies widely according to the cause. The underlying disorder should be treated whenever possible. Patients who are pregnant may be counseled regarding the options for continued care. When thyroid abnormalities are discovered, thyroid hormone, radioactive iodine, or antithyroid drugs may be administered as appropriate. When hyperprolactinemia is discovered, treatment may include discontinuation of contributing medications, treatment with dopamine agonists such as *bromocriptine* or *cabergoline* and, rarely, surgery for particularly large pituitary tumors. When ovarian failure causes amenorrhea, hormone replacement is prescribed for prevention of osteoporosis and to diminish menopausal symptoms. Gonadectomy is required when a Y cell line is present.

Surgical removal, radiation therapy, or a combination of both is generally advocated for treatment of central nervous system tumors other than prolactinomas. It may be necessary to treat individuals who have panhypopituitarism with various replacement regimens once all the deficits have been elucidated. These regimens include estrogen replacement for lack of gonadotropins, corticosteroid replacement for lack of ACTH, thyroid hormone for lack of TSH, and *desmopressin acetate (1-deamino-8-D-AVP [DDAVP])* to replace vasopressin.

The treatment of amenorrhea associated with hypothalamic dysfunction also depends on the underlying cause:

1. Hormonally active ovarian tumors are surgically removed.
2. Obesity, malnutrition or chronic disease, Cushing's syndrome, and acromegaly should be specifically treated.
3. Pseudocyesis and stress-induced amenorrhea may respond to psychotherapy.
4. Exercise-induced amenorrhea may improve with moderation of activity and weight gain when appropriate.
5. Anorexia nervosa generally demands a multidisciplinary approach, with severe cases requiring hospitalization.
6. Chronic anovulation or PCO syndrome may be treated after identifying the desires of the patient. Patients often are concerned about their lack of menstruation but not about hirsutism or infertility. The endometrium of these individuals should be protected from the environment of unopposed estrogen that accompanies the anovulatory state. An oral contraceptive is a good alternative for those patients who also require contraception. For those patients who are not candidates for oral contraceptives, cyclic administration of progestin is advised. This treatment option presumes an adequate estrogenic environment to induce proliferation of the endometrium and is not sufficient to cause withdrawal bleeding in patients who are hypoestrogenic (i.e., anorexia nervosa). In these individuals, estrogen replacement must be added to the progestin regimen for successful menstrual regulation and prevention of osteoporosis. The most common progestin used to induce withdrawal bleeding and thus protect the endometrium from hyperplastic transformation is *medroxyprogesterone acetate* (10 mg for 10 days per month). Occasionally, ovulation may occur; therefore, patients should be made aware that pregnancy is possible and appropriate contraceptive measures should be used. There is concern that medroxyprogesterone acetate used in early pregnancy may increase the incidence of pseudohermaphroditism (80). Alternatively, *progesterone* suppositories (50 to 100 mg) or *micronized progesterone* (200 mg) could be given for 10 days to induce withdrawal bleeding. No increased incidence of birth defects has been associated with the use of these natural progesterones (81).

7. When chronic anovulation is caused by attenuated congenital adrenal hyperplasia, glucocorticoid administration (i.e., *dexamethasone* 0.5 mg at bedtime) is sometimes successful in restoring the normal feedback mechanisms, thereby permitting regular menstruation and ovulation.

Hirsutism

Patients who have oligomenorrhea or amenorrhea resulting from chronic anovulation may have hirsutism (Chapter 25). After ruling out androgen-secreting tumors and congenital adrenal hyperplasia, treatment may be aimed at decreasing coarse hair growth.

Oral Contraceptives Oral contraceptives may be effective by decreasing ovarian androgen production as well as increasing circulating levels of sex hormone–binding globulin, leading to decreased free androgen circulation.

Antiandrogens *Spironolactone* has also been used because of its ability to decrease androgen production as well as compete with androgens at the androgen receptor level. Side effects include limited diuresis and dysfunctional uterine bleeding.

Flutamide is approved by the U.S. Food and Drug Administration for adjuvant therapy in prostatic cancer, and in the treatment of hirsutism it has effects similar to *spironolactone* with fewer side effects (82). Liver function should be monitored because of the rare complication of hepatotoxicity.

Cyproterone acetate, a strong progestin and antiandrogen, is used widely abroad but is not currently available in the United States. It is usually administered in combination with *ethinyl estradiol* in an oral contraceptive. By decreasing circulating androgen and LH levels, and by inducing antagonism of androgen effects at the peripheral level, *cyproterone acetate* is effective in treating hirsutism (83).

GnRH Agonist GnRH agonist administration with add-back therapy is increasingly being used in the United States. Administration of GnRH agonist agents virtually eliminates ovarian steroid production, and estrogen-progestin add-back therapy allows long-term administration and protection against osteoporosis.

5α-Reductase Inhibitors *Finasteride,* a 5α-reductase inhibitor, is approved by the U.S. Food and Drug Administration for the treatment of benign prostatic hypertrophy (*Proscar*) and male pattern baldness (*Propecia*). It is effective in treating hirsutism, although perhaps no more effective than other available agents (84,85). *Finasteride* has significant teratogenic potential, which precludes its use in any woman who may become pregnant. Its major advantage is that it is exceptionally well tolerated and may be used when side effects preclude the use of other therapeutic options for hirsutism.

Eflornithine hydrochloride, a topical cream, has been approved by the U.S. Food and Drug Administration for use on the face and chin. Improvements in facial hirsutism may be seen in 4 to 8 weeks of twice-daily applications.

Ovulation Induction

A large subset of patients with amenorrhea or oligomenorrhea and chronic anovulation seek care because they are unable to conceive (Chapter 27). Ovulation induction therapy is generally the treatment of choice for such patients, but pretreatment counseling should be provided in sufficient detail to ensure realistic expectations. The patient should be provided with information regarding the chances of a successful pregnancy (considering age of the patient and treatment modality), potential complications (hyperstimulation and multiple gestation), expense, time, and psychological impact involved in completing the course of therapy (86). **Patients may be advised that there is no increase in congenital anomalies in children born following ovulation induction** (87).

Recent studies have raised the possibility of a relationship between ovulation induction and the risk of ovarian cancer (88,89). Ongoing studies are attempting to address this issue conclusively, but data support an increase of approximately 2.5-fold in ovarian cancer in patients treated for infertility, which appears unrelated to the use of ovulation-inducing drugs (90,91). No change in ovulation induction practices seems warranted at the present time. Pregnancy and treatment with oral contraceptives before or after childbearing may protect against ovarian cancer.

***Clomiphene citrate* is the usual first choice for ovulation induction in most patients because of its relative safety, efficacy, route of administration (oral), and relatively low cost** (92). *Clomiphene citrate* is indicated primarily in patients with adequate levels of estrogen and normal levels of FSH and prolactin. It is generally ineffective in hypogonadotropic patients who already have a poor estrogen supply (93). Patients with inappropriate gonadotropin release (an increased LH-to-FSH ratio), such as that which occurs in PCO syndrome, are also candidates for therapy with *clomiphene citrate.* Up to 80% of certain patients can be expected to ovulate after clomiphene citrate therapy, and pregnancy rates approach 40% (86). Contraindications to the use of *clomiphene citrate* include pregnancy, liver disease, and preexisting ovarian cysts. Side effects include hot flashes (>11% of patients) and poorly understood visual symptoms, which generally have been viewed as an indication to discontinue subsequent *clomiphene citrate* use. The incidence of multiple gestation ranges from 6.25% to 12.3% (86). The most commonly recommended treatment regimen is 50 mg daily for 5 days, beginning on the third to fifth day of menstrual or withdrawal bleeding. Cycles are easily monitored by measuring midcycle estradiol levels and midluteal progesterone levels to assess folliculogenesis and ovulation. Ultrasonographic monitoring may also be helpful, especially for ovulation triggering with hCG. With these data, it is possible to adjust immediately the dose for the subsequent cycle if a given regimen is ineffective. Dosage increases of 50 mg/day are usually used, and more than 70% of conceptions occur at doses no higher than 100 mg/day for 5 days (94). Dosages higher than 150 mg/day for 5 days are usually ineffective, and patients who remain anovulatory with this dosage should undergo further evaluation accompanied by changes in the therapeutic plan. Longer courses of *clomiphene citrate* therapy, as well as adjunctive therapy with glucocorticoids and hCG, have been recommended (93). Patients with PCO syndrome, especially those with insulin resistance, may benefit from the use of insulin-sensitizing agents either as primary or adjunctive therapy (95). These include the biguanide *metformin* and thiazolidinediones (*rosiglitazone* and *pioglitazone*).

Women who do not ovulate or become pregnant with *clomiphene citrate,* as well as women with hypogonadotropic hypoestrogenic anovulation, may be candidates for therapy with injectable gonadotropins. Much higher pregnancy rates (up to 90%) occur in the latter category. Available preparations include recombinant FSH or products purified from the urine of menopausal women (FSH or FSH-LH combinations). Oral gonadotropin therapy is currently in research and development. Administration protocols and dosages vary widely and should be adjusted to individual needs. Safe administration requires careful monitoring of ovarian response with ultrasonography and serial estradiol measurements. In general, gonadotropins are administered at a dose of 75 to 150 IU/day by subcutaneous or intramuscular injection for 3 to 5 days, after which estradiol and follicular monitoring commence. In most cycles, gonadotropin administration lasts from 7 to 12 days. Ovulation is triggered by subcutaneous or intramuscular injection of 5,000 to 10,000 IU hCG once the lead follicle reaches 16 to 20 mm in diameter based on ultrasonographic assessments. Ovulation generally occurs approximately 36 hours after hCG administration. Luteal phase support is sometimes given with additional injections of hCG or with progesterone supplementation.

The two major complications associated with induction of ovulation with gonadotropins are multiple pregnancy (10% to 30%) and ovarian hyperstimulation syndrome. The incidence of both of these complications can be lowered by careful monitoring. Cycles complicated by the recruitment of numerous follicles or by estradiol levels approaching or exceeding

2,000 pg/ml may be canceled by withholding the ovulatory dose of hCG. Selected patients may be converted safely to *in vitro* fertilization. Because severe ovarian hyperstimulation syndrome is life-threatening and may lead to prolonged hospitalization, ovulation induction with gonadotropins generally is performed by experienced practitioners who devote a significant portion of their practice to the treatment of infertility.

Ovulation induction with GnRH may be effective in patients with chronic anovulation associated with low levels of estrogen and gonadotropins. In order for therapy to be successful, a functional ovary and pituitary gland must be present. Therefore, patients with ovarian or pituitary failure do not respond to GnRH therapy. To be effective, GnRH must be administered in a pulsatile fashion either intravenously or subcutaneously by a programmable pump. Ovulation induction with GnRH, as compared with gonadotropins, is associated with a relatively low incidence of ovarian hyperstimulation and multiple births. In addition, the need for appropriate timing of the ovulatory dose of hCG is avoided because patients treated with pulsatile GnRH have an appropriately timed endogenous LH surge. Disadvantages are mainly related to maintaining the programmable pump and injection site. After ovulation, luteal phase support is necessary and may be provided with hCG, progesterone, or continuation of the GnRH therapy.

Patients who lack oocytes (ovarian failure) and desire pregnancy may be candidates for oocyte donation. Oocytes may be harvested after ovulation induction from appropriate donors, fertilized with sperm from the recipient's husband, and transferred into the recipient's uterus after the endometrium has been appropriately prepared with hormonal regimens. Estrogen and progesterone are used to prepare the endometrium for implantation of the transferred embryo(s).

References

1. **Rosen GF, Kaplan B, Lobo RA.** Menstrual function and hirsutism in patients with gonadal dysgenesis. *Obstet Gynecol* 1988;17:677–680.
2. **Turner HH.** A syndrome of infantilism, congenital webbed neck, and cubitus-valgus. *Endocrinology* 1938;23:566–574.
3. **Baughman FA, Kolk KJ, Mann JD, et al.** Two cases of primary amenorrhea with deletion of the long arm of X chromosome (46,XXq−) *Am J Obstet Gynecol* 1968;102:1065–1069.
4. **Hsu LYF, Hirschhorn K.** Genetic and clinical consideration of long arm deletion of the X chromosome. *Pediatrics* 1970;45:656–664.
5. **Rimoin DL, Schimke NR.** *Genetic disorders of the endocrine glands.* St Louis: Mosby, 1971:285–292.
6. **Ferguson-Smith MA.** Karyotype-phenotype correlations in gonadal dysgenesis and their bearing on the pathogenesis of malformations. *J Med Genet* 1965;2:142–155.
7. **Hawkins JR.** Mutational analysis of SRY in XY females. *Hum Mutat* 1993;2:347–350
8. **Bose HS, Sugawara T, Strauss J, et al.** The pathophysiology and genetics of congenital lipoid adrenal hyperplasia. *N Engl J Med* 1996;335:1870–1878.
9. **Goldsmith O, Soloman DH, Horton R.** Hypogonadism and mineralocorticoid excess: the 17-hydroxylase deficiency syndrome. *N Engl J Med* 1967;277:673–677.
10. **Adashi EY, Hennebold JD.** Mechanisms of disease: single gene mutations resulting in reproductive dysfunction in women. *N Engl J Med* 1999;340:709–718.
11. **Zachman M, Werder EA, Prader A.** Two types of male pseudohermaphroditism due to 17,20-desmolase deficiency. *J Clin Endocrinol Metab* 1982;55:487–490.
12. **Bulun, SE.** Clinical review 78: aromatase deficiency in women and men: would you have predicted the phenotypes? *J Clin Endocrinol Metab* 1996;81:867–871.
13. **Mullis PE, Yoshimura N, Kuhlmann B, et al.** Aromatase deficiency in a female who is compound heterozygote for two new point mutations in the P450 arom gene: impact of estrogens on hypergonadotropic hypogonadism, multicystic ovaries and bone densitometry in childhood. *J Clin Endocrinol Metab* 1997;82:1739–1745.
14. **Latronico AC, Anasti M, Arnhold I, et al.** Testicular and ovarian resistance to luteinizing hormone caused by inactivating mutations of the luteinizing hormone-receptor gene. *N Engl J Med* 1996;334:507–512.

15. **Tapanainen JS, Vaskivup T, Aittomaki K, et al.** Inactivating FSH receptor mutations and gonadal dysfunction. *Mol Cell Endocrinol* 1998;145:129–135.

16. **Barrett A, Nicholls J, Gibson B.** Late effects of total body irradiation. *Radiother Oncol* 1987;9:131–135.

17. **Ahmed SR, Shalet SM, Campbell RH, et al.** Primary gonadal damage following treatment of brain tumors in childhood. *J Pediatr* 1983;103:562–565.

18. **Styne DM, Grumbach MM.** Disorders of puberty in the male and female. In: **Yen SSC, Jaffe RB,** eds. *Reproductive endocrinology,* 3rd ed. Philadelphia: WB Saunders, 1991:511–554.

19. **Banna M.** Craniopharyngioma: based on 160 cases. *Br J Radiol* 1976;49:206–223.

20. **Thomsett JJ, Conte FA, Kaplan SL, et al.** Endocrine and neurologic outcome in childhood craniopharyngioma: review of effective treatment in 42 patients. *J Pediatr* 1980;97:728–735.

21. **Peterson RE, Imperato-McGinley J, Gautier T, et al.** Male pseudohermaphroditism due to steroid 5α reductase deficiency. *Am J Med* 1977;62:170–191.

22. **deRoux N, Young J, Misrahi M, et al.** A family with hypogonadotropic hypogonadism and mutations in the gonadotropin-releasing hormone receptor. *N Engl J Med* 1997;337:1597–1602.

23. **Layman LC.** Mutations in human gonadotropin genes and their physiologic significance in puberty and reproduction. *Fertil Steril* 1999;71:201–218.

24. **Layman LC, Lee EJ, Peak DB, et al.** Brief report: delayed puberty and hypogonadism caused by mutations in the follicle-stimulating hormone (β)-subunit gene. *N Engl J Med* 1997;337:607–611.

25. **Matthews CH, Borgato S, Beck-Peccoz P, et al.** Primary amenorrhea and infertility due to a mutation in the β-subunit of follicle-stimulating hormone. *Nat Genet* 1993;5:83–86.

26. **Kulin HE, Bwibo N, Mutie D, et al.** Gonadotropin excretion during puberty in malnourished children. *J Pediatr* 1984;105:325–328.

27. **Cumming DC, Rebar RW.** Exercise in reproductive function in women. *Am J Intern Med* 1983;4:113–125.

28. **Ferraris J, Saenger P, Levine L, et al.** Delayed puberty in males with chronic renal failure. *Kidney Int* 1980;18:344–350.

29. **Siris ES, Leventhal BG, Vaitukaitis JL.** Effects of childhood leukemia and chemotherapy on puberty and reproductive function in girls. *N Engl J Med* 1976;294:1143–1146.

30. **Copeland KC, Underwood LE, Van Wyk JJ.** Marijuana smoking and pubertal arrest. *Pediatrics* 1980;96:1079–1080.

31. **Patton ML, Woolf PD.** Hyperprolactinemia and delayed puberty: a report of three cases and their response to therapy. *Pediatrics* 1983;71:572–575.

32. **Asherson RA, Jackson WPU, Lewis B.** Abnormalities of development associated with hypothalamic calcification after tuberculous meningitis. *BMJ* 1965;2:839–843.

33. **Davajan V, Kletzky OA.** Primary amenorrhea: phenotypic female external genitalia. In: **Mishell DR, Davajan V, Lobo RA,** eds. *Infertility contraception and reproductive endocrinology,* 3rd ed. Cambridge, MA: Blackwell Science, 1991:356–371.

34. **Grumbach MM, Styne DM.** Puberty: ontogeny, neuroendocrinology, physiology and disorders. In: **Wilson JB, Foster DW,** eds. *Williams textbook of endocrinology,* 8th ed. Philadelphia: WB Saunders, 1992.

35. **Lichter AS, Wara WM, Sheline GE, et al.** The treatment of craniopharyngiomas. *Int J Radiat Oncol Biol Phys* 1977;2:675–683.

36. **Wara WM, Fellows FC, Sheline GE, et al.** Radiation therapy for pineal tumors and suprasellar germinomas. *Radiology* 1977;124:221–223.

37. **Koenig MP, Suppinger K, Leichti B.** Hypoprolactinemia as a cause of delayed puberty: successful treatment with bromocriptine. *J Clin Endocrinol Metab* 1977;45:825–828.

38. **Speroff L, Glass RH, Kase NG.** *Clinical gynecologic endocrinology and infertility,* 5th ed. Baltimore, MD: Williams & Wilkins, 1994.

39. **Rosen GF, Vermesh M, d'Ablain GG, et al.** The endocrinologic evaluation of a 45X true hermaphrodite. *Am J Obstet Gynecol* 1987;157:1272–1273.

40. **Buttram VC Jr, Gibbons WE.** Müllerian anomalies: a proposed classification. *Fertil Steril* 1979;32:40–46.

41. **Cramer DW, Goldstein DP, Fraer C, et al.** Vaginal agenesis (Mayer-Rokitansky-Küster-Hauser syndrome) associated with the N314D mutation of galactose-1-phosphate uridyl transferase (GALT). *Mol Hum Reprod* 1996;2:145–148.

42. **Fore SR, Hammond CB, Parker RT, et al.** Urology and genital anomalies in patients with congenital absence of the vagina. *Obstet Gynecol* 1975;46:410–416.

43. **Griffin JE, Edwards C, Madden JD, et al.** Congenital absence of the vagina. *Ann Intern Med* 1976;85:224–236.

44. **Klein SM, Garcia CR.** Asherman's syndrome: a critique and current review. *Fertil Steril* 1973;24:722–735.

45. **Amrhein JA, Meyer WJ III, Jones HW Jr, et al.** Androgen insensitivity in man: evidence of genetic heterogeneity. *Proc Natl Acad Sci U S A* 1976;73:891–894.

46. **Rock JA.** Anomalous development of the vagina. *Semin Reprod Endocrinol* 1986;4:1–28.

47. **Frank RT.** The formation of an artificial vagina. *Am J Obstet Gynecol* 1938;35:1053–1055.

48. **Rock JA, Zacur HA, Diugi AM, et al.** Pregnancy success following surgical correction of imperforate hymen and complete transverse vaginal septum. *Obstet Gynecol* 1982;59:448–451.

49. **Williams EA.** Uterovaginal agenesis. *Ann R Coll Surg Engl* 1976;58:266–277.

50. **Ingram JN.** The bicycle seat stool in the treatment of vaginal agenesis and stenosis: a preliminary report. *Am J Obstet Gynecol* 1982;140:867–873.

51. **McIndoe A.** The treatment of congenital absence and obliterative condition of the vagina. *Br J Plast Surg* 1950;2:254–267.

52. **Rock JA.** Surgery for anomalies of the Müllerian ducts. In: **Thompson JD, Rock JA,** eds. *TeLinde's operative gynecology,* 7th ed. Philadelphia: JB Lippincott, 1992:603–646.

53. **Conte FA, Grumbach MM.** Pathogenesis, classification, diagnosis, and treatment of anomalies of sex. In: **De Groot LJ,** ed. *Endocrinology.* Philadelphia: WB Saunders, 1989:1810–1847.

54. **Manuel M, Katayama KP, Jones HW Jr.** The age of occurrence of gonadal tumors in intersex patients with a Y chromosome. *Am J Obstet Gynecol* 1976;124:293–300.

55. **Doody KM, Carr BR.** Amenorrhea. *Obstet Gynecol Clin North Am* 1990;17:361–387.

56. **Aiman J, Smentek C.** Premature ovarian failure. *Obstet Gynecol* 1984;66:9–14.

57. **Rebar RW, Cedars MI.** Hypergonadotropic forms of amenorrhea in young women. *Reprod Endocrinol* 1992;21:173–191.

58. **Jick H, Porter J, Morrison AS.** Relation between smoking and age of natural menopause. *Lancet* 1977;1:1354–1355.

59. **Mattison DR.** The effects of smoking on fertility from gametogenesis to implantation. *Environ Res* 1982;28:410–433.

60. **Sharara FI, Beatse SN, Leonardi MR, et al.** Cigarette smoking accelerates the development of diminished ovarian reserve as evidenced by the clomiphene citrate challenge test. *Fertil Steril* 1994;62:257–262.

61. **Singh RP, Carr DH.** The anatomy and histology of XO human embryos and fetuses. *Anat Rec* 1966;155:369–383.

62. **Krauss CM, Tarskoy RN, Atkins L, et al.** Familial premature ovarian failure due to interstitial deletion of the long arm of the X chromosome. *N Engl J Med* 1987;317:125–131.

63. **Mattison DR, Evan MI, Schwimmer WB.** Familial premature ovarian failure *Am J Hum Genet* 1984;36:1341–1348.

64. **Stillman RJ, Schinfeld JS, Schiff I, et al.** Ovarian failure in long term survivors of childhood malignancy. *Am J Obstet Gynecol* 1981;139:62–66.

65. **Mignot MH, Shoemaker J, Kleingel M, et al.** Premature ovarian failure. I: the association with autoimmunity. *Eur J Obstet Gynecol Reprod Biol* 1989;30:59–66.

66. **Jones GS, de Moraes-Ruehsen M.** A new syndrome of amenorrhea in association with hypergonadotropism and apparently normal ovarian follicular apparatus. *Am J Obstet Gynecol* 1969;104:597–600.

67. **Kim MH.** "Gonadotropin-resistant ovaries" syndrome in association with secondary amenorrhea. *Am J Obstet Gynecol* 1974;120:257–263.

68. **de Moraes-Ruehsen M, Blizzard RM, Garcia-Bunuel R, et al.** Autoimmunity and ovarian failure. *Am J Obstet Gynecol* 1972;112:693–703.

69. **Kaufman FR, Kogut MD, Donnell GN, et al.** Hypergonadotropic hypogonadism in female patients with galactosemia. *N Engl J Med* 1981;304:994–998.

70. **Cramer DW, Harlow BL, Barbieri RL, et al.** Galactose-1-phosphate uridyl transferase activity associated with age at menopause and reproductive history. *Fertil Steril* 1989;51:609–615.

71. **Coulam CB.** Premature gonadal failure. *Fertil Steril* 1982;38:645–655.

72. **Genazzani AR, Petragtia F, DeRamundo BM, et al.** Neuroendocrine correlates of stress-related amenorrhea. *Ann N Y Acad Sci* 1991;626:125–129.

73. **Herzog DB, Copeland PM.** Eating disorders. *N Engl J Med* 1985;313:295–303.

74. **Olson BR.** Exercise induced amenorrhea. *Am Fam Physician* 1989;39:213–221.

75. **Desouza MJ, Metzger DA.** Reproductive dysfunction in amenorrheic athletic and anorexic patients: a review. *Med Sci Sports Exerc* 1991;23:995–1007.

76. **Frisch RE, McArthur JW.** Menstrual cycles: fatness as a determinant of minimum weight for height necessary for their maintenance or onset. *Science* 1974;185:949–995.

77. **Laughlin GA, Yen SS.** Nutritional and endocrine-metabolic aberrations in amenorrheic athletes. *J Clin Endocrinol Metab* 1997;81:4301–4309.

78. **Highet R.** Athletic amenorrhea: an update on a etiology, complications and management. *Sports Med* 1989;7:82–108.

79. **Medlej R, Laboaccaro JM, Berta P, et al.** Screening for Y-derived sex determining gene SRY in 40 patients with Turner syndrome. *J Clin Endocrinol Metab* 1992;75:1289–1292.

80. **Schardein JL.** Congenital abnormalities and hormones during pregnancy: a clinical review. *Teratology* 1980;22:251–270.

81. **Resseguie LJ, Hick JF, Bruen JA, et al.** Congenital malformations among offspring exposed in utero to progestins, Olmsted County, Minnesota, 1936–1974. *Fertil Steril* 1985;43:514–519.

82. **Cusan L, Dupont A, Gomez JL, et al.** Comparison of flutamide and spironolactone in the treatment of hirsutism: a randomized controlled trial. *Fertil Steril* 1994;61:281–287.

83. **Belisle S, Love EJ.** Clinical efficacy and safety of cyproterone acetate in severe hirsutism results of a multicentered Canadian study. *Fertil Steril* 1986;46:1015–1020.

84. **Rittmaster RS.** Finasteride. *N Engl J Med* 1994;330:120–125.

85. **Price TM.** Finasteride for hirsutism. *Contemp Obstet Gynecol* 1999;44:73–84.

86. **Adashi EY, McClamrock HD.** ACOG technical bulletin. Washington, DC: American College of Obstetricians and Gynecologists, 1994, Number 197.

87. **Scialli AR.** The reproductive toxicity of ovulation induction. *Fertil Steril* 1986;45:315–323.

88. **Whittemore AS, Harris R, Itnyre J, et al.** Characteristics relating to ovarian cancer risk: collaborative analysis of 12 US case-control studies. *Am J Epidemiol* 1992;136:1184–1203.

89. **Rossing MA, Daling JR, Weiss NL, et al.** Ovarian tumors in a cohort of infertile women. *N Engl J Med* 1994;331:771–776.

90. **Venn A, Watson L, Lumley J, et al.** Breast and ovarian cancer incidence after infertility and in vitro fertilisation. *Lancet* 1995;346:995–1000.

91. **Mosgaard BJ, Lidegaard O, Kjaer SK, et al.** Infertility, fertility drugs, and invasive ovarian cancer: a case-control study. *Fertil Steril* 1997;67:1005–1012.

92. **Adashi EY.** Clomiphene citrate-initiated ovulation: a clinical update. *Semin Reprod Endocrinol* 1986;4:255–276.

93. **McClamrock HD, Adashi EY.** Ovulation induction. I: appropriate use of clomiphene citrate. *Fem Pat* 1988;13:92–106.

94. **Rust LA, Israel R, Mishell DR Jr.** An individualized graduated therapeutic regimen for clomiphene citrate. *Am J Obstet Gynecol* 1974;120:785–790.

95. **Nestter, JE, Jakubowitcz, DJ.** Decrease in ovarian extocrone, p450 17-α hydroxylase activity and serum free testosterone after reduction in insulin secretion in polycystic ovary syndrome. *N Engl J Med* 1996;335:617–623.

25 Endocrine Disorders

Avner Hershlag
C. Matthew Peterson

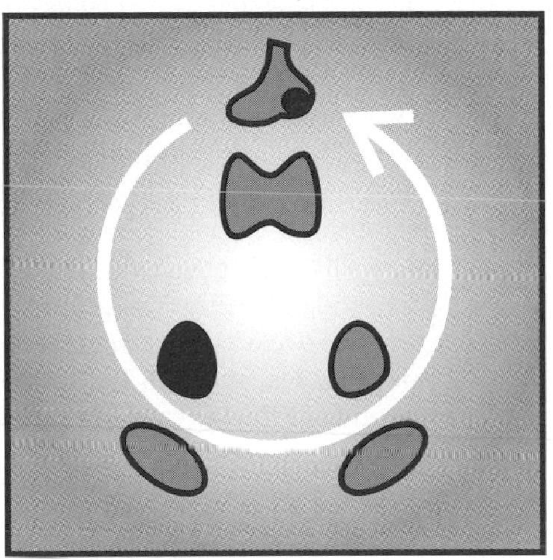

The endocrine disorders encountered most frequently in gynecologic patients are those related to androgen excess, including what is arguably the most common endocrinopathy in women—polycystic ovary syndrome (PCOS). Rare causes of virilization in women include tumors of the ovary and the adrenal gland. These conditions, as well as common disorders of the pituitary and thyroid glands, are reviewed in this chapter.

Hyperandrogenism

Diseases that reflect a state of hyperandrogenism result from either excess production of androgen such as from an adrenal or ovarian tumor, from metabolic derangements such as PCOS, or from increased end-organ sensitivity.

Hirsutism

Hirsutism, which is the most frequent manifestation of androgen excess in women, is defined as excessive growth of terminal hair in a malelike pattern. This refers particularly to midline hair, side burns, moustache, beard, chest or intermammary hair, and inner thigh and midline lower back hair entering the intergluteal area. The response of the pilosebaceous unit to androgens causes vellus hair to transform into terminal hair in androgen-dependent areas. The resulting terminal hair is coarse, stiff, pigmented, and long.

Androgens affect various types of hair differently. Hair that shows no androgen dependence includes lanugo, eyebrows, and eyelashes. Hair that is more dependent on adrenal androgens includes axillary and pubic hair. Hair that depends significantly on gonadal androgens includes midline, facial, and intermammary hair. Scalp hair is inhibited by gonadal androgens, resulting in the common temporal balding seen in males and in virilized females. Hirsutism results from both increased androgen production and skin sensitivity to androgens. Skin sensitivity depends on the local activity of 5α-reductase, the enzyme that converts testosterone to dihydrotestosterone (DHT), the active androgen in hair follicles.

Hair demonstrates cyclic activity between growth (anagen), involution (catagen), and resting (telogen) phases. Both the growth and resting phases vary in length for different areas of hair growth. Much of the influence of androgens or pharmaceutical agents depends on the phase of hair growth. Synchronization in the hair growth phase may lead to dramatic consequences, such as the hair loss occasionally encountered during pregnancy.

Social and clinical reactions to hirsutism may vary significantly. Androgen-dependent hair (excluding pubic and axillary hair) occurs in only 5% of premenopausal Caucasian women and is considered abnormal in white women of North America. The presence of sexual hair in other locations is viewed as normal, however, and is socially acceptable in some ethnic groups, such as Eskimos and women of Mediterranean origin.

Two conditions should be distinguished from hirsutism. **Hypertrichosis is the term reserved for androgen-independent growth of hair that is prominent in nonsexual areas, such as the trunk and extremities.** This may be either an autosomal-dominant congenital disorder or may be caused by metabolic disorders (such as anorexia nervosa, hyperthyroidism, porphyria cutanea tarda) or medications (phenytoin, minoxidil, cyclosporine, diazoxide). **Virilization is characterized by male-pattern baldness (crown routinely and temples occasionally), coarsening of the voice, decrease in breast size, increase in muscle mass, loss of female body contour (obesity, particularly of the upper segment, and alteration of the waist-to-hip ratio), and enlargement of the clitoris (the mean transverse diameter of the glans is 3.4 ± 1 mm and the longitudinal diameter is 5.1 ± 1.4 mm)** (1).

The history should focus on the age of onset and rate of progression of hirsutism or virilization. A fast rate of progression is associated with a more severe degree of hyperandrogenism and should raise suspicion of ovarian and adrenal neoplasms or Cushing's syndrome. The same is true of rapid progression or onset of symptoms before or after adolescence. Anovulation, manifesting as amenorrhea or oligomenorrhea, increases the probability of hyperandrogenism. Hirsutism in women with regular cycles may be associated with normal androgen levels and is considered *idiopathic hirsutism.*

A sensitive and tactful approach by the physician is mandatory and should include questioning of the patient regarding whether she shaves or removes hair chemically or mechanically and, if so, how frequently. A family history should be obtained to disclose evidence of idiopathic hirsutism, PCOS, congenital adrenal hyperplasia (CAH), diabetes mellitus, and cardiovascular disease. A history of drug use should also be obtained. In addition to drugs that commonly cause hypertrichosis, anabolic steroids and testosterone derivatives may cause virilization. During the physical examination, attention should be directed to obesity, hypertension, galactorrhea, male-pattern baldness, acne (face and back), and hyperpigmentation. The presence of an androgen-producing ovarian neoplasm or Cushing's syndrome should be considered. In many cases of Cushing's syndrome, the patient's initial symptom is hirsutism. The physician should search for the physical signs of the syndrome such as "moon face," plethora, purple striae, dorsocervical and supraclavicular fat pads, and proximal muscle weakness. The type, pattern, and extent of hair growth are next evaluated.

Typically, clinical evaluation of the degree of hirsutism is subjective. Most physicians arbitrarily classify the degree of hirsutism as mild, moderate, or severe. Objective assessment is helpful, however, especially in establishing a baseline from which therapy can be evaluated. A hirsutism scoring scale of androgen-sensitive hair in nine body areas rated on a scale of 0 to 4 has been used (2). A score higher than 8 is defined as hirsutism.

Role of Androgens

Androgens and their precursors are produced by both the adrenal glands and the ovaries in response to their respective trophic hormones, luteinizing hormone (LH) and adrenocorticotropic hormone (ACTH) (Fig. 25.1). Biosynthesis begins with the rate-limiting conversion of cholesterol to pregnenolone by side-chain cleavage enzyme. Thereafter, pregnenolone undergoes a two-step conversion to the 17-ketosteroid dehydroepiandrosterone (DHEA) along the Δ-5 steroid pathway. This conversion is accomplished by CYP17, an enzyme

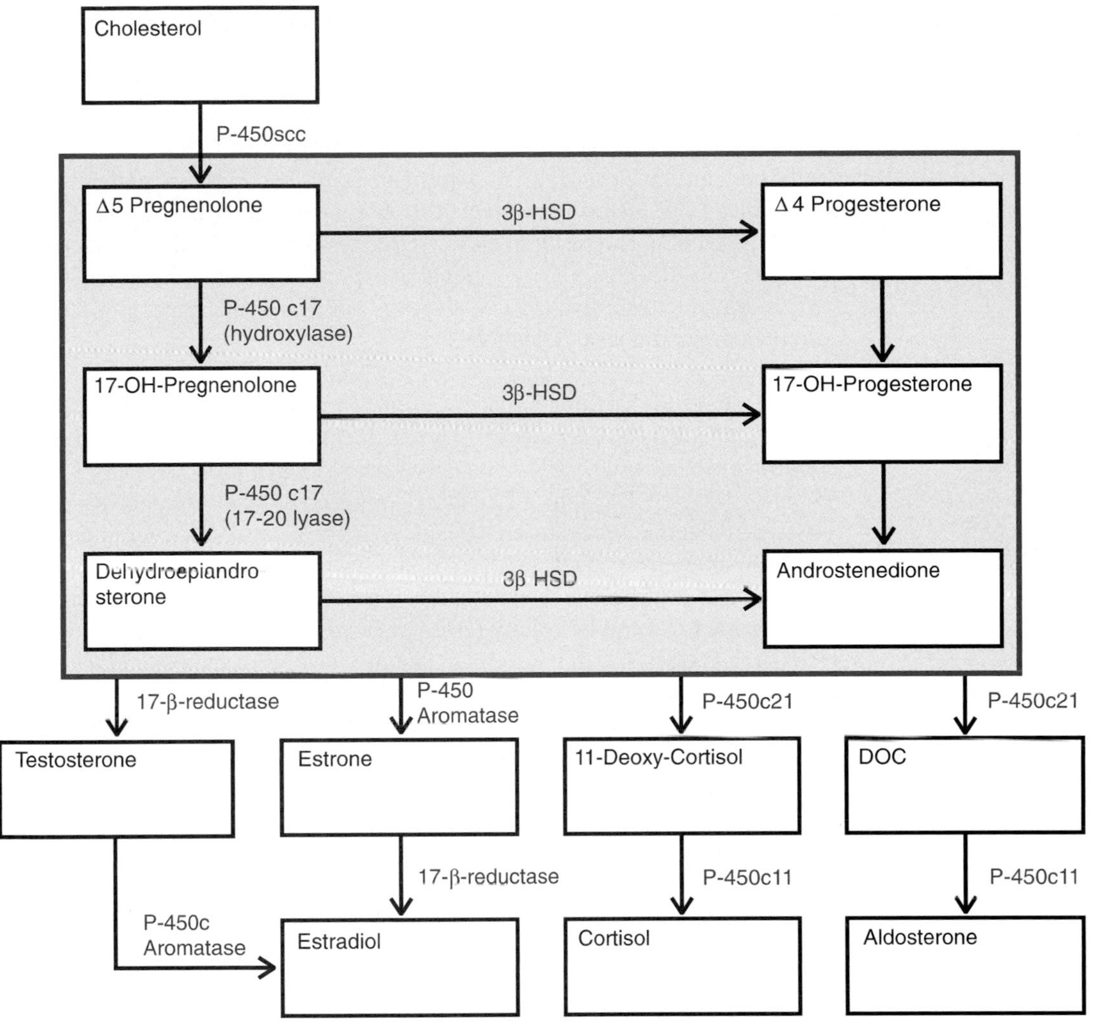

Figure 25.1 Major steroid biosynthesis pathway.

with both 17α-hydroxylase and 17,20-lyase activities. In a parallel fashion, progesterone undergoes transformation to androstenedione in the Δ-4 steroid pathway. The metabolism of Δ-5 to Δ-4 intermediate is accomplished via a Δ-5-isomerase, 3β-hydroxysteroid dehydrogenase (3β-HSD).

Adrenal 17-Ketosteroids

Secretion of adrenal 17-ketosteroids begins prepubertally (adrenarche) with a dramatic change in the response of the adrenal cortex to ACTH and with preferential secretion of Δ-5 steroids, including 17-hydroxypronenolone, DHEA, and dehydroepiandrosterone sulfate (DHEAS). The basis for this action is related to the increase in the zona reticularis and in the increased activity of the 17-hydroxylase and the 17,20-lyase enzymes.

Testosterone

Approximately one-half of a woman's serum testosterone is derived from peripheral conversion of secreted androstenedione, and the other one-half is derived from direct glandular secretion. The ovaries and adrenal glands contribute about equally to the direct glandular testosterone production in women.

Approximately 66% to 78% of circulatory testosterone is bound to sex hormone–binding globulin (SHBG) and is considered biologically inactive. Most of the proportion of serum testosterone that is not bound to SHBG is associated with albumin (20% to 32%). Finally, a small percentage (1% to 2%) of testosterone is entirely unbound or free.

The concentration of free testosterone has an inverse relationship with the SHBG concentration. Increased SHBG levels are noted in conditions associated with high estrogen levels. Thus, pregnancy and the luteal phase, use of estrogen (including oral contraceptives), and conditions causing elevated thyroid hormone levels and cirrhosis of the liver are associated with reduced free testosterone levels caused by elevated SHBG levels. Conversely, levels of SHBG decrease and result in elevated free testosterone levels in response to androgens, androgenic medications (progestational agents with androgenic biologic activities, danazol), androgenic disorders (PCOS, CAH, Cushing's syndrome), glucocorticoids, growth hormone, prolactin, insulin, and obesity.

Because nearly all practitioners measure some form of testosterone level, a basic understanding of the methods and accuracy of various techniques is critical. Testosterone nonspecifically bound to albumin (AT) is linearly related to free testosterone (FT) by the equation $AT = K_a [A] \times FT$, where AT is the albumin-bound testosterone, K_a is the association constant of albumin for testosterone, and [A] is the albumin concentration. In most cases of hirsutism, albumin levels are within a tight physiologic range and thus do not significantly affect the free testosterone concentration. **Therefore, in most cases of hirsutism, the free testosterone level can be calculated by measuring the total testosterone as well as the SHBG concentration.** A physiologic albumin level is assumed, and the free testosterone level is calculated with good reliability when compared with equilibrium dialysis. This method provides a rapid, simple, and accurate determination of the total and calculated free testosterone level as well as the concentration of SHBG.

The bioavailable testosterone level is also based on the relationship of albumin and free testosterone but incorporates the actual measurement of albumin levels with the total testosterone and SHBG. The assessment of free testosterone by methods other than the direct immunoassay of total testosterone, SHBG, and albumin in the case of bioavailable testosterone is unreliable (3).

A notable exception to the accuracy of the aforementioned measurements is pregnancy. During pregnancy estradiol occupies a large proportion of SHBG binding sites, resulting in an overestimation of the actual binding capacity of SHBG. Testosterone is unable to bind all the SHBG sites because they are occupied by estradiol; thus, an underestimation of free testosterone level occurs. Therefore, during pregnancy a total testosterone level is the only clinically reliable measurement and can be used to help rule out a testosterone-secreting tumor.

For testosterone to exert its biologic effects on many target tissues, it must be converted into its active metabolite, DHT, by 5α-reductase (a cytosolic enzyme that reduces testosterone and androstenedione levels). Two isozymes of 5α-reductase exist: type 1, which predominates in the skin, and type 2, or acidic 5α-reductase, which is found in the liver, prostate, seminal vesicles, and genital skin. The type 2 isozyme has a 20-fold higher affinity for testosterone than type 1. Both type 1 and 2 deficiencies in males result in ambiguous genitalia, and both isozymes may play a role in androgen effects on hair growth. Dihydrotestosterone is more potent than testosterone, primarily because of its higher affinity and slower dissociation from the androgen receptor. The relative androgenicity of androgens is as follows: DHT = 300, testosterone = 100, androstenedione = 10, and DHEAS = 5.

Until adrenarche, androgen levels remain low. Around 8 years of age, adrenarche is heralded by a marked increase in DHEA and DHEAS. The half-life of free DHEA is extremely short (about 30 minutes) but extends to several hours if DHEA is sulfated. Although no clear role is identified for DHEAS, it is associated with stress and level is inversely related to aging.

With age, the adrenal glands produce less DHEA and DHEAS. Once the ovaries cease production of estrogen during menopause, the production of testosterone and androstenedione

Table 25.1. Normal Values for Serum Androgens[a]

Testosterone (total)	20–80 ng/dl
Free testosterone (calculated)	0.6–6.8 pg/ml
Percent free testosterone	0.4–2.4%
Bioavailable testosterone	1.6–19.1 ng/dl
SHBG	18–114 nmol/L
Albumin	3300–4800 mg/dl
Androstenedione	20–250 ng/dl
Dehydroepiandrosterone sulfate	100–350 μg/dl
17-hydroxyprogesterone (follicular phase)	30–200 ng/dl

SHBG, sex hormone–binding globulin.
[a]Normal values may vary among different laboratories. Free testosterone is calculated using measurements for total testosterone and sex hormone–binding globulin, while bioavailable testosterone is calculated using measured total testosterone, sex hormone–binding globulin, and albumin. Calculated values for free and bioavailable testosterone compare well with equilibrium dialysis methods of measuring unbound testosterone. Bioavailable testosterone includes free plus very weakly bound (non-SHBG, nonalbumin) testosterone. Bioavailable testosterone is an assessment of bioactive testosterone in the serum.

increases. The diurnal variation is maintained by the adrenal contribution. These androgens are ultimately converted to estrone (E_1) and estradiol (E_2) via extragonadal aromatization.

Laboratory Evaluation

Critical laboratory testing for the assessment of hirsutism should include total testosterone, SHBG, calculated free or bioavailable testosterone (includes actual albumin concentration measurement), DHEAS, and 17-hydroxyprogesterone (17-OHP) measurements (Table 25.1). If a patient is oligomenorrheic, LH, follicle-stimulating hormone (FSH), prolactin, and thyroid-stimulating hormone (TSH) values are useful in the initial evaluation. Hyperthyroidism and hyperprolactinemia may result in reduced levels of SHBG and may significantly increase free testosterone levels resulting in hirsutism. Elevated LH-to-FSH ratios are noted in over one-half of women with PCOS and are occasionally helpful in establishing the diagnosis of PCOS. In cases of suspected Cushing's syndrome, patients should undergo screening with a 24-hour urinary cortisol (most sensitive) assessment or an overnight dexamethasone suppression test. For this test, the patient takes 1 mg of dexamethasone at 11:00 PM, and a blood cortisol assessment is performed at 8:00 AM the next day. **Cortisol levels of 2 mg/ml or higher require a further workup for evaluation of Cushing's syndrome.**

Some hirsute women manifest testosterone levels above normal (20 to 80 ng/dl [0.723 nmol/L]). However, there is no direct correlation between the level of hirsutism and the total testosterone concentration because hirsutism is caused by the action of the testosterone metabolite DHT, which in turn is related to the concentration of SHBG. Low SHBG levels, which frequently occur in the presence of elevated androgen and insulin levels, increase free testosterone levels. The result is hirsutism in the absence of an increase in total testosterone. Therefore, the total serum testosterone concentration is subject to wide variation in the concentration of binding proteins, and therefore is not a reliable index of bioavailable testosterone. It does, however, serve as a marker for androgen-producing neoplasms. **Total testosterone levels >200 ng/dl should prompt a workup for ovarian or adrenal tumors.**

In the past, testing for androgen conjugates (e.g., 3α-androstenediol G [3α-diol G] and androsterone G [AOG] as markers for 5α-reductase activity in the skin) has been advocated. However, routine determination of androgen conjugates to assess hirsute patients is not recommended, because hirsutism itself is an excellent bioassay of free testosterone action on the hair follicle and because these androgen conjugates arise from adrenal precursors and are likely markers of only adrenal and not ovarian steroid production (4).

In most laboratories, the upper limit of a DHEAS level is 350 μg/dl (9.5 nmol/L). A random sample is sufficient because the level of variation is minimized as a result of the long half-life of the sulfated form. A normal level essentially rules out adrenal disease, and moderate elevations are a common finding in the presence of PCOS. As a rule, a DHEAS level of over 700 μg/dl (20 nmol/L) indicates the need to rule out an adrenal tumor or Cushing's syndrome. Occasionally, ovarian tumors are associated with high DHEAS levels.

Because the 17-OHP level varies significantly in the cycle, standardized testing requires evaluation in the morning during the follicular phase. A baseline follicular phase 17-OHP level should be less than 200 ng/dl (6 nmol/L). When levels are greater than 200 ng/dl but less than 800 ng/dl (24 nmol/L), ACTH testing should be performed. Levels greater than 800 ng/dl (24 nmol/L) also warrant ACTH testing but are virtually diagnostic of 21-hydroxylase deficiency.

Polycystic Ovary Syndrome

The most common cause of hyperandrogenism and hirsutism is PCOS. The association of amenorrhea with bilateral polycystic ovaries was first described in 1935 by Stein and Leventhal (5) and was known for decades as the Stein-Leventhal syndrome. In the past the clinical diagnosis rested on the triad of hirsutism, amenorrhea, and obesity. **Subsequently it has been recognized that PCOS has an extremely heterogenous clinical picture and is multifactorial in etiology** (6). Following are diagnostic criteria based on the modified consensus of the National Institutes of Health and Child Health and Human Development.

- **Major**
  Chronic anovulation
  Hyperandrogenemia
  Clinical signs of hyperandrogenism
  Other etiologies excluded
- **Minor**
  Insulin resistance
  Perimenarchal onset of hirsutism and obesity
  Elevated LH-to-FSH ratio
  Intermittent anovulation associated with hyperandrogenemia (free testosterone, DHEAS)

In this schema, there are only two major criteria for PCOS: anovulation and the presence of laboratory or clinical evidence or both of hyperandrogenism in the absence of other pathologies such as ovarian and adrenal neoplasms, pituitary disease, or CAH.

All other frequently encountered manifestations are less consistent findings and therefore qualify only as minor criteria. They include insulin resistance, perimenarchal onset of hirsutism and obesity, elevated LH-to-FSH ratio, ultrasonographic evidence of PCOS, and oligoovulation.

Hirsutism occurs in approximately 70% of patients in the United States with PCOS (7) and in only 10% to 20% of Japanese patients with PCOS (8). A likely explanation for this discrepancy is the genetically determined differences in skin 5α-reductase activity (9,10).

Menstrual dysfunction typically occurs in PCOS, ranging from oligomenorrhea to amenorrhea. As a rule, patients with PCOS exhibit anovulation. Even in hyperandrogenic women with regular menstrual cycles, the rate of anovulation is 21% (11). Severe acne in the teenage years appears to be an accurate predictor of PCOS (12).

Obesity is found in over 50% of patients with PCOS. The body fat is usually deposited centrally (android obesity), and a higher waist-to-hip ratio indicates an increased risk of diabetes mellitus and cardiovascular disease (13).

Insulin resistance and hyperinsulinemia are commonly exhibited in PCOS. Insulin resistance is now recognized as a major risk factor for the development of type 2 diabetes mellitus (14). About one-third of obese PCOS patients have impaired glucose tolerance (IGT), and 7.5% to 10% have type 2 diabetes mellitus (15,16). These rates are mildly increased even in nonobese women who have PCOS (10% IGT; 1.5% diabetes, respectively) (16), compared with the general population of the United States (7.8% IGT; 1% diabetes, respectively) (17).

Abnormal lipoproteins are common in PCOS and include elevated total cholesterol, triglycerides, and low-density lipoproteins (LDL), and low levels of high-density lipoproteins (HDL) and apoprotein A-I (13,18). According to one report, the most characteristic lipid alteration is decreased levels of $HDL_{2\alpha}$ (19).

Other observations in women with PCOS include impaired fibrinolysis as shown by elevated circulating levels of plasminogen activator inhibitor (20), an increased incidence of hypertension over the years that reaches a 40% incidence by perimenopause (18), a greater prevalence of atherosclerosis and cardiovascular disease (21,22), and an estimated sevenfold increased risk for myocardial infarction (23).

Pathology

Macroscopically, ovaries in women with PCOS are 2 to 5 times the normal size. A cross-section of the surface of the ovary discloses a white, thickened cortex with multiple cysts that are typically less than a centimeter in diameter (24). Microscopically, the superficial cortex is fibrotic and hypocellular and may contain prominent blood vessels. In addition to smaller atretic follicles, there is an increase in the number of follicles with luteinized theca interna. The stroma may contain luteinized stromal cells (24).

Pathophysiology and Laboratory Findings

The hyperandrogenism and anovulation that accompany PCOS may be caused by abnormalities in four endocrinologically active compartments, (a) the ovaries, (b) the adrenal glands, (c) the periphery (fat), and (d) the hypothalamus-pituitary compartment.

In patients with PCOS, the ovarian compartment is the most consistent contributor of androgens. Dysregulation of CYP17, the androgen-forming enzyme in both the adrenals and the ovaries, may be one of the central pathogenetic mechanisms underlying hyperandrogenism in PCOS (25). The ovarian stroma, theca, and granulosa contribute to ovarian hyperandrogenism and are stimulated by LH (26). This hormone relates to ovarian androgenic activity in PCOS in a number of ways.

1. Total and free testosterone levels correlate directly with LH levels (27).
2. The ovaries are more sensitive to gonadotropic stimulation, possibly as a result of CYP17 dysregulation (25).
3. Treatment with a gonadotropin-releasing hormone (GnRH) agonist effectively suppresses serum testosterone and androstenedione levels (28).
4. Larger doses of a GnRH agonist are required for androgen suppression than for estrogen suppression (29).

The increased testosterone levels in patients with PCOS are considered ovarian in origin. The serum total testosterone levels are usually no more than twice the upper normal range (20 to 80 ng/dl). However, in ovarian hyperthecosis, values may reach

200 ng/dl or more (30). High intraovarian androgen concentrations inhibit follicular maturation. Although ovarian theca cells are hyperactive, the retarded follicular maturation results in inactive granulosa cells with minimal aromatase activity for conversion to estrogens.

The adrenal compartment also plays a role in the development of PCOS. Although the hyperfunctioning CYP17 androgen-forming enzyme coexists in both the ovaries and the adrenal glands (30), DHEAS is increased in only about 50% of patients with PCOS (31,32). The hyperresponsiveness of DHEAS to stimulation with ACTH (30), the onset of symptoms around puberty, and the observation that 17,20-lyase activation (one of the two CYP17 enzymes) is a key event in adrenarche have led to the concept of PCOS as an exaggerated adrenarche.

The peripheral compartment, defined as the skin and the adipose tissue, manifests its contribution to the development of PCOS in several ways.

1. The presence and activity of 5α-reductase in the skin largely determines the presence or absence of hirsutism (9,10).
2. Aromatase and 17β-hydroxysteroid dehydrogenase activities are increased in fat cells (33), and peripheral aromatization is increased with body weight (34).
3. The metabolism of estrogens, by way of reduced 2-hydroxylation and 17α-oxidation, is decreased (35).
4. Whereas E_2 is at a follicular phase level in patients with PCOS, E_1 levels are increased as a result of peripheral aromatization of androstenedione (36).
5. A chronic hyperestrogenic state results with reversal of the E_1-to-E_2 ratio.

The hypothalamic-pituitary compartment also participates in aspects critical to the development of PCOS.

1. An increase in LH pulse frequency is the result of increased GnRH pulse frequency (37).
2. This increase in LH pulse frequency typically results in elevated LH and LH-to-FSH ratio.
3. FSH is not increased with LH, probably because of the synergistic negative feedback of chronically elevated estrogen levels and normal follicular inhibin.
4. About 25% of patients with PCOS exhibit elevated prolactin levels. The hyperprolactinemia may result from abnormal estrogen feedback to the pituitary gland. In some patients with PCOS, *bromocriptine* has reduced LH levels and restored ovulatory function (38).

Genetic association and linkage analysis studies presently under way suggest an oligogenic origin for PCOS.

Insulin Resistance

Patients with PCOS are at risk for hyperinsulinemia and insulin resistance. The most common cause of insulin resistance and compensatory hyperinsulinemia is obesity. The insulin resistance seen in PCOS seems to be independent of the expected insulin resistance that occurs with obesity alone (38). The following observations provide evidence that the insulin resistance associated with PCOS is not the result of hyperandrogenism:

1. Hyperinsulinemia is not a characteristic of hyperandrogenism in general but is uniquely associated with PCOS (39).

2. In obese women with PCOS, 30% to 45% have glucose intolerance or frank diabetes mellitus, whereas ovulatory hyperandrogenic women have normal insulin levels and glucose tolerance (39). It seems that the negative effects of PCOS and obesity on the action of insulin are synergistic.

3. Treatment with long-acting GnRH analogs does not change insulin levels or insulin resistance (40).

4. Oophorectomy in patients with hyperthecosis accompanied by hyperinsulinemia and hyperandrogenemia does not change insulin resistance, despite a decrease in androgen levels (41).

Acanthosis nigricans is considered a marker for insulin resistance in hirsute women. This thickened, pigmented, velvety skin lesion is most often found in the vulva and may be present on the axilla, over the nape of the neck, below the breast, and on the inner thigh (42). **Women with severe insulin resistance sometimes develop HAIR-AN syndrome** (43), **consisting of hyperandrogenism (HA), insulin resistance (IR), and acanthosis nigricans (AN).** These patients usually have high testosterone levels (>150 ng/dl), fasting insulin levels of greater than 25 μIU/ml (normal <20 to 24 μIU/ml), and maximal serum insulin responses to glucose load exceeding 300 μIU/ml (normal is <160 μIU/ml at 2 hours post–glucose load).

Insulin alters ovarian steroidogenesis independent of gonadotropin secretion in PCOS. Insulin and insulin-like growth factor I (IGF-I) receptors are present in the ovarian stromal cells. A specific defect in the early steps of insulin receptor–mediated signaling (diminished autophosphorylation) has been identified in 50% of women with PCOS (44).

Clinically, it is important to realize that patients with PCOS are at increased risk for glucose intolerance or frank diabetes mellitus early in life. Therefore, it is appropriate to screen obese women with PCOS for glucose intolerance on a regular basis, once or twice a year. Abnormal glucose metabolism may be significantly improved with weight reduction, which may also reduce hyperandrogenism and restore ovulatory function (45). In obese, insulin-resistant women, caloric restriction that results in weight reduction will reduce the severity of insulin resistance (a 40% decrease in insulin level with a 10-kg weight loss) (46). This decrease in insulin levels should result in a marked decrease in androgen production (a 35% decrease in testosterone levels with a 10-kg weight loss) (46).

Radiologic Studies

Ultrasonographic examination may be a useful method for the early detection and subsequent follow-up of PCOS (47). Generally, ovarian size is increased (48,49). The most important ultrasonographic finding is a bilaterally increased number of microcysts measuring 0.5 to 0.8 cm with generally more than five microcysts in each ovary. As the number of microcysts increases and the ovarian volume enlarges, clinical and endocrine abnormalities become more obvious, and the condition becomes more severe.

Long-term Risks

In chronic anovulatory patients with PCOS, persistently elevated estrogen levels, uninterrupted by progesterone, increase the risk of endometrial carcinoma (50). These neoplasms are usually well differentiated, stage I lesions with a cure rate of more than 90% (see Chapter 30). Likewise, the hyperestrogenic state is associated with an increased risk of breast cancer (51). **The risk is greater in nonobese women and patients who have not been taking oral contraceptives (OCs). The risk of ovarian cancer also is increased two- to threefold in women with PCOS** (52). The risk is greater in nonobese women and patients who have not been taking OCs.

Table 25.2. Treatment of Hirsutism

Treatment Category	*Specific Regimens*
Weight loss	—
Hormonal suppression	Oral contraceptives *Medroxyprogesterone* Gonadotropin-releasing hormone analogs Glucocorticoids
Steroidogenic enzyme inhibitors	*Ketoconazole*
5α-reductase inhibitors	*Finasteride*
Antiandrogens	*Spironolactone* *Cyproterone acetate* *Flutamide*
Mechanical	Temporary Permanent Electrolysis Laser hair removal

Treatment of Hyperandrogenism and PCOS

Treatment depends on a patient's goals. Some patients require hormonal contraception, whereas others desire ovulation induction. Interruption of the steady state of hyperandrogenism and control of hirsutism usually can be accomplished simultaneously. An exception is those patients desiring pregnancy, in whom effective control of hirsutism may not be possible. Treatment regimens for hirsutism are listed in Table 25.2. The induction of ovulation and treatment of infertility are discussed in Chapter 27.

Weight Reduction

Weight reduction in obese patients is the initial recommendation, because it reduces insulin, SHBG, and androgen levels (mainly calculated or bioavailable testosterone), and may restore ovulation either alone or combined with ovulation-induction agents (52). **Weight loss of as little as 5% to 7% over a 6-month period can reduce the calculated or bioavailable free testosterone significantly and restore ovulation and fertility in over 75% of women** (53).

Oral Contraceptives

Combination OCs decrease adrenal and ovarian steroid production (55–58) and reduce hair growth in nearly two-thirds of hirsute patients. Treatment with OCs offers the following benefits:

1. The progestin component suppresses LH, resulting in diminished ovarian androgen production.
2. The estrogen increases hepatic production of SHBG, resulting in decreased free testosterone concentration (59,60).
3. Circulating androgen levels are reduced, which to some extent is independent of the effects of both LH and SHBG (13).
4. Estrogens decrease conversion of testosterone to DHT in the skin by inhibition of 5α-reductase.
5. Adrenal androgen secretion is reduced (61).

When an OC is used to treat hirsutism, a balance must be maintained between the decrease in free testosterone levels and the intrinsic androgenicity of the progestin. Three progestin compounds that are present in OCs (*norgestrel, norethindrone,* and *norethindrone acetate*) are believed to be androgen dominant. The androgenic bioactivity of these steroids may be a factor of their shared structural similarity with 19-nortestosterone steroids (62). Oral contraceptives containing the so-called new progestins (*desogestrel, gestodene, norgestimate,* and *drospirenone*) have minimized androgenic activity.

The use of OCs alone may be relatively ineffective (<10% success rate) in the treatment of hirsutism in women with PCOS (63). Insulin resistance may also be enhanced by OCs in these patients (64).

Medroxyprogesterone Acetate

Oral or intramuscular administration of *medroxyprogesterone acetate* has been used successfully for treatment of hirsutism (65). It directly affects the hypothalamic–pituitary axis by decreasing GnRH production and the release of gonadotropins, thereby reducing testosterone and estrogen levels. Despite a decrease in SHBG, total and free androgen levels are decreased significantly (66). **The recommended oral dosage is 20 to 40 mg daily in divided doses or 150 mg given intramuscularly every 6 weeks to 3 months in the depot form.** Hair growth is reduced in up to 95% of patients (67). Side effects of the treatment include amenorrhea, headaches, fluid retention, weight gain, hepatic dysfunction, and depression.

Gonadotropin-releasing Hormone Agonists

Administration of GnRH agonists may allow the differentiation of androgen produced by adrenal sources from that of ovarian sources (29). It has been shown to suppress ovarian steroids to castration levels in patients with PCOS (68). Treatment with *leuprolide acetate* given intramuscularly every 28 days decreases hirsutism and hair diameter in both idiopathic hirsutism and hirsutism secondary to PCOS (69). Ovarian androgen levels are significantly and selectively suppressed. The addition of OC or estrogen replacement therapy to GnRH agonist treatment (add-back therapy) prevents bone loss and other side effects of menopause, such as hot flushes and genital atrophy. The hirsutism-reducing effect is retained (66,70). Suppression of hirsutism is not potentiated by the addition of estrogen replacement therapy to GnRH agonist treatment (71).

Glucocorticoids

Dexamethasone may be used to treat patients with PCOS who have either adrenal or mixed adrenal and ovarian hyperandrogenism. Doses of *dexamethasone* as low as 0.25 mg nightly or every other night are used initially to suppress DHEAS concentrations to less than 400 μg/dl. **Because *dexamethasone* has 40 times the glucocorticoid effect of cortisol, daily doses greater than 0.5 mg every evening should be avoided to prevent the risk of adrenal suppression and severe side effects that resemble Cushing's syndrome.** To avoid oversuppression of the pituitary–adrenal axis, morning serum cortisol levels should be monitored intermittently (maintain at >2 μg/dl). Reduction in hair growth rate has been reported (72), as well as significant improvement in acne associated with adrenal hyperandrogenism.

Ketoconazole

Ketoconazole inhibits the key steroidogenic cytochromes. Administered at a low dose (200 mg/day), it can significantly reduce the levels of androstenedione, testosterone, and calculated free testosterone (73).

Spironolactone

Spironolactone is a specific antagonist of aldosterone, which competitively binds to the aldosterone receptors in the distal tubular region of the kidney. It is, therefore, an effective potassium-sparing diuretic, which was originally used for treatment of hypertension. The effectiveness of *spironolactone* in the treatment of hirsutism is based on the following mechanisms:

1. Competitive inhibition at the intracellular receptor level for DHT (74).

2. Suppression of testosterone biosynthesis by a decrease in the CYP enzymes (75).

3. Increase in androgen catabolism (with increased peripheral conversion of testosterone to estrone).

4. Inhibition of skin 5α-reductase activity (74).

Although total and free testosterone levels are significantly reduced in patients with both PCOS and idiopathic hirsutism (hyperandrogenism with regular menses) after treatment with *spironolactone,* total and free testosterone levels in patients with PCOS remain higher than those with idiopathic hirsutism (hyperandrogenism with regular menses) (76). In both groups, SHBG levels are unaltered. The reduction in circulating androgen levels observed within a few days of *spironolactone* treatment partially accounts for the progressive regression of hirsutism.

At least a modest improvement in hirsutism can be anticipated in 70% to 80% of women using at least 100 mg of *spironolactone* per day for 6 months (77). Spironolactone reduces the daily linear growth rate of sexual hair, hair shaft diameters, and daily hair volume production (78). **The most common dosages is 25 to 100 mg twice daily. Women treated with 200 mg/day show a greater reduction in hair shaft diameter than women receiving 100 mg/day** (79). Maximal effect on hair growth is noted between 3 and 6 months but continues for 12 months. Electrolysis can be recommended 9 to 12 months after the initiation of *spironolactone* for permanent hair removal.

The most common side effect of *spironolactone* is menstrual irregularity (usually metrorrhagia), which may occur in over 50% of patients with a dosage of 200 mg/day (79). Normal menses may resume with reduction of the dosage. Infrequently, other side effects such as urticaria, mastodynia, or scalp hair loss occur (79). Nausea and fatigue can occur with high doses (77). Because spironolactone can increase serum potassium levels, its use is not recommended in patients with renal insufficiency or hyperkalemia. Periodic monitoring of potassium and creatinine levels is suggested.

Return of normal menses in amenorrheic patients is reported in up to 60% of cases (76). Patients must be counseled to use contraception while taking *spironolactone* because it theoretically can feminize a male fetus.

Cyproterone Acetate

Cyproterone acetate is a synthetic progestin derived from 17-OHP that has potent antiandrogenic properties. The primary mechanism of *cyproterone acetate* is competitive inhibition of testosterone and DHT at the level of androgen receptors (80). This agent also induces hepatic enzymes and may increase the metabolic clearance rate of plasma androgens (81).

The combination of *ethinyl estradiol* with *cyproterone acetate,* which was commonly used in Europe for many years, significantly reduces plasma testosterone and androstenedione levels, suppresses gonadotropins, and increases SHBG levels (82). *Cyproterone acetate* also shows mild glucocorticoid activity (83) and may reduce DHEAS levels (84). Administered in a reverse sequential regimen (cyproterone acetate 100 mg/day on days 5 to 15, and *ethinyl estradiol* 30 to 50 mg/day on cycle days 5 to 26), this cyclic schedule allows regular menstrual bleeding, provides excellent contraception, and is effective in the treatment of even severe hirsutism and acne (85). When a desired clinical response is achieved, the dose of *cyproterone acetate* may be tapered gradually at 3- to 6-month intervals.

Side effects of *cyproterone acetate* include fatigue, weight gain, decreased libido, irregular bleeding, nausea, and headaches. These symptoms occur less often when *ethinyl estradiol* is added. *Cyproterone acetate* administration has been associated with liver tumors in beagles and is not approved by the U.S. Food and Drug Administration for use in the United States.

Flutamide

Flutamide, a pure nonsteroidal antiandrogen, is approved for treatment of advanced prostate cancer. Its mechanism of action is inhibition of nuclear binding of androgens in target tissues. Although it has a weaker affinity to the androgen receptor than spironolactone or *cyproterone acetate,* larger doses (250 mg given 2 or 3 times daily) may compensate for the reduced potency. *Flutamide* is also a weak inhibitor of testosterone biosynthesis.

In a single, 3-month study of *flutamide* alone, most patients demonstrated significant improvement in hirsutism with no change in androgen levels (86). Significant improvement in hirsutism with a significant drop in androstenedione, DHT, LH, and FSH levels was observed in an 8-month follow-up of *flutamide* and low-dose OCs in women who did not respond to OCs alone (87). The side effects of *flutamide* treatment combined with a low-dose OC included dry skin, hot flashes, increased appetite, headaches, fatigue, nausea, dizziness, decreased libido, liver toxicity, and breast tenderness (88). Many patients taking *flutamide* (50% to 75%) report dry skin or a blue-green discoloration of urine. The risk of liver toxicity precludes flutamide as a routine option for the treatment of hirsutism.

Cimetidine

Cimetidine is a histamine H_2 receptor antagonist that has demonstrated a weak antiandrogenic effect as a result of its ability to occupy androgen receptors and inhibit DHT binding at the level of the hair follicles. Although *cimetidine* has been reported to reduce hair growth in women with hirsutism (89), two later studies show no beneficial effect (90,91).

Finasteride

Finasteride is a specific inhibitor of type 2 5α-reductase enzyme activity that has been approved in the United States at a 5-mg dose for the treatment of benign prostatic hyperplasia and at a 1-mg dose to treat male-pattern baldness. In a study in which *finasteride* (5 mg daily) was compared with *spironolactone* (100 mg daily) (92), both drugs resulted in similar significant improvement in hirsutism despite differing effects on androgen levels. Most of the improvement in hirsutism occurred after 6 months of therapy with 7.5 mg of *finasteride* daily (93). The improvement in hirsutism in the presence of rising testosterone levels serves as convincing evidence that it is the binding of DHT and not testosterone to the androgen receptor that is responsible for hair growth. *Finasteride* does not prevent ovulation or cause menstrual irregularity. The increase in SHBG caused by OCs further decreases free testosterone levels; OCs in combination with *finasteride* are more effective in reducing hirsutism than *finasteride* alone. As with *spironolactone, finasteride* could theoretically feminize a male fetus; therefore, both of these agents are used only with additional contraception.

Ovarian Wedge Resection

Bilateral ovarian wedge resection is associated with only transient reduction in androstenedione levels and a prolonged minimal decrease in plasma testosterone (94,95). In patients with hirsutism and PCOS who have had wedge resection, hair growth was reduced by approximately 16% (96,97). Although Stein's original report cited a pregnancy rate of 85% following wedge resection and maintenance of ovulatory cycles, subsequent reports show lower pregnancy rates and a concerning incidence of periovarian adhesions (98).

Laparoscopic Electrocautery

Laparoscopic ovarian electrocautery is used as an alternative to wedge resection in patients with severe PCOS whose condition is resistant to *clomiphene citrate.* In a recent series (99), ovarian drilling was achieved laparoscopically with an insulated electrocautery needle, using 100-W cutting current to aid in entry and 40-W coagulating current to treat each microcyst over 2 seconds (8-mm needle in ovary). In each ovary, 10 to 15 punctures were created. This led to spontaneous ovulation in 73% of patients, with 72% conceiving within 2 years. Of those who had undergone a follow-up laparoscopy, 11 of 15 were adhesion free. To reduce adhesion formation, a technique that cauterized the ovary only in four points led to a similar pregnancy rate (100), with a miscarriage rate of 14% (much lower than the usual miscarriage rate of 30% to 40% for patients with PCOS). Most series report a decrease in both androgen and LH concentrations and an increase in FSH concentrations (101,102). Unilateral diathermy has been shown to result in bilateral ovarian activity (103). Further studies are anticipated to define candidates who may benefit most from such a procedure. The risk of adhesion formation should be discussed with the patient.

Physical Methods of Hair Removal

Depilatory creams remove hair only temporarily. They break down and dissolve hair by hydrolyzing disulfide bonds. Although depilatories can have a dramatic effect, many women cannot tolerate these irritative chemicals. The topical use of corticosteroid cream may prevent contact dermatitis. *Eflornithine hydrochloride* cream also know as *difluoromethylornithine* (*DMFO*), irreversibly blocks ornithine decarboxylase (ODC), the enzyme in hair follicles that is important in regulating hair growth. It also has proved effective in the treatment of unwanted facial hair (104).

Shaving is effective. Contrary to common belief, it does not change the quality, quantity, or texture of hair (105). However, plucking, if done unevenly and repeatedly, may cause inflammation and damage to hair follicles and render them less amenable to electrolysis. Waxing is a grouped method of plucking in which hairs are plucked out from under the skin surface. The results of waxing last longer (up to 6 weeks) than shaving or depilatory creams (105).

Bleaching removes the hair pigment through the use of hydrogen peroxide (usually 6% strength), which is sometimes combined with ammonia. Although hair lightens and softens during oxidation, this method is frequently associated with hair discoloration, or skin irritation, and is not always effective (104).

Electrolysis and laser hair removal are the only permanent means recommended for hair removal. Under magnification, a trained technician destroys each hair follicle individually. When a needle is inserted into a hair follicle, galvanic current, electrocautery, or both used in combination (blend) destroy the hair follicle. After the needle is removed, a forceps is used to remove the hair. Hair regrowth ranges from 15% to 50%. Problems with electrolysis include pain, scarring, and pigmentation. Cost can also be an obstacle (106). Laser hair removal destroys the hair follicle through photoablation.

Insulin Sensitizers

Because hyperinsulinemia appears to play a role in PCOS-associated anovulation, treatment with insulin sensitizers may shift the endocrine balance toward ovulation and pregnancy, either alone or in combination with other treatment modalities.

Metformin (*Glucophage*) is an oral biguanide antihyperglycemic drug used extensively in Europe for non–insulin-dependent diabetes. Given its category B status, there has been limited use of the drug in pregnant women with diabetes. Preliminary studies evaluating *metformin* use in pregnancy suggest no teratogenicity and a reduced miscarriage rate but a potential increased risk of preeclampsia and perinatal mortality (107,108).

Metformin lowers blood glucose mainly by inhibiting hepatic glucose production and by enhancing peripheral glucose uptake. *Metformin* enhances insulin sensitivity at the postreceptor level and stimulates insulin-mediated glucose disposal (109).

The hyperandrogenism of PCOS is substantially relieved with metformin therapy, which leads to a drop in insulin levels and improved reproductive function (110–112). *Metformin* (500 mg 3 times daily) increases ovulation rates both spontaneously and when used in combination with *clomiphene citrate* in obese patients with PCOS. In this group, a 90% ovulation rate has been achieved (113).

The most common side effects are gastrointestinal, including nausea, vomiting, diarrhea, bloating, and flatulence. Because the drug has caused fatal lactic acidosis in men with diabetes who have renal insufficiency, baseline renal function testing is suggested. The drug should not be given to women with elevated serum creatinine levels (109).

Troglitazone, another insulin sensitizer, has been reported to enhance the number of ovulatory cycles when used alone or with clomiphene citrate (114). The drug has been withdrawn from the market because of liver toxicity and other adverse effects.

A step-by-step approach to ovulation induction in women with PCOS has been suggested (109). This algorithm offers a practical way to integrate insulin sensitizers and ovulation induction in the treatment of PCOS. This regimen may need to be modified as knowledge of the disorder and its treatment continues to evolve. The step approach is: If body-mass index is elevated, loss of at least 5% of current body weight, Ovulation induction with clomiphene (with or without glucocorticoid if DHEAS is elevated), Insulin sensitizer as a single agent, Insulin sensitizer in combination with *clomiphene citrate,* Gonadotropin therapy, Insulin sensitizer in combination with gonadotropin therapy, Ovarian surgery, and *In vitro* fertilization (IVF).

Current concepts regarding the role of obesity and insulin resistance/hyperinsulinemia in PCOS suggest that the primary intervention should be to recommend and assist with weight loss (5–10% of body weight). In those with an elevated BMI, *orlistat* has proven to be helpful in initiating and maintaining weight loss. A percentage of PCOS patients will respond to weight loss with spontaneous ovulation. In those who do not respond to weight loss alone or who are unable to lose weight, the sequential addition of *chomiphene citrate* followed by an insulin sensitizer alone, followed by the combination of these agents may promote ovulation without the need to proceed to injectable gonadotropins.

A prevailing concern over the increased incidence of spontaneous abortions in women with PCOS and the potential reduction afforded by insulin sensitizers suggest that insulin sensitizers may be beneficial in combination with gonadotropin therapy for ovulation induction or *in vitro* fertilization (115).

Cushing's Syndrome

The adrenal cortex produces three classes of steroid hormones—glucocorticoids, mineralocorticoids, and sex steroids (androgen and estrogen precursors). Hyperfunction of the adrenal gland can produce clinical signs of increased activity of any or all of these hormones. Increased glucocorticoid action results in nitrogen wasting and a catabolic state. This causes muscle weakness, osteoporosis, atrophy of the skin with striae, nonhealing ulcerations and ecchymoses, reduced immune resistance that increases the risk of bacterial and fungal infections, and glucose intolerance resulting from enhanced gluconeogenesis and antagonism to insulin action.

Although most patients with Cushing's syndrome gain weight, some lose it. Obesity is typically central, with characteristic redistribution of fat over the clavicles around the neck and on the trunk, abdomen, and cheeks. Cortisol excess may lead to insomnia, mood disturbances, depression, and even overt psychosis. With overproduction of sex steroid precursors, women may develop some degree of masculinization (hirsutism, acne, oligomenorrhea or amenorrhea, thinning of scalp hair), and men may manifest some degree of feminization

Table 25.3. Causes of Cushing's Syndrome

Category	Cause	Relative Incidence
ACTH-dependent	Cushing's syndrome	60%[a]
	Ectopic ACTH-secreting tumors	15%
	Ectopic CRH-secreting tumors	Rare
ACTH-independent	Adrenal cancer	15%
	Adrenal adenoma	10%
	Micronodular adrenal hyperplasia	Rare
	Iatrogenic/factitious	Common

ACTH, adrenocorticotropic hormone; CRH, corticotropin-releasing hormone.
[a]ACTH-dependent Cushing's syndrome may be caused by pituitary adenoma, basophil hyperplasia, nodular adrenal hyperplasia, or cyclic Cushing's syndrome.

(gynecomastia and impotence). With overproduction of mineralocorticoids, patients may manifest arterial hypertension and hypokalemic alkalosis. The associated fluid retention may cause pedal edema.

The characteristic laboratory findings associated with hypercortisolism are confined mainly to a complete blood count showing evidence of granulocytosis and reduced levels of lymphocytes and eosinophils. Increased urinary calcium secretion may be present.

Causes

The six recognized noniatrogenic causes of Cushing's syndrome can be either ACTH dependent or ACTH independent (Table 25.3). **The ACTH-dependent causes can result from ACTH secreted by pituitary adenomas or from an ectopic source. The hallmark of ACTH-dependent forms of Cushing's syndrome is the presence of normal or high plasma ACTH concentrations with increased cortisol levels. The adrenal glands are hyperplastic bilaterally. Pituitary ACTH-secreting adenoma, or Cushing's disease, is the most common cause of Cushing's syndrome.** These pituitary adenomas are usually microadenomas (<10 mm in diameter) that may be as small as 1 mm. They behave as if they are resistant, to a variable degree, to the feedback effect of cortisol. Like the normal gland, these tumors secrete ACTH in a pulsatile fashion; unlike the normal gland, the diurnal pattern of cortisol secretion is lost. **Ectopic ACTH syndrome most often is caused by malignant tumors.** About one-half of these tumors are small-cell carcinomas of the lung (116). Other tumors include bronchial and thymic carcinomas, carcinoid tumors of the pancreas, and medullary carcinoma of the thyroid.

Ectopic corticotropin-releasing hormone (CRH) tumors are rare and include such tumors as bronchial carcinoids, medullary thyroid carcinoma, and metastatic prostatic carcinoma (116). The presence of an ectopic CRH-secreting tumor should be suspected in patients who react biochemically similar to those with pituitary ACTH-dependent disease but who have rapid disease progression and very high plasma ACTH levels.

The most common cause of ACTH-independent Cushing's syndrome is exogenous or iatrogenic (i.e., superphysiologic therapy with corticosteroids) or factitious (self-induced). Corticosteroids are used in pharmacologic quantities to treat a variety of diseases with an inflammatory component. Over time, this practice will result in Cushing's syndrome. When corticosteroids are taken by the patient but not prescribed by a physician, the diagnosis may be especially challenging. The diagnostic workup for Cushing's syndrome is summarized in Fig. 25.2 and Tables 25.4 and 25.5 (117–119).

Figure 25.2 The workup of Cushing's syndrome.

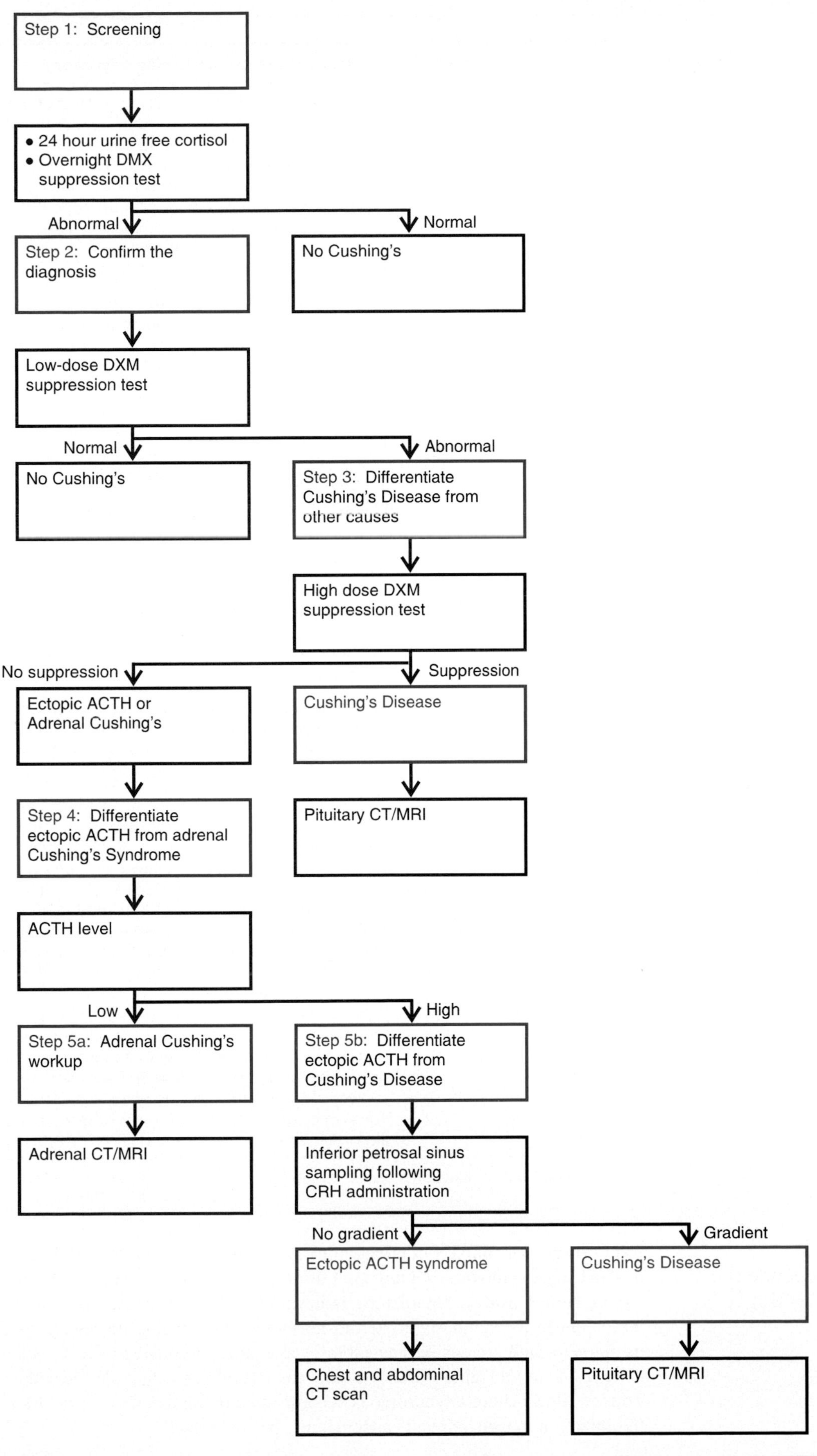

Step 1: Screening
• 24 hour urine free cortisol
• Overnight DMX suppression test
Abnormal
Normal
Step 2: Confirm the diagnosis
No Cushing's
Low-dose DXM suppression test
Normal
Abnormal
No Cushing's
Step 3: Differentiate Cushing's Disease from other causes
High dose DXM suppression test
No suppression
Suppression
Ectopic ACTH or Adrenal Cushing's
Cushing's Disease
Step 4: Differentiate ectopic ACTH from adrenal Cushing's Syndrome
Pituitary CT/MRI
ACTH level
Low
High
Step 5a: Adrenal Cushing's workup
Step 5b: Differentiate ectopic ACTH from Cushing's Disease
Adrenal CT/MRI
Inferior petrosal sinus sampling following CRH administration
No gradient
Gradient
Ectopic ACTH syndrome
Cushing's Disease
Chest and abdominal CT scan
Pituitary CT/MRI

Table 25.4. Diagnostic Workup for Cushing's Syndrome

Screening	**Women with hirsutism who are suspected of having Cushing's syndrome should be tested for urinary free cortisol in a 24-hour collection and should undergo an overnight *dexamethasone* suppression test.** Two consecutive collections are recommended with creatinine determination. Normal urinary free cortisol should range from 30 to 80 μg/day. The overnight *dexamethasone* suppression test is an 8:00 AM cortisol determination after the patient is given 1 mg of *dexamethasone* at 11:00 PM the previous night.
Confirmation of diagnosis	**Confirmation of diagnosis at this stage can be performed by the 2-day, low-dose *dexamethasone* suppression test of Liddle** (117). The patient is given 0.5 mg of *dexamethasone* every 6 hours for 2 days. A 24-hour urine specimen is collected during the second day. Cushing's syndrome is ruled out if there is suppression of urinary 17-hydroxycorticosteroids to <3 mg/24 hr (or to 0% of baseline), suppression of plasma cortisol to <4 μg/day, or suppression of urinary free cortisol to <25 μg/24 hr.
Differentiation of Cushing's syndrome	**The high-dose *dexamethasone* suppression test is used to differentiate Cushing's syndrome from other causes (2 mg every 6 hours).** Normally, urinary 17-hydroxycorticoids should be 40% of baseline after 2 days. This test partially suppresses adrenocorticotropic hormone (ACTH) section with a resulting decrease in cortisol production in most patients with Cushing's syndrome; however, it has no effect on the majority of patients with ectopic or adrenal Cushing's syndrome.
Differentiation of ectopic ACTH syndrome	**High plasma ACTH (>4.5 pmol/L or >20 pg/ml) is consistent with ectopic ACTH production from adrenal glands.** A low ACTH level (<1.1 pmol/L or <5 pg/ml) identifies a patient who most likely has adrenal Cushing's syndrome.
ACTH-independent and -dependent	**A patient with ACTH-independent Cushing's syndrome should undergo an adrenal scan by MRI and should be prepared for adrenal surgery.** A patient with ACTH-dependent Cushing's syndrome should initially receive an administration of cortical-releasing hormone (1 ug/kg IV over 1 minute), which is followed 3–5 minutes later by simultaneous sampling of both the inferior petrosal sinuses and of the peripheral vein. The ratio of ACTH levels from the inferior petrosal sinuses to peripheral plasma is then calculated. An inferior petrosal sinus is virtually diagnostic of a pituitary tumor. Moreover, 95% of patients with Cushing's syndrome are found to have ratios over 2. If the test indicates a patient has Cushing's syndrome, a pituitary MRI with gadolinium enhancement should be obtained in preparation for transsphenoidal surgery. If the results indicate ectopic ACTH secretion, a computed tomography scan of the chest and possibly the abdomen should be performed (118, 119).

IV, intravenous; MRI, magnetic resonance imaging.

Treatment of ACTH-independent Forms of Cushing's Syndrome

Excluding cases that are of iatrogenic or factitious etiology, ACTH-independent forms of Cushing's syndrome are adrenal in origin. Adrenal cancers are usually very large by the time Cushing's syndrome is manifest. This is because the tumors are relatively inefficient in the synthesis of steroid hormones. In general, tumors are larger than 6 cm in diameter and are easily detectable by computed tomography (CT) scanning or magnetic resonance imaging (MRI). Adrenal cancers often produce steroids other than cortisol. Thus, when Cushing's syndrome is accompanied by hirsutism or virilization in women or feminization in men, adrenal cancer should be suspected.

Table 25.5. Laboratory Diagnosis of Cushing's Syndrome

Diagnosis	*24-Hour Urinary Cortisol*	*DEX Low Dose*	*DEX High Dose*	*ACTH*
ACTH-dependent				
Cushing's syndrome (60%) Pituitary adenoma Basophil hyperplasia Nodular adrenal hyperplasia Cyclic Cushing's syndrome	Increased	Increased	Decreased	Normal
Ectopic ACTH (15%)	Increased	Increased	Increased	Increased
Ectopic CRH (rare)	Increased	Increased	Increased or decreased	Increased
ACTH-independent				
Adrenal neoplasia Adenoma (10%) Carcinoma (15%) Primary adrenocorticoid nodular dysplasia (<1%)	Increased	Increased	Increased	Decreased
Pseudo-Cushing's syndrome (alcohol-related, <1%)	Increased	Increased	Decreased	Normal
Exogenous glucocorticoids/factitious (not cortisol)	Increased or decreased	Decreased	Decreased	Decreased

DEX, dexamethasone; ACTH, adrenocorticotropic hormone; CRH, corticotropin-releasing hormone.

An adrenal tumor that appears large and irregular on radiologic imaging is suggestive of carcinoma. In these cases, a unilateral adrenalectomy through an abdominal exploratory approach is preferable. In most malignant tumors, complete resection is virtually impossible. However, a partial response to postoperative chemotherapy or radiation may be achieved. Most patients with malignancy die within 1 year. When administered immediately after surgery, mitotane (O,P-DDD, adrenocorticolytic drug) may be of benefit in preventing or delaying recurrent disease (124). Manifestations of Cushing's syndrome in these patients are controlled by adrenal enzyme inhibitors.

Adrenal adenomas are smaller than carcinomas and average 3 cm in diameter. These tumors are usually unilateral and infrequently are associated with other steroid-mediated syndromes. Micronodular adrenal disease is a disorder of children, adolescents, and young adults. The adrenal glands contain numerous small (>3 mm) nodules, which often are pigmented and secrete sufficient cortisol to suppress pituitary ACTH. This condition can be sporadic or familial.

Surgical removal of a neoplasm is the treatment of choice (127,128). If a unilateral, well-circumscribed adenoma is identified by MRI or CT scanning, the flank approach may be the most convenient. The cure rate following surgical removal of adrenal adenomas approaches 100%. Several months of corticosteroid replacement therapy usually is required.

Treatment of Cushing's Disease

The treatment of choice for Cushing's disease is transsphenoidal resection. The cure rate is approximately 80% in patients with microadenomas who undergo surgery by an experienced surgeon (120) and is less than 50% in patients with macroadenomas (121). Transient diabetes insipidus is common (122).

Radiation Therapy

High-voltage external pituitary radiation (4,200 to 4,500 cGy) is given at a rate not exceeding 200 cGy/day. Although only 15% to 25% of adults show total improvement (122), approximately 80% of children respond (123).

Medical Therapy

Mitotane can be used to induce medical adrenalectomy during or after pituitary radiation (124). The role of medical therapy is to prepare the severely ill patient for surgery and to maintain normal cortisol levels while a patient awaits the full effect of radiation. Occasionally, medical therapy is used for patients who respond to therapy with only partial remission. Adrenal enzyme inhibitors include *aminoglutethimide, metyrapone, trilostane,* and *etomidate.*

A combination of *aminoglutethimide* and *metyrapone* may cause a total adrenal enzyme block requiring corticosteroid-replacement therapy. *Ketoconazole,* an FDA-approved antifungal agent, also inhibits adrenal steroid biosynthesis at the side arm cleavage and 11β-hydroxylation steps. The dose of *ketoconazole* for adrenal suppression is 600 to 800 mg/day for 3 months to 1 year (125). *Ketoconazole* is effective for long-term control of hypercortisolism of either pituitary or adrenal origin.

Nelson's syndrome is an ACTH-secreting pituitary adenoma that develops after bilateral adrenalectomy for Cushing's disease (126). This syndrome reportedly complicates 10% to 50% of bilateral adrenalectomy cases. Nelson's syndrome is less common today because bilateral adrenalectomy is less frequently used as initial treatment. Present medical management produces such an effective block to steroid overproduction that it is used primarily as well as after the failure of surgical and radiation therapy. This syndrome is usually caused by a macroadenoma that produces sellar pressure symptoms of headaches, visual field disturbances, and ophthalmoplegia. Extremely high ACTH levels are associated with severe hyperpigmentation (melanocyte-stimulating hormone activity). The treatment is surgical removal or radiation.

Congenital Adrenal Hyperplasia

CAH is transmitted as an autosomal recessive disorder. Several adrenocortical enzymes necessary for cortisol biosynthesis may be affected. Failure to synthesize the fully functional enzyme has the following effects:

1. A relative decrease in cortisol production
2. A compensatory increase in ACTH levels
3. Hyperplasia of the zona reticularis of the adrenal cortex
4. An accumulation of the precursors of the affected enzyme in the bloodstream.

21-Hydroxylase Deficiency

Deficiency of 21-hydroxylase is responsible for over 90% of all cases of CAH. The disorder produces a spectrum of conditions. Salt-wasting CAH, which is the most severe form, affects 75% of patients in whom, during the first 2 weeks of life, a hypovolemic salt-wasting crisis is manifest, accompanied by hyponatremia, hyperkalemia, and acidosis. The salt-wasting crisis results from ineffective aldosterone synthesis. The condition is usually diagnosed earlier in affected women than in men because it causes genital virilization (e.g., clitoromegaly, labioscrotal fusion, and abnormal urethral course).

In simple virilizing CAH, affected patients are diagnosed as virilized newborn females or as rapidly growing masculinized boys at 3 to 7 years of age.

1. Basal follicular phase 17-OHP <200 ng/dl virtually excludes the disorder; no further testing is required.

2. Basal 17-OHP >500 ng/dl establishes the diagnosis; there is no need for further testing (125).

3. Basal 17-OHP >200 ng/dl and <500 ng/dl requires ACTH stimulation testing.

4. In the ACTH stimulation test, plasma levels of 17-OHP are checked 1 hour following intravenous administration of a bolus of 0.25 mg ACTH 1-24 (*cosyntropin* [*Cortrosyn*]) (Fig. 25.3). 17-OHP levels after ACTH stimulation in adult-onset adrenal hyperplasia are generally >1,000 ng/dl (129) (Fig. 25.3).

5. Individuals who are heterozygous (carriers) for both adult-onset adrenal hyperplasia and CAH reveal stimulated 17-OHP values <1,000 ng/dl. In many cases, an overlap with the values seen in the normal population is observed (130) (Fig. 25.3).

Nonclassic Congenital Adrenal Hyperplasia

The nonclassic type 21-hydroxylase deficiency represents partial deficiency in 21-hydroxylation, which produces a late-onset, milder hyperandrogenemia. Some women with a mild gene defect demonstrate elevated circulating 17-OHP concentrations but no clinical symptoms or signs.

Figure 25.3 Basal and stimulated 17-hydroxyprogesterone concentration.

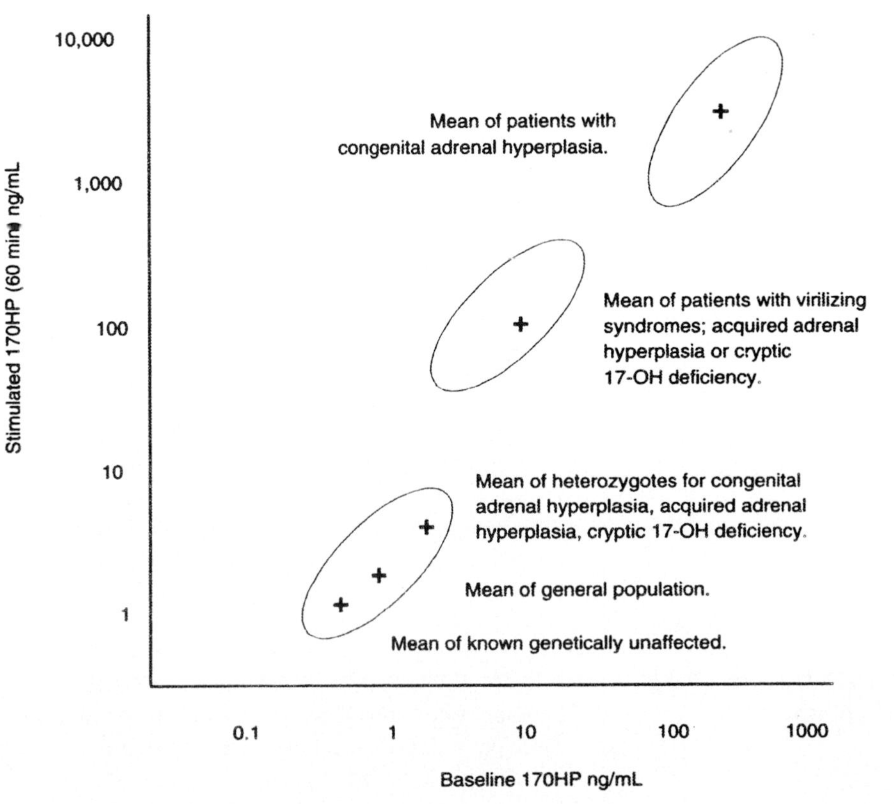

The hyperandrogenic symptoms of adult-onset CAH are mild and typically present at or after puberty. Following are the three phenotypic varieties (129):

1. PCOS (39%)
2. Hirsutism alone without oligomenorrhea (39%)
3. Cryptic (22%) (hyperandrogenism but no hyperandrogenic symptoms).

The need for screening patients with hirsutism for adult-onset adrenal hyperplasia depends on the patient population. The disease frequency is estimated to occur in 0.1% of the general population, 1% to 2% of Hispanics and Yugoslavs, and 3% to 4% of Ashkenazi Jews (131).

Genetics of 21-Hydroxylase Deficiency

1. The 21-hydroxylase gene is located on the short arm of chromosome 6, in the midst of the HLA region.
2. The 21-hydroxylase gene is now termed *CYP21*. Its homologue is the pseudogene *CYP21P* (132).
3. Because *CYP21P* is a pseudogene, the lack of transcription renders it nonfunctional. The *CYP21* is the active gene.
4. The *CYP21* gene and the *CYP21P* pseudogene alternate with two genes called *C4B* and *C4A,* both of which encode for the fourth component (C4) of serum complement (132).
5. The close linkage between the 21-hydroxylase genes and HLA alleles has allowed the study of 21-hydroxylase inheritance patterns in families through blood HLA typing (e.g., linkage of HLA-B14 was found in Ashkenazi Jews, Hispanics, and Italians) (133).

Prenatal Diagnosis and Treatment

In families at risk for CAH, first-trimester prenatal screening is advocated (132). Currently, the fetal DNA is used for specific amplification of the *CYP21* gene using polymerase chain reaction (PCR) amplification (134). An aggressive and still controversial approach involves the use of *dexamethasone* treatment for all pregnant women at risk of having a child with CAH. The dosage is 20 mg/kg in three divided doses administered as soon as pregnancy is recognized and no later than 9 weeks of gestation. This is done prior to performing chorionic villus sampling or amniocentesis in the second trimester. *Dexamethasone* crosses the placenta and suppresses ACTH in the fetus. If the fetus is determined to be an unaffected female or a male, treatment is discontinued. If the fetus is an affected female, dexamethasone therapy is continued. When *dexamethasone* is administered before 9 weeks of gestation and is continued to term, it effectively reduces genital ambiguity in genetic females (132). However, at least two-thirds of treated females still require surgical repair of the genitalia. Although prenatal treatment reduces virilization in females, the efficacy and safety to both mother and baby have not been verified. The unnecessary treatment in seven out of every eight pregnancies poses a serious ethical dilemma (135).

11β-Hydroxylase Deficiency

In a small percentage of patients with CAH, hypertension rather than mineralocorticoid deficiency develops. The hypertension responds to corticosteroid replacement (136). Most of these patients have a deficiency in 11β-hydroxylase. In most populations, 11β-hydroxylase deficiency accounts for 5% to 8% of the cases of CAH, or 1 in 100,000 births (137). A much higher incidence, 1 in 5,000 to 7,000, has been described in Moroccan Jewish immigrants (138).

Two 11β-hydroxylase isoenzymes are responsible for cortisol and aldosterone synthesis, respectively, CYP11-B1 and CYP11-B2. They are encoded by two genes on the middle of the long arm of chromosome 8 (139,140). No HLA linkage has been identified.

Inability to synthesize a fully functional 11β-hydroxylase enzyme causes a decrease in cortisol production, a compensatory increase in ACTH secretion, and increased production of 11-deoxycortisol, 11-deoxycorticosterone, DHEA, and androstenedione. The diagnosis of 11β-hydroxylase–deficient late-onset adrenal hyperplasia is determined when 11-deoxycortisol levels are higher than 25 ng/ml 60 minutes after ACTH 1-24 stimulation (141).

Patients with 11β-hydroxylase deficiency may present with either a classic pattern of the disorder or symptoms of a mild deficiency. The severe, classic form occurs in about two-thirds of the patients with mild-to-moderate hypertension during the first years of life. In about one-third of the patients it is associated with left ventricular hypertrophy, with or without retinopathy, and death is occasionally reported from cerebrovascular accident (136). Signs of androgen excess are common in the severe form and are similar to those seen in the 21-hydroxylase deficiency.

In the mild, nonclassic form, children are found to have virilization or precocious puberty but not hypertension. Adult women will seek treatment for postpubertal onset of hirsutism, acne, and amenorrhea.

3β-Hydroxysteroid Dehydrogenase Deficiency

Deficiency of 3β-hydroxysteroid dehydrogenase occurs with varying frequency in hirsute patients (142,143). The enzyme is found in both the adrenal glands and ovaries (unlike 21- and 11-hydroxylase) and is responsible for transforming Δ-5 steroids into the corresponding Δ-4 compounds. The diagnosis of this disorder relies on the relationship of Δ-5 and Δ-4 steroids. A marked elevation of DHEA and DHEAS in the presence of normal or mildly elevated testosterone or androstenedione may be a signal to initiate a screening protocol for 3β-hydroxysteroid dehydrogenase deficiency using exogenous ACTH stimulation (142). Following intravenous administration of a 0.25-mg ACTH 1-24 bolus, 17-hydroxypregnenolone levels rise significantly within 60 minutes in women with 3β-hydroxysteroid dehydrogenase deficiency compared with normal women (2,276 ng/dl compared with normal of 1,050 ng/dl). The mean poststimulation ratio between 17-hydroxypregnenolone and 17-OHP was markedly elevated (mean ratio of 11 compared with 3.4 in normal controls and 0.4 in 21-hydroxylase deficiency). Because of the rarity of this disorder, routine screening of hyperandrogenic patients is not justified(142,143).

Treatment of Adult-onset Congenital Adrenal Hyperplasia

In adults with CAH, *dexamethasone* has been shown to suppress the hypothalamic–pituitary axis better than cortisone acetate or hydrocortisone administered in equivalent doses and to possibly induce less fluid retention than other corticosteroids. Evening administration with a dosage of 0.25 to 0.5 mg is most effective (144). In some patients, alternate-day therapy using the same dosage is sufficient. Periodic evaluation of serum cortisol is recommended. If morning serum cortisol concentrations are maintained at greater than 2 μg/dl, oversuppression is unlikely (145).

Androgen-secreting Ovarian and Adrenal Tumors

Patients with severe hirsutism, virilization, or recent and rapidly progressing signs of androgen excess require careful investigation for the presence of an androgen-secreting neoplasm. In prepubertal girls, virilizing tumors may cause signs of heterosexual precocious puberty in addition to hirsutism, acne, and virilization. A markedly elevated total testosterone level (2.5 times the upper normal range or over 200 ng/dl) is typical of an ovarian androgen-secreting tumor, and a DHEAS level greater than 800 μg/dl is typical of an adrenal tumor. An adrenal tumor is unlikely when serum DHEAS and urinary 17-ketosteroid excretion measurements are in the normal basal range and the serum cortisol concentration is greater than 3.3 μg/dl after dexamethasone administration (146). The results of other dynamic tests, especially testosterone suppression and stimulation, are unreliable (147).

A vaginal and abdominal ultrasonographic examination is the first step in the evaluation of an ovarian neoplasm. Duplex Doppler scanning may increase the accuracy of tumor localization (148).

CT scanning can reveal tumors larger than 10 mm (1 cm) in the adrenal gland but may not help to distinguish among different types of solid tumors (149). In the ovaries, CT scanning cannot help differentiate hormonally active from functional tumors (148,149).

MRI is comparable, if not superior, to CT scanning in detecting ovarian neoplasms. When CT and selective venous catheterization fail, nuclear medicine scanning of the abdomen and pelvis after injection with NP-59 ((131-iodine) 6-beta-iodomethyl-19-norcholesterol), preceded by adrenal and thyroid suppression, may facilitate tumor localization (150).

If all four vessels are catheterized transfemorally, selective venous catheterization allows direct localization of the tumor. Samples are obtained for hormonal analysis, with positive localization defined as a 5:1 testosterone gradient compared with lower vena cava values (151). Under such circumstances specificity approaches 80%, but this rate should be weighed against the 5% rate of significant complications such as adrenal hemorrhage and infarction, venous thrombosis, hematoma, and radiation exposure (152).

Androgen-producing Ovarian Neoplasms

Ovarian neoplasms are the most frequent androgen-producing tumors. *Granulosa cell tumors* constitute 1% to 2% of all ovarian tumors and occur mostly in adult women (in postmenopausal more frequently than in premenopausal women) (see Chapter 32). Usually associated with estrogen production, they are the most common functioning tumors in children and lead to isosexual precocious puberty (153). Total abdominal hysterectomy and bilateral salpingo-oophorectomy are the treatments of choice. If fertility is desired, in the absence of contralateral or pelvic involvement, unilateral salpingo-oophorectomy is justifiable. The 10-year survival rates vary from 60% to 90%, depending on the stage, tumor size, and histologic atypia (153).

Thecomas are rare and occur in older patients (153). In one study only 11% were found to be androgenic, even in the presence of steroid-type cells (luteinized thecomas) (154). The tumor is rarely malignant and rarely bilateral, and a simple oophorectomy is sufficient treatment.

Sclerosing stromal tumors are benign neoplasms that usually occur in patients younger than 30 years (153). A few cases with estrogenic or androgenic manifestations have been reported.

Sertoli-Leydig cell tumors, previously classified as androblastoma or arrhenoblastoma, account for 11% of solid ovarian tumors. They contain various proportions of Sertoli cells, Leydig cells, and fibroblasts (153). Sertoli-Leydig cell tumors are the most common virilizing tumors in women of reproductive age; however, masculinization occurs in only one-third of patients. The tumor is bilateral in 1.5%. In 80% of cases, it is diagnosed at stage IA (153). Treatment with unilateral salpingo-oophorectomy is justified in patients with stage IA disease who desire fertility. Total abdominal hysterectomy, bilateral salpingo-oophorectomy, and adjuvant therapy are recommended for postmenopausal women who have advanced-stage disease.

Pure Sertoli cell tumors are usually unilateral. For a premenopausal woman with stage I disease, a unilateral salpingo-oophorectomy is the treatment of choice. Malignant tumors are rapidly fatal (155).

Gynandroblastomas are benign tumors with well-differentiated ovarian and testicular elements. A unilateral oophorectomy or salpingo-oophorectomy is sufficient treatment.

Sex cord tumors with annular tubules (SCTAT) are frequently associated with Peutz-Jeghers syndrome (gastrointestinal polyposis and mucocutaneous melanin pigmentation) (156). Their morphologic features range between those of the granulosa cell and Sertoli cell tumors.

Whereas SCTAT with Peutz-Jeghers syndrome tend to be bilateral and benign, SCTAT without Peutz-Jeghers syndrome are almost always unilateral and are malignant in one-fifth of cases (153).

Steroid Cell Tumors

According to Young and Scully, steroid cell tumors are composed entirely of steroid-secreting cells subclassified into stromal luteoma, Leydig cell tumors (hilar and nonhilar), and steroid cell tumors that are not otherwise specific (153). Virilization or hirsutism is encountered with three-fourths of Leydig cell tumors, with one-half of steroid cell tumors that are not otherwise specific, and with 12% of stromal luteomas.

Nonfunctioning Ovarian Tumors

Ovarian neoplasms, which are usually non–steroid-producing, are occasionally associated with androgen excess and include serous and mucinous cystadenomas, Brenner tumors, Krukenberg tumors, benign cystic teratomas, and dysgerminomas (157). Gonadoblastomas arising in the dysgenetic gonads of patients with a Y chromosome are associated with androgen and estrogen secretion (158,159).

Stromal Hyperplasia and Stromal Hyperthecosis

Stromal hyperplasia is a nonneoplastic proliferation of ovarian stromal cells. Stromal hyperthecosis is defined as the presence of luteinized stromal cells at a distance from the follicles (160). Stromal hyperplasia, which is typically seen in patients between 60 and 80 years of age, may be associated with hyperandrogenism, endometrial carcinoma, obesity, hypertension, and glucose intolerance (160). *Hyperthecosis* also is seen in a mild form in older patients. In patients of reproductive age, hyperthecosis may demonstrate severe clinical manifestations of virilization, obesity, and hypertension. Hyperinsulinemia and glucose intolerance may occur in up to 90% of patients with hyperthecosis and probably play a role in the etiology of stromal luteinization and hyperandrogenism (161). Hyperthecosis is found in many patients with hyperandrogenemia, insulin resistance, and acanthosis nigricans (HAIR-AN syndrome).

In patients with hyperthecosis, levels of ovarian androgens, including testosterone, DHT, and androstenedione are increased, usually in the male range. The predominant estrogen, as in PCOS, is estrone, which is derived from peripheral aromatization. The E_1-to-E_2 ratio is increased. Unlike in PCOS, gonadotropin levels are normal (162).

Wedge resection for the treatment of mild hyperthecosis has been successful and has resulted in resumption of ovulation and even in a pregnancy (163). However, in cases of more severe hyperthecosis and high free testosterone levels (1 to 3 ng/dl), the ovulatory response to wedge resection is only transient (162). In a study in which bilateral oophorectomy was used to control severe virilization, hypertension and glucose intolerance sometimes disappeared (164). Moreover, when a GnRH agonist was used to treat patients with severe hyperthecosis, ovarian androgen production was dramatically suppressed (165).

Virilization During Pregnancy

Luteomas of pregnancy are frequently associated with maternal and fetal masculinization. This is not a true neoplasm but rather a reversible hyperplasia, which usually regresses postpartum. A review of the literature reveals a 30% incidence of maternal virilization and a 65% incidence of virilized females in the presence of a pregnancy luteoma and maternal masculinization (166).

Other tumors causing virilization in pregnancy include (in descending order of frequency) Krukenberg tumors, mucinous cystic tumors, Brenner tumors, serous cystadenomas, endodermal sinus tumors, and dermoid cysts. Five cases of virilization of a female child have been reported (153).

Virilizing Adrenal Neoplasms

High testosterone levels (in the tumor range), accompanied by normal or only moderately elevated DHEAS levels, should not divert attention from the adrenal gland to the ovary. In fact, patients with these adenomas manifest increased testosterone production following stimulation with human chorionic gonadotropin (hCG) or LH and decreased testosterone secretion following LH suppression.

Of the fewer than 100 reported cases of pure virilizing adrenal neoplasms, 90% were benign. Although the peak age for the diagnosis of adenomas was 20 to 40 years, most of the pure testosterone-producing tumors occurred in menopausal women. With one exception, all cases of adenomas and carcinomas were unilateral. Fifty percent were palpable abdominally in children; in adults, none was detected solely by physical examination (167).

Prolactin Disorders

Prolactin was first identified as a product of the anterior pituitary in 1933 (168). Since that time, it has been found in nearly every vertebrate species. The specific activities of human prolactin (hPRL) have been further defined by the separation of its activity from growth hormone (169) and subsequently by the development of radioimmunoassays (170–172). Although the initiation and maintenance of lactation is the primary function of prolactin, many studies have documented a significant role for prolactin activity both within and beyond the reproductive system.

Prolactin Secretion

There are 199 amino acids within human prolactin, with a molecular weight (MW) of 23,000 daltons (Fig. 25.4). Although human growth hormone and placental lactogen have significant lactogenic activity, they have only a 16% and 13% amino acid sequence homology with prolactin, respectively.

In the basal state three forms are released, a monomer, a dimer, and a multimeric species, called *little, big, and big-big prolactin,* respectively (173–175). The two larger species can be degraded to the monomeric form by reducing disulfide bonds (176). The proportions of each of these prolactin species vary with physiologic, pathologic, and hormonal stimulation (176–179). The heterogeneity of secreted forms remains an active area of research. Overall, studies thus far indicate that little prolactin (MW 23,000 daltons) constitutes more than 50% of all combined prolactin production and is most responsive to extrapituitary stimulation or suppression (175,178,179). The bioactivity and immunoreactivity of little prolactin is influenced by glycosylation (180–183). It appears that the glycosylated form is the predominant species secreted, but the most potent biologic form appears to be the 23,000-dalton nonglycosylated form of prolactin (182). To some degree, the physical heterogeneity of prolactin may explain the biologic heterogeneity of this hormone, but it further complicates the physiologic evaluation of prolactin's myriad effects.

In contrast to other anterior pituitary hormones, which are controlled by hypothalamic-releasing factors, prolactin secretion is primarily under inhibitory control mediated by dopamine. **Multiple lines of evidence suggest that dopamine, which is secreted by the tuberoinfundibular dopaminergic neurons into the portal hypophyseal vessels, is the primary prolactin-inhibiting factor.** Dopamine receptors have been found on pituitary lactotrophs (184), and treatment with dopamine or dopamine agonists suppresses prolactin secretion (185–190). The dopamine antagonist metaclopramide abolishes the pulsatility

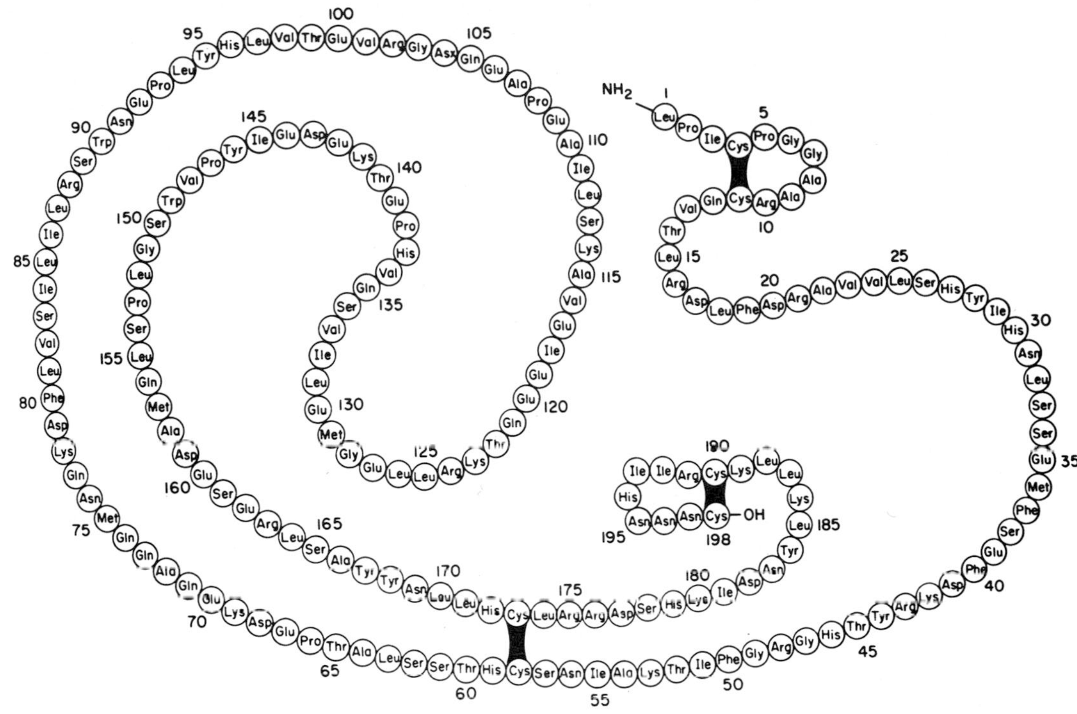

Figure 25.4 Amino acid sequence of prolactin. Three cysteine disulfide bands are located within the molecule. (From **Bondy PK.** *Rosenberg leukocyte esterase: metabolic control and disease,* 8th ed. Philadelphia: WB Saunders, 1980, with permission.)

of prolactin release and increases serum prolactin levels (186,187,191). Interference with dopamine release from the hypothalamus to the pituitary routinely increases serum prolactin levels. γ-Aminobutyric acid (GABA) and other neuropeptides also may function as prolactin-inhibiting factors (Table 25.6) (192–195). Several hypothalamic polypeptides that increase prolactin-releasing activity are listed in Table 25.6.

Hyperprolactinemia

Physiologic alterations or conditions may result in transient as well as persistent elevations in prolactin levels. Drug-related and physiologic conditions resulting in hyperprolactinemia do not always require intervention.

Evaluation

Plasma levels of immunoreactive prolactin are 5 to 27 ng/ml throughout the normal menstrual cycle. Samples should not be drawn soon after the patient awakes or after procedures. Prolactin is secreted in a pulsatile fashion with a pulse frequency ranging from about 14 pulses per 24 hours in the late follicular phase to about nine pulses per 24 hours in the late luteal phase. There also is a diurnal variation, with the lowest levels occurring in midmorning. Levels rise 1 hour after the onset of sleep and continue to rise until peak values are reached between 5:00 and 7:00 AM (196,197). The pulse amplitude of prolactin appears to increase from early to late follicular and luteal phases (198–200). Because of the variability of secretion and inherent limitations of radioimmunoassay, an elevated level should always be rechecked. This sample preferably is drawn midmorning and not after stress, previous venipuncture, breast stimulation, or physical examination, which increase prolactin levels.

Prolactin and TSH determinations are basic evaluations in infertile women. Infertile men with hypogonadism also should be tested. Likewise, prolactin levels should be measured in the evaluation of amenorrhea, galactorrhea, amenorrhea with galactorrhea, hirsutism with amenorrhea, anovulatory bleeding, and delayed puberty (Fig. 25.5).

Table 25.6. Chemical Factors Modulating Prolactin Release and Conditions That Result in Hyperprolactinemia

Inhibitory factors
Dopamine
γ-Aminobutyric acid
Histidyl-proline diketopiperazine
Pyroglutamic acid
Somatostatin
Stimulatory factors
β-Endorphin
17β-Estradiol
Enkephalins
Gonadotropin-releasing hormone
Histamine
Serotonin
Substance P
Thyrotropin-releasing hormone
Vasoactive intestinal peptide
Physiologic conditions
Anesthesia
Empty sella syndrome
Idiopathic
Intercourse
Major surgery and disorders of chest wall (burns, herpes, chest percussion)
Newborns
Nipple stimulation
Pregnancy
Postpartum (nonnursing: days 1–7; nursing: with suckling)
Sleep
Stress
Postpartum
Hypothalamic conditions
Arachnoid cyst
Craniopharyngioma
Cystic glioma
Cysticercosis
Dermoid cyst
Epidermoid cyst
Histiocytosis
Neurotuberculosis
Pineal tumors
Pseudotumor cerebri
Sarcoidosis
Suprasellar cysts
Tuberculosis
Pituitary conditions
Acromegaly
Addison's disease
Craniopharyngioma
Cushing's syndrome
Hypothyroidism
Histiocytosis
Lymphoid hypophysitis
Metastatic tumors (especially of the lungs and breasts)
Multiple endocrine neoplasia
Nelson's syndrome
Pituitary adenoma (microadenoma or macroadenoma)
Post–oral contraception
Sarcoidosis
Thyrotropin-releasing hormone administration

Table 25.6.—*continued*
Trauma to stalk Tuberculosis
Metabolic dysfunction
Ectopic production (hypernephroma, bronchogenic sarcoma) Hepatic cirrhosis Renal failure Starvation refeeding
Drug conditions
α Methyldopa Antidepressants (*amoxapine, imipramine, amitriptyline*) *Cimetidine* Dopamine antagonists (phenothiazines, thioxanthenes, *butyrophenone, diphenylbutylpiperidine, dibenzoxazepine, dihydroindolone, procainamide, metaclopramide*) Estrogen therapy Opiates *Reserpine* *Sulpiride* *Verapamil*

Physical Signs

Amenorrhea without galactorrhea is associated with hyperprolactinemia in approximately 15% of women (201–203). The cessation of normal ovulatory processes attributed to elevated prolactin levels may be related to the following gonadal and hypothalamic-pituitary effects: reduction in granuosa cell number and FSH binding (204), inhibition of granulosa cell 17β-estradiol production by interfering with FSH action (204–206), inadequate luteinization and reduced progesterone (207–209), and the suppressive effects of prolactin on GnRH pulsatile release, which may mediate most of the anovulatory effects (210–222).

Although isolated galactorrhea commonly is considered indicative of hyperprolactinemia, prolactin levels are within the normal range in nearly 50% of such patients (223–225) (Fig. 25.5). In these cases, an earlier transient episode of hyperprolactinemia may have existed, that triggered galactorrhea. This situation is very similar to nursing mothers in whom milk secretion, once established, continues despite normal prolactin levels. Repeat testing is occasionally helpful in detecting hyperprolactinemia. Approximately one-third of women with galactorrhea have normal menses. Conversely, hyperprolactinemia commonly occurs in the absence of galactorrhea (66%), which may result from inadequate estrogenic or progestational priming of the breast.

In patients with both galactorrhea and amenorrhea (including the syndromes described and named by Forbes, Henneman, Griswold, and Albright in 1951, Argonz and del Castilla in 1953, and Chiari and Frommel in 1985), **approximately two-thirds will have hyperprolactinemia; in that group, approximately one-third will have a pituitary adenoma** (226). In anovulatory women, 3% to 10% of women diagnosed with polycystic ovary disease have hyperprolactinemia (227,228) (Fig. 25.6).

In all cases of delayed puberty, pituitary abnormalities, including craniopharyngiomas and adenomas, must be considered. Additionally, the multiple endocrine neoplasia type 1 syndrome should be considered, particularly in patients with a family history of multiple adenomas (229). Prolactinomas are noted in approximately 20% of patients with multiple endocrine neoplasia type 1 (MEN-1). The *MEN-1* gene is localized to chromosome 11q13 and appears to act as a constitutive tumor suppressor gene. An inactivating mutation results in development of the tumor. It is thought that prolactinomas that occur in patients with MEN-1 may be more aggressive than sporadic prolactinomas (230). Prolactin and TSH levels should be measured in all patients with delayed puberty.

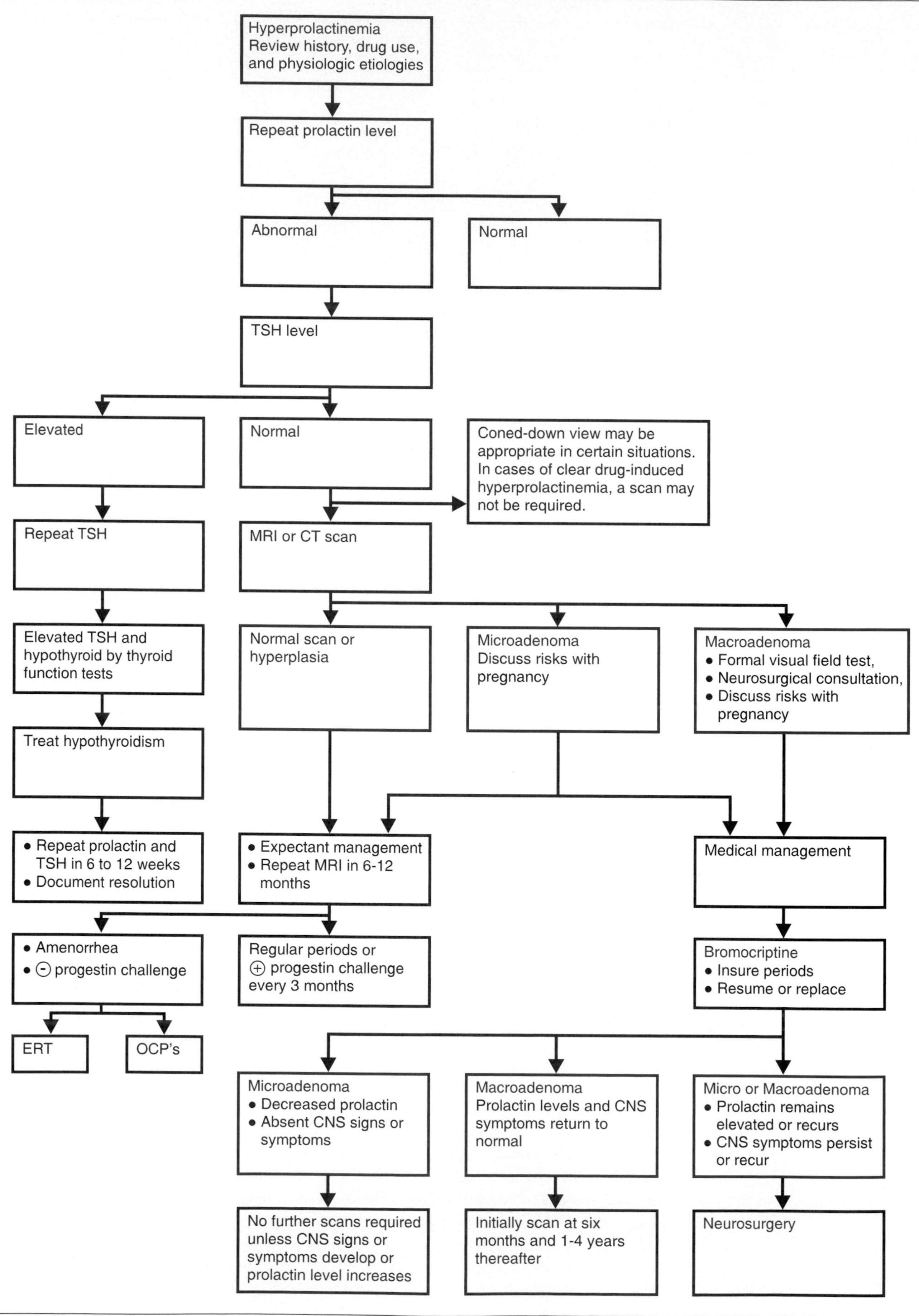

Hyperprolactinemia
Review history, drug use, and physiologic etiologies
Repeat prolactin level
Abnormal
Normal
TSH level
Elevated
Normal
Coned-down view may be appropriate in certain situations. In cases of clear drug-induced hyperprolactinemia, a scan may not be required.
Repeat TSH
MRI or CT scan
Elevated TSH and hypothyroid by thyroid function tests
Normal scan or hyperplasia
Microadenoma
Discuss risks with pregnancy
Macroadenoma
• Formal visual field test,
• Neurosurgical consultation,
• Discuss risks with pregnancy
Treat hypothyroidism
• Repeat prolactin and TSH in 6 to 12 weeks
• Document resolution
• Expectant management
• Repeat MRI in 6-12 months
Medical management
• Amenorrhea
• ⊖ progestin challenge
Regular periods or ⊕ progestin challenge every 3 months
Bromocriptine
• Insure periods
• Resume or replace
ERT
OCP's
Microadenoma
• Decreased prolactin
• Absent CNS signs or symptoms
Macroadenoma
Prolactin levels and CNS symptoms return to normal
Micro or Macroadenoma
• Prolactin remains elevated or recurs
• CNS symptoms persist or recur
No further scans required unless CNS signs or symptoms develop or prolactin level increases
Initially scan at six months and 1-4 years thereafter
Neurosurgery

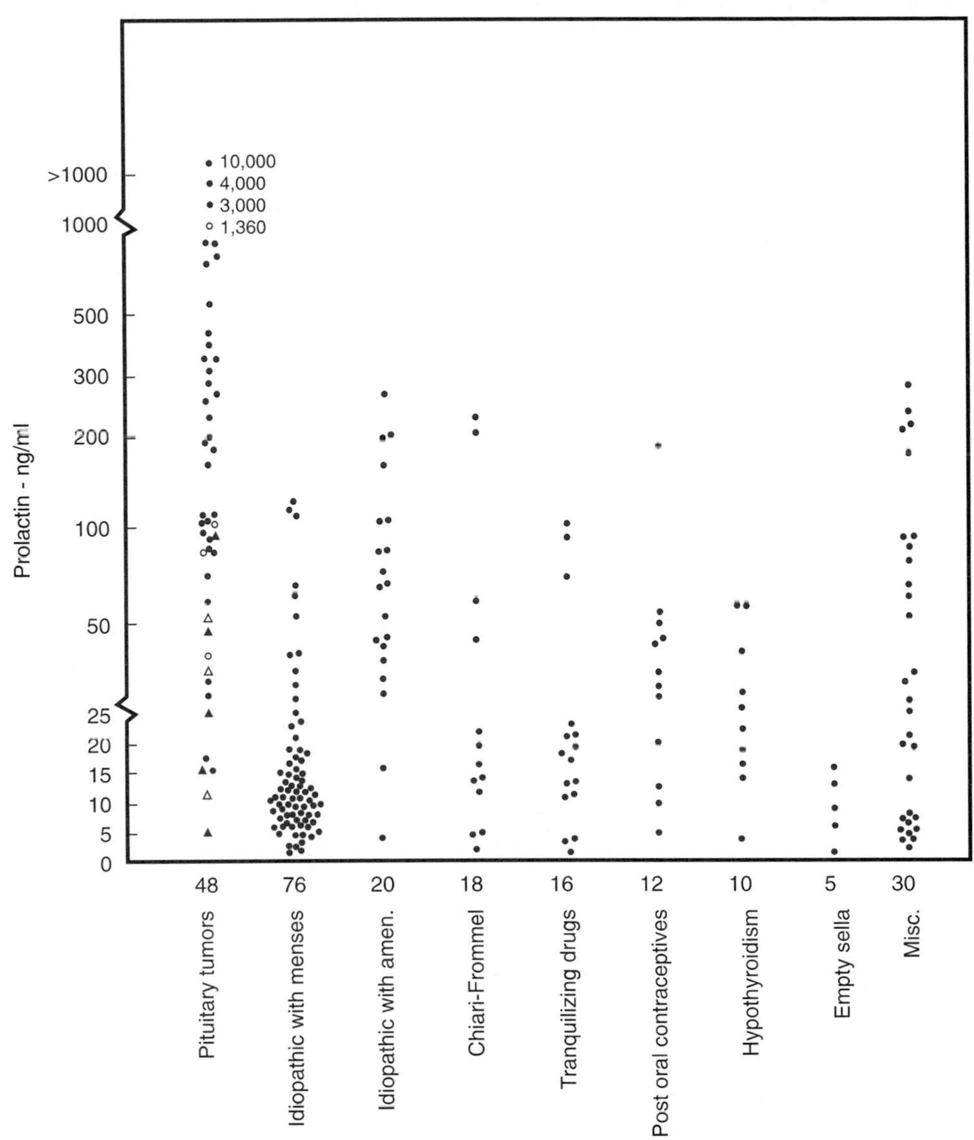

Figure 25.6 Prolactin levels in 235 patients with galactorrhea. Among patients with a tumor, open triangles denote associated acromegaly, and solid circles and solid triangles denote previous radiotherapy or surgical resection, respectively. (From **Kleinberg DL, Noel GL, Frantz AG.** Galactorrhea: a study of 235 cases, including 48 with pituitary tumors. *N Engl J Med* 1977;296:589–600.)

Once an elevated prolactin level is documented, knowledge of neuroanatomy as well as imaging techniques and their interpretation is essential to further management (see Chapter 7). Patients can be reassured that hyperprolactinemia usually is associated with a relatively benign condition (pituitary microadenoma or release of pituitary stem cell growth inhibition through activation or loss of function mutations in the pituitary lactotroph) that requires only periodic monitoring. However, it is critical for the physician to exercise vigilance and to consider other potential etiologies, particularly sellar and suprasellar tumors. Levels of TSH should be measured in all cases of hyperprolactinemia (Fig. 25.5)

Figure 25.5 Workup for hyperprolactinemia.

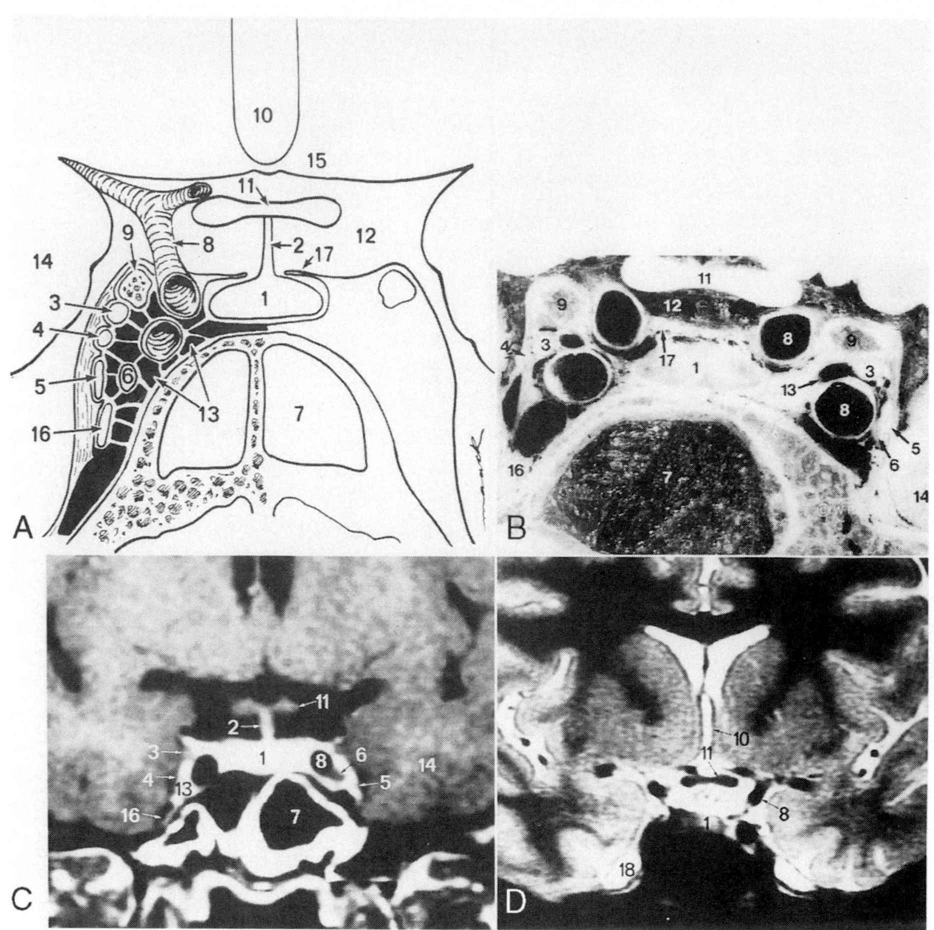

Figure 25.7 Anatomy of the intrasellar region and cavernous sinus by: (A) anatomic diagram, **(B)** coronal cytomicrosome section, **(C)** coronal postcontrast T1-weighted MRI, and **(D)** coronal postcontrast T2-weighted MRI. (1, pituitary gland; 2, infundibular stalk; 3, cranial nerve (CN) III; 4, CN IV; 5, CN VI; 6, CN VI; 7, sphenoid sinus; 8, internal carotid artery; 9, anterior clinoid process; 10, third ventricle; 11, optic chiasm; 12, suprasellar cistern; 13, venous spaces of cavernous sinus; 14, temporal lobe; 15, hypothalamus; 16, CN V_2; 17, diaphragma sellae; 18, Meckel's cave.)

Imaging Techniques

In patients with larger microadenomas and macroadenomas prolactin levels usually are higher than 100 ng/ml. However, levels lower than 100 ng/ml may be associated with smaller microadenomas and other suprasellar tumors that may be easily missed on a "coned-down" view of the sella turcica. In patients with a clearly identifiable drug-induced or physiologic hyperprolactinemia, scanning may not be necessary. MRI imaging of the sella and pituitary gland with gadolinium enhancement appears to provide the best anatomic detail (231) (Fig. 25.7). The cumulative radiation dose from multiple CT scans may cause cataracts, and the "coned-down" views or tomograms of the sella are very insensitive and likewise expose the patient to radiation. Even modest elevations of prolactin can be associated with microadenomas or macroadenomas, nonlactotroph pituitary tumors, and other central nervous system abnormalities; thus, imaging of the pituitary gland must be considered (Table 25.7). For patients with hyperprolactinemia who desire future fertility, MRI is indicated to differentiate a pituitary microadenoma from a macroadenoma as well as to identify other potential sellar-suprasellar masses. Although rare, when pregnancy-related complications of a pituitary adenoma occur, they occur more frequently in the presence of macroadenomas (Table 25.7).

Table 25.7. Sellar and Suprasellar Tumors and Conditions That May Result in Hyperprolactinemia

Abscess	Lipoma
Aneurysm	Lymphoma
Arachnoid cyst	Meningioma
Cephalocele	Meningitis (bacterial, fungal, granulomatous)
Chloroma (granulocytic sarcoma)	Metastasis
Colloid cyst	Mucocele
Craniopharyngioma	Nasopharyngeal carcinoma
Dermoid	Opticochiasmatic-hypothalamic glioma
Ectopic neurohypophysis	Osteocartilaginous tumor
"Empty" sella	Paracytic cyst
Epidermoid tumor	Pars intermedia cysts
Germinoma	Pituitary adenoma
Hamartoma (tuber cinereum/hypothalmus)	Rathke's cleft cyst
Histiocytosis	Sarcoidosis
Hyperplasia	
Hypophysitis	

In over 90% of untreated women, microprolactinomas do not enlarge over a 4- to 6-year period. For that reason, the argument that medical therapy will prevent a microadenoma from growing is false. Whereas prolactin levels correlate with tumor size, both elevations and reductions in prolactin levels may occur without any change in tumor size. If during follow-up a prolactin level rises significantly or central nervous system symptoms (headache, visual changes) are noted, repeat scanning may be indicated.

Hypothalamic Disorders

Dopamine was the first of many substances demonstrated to be produced in the arcuate nucleus. Dopamine-releasing neurons innervate the external zone of the median eminence. When released into the hypophyseal portal system, dopamine inhibits prolactin release in the anterior pituitary. Lesions that disrupt dopamine release can result in hyperprolactinemia. Such lesions may arise from the suprasellar area, pituitary gland, and infundibular stalk, as well as from adjacent bone, brain, cranial nerves, dura, leptomeninges, nasopharynx, and vessels. Numerous pathologic entities and physiologic conditions in the hypothalamic-pituitary region can disrupt dopamine release and cause hyperprolactinemia (Table 25.7).

Pituitary Disorders

Microadenoma

In over one-third of women with hyperprolactinemia, a radiologic abnormality consistent with a microadenoma is found. Release of pituitary stem cell growth inhibition via activation or loss-of-function mutations results in cell cycle dysregulation and is critical to the development of pituitary microadenomas and macroadenomas. Microadenomas (<1 cm) are monoclonal in origin. Genetic mutations are thought to release stem cell growth inhibition and result in autonomous anterior pituitary hormone production, secretion, and cell proliferation. Additional anatomic factors that may contribute to adenoma formation include reduced dopamine concentrations in the hypophyseal portal system and vascular isolation of the tumor or both. Recently, the heparin-binding secretory transforming *(HST)* gene has been noted in a variety of cancers as well as in prolactinomas (232). **Patients with microadenomas (<1 cm) can generally be reassured of a benign course** (233,234).

Both microadenomas and macroadenomas (>1 cm) are monoclonal in origin. Pituitary prolactinomas or lactotrope adenomas are sparely or densely granulated histologically. The sparsely granulated lactotrope adenomas have trabecular, papillary, or solid patterns. Calcification of these tumors may take the form of a psammoma body or a pituitary stone.

Densely granulated lactotrope adenomas are strongly acidophilic tumors and appear to be more aggressive than sparsely granulated lactotrope adenomas. Unusual acidophil stem cell adenomas can be associated with hyperprolactinemia with some clinical or biochemical evidence of growth hormone excess.

Microadenomas rarely progress to macroadenomas. Six large series of patients with microadenomas reveal that, with no treatment, the risk of progression for microadenoma to a macroadenoma is only approximately 7% (235). Treatments include expectant, medical or, rarely, surgical therapy. All affected women should be advised to notify their physicians of chronic headaches, visual disturbances (particularly tunnel vision consistent with bitemporal hemianopsia), and extraocular muscle palsies. Formal visual field testing is rarely necessary.

Expectant Management In women who do not desire fertility, expectant management can be used for both microadenomas and hyperprolactinemia without an adenoma if menstrual function remains intact. Hyperprolactinemia-induced estrogen deficiency, rather than prolactin itself, is the major factor in the development of osteopenia (236). Therefore, estrogen replacement or OCs are indicated for patients with amenorrhea or irregular menses. Patients with drug-induced hyperprolactinemia can also be managed expectantly with attention to the risks of osteoporosis. In the absence of symptoms, imaging may be repeated in 12 months to assess further growth of the microadenoma.

Medical Treatment Ergot alkaloids are the mainstay of therapy. In 1985, bromocriptine was approved for use in the United States to treat hyperprolactinemia caused by a pituitary adenoma. Ergot alkaloids increase dopamine levels, thus decreasing prolactin levels. *Bromocriptine* decreases prolactin synthesis, DNA synthesis, cell multiplication, and tumor growth. Bromocriptine treatment results in normal prolactinemia or return of ovulatory menses in 80% to 90% of patients.

Because ergot alkaloids, like *bromocriptine,* are excreted via the biliary tree, caution is required using it in the presence of liver disease. The major adverse effects include nausea, headaches, hypotension, dizziness, fatigue and drowsiness, vomiting, headaches, nasal congestion, and constipation. **Many patients tolerate the drug on the following regimen: one-half tablet every evening (1.25 mg) for 1 week, one-half tablet morning and evening (1.25 mg) during the second week, one-half tablet in the morning (1.25 mg) and a full tablet every evening (2.5 mg) during the third week, and one tablet every morning and early evening during the fourth week and thereafter (2.5 mg twice a day).** The lowest dose that maintains the prolactin level in the normal range is continued. Pharmacokinetic studies show peak serum levels occur 3 hours after an oral dose with a nadir at 7 hours. There is little detectable *bromocriptine* in the serum by 11 to 14 hours. Therefore, twice-a-day administration is required. Prolactin levels can be checked soon (6 to 24 hours) after the last dose.

One rare, but notable, adverse effect of *bromocriptine* is a psychotic reaction. Symptoms include auditory hallucinations, delusional ideas, and changes in mood that quickly resolve after discontinuation of the drug (237).

Many investigators report no difference in fibrosis, calcification, prolactin immunoreactivity, or the surgical success in patients pretreated with *bromocriptine* compared to those not receiving *bromocriptine* (238).

An alternative to oral administration is the vaginal administration of *bromocriptine* tablets, which is well tolerated (239). *Cabergoline,* another ergot alkaloid, has a very long half-life and can be given orally once per week. Its long duration of action is attributable to slow elimination by pituitary tumor tissue, high affinity binding to pituitary dopamine receptors, and extensive enterohepatic recirculation.

Cabergoline, which appears to be as effective as *bromocriptine* in lowering prolactin levels and in reducing tumor size, has substantially fewer adverse effects than bromocriptine. Very rarely, patients experience nausea and vomiting with cabergoline; they may be treated with intravaginal *cabergoline* just as with *bromocriptine.* Although *cabergoline* appears to be safe to use during pregnancy, more extensive data regarding the use of *bromocriptine* in pregnancy is available; therefore *bromocriptine* is preferred for pregnant patients.

When *bromocriptine* or *cabergoline* cannot be used, other medications such as *pergolide* or *methergoline* may be used. In patients with a microadenoma who are receiving *bromocriptine* therapy, a repeat MRI scan may be performed 6 to 12 months after prolactin levels are normal. Normal prolactin levels and resumption of menses should not be considered absolute proof of tumor response to treatment. Further MRI scans should be performed if new symptoms appear.

Discontinuation of *bromocriptine* therapy after 2 to 3 years may be attempted because some adenomas undergo hemorrhagic necrosis and cease to function.

Macroadenomas

Macroadenomas are pituitary tumors that are larger than 1 cm in size. *Bromocriptine* is the best initial and potentially long-term treatment option, but transsphenoidal surgery may be required. Evaluation for pituitary hormone deficiencies may be indicated. Symptoms of macroadenoma enlargement include severe headaches, visual field changes and, rarely, diabetes insipidus and blindness. After prolactin has reached normal levels following ergot alkaloid treatment, a repeat MRI is indicated within 6 months to document shrinkage or stabilization of the size of the macroadenoma. This examination may be performed earlier if new symptoms develop or if there is no improvement in previously noted symptoms. Normalized prolactin levels or resumption of menses should not be taken as absolute proof of tumor response to treatment.

Medical Treatment Macroadenomas treated with *bromocriptine* routinely show a decrease in prolactin levels and size; nearly one-half show a 50% reduction in size, and another one-fourth show a 33% reduction after 6 months of therapy. Because tumor regrowth occurs in over 60% of cases after discontinuation of *bromocriptine* therapy, long-term therapy is required.

After stabilization of tumor size is documented, the MRI scan is repeated 6 months later and, if stable, yearly for several years. Serum prolactin levels are measured every 6 months. Because tumors may enlarge despite normalized prolactin values, a reevaluation of symptoms at regular intervals (6 months) is required.

Surgical Intervention Tumors that are unresponsive to *bromocriptine* or that cause persistent visual field loss require surgical intervention. Some neurosurgeons have noted that a short (2- to 6-week) preoperative course of bromocriptine increases the efficacy of surgery in patients with larger adenomas (239). Unfortunately, despite surgical resection, recurrence of hyperprolactinemia and tumor growth is common. Complications of surgery include cerebral carotid artery injury, diabetes insipidus, meningitis, nasal septal perforation, partial or panhypopituitarism, spinal fluid rhinorrhea, and third nerve palsy. Periodic MRI scanning after surgery is indicated, particularly in patients with recurrent hyperprolactinemia.

Metabolic Dysfunction

Occasionally, patients with hypothyroidism exhibit hyperprolactinemia with remarkable pituitary enlargement caused by thyrotroph hyperplasia. These patients respond to thyroid replacement with reduction in pituitary enlargement and normalization of prolactin levels (240).

Hyperprolactinemia occurs in 20% to 75% of women with chronic renal failure. Prolactin levels are not normalized through hemodialysis but are normalized after transplantation (241–244). Occasionally, women with hyperandrogenemia also have hyperprolactinemia. Elevated prolactin levels may alter adrenal function by enhancing the release of adrenal androgens such as DHEAS (245).

Drug-induced Hyperprolactinemia

Numerous drugs interfere with dopamine secretion (Table 25.6). The same principles used in the management of pituitary microadenomas or hyperplasia can be applied in these situations. If medication can be discontinued, resolution of hyperprolactinemia is uniformly prompt.

Use of Estrogen in Hyperprolactinemia

In rodents, rapid pituitary prolactin-secreting adenoma (prolactinoma) occurs with high-dose estrogen administration (246). However, even conditions associated with high estrogen levels, such as pregnancy, do not cause prolactinomas in humans. Indeed, pregnancy may have a favorable influence on preexisting prolactinomas (247,248). Studies (249–251) and autopsy surveys (228) indicate that estrogen administration is not associated with clinical, biochemical, or radiologic evidence of growth of pituitary microadenomas or the progression of idiopathic hyperprolactinemia to an adenoma status. For these reasons, estrogen replacement or OC use is appropriate for hypoestrogenic patients with hyperprolactinemia secondary to microadenoma or hyperplasia.

Monitoring Pituitary Adenomas During Pregnancy

Prolactin-secreting microadenomas rarely create complications during pregnancy. However, monitoring of patients with serial gross visual field examinations and funduscopic examination is recommended. If persistent headaches, visual field deficits, or visual or funduscopic changes occur, MRI scanning is advisable. Because serum prolactin levels are elevated throughout pregnancy, prolactin measurements are of no value.

Although not recommended, bromocriptine use during pregnancy in women with symptomatic (visual field defects, headaches) microadenoma enlargement has resulted in resolution of deficits and symptoms (253–256).

Pregnant women with previous transsphenoidal surgery for microadenomas or macroadenomas may be monitored additionally with monthly Goldman perimetry visual field testing. Periodic MRI scanning may be necessary in women with symptoms or visual changes. Bromocriptine has been used on a temporary basis to resolve symptoms and visual field deficits in symptomatic patients with macroadenoma to allow completion of pregnancy before initiation of definitive therapy. **Breast feeding is not contraindicated in the presence of microadenomas or macroadenomas** (253–256).

Thyroid Disorders

Thyroid disorders are 10 times more common in women than men (233). Approximately 1% of the female population of the United States will develop overt hypothyroidism. Even prior to the discovery of the long-acting thyroid stimulator (LATS) in women with Graves' disease in 1956, numerous investigations demonstrated a link between these autoimmune thyroid disorders and reproductive physiology and pathology (258).

Thyroid Hormones

Iodide is actively transported into the thyroid follicular cell. Sodium-iodide symporter (NIS) is a key molecule in thyroid function. It allows the accumulation of iodide from the circulation into the thyrocyte against an electrochemical gradient. This subtype requires energy that is supplied by Na-K ATPase. Uptake is stimulated by TSH. The enzyme thyroid peroxidase (TPO) then oxidizes iodide near the cell-colloid surface and incorporates it into tyrosyl residues within the thyroglobulin molecule, which results in the formation of monoiodotyrosine (MIT) and diiodotyrosine (DIT). Triiodothyronine (T_3) and thyroxine (T_4), formed by secondary coupling of MIT and DIT, are also catalyzed by TPO. Thyroglobulin, the major protein formed in the thyroid gland, has an iodine content of 0.1% to 1.1% by weight. About 33% of the iodine is present in thyroglobulin in the form of T_3 and T_4, and the remainder is present in the iodotyrosines (MIT and DIT) and unbound iodine. Thyroglobulin provides a storage capacity capable of maintaining a euthyroid state for nearly 2 months without the formation of new thyroid hormones. The membrane-bound, heme-containing oligomer TPO is localized in the rough endoplasmic reticulum, Golgi vesicles, lateral and apical vesicles, and the follicular cell surface. The thyroid antimicrosomal antibodies found in patients with autoimmune thyroid disease are directed against the TPO enzyme (259,260).

Thyroid-stimulating hormone regulates thyroidal iodine metabolism by activation of adenylate cyclase. This facilitates endocytosis, digestion of thyroglobulin-containing colloid, and the release of thyroid hormones T_4, T_3, and reverse T_3. T_4 is released from the thyroid at 40 to 100 times the concentration of T_3. The reverse T_3 concentration, a histologically inactive metabolite, is 30% to 50% of T_3 secretion and 1% of T_4 concentration. Of thyroid hormones released, 70% are bound. Although T_4 is present in the circulating storage pool and has a slow turnover rate (about 7 days), T_3 concentration is lower and has a higher turnover rate. Approximately 30% of T_4 is converted to T_3 in the periphery. Reverse T_3 levels may help regulate the conversion of T_4 to T_3. T_3 is the primary physiologically functional thyroid hormone, which binds the nuclear receptor at 10 times the affinity of T_4. Thyroid hormone effects on cells include increased oxygen consumption, heat production, and metabolism of fats, proteins, and carbohydrates. Systemically, thyroid hormone activity is responsible for the basal metabolic rate and balances fuel efficiency with performance, much as a carburetor functions in an engine. Hyperthyroid states result in excessive fuel consumption with marginal performance.

Iodide Metabolism

Normal function of the thyroid gland is dependent on iodine. The present recommended daily allowance by the U.S. National Research Council is 150 to 300 mg/day. Present daily consumption in the United States averages 200 to 600 mg/day. Iodine is usually ingested in the form of iodized salt (100 mg of potassium iodine/kg of salt) (261).

Although the thyroid gland depends on iodine, sufficiency of iodine also appears to be associated with the development of autoimmune thyroid disorders (262,263) and reduced remission rates in patients treated for Graves' disease (264). Animal studies suggest that iodine stimulates immunoglobulin production by B lymphocytes, activates macrophages, and increases the immunogenic potential of thyroglobulin because of the higher iodide content (265–268).

Factors Affecting Thyroid Function

Other potential causes of autoimmune thyroid diseases include pollutants (plasticizers, polychlorinated biphenyls, and coal-processing pollutants) (269,270) and antibodies to *Yersinia enterocolitica* (271). The female hormonal milieu and its potential effects on immune surveillance undoubtedly play a role in the increased risk (10-fold) of women to develop autoimmune thyroid disease. The immunoglobulins produced against the thyroid are polyclonal, and the multiple combinations of various antibodies present (stimulating versus blocking, complement fixing, and noncytotoxic) combine to create the clinical spectrum of autoimmune thyroid diseases that affect successful reproductive function.

Evaluation

Thyroid Function

Total serum T_4 is measured by radioimmunoassay. Conditions that elevate the levels of thyroid-binding globulin (TBG) (pregnancy, OC use, estrogen replacement, hepatitis, and genetic abnormalities of TBG) necessitate measuring T_3 resin uptake for clarification.

The T_3 resin uptake determines the concentration of radiolabeled T_3 bound to serum TBG and an artificial resin. The number of binding sites available in TBG is inversely proportional to the amount of labeled T_3 bound to the artificial resin. Therefore, high TBG T_3 receptor site availability results in a low T_3 resin uptake.

The free T_4 index (FTI) is obtained by multiplying the serum T_4 concentration by the T_3 resin uptake percentage, yielding an indirect measurement of free T_4:

$$\%\mathbf{freeT_4} \times \mathbf{T_4\ total} = \mathbf{freeT_4}.$$

Equilibrium dialysis may be used to determine the percentage of free T_4. Free T_4 and T_3 may also be determined by radioimmunoassay.

TSH receptor antibodies (TSHR-Ab or TRAb) are pathogenic and capable of activating or blocking TSH receptor functions. TSHR-Ab are detected using two approaches—competitive and functional assays. The competition between antibody and TSH for binding to the TSH receptor is the basis for the measurement of TSH-binding inhibitory immunoglobulin (TSII). The functional assay approach is based on the status of the receptor induced by the antibody-receptor interaction. This functional assay measures the production and accumulation of cyclic (AMP), thyroid hormone or thyroglobulin secretion, or iodide uptake in thyroid epithelial cells or Chinese hamster ovary cells transfected with the human TSH receptor. Whereas the competitive assay does not indicate any functional activity of the antibody, the functional assay identifies whether the antibody is agonistic (thyroid-stimulating antibody [TSAb] or antagonistic TSH stimulation–blocking antibody [TSBAb or TSHBAb]). Both types of antibodies may be present in the same patient, and the effect is the algebraic sum of the two levels of activity (agonistic and antagonistic) (Fig. 25.8).

The present TSH sandwich immunoassays are extremely sensitive and are capable of differentiating low-normal from pathologic or iatrogenically subnormal values and elevations. Thus, TSH measurements provide the best single screen for thyroid dysfunction (272) and accurately predict thyroid hormone dysfunction in about 80% of cases.

Immunologic Abnormalities

Many antigen-antibody reactions affecting the thyroid gland can be detected. A number of recognized thyroid autoantigens are listed in Table 25.8. Antibody production to thyroglobulin obviously depends on a breach in normal immune surveillance (273,274). The incidence of thyroid autoantibodies in various autoimmune thyroid disorders is shown in Table 25.9.

Antibodies to thyroglobulin are restricted to one minor and two major epitopes. Antibodies are mainly noncomplement-fixing immunoglobulin G (IgG) polyclonal antibodies (275). Antithyroglobulin antibodies are found in patients with Hashimoto's thyroiditis, Graves' disease, acute thyroiditis, nontoxic goiter, and thyroid cancer. They also appear in normal women.

Antimicrosomal antibodies directed against TPO are found in Hashimoto's thyroiditis, Graves' disease, and postpartum thyroiditis. The antibodies produced are characteristically

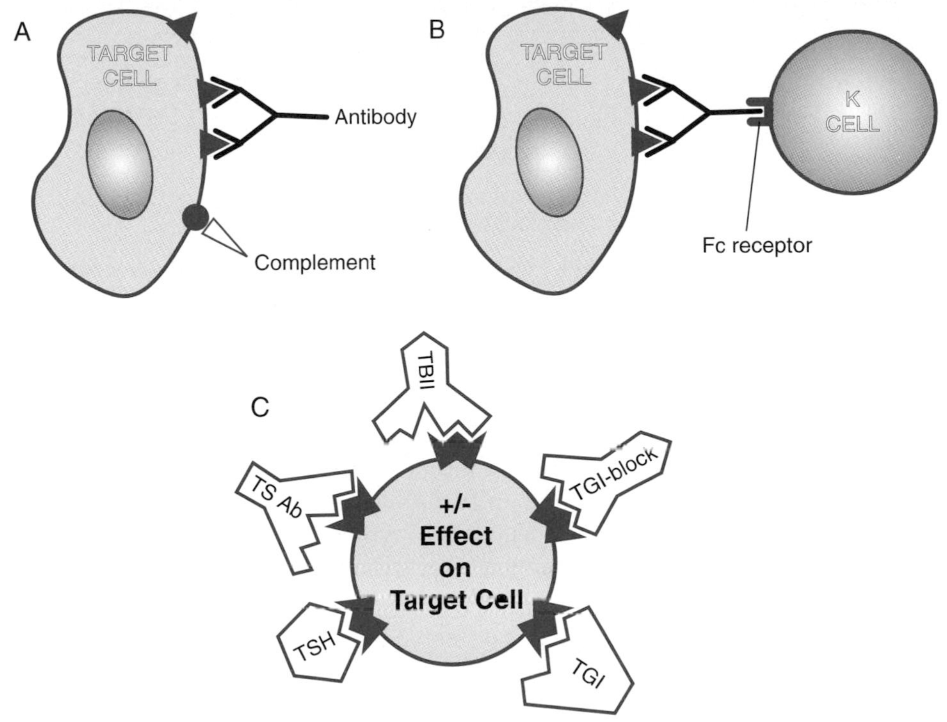

Figure 25.8 Types of autoimmune injury found in Hashimoto's thyroiditis. A: Complement-mediated cytotoxicity, which can be abolished by inactivating the complement system. **B:** Antibody-dependent cell-mediated cytotoxicity (ADCC) function through killer T cells, monocytes, and natural killer cells that have immunoglobulin G fragment receptors. **C:** Stimulation of blockade of hormone receptors leading to hyperfunction or hypofunction or growth, depending on the types of immunoglobulins acting on the target cell. (TBII, TSH-binding inhibitor immunoglobulin; TGI, thyroid growth–promoting immunoglobulin; TSAb, thyroid-stimulating antibodies; TSH, thyroid-stimulating hormone.) (From **Coulam CB, Faulk WP, McIntyre JA.** *Immunologic obstetrics.* New York: Norton Medical Books, 1992:658, with permission.)

cytotoxic, complement-fixing IgG antibodies. Antimicrosomal antibodies correlate with the histologic appearance of lymphocytic thyroiditis (259,260).

Antibodies to T_3 and T_4 are present in some patients with Hashimoto's thyroiditis and Graves' disease who have antithyroglobulin antibodies (276). These antibodies can cause artifacts in the measurement of thyroid hormone levels.

Table 25.8. Thyroid Autoantigens

Antigen	*Location*	*Function*
Thyroglobulin (Tg)	Thyroid	Thyroid hormone storage
Thyroid peroxidase (TPO) (microsomal antigen)	Thyroid	Transduction of signal from TSH
TSH receptor (TSHR)	Thyroid, lymphocytes, fibroblasts, adipocytes (including retroorbital)	Transduction of signal from TSH
Na^+/I^- symporter (NIS)	Thyroid, breast, salivary or lacrimal gland, gastric or colonic mucosa, thymus, pancreas	ATP-driven uptake of I^- along with Na^+

TSH, thyroid-stimulating hormone; ATP, adenosine triphosphate.

Table 25.9. Prevalence of Thyroid Autoantibodies and Their Role in Immunopathology

Antibody	*General Population*	*Hypothyroid Autoimmune Thyroiditis*	*Graves' Disease*
Antithyroglobulin (anti-Tg)	3%	35% to 60%	12% to 30%
Antimicrosomal thyroid peroxidase (anti-TPO)	10% to 15%	80% to 99%	45% to 80%
Anti-TSH receptor (anti-TSHR)	1% to 2%	6% to 60%	70% to 100%
Anti-Na^+/I^- symporter (anti-NIS)	0%	25%	20%

TSH, thyroid stimulating hormone.

Another group of antibodies important in autoimmune thyroid disease binds the TSH receptor. These antibodies often create the signs and symptoms that lead to an evaluation. TSAb or thyroid-stimulating immunoglobulin (TSI) activates the TSH receptor (Table 25.10). Long-acting thyroid stimulators are monoclonal or limited polyclonal TSAb, which mimic TSH action. They are quantified by their ability to stimulate human thyroid cell cultures to produce cyclic adenosine monophosphate or to release T_3.

TBII is detectable in two varieties, those that block TSH binding and those that block both pre- and postreceptor processes. Several investigators have detected such blocking antibodies in patients with primary hypothyroidism who have atrophic thyroid glands (277–279). The nomenclature and detection assay of TSH receptor antibodies are listed in Table 25.10.

Thyroid growth-promoting immunoglobulins (TGI) stimulate growth but not hormone release (250–259). Their immunologic antagonists are the TGI-blocking antibodies that are capable of inhibiting TSH-mediated growth responses in patients who may have had thyroid damage by immune destruction (277–280).

Table 25.10. Nomenclature of Anti-TSH Receptor Antibodies

Abbreviation	*Term*	*Assay Used*	*Refers To*
LATS	Long-acting thyroid stimulator	*In vivo* assay of stimulation of mouse thyroid	Original description of serum molecule able to stimulate mouse thyroid; no longer used
TSHR-Ab, TRAb	TSH receptor antibodies	Any	All antibodies recognizing the TSH receptor
TBII	TSH-binding inhibitory immunoglobulin	Competitive binding assays with TSH	Antibodies able to compete with TSH for TSH receptor binding irrespective of biologic activity
TSAb	Thyroid-stimulating antibodies	Bioassays of TSH receptor activation	TSH receptor-stimulating antibodies
TSI	Thyroid-stimulating immunoglobulins	As TSAb	Identical to TSAb
TSBAb, TSHBAb	TSH stimulation-blocking antibodies	Competition with TSH in bioassays of TSH receptor activation	Antibodies able to block activation of the TSH receptor by TSH

TSH, thyroid-stimulating hormone.

Antibodies to the NIS are prevalent in a number of thyroid conditions. Increased expression of NIS protein and NIS mRNA is found in patients with autonomous thyroid adenomas and in Graves' disease. They are decreased in Hashimoto's thyroiditis, cold nodules, and thyroid carcinoma.

Autoimmune Thyroid Disease

The most common thyroid abnormalities in women, autoimmune thyroid disorders, represent the combined effects of the multiple antibodies produced (281). The various antigen-antibody reactions result in the wide clinical spectrum of these disorders. The transmission of these immunoglobulins transplacentally potentially complicates thyroid function in the fetus. The presence of autoimmune thyroid disorders, particularly Graves' disease, is associated with other autoimmune conditions. Other autoimmune conditions associated with Graves' disease are Hashimoto's thyroiditis, Addison's disease, ovarian failure, rheumatoid arthritis, Sjögren's syndrome, diabetes mellitus (type I), vitiligo, pernicious anemia, myasthenia gravis, and idiopathic thrombocytopenic purpura.

Certain groups of individuals require assessment of thyroid function at least once. Such individuals include women with atrial fibrillation, hyperemesis gravidarum, and hyperlipidemia. Periodic assessment of thyroid function is indicated in patients who receive amiodarone and lithium. Epidemiologists recommend that all women with diabetes be annually screened for thyroid dysfunction. Women with type 1 diabetes are 3 times more likely to experience postpartum thyroid dysfunction, and it is recommended that all women with diabetes be screened in their first trimester with TSH. Any woman with a history of postpartum thyroiditis should also be offered annual surveillance of thyroid function. Because there is a high prevalence of hypothyroidism in women with Turner's and Down's syndrome, an annual check of thyroid function is recommended. Periodic TSH screening in mature women is advisable.

Hashimoto's Thyroiditis

Hashimoto's thyroiditis or chronic lymphocytic thyroiditis, which was first described in 1912, can manifest as hyperthyroidism, hypothyroidism, euthyroid goiter, or diffuse goiter. High levels of antimicrosomal and antithyroglobulin antibody are usually present. Typically, glandular hypertrophy is found, but atrophic forms are also present. The composition of various antibodies (i.e., TBII, causing the atrophic form and congenital hypothyroidism in some neonates, and TGI, causing the goitrous variety) results in varied physical findings.

Three classic types of autoimmune injury are found in Hashimoto's thyroiditis, (a) complement-mediated cytotoxicity, (b) antibody-dependent cell-mediated cytotoxicity, and (c) stimulation or blockade of hormone receptors, which results in hyper- or hypofunction or growth (Fig. 25.8).

The histologic picture of Hashimoto's thyroiditis includes cellular hyperplasia, disruption of follicular cells, and infiltration of the gland by lymphocytes, monocytes, and plasma cells. Occasionally, adjacent lymphadenopathy may be noted. Some epithelial cells are enlarged and demonstrate oxyphilic changes in the cytoplasm (Askanazy cells or Hürthle cells, which are not specific to this disorder). The interstitial cells show fibrosis and lymphocytic infiltration. Graves' disease and Hashimoto's thyroiditis may cause very similar histologic findings manifested by a similar mechanism of action. Nearly all patients with Hashimoto's thyroiditis and about two-thirds of patients with Graves' disease have sera demonstrating antibody-dependent cell-mediated cytotoxicity.

Clinical Characteristics and Diagnosis of Hashimoto's Thyroiditis

Most patients with Hashimoto's thyroiditis are relatively asymptomatic with painless goiter and hypothyroidism. The goiter can also involve the pyramidal lobe. At later stages of the disease, hypothyroidism can be found without a goiter. Notable manifestations of hypothyroidism include cold intolerance, constipation, carotene deposition in the periorbital region, carpal tunnel syndrome, dry skin, fatigue, hair loss, lethargy, and weight gain.

Table 25.11. Potential Causes of Hypothyroidism

Primary
Congenital absence of thyroid gland
External thyroid gland radiation
Familial disorders and thyroxine synthesis
Hashimoto's thyroiditis
Iodine-131 ablation for Graves' disease
Ingestion of antithyroid drugs
Iodine deficiency
Idiopathic myxedema (autoimmune)
Surgical removal of thyroid gland
Secondary
Hypothalamic thyrotropin-releasing hormone deficiency
Pituitary or hypothalamic tumors or disease

Hashitoxicosis, the hyperthyroid manifestation of autoimmune thyroid disease, may represent a variant of Graves' disease. This form is estimated to occur in 4% to 8% of patients with Hashimoto's thyroiditis. These patients often become hypothyroid during the course of treatment.

In many cases, an elevated serum level of TSH is noted during routine screening. Elevated serum antithyroglobulin and antimicrosomal antibody elevation confirm the diagnosis. The sedimentation rate may be elevated, depending on the course of the disease at the time of recognition. Other causes of hypothyroidism should be considered as listed in Table 25.11.

Most clinicians treat women who have elevated serum TSH concentrations and positive thyroid antibody tests, even in the absence of symptoms, in view of the annual risk for hypothyroidism of approximately 5% (282). If the serum TSH alone is elevated, without positive thyroid antibody titers, the annual risk for hypothyroidism drops to approximately 3% per year.

Treatment

Thyroxine replacement is initiated in patients with symptomatic hypothyroidism, patients who have a goiter that is cosmetically or physically bothersome and are subclinically hypothyroid, and patients who are undergoing fertility therapy and are subclinically hypothyroid. Regression of gland size usually does not occur, but treatment prevents further growth. Pregnant patients with an elevated TSH level should be treated with *levothyroxine*. Treatment does not slow progression of the disease. Replacement therapy is monitored by TSH determinations at least 6 weeks after a change in dose. *Aluminum hydroxide* (antacids), *cholestyramine,* iron, and *sucralfate* may interfere with absorption. The half-life of *levothyroxine* is nearly 7 days; therefore, nearly 6 weeks of treatment are necessary before the effects of a dose change can be evaluated.

Hypothyroidism appears to be associated with decreased fertility resulting from ovulatory difficulties and not with spontaneous abortion (283–286). Studies also suggest that early subclinical hypothyroidism may be associated with menorrhagia (287).

Severe primary hypothyroidism is associated with amenorrhea or anovulation (283,288–290). Enhanced sensitivity of the prolactin-secreting cells to thyrotropin-releasing hormone (TRH) and defective dopamine turnover resulting in hyperprolactinemia associated with a deficiency of thyroid hormone are the apparent explanations for the hyperprolactinemia (291–294). Hyperprolactinemia-induced luteal phase defects also are associated with less severe forms of hypothyroidism (273–275). Replacement therapy appears to reverse the hyperprolactinemia and correct ovulatory defects (295–297).

Graves' Disease

Graves' disease is characterized by exophthalmos, goiter, and hypothyroidism. A heritable specific defect in immunosurveillance by suppressor T lymphocytes is believed to result in the development of a helper T-cell population that reacts to thyroid antigens and induces a B-cell–mediated response (301), resulting in the clinical features of Graves' disease. TSAb are detected in the serum of 90% of patients with Graves' disease. Human leukocyte antigen (HLA) class II antigens DR, DP, DQ, and DS can present antigens to T cells and are expressed on thyroid epithelial cells. Antibodies to the TSH receptor are produced when this immunogen (TSH receptor) is presented to helper T lymphocytes with the D locus antigens (302).

The class II antigens are upregulated by chronic stimulation of the TSH receptor, reduction in the iodinating capacity of thyroid tissue, viral transformation, and interferon-α (302,303). The clinical use of *interferon-α* has been associated with autoimmune thyroid disease. Graves' disease is a complex autoimmune disorder in which several genetic susceptibility loci and environmental factors are likely to play a role in the development of the disease. HLA and the CTLA-4 gene region have been established as susceptibility loci; however, the magnitude of their contributions seems to vary among patient populations and study groups. Additional loci are likely to be identified by a combination of genome-wide linkage analyses and allelic association analyses of candidate genes.

Clinical Characteristics and Diagnosis

The classic triad of exophthalmos, goiter, and hyperthyroidism may be associated with frequent bowel movements, heat intolerance, irritability, nervousness, palpitations or tachycardia, tremor, weight loss, and lower extremity swelling. Physical findings include lid lag, nontender thyroid enlargement (2- to 4-times normal), onycholysis, palmar erythema, proptosis, staring gaze, and thick skin. A cervical venous bruit and tachycardia are usually noted. The tachycardia does not respond to increased vagal tone produced with a Valsalva maneuver. Severe cases may demonstrate acropachy, chemosis, clubbing, dermopathy, exophthalmos with ophthalmoplegia, follicular conjunctivitis, pretibial myxedema, and vision loss.

Approximately 40% of patients with new onset of Graves' disease and many of those who have received treatment have elevated T_3 and normal T_4 levels. Therefore, assessment of T_4, T_3, and TSH values is indicated. The TSH value may remain undetectable for some time even after the initiation of treatment. In most patients, antimicrosomal antibodies are present. Measurement of TSAb is useful in evaluating medical treatment, prognosis, and potential fetal complications such as neonatal thyrotoxicosis. Autonomously functioning, benign thyroid neoplasias that exhibit a similar clinical picture include toxic adenomas and toxic multinodular goiter. Very rare conditions causing thyrotoxicosis include hCG-secreting choriocarcinoma, TSH-secreting pituitary adenomas, and struma ovarii. Factitious ingestion of thyroxine or desiccated thyroid must be considered in patients with eating disorders. Other potential causes of hyperthyroidism are listed in Table 25.12.

Treatment

Iodine-131 Ablation Treatment of women with hyperthyroidism of an autoimmune origin presents unique challenges to the physician who must consider the patient's needs and her reproductive plans. Because the drugs used to treat this disorder have potentially harmful effects on the fetus, special attention must be given to the use of contraception and the potential for pregnancy.

A single dose of radioactive iodine-131 (^{131}I) is an effective cure in about 80% of cases and is the most commonly used definitive treatment in nonpregnant women. Any woman of childbearing age should be tested for pregnancy before undergoing diagnostic or therapeutic administration of ^{131}I. Ablation of a second-trimester fetal thyroid

Table 25.12. Potential Causes of Hyperthyroidism
Factitious hyperthyroidism
Graves' disease
Metastatic follicular cancer
Pituitary hyperthyroidism
Postpartum thyroiditis
Silent hyperthyroidism (low radioiodine uptake)
Struma ovarii
Subacute thyroiditis
Toxic multinodular goiter
Toxic nodule
Tumors secreting human chorionic gonadotropin (molar pregnancy, choriocarcinoma)

gland and congenital hypothyroidism from treatment during the first trimester have been reported (304,305). Nuclear medicine professionals provide expertise in the administration of the radioactive isotope, and the endocrinologist continues to provide suppressive medical treatment for 6 to 12 weeks after administration of ^{131}I. Therefore, medical therapy is the backbone of therapy even when radioactive ^{131}I or surgery is eventually planned. Postablative hypothyroidism develops in 50% of patients within the first year after ^{131}I therapy and in more than 2% of patients per year thereafter.

Thyroid-stimulating Receptor Antibody in Graves' Disease The level of TSHR-Ab (TBII) grossly parallels the degree of hyperthyroidism as assessed by the serum levels of thyroid hormones and total thyroid volume. Recent studies suggest that the combination of a small goiter volume (<40 ml) and a low TBII level (<30 units/L) results in a 45% chance of remission during the 5 years after completion of a 12- to 24-month course of antithyroid drug therapy (306). In contrast, the overall rate of relapse exceeded 70% in patients with a large goiter volume (>70 ml) and a higher TBII level (>30 units/L). Thus, the subgroup of patients with larger goiters and higher TBII levels had less than a 10% chance to remain in remission in the 5 years after treatment. Therefore, although it is not necessary for the diagnosis of Graves' disease, except in some cases of multinodular goiter, a TSHR-Ab measurement may be a useful marker of disease severity and, in combination with other clinical factors, may contribute to the initial decisions regarding treatment. See table 25.10 to review the nomenclature and assay methods for TSHR-Ab.

TSHR-Ab measurements (TBII) during treatment with antithyroid drugs also are predictive of subsequent outcome. In one series, 73% of TBII-negative patients had remission compared with only 28% of TBII-positive patients who had achieved remission after 12 months of antithyroid drug therapy (307). Furthermore, the duration of a course of antithyroid drug therapy can be modified according to the TSHR-Ab status. In patients whose TSHR-Ab (TSAb) status became negative and antithyroid drug therapy was discontinued, the relapse rate was 41% compared with a rate of 92% for those patients who remained TSAb-positive (308). Regardless of the rapidity of the disappearance of TSAb, it does seem that antithyroid drug therapy should be maintained for 9 to 12 months to minimize the risk of relapse. TSHR-Ab status also appears to determine in an inverse relationship the reduction in thyroid volume after radioactive iodine therapy.

Antithyroid Drugs Antithyroid drugs of the thioamide class include *propylthiouracil (PTU)* and *methimazole.* Low doses of these agents block the secondary coupling reactions that form T_3 and T_4 from MIT and DIT. At higher doses, they also block iodination of tyrosyl residues in thyroglobulin. Approximately one-third of patients treated by this modality alone go into remission and become euthyroid (309).

PTU causes a reduction of hyperthyroid symptoms at a dose of 100 mg taken every 8 hours over 1 month. It blocks the intrathyroid synthesis of T_3 and the peripheral conversion of T_4 to T_3 but does not cross the placenta as easily as *methimazole,* and therefore is the drug of choice during pregnancy. Drug efficacy is monitored weekly by evaluation of appetite, emotional lability, insomnia, and tremor. A general rule is to lower the dosage by 50% when thyroid function returns to normal, which frequently correlates with the return to a normal heart rate and, subsequently, normalization of TSH levels. Thyroxine is usually the first value to become normal.

Pruritus affects 3% to 5% of treated patients. Serious adverse reactions include agranulocytosis (occurring 1 to 2 months after therapy in 0.02%) and a generalized drug eruption accompanied by arthralgia, fever, and sore throat. A complete blood count determination is performed if the patient develops an upper respiratory tract infection. If adverse reactions occur, methimazole may be used.

Methimazole (10 mg) is given every 8–24 hours. Its dosage is reduced, as with *PTU.* It is not the drug of choice in pregnant women because it does not block peripheral conversion and crosses the placenta more readily than *PTU.* It does, however, have fewer adverse reactions, a longer dosing interval, and a lower cost than *PTU;* therefore, it is most often prescribed in nonpregnant women.

Other medical therapies include *iodide* and *lithium,* both of which reduce thyroid hormone release and inhibit the organification of iodine. *Iodide* also leads to the secondary coupling of T_3 and T_4. These medications are rarely used in women of reproductive age because of their risks to the fetal thyroid and to fetal development (*iodine* causes congenital goiter; *lithium* causes Ebstein's anomaly).

Surgery A subtotal thyroidectomy is less commonly used primarily but is used routinely if medical treatment fails or if a patient is hypersensitive to medical therapy. Surgery is the most rapid and consistent method of achieving a euthyroid state in Graves' disease that avoids the possible long-term risks of radioactive iodine. Children, young women, pregnant women, and patients with coexistent thyroid nodules are potential candidates for thyroidectomy. It is felt to be the treatment of choice for a patient with significant Graves' ophthalmology. Patients should be rendered euthyroid before a thyroidectomy. The risks of surgery include postoperative hypoparathyroidism, recurrent laryngeal nerve paralysis, routine anesthetic and surgical risks, hypothyroidism, and failure to relieve thyrotoxicosis.

β-Blockers *Propranolol* is occasionally used prior to surgery in patients who prove to be hypersensitive to other medical therapy and to provide symptomatic relief while awaiting a reduction in T_4 caused by *PTU* or *methimazole.*

Reproductive Effects of Hyperthyroidism

High levels of TSAb in women with Graves' disease have been associated with fetal-neonatal hyperthyroidism (310,311). Despite both the inhibition and elevation of gonadotropins seen in thyrotoxicosis (312), most women remain ovulatory and fertile (313). Severe thyrotoxicosis can result in weight loss, menstrual cycle irregularities, and amenorrhea. An increased risk of spontaneous abortion is noted in women with thyrotoxicosis (313). In those who deliver, an increased incidence of congenital anomalies (6%) is noted in their offspring (287). Effective treatment appears to reduce this risk.

Autoimmune hyperthyroid Graves' disease may improve spontaneously, in which case antithyroid drug therapy may be reduced or stopped. Nevertheless, TSHR-Ab production may persist for several years after radical radioactive iodine therapy or surgical treatment for hyperthyroid Graves' disease. In this circumstance there is a risk of exposing a fetus to TSHR-Ab. Fetal-neonatal hyperthyroidism is observed in 2% to 10% of pregnancies occurring in mothers with a current or previous diagnosis of Graves' disease, secondary to the transplacental passage of maternal TSHR-Ab. This is a serious condition with a 16% neonatal mortality rate as well as a risk of intrauterine fetal death, stillbirth, and skeletal developmental abnormalities such as craniosynostosis. Guidelines for TSHR-Ab testing during pregnancy in women with previously treated Graves' disease are found in Table 25.13.

Postpartum Thyroid Dysfunction

This clinical entity is often difficult to diagnose, because its symptoms appear 1 to 8 months postpartum and are often attributed to postpartum depression and difficulties adjusting to the demands of the neonate and infant. Following are criteria for the diagnosis of postpartum thyroiditis: (a) no history of thyroid hormonal abnormalities either before or during pregnancy, (b) documented abnormal TSH level (either depressed or elevated) during the first year postpartum, and (c) absence of a positive TSH-receptor antibody titer (Graves' disease) or a toxic nodule. Amino and others, who alerted clinicians to this condition,

Table 25.13. Guidelines for TSHR-Ab Testing During Pregnancy With Previously Treated Graves' Disease

1. In the woman with antecedent Graves' disease in remission after ATD treatment, the risk for fetal-neonatal hyperthyroidism is negligible, and systematic measurement of TSHR-Ab is not necessary. Thyroid function should be evaluated during pregnancy to detect an unlikely but possible recurrence. In that case, TSHR-Ab assay is mandatory.
2. In the woman with antecedent Graves' disease previously treated with radioiodine or thyroidectomy and regardless of the current thyroid status (euthyroidism with or without thyroxine substitution), TSHR-Ab should be measured early in pregnancy to evaluate the risk for fetal hyperthyroidism. If the TSHR-Ab level is high, careful monitoring of the fetus is mandatory for the early detection of signs of thyroid overstimulation (tachycardia, impaired growth rate, oligohydramnios, goiter). Cardiac echography and measurement of circulatory velocity may be confirmatory. Ultrasonographic measurements of the fetal thyroid have been defined from 20 weeks gestational age but require a well-trained operator, and thyroid visibility may be hindered due to fetal head position. Color Doppler ultrasonography is helpful in evaluating thyroid hypervascularization. Because of the potential risks of fetal-neonatal hyperthyroid cardiac insufficiency and the inability to measure the degree of hyperthyroidism in the mother because of previous thyroid ablation, it may be appropriate to consider direct diagnosis in the fetus. Fetal blood sampling through cordocentesis is feasible as early as 25 to 27 weeks gestation with less than 1% adverse effects (fetal bleeding, bradycardia, infection, spontaneous abortion, in utero death) when performed by experienced clinicians. ATD administration to the mother may be considered to treat the fetal hyperthyroidism.
3. In the woman with concurrent hyperthyroid Graves' disease, regardless of whether it has preceded the onset of pregnancy, ATD treatment should be monitored and adjusted to keep free T_4 in the high-normal range to prevent fetal hypothyroidism. TSHR-Ab should be measured at the beginning of the last trimester, especially if the required ATD dosage is high. If the TSHR-Ab assay is negative or the level low, fetal-neonatal hyperthyroidism is rare. If antibody levels are high (TBII $\geq$ 40 U/L or TSAb $\geq$ 300%), evaluation of the fetus for hyperthyroidism is required. In this condition, there is usually a fair correlation between maternal and fetal thyroid function such that monitoring the ATD dosage according to the mother's thyroid status is appropriate for the fetus. In some cases in which a high dose of ATD (>300 mg/d of propylthiouracil [PTU] or >20 mg/d of methimazole) is necessary, there is a risk of goitrous hypothyroidism in the fetus, which might be indistinguishable from goitrous Graves' disease. The correct diagnosis relies on the assay of fetal thyroid hormones and TSH, which allows for optimal treatment.
4. In any woman who has previously given birth to a newborn with hyperthyroidism, a TSHR-Ab assay should be performed early in the course of pregnancy.

ATD, autoimmune thyroid disease; TSHR-Ab, thyroid-stimulating hormone receptor antibodies; TBII, TSH-binding inhibitory immunoglobulin; TSAb, thyroid-stimulating antibody; T_4, thyroxine.

documented an incidence of approximately 5% in their population (316). A number of studies now describe clinical and biochemical evidence of postpartum thyroid dysfunction in 5% to 10% (317). These women have a 25% chance of becoming permanently hypothyroid.

Histologically, lymphocytic infiltration and inflammation are found. Antimicrosomal antibodies are also found in this disorder (318,319). Women who are at greatest risk of developing this disorder are those with a personal or family history of the disorder, those with an autoimmune thyroid disorder, or those with an autoimmune disease.

Clinical Characteristics and Diagnosis

Postpartum thyroiditis usually begins with a transient hyperthyroid phase between 6 weeks and 6 months postpartum followed by a hypothyroid phase. However, only one-fourth of the cases follow this classic clinical picture, whereas over one-third have either hyperthyroidism or hypothyroidism alone. Individuals with type 1 diabetes are 3 times more likely to develop postpartum thyroiditis, and women with a history of postpartum thyroiditis in a previous pregnancy have nearly a 70% chance of recurrence in a subsequent pregnancy. Numerous case reports demonstrate a possible association between postpartum thyroiditis and other autoimmune disorders. Postpartum thyroiditis appears to be caused by the combination of a rebounding immune system in the postpartum state with the presence of thyroid autoantibodies. Although psychotic episodes are rare, postpartum thyroid dysfunction should be considered in all women with postpartum psychosis. The thyrotoxic phase may be subclinical and overlooked, particularly in areas where iodine intake is low (320). In contrast to patients with Graves' disease, those with the hyperthyroid form have a low level of radioactive isotope uptake.

The absence of thyroid tenderness, pain, fever, elevated sedimentation rate, and leukocytosis helps to rule out subacute thyroiditis (de Quervain thyroiditis). Evaluation of TSH, T_4, T_3, T_3 resin uptake, and antimicrosomal antibody titer confirm the diagnosis.

Treatment

Most patients are diagnosed during the hypothyroid phase and require 6 to 12 months of T_4 replacement if they are symptomatic. Because approximately 10% to 30% of women develop permanent hypothyroidism, TSH should be evaluated following discontinuation of replacement therapy.

Rarely, patients are diagnosed during the hyperthyroid phase (321). Antithyroid medications are not routinely used for these women. *Propranolol* may be used for symptomatic relief. Approximately two-thirds of these patients return to a euthyroid state, and one-third return to a hypothyroid state.

Positive Antithyroid Antibody Status

Women who have thyroid autoantibodies before and after conception appear to be at an increased risk for spontaneous abortion (322,323). Non–organ-specific antibody production and pregnancy loss are documented in cases of antiphospholipid abnormalities (324). The concurrent presence of organ-specific thyroid antibodies and non–organ-specific autoantibody production is not uncommon (325,326). In cases of recurrent pregnancy loss, thyroid autoantibodies may serve as peripheral markers of abnormal T-cell function and further implicate an immune component as the cause of reproductive failure (327).

Thyroid Nodules

Thyroid nodules are a common finding on physical examination and are demonstrated by ultrasonography in more than 50% of patients (328). Fine-needle biopsy and aspiration are required to rule out malignancy. In the case of indeterminate aspirates, 2% to 20% are malignant; therefore, surgical biopsy is often indicated (329).

Turner's Syndrome and Down's Syndrome

Patients with Turner's syndrome, characterized by a 45,XO karyotype (or other alterations in the X chromosome), have a short stature, primary amenorrhea, and other abnormalities. In this syndrome a high prevalence of autoimmune thyroid disorders is noted. Approximately 50% of adult patients with Turner's syndrome have antithyroid peroxidase (anti-TPO) and antithyroglobulin (anti-TG) autoantibodies. Of these patients, approximately 30% will develop subclinical or clinical hypothyroidism. The disorder is indistinguishable from Hashimoto's thyroiditis. A susceptibility locus for Graves' disease is noted on chromosome X (330).

Down's syndrome, caused by an extra chromosome 21, is characterized by an atypical body habitus, mental retardation, cardiac malformations, an increased risk for leukemia, and a reduced life expectancy. The extra chromosome is almost always of maternal origin. Autoimmune thyroid disorders are more common in patients with Down's syndrome than in the general population. The gene for autoimmune polyglandular syndrome I (APECED) has been mapped to chromosome 21 and is thought to be a transcription factor involved in immune regulation (AIRE) and may play a role in the development of autoimmune thyroid disease in these patients (331). Hashimoto's thyroiditis is the most common abnormality associated with Down's syndrome. Hypothyroidism develops in as many as 50% of patients over age 40 with Down's syndrome. These clinical syndromes and other evidence suggest part of the genetic susceptibility to Hashimoto's thyroiditis may reside on chromosomes X and 21.

References

1. **Verkauf BS, Von Thron J, O'Brien WF.** Clitoral size in women. *Obstet Gynecol* 1992;80:41–44.
2. **Ferrimann D, Gallway JD.** Clinical assessment of body hair growth in women. *J Clin Endocrinol Metab* 1961;21:1440.
3. **Vermeulen A, Verdonek L, Kaufman JM.** A critical evaluation of simple methods for the estimation of free testosterone in the serum. *J Clin Endocrinol Metab* 1999;84:3666–3672.
4. **Rittmaster RS.** Clinical relevance of testosterone and dihydrotestosterone metabolism in women. *Am J Med* 1995;98[Suppl]:17S–21S.
5. **Stein IF, Leventhal ML.** Amenorrhea associated with bilateral polycystic ovaries. *Am J Obstet Gynecol* 1935;29:181–191.
6. **Zawadzki JK, Dunaif A.** Diagnostic criteria for polycystic ovary syndrome towards a rational approach. In: **Dunaif A, Givens JR, Haseltine FP, et al.,** eds. *Polycystic ovary syndrome.* Cambridge: Blackwell Science, 1992:377–384.
7. **Goldzieher JW, Axelrod LR.** Clinical and biochemical features of polycystic ovarian disease. *Fertil Steril* 1963;14:631.
8. **Aono T, Miyazaki M, Miyoke A, et al.** Responses of serum gonadotropins to LH-releasing hormone and estrogens in Japanese women with polycystic ovaries. *Acta Endocrinol (Copenh)* 1977;85: 840–849.
9. **Serafini P, Alban F, Lobo RA.** 5α-reductase activity in the genital skin of hirsute women. *J Clin Endocrinol Metab* 1985;60:349–355.
10. **Lobo RA, Goebelsmann U, Horton R.** Evidence for the importance of peripheral tissue events in the development of hirsutism in polycystic ovary syndrome. *J Clin Endocrinol Metab* 1983;57: 393–397.
11. **Carmina E, Lobo RA.** Do hyperandrogenic women with normal menses have polycystic ovary syndrome? *Fertil Steril* 1999;71:319–322.
12. **Peserico A, Angeloni G, Bertoli P, et al.** Prevalence of polycystic ovaries in women with acne. *Arch Dermatol Res* 1989;281:502–503.
13. **Wild RA.** Obesity, lipids, cardiovascular risk, and androgen excess. *Am J Med* 1995;98[Suppl]:27S–32S.
14. **Kenny SJ, Aubert RE, Geiss LS.** Prevalence and incidence of non–insulin-dependent diabetes. In:

Harris, et al., eds. *Diabetes in America*, 2nd ed. Washington, DC: US National Institutes of Health, NIH 34, Pub. No. 95:1468.

15. **Ehrmann DA, Barnes RB, Rosenfield RL, et al.** Prevalence of impaired glucose tolerance and diabetes in women with polycystic ovary syndrome. *Diabetes Care* 1999;22:141–146.
16. **Legro RS, Kumselman AR, Dodson WC, et al.** Prevalence and predictors of risk for type 2 diabetes mellitus and impaired glucose tolerance in polycystic ovary syndrome: a prospective, controlled study in 254 affected women. *J Clin Endocrinol Metab* 1999;84:165–169.
17. **Harris MI, Hadden WC, Knowler WC, et al.** Prevalence of diabetes and impaired glucose tolerance and plasma glucose levels in United States population aged 20 to 74 years. *Diabetes* 1987;36:523–534.
18. **Dahlgren E, Johansson S, Lindstedt G, et al.** Women with polycystic ovary wedge resected in 1956 to 1965: a long-term follow-up focusing on natural history and circulating hormones. *Fertil Steril* 1992;57: 505–513.
19. **Conway GS, Agrawal R, Betteridge DJ, et al.** Risk factors for coronary artery disease in lean and obese women with the polycystic ovary syndrome. *Clin Endocrinol (Oxf)* 1992;37:119–125.
20. **Anderson P, Selje Flot I, Abdelnoor M.** Increased insulin sensitivity and fibrinolytic capacity after dietary intervention in obese women with polycystic ovary syndrome. *Metabolism* 1995;44:611–616.
21. **Guzick DS, Talbott EO, Suton-Tyrrell K, et al.** Carotid atherosclerosis in women with polycystic ovary syndrome: initial results from a case-control study. *Am J Obstet Gynecol* 1996;174:1224–1229.
22. **Birdsall MA, Farquhar CM, White HD.** Association between polycystic ovaries and extent of coronary artery disease in women having cardiac catheterization. *Ann Intern Med* 1997;126:32–35.
23. **Danigren E, Janson PO, Johansson S, et al.** Polycystic ovary syndrome and risk for myocardial infarction. Evaluated from a risk factor model based on a prospective population study of women. *Acta Obstet Gynecol Scand* 1992;71:559–604.
24. **Clement PB.** Nonneoplastic lesions of the ovary. In: **Kurman RJ**, ed. *Blaustein's pathology of the female genital tract,* 4th ed. New York: Springer-Verlag, 1994:597–645.
25. **Rosenfield RL, Barnes RB, Cara JF, et al.** Dysregulation of cytochrome P450-17 α as the cause of polycystic ovarian syndrome. *Fertil Steril* 1990;53:785–791.
26. **McNatty KP, Makris A, De-Grazia C, et al.** The production of progesterone, androgens, and estrogens by granulosa cells, theca tissue and stromal tissue from human ovaries in vitro. *J Clin Endocrinol Metab* 1979;49:687–699.
27. **Lobo RA, Kletzky OA, Campeau JD, et al.** Elevated bioactive luteinizing hormone in women with polycystic ovarian disease. *Fertil Steril* 1983;39:674–678.
28. **Chang RJ, Laufer LR, Meldrum DR, et al.** Steroid secretion in polycystic ovarian disease after ovarian suppression by a long-acting gonadotropin-releasing hormone agonist. *J Clin Endocrinol Metab* 1983;56:897–903.
29. **Biffignandi P, Massucchetti C, Molinetti GM.** Female hirsutism: pathophysiological considerations and therapeutic options. *Endocr Rev* 1984;5:498–513.
30. **Rittmaster RS.** Differential suppression of testosterone and estradiol in hirsute women with the superactive gonadotropin-releasing hormone agonist leuprolide. *J Clin Endocrincol Metab* 1988;67:651–655.
31. **Lobo RA.** Hirsutism in polycystic ovary syndrome: current concepts. *Clin Obstet Gynecol* 1991;34:817–826.
32. **Hoffman DI, Klove K, Lobo RA.** The prevalence and significance of elevated dehydroepiandrosterone sulfate levels in anovulatory women. *Fertil Steril* 1984;42:76–81.
33. **Lobo RA.** The role of the adrenal in polycystic ovary syndrome. *Semin Reprod Endocrinol* 1984;2:251–264.
34. **Deslypere JP, Verdnock L, Vermeulen A.** Fat tissues: a steroid reservoir and site of steroid metabolism. *J Clin Endocrinol Metab* 1985;61:564–570.
35. **Edman CD, MacDonald PC.** Effect of obesity on conversion of plasma androstenedione to estrone in ovulatory and anovulatory young women. *Am J Obstet Gynecol* 1978;130:456–461.
36. **Schneider J, Bradlow HL, Strain G, et al.** Effect of obesity on estradiol metabolism. Decreased formation of nonuterotropic metabolites. *J Clin Endocrinol Metab* 1983;56:973–978.
37. **Judd HL.** Endocrinology of polycystic ovarian disease. *Clin Obstet Gynecol* 1978;21:99–114.
38. **Hall JE, Whitcomb RW, Rivier JE, et al.** Differential regulation of luteinizing hormone, follicular stimulating hormone and free α sub-unit secretion from the gonadotrope by gonadotropin-releasing hormone (GnRH): evidence from use of two GnRH antagonists. *J Clin Endocrinol Metab* 1990;70:328–335.
39. **Seibel MM.** Toward understanding the pathophysiology and treatment of polycystic ovary disease. *Semin Reprod Endocrinol* 1984;2:297.
40. **Dunaif A, Graf M, Mandeli J, et al.** Characterization of groups of hyperandrogenic women with acanthosis nigricans, impaired glucose tolerance, and/or hyperinsulinemia. *J Clin Endocrinol Metab* 1987;65:499–507.

41. **Dunaif A, Green G, Futterweit W, et al.** Suppression of hyperandrogenism does not improve peripheral or hepatic insulin resistance in the polycystic ovary syndrome. *J Clin Endocrinol Metab* 1990;70:699–704.

42. **Nagamani M, Van Dinh T, Kelver ME.** Hyperinsulinemia in hyperthecosis of the ovaries. *Am J Obstet Gynecol* 1986;154:384–389.

43. **Grasinger CC, Wild RA, Parker IJ.** Vulvar acanthosis nigricans: a marker for insulin resistance in hirsute women. *Fertil Steril* 1993;59:583–586.

44. **Barbieri RL, Ryan KJ.** Hyperandrogenism, insulin resistance and acanthosis nigricans syndrome: a common endocrinopathy with unique pathophysiological features. *Am J Obstet Gynecol* 1983;147:90–101.

45. **Dunaif A.** Hyperandrogenic anovulation (PCOS): a unique disorder of insulin action associated with an increased risk of non–insulin-dependent diabetes mellitus. *Am J Med* 1995;98:33S–39S.

46. **Kiddy DS, Hamilton-Fairley D, Bush A, et al.** Improvement of endocrine and ovarian function during dietary treatment of obese women with polycystic ovary syndrome. *Clin Endocrinol* 1992;36:105–111.

47. **Pasquali R, Antenucci D, Casimirri F, et al.** Clinical and hormonal characteristics of obese and amenorrheic hyperandrogenic women before and after weight loss. *J Clin Endocrinol Metab* 1989;68:173–179.

48. **Comparetto G, Gullo D, Venezia R, et al.** Proposal for a purely echographic classification of polycystic ovary syndrome. *Acta Steril Fertil* 1982;13:79–94.

49. **Farquhan CM, Birdsall M, Manning P.** The prevalence of polycystic ovaries on ultrasound scanning in a population of randomly selected women. *Aust N Z J Obstet Gynaecol* 1994;34:67–72.

50. **Jafari K, Tavaheri C, Ruiz G.** Endometrial adenocarcinoma and the Stein-Leventhal syndrome. *Obstet Gynecol* 1978;51:97–100.

51. **Cowan LD, Gordis L, Tonascia JA, et al.** Breast cancer incidence in women with a history of progesterone deficiency. *Am J Epidemiol* 1981;114:209–217.

52. **Schildkraut JM, Schwinge PJ, Bostos E, et al.** Epithelial ovarian cancer risk among women with polycystic ovary syndrome. *Obstet Gynecol* 1996;88:554–559.

53. **Futterweit W.** An endocrine approach to obesity. In: **Simopoulos AP, VanItallie TB, Gullo SP, et al.,** eds. *Obesity: new directions in assessment and management.* New York: Charles Press, 1994:96–121.

54. **Kiddy DS, Hamilton-Fairley D, Bush A, et al.** Improvement in endocrine and ovarian function during dietary treatment of obese women with polycystic ovary syndrome. *Clin Endocrinol (Oxf)* 1992;36:105–111.

55. **Givens JR, Andersen RN, Wiser WL, et al.** The effectiveness of two oral contraceptives in suppressing plasma androstenedione, testosterone, LH, and FSH and in stimulating plasma testosterone binding capacity in hirsute women. *Am J Obstet Gynecol* 1976;124:333–339.

56. **Raji SG, Raj MHG, Talbert LM, et al.** Normalization of testosterone levels using a low estrogen-containing oral contraceptive in women with polycystic ovary syndrome. *Obstet Gynecol* 1982;60:15–19.

57. **Wiebe RH, Morris CV.** Effect of an oral contraceptive on adrenal and ovarian androgenic steroids. *Obstet Gynecol* 1984;63:12–14.

58. **Wild RA, Umstot ES, Andersen RN, et al.** Adrenal function in hirsutism: II. Effect of an oral contraceptive. *J Clin Endocrinol Metab* 1982;54:676–681.

59. **Marynick SP, Chakmakjian ZH, McCaffree DL, et al.** Androgen excess and acne. *N Engl J Med* 1983;308:981–986.

60. **Schiavone FE, Rietschel RL, Sgoutas D, et al.** Elevated free testosterone levels in women with acne. *Arch Dermatol* 1983;119:799–802.

61. **Amin E, El-Sayed MM, El-Gamel BA, et al.** Comparative study of the effect of oral contraceptives containing 50 μg of estrogen on adrenal cortical function. *Am J Obstet Gynecol* 1980;137:831–833.

62. **Goldzieher JW.** Polycystic ovarian disease. *Fertil Steril* 1981;35:371–394.

63. **Rittmaster RS.** Medical treatment of androgen dependent hirsutism. *J Clin Endocrinol Metab* 1995;80:2559–2563.

64. **Godsland IF, Walton C, Felton C, et al.** Insulin resistance, secretion, and metabolism in users of oral contraceptives. *J Clin Endocrinol Metab* 1992;74:64–70.

65. **Ettinger B, Goldtich IM.** Medroxyprogesterone acetate for the evaluation of hypertestosteronism in hirsute women. *Fertil Steril* 1977;28:1285–1288.

66. **Jeppsson S, Gershagen S, Johannsson ED, et al.** Plasma levels of medroxyprogesterone acetate (MPA), sex-hormone binding globulin, gonadal steroids, gonadotrophins and prolactin in women during long-term use of depo MPA (Depo-Provera) as a contraceptive agent. *Acta Endocrinol (Copenh)* 1982;99:339–343.

67. **Gordon GG, Southern AL, Calanog A, et al.** The effect of medroxyprogesterone acetate on androgen metabolism in the polycystic ovary syndrome. *J Clin Endocrinol Metab* 1972;35:444–447.

68. **Meldrum DR, Chang RJ, Lu J, et al.** "Medical oophorectomy" using a long-acting GnRH agonist—a possible new approach to the treatment of endometriosis. *J Clin Endocrinol Metab* 1982;54:1081–1083.

69. **Falsetti L, Pasinetti E.** Treatment of moderate and severe hirsutism by gonadotropin-releasing hormone agonists in women with polycystic ovary syndrome and idiopathic hirsutism. *Fertil Steril* 1994;61:817–822.

70. **Morcos RN, Abdul-Malak ME, Shikora E.** Treatment of hirsutism with a gonadotropin-releasing hormone agonist and estrogen replacement therapy. *Fertil Steril* 1994;61:427–431.

71. **Tiitinen A, Simberg N, Stenman UH, et al.** Estrogen replacement does not potentiate gonadotropin-releasing hormone agonist-induced androgen suppression in the treatment of hirsutism. *J Clin Endocrinol Metab* 1994;79:447–451.

72. **Cunningham SK, Loughlin T, Culliton M, et al.** Plasma sex hormone–binding globulin and androgen levels in the management of hirsute patients. *Acta Endocrinol (Copenh)* 1973;104:365–371.

73. **Gal M, Orly J, Barr I, et al.** Low dose ketoconazole attenuates serum androgen levels in patient with polycystic ovary syndrome and inhibits ovarian steroidogenesis in vitro. *Fertil Steril* 1994;61: 823–832.

74. **Serafini PC, Catalino J, Lobo RA.** The effect of spironolactone on genital skin 5α-reductase activity. *J Steroid Biochem Mol Biol* 1985;23:191–194.

75. **Menard RH, Guenther TM, Kon H.** Studies on the destruction of adrenal and testicular cytochrome P-450 by spironolactone. *J Biol Chem* 1979;254:1726–1733.

76. **Cumming DC, Yang JC, Rebar RW, et al.** Treatment of hirsutism with spironolactone. *JAMA* 1982;247:1295–1298.

77. **Rittmaster R.** Evaluation and treatment of hirsutism. *Infert Reprod Med Clin North Am* 1991;2:511–545.

78. **Barth JH, Cherry CA, Wojnarowska F, et al.** Spironolactone is an effective and well tolerated systemic antiandrogen therapy for hirsute women. *J Clin Endocrinol Metab* 1989;68:966–970.

79. **Lobo RA, Shoupe D, Serafini P, et al.** The effects of two doses of spironolactone on serum androgens and anagen hair in hirsute women. *Fertil Steril* 1985;43:200–205.

80. **Garner PR, Poznanski N.** Treatment of severe hirsutism resulting from hyperandrogenism with the reverse sequential cyproterone acetate regimen. *J Reprod Med* 1984;29:232–236.

81. **Helfer EL, Miller JL, Rose LI.** Side effects of spironolactone therapy in the hirsute woman. *J Clin Endocrinol Metab* 1988;66:208–211.

82. **Miller JA, Jacobs HS.** Treatment of hirsutism and acne with cyproterone acetate. *J Clin Endocrinol Metab* 1986;15:373–389.

83. **Mowszowicz I, Wright F, Vincens M, et al.** Androgen metabolism in hirsute patients treated with cyproterone acetate. *J Steroid Biochem Mol Biol* 1984;20:757–761.

84. **Calaf-Alsina J, Rodriguez-Espinosa J, Cabero-Roura A, et al.** Effects of a cyproterone-containing oral contraceptive on hormonal levels in polycystic ovarian disease. *Obstet Gynecol* 1987;69:255–258.

85. **Girard J, Baumann J, Buhler U, et al.** Cyproterone acetate and ACTH adrenal function. *J Clin Endocrinol Metab* 1978;47:581–586.

86. **Marcondes JA, Minnani SL, Luthold WW.** Treatment of hirsutism in women with flutamide. *Fertil Steril* 1992;57:543–547.

87. **Ciotta L, Cianci A, Marletta E, et al.** Treatment of hirsutism with flutamide and a low-dosage oral contraceptive in polycystic ovarian disease patients. *Fertil Steril* 1994;62:1129–1135.

88. **Cusan L, Dupont A, Belanger A, et al.** Treatment of hirsutism with the pure antiandrogen flutamide. *J Am Acad Dermatol* 1990;23:462–469.

89. **Vigersky RA, Mehlman I, Glass AR, et al.** Treatment of hirsute women with cimetidine. *N Engl J Med* 1980;303:1042.

90. **Lissak A, Sorokin Y, Carderon I, et al.** Treatment of hirsutism with cimetidine: a prospective randomized controlled trial. *Fertil Steril* 1989;51:247–250.

91. **Golditch IM, Price VH.** Treatment of hirsutism with cimetidine. *Obstet Gynecol* 1990;75:911–913.

92. **Wong L, Morris RS, Chang L, et al.** A prospective randomized trial comparing finasteride to spironolactone in the treatment of hirsute women. *J Clin Endocrinol Metab* 1995;80:233–238.

93. **Ciotta L, Cianci A, Cologen AE, et al.** Clinical and endocrine effects of finasteride, a 5α-reductase inhibitor, in women with idiopathic hirsutism. *Fertil Steril* 1995;64:299–306.

94. **Judd HL, Rigg LA, Anderson DC, et al.** The effects of ovarian wedge resection on circulating gonadotropin and ovarian steroid levels in patients with polycystic ovary syndrome. *J Clin Endocrinol Metab* 1976;43: 347–355.

95. **Katz M, Carr PJ, Cohen BM, et al** Hormonal effects of wedge resection of polycystic ovaries. *Obstet Gynecol* 1978;51:437–444.

96. **Goldzieher JW, Green JA.** The polycystic ovary. I. Clinical and histologic features. *J Clin Endocrinol Metab* 1962;22:325–338.

97. **Stein I.** Duration of fertility following ovarian wedge resection. Stein-Leventhal syndrome. *West J Surg Obstet Gynecol* 1964;78:124–127.

98. **Adashi EY, Rock JA, Guzick D, et al.** Fertility following bilateral ovarian wedge resection: a critical analysis of 90 consecutive cases of the polycystic ovary syndrome. *Fertil Steril* 1981;36:320–325.

99. **Felemban A, Lin Tan S, Tulandi T.** Laparoscopic treatment of polycystic ovaries with insulated needle cauterization: a reappraisal. *Fertil Steril* 2000;73:266–269.

100. **Armar NA, Lachelin GCL.** Laparoscopic ovarian diathermy: an effective treatment for anti-oestrogen resistant anovulatory infertility in women with polycystic ovary syndrome. *Br J Obstet Gynaecol* 1993;100:161–164.

101. **Armar NA, McGarrigle HHG, Honour JW, et al.** Laparoscopic ovarian diathermy in the management of anovulatory infertility in women with polycystic ovaries: endocrine change and clinical outcome. *Fertil Steril* 1990;53:45–49.

102. **Rossmanith WG, Keckstein J, Spatzier K, et al.** The impact of ovarian laser surgery on the gonadotropin secretion in women with polycystic ovarian disease. *Clin Endocrinol* 1991;34:223–230.

103. **Balen AH, Jacobs HS.** A prospective study comparing unilateral and bilateral laparoscopic ovarian diathermy in women with the polycystic ovary syndrome. *Fertil Steril* 1994;62:921–925.

104. **Schrode K, Huber F, Staszak J, et al.** Randomized, double blind, vehicle controlled safety and efficacy evaluation of eflornithine 15% cream in the treatment of women with excessive facial hair. Presented at: American Academy of Dermatology Annual Meeting. March 11–14, 2000; San Francisco, California.

105. **Lynfield YL, Mac Williams P.** Shaving and hair growth. *J Invest Dermatol* 1970;55:170–172.

106. **Wagner RF.** Physical methods for the management of hirsutism. *Cutis* 1990;45:319–321, 325–326.

107. **Hellmuth E, Damm P, Molsted-Pedersen L.** Oral hypoglycemic agents in 118 diabetic pregnancies. *Diabet Med* 2000;17:507–511.

108. **Glueck CJ, Phillips H, Camercon D, et al.** Continuing metformin throughout pregnancy in women with polycystic ovary syndrome appears to safely reduce first-trimester spontaneous abortion: a pilot study. *Fertil Steril* 2001;75:46–52.

109. **Kim LH, Taylor AE, Barbieri RL.** Insulin sensitizers and polycystic ovary syndrome: can a diabetes medication treat infertility? *Fertil Steril* 2000;73:1097–1098.

110. **Velazquez EM, Mendoza S, Hamer T, et al.** Metformin therapy in polycystic ovary syndrome reduces hyperinsulinemia, insulin resistance, hyperandrogenemia, and systolic blood pressure, while facilitating normal menses and pregnancy. *Metabolism* 1994;43:647–654.

111. **Nestler JE, Jakubowicz DJ.** Decreases in ovarian cytochrome P450c17 activity and serum free testosterone after reduction in insulin secretion in women with polycystic ovary syndrome. *N Engl J Med* 1996;335:617–623.

112. **Diamanti-Kandarakis E, Kouli C, Tsianateli T, et al.** Therapeutic effects of metformin on insulin resistance and hyperandrogenism in polycystic ovary syndrome. *Eur J Endrocrinol* 1998;138:269–274.

113. **Nestler JE, Jakubowicz DJ, Evans WS, et al.** Effects of metformin on spontaneous and clomiphene-induced ovulation in the polycystic ovary syndrome. *N Engl J Med* 1998;338:1876–1880.

114. **Hasegawa I, Murakawa H, Suzuki M, et al.** Effect of troglitazone on endocrine and ovulatory performance in women with insulin resistance-related polycystic ovary syndrome. *Fertil Steril* 1999;71:323–327.

115. **Stadtmauer LA, Toma SK, Riehl RM, et al.** Metformin treatment of patients with polycystic ovary syndrome undergoing in vitro fertilization improves outcomes and is associated with modulation of the insulin-like growth factors. *Fertil Steril* 2001;75:505–509.

116. **Orth DN.** Ectopic hormone production. In: **Felig P, Baster JD, Broadus AE, et al.,** eds. *Endocrinology and metabolism.* New York: McGraw-Hill, 1987:1692–1735.

117. **Liddle GW.** Test of pituitary-adrenal suppressibility in the diagnosis of Cushing's syndrome. *J Clin Endocrinol Metab* 1960;20:1539.

118. **Oldfield EH, Doppman JL, Nieman LK, et al.** Petrosal sinus sampling with and without corticotropin-releasing hormone for the differential diagnosis of Cushing's syndrome. *N Engl J Med* 1991;325:897–905.

119. **Gold EM.** The Cushing's syndrome: changing views of diagnosis and treatment. *Ann Intern Med* 1979;90:829–844.

120. **Boggan JE, Tyrell JB, Wilson CB.** Transsphenoidal microsurgical management of Cushing's disease. Report of 1,090 cases. *J Neurosurg* 1983;59:195–200.

121. **Bigos ST, Somma M, Rasia E, et al.** Cushing's disease: management by transsphenoidal pituitary microsurgery. *J Clin Endocrinol Metab* 1980;50:348–354.

122. **Aron DC, Findling JW, Tyrell JB.** Cushing's disease. *J Clin Endocrinol Metab* 1987;16:705–730.

123. **Jennings AS, Liddle GW, Orth DN.** Results of treating childhood Cushing's disease with pituitary irradiation. *N Engl J Med* 1977;297:957–962.

124. **Schteingart DE, Tsao HS, Taylor CI, et al.** Sustained remission of Cushing's disease with mitotane and pituitary irradiation. *Ann Intern Med* 1980;92:613–619.

125. **Loli L, Berselli ME, Tagliaterri M.** Use of ketoconazole in the treatment of Cushing's syndrome. *J Clin Endocrinol Metab* 1986;63:1365–1371.

126. **Nelson DH, Meakin JW, Dealy JB, et al.** ACTH-producing tumor of the pituitary gland. *N Engl J Med* 1958;85:731–734.

127. **Ortho DN, Liddle GW.** Results of treatment in 108 patients with Cushing's syndrome. *N Engl J Med* 1971;285:243–247.

128. **Valimaki M, Pelkonen R, Porkka L, et al.** Long-term results of adrenal surgery in patients with Cushing's syndrome due to adrenocortical adenoma. *Clin Endocrinol (Oxf)* 1984;20:229–236.

129. **Azziz R, Zacur HA.** 21-Hydroxylase deficiency in female hyperandrogenism: screening and diagnosis. *J Clin Endocrinol Metab* 1989;69:577–583.

130. **DeWailly D, Vantyghem-Handiquet MC, Sainsard D, et al.** Clinical and biological phenotypes in late-onset 21-hydroxylase deficiency. *J Clin Endocrinol Metab* 1986;63:418–423.

131. **New MI, Lorenzen F, Lerner AJ, et al.** Genotyping steroid 21-hydroxylase deficiency: hormonal reference data. *J Clin Endocrinol Metab* 1983;57:320–326.

132. **Speiser PW, Dupont B, Rubenstein P, et al.** High frequency of nonclassical steroid 21-hyroxylase deficiency. *Am J Hum Genet* 1985;37:650–657.

133. **New MI.** Steroid 21-hydroxylase deficiency (congenital adrenal hyperplasia). *Am J Med* 1995;98:2S–8S.

134. **Speiser PW, New MI, White PC.** Molecular genetic analysis of nonclassic steroid 21-hydroxylase deficiency associated with HLA-B14, DRI. *N Engl J Med* 1988;319:19–23.

135. **Owerback D, Ballard AL, Draznin AB.** Salt-wasting congenital adrenal hyperplasia: detection and characterization of mutations in the steroid 21-hydroxylase gene, *CYP21*, using the polymerase chain reaction. *J Clin Endocrinol Metab* 1992;74:553–558.

136. **White PC.** Steroid 11β-hydroxylase deficiency and related disorders. *Endocrinol Metab Clin North Am* 2001;30:61–79.

137. **White PC, Curnow KM, Pascoe L.** Disorders of steroid 11β-hydroxylase isozymes. *Endocr Rev* 1994;15:421–438.

138. **Rosler A, Leiberman E, Cohen T.** High frequency of congenital adrenal hyperplasia (classic 11β-hydroxylase deficiency) among Jews from Morocco. *Am J Med Genet* 1992;42:827–834.

139. **Mornet E, Dupont J, Vitek A, et al.** Characterization of two genes encoding human steroid 11β-hydroxylase (P-450(11) β). *J Biol Chem* 1989;264:20961–20967.

140. **Taymans SE, Pack S, Pak E, et al.** Human CYP11B2 (aldosterone synthase) maps to chromosome 8q24.3. *J Clin Endocrinol Metab* 1998;83:1033–1036.

141. **Azziz R, Boots LR, Parker CR Jr, et al.** 11-Hydroxylase deficiency in hyperandrogenism. *Fertil Steril* 1991;55:733–741.

142. **Pang S, Lerner AJ, Stoner E, et al.** Late-onset adrenal steroid 3β-hydroxysteroid dehydrogenase deficiency. I. A cause of hirsutism in pubertal and postpubertal women. *J Clin Endocrinol Metab* 1985;60: 428–439.

143. **Azziz R, Bradley EL, Potter HD, et al.** 3β-Hydroxysteroid dehydrogenase deficiency in hyperandrogenism. *Am J Obstet Gynecol* 1993;168:889–895.

144. **Nichols T, Nugent CA.** Tyler fundal height. Diurnal variation in suppression of adrenal function by glucocorticoids. *J Clin Endocrinol Metab* 1965;25:343–349.

145. **Boyers SP, Buster JE, Marshall JR.** Hypothalamic-pituitary-adrenocortical function during long-term low-dose dexamethasone therapy in hyperandrogenized women. *Am J Obstet Gynecol* 1982;142:330–339.

146. **Derksen J, Naggesser SK, Meinders AE.** Identification of virilizing adrenal tumors in hirsute women. *N Engl J Med* 1994;331:968–973.

147. **Ettinger B, Von Werder K, Thenaurs GC, et al.** Plasma testosterone stimulation-suppression dynamics in hirsute women. *Am J Med* 1971;51:170–175.

148. **Surrey ES, de Ziegler D, Gambone JC, et al.** Preoperative localization of androgen-secreting tumors: clinical, endocrinologic and radiologic evaluation of ten patients. *Am J Obstet Gynecol* 1988;158:1313–1322.

149. **Korobkin M.** Overview of adrenal imaging/adrenal CT. *Urol Radiol* 1989;11:221–226.

150. **Taylor L, Ayers JW, Gross MD, et al.** Diagnostic considerations in virilization: iodomethyl-norcholesterol scanning of androgen secreting tumors. *Fertil Steril* 1986;46:1005–1010.

151. **Moltz L, Pickartz H, Sorensen R, et al.** Ovarian and adrenal vein steroids in seven patients with androgen-secreting ovarian neoplasms: selective catheterization findings. *Fertil Steril* 1984;42:585–593.

152. **Wentz AC, White RI, Migeon CJ, et al.** Differential ovarian and adrenal vein catheterization. *Am J Obstet Gynecol* 1976;125:1000–1007.

153. **Young RH, Scully RE.** Sex-cord stromal steroid cell and other ovarian tumors with endocrine, paraendocrine, and paraneoplastic manifestations. In: **Kurman RJ,** ed. *Blaustein's pathology of the female genital tract,* 4th ed. New York: Springer-Verlag, 1994:783–847.

154. **Zhang J, Young RH, Arseneau J, et al.** Ovarian stromal Leydig cells (luteinized thecomas and stromal Leydig cell tumors): a clinicopathological analysis of 50 cases. *Int J Gynecol Pathol* 1982;1:270–285.

155. **Young RH, Scully RE.** Ovarian Sertoli cell tumors: a report of 10 cases. *Int J Gynecol Pathol* 1984;2:349–363.

156. **Young RH, Welch WR, Dickersin GR, et al.** Ovarian sex cord tumor with annular tubules: review of 74 cases including 27 with Peutz-Jeghers syndrome and four with adenoma malignum of the cervix. *Cancer* 1982;50:1384–1402.

157. **Aiman J.** Virilizing ovarian tumors. *Clin Obstet Gynecol* 1991;34:835–847.

158. **Scully RE.** Gonadoblastoma. A review of 74 cases. *Cancer* 1970;25:1340–1356.

159. **Ireland K, Woodruff JD.** Masculinizing ovarian tumors. *Obstet Gynecol Surv* 1976;31:83–111.

160. **Boss JH, Scully RE, Wegner KH, et al.** Structural variations in the adult ovary—clinical significance. *Obstet Gynecol* 1965;25:747–763.

161. **Nagamani M, Van Dinh T, Kelver ME.** Hyperinsulinemia in hyperthecosis of the ovaries. *Am J Obstet Gynecol* 1986;154:384–389.

162. **Judd HL, Scully RE, Herbst AL, et al.** Familial hyperthecosis: comparison of endocrinologic and histologic findings with polycystic ovarian disease. *Am J Obstet Gynecol* 1973;117:976–982.

163. **Karam K, Hajis I.** Hyperthecosis syndrome. *Acta Obstet Gynecol Scand* 1979;58:73–79.

164. **Braithwaite SS, Erkman-Balis B, Avila TD.** Post-menopausal virilization due to ovarian stromal hyperthecosis. *J Clin Endocrinol Metab* 1978;46:295–300.

165. **Steingold KA, Judd HL, Nieberg RK, et al.** Treatment of severe androgen excess due to ovarian hyperthecosis with a long-acting gonadotropin-releasing hormone agonist. *Am J Obstet Gynecol* 1986;154:1241–1248.

166. **Garcia-Bunuel R, Berek JS, Woodruff JD.** Luteomas of pregnancy. *Obstet Gynecol* 1975;154:407–414.

167. **Pittaway DE.** Neoplastic causes of hyperandrogenism. *Infert Reprod Med Clin North Am* 1991;2:531–545.

168. **Riddle O, Bates RW, Dykshorn S.** The preparation, identification and assay of prolactin. A hormone of the anterior pituitary. *Am J Physiol* 1933;105:191–196.

169. **Frantz AG, Kleinberg DL.** Prolactin: evidence that it is separate from growth hormone in human blood. *Science* 1970;170:745–747.

170. **Lewis UJ, Singh RNP, Sinha YN, et al.** Electrophoretic evidence for human prolactin. *J Clin Endocrinol Metab* 1971;33:153–156.

171. **Hwang P, Guyda H, Friesen H.** A radioimmunoassay for human prolactin. *Proc Natl Acad Sci U S A* 1971;68:1902–1906.

172. **Hwang P, Guyda H, Friesen H.** Purification of human prolactin. *J Biol Chem* 1972;247:1955–1958.

173. **Suh HK, Frantz AG.** Size heterogeneity of human prolactin in plasma and pituitary extracts. *J Clin Endocrinol Metab* 1974;39:928–935.

174. **Guyda HJ, Whyte S.** Heterogeneity of human growth hormone and prolactin secreted in vitro: immunoassay and radioreceptor assay correlations. *J Clin Endocrinol Metab* 1975;41:953–967.

175. **Farkough NH, Packer MG, Frantz AG.** Large molecular size prolactin with reduced receptor activity in human serum: high proportion in basal state and reduction after thyrotropin-releasing hormone. *J Clin Endocrinol Metab* 1979;48:1026–1032.

176. **Benveniste R, Helman JD, Orth DN, et al.** Circulating big human prolactin: conversion to small human prolactin by reduction of disulfide bonds. *J Clin Endocrinol Metab* 1979;48:883–886.

177. **Jackson RD, Wortsman J, Malarkey WB.** Characterization of a large molecular weight prolactin in women with idiopathic hyperprolactinemia and normal menses. *J Clin Endocrinol Metab* 1985;61:258–264.

178. **Fraser IS, Lun ZG, Zhou JP, et al.** Detailed assessment of big prolactin in women with hyperprolactinemia and normal ovarian function. *J Clin Endocrinol Metab* 1989;69:585–592.

179. **Larrea F, Escorza A, Valero A, et al.** Heterogeneity of serum prolactin throughout the menstrual cycle and pregnancy in hyperprolactinemia women with normal ovarian function. *J Clin Endocrinol Metab* 1989;68:982–987.

180. **Lewis UJ, Singh RNP, Sinha YN, et al.** Glycosylated human prolactin. *Endocrinology*1985;116:359–363.

181. **Markoff E, Lee DW.** Glycosylated prolactin is a major circulating variant in human serum. *J Clin Endocrinol Metab* 1985;65:1102–1106.

182. **Markoff E, Lee DW, Hollingsworth DR.** Glycosylated and nonglycosylated prolactin in serum during pregnancy. *J Clin Endocrinol Metab* 1988;67:519–523.

183. **Pellegrini I, Gunz G, Ronin C, et al.** Polymorphism of prolactin secreted by human prolactinoma cells: immunological, receptor binding, and biological properties of the glycosylated and nonglycosylated forms. *Endocrinology* 1988;122:667–674.

184. **Goldsmith PC, Cronin MJ, Weiner RI.** Dopamine receptor sites in the anterior pituitary. *J Histochem Cytochem* 1979;27:1205–1207.

185. **Quigley ME, Judd SJ, Gilliland GB, et al.** Effects of a dopamine antagonist on the release of gonadotropin and prolactin in normal women and women with hyperprolactinemic anovulation. *J Clin Endocrinol Metab* 1979;48:718–720.

186. **Quigley ME, Hudd SJ, Gilliland GB, et al.** Functional studies of dopamine control of prolactin secretion in normal women and women with hyperprolactinemic pituitary microadenoma. *J Clin Endocrinol Metab* 1980;50:994–998.

187. **DeLeo V, Petraglia F, Bruno MG, et al.** Different dopaminergic control of plasma luteinizing hormone, follicle-stimulating hormone and prolactin in ovulatory and postmenopausal women: effect of ovariectomy. *Gynecol Obstet Invest* 1989;27:94–98.

188. **Lachelin GCL, Leblanc H, Yen SSC.** The inhibitory effect of dopamine agonists on LH release in women. *J Clin Endocrinol Metab* 1977;44:728–732.

189. **Hill MK, Macleod RM, Orcutt P.** Dibutyryl cyclic AMP, adenosine and guanosine blockade of the dopamine, ergocryptine, and apomorphine inhibition of prolactin release in vitro. *Endocrinology* 1976;99:1612–1617.

190. **Lamberger L, Crabtree RE.** Pharmacologic effects in man of a potent long-acting dopamine receptor agonist. *Science* 1979;205:1151–1152.

191. **Braund W, Roeger DC, Judd SJ.** Synchronous secretion of luteinizing hormone and prolactin in the human luteal phase: neuroendocrine mechanisms. *J Clin Endocrinol Metab* 1984;58:293–297.

192. **Grossman A, Delitala G, Yeo T, et al.** GABA and muscimol inhibit the release of prolactin from dispersed rat anterior pituitary cells. *Neuroendocrinology* 1981;32:145–150.

193. **Gudelsky GA, Apud JA, Masotto C, et al.** Ethanolamine-O-sulfate enhances γ-aminobutyric acid secretion into hypophysial portal blood and lowers serum prolactin concentrations. *Neuroendocrinology* 1983;37:397–399.

194. **Melis GB, Paoletti AM, Mastrapasqua NM, et al.** The effects of the GABAergic drug, sodium valproate, on prolactin section in normal and hyperprolactinemic subjects. *J Clin Endocrinol Metab* 1982;54:485–489.

195. **Melis GB, Fruzetti F, Paoletti M, et al.** Pharmacological activation of δ-aminobutyric acid system blunts prolactin response to mechanical breast stimulation in puerperal women. *J Clin Endocrinol Metab* 1984;58:201–205.

196. **Sassin JF, Frantz AG, Weitzman ED, et al.** Human prolactin: 24-hour pattern with increased release during sleep. *Science* 1972;177:1205–1207.

197. **Sassin JE, Frantz AG, Kapen S, et al.** The nocturnal rise of human prolactin is dependent on sleep. *J Clin Endocrinol Metab* 1973;37:436–440.

198. **Carandente F, Angeli A, Candiani GB, et al.** Rhythms in the ovulatory cycle. 1st: prolactin. Chronobiological Research Group on Synthetic Peptides in Medicine. *Chronobiologia* 1989;16:35–44.

199. **Pansini F, Bianchi A, Zito V, et al.** Blood prolactin levels: influence of age, menstrual cycle and oral contraceptives. *Contraception* 1983;28:201–207.

200. **Pansini F, Bergamini CM, Cavallini AR, et al.** Prolactinemia during the menstrual cycle. *Gynecol Obstet Invest* 1987;23:172–176.

201. **Bohnet HG, Dahlen HG, Wuhjke W, et al.** Hyperprolactinemic anovulatory syndrome. *J Clin Endocrinol Metab* 197;42:132–143.

202. **Franks S, Murray MAF, Jequier AM, et al.** Incidence and significance of hyperprolactinemia in women with amenorrhea. *Clin Endocrinol (Oxf)* 1975;4:597–607.

203. **Jacobs HS, Hull MGR, Murray MAF, et al.** Therapy oriented diagnosis of secondary amenorrhea. *Horm Res* 1975;6:268–277.

204. **McNatty KP.** Relationship between plasma prolactin and the endocrine microenvironment of the developing human antral follicle. *Fertil Steril* 1979;32:433–438.

205. **Dorrington J, Gore-Lanton RE.** Prolactin inhibits oestrogen synthesis in the ovary. *Nature* 1981;290:600–602.

206. **Cutie RE, Andino NA.** Prolactin inhibits the steroidogenesis in midfollicular phase human granulosa cells cultured in a chemically defined medium. *Fertil Steril* 1988;49:632–637.

207. **Adashi EY, Resnick CE.** Prolactin as an inhibitor of granulosa cell luteinization: implications for hyperprolactinemia-associated luteal phase dysfunction. *Fertil Steril* 1987;48:131–139.

208. **Soto EA, Tureck RW, Strauss JF III.** Effects of prolactin on progestin secretion by human granulosa cells in culture. *Biol Reprod* 1985;32:541–545.

209. **Demura R, Ono M, Demura H, et al.** Prolactin directly inhibits basal as well as gonadotropin-stimulated secretion of progesterone and 17β-estradiol in the human ovary. *J Clin Endocrinol Metab* 1985;54:1246–1250.

210. **Boyar RM, Kapen S, Finkelstein JW, et al.** Hypothalamic-pituitary function in diverse hyperprolactinemic states. *J Clin Invest* 1974;53:1588–1598.

211. **Bohnet HG, Dahlen HG, Wuttke W, et al.** Hyperprolactinaemic anovulatory syndrome. *J Clin Endocrinol Metab* 1976;42:132–144.

212. **Franks S, Murray MAF, Jequier AM, et al.** Incidence and significance of hyperprolactinemia in women with amenorrhea. *Clin Endocrinol (Oxf)* 1975;4:597–607.

213. **Moult PJA, Rees LH, Besser GM.** Pulsatile gonadotrophin secretion in hyperprolactinaemic amenorrhoea and the response to bromocriptine therapy. *Clin Endocrinol* 1982;16:153–162.

214. **Buckman MT, Peake GT, Srivastava L.** Patterns of spontaneous LH release in normo- and hyperprolactinaemic women. *Acta Endocrinol (Copenh)* 1981;97:305–310.

215. **Aono T, Miyake A, Yasuda T, et al.** Restoration of oestrogen positive feedback on LH release by bromocriptine in hyperprolactinemic patients with galactorrhea-amenorrhea. *Acta Endocrinol (Copenh)* 1979;91:591–600.

216. **Travaglini P, Ambrosi B, Beck-Pecoz P, et al.** Hypothalamic-pituitary-ovarian function in hyperprolactinemic women. *J Clin Invest* 1978;1:39–45.

217. **Glass MR, Shaw RW, Butt WR, et al.** An abnormality of oestrogen feedback in amenorrhea galactorrhea. *BMJ* 1975;111:274–275.

218. **Koike K, Aono T, Tsutsumi H, et al.** Restoration of oestrogen-positive feedback effect on LH release in women with prolactinoma by transsphenoidal surgery. *Acta Endocrinol (Copenh)* 1982;100:492–498.

219. **Quigley ME, Judd SJ, Gilliland GB, et al.** Effects of a dopamine antagonist on the release of gonadotropin and prolactin in normal women with hyperprolactinemic anovulation. *J Clin Endocrinol Metab* 1979;48:718–720.

220. **Boyar RM, Kapen S, Finkelstein JW, et al.** Hypothalamic-pituitary function in diverse hyperprolactinemic states. *J Clin Invest* 1974;53:1588–1598.

221. **Rakoff J, VandenBerg G, Siler TM, et al.** An integrated direct functional test of the adenohypophysis. *Am J Obstet Gynecol* 1974;119:358–368.

222. **Zarate A, Jacobs S, Canales ES, et al.** Functional evaluation of pituitary reserve in patients with the amenorrhea-galactorrhea syndrome utilizing luteinizing hormone-releasing hormone (LH-RH), L-dopa and chlorpromazine. *J Clin Endocrinol Metab* 1973;37:855–859.

223. **Kleinberg DL, Noel GL, Frantz AG.** Galactorrhea: a study of 235 cases, including 48 with pituitary tumors. *N Engl J Med* 1977;296:589–600.

224. **Tolis G, Somma M, Van Campenhout J, et al.** Prolactin secretion in 65 patients with galactorrhea. *Am J Obstet Gynecol* 1974;118:91–101.

225. **Boyd AE III, Reichlin S, Tuskoy RN.** Galactorrhea-amenorrhea syndrome: diagnosis and therapy. *Ann Intern Med* 1977;87:165–175.

226. **Schlechte J, Sherman B, Halmi N, et al.** Prolactin-secreting pituitary tumors. *Endocr Rev* 1980;1:295–308.

227. **Minakami H, Abe N, Oka N, et al.** Prolactin release in polycystic ovarian syndrome. *Endocrinol Jpn* 1988;35:303–310.

228. **Murdoch AP, Dunlop W, Kendall-Taylor P.** Studies of prolactin secretion in polycystic ovary syndrome. *Clin Endocrinol* 1986;24:165–175.

229. **Lythgoe K, Dotson R, Peterson CM.** Multiple endocrine neoplasia I presenting as primary amenorrhea. A case report. *Obstet Gynecol* 1995;86:683–686.

230. **Burgess JR, Shepherd JJ, Parameswaran V, et al.** Spectrum of pituitary disease in multiple endocrine neoplasia type 1 (MEN-1): clinical, biochemical, and radiologic features of pituitary disease in a large MEN-1 kindred. *J Clin Endocrinol Metab* 1996;81:2642–2646.

231. **Bohler HCL Jr, Jones EE, Briner ML.** Marginally elevated prolactin levels require magnetic imaging and evaluation for acromegaly. *Fertil Steril* 1994;61:1168–1170.

232. **Gonsky R, Herman V, Melmed S, et al.** Transforming DNA sequences present in human prolactin-secreting pituitary tumors. *Mol Endocrinol* 1991;5:1687–1695.

233. **Sisan DA, Sheehan JP, Sheeler LR.** The natural history of untreated microprolactinomas. *Fertil Steril* 1987;48:67–71.

234. **Schlechte J, Dolan K, Sherman B, et al.** The natural history of untreated hyperprolactinemia: a prospective analysis. *J Clin Endocrinol Metab* 1989;68:412–418.

235. **Weiss MH, Teal J, Gott P, et al.** Natural history of microprolactinomas: six-year follow-up period. *Neurosurgery* 1983;12:180–183.

236. **Klibanski A, Biller BMK, Rosenthal DI, et al.** Effects of prolactin and estrogen deficiency in amenorrheic bone loss. *J Clin Endocrinol Metab* 1988;67:124–130.

237. **Turner TH, Cookson JC, Wass JAH, et al.** Psychotic reactions during treatment of pituitary tumors with dopamine agonists. *BMJ Clin Res Ed* 1984;289:1101–1103.

238. **Weiss MH, Wycoff RR, Yadley R, et al.** Bromocriptine treatment of prolactin-secreting tumors: surgical implications. *Neurosurgery* 1983;12:640–642.

239. **Katz E, Weiss BE, Hassell A, et al.** Increased circulating levels of bromocriptine after vaginal compared to oral administration. *Fertil Steril* 1991;55:882–884.

240. **Abram M, Brue T, Marange I, et al.** Pituitary tumor syndrome and hyperprolactinemia in peripheral hypothyroidism. *Ann Endocrinol (Paris)* 1992;53:215–223.

241. **Chirito E, Bonda A, Friesen HG.** Prolactin in renal failure. *Clin Res* 1972;20:423.

242. **Nagel TC, Freinkel N, Bell RH, et al.** Gynecomastia, prolactin, and other peptide hormones in patients undergoing chronic hemodialysis. *J Clin Endocrinol Metab* 1973;36:428–432.

243. **Olgaard K, Hagen C, McNeilly AS.** Pituitary hormones in women with chronic renal failure: the effect of chronic haemo- and peritoneal dialysis. *Acta Endocrinol* 1975;80:237–246.

244. **Hagen C, Olgaard K, McNeilly AS, et al.** Prolactin and the pituitary-gonadal axis in male uremic patients on regular dialysis. *Acta Endocrinol* 1976;82:29–38.

245. **Thorner MO, Edwards CRW, Hanker JP.** Prolactin and gonadotropin interaction in the male. In: **Troen P, Nankin H,** eds. *The testis in normal and infertile men.* New York: Raven Press, 1977:351–366.

246. **Lloyd RV.** Estrogen-induced hyperplasia and neoplasia in the rat anterior pituitary gland; an immunohistochemical study. *Am J Pathol* 1983;113:198–206.

247. **Scheithauer BW, Sano T, Kovacs KT, et al.** The pituitary gland in pregnancy: a clinico-pathologic and immunohistochemical study of 69 cases. *Mayo Clin Proc* 1990;65:461–474.

248. **Weil C.** The safety of bromocriptine in hyperprolactinemic female infertility; a literature review. *Curr Med Res Opin* 1986;10:172–195.

249. **Shy KK, McTiernan AM, Daling JR, et al.** Oral contraceptive use and the occurrence of pituitary prolactinoma. *JAMA* 1983;249:2204–2207.

250. **Corenblum B, Taylor PJ.** Idiopathic hyperprolactinemia may include a distinct entity with a natural history different from that of prolactin adenomas. *Fertil Steril* 1988;49:544–546.

251. **Corenblum B, Donovan L.** The safety of physiological estrogen plus progestin replacement therapy and with oral contraceptive therapy in women with pathological hyperprolactinemia. *Fertil Steril* 1993;59:671–673.

252. **Scheithauer BW, Kovacs KT, Randall RV, et al.** Effects of estrogen on the human pituitary: a clinicopathologic study. *Mayo Clin Proc* 1989;64:1077–1084.

253. **Krupp P, Monka C.** Bromocriptine in pregnancy: safety aspects. *Klin Wochenschr* 1987;65:823–827.

254. **Raymond JP, Golstein E, Konopka P.** Follow-up of children born of bromocriptine-treated mothers. *Horm Res* 1985;22:239–246.

255. **Ruiz-Velasco V, Tolis G.** Pregnancy in hyperprolactinemic women. *Fertil Steril* 1984;41:793–805.

256. **Turkalj I, Braun P, Krupp P.** Surveillance of bromocriptine in pregnancy. *JAMA* 1982;247:1589–1591.

257. **Tunbridge WM, Evered DC, Hall R, et al.** The spectrum of thyroid disease in a community: the Whickham survey. *Clin Endocrinol* 1977;7:481–493.

258. **Whartona T.** Adenographia: sive glandularum totius corporis descripto. London, 1659.

259. **Portmann L, Hamada N, Heinrich G, et al.** Antithyroid peroxidase antibody in patients with autoimmune thyroid disease: possible identity with antimicrosomal antibody. *J Clin Endocrinol Metab* 1985;61:1001–1003.

260. **Czarnocka B, Ruf J, Ferrand M, et al.** Purification of the human thyroid peroxidase and its identification as the microsomal antigen involved in autoimmune thyroid disease. *FEB S Lett* 1985;190:147–152.

261. **Norman AW, Litwack G.** Thyroid hormones. In: **Norman AW, Litwack G,** eds. *Hormones.* San Diego: Academic Press, 1987:221.

262. **Boukis MA, Koutrar DA, Souvatzoglou A, et al.** Thyroid hormone and immunological studies in endemic goiter. *J Clin Endocrinol Metab* 1983;57:859–862.

263. **Asamer H, Riccabona G, Holthaus N, et al.** Immunohistologic findings in thyroid disease in an endemic goiter area. *Arch Klin Med* 1968;215:270–284.

264. **Greer MA.** Antithyroid drugs in the treatment of thyrotoxicosis. *Thyroid Today* 1980;3.

265. **McGregor MA, Weetman AP, Ratanchaiyavong S, et al.** Iodine: an influence on the development of autoimmune thyroid disease. In: **Hall R, Kobberling J,** eds. *Thyroid disorders associated with iodine deficiency and excess.* New York: Raven Press, 1985:209–216.

266. **Weetman AP, McGregor AM, Campbell H, et al.** Iodide enhances Ig synthesis by human peripheral blood lymphocytes in vitro. *Acta Endocrinol (Copenh)* 198;103:210–215.

267. **Allen EM, Appel MC, Braverman LM.** The effect of iodide ingestion on the development of spontaneous lymphocytic thyroiditis in the diabetes prone BB/W rat. *Endocrinology* 1986;118:1977–1981.

268. **Sundick RS, Herdegen D, Brown TR.** Thyroiditis induced by dietary iodine may be due to the increased immunogenicity of highly iodinated thyroglobulin. In: **Drexhage HA, Wiersinga WM,** eds. *The thyroid and autoimmunity.* Amsterdam, New York: Elsevier Science, 1986:213.

269. **Bahn AK, Mills JL, Snyder PJ, et al.** Hypothyroidism in workers exposed to polybrominated biphenols. *N Engl J Med* 1980;302:31–33.

270. **Gaitan E, Cooksey RC, Legan J.** Simple goiter and autoimmune thyroiditis: environmental and genetic factors. *Clin Ecol* 1985;3:158–162.

271. **Wenzel BE, Hessemann J.** Antigenic homologies between plasmid encoded proteins from enteropathogenic *Yersinia* and thyroid autoantigen. *Horm Metab Res Suppl* 1987;17:77–78.

272. **Caldwell G, Kellett HA, Gow SM, et al.** A new strategy for thyroid function testing. *Lancet* 1985;1:1117–1119.

273. **DelPozo E, Wyss H, Tolis G, et al.** Prolactin and deficient luteal function. *Obstet Gynecol* 1979;53:282–286.

274. **Van Hearle AJ, Uller RP, Matthews NL, et al.** Radioimmunoassay for measurement of thyroglobulin in human serum. *J Clin Invest* 1973;52:1320–1327.

275. **Nye L, Pontes de Carvalho LC, Roitt IM.** Restrictions in the response to autologous thyroglobulin in the human. *Clin Exp Immunol* 1980;41:252–263.

276. **Permachandra BN, Blumenthal HT.** Abnormal binding of thyroid hormone in sera of patients with Hashimoto's thyroiditis. *J Clin Endocrinol Metab* 1967;27:931–936.

277. **Drexhage HA, Bottazzo GF, Bitensky L, et al.** Thyroid growth-blocking antibodies in primary myxedema. *Nature* 1981;239:594–595.

278. **Konishi J, Iida Y, Endo K, et al.** Inhibition of thyrotropin-induced adenosine 3′5′-monophosphate increase by immunoglobulins from patients with primary myxedema. *J Clin Endocrinol Metab* 1983;57:544–549.

279. **Steel NR, Bingle JP, Ramsey ID.** Myxedema followed by TSAb induced hyperthyroidism: report of two cases. *Postgrad Med J* 1985;61:25–27.

280. **Drexhage HA, Bottazzo GF, Doniach D, et al.** Evidence for thyroid-growth-stimulating immunoglobulins in some goitrous thyroid disease. *Lancet* 1980;2:287–292.

281. **Niswander RR, Gordon M, Berendes HW.** *The women and their pregnancies: the collaborative perinatal study of the National Institute of Neurologic Disease and Stroke.* Philadelphia: WB Saunders, 1972:246.

282. **Vanderpump MPJ, Tunbridge WMG.** *The thyroid: a fundamental and clinical text,* 7th ed. Philadelpha: Lippincott-Raven Publishers, 1996:474–482.

283. **Albright F.** Metropathia hemorrhagica. *Maine MJ* 1938;29:235–238.

284. **Lao TTH, Chin RKH, Panesar NS, et al.** Observations on thyroid hormones in hyperemesis gravidarum. *Asia Oceania J Obstet Gynaecol* 1988;14:449–452.

285. **Morimoto C, Reinherz EL, Schlossman SF, et al.** Alterations in immunoregulatory T cell subsets in active systemic lupus erythematosus. *J Clin Invest* 1990;66:1171–1174.

286. **Grodstein F, Goldman MB, Ryan L, et al.** Self-reported use of pharmaceuticals and primary ovulatory infertility. *Epidemiology* 1993;4:151–165.

287. **Wilansky DL, Greisman B.** Early hypothyroidism in patients with menorrhagia. *Am J Obstet Gynecol* 1989;160:673–677.

288. **Honbo KS, Van Herle AJ, Kellet KA.** Serum prolactin in untreated primary hypothyroidism. *Am J Med* 1978;64:782–787.

289. **Kleinberg DL, Noel G, Frantz AG.** Galactorrhea: a study of 235 cases. *N Engl J Med* 1977;296:589–601.

290. **Yamada T, Tsukui T, Ikejiri K, et al.** Volume of sella turcica in normal patients and in patients with primary hypothyroidism. *J Clin Endocrinol Metab* 1976;42:817–822.

291. **Feek CM, Sawers JSA, Brown NS, et al.** Influence of thyroid status on dopaminergic inhibition of thyrotropin and prolactin secretion. *J Clin Endocrinol Metab* 1980;51:585–589.

292. **Kramer M, Kauschansky A, Genel M.** Adolescent secondary amenorrhea: association with hypothalamic hypothyroidism. *Pediatrics* 1979;94:300–303.

293. **Scanlon MF, Chan V, Heath M, et al.** Dopaminergic control of thyrotropin α-subunit, thyrotropin β-subunit and prolactin in euthyroidism and hypothyroidism. *J Clin Endocrinol Metab* 1981;53:360–365.

294. **Thomas R, Reid RL.** Thyroid disease and reproductive dysfunction. *Obstet Gynecol* 1987;70:789–798.

295. **Bohnet HG, Fieldler K, Leidenberger FA.** Subclinical hypothyroidism and infertility. *Lancet* 1981;2:1278.

296. **DelPozo E, Wyss H, Tolis G, et al.** Prolactin and deficient luteal function. *Obstet Gynecol* 1979;53:282–286.

297. **Warfel W.** Thyroid regulation pathways and its effect on human luteal function. *Gynakol Geburtshilfliche Rundsch* 1992;32:145–150.

298. **Frantz AG.** Hyperprolactinemia. In: **Collu R, Brown Gm, Van Loon GR,** eds. *Clinical neuroendocrinology.* Cambridge: Blackwell Science, 1986:311–332.

299. **Keye WR, Ho Yuen B, Knopf R, et al.** Amenorrhea, hyperprolactinemia, and pituitary enlargement secondary to primary hypothyroidism. *Obstet Gynecol* 1976;48:697–702.

300. **Natori S, Karashima T, Koga S, et al.** A case report of idiopathic myxedema with secondary amenorrhea and hyperprolactinemia: effect of thyroid hormone replacement on reduction of pituitary enlargement and restoration of fertility. *Fukuoka Igaku Zasshi* 1991;82:461–463.

301. **Volpe R.** The immunologic basis of Graves' disease. *N Engl J Med* 1972;287:463–464.

302. **Bottazzo GF, Dean BM.** Autoimmune thyroid disease. *Annu Rev Med* 1986;37:353–354.

303. **Wenzel BE, Gutekunst R, Schulte K, et al.** In vitro induction of class II and autoantigen expression of human thyroid monolayers stimulates autologous T-lymphocytes in co-cultures. *Ann Endocrinol* 1986;47:15–18.

304. **Burrow CN.** Thyroid disease. In: **Burrow GN, Ferris TF,** eds. *Medical complications during pregnancy.* Philadelphia: WB Saunders, 1982:205.

305. **Stoffer SS, Hamburger JI.** Inadvertent ^{131}I therapy for hyperthyroidism in the first trimester of pregnancy. *J Nucl Med* 1976;17:146–148.

306. **Vitti P, Rago T, Chiovato L, et al.** Clinical features of patients with Graves' disease undergoing remission after antithyroid drug treatment. *Thyroid* 1997;3:369–375.

307. **Michelangeli V, Poon C, Taft J, et al.** The prognostic value of thyrotropin receptor antibody measurement in the early stages of treatment of Graves' disease with antithyroid drugs. *Thyroid* 1998;8:119–124.

308. **Edan G, Massart C, Hody B, et al.** Optimum duration of antithyroid drug treatment determined by assay of thyroid-stimulating antibody in patients with Graves' disease. *BMJ* 1989;298:359–361.

309. **McKenzie JM, Zakarija M.** Hyperthyroidism. In: **DeGroot LJ, Cahill GF, Martini L,** eds. *Endocrinology.* New York: Grune & Stratton, 1979:647.

310. **Zakarija M, Garcia M, McKenzie JM.** Studies on multiple thyroid cell membrane directed antibodies in Graves' disease. *J Clin Invest* 1985;76:1885–1898.

311. **Zakarija M, McKenzie JM.** Pregnancy associated changes in the thyroid stimulating antibodies of Graves' disease and the relationship to neonatal hyperthyroidism. *J Clin Endocrinol Metab* 1983;57:1036–1040.

312. **Tanaka T, Tamai H, Kuma K, et al.** Gonadotropin response to luteinizing hormone–releasing hormone in hyperthyroid patients with menstrual disturbances. *Metabolism* 1981;30:323–325.

313. **Thomas R, Reid RL.** Thyroid disease and reproductive dysfunction. *Obstet Gynecol* 1987;70:789–798.

314. **Laurberg P, Nygaard B, Glinoer D, et al.** Guidelines for TSH-receptor antibody measurements in pregnancy: results of an evidence-based symposium organized by the European Thyroid Association. *Eur J Endocrinol* 1998;139:584–586.

315. **McKenzie JM, Zakarija M.** Fetal and neonatal hyperthyroidism and hypothyroidism due to maternal TSH receptor antibodies. *Thyroid* 1992;2:155–159.

316. **Amino N, Mori H, Iwatani Y, et al.** High prevalence of transient postpartum thyrotoxicosis and hypothyroidism. *N Engl J Med* 1982;306:849–852.

317. **Hayslip CC, Fein HG, O'Donnell VM, et al.** The value of serum antimicrosomal antibody testing in screening for symptomatic postpartum thyroid dysfunction. *Am J Obstet Gynecol* 1988;159:203–209.

318. **Iwatani Y, Amino N, Tamaki H, et al.** Increase in peripheral large granular lymphocytes in postpartum autoimmune thyroiditis. *Endocrinol Jpn* 1988;35:447–453.

319. **Vargas MT, Briones-Urbina R, Gladman D, et al.** Antithyroid microsomal autoantibodies and HLA-DR5 are associated with postpartum thyroid dysfunction: evidence supporting an autoimmune pathogenesis. *J Clin Endocrinol Metab* 1988;67:327–333.

320. **Jansson R, Karlson A.** Autoimmune thyroid disease in pregnancy and the postpartum period. In: **McGregory AM,** ed. *Immunology of endocrine disease.* Lancaster, UK: MTP Press, 1986:181–188.

321. **Walfish PG, Chan JYC.** Post-partum hyperthyroidism. *J Clin Endocrinol Metab* 1985;14:417–447.

322. **Glinoer D, Soto MF, Bourdoux P, et al.** Pregnancy in patients with mild thyroid abnormalities: maternal and neonatal repercussions. *J Clin Endocrinol Metab* 1991;73:421–427.

323. **Stagnaro-Green A, Roman SH, Cobin RH, et al.** Detection of at-risk pregnancy by means of highly sensitive assays for thyroid autoantibodies. *JAMA* 1990;264:1422–1425.

324. **Maier DB, Parke A.** Subclinical autoimmunity and recurrent aborters. *Fertil Steril* 1989;51:280–285.

325. **Magaro M, Zoli A, Altomonte L, et al.** The association of silent thyroiditis and active systemic lupus erythematosus. *Clin Exp Rheumatol* 1992;10:67–70.

326. **LaBarbera A, Miller MM, Ober C, et al.** Autoimmune etiology in premature ovarian failure. *Am J Reprod Immunol* 1988;16:114–118.

327. **Peterson CM.** Thyroid disease and fertility. In: **Gleicher N,** ed. *Autoimmunity in reproduction. Immunol Allergy Clin NA* 1995;14:725–738.

328. **Ezzat S, Sarti DA, Cain DR, et al.** Thyroid incidentalomas: prevalence by palpitation and ultrasonography. *Arch Intern Med* 1994;154:1838–1840.

329. **McHenry CR, Walfish PG, Rosen IB.** Non-diagnostic fine needle aspiration biopsy: a dilemma in management of nodular thyroid disease. *Am Surgeon* 1993;59:415–419.

330. **Barbesino G, Tomer Y, Concepcion E, et al.** Linkage analysis of candidate genes in autoimmune thyroid disease: 1. Selected immunoregulatory genes. International Consortium for the Genetics of Autoimmune Thyroid Disease. *J Clin Endocrinol Metab* 1998;83:1580–1584.

331. **Aaltonen J, Bjorses P, Sandkujil L, et al.** An autosomal locus causing autoimmune disease: autoimmune polyglandular disease type I assigned to chromosome 21. *Nat Genet* 1994;8:83–87.

26 Endometriosis

Thomas M. D'Hooghe
Joseph A. Hill

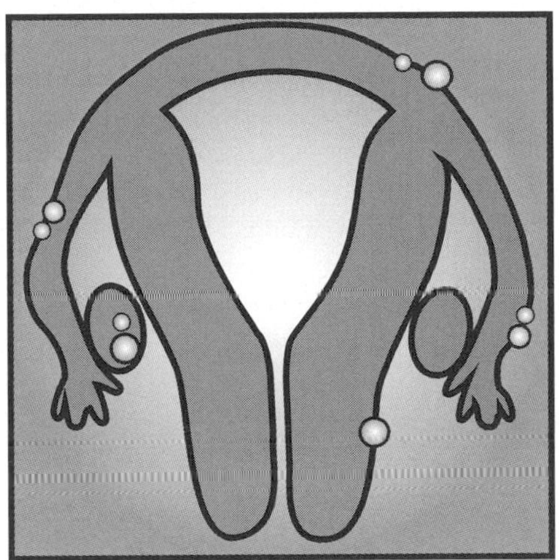

Endometriosis is defined as the presence of endometrial tissue (glands and stroma) outside the uterus. The most frequent sites of implantation are the pelvic viscera and the peritoneum. Endometriosis varies in appearance from a few minimal lesions on otherwise intact pelvic organs to massive ovarian endometriotic cysts that distort tuboovarian anatomy and extensive adhesions often involving bowel, bladder, and ureter. It is estimated to occur in 7% of reproductive age women in the United States and often is associated with pelvic pain and infertility. Considerable progress has been made in understanding the pathogenesis, spontaneous evolution, diagnosis, and treatment of endometriosis.

Etiology

Although signs and symptoms of endometriosis have been described since the 1800s, its widespread occurrence was acknowledged only during this century. Endometriosis is an estrogen-dependent disease. Three theories have been proposed to explain the histogenesis of endometriosis:

1. Ectopic transplantation of endometrial tissue
2. Coelomic metaplasia
3. The induction theory

No single theory can account for the location of endometriosis in all cases.

Transplantation Theory The transplantation theory, originally proposed by Sampson in the mid-1920s, is based on the assumption that endometriosis is caused by the seeding or implantation of endometrial cells by transtubal regurgitation during menstruation (1). Substantial clinical and experimental data support this hypothesis (2,3). Retrograde menstruation occurs in 70% to 90% of women (4,5), and it may be more common in women with endometriosis than in those without the disease (5). The presence of endometrial cells in the peritoneal fluid, indicating retrograde menstruation, has been reported in 59% to 79% of women during menses or in the early follicular phase (6,7), and these cells can be cultured *in vitro* (7). Evidence supporting retrograde menstruation is the presence of endometrial cells in the dialysate of women undergoing peritoneal dialysis during menses (8). Also, endometriosis is most often found in dependent portions of the pelvis—the ovaries, the anterior and posterior cul-de-sac, the uterosacral ligaments, the posterior uterus, and the posterior broad ligaments (9).

Endometrium obtained during menses can grow when injected beneath abdominal skin or into the pelvic cavity of animals (10,11). Endometriosis has been found in 50% of Rhesus monkeys after surgical transposition of the cervix to allow intraabdominal menstruation (12). Increased retrograde menstruation by obstruction of the outflow of menstrual fluid from the uterus is associated with a higher incidence of endometriosis in women (13,14) and in baboons (15). Women with shorter intervals between menstruation and longer duration of menses are more likely to have retrograde menstruation and are at higher risk for endometriosis (16).

Ovarian endometriosis may be caused by either retrograde menstruation or by lymphatic flow from the uterus to the ovary (17). Extrapelvic endometriosis, although rare (1% to 2%), potentially may result from vascular or lymphatic dissemination of endometrial cells to many gynecologic (vulva, vagina, cervix) and nongynecologic sites. The latter include bowel (appendix, rectum, sigmoid colon, small intestine, hernia sacs), lungs and pleural cavity, skin (episiotomy or other surgical scars, inguinal region, extremities, umbilicus), lymph glands, nerves, and brain (18).

Coelomic Metaplasia The transformation (metaplasia) of coelomic epithelium into endometrial tissue has been proposed as a mechanism for the origin of endometriosis. This theory has not been supported by either strong clinical or experimental data, however. In contrast, a recent study evaluating structural and cell surface antigen expression in the rete ovarii and epoophoron reported little commonality between endometriosis and ovarian surface epithelium, suggesting that serosal metaplasia is unlikely in the ovary (19).

Induction Theory The induction theory is, in principle, an extension of the coelomic metaplasia theory. It proposes that an endogenous (undefined) biochemical factor can induce undifferentiated peritoneal cells to develop into endometrial tissue. This theory has been supported by experiments in rabbits (20,21) but has not been substantiated in women and primates.

Genetic Factors

Population Studies

The risk or endometriosis is 7 times greater if a first-degree relative has been affected by endometriosis (22). Because no specific mendelian inheritance pattern has been identified, multifactorial inheritance has been postulated. A relative risk for endometriosis of 7.2 has been found in mothers and sisters, and a 75% (6 of 8) incidence has been noted in homozygotic twins of patients with endometriosis (23). In another twin study, 51% of the variance of the latent liability to endometriosis may be attributable to additive genetic influences (24). Other investigators reported that 14 monozygotic twin pairs were concordant for endometriosis, and 2 pairs were discordant (25). Of these twin pairs, 9 had moderate to severe endometriosis.

A relationship has been shown between endometriosis and systematic lupus erythematosus (26), dysplastic nevi, and a history of melanoma in women of reproductive age (27). Endometriosis also is linked to the presence of individual human leukocyte antigens (28–30).

Mutations

In women with endometriosis, no mutations were found in the *TP53* and *RASK* genes (31). No significant differences were observed in *N314D* (galactose-1-phosphate uridyl transferase) mutation frequency between women with endometriosis (18%) and controls (17%) (32).

Steroid Receptor Genetics

An association of estrogen receptor gene polymorphisms (two-allele and multiallele polymorphism) with endometriosis has been reported (33). Furthermore, various exon-deleted progesterone-receptor messenger RNAs (mRNAs) have been documented in human endometrium and ovarian endometriosis (34).

Aneuploidy

Epithelial cells of endometriotic cysts are monoclonal on the basis of phosphoglycerate kinase gene methylation, but normal endometrial glands are monoclonal (35,36). In a comparison of endometriotic tissue with normal tissue from the endometrium flow, cytometric DNA analysis failed to show aneuploidy (37). However, more recent studies using comparative genomic hybridization (38) or multicolor *in situ* hybridization (39) showed aneuploidy for chromosomes 11, 16, and 17 (39), increased heterogeneity of chromosome 17 aneuploidy (40), and losses of 1p and 22q (50%), 5p (33%), 6q (27%), 70 (22%), 9q (22%), and 16 (22%) of 18 selected endometriotic tissues (38).

Loss of Heterozygosity

Microsatellite DNA assays reveal an allelic imbalance (loss of heterozygosity) in *p16 (Ink4), GALT, p53,* and *APOA2* loci in patients with endometriosis, even in stage II of endometriosis (41). Another report (36) found in 28% of endometriotic lesions a loss of heterozygosity at one or more sites: chromosomes 9p (18%), 11q (18%), and 22q (15%).

Immunologic Factors and Inflammation

Although retrograde menstruation appears to be a common event in women, not all women who have retrograde menstruation develop endometriosis. The immune system may be altered in women with endometriosis, and it has been hypothesized that the disease may develop as a result of reduced immunologic clearance of viable endometrial cells from the pelvic cavity (42,43). Endometriosis can be caused by decreased clearance of peritoneal fluid endometrial cells due to reduced natural killer (NK) cell activity, or decreased macrophage activity (45). Decreased cell-mediated cytotoxicity toward autologous endometrial cells has been associated with endometriosis (44–48). However, these studies used techniques that have considerable variability in target cells and methods (49,50). Whether NK cell activity is lower in patients who have endometriosis than in those without endometriosis is controversial. Some reports demonstrate reduced NK activity (51–54,57), whereas others have found no increase in NK activity, even in women with moderate to severe disease (46–48,55). There also is great variability in NK cell activity among normal individuals that may be related to variables such as smoking, drug use, and exercise (49).

In contrast, endometriosis can also be considered a condition of immunologic tolerance, as opposed to ectopic endometrium, which essentially is self-tissue (42). It can be questioned why viable endometrial cells in the peritoneal fluid would be a target for NK cells or macrophages. Autotransplantation of blood vessels, muscles, skin grafts, and other tissues is known to be extremely successful in (45–47). Furthermore, there is no *in vitro* evidence that peritoneal fluid macrophages actually attack and perform phagocytosis of viable peritoneal fluid endometrial cells. High-dose immunosuppression can slightly increase the progression of spontaneous endometriosis in baboons (56). There is no clinical evidence, however, that the prevalence of endometriosis is increased in immunosuppressed patients. The fact that women with kidney transplants, who undergo chronic immunosuppression, are not known to have increased infertility problems can be considered indirect evidence that these patients do not develop extensive endometriosis.

Substantial evidence suggests that endometriosis is associated with a state of subclinical peritoneal inflammation, marked by an increased peritoneal fluid volume, increased peritoneal fluid white blood cell concentration (especially macrophages with increased activation status), and increased inflammatory cytokines, growth factors, and angiogenesis-promoting substances. It has been reported in baboons that subclinical peritoneal inflammation occurs both during menstruation and after intrapelvic injection of endometrium (57). A higher basal activation status of peritoneal macrophages in women with endometriosis may impair fertility by reducing sperm motility, increasing sperm phagocytosis, or interfering with fertilization (58,59), possibly by increased secretion of cytokines such as tumor necrosis factor-α (TNF-α) (60–62). TNF also may facilitate the pelvic implantation of ectopic endometrium (63,64). The adherence of human endometrial stromal cells to mesothelial cells *in vitro* has been increased by the pretreatment of mesothelial cells with physiologic doses of TNF-α (63). Macrophages or other cells may promote the growth of endometrial cells (65,66) by secretion of growth and angiogenetic factors such as epidermal growth factor (EGF) (63), macrophage-derived growth factor (MDGF) (67), fibronectin (68), and adhesion molecules such as integrins (69). After attachment of endometrial cells to the peritoneum, subsequent invasion and growth appears to be regulated by matrix metalloproteinases (MMPs) and their tissue inhibitors (70,71).

There is increasing evidence that local inflammation and secretion of prostaglandins (PG) is related to differences in endometrial aromatase activity between women with and without endometriosis. Expression of aromatase cytochrome P450 protein and mRNA was observed in human endometriotic implants but not in normal endometrium, suggesting that ectopic endometrium produces estrogens, which may be involved in the tissue growth interacting with the estrogen receptor (72). Inactivation of 17β-estradiol has been reported to be impaired in endometriotic tissues because of deficient expression of 17β-hydroxysteroid dehydrogenase type 2, which is normally expressed in eutopic endometrium in response to progesterone (73). Finally, the inappropriate aromatase expression in endometriosis lesions can be stimulated by prostaglandin E_2 (PGE_2). This also leads to local production of E_2, which also stimulates PGE_2 production, resulting in a positive-feedback system between local inflammation and estrogen-driven local growth of ectopic endometrium (74).

Environmental Factors and Dioxin

There is an increasing awareness of potential links between reproductive health, infertility, and environmental pollution. Attention has been directed to the potential role of dioxins in the pathogenesis of endometriosis, but the issue remains controversial.

A 1976 explosion of a factory in Seveso (Italy) resulted in the highest levels of dioxin exposure recorded in humans (75), but so far no data have been published. The Seveso Women's Health Study will correlate prospective individual data on exposure to dioxin with reproductive endpoints such as the incidence of endometriosis, infertility, and decreased sperm quality. Thus far, one case-control study has failed to show in the general population an association between endometriosis and exposure to polychlorinated biphenyl and chlorinated pesticides during adulthood: no differences in mean plasma concentrations of 14 polychlorinated biphenyl and 11 chlorinated pesticides were found between women with and without endometriosis (76).

Genetic mechanisms may play a role in dioxin exposure and the development of endometriosis. Transcripts of the *CYP1A1* gene, a dioxin-induced gene, have been reported to be significantly higher (9 times higher) in endometriotic tissues than in eutopic endometrium (77). Other investigators have reported a similar expression of arylhydrocarbon receptor and dioxin-related genes (using semiquantitative reverse transcriptase polymerase chain reaction) in the endometrium from women with or without endometriosis (78). In Japanese subjects, no association was found between endometriosis prevalence or severity and polymorphisms for arylhydrocarbon receptor repressor, arylhydrocarbon (x2) receptor, and arylhydrocarbon nuclear translocator or *CYP1A1* genes (79). Based on these data, there is insufficient evidence supporting the association between endometriosis and dioxin exposure in humans.

Primates

An initial retrospective case-control study reported that the prevalence of endometriosis was not statistically different (Fisher exact test, $p = 0.08$) between monkeys chronically exposed to dioxin during 4 years (11 of 14, 79%) and in nonexposed animals (2 of 6, 33%) after a period of 10 years. However, a positive correlation was found between the severity of endometriosis and dioxin dose, serum levels of dioxin, and dioxin-like chemicals (80,81). Two prospective studies have evaluated the association between dioxin exposure and development of endometriosis in Rhesus monkeys. In the most recent study (82), monkeys exposed over 12 months to low-dose dioxin (0.71 ng/kg/d) had endometriosis implants with smaller maximal and minimal diameters and similar survival rate when compared with endometriotic lesions in unexposed controls, suggesting no effect of dioxin on endometriosis. However, after 12 months of exposure to high-dose dioxin (17.86 ng/kg/d), larger diameters and a higher survival rate of endometriosis implants were observed in exposed Rhesus monkeys compared with nonexposed controls. The second randomized controlled study performed in 80 Rhesus monkeys compared those with no treatment with those treated with 0, 5, 20, 40, and 80 μg of *Aroclor* (1,254/kg/d) for 6 years. Endometriosis occurred in 37% of controls and in 25% of treated monkeys as determined by laparoscopy and necropsy data (83). No association was observed between endometriosis severity and polychlorinated biphenyl exposure. These data question the importance of dioxin exposure in the development of endometriosis in primates, except at high doses.

Rodents

Continuous exposure to 2,3,7,8-tetrachlorodibenzo-P-dioxin inhibited the growth of surgically induced endometriosis in ovariectomized mice treated with high-dose estradiol. No correlation was observed between the dose of dioxin and survival of endometrial implants, adhesions, and serum E_2 levels (84). In ovariectomized mice induced with endometriosis, similar stimulating effects of estrone and 4-chlorodiphenyl ether (4-CDE) were observed on survival rates of endometriotic mice, suggesting an estrogen-like effect of 4-CDE (85). Potential mechanisms mediating dioxin action to promote endometriosis in rodents are complex and probably different in rats and mice, not to mention women. The mouse appears to be a better model to elucidate these mechanisms (86), but both models have important limitations.

Future Research

The study of endometriosis is compounded by the need to exclude other causes and to assess symptoms within the context of the pelvic condition (i.e., the presence or absence of pathology). The pathogenesis of endometriosis, the pathophysiology of related infertility, and the spontaneous evolution of endometriosis are still being investigated. At the time of diagnosis, most patients with endometriosis have had the disease for an unknown period, making it difficult to initiate any clinical experiments that would determine definitely the etiology or progression of the disease (3). Because endometriosis occurs naturally only in women and primates and invasive experiments cannot be performed easily, it is difficult to undertake properly controlled studies. Thus, there is a need for the development of a good animal model with spontaneous endometriosis.

The main advantage of the rat and rabbit animal models used to study endometriosis is their low cost relative to primates. The disadvantages are numerous, however. Rodents lack a menstrual cycle comparable to that of primates and do not have spontaneous endometriosis. Whereas the rat ovulates spontaneously, it has a shorter luteal phase than humans. The reproductive pattern of the rabbit lacks a luteal phase. There is a wide phylogenetic gap between these two species and the human. In both rodent models, the type of lesions appear to be quite different from the variety of pigmented and nonpigmented lesions observed in women (88–90).

Primates, conversely, are phylogenetically close to humans, have a comparable menstrual cycle, are afflicted with spontaneous endometriosis, and when induced with endometriosis, develop macroscopic lesions that are similar to those found in human disease (12,91–95). Although the great apes are closest to humans in many anatomic and physiologic aspects of reproduction, they are not practical models for study; therefore, Rhesus and cynomolgus monkeys have been used. Baboons may be a better choice for study because they are continuous breeders, are phylogenetically very close to humans, and have similar reproductive anatomy and physiology with regard to menstrual cycle characteristics and regularity, embryo implantation, and fetal development (91). In addition, spontaneous endometriosis in the baboon has been found to be both minimal and disseminated, similar to the different stages of endometriosis in women (91,96,97). Experimental endometriosis can be successfully induced by the intrapelvic injection of menstrual endometrium (11). In recent years, the baboon has been established in about 30 peer reviewed articles as an excellent model for endometriosis research (98).

Prevalence

Endometriosis is predominantly found in women of reproductive age but has been reported in adolescents and in postmenopausal women receiving hormonal replacement (99). It is found in women of all ethnic and social groups. In women with pelvic pain or infertility, a high prevalence of endometriosis (from a low of 20% to a high of 90%) has been reported (2,100). In asymptomatic women having tubal ligation (women of proven fertility), the prevalence of endometriosis ranges from 3% to 43% (5,101–105). This great variation in the reported prevalence may be explained by several factors. First, it may vary with the diagnostic method used: laparoscopy, the operation of choice for diagnosis, is generally accepted to be a better method than laparotomy for diagnosing minimal to mild endometriosis. Second, minimal or mild endometriosis may be more thoroughly noted in a symptomatic patient being given general anesthesia than in an asymptomatic patient during tubal sterilization. Third, the experience of the surgeon is important because there is a wide variation in the appearance of subtle endometriosis implants, cysts, and adhesions. Most studies that evaluate the prevalence of endometriosis in women of reproductive age lack histologic confirmation (5,101,102,105–110).

Diagnosis

Clinical Presentation

Endometriosis should be suspected in women with subfertility, dysmenorrhea, dyspareunia, or chronic pelvic pain. However, endometriosis may be asymptomatic.

Risk factors for endometriosis include short cycle length (111), heavier menstruation, and longer flow duration (16,112), probably related to a higher incidence of retrograde menstruation. Patient height and weight are positively and negatively, respectively, associated with the risk for endometriosis (113).

Endometriosis can be associated with significant gastrointestinal symptoms (pain, nausea, vomiting, early satiety, bloating and distention, altered bowel habits). A characteristic motility change (ampulla of Vater–duodenal spasm, a seizure equivalent of the enteric nervous system), along with bacterial overgrowth, has been documented in most women with the disease (114). Women of reproductive age with endometriosis are not osteopenic (115).

The average delay between onset of pain symptoms and surgically confirmed endometriosis is quite long: ±8 years in the United Kingdom and ±9 to 12 years in the United States (116). A delay in diagnosis of endometriosis of 6 and 3 years in women with pain and women with infertility, respectively, has been reported. Over the past two decades, there has been a steady decrease in the delay in diagnosis and a decline in the prevalence of advanced endometriosis at first diagnosis (117). At the same time, patient awareness of endometriosis has increased. For many patients, endometriosis becomes a chronic disease, affecting quality of life resulting from pain, emotional impact of subfertility, anger about disease recurrence, and uncertainty about the future regarding repeated surgeries or long-term medical therapy and its side effects. Therefore, there is a need to look at endometriosis, at least in a subset of highly symptomatic women, as a chronic disease. Quality-of-life issues should, therefore, be addressed and studied using reliable and valid questionnaires (118).

Pain

In adult women, dysmenorrhea may be especially suggestive of endometriosis if it begins after years of pain-free menses. Dysmenorrhea often starts before the onset of menstrual bleeding and continues throughout the menstrual period. In adolescents, the pain may be present after menarche without an interval of pain-free menses. The distribution of pain is variable but most often is bilateral.

Local symptoms can arise from rectal, ureteral, and bladder involvement. Lower back pain can occur. Most studies have failed to detect a correlation between the degree of pelvic pain and the severity of endometriosis (103). Some women with extensive disease have no pain, whereas others with only minimal disease may experience severe pelvic pain. Severe pelvic pain and dyspareunia may be associated with deep infiltrating subperitoneal endometriosis (100,110). Possible mechanisms causing pain in patients with endometriosis include local peritoneal inflammation, deep infiltration with tissue damage, adhesion formation, fibrotic thickening, and collection of shed menstrual blood in endometriotic implants, resulting in painful traction with the physiologic movement of tissues (110,119).

In rectovaginal endometriotic nodules, a close histologic relationship has been observed between nerves and endometriotic foci and between nerves and the fibrotic component of the nodule (120).

Subfertility

An association between endometriosis and subfertility is generally accepted, but most of the studies suggesting this link have been based on retrospective or cross-sectional analysis. When endometriosis is moderate or severe, involving the ovaries and causing adhesions that block tuboovarian motility and ovum pickup, it is associated with subfertility (121). This effect has also been shown in primates, including cynomolgus monkeys and baboons (94,122). Although numerous mechanisms (ovulatory dysfunction, luteal insufficiency, luteinized unruptured follicle syndrome, recurrent abortion, altered immunity, and intraperitoneal inflammation) have been proposed (123), the association between fertility and minimal or mild endometriosis remains controversial (121).

Infertility **Based on the number of asymptomatic women who are found to have endometriosis during tubal ligation, it would appear that the prevalence of endometriosis is not necessarily higher in infertile than in fertile women with endometriosis** (5). **In fertile women, endometriosis has been reported to be minimal or mild in 80% and moderate or severe in 20%** (5,101–105).

In women with mild disease, some studies have reported a lower spontaneous *monthly fecundity rate* (MFR), which is the total number of pregnancies divided by the number of months of pregnancy exposure (i.e., 5% to 11% compared with 25% in a normally fertile population) (123). Other studies using artificial insemination with donor semen have reported that the MFR in women with minimal and mild endometriosis is either reduced (4%) or normal (20%) (124–127). Fertility is not reduced in baboons with spontaneous minimal endometriosis (122,128). In one study, the fecundity rate (probability of becoming pregnant in the first 36 weeks after laparoscopy and carrying the pregnancy to ≥20 weeks) was 18% in infertile women with minimal to mild endometriosis and 23.7% in women with unexplained infertility (no significant difference). None of these women had been surgically treated for endometriosis during the diagnostic laparoscopy. However, 10% of women in each group had been treated with intrauterine insemination, *in vitro* fertilization (IVF) or cystectomy-myomectomy (129). It remains unclear whether the mere presence of peritoneal endometriosis directly correlates with infertility.

Spontaneous Abortion A possible association between endometriosis and spontaneous abortion has been suggested in mostly uncontrolled or retrospective studies. Some controlled studies evaluating the association between endometriosis and spontaneous abortion have important methodologic shortcomings: heterogeneity between cases and controls, analysis of the abortion rate before the diagnosis of endometriosis, and selection bias of study and control groups (357). Based on controlled prospective studies, there is no evidence that endometriosis is associated with (recurrent) pregnancy loss (132), or that medical or surgical treatment of endometriosis reduces the spontaneous abortion rate (133,134).

Endocrinologic Abnormalities

Endometriosis has been associated with anovulation, abnormal follicular development with impaired follicle growth, reduced circulating E_2 levels during the preovulatory phase, disturbed luteinizing hormone (LH) surge patterns, premenstrual spotting, the luteinized unruptured follicle syndrome, and galactorrhea and hyperprolactinemia (135). Increased incidence and recurrence of the luteinized unruptured follicle syndrome has been reported in baboons with mild endometriosis, but not in primates with minimal endometriosis or a normal pelvis (136). Luteal insufficiency with reduced circulating E_2 and progesterone levels, out-of-phase endometrial biopsies, and aberrant integrin expression has been reported in the endometrium of women with endometriosis by some researchers (135,137), but these findings have not been confirmed by other investigators (138). Therefore, no convincing data exist to conclude that the incidence of these endocrinologic abnormalities is increased in women who have endometriosis.

Extrapelvic Endometriosis

Extrapelvic endometriosis, although often asymptomatic, should be suspected when symptoms of pain or a palpable mass occur outside the pelvis in a cyclic pattern. Endometriosis involving the intestinal tract (especially colon and rectum) is the most common site of extrapelvic disease and may cause abdominal and back pain, abdominal distention, cyclic rectal bleeding, constipation, and obstruction. Ureteral involvement can lead to obstruction and result in cyclic pain, dysuria, and hematuria. Pulmonary endometriosis can manifest as pneumothorax, hemothorax, or hemoptysis during menses. Umbilical endometriosis should be suspected when a patient has a palpable mass and cyclic pain in the umbilical area (18).

Clinical Examination

In many women with endometriosis, no abnormality is detected during the clinical examination. The vulva, vagina, and cervix should be inspected for any signs of endometriosis, although the occurrence of endometriosis in these areas is rare (e.g., episiotomy scar).

Other possible signs of endometriosis include uterosacral or cul-de-sac nodularity, lateral or cervical displacement due to uterosacral scarring (139), painful swelling of the rectovaginal septum, and unilateral ovarian (cystic) enlargement. In more advanced disease, the uterus is often in fixed retroversion, and the mobility of the ovaries and fallopian tubes is reduced. Evidence of deeply infiltrative endometriosis (deeper than 5 mm under the peritoneum) in the rectovaginal septum with cul-de-sac obliteration or cystic ovarian endometriosis should be suspected by clinical documentation of uterosacral nodularities during menses, especially if CA125 serum levels are higher than 35 IU/mL (140–142).

The clinical examination may have false-negative results. Therefore, the diagnosis of endometriosis should always be confirmed by biopsy of suspicious lesions that are obtained laparoscopically.

Imaging and Endometriosis

When filling defects (presence of hypertrophic or polypoid endometrium) are observed at hysterosalpingography (143), there is a significant positive correlation with endometriosis with a positive predictive value of 84% and negative predictive value of 75%.

Gynecologic transvaginal (144) or transrectal ultrasonography (145) is an important diagnostic tool in the assessment of ovarian endometriotic cysts (differentiation from other adnexal masses) and of rectovaginal endometriosis (sensitivity, 97%; specificity, 96%).

Other imaging techniques, including computed tomography (CT) and magnetic resonance imaging (MRI), can be used to provide additional and confirmatory information, but they cannot be used for determining the primary diagnosis (146). These techniques are more costly than ultrasound, and their added value is not clear.

CA125

There is no blood test available for the diagnosis of endometriosis. Levels of CA125, a marker found on derivatives of the coelomic epithelium and common to most nonmucinous epithelial ovarian carcinomas, have been found to be significantly higher in women with moderate or severe endometriosis and normal in women with minimal or mild disease (147,148). During menstruation, an increase in CA125 levels has been shown in women with and without endometriosis (149–153). Other studies have not found an increase during menses (154,155) or have found an increase only with moderate to severe endometriosis (156,157). The levels of CA125 vary widely, not only in patients without endometriosis (8 to 22 U/mL in the nonmenstrual phase), but also in those with minimal to mild endometriosis (14 to 31 U/mL in the nonmenstrual phase) and in those with moderate to severe disease (13 to 95 U/mL in the nonmenstrual phase).

The reason CA125 levels are increased in moderate to severe endometriosis is unclear. It has been hypothesized that endometriosis lesions contain a greater amount of CA125 than normal endometrium and that the associated inflammation could lead to an increased shedding of CA125 (148).

The specificity of CA125 has been reported to be higher than 80% in most studies. This high level of specificity is achieved in selected women with infertility or pain who are known to be at risk for endometriosis. The low level of sensitivity of CA125 (20% to 50% in most studies) poses limitations for the clinical use of this test for diagnosis of endometriosis. Theoretically, the sensitivity might increase during the menstrual period, when the increase in CA125 levels is more pronounced in women who have endometriosis. However, studies using cutoff levels of 35 U/mL (156,157) or 85 U/mL (158) have not found a significant improvement in sensitivity. A sensitivity of 66% was found when CA125 was determined during both the follicular phase and the menstrual phase in each patient and when the ratio of menstrual versus follicular values (>1.5) was used instead of one CA125 level (157). More recent studies reported that the value of CA125 in diagnosis of endometriosis is limited but higher for moderate to severe disease, especially if serum CA125 concentrations are measured during the midfollicular phase (159,160).

Serial CA125 determinations may be useful to predict the recurrence of endometriosis after therapy (161,162). CA125 levels decrease after combined medical and surgical therapy or during medical treatment of endometriosis with danazol, gonadotropin-releasing hormone (GnRH) analogues, or gestrinone, but not with medroxyprogesterone acetate (MPA) or placebo (163–165). CA125 levels have been reported to increase to pretreatment levels as early as 3, 4, or 6 months after the cessation of therapy with danazol, GnRH analogs, or gestrinone (153,164–168). Posttreatment increases in CA125 levels have been reported to correlate with endometriosis recurrence (152,162,169). However, other studies have not substantiated a correlation between posttreatment CA125 levels and disease recurrence (163,166,170).

Laparoscopic Findings

During diagnostic laparoscopy, the pelvic and abdominal cavity should be systematically investigated for the presence of endometriosis. This examination should include

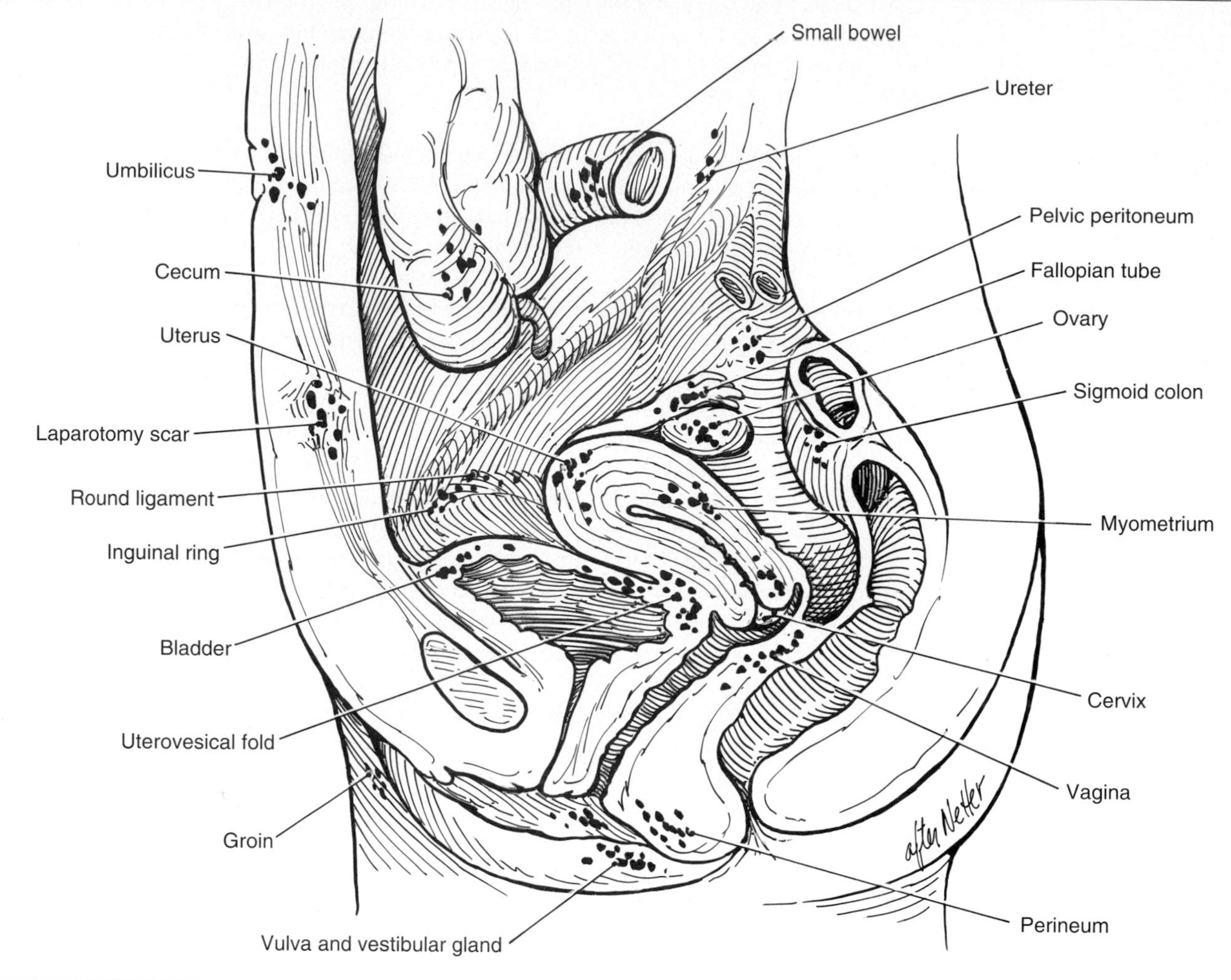

Figure 26.1 Pelvic localization of endometriosis.

a complete inspection and palpation in a clockwise or counterclockwise fashion with a blunt probe of the bowel, bladder, uterus, tubes, ovaries, cul-de-sac, and broad ligament (Fig. 26.1).

Characteristic findings include typical ("powder-burn," "gunshot") lesions on the serosal surfaces of the peritoneum. These are black, dark brown, or bluish nodules or small cysts containing old hemorrhage surrounded by a variable degree of fibrosis (Fig. 26.2). Endometriosis can appear as subtle lesions (Fig. 26.3), including red implants (petechial, vesicular, polypoid, hemorrhagic, red flamelike), serous or clear vesicles, white plaques or scarring, yellow-brown discoloration of the peritoneum, and subovarian adhesions (89–91,171,172). Histologic confirmation of the laparoscopic impression is essential for the diagnosis of endometriosis (173), not only for subtle lesions but also for typical lesions reported to be histologically negative in 24% of cases (174).

Mild forms of deep endometriosis may only be detected by palpation under an endometriotic lesion or by discovery of a palpable mass beneath visually normal peritoneum, most notably in the posterior cul-de-sac (141) (Fig. 26.4). Reduced Douglas depth and volume in women with deep endometriosis suggest that such lesions develop not in the rectovaginal septum but intraperitoneally and that burial by anterior rectal wall adhesions creates a false bottom, giving an erroneous impression of extraperitoneal origin (175).

The diagnosis of ovarian endometriosis is facilitated by careful inspection of all sides of both ovaries, which may be difficult when adhesions are present in more advanced stages of disease (Fig. 26.5). With superficial ovarian endometriosis, lesions can be both typical and subtle. Larger ovarian endometriotic cysts (endometrioma) are usually located on the anterior surface of the ovary and are associated with retraction, pigmentation, and adhesions to the posterior peritoneum. These ovarian endometriotic cysts often contain a thick, viscous dark brown fluid ("chocolate fluid") composed of hemosiderin derived from previous intraovarian hemorrhage. Because this fluid may also be found in other conditions, such as in hemorrhagic corpus luteum cysts or neoplastic cysts, biopsy and preferably removal of the ovarian cyst for histologic confirmation are necessary for the diagnosis in the revised endometriosis classification of the American Society for Reproductive Medicine. If that is not possible, the presence of an ovarian endometriotic cyst should be confirmed by the following features: cyst diameter of less than 12 cm, adhesion to pelvic sidewall or broad ligament, endometriosis on surface of ovary, and tarry, thick, chocolate-colored fluid content (176). Ovarian endometriosis appears to be a marker for more extensive pelvic and intestinal disease. Exclusive ovarian disease is found in only 1% of endometriosis patients, with the remaining patients having mostly extensive pelvic or intestinal endometriosis (177).

Histologic Confirmation

Histologic confirmation is essential in the diagnosis of endometriosis. In a study of 44 patients with chronic pelvic pain, endometriosis was laparoscopically diagnosed in 36%, but histologic confirmation was obtained in only 18%. This resulted in a low diagnostic accuracy of laparoscopic inspection with a positive predictive value of only 45%, explained by a specificity of only 77% (178).

Microscopically, endometriotic implants consist of endometrial glands and stroma with or without hemosiderin-laden macrophages (Fig. 26.6). It has been suggested, however, that using these stringent and unvalidated histologic criteria may result in significant underdiagnosis of endometriosis (2). Furthermore, problems in obtaining biopsies (especially small vesicles) and variability in tissue processing (step or partial instead of serial sectioning) may contribute to false-negative results. Endometrioid stroma may be more characteristic of endometriosis than endometrioid glands (179). Stromal endometriosis, which contains endometrial stroma with hemosiderin-laden macrophages or hemorrhage, has been reported in women (173,174) and in baboons (97) and may represent a very early event in the pathogenesis of endometriosis. Isolated endometrial stromal cell nodules, immunohistochemically positive for vimentin and estrogen receptor, can be found without endometrial glands along blood or lymphatic vessels (180).

Different types of lesions may have different degrees of proliferative or secretory glandular activity (179). Vascularization, mitotic activity, and the three-dimensional structure of endometriosis lesions are key factors (181–183). Deep endometriosis has been described as a specific type of pelvic endometriosis characterized by proliferative strands of glands and stroma in dense fibrous and smooth muscle tissue (110). However, smooth muscles are also frequent components of endometriotic lesions on the peritoneum, ovary, rectovaginal septum, and uteroasacral ligaments (184).

Microscopic endometriosis is defined as the presence of endometrial glands and stroma in macroscopically normal pelvic peritoneum. It is believed to be important in the histogenesis of endometriosis and its recurrence after treatment (185,186). The clinical relevance of microscopic endometriosis is controversial because it has not been observed uniformly. Using undefined criteria for what constitutes normal peritoneum, peritoneal biopsy specimens of 1 to 3 cm were obtained during laparotomy from 20 patients with moderate to severe endometriosis (186). Examination of the biopsy results with low-power scanning electron microscopy revealed unsuspected microscopic endometriosis in 25% of cases not confirmed by light microscopy. Peritoneal endometriotic foci have been demonstrated by

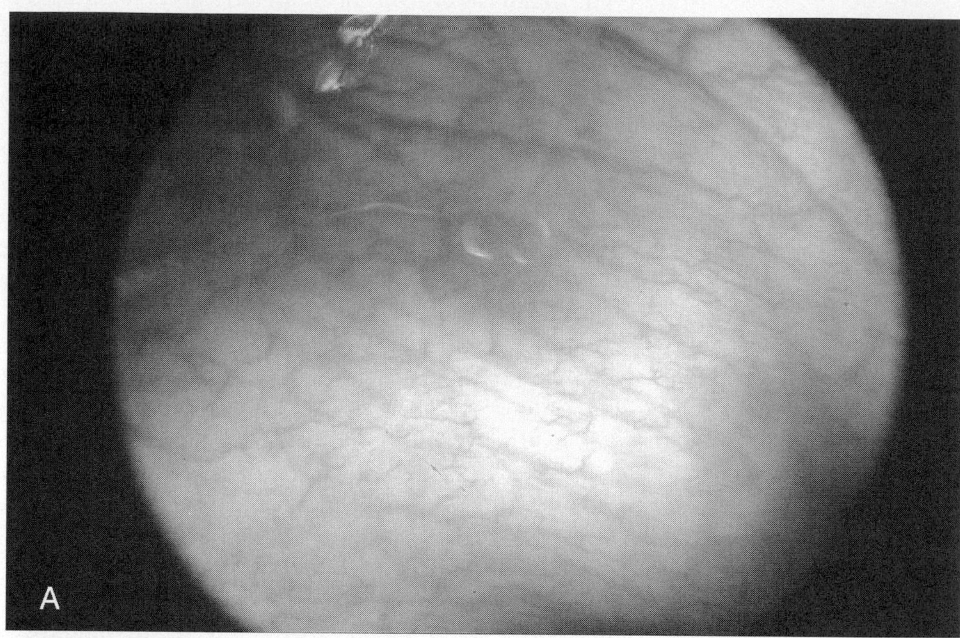

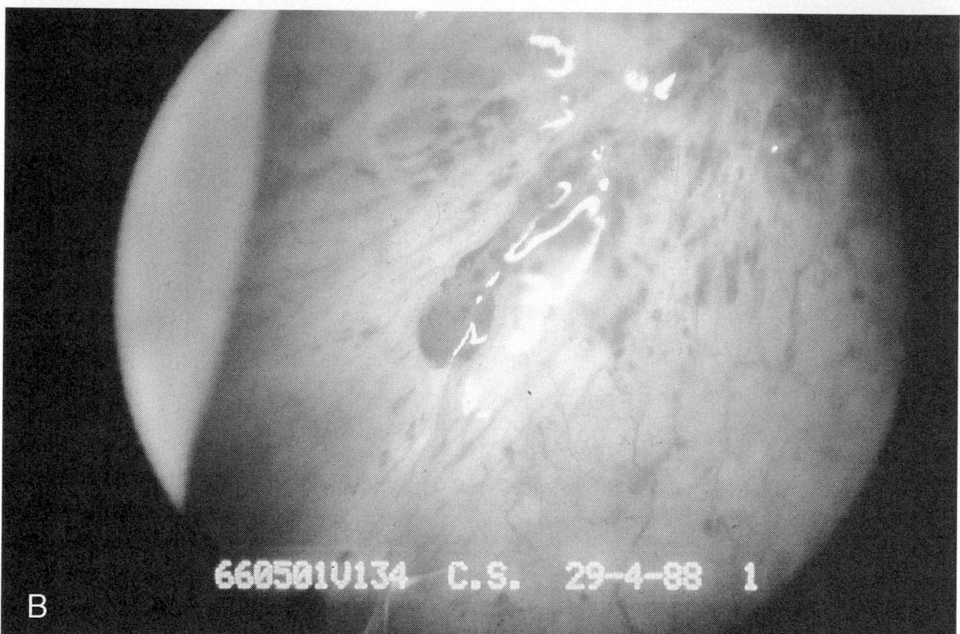

Figure 26.2 Subtle and typical endometriotic lesions. A: Clear translucent vesicle on pelvic peritoneum. **B:** Red polypoid lesions and petechial and hemorrhagic areas on pelvic peritoneum.

light microscopy in areas that show no obvious evidence of disease (187). In serial sections of laparoscopic biopsies of normal peritoneum, 10% to 15% of women were shown to have microscopic endometriosis, and endometriosis was found in 6% of those without macroscopic disease (172,188,189).

In contrast, other studies have been unable to detect microscopic endometriosis in 2-mm biopsy specimens of visually normal peritoneum (88,190–192). Examination of larger samples (5 to 15 mm) of visually normal peritoneum has revealed microscopic endometriosis in only 1 of 55 patients studied (193). Similarly, a histologic study of serial sections through the entire pelvic peritoneum of visually normal peritoneum from baboons with and without

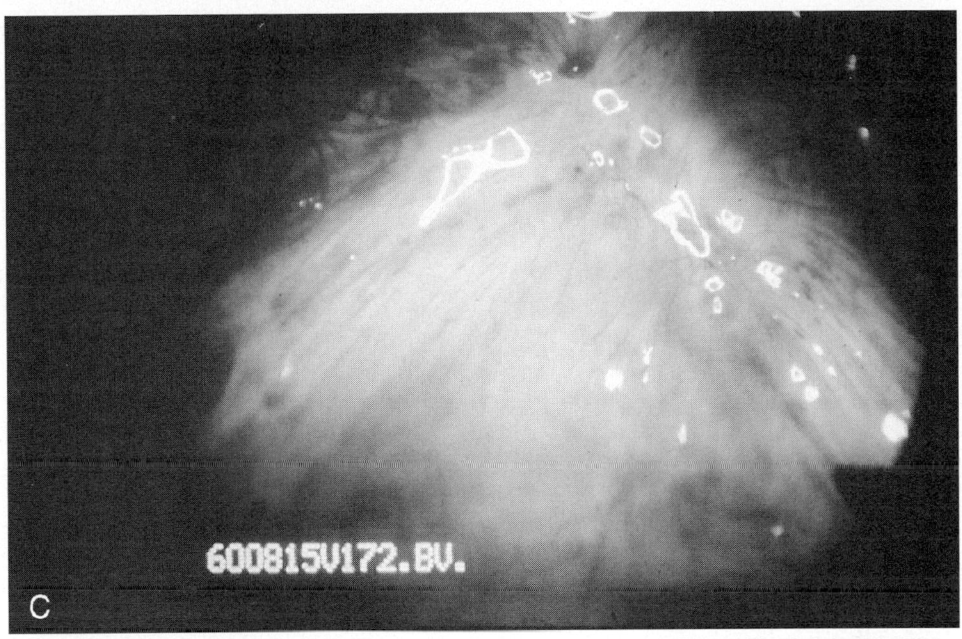

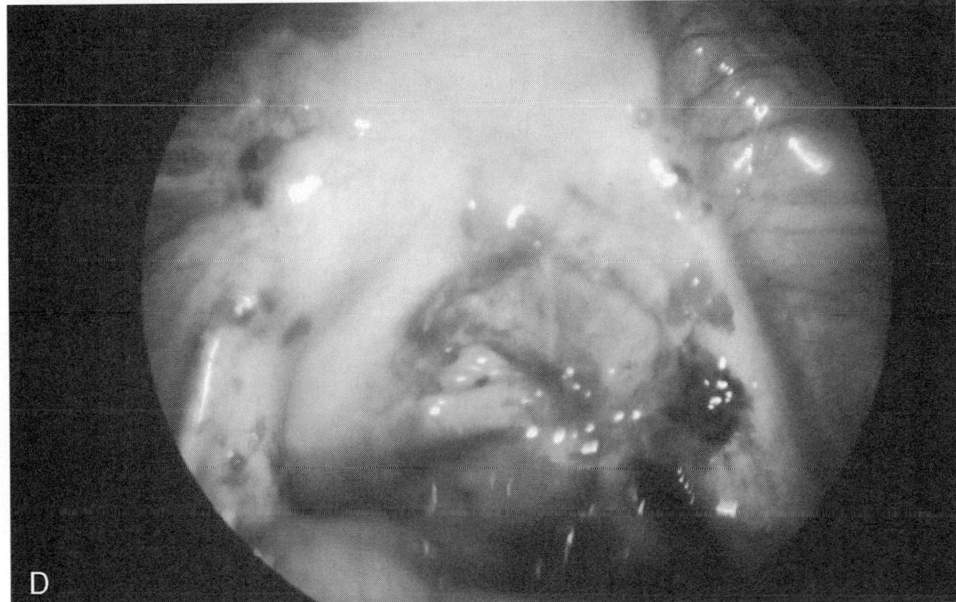

Figure 26.2 **C:** Typical black-puckered lesions on uterosacral ligaments. **D:** Combination of typical black-puckered lesions on left uterosacral ligament and red polypoid lesions in cul-de-sac.

disease indicated that microscopic endometriosis is a rare occurrence (194). Therefore, it appears that macroscopically appearing normal peritoneum rarely contains microscopic endometriosis (193).

Classification

The current classification system of endometriosis is the former American Fertility Society (AFS) system (Fig. 26.5), which has been revised without major changes (121). It is based on the appearance, size, and depth of peritoneal and ovarian implants; the presence, extent, and type of adnexal adhesions; and the degree of cul-de-sac obliteration. **In the new classification system, the morphology of peritoneal and ovarian implants should be categorized as red (red, red-pink, and clear lesions), white (white, yellow-brown, and peritoneal defects), and black (black and blue lesions).**

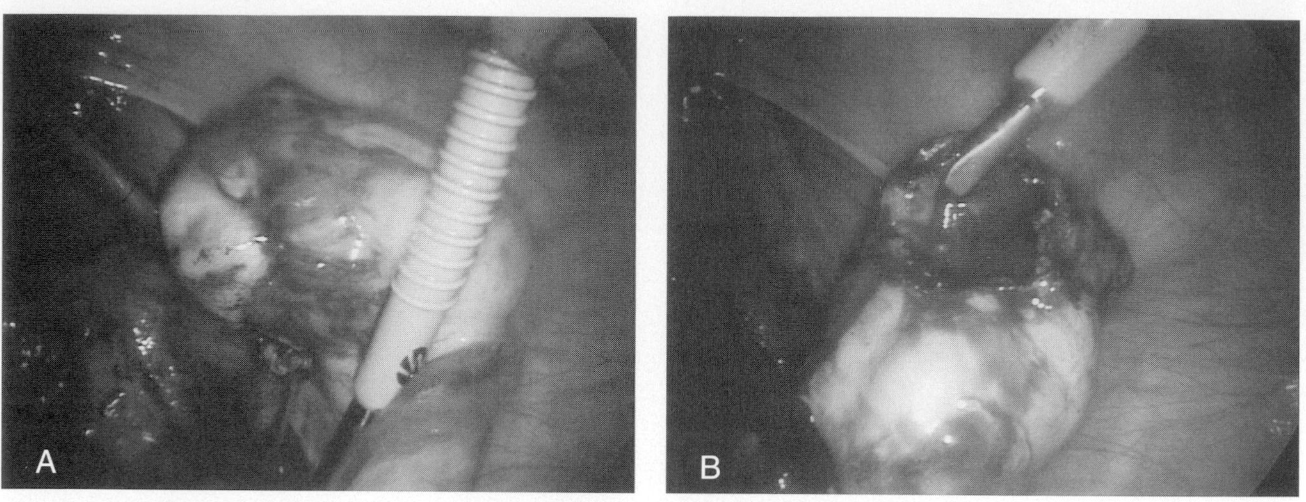

Figure 26.3 Ovarian endometriosis: endometriotic cyst (endometrioma) on the left ovary.

Figure 26.4 Laparoscopic excision of deep endometriosis from the cul-de-sac.

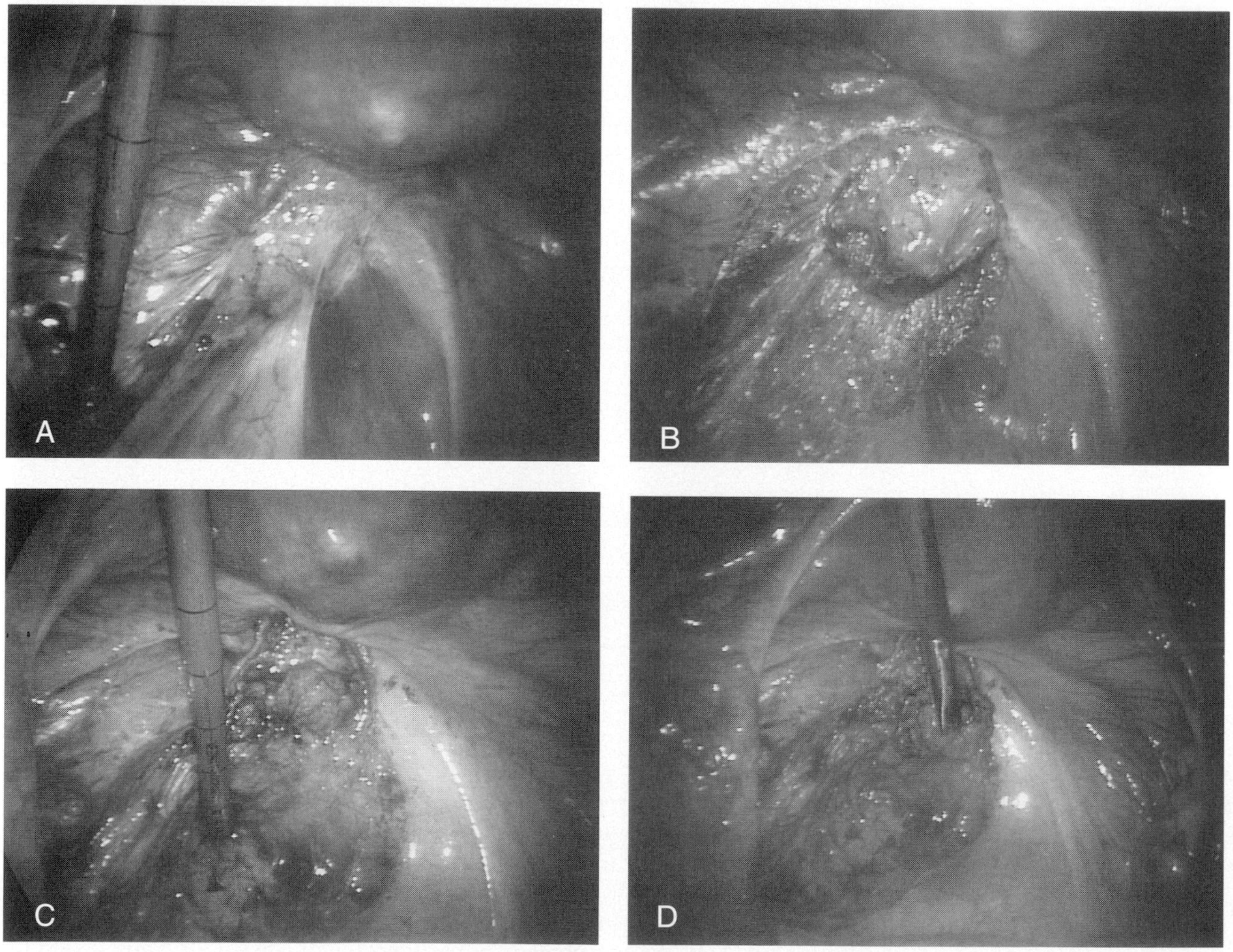

Revised American Fertility Society Classification of Endometriosis: 1985

Patient's Name ________________ Date ________________

Stage I (Minimal) - 1-5
Stage II (Mild) - 6-15
Stage III (Moderate) - 16-40
Stage IV (Severe) - >40
Total ________________

Laparoscopy ________ Laparotomy ________ Photography ________
Recommended Treatment ________________

Prognosis ________________

	ENDOMETRIOSIS	<1cm	1-3cm	>3cm
PERITONEUM	Superficial	1	2	4
	Deep	2	4	6
OVARY	R Superficial	1	2	4
	Deep	4	16	20
	L Superficial	1	2	4
	Deep	4	16	20

POSTERIOR CULDESAC OBLITERATION	Partial	Complete
	4	40

	ADHESIONS	<1/3 Enclosure	1/3-2/3 Enclosure	>2/3 Enclosure
OVARY	R Filmy	1	2	4
	Dense	4	8	16
	L Filmy	1	2	4
	Dense	4	8	16
TUBE	R Filmy	1	2	4
	Dense	4*	8*	16
	L Filmy	1	2	4
	Dense	4*	8*	16

*If the fimbriated end of the fallopian tube is completely enclosed, change the point assignment to 16.

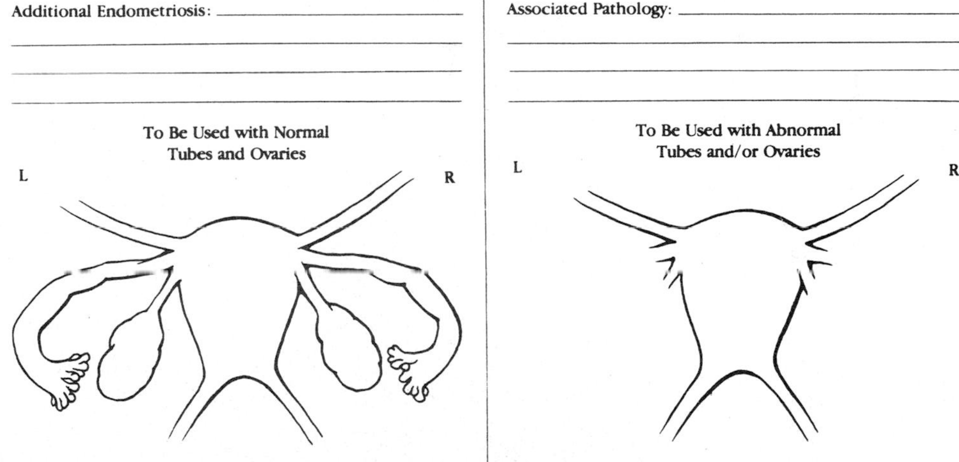

Figure 26.5 Revised American Fertility Society Classification, 1985. (From the America Fertility Society. Revised American Fertility Society classification of endometriosis. *Fertil Steril* 1985;43:351–235, with permission.)

This system reflects the extent of endometriotic disease but has considerable intraobserver and interobserver variability (195,196). Because the revised classification of endometriosis is the only internationally accepted system, it appears to be the best available tool to describe objectively the extent of endometriosis and relate it to spontaneous evolution and to therapeutic outcomes (pain relief, enhancement of fertility).

The classification system has also been criticized because several investigators failed to find a correlation between it and endometriosis-related pain or infertility, as will be reviewed in the section, Results of Surgical Treatment.

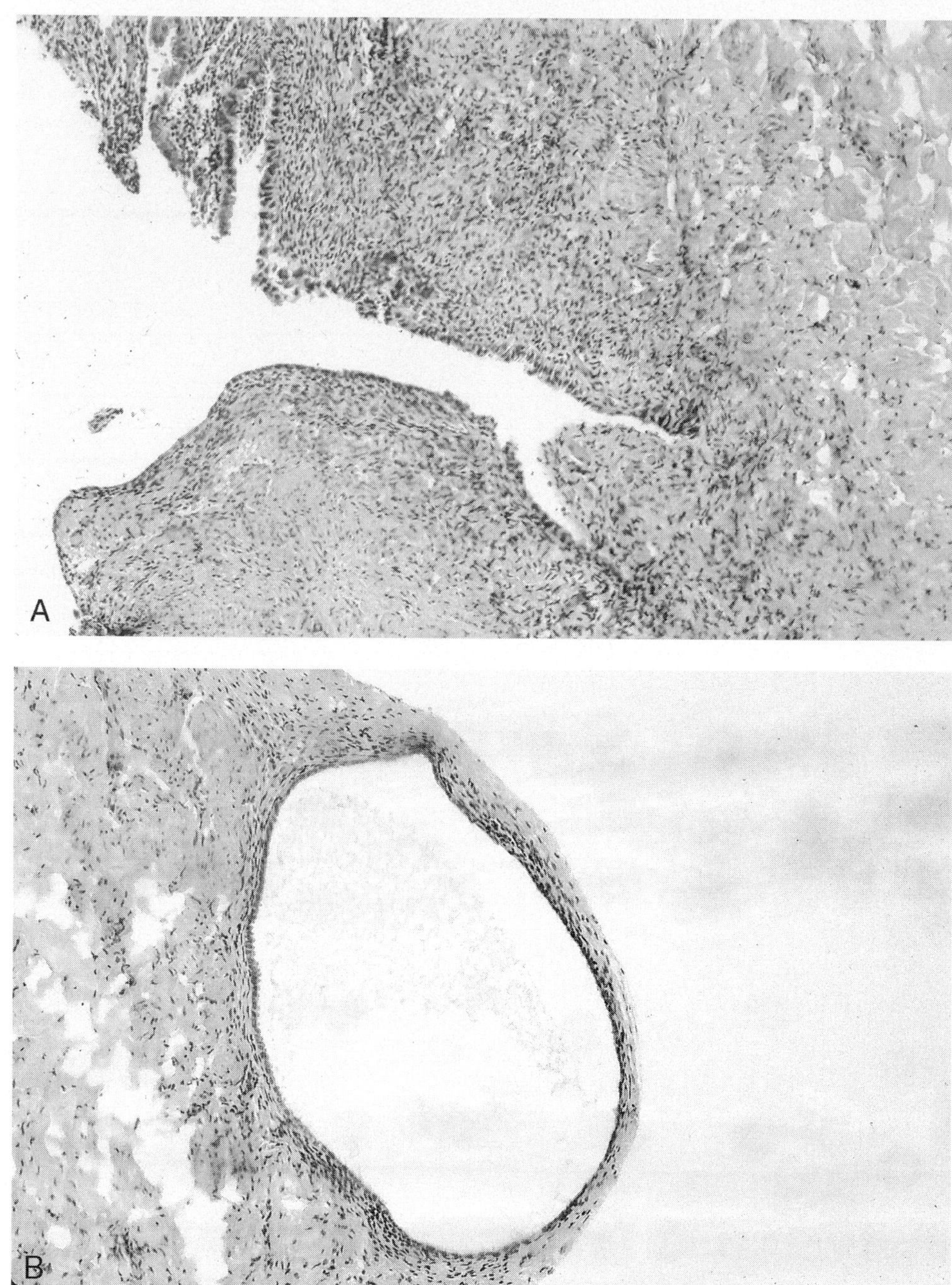

Figure 26.6 Histologic appearance of endometriosis: endometrial glandular epithelium, surrounded by stroma in (A) typical lesion and (B) clear vesicle.

Spontaneous Evolution

Endometriosis appears to be a progressive disease in a significant proportion (30% to 60%) of patients. During serial observations, deterioration (47%), improvement (30%), or elimination (23%) was documented over a 6-month period (197). In another study, endometriosis progressed in 64%, improved in 27%, and remained unchanged in 9% of patients over 12 months (198). A third study of 24 women reported 29% with disease progression, 29% with disease regression, and 42% with no change over 12 months. Follow-up studies in both baboons and women (200,201) with spontaneous endometriosis over 24 months have demonstrated disease progression in all baboons and in 6 of 7 women. Several studies have reported that subtle lesions and typical implants may represent younger and older types of endometriosis, respectively. In a cross-sectional study, the incidence of subtle lesions decreased with age (203). This was recently confirmed by a 3-year prospective study that reported that the incidence, overall pelvic area involved, and volume of subtle lesions decreased with age, but in typical lesions, these parameters and the depth of infiltration increased with age (100). Remodeling of endometriotic lesions (transition between typical and subtle subtypes) has been reported to occur in women and in baboons, indicating that endometriosis is a dynamic condition (202,204). Several studies in women, cynomolgus monkeys, and rodents have shown that endometriosis is ameliorated after pregnancy (204,205).

The characteristics of endometriosis are variable during pregnancy, and lesions tend to enlarge during the first trimester but regress thereafter (208). Studies in baboons have revealed no change in the number or surface area of endometriosis lesions during the first two trimesters of pregnancy (209). These results do not exclude a beneficial effect that potentially may occur during the third trimester or in the immediate postpartum period. Establishment of a "pseudopregnant state" with exogenously administered estrogen and progestins was based on the belief that symptomatic improvement may result from decidualization of endometrial implants during pregnancy (210). This hypothesis, however, has not been substantiated.

Treatment

Prevention

No strategies to prevent endometriosis have been uniformly successful. Although a reduced incidence of endometriosis has been reported in women who engaged in aerobic activity from an early age (16), the possible protective effect of exercise has not been investigated thoroughly. There also is insufficient evidence that oral contraceptive use offers protection against the development of endometriosis. In contrast, a recent report (211) showed an increased risk for endometriosis development in a select population of women taking oral contraceptives.

Regardless of the clinical profile (subfertility, pain, asymptomatic findings), treatment of endometriosis may be justified because endometriosis appears to progress in 30% to 60% of patients within a year of diagnosis and because it is not possible to predict in which patients it will progress (198). **Unfortunately, elimination of the endometriotic implants by surgical or medical treatment often provides only temporary relief. Therefore, the goal should be to eliminate the endometriotic lesions and, more importantly, to treat the sequelae (pain and subfertility) often associated with this disease.**

Surgical Treatment

In most women with endometriosis, preservation of reproductive function is desirable. Therefore, the least invasive and least expensive approach that is effective should be used. The goal of surgery is to excise or coagulate all visible endometriotic lesions and associated adhesions—peritoneal lesions, ovarian cysts, deep rectovaginal endometriosis—and to restore normal anatomy. Laparoscopy can be used in most women, and this technique decreases cost, morbidity, and the possibility of recurrence of adhesions postoperatively. **Laparotomy should be reserved for patients with advanced-stage disease who cannot undergo a laparoscopic procedure and for those in whom fertility conservation is not necessary.**

Peritoneal Endometriosis Endometriosis lesions can be removed during laparoscopy by surgical excision with scissors, bipolar coagulation, or laser methods (CO_2 laser, potassium-titany-phosphate laser, or argon laser). Although some surgeons claim that the CO_2 laser is superior because it causes only minimal thermal damage, no evidence is available to show that one technique is better than the other. Comparable cumulative pregnancy rates have been reported after treatment of mild endometriosis with laparoscopic excision and electrocoagulation (212).

Ovarian Endometriosis **Superficial ovarian lesions can be vaporized. Small ovarian endometrioma (<3 cm in diameter) can be aspirated, irrigated, and inspected with ovarian cystoscopy for intracystic lesions; their interior wall can be vaporized to destroy the mucosal lining of the cyst (213). Large (>3 cm in diameter) ovarian endometrioma should be aspirated, followed by incision and removal of the cyst wall from the ovarian cortex. To prevent recurrence, the cyst wall of the endometrioma must be removed, and normal ovarian tissue must be preserved.**

Although as little as one tenth of an ovary is enough to preserve function and fertility (214), there is increasing concern that ovarian cystectomy with concomitant removal or destruction of primordial follicles may reduce ovarian volume and reserve and diminish fertility. A recent study reported reduced follicular response in natural and clomiphene citrate-stimulated cycles, but not in gonadotropin-stimulated cycles, in women younger than 35 years of age who underwent cystectomy compared with controls of similar age with normal ovaries (215). Therefore, it has been proposed to replace cystectomy by fenestration and coagulation of the inner wall of the endometriotic ovarian cyst. In one study, cumulative clinical pregnancy rates and recurrence rates were comparable in women treated with cystectomy and with fenestration and coagulation after 36 months, but conception occurred more quickly in the fenestration and coagulation group (216). A more recent case-control study in 231 patients reported a lower cumulative reoperation rate in the cyst excision group than in the fenestration and coagulation group after 18 (6% versus 22%) and 42 (24% versus 59%) months of follow-up (217). A randomized controlled trial demonstrated that pain and subfertility caused by ovarian endometrioma were improved more by cystectomy than by fenestration and coagulation (218). A reduced recurrence of pain after 2 years [odds ratio (OR), 0.2; confidence interval (CI), 0.05 to 0.77], an increased pain-free interval after operation (19 months versus 9.5 months), and an increased pregnancy rate (67% versus 23%) were found in the cystectomy group when compared with the fenestration and coagulation group (218). Therefore, based on the current evidence, ovarian cystectomy appears to be the method of choice.

Adhesiolysis The removal of endometriosis-related adhesions (adhesiolysis) should be performed carefully as described in Chapter 21. Routine use of pharmacologic or liquid agents to prevent postoperative adhesions after fertility surgery cannot be recommended based on evidence from randomized controlled trials (219).

Preoperative Hormonal Treatment In patients with severe endometriosis, it has been recommended that surgical treatment be preceded by a 3-month course of medical treatment to reduce vascularization and nodular size (141). However, a recent randomized study comparing 3 months of preoperative treatment with GnRH and no treatment in 75 women with moderate to severe endometriosis failed to show a significant difference in ease of surgery between the two groups (220).

Deep Rectovaginal and Rectosigmoidal Endometriosis The surgical excision of deep rectovaginal and rectosigmoidal endometriosis is difficult and can be associated with major complications. Postoperative bowel perforations with peritonitis have been reported in 2% to 3% of cases (221).

Preoperative investigations, including gynecologic ultrasound, intravenous pyelography (to exclude ureteral endometriosis), and colon contrast radiography (to exclude transmural rectosigmoidal endometriosis), are essential. Preoperative laxatives, starch-free diet, and full bowel preparation are needed to allow perioperative bowel suturing, if needed. To allow complete excision of rectovaginal endometriosis, 6% of patients needed bowel wall resection, and 14% required partial resection of the posterior vaginal fornix (221). Segmental rectosigmoid resection can be performed by laparotomy, laparoscopy with intracorporeal suturing, or by laparoscopically assisted vaginal technique (222). The latter technique appears to be faster than laparoscopy with intracorporeal suturing and cheaper than laparotomy because of decreased hospital stay and lower operating room charges (222). Ureter stents may be required before excision of peritoneal endometriosis surrounding the ureter. A multidisciplinary approach involving gynecologic and gastroenterologic surgeons and urologists is desirable.

Oophorectomy and Hysterectomy Radical procedures such as oophorectomy or total hysterectomy are indicated only in severe situations and can be performed either laparoscopically or, more commonly, by laparotomy. However, it is important to note that women aged 30 years or younger at the time of hysterectomy for endometriosis-associated pain are more likely than older women to have residual symptoms, to report a sense of loss, and to report more disruption from pain in different aspects of their lives (223).

Postoperative Hormone Replacement Postoperative hormone replacement with estrogen is required after bilateral oophorectomy, and there is a negligible risk for renewed growth of residual endometriosis. To reduce this risk, hormone replacement therapy should be withheld until 3 months after surgery. The addition of progestins to this regimen protects the endometrium. Some cases of adenocarcinoma have been reported, presumably arising from endometriosis lesions left in women treated with unopposed estrogen (214).

Results of Surgical Treatment

Pain

The outcome of surgical therapy in patients with endometriosis and pain is influenced by many psychological factors relating to personality, depression, and marital and sexual problems. **There is a significant placebo response to surgical therapy: diagnostic laparoscopy without complete removal of endometriosis may alleviate pain in 50% of patients** (224–226). Similar results have been reported using oral placebos (227). Although some reports have claimed pain relief with laser laparoscopy in 60% to 80% of patients with very low morbidity, none was prospective or controlled and, thus, did not allow a definitive conclusion regarding treatment efficacy (141,228–231).

Endometriosis Stage and Pain Relief after Surgery **In patients with pain, the endometriosis stage was not related to pain symptoms in several studies** (232,233). **However, more recent studies reported a positive correlation between endometriosis stage and endometriosis-related dysmenorrhea or chronic pelvic pain** (234,235).

In a prospective, controlled, randomized, double-blind study, surgical therapy has been shown to be superior to expectant management 6 months after treatment of mild and moderate endometriosis (224). In women with mild and moderate disease treated with laser, 74% achieved pain relief. Treatment was least effective in women with minimal disease. There were no reported operative or laser complications (224). One year later, symptom relief was still present in 90% of those who initially responded (199). Patients with severe disease were not included because it had previously been shown that surgery resulted in pain relief in 80% of patients who did not respond to medical therapy (236).

These results suggest that laser laparoscopy may be effective for the treatment of pain associated with mild to severe endometriosis. In women with minimal endometriosis, laser treatment may limit progression of disease.

Effects of Postoperative Hormonal Treatment on Pain **Substantial evidence from randomized controlled trials supports the postoperative medical treatment of endometriosis-associated pain for 6 to 12 months.** Postoperative GnRH treatment resulted in reduced pain scores and in a delay of pain recurrence for more than 12 months if the agonists were given for 6 months but not if they were only administered for 3 months (237–239). Similarly, postoperative hormonal treatment with *danazol,* 100 mg/d (low dose), for 12 months after surgery for moderate to severe endometriosis resulted in a significantly lower pain score in the treated group when compared with the placebo group. In contrast, postoperative high-dose *danazol,* 600 mg/d for 3 months, was not superior to expectant management with respect to pain recurrence in an identical patient population (240).

Subfertility

Endometriosis Stage and Pregnancy Outcome after Surgery When endometriosis causes mechanical distortion of the pelvis, surgery should be performed if reconstruction of normal pelvic anatomy can be achieved. The success of surgery in relieving infertility is probably related to the severity of endometriosis. A recent retrospective multicenter analysis (241) reported cumulative pregnancy rates of 39%, 31%, 30%, and 25% in patients with endometriosis stages I, II, III, and IV, respectively, 12 months after surgical treatment. Although there appeared to be a negative correlation between stage of endometriosis and fertility outcome, no significant difference was found between the four groups in this study. However, the study had many limitations, including retrospective design, lack of well-defined definition of male factor infertility as potential bias, multicenter data with significant interobserver variability, inclusion of only a limited number of patients with substantial adhesive disease, variable infertility treatment after 6 months of follow-up, and absence of a control group. A somewhat higher cumulative intrauterine pregnancy rate has been reported in 30 women with deep uterosacral endometriosis after surgery: 48% after 12 months (47% for AFS stages I to II and 46% for AFS stages III to IV) (242). A cumulative pregnancy rate of 24% was reported in patients 9 months after undergoing reoperation for stage III to IV endometriosis (243).

Other investigators reported a negative correlation between stage of endometriosis and fertility after surgical treatment. In an older study, using an older classification system, a significant decrease in fecundability was seen in women with severe or extensive endometriosis compared with women with mild or moderate disease (244,245). Other studies have reported a significant negative correlation between endometriosis stage and pregnancy rate and decreased pregnancy rates when the revised scores exceeded 70 (246,247).

Preoperative and Postoperative Medical Treatment Preoperative medical treatment with danazol, GnRH agonists, or progestins may be useful to reduce the extent of endometriosis in patients with advanced disease. Postoperative medical treatment is rarely indicated because it does not work based on randomized trials, because it prevents pregnancy, and because the highest pregnancy rates occur during the first 6 to 12 months after conservative surgery (238,239). If pregnancy does not occur within 2 years of surgery, there is little chance of subsequent fertility (248).

Minimal to Mild Endometriosis and Fertility after Surgery Surgical management of infertile women with minimal to mild endometriosis is controversial. The cumulative pregnancy rate after 5 years without therapy has been reported to be as high as 90% in women with minimal or mild endometriosis (249). This is comparable to the 93% rate reported in women who do not have endometriosis. Laparoscopic destruction of endometriosis has been reported to improve fertility in patients with minimal to mild disease (250–252), but not all investigators share this conclusion (253–255). It has been hypothesized that the MFR is higher during the first 6 to 12 months after laparoscopic surgery than with expectant management (256,257).

Two randomized controlled studies have evaluated the effect of surgical treatment of endometriosis on fertility parameters (133,134). Marcoux and coworkers (133) reported that laparoscopic surgery enhanced fecundity in infertile women with minimal or mild endometriosis. They studied 341 infertile women, 20 to 39 years of age, with minimal or mild endometriosis. During diagnostic laparoscopy, the women were randomly assigned to undergo resection or ablation of visible endometriosis or diagnostic laparoscopy only. They were followed for 36 weeks after the laparoscopy or, for those who became pregnant during that interval, for up to 20 weeks of pregnancy. The study objects were recruited among infertile women scheduled for diagnostic laparoscopy with strict eligibility criteria. There was no previous surgical treatment for endometriosis and no medical treatment for endometriosis in the previous 9 months. There was no other medical or surgical treatment for infertility in the previous 3 months. They had no history of pelvic inflammatory disease and no severe pelvic pain precluding expectant management. The diagnosis of endometriosis required the presence of one or more typical bluish or black lesions. The stage of endometriosis was determined according to the revised AFS classification. During the diagnostic laparoscopy, the women were randomly assigned to undergo resection or ablation of visible endometriosis or diagnostic laparoscopy only. They found that resection or ablation of minimal and mild endometriosis increased the likelihood of pregnancy in infertile women. In the treated group, 31% of the patients became pregnant, compared with 18% in the nontreated group ($p = 0.006$).

In a multicenter Italian study, a similar study design was used to compare the effect of diagnostic laparoscopy with surgical resection and ablation of visible endometriosis (on fertility parameters) in infertile women with minimal to mild endometriosis (134). Eligible patients were women aged less than 36 years who were trying to conceive and had a laparoscopically confirmed diagnosis of minimal or mild endometriosis, according to the revised AFS classification system. None of the women had had therapy for endometriosis or infertility. Treatment was randomly allocated during laparoscopy. There was a follow-up period of 1 year after the laparoscopy. The results of this study did not show a beneficial effect of surgery regarding fertility. During the follow-up period after laparoscopy, no statistically significant differences in conception and live-birth rates were observed in the treated group (24% and 20%, respectively) and in the control group (29% and 22%, respectively).

Based on these studies, and taking into account the larger patient population in the Canadian multicenter study, **surgical treatment of minimal to mild endometriosis appears to offer a small but significant benefit with regard to fertility outcome.** Furthermore, the surgical removal of peritoneal endometriosis may also be important to prevent progression of endometriosis. However, care is needed to prevent adhesion formation that could result as a consequence of overenthusiastic excision of minimal to mild endometriosis.

Medical Treatment

Because estrogen is known to stimulate the growth of endometriosis, hormonal therapy has been designed to suppress estrogen synthesis, thereby inducing atrophy of ectopic endometrial implants or interrupting the cycle of stimulation and bleeding. Implants of endometriosis react to gonadal steroid hormones in a manner similar but not identical to normally stimulated ectopic endometrium. Ectopic endometrial tissue displays histologic and biochemical differences from normal ectopic endometrium in characteristics such as glandular activity (proliferation, secretion), enzyme activity (17β-hydroxysteroid dehydrogenase), and steroid (estrogen, progestin, and androgen) hormone receptor levels. The use of *diethylstilbestrol, methyltestosterone,* or other androgens is no longer advocated because they lack efficacy, have significant side effects, and pose risks to the fetus if pregnancy occurs during therapy. A new generation of aromatase inhibitors, estrogen receptor modulators, and progesterone antagonists may offer new hormonal treatment options in the future. Recent progress in the understanding of the pathogenesis of endometriosis has led to the expectation that new pharmaceutical agents affecting inflammation, angiogenesis, and MMP activity may prevent or inhibit the development of endometriosis.

Oral Contraceptives

Continuous Administration Manipulation of the endogenous hormonal milieu is the basis for the medical management of endometriosis. The treatment of endometriosis with continuous low-dose monophasic combination contraceptives (one pill per day for 6 to 12 months) was originally used to induce pseudopregnancy caused by the resultant amenorrhea and decidualization of endometrial tissue (210). Kistner was the first to introduce the concept of an adynamic endometrium through elimination of the normal cyclic hormonal changes characteristic of the menstrual cycle (258). This induction of a pseudopregnancy state with combination oral contraceptive pills has been shown to be effective in reducing dysmenorrhea and pelvic pain. In addition, the subsequent amenorrhea induced by oral contraceptives could potentially reduce the amount of retrograde menstruation (one of the many risk factors proposed in the etiology of endometriosis), decreasing the risk for disease progression. Pathologically, oral contraceptive use is associated with decidualization of endometrial tissue, necrobiosis, and possibly absorption of the endometrial tissue (259). Unfortunately, there is no convincing evidence that medical therapy with oral contraceptives offers definitive therapy. Instead, the endometrial implants survive the induced atrophy and, in most patients, reactivate after termination of treatment.

Any low-dose combination oral contraceptive containing 30 to 35 mg of ethinyl estradiol used continuously can be effective in the management of endometriosis. The objective of the treatment is the induction of amenorrhea, which should be continued for 6 to 12 months. Symptomatic relief of dysmenorrhea and pelvic pain is reported in 60% to 95% of patients (260,261). After a first-year recurrence rate of 17% to 18%, a 5% to 10% annual recurrence rate has been observed. In addition, a posttreatment pregnancy rate of up to 50% can be expected. Although oral contraceptives are effective in inducing a decidualized endometrium, the estrogenic component in oral contraceptives may potentially stimulate endometrial growth and increase pelvic pain in the first few weeks of treatment. The long-term significance of this effect remains to be determined. Oral contraceptives are less costly than other treatments and may be helpful in the short-term management of endometriosis with potential long-term benefits in some women.

Cyclic Administration There is no convincing evidence that cyclic use of combination oral contraceptives provides prophylaxis against either the development or recurrence of endometriosis. Estrogens in oral contraceptives potentially may stimulate the proliferation of endometriosis. The reduced menstrual bleeding that often occurs in women taking oral contraceptives may be beneficial to women with prolonged, frequent menstrual bleeding, which is a known risk factor for endometriosis (16). Further research is warranted to assess the effect of low-dose oral contraceptives in preventing endometriosis and in treating associated pain. In a recent randomized controlled study, a cyclic 2-day oral contraceptive (*ethinyl estradiol* 20 gamma + *desogestrel* 0.15 mg) combined with very-low-dose danazol (50 mg/d) was less effective in relief of dysmenorrhea than depot *medroxyprogesterone* acetate (150 mg every 3 months) (262).

Progestins

Progestins may exert an antiendometriotic effect by causing initial decidualization of endometrial tissue followed by atrophy. They can be considered as the first choice for the treatment of endometriosis because they are as effective as *danazol* or GnRH analogues and have a lower cost and a lower incidence of side effects than these agents (263).

There is no evidence that any single agent or any particular dose is preferable to another. The effective doses of several progestins are summarized in Table 26.1. In most studies, the effect of treatment has been evaluated after 3 to 6 months of therapy. *MPA* has been the most studied agent. It is effective in relieving pain starting at a dose of 30 mg/d and increasing the dose based on the clinical response and bleeding patterns (264,265). However, a recent randomized placebo controlled study reported a significant reduction in stages and scores of endometriosis in both the placebo group and the group treated with *MPA,* 50 mg/d, and placebo at laparoscopy within 3 months after cessation of therapy (266). These findings raise questions about the need for medical therapy.

Medroxyprogesterone acetate (150 mg) given intramuscularly every 3 months is also effective for the treatment of pain associated with endometriosis, but it is not indicated in infertile women because it induces profound amenorrhea and anovulation, and a varying

Table 26.1. Medical Treatment of Endometriosis-Associated Pain: Effective Regimens (Usual Duration: 6 Months)

	Administration	*Dose*	*Frequency*
Progestogens			
Medroxyprogesterone acetate	PO	30 mg	Daily
Megestrol acetate	PO	40 mg	Daily
Lynoestrenol	PO	10 mg	Daily
Dydrogesterone	PO	20–30 mg	Daily
Antiprogestins			
Gestrinone	PO	1.25 or 2.5 mg	Twice weekly
Danazol	PO	400 mg	Daily
Gonodotropin-Releasing Hormone			
Leuprolide	SC	500 mg	Daily
	IM	3.75 mg	Monthly
Goserelin	SC	3.6 mg	Monthly
Buserelin	IN	300 μg	Daily
	SC	200 μg	Daily
Nafarelin	IN	200 μg	Daily
Triptorelin	IM	3.75 mg	Monthly

PO, oral; SC, subcutaneous; IM, intramuscular; IN, intranasal.

length of time is required for ovulation to resume after discontinuation of therapy. *Megestrol acetate* has been administered in a dose of 40 mg/d with good results (276). Other treatment strategies have included *dydrogesterone* (20 to 30 mg/d, either continuously or on days 5 to 25) and *lynestrenol* (10 mg/d). The effectiveness of natural progesterone has not been evaluated.

Side effects of progestins include nausea, weight gain, fluid retention, and breakthrough bleeding due to hypoestrogenemia. Breakthrough bleeding, although common, is usually corrected by short-term (7-day) administration of estrogen. Depression and other mood disorders are a significant problem in about 1% of women taking these medications.

Local progesterone treatment of endometriosis-associated dysmenorrhea with a *levonorgestrel*-releasing intrauterine system for 12 months has resulted in a significant reduction in dysmenorrhea, pelvic pain, and dyspareunia; a high degree of patient satisfaction; and a significant reduction in the volume of rectovaginal endometriotic nodules (267,268). Although the results are promising, none of these pilot studies included a control group. Further randomized evidence is needed to determine whether intrauterine progesterone treatment is effective in the suppression of endometriosis.

Progesterone Antagonists

Progesterone antagonists and progesterone receptor modulators may suppress endometriosis based on their antiproliferative effects on the endometrium, without the risk for hypoestrogenism or bone loss that occurs with GnRH treatment. These products are soon to be introduced in the United States, but their clinical effectiveness remains to be proved.

Mifepristone Mifepristone (RU-486) is a potent antiprogestagen with a direct inhibitory effect on human endometrial cells and, in high doses, an antiglucocorticoid action (269). The recommended dose for endometriosis is 25 to 100 mg/d. In uncontrolled studies, *mifepristone,* 50 to 100 mg/d, reduced pelvic pain and induced 55% regression of the lesions without significant side effects (270,271). In an uncontrolled pilot study, *mifepristone,* 5 mg/d, resulted in pain improvement, but there was no change in endometriosis lesions, suggesting that this dosage is probably too low (272).

Onapristone Progesterone antagonists *onapristone* (*ZK98299*) and *ZK136799,* used in the treatment of rats with surgically induced endometriosis, resulted in a remission in 40% to 60% of treated animals. In animals with persistent endometriosis, growth inhibition was obtained in 48% and 85% of endometriotic lesions after therapy with *onapristone* and *ZK136799*, respectively (273).

Other Progesterone Antagonists The chemical synthesis and pharmacologic characterization of a highly potent progesterone antagonist, *ZK230211*, have been reported, with little or no other endocrinologic effects. *ZK230211* is active on both progesterone receptors A and B (274). In primates, this drug has been reported to block ovulation and menstruation at all effective doses (275), whereas another progesterone antagonist, *ZK137316*, allowed ovulation but blocked menstruation in a dose-dependent fashion. All progesterone antagonist–treated animals maintained normal follicular phase concentration of estradiol and returned to menstrual cyclicity within 15 to 41 days after treatment (275). Both progesterone antagonists block unopposed estrogen action on the endometriosis through their antiproliferative effect.

Gestrinone

Gestrinone is a 19-nortestosterone derivative with androgenic, antiprogestagenic, antiestrogenic, and antigonadotropic properties. It acts centrally and peripherally to increase free testosterone and reduce sex hormone–binding globulin levels (androgenic effect), reduce serum estradiol values to early follicular phase levels (antiestrogenic effect), reduce mean LH levels, and obliterate the LH and follicle-stimulating hormone (FSH) surge (antigonadotropic effect). *Gestrinone* causes cellular inactivation and degeneration of endometriotic implants but not their disappearance (277). Amenorrhea occurs in 50% to 100% of women and is dose dependent.

Resumption of menses generally occurs 33 days after discontinuing the medication (278,279). An advantage of gestrinone is its long half-life (28 hours) when given orally. The standard dose has been 2.5 mg twice a week. Although it has been reported that 1.25 mg twice weekly is equally effective (280), a more recent randomized study demonstrated in women with mild to moderate endometriosis that 2.5 mg *gestrinone,* twice weekly for 24 weeks, is more effective and has a better effect on bone mass (+7% versus −7%) when compared with 1.25 mg *gestrinone,* 2 times weekly for 24 weeks (281).

The clinical side effects of gestrinone are dose dependent and similar to but less intense than those caused by *danazol* (278). They include nausea, muscle cramps, and androgenic effects such as weight gain, acne, seborrhea, and oily hair and skin.

In a multicenter, randomized, double-blind study, *gestrinone* was as effective as GnRH for the treatment of pelvic pain associated with endometriosis (282). However, *gestrinone* has fewer side effects and has the added advantage of twice-weekly administration. Pregnancy is contraindicated while taking gestrinone because of the risk for masculinization of the fetus.

Danazol

Danazol is not more effective than other available medications to treat endometriosis. Recognized pharmacologic properties of *danazol* include suppression of GnRH or gonadotropin secretion, direct inhibition of steroidogenesis, increased metabolic clearance of estradiol and progesterone, direct antagonistic and agonistic interaction with endometrial androgen and progesterone receptors, and immunologic attenuation of potentially adverse reproductive effects (283,284). The multiple effects of *danazol* produce a high-androgen, low-estrogen environment (estrogen levels in the early follicular to postmenopausal range) that does not support the growth of endometriosis, and the amenorrhea that is produced prevents new seeding of implants from the uterus into the peritoneal cavity.

The immunologic effects of danazol have been studied in women with endometriosis and adenomyosis and include a decrease in serum immunoglobulins, a decrease in serum C3, a rise in serum C4 levels, decreased serum levels of autoantibodies against various phospholipid antigens, and decreased serum levels of CA125 during treatment

(152,153,165–168,285,286). *Danazol* inhibits peripheral blood lymphocyte proliferation in cultures activated by T-cell mitogens but does not affect macrophage-dependent T-lymphocyte activation of B lymphocytes (284). *Danazol* inhibits interleukin-1 and TNF production by monocytes in a dose-dependent manner, and suppresses macrophage- and monocyte-mediated cytotoxicity of susceptible target cells in women with mild endometriosis (287). These immunologic findings may be important in the remission of endometriosis with danazol treatment and may offer an explanation of the effect of *danazol* in the treatment of a number of autoimmune diseases, including hereditary angioedema (289), autoimmune hemolytic anemia (290), systemic lupus erythematosus (291), and idiopathic thrombocytopenic purpura (292,293). Doses of 800 mg/d are frequently used in North America, whereas 600 mg/d is commonly prescribed in Europe and Australia. It appears that the absence of menstruation is a better indicator of response than drug dose. A practical strategy for the use of *danazol* is to start treatment with 400 mg daily (200 mg twice a day) and increase the dose, if necessary, to achieve amenorrhea and relieve symptoms (279).

The significant adverse side effects of *danazol* are related to its androgenic and hypoestrogenic properties. The most common side effects include weight gain, fluid retention, acne, oily skin, hirsutism, hot flashes, atrophic vaginitis, reduced breast size, reduced libido, fatigue, nausea, muscle cramps, and emotional instability. Deepening of the voice is another potential side effect that is nonreversible. Although *danazol* can cause increased cholesterol and low-density lipoprotein levels and decreased high-density lipoproteins levels, it is unlikely that these short-term effects are clinically important. *Danazol* is contraindicated in patients with liver disease because it is largely metabolized in the liver and may cause hepatocellular damage. *Danazol* is also contraindicated in patients with hypertension, congestive heart failure, or impaired renal function because it can cause fluid retention. The use of danazol is contraindicated in pregnancy because of its androgenic effects on the fetus.

Because the many side effects of oral *danazol* limit its use, alternative routes of administration have been studied. In an uncontrolled pilot study, local *danazol* treatment using a vaginal *danazol* ring (1,500 mg) has been shown to be effective for pain relief in deeply infiltrative endometriosis without the classic *danazol* side effects, or detectable serum *danazol* levels, while allowing ovulation and conception (294).

Gonadotropin-releasing Hormone Agonists

GnRH agonists bind to pituitary GnRH receptors and stimulate LH and FSH synthesis and release. However, the agonists have a much longer biologic half-life (3 to 8 hours) than endogenous GnRH (3.5 minutes), resulting in the continuous exposure of GnRH receptors to GnRH agonist activity. This causes a loss of pituitary receptors and downregulation of GnRH activity, resulting in low FSH and LH levels. Consequently, ovarian steroid production is suppressed, providing a medically induced and reversible state of pseudomenopause. A direct effect of GnRH agonists on ectopic endometrium is also possible because expression of the GnRH receptor gene has been documented in ectopic endometrium and because direct inhibition of endometriosis cells has been demonstrated *in vitro* (295). Furthermore, in rat models for surgical adhesion formation and endometriosis, GnRH agonist therapy decreased activity of plasminogen activators and matrix MMPs and increased the activity of their inhibitors, suggesting potential GnRH agonist–regulated mechanisms for reducing adhesion formation (296).

Various GnRH agonists have been developed and used in treating endometriosis. These agents include *leuprolide, buserelin, nafarelin, histrelin, goserelin, deslorelin,* and *triptorelin*. These drugs are inactive orally and must be administered intramuscularly, subcutaneously, or by intranasal absorption. The best therapeutic effect is often associated with an *estradiol* dose of 20 to 40 pg/mL (75 to 150 pmol/L). These so-called depot formulations are attractive because of the reduced frequency of administration and because nasal administration can be complicated by variations in absorption rates and problems with patient compliance (279). The results with GnRH agonists are similar to those with *danazol* or progestin therapy.

Although GnRH agonists do not have an adverse effect on serum lipids and lipoproteins, their side effects are caused by hypoestrogenism and include hot flashes, vaginal dryness, reduced libido, and osteoporosis (6% to 8% loss in trabecular bone density after 6 months of therapy). Reversibility of bone loss is equivocal and therefore of concern (297,298), especially because treatment periods of longer than 6 months may be required. The goal is to suppress endometriosis and maintain serum estrogen levels of 30 to 45 pg/mL. More extreme estradiol suppression will induce bone loss (297). The dose of daily GnRH agonist can be regulated by monitoring estradiol levels, by the addition of low-dose progestin or estrogen-progestin in an add-back regimen, or by draw-back therapy. The goal of add-back therapy is to treat endometriosis and endometriosis-associated pain effectively, while preventing vasomotor symptoms and bone loss related to the hypoestrogenic state induced by GnRH analogues. Add-back therapy can be achieved by administering progestogens only, including *norethisterone,* 1.2 mg, and *norethindrone acetate,* 5 mg, but bone loss is not prevented by *medrogestone,* 10 mg/d (298–300). Add-back therapy can also be achieved by tibolone, 2.5 mg/d (301,302), or by an estrogen-progestin combination (i.e., conjugated estrogens, 0.625 mg, combined with *medroxyprogesterone acetate,* 2.5 mg, or with *norethindrone acetate,* 5 mg, estradiol, 2 mg, and *norethisterone acetate,* 1 mg) (299–303). However, some concern remains about the long-term effects of GnRH analogues on bone loss. In one report, bone mineral density reduction occurred during long-term GnRH agonist use and was not fully recovered up to 6 years after treatment (304). Use of add-back therapy (2 mg *estradiol* and 1 mg *norethisterone acetate*) did not affect this process (304).

Draw-back therapy has recently been suggested as an alternative in a study showing that 6 months of intake of 400 μg/d of *nafarelin* was as effective as a draw-back regimen consisting of 1 month of intake of 400 μg/d of *nafarelin* followed by 5 months of 200 μg/d of *nafarelin,* with similar estradiol levels (30 pg/mL) but less loss of bone mineral density (305).

Aromatase Inhibitors

Treatment of rats with induced endometriosis using the nonsteroidal aromatase inhibitor *fadrozole hydrochloride* (306) or YM511 (307) resulted in a dose-dependent volume reduction of endometriosis transplants, but these products have so far not been used in published human studies. Treatment of severe postmenopausal endometriosis with an aromatase inhibitor, *anastrozole,* 1 mg/d, and elemental *calcium,* 1.5 g/d for 9 months, resulted in hypoestrogenism, pain relief after 2 months, and after 9 months a 10-fold reduction in the 30-mm diameter size of red, polypoid vaginal lesions, along with remodeling to gray tissue. No other data are available, except this case report (308).

Selective Estrogen Receptor Modulators

Raloxifen In animal models, *raloxifene* therapy resulted in regression of endometriosis. The effect was seen in both a surgically prepared, rat uterine explant model and in Rhesus macaques diagnosed with spontaneous endometriosis before exposure (309).

Nonhormonal Medical Therapy

Modulation of Cytokines In rats with experimental endometriosis, recombinant human TNF-α–binding protein can reduce 64% of the size of endometriosis-like peritoneal lesions (310). Similarly, a recent prospective randomized placebo- and drug-controlled study in baboons showed that recombinant human TNF-α–binding protein effectively inhibits the development of endometriosis and endometriosis-related adhesions (311).

In mice with experimental endometriosis, a placebo-controlled double-blind study showed that intraperitoneal or subcutaneous injection of recombinant interferon-α2B resulted in smaller endometriotic lesions when compared with the placebo control group (312). In rats with experimental endometriosis, regression of endometrial explants was observed after treatment with immune-enhancing modulators *loxoribine* and *levamisole* (313).

Antiinflammation In the future, leukotriene receptor antagonists could be of use in patients with endometriosis who do not respond to prostaglandin synthetase inhibitors (314).

In humans, a randomized placebo-controlled trial of oral *pentoxifylline,* 800 mg/d for 12 months, reported after life-table analysis a similar overall pregnancy rate in treated patients (31%) and in controls (18.5%) (315).

Inhibition of Matrix Metalloproteinase In nude mice, suppression of MMPs by progesterone or by a natural inhibitor slows the establishment of ectopic lesions by human endometrium (316). Thus far, no clinical reports have been published.

Efficacy of Medical Treatment

Pain Medical treatment with progestins, *danazol, gestrinone,* or GnRH agonists is effective in treating pain associated with endometriosis, as shown in several prospective, randomized, placebo-controlled double-blind studies (197,226,317,318). Based on published studies, *medroxyprogesterone acetate, danazol, gestrinone,* and GnRH agonists have similar efficacy in resolution of the laparoscopically documented disease and in pain alleviation (278). Postoperative medical therapy may be required in patients with incomplete surgical resection and persistent pain. Treatment should last at least 3 to 6 months, and pain relief may be of short duration, presumably because endometriosis recurs. Disadvantages of medical therapy over surgical therapy include the high cost of hormone preparations, the high prevalence of side effects, and the higher recurrence rate of endometriosis.

Subfertility Conception is either impossible or contraindicated during medical treatment of endometriosis. There is no evidence that medical treatment of minimal to mild endometriosis leads to better chances of pregnancy than expectant management (197,249, 317–323).

Adolescent Endometriosis The incidental finding of minimal to mild endometriosis in a young woman without immediate interest in pregnancy is a common clinical problem. Seventy percent of girls with chronic pelvic pain unresponsive to oral contraceptives (OAC) or nonsteroidal antiinflammatory drugs are affected by endometriosis (324). Mild disease can be treated by surgical removal of implants at the time of diagnosis, followed by administration of continuous low-dose combination oral contraceptives to prevent recurrence. More advanced disease can be treated medically for 6 months, followed by continuous oral contraceptives to prevent progression of disease. GnRH agonists with add-back therapy can be considered for adolescents older than 16 years of age who have completed pubertal maturation (324).

Recurrence

Endometriosis tends to recur unless definitive surgery is performed. The recurrence rate is about 5% to 20% per year, reaching a cumulative rate of 40% after 5 years. The rate of recurrence increases with the stage of disease, the duration of follow-up, and the occurrence of previous surgery (325–329). The likelihood of recurrence appears to be lower when endometriosis is located only on the right side of the pelvis than when the left side is involved (330).

In a recent randomized controlled trial, postoperative low-dose cyclic oral contraceptive use resulted in a significantly lower cumulative recurrence rate after 1 year, but not after 2 to 3 years (331). In women treated with a second operation for recurrent endometriosis, the cumulative recurrence rate was comparable to those rates after laparoscopy or laparotomy (332).

The recurrence rates reported in women 5 years after therapy with various GnRH agonists were 37% for minimal disease and 74% for severe disease (325). In women treated with GnRH agonists or *danazol* for endometriosis associated with pelvic pain, the recurrence rates of endometriosis were similar, and associated pain symptoms usually returned after cessation of therapy (333). Pain recurs within 5 years in about one in five patients with pelvic pain treated by complete laparoscopic excision of visible endometriotic lesions (334).

Assisted Reproduction and Endometriosis

The treatment of endometriosis-related infertility is dependent on the age of the woman, the duration of infertility, the stage of endometriosis, the involvement of ovaries, tubes, or both in the endometriosis process, previous therapy, associated pain symptoms, and the priorities of the patient, taking into account her attitude toward the disease, the cost of treatment, her financial means, and the expected results. Assisted reproduction, including controlled ovarian hyperstimulation with intrauterine insemination, IVF, and gamete intrafallopian transfer, may be options for infertility treatment in addition to surgical reconstruction and expectant management. IVF is the method of choice when distortion of the tuboovarian anatomy contraindicates the use of superovulation with intrauterine insemination or gamete intrafallopian transfer.

Intrauterine Insemination

Endometriosis-associated infertility can be successfully treated with intrauterine insemination. A recent randomized study (335) compared controlled ovarian hyperstimulation with FSH and intrauterine insemination with no treatment during 311 cycles in 103 couples with minimal to mild endometriosis as the only infertility factor. This study reported a significantly higher live-birth rate per cycle in the treated group (11%) than in the control group (2%) (OR, 5.6; 95% CI, 1.8 to 17.4). However, there is clear evidence that the pregnancy rate in an insemination program is lower in women with endometriosis than in women with unexplained infertility (336,337). In a recent metaanalysis of 5,214 cycles by stepwise logistic regression (338), evaluating the effectiveness of ovulation induction and intrauterine insemination in the treatment of persistent infertility, the OR for pregnancy associated with endometriosis was 0.45 (95% CI, 0.27 to 0.76) and for male factor was 0.48 (95% CI, 0.37 to 0.61).

In Vitro Fertilization

Based on several retrospective studies, several investigators (130,135) have suggested that the pregnancy rate after IVF may be lower in women with endometriosis than in women without the disease. In earlier studies, this had been ascribed to a reduced oocyte quality and decreased fertilization rate in women with endometriosis. However, these findings were not confirmed in more recent studies that reported a normal fertilization rate but a reduced implantation rate per embryo transferred also in women obtaining oocytes from oocyte donors with endometriosis (339,340). This reduced implantation rate could possibly be related to increased interleukin-6 levels in follicular fluid of women with endometriosis when compared with controls (341). However, in a more recent case-control study in an IVF egg-donation program comparing oocyte receptors in patients with endometriosis stage III or IV (cases) with oocyte receptors in patients without endometriosis (controls), a similar implantation rate, miscarriage rate, and pregnancy rate was observed in cases and controls, suggesting that there is no endometrial implantation problem in women with endometriosis stage III or IV treated with IVF (342). In another case-control study, the cumulative pregnancy rate and live-birth rate was comparable after five cycles of IVF in women with ovarian endometriosis and those with tubal infertility: 63% versus 63% (CPR) and 47% versus 51% (CLBR), but women with ovarian endometriosis had poorer responses and needed higher gonadotropin therapy (343).

When endometriosis was assigned a stage, the pregnancy rate after IVF was decreased in patients with stage IV endometriosis but normal in women with less advanced disease (344–350). However, some studies have been unable to demonstrate a significant negative correlation between either the presence or stage of endometriosis and the pregnancy rate per cycle (351,352). The use of *danazol, gestrinone,* or GnRH agonists in women with endometriosis before IVF has been reported to improve the pregnancy rate by some (350,354) but not all investigators (352).

Intracytoplasmic Sperm Injection

A recent well-controlled study in intracytoplasmic sperm injection (ICSI) patients (353) reported a reduced number of oocytes recovered after ovarian aspiration but a normal fertilization rate, implantation rate, and pregnancy rate in women with endometriosis when compared with controls. These normal fertilization, implantation, and pregnancy rates also were reported in another recent ICSI study (355).

Gamete Intrafallopian Transfer

The use of gamete intrafallopian transfer in patients with endometriosis is reported to result in a higher monthly fecundity rate (25%) than with IVF (14%), but this difference may be related to selection bias because less severe forms of endometriosis may have been more likely to be treated with gamete intrafallopian transfer, reserving IVF for more advanced stages of disease (257). In one study, the gamete intrafallopian transfer pregnancy rate in patients with a primary diagnosis of endometriosis (32.5%) was lower than in matched controls (356).

The current evidence suggests that patients with endometriosis have a poorer ovarian response and need a higher dose of gonadotropin therapy in IVF or ICSI programs, but no reduced endometrial implantation. It remains unclear whether the presence or degree of endometriosis is associated with impaired oocyte quality, fertilization rate, and implantation rate. Future studies evaluating the association between endometriosis and reproductive outcome after assisted reproduction should be prospective and should include the following components (131):

- Accurate and recent laparoscopic description of the stage of endometriosis
- Date, number of procedures, and interval between surgery
- Ultrasonographic evidence of endometriosis, confirmed by cytology or histology when endometriotic cysts are aspirated during oocyte aspiration
- Effectiveness of interim suppressive therapy between diagnosis and treatment with assisted reproduction
- Reliability and date of negative diagnosis
- Clear definition of implantation rate, pregnancy rate, abortion rate, and live-birth rate per started cycle, per oocyte aspiration, and per embryo transfer

References

1. **Sampson JA.** Peritoneal endometriosis due to menstrual dissemination of endometrial tissue into the pelvic cavity. *Am J Obstet Gynecol* 1927;14:422–469.
2. **Haney AF.** Endometriosis: pathogenesis and pathophysiology. In: **Wilson EA,** ed. *Endometriosis.* New York: AR Liss, 1987:23–51.
3. **Ramey JW, Archer DF.** Peritoneal fluid: its relevance to the development of endometriosis. *Fertil Steril* 1993;60:1–14.
4. **Halme J, Becker S, Hammond MG, et al.** Retrograde menstruation in healthy women and in patients with endometriosis. *Obstet Gynecol* 1984;64:151–154.
5. **Liu DTY, Hitchcock A.** Endometriosis: its association with retrograde menstruation, dysmenorrhoea and tubal pathology. *Br J Obstet Gynaecol* 1986;93:859–862.
6. **Koninckx PR, De Moor P, Brosens IA.** Diagnosis of the luteinized unruptured follicle syndrome by steroid hormone assays in peritoneal fluid. *Br J Obstet Gynaecol* 1980b;87:929–934.
7. **Kruitwagen RFPM, Poels LG, Willemsen WNP, et al.** Endometrial epithelial cells in peritoneal fluid during the early follicular phase. *Fertil Steril* 1991;55:297–303.
8. **Blumenkrantz MJ, Gallagher N, Bashore RA, et al.** Retrograde menstruation in women undergoing chronic peritoneal dialysis. *Obstet Gynecol* 1981;57:667–670.
9. **Jenkins S, Olive DL, Haney AG.** Endometriosis: pathogenetic implications of the anatomic distribution. *Obstet Gynecol* 1986;67:355–358.
10. **Scott RB, TeLinde RW, Wharton LR Jr.** Further studies on experimental endometriosis. *Am J Obstet Gynecol* 1953;66:1082–1099.
11. **D'Hooghe TM, Bambra CS, Isahakia M, Koninckx PR.** Intrapelvic injection of menstrual endometrium causes endometriosis in baboons (Papio cynocephalus, Papio anubis). *Am J Obstet Gynecol* 1995;173: 125–134.
12. **TeLinde RW, Scott RB.** Experimental endometriosis. *Am J Obstet Gynecol* 1950;60:1147–1173.

13. **Olive DL, Henderson DY.** Endometriosis and müllerian anomalies. *Obstet Gynecol* 1987;69:412–415.

14. **Pinsonneault O, Goldstein DP.** Obstructing malformations of the uterus and vagina. *Fertil Steril* 1985;44:241–247.

15. **D'Hooghe TM, Bambra CS, Suleman MA, et al.** Development of a model of retrograde menstruation in baboons (Papio anubis). *Fertil Steril* 1994:62:635–638.

16. **Cramer DW, Wilson E, Stillman RJ, et al.** The relation of endometriosis to menstrual characteristics, smoking and exercise. *JAMA* 1986;355:1904–1908.

17. **Ueki M.** Histologic study of endometriosis and examination of lymphatic drainage in and from the uterus. *Am J Obstet Gynecol* 1991;165:201–209.

18. **Rock JA, Markham SM.** Extra pelvic endometriosis. In: **Wilson EA,** ed. *Endometriosis*. New York: AR Liss, 1987:185–206.

19. **Russo L, Woolmough E, Heatley MK.** Structural and cell surface antigen expression in the rete ovarii and epoophoron differs from that in the fallopian tube and in endometriosis. *Histopathology* 2000;37:64–69.

20. **Levander G, Normann P.** The pathogenesis of endometriosis: an experimental study. *Acta Obstet Gynecol Scand* 1955;34:366–398.

21. **Merrill JA.** Endometrial induction of endometriosis across millipore filters. *Am J Obstet Gynecol* 1966;94:780–789.

22. **Simpson JL, Elias S, Malinak LR, et al.** Heritable aspects of endometriosis. I. Genetics studies. *Am J Obstet Gynecol* 1980;137:327–331.

23. **Moen MH, Magnus P.** The familial risk of endometriosis. *Acta Obstet Gynecol Scand* 1993;72:560–564.

24. **Treloar SA, O'Connor DT, O'Connor VM, et al.** Genetic influences on endometriosis in an Australian twin sample. *Fertil Steril* 1999;71:701–710.

25. **Hadfield RM, Mardon HJ, Barlow DH, et al.** Endometriosis in monozygotic twins. *Fertil Steril* 1997;68:941–942.

26. **Grimes DA, LeBolt SA, Grimes KR, et al.** Systemic lupus erythematosis and reproductive function: a case-control study. *Am J Obstet Gynecol* 1985;153:179–186.

27. **Hornstein MD, Thomas PP, Sober AJ, et al.** Association between endometriosis, dysplastic naevi and history of melanoma in women of reproductive age. *Hum Reprod* 1997b;12:143–145.

28. **Simpson JL, Malinak LR, Elias S, et al.** HLA associations in endometriosis. *Am J Obstet Gynecol* 1984;148:395–397.

29. **Moen M, Bratlie A, Moen T.** Distribution of HLA-antigens among patients with endometriosis. *Acta Obstet Gynecol Scand Suppl* 1984;123:25–27.

30. **Maxwell C, Kilpatrick DC, Haining R, et al.** No HLA-DR specificity is associated with endometriosis. *Tissue Antigens* 1989;34:145–147.

31. **Thomas EJ, Campbell IG.** Molecular genetic defects in endometriosis. *Gynecol Obstet Invest Suppl* 2000;50:44–50.

32. **Morland SH, Jiang X, Hitchcock A, et al.** Mutation of galactose-1-phosphate uridyl transferat and its association with ovarian cancer and endometriosis. *Int J Cancer* 1998;77:825–827.

33. **Georgiou I, Syrrou M, Bouba I, et al.** Association of estrogen receptor gene polymorphisms with endometriosis. *Fertil Steril* 1999;72:164–166.

34. **Misao R, Sun WS, Iwagaki S, et al.** Identification of various exon-deleted progesterone-receptor mRNAs in human endometrium and ovarian endometriosis. *Biochem Biophys Res Commun* 1998;252:302–306.

35. **Tamura M, Fukaya T, Murakami T, et al.** *Lab Invest* 1998;78:213–218.

36. **Jiang X, Hitchcock A, Bryan E, et al.** Microsatellite analysis of endometriosis reveals loss of heterozygosity at candidate ovarian tumor suppressor gene loci. *Cancer Res* 1996;56:3534–3539.

37. **Bergqvist A, Baldetorp B, Ferno M.** Flow cytometric DNA analysis in endometriotic tissue compared to normal tissue EM. *Hum Reprod* 1996;11:1731–1735.

38. **Gogusev J, Bouquet de Joliniere J, Telvi L, et al.** Detection of DNA copy number changes in human endometriosis by comparative genomic hybridisation. *Hum Genet* 1999;105:444–451.

39. **Shin JC, Ross HL, Elias S, et al.** Detection of chromosomal aneuploidy in endometriosis by multicolor in situ hybridization. *Hum Genet* 1997;100:401–406.

40. **Kosugi Y, Elias S, Malinak LR, et al.** Increased heterogeneity of chromosome 17 aneuploidy in endometriosis. *Am J Obstet Gynecol* 1999;180:792–797.

41. **Goumenou AG, Arvanitis DA, Matalliotakis IM, et al.** Microsatellite DNA assays reveal an allelic imbalance in p16Ink4, GALT, p53, and APOA2 loci in patients with endometriosis. *Fertil Steril* 2001;75:160–165.

42. **D'Hooghe TM, Hill JA.** Immunobiology of endometriosis. In: **Bronston R, Anderson DJ,** eds. *Immunology of reproduction.* Cambridge, MA: Blackwell Scientific, 1996:322–356.

43. **Dmowski WP, Steele RN, Baker GF.** Deficient cellular immunity in endometriosis. *Am J Obstet Gynecol* 1981;141:377–383.

44. **Steele RW, Dmowski WP, Marmer DJ.** Immunologic aspects of endometriosis. *Am J Reprod Immunol* 1984;6:33–36.

45. **Oosterlynck D, Cornillie FJ, Waer M, et al.** Women with endometriosis show a defect in natural killer cell activity resulting in a decreased cytotoxicity to autologous endometrium. *Fertil Steril* 1991;56:45–51.

46. **Vigano P, Vercillini P, Di Blasio AM, et al.** Deficient antiendometrium lymphocyte-mediated cytotoxicity in patients with endometriosis. *Fertil Steril* 1991;56:894–899.

47. **Melioli G, Semino C, Semino A, et al.** Recombinant interleukin-2 corrects *in vitro* the immunological defect of endometriosis. *Am J Reprod Immunol* 1993;30:218–277.

48. **D'Hooghe TM, Scheerlinck JP, Koninckx PR, et al.** Anti-endometrial lymphocytotoxicity and natural killer activity in baboons with endometriosis. *Hum Reprod* 1995;10:558–562.

49. **Hill JA.** Immunology and endometriosis. *Fertil Steril* 1992;58:262–264.

50. **Hill JA.** "Killer cells" and endometriosis. *Fertil Steril* 1993;60:928–929.

51. **Oosterlynck DJ, Meuleman C, Waer M, et al.** The natural killer activity of peritoneal fluid lymphocytes is decreased in women with endometriosis. *Fertil Steril* 1992;58:290–295.

52. **Iwasaki K, Makino T, Maruyama T, et al.** Leukocyte subpopulations and natural killer activity in endometriosis. *Int J Fertil Menopausal Stud* 1993;38:229–234.

53. **Garzetti GG, Ciavattini A, Provinciali M, et al.** Natural killer activity in endometriosis: correlation between serum estradiol levels and cytotoxicity. *Obstet Gynecol* 1993;81:665–668.

54. **Tanaka E, Sendo F, Kawagoe S, et al.** Decreased natural killer activity in women with endometriosis. *Gynecol Obstet Invest* 1992;34:27–30.

55. **Hirata J, Kikuchi Y, Imaizumi E, et al.** Endometriotic tissues produce immunosuppressive factors. *Gynecol Obstet Invest* 1993;37:43–47.

56. **D'Hooghe TM, Bambra CS, De Jonge I, et al.** A serial section study of visually normal posterior pelvic peritoneum from baboons with and without spontaneous endometriosis. *Fertil Steril* 1995;63:1322–1325.

57. **D'Hooghe TM, Nugent N, Cuneo S, et al.** *Recombinant human TNF binding protein (r-hTBP-1) inhibits the development of endometriosis in baboons: a prospective, randomized, placebo- and drug-controlled study.* Accepted for oral presentation at the Annual Meeting of the American Society for Reproductive Medicine, Orlando, USA, October 22nd-24th 2001.

58. **Zeller JM, Henig I, Radwanska E, et al.** Enhancement of human monocyte and peritoneal macrophage chemiluminescence activities in women with endometriosis. *Am J Reprod Immunol Microbiol* 1987;13: 78–82.

59. **Halme J, Becker S, Haskill S.** Altered maturation and function of peritoneal macrophages: possible role in pathogenesis of endometriosis. *Am J Obstet Gynecol* 1987;156:783–789.

60. **Hill JA, Haimovici F, Politch JA, et al.** Effects of soluble products of activated macrophages (lymphokines and monokines) on human sperm motion parameters. *Fertil Steril* 1987;47:460–465.

61. **Halme J.** Release of tumor necrosis factor-a by human peritoneal macrophages in vivo and *in vitro*. *Am J Obstet Gynecol* 1989;161:1718–1725.

62. **Hill JA, Cohen J, Anderson DJ.** The effects of lymphokines and monokines on human sperm fertilizing ability in the zona-free hamster egg penetration test. *Am J Obstet Gynecol* 1989;160:1154–1159.

63. **Zhang R, Wild RA, Ojago JM.** Effect of tumor necrosis factor-alpha on adhesion of human endometrial stromal cells to peritoneal mesothelial cells: an *in vitro* system. *Fertil Steril* 1993;59:1196–1201.

64. **Sillem M, Prifti S, Monga B, et al.** Integrin-mediated adhesion of uterine endometrial cells from endometriosis patients to extracellular matrix proteins is enhanced by TNFalpha and IL-1. *Eur J Obstet Gynecol* 1999;87:123–127.

65. **Olive DL, Montoya I, Riehl RM, et al.** Macrophage-conditioned media enhance endometrial stromal cell proliferation *in vitro*. *Am J Obstet Gynecol* 1991;164:953–958.

66. **Sharpe KL, Zimmer RL, Khan RS, et al.** Proliferative and morphogenic changes induced by the coculture of rat uterine and peritoneal cells: a cell culture model for endometriosis. *Fertil Steril* 1992;58:1220–1229.

67. **Halme J, White C, Kauma S, et al.** Peritoneal macrophages from patients with endometriosis release growth factor activity *in vitro*. *J Clin Endocrinol Metab* 1988;66:1044–1049.

68. **Kauma S, Clark MR, White C, et al.** Production of fibronectin by peritoneal macrophages and concentration of fibronectin in peritoneal fluid from patients with or without endometriosis. *Obstet Gynecol* 1988;72:13–18.

69. **van der Linden PJQ, de Goeij APFM, et al.** Expression of integrins and E-cadherin in cells from menstrual effluent, endometrium, peritoneal fluid, peritoneum, and endometriosis. *Fertil Steril* 1994;61:85–90.

70. **Sharpe-Timms KL, Keisler LW, McIntush EW, et al.** Tissue inhibitor of metalloproteinase-1 concentrations are attenuated in peritoneal fluid and sera of women with endometriosis and restored in sera by gonadotropin-releasing hormone agonist therapy. *Fertil Steril* 1998;69:1128–1134.

71. **Kokorine I, Nisolle M, Donnez J, et al.** Expression of interstitial collagenase (MMP-1) is related to the activity of human endometriotic lesions. *Fertil Steril* 1997;68:246–251.

72. **Kitawaki J, Noguchi T, Amatsu T, et al.** Expression of aromatase cytochrome P450 protein and messenger ribonucleic acid in human endometriotic and adenomyotic tissues but not in normal endometrium. *Biol Reprod* 1997;57:514–519.

73. **Zeitoun K, Takayama K, Sasano H, et al.** *J Clin Endocrinol Metab* 1998;83:4474–4480.

74. **Bulun SE, Zeitoun K, Takayama K, et al.** Molecular basis for treating endometriosis with aromatase inhibitors. *Hum Reprod Update* 2000;6:413–418.

75. **Eskenazi B, Mocarelli P, Warner M, et al.** Seveso Women's Health Study: a study of the effects of 2,3,7,7-tetrachlorodibenzo-p-dioxin on reproductive health. *Chemosphere* 2000;40:1247–1253.

76. **Lebel G, Dodin S, Ayotte P, et al.** Organochlorine exposure and the risk of endometriosis. *Fertil Steril* 1998;69:221–228.

77. **Bulun S, Zeitoun KM, Kilic G.** Expression of dioxin-related transactivating factors and target genes in human eutopic endometrial and endometriotic tissues. *Am J Obstet Gynecol* 2000:182:767–775.

78. **Igarashi T, Osuga Y, Tsutsumi O, et al.** *Endocr J* 1999;46:765–772.

79. **Watanabe T, Imoto I, Losugi Y, et al.** Human arylhydrocarbon receptor repressor (AHRR) gene: genomic structure and analysis of polymorphism in endometriosis. *J Hum Genet* 2001;46:342–346.

80. **Rier SE, Martin DC, Bowman RE, et al.** Endometriosis in rhesus monkeys (Macaca Mulatta) following chronic exposure to 2,3,7,8-tetrachlorodibenzo-p-dioxin. *Fund Appl Toxicol* 1993;21:433–441.

81. **Rier SE, Turner WE, Martin DC, et al.** Serum levels of TCDD and dioxin-like chemicals in rhesus monkeys chronically exposed to dioxin: correlation of increased serum PCB levels with endometriosis. *Toxicol Sci* 2001;59:147–159.

82. **Yang Y, Degranpre P, Kharfi A, et al.** Identification of macrophage migration inhibitory factor as a potent endothelial cell growth promoting agent released by ectopic human endometrial cells. *J Clin Endocrinol Metab* 2000;85:4721–4727.

83. **Arnold DL, Nera EA, Stapley R, et al.** Prevalence of endometriosis in rhesus (Macacca Mulatta) monkeys ingesting PCB (Aroclor 1254): review and evaluation. *Fund Appl Toxicol* 1996;31:42–55.

84. **Yang JZ, Foster WG.** Continuous exposure of 2,3,7,8 tetrachlorodibenzo-p-dioxin inhibits the growth of surgically induced endometriosis in the ovariectomized mouse treated with high dose estradiol. *Toxicol Ind Health* 1997;13:15–25.

85. **Yang JZ, Yagminas AL, Foster WG.** Stimulating effects of 4-chlorodiphenyl ether on surgically induced endometriosis in the mouse. *Reprod Toxicol* 1997;11:69–75.

86. **Cummings AM, Metcalf JL, Birnbaum L.** Promotion of endometriosis by 2,3,7,8-tetrachlorodibenzo-p-dioxin in rats and mice: time-dose dependence and species comparison. *Toxicol Appled Pharmacol* 1996;138:131–139.

87. **Smith EM, Hammonds EM, Clark MK, et al.** Occupational exposures and risk of female infertility. *J Occup Environ Med* 1997;39:138–147.

88. **Jansen RPS, Russell P.** Nonpigmented endometriosis: clinical, laparoscopic and pathologic definition. *Am J Obstet Gynecol* 1986;155:1160–1163.

89. **Stripling MC, Martin DC, Chatman DL, et al.** Subtle appearance of pelvic endometriosis. *Fertil Steril* 1988;49:427–431.

90. **Martin DC, Hubert GD, Vander Zwaag R, et al.** Laparoscopic appearances of peritoneal endometriosis. *Fertil Steril* 1989;51:63–67.

91. **D'Hooghe TM, Bambra CS, Cornillie FJ, et al.** Prevalence and laparoscopic appearances of endometriosis in the baboon (Papio cynocephalyus, Papio anubis). *Biol Reprod* 1991;45:411–416.

92. **Schenken RS, Williams RF, Hodgen GD.** Experimental endometriosis in primates. *Ann N Y Acad Sci* 1991;622:242–255.

93. **Dizerega GS, Barber DL, Hodgen GD.** Endometriosis: role of ovarian steroids in initiation, maintenance and suppression. *Fertil Steril* 1980;649–653.

94. **Schenken RS, Asch RH, Williams RF, et al.** Etiology of infertility in monkeys with endometriosis: luteinized unruptured follicles, luteal phase defects, pelvic adhesions, and spontaneous abortions. *Fertil Steril* 1984;41:122–130.

95. **Mann DR, Collins DC, Smith MM, et al.** Treatment of endometriosis in Rhesus monkeys: effectiveness

of a gonadotropin-releasing hormone agonist compared to treatment with a progestational steroid. *J Clin Endocrinol Metab* 1986;63:1277–1283.

96. **Da Rif CA, Parker RF, Schoeb TR.** Endometriosis with bacterial peritonitis in a baboon. *Lab Anim Sci* 1984;34:491–493.

97. **Cornillie FJ, D'Hooghe TM, Lauweryns JM, et al.** Morphological characteristics of spontaneous pelvic endometriosis in the baboon (Papio anubis and Papio cynocephalus). *Gynecol Obstet Invest* 1992;34:225–228.

98. **D'Hooghe TM.** Clinical relevance of the baboon as a model for the study of endometriosis. *Fertil Steril* 1997;68:613–625.

99. **Sanfilippo JS, Williams RS, Yussman MA, et al.** Substance P in peritoneal fluid. *Am J Obstet Gynecol* 1992;166:155–159.

100. **Koninckx PR, Meuleman C, Demeyere S, et al.** Suggestive evidence that pelvic endometriosis is a progressive disease, whereas deeply infiltrating endometriosis is associated with pelvic pain. *Fertil Steril* 1991;55:759–765.

101. **Moen MH.** Endometriosis in women at interval sterilization. *Acta Obstet Gynecol Scand* 1987;66:451–454.

102. **Kirshon B, Poindexter AN, Fast J.** Endometriosis in multiparous women. *J Reprod Med* 1989;215–217.

103. **Mahmood TA, Templeton A.** Prevalence and genesis of endometriosis. *Hum Reprod* 1991;6:544–549.

104. **Moen MH, Muus KM.** Endometriosis in pregnant and non-pregnant women at tubal sterilization. *Hum Reprod* 1991;6:699–702.

105. **Waller KG, Lindsay P, Curtis P, et al.** The prevalence of endometriosis in women with infertile partners. *Eur J Obstet Gynecol Reprod Biol* 1993;48:135–139.

106. **Strathy JH, Molgaard CA, Coulam CB, et al.** Endometriosis and infertility: a laparoscopic study of endometriosis among fertile and infertile women. *Fertil Steril* 1982;38:667–672.

107. **Fakih HN, Tamura R, Kesselman A, et al.** Endometriosis after tubal ligation. *J Reprod Med* 1985;30:939–941.

108. **Dodge ST, Pumphrey RS, Miyizawa K.** Peritoneal endometriosis in women requesting reversal of sterilization. *Fertil Steril* 1986;45:774–777.

109. **Trimbos JB, Trimbos-Kemper GCM, Peters AAW, et al.** Findings in 200 consecutive asymptomatic women having a laparoscopic sterilization. *Arch Gynecol Obstet* 1990;247:121–124.

110. **Cornillie FJ, Oosterlynck D, Lauweryns JM, et al.** Deeply infiltrating pelvic endometriosis: histology and clinical significance. *Fertil Steril* 1990;53:978–983.

111. **Arumugam K, Lim JMH.** Menstrual characteristics associated with endometriosis. *Br J Obstet Gynecol* 1997;104:948–950.

112. **Vercellini P, De Giorgi O, Aimi G, et al.** Menstrual characteristics in women with and without endometriosis. *Obstet Gynecol* 1997;90:264–268.

113. **Signorello LB, Harlow BL, Cramer DW, et al.** Epidemiologic determinants of endometriosis: a hospital-based control study. *Ann Epidemiol* 1997;7:267–274.

114. **Mathias JR, Franklin R, Quast DC, et al.** Relation of endometriosis and neuromuscular disease of the gastrointestinal tract: new insights. *Fertil Steril* 1998;70:81–88.

115. **Ulrich U, Murano R, Skinner MA, et al.** Women of reproductive age with endometriosis are not osteopenic. *Fertil Steril* 1998;69:821–825.

116. **Hadfield RM, Mardon H, Barlow D, et al.** Delay in the diagnosis of endometriosis: a survey of women from the USA and the UK. *Hum Reprod* 1996;11:878–880.

117. **Dmowski WP, Lesniewicz R, Rana N, et al.** Changing trends in the diagnosis of endometriosis: a comparative study of women with endometriosis presenting with chronic pain or infertility. *Fertil Steril* 1997;67:238–243.

118. **Colwell HH, Mathias SD, Pasta DJ, et al.** A health-related quality-of-life instrument for symptomatic patients with endometriosis: a validation study. *Am J Obstet Gynecol* 1998;179:47–55.

119. **Barlow DH, Glynn CJ.** Endometriosis and pelvic pain. *Baillieres Clin Obstet Gynaecol* 1993;7:775–790.

120. **Anaf V, Simon Ph, El Nakadi I, et al.** Relationship between endometriotic foci and nerves in rectovaginal endometriotic nodules. *Hum Reprod* 2000a;15:1744–1750.

121. **American Fertility Society.** Revised American Fertility Society Classification of Endometriosis. *Fertil Steril* 1985;43:351–352.

122. **D'Hooghe TM, Bambra CS, Raeymaekers BM, et al.** A prospective controlled study over 2 years shows a normal monthly fertility rate (MFR) in baboons with stage I endometriosis and a decreased MFR in primates with stage II-IV disease. *Fertil Steril* 1994;5[Suppl]:1–113.

123. **Haney AF.** Endometriosis-associated infertility. *Baillieres Clin Obstet Gynaecol* 1993;7:791–812.

124. **Jansen RPS.** Minimal endometriosis and reduced fecundability; prospective evidence from an artificial insemination by donor program. *Fertil Steril* 1986;46:141–143.

125. **Hammond MG, Jordan S, Sloan CS.** Factors affecting pregnancy rates in a donor insemination program using frozen semen. *Am J Obstet Gynecol* 1986;155:480–485.

126. **Portuondo JA, Echanojauregui AD, Herran C, et al.** Early conception in patients with untreated mild endometriosis. *Fertil Steril* 1983;39:22–25.

127. **Rodriguez-Escudero FJ, Negro JL, Corcosstegui B, et al.** Does minimal endometriosis reduce fecundity? *Fertil Steril* 1988;50:522–524.

128. **D'Hooghe TM, Bambra CS, Koninckx PR.** Cycle fecundity in baboons of proven fertility with minimal endometriosis. *Gynecol Obstet Invest* 1994;37;63–65.

129. **Berube S, Marcoux S, Langevin M, et al.,** and the Canadian Collaborative Group on Endometriosis. Fecundity of infertile women with minimal or mild endometriosis and women with unexplained infertility. *Fertil Steril* 1998;69:1034–1041.

130. **D'Hooghe TM, Hill JA.** Immunobiology of endometriosis. In: **Bronson RA, Alexander NJ, Anderson DJ, et al,** eds. *Immunology of reproduction.* Blackwell Science, 1996;322–358.

131. **Vercammen E, D'Hooghe TM, Hill JA.** Endometriosis and recurrent miscarriage. *Semin Reprod Med* 2000;18:363–368.

132. **Matorras R, Rodriguez F, Gutierrez de Teran G, et al.** Endometriosis and spontaneous abortion rate: a cohort study in infertile women. *Eur J Obstet Gynecol Reprod Biol* 1998;77:101–105.

133. **Marcoux S, Maheux R, Bérubé S, and the Canadian Collaborative Group on Endometriosis.** Laparoscopic surgery in infertile women with minimal or mild endometriosis. *N Engl J Med* 1997;337: 217–222.

134. **Gruppo Italiano per lo Studio dell' Endometriosi.** Ablation of lesions or no treatment in minimal-mild endometriosis in infertile women: a randomized trial. *Hum Reprod* 1999;14:1332–1334.

135. **Cahill DJ, Hull MGR.** Pituitary-ovarian dysfunction and endometriosis. *Hum Reprod Update* 2000;6: 56–66.

136. **D'Hooghe TM, Bambra CS, Raeymaekers BM, et al.** Increased incidence and recurrence of recent corpus luteum without ovulation stigma (luteinized unruptured follicle-syndrome?) in baboons (Papio anubis, Papio cynocephalus) with endometriosis. *J Soc Gynecol Invest* 1996;3:140–144.

137. **Lessey BA, Castelbaum AJ, Sawin SW, et al.** Aberrant integrin expression in the endometrium of women with endometriosis. *J Clin Endocrinol Metab* 1994;79:643–649.

138. **Matorras R, Rodriguez F, Perez C, et al.** Infertile women with and without endometriosis: a case-control study of luteal phase and other infertility conditions. *Acta Obstet Gynecol Scand* 1996;75:826–831.

139. **Propst AM, Storti K, Barbieri RL.** Lateral cervical displacement is associated with endometriosis. *Fertil Steril* 1998;70:568–570.

140. **Koninckx PR, Martin DC.** Deep endometriosis: a consequence of infiltration or retraction or possibly adenomyosis externa? *Fertil Steril* 1992;58:924–928.

141. **Koninckx PR, Oosterlynck D, D'Hooghe TM, et al.** Deeply infiltrating endometriosis is a disease whereas mild endometriosis could be considered a non-disease. *Ann N Y Acad Sci* 1994;734:333–341.

142. **Koninckx PR, Meuleman C, Oosterlynck D, et al.** Diagnosis of deep endometriosis by clinical examination during menstruation and plasma CA 125 concentration. *Fertil Steril* 1996;65:280–287.

143. **McBean JH, Gibson M, Brumsted JR.** The association of intrauterine filling defects on HSG with endometriosis. *Fertil Steril* 1996;66:522–526.

144. **Guerriero S, Paoletti AM, Mais V, et al.** Transvaginal ultrasonography combined with CA125 plasma levels in the diagnosis of endometrioma. *Fertil Steril* 1996;65:293–298.

145. **Fedele L, Bianchi S, Portuese A, et al.** Transrectal ultrasonography in the assessment of rectovaginal endometriosis. *Obstet Gynecol* 1998;91:444–448.

146. **Kinkel K, Chapron C, Balleyguier C, et al.** Magnetic resonance imaging characteristics of deep endometriosis. *Hum Reprod* 1999;14:1080–1086.

147. **Bast RC, Klug TL, St. John E, et al.** A radio-immunoassay using a monoclonal antibody to monitor the course of epithelial ovarian cancer. *N Engl J Med* 1983;309:883–887.

148. **Barbieri RL, Niloff JM, Bast RC Jr, et al.** Elevated serum concentrations of CA125 in patients with advanced endometriosis. *Fertil Steril* 1986;45:630–634.

149. **Pittaway DE, Fayez JA.** The use of CA125 in the diagnosis and management of endometriosis. *Fertil Steril* 1986;46:790–795.

150. **Pittaway DE, Fayez JA.** Serum CA125 levels increase during menses. *Am J Obstet Gynecol* 1987;156: 75–76.

151. **Masahashi T, Matsuzawa K, Ohsawa M, et al.** Serum CA125 levels in patients with endometriosis: changes in CA125 levels during menstruation. *Obstet Gynecol* 1988;72:328–331.

152. **Takahashi K, Yoshino K, Kusakari M, et al.** Prognostic potential of serum CA125 levels in danazol-treated patients with external endometriosis: a preliminary study. *Int J Fertil* 1990;35:226–229.

153. **Franssen AMHW, van der Heijden PFM, Thomas CMG, et al.** On the origin and significance of serum CA125 concentrations in 97 patients with endometriosis before, during, and after buserelin acetate, nafarelin, or danazol. *Fertil Steril* 1992;57:974–979.

154. **Moloney MD, Thornton JG, Cooper EH.** Serum CA125 antigen levels and disease severity in patients with endometriosis. *Obstet Gynecol* 1989;73:767–769.

155. **Nagamani M, Kelver ME, Smith ER.** CA125 levels in monitoring therapy for endometriosis and in prediction of recurrence. *Int J Fertil* 1992;37:227–231.

156. **Hornstein M, Thomas PP, Gleason RE, et al.** Menstrual cyclicity of CA125 in patients with endometriosis. *Fertil Steril* 1992;58:279–283.

157. **O'Shaughnessy A, Check JH, Nowroozi K, et al.** CA125 levels measured in different phases of the menstrual cycle in screening for endometriosis. *Obstet Gynecol* 1993;81:99–103.

158. **Pittaway DE, Douglas JW.** Serum CA125 in women with endometriosis and chronic pain. *Fertil Steril* 1989;51:68–70.

159. **Mol BWJ, Bayram N, Lijmer JG, et al.** The performance of CA-125 measurement in the detection of endometriosis: a meta-analysis. *Fertil Steril* 1998;70:1101–1108.

160. **Hompes PGA, Koninckx PR, Kennedy S, et al.** Serum CA-125 concentrations during midfollicular phase, a clinically useful and reproducible marker in diagnosis of advanced endometriosis. *Clin Chem* 1996;42: 1871–1874.

161. **Pittaway DE.** CA125 in women with endometriosis. *Obstet Gynecol Clin North Am* 1989;16: 237–252.

162. **Pittaway DE.** The use of serial CA125 concentrations to monitor endometriosis in infertile women. *Am J Obstet Gynecol* 1990;163:1032–1037.

163. **Kauppila A, Telimaa S, Ronnberg L, et al.** Placebo-controlled study on serum concentrations of CA125 before and after treatment with danazol or high-dose medroxyprogesterone acetate alone or after surgery. *Fertil Steril* 1988;49:37–41.

164. **Dawood MY, Khan-Dawood FS, Wilson L Jr.** Peritoneal fluid prostaglandins and prostanoids in women with endometriosis, chronic pelvic inflammatory disease, and pelvic pain. *Am J Obstet Gynecol* 1984;148:391–395.

165. **Bischof P, Galfetti MA, Seydoux J, et al.** Peripheral CA125 levels in patients with uterine fibroids. *Hum Reprod* 1992;7:35–38.

166. **Ward BG, McGuckin MA, Ramm L, et al.** Expression of tumour markers CA125, CASA and OSA in minimal/mild endometriosis. *Aust N Z J Obstet Gynaecol* 1991;31:273–275.

167. **Fraser IS, McCarron G, Markham R.** Serum CA125 levels in women with endometriosis. *Aust N Z J Obstet Gynecol* 1989;29:416–420.

168. **Acien P, Shaw RW, Irvine L, et al.** CA125 levels in endometriosis patients before, during and after treatment with danazol or LHRH agonists. *Eur J Obstet Gynecol* 1989;32:241–246.

169. **Takahashi K, Abu Musa A, Nagata H, et al.** Serum CA125 and 17-b-estradiol in patients with external endomettriosis on danazol. *Gynecol Obstet Invest* 1990;29:301–304.

170. **Fedele L, Arcaini L, Vercellini P, et al.** Serum CA125 measurements in the diagnosis of endometriosis recurrence. *Obstet Gynecol* 1988;72:19–22.

171. **Vasquez G, Cornillie F, Brosens IA.** Peritoneal endometriosis: scanning electron microscopy and histology of minimal pelvic endometriotic lesions. *Fertil Steril* 1984;42:696–703.

172. **Nisolle M, Paindaveine B, Bourdin A, et al.** Histological study of peritoneal endometriosis in infertile women. *Fertil Steril* 1990;53:984–948.

173. **Clement PB.** Pathology of endometriosis. *Pathol Annu* 1990;245–295.

174. **Moen MH, Halvorsen TB.** Histologic confirmation of endometriosis in different peritoneal lesions. *Acta Obstet Gynecol Scand* 1992;71:337–342.

175. **Vercellini P, Aimi G, Panazza S, et al.** Deep endometriosis conundrum: evidence in favor of a peritoneal origin. *Fertil Steril* 2000;73:1043–1046.

176. **Vercellini P, Vendola N, Bocciolone L, et al.** Reliability of the visual diagnosis of endometriosis. *Fertil Steril* 1991;56:1198–2000.

177. **Redwine DB.** Ovarian endometriosis: a marker for more extensive pelvic and intestinal disease. *Fertil Steril* 1999;72:310–315.

178. **Walter AJ, Hentz JG, Magtibay PM, et al.** Endometriosis: correlation between histologic and visual findings at laparoscopy. *Am J Obstet Gynecol* 2001;184:1407–1413.

179. **Czernobilsky B.** Endometriosis. In: **Fox H,** ed. *Obstetrical and gynecological pathology.* New York: Churchill Livingstone, 1987:763–777.

180. **Mai KT, Yazdi HM, Perkins DG, et al.** Pathogenetic role of the stromal cells in endometriosis and adenomyosis. *Histopathology* 1997;30:430–442.

181. **Cornillie FJ, Vasquez G, Brosens IA.** The response of human endometriotic implants to the anti-progesterone steroid R2323: a histologic and ultrastructural study. *Pathol Res Pract* 1990;180:647–655.

182. **Donnez J, Nisolle M, Casanas-Roux F.** Three-dimensional architectures of peritoneal endometriosis. *Fertil Steril* 1992;57:980–983.

183. **Nisolle M, Casanas-Roux F, Anaf V, et al.** Morphometric study of the stromal vascularization in peritoneal endometriosis. *Fertil Steril* 1993;59:681–684.

184. **Anaf V, Simon Ph, Fayt I, et al.** Smooth muscles are frequent components of endometriotic lesions. *Hum Reprod* 2000;15:767–771.

185. **Wardle PG, Hull MGR.** Is endometriosis a disease? *Baillieres Clin Obstet Gynecol* 1993;7:673–685.

186. **Murphy AA, Green WR, Bobbie D, et al.** Unsuspected endometriosis documented by scanning electron microscopy in visually normal peritoneum. *Fertil Steril* 1986;46:522–524.

187. **Steingold KA, Cedars M, Lu JKH, et al.** Treatment of endometriosis with a long-acting gonadotropin-releasing hormone agonist. *Obstet Gynecol* 1987;69:403–411.

188. **Nezhat F, Allan CJ, Nezhat F, et al.** Nonvisualized endometriosis at laparoscopy. *Int J Fertil* 1991;36:340–343.

189. **Balasch J, Creus M, Fabregeus F, et al.** Visible and non-visible endometriosis at laparoscopy in fertile and infertile women and in patients with chronic pelvic pain: a prospective study. *Hum Reprod* 1996;11:387–391.

190. **Hayata T, Matsu T, Kawano Y, et al.** Scanning electron microscopy of endometriotic lesions in the pelvic peritoneum and the histogenesis of endometriosis. *Int J Gynecol Obstet* 1992;39:311–319.

191. **Murphy AA, Guzick DS, Rock JA.** Microscopic peritoneal endometriosis. *Fertil Steril* 1989;51:1072–1074.

192. **Redwine DB.** Is "microscopic" peritoneal endometriosis invisible? *Fertil Steril* 1988;50:665–666.

193. **Redwine DB, Yocom LB.** A serial section study of visually normal pelvic peritoneum in patients with endometriosis. *Fertil Steril* 1990;54:648–651.

194. **D'Hooghe TM, Bambra CS, De Jonge I, et al.** A serial section study of visually normal posterior pelvic peritoneum from baboons with and without spontaneous endometriosis. *Fertil Steril* 1995;63:1322–1325.

195. **Hornstein MD, Gleason RE, Orav J, et al.** The reproducibility of the revised American Fertility Society classification of endometriosis. *Fertil Steril* 1993;59:1015–1021.

196. **Lin SY, Lee RKK, Hwu YM, et al.** Reproducibility of the revised American Fertility Society classification of endometriosis during laparoscopy or laparotomy. *Int J Gynecol Obstet* 1998;60:265–269.

197. **Thomas EJ, Cooke ID.** Impact of *gestrinone* on the course of asymptomatic endometriosis. *BMJ* 1987;294:272–274.

198. **Mahmood TA, Templeton A.** The impact of treatment on the natural history of endometriosis. *Hum Reprod* 1990;5:965–970.

199. **Sutton CJG, Pooley AS, Ewen SP, et al.** Follow-up report on a randomized controlled trial of laser laparoscopy in the treatment of pelvic pain associated with minimal to moderate endometriosis. *Fertil Steril* 1997;68:1070–1074.

200. **D'Hooghe TM, Bambra CS, Raeymaekers BM, et al.** Serial laparoscopies over 30 months show that endometriosis is a progressive disease in captive baboons (Papio anubis, Papio cynocephalus). *Fertil Steril* 1996;65:645–649.

201. **Hoshiai H, Ishikawa M, Yoshiharu S, et al.** Laparoscopic evaluation of the onset and progression of endometriosis. *Am J Obstet Gynecol* 1993;169:714–719.

202. **D'Hooghe TM, Bambra CS, Isahakia M, et al.** Evolution of spontaneous endometriosis in the baboon (Papio anubis, Papio Cynocephalus) over a 12-month period. *Fertil Steril* 1992;58:409–412.

203. **Redwine DB.** Age-related evolution in color appearance of endometriosis. *Fertil Steril* 1987;48:1062–1063.

204. **Wiegerinck MAHM, Van Dop PA, Brosens IA.** The staging of peritoneal endometriosis by the type of active lesion in addition to the revised American Fertility Society classification. *Fertil Steril* 1993;60:461–464.

205. **Hanton EM, Malkasian GD Jr, Dockerty MB, et al.** Endometriosis associated with complete or partial obstruction of menstrual egress. *Obstet Gynecol* 1966;28:626–629.

206. **Schenken RS, Williams RF, Hodgen G.** Effect of pregnancy on surgically induced endometriosis in cynomolgus monkeys. *Am J Obstet Gynecol* 1987;157:1392–1396.

207. **Vernon MW, Wilson EA.** Studies on the surgical induction of endometriosis in the rat. *Fertil Steril* 1985;44:684–694.

208. **McArthur JW, Ulfelder H.** The effect of pregnancy upon endometriosis. *Obstet Gynecol Surv* 1965;20:709–733.

209. **D'Hooghe TM, Bambra CS, De Jonge I, et al.** Pregnancy does not affect endometriosis in baboons (Papio anubis, Papio cynocephalus). *Arch Gynecol Obstet* 1997;261:15–19.

210. **Kistner RW.** The treatment of endometriosis by inducing pseudopregnancy with ovarian hormones: a report of fifty-eight cases. *Fertil Steril* 1959;10:539–556.

211. **Italian Endometriosis Study Group.** Oral contraceptive use and risk of endometriosis. *Br J Obstet Gynecol* 1999;106:695–699.

212. **Tulandi T, Al Took S.** Reproductive outcome after treatment of mild endometriosis with laparoscopic excision and electrocoagulation. *Fertil Steril* 1998;69:229–231.

213. **Brosens IA, Puttemans PJ.** Double-optic laparoscopy. Salpingoscopy, ovarian cystoscopy, and endoovarian surgery with the argon laser. *Baillieres Clin Obstet Gynaecol* 1989;3:595–608.

214. **Heaps JM, Berek JS, Nieberg RK.** Malignant neoplasms arising in endometriosis. *Obstet Gynecol* 1990;75:1023–1028.

215. **Loh FH, Tan AT, Kumar J, Ng SC.** Ovarian response after laparoscopic ovarian cystectomy for endometriotic cysts in 132 monitored cycles. *Fertil Steril* 1999;72:316–321.

216. **Hemmings R, Bissonnette F, Bouzayen R.** Results of laparoscopic treatments of ovarian endometriomas: laparoscopic ovarian fenestration and coagulation. *Fertil Steril* 1998;70:527–529.

217. **Saleh A, Tulandi T.** Reoperation after laparoscopic treatment of ovarian endometrioma by excision and by fenestration. *Fertil Steril* 1999;72:322–324.

218. **Beretta P, Franchi M, Ghezzi F, et al.** Randomized clinical trial of two laparoscopic treatments of endometriosis: cystectomy versus drainage and coagulation. *Fertil Steril* 1998;70:1176–1180.

219. **Watson A, Vandekerckhove P, Lilford R.** Liquid and fluid agents for preventing adhesions after surgery for subfertility. *Cochrane Database Syst Rev* 2000;3:CD001298.

220. **Audebert A, Descampes P, Marret H, et al.** Pre or post operative medical treatment with nafarelin in stage III-IV endometriosis: a French multicentered study. *Eur J Obstet Gynecol Reprod Biol* 1998;79:145–148.

221. **Koninckx PR, Timmermans B, Meuleman C, et al.** Complications of CO-2 laser endoscopic excision of deep endometriosis. *Hum Reprod* 1996;11:2263–2268.

222. **Redwine DB, Koning M, Sharpe DR.** Laparoscopically assisted transvaginal segmental resection of the rectosigmoid colon for endometriosis. *Fertil Steril* 1996;65:193–197.

223. **MacDonald SR, Klock SC, Milad MP.** Long-term outcome of nonconservative surgery (hysterectomy) for endometriosis-associated pain in women < 30 years old. *Am J Obstet Gynecol* 1999;180:1360–1363.

224. **Sutton CJG, Ewen SP, Whitelaw N, et al.** Prospective, randomized, double-blind, controlled trial of laser laparoscopy in the treatment of pelvic pain associated with minimal, mild, and moderate endometriosis. *Fertil Steril* 1994;62:696–700.

225. **Candiani GB, Fedele L, Vercellini P, et al.** Presacral neurectomy for the treatment of pelvic pain associated with endometriosis: a controlled study. *Am J Obstet Gynecol* 1992;167:100–103.

226. **Fedele L, Bianchi S, Bocciolone L, et al.** Buserelin acetate in the treatment of pelvic pain associated with minimal and mild endometriosis: a controlled study. *Fertil Steril* 1993;59:516–521.

227. **Overton CE, Lindsay PC, Johal B, et al.** A randomized, double-blind, placebo-controlled study of luteal phase dydrogesterone (Duphaston) in women with minimal to mild endometriosis. *Fertil Steril* 1994;62:701–707.

228. **Feste JR.** Laser laparoscopy: a new modality. *J Reprod Med* 1985;30:413–417.

229. **Nezhat C, Winer W, Crowgey S, et al.** Videolaparoscopy for the treatment of endometriosis associated with infertility. *Fertil Steril* 1989;51:237–240.

230. **Sutton CJG, Hill D.** Laser laparoscopy in the treatment of endometriosis: a 5 year study. *Br J Obstet Gynaecol* 1990;97:181–185.

231. **Daniell JF.** Fiberoptic laser laparoscopy. *Baillieres Clin Obstet Gynaecol* 1989;3:545–562.

232. **Fedele L, Bianchi S, Bocciolone L, et al.** Pain symptoms associated with endometriosis. *Obstet Gynecol* 1992;79:767–769.

233. **Vercellini P, Cortesi I, Trespidi L, et al.** Endometriosis and pelvic pain: relation to disease stage and localization. *Fertil Steril* 1996;65:299–304.

234. **Muzii L, Marano R, Pedulla S, et al.** Correlation between endometriosis-associated dysmenorrhea and the presence of typical and atypical lesions. *Fertil Steril* 1997;68:19–22.

235. **Stovall DW Bowser LM, Archer DF, et al.** Endometriosis-associated pain: evidence for an association between the stage of disease and a history of chronic pelvic pain. *Fertil Steril* 1997;68: 13–18.

236. **Sutton CJG, Hill D.** Laser laparoscopy in the treatment of endometriosis: a 5 year study. *Br J Obstet Gynaecol* 1990;97:181–185.

237. **Hornstein MD, Hemmings R, Yuzpe AA, et al.** Use of nafarelin versus placebo after reductive laparoscopic surgery for endometriosis. *Fertil Steril* 1997;68:860–864.

238. **Vercellini P, Crosignani PG, Fadini R, et al.** A gonadotropin-releasing hormone agonist compared with expectant management after conservative surgery for symptomatic endometriosis. *Br J Obstet Gynaecol* 1999;106:672–677.

239. **Parazzini F, Fedele L, Busacca M, et al.** Postsurgical treatment of advanced endometriosis: results of a randomized clinical trial. *Am J Obstet Gynecol* 1994;171:1205–1207.

240. **Bianchi S, Busacca M, Agnoli B, et al.** Effects of 3 month therapy with danazol after laparoscopic surgery for stage III/IV endometriosis: a randomized study. *Fertil Steril* 1999;14:1334–1337.

241. **Guzick DS, Canis M, Silliman NP, et al.** Prediction of pregnancy in infertile women based on the ASRM's revised classification for endometriosis. *Fertil Steril* 1997;67:822–836.

242. **Chapron C, Fritel X, Dubuisson JB.** Fertility after laparoscopic management of deep endometriosis infiltrating the uterosacral ligaments. *Hum Reprod* 1999;14:329–332.

243. **Pagidas K, Falcone T, Hemmings R, et al.** Comparison of reoperation for moderate (stage III) and severe (stage IV) endometriosis-related infertility. *Fertil Steril* 1996;65:791–795.

244. **Rock JA, Guzick DS, Dengos C, et al.** The conservative surgical treatment of endometriosis: evaluation of pregnancy success with respect to the extent of disease as categorized using contemporary classification systems. *Fertil Steril* 1981;35:131–137.

245. **American Fertility Society.** Classification of endometriosis. *Fertil Steril* 1979;32:633–634.

246. **Adamson GD, Hurd SJ, Pasta DJ, et al.** Laparoscopic endometriosis treatment: is it better? *Fertil Steril* 1993;59:35–44.

247. **Canis M, Pouly JL, Wattiez A, et al.** Incidence of bilateral adnexal disease in severe endometriosis (revised American Fertility Society (AFS) stage IV): should a stage V be included in the AFS classification. *Fertil Steril* 1992;691–692.

248. **Olive DL, Lee KL.** Analysis of sequential treatment protocols for endometriosis-associated infertility. *Am J Obstet Gynecol* 1986;154:613–619.

249. **Badawy SZA, El Bakry MM, Samuel D, et al.** Cumulative pregnancy rates in infertile women with endometriosis. *J Reprod Med* 1988;33:757–760.

250. **Nowroozi K, Chase JS, Check JH, et al.** The importance of laparoscopic coagulation of mild endometriosis in infertile women. *Int J Fertil* 1987;32:442–444.

251. **Paulson JD, Asmar P, Saffan DS.** Mild and moderate endometriosis: comparison of treatment modalities for infertile couples. *J Reprod Med* 1991;36:151–155.

252. **Tulandi T, Mouchawar M.** Treatment-dependent and treatment-independent pregnancy in women with minimal and mild endometriosis. *Fertil Steril* 1991;56:790–791.

253. **Schenken RS, Malinak LR.** Conservative versus expectant management for the infertile patient with mild endometriosis. *Fertil Steril* 1982;37:183–186.

254. **Arumugam K, Urquhart R.** Efficacy of laparoscopic electrocoagulation in infertile patients with minimal or mild endometriosis. *Acta Obstet Gynecol Scand* 1991;70:125–127.

255. **Adamson S, Edwin SS, LaMarche S, et al.** Actions of interleukin-4 on prostaglandin biosynthesis at the chorion-decidual interface. *Am J Obstet Gynecol* 1993;169:1442–1447.

256. **Olive DL, Martin DC.** Treatment of endometriosis-associated infertility with CO_2 laser laparoscopy: the use of one- and two-parameter exponential models. *Fertil Steril* 1987;48:18–23.

257. **Rosen GF.** Treatment of endometriosis-associated infertility. *Infert Reprod Med Clin North Am* 1992;3: 721–730.

258. **Kistner RW.** The use of progestins in the treatment of endometriosis. *Am J Obstet Gynecol* 1958;75: 264–278.

259. **Moghissi KS.** Pseudopregnancy induced by estrogen-progestogen or progestogens alone in the treatment of endometriosis. *Prog Clin Biol Res* 1990;323:221–232.

260. **Dawood MY.** Endometriosis. In: **Gold JJ, Josimovich JB,** eds. *Gynecologic endocrinology.* New York: Plenum, 1987:387–404.

261. **Dmowski WP.** Endometriosis. In: **Glass RH**, ed. *Office gynecology.* Baltimore: Williams & Wilkins, 1987:317–336.

262. **Vercellini P, De Giorgi O, Oldani S, et al.** Depot medroxyprogesterone acetate versus an oral contraceptive combined with very-low-dose danazol for long-term treatment of pelvic pain associated with endometriosis. *Am J Obstet Gynecol* 1996;175:396–341.

263. **Vercellini P, Cortesi I, Crosignani PG.** Progestins for symptomatic endometriosis: a critical analysis of the evidence. *Fertil Steril* 1997;68:393–341.

264. **Moghissi KS, Boyce CR.** Management of pelvic endometriosis with oral medroxyprogesterone-acetate. *Obstet Gynecol* 1976;47:265–267.

265. **Luciano AA, Turksoy RN, Carleo J.** Evaluation of oral medroxyprogesterone acetate in the treatment of endometriosis. *Obstet Gynecol* 1988;72:323–327.

266. **Harrison RF, Barry-Kinsella C.** Efficacy of medroxy-progesterone treatment in infertile women with endometriosis: a prospective, randomized, placebo-controlled study. *Fertil Steril* 2000;74:24–30.

267. **Vercellini P, Aimi G, Panazza S, et al.** A levonorgestrel-releasing intrauterine system for the treatment of dysmenorrhea associated with endometriosis: a pilot study. *Fertil Steril* 1999;72:505–508.

268. **Fedele L, Bianchi S, Zanconato G, et al.** Use of a levonorgestrel-releasing intrauterine device in the treatment of rectovaginal endometriosis. *Fertil Steril* 2001;75:485–488.

269. **Murphy AA, Zhou MH, Malkapuram S, et al.** RU486-induced growth inhibition of human endometrial cells. *Fertil Steril* 2000;74:1014–1019.

270. **Koide SS.** Mifepristone: auxilliary therapeutic use in cancer and related disorders. *J Reprod Med* 1998;43:551–560.

271. **Kettel LM, Murphy AA, Morales AJ, et al.** Treatment of endometriosis with the antiprogesterone mifepristone (RU486). *Fertil Steril* 1996;65:23–28.

272. **Kettel LM, Murphy AA, Morales AJ, et al.** Preliminary report on the treatment of endometriosis with low-dose mifepristone (RU486). *Am J Obstet Gynecol* 1998;178:1151–1156.

273. **Stoeckemann K, Hegele-Hartung C, Chwalisz K.** Effects of the progesterone antagonists onapristone (ZK 98 299) and ZK 136 799 on surgically induced endometriosis in intact rats. *Hum Reprod* 1995;10: 3264–3271.

274. **Fuhrmann U, Hess Stummp H, Cleve A, et al.** Synthesis and biological activity of a novel, highly potent progesterone receptor antagonist. *J Med Chem* 2000;43:5010–5016.

275. **Slayden OD, Chwalisz K, Brenner RM.** Reversible suppression of menstruation with progesterone antagonists in rhesus macaques. *Hum Reprod* 2001;8:1562–1574.

276. **Schlaff WD, Dugoff L, Damewood MD, et al.** Megestrol acetate for treatment of endometriosis. *Obstet Gynecol* 1990;75:646–648.

277. **Brosens IA, Verleyen A, Cornillie FJ.** The morphologic effect of short-term medical therapy of endometriosis. *Am J Obstet Gynecol* 1987;157:1215–1221.

278. **Fedele L, Bianchi S, Viezzoli T, et al.** Gestrinone versus danazol in the treatment of endometriosis. *Fertil Steril* 1989;51:781 785.

279. **Wingfield M, Healy DL.** Endometriosis: medical therapy. *Baillieres Clin Obstet Gynecol* 1993;7: 813–838.

280. **Hornstein MD, Gleason RE, Barbieri RL.** A randomized double-blind prospective trial of two doses of *gestrinone* in the treatment of endometriosis. *Fertil Steril* 1990;53:237–241.

281. **Dawood MY, Obasiulu CW, Ramos J, et al.** Clinical, endocrine, and metabolic effects of two doses of *gestrinone* in treatment of pelvic endometriosis. *Am J Obstet Gynecol* 1997;176:387–394.

282. **Gestrinone Italian Study Group.** *Gestrinone* versus a GnRHa for the treatment of pelvic pain associated with endometriosis: a multicenter, randomized, double-blind study. *Fertil Steril* 1996;66:911–919.

283. **Barbieri RL, Ryan KJ.** Danazol: endocrine pharmacology and therapeutic applications. *Am J Obstet Gynecol* 1981;141:453–463.

284. **Hill JA, Barbieri RL, Anderson DJ.** Immunosuppressive effects of danazol in vitro. *Fertil Steril* 1987;48:414–418.

285. **El-Roeiy A, Dmowski WP, Gleicher N, et al.** Danazol but not gonadotropin-releasing hormone agonists suppresses autoantibodies in endometriosis. *Fertil Steril* 1988:50;864–871.

286. **Ota H, Maki M, Shidara Y, et al.** Effects of danazol at the immunologic level in patients with adenomyosis, with special reference to autoantibodies: a multi-center cooperative study. *Am J Obstet Gynecol* 1992;167:481–486.

287. **Mori H, Nakagawa M, Itoh N, et al.** Danazol suppresses the production of interleukin-1b and tumor necrosis factor by human monocytes. *Am J Reprod Immunol* 1990;24:45–50.

288. **Braun DP, Gebel H, Rotman C, et al.** The development of cytotoxicity in peritoneal macrophages from women with endometriosis. *Fertil Steril* 1992;1203:1203–1210.

289. **Gelfand JA, Sherins RJ, Alling DW, et al.** Treatment of hereditary angioedema with danazol. *N Engl J Med* 1976;295:1444–1448.

290. **Ahn YS, Harrington WJ, Mylvaganam R, et al.** Danazol therapy for autoimmune hemolytic anemia. *Ann Intern Med* 1985;102:298–301.

291. **Agnello V, Pariser K, Gell J, et al.** Preliminary observations on danazol therapy of systemic lupus erythematosus: effect on DNA antibodies, thrombocytopenia and complement. *J Rheumatol* 1983;10:682–687.

292. **Schreiber AD, Chien P, Tomaski A, et al.** Effect of danazol in immune thrombocytopenic purpura. *N Engl J Med* 1987;316:503–508.

293. **Mylvaganam R, Ahn YS, Harrington WJ, et al.** Immune modulation by danazol in autoimmune thrombocytopenia. *Clin Immunol Immunopathol* 1987;42:281–287.

294. **Igarashi M, Iizuka M, Abe Y, et al.** Novel vaginal danazol ring therapy for pelvic endometriosis, in particular deeply infiltrating endometriosis. *Hum Reprod* 1998;13:1952–1956.

295. **Borroni R, Di Blasio AM, Gaffuri B, et al.** Expression of GnRH receptor gene in human ectopic endometrial cells and inhibition of their proliferation by leuprolide acetate. *Mol Cell Endocrinol* 2000;159:37–43.

296. **Sharpe-Timms KL, Zimmer RL, Jolliff WJ, et al.** GnRHa therapy alters activity of plasminogen activators, matrix metalloproteinases, and their inhibitors in rat models for adhesion formation and endometriosis: potential GnRHa regulated mechanisms reducing adhesion formation. *Fertil Steril* 1998;68:916–923.

297. **Barbieri RL.** Hormone treatment of endometriosis: the estrogen threshold hypothesis. *Am J Obstet Gynecol* 1992;166:740–745.

298. **Riis BJ, Christiansen C, Johansen JS, et al.** Is it possible to prevent bone loss in young women treated with luteinizing hormone-releasing agonists? *J Clin Endocrinol Metab* 1990;70:920–924.

299. **Hornstein MD, Surrey ES, Weisberg GW, et al.** Leuprolide acetate depot and hormonal add-back in endometriosis: a 12-month study. *Obstet Gynecol* 1998;91:16–24.

300. **Sillem M, Parviz M, Woitge HW, et al.** Add-back medrogestone does not prevent bone loss in premenopausal women treated with goserelin. *Exp Clin Endocrinol Diabetes* 1999;107:379–385.

301. **Taskin O, Uryan I, Yalcinoglu I, et al.** Effectiveness of tibolone on hypoestrogenic symptoms induced by goserelin treatment in patients with endometriosis. *Fertil Steril* 1997;67:40–45.

302. **Lindsay PC, Shaw RW, Bennink HJC, et al.** The effect of add-back treatment with tibolone (Livial) on patients treated with the GnRHa triptoreling (Decapeptyl). *Fertil Steril* 1996;65:342–348.

303. **Franke HR, van de Weijere PHM, Pennings TMM, et al.** Gonadotropin-releasing hormone agonist plus "add-back" hormone replacement therapy for treatment of endometriosis: a prospective randomized placebo-controlled double-blind trial. *Fertil Steril* 2000;74:534–539.

304. **Pierce SJ, Gazvani MR, Farquharson RG.** Long-term use of gonadotropin-releasing hormone analogs and hormone replacement therapy in the management of endometriosis: a randomized trial with a 6-year follow-up. *Fertil Steril* 2000;74:964–968.

305. **Tahara M, Matsuoka T, Yokoi T, et al.** Treatment of endometriosis with a decreasing dosage of gonadotropin-releasing hormone agonist (nafarelin): a pilot study with low-dose agonist therapy ("draw-back" therapy). *Fertil Steril* 2000;73:799–804.

306. **Yano S, Ikegami Y, Nakao K.** Studies on the effect of the new non-steroidal aromatase inhibitor fadrozole hydrochloride in an endometriosis model in rats. *Arzneimittelforschung* 1996;46:192–195.

307. **Kudoh M, Susaki Y, Ideyama Y, et al.** Inhibitory effects of a novel aromatase inhibitor, YM511, in rats with experimental endometriosis. *J Steroid Biochem Mol Biol* 1997;63:1–3.

308. **Takayama K, Zeitoun K, Gunby RT, et al.** Treatment of severe postmenopausal endometriosis with an aromatase inhibitor. *Fertil Steril* 1998;69:709–713.

309. **Buelke SJ, Bryant HU, Francis PC.** The selective estrogen receptor modulator, raloxifene: an overview of nonclinical pharmacology and reproductive and developmental testing. *Reprod Toxicol* 1998;12:217–221.

310. **D'Antonio M, Martelli F, Peano S, et al.** Ability of recombininant human TNF binding protein-1 (r-hTBP-1) to inhibit the development of experimentally induced endometriosis in rats. *J Reprod Immunol* 2000;48:81–98.

311. **D'Hooghe TM, Nugent N, Cuneo S, et al.** *Recombinant human TNF binding protein (r-hTBP-1) inhibits the development of endometriosis in baboons: a prospective, randomized, placebo- and drug-controlled study.* Accepted for oral presentation at the Annual Meeting of the American Society for Reproductive Medicine, Orlando, USA, October 22nd-24th 2001.

312. **Ingelmo JM, Quereda F, Acien P.** Intraperitoneal and subcutaneous treatment of experimental endometriosis with recombinant human interferon-alpha-2b in a murine model. *Fertil Steril* 1999;71:907–911.

313. **Keenan JA, Williams-Boyce PK, Massey PJ, et al.** Regression of endometrial explants in a rat model of endometriosis treated with immune modulators loxoribine and levamisole. *Fertil Steril* 2000;72:135–141.

314. **Abu JI, Konje JC.** Leukotrienes in gynaecology: the hypothetical value of anti-leukotriene therapy in dysmenorrhea and endometriosis. *Hum Reprod Update* 2000;6:200–205.

315. **Balasch J, Creus M, Fabregues F, et al.** Pentoxifylline versus placebo in the treatment of infertility associated with minimal or mild endometriosis: a pilot randomized clinical trial. *Hum Reprod* 1997;12:2046–2050.

316. **Bruner KL, Matrisian LM, Rodgers WH, et al.** Suppression of matrix metalloproteinases inhibits establishment of ectopic lesions by human endometrium in nude mice. *J Clin Invest* 1997;99:2851–2857.

317. **Telimaa S, Puolakka J, Ronnberg L, et al.** Placebo-controlled comparison of danazol and high-dose medroxyprogesterone acetate in the treatment of endometriosis. *Gynecol Endocrinol* 1987;1:13–23.

318. **Dlugi AM, Miller JD, Knittle J, and the Lupron Study Group.** Lupron depot (leuprolide acetate for depot suspension) in the treatment of endometriosis: a randomized, placebo-controlled, double-blind study. *Fertil Steril* 1990;54:419–427.

319. **Evers JLH.** The pregnancy rate of the no-treatment group in randomized clinical trials of endometriosis therapy. *Fertil Steril* 1989;52:906–909.

320. **Bayer SR, Seibel MM, Saffan DS, et al.** Efficacy of danazol treatment for minimal endometriosis in infertile women: a prospective randomized study. *J Reprod Med* 1988;33:179–183.

321. **Fedele L, Bianchi S, Marchini M, et al.** Superovulation with human menopausal gonadotrophins in the treatment of infertility associated with minimal or mild endometriosis: a controlled randomized study. *Fertil Steril* 1992;58:28–31.

322. **Thomas EJ, Cooke ID.** Successful treatment of asymptomatic endometriosis: does it benefit infertile women? *BMJ* 1987;294:1117–1119.

323. **Fedele L, Parazzini F, Radici E, et al.** Buserelin acetate versus expectant management in the treatment of infertility associated with endometriosis: a randomized clinical trial. *Am J Obstet Gynecol* 1992;166:1345–1350.

324. **Propst AM, Laufer M.** Endometriosis in adolescents. Incidence, diagnosis and treatment. *J Reprod Med* 1999;44:751–758.

325. **Fedele L, Bianchi S, DiNola G, et al.** The recurrence of endometriosis. *Ann N Y Acad Sci* 1994;734:358–364.

326. **Busacca M, Marana R, Caruana P, et al.** Recurrence of ovarian endometrioma after laparoscopic excision. *Am J Obstet Gynecol* 1999;180:519–523.

327. **Schindler AE, Foertig P, Kienle E, et al.** Early treatment of endometriosis with GnRH-agonists: impact on time to recurrence. *Eur J Obstet Gynecol* 2000;93:123–125.

328. **Waller KG, Shaw MD.** Gonadotropin-releasing hormone analogues for the treatment of endometriosis: long term follow-up. *Fertil Steril* 1993;59:511–515.

329. **Dmowski WP, Cohen MR.** Antigonadotropin (danazol) in the treatment of endometriosis: evaluation of posttreatment fertility and three-year follow-up data. *Am J Obstet Gynecol* 1978;130:41–48.

330. **Ghezzi F, Beretta P, Franchi M, et al.** Recurrence of endometriosis and anatomical location of the primary lesion. *Fertil Steril* 2001;75:136–140.

331. **Muzii L, Marana R, Caruana P, et al.** Postoperative administration of monophasic combined oral contraceptives after laparoscopic treatment of ovarian endometriomas: a prospective, randomized trial. *Am J Obstet Gynecol* 2000;183:588–592.

332. **Busacca M, Fedele L, Bianchi S, et al.** Surgical treatment of recurrent endometriosis. *Hum Reprod* 1998;13:2271–2274.

333. **Vercellini P, Trespidi L, Colombo A, et al.** A gonadotropin-releasing hormone agonist versus a low-dose oral contraceptive for pelvic pain associated with endometriosis. *Fertil Steril* 1993;60:75–79.

334. **Redwine DB.** Conservative laparoscopic excision of endometriosis by sharp dissection: life table analysis of reoperation and persistent of recurrent disease. *Fertil Steril* 1991;56:628–634.

335. **Tummon IS, Asher LS, Martin JRB, et al.** Randomized controlled trial of superovulation and insemination for infertility associated with minimal or mild endometriosis. *Fertil Steril* 1997;68:8–12.

336. **Nuojua HS, Tomas C, Bloigu R, et al.** Intrauterine insemination treatment in subfertility: an analysis of factors affecting outcome. *Hum Reprod* 1999;14:698–703.

337. **Omland AK, Tanbo T, Dale PO, et al.** Artificial insemination by husband in unexplained infertility compared with infertility associated with peritoneal endometriosis. *Hum Reprod* 1998;13:2602–2605.

338. **Hughes EG.** The effectiveness of ovulation induction and intrauterine insemination in the treatment of persistent infertility: a meta-analysis. *Hum Reprod* 1997;1865–1872.

339. **Simon C, Guttierez A, Vidal A, et al.** Outcome of patients with endometriosis in assisted reproduction: results from in-vitro fertilization and oocyte donation. *Hum Reprod* 1994;9:725–729.

340. **Arici A, Oral E, Bukulmez O, et al.** The effect of endometriosis on implantation: results from the Yale University *in vitro* fertilization and embryo transfer program. *Fertil Steril* 1996;65:603–607.

341. **Pellicer A, Valbuena D, Bauset C, et al.** The follicular endocrine environment in stimulated cycles of women with endometriosis: steroid levels and embryo quality. *Fertil Steril* 1998;69:1135–1141.

342. **Diaz I, Navarro J, Blasco L, et al.** Impact of stage III-IV endometriosis on recipients of sibling oocytes: matched case-control study. *Fertil Steril* 2000;74:31–34.

343. **Al Azemi M, Lopez BA, Steele J, et al.** Ovarian response to repeated controlled stimulation in IVF cycles in patients with ovarian endometriosis. *Hum Reprod* 2000;15:72–75.

344. **Chillik CF, Acosta AA, Garcia JE, et al.** The role of *in vitro* fertilization in infertile patients with endometriosis. *Fertil Steril* 1985;44:56–59.

345. **Matson PL, Yovich JL.** The treatment of infertility associated with endometriosis by *in vitro* fertilization. *Fertil Steril* 1986;46:432–434.

346. **Molloy D, Martin M, Speirs A, et al.** Performance of patients with a "frozen pelvis" in an *in vitro* fertilization program. *Fertil Steril* 1987;47:450–455.

347. **Yovich JL, Matson PL, Richardson PA, et al.** Hormone profiles and embryo quality in women with severe endometriosis treated by *in vitro* fertilization and embryo transfer. *Fertil Steril* 1988;50:249–256.

348. **Oehninger S, Acosta AA, Kreiner D, et al.** *In vitro* fertilization and embryo transfer (IVF/ET): an established and successful therapy for endometriosis. *J In Vitro Fertil Embryo Transf* 1988;5:248–256.

349. **Redwine DB.** Conservative laparoscopic excision of endometriosis by sharp dissection: life table analysis of reoperation and persistent of recurrent disease. *Fertil Steril* 1991;56:628–634.

350. **Dicker D, Goldman JA, Levy T, et al.** The impact of long-term gonadotrophin-releasing hormone analogue treatment on preclinical abortions in patients with severe endometriosis undergoing *in vitro* fertilization-embryo transfer. *Fertil Steril* 1992;57:597–600.

351. **Inoue M, Kobayashi Y, Honda I, et al.** The impact of endometriosis on the reproductive outcome of infertile patients. *Am J Obstet Gynecol* 1992;167:278–282.

352. **Tummon IS, Colwell KA, Mackinnon CJ, et al.** Abbreviated endometriosis-associated infertility correlates with *in vitro* fertilization success. *J In Vitro Fertil Embryo Transf* 1991;8:149–153.

353. **Wardle PG, Foster PA, Mitchell JD, et al.** Endometriosis and IVF: effect of prior therapy. *Lancet* 1986:276–277.

354. **Minguez Y, Rubio C, Bernal A, et al.** The impact of endometriosis in couples undergoing intracytoplasmic sperm injection. *Hum Reprod* 1997;12:2282–2285.

355. **Bukulmez O, Yarali H, Gurgan T.** The presence and extent of endometriosis do not effect clinical pregnancy rate and implantation rates in patients undergoing ICSI. *Eur J Obstet Gynecol Reprod Biol* 2001;96:102–107.

356. **Guzick DS, Yao YAS, Berga SL, et al.** Endometriosis impairs the efficacy of gamete intrafallopian transfer: results of a case-control study. *Fertil Steril* 1994;62:1186–1191.

357. **Metzger DA, Olive DL, Stohs GF, et al.** Association of endometriosis and spontaneous abortion: effect of control group selection. *Fertil Steril* 1986;45:18–22.

Novak's Gynecology, 13th Edition. Edited by J.S. Berek. Lippincott Williams & Wilkins, Philadelphia © 2002

27 Infertility

Mylene W. M. Yao
Daniel J. Schust

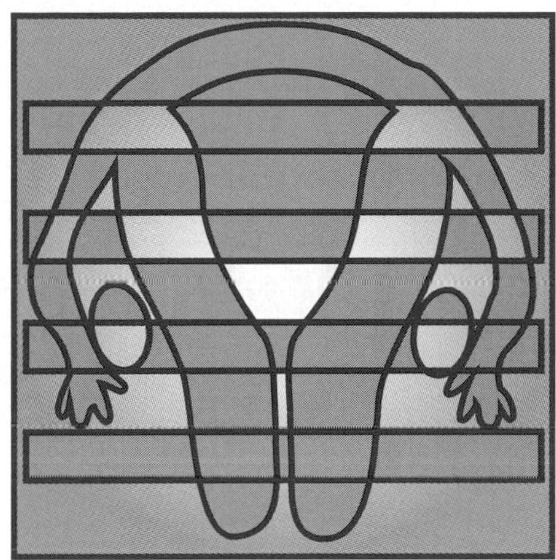

Infertility is defined as 1 year of unprotected intercourse without pregnancy. This condition may be further classified as *primary infertility,* in which no previous pregnancies have occurred, and *secondary infertility,* in which a prior pregnancy, although not necessarily a live birth, has occurred. *Fecundability* is the probability of achieving pregnancy within a single menstrual cycle, and *fecundity* is the probability of achieving a live birth within a single cycle. The fecundability of a normal couple has been estimated at 20% to 25% (1). **On the basis of this estimate, about 90% of couples should conceive after 12 months of unprotected intercourse.**

Infertility affects about 10% to 15% of reproductive-age couples in the United States. Despite the relatively stable prevalence of infertility in the United States, the use of infertility services has increased significantly. Between 1968 and 1984, the number of office visits for infertility increased nearly threefold to the current 1.6 million visits annually (2). There are several reasons for this increase. Recent media coverage of assistive reproductive technology (ART) and other fertility treatments has heightened awareness of the problem and its treatment; the aging of the post–World War II "baby boomers" has led to an increase in the number of reproductive-age women; and sociologic changes have led to delayed marriage with a consequent postponement of childbearing. Still, despite an increased awareness of available therapies, only 43% of infertile couples seek treatment, and only 24% seek specialized care. Fewer than 2% use *in vitro* fertilization (IVF) or other ART methods. The women most likely to obtain specialized treatment are 30 years of age or older, white, married, and of relatively high socioeconomic status (3).

Epidemiology

Data from the U.S. National Survey of Family Growth indicate that the prevalence of infertility among women who had not been surgically sterilized was 13.3% in 1965, 13.9% in 1982, and 13.7% in 1988 (4). In 1990, about 1 in 3 women in the United States reported 12 consecutive months of unprotected coitus without pregnancy at some time in her life (5).

A number of demographic variables, including age and socioeconomic status, have been associated with infertility. The delay in childbearing in the United States population has led to attempts to conceive by a higher percentage of women in the older reproductive age groups. **As a result, although the overall prevalence of infertility has not changed in the United States since 1965, the percentage of women with primary infertility has increased significantly.** In 1965, only one of six infertile women was nulliparous, whereas in 1988, more than half of infertile women had never been pregnant (6). The prevalence of infertility does not differ significantly among racial and ethnic groups. Although patients seeking treatment for infertility are predominantly of high socioeconomic status, infertility is more common among groups of relatively low socioeconomic status (6). Improved familiarity with and access to infertility services among the affluent and better-educated patients probably accounts for their greater use of these medical resources.

The Infertile Couple

Initial Visit

The physician's initial encounter with the infertile couple is the most important one because it sets the tone for subsequent evaluation and treatment. **The male partner should be present at this first visit because his history is a key component in the selection of diagnostic and therapeutic plans. It cannot be overemphasized that infertility is a problem of the couple. The presence of the male partner beginning with the initial evaluation involves him in the therapeutic process.** This essential involvement demonstrates that the physician is receptive to the male partner's needs as well as to those of the female partner, while allowing the male partner an opportunity to ask questions and to voice any concerns.

The physician should obtain a complete medical, surgical, and gynecologic history from the woman. Specifically, information regarding menstrual cyclicity, pelvic pain, and obstetric history is important. Risk factors for infertility, such as a history of pelvic inflammatory disease (PID), intrauterine device use, or pelvic surgery, should be reviewed. A history of intrauterine exposure to diethylstilbestrol (DES) is significant. In addition, questions should be asked about pituitary, adrenal, and thyroid function. A directed history, including past genital surgery, infections (including mumps orchitis), and previous genital trauma, should be obtained from the male partner. A history of occupational exposures that might affect the reproductive function of either partner is also important. Additionally, the interviewer should obtain information about coital frequency, dyspareunia, and sexual dysfunction.

The initial interview provides the physician with the opportunity to assess the emotional impact of infertility on the couple. It further gives the physician a chance to emphasize the emotional support available to the couple as they proceed with the diagnostic evaluation and suggested treatments. In some cases, referral to a trained social worker or psychologist at this point may be beneficial.

The physical examination of the female should be thorough, with particular attention given to height, weight, body habitus, hair distribution, thyroid gland, status with regard to galactorrhea, and findings of the pelvic examination. Referral of the male to a urologist for examination is often beneficial if historic information or subsequent evaluation suggests an abnormality. The initial encounter also gives the doctor the opportunity to outline the general causes of infertility and to discuss subsequent diagnostic and treatment plans. (Figs. 27.1 to 27.5).

Causes of Infertility

The main causes of infertility include the following:

1. Male factor

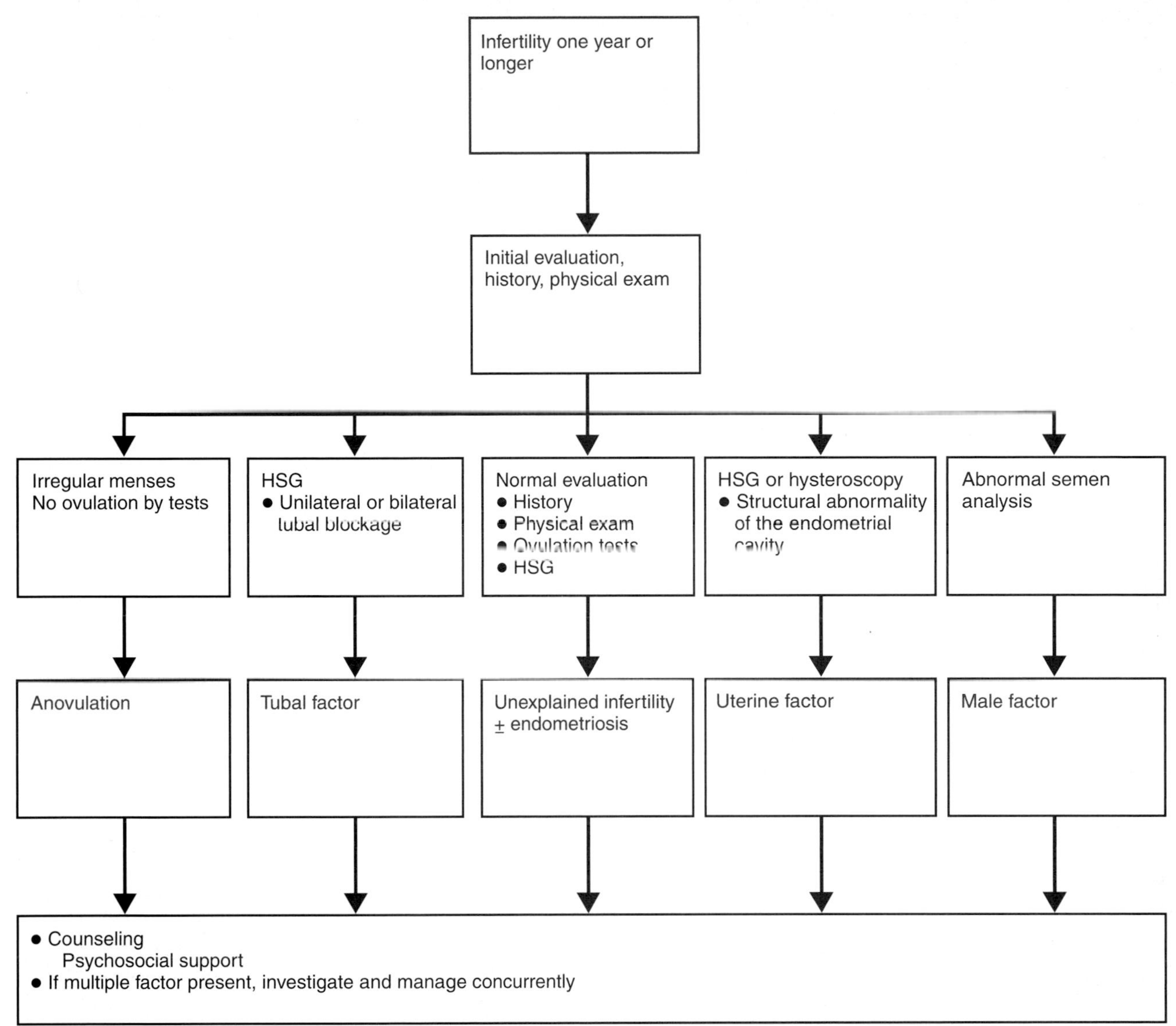

Figure 27.1 Diagnostic and treatment algorithm: infertility. (From **Yao M.** Clinical management of infertility. Washington, DC: The Advisory Board: 2000, with permission.)

2. Decreased ovarian reserve
3. Ovulatory disorders (ovulatory factor)
4. Tubal injury, blockage, or paratubal adhesions (including endometriosis with evidence of tubal or peritoneal adhesions)
5. Cervical and immunologic factors
6. Uterine factors
7. Conditions such as immunologic aberrations, infections, and serious systemic illnesses
8. Unexplained factors (including endometriosis with no evidence of tubal or peritoneal adhesions)

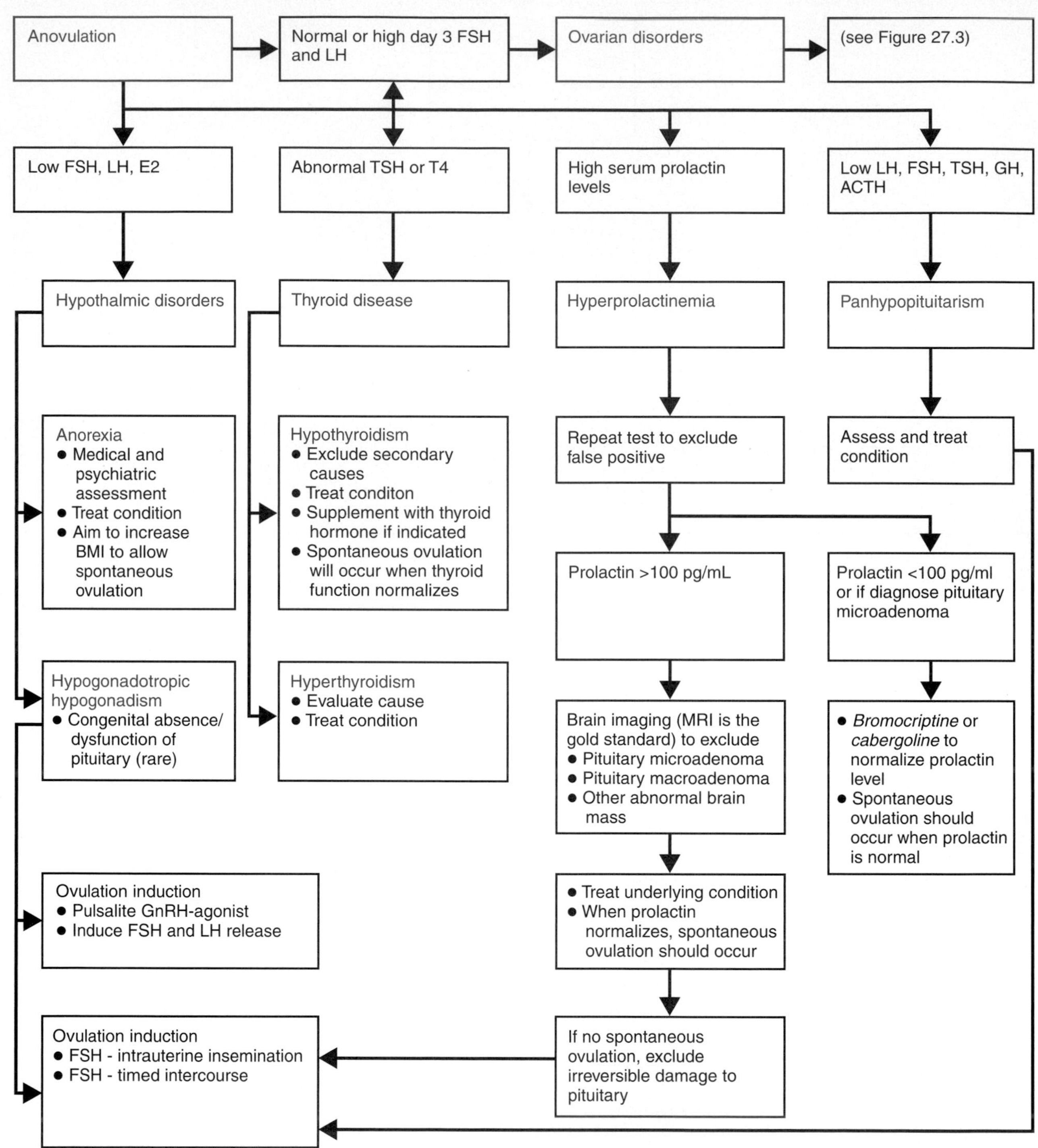

Figure 27.2 Diagnostic and treatment algorithm: anovulation. (From **Yao M.** Clinical management of infertility. Washington, DC: The Advisory Board: 2000, with permission.)

Factors from either or both partners may contribute to difficulties in conceiving; therefore, it is important to consider all possible diagnoses before pursuing invasive treatment. In some cases, no specific cause is detected despite an extensive and complete evaluation. The relative prevalence of the different causes of infertility varies widely among patient populations (Table 27.1).

Very few couples have absolute infertility, which can result from congenital or acquired irreversible loss of functional gametes in either partner or the absence of a uterus in the

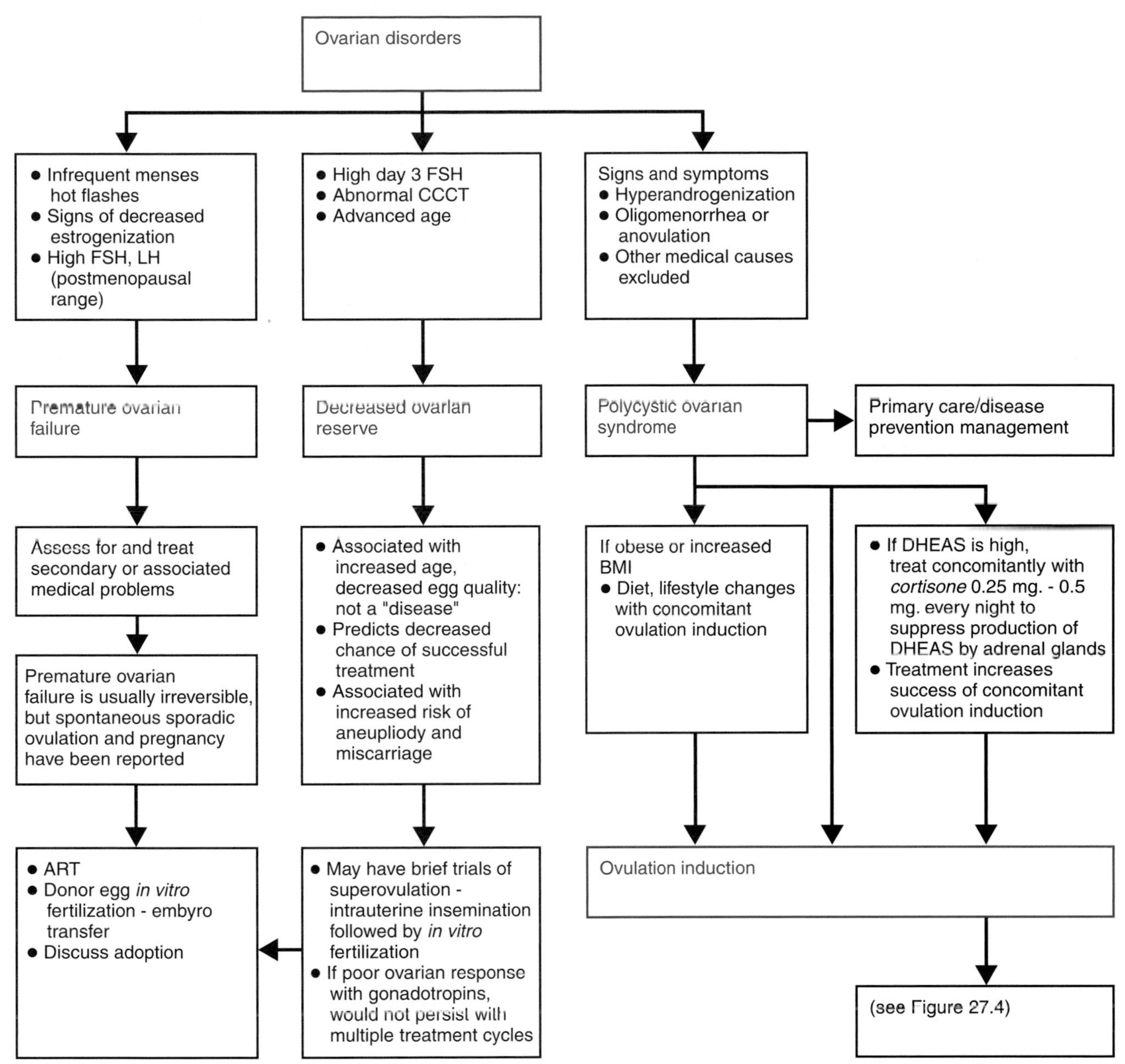

Figure 27.3 Diagnostic and treatment algorithm: ovarian disorders. (From **Yao M.** Clinical management of infertility. Washington, DC: The Advisory Board: 2000, with permission.)

female. These specific couples should be counseled regarding their options of adoption, the use of donor gametes, or surrogacy. Rather, most couples who have difficulty conceiving have subfertility. According to this fundamental concept, most couples could conceive spontaneously in time, but because of known or unidentifiable causes, their spontaneous fecundity rate is so low that medical management is warranted. Another reason to seek medical attention, particularly among older women, is that as time passes during unsuccessful spontaneous attempts, fecundability will be further compromised by increasing age and concomitantly decreasing ovarian reserve. Although identification of apparent causes of subfertility (such as anovulation or oligospermia) allows treatment to be targeted, effective empiric treatments greatly increase the chance of a pregnancy even when no distinct cause is identified. Overall, these treatments aim at increasing the probability of conception and implantation by optimizing gamete (sperm and oocyte) and uterine factors.

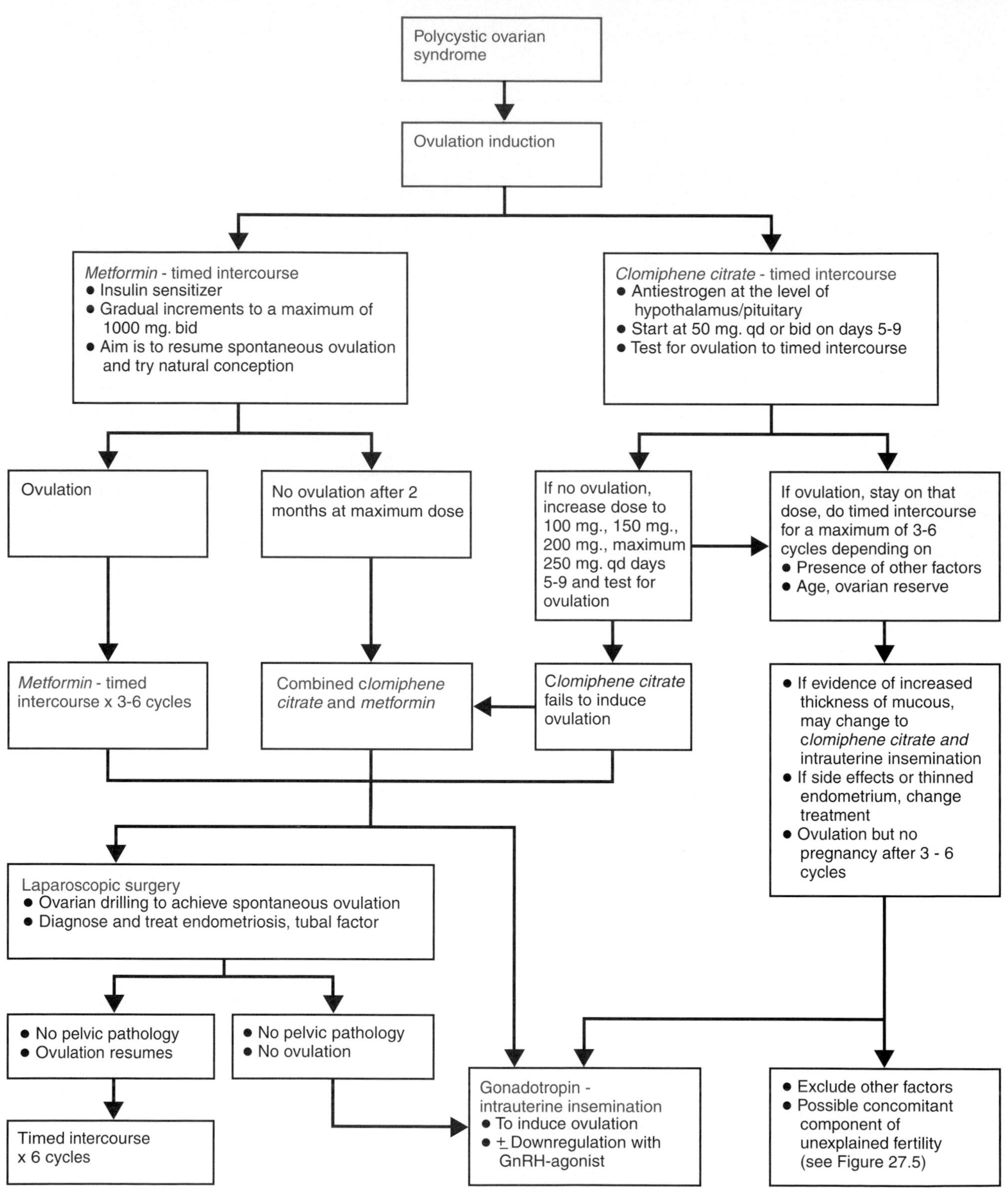

Figure 27.4 Diagnostic and treatment algorithm: polycystic ovarian syndrome. (From **Yao M.** Clinical management of infertility. Washington, DC: The Advisory Board: 2000, with permission.)

The next section of this chapter outlines causes of male and female infertility, their methods of diagnosis, and the specific treatments for these conditions. The basic investigations that should be performed before starting any infertility treatment are semen analysis, confirmation of ovulation, and the documentation of tubal patency by hysterosalpingography (HSG). Some treatments, especially ART, are indicated for more than one diagnosis

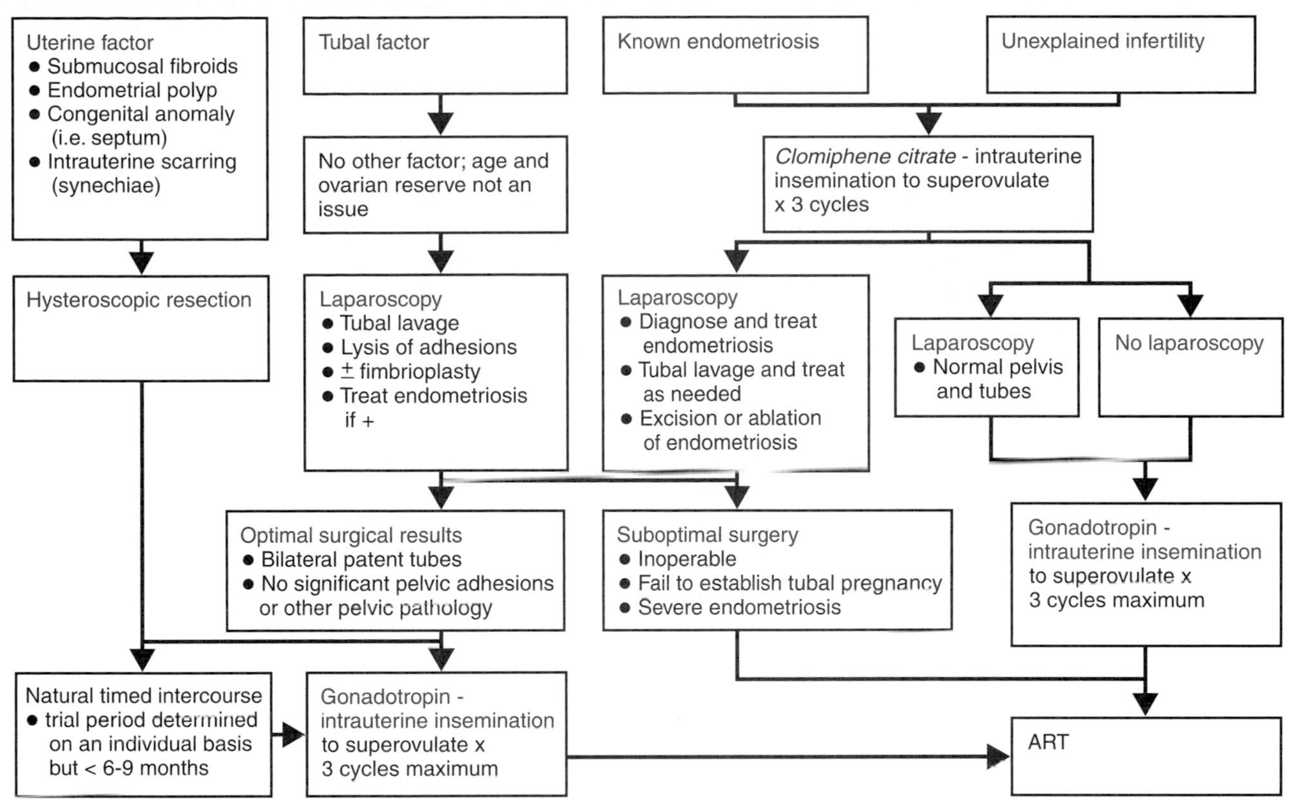

Figure 27.5 Diagnostic and treatment algorithm: tubal factor. (From **Yao M.** Clinical management of infertility. Washington, DC: The Advisory Board: 2000, with permission.)

and are discussed in greater detail. Often, more than one cause is identified in a couple. For this reason, multiple directions of investigation and treatment may be undertaken in parallel.

Male Factor

The combined effects of our increased understanding of genetic causes in male factor infertility and the efficacy of intracytoplasmic sperm injection (ICSI) in ART have revolutionized modern treatment of male factor infertility. For men, semen analysis as the initial step in their diagnostic evaluation for infertility is a fairly simple one. Semen analysis is inexpensive and noninvasive, and it should be included at the initiation of every infertility workup. The assessment of semen parameters, however, is confounded by controversies regarding the proper range of normal values. Semen parameters in normal fertile men vary considerably over time and may even drop below established norms; this situation makes evaluation of the male patient more difficult. The value and interpretation of the semen analysis and

Table 27.1. Causes of Infertility

Relative prevalence of the etiologies of infertility (%)	
Male factor:	25–40
Both male and female factors:	10
Female factor:	40–55
Unexplained infertility:	10
Approximate prevalence of the causes of infertility in the female (%)	
Ovulatory dysfunction:	30–40
Tubal or periotoneal factor:	30–40
Unexplained infertility:	10–15
Miscellaneous causes:	10–15

other tests for male infertility should be considered within the context of male reproductive physiology.

Physiology

The male reproductive tract consists of the testis, epididymis, vas deferens, prostate, seminal vesicles, ejaculatory duct, bulbourethral glands, and urethra. The testes contain two cell types: the Sertoli cells, which line the seminiferous tubules (the site of spermatogenesis), and the Leydig cells (the site of androgen synthesis). In the male, the pituitary gland secretes luteinizing hormone (LH) and follicle-stimulating hormone (FSH), which act on the testes. LH stimulates the synthesis and secretion of testosterone by the Leydig cells, and FSH stimulates the Sertoli cells to secrete inhibin. FSH and testosterone act on the seminiferous tubules to stimulate spermatogenesis. In humans, it takes about 75 days for spermatogonia to develop into mature sperm cells. The immature spermatogonia undergo mitotic division, giving rise to spermatocytes. These spermatocytes subsequently undergo meiosis, or reduction division, which gives rise to spermatids containing 23 (rather than 46) chromosomes. Upon maturation, spermatids become spermatozoa, which enter the epididymis, where they continue to mature and become progressively more motile during the 12 to 21 days that is required to traverse this tortuous structure.

During ejaculation, mature spermatozoa are released from the vas deferens along with fluid from the prostate, seminal vesicles, and bulbourethral glands. The semen released is a gelatinous mixture of spermatozoa and seminal plasma; however, it thins out 20 to 30 minutes after ejaculation by a process called *liquefaction.* Liquefaction occurs secondary to the presence of proteolytic enzymes within the prostatic fluid. The released spermatozoa are not usually capable of fertilization. Instead, a series of complex biochemical and electrical events, termed *capacitation,* must take place within the sperm's outer surface membrane before fertilization can occur. Normally, capacitation occurs in the cervical mucus; however, it can occur in physiologic media *in vitro*. Finally, as part of fertilization, the sperm must undergo the acrosome reaction, in which the release of enzymes of the inner acrosomal membrane results in the breakdown of the outer plasma membrane and its fusion with the outer acrosomal membrane (7). Several of the enzymes within the acrosome appear to be important to the sperm's penetration of the egg's zona pellucida. As the sperm penetrates the egg, it initiates a hardening of the zona pellucida (cortical reaction), which prevents penetration by additional sperm (8).

Semen Analysis

The basic semen analysis measures semen volume, sperm concentration, sperm motility, and sperm morphology. In addition, many laboratories measure pH, fructose levels, and white blood cell counts within the semen. Normal values suggested by the World Health Organization (WHO) are listed in Table 27.2 (18). These values represent only general guidelines, and normal values should be separately established by individual andrology laboratories.

Specimen Collection The method used for semen specimen collection is important to the achievement of accurate results. The optimal period of abstinence before semen collection

Table 27.2. Normal Values for a Semen Analysis

Volume	>2.0 mL
Sperm concentration	>20 million/mL
Motility	>50%
Morphology	>30% normal forms

From **World Health Organization.** *Laboratory manual for the examination of human semen and sperm-cervical interaction.* Cambridge, England: Cambridge University Press, 1992, with permission.

is unknown; however, because a decrease in sperm concentration is associated with frequent ejaculation, a period of 2 to 3 days usually is recommended. The specimen should be obtained by masturbation and collected in a clean container. Because of the presence of spermicidal agents, collection into condoms is generally unacceptable, although special sheaths that do not contain spermicides are available for semen collection. All semen specimens should be taken to the laboratory within 1 to 2 hours of collection. Even when collection is done under optimal circumstances, interpretation of the results of the semen analysis is complicated by wide differences in normal semen parameters (9), seasonal variability (10), variations among laboratories or technicians (11), and inconsistent correlation with fertility outcome. Semen parameters also may vary widely from one man to another and among men with proven fertility. In many circumstances, several specimens are necessary to verify an abnormality.

Sperm Volume **The normal ejaculated volume of semen is 2 to 6 mL.** Volumes may be abnormally low in cases of retrograde ejaculation, and high volumes usually reflect relatively long periods of abstinence or inflammation of the accessory glands. Absence of fructose or high pH may be associated with ejaculatory tract obstruction or seminal vesicle dysfunction.

Sperm Concentration **Sperm concentration or density is defined as the number of sperm per milliliter in the total ejaculate.** Establishing a lower limit of normal for sperm concentration is difficult. Historically, cutoffs of 60 million sperm per milliliter for normal fertility have been advocated, but most WHO laboratories recognize the value of 20 million sperm per milliliter as a lower limit of normal (12). Some have advocated concentrations of 5 million sperm per milliliter as a lower limit of normal (13,14).

Sperm Motility **An equally important parameter in the semen analysis is sperm motility, which is defined as the percentage of progressively motile sperm in the ejaculate.** Lower limits of normal vary considerably and depend on the local laboratory's experience. The WHO and many laboratories use a cutoff of 50% motility as the lower limit of normal; whereas others requires 40% motility as a criterion for defining male factor infertility (15). Computer-assisted semen analysis, in which computer-generated images of sperm specimens quantitate both sperm counts and sperm motility, may yield results very different from those of nonautomated semen analyses. Regardless of how motility is assessed, the interpretation of sperm motility—as with sperm concentration—is hampered by both significant variability among repeat samples obtained from a single individual and poor correlation of motility with fertility.

Sperm Morphology The WHO uses a fairly permissive visual assessment of sperm within a semen specimen to assess morphology values; greater than 30% normal forms is defined as acceptable. More stringent criteria have evolved from other sources. The strict Tygerberg criteria were introduced by Kruger and Menkveld in 1986 to assess sperm morphology (16). Using this system, the entire spermatozoon—including the head, midpiece, and tail—is assessed, and even mild abnormalities in head forms are classified as abnormal. Most sperm from normal men exhibit minor abnormalities when subjected to Tygerberg standards. One advantage of these strict criteria, however, is that the Tygerberg classification correlates with prognosis in IVF treatment. For example, greater than 14% normal morphology is associated with normal rates of fertilization in IVF programs; 4% to 14% normal morphology is associated with a "good prognosis." Values of less than 4% normal sperm morphology are associated with poor prognosis for fertilization and pregnancy in IVF (17). In some studies, this sperm morphology classification has also been found to be predictive of pregnancy outcomes after intrauterine insemination (IUI) treatment, especially when the total motile sperm count is less than 1×10^6 (18). The disparity in assessment criteria for semen morphology mandates that to interpret semen analysis results properly, the clinician must thoroughly understand the methodology used by the local andrology laboratory.

White Blood Cells Although measurements of semen volume, sperm concentration, sperm motility, and sperm morphology make up the standard semen analysis, some laboratories also report numbers of round cells. These cells, which may be lymphocytes, can signify the presence of prostatitis or, alternatively, may actually be immature germ cells. These two cell types can be distinguished by an immunoperoxidase staining technique that identifies leukocytes (Endtz test) (19). The WHO views ejaculates with more than 5 million round cells per milliliter or more than 1 million leukocytes per milliliter as abnormal (20); however, the prognostic significance of leukocytes in the semen is controversial. The presence of immature sperm cells in the ejaculate suggests a defect in spermatogenesis and, therefore, may signify a relatively poor prognosis for fertilization (21). Although the standard semen analysis and associated tests provide a fairly reasonable picture of semen quality, they yield little information about sperm function. Consequently, several tests of sperm function have been devised in an effort to assess the physiologic properties of sperm and thereby predict the likelihood of fertilization of normal oocytes.

Sperm Penetration Assay The most commonly used test of sperm function is the *sperm penetration assay* (SPA), or hamster egg penetration test (22). This test attempts to measure the ability of an individual patient's sperm to undergo capacitation (i.e., the acrosome reaction), to fuse with and penetrate the oocyte membrane, and to undergo nuclear decondensation. In the SPA, golden hamsters are superovulated, and their eggs are collected and treated with enzymes to remove the cumulus and zona pellucida. Meanwhile, sperm are isolated from the patient's semen and placed in a protein-rich environment that promotes capacitation. Sperm from normal fertile men are used as positive controls. After this incubation, the zona-free eggs are exposed to patient and control sperm. The presence of one or more swollen sperm heads within the hamster oocyte after exposure to sperm demonstrates penetration. Most laboratories report the percentage of eggs successfully penetrated; however, some laboratories count the number of penetrations per egg (usually two or more is considered normal). Cutoff values for the lower limit of normal in the SPA differ remarkably among laboratories.

The prognostic value of the SPA has been controversial almost since its inception. On the basis of a metaanalysis of the SPA, the test does not discriminate between fertile and infertile men (23). The value of the test as a predictor of success in IVF has been no less controversial. In most evaluations of the male partner, the SPA offers little definitive information; however, it may uncover sperm abnormalities in couples with otherwise unexplained infertility.

Several other tests attempt to correlate sperm function with fertility prognosis. The human zona-binding assay (the *Hemizona test*) examines the ability of the sperm to bind to zona. In this assay, human zona are bisected; half of the zona is exposed to the patient's sperm, and half is exposed to sperm from a known fertile donor control (24). Results compare the binding ability of samples of patients to those of controls. The hypoosmotic swelling test examines the normality of the sperm tail. When placed in a hypoosmotic solution of sodium citrate and fructose, the normal sperm tail swells and coils; when there is an abnormality in fluid transport across the tail membrane, the sperm tail fails to swell (25). To detect the acrosome reaction, some investigators have used monoclonal antibodies (26), whereas others have measured adenosine triphosphate (ATP) content in the semen (27). These functional tests should be considered experimental until more definitive evidence demonstrates their utility in clinical settings.

Further Evaluation If abnormalities in the semen are detected, further evaluation of the male partner by a urologist is indicated to diagnose the defect. Table 27.3 lists the differential diagnoses for male factor infertility (40). Several groups have attempted to assess the distribution of male infertility diagnoses; two such distributions are shown in Table 27.4 (24,28). The first is the result of a WHO study of 7,057 men with complete diagnoses based on the WHO standard investigation of the infertile couple (28). The figures include data from cases in which the male partner was normal and the presumed cause of the couple's infertility was a female factor. The second distribution is the result of a

Table 27.3. Etiologic Factors in Male Infertility

Pretesticular	Testicular
Endocrine	*Genetic*
Hypogonadotropic hypogonadism	Klinefelter's syndrome
Coital disorders	Y chromosome deletions
Erectile dysfunction	Immotile cilia syndrome
Psychosexual	*Congenital*
Endocrine, neural, or vascular	Cryptorchidism
Ejaculatory failure	*Infective (orchitis)*
Psychosexual	*Antispermatogenic agents*
After genitourinary surgery	Heat
Neural	Chemotherapy
Drug related	Drugs
	Irradiation
Posttesticular	*Vascular*
Obstructive	Torsion
Epididymal	Varicocele
Congenital	*Immunologic*
Infective	*Idiopathic*
Vasal	
Genetic: cystic fibrosis	
Acquired: vasectomy	
Epididymal hostility	
Epididymal asthenozoospermia	
Accessory gland infection	
Immunologic	
Idiopathic	
Postvasectomy	

From **De Kretser DM.** Male infertility. *Lancet* 1997;349:787–790, with permission.

study of 425 subfertile male patients (24). Although the two studies represent different populations (one is from a study of couples, the other from a urologic practice) and differ in their distribution of male infertility diagnoses, idiopathic male factor and varicocele predominate. Other anatomic and endocrine causes occur less frequently.

The widely accepted concept of a global decline in sperm counts needs to be reassessed (9,30). A number of recent analyses reported no decrease in sperm counts over time (31–33). Geographic differences in the results of semen analyses do seem to exist, but a global trend toward decreasing semen quality does not (34–36). Furthermore, the rate of male factor infertility has not increased significantly in recent decades. Thus, even if semen

Table 27.4. Frequency of Some Etiologies in Male Factor Infertility

Cause	Percentage	Cause	Percentage
No demonstrable cause	48.5	Varicocele	37.4
Idiopathic abnormal semen	26.4	Idiopathic	25.4
Varicocele	12.3	Testicular failure	9.4
Infectious factors	6.6	Obstruction	6.1
Immunologic factors	3.1	Cryptorchidism	6.1
Other acquired factors	2.6	Low semen volume	4.7
Congenital factors	2.1	Semenagglutination	3.1
Sexual factors	1.7	Semen viscosity	1.9
Endocrine disturbances	0.6	Other	5.9
TOTAL	103.9[a]		100

[a] More than 100% because of multiple factors.

From **The ESHRE CAPRI Workshop Group.** Male sterility and subfertility: guidelines for management. *Hum Reprod* 1994;9:1260–1264, and **Burkman LJ, Cobbington CC, Franken DR, et al.** The hemizona assay (HZA): development of a diagnostic test for the binding of human spermatozoa to the human hemizona pellucida to predict fertilization potential. *Fertil Steril* 1988;49:688–697, with permission.

characteristics are changing, these changes do not appear to be having a dramatic clinical effect. Nevertheless, exposures to environmental toxins may certainly be harmful to sperm, and the incidence of some exposures (e.g., phytoestrogens) may be on the rise. Marijuana and cocaine use can reduce sperm concentration (37,38). Certain drugs, such as anabolic steroids, chemotherapeutic agents, cimetidine, erythromycin, nitrofurans, spironolactone, sulfasalazine, and tetracycline, also may reduce semen parameters. Finally, commonly ingested agents present in cigarettes and coffee have been associated with diminished semen quality (39).

Treatment

Treatment of male factor infertility may be classified as medical, surgical, or ART-related therapies. Further, the diagnosis and treatment of azoospermia (no sperm on semen analysis) will be discussed separately from other forms of male factor infertility.

Medical therapies for male factor infertility are severely limited. Medical correction of underlying treatable endocrine or infectious causes of subfertility tends to be efficacious. These conditions may include sexually transmitted diseases, thyroid disorders, and other rare causes of male infertility. Clomiphene citrate, an estrogen agonist and partial antagonist, has often been used to treat male infertility of idiopathic origin. Clomiphene citrate acts on the hypothalamic–pituitary axis and, in men, increases serum levels of LH, FSH, and testosterone (41). Although efficacy of clomiphene for male factor infertility is controversial, most studies have shown little improvement in semen parameters and no improvement in pregnancy rates (42). However, severe idiopathic male factor infertility has been treated with pure FSH, with no notable improvement in semen parameters but a significant increase in fertilization rates during ART (43).

Surgical approaches to male factor infertility include procedures to correct varicocele, artificial insemination, and ART.

Varicocele

A varicocele is an abnormal dilation of the veins within the spermatic cord. Varicoceles nearly always occur on the left side, presumably because of the direct insertion of the spermatic vein into the renal vein on that side. The pathophysiologic effects of varicocele on testicular function are uncertain but appear to be mediated by an associated rise in testicular temperature or a reflux of toxic metabolites from the left adrenal or renal veins (44). In either event, the effect on sperm production is bilateral. Our understanding of the role of varicoceles in infertility is complicated by two issues: the prevalence of varicoceles in the normal male population and the efficacy of varicocele repair in infertile men. One WHO study found varicocele to be present in 25.4% of men with abnormal semen analyses, as opposed to 11.7% of men with normal semen (45). This study failed to demonstrate a difference in the frequency of spontaneous pregnancies among couples in which the men did or did not have varicoceles. The presence of a varicocele was, however, associated with decreased testicular volume, impaired semen quality, and a reduction in serum testosterone levels.

Varicocele repair involves interruption of the internal spermatic vein and is commonly performed in the 40% of infertile men with clinically evident varicoceles. Currently, it is performed as an outpatient procedure and may involve laparoscopy, open surgery, or the injection of embolizing agents. Despite its widespread use, the therapeutic benefits of varicocele repair have remained controversial. Two multicenter trials have shown that pregnancy rates are significantly increased after varicocelectomy (46,47). However, the validity of the control groups in each of these trials has been criticized (48). A more recent metaanalysis on four randomized, controlled trials involving a total of 385 patients failed to demonstrate significantly altered pregnancy rates after varicocelectomy (48–52).

Artificial Insemination

Artificial insemination encompasses a variety of procedures. All involve the placement of whole semen or processed sperm into the female reproductive tract, which permits sperm–oocyte interaction in the absence of intercourse. The placement of whole semen into the vagina as a mode of fertility treatment is now rarely performed. Exceptions include cases of severe coital dysfunction, including those involving severe hypospadias, retrograde ejaculation, erectile abnormalities, and psychosocial dysfunction precluding intercourse. Currently, all of the common forms of artificial insemination involve processed sperm obtained from the male partner or a donor before its use. Artificial insemination has mainly been used to treat unexplained infertility (usually combined with superovulation) and male factor infertility. The efficacy of each type of insemination method should be assessed separately for each of these two diagnoses.

Types of Insemination for Unexplained Infertility Many techniques for artificial insemination have been described. Of intracervical, intrauterine, intraperitoneal, and intrafollicular insemination and fallopian tube sperm perfusion, only the first two methods have been routinely employed. **Intrauterine insemination (IUI) is the best studied and most widely practiced of all the insemination techniques.** It involves placement of about 0.3 mL of washed, processed, and concentrated sperm into the intrauterine cavity by transcervical catheterization. In contrast with IUI, intracervical insemination may be performed either with unwashed or with processed specimens. The success rates with intracervical insemination are consistently lower than those with IUI (53).

Fallopian tube sperm perfusion (FSP) differs from IUI in that a large volume of washed sperm (about 4 mL) is injected into the intrauterine cavity. This is a more expensive procedure because larger volumes of media are required during sperm processing. Technical performance of FSP may be complicated by efflux of sperm through the vagina during the intrauterine injection of such large volumes of fluid. Among several techniques of efflux prevention, use of an intrauterine Foley catheter with balloon inflation is most commonly described. Although many have demonstrated that fallopian sperm perfusion does not offer any general advantage over IUI (54–57), its benefit in the treatment of unexplained infertility remains controversial. Several prospective randomized trials have reported higher pregnancy rates among patients with unexplained infertility in cycles treated with FSP compared with those using IUI (58–61). One recent metaanalysis found that FSP significantly improves pregnancy rates in patients with unexplained infertility undergoing controlled ovarian hyperstimulation (COH)/insemination with an odds ratio (OR) of 1.9 and a 95% confidence interval (CI) of 1.2 to 3 (60) (see *Controlled Ovarian Hyperstimulation*).

Direct intraperitoneal insemination involves the injection of washed, processed sperm into the intraperitoneal cavity by puncture of the posterior vaginal cul-de-sac. Evidence from prospective randomized trials showed that direct intraperitoneal insemination offers no advantage over IUI (62–65). Intrafollicular insemination as a treatment of male factor infertility has also been reported (66), but in a series of 50 patients with unexplained infertility, only one intrauterine pregnancy resulted (67). Its low efficacy has deterred further investigation of this technique. In summary, IUI is the best-studied insemination technique, with proven superiority to intracervical insemination in the treatment of unexplained infertility (53). FSP appears to be a viable alternative to IUI with COH/insemination in couples with unexplained infertility. However, the potential increase in pregnancy rates using FSP over IUI is unlikely to be as great as that of IVF/ICSI over IUI. Therefore, although COH/FSP may be chosen instead of COH/IUI in a center where FSP gives a higher pregnancy rate, there is no benefit to switch from COH/IUI to COH/FSP after three cycles of failed COH/IUI in patients with unexplained infertility. IVF/ICSI remains the best available treatment option in patients with unexplained infertility who have not become pregnant with COH/IUI treatment.

Processing Semen Two important issues regarding the use of artificial insemination procedures are the mode of semen processing and the number and timing of inseminations. Many protocols have been developed for sperm preparation. Seminal fluid usually is prevented from reaching the intrauterine cavity and intraabdominal space by the cervical barrier. The introduction of seminal fluid past this barrier may be associated with severe uterine cramping or anaphylactoid reactions, possibly mediated by seminal factors such as prostaglandins. Thus, protocols for processing whole semen include the washing of specimens to remove seminal factors and to isolate pure sperm. Some semen preparation methods attempt to enhance sperm motility or morphology further by using additional separation protocols. These methods include centrifugation through density gradients, sperm migration protocols, and differential adherence procedures. Finally, phosphodiesterase inhibitors, such as pentoxiphylline, have been used during semen processing in an attempt to enhance sperm motility, fertilization capacity, and acrosome reactivity for IVF procedures (68).

IUI as Treatment of Male Factor Infertility Studies of the efficacy of IUI in the treatment of male factor infertility have been generally difficult to assess because of variations in inclusion criteria. Further, sperm function tests are not consistently used in these studies, nor is their use standardized. Considering these limitations, the benefits of IUI in male factor infertility have been accepted because IUI appears to result in higher pregnancy rates than natural intercourse or intracervical insemination (OR, 2.20;95% CI, 1.43 to 3.39) (69). However, the IUI pregnancy rates are generally lower in couples with male factor infertility than in couples with unexplained infertility (4.8% versus 11.6%) (69). In a retrospective analysis of 1,841 couples undergoing 4,056 cycles of IUI for male factor infertility, pregnancy rates were found to be related to total motile sperm count. Optimal pregnancy rates (>8.2% per cycle) were reached with initial total motile sperm counts of greater than or equal to 5.0×10^6. Higher counts did not necessarily yield higher pregnancy rates. The minimal total motile sperm count that resulted in a pregnancy was 1.6×10^6 (70).

Some couples with male factor infertility fail treatment with artificial insemination, and some have initial semen parameters that make insemination a suboptimal approach. In these couples, use of ART, especially with ICSI, may be superior treatment options. The efficacy of ICSI in ART allows almost all cases of male factor infertility to be highly treatable. ICSI only requires that viable sperm be present. Therefore, ICSI should be considered if the total motile sperm count is less than 0.5×10^6 because the IUI success rates are extremely low with such sperm counts (71). Finally, ICSI should be recommended after a maximum of three IUI cycles have failed in a couple with male factor infertility.

Azoospermia: Classification and Treatment

Azoospermia is the absence of spermatozoa in the ejaculate. Azoospermia is found on semen analysis in about 5% of all couples being investigated for infertility (72), and its incidence is 10% to 20% among infertile men who have abnormal semen analysis (73). Traditionally, azoospermia has been classified as obstructive or nonobstructive. However, an increased understanding of the various etiologies of azoospermia and treatment advances using surgical sperm retrieval and ART have prompted a reclassification. The new classification system, advocated by Sharif and others, may better reflect the etiology, prognosis, and treatment of azoospermia (74–76). It separates azoospermic patients into those with pretesticular, testicular, and posttesticular causes.

Pretesticular Azoospermia

Pretesticular azoospermia represents those conditions in which the hypothalamic–pituitary axis fails to stimulate spermatogenesis within the testis. Congenital, acquired, and idiopathic etiologies of hypogonadotropic hypogonadism are included in this category. A full endocrine history, including information on puberty and growth and a review of endocrine systems, should guide the physician in the evaluation of the hypogonadotropic hypogonadal patient. Laboratory investigations of particular benefit in this population include measurement of serum LH, FSH, testosterone, and prolactin levels and imaging of the pituitary gland. Low levels of gonadotropins (LH and FSH) and low serum levels of testosterone are characteristic.

Hormonal treatment of hypogonadotropic hypogonadism has been conclusively demonstrated to be efficacious. In fact, pulsatile gonadotropin-releasing hormone (GnRH) therapy is both conceptually indicated and effective in infertile men with hypothalamic dysfunction (77), including those patients with Kallmann's syndrome. Infertile males with hypogonadotropic hypogonadism secondary to panhypopituitarism also may respond to GnRH therapy (78). An alternative treatment uses human chorionic gonadotropin (hCG), 1,000 to 2,500 IU twice a week, with the dose titrated to maintain serum testosterone and estradiol levels within the normal range. Treatment with hCG is then combined with human menopausal gonadotropin (hMG), which is given at a dose of 150 IU three times weekly (79,80). Spermatogenesis and pregnancy can be achieved in up to 80% to 88% of patients after 1 year of therapy (79,80).

Testicular Azoospermia

Gonadal failure is the hallmark of testicular azoospermia. Causes of this condition may be congenital or genetic (e.g., Klinefelter's syndrome, microdeletion of Y chromosome), acquired (e.g., radiation therapy, chemotherapy, testicular torsion, or mumps orchitis), or developmental (e.g., testicular maldescent). The latter disorder may be associated most closely with male factor infertility in the absence of complete testicular azoospermia. A large observational cohort study suggested that infertility was, in fact, associated with congenital bilaterally maldescended testes, but that men with congenital unilaterally maldescended testes did not have decreased fertility when compared with controls (81).

Men with hypergonadotropic hypogonadism (elevated levels of LH and FSH with low serum levels of testosterone) **generally have primary gonadal failure.** A karyotype should be obtained in such cases to detect chromosomal abnormalities such as Klinefelter's syndrome (47,XXY). Acquired causes of primary gonadal failure are usually evident on history, but they should be confirmed by assessment of the serum hormonal profile and biopsy. If the diagnosis of gonadal failure is confirmed on biopsy, endocrine therapy is contraindicated.

It is becoming increasingly evident that some cases of male factor infertility that have previously been categorized as idiopathic are actually the result of genetic defects on the Y chromosome. The two most commonly implicated candidate gene families are the RNA-binding motif (RBM) and the "deleted in azoospermia" (DAZ) families, but microdeletions at various loci on the Y chromosome have been described. For example, microdeletions in Yq11.23 have been found in 10% to 20% of men with idiopathic azoospermia or severe oligospermia (82,83). In another study involving 200 infertile men, 7% were found to have microdeletions in the Y chromosome (84). Semen analyses in affected men varied between oligospermia and azoospermia. Interestingly, 2% of fertile men also have microdeletions in the Y chromosome. These microdeletions can be transmitted to the male offspring, who may then also suffer from infertility. Therefore, screening for genetic causes is indicated in nonacquired cases of testicular azoospermia so that proper genetic counseling can be provided before treatment. Treatment is focused on surgical retrieval of spermatozoa with subsequent fertilization of the oocyte by ICSI. These approaches have made fertility possible for some men with testicular azoospermia.

Intracytoplasmic Sperm Injection ICSI is a micromanipulation technique commonly used in some ART procedures. It was first reported to result in human pregnancies in 1992 (85). ICSI is performed to increase the fertilization rate of oocytes retrieved during ART. The procedure involves stripping the aspirated cumulus complex of all surrounding granulosa cells, so that micromanipulation can be performed on the egg itself. A holding pipette is used to stabilize the egg while an injection pipette is used to insert a viable sperm into the cytoplasm of the egg (ooplasm). This procedure is thought to bypass some of the physiologic events, such as capacitation and the acrosome reaction, that are normally required for fertilization *in vivo*.

In general, ICSI has allowed couples with male factor infertility to achieve ART pregnancy outcomes that are comparable with those of couples with non–male factor infertility using conventional IVF treatment. The indications of ICSI have evolved since its introduction. They will most likely continue to evolve as more is learned about risks and benefits of ICSI. One absolute indication for ICSI is severe male factor infertility as demonstrated by total progressively motile sperm counts (0.5×10^6/mL and <3% normal morphology according to strict Tygerberg criteria) (71). Sperm counts of less than 0.5×10^6/mL are associated with poor fertilization rates in IVF, and this finding alone is also an indication for ICSI (86). Other indications for ICSI include the sole presence of spermatozoa lacking an acrosome or those that are completely immotile, as well as the use of surgically recovered epididymal or testicular sperm. Other absolute indications for ICSI are non–male factor–related and include a history of two previous fertilization failures with conventional IVF and the fertilization of oocytes before preimplantation genetic diagnosis (87). The benefit of combined IVF/ICSI in ART for unexplained infertility also is described under *Unexplained Infertility*.

Micromanipulation is a highly skilled technique. When performed by specially trained embryologists, the immediate risk for damaging the manipulated oocyte is less than 10% (71). Normal physiologic processes—capacitation, zona binding, and penetration of the oolemma—are bypassed by the spermatozoa used in ICSI. Because the particular spermatazoa used for ICSI might otherwise be incapable of fertilization, concerns have been voiced regarding possible increased risks for congenital abnormalities among ICSI offspring. Several large series have followed 1,987 (88), 1,139 (89), and 730 (90) children born after ICSI. Each has reported no increase in major or minor congenital malformations among offspring produced by ICSI when compared with the general population (88–90) and when adjusted for multiple gestation (89). However, an increased incidence of sex chromosome karyotypic abnormalities (88,91) and hypospadias (89) has been suggested. Because the prevalence of sex chromosome karyotypic abnormalities and other genetic etiologies is increased in infertile men with severe oligospermia or azoospermia, genetic counseling should be offered before treatment with ART (92).

Posttesticular Azoospermia

In posttesticular azoospermia, the hypothalamic–pituitary axis and spermatogenesis are normal. No sperm appear in the ejaculate secondary to congenital absence or obstruction of the vas deferens or ejaculatory ducts, acquired obstruction of these ducts, or ductal dysfunctions, including retrograde ejaculation. Although low seminal pH (6.7 to 8.0) or low seminal fructose may signal the congenital absence or obstruction of the vas deferens, the diagnosis is confirmed by vasography. In some cases, testicular biopsy may be indicated to differentiate between primary testicular damage and outflow obstruction. Congenital bilateral absence of the vas deferens (CABVD) is found in 1% to 2% of infertile men and 95% of men with cystic fibrosis (93). Common mutations of the cystic fibrosis transmembrane conductance regulator gene *(CFTR),* which encodes a cyclic adenosine monophosphate (cAMP)-regulated chloride channel, can be found in some infertile men with CABVD, despite the absence of clinical symptoms of cystic fibrosis. Therefore, screening for mutations in the *CFTR* gene is indicated if men with CABVD plan to undergo sperm retrieval and ICSI in order to conceive using their own sperm. One cost-effective screening method addressing this problem involves screening the female partner for the three most common mutations in the *CFTR* gene. If negative, the couple has a risk of less than 1 in 1,500 for conceiving a child with cystic fibrosis, regardless of the paternal genotype (40).

Prior vasectomy is probably the most common cause of posttesticular azoospermia in infertile men. The reversal of vasectomy by microsurgical vasovasostomy is quite effective. In one study, vas deferens patency was obtained in 86% of cases, and pregnancy was achieved in 52% of cases after primary procedures (94). Rates of patency and pregnancy vary inversely with the length of time from vasectomy. For those patients with azoospermia 3 months after the reversal procedure, either the reanastomosis has failed or the epididymis is obstructed. Repeat vasovasostomy is associated with patency rates of 75% and pregnancy rates of 43% (94).

Epididymal obstruction is best diagnosed by vasography or documentation of normal spermatogenesis on testicular biopsy. There are two approaches to the treatment of posttesticular obstruction if the use of donor sperm is not being considered. Epididymal aspiration proximal to the obstruction may be used in cases of epididymal or vas deferens obstruction in order to obtain sperm for use in ART. Alternatively, microsurgical vasoepididymostomy is associated with patency rates of 70% and postoperative pregnancy rates of 44% at 1 year if no other infertility factor is present (95).

Some men with reduced semen volume may have retrograde ejaculation, in which sperm is propelled into the bladder during ejaculation rather than through the urethra. This diagnosis can be confirmed by examination of a postejaculatorily voided or catheterized urine specimen. This condition occurs in rare cases of patients with diabetes mellitus, in certain neurologic conditions, and after bladder or prostatic surgery. For subfertile men with retrograde ejaculatory dysfunction, α-adrenergic agonists such as phenylephrine have been reported to strengthen internal urethral sphincter tone (96). Sperm may also be isolated from the neutralized urine of men with retrograde ejaculation and processed for insemination or for ART (97).

Surgical Sperm Recovery for ICSI Among the many surgical methods for sperm recovery, the most widely described are microsurgical epididymal sperm aspiration (MESA), percutaneous epididymal sperm aspiration (PESA), testicular sperm extraction (TESE), and percutaneous testicular sperm fine-needle aspiration (TESA, also called *fine-needle aspiration,* or FNA) (98). The choice of surgical sperm recovery method depends on the underlying diagnosis, whether the goal of the procedure is diagnostic or therapeutic, and whether isolated sperm will be used immediately or will be cryopreserved.

TESA may be used to recover sperm in cases of posttesticular azoospermia (in which spermatogenesis is expected to be normal), with a successful sperm recovery in 96% of patients (99). TESA is usually well tolerated by patients. It is typically performed with a 21-gauge needle with no anesthesia or with a 19-gauge needle or biopsy gun using local anesthesia. Fertilization and implantation rates have been reported to be similar in a retrospective analysis comparing TESA with open biopsy using TESE (99). Alternatively, if the nature of the obstruction needs to be investigated by a full scrotal exploration, or if attempted surgical correction of the obstruction will be performed at the time of sperm recovery, MESA may be the preferred procedure. MESA is performed with general or regional anesthesia using a microsurgical approach. One advantage of MESA is that a very large number of spermatozoa are usually retrieved, so that cryopreservation and avoidance of repeat surgery may be possible (100). Fresh and frozen-thawed epididymal (101) or testicular spermatozoa (102) appear to have comparable fertilization and ongoing pregnancy rates when used for ICSI.

Sperm retrieval using PESA is another option for the treatment of posttesticular azoospermia. PESA is performed using a 19-gauge needle with local or regional anesthesia. A sperm recovery rate of greater than 80% has been reported with 55% fertilization and 33% ongoing pregnancy rates after ICSI (103). Although this procedure appears less invasive than some of its alternatives, it is performed blindly. Bleeding and epididymal injury are possible, and postsurgical fibrosis may result (104). In contrast, men with testicular azoospermia or gonadal failure require TESE, and possibly multiple biopsies, to retrieve sperm (105). TESE followed by ICSI has resulted in ongoing pregnancies, even for patients with 47,XXY Klinefelter's syndrome (106,107). However, the sperm recovery rate with TESE is only about 50%, and clinical outcomes for ICSI after TESE among patients with testicular azoospermia are variable.

Lower fertilization rates but comparable ongoing pregnancy rates have been reported for ICSI using testicular spermatozoa recovered from testicular azoospermia, compared with epididymal spermatozoa, posttesticular azoospermia (91,108). In addition, if an associated histologic diagnosis of testicular aplasia, Sertoli cell–only syndrome, or spermatogenesis arrest is noted, all measures of success are reduced when compared with patients who have normal testicular histology (109). These measures of success include the following: lower sperm recovery rates (110), lower ongoing pregnancy rates (18% to 19% versus 33.5%), and lower implantation rates (5% to 9% versus 12%) (107,109). Despite these findings, the histologic diagnosis alone should not be used to exclude patients from ICSI treatment. Among patients with testicular azoospermia, surgically recovered sperm may be at various stages of maturation arrest (i.e., round spermatid, elongated spermatid, and motile and immotile spermatozoa). Sperm at all stages have been used to establish successful pregnancies using ICSI (71,111). However, the fertilization and pregnancy rates associated with maturation-arrested spermatid are very low, and couples should be properly counseled regarding their prognosis and alternative options (112–114). Finally, cryopreservation of testicular tissues and of spermatozoa for use in subsequent ICSI treatment cycles has been reported (115). Fertilization rates of 48%, ongoing pregnancy rates of 16%, and implantation rates of 9% were documented using cryopreservation in a mixed population of 246 patients diagnosed with testicular and posttesticular azoospermia (115).

Donor Insemination **For men with azoospermia, couples with significant male factor infertility who do not desire ART, or women seeking pregnancy without a male partner, therapeutic donor insemination offers an effective option.** A number of important issues surround the use of this form of artificial insemination. First, despite reports that the use of fresh donor semen is associated with higher pregnancy rates than the use of frozen specimens (116), both the Centers for Disease Control and Prevention (CDC) and the American Society for Reproductive Medicine recommend the use of frozen samples (117). This recommendation stems from the increasing incidence of human immunodeficiency virus (HIV) infection in the general population and the lag time between HIV infection and seroconversion. Currently, semen donors are screened for HIV infection, hepatitis B, hepatitis C, syphilis, gonorrhea, chlamydia, and cytomegalovirus infections, all of which may be transmitted through the semen vector. All cryopreserved samples are quarantined for 6 months, and the donor is retested for HIV before clinical use of the specimen. Donors are likewise questioned about any family history of genetically transmitted disorders, including both mendelian (e.g., hemophilia, Tay-Sachs disease, thalassemia, cystic fibrosis, congenital adrenal hyperplasia, Huntington's disease) and polygenic-multifactorial (e.g., mental retardation, diabetes, heart malformation, spina bifida) conditions. Those with positive family histories conditions are eliminated as donor candidates.

A second issue surrounding the use of therapeutic donor insemination—that which is most important to the patient—is the success rate of treatment. In patients younger than 30 years of age who have no other infertility factors, conception rates approach 62% after 12 cycles of treatment with frozen sperm (118).

IUI was superior to intracervical insemination for donor insemination in several prospective randomized or crossover trials. Overall, the cycle fecundity rates ranged from 9.7%% to 24% for IUI to 3.9%% to 17.9% for intracervical insemination (119–125). A metaanalysis concluded that IUI had a significantly higher cycle fecundity rate when compared with ICSI (OR, 2.4; 95% CI, 1.5% to 3.8) (126). Moreover, the concomitant use of clomiphene citrate or gonadotropin (hMG) for COH did not result in higher fecundity rates (126).

The length of recommended treatment also should be considered. When frozen donor semen is used, more than 80% of consequent pregnancies will occur during the first 12 months of treatment (127). Thus, patients who do not conceive within 6 to 12 months should be assessed for female factors and encouraged to terminate treatment or move to alternative forms of therapy.

Last, but not least, one must consider the psychosocial aspects of pregnancies involving donor gametes. Among patients without a male partner, the potential repercussions of becoming a single mother and the issue of telling others about the father of the child must be discussed. If the couple is married, it is imperative that the husband be aware of the process of using donor gametes, and most programs require that the husband sign a consent form. A skilled infertility social worker or psychologist can be immeasurably helpful in addressing these concerns.

Age and Decreased Ovarian Reserve

An association between the age of the woman and reduced fertility has been well documented, with the decline in fecundability beginning in the early 30s but accelerating during the late 30s and early 40s. Chronologic age is the strongest determinant of reproductive success in spontaneous and ART cycles because it is a predictor of ovarian reserve (128,129). However, age has traditionally not been considered a "cause" of infertility, probably because it represents a physiologic rather than a pathologic state.

Data from rural Senegal, in which each female gives birth to an average of 7.9 children, show declining fertility rates with a peak of fertility at 25 years of age and a steep decline after 35 years of age (130) (Fig. 27.6). Similarly, among the Hutterites, a communal sect living in the Dakotas and Montana that practices no contraception and has large families, fertility peaks by 25 years of age, and one third of women are no longer fertile by 40 years of age (131). The fecundability of women undergoing donor insemination whose husbands are azoospermic provides insight into the effects of age on the fertility of the female alone. A French group that studied women enrolled in artificial insemination programs found that fertility rates begin to drop after 30 years of age. The pregnancy rate after 1 year of inseminations was 74% in women aged 30 years and younger, 62% in women aged 30 to 35 years, and 54% in women older than 35 years of age (132).

The physiology of declining fertility in older women is better understood in light of data from oocyte donation programs. When embryos produced from oocytes retrieved from younger women are transferred into older women, the pregnancy rates among the older women approximate those of the younger women (133), and variations in pregnancy rates are directly dependent on the age of the donors, not that of the recipients (133–135). In fact, among 260 egg donors (mean age of 30 years) who underwent controlled ovarian stimulation (COH with exogenous gonadotropins), the number of oocytes retrieved per cycle decreased steadily at the rate of 0.24 oocyte per year of increasing age (135). In another study, the use of oocytes from young donors provided cycle fecundity rates of 50% per cycle. The accumulated pregnancy and live birth rates in this investigation reached 95% and 89%, respectively, after up to four cycles of ART (136). **These observations strongly support that it is the age of the oocyte, rather than the age of the endometrium, that accounts for the age-related decline in female fertility.**

This oocyte-related decline in fertility is also known as *decreased ovarian reserve.* Absolute evidence of decreased ovarian reserve often can be ascertained only after ART treatment shows decreased ovarian responsiveness to COH. In ART, decreased ovarian reserve is reflected by an increased requirement for gonadotropins (FSH ± LH), small numbers of ovarian follicles and oocytes, and low serum estradiol levels during exogenous stimulation of folliculogenesis. These clinical outcomes probably reflect a decreased number of ovarian antral follicles as well as poor quality of granulosa cells and oocytes (137). Although age is the best predictor of ovarian reserve as reflected by ovarian responsiveness to COH, there

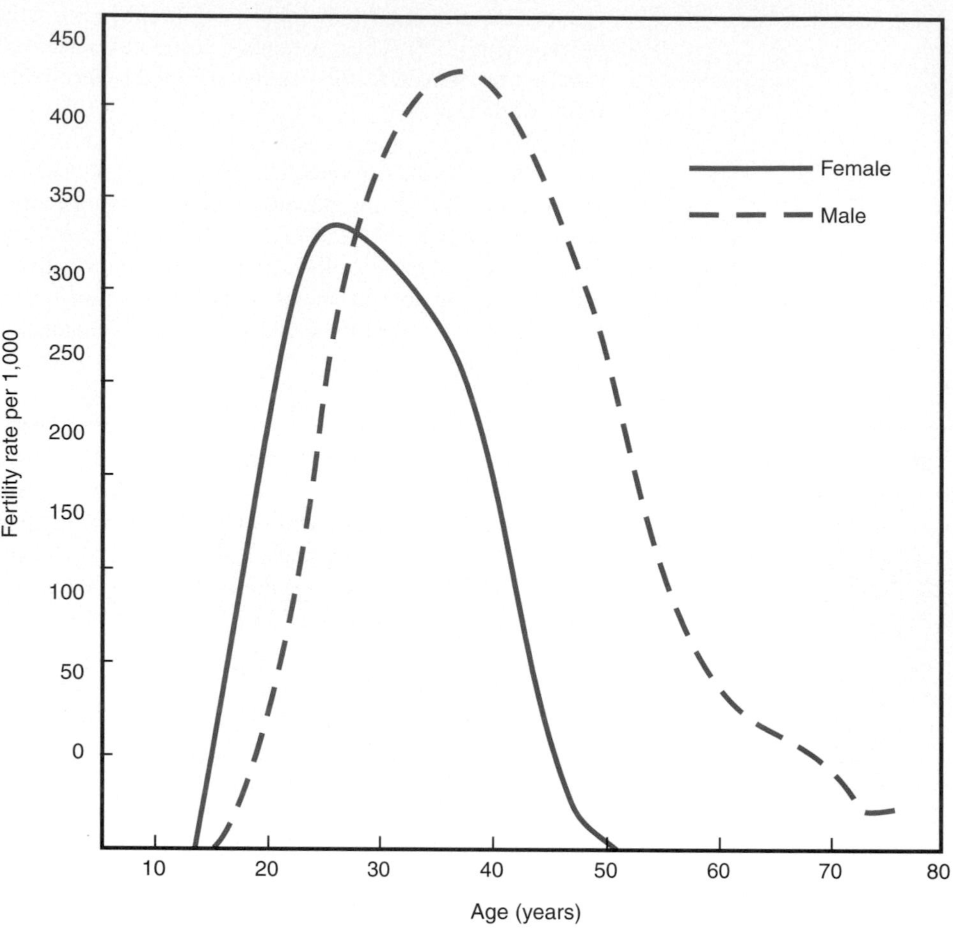

Figure 27.6 Age pattern of male and female fertility in a transitional society (Senegal).

is a subset of women who demonstrate an ovarian reserve that is prematurely diminished based on their chronologic age. Similarly, there are women who respond well to COH and achieve pregnancies despite their advanced age. Therefore, tremendous efforts have been expended to identify an ovarian reserve test that can be used to counsel patients and to guide their management.

Ovarian reserve screening tests that have been proposed include serum day 3 FSH, *clomiphene citrate* challenge test (CCCT), serum inhibin B, and transvaginal ultrasound to assess antral follicle number or ovarian size (138–140). Measurement of day 3 FSH is based on evidence that small increases in basal serum FSH levels correlate with the decreased fecundability seen among women in their late 30s. *Clomiphene citrate* is thought to have antiestrogenic effects in the hypothalamic–pituitary axis, resulting in a decrease in suppression of FSH production by the pituitary. In the CCCT, serum FSH is drawn on day 3, and again on day 10 after administration of *clomiphene citrate* (100 mg orally each day) from days 5 to 9. FSH levels vary depending on the assay used and the population being screened; therefore, each ART center typically sets its own reference range for evaluating the results of a CCCT. In a general infertility patient population, the incidence of an abnormal CCCT rises from less than 10% in patients younger than 35 years of age to 26% in patients older than 40 years of age (141). However, the results of day 3 FSH levels and CCCT must be interpreted with caution. These tests have mainly been studied in women with subfertility. Among these patients, day 3 FSH testing has a sensitivity of 8% in identifying women who will not conceive with subsequent IVF treatment. Day 3 FSH and

CCCT each displays a high specificity (96%) in predicting IVF outcome; however, addition of the CCCT to a day 3 FSH assessment only increases the sensitivity of prediction to 26% (142–144). Although abnormal CCCT results portend poor prognosis for pregnancy independent of age, older patients with normal CCCT still have significantly decreased pregnancy rates. Because among older patients even a normal CCCT is not reassurance of good prognosis, chronologic age must still be considered a salient, independent predictor of treatment outcome (129).

A great deal of emotional, physical, temporal, and financial effort is involved in the process of fertility treatments involving ART. Day 3 FSH and CCCT results can be used to counsel patients regarding their potential for pregnancy with IVF treatment. In one study, 5% of 435 women beginning their first IVF cycle had a day 3 FSH level greater than 15 IU/L (145). These women were 3.9 times more likely to have an unsuccessful treatment cycle. Similarly, among 175 IVF cycles involving women older than 40 years of age, no pregnancies resulted when testing revealed a day 3 FSH greater than 11.1 mIU/mL or a day 10 FSH greater than 13.5 mIU/mL after CCCT (146). Therefore, it is reasonable to advise women with advanced age (>40 years) and abnormal day 3 FSH or CCCT results to strictly limit the number of IVF cycle attempts because of their overall poor prognosis. These tests should not, however, be used as the sole basis to exclude women from IVF treatment (142).

Recently, serum inhibin B has also been proposed as a potential screening test for ovarian reserve. Inhibin B is produced by ovarian granulosa cells predominantly during the follicular phase of the menstrual cycle. Inhibin B suppresses the production of FSH by the pituitary gland. The normal rise in circulating levels of FSH associated with menopause is thought to be secondary to the decrease in inhibin B production accompanying the age-related depletion of functional ovarian follicles. In fact, in the CCCT, the main mechanism by which FSH is normally suppressed is via inhibin B production by granulosa cells. Women with decreased ovarian reserve have a lower rise in the day 10 serum inhibin B levels in response to the CCCT (147). In addition, women who have clinical evidence of diminished ovarian reserve and normal day 3 FSH levels have been found to have decreased day 3 inhibin B levels. This observation suggests that a decrease in day 3 serum inhibin B levels may precede detectable changes in day 3 FSH levels (140). Although the degree of elevation in serum inhibin B levels 24 hours after administration of exogenous FSH appears to be positively predictive of good ovarian response (148), clinical application of serum inhibin B still requires further evaluation. In particular, basal inhibin B levels do not provide additional age-independent prognostic value for predicting pregnancy outcomes after ART (128). One possible reason for this is that levels of inhibin B may reflect granulosa cell function and thereby only forecast ovarian response in ART. Although granulosa cell competence is certainly associated with oocyte quality, clinical application of serum inhibin B testing will also depend on whether levels are predictive of normal meiotic division of the oocyte because fetal karyotype is an important determinant of pregnancy outcome (149).

Spontaneous Abortion

Another factor contributing to the decreased fecundity among older reproductive-age women is the increased risk for spontaneous abortion in this population. A large study based on the Danish national registry estimated the rates of clinically recognized spontaneous abortion for various age groups to be 13.3% (12 to 19 years), 11.1% (20 to 24 years), 11.9% (25 to 29 years), 15.0% (30 to 34 years), 24.6% (35 to 39 years), 51.0% (40 to 44 years), and 93.4% (>45 years) (150). In addition, using sensitive hCG assays in women during their reproductive years, 22% of all pregnancies were found to be lost before they could be clinically diagnosed (151). One might predict that this proportion would be increased among older women attempting pregnancy, making subclinical spontaneous pregnancy loss a significant consideration among older women who are thought to be having difficulty conceiving.

One major cause for the increase in spontaneous losses among older women is their increased incidence of chromosomally abnormal fetuses. A cytogenetic analysis of

750 spontaneous abortions revealed that the increase in chromosomally abnormal conceptuses seen with increased maternal age was mainly due to an increase in chromosomal trisomies. In particular, the incidence of trisomies 16, 21, 22, 18, and 20 were significantly increased, with 18 and 20 being the most dramatic. In contrast, the risk for monosomy X and polypoidy did not increase with advanced maternal age (152). In conclusion, an increased spontaneous loss rate, coupled with a reduced conception rate, significantly decreases the chance of a live birth among women older than 40 years of age.

Age of Male Partner

There is little doubt that increasing age is accompanied by reduced female fecundity; however, the age-related decline in fecundity for men is more controversial. Male fertility peaks at about 35 years of age and declines sharply after 45 years of age; however, men have reportedly fathered children into their 80s (6). Also, the risk for chromosomal trisomies appears to be related, at least in part, to increased paternal age (153). Recent observations have demonstrated an increase in the rate of autosomal recessive disorders among the progeny of men 35 years of age and older (154,155). These findings suggest an age-related decline in gamete quality among men, albeit one that is more subtle than that experienced by women.

Ovulatory Factor

Disorders of ovulation account for about 30% to 40% of all cases of female infertility. These disorders are generally among the most easily diagnosed and most treatable causes of infertility. The normal length of the menstrual cycle in reproductive-age women varies from 25 to 35 days; most women have cycle lengths of 27 to 31 days. Figure 27.7 shows the fluctuations of estradiol, progesterone, FSH and LH in a normal, 28-day ovulatory cycle. Women who have regular monthly menses (about every 4 weeks) with moliminal symptoms, such as premenstrual breast swelling and dysmenorrhea, almost invariably have ovulatory cycles. Because ovulation is an obligatory prerequisite to conception, ovulation must be documented as part of the basic assessment of the infertile couple. Initial diagnoses among women with ovulatory factor infertility may include anovulation (complete absence of ovulation) or oligoovulation (infrequent ovulation).

Figure 27.7 Relative hormonal fluctuations in a normal, ovulatory, 28-day menstrual cycle.

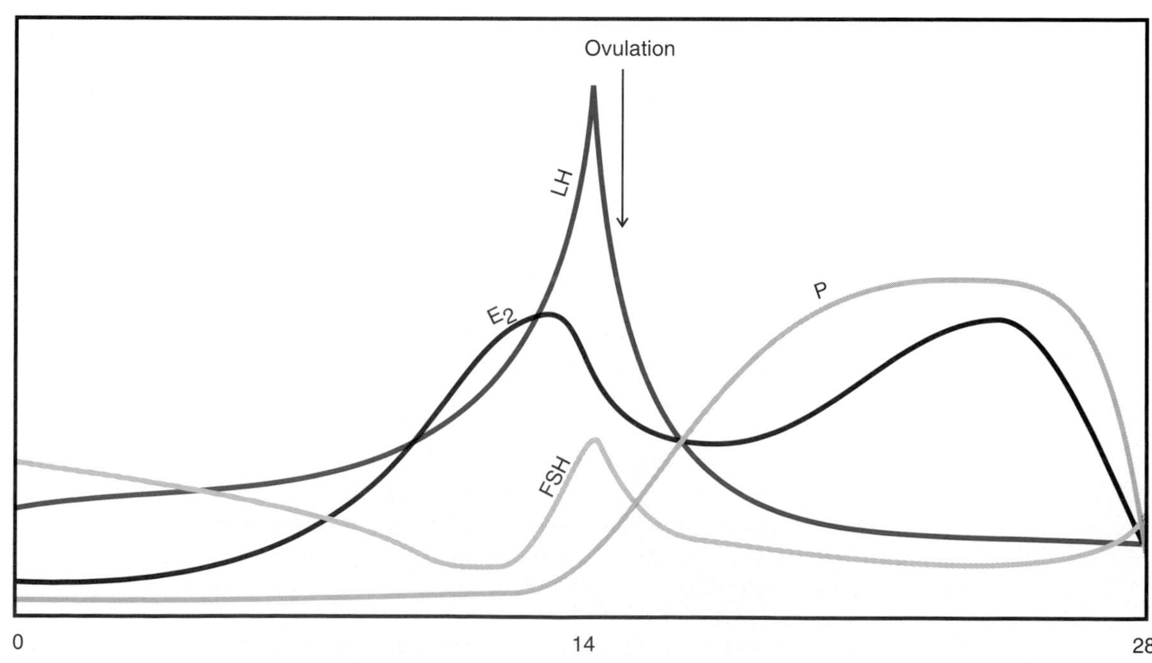

Methods to Document Ovulation

Luteinizing Hormone Monitoring **Documentation of the LH surge represents a remarkably reproducible method of predicting ovulation. Ovulation occurs 34 to 36 hours after the onset of the LH surge and about 10 to 12 hours after the LH peak** (156,157). Commercially available kits for documenting the LH surge are generally accurate, quick, convenient, and relatively inexpensive enzyme-linked immunosorbent assays (ELISAs) using 40 mIU/mL as the threshold for detection (158,159). The positive and negative predictive values of these kits have been described to be 90% and 96%, respectively (160). A 100% correlation between urinary LH prediction of ovulation and transvaginal ultrasound diagnosis of ovulation has further confirmed the value of urine LH detection kits for home ovulation detection (161). Still, there may be up to 5% to 10% of women for whom this ELISA test cannot detect urinary LH, probably either because of failed recognition by the antibody used or because their peak urinary LH concentration does not rise above the threshold set by the kit manufacturers. Serum LH measurements may be necessary to predict ovulation in such cases.

Basal Body Temperature **The least expensive method of confirming ovulation is for the patient to record her temperature each morning on a basal body temperature (BBT) chart.** The oral or rectal temperature should be determined before the patient arises, eats, or drinks. Smoking is forbidden before temperature measurement, and irregular sleep patterns can interfere with the test results. Patients monitoring BBT record their temperature daily but also record times when coitus occurs. Use of a BBT is preferred to use of a conventional thermometer because of the BBT instrument's precision in the temperature range under consideration. The principle behind temperature charting as a means to document ovulation is simple. Significant progesterone secretion by the ovary generally occurs only after ovulation. Progesterone is a thermogenic hormone. The secretion of progesterone causes a temperature increase of about 0.58°F over the baseline temperature of 97° to 98.8°F typically recorded during the follicular phase of the menstrual cycle. Charting of daily BBTs produces a characteristic biphasic pattern in women with ovulatory cycles. Frequently, a nadir in charted BBT is noted at the time of the LH surge, but this finding is inconsistent. A normal luteal phase is characterized by a documented temperature elevation lasting at least 10 days.

BBT charting for documentation of ovulation, although simple, has several drawbacks. Presumptive ovulation can be identified only retrospectively (i.e., the test merely confirms rather than predicts ovulation). Even retrospectively, the exact time of ovulation is difficult to determine using BBTs, although in most instances, it is probably 1 day before documented temperature elevation. An unequivocal temperature rise generally occurs 2 days after the LH surge and correlates with serum progesterone levels of 0.4 ng/mL (162). Also, in a small percentage of patients, BBT charts are monophasic, despite the documentation of ovulation by other methods. Further, BBT charting is correlated with transvaginal ultrasound evidence of ovulation in only 30.4% of cases (161). Despite its limitations, for many patients, BBT charting is a simple way to document ovulation, and unequivocal biphasic cycles are almost certainly ovulatory. Patients with monophasic cycles require confirmation of ovulation using alternative methods.

Midluteal Serum Progesterone Elevations in serum levels of progesterone constitute indirect evidence of ovulation. When used to document ovulation, serum progesterone measurement should coincide with peak progesterone secretion in the midluteal phase (typically on days 21 to 23 of an ideal 28-day cycle). The lower limit of progesterone levels in the luteal phase varies among laboratories, but a level above 3 ng/mL (10 nmol/L) typically confirms ovulation. However, an appropriate interpretation of isolated luteal-phase measurements of serum progesterone is complicated by the frequent pulses that characterize the secretion of this hormone (163). Although ovulatory levels are often considerably higher than 3 ng/mL, low midluteal serum levels of progesterone are not necessarily diagnostic of anovulation.

Ultrasound Monitoring **Ovulation can also be documented by monitoring the development of a dominant follicle by ultrasound until ovulation takes place.** Ovulation

identified. In humans, abnormalities in leptin receptor function lead to early-onset morbid obesity and absent pubertal development, presumably secondary to defective hypothalamic function (210).

Low BMI also can cause anovulation and infertility in women, possibly by disrupting hypothalamic function (211). Examples of conditions characterized by low BMI include anorexia nervosa, professional athletic training, and malnutrition. In most patients with these conditions, weight gain is the ideal treatment for ovulatory dysfunction, avoiding the use of ovarian stimulatory medications and their complications. Other health benefits, including the reduction of complications from pregnancy and osteoporosis, can result from correction of an abnormally low BMI. In one study, increased caloric intake and weight gain alone resulted in the resumption of menses in 90% patients with amenorrhea related to low BMI; 73% had spontaneous conception (212). In another study, a mean weight gain of 3.6 kg was sufficient to promote the resumption of spontaneous ovulation (213).

Other conditions of hypothalamic dysfunction, such as congenital hypothalamic failure (*Kallmann's syndrome*), can be treated using pulsatile GnRH therapy if the pituitary–ovarian axis is intact. Gonadotropin therapy should be chosen for patients in whom pituitary dysfunction is present, such as those with empty sella syndrome. Each of these treatment modalities is discussed in greater detail under *Gonadotropin Therapy*.

Hypothyroidism The prevalence of abnormal TSH levels in the general infertility population has been reported to be 6.3%, 4.8%, 2.6%, and 1.5% for women from couples diagnosed with anovulatory infertility, unexplained infertility, tubal infertility, and male infertility, respectively (214). This diagnosis is significant in the management of infertility. For instance, one study reported that among 171 women with hypothyroidism, 23% had irregular menses, likely resulting from anovulation (215). Spontaneous ovulatory cycles typically resume when euthyroid status is achieved using *thyroxine* supplementation.

In contrast to the causal relationship between hypothyroidism and anovulation, the association between hypothyroidism or thyroid antibodies and spontaneous abortion is still unclear. Although hypothyroidism has been associated with increased fetal wastage in some studies (216,217), thyroid antibody status was not associated with pregnancy loss in women with unexplained recurrent miscarriage (218), nor did it affect pregnancy rates with IVF treatment (219). Others, however, have reported conflicting results, indicating that thyroid antibodies occur at a higher than average frequency in women with recurrent pregnancy loss, but not among women undergoing ART for infertility (220,221).

Tubal, Paratubal, and Peritoneal Factors

Tubal and peritoneal factors account for 30% to 40% of cases of female infertility. Tubal factors include damage or obstruction of the fallopian tubes and are usually associated with previous PID or previous pelvic or tubal surgery. Peritoneal factors include peritubal and periovarian adhesions, which generally result from PID, surgery, or endometriosis. The risk for infertility after a single bout of PID is surprisingly high and increases rapidly with subsequent episodes. In fact, the incidence of tubal infertility has been reported to be 12%, 23%, and 54% after one, two, and three episodes of PID, respectively (222). Still, about half of patients with documented tubal damage have no identifiable risk factors for tubal disease (223). Most of these women are presumed to have had subclinical chlamydial infections.

Hysterosalpingography **HSG is the initial diagnostic test used to assess tubal patency because it has a sensitivity of 85% to 100% in identifying tubal occlusion.** The particular specificity of HSG in identifying PID-related tubal occlusion approaches 90% (224,225). Other causes of apparent tubal blockage include salpingitis, isthmica nodosa, benign polyps within the tubal lumen, tubal endometriosis, tubal spasm, and intratubal mucous debris (226). Bilateral tubal pathology documented on HSG is associated with significantly reduced fecundity rates and warrants further evaluation using falloscopy, selective salpingography, or laparoscopy.

HSG is usually performed between cycle days 6 and 11. To reduce the chance of iatrogenic infection, HSG should ideally follow the cessation of menstrual flow; to avoid possible fetal irradiation and interference with conception, HSG should precede ovulation. It is estimated that infection follows 1% to 3% of HSG procedures and occurs almost exclusively in women with hydrosalpinges or with current or prior pelvic infection. Therefore, known hydrosalpinges, current PID or cervicitis, and palpable adnexal masses or tenderness on bimanual examination all constitute contraindications to HSG. Because there is a high prevalence of current or past chlamydial infection among infertile women and complications of HSG-associated pelvic infection could further compromise fertility, it is reasonable to prescribe antibiotic prophylaxis to patients scheduled for HSG. One typical regimen uses *doxycycline,* 100 mg twice daily, beginning the day before HSG and continuing for 3 to 5 days. Other rare complications of HSG include uterine perforation, hemorrhage, and allergic reaction to the contrast dye. HSG often causes uterine cramping, and prophylaxis with a nonsteroidal antiinflammatory drug may minimize this discomfort.

Performing the HSG procedure itself is fairly straightforward. After a bimanual examination and vaginal cleansing, an acorn (Jarcho) cannula, a pediatric Foley catheter, or some other injection device is introduced into the uterine cervix. A paracervical anesthetic block is not routinely needed but may be used in selected patients. Either a water-soluble contrast medium, such as meglumine *diatrizoate* (*Renografin-60*), or a low-viscosity oil-based dye, such as *ethiodized oil* (*Ethiodol*), may be used for the procedure. Each contrast material has advantages. Water-soluble contrast material is more rapidly absorbed than oil-based dyes and does not carry the risk for either lipid embolism due to dye extravasation or lipid granuloma formation. Oil-based dyes are associated with less uterine cramping, better resolution of tubal architecture, and a higher postprocedure pregnancy rate (227). A recent update of a 1994 metaanalysis has found that the use of oil-soluble media to flush the tubes during HSG significantly increases subsequent pregnancy rates (OR, 1.8; 95% CI, 1.29 to 2.50). Similar therapeutic benefit has not been demonstrated using water-soluble contrast media (228).

HSG should be performed using fluoroscopy, with care taken to minimize ovarian exposure to x-rays. Careful and slow initial injection of 3 to 4 mL of contrast media should give a clear outline of the uterine cavity. Further injection of about 5 to 10 mL of contrast media is usually sufficient to demonstrate bilateral tubal patency or tubal obstruction. Generally, only two radiographic views are needed, one demonstrating the filling of the uterine cavity and the other (at the completion of the procedure) showing tubal findings. The radiation exposure required for the completion of an HSG examination has been shown to be well below the documented limiting ovarian dose of 10 cGy (229).

Laparoscopy **The best technique for diagnosing tubal and peritoneal disease is laparoscopy.** It allows visualization of all pelvic organs and permits detection of intramural and subserosal uterine fibroids, peritubal and periovarian adhesions, and endometriosis. Abnormal findings on HSG can be verified by direct visualization on laparoscopy. For instance, tubal patency may be confirmed at laparoscopy by observation of the passage of a dye, such as methylene blue or indigo carmine, through the fimbrial openings of the tubes. Unlike HSG, laparoscopy allows careful assessment of the external architecture of the tubes and, in particular, visualization of the fimbria. Identified abnormalities, including tubal obstruction, pelvic adhesions, and endometriosis, can be treated laparoscopically at the time of diagnosis.

Other Diagnostic Modalities Successful evaluation of proximal tubal obstruction using selective *salpingography* and *falloposcopy* has been described. Based on techniques derived from coronary angioplasty, salpingography uses small guidewires to permit selective tubal cannulization and radiographic visualization under fluoroscopy. Falloposcopy is based on similar principles, but allows direct fiberoptic visualization of tubal ostia and intratubal architecture. Falloposcopy allows the visual identification of tubal ostial spasm, abnormal tubal mucosal patterns, and even intraluminal debris causing tubal obstruction. In fact, a tubal disease scoring system based on falloposcopic examination has been suggested to identify patients with poor prognoses for spontaneous conception (230). Complications associated with falloposcopy include a 5.1% rate of pinpoint perforations of the tube.

Abdominal and transvaginal, ultrasound-guided tubal cannulations have also been used to identify tubal blockage. Each reports high diagnostic sensitivity and specificity. Alternatively, sonohysterography with contrast media offers a much less invasive method of diagnosing fallopian tubal obstruction while maintaining a sensitivity and specificity similar to that of laparoscopic chromotubation (231). Further prospective evaluation and cost analyses are necessary to determine the utility of tubal cannulation and sonohysterography with contrast media.

Treatment of Tubal Factor Infertility

Therapies that directly address correcting tubal factor infertility are entirely surgical and include (a) correction of periadnexal disease; (b) correction of proximal, distal, or combined tubal disease; and (c) correction of iatrogenic tubal abnormalities (e.g., tubal sterilization). **As success rates continue to improve in ART, the indications for surgical approaches in the treatment of tubal factor infertility may become increasingly limited.** Still, a number of the principles underlying surgical management remain important. Surgical treatment of periadnexal disease causing tubal factor infertility has been proved effective, regardless of whether the approach is by laparotomy (232) or laparoscopy (233). Adhesion prevention, however, becomes particularly vital when surgery is used to address prior adhesive disease causing infertility. The relative value of laparotomy versus laparoscopy for the treatment of tubal infertility has received considerable attention, as have their respective effects on postoperative adhesion formation. For example, one study comparing laparoscopy and laparotomy for the treatment of ectopic pregnancy demonstrated that adhesion formation occurred more frequently after laparotomy, even when meticulous technique was maintained during all procedures (234). Many adjuncts for postoperative adhesion prevention have been proposed, including the use of antiinflammatory agents, barrier agents, fibrinolytic substances, and anticoagulants. However, none of these interventions has consistently altered postoperative adhesive complications. Thus, careful hemostatic surgical technique and judicious use of the laparoscopic approach remain the only generally recommended principles guiding surgical treatment of tubal factor infertility.

Proximal Tubal Occlusion Correction of proximal tubal occlusion may involve the use of those same techniques employed in establishing its diagnosis. For instance, selective salpingography performed under fluoroscopy may be used to inject contrast media directly into the tubal lumen in an attempt to overcome obstruction resulting from mucous plugging. If selective salpingography fails to create tubal patency, proximal tubal cannulation can be performed using a guidewire under direct visualization or using radiologic guidance. Proximal tubal cannulation has a reported a success rate of 85% in establishing tubal patency. Reocclusion occurs in 30% of cases. The risk for tubal perforation with cannulation is reported to be 3% to 11%, but tubal damage is usually mild and heals spontaneously (226).

Until the mid-1970s, tubal implantation was considered the best approach for treating proximal tubal obstruction. Since that time, microsurgical tubocornual anastomosis has become the preferred surgical approach, with postsurgical ongoing pregnancy rates averaging 47.4% in five reported series involving 175 patients (226,235–238). Hysteroscopic cannulation appears to have similar efficacy, with a 48.9% ongoing pregnancy rate among 133 patients treated in four series (226,239–242). Although ongoing pregnancy rates with microsurgical tubocornual anastomosis and hysteroscopic cannulation appear comparable, cannulation is significantly less invasive and has fewer morbid complications. Microsurgery, however, provides access to other pelvic structures, allowing the surgeon to assess the distal fimbriae and to lyse any periadnexal adhesions that may be present. In contrast to both microsurgical anastomosis and hysteroscopic cannulation, the ongoing pregnancy rates for selective salpingography and fluoroscopic tubal cannulation have averaged only 26% (226,243–247).

Distal Tubal Occlusion Treatment of distal tubal disease involves surgical correction by fimbrioplasty or neosalpingostomy. By definition, *fimbrioplasty* is the lysis of fimbrial adhesions or the dilation of fimbrial phimosis, whereas *neosalpingostomy* involves the creation of a new tubal opening in an occluded fallopian tube (248). Distal tubal disease can be treated either laparoscopically or by laparotomy using conventional microsurgical techniques. Regardless of the method used, the efficacy of neosalpingostomy or fimbrioplasty as treatment for distal tubal occlusion rests largely on the extent of tubal and peritubal disease, as assessed by HSG and laparoscopy. Poor prognostic factors for a successful pregnancy after neosalpingostomy include hydrosalpinx greater than 30 mm in diameter, absence of visible fimbriae, and dense pelvic or adnexal adhesions (249). The appearance of the tubal mucosa has added prognostic significance for the fertility outcome of laparoscopic tuboplasty for distal tubal occlusion (250). In one study, laparoscopic distal tuboplasty produced an overall pregnancy rate of 27% and an ectopic pregnancy rate of 4.5% among 44 patients (251). Fimbrioplasty appeared to be more successful than neosalpingostomy; however, the choice of surgery might have been influenced by the extent of disease. Similarly, a more recent study on a series of 194 cases of laparoscopic fimbrioplasty and neosalpingostomy resulted in an intrauterine pregnancy rate of 27.3% and an ectopic pregnancy rate of 4.1% (252). Patients with both proximal and distal tubal disease represent the poorest candidates for surgical management of tubal infertility. Studies of surgical treatment for these patients have had small numbers of patients but have consistently yielded poor results (253). This select group of patients should benefit most from IVF.

Sterilization Reversal About 0.2% of women who choose surgical tubal sterilization request reversal procedures (254,255). The success of tubal reanastomosis is dependent on the method of sterilization, the site of anastomosis, and the presence of other infertility factors. Pregnancy rates are lowest (49%) after the reversal of sterilization procedures involving unipolar electrocautery. In contrast, postprocedure pregnancy rates rose to 67% when the sterilization technique involved Fallope rings or spring-loaded clips and 75% when Pomeroy tubal ligation was employed. The prognosis is best when anastomotic sites have no significant differences in tubal diameter (e.g., isthmic–isthmic or cornual–isthmic anastomoses). Tubal length is also an important prognostic consideration: final anastomosed tubal lengths of less than 4 cm are associated with low pregnancy rates (256). Pregnancy rates higher than 40% have been reported after microsurgical fimbriectomy correction (257). Laparoscopy to assess surgical prognostic factors such as potential final tubal length, site of reanastomosis, method of sterilization (if not previously known), and presence of associated pelvic pathology, is often performed before microsurgical fallopian tubal reanastomosis by laparotomy.

Historically, all sterilization reversal procedures have involved laparotomy. More recently, excellent pregnancy rates have been reported after laparoscopic tubal anastomosis. In one study of 186 patients followed after laparoscopic tubal anastomosis with a two-layer closure, cumulative pregnancy postprocedure rates were 60.3%, 79.4%, and 83.3% at 6, 12, and 18 months, respectively (258). In another study, laparoscopic tubal reanastomosis was performed on 102 women, of whom 70% conceived and 65% had ongoing intrauterine pregnancies during the 15-month follow-up period (259). Rates of ectopic pregnancy were similar (3% and 7%) in both series (258,259). The surgical time of laparoscopic tubal reanastomosis most certainly depended on the surgeon's experience as well as the number of layers involved in tubal closure. Reported operative duration ranged from 71.35 minutes to 140.2 minutes, ±53.3 minutes (258,259).

Recently, successful robotic-assisted laparoscopic microsurgical tubal anastomosis has been reported in humans. The reported procedures had a mean duration of 159 ± 33.8 minutes and were performed solely using robotic arms that were remotely controlled by surgeons with previous extensive experience with microsurgical tubal anastomosis by laparotomy. The reported postprocedure tubal patency rate was 89% at 6 weeks, and the ongoing pregnancy rate was 50% (260). Despite advances in surgical technology, however, IVF should be considered for patients with prior sterilization and poor prognostic characteristics. Likewise, IVF is indicated for those patients whose tubal reanastomoses have not yielded a pregnancy by 12 to 18 months after surgery.

Cervical and Immunologic Factors

Postcoital Test **Cervical factor is a cause of infertility in no more than 5% of infertile couples.** The classic test for evaluation of the potential role of cervical factor in infertility is the postcoital test (PCT). The PCT is designed to assess the quality of cervical mucus, the presence and number of motile sperm in the female reproductive tract after coitus, and the interaction between cervical mucus and sperm. The PCT does not yield sufficient information on sperm count, motility, or morphology to allow assessment of semen quality. The PCT should be performed just before ovulation because its proper interpretation requires the examination of cervical mucus at a time of sufficient estrogen exposure. Serum estrogen levels peak just before ovulation, providing optimal stimulation to the estrogen-sensitive, mucus-producing cervical glands. Therefore, the PCT should be performed 1 or 2 days before the anticipated time of ovulation. For patients with irregular cycles, the patient's urinary LH surge may be helpful in scheduling the test.

Use and interpretation of treatment recommendations based on the PCT are all controversial. Even the appropriate timing of coitus preceding examination of the cervical mucus is unclear. Although an optimal interval may be less than 2 hours from intercourse to PCT, an adequate test can be performed within 24 hours of intercourse. Although the data are not definitive, intercourse after 2 days of abstinence and about 2 to 12 hours before the PCT is performed should yield adequate information. Couples should be reminded not to use lubricants that may contain spermicidal agents.

The PCT is inexpensive and easily performed. A small amount of cervical mucus is withdrawn by means of long oval forceps with small apertures at the tip. Alternatively, an angiocatheter syringe or tuberculin syringe may be used to withdraw mucus from the endocervical canal. The mucus is placed on a glass slide and covered with a cover slip. A small trail of mucus may be left to dry outside the cover slip so that ferning can be assessed. Many infertility specialists also take a "vaginal pool" specimen from the posterior vaginal fornix to document the presence of sperm in the vagina. Cervical mucus is rapidly evaluated for spinnbarkeit (i.e., stretchability), ferning, and clarity. The presence of, number per high-power field, and motility of sperm should be carefully assessed by the examination of several microscopic fields.

Normal estrogen-stimulated mucus should stretch 8 to 10 cm when it is pulled from the cervix with forceps or when the cover slip is lifted off the slide, should demonstrate a highly characteristic ferning pattern similar to that seen on examination of amniotic fluid, and should be clear and watery. The characteristics of cervical mucus change under the influence of progesterone after ovulation. At that time, the cervical mucus appears thick and opaque and lacks ferning. Although the number of motile sperm per high-power field should be documented, normal values have not been established. Some authors suggest that virtually any number of motile sperm seen on the PCT is normal (261), whereas others require greater than 20 sperm per high-power field (262).

There are several potential causes for an abnormal PCT. The most common is incorrect timing of the test within the menstrual cycle, leading to the production of cervical mucus that is suboptimal for sperm penetration. Other causes of poor mucus quality include anovulation, anatomic factors (e.g., prior cervical conization or cryotherapy), infection, and certain medications. Clomiphene citrate may exert detrimental effects on cervical mucus by its antiestrogenic action on cervical glands. This is one reason why clomiphene citrate should be offered to patients with unexplained infertility only when coupled with IUI. Abnormal semen characteristics are often reflected in the PCT and may be responsible for abnormal PCT results. An independent semen analysis is required for proper assessment for male factor infertility. Poor PCT results may, of course, reflect suboptimal mucus–sperm interactions. The observation of shaking or uniformly dead sperm on PCT suggests the presence of antisperm antibodies.

Although there is plausible biologic rationale behind the PCT, this test has been accepted without critical review of its prognostic value or of its impact on the overall management plan of the subfertile couple. The PCT lacks reproducibility, standard methodology, and uniform criteria for assessment. These factors, in conjunction with poor correlation between PCT results and pregnancy outcome, argue against use of the PCT as a standard investigational tool in infertility patients (262–265). For example, one study reported no difference in pregnancy outcomes among women whose cervical mucus contained 0 to 11 motile sperm per high-power field (263), whereas another reported abnormal PCTs in 20% of fertile couples (262). A review of the world's English-language literature challenged the validity of the PCT and found that the sensitivity and specificity of the test ranged from 0.09 to 0.71 and from 0.62 to 1.00, respectively (264).

Couples seeking reproductive medical intervention undergo many tests that are considered necessary, although they are costly from physical, emotional, and financial perspectives. Therefore, any test performed should have proven value in determining the prognosis or the course of treatment. Management decisions based on testing should affect the treatment outcome. This is not the case for the PCT, for which the results seldom alter the management of patients with unexplained infertility because the accepted treatment of superovulation/IUI bypasses the cervical mucus. In a prospective, randomized controlled study, couples who underwent PCT had cumulative pregnancy rates after 24 months of therapy identical to those of a control group not using PCT (266). Therefore, PCT testing has no effect on treatment outcome. Finally, although the PCT may screen for the presence of antisperm antibodies, no proven treatment is accepted for this diagnosis. PCT is therefore not indicated for this application.

Antisperm Antibodies Injection of sperm from one animal into another can elicit an antibody response (267). Spermatozoa can also be autoantigenic. Thus, both males and females have the capacity to produce humoral response to sperm. Either allogenic or autoimmune response could, in turn, adversely affect fertility. Antisperm antibodies are most commonly limited to immunoglobulin G (IgG), IgM, and IgA isotypes, and each subclass has characteristic anatomic localization. Systemically produced IgG molecules may be found in serum as well as in cervical mucus and semen. Agglutinating antibodies of the IgA class are typically found in cervical mucus and seminal plasma. The larger IgM antibodies have difficulty traversing the genital tract mucosa and therefore are found exclusively in serum. In addition to subclassification by isotype, antisperm antibodies can be free, agglutinating, bound to sperm that is motile, or bound to sperm that is immobilized. Further complexity arises in that sperm-bound antisperm antibodies can bind to different parts of the outer sperm plasma membrane, including the head, body, or tail. One major challenge in understanding antisperm antibodies is to determine the relative importance of each of these factors with respect to disease pathogenesis, impact on fertility, and prognosis.

Many etiologies have been proposed to explain the formation of antisperm antibodies (268). In women, coital trauma that disrupts the vaginal epithelium could theoretically expose immune effector cells to sperm antigens, thereby leading to antisperm antibody formation. However, it remains unclear why most women, who are repeatedly exposed to billions of spermatozoa, do not exhibit this immune response. In men, the blood–testis barrier normally shields the serum from exposure to sperm and their antigens. Conditions that cause breaks in this barrier could activate autoimmunity. Testicular trauma or torsion, occlusion of the vas deferens secondary to childhood inguinal herniorrhaphy or cystic fibrosis, vasectomy reversal, and genital tract infections have all been suggested to elicit antisperm antibody formation.

The mechanisms by which antisperm antibodies might adversely affect fertility continue to be contested. Many mechanisms have been proposed. One or more of these could be involved in a particular infertile couple. Distinct mechanisms might be operative under specific circumstances. Adverse antibody-mediated effects on semen quality (either before ejaculation or upon contact of ejaculate with the female reproductive tract) present obvious potential for subfertility. Other, more specific, proposed mechanisms include antisperm antibody–mediated interference with capacitation, with the acrosome reaction, with sperm–egg recognition and fusion, and with cleavage of the early embryo (268). Although some investigators have demonstrated that the presence and amount of antisperm antibodies is associated with fertilization failure during IVF or subzonal sperm insemination (269–271), others have failed to identify a link between reduced fertility and antibody positivity (272,273).

Myriad tests presently are available for the detection of antisperm antibodies, making the appropriate evaluation of immunologic infertility even more bewildering. Sperm agglutination tests (Kibrick's or Franklin-Dukes) and sperm complement-dependent immobilization tests (Isojoma's) have largely been replaced by the immunobead or mixed agglutination tests (Fig. 27.8). The immunobead test uses commercially available anti-IgG–, anti-IgA–, or

Figure 27.8 The mixed agglutination reaction (MAR) to evaluate immunologic infertility by assessment of antisperm antibodies. (Redrawn and adapted from **Garenne ML, Frisch RE.** Natural fertility. *Infertil Reprod Med Clin North Am* 1994;259–282, with permission.)

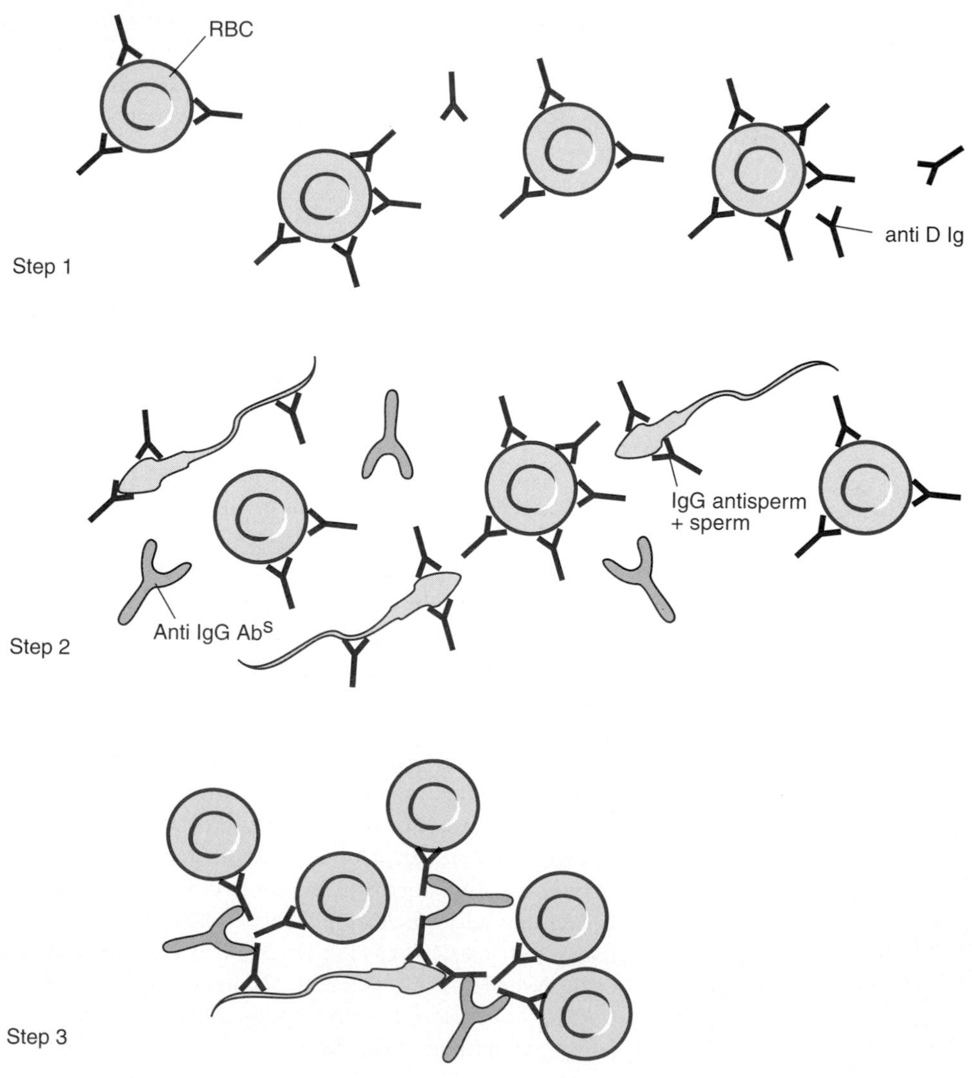

anti-IgM–coated polyacrylamide beads. Washed spermatozoa are exposed to the labeled beads, and sperm binding is assessed. The test yields specific information on both the immunoglobulin class of the antisperm antibody and the site of binding to the involved sperm (274). In the mixed agglutination reaction, human red blood cells sensitized with human IgG are mixed with "patient" semen. The presence of antibody-coated spermatozoa results in the formation of mixed agglutinates with the red blood cells (275). A comparison of these two methods demonstrates good correlation of results; however, the latter test is easier to perform (276).

Despite recent improvements in techniques for the identification of antisperm antibodies, the clinical utility of these tests should be limited to very special cases until their prognostic value, impact on infertility management, or effectiveness in treatment can be demonstrated in prospective trials. Corticosteroid therapy for men with antisperm antibodies has been studied in a prospective, double-blind, placebo-controlled trial. This trial did demonstrate decreased antisperm IgG in response to corticosteroid therapy; however, no improvement in sperm-bound IgA or pregnancy outcomes could be documented (277). In fact, there is currently no support for the use of corticosteroid therapy in antisperm antibody–positive patients because IUI alone has been shown to result in higher pregnancy rates than the combination of corticosteroids and timed intercourse (272). In summary, in a couple with no identifiable cause of infertility, a positive or negative antisperm antibody test will not alter their proposed therapeutic plan: superovulation and IUI followed by IVF or ICSI (278). One potential use of antisperm antibody testing that warrants investigation is the identification of those couples predicted to have high fertilization failure rates with IVF who might benefit more from immediate use of ICSI.

Uterine Factors

Uterine anatomy and function are both critical determinants governing implantation of the embryo and subsequent fetal growth and development. Of course, these two elements are not distinct entities. They are intimately related; thus, most of the uterine factors implicated in infertility have defects in both structure and function. For example, the endometrial lining of uteri with congenital anatomic abnormalities exhibits functional aberrations. Endometrial molecular mechanisms of implantation and gestation are exquisitely controlled and remarkably complex; thus, even subtle defects in endometrial progression from the periimplantation, luteal phase to the mature decidua supporting a placenta and fetus can result in infertility or early pregnancy loss.

Diagnostic Imaging for Uterine Pathology

Uterine abnormalities that have been implicated in infertility include congenital malformations, luteal-phase defects, and other acquired conditions such as leiomyomas, endometrial polyps, and intrauterine synechiae. For infertility patients who have had no recent imaging tests, it is reasonable to begin the workup with HSG because it has an 85% to 100% sensitivity for detecting tubal pathology among infertility patients (224,225). However, HSG has only 44% and 75% sensitivity rates in documenting uterine malformations and intrauterine adhesions, respectively (279).

Sonohysterography appears to be superior to HSG in the detection of uterine malformations, correctly identifying 90% of abnormalities among infertile patients (280). These data are consistent with those observed in patients with abnormal uterine bleeding in the general gynecologic setting, where sonohysterography has sensitivities of 87% and 93% in detecting any intrauterine pathology and endometrial polyps, respectively (281,282). In women with abnormal bleeding, compared with conventional transvaginal ultrasound, sonohysterography has both higher sensitivity (93% versus 65%) and specificity (94% versus 76%) for the detection of endometrial polyps. Sonohysterography also decreases the false-positive and false-negative rates from 25% to 5.4% and from 36% to 8%, respectively (282).

In most practices, diagnostic hysteroscopy is the preferred procedure for the diagnosis of uterine pathology in infertility patients. However, the ideal imaging test employed during an infertility workup would be one that is relatively noninvasive and has high sensitivity and specificity in the detection of uterine abnormalities as well as tubal blockage. The use of contrast media (i.e., Echovist) instead of saline during sonohysterography has been reported to have sensitivity comparable to that of HSG and laparoscopic chromotubation in the detection of tubal blockage (225). This test has great potential for generalized use in infertility investigations but presently lacks prospective comparison with the combined use of HSG and diagnostic hysteroscopy in the infertile population.

Congenital Anomalies of the Uterus

Congenital uterine anomalies may be associated with infertility, spontaneous pregnancy loss in the first or second trimester, or late-trimester pregnancy complications. In women with didelphic, unicornuate, and septate uteri, the rates of spontaneous abortion and preterm delivery are highly increased at 25% to 38% and 25% to 47%, respectively (283). Endometrial dysfunction during the luteal phase may result in infertility, whereas dysfunction occurring after implantation results in pregnancy loss. Further, pregnancy outcome in the presence of a uterine anomaly may depend on the location of blastocyst implantation in a particular cycle. This may explain why a woman with a septate uterus might encounter recurrent pregnancy loss even after having delivered a term infant.

With the exception of a septate uterus, infertility associated with most congenital uterine anomalies is not amenable to surgical treatment (284,285). Hysteroscopic septoplasty has been demonstrated to decrease significantly the risk for spontaneous abortion in women with septate uteri, and surgical therapy is indicated in patients with known uterine septi and who have recurrent spontaneous abortion (286). Indications for surgical correction of congenital uterine anomalies when the presenting complaint is infertility are less obvious. Among seven series of hysteroscopic metroplasties performed for infertility, the overall pregnancy rate after treatment was 48% (286). It is still reasonable to consider surgical options in some infertile patients with uterine septi because septoplasty may maximize the chance of having a live birth by decreasing the associated risks for spontaneous abortion and preterm labor.

In Utero Exposure to Diethylstilbestrol

Exposure to *DES in utero* increases a woman's risk for congenital reproductive tract malformations and obstetric complications, including preterm labor and cervical incompetence (287). In one study, almost 70% of women exposed to *DES in utero* were noted to have uterine malformations on HSG. The most common malformation was the T-shaped uterus (288). Whether *DES*-exposed women also have higher rates of infertility remains unclear (289,290). One investigator reported that decreased fertility in these women was particularly prevalent when constriction of the upper segment of the reproductive tract was present (291). This question is difficult to study; however, since there is great variation in the degree of congenital uterine, tubal, and cervical anomalies associated with exposure (287). Furthermore, some abnormalities may promote other infertility factors. For instance, cervical anomalies may promote production of suboptimal cervical mucous, or cervical stenosis may promote retrograde menstruation and the subsequent development of endometriosis. Finally, some *DES*-exposed infertile patients will also have unrelated but additional reasons for their infertile state. Overall, when a *DES*-exposed woman has uterine anomalies on HSG and greater than 1 to 2 years of primary infertility, her prognosis for future pregnancy is extremely poor (292). Metroplasty for correction of T-shaped and hypoplastic *DES*-exposed uteri has unproven value and is not recommended. Results of IVF treatment are generally poor in infertile, *DES*-exposed women. Although ovarian response rates to COH are comparable in *DES*-exposed women and nonexposed women with unexplained infertility, *DES* exposure is associated with significantly lower implantation rates in IVF (293).

Acquired Abnormalities of the Uterus

Leiomyomas Among women with infertility and uterine leiomyomas, many variables may affect pregnancy rates, including leiomyoma size, location, and number (solitary versus multiple) as well as the presence of symptoms associated with these tumors. **Leiomyomas**

have never been shown to be a direct cause of infertility. It has been suggested, however, that uterine leiomyomas might alter uterine contractility and thereby disrupt normal sperm migration. Alternatively, the presence of leiomyomas might adversely affect vascular and molecular profiles of sites of implantation (294). No prospective, randomized trial comparing expectant management with myomectomy in infertile patients with uterine leiomyomas has yet been conducted. However, one recent case-control study compared pregnancy outcomes among 106 women who had laparoscopic myomectomy for fibroids, 106 women with uterine fibroids who did not have surgery, and 106 women who had unexplained infertility but no fibroids. Reported live birth rates were significantly different among the study populations: 42% for the laparoscopic surgery group, 11% for the group with myomas but no surgery, and 25% for the unexplained infertility group (295). A metaanalysis of 12 prospective series involving a total of 138 women who underwent abdominal myomectomy for infertility showed that cumulative postprocedure pregnancy rates at 1 year were 57% to 67%. Not surprisingly, pregnancy rates for those women who had no other factor contributing to their infertility were higher than for women with additional causes of infertility (61% versus 38%). Women who had treatment for submucous fibroids had a postoperative pregnancy rate of 70% at 1 year (296). Vercellini and colleagues reported 24-month cumulative conception rates of 87%, 66%, and 47% in patients younger than 30 years of age, 30 to 35 years of age, and older than 35 years, respectively, after abdominal myomectomy in 138 infertile women (297). The presence of other causes of infertility and duration of infertility were associated with worse prognosis, whereas the size, number, or site of fibroids did not affect pregnancy outcomes. Others have reported success rates after abdominal myomectomy that are comparable to the 65% pregnancy rate and 50% live delivery rate reported for laparoscopic myomectomy (298). Successful laparoscopic myomectomy, however, is contingent on a number of factors, including stringent criteria for patient selection and the surgeon's experience with the procedure. In addition, appropriate closure of the created uterine defect is essential to minimize the complication of uterine rupture during subsequent pregnancy (299,300). In short, both myomectomy and superovulation/IUI are reasonable treatment options for women with uterine fibroids and otherwise unexplained infertility, particularly if the leiomyomas are large, submucous, solitary, or distorting the uterine cavity.

Endometrial Polyps Even in the absence of symptomatic uterine bleeding abnormalities, endometrial polyps may be discovered in women with infertility. The incidence of asymptomatic endometrial polyps in women with infertility has been reported to be about 10% (301). The value of routine hysteroscopic removal of endometrial polyps before infertility treatment and the rate of polyp recurrence during therapy are not known. It is intriguing that of 83 patients who were diagnosed with an endometrial polyp during COH for IVF and who underwent hysteroscopy immediately after oocyte retrieval, only 58% had histopathologic confirmation of the diagnosis (302). Although pregnancy rates in these women were similar to those of other IVF patients, spontaneous abortion rates appeared higher in those patients with polyps (302).

Intrauterine Synechiae or Asherman's Syndrome About 13% of 78 infertile women scheduled for IVF treatment were found to have intrauterine adhesions when evaluated with diagnostic hysteroscopy (301). Causes of intrauterine adhesions are often iatrogenic, with typical patient histories involving intraoperative or postoperative complications of uterine evacuations for menorrhagia or pregnancy termination. Other cases of Asherman's syndrome have been associated with intrauterine infection with pathogens including schistosoma and mycobacteria. In some Third World countries, tuberculous endometritis may be an important cause of uterine factor infertility (303). Tuberculous endometritis differs from most other types of chronic bacterial or viral endometritis in that its treatment is followed by significant uterine scarring and low pregnancy rates (304). In its severe forms, Asherman's syndrome has been associated with amenorrhea, menstrual irregularities, and spontaneous abortion. As with submucous myomas and uterine septi, intrauterine adhesions may interfere with embryo implantation.

Intrauterine synechiae can be treated with lysis of adhesions by either dilation and curettage or hysteroscopic resection. In many cases, it is important that postsurgical management include efforts to avoid reformation of adhesive disease. Regimens addressing this problem include intraoperative placement of an intrauterine pediatric Foley catheter or an intrauterine device. These mechanical solutions are typically left in place for about 1 week postoperatively. Postsurgical estrogen therapy may be administered in addition to or in lieu of mechanical devices. It is thought that estrogens will rapidly rebuild the endometrial lining after surgery and thereby prevent the reformation of scar tissue. A typical regimen consists of conjugated estrogen at a dosage of 2.5 mg/d for 1 to 2 months. Surgical treatment of intrauterine synechiae can yield very satisfying results; pregnancy rates above 80% have been reported among patients with mild to moderate disease (305).

Disorders of Endometrial Function and Luteal-phase Defect

There are probably few areas of greater controversy in the field of infertility than those surrounding the existence, diagnosis, and treatment of inadequate luteal phase or luteal-phase defect. The controversy has been fueled by disagreements about both the definition of this entity and the efficacy of its treatment. Although variously defined, **most agree that luteal-phase defect is present when two endometrial biopsies demonstrate a delay in the histologic development of the endometrium of more than 2 days beyond the actual cycle day** (306). Thus, if a luteal-phase lag is found on an initial endometrial biopsy, it must be confirmed on a subsequent biopsy to meet criteria for the diagnosis. The actual cycle day has conventionally been calculated by assigning the onset of the menses following biopsy as day 28 and counting backward to the day of biopsy. However, the use of the day of ovulation as a reference point may be more meaningful physiologically.

In addition to delayed endometrial maturation, luteal-phase defect can also be characterized by histologic asynchrony between endometrial epithelial and stromal compartments. A variety of factors could be responsible for such histologic alterations, including inadequate follicular development, inadequate FSH or LH secretion, hyperprolactinemia, and an inappropriate progesterone production by the corpus luteum (307). Regardless of its primary cause, LPD probably is marked by an aberrant molecular profile within the endometrium, which, in turn, can adversely affect endometrial receptivity to blastocyst implantation (308,309). Using murine gene knockout models, the genes *Hoxa-10, Hoxa-11, leukemia-inhibiting factor (Lif), Lif receptor,* and *cyclooxygenase-2 (Cox 2)* have each been determined to have a critical functional role in implantation in mice (310–314). The cycle-dependent expression patterns of these genes in the human endometrium and their high degree of conservation between mouse and human both serve to support their potential importance in human implantation (315). Thus, these mouse models serve as valuable tools in the dissection of molecular genetic pathways that are potentially relevant in human implantation.

In recent years, a temporal and functional "implantation window" has been proposed to occur during the midluteal phase of the human menstrual cycle. This concept has been offered to help synthesize a growing body of data suggesting a defined period of optimal receptivity of the uterus for the implanting blastocyst. That an implantation window exists is supported by the finding that embryos implanting on postovulation days 8 to 10 have maximal viability, whereas the risk for early pregnancy loss increases with later implantation. Using a ratio of urinary estrogen metabolites to progesterone metabolites to time ovulation, the percentage of pregnancy losses associated with implantation on postovulation days 9, 10, 11, and beyond day 11 were 13%, 26%, 52%, and 82%, respectively (316). Although the implantation window has been defined by the temporal expression pattern of endometrial β_3, α_4, and α_1 integrins, there is controversy over length of this proposed window—between days 20 and 24 or much narrower, between days 22 and 23 of a 28-day cycle (317,318). At present, the diagnosis of luteal-phase defect based on testing for the expression of these integrins has not become standard clinical practice because endometrial integrin expression may be characterized by significant intercycle variability. Further, the value of assessing integrin expression levels in predicting pregnancy outcome is not yet known (319).

Perhaps the most crucial question is whether luteal-phase defect exists at all. In a collection of serial luteal-phase endometrial biopsy specimens from normally fertile women, investigators documented isolated out-of-phase specimens in 31.4% of normally cycling participants and sequential out-of-phase specimens in 6.6%, suggesting that normal women often have out-of-phase endometria (320). Other authors have reported that the frequency of out-of-phase endometrial specimens among infertile patients is no greater than the rate that would occur by chance alone (321,322).

Because of the discomfort and inconvenience associated with the multiple endometrial biopsies needed to confirm the diagnosis of luteal-phase defect, several investigators have attempted to identify alternative luteal-phase markers for this diagnosis. One possibility would involve definition of a luteal-phase serum progesterone level that would correlate sufficiently with endometrial biopsy results to allow its use as a screening tool for luteal-phase defect. Although some studies have advocated such testing, data that convincingly associate single midluteal phase serum progesterone levels with proposed luteal-phase abnormalities are lacking. The characteristic pulsatile secretion of progesterone further reduces the utility of such testing (323). Given the current uncertainties about the diagnosis and treatment of luteal-phase defect, attempts to diagnose this disorder should be confined to infertile patients who lack other identifiable diagnoses and to those in whom treatment specifically directed at luteal-phase defect is being contemplated.

Current treatments for presumed luteal-phase defect among infertile patients are empiric and reflect the hypothesis that progesterone insufficiency is causal. Treatment, therefore, involves the administration of vaginal or intramuscular progesterone (50 to 100 mg/d) beginning 3 days after documentation of an LH surge. Progesterone supplementation is typically continued until the first day of the next menstrual cycle or until documentation of a negative serum quantitative hCG value. If a patient becomes pregnant while on therapy, progesterone is continued until 8 to 10 weeks of gestation.

If one accepts both that luteal-phase defect does exist and that it is a reflection of luteal progesterone insufficiency, then it would seem prudent to begin therapeutic progesterone supplementation soon after ovulation and before implantation. Initiating therapy only after pregnancy is confirmed may be misguided. In fact, among patients with proposed luteal-phase defect, those pregnancies that survive to the point of confirmation by hCG may not require any treatment because they have already persisted beyond the periimplantation period. Studies supporting progesterone supplementation for luteal-phase defect have reported pregnancy rates after intervention of 50% to 80%. All of these studies have been small and poorly controlled (324). A prospective, randomized trial studying the impact of progesterone supplementation on pregnancy rates and outcomes in infertility patients diagnosed with luteal-phase defect is warranted.

Infectious Factors

The relationship between subclinical infection and fertility has received considerable attention. Particular interest has focused on two potential pathogens: *Chlamydia trachomatis* and *Mycoplasma* species. The association of chlamydia with PID has been well established. Chlamydia is the predominant pathogen detected in about 20% of cases of acute salpingitis in the United States. Chlamydia may produce asymptomatic infection in the female genital tract, and it is likely that some women experience silent tubal infection. Despite few if any symptoms, these infections may result in tubal damage. A possible link between infection and infertility is suggested by evidence that the prevalence of positive chlamydial cultures may be higher among infertile patients than among controls (325). In a study of 286 women undergoing 344 oocyte retrievals, seropositivity for chlamydia and the presence of bacterial vaginosis were highly associated with tubal disease. Reproductive outcomes of IVF, however, were no different than those of controls (326).

In another recent study, the incidence of bacterial vaginosis among 771 current IVF patients was 25%. Although their pregnancy rates were not affected, those IVF patients with bacterial

downregulation (360). However, the same study found that there was no difference in clinical outcomes between the two types of gonadotropins in IVF protocols using GnRH agonist downregulation. Because GnRH agonist downregulation is not included in most COH/IUI cycles, FSH preparations may be particularly beneficial in these regimens.

Another metaanalysis of 12 randomized, controlled trials comparing urinary FSH (purified FSH and highly purified FSH) and recombinant FSH in ART cycles concluded that higher pregnancy rates resulted from recombinant FSH use (OR, 1.20; 95% CI, 1.02 to 1.42) (361). However, there is no evidence to suggest a difference in clinical outcomes between the two available recombinant FSH preparations. Overall, recombinant FSH appears to be superior to other gonadotropin preparations and is preferred in COH cycles, with or without ART. Nonetheless, there may be subsets of patients who respond better to hMG, perhaps because they need the LH component. Alternatively, the recombinant forms may not elicit optimal response in patients with particular FSH receptor variants. Therefore, if the ovarian response is poor with recombinant FSH, a trial of hMG should be considered.

Regardless of the indication, regimens involving gonadotropin therapy for ovulation induction or COH follow fairly similar protocols. All include close monitoring of folliculogenesis using transvaginal ultrasonography and serum estradiol levels. Such monitoring allows informed adjustment of gonadotropin dosages, timed hCG injection and IUI, and most importantly, limitation of complications such as OHSS and multiple gestation. Patient age, ovarian reserve, and infertility diagnosis help to individualize the initial gonadotropin dose, the maximum allowable number of follicles, and the speed of ovarian stimulation (or cycle length). Of the many protocols that have been proposed, the following sections illustrate the key points for gonadotropin stimulation in non-IVF/ICSI cycles.

Baseline Transvaginal Ultrasound Scan

Patients begin therapy on day 2 or 3 after the onset of a spontaneous or induced menses. (Day 1 is the first day of menses.) A baseline transvaginal ultrasound is performed on day 1 or 2, before the start of therapy, to identify uterine abnormalities such as endometrial polyps, submucosal fibroids, or congenital defects. Hormonally responsive pathology, including endometrial polyps and submucosal fibroids, may not be apparent at this point in the menstrual cycle, when tissues are in a hypoestrogenic state. Therefore, a systematic survey should be repeated in subsequent ultrasound examinations throughout the course of the stimulation protocol (363). The two-hand transvaginal ultrasound technique often allows better visualization over the one-hand technique. This technique combines current technology with the traditional bimanual pelvic examination. The nondominant hand of the ultrasonographer can be used to apply gentle abdominal pressure to improve the definition of pelvic structures (363). The findings of a thin endometrium (<4 mm) and quiescent ovaries on the baseline scan reflect the hypoestrogenic state of the early follicular phase, which provide the optimal conditions with which to commence treatment. Conversely, a thick endometrium represents endogenous hormonal stimulation above normal basal levels and indicates that the patient should not initiate the cycle.

Unilocular, clear cysts may represent functional cysts or unruptured luteinized cysts. Complex ovarian cysts detected at baseline usually reflect old hemorrhagic corpus luteae and are commonly seen if the patient has been treated with gonadotropins in the previous cycle. Nevertheless, the differential diagnoses, including endometrioma, benign ovarian tumor, or malignancy, must be considered. The management of ovarian cysts present at baseline is controversial. In 174 prospective, non-IVF, COH cycles, a significantly lower cycle fecundity rate was observed with a baseline ovarian cyst larger than 10 mm (364). Confusion may have arisen because several IVF studies have reported no adverse effect on pregnancy outcomes associated with presence of a baseline ovarian cyst (365–367). Extrapolation of results from IVF studies to non-IVF, COH cycles is not appropriate; this issue is debatable even among IVF studies (368). More importantly, these ovarian cysts tend to resolve spontaneously within 1 to 2 months. Low-dose oral contraceptive has a lower efficacy than older, high-dose oral contraceptive in preventing the formation of new cysts (369,370). Since oral contraceptives do not affect the speed of resolution of old cysts, they are not necessary in this scenario.

Starting Dose of Gonadotropin

Gonadotropin dosages can be administered each day in the evening, allowing morning measurements of serum estradiol to reflect the steady state. If the patient has had previous gonadotropin treatment, the starting dose should be based on review of ovarian response in previous cycles. The following guidelines can be used for determining the starting dose of gonadotropins in the first COH or ovulation induction cycle:

- In unexplained infertility, the patient's ovarian response is usually dependent on her age, and it may be difficult to predict. There are no strict guidelines; however, one should always start at lower doses and increase the dose on day 6, if necessary. For example, a maximum of 1 to 1.5 ampules of gonadotropin per day should be used for women younger than 30 years of age, whereas women older than 40 years of age can be started at a maximum of 2 to 3 ampules per day.
- Anovulatory PCOS patients should start at 1 ampule of gonadotropin per day. A smaller dose of 0.5 ampule per day is sometimes necessary to minimize the risk for OHSS.
- Patients with hypogonadotropic hypogonadism usually begin with 1 ampule per day.

Monitoring and Adjustment of Dosage

The chosen initial daily dosage of gonadotropins is maintained until day 6 or 7, when the serum estradiol level is first measured to document ovarian response. Transvaginal ultrasound also is done at this time to determine follicular response.

- If no response has occurred by these measurements, the gonadotropin dosage is increased by 1 or 2 ampules per day every 3 or 4 days until a response is evident by rising estradiol levels (or until the maximal dosage is reached). The maximal dosage is usually 6 to 8 ampules per day because an increase in ovarian response is not seen with higher dosages (371).
- Once an ovarian response is obtained, treatment typically is continued without further increase in dose.

Cycle Progression and Monitoring

Transvaginal ultrasound and serum estradiol measurements are performed every 1 to 3 days to evaluate follicular size, number, and quality. Follicles can be predicted to grow 1 to 2 mm per day, and follicular development is believed to be adequate when maximal follicular diameter exceeds 18 to 19 mm. When hMG is used, the serum estradiol level roughly corresponds to 150 to 250 pg/mL per mature follicle. However, serum estradiol levels may not be as closely correlated with the number of mature follicles when recombinant FSH is used. In general, the serum estradiol level can be expected to double every 24 hours if the same dosage of gonadotropins is maintained. Therefore, the main reasons for following the estradiol levels are as follows:

1. To detect missed spontaneous ovulation or premature luteinization, which may be reflected by a drop in serum estradiol levels

2. To identify patients at risk for OHSS:
   - Estradiol levels approaching 800 to 1000 pg/mL indicate increased risk for OHSS. A decrease in gonadotropin dosage should be considered, and monitoring is mandated in 24 hours. Withholding gonadotropin in this situation is referred to as "coasting" and is usually followed by a more than 25% decrease in serum estradiol while the follicle numbers and diameters increase. If follicle numbers increase and are excessive, the cycle should be cancelled (372–374).

- Estradiol levels in the range of 1,500 to 2,000 pg/mL indicate that treatment should absolutely be stopped because of the high risk for OHSS. All medications should be discontinued, and hCG should not be administered. The patient should be asked to abstain from intercourse until menses occurs because she may spontaneously ovulate. Under these conditions, ovulation and intercourse may lead to increased risk for multiple gestation.

Human Chorionic Gonadotropin Administration

When the largest measured follicle reaches a maximum diameter of 18 to 19 mm or more, 10,000 IU of hCG is administered intramuscularly. Recombinant hCG is also available now for subcutaneous injection. Optimal pregnancy rates are achieved with IUI performed at 12 and 34 to 36 hours after the hCG injection. If the plan is to have natural intercourse, it can be timed within 12 to 36 hours of hCG administration as well.

Pregnancy Test or Plans for Next Cycle

If menses does not ensue after a treatment cycle, testing for pregnancy should be performed about 15 or 16 days after hCG administration. Testing for serum or urinary levels of β-hCG should not be affected by prior administration of exogenous hCG at this point, and β-hCG should be detectable by either method. If pregnancy does not occur, the cycle should be reviewed. If appropriate follicle size, number, and estradiol levels have been reached, then there is no need to change the gonadotropin dosage. The dosage should be changed if COH was inadequate or excessive. If the length of the stimulated cycle was too short (i.e., the follicular stimulation was too fast), endometrial maturation could have been suboptimal, and gonadotropin dosage should be decreased in a subsequent cycle.

Special Issues of COH and IUI in PCOS PCOS patients represent one of the most challenging subpopulations to treat safely and successfully using COH/IUI. The multiple small ovarian antral follicles characteristic of these patients may be very resistant to stimulation, but they are equally likely to respond and grow with minimal increases in gonadotropin dosage. The incidence of multiple pregnancy and OHSS is increased in these patients (375). Up to 30% or more of COH cycles may be cancelled as a result of excessive follicular development. Several approaches that have been proposed to avoid complications of COH and cycle cancellation include downregulation with gonadotropin-releasing hormone GnRH agonists, dual suppression with oral contraceptives and GnRH agonists, pretreatment with metformin, and surgical ovarian diathermy (205,376–379).

A dual suppression protocol described for PCOS hyperresponders in IVF treatment could also be used to lower ovarian response in COH/IUI cycles. In this protocol, low-dose oral contraceptives were taken for 25 days, the last 5 of which utilized concurrent administration of the GnRH agonist leuprolide acetate (1 mg/d by subcutaneous injection). Low-dose gonadotropin was then started on day 3 of GnRH agonist treatment. This protocol resulted in significant improvements in clinical pregnancy rates, a decrease in cancellation as a result of excessive ovarian response, and a decrease in the incidence of OHSS (378).

Alternatively, PCOS patients can be pretreated for at least 1 month with metformin at the full dose of 1,500 mg/d, before COH/IUI with gonadotropins. In a randomized, prospective trial, pretreatment with metformin resulted in fewer ovarian follicles, lower serum estradiol levels, and no cycle cancellations due to excessive ovarian response during gonadotropin COH (378).

Hypogonadotropic Hypogonadism **Therapy with hMG is most successful in patients with hypogonadotropic hypogonadism, yielding cumulative pregnancy rates of 91.2% after six treatment cycles using hMG alone** (380). In this particular group of patients, hMG is recommended over purified FSH for ovulation induction because purified FSH has been associated with a significantly higher total dosage requirement, lower estradiol, and decreased number of lead follicles (381). Prior to ovulation induction in these patients, one must first determine on baseline transvaginal ultrasound whether the ovaries appear

PCO-like, with multiple small antral follicles, thick stroma, or enlarged ovarian volume. A subset of patients with isolated hypogonadotropic hypogonadism has been described to have PCO-like ovaries and respond to gonadotropins much like PCOS patients, exhibiting higher serum estradiol levels and a greater number of follicles (382). This finding, in conjunction with the fact that patients with hypogonadotropic hypogonadism typically are younger and have better ovarian reserve than patients with unexplained infertility, make it prudent to start with small doses of hMG in this population. This practice should help to avoid complications of OHSS and multiple gestation.

Hypothalamic Failure Most patients with acquired hypogonadotropic hypogonadism secondary to cranial surgery, or radiotherapy for various cranial tumors have hypothalamic failure as the source of their dysfunctional hypothalmic–pituitary axis (383). In these patients, GnRH stimulation testing and the assessment of endogenous pulsatile LH secretion often can confirm whether the hypothalamic–pituitary axis is intact. Patients with hypothalamic failure and subsequent ovulatory factor infertility represent the best candidates for ovulation induction with GnRH agonists. To mimic physiologic hypothalamic–pituitary interactions, GnRH agonists must be administered in a pulsatile fashion, thereby avoiding the downregulation of the GnRH receptors that accompanies continuous GnRH agonist stimulation. Coexistent growth hormone deficiency or prolactin abnormalities do not affect the efficacy of pulsatile GnRH agonist therapy (383). Because GnRH agonists are rapidly degraded by gastric enzymes (and thus ineffective when administered orally), pulsatile GnRH agonists are administered either intravenously or subcutaneously with a minipump delivery system. Adverse effects of pulsatile GnRH agonist therapy are mainly related to pump function and route of delivery (i.e., phlebitis at the needle site). The intravenous route is superior (384), but it is recommended that women with a history of bacterial endocarditis be offered only subcutaneous therapy.

In hypothalamic hypogonadotropic hypogonadism, normal pituitary negative and positive feedback mechanisms are functional upon treatment with pulsatile GnRH agonists. In this situation, pulsatile GnRH agonist therapy simulates normal physiology and offers some advantages over hMG as a treatment for ovulatory infertility. More than two dominant follicles are seen in only 18.9% of patients with hypogonadotropic infertility who are treated with pulsatile GnRH, and more than three follicles are seen in only 5.4% of patients (385). Because OHSS is a rare occurrence, less intensive monitoring is required during GnRH agonist treatment cycles. Moreover, the risk for multiple gestation approximates that associated with *clomiphene citrate* therapy—only 8% (385). These are important advantages when compared with gonadotropin therapies. Cumulative pregnancy rates among women with hypothalamic hypogonadism approach 80% after 6 treatment cycles and 93% after 12 GnRH agonist treatment cycles (386), with no documented increase in the rates of spontaneous abortion (387).

The optimal dosing interval for pulsatile GnRH agonist therapy is 60 to 90 minutes, and the usual recommended dosage is 75 to 100 ng/kg/pulse (381,382). Increased dosage of up to 250 ng/kg/pulse has been reported to be required in the successful treatment of a patient with known GnRH receptor mutation (388). With typical regimens of pulsatile GnRH, ovulation occurs on day 14 and can be documented by standard LH testing. Patients treated with pulsatile GnRH usually benefit from luteal-phase support through continuation of the GnRH pump, administration of hCG, or progesterone supplementation.

Assisted Reproductive Technologies

All methods of ART, by definition, involve interventions to retrieve oocytes. These techniques include IVF, ICSI, gamete intrafallopian transfer (GIFT), zygote intrafallopian transfer (ZIFT), cryopreserved embryo transfers, and the use of donor oocytes. A typical ART cycle has the following main components:

- Downregulation using GnRH agonist
- COH using gonadotropins with folliculogenesis monitoring using transvaginal ultrasound and assessment of serum estradiol levels

- Oocyte maturation using hCG
- Oocyte retrieval
- Fertilization by IVF, ICSI, or GIFT
- *In vitro* embryo culture (except in GIFT)
- Luteal support or endometrial preparation using progesterone supplementation
- Transfer of fresh embryos with possible cryopreservation of excess embryos
- First-trimester pregnancy monitoring

Folliculogenesis in the Spontaneous Cycle In unassisted ovulation, the cohort of follicles destined to begin folliculogenesis in any particular menstrual cycle are recruited in the previous cycle's luteal phase. By about the middle of the next follicular phase, one of these follicles will become dominant, and further development of this dominant follicle suppresses maturation of other follicles within the selected cohort of that particular cycle. Follicular-phase growth of a single dominant follicle in nonstimulated cycles induces an intricate series of hormonally regulated feedback loops, resulting in the midcycle LH surge, which is critical for maturation of the oocyte and ovulation. Progesterone production commences just before ovulation and becomes significantly increased after ovulation. Estradiol production during the follicular phase causes proliferation of the endometrial epithelium. However, progesterone is critical in the final maturation of the endometrial glands and stroma required for implantation of the blastocyst. In the presence of successful implantation, the hCG-stimulated corpus luteum will continue to be the critical source of progesterone until the placenta independently produces sufficient amounts of progesterone at 8 to 10 weeks of gestation.

Downregulation Using GnRH Agonist The use of GnRH agonist has become standard in ART protocols. It prevents spontaneous ovulation, decreases treatment complications, and allows the control of ovulation to rest exclusively on administration of exogenous medications. Commercial preparations of GnRH agonist consist of decapeptides that differ from the endogenous GnRH agonist at 2 amino acid residues. This modification increases both the half-life and the receptor binding affinities of GnRH agonist. When used in a nonpulsatile fashion, GnRH agonist causes an initial agonist effect that is accompanied by upregulation of GnRH receptors within the pituitary gland. This initial activity may be manifested as increased gonadotropin effects, which are referred to as the *flare response.* However, continued administration of GnRH agonist downregulates GnRH receptors, resulting in minimal basal production of LH and FSH and no stimulation of the ovarian follicles. Therefore, GnRH agonist induces a quiescent hypothalamic–pituitary–ovarian axis and a menopause-like state characterized by low estradiol levels. Consequently, in addition to rash or skin irritation at the subcutaneous injection site, it is not uncommon for patients using GnRH agonist to experience side effects such as hot flashes and moodiness.

The most commonly used regimen for superovulation in ART is called the *long,* or *luteal, downregulation protocol.* In this protocol, GnRH agonist is started in the luteal phase (day 21) of the previous cycle, which minimizes its flare effect and prevents the follicular recruitment that is thought to begin in the luteal phase. The couple undergoing treatment is advised to abstain from intercourse during the cycle before the start of COH; however, concomitant use of GnRH agonist in the presence of an unsuspected pregnancy has not been reported to be associated with increased spontaneous abortion, congenital abnormalities, or pregnancy complications.

Before the adoption of GnRH agonist as a standard part of ART cycles, premature luteinization and spontaneous ovulation presented significant challenges to the success of ART. Prospective, randomized trials indicate that use of GnRH agonist under the long protocol offers many benefits when compared with either no GnRH agonist use or use commencing in the follicular phase of the ART cycle (called the *short,* or *flare, protocol*). GnRH agonist in the long protocol significantly lowered the incidence of premature luteinization and spontaneous ovulation, resulting in reduced cycle cancellation rates (389–391). Significantly more oocytes and embryos were yielded using the long protocol, whereas the rate of OHSS decreased (389,391,391). For logistical reasons, patients preferred the convenience of the long protocol because it requires less frequent monitoring (393). Most importantly, clinical pregnancy rates (389) and live birth rates per retrieval (394) were significantly higher using the long protocol. The benefits of using the long protocol GnRH agonist greatly outweigh its disadvantages: daily administration (for most preparations, e.g., leuprolide acetate), increased requirement for gonadotropins, and an overall increase in the costs of medication. A metaanalysis reviewing the efficacy of various GnRH agonist regimens concluded that the addition of GnRH agonist downregulation to ovulation induction regimens for ART was advantageous (395). They noted an improvement in pregnancy rates and a decrease in cancellation rates with no associated increase in spontaneous abortion rates.

The controversy over the choice of long or short GnRH agonist protocols was put to rest by a large, prospective, observational, multicenter study involving 1,244 couples receiving their first IVF or GIFT treatment. Although serum estradiol levels were higher in patients on short protocols, these patients had 11% fewer oocytes retrieved. Further, the clinical pregnancy rate was 35% lower using the short protocol when compared with the long protocol, even after adjusting for factors such as age, infertility diagnosis, IVF or GIFT therapy, and year of treatment (396). Currently, the long GnRH agonist protocol is generally recommended for most patients, and use of the short protocol in ART patients with poor ovarian response has not been proven beneficial (396).

Many other regimens have been suggested for the administration of GnRH agonists in gonadotropin-stimulated cycles. Some of the more commonly used ones are summarized in Fig. 27.9 and Table 27.8. Recently, GnRH antagonists (*Cetrorelix* by Asta Medica and *Ganirelix* by Organon) have been proposed to have advantages over traditional GnRH agonists. GnRH antagonists bind to gonadotropin receptors and cause immediate downregulation of gonadotropin release by the pituitary gland. Because they avoid the flare effect associated with the use of GnRH agonists, they can be started concurrently with gonadotropins and do not require additional time for downregulation. GnRH antagonists also have the theoretic potential to decrease the risk for OHSS. However, more studies need to be conducted to identify the optimal dosage and the effects of GnRH antagonists on IVF pregnancy outcomes (397).

Controlled Ovarian Hyperstimulation Typical use of gonadotropins for COH in ART is similar to the superovulation protocol used in COH/IUI for unexplained infertility. There are several key differences:

- When the GnRH agonist luteal downregulation protocol is used, ovarian suppression should be confirmed by a baseline transvaginal ultrasound showing no ovarian cysts larger than 5 cm (365), a thin endometrium, serum estradiol level of less than 50 pg/mL, and serum progesterone level of less than 1.0 ng/mL. Ovarian suppression is usually achieved after about 10 days of GnRH agonist therapy. Once ovarian suppression is confirmed, COH using gonadotropins can be initiated.
- The aim of COH in ART is to recruit more follicles than in COH/IUI. Unlike COH/IUI, the risk for multiple gestation under ART regimens is strictly dependent on the number of embryos that are transferred and not on the number of follicles.
- In general, the monitoring during COH for ART is slightly less frequent than in COH/IUI. Spontaneous ovulation is prevented by the routine use of GnRH agonist, and slightly greater flexibility can be exercised on the day of hCG administration without affecting the pregnancy outcomes (398).
- The removal of granulosa cells during aspiration of each developing follicle with ART is believed to decrease the risk for subsequent OHSS (399). Thus, higher serum estradiol levels and larger follicular sizes are typically allowed before hCG administration in ART protocols. OHSS does, however, remain a major concern (400).

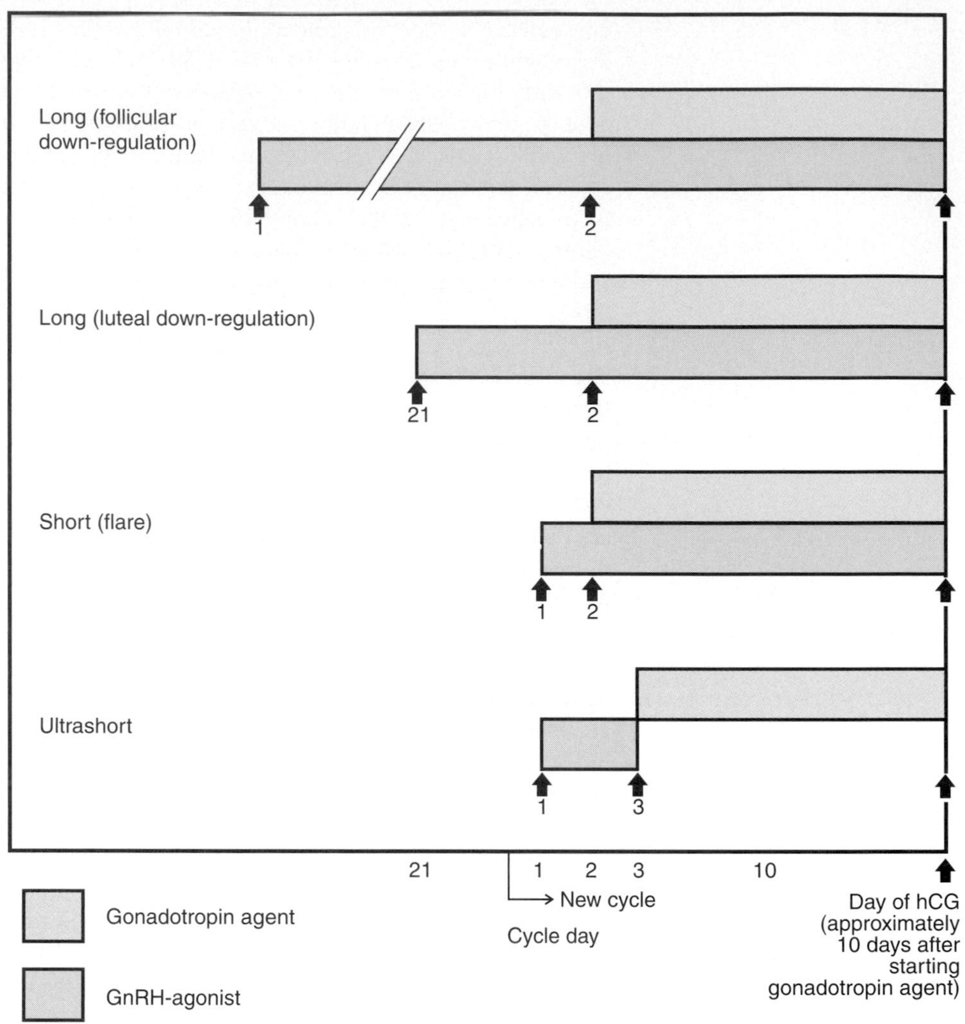

Figure 27.9 Protocols for using gonadotropin-releasing hormone (GnRH) agonist with gonadotropins in controlled ovarian hyperstimulation.

Choice of Gonadotropins In recent years, improved clinical pregnancy rates have been accompanied by progress in all facets of ART. Concurrent with improvements in embryo culture and embryo transfer techniques has been the introduction of several generations of gonadotropin formulations. The main theme of this pharmaceutical progress has been that of increasing the purity of the FSH component in novel preparations. As a result, current recombinant FSH preparations contain absolutely no LH and no other protein contaminants.

Although no difference in pregnancy rates can be shown between use of urinary FSH and hMG in downregulated ART cycles, urinary FSH has been linked to higher pregnancy rates in nondownregulated ART cycles (360). Further, purified FSH appears to be superior to hMG in the COH of clomiphene citrate–resistant PCOS patients in that it reduces the incidence of moderate to severe OHSS without affecting pregnancy rates (359).

In contrast to the comparisons between purified FSH and hMG, the efficacy of recombinant FSH relative to purified FSH or highly purified FSH has not been as certain. In addition to the benefits discussed under the section on COH and IUI, the impact on clinical outcomes of recombinant FSH relative to purified FSH or highly purified FSH has been studied in many prospective, randomized trials involving predominantly IVF or ICSI treatment or both. The

Table 27.8. Protocols for Using Gonadotropin-Releasing Hormone (GnRH) Agonist with Gonadotropins in Controlled Ovarian Hyperstimulation

Protocol	*Time of GnRH-α Start*	*Time of GnRH-α Discontinuation*	*Comments*
Long (follicular downregulation) (389)	Follicular phase of previous cycle or earlier	Day of hCG injection	Theoretical benefit for patients at high risk for OHSS due to increased suppression
Long (luteal downregulation)	Luteal phase of previous cycle (day 21)	Day of hCG injection	Most common protocol (see text)
Short (flare)	Follicular phase of ART cycle (started concurrently with, or just before, gonadotropins)	Day of hCG injection	Flare effect is hypothesized to cause additional stimulatory effects on follicles Theoretical enhancement of ovarian response in poor responders
Ultrashort (390,391)	Day 2 of ART cycle	GnRH-α is given for 3 days only	
Discontinuous (542)	Luteal phase of previous cycle (day 21)	Start day of gonadotropin injection	Theoretically decreased suppression, which may be desired in poor responders
OCP/microdose (543,544)	Low-dose OCP started on day 1 of previous cycle *Leuprolide acetate* 40 μg SC b.i.d started in luteal phase of previous cycle or concurrently with gonadotropins	Day of hCG injection	Reported to enhance ovarian response in poor responders

data are conflicting. Some studies have reported no differences among preparations with regard to number of follicles, eggs, embryos, fertilization rate, or total dosage requirement (401,402). Others have found recombinant FSH to be associated with shorter duration of stimulation (403–405), decreased total dosage requirements (403,405,406), greater numbers of follicles and oocytes (403,404), and greater number of embryos (405,406). Importantly, pregnancy rates per cycle have not increased significantly with use of recombinant FSH (401–408). Of course, this lack of demonstrable difference could be attributed to inadequate power in each individual study. A recent metaanalysis reported that recombinant FSH improved pregnancy rates when compared with studies using purified FSH or highly purified FSH with OR, 1.20 (95% CI, 1.02 to 1.42) (361).

Whether recombinant FSH affects the incidence of therapeutic complications in women undergoing ART deserves attention as well. Several randomized, controlled trials have reported a trend toward an elevated incidence of OHSS with the use of recombinant FSH, although this effect has not reached statistical significance (403–405). Taken together, results suggest an important role for recombinant FSH in ART regimens. This is based on its characteristic batch-to-batch consistency and subcutaneous route of administration, its possible superiority in outcomes over other gonadotropin preparations used in typical COH, its documented benefits over hMG in PCOS patients, and the small increase in ART pregnancy rates as determined by metaanalysis. Whether new metaanalyses that include recently published studies (401–404,406) will change current recommendations remains to be seen.

Role of Low-Dose Aspirin in ART A recent prospective, randomized trial demonstrated that the use of *aspirin* at a dose of 100 mg/d, initiated at the time of GnRH agonist luteal downregulation and continued throughout COH, resulted in an improvement in ovarian response, implantation, and pregnancy rates in IVF (409). Although low-dose *aspirin* has not become a standard part of the ART protocol, many patients are now taking it with or without recommendation. Significant complications have yet to be reported with the use of low-dose *aspirin* in ART. Still, the safety of this adjunctive therapy warrants close examination before its wide acceptance in ART.

Recombinant Human Luteinizing Hormone According to the two-cell theory of ovarian hormone production, stimulation of the theca lutein cells by LH is critical to the overall development of the ovarian follicle. Highly purified FSH contains minimal amounts of LH (<0.1%), and GnRH agonist suppresses endogenous pituitary LH and FSH production. Therefore, it has been suggested that supplemental LH might improve folliculogenesis and pregnancy rates when highly purified or recombinant FSH is used for COH in ART. A prospective, randomized trial comparing highly purified FSH and highly purified FSH combined with supplemental rhLH has reported a trend toward lower implantation and pregnancy rates when rhLH was added to GnRH agonist–downregulated ovulation induction cycles (410). Although it is possible that some yet-to-be determined subset of infertility patients might benefit from rhLH supplementation, the generalized use of this hormone in ART currently appears to be limited.

hCG Injection The injection of hCG serves to induce oocyte maturation before oocyte retrieval. The dosage of hCG is typically 10,000 IU given intramuscularly. Different criteria for hCG injection during COH for ART have been described, but all usually include the presence of one or two leading follicles with mean diameters larger than 16 to 18 mm, at least two other follicles with mean diameters larger than 14 mm, and serum estradiol levels above defined threshold levels of 300 to 500 pg/mL. Each IVF center sets site-specific criteria based on its own experience and pregnancy outcomes. The overall goal, however, is to avoid performing surgery (oocyte retrieval) on patients who have zero to minimal chance of conceiving because of poor ovarian response. In the past, serial hCG injections were given for induction of luteal support; however, that approach can lead to an increased incidence and severity of OHSS. Luteal-phase support now relies solely on exogenous progesterone supplementation.

Oocyte Retrieval Oocyte retrieval is typically performed 36 hours after the hCG injection. Although historically performed by laparoscopy, laparoscopic oocyte retrieval has now been replaced by the transvaginal ultrasound-guided approach. Transvaginal ultrasound-guided retrieval is markedly less invasive than its laparoscopic counterpart, and the use of ultrasound permits the surgeon to visualize the location of the needle within each ovarian follicle. Intravenous sedation is commonly used for transvaginal ultrasound–guided oocyte retrieval; however, spinal anesthesia may offer an advantage in certain cases, especially when the patient has numerous follicles or the retrieval is anticipated to be anatomically challenging (411–413).

Because the vaginal canal and wall are traversed using transvaginal ultrasound-guided oocyte aspiration, the possibility of iatrogenically infecting the patient or her oocytes deserves particular consideration. Sterile normal saline typically is used for surgical preparation during oocyte retrieval. In one prospective, randomized trial comparing sterile normal saline to 1% *povidone-iodine* for this application, the former had higher associated pregnancy rates while maintaining low infection rates (414). Although the exact mechanism for this finding is unclear, it is hypothesized that contact with *povidone-iodine* could potentially harm oocytes. Therefore, if povidone-iodine is used, it is recommended that the vagina be lavaged with normal saline after preparation. In addition, routine antibiotic prophylaxis is recommended for transvaginal ultrasound procedures. Such prophylaxis reduces the incidence of postprocedure positive microbiology cultures of embryo catheter tips in 78% of patients undergoing embryo transfer. The importance of this effect is suggested by the fact that lower implantation and pregnancy rates are associated with positive microbial catheter-tip cultures (415).

Performance of the retrieval itself often is fairly simple. A long, 16-gauge needle, secured by a guide onto the transvaginal ultrasound probe, is used to traverse the upper vaginal wall and enter into a follicle under direct, real-time transvaginal ultrasound guidance. Follicular fluid is then aspirated using about 100 mm Hg of vacuum. Higher pressures may traumatize the oocyte. When the entire follicular fluid content has been aspirated into sterile, prewarmed culture tubes, the inner wall of the follicle is gently curetted with the needle. This process is repeated until all the follicles are aspirated. At the end of the procedure, a speculum is inserted into the vagina, and the cervix and vaginal walls are inspected for bleeding. Although transvaginal ultrasound-guided oocyte retrieval is both rapid and minimally invasive, all potential risks, albeit rare, should be clearly explained to the patient before IVF treatment begins. These risks include the following:

- Excessive bleeding, possibly requiring blood transfusion
- Potential needle-induced injury to structures in proximity to the ovaries, including bowel, bladder, and major blood vessels, may require repair by emergency laparotomy, resulting in an abdominal surgical scar.
- Late infectious complications, such as abscesses in the peritoneum, bowel, ovary, or uterus, may require hospitalization for intravenous antibiotics or surgical interventions. In the specific case of iatrogenic tuboovarian abscess, failure of medical treatment may necessitate surgical removal of the tubes and ovaries.
- Risks associated with intravenous sedation or general anesthesia
- A remote risk that no oocytes will be obtained or fertilized

IVF, ICSI, GIFT, and ZIFT Fertilization of the human oocyte by human sperm *in vivo* requires the interaction of capacitated spermatozoa with ovulated oocytes, most often within the ampullary portion of the fallopian tube. Capacitation of sperm takes place in the female reproductive tract and involves both changes in sperm motility and changes in the sperm cell membrane that allow the acrosome reaction. Acrosome-reacted sperm are able to penetrate the oocyte's cumulus oophorus and zona pellucida, binding to the oocyte cell membrane and promoting fertilization. The interaction of spermatozoa and oocyte is not a chance occurrence as Complex oocyte–sperm intercommunications appear to play an important role in this process (416).

The mandate of the ART team is to attempt to re-create precisely those processes known to occur in unassisted conception. In all ART procedures, male gametes are initially collected directly by ejaculation into a sterile cup. They are then processed, concentrated, and incubated in protein-supplemented media for 3 to 4 hours before being used for fertilization. This final incubation allows for sperm capacitation. Before fertilization, retrieved oocytes are also cultured in protein-supplemented media for about 6 to 8 hours. For IVF purposes, 50,000 to 100,000 capacitated sperm are placed in culture with a single oocyte; 16 to 18 hours later, fertilization is documented by the presence of two pronuclei within the developing embryo.

Indications for ICSI are discussed under Male Factor Infertility. The procedure itself begins by stripping all granulosa cells from the aspirated cumulus complex (oocyte and surrounding cells). This is followed by micromanipulation of egg and sperm under magnification. More specifically, a holding pipette is used to stabilize the egg while an injection pipette is used to insert a viable sperm into the ooplasm of the egg.

Techniques such as GIFT and ZIFT use the tubal microenvironment as the initial point of germ cell contact after transfer. As in standard IVF, all regimens typically involve GnRH agonist downregulation followed by COH with gonadotropins. GIFT and ZIFT differ both in the duration that the gametes remain *in vitro* and their time of transfer. In the GIFT procedure, oocyte retrieval can be performed transvaginally or laparoscopically. Aspirated oocytes and freshly processed sperm are then resuspended in a small amount of media and rapidly transferred into the fallopian tube by laparoscopy. Historically, GIFT was initially preferred over IVF for two reasons. The limited quality of transvaginal ultrasound at the time precluded reliable transvaginal ultrasound-guided oocyte retrieval and required laparoscopic approaches. At the same time, *in vitro* embryo culture techniques had significant limitations, and it was felt that minimization of the duration of *in vitro* gamete exposure was desirable. Today, however, transvaginal ultrasound quality is excellent, and dramatic improvements have been made in gamete and embryo culture techniques. To its detriment, GIFT requires normally functioning fallopian tubes and precludes the assessment of fertilization. Taken together, there remain very few primary medical indications for GIFT; nearly all are social or religious. ZIFT also requires normally functioning fallopian tubes; unlike GIFT, however, the ZIFT procedure involves *in vitro* fertilization of retrieved oocytes and overnight culture. Zygote-stage embryos are then laparoscopically transferred to the fallopian tubes about 24 hours after oocyte retrieval. Fertilization can be assessed with ZIFT.

Luteal Support Because the act of retrieving oocytes and associated granulosa cells may adversely affect subsequent corpus luteal function, retrieval poses the possible risk of subsequent progesterone insufficiency. Therefore, the requirement for luteal support represents yet another way in which ART cycles differ from COH/IUI protocols. Luteal support is usually initiated on the day after oocyte retrieval for ART. Commonly used regimens include the following:

- *Progesterone* in oil 50 mg, once a day, intramuscularly
- Vaginal *progesterone* suppositories, 200 mg twice a day.
- Oral micronized *progesterone,* 200 mg twice a day

Despite similar levels of circulating progesterone, the last regimen is associated with decreased per-embryo implantation rates when compared with use of intramuscular progesterone (417).

Embryo Transfer In unassisted conception, the fertilized oocyte traverses through the fallopian tube for 2 to 3 days before entry into the uterus for implantation. This transport is largely dependent on directional ciliary movement within the fallopian tube, although tubal muscular contractions may be involved (418). The embryo is normally at the morular or early blastocyst stage of development when it reaches the uterine cavity. By this time, and under the influence of luteal-phase levels of progesterone, the endometrium has undergone the decidual changes that prepare it for implantation. The embryo resides in the intrauterine cavity for 2 to 3 days before implantation. During this period, the zona pellucida detaches, allowing implantation to occur 5 to 7 days after fertilization.

ART protocols for *in vitro* embryo culture and development attempt to recapitulate the timing and conditions of these events, albeit in an incredibly simplified fashion. The development of sequential media has allowed embryos to be grown *in vitro* until about 72 hours (or day 3 after oocyte retrieval), when they are transferred back into the cavity of the uterus. Embryo morphologic criteria—including such parameters as cell number, symmetry, fragmentation, and granularity—are used in most centers to judge the quality of a particular embryo; however, these methods of assessment do not correlate well with embryonic developmental potential (419).

In an effort to better assess and select for transfer those embryos that will result in successful pregnancy, investigators have recently evaluated the advantages of extending the *in vitro* embryo culture period before transfer. *In vitro* culture to day 5 postretrieval allows the evaluation and selection of embryos at the blastocyst stage. It is possible that this extended culture does, in fact, increase the ability to judge appropriately the quality of an embryo. For instance, grading of the blastocyst according to the morphology of the inner cell mass and trophectoderm has been correlated with implantation and pregnancy rates (420). Because of its increased implantation rate, extended embryo culture may offer the advantage of limiting the number of transferred embryos while maintaining clinical pregnancy rates. The true value of blastocyst transfer may therefore lie in its potential to decrease the rates of high-order multiple gestation resulting from ART. However, for reasons that are unclear, there appears to be an increased risk for monozygotic twinning of embryos cultured to the blastocyst stage, which can lead to increased obstetric complications (421).

Pregnancy rates resulting from blastocyst transfer range between 44% for low-scoring blastocysts and 87% for top-scoring ones. Another predictor of the success rate of day 5 transfer is the number of eight-cell embryos on day 3 (421). Extended culture to the blastocyst stage (day 5) has been advocated by some to be beneficial for all IVF patients, with overall pregnancy rates of up to 43.8% (420,422). Others recommend it only if there are three or more eight-cell embryos on day 3 of *in vitro* culture (422). Still others do not recommend it at all (423). The true application of extended embryo culture and blastocyst transfer remains to be determined.

Technical Aspects of Embryo Transfer Despite its theoretic simplicity, transcervical embryo transfer into the intrauterine cavity is a procedure that requires a significant amount of skill. Correct performance of the procedure is thought to exert significant impact on clinical outcome. Apart from the skill and experience of the operator, variables such as aspiration of cervical mucus (424), visualization by ultrasound guidance (425), duration of supine position immediately after embryo transfer (426), and type of bacteria cultured from the transfer catheter-tip postprocedure (427) have all been suggested to affect clinical pregnancy outcomes. Microbial contamination of the embryo transfer is especially relevant because it may be prevented by antibiotic prophylaxis at the time of oocyte retrieval and careful handling of the catheter. Clinical pregnancy rates are reduced by half in women with positive catheter-tip cultures (428).

Many different types of catheters have been used to perform embryo transfers, including hard catheters (Erlangen, Tefcat, Tom Cat, Norfolk) and soft catheters (Frydman, Wallace). The Frydman and Wallace catheters are currently the most popular because they are thought to be the least traumatic to the endometrium; however, no catheter has been demonstrated to be definitively superior (429,430).

In women with a history of tubal disease, the difficulty of embryo transfer has been associated with an increased risk for ectopic pregnancy (431). The number of transfer attempts, the time required for embryo transfer procedures, and the presence of blood inside the transfer catheter after the procedure do not affect clinical outcomes (432). In a series of more than 800 consecutive embryo transfer procedures, 85.9% were easy, 8.4% were difficult, 3.2% needed to be repeated, and 2.5% required cervical dilation. Technical difficulties, repeated embryo transfers due to retained embryos, and cervical dilation for stenosis did not affect the pregnancy rates in this study (433). The timing of the correction of cervical hindrances to embryo transfers may be crucial. Specifically, although it markedly facilitated the embryo transfers itself, cervical dilation at the time of oocyte retrieval in patients with a history of very difficult embryo transfer was associated with poor pregnancy outcome (1 in 41 cycles) (434). In contrast, if performed before commencement of IVF/embryo transfer, surgical treatments for anticipated problems with embryo transfer yield good pregnancy rates. For example, hysteroscopic examination of the cervical canal may reveal a ridge, which can be resected (435). Alternatively, transcervical placement of a Malecot catheter at the time of hysteroscopy has been successful in allowing facile entry into the uterine cavity during subsequent embryo transfer or IUI. The Malecot catheter can be left in place for several weeks after hysteroscopy, as long as *doxycycline* 100 mg twice daily is taken; it is easily removed using gentle traction in the office as the day of embryo transfer approaches (436). Good clinical pregnancy outcomes have been reported for both techniques.

Cryopreservation of Embryos The success of modern ovulation induction and fertilization regimens often results in embryos in excess of the number appropriate for transfer in a single cycle. Cryopreservation of these embryos permits embryo transfer to the same patient in nonstimulated cycles in the future. Some patients receive cryopreserved embryos during "natural" cycles; others undergo endometrial preparation with sequential exogenous estrogen and progesterone. Either regimen is significantly less expensive than a gonadotropin-stimulated cycle. More importantly, the risks of surgical complications and OHSS are nonexistent in cycles using cryopreserved embryos. Therefore, pregnancies resulting from transfer of cryopreserved embryos effectively reduce both the financial and medical costs of pregnancy per ovulation stimulation. There is, of course, a perceived downside to cryopreserved cycles because not all embryos survive thawing and pregnancy rates are lower than those using fresh embryos. In transfers of cryopreserved embryos using nondonor eggs (eggs from the intended recipient), 90% of thawing procedures resulted in viable embryos for transfer. The rates of clinical pregnancy and delivery were 23.8% and 18.8%, respectively, for cryopreserved embryo transfer procedures (437). These are only perceived disadvantages, however, because the risk for cryocycles is minimal and excess embryos would otherwise not be used.

Pregnancy Testing and Follow-up of Early Pregnancy The uncertainties surrounding ART treatment and its outcomes can be highly stressful and treated couples are understandably anxious to obtain a pregnancy test as early as possible (438). Serial quantitative hCG levels can be done starting on day 16 after oocyte retrieval. Serum hCG levels taken earlier than this day may give false-negative or false-positive results. The latter may reflect the use of intramuscular hCG to trigger ovulation because this exogenous hCG can be detected for up to 14 days after injection (439). Day 16 serum quantitative hCG levels lower than 50 IU/L are associated with a 35% chance of an ongoing intrauterine pregnancy; levels greater than 500 IU/L are predictive of successful outcome in more than 95% of cases (440). In this same study, a single serum progesterone level on day 16 did not provide further prognostic value and is therefore not recommended (440).

Patients are usually followed with serial serum hCG levels early in pregnancy, followed by transvaginal ultrasound at 5 to 6 weeks of gestation to document intrauterine location of the pregnancy and the number of gestational sacs. This is especially important for patients with risk factors for ectopic pregnancy, those who are experiencing vaginal bleeding, and those at high risk for higher-order multiple gestation. In addition, such close follow-up in early pregnancy is both indicated and necessary among ART patients because an ongoing pregnancy requires patients to continue daily self-administration of supplemental progesterone (until the luteal-placental shift at about 9 to 10 weeks of gestation). Transvaginal ultrasound at 7 to 8 weeks for identification of fetal cardiac activity can provide further reassurance.

Success Rates Success rates of IVF vary from program to program; within a program, the rates of success vary with the patient's diagnosis and age. The most comprehensive assessment of the efficacy of ART in North American programs comes from the database of the Society for Assisted Reproductive Technology (SART) (437). The society's data collection began in 1985, and its annual summary is published in an effort to improve the quality of statistical reporting on ART. The database attempts to eliminate the effects of interprogram variation. The most recently published report of the society summarizes the results of ART in the United States and Canada for 1997, which are shown in Table 27.9 (437). **Information on SART and registered ART clinics are accessible by the public at http://www.sart.org.** Significant improvements in the overall ART outcomes have been made when compared with the last published results. In 1997, a 28.4% (16.8% in 1992) rate of delivered pregnancies was reported per oocyte retrieval for standard IVF, with a cancellation rate of 21.7% (15.4% in 1992), a pregnancy loss rate of 18.1% (20% in 1992), and an ectopic pregnancy rate of 0.9% (1.2% in 1992) per transfer. The delivered-pregnancy rate for cryopreserved embryo transfer was 18.8% in 1997 (11.6% in 1992). Although the rates of birth defects did not appear to be different from that of the general population, the SART reporting system was not designed to specifically address this issue.

The age of the woman was a significant determinant of success in ART (437) (Table 27.10). Women aged 41 years and older had a delivery rate per retrieval of only 9.4%. The increase in cancellation rates with age—most likely the result of poor ovarian response–was consistent

Table 27.9. Reported Outcomes for Assisted Reproductive Technology Procedures Performed in 1997 in the United States[a]

	Standard IVF	*IVF Plus ICSI*	*GIFT*	*ZIFT*	*Donor Oocyte Transfer[c]*	*CPE Transfer*	*CPE Transfer with Donor Oocyte*	*Host Uterus Transfer*
No. of cyles or procedures[b]	33,032	18,312	1,943	1,104	4,616	10,181	1,584	600
Cancellations (%)	21.7	NA	14.4	10.4	6.2	6.0	4.3	6.2
No. of retrievals	25,878	18,292	1,663	989	NA	NA	NA	563
No. of transfers	24,027	17,243	1,640	911	4,122	9,165	1,467	540
Transfers per retrieval (%)	92.8	94.3	98.6	92.1	NA	NA	NA	95.9
No. of clinical pregnancies	8,975	6,072	627	346	1,978	2,185	400	226
Pregnancy loss (%)	18.1	18.5	20.4	19.9	16.6	21.3	18.8	17.3
No. of deliveries	7,353	4,949	499	277	1,650	1,719	325	187
Deliveries per retrieval (%)	28.4	27.1	30.0	28.0	NA	NA	NA	33.2
Singelton (%)	59.6	62.9	66.9	66.4	56.5	74.4	65.8	83.3
No. of ectopic pregnancies (EP)	220	102	16	11	21	60	10	1
EP transfer (%)	0.9	0.6	1.0	1.2	0.5	0.7	0.7	0.2
Abnormal neonates (%)[e]	1.6	1.7	1.9	1.6	1.9	1.8	2.0	1.9

IVF, *in vitro* fertilization; ICSI, intracytoplasmic sperm injection; GIFT, gamete intrafallopian transfer; ZIFT, zygote intrafallopian transfer; CPE, cryopreserved embryo; NA, not applicable. See text for discussion.
[a] Except combination (n = 1,173), research (n = 40), embryo banking (n = 258), and other (n = 226) cycles.
[b] Includes all cycles regardless of maternal age and infertility diagnosis.
[c] Includes known or anonymous but not host uterus transfer or surrogate.
[d] Cryopreserved embryo transfer cycles not done in combination with fresh embryo transfer and not with donor egg or embryo.
[e] Reporting of structural and functional abnormality is problematic. See text for discussion.
From **Adamson D.** ASRM/SART registry 1997 results. *Fertil Steril* 2000;74:641–653, with permission.

with significantly decreased ovarian reserve in older women. With the high efficacy of ICSI as a treatment for male factor infertility, the delivery rates per retrieval among couples with male factor infertility were comparable to those achieved in couples without male factor for a given female age group.

Treatment with Donor Oocytes Women with premature ovarian failure have very few reproductive options. The use of donor oocytes may represent the only proven method by which most of these patients can become pregnant. Other patients to be considered for donor oocyte technology may include those with poor oocyte quality (including some patients with failed fertilization), those with poor ovarian response to stimulation, and those with a history of multiple failed ART cycles. Using embryos fertilized from donor eggs in 418 fresh embryo transfer involving 276 recipients, clinical pregnancy and delivery rates were 36.2% and 29.3%, respectively. The cumulative pregnancy rate after four cycles reached 87.9% (441).

Treatment with donor oocytes is available in most ART programs. The method of donor selection is an important consideration. Some patients may wish to find their own donor in a sister or friend; others may choose to use a matching service to identify a donor, who can remain anonymous. Although some ART programs may choose to be excluded from the matching process, most will assume the responsibility of screening the donor for medical, reproductive, and psychological fitness. Like semen donors, potential oocyte donors must

Table 27.10. *In Vitro* Fertilization (IVF) Procedures[a] by Maternal Age Group and Infertility Diagnosis

Patient Category	*No. of Retrievals*	*Cancelled Cycles (%)*	*Transfers per Retrieval (%)*	*No. of Pregnancies*	*No. of Deliveries*	*Deliveries per Retriveal (%)*	*Multiple Births per Delivery (%)*
1997 IVF procedures without ICSI							
Women ≤ 34 years of age, no male factor infertility	24,725	10.2	93.9	5,802	4,988	33.9	44.7
Women 35–37 years of age, no male factor infertility	7,513	14.8	94.4	2,716	2,206	29.4	38.4
Women 38–40 years of age, no male factor infertility	6,257	19.3	93.0	1,763	1,326	21.2	28.6
Women ≥ 41 years of age, no male factor infertility	3,682	24.4	90.0	591	345	9.4	28.8

[a] With and without intracytoplasmic sperm injection (ICSI).
From **Adamson D.** ASRM/SART registry 1997 results. *Fertil Steril* 2000;74:641–653, with permission.

be stringently assessed, including screening for transmittable infectious or genetic diseases. Unlike semen, however, oocytes cannot presently be cryopreserved and quarantined; hence, the risk for transmission of infectious agents cannot be completely averted. Moreover, because oocyte donation involves COH, a donor is exposed to the same intensive monitoring and significant potential complications inherent to this intervention. Potential donors must be provided with detailed educational information and meticulous informed consent is mandatory. In addition to undergoing medical screening, oocyte donors are subjected to a comprehensive psychosocial evaluation before being accepted as program participants. Even with such extensive screening and preparation, there is a significant dropout rate for both anonymous and directed oocyte donors (442). It is advisable to obtain legal counsel in the development of any ovum donation center because many potentially litigious issues arise in the administration of such a program.

Oocyte cryopreservation is not generally available or successful and embryo cryopreservation reduces subsequent pregnancy rates. Considerable coordination is required to ensure that the recipient's endometrium is appropriately prepared when embryos freshly fertilized from the donor oocytes are ready to be transferred (443). Regimens for ovulation induction and oocyte retrieval for the oocyte donor follow those of standard IVF protocols (Fig. 27.10). Although the oocyte donor is exposed to many of the adverse effects of COH protocols (OHSS, postoperative pelvic discomfort, surgical and anesthesia risks, and medication side effects), her risk for multiple gestation and ectopic pregnancy can be virtually eliminated if she abstains from intercourse during her stimulation cycle.

To ensure adequate endometrial preparation, most recipients of donor oocytes are taken through a "mock" cycle before their actual treatment cycle. During the mock cycle, all hormonal agents are administered, and endometrial adequacy is documented by timed endometrial biopsies. The impact that the completion of a mock cycle might have on the pregnancy rates of subsequent ART cycles with donor eggs has not been studied in a randomized trial. However, important factors such as patient compliance, histologic evidence of endometrial response to exogenous hormones, and the ease of embryo transfer can be

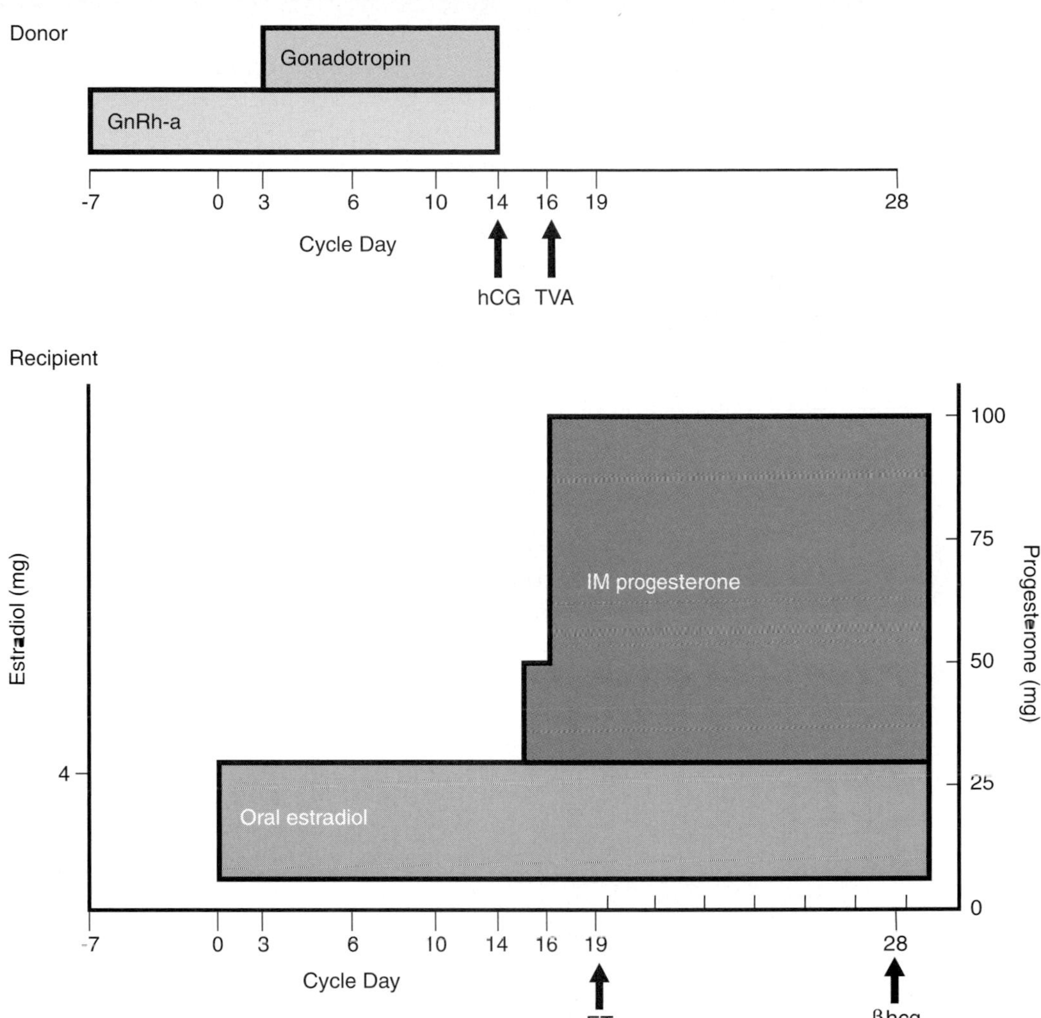

Figure 27.10 Regimens of ovarian stimulation and hormone replacement used to synchronize the development of ovarian follicles in the oocyte donor and the endometrial cycle in the recipient. (hMG, human menopausal gonadotropin; hCG, human chorionic gonadotropin; β-hCG, the β subunit of hCG; OHSS, ovarian hyperstimulation syndrome; OCP, oral contraceptive pill; ART, assistive reproductive technology.) *Reproduced with permission from:* **Chang PL, Sauer MY**. Assisted reproductive techniques. Stenchever MA, ed. *Atlas of Clinical Gynecology,* Mishell DR, ed, *Reproductive Endocrinology*. Vol. 3. Philadelphia: Current Sciences Group, 1998.

assessed (444). Many regimens for endometrial preparation have been described, although successful pregnancies have also been reported after embryo transfer in natural cycles. The following is a typical regimen for endometrial preparation in recipients of donor oocytes:

- **If the recipient has no baseline ovarian function, no downregulation or baseline testing is required.** However, if the recipient has endogenous ovarian function, GnRH agonist is started on day 21 in the luteal phase of the previous cycle. At onset of menses, downregulation is confirmed with serum estradiol levels of less than 50 pg/mL and progesterone levels of less than 1.0 ng/mL. If confirmed, the dose of GnRH agonist is reduced.
- Start *estradiol:* (*Estraderm* patches 0.2 mg every 48 hours or *Vivelle* patches 0.2 mg every 48 hours or *Estrace,* 1.0 mg orally once per day).
- Monitor serum estradiol levels every 3 to 7 days and adjust dosage to maintain serum estradiol levels of 150 to 300 pg/mL, or continue fixed dose.
- Continue supplementation at dosages that maintain these estrogen levels for at least 21 days.

- The progesterone start day is scheduled according to the day of embryo transfer (in a therapeutic cycle) or the day of endometrial biopsy (in the mock cycle).
- Start *progesterone*, 25–50 mg intramuscularly (day 1), then increase to 50–100 mg/d intramuscularly the following day.
- Discontinue GnRH agonist on day 2 of *progesterone*.
- Mock cycle: perform endometrial biopsy 10 to 12 days after *progesterone* is started. Therapeutic cycle: perform embryo transfer on day 4 of *progesterone*.
- Measure quantitative hCG 16 days or more after the day of donor oocyte retrieval.

Many controversial issues and much ethical debate surround oocyte donation. Donors' expectations regarding the process itself, the quality of their medical care, and their level of involvement in decisions can be addressed by a conscientious ART team (445). Other topics, such as methods of donor recruitment and amounts of financial compensation, are much more challenging issues (446,447). Further effort is warranted to help clarify these issues and provide access to this highly efficacious ART treatment.

Complications of ART

Twins and Higher-order Multiple Gestation

Multiple gestation, especially higher-order multiple gestation, is a serious complication of infertility treatment and has tremendous medical, psychological, social, and financial implications. In recent years, it has been reported that only 20% of higher-order multiple gestations are the result of spontaneous conceptions. The remaining 80% are attributable to reproductive interventions. Of these multiple gestations, half are attributable to ART and half to the use of ovulation drugs in non-ART cycles (448). Because the average age of women attempting pregnancy has risen during recent decades and increased maternal age affects the incidence of multiple gestation, rates of higher-order multiple gestation must be adjusted for maternal age when compared across time (449). For decades before 1971, higher-order multiple gestation occurred at a maternal age–adjusted incidence of about 30 per 100,000 live births from spontaneous conceptions (449,450). This incidence rose to 173.6 per 100,000 live births in 1997 (449) (Table 27.11). Because higher-order multiple gestations are predominantly triplets (91.2% were triplets in 1997) (448), this rate represents 6,737 triplets born in the United States in 1997 alone (Table 27.12).

Significant medical risks accompany higher-order multiple gestation. There is an increased incidence of potentially life-threatening obstetric conditions such as acute fatty liver (452)

Table 27.11. Rate[a] of Triplet and Higher-order Multiple Births, by Mother's Age; United States, 1980–1997

	Triplet and Higher-order Multiple Births	
Age group (yr)	*1980*	*1997*
<20	14.8	20.7
20–24	31.4	46.8
25–29	42.8	151.0
30–34	58.3	293.6
35–39	47.6	403.2
40–44	[b]	315.4
45–49	[b]	2,100.2
All ages	37.0	173.6

[a] Per 100,000 live-born infants.
[b] Numbers do not meet standards of reliability or precision.
From Contribution of assisted reproductive technology and ovulation-inducing drugs to triplet and higher-order multiple births—United States, 1980–1997. *MMWR Morb Mortal Wkly Rep* 2000;49:535–538, with permission.

Table 27.12. Contribution of Assisted Reproductive Technology (ART) to Triplet and Higher-order Multiple Births (≥Triplets)—United States, 1989–1997

Year	*Total No. Live-born Infants*	*No. of ≥Triplets*	*Percentage of ≥ Triplets of Total No. Live-born Infants*	*≥Triplets Ratio*[a]	*Percentage of ≥ Triplets by Spontaneous Conception*	*Percentage of ≥Triplets Using ART*	*Estimated Percentage of ≥Triplets Using Ovulation Drugs*
1989	4,040,958	2,798	0.07	69.2	—	—	—
1990	4,158,212	3,028	0.07	72.8	—	22.0[c]	—
1991	4,110,907	3,346	0.08	81.4	—	22.0[c]	—
1992	4,065,014	3,883	0.09	95.6	—	—	—
1993	4,000,240	4,168	0.10	104.2	—	—	—
1994	3,952,767	4,594	0.12	116.2	—	—	
1995	3,899,589	4,973	0.13	127.2	—	—	—
1996[b]	3,891,494	5,939	0.15	152.6	20.9	38.7	40.4
1997[b]	3,880,894	6,737	0.17	173.6	18.4	43.4	38.2

[a] Number of ≥triplets per 100,000 live-born infants.
[b] Based on number of ART-associated ≥triplets and total number of ≥triplets, 1990 and 1991 (3).
[c] Percentage of ≥triplets by spontaneous conception, percentage of ≥triplets using ART, and estimated percentage of ≥triplets using ovulation durgs add up to 100% overall ≥triplet ratio.
From Contribution of assisted reproductive technology and ovulation-inducing drugs to triplet and higher-order multiple births—United States, 1980–1997. *MMWR Morb Mortal Wkly Rep* 2000;49:535–538, with permission.

and severe preeclampsia (452). The rate of fetal death during the third trimester is also unacceptably high at almost 17% (454). Obstetrically, triplets are at increased risk for preterm birth, low birth weight (<2,500 g), and very low birth weight (<1,500 g) compared with singletons or twins (451,455). When adjusted for gestational age at birth, triplets have the same rates of neonatal morbidity and mortality as twins and singletons (456,457), but triplets typically deliver much earlier. One exception to this equalization is that premature triplets are at significantly greater risk for severe retinopathy of prematurity even when delivered at the same gestational age as a matched singleton or twin (457). Because of the extensive obstetric and neonatal intensive care required in higher-order multiple gestation pregnancies, enormous expenditures are required to provide medical care to these families (458). Finally, although not fully described, the immediate and long-term emotional and psychological impact on the mother, her partner, and the family unit, including other siblings, is likely to be daunting.

To rectify this trend in higher-order multiple gestations, a number of medical and nonmedical causes are being identified. Non-ART COH with gonadotropins is a highly efficacious and commonly used treatment modality for infertile couples. It is significantly less expensive than ART and thereby more accessible to many patients. Unfortunately, it is associated with a 20% incidence of twin gestations and 10% incidence of higher-order multiple gestation (459). Current monitoring protocols for non-ART COH, based on serum estradiol levels and the number of large follicles on ultrasound cannot entirely predict the risk for higher-order multiple gestation (460). The risk for higher-order multiple gestation is significantly increased with younger age, peak serum estradiol levels greater than 1,385 pg/mL, and a total number of follicles of seven or more (460). It is difficult to glean the significance of this latter measurement, however, because total follicle number depends on which follicles are measured, and it is unclear what should be the smallest reportable size. Further, a high total number of follicles may result from overstimulation of a patient with normal ovaries but unexpectedly high ovarian response or from treatment of a patient with PCO-like ovaries. Because the prevention and management strategies would differ for these two conditions, further stratification of patients and characterization of the COH cycles may clarify relative risks and direct more efficacious prevention of multiple gestation and OHSS.

Suggestions to address non-ART COH as a cause of higher-order multiple gestation are being explored. None is without cost. One option would promote lowering the dosage of gonadotropins used in COH to aim at a lesser degree of ovarian response. This approach will almost certainly lower pregnancy rates. An alternative would be fewer interventions with non-ART COH and substitution with ART. In ART, the rate of higher-order multiple gestation is determined by the number of embryos transferred, not the ovarian response, so that there is a greater control of the higher-order multiple gestation rate by physicians. This approach, however, would require a dramatic change in the guidelines for insurance company reimbursement of infertility treatments or would necessitate the financing of such treatment by the couple. Currently, there are no accepted criteria guiding when a non-ART cycle should be cancelled in an attempt to reduce the risk for higher-order multiple gestation. Informed recommendations for such standardization might be helpful.

More progress is being made toward reduction of higher-order multiple gestation in the area of ART. One approach, discussed under Embryo Transfer, would involve greater use of extended embryo culture, in which embryos are allowed to grow to the blastocyst stage *in vitro*. Blastocysts have been shown to have greater developmental potential and higher implantation rates than day 3 embryos, so that even if fewer (a maximum of one to two) blastocysts are transferred, pregnancy rates remain high (420). Another approach would follow the lead of countries outside the United States that have defined set limits for the maximum number of embryos transferred in a given ART cycle. The American Society of Reproductive Medicine has recently addressed this issue by publishing guidelines for embryo transfer during ART. Briefly, a maximum of three, four, and five embryos can be transferred to women with above-average prognosis (age < 35 years), average prognosis (age between 30 and 40 years), and below-average prognosis (age > 40 years or multiple failed ART cycles), respectively (461). In donor oocyte cycles, the age of the donor (not the recipient) should be used to determine the number of embryos to be transferred (461). Data on the efficacy of this protocol is expected to be available in a few years. Meanwhile, Templeton and Morris advocated even more stringent guidelines, promoting the transfer of a maximum of two embryos in ART cycles to minimize the risk for higher-order multiple gestation (462). Cryopreservation of excess embryos should certainly be encouraged further in order to promote more cycles involving transfer of cryopreserved embryos. Universal application of such changes will force patients and doctors to emphasize cumulative birth rates rather than pregnancy rate per cycle. By focusing on cumulative birth rates, patients can have more realistic expectations, and the demand to have an excessive number of embryos transferred would decrease (463,464). As discussed for non-ART COH, these changes will involve alterations in the entire financial reimbursement structure for ART services. There is no doubt that this approach will present many challenges.

Other factors contributing to the increased rates of higher-order multiple gestation have been identified. It has been suggested that government-mandated annual reporting of clinic-specific pregnancy rates places undue emphasis on pregnancy rate per cycle. This may encourage the promotion of higher pregnancy rates at the expense of higher multiple pregnancy rates. If our goal in infertility therapy is the delivery of a healthy baby, both pregnancy rates and incidence of multiple gestation must be considered in determining treatment efficacy. Financial reimbursement schedules by insurance companies, lack of federal support for IVF research, and insufficient patient education regarding the true risk for higher-order multiple gestation are all being examined (465–468).

On the scientific front, new technologies, such as preimplantation genetic diagnosis, may ultimately eliminate the risk for higher-order multiple gestation. Preimplantation genetic diagnosis is a clinical diagnostic procedure that can be performed on the embryo itself in order to determine whether a particular genetic abnormality is present before its transfer into the uterus (469). Preimplantation genetic diagnosis has been developed in an effort to improve the chances of having healthy infants among families at high risk for a particular genetic disease. It is most frequently performed using blastomere (a cell from a day 3 embryo containing six to eight cells) biopsy, followed by genetic testing on the cell obtained. The technique chosen for diagnostic testing depends on the type of genetic defect being investigated. For example, fluorescence *in situ* hybridization (FISH) can be used to assess aneuploidy, translocation, and other chromosomal structural defects (470). FISH can also be used to exclude transmittal of X-linked diseases by identification X and Y chromosomes, thus allowing transfer of female embryos only (471). Alternatively, familial single gene mutations can be identified by extracting blastomere DNA, followed by polymerase chain reaction, restriction enzyme digest, or sequencing. In a recent study involving 262 ART cycles, the embryos obtained from women with a poor prognosis (characterized by age older than 35 years with previous IVF failures and karyotypic defects) were randomized to preimplantation genetic diagnosis for aneuploidy or a control procedure. Those chromosomes commonly involved in aneuploidies (X, Y, 13, 14, 15, 16, 18, 21, and 22) were assessed using FISH in the study group. Although fewer embryos were transferred in the preimplantation genetic diagnosis group, higher clinical pregnancy rates (37% versus 27%) and implantation rates (22.5% versus 10.2%) were reported when compared with controls (472). Therefore, preimplantation genetic diagnosis may assist in the selection of euploidic embryos, relegating to this technique a tremendous potential in lowering the risk of higher-order multiple gestation.

As progress is being made to eradicate the complication of higher-order multiple gestation, others have suggested ways to reduce subsequent risks once higher-order multiple gestation has occurred. One option for preventing some of the maternal and fetal complications of higher-order multiple gestation involves the judicious use of selective pregnancy termination or multifetal reduction. Although any high order multiple gestation is a candidate for this procedure, the reduction of triplet to twin pregnancies is most common and best studied. Overall, about 14% of triplet pregnancies reduce spontaneously to twin pregnancies after fetal heart activity is documented on transvaginal ultrasound at 8 to 9 weeks (473,474). Although some studies have not found multifetal reduction to result in significant improvement in gestational length or intrauterine growth restriction (474,475), many centers have reported improved outcomes after reductions to twin gestations. Twin gestations after reduction have similar outcomes when compared with spontaneous twin gestations (476,477). Reduction of triplet to twin gestation has been reported to decrease the risk for preterm birth (478), low birth weight (478), preeclampsia (477), and delivery before 36 weeks (477). Specifically, preterm birth before 28, 32, and 34 weeks of gestation, as well as birth weights of less than 1,000, 1,500, and 2,000 g were significantly lower in twins after reduction from triplet pregnancy compared with triplets who did not undergo reduction (479). However, any benefits achieved for newborn health often incur tremendous emotional, psychological, and physical costs. The major complications of fetal reduction include a 13% risk for premature rupture of the membranes for triplet to twin reduction (480). There is a 5% to 10% risk for losing the entire pregnancy (481) after reduction has occurred. Further, major depression occurs in 80% of women who lose the pregnancy as a complication of fetal reduction and in one third of women who have live twins after fetal reduction (482).

Ovarian Hyperstimulation Syndrome

OHSS is a medical complication that is both completely iatrogenic and unique to the treatment of infertility. Although the pathophysiology of OHSS is not well understood, the signs and symptoms of this disease can be attributed to local and systemic increase in capillary permeability. These changes, in turn, result in the depletion of intravascular volume at the expense of third-space fluid accumulation.

OHSS has been directly associated with increasing numbers of stimulated follicles and retrieved oocytes (483,484), the presence of PCOS (485–487) and high serum estradiol levels (483,488,489). Despite these associations, however, hyperestrogenemia is not currently thought to be the main cause of OHSS (490–493). Rather, the increased production of vasoactive substances, such as prorenin, renin, angiotensin-converting enzyme, angiotensin I, angiotensin II, and angiotensinogen, by the hyperstimulated ovaries has been implicated in this disease (494–502). Still, it remains possible that hyperestrogenemia, especially in the presence of hemoconcentration, has important effects on the thromboembolic risks demonstrated with OHSS.

Inflammatory responses are certainly present in OHSS patients, with possible roles for cytokines, histamine, and prostaglandins in the disease pathogenesis (503–509). In particular, the link between vascular endothelial growth factor (VEGF) and OHSS has been extensively studied. VEGF has been shown to exhibit a dose-related expression in human granulosa cells upon stimulation by hCG (510). Further, serum VEGF levels correlate with OHSS severity (511,512) demonstrating a sensitivity and specificity of 100% and 60%, respectively (512). The central role of an inflammatory response is supported by a number of other findings. For instance, mast cells are abundant in ovulatory follicles (513), and histamine blockade has been reported to ameliorate and, in some cases, even prevent OHSS in animal models (505–507,514). Further, it is clinically well recognized that allergy or hypersensitivity act as risk factors for the development of OHSS (483). However, to date, scientific evidence for these factors is still considered preliminary, and further investigation is warranted to clarify their true role in OHSS (493).

Recently, a distinction between early- and late-onset OHSS has been described (515). Early OHSS, with onset arbitrarily set within 9 days of oocyte retrieval, is associated with higher serum estradiol levels and follicle numbers during COH. In contrast, late OHSS has onset more than 9 days after oocyte retrieval. Late-onset OHSS has been associated, not with measures of follicular response, but rather with multiple gestation. Early and late OHSS may even reflect somewhat distinct pathophysiologic mechanisms. It has been proposed that early OHSS may result from ovarian stimulation by the exogenous hCG given to trigger ovulation, whereas late OHSS may be more closely linked to the endogenous hCG produced when pregnancy ensues (515).

OHSS has a varied spectrum of clinical presentation. An attempt to better understand this heterogeneity led to the development of a staging system for OHSS that would reflect symptom severity. This classification categorizes patients into mild, moderate, and severe disease (516). In mild OHSS, patients often complain of mild abdominal distention and soreness, nausea, and vomiting. Ovarian enlargement can be 5 to 12 cm. Moderate disease is marked by the presence of abdominal ascites on ultrasound examination. Severe disease is diagnosed when there are clinical signs of tense ascites, hydrothorax, shortness of breath, hemoconcentration, hypercoagulability, or any complications of OHSS such as renal failure, thromboembolism, or acute respiratory distress syndrome (ARDS).

This classification may serve as a useful guide; however, its application may sometimes be misleading. For example, ovarian enlargement is common after COH and, by itself, is not informative. Further, many patients experience mild pelvic soreness and abdominal bloating after COH, and their ovaries may be enlarged when viewed on transvaginal ultrasound. Whether these patients reflect an abnormal response to COH or merely represent a subset of normal responders is debatable. The fact that reported incidence of OHSS after COH has ranged from 7.3% (mild or moderate disease) and 4.2% (severe disease) to 33% overall may suggest that the staging system is itself open to interpretation (483,516).

Management of OHSS Patients undergoing COH with or without ART should be educated about the signs and symptoms of OHSS. They should be instructed to contact their health care provider if they experience abdominal bloating, abdominal discomfort or pain, early satiety, nausea, vomiting, decreased urine output, or weight gain of more than 2 lb per day. Patients with these initial symptoms should be fully assessed to establish their baseline condition for future comparisons, if that should become that necessary. Following are those points most pertinent in the assessment of patients with OHSS potential:

History

- Age, history of OHSS in previous infertility treatment, history of PCOS
- Characteristics of COH (dose of gonadotropins, number of follicles, number of eggs for an ART cycle, peak serum estradiol level, date of hCG administration, date of oocyte retrieval, date of embryo transfer, number of embryos transferred at embryo transfer)
- Onset of symptoms, their progression (stable versus rapidly worsening), and their severity

Specific questions should address the presence of the following symptoms:

- Abdominal discomfort, pain, bloating; increased abdominal girth; early satiety
- Shortness of breath, chest pain
- Nausea, vomiting
- Weight gain (total amount gained since start of COH and pounds gained per day)
- Decreased urine output

A complete physical examination should be performed, with specific attention to the following areas:

- Signs of hypotension, hemodynamic instability, and dehydration
- Chest: evidence of pleural effusion, congestive heart failure, limited chest expansion because of ascites
- Abdomen: ascites (mild, moderate, tense), peritoneal signs
- Peripheral exam: pitting edema
- Pelvic exam is **contraindicated** because enlarged ovaries can be fragile

Investigations

- Complete blood count, prothrombin time, partial thromboplastin time, serum electrolytes, liver function tests, creatinine, blood urea nitrogen
- Chest x-ray if there is significant shortness of breath or abnormalities on chest exam (shielding the pelvis can protect potential pregnancy from irradiation)
- Transvaginal ultrasound to document the baseline amount of ascites and size of ovaries
- Documentation of oxygen saturation is indicated if there is evidence of respiratory compromise
- Serum hCG on day 16 after oocyte retrieval if embryo transfer has occurred

This initial assessment should enable the clinician to decide whether the OHSS patient needs to be admitted to the hospital for observation and supportive care. Accepted indications for hospitalization include inability to tolerate oral hydration, hemodynamic instability, respiratory compromise, tense ascites, hemoconcentration, leukocytosis, hyponatremia, hyperkalemia, abnormal renal or liver function, and decreased oxygen saturation. If the diagnosis and its severity remain in doubt after initial assessment, it is reasonable to observe patients overnight while further assessing fluid balance and the presence of oliguria. The need for more prolonged hospitalization often becomes rapidly evident. The presence of peritoneal signs, such as abdominal rebound tenderness or guarding, in a patient with possible OHSS may indicate ovarian torsion, hemorrhage, or rupture of enlarged ovarian cysts. These signs may also represent those rare cases of postoocyte retrieval tuboovarian abscess. Further, admission to hospital is mandatory, and admission to an intensive care setting should be seriously considered if the patient has complications of OHSS such as renal failure, ARDS, thromboembolic disease, or severe hydrothorax.

The onset of OHSS soon after hCG administration or oocyte retrieval is associated with an increased risk for progression to severe disease. Pregnancy is also known to cause worsening of OHSS, most likely due to ovarian stimulation by endogenous hCG. Therefore, in cases of very-early-onset OHSS, the benefits of withholding embryo transfer, cryopreserving these embryos, and performing ET in a future unstimulated cycle should be considered and discussed.

Outpatient Management If hospitalization is not indicated by initial assessment and the patient can be managed as an outpatient, she should be instructed to limit her activity, to weigh herself daily, and to monitor her fluid intake (at least 1 L/d of mostly electrolyte-balanced fluid) and output. Daily follow-up by telephone or visit is important because the severity of OHSS may change any time. The patient should contact her health care provider if she notes worsening of the symptoms or if her weight gain increases to more than 2 lb per day. Reassessment is indicated in these situations.

Inpatient Management Inpatient management of patients with OHSS is composed of meticulous vital sign and fluid balance monitoring as well as supportive care. This typically involves use of intravenous hydration and prevention of complications such as thromboembolic prophylaxis, although more invasive interventions, such as paracentesis, may become necessary. The following is a typical inpatient protocol used for management of the patient with moderate to severe OHSS:

Perform the initial assessment as outlined previously.

- Vital signs (including oxygen saturation monitoring if respiratory compromise is present) every 4 hours initially
- Fluid intake and output measurements
- Daily weights and abdominal girth
- Daily hematocrit, leukocyte count, serum electrolytes, renal function tests
- Liver function tests, prothrombin time, partial thromboplastin time on admission and then repeated only as necessary

Supportive Care

- If there is hypotension or oliguria, give a bolus of 1 L of normal saline (NS) over 1 hour, then maintain with D5NS (or $D5_{1/2}NS$) at 150 mL/h. If there is no hypotension or oliguria, but the hematocrit is greater than 45%, start maintenance at D5NS at 150 mL/h. The maintenance rate for intravenous fluids can be lowered if the hematocrit is normal. Although administration of intravenous fluids will certainly lead to an increase in third spacing, it is important to maintain adequate intravascular volume and urine output. The hematocrit may need to be monitored twice a day initially; the intravenous fluid maintenance can be titrated downward as the hematocrit normalizes. This should help to minimize third-spacing side effects. Lactated Ringer's solution should not be used for intravenous hydration in patients with OHSS.
- If oliguria persists, a small bolus of 250 to 500 mL of NS can be given to increase urine output. The efficacy of albumin (or other plasma expanders) in the treatment or resolution of OHSS has not been studied in a prospective, randomized fashion. However, it is reasonable to attempt gentle diuresis in a patient who has normal blood pressure and hematocrit but in whom oliguria or weight gain persists. This may be accomplished using sequential administration of 50 mL of 25% albumin followed by *furosemide,* 10 mg given intravenously. This combination can be repeated 3 to 4 times per 24 hours as necessary. Serum sodium, potassium, and creatinine must be monitored closely when employing albumin or furosemide diuresis.
- Small amounts of fluid can be taken orally. As the OHSS improves, amount of intake can be increased as the intravenous fluid maintenance decreases. During the

resolution of OHSS, a maximum total input of 1 L/d has been recommended to prevent increases in third spacing (493).

- Paracentesis is indicated if the patient has severe abdominal discomfort and respiratory compromise due to large volumes of ascites. Hydrothoraces have also been reported to resolve after paracentesis. Presence of massive ascites combined with persistent oliguria or hypotension despite medical therapy is also an indication for paracentesis because diuresis often results after the severe abdominal pressure is relieved. Both abdominal paracentesis under ultrasound guidance and transvaginal ultrasound-guided transvaginal paracentesis are described and acceptable practices (517,518).
- If embryo transfer has already been performed or is scheduled, progesterone supplementation should be given as indicated by the ART protocol. Administration of progesterone is not thought to affect OHSS adversely. However, pregnancy may cause worsening of OHSS as a result of the stimulation of the ovaries by increasing levels of endogenous hCG.
- Antiemetics and analgesics (i.e., *acetaminophen*) can be given symptomatically.
- Complications of OHSS, such as ARDS, thromboembolism, and renal failure, should be treated in the intensive care setting when indicated.

Preventative Measures

- Hemoconcentration and severe leukocytosis are considered risk factors for thromboembolic disease among OHSS patients (493). Therefore, *heparin,* 5,000 IU subcutaneously twice a day, should be given to all OHSS inpatients to prevent thromboembolism. In addition, high-high vascular support stockings should be used in ambulatory patients. Intermittent compression stockings should be used for patients who are not ambulating.

Prevention of OHSS Because OHSS has the potential to cause severe and sometimes life-threatening complications, it is prudent to aim toward disease prevention. It is usually not possible to identify patients who are at risk for OHSS during COH. However, when high estradiol levels (≥3,000 pg/mL) are noted before hCG administration, prevention of OHSS can be attempted using a technique called coasting. Coasting involves withholding gonadotropin and delaying hCG until serum estradiol levels decrease or follicular diameter of greater than or equal to 18 mm is seen on transvaginal ultrasound (372–374). Coasting does not completely prevent the risk for severe OHSS or cycle cancellation, but it does minimize the risk for severe OHSS while maintaining high pregnancy rates. An alternative strategy to minimize OHSS risk would cryopreserve embryos (or prezygotes) at the pronucleate stage and transfer thawed embryos to the uterus in a subsequent cycle using endometrial preparation without COH. The strategy of prezygote cryopreservation results in excellent pregnancy and live birth rates comparable to similar cycles with fresh embryo transfer. The incidence of severe OHSS appears to be decreased, but more importantly, the duration of severe OHSS may be shortened when cryopreservation strategies are used (519–521).

Unfortunately, even with close monitoring and use of the lowest possible doses of gonadotropins during COH, it is still often difficult to prevent OHSS. One novel strategy that may address these difficulties involves the *in vitro* maturation (IVM) of oocytes. IVM has been performed with success in some centers. Using IVM, immature follicles are aspirated and the retrieved oocytes are grown *in vitro* until mature. This is potentially advantageous because IVM completely obviates the need to stimulate the ovaries with gonadotropins. ICSI is performed on IVM oocytes, and embryos are transferred to a uterus that has been hormonally prepared. This technology is especially promising and appropriate in women with PCOS. IVM is particularly applicable to women with PCOS, who have a known increased risk for OHSS; further, their ovaries are characterized by multiple small follicles that can be aspirated in the absence of stimulation. IVM has been reported to yield pregnancy rates of 27.1% to 38% in women with PCOS (522–524).

Ectopic and Heterotopic Pregnancies

The incidence of ectopic pregnancy is 2% in the general population (525). However, its incidence is increased in IVF and can be as high as 4% (526). The main risk factors for ectopic pregnancy in IVF treatment are tubal factor infertility and possibly, previous myomectomy (526). The incidence of heterotopic pregnancy, which is normally rare, is particularly high (1%) after IVF treatment. Multiple gestation and high hormonal levels during COH and early pregnancy have been suggested to be possible causes. It is important to have a high index of suspicion for the occurrence of heterotopic pregnancies because only 40% to 84% of cases can be diagnosed on transvaginal ultrasound at the initial presentation (527,528). After treatment of the heterotopic gestation with laparoscopy, laparotomy, or ultrasound-guided KCl injection into the extrauterine pregnancy, the overall delivery rate for the intrauterine pregnancy is 66% (527).

Risk for Cancer after Fertility Therapy

The possibility that ovulation-inducing medications might promote the development of cancers of the reproductive tract was first introduced in the early 1990s by Whittenmore and colleagues, specifically with regard to ovarian cancer (529). One theory behind this proposed risk is that ovarian cancer may arise, in some cases, as the result of damage to the ovarian epithelium during ovulation. Lactation, oral contraceptives, late onset of menarche, early menopause, and multiparity are known to protect against ovarian cancer. Moreover, each is associated with a reduction in the total lifetime number of ovulatory cycles. The decreased risk for ovarian cancer noted among women with increased length of anovulation begged the question of whether dramatic increase in the number of eggs ovulated during superovulation therapy would, in turn, increase the risk for ovarian cancer. Alternatively, some believe that because gonadotropins (FSH and LH) increase cellular proliferation and division within ovarian follicles, their use might create a predisposition toward the occurrence of cancer cells. Both of the most common hormonal therapies used for induction of ovulation—clomiphene citrate and exogenous gonadotropins—result in increased gonadotropin stimulation to the ovary. These therapies might therefore increase the incidence of ovarian cancer in treated infertility patients. Concern about this potential risk for cancer after fertility therapy has also been extended to other organs, including the uterus and breast.

Currently, several factors prevent an accurate calculation of the true risk for developing cancer of the breast, uterus, or ovary after treatment with ovulation-inducing agents. First, contemporary fertility treatments and their dosages remain relatively new and are usually used in women younger than 40 to 45 years of age. Because ovarian, uterine, and some breast cancers typically occur in older women, the number of patients who were treated with fertility drugs and are now in their middle to late 60s may still be too small to allow us to detect elevations in cancer risk. Second, it is hard to differentiate the effect of fertility treatment from the effect that being infertile might itself have on future development of malignancies of the breast, uterus, or ovary. Finally, most of the studies addressing these risks are clouded by small numbers, intake of a variety of medications, and recall bias. All these factors make the interpretation of data difficult (530).

Two of the most recent studies failed to attribute an increased risk for breast, uterine, or ovarian cancer to medications used for superovulation in the treatment of infertility (531,532). One study evaluated more than 20,000 women with exposure to fertility drugs used for IVF and compared them to nearly 10,000 infertile controls. The authors reported no overall increased incidence of uterine, breast, or ovarian cancers in women exposed to medications used for IVF (532). Two other interesting findings represent some of the limitations to these types of studies. The authors reported that the risk for ovarian and uterine cancer was higher in women with unexplained infertility, regardless of whether they had received ovulation induction medications. This may suggest risks associated with the unexplained infertility itself, or the possibility of undiagnosed cancers causing infertility. In addition, the authors reported an increase in the risk for breast and uterine cancer only within the first year after receiving infertility medications for IVF. Again this result is confusing.

Patients undergoing IVF are followed closely and may therefore be more likely to report early signs or symptoms of these cancers to their physicians. Alternatively, rather than causing these cancers, fertility medications may only stimulate the growth and subsequent diagnosis of preexisting tumors.

Psychological Support

Stress, as manifested by anxiety or depression, is thought to be increased in women experiencing infertility. The relationship between stress and infertility is complex and may represent a vicious cycle in which infertility results in stress, which results in further difficulty in conceiving (533–535). Results from a recent prospective, randomized trial support the value of group cognitive-behavioral therapy among infertile couples (536). This therapy uses a variety of approaches, including relaxation training such as yoga, cognitive restructuring, methods for emotional expression, and information on nutrition and exercise with respect to infertility. Although the mechanism by which relaxation therapies aid fertility is unknown and issues such as high dropout rates need to be addressed by further research, the option of psychological support and counseling, on an individual or group basis, should be offered to patients experiencing infertility (537).

Other Considerations

One of the most important aspects of the treatment of patients with subfertility or infertility is the process of deciding when no further treatment will be pursued. This crucial topic must be addressed early in infertility therapy. Patients must be accurately informed of estimated success rates and reasonable expectations for all therapeutic interventions. It is equally important to identify an end point to medical intervention at the outset of treatment. This end point offers patients a mental time frame in which they can make both medical and personal decisions. One viable alternative for many couples is adoption, although the process of adoption has recently become increasingly complex. Many patients may want to explore simultaneously infertility therapy and adoption. The choice of which course to pursue is a very difficult decision that may be facilitated by both physician input and strong psychosocial counseling and support.

Preservation of Fertility in Cancer Patients

Aside from helping subfertile couples build families, technologic advances in tissue and gamete cryopreservation, in combination with ART, have made future fertility possible for some men and women who are faced with surgery, radiotherapy, or chemotherapy for cancer treatment. Sperm cryopreservation has become a widely available option to allow fertility preservation in young men whose cancer treatment may render them infertile. The wide range of neoplastic disorders for which sperm cryopreservation have been successful include leukemia, lymphoma, Hodgkin's lymphoma, non-Hodgkin's lymphoma, and testicular cancer (538). Although most patients with these disorders are systemically ill and therefore exhibit decreased total motile sperm counts when compared with patients who do not have cancer, less than 20% have azoospermia, and cryopreservation is possible in most patients (538). Further, cryopreserved sperm from cancer patients tolerate thawing as well as samples obtained from patients without cancer (539).

Unfortunately, the efficacy of oocyte cryopreservation lags far behind that of sperm preservation. Married women who are scheduled to undergo sterility-inducing cancer treatments may take the option of completing an IVF cycle so that oocytes can be fertilized and the resulting embryos can be cryopreserved for transfer later in life. However, an IVF cycle may require 2 weeks to complete, rendering this option unrealistic for patients in whom a delay in cancer treatment would compromise their prognosis. Even patients who are able to undergo IVF treatment usually do not have the time necessary for use of a downregulation protocol. Consequently, these women are usually prescribed the shorter, flare protocol, which may give suboptimal response (396). GnRH antagonists may have a special advantage in this situation. GnRH antagonists can induce hypothalamic–pituitary downregulation after being started on day 6 of gonadotropin treatment, which obviates the need for the more time-consuming use of GnRH agonists (540).

Patients who are single or who have medical contraindications to IVF treatment may be candidates for ovarian tissue cryopreservation. Ovarian cortical biopsy specimens containing numerous primordial follicles have been successfully retrieved by a laparoscopic approach in healthy volunteers and in cancer patients (541–543). It remains to be determined whether this promising technology creates a risk for reintroduction of malignant cells after autotransplantation of ovarian tissue and whether thawed immature oocytes should be used in *in vitro* maturation protocols.

References

1. **Cramer DW, Walker Am, Schiff I.** Statistical methods in evaluating the outcome of infertility therapy. *Fertil Steril* 1979;32:80–86.
2. **Office of Technology Assessment, United States Congress.** Infertility: medical and social choices. Publication No. OTA-BA-358. Washington, DC: U.S. Government Printing Office, May 1988.
3. **Wilcox LS, Mosher WD.** Use of infertility services in the United States. *Obstet Gynecol* 1993;82:122–127.
4. **Mosher WD, Pratt WF.** The demography of infertility in the United States. In: **Asch RH, Stubb JWW,** eds. *Annual progress in reproductive medicine.* Park Ridge, NJ: The Parthenon Publishing Group, 1993: 37–43.
5. **Cates W Jr, Rolfs AT, Arel SO.** Sexually transmitted diseases, pelvic inflammatory disease and infertility: an epidemiologic update. *Epidemiol Rev* 1990;12:199–220.
6. **Chandra A, Mosher WD.** The demography of infertility and the use of medical care for infertility. *Infert Reprod Med Clin North Am* 1994;5:283–296.
7. **Barros C, Yanagimachi R.** Induction of the zona reaction in golden hamster eggs by cortical granule material. *Nature* 1971;233:268–269.
8. **Bordson BL, Leonardo VS.** The appropriate upper age limit for semen donors: a review of the genetic effects of potential age. *Fertil Steril* 1991;56:397–401.
9. **Carlsen E, Giwercman A, Keiding N, et al.** Evidence for decreasing quality of semen during the past 50 years. *BMJ* 1992;305:609–613.
10. **Politoff L, Birkhausen M, Almendral A, et al.** New data confirming a circannual rhythm in spermatogenesis. *Fertil Steril* 1989;52:486–489.
11. **Jequier AM, Ukombre EB.** Errors inherent in the performance of a routine semen analysis. *Br J Urol* 1983;55:434–436.
12. **MacLeod J.** The semen examination. *Clin Obstet Gynecol* 1965;8:115–127.
13. **Smith KD, Rodriguez-Rigau LJ, Steinberger E.** Relation between indices of semen analysis and pregnancy rate in infertile couples. *Fertil Steril* 1977;28:1314–1319.
14. **Bostofte E, Serup J, Rebbe H.** Relation between number of immobile spermatozoa and pregnancies obtained during a twenty-year follow-up period. *Int J Androl* 1982;5:379–386.
15. **The American Fertility Society and Society for Assisted Reproductive Technology.** *Clinic-specific outcome assessment for the year 1992.* Birmingham, Alabama: The American Fertility Society, 1994.
16. **Kruger TF, Menkveld R, Stander FS, et al.** Sperm morphologic features as a prognostic factor in in vitro fertilization. *Fertil Steril* 1986;46:1118–1123.
17. **Kruger TF, Acosta AA, Simmons KF, et al.** Predictive value of abnormal sperm morphology in in vitro fertilization. *Fertil Steril* 1988;49:112–117.
18. **Ombelet W, Vandeput H, Van de Putte G, et al.** Intrauterine insemination after ovarian stimulation with clomiphene citrate: predictive potential of inseminating motile count and sperm morphology. *Hum Reprod* 1997;12:1458–1463.
19. **Wolff H, Anderson DJ.** Immunohistologic characterization and quantitation of leukocyte subpopulations in human semen. *Fertil Steril* 1988;49:497–504.
20. **World Health Organization.** *Laboratory manual for the examination of human semen and sperm-cervical mucus interaction.* Cambridge, England: Cambridge University Press, 1992.
21. **Tomlinson MJ, Barratt CLR, Bolton AE, et al.** Round cells and sperm fertilizing capacity: the presence of immature germ cells but not seminal leukocytes are associated with reduced success of in vitro fertilization. *Fertil Steril* 1992;58:1257–1259.
22. **Yanagimachi R, Yanagimachi H, Rogers BJ.** The use of zone-free animal ova as a test for assessment of fertilizing capacity of human spermatozoa. *Biol Reprod* 1976;15:471–476.
23. **Mao C, Grimes DA.** The sperm penetration assay: can it discriminate between fertile and infertile men? *Am J Obstet Gynecol* 1988;159:279–286.
24. **Burkman LJ, Cobbington CC, Franken DR, et al.** The hemizona assay (HZA): development of a

diagnostic test for the binding of human spermatozoa to the human hemizona pellucida to predict fertilization potential. *Fertil Steril* 1988;49:688–697.

25. **Jeyrendran RS, Van der Ven HH, Perez-Pelaez M, et al.** Development of an assay to assess the functional integrity of the human sperm membrane and its relationship to other semen characteristics. *J Reprod Fertil* 1984;70:219–228.

26. **Wolf D, Boldt J, Byrd W, et al.** Acrosomal status evaluation in normal ejaculated sperm with monoclonal antibodies. *Biol Reprod* 1985;32:1157–1162.

27. **Comhaire FH, Vermeolen L, Schoonjans F.** Reassessment of the accuracy of traditional sperm characteristics and adenosine triphosphate (ATP) in estimating the fertilizing potential of human semen in vivo. *Int J Androl* 1987;10:653–662.

28. **The ESHRE CAPRI Workshop Group.** Male sterility and subfertility: guidelines for management. *Hum Reprod* 1994;9:1260–1264.

29. **Greenberg SH, Lipshultz LI, Wein AJ.** Experience with 425 subfertile male patients. *J Urol* 1978;119:507–510.

30. **Auger J, Kunstmann JM, Czyglik F, et al.** Decline in semen quality among fertile men in Paris during the past 20 years. *N Engl J Med* 1995;332:281–285.

31. **Olsen GW, Bodner KM, Ramlow JM, et al.** Have sperm counts been reduced 50% in 50 years? A statistical model revisited. *Fertil Steril* 1995;63:887–893.

32. **Rasmussen PE, Erb K, Westergaard LG, et al.** No evidence for decreasing semen quality in four birth cohorts of 1055 Danish men born between 1950 and 1970. *Fertil Steril* 1997;68:1059–1064.

33. **Fisch H, Goluboff ET, Olson JH, et al.** Semen analyses in 1283 men from the United States over a 25-year period: no decline in quality. *Fertil Steril* 1996;65:1009–1014.

34. **Swan SH, Elkin EP.** Declining semen quality: can the past inform the present? *Bioessays* 1999;21:614–621.

35. **Saidi JA, Chang DT, Goluboff ET, et al.** Declining sperm counts in the United States? A critical review. *J Urol* 1999;161:460–462.

36. **Fisch H, Ikeguchi EF, Goluboff ET.** Worldwide variations in sperm counts. *Urology* 1996;48:909–911.

37. **Close CE, Roberts PL, Berger RE.** Cigarettes, alcohol and marijuana are related to pyospermia in infertile men. *J Urol* 1990;144:900–903.

38. **Bracken MB, Eskenazi B, Sachse K, et al.** Association of cocaine use with sperm concentration, motility, and morphology. *Fertil Steril* 1990;53:315–322.

39. **Marshburn PB, Sloan CS, Hammond MG.** Semen quality and association with coffee drinking, cigarette smoking, and ethanol consumption. *Fertil Steril* 1989;52:162–165.

40. **de Kretser DM. Male infertility.** *Lancet* 1997;349:787–790.

41. **Sokol RZ, Steiner BS, Bustillo M, et al.** A controlled comparison of the efficacy of clomiphene citrate in male infertility. *Fertil Steril* 1988;49:865–870.

42. **World Health Organization.** A double-blind trial of clomiphene citrate for the treatment of idiopathic male infertility. *Int J Androl* 1992;7:1067–1072.

43. **Acosta AA, Khalifa E, Oehninger S.** Pure human follicle stimulating hormone has a role in the treatment of severe male factor infertility by assisted reproduction: Norfolk's total experience. *Hum Reprod* 1992;7:1067–1072.

44. **Takihara H, Sakatoku J, Cockett ATK.** The pathophysiology of varicocele male infertility. *Fertil Steril* 1991;55:861–868.

45. **World Health Organization.** The influence of varicocele on parameters of fertility in a large group of men presenting to infertility clinics. *Fertil Steril* 1992;57:1289–1293.

46. **Madgar I, Weissenberg R, Lunenfeld B, et al.** Controlled trial of high spermatic vein ligation for varicocele in infertile men. *Fertil Steril* 1995;63:120–124.

47. **Hargreave TB.** Varicocele: overview and commentary on the results of the World Health Organization varicocele trial. In: **Waites GMH, Firck J, Baker GWH,** eds. *Current advances in andrology. (Proceedings of the VIth International Congress of Andrology).* Bologna, Italy: Monduzzi Editore, 31–44.

48. **Kamishke A, Nieschlag E.** Analysis of medical treatment of male infertility. *Hum Reprod* 1999;14 [Suppl 1]:1–23.

49. **Nilsson S, Edvinsson A, Nilsson B.** Improvement of semen and pregnancy rate after ligation and division of the internal spermatic vein: fact or fiction? *Br J Urol* 1979;51:591–596.

50. **Breznik R, Vlaisavljevic V, Borko E.** Treatment of varicocele and male infertility. *Arch Androl* 1993;30:157–160.

51. **Yamamoto M, Hibi H, Hirata Y et al.** Effects of varicocelectomy on sperm parameters and pregnancy rate in patients with subclinical varicocele: a randomized prospective controlled study. *J Urol* 1996;155:1636–1638.

52. **Nieschlag E, Hertle L, Fischedick A, et al.** Update on treatment of varicocele: counselling as effective as occlusion of the vena spermatica. *Hum Reprod* 1998;13:2147–2150.

53. **Guzick DS, Carson SA, Coutifaris C, et al.** Efficacy of superovulation and intrauterine insemination in the treatment of infertility. National Cooperative Reproductive Medicine Network. *N Engl J Med* 1999;340:177–183.

54. **Karande VC, Rao R, Pratt DE, et al.** A randomized prospective comparison between intrauterine insemination and fallopian sperm perfusion for the treatment of infertility. *Fertil Steril* 1995;64:638–640.

55. **El Sadek MM, Amer MK, Abdel-Malak G.** Questioning the efficacy of fallopian tube sperm perfusion. *Hum Reprod* 1998;13:3053–3056.

56. **Nuojua-Huttunen S, Tuomivaara L, Juntunen K, et al.** Comparison of fallopian tube sperm perfusion with intrauterine insemination in the treatment of infertility. *Fertil Steril* 1997;67:939–942.

57. **Gregoriou O, Pyrgiotis E, Konidaris S, et al.** Fallopian tube sperm perfusion has no advantage over intrauterine insemination when used in combination with ovarian stimulation for the treatment of unexplained infertility. *Gynecol Obstet Invest* 1995;39:226–228.

58. **Kahn JA, Sunde A, Koskemies A, et al.** Fallopian tube sperm perfusion (FSP) versus intrauterine insemination (IUI) in the treatment of unexplained infertility: a prospective randomized study. *Hum Reprod* 1993;8:890–894.

59. **Fanchin R, Olivennes F, Righini C, et al.** A new system for fallopian tube sperm perfusion leads to pregnancy rates twice as high as standard intrauterine insemination. *Fertil Steril* 1995;64:505–510.

60. **Trout SW, Kemmann E.** Fallopian sperm perfusion versus intrauterine insemination: a randomized controlled trial and metaanalysis of the literature. *Fertil Steril* 1999;71:881–885.

61. **Mamas L.** Higher pregnancy rates with a simple method for fallopian tube sperm perfusion, using the cervical clamp double nut bivalve speculum in the treatment of unexplained infertility: a prospective randomized study. *Hum Reprod* 1996;11:2618–2622.

62. **Tiemessen CH, Bots RS, Peeters MF, et al.** Direct intraperitoneal insemination compared to intrauterine insemination in superovulated cycles: a randomized cross-over study. *Gynecol Obstet Invest* 1997;44:149–152.

63. **Ajossa S, Melis GB, Cianci A, et al.** An open multicenter study to compare the efficacy of intraperitoneal insemination and intrauterine insemination following multiple follicular development as treatment for unexplained infertility. *J Assist Reprod Genet* 1997;14:15–20.

64. **Gregoriou O, Papadias C, Konidaris S, et al.** A randomized comparison of intrauterine and intraperitoneal insemination in the treatment of infertility. *Int J Gynaecol Obstet* 1993;42:33–36.

65. **Hovatta O, Kurunmaki H, Tiitinen A, et al.** Direct intraperitoneal or intrauterine insemination and superovulation in infertility treatment: a randomized study. *Fertil Steril* 1990;54:339–341.

66. **Abella EA, Tarantino S, Wade R.** Intrafollicular insemination for male factor infertility. *Fertil Steril* 1992;58:442–443.

67. **Nuojua-Huttunen S, Tuomivaara L, Juntunen K, et al.** Intrafollicular insemination for the treatment of infertility. *Hum Reprod* 1995;10:91–93.

68. **Yovich JL.** Pentoxifylline: actions and applications in assisted reproduction. *Hum Reprod* 1993;8:1786–1791.

69. **Ford WC, Mathur RS, Hull MG.** Intrauterine insemination: is it an effective treatment for male factor infertility? *Baillieres Clin Obstet Gynaecol* 1997;11:691–710.

70. **Dickey RP, Pyrzak R, Lu PY, et al.** Comparison of the sperm quality necessary for successful intrauterine insemination with World Health Organization threshold values for normal sperm. *Fertil Steril* 1999;71:684–689.

71. **Palermo GD, Cohen J, Rosenwaks Z.** Intracytoplasmic sperm injection: a powerful tool to overcome fertilization failure. *Fertil Steril* 1996;65(5):899–908.

72. **Irvine DS.** Epidemiology and aetiology of male infertility. *Hum Reprod* 1998;13[Suppl 1]:33–44.

73. **Stanwell-Smith RE, Hendry WF.** The prognosis of male subfertility: a survey of 1025 men referred to a fertility clinic. *Br J Urol* 1984;56:422–428.

74. **Sharif K.** Reclassification of azoospermia: the time has come? *Hum Reprod* 2000;15:237–238.

75. **Berkow R, Fletcher AJ.** *The Merck manual of diagnosis and therapy.* Rahway, NJ: Merck Sharp & Dohme Research Laboratories, 1992.

76. **Mak V, Jarvi KA.** The genetics of male infertility. *J Urol* 1996;156:1245–1256.

77. **Whitcomb RW, Crowley WF Jr.** Male hypogonadotropic hypogonadism. *Endocrinol Metab Clin North Am* 1993;22:125–143.

78. **Van de Berk D, Wijnberg M, Van Dop PA.** Initiation of spermatogenesis and successful in vitro fertilization in an infertile male with panhypopituitarism; superiority of pulsatile LH-RH over gonadotropins? A case report. *Eur J Obstet Gynecol Reprod Biol* 1991;40:153–157.

79. **Burgues S, Calderon MD, for the Spanish Collaborative Group on male hypogonadotropic hypogonadism.** Subcutaneous self-administration of highly purified follicle-stimulating hormone and human chorionic gonadotrophin for the treatment of male hypogonadotrophic hypogonadism. *Hum Reprod* 1997;12:980–986.

80. **Buchter D, Behre HM, Kliesch S, et al.** Pulsatile GnRH or hCG/HMG as effective treatment for men with hypogonadotropic hypogonadism: a review of 42 cases. *Eur J Endocrinol* 1998;139:298–303.

81. **Coughlin MT, O'Leary LA, Songer NJ, et al.** Time to conception after orchidopexy: evidence for subfertility? *Fertil Steril* 1997;67:742–746.

82. **Reijo R, Lee TY, Salo P, et al.** Diverse spermatogenic effects in humans caused by Y chromosome deletions encompassing a novel RNA-binding protein gene. *Nat Genet* 1995;10:383–393.

83. **Ma K, Inglis JD, Sharkey A, et al.** A Y chromosome gene family with RNA-binding protein homology: candidates for the azoospermia factor AZF controlling human spermatogenesis. *Cell* 1993;73:1287–1295.

84. **Pryor JL, Kent-First M, Muallem A, et al.** Microdeletions in the Y chromosome of infertile men. *N Engl J Med* 1997;336:534–539.

85. **Palermo G, Joris H, Devroey P, et al.** Pregnancies after intracytoplasmic injection of single spermatozoon into an oocyte. *Lancet* 1992;340:17–18.

86. **Jovich JL, Stanger JD.** The limitations of in-vitro fertilization from male with severe oligospermia and abnormal sperm morphology. *J In Vitro Fertil Embryo* Transf 1984;1:172–179.

87. **Hamberger L, Lundin K, Sjogren A, et al.** Indications for intracytoplasmic sperm injection. *Hum Reprod* 1998;13[Suppl 1]:128–133.

88. **Bonduelle M, Camus M, De Vos A, et al.** Seven years of intracytoplasmic sperm injection and follow up of 1987 subsequent children. *Hum Reprod* 1999;14[Suppl 1]:243–64.

89. **Wennerholm UB, Bergh C, Hamberger L, et al.** Incidence of congenital malformations in children born after ICSI. *Hum Reprod* 2000;15:944–948.

90. **Loft A, Petersen K, Erb K, et al.** A Danish national cohort of 730 infants born after intracytoplasmic sperm injection (ICSI) 1994-1997. *Hum Reprod* 1999;14:2143–2148.

91. **Tarlatzis BC, Bili H.** Intracytoplasmic sperm injection: survey of world results. *Ann N Y Acad Sci* 2000; 900:336–344.

92. **Johnson MD.** Genetic risks of intracytoplasmic sperm injection in the treatment of male infertility: recommendations for genetic counseling and screening. *Fertil Steril* 1998;70:397–411.

93. **Jequier AM, Ansell ID, Bullimore NJ.** Congenital absence of the vasa deferentia presenting with infertility. *J Androl* 1985;6:15–19.

94. **Belker AM, Thomas AJ Jr, Fuchs EF, et al.** Results of 1469 microsurgical vasectomy reversals by the Vasovasostomy Study Group. *J Urol* 1991;145:505–511.

95. **Schlegel PN, Goldstein M.** Microsurgical vasoepididymostomy: refinements and results. *J Urol* 1993;150:1165–1168.

96. **Stockamp K, Schreiter F, Altwein JE.** α-Adrenergic drugs in retrograde ejaculation. *Fertil Steril* 1974;25:817–820.

97. **Shangold GA, Cantor B, Schreiber JR.** Treatment of infertility due to retrograde ejaculation: a simple, cost-effective method. *Fertil Steril* 1990;54:175–177.

98. **Tournaye H.** Surgical sperm recovery for intracytoplasmic sperm injection: which method is to be preferred? *Hum Reprod* 1999;14[Suppl 1]:71–81.

99. **Tournaye H, Clasen K, Aytoz A, et al.** Fine needle aspiration versus open biopsy for testicular sperm recovery: a controlled study in azoospermic patients with normal spermatogenesis. *Hum Reprod* 1998;13: 901–904.

100. **Devroey P, Liu J, Nagy Z, et al.** Ongoing pregnancies and birth after intracytoplasmic sperm injection with frozen-thawed epididymal spermatozoa. *Hum Reprod* 1995;10:903–906.

101. **Tournaye H, Meedad T, Silber S, et al.** No differences in outcome after intracytoplasmic sperm injection with fresh or frozen-thawed epididymal spermatozoa. *Hum Reprod* 1999;14:90–96.

102. **Habermann H, Seo R, Cieslak J, Niederberger C, et al.** In vitro fertilization outcomes after intracytoplasmic sperm injection with fresh or frozen-thawed testicular spermatozoa. *Fertil Steril* 2000;73:955–960.

103. **Meniru G, Bortha S, Podsindly B, et al.** ICSI: with epididymal sperm-percutaneous retrieval. In: **Filicori M,** ed. *Proceedings of the Symposium: Treatment of infertility—the new frontiers.* Boca Raton, FL: 1998:363–374.

104. **Girardi SK, Schlegel P.** MESA: review of techniques, preoperative considerations and results. *J Androl* 1996;17:5–9.

105. **Tournaye H, Staessen C, Liebaers I, et al.** Testicular sperm recovery in 47XXY Klinefelter patients. *Hum Reprod* 1996;11:1644–1649.

106. **Palermo GD, Schlegel PN, Sills ES, et al.** Births after intracytoplasmic injection of sperm obtained by testicular extraction from men with nonmosaic Klinefelter's syndrome. *N Engl J Med* 1998;338: 588–590.

107. **Tournaye H, Camus M, Vandervorst M, et al.** Sperm retrieval for ICSI. *Int J Androl* 1997;20(S3):69–73.

108. **Palermo GD, Schlegel N, Hariprashad JJ, et al.** Fertilization and pregnancy outcome with intracytoplasmic sperm injection for azoospermic men. *Hum Reprod* 1999;14:741–748.

109. **Tournaye H, Liu J, Nagy Z, et al.** Correlation between testicular histology and outcome after intracytoplasmic sperm injection using testicular sperm. *Hum Reprod* 1996;11:127–132.

110. **Meng MV, Cha I, Ljung BM, et al.** Relationship between classic histological pattern and sperm findings on fine needle aspiration map in infertile men. *Hum Reprod* 2000;15:1973–1977.

111. **Lundin K, Sjogren A, Nilsson L, et al.** Fertilization and pregnancy after intracytoplasmic sperm microinjection of acrosomeless spermatozoa. *Fertil Steril* 1994;62:1266–1267.

112. **Devroey P.** Are spermatid injections of any clinical value? Testicular sperm extraction and intracytoplasmic sperm injection. *Hum Reprod* 1998;13:2045–2046.

113. **Al-Hasani S, Ludwig M, Palermo I, et al.** Intracytoplasmic injection of round and elongated spermatids from azoospermic patients: results and review.

114. **Silber SJ, Johnson L, Verheyen G, et al.** Round spermatid injection. *Fertil Steril* 2000;73:897–900.

115. **Fischer R, Barkloh V, Naethere D, et al.** Use of cryopreserved testicular sperm. In: **Filicori M,** ed. *Proceedings of the Symposium: treatment of infertility—the new frontiers.* Boca Raton, FL: 1998:403–412.

116. **Subak LL, Adamson GD, Boltz NL.** Therapeutic donor insemination: a prospective, randomized trial of fresh versus frozen sperm. *Am J Obstet Gynecol* 1992;166:1597–1604.

117. **The American Fertility Society.** Guidelines for gamete donation: 1993. *Fertil Steril* 1993;59[Suppl 1]: 1S—9S.

118. **Shenfield F, Doyle P, Valentine A, et al.** Effects of age, gravidity, and male infertility status on cumulative conception rates following artificial insemination with cryopreserved donor semen: analysis of 2998 cycles of treatment in one center over 10 years. *Hum Reprod* 1993;8:60–64.

119. **Byrd W, Bradshaw K, Carr B, et al.** A prospective randomized study of pregnancy rates following intrauterine and intracervical insemination using frozen donor sperm. *Fertil Steril* 1990;53:521–527.

120. **Patton PE, Burry KA, Thurmond A, et al.** Intrauterine insemination outperforms intracervical insemination in a randomized, controlled study with frozen, donor semen. *Fertil Steril* 1992;57:559–564.

121. **Hurd WW, Randolph JFJ, Ansbacher R, et al.** Comparison of intracervical, intrauterine, and intratubal techniques for donor insemination. *Fertil Steril* 1993;59:339–342.

122. **Peters AJ, Hecht B, Wentz AC, et al.** Comparison of the methods of artificial insemination on the incidence of conception in single unmarried women. *Fertil Steril* 1993;59:121–124.

123. **Williams DB, Moley KH, Cholewa C, et al.** Does intrauterine insemination offer an advantage to cervical cap insemination in a donor insemination program? *Fertil Steril* 1995;63:295–298.

124. **Wainer R, Merlet F, Ducot B, et al.** Prospective randomized comparison of intrauterine and intracervical insemination with donor spermatozoa. *Hum Reprod* 1995;10:2919–2922.

125. **Matorras R, Gorostiaga A, Diez J, et al.** Intrauterine insemination with frozen sperm increases pregnancy rates in donor insemination cycles under gonadotropin stimulation. *Fertil Steril* 1996;65:620–625.

126. **Goldberg JM, Masch E, Falcone T, et al.** Comparison of intrauterine and intracervical insemination with frozen donor sperm: a meta-analysis. *Fertil Steril* 1999;72:792–795.

127. **Speroff L, Glass RH, Kase N.** *Clinical gynecologic endocrinology and fertility.* 5th ed. Baltimore: Williams & Wilkins, 1994:890.

128. **Hall JE, Welt CK, Cramer DW.** Inhibin A and inhibin B reflect ovarian function in assisted reproduction but are less useful at predicting outcome. *Hum Reprod* 1999;14:409–415.

129. **Scott RT, Opsahl MS, Leonardi MR, et al.** Life table analysis of pregnancy rates in a general infertility population relative to ovarian reserve and patient age. *Hum Reprod* 1995;10:1706–1710.

130. **Garenne ML, Frisch RE.** Natural fertility. *Infert Reprod Med Clin North Am* 1994;5:259–282.

131. **Tietze C.** Reproductive span and role of reproduction among Hutterite women. *Fertil Steril* 1957;8:89–97.

132. **Federation CECOS, Schwartz D, Mayaux MJ.** Female fecundity as a function of age: results of artificial insemination in 2193 nulliparous women with azoospermic husbands. *N Engl J Med* 1982;306: 404–406.

133. **Navot D, Drews MR, Bergh PA, et al.** Age-related decline in female fertility is not due to diminished capacity of the uterus to sustain embryo implantation. *Fertil Steril* 1994;61:97–101.

134. **Sauer MV, Paulson RJ, Lobo RA.** Reversing the natural decline in human fertility: an extended clinical trial of oocyte-donation to women of advanced reproductive age. *JAMA* 1992;268:1275–1279.

135. **Stolwijk AM, Zielhuis GA, Sauer MV, et al.** The impact of the woman's age on the success of standard and donor in vitro fertilization. *Fertil Steril* 1997;67:702–710.

136. **Remohf J, Gartner B, Gallardo E, et al.** Pregnancy and birth rates after oocyte donation. *Fertil Steril* 1997;67:717–712.

137. **Sadraie SH, Saito H, Kaneko T, et al.** Effects of aging on ovarian fecundity in terms of the incidence of apoptotic granulosa cells. *J Assist Reprod Genet* 2000;17:168–173.

138. **Navot D, Rosenwaks Z, Margalioth EJ.** Prognostic assessment of female fecundity. *Lancet* 1987;2:645–647.

139. **Syrop CH, Dawson JD, Husman KJ, et al.** Ovarian volume may predict assisted reproductive outcomes better than follicle stimulating hormone concentration on day 3. *Hum Reprod* 1999;14(7):1752–1756.

140. **Seifer DB, Scott RT, Bergh PA, et al.** Women with declining ovarian reserve may demonstrate a decrease in day 3 serum inhibin B before a rise in day 3 follicle-stimulating hormone. *Fertil Steril* 1999;72: 63–65.

141. **Scott RT, Leonardi MR, Hofmann GE, et al.** A prospective evaluation of clomiphene citrate challenge test screening of the general infertility population. *Obstet Gynecol* 1993;82:539–544.

142. **Barhnart K, Osheroff J.** We are overinterpreting the predictive value of serum follicle-stimulating hormone levels. *Fertil Steril* 1999;72:8–9.

143. **Wassertheil-Smoller S.** Mostly about screening tests. In: *Biostatistics and epidemiology: a primer for health professionals.* 2nd ed. New York: Springer-Verlag, 1995:118–125.

144. **Barnhart K, Osheroff J.** Follicle stimulating hormone as a predictor of fertility. *Curr Opin Obstet Gynecol* 1998;19:227–232.

145. **Bancsi LFJMM, Huijs AM, den Ouden CT, et al.** Basal follicle-stimulating hormone levels are of limited value in predicting ongoing pregnancy rates after in vitro fertilization. *Fertil Steril* 2000;73:552–557.

146. **Watt AH, Legedza AT, Ginsburg ES, et al.** The prognostic value of age and follicle-stimulating hormone levels in women over forty years of age undergoing in vitro fertilization. *J Assist Reprod Genet* 2000;17:264–268.

147. **Hofmann GE, Danforth DR, Seifer DB.** Inhibin-B: the physiologic basis of the clomiphene citrate challenge test for ovarian reserve screening. *Fertil Steril* 1998;69:474–477.

148. **Dzik A, Lambert-Messerlian G, Izzo VM, et al.** *Fertil Steril* 2000;74:1114–1117.

149. **Driancourt MA, Thuel B.** Control of oocyte growth and maturation by follicular cells and molecules present in follicular fluid: a review. *Reprod Nutr Dev* 1998;38(4):345–362.

150. **Andersen A-M N, Wohlfahrt J, Christens P, et al.** Maternal age and fetal loss: population based register linkage study. *BMJ* 2000;320:1708–1712.

151. **Wilcox AJ, Weinberg CR, O'Connor JF, et al.** Incidence of early loss of pregnancy. *N Engl J Med* 1988;319:189–194.

152. **Eiben B, Bartels I, Bahr-Porsch S, et al.** Cytogenetic analysis of 750 spontaneous abortions with the direct preparation method of chorionic villi and its implications for studying genetic causes of pregnancy wastage. *Am J Hum Genet* 1990;47:656–663.

153. **Griffin DK, Abruzzo MA, Millie EA, et al.** Non-disjunction in human sperm: evidence for an effect of increasing paternal age. *Hum Mol Genet* 1995;4:2227–232.

154. **Stene J, Fischer G, Stene E, et al.** Paternal age affect in Down's syndrome. *Ann Hum Genet* 1977;40:299–306.

155. **Bedford JM.** Sperm capacitation and fertilization in mammals. *Biol Reprod* 1970;2[Suppl]:128–158.

156. **World Health Organization.** Temporal relationships between ovulation and defined changes in the concentration of plasma estradiol 17b luteinizing hormone, follicle stimulating hormone and progesterone. *Am J Obstet Gynecol* 1980;138:383–390.

157. **Hoff JD, Quigley ME, Yen SSC.** Hormonal dynamics at midcycle: a reevaluation. *J Clin Endocrinol Metab* 1987;57:792–796.

158. **Elkind-Hirsch K, Goldzieher JW, Gibbons WE, et al.** Evaluation of the Ovu-Stick urinary luteinizing hormone kit in normal and stimulated menstrual cycles. *Obstet Gynecol* 1986;67:450–453.

159. **Rybak EA.** The fertile window: updated perspectives on the physiology, epidemiology, and prevailing methods for personal detection of ovulation. *Postgrad Obstet Gynecol* 2000;20:1–7.

160. **Grinsted J, Jacobsen JD, Grinsted L, et al.** Prediction of ovulation. *Fertil Steril* 1989;52:388–393.

161. **Guida M, Tommaselli GA, Palomba S, et al.** Efficacy of methods for determining ovulation in a natural family planning program. *Fertil Steril* 1999;72:900–904.

162. **Luciano AA, Peluso J, Koch EI, et al.** Temporal relationship and reliability of the clinical, hormonal, and ultrasonographic indices of ovulation in infertile women. *Obstet Gynecol* 1990;75:412–416.

163. **Filcori M, Butler JP, Crowley WF.** Neuroendocrine regulation of the corpus luteum in the human: evidence for pulsatile progesterone secretion. *J Clin Invest* 1984;73:1638–1647.

164. **Katz E.** The luteinized unruptured follicle and other ovulatory dysfunctions. *Fertil Steril* 1988;50:839–850.

165. **Kerin JF, Edmonds DK, Warner GM, et al.** Morphological and functional relations of graafian follicle growth to ovulation in women using ultrasonic, laparoscopic and biochemical measurements. *Br J Obstet Gynaecol* 1981;88:81–90.

166. **O'Herlihy C, de Crespigny LC, Lopata A, et al.** Preovulatory follicle size: comparison of ultrasound and laparoscopic measurements. *Fertil Steril* 1980;34:24–26.

167. **Bates GW, Whitworth NS.** Effect of body weight reduction on plasma androgens in obese infertile women. *Fertil Steril* 1982;38:406–409.

168. **Pasquali R, Antenucci D, Casimirri F, et al.** Clinical and hormonal characteristics of obese and amenorrheic women before and after weight loss. *J Clin Endocrinol Metab* 1989;68:173–179.

169. **Clark AM, Thornley B, Tomlinson L, et al.** Weight loss in obese infertile women results in improvement in reproductive outcome for all forms of fertility treatment. *Hum Reprod* 1998;13:1502–1505.

170. **Pi-Sunyer FX.** Medical hazards of obesity. *Ann Intern Med* 1993;119:665.

171. **Clark JH, Markaverich BM.** The agonist-antagonist properties of clomiphene. *Pharmacol Ther* 1981;15:467–519.

172. **Kettel LM, Roseff SH, Berga SL, et al.** Hypothalamic–pituitary–ovarian response to clomiphene citrate in women with polycystic ovarian syndrome. *Fertil Steril* 1993;59:532–538.

173. **Adashi EY.** Clomiphene citrate-initiated ovulation: a clinical update. *Semin Reprod Endocrinol* 1986;4:255–276.

174. **Kessel B, Hsueh AJW.** Clomiphene citrate augments follicle-stimulating hormone-induced luteinizing hormone receptor content in cultured rat granulosa cells. *Fertil Steril* 1987;47:334–340.

175. **Hammerstein J.** Mode of action of clomiphene. *Acta Endocrinol* 1969;60:635–644.

176. **Eden JA, Place J, Carter GD, et al.** The effect of clomiphene citrate on follicular phase increase in endometrial thickness and uterine volume. *Obstet Gynecol* 1989;73:187–990.

177. **Van Campenhout J, Simiard R, Leduc B.** Antiestrogenic effects of clomiphene in the human being. *Fertil Steril* 1968;19:700–706.

178. **Li TC, Warren MA, Murphe C, et al.** A prospective, randomized, crossover study comparing the effects of clomiphene citrate and cyclofenil on endometrial morphology in the luteal phase of normal, fertile women. *Br J Obstet Gynaecol* 1992;99:10008–10013.

179. **Thompson LA, Barrett CLR, Thornton SJ, et al.** The effects of clomiphene citrate and cyclofenil on cervical mucus volume and receptivity over the periovulatory period. *Fertil Steril* 1993;59:125–129.

180. **Gysler M, March CM, Mishell DR Jr, et al.** A decade's experience with an individualized clomiphene treatment regimen including its effects on the postcoital test. *Fertil Steril* 1982;37:161–167.

181. **Hammond MG, Halme JK, Talbert LM.** Factors affecting pregnancy rate in clomiphene citrate induction of ovulation. *Obstet Gynecol* 1983;62:196–202.

182. **Ritchie WGM.** Ultrasound in the evaluation of normal and induced ovulation. *Fertil Steril* 1985;43:167–181.

183. **Shoham Z, Zosmer A, Insler V.** Early miscarriage and fetal malformation after induction of ovulation (by clomiphene citrate and/or human menotropins), in vitro fertilization, and gamete intrafallopian transfer. *Fertil Steril* 1991;55:1051–1056.

184. **Biljan MM, Mahutte NG, Tulandi T, et al.** Prospective randomized double-blind trial of the correlation between time of administration and antiestrogenic effects of clomiphene citrate on reproductive end organs. *Fertil Steril* 1999;71:633–638.

185. **Trott EA, Plouffe Jr L, Hansen K, et al.** Ovulation induction in clomiphene-resistant anovulatory women with normal dehydroepiandrosterone sulfate levels: beneficial effects of the addition of dexamethasone during the follicular phase. *Fertil Steril* 1996;66:484.

186. **Barbieri RL.** Induction of ovulation in infertile women with hyperandrogenism and insulin resistance. *Am J Obstet Gynecol* 2000;183:1412–1418.

187. **Nestler JE, Stovall D, Akhter N, et al.** Strategies for the use of insulin-sensitizing drugs to treat infertility in women with polycystic ovary syndrome. *Fertil Steril* 2002;77:209–215.

188. **Nestler JE, Jakubowicz DJ.** Lean women with polycystic ovary syndrome respond to insulin reduction with decreases in ovarian P450c17alpha activity and serum androgens. *J Clin Endocrinol Metab* 1997;82:4075–4079.

189. **Bailey CJ, Turner RC.** Metformin drug therapy. *N Engl J Med* 1996;334:574–579.

190. **Kolodziejczyk B, Duleba AJ, Spaczynski RZ, et al.** metformin therapy decreases hyperandrogenism and hyperinsulinemia in women with polycystic ovary syndrome. *Fertil Steril* 2000;73:1149–1154.

191. **Nestler JE, Jakubowicz DJ, Evans WS, et al.** Effects of Metformin on spontaneous and clomiphene-induced ovulation in the polycystic ovary syndrome. *N Engl J Med* 1998;338:1876–1880.

192. **Haesgawa I, Murakawa H, Suzuki M, et al.** Effect of troglitazone on endocrine and ovulatory performance in women with insulin resistance-related polycystic ovary syndrome. *Fertil Steril* 1999;71:323–327.

193. **Dunaif A, Scott D, Finegood D, et al.** The insulin-sensitizing agent troglitazone improves metabolic and reproductive abnormalities in the polycystic ovary syndrome. *J Clin Endocrinol Metab* 1996;81:3299–3306.

194. **Glueck CJ, Phillips H, Cameron D, et al.** Continuing metformin throughout pregnancy in women with polycystic ovary syndrome appears to safely reduce first-trimester spontaneous abortion: a pilot study. *Fertil Steril* 2001;75:46–52.

195. **Stein IF, Leventhal ML.** Amenorrhea associated with bilateral polycystic ovaries. *Am J Obstet Gynecol* 1935;29:181–191.

196. **Judd HL, Rigg LA, Anderson DC, et al.** The effects of ovarian wedge resection on circulating gonadotropin and ovarian steroid levels in patients with polycystic ovarian syndrome. *J Clin Endocrinol Metab* 1976;43:347–355.

197. **Adashi EY, Rock JR, Guzick D, et al.** Fertility following bilateral ovarian wedge resection: a critical analysis of 90 consecutive cases of the polycystic ovarian syndrome. *Fertil Steril* 1981;36:320–325.

198. **Weinstein D, Polishuk WZ.** The role of wedge resection of the ovary as a cause for mechanical sterility. *Surg Gynecol Obstet* 1975;141:417–423.

199. **De Waart MJ, Boeckx W, Brosens I.** Pelvic adhesions following microsurgical wedge resection compared to laparoscopic electrocoagulation of the rabbit ovaries. *Infertility* 1987;10:33 39.

200. **Naether OGJ, Fischer R.** Adhesion formation after laparoscopic electrocoagulation of the ovarian surface in the polycystic ovary patients. *Fertil Steril* 1993;60:95–98.

201. **Campo S, Felli A, Lamanna MA, et al.** Endocrine changes and clinical outcome after laparoscopic ovarian resection in patients with polycystic ovaries. *Human Reprod* 1993;8:359–363.

202. **Aakvaag A, Gjonnaess H.** Hormonal response to electrocautery of the ovary in patients with polycystic ovarian disease. *Br J Obstet Gynaecol* 1985;92:1258–1264.

203. **Daniell JF, Miller W.** Polycystic ovaries treated by laparoscopic laser vaporization. *Fertil Steril* 1989;51:232–236.

204. **Armar NA, McGarrigle HHG, Honour J, et al.** Laparoscopic ovarian diathermy in the management of anovulatory infertility in women with polycystic ovaries; endocrine changes and clinical outcome. *Fertil Steril* 1990;53:45–49.

205. **Felemban A, Tan SL, Tulandi T.** Laparoscopic treatment of polycystic ovaries with insulated needle cautery: a reappraisal. *Fertil Steril* 2000;73:266–269.

206. **Colacurci N, Zullo F, De Franciscis P, et al.** In vitro fertilization following laparoscopic ovarian diathermy in patients with polycystic ovarian syndrome. *Acta Obstet Gynecol Scand* 1997;76:555–558.

207. **Li TC, Saravelos H, Chow MS, et al.** Factors affecting the outcome of laparoscopic ovarian drilling for polycystic ovarian syndrome in women with anovulatory infertility. *Br J Obstet Gynaecol* 1998;105:338–344.

208. **Blacker CM.** Ovulation stimulation and induction. *Endocrinol Metab Clin North Am* 1992;21:57–84.

209. **Devane GW, Guzick DS.** Bromocriptine therapy in normoprolactinemic women with unexplained infertility and galactorrhea. *Fertil Steril* 1986;46:1026–1031.

210. **Clement K, Vaisse C, Lahlou N, et al.** A mutation in the human leptin receptor gene causes obesity and pituitary dysfunction. *Nature* 1998;392:398–401.

211. **Frisch RE.** The right weight: body fat, menarche and ovulation. *Baillieres Clin Obstet Gynaecol* 1990;4:419–439.

212. **Bates GW, Bates SR, Whitworth NS.** Reproductive failure in women who practice weight control. *Fertil Steril* 1982;37:373–378.

213. **Knuth UA, Hull MG, Jacobs HS.** Amenorrhoea and loss of weight. *Br J Obstet Gynaecol* 1977;84:801–807.

214. **Arojoki M, Jokimaa V, Juuti A, et al.** Hypothyroidism among infertile women in Finland. *Gynecol Endocrinol* 2000;14:127–131.

215. **Krassas GE, Pontikides N, Kaltsas TH, et al.** Disturbances of menstruation in hypothyroidism. *Clin Endocrinol* 1999;50:655–659.

216. **Thomas R, Reid RL.** Thyroid disease and reproductive dysfunction: a review. *Obstet Gynecol* 1987;70:789–798.

217. **Davis LE, Leveno KJ, Cunningham FG.** Hypothyroidism complicating pregnancy. *Obstet Gynecol* 1988;72:108–112.

218. **Rushworth FH, Backos M, Rai R, et al.** Prospective pregnancy outcome in untreated recurrent miscarriers with thyroid autoantibodies. *Hum Reprod* 2000;15:1637–1639.

219. **Muller AF, Verhoeff A, Mantel MJ, et al.** Thyroid autoimmunity and abortion: a prospective study in women undergoing in vitro fertilization. *Fertil Steril* 1999;71:30–34.

220. **Kutteh WH, Yetman DL, Carr AC, et al.** Increased prevalence of antithyroid antibodies identified in women with recurrent pregnancy loss but not in women undergoing assisted reproduction. *Fertil Steril* 1999;71:843–848.

221. **Kutteh WH, Schoolcraft WB, Scott RT Jr.** Antithyroid antibodies do not affect pregnancy outcome in women undergoing assisted reproduction. *Hum Reprod* 1999;14:2886–2890.

222. **Westrom L.** Incidence, prevalence and trends of acute pelvic inflammatory disease and its consequences in industrialized countries. *Am J Obstet Gynecol* 1980;138:880–892.

223. **Rosenfeld DL, Seidman SM, Bronson RA, et al.** Unsuspected chronic pelvic inflammatory disease in the infertile female. *Fertil Steril* 1983;39:44–48.

224. **Krynicki E, Kaminski P, Szymanski R, et al.** Comparison of hysterosalpingography with laparoscopy and chromopertubation. *J Am Assoc Gynecol Laparosc* 1996;3[4 Suppl]:S22–23.

225. **Reis MM, Soares SR, Cancado ML, et al.** Hysterosalpingo contrast sonography (HyCoSy) with SHU 454 (Echovist) for the assessment of tubal patency. *Hum Reprod* 1998;13:3049–3052.

226. **Honore GM, Holden AEC, Schenken RS.** Pathophysiology and management of proximal tubal blockage. *Fertil Steril* 1999;71:785–795.

227. **Watson A, Vanderkerckhove P, Lilford R, et al.** A meta-analysis of the therapeutic role of oil-soluble contrast media at hysterosalpingography: a surprising result? *Fertil Steril* 1994;61:470–477.

228. **Vandekerckhove P, Watson A, Lilford R, et al.** Oil-soluble versus water-soluble media for assessing tubal patency with hysterosalpingography or laparoscopy in subfertile women. *Cochrane Database Syst Rev* 2000;2:CD000092.

229. **Karande VC, Pratt DE, Balin MS, et al.** What is the radiation exposure to patients during a gynecoradiologic procedure? *Fertil Steril* 1997;67:401–403.

230. **Dechaud H, Daures JP, Hedon B.** Prospective evaluation of falloposcopy. *Hum Reprod.* 1998;13(7):1815–1818.

231. **Holz K, Becker R, Schurmann R.** Ultrasound in the investigation of tubal patency: a meta-analysis of three comparative studies of Echovist-200 including 1007 women. *Zentralbl Gynakol* 1997;119:366–373.

232. **Tulandi T, Collins JA, Burrows E, et al.** Treatment-dependent and treatment-independent pregnancy among women with periadnexal adhesions. *Am J Obstet Gynecol* 1992;162:354–357.

233. **Gomel V.** Salpingoovariolysis by laparoscopy in infertility. *Fertil Steril* 1983;40:607–611.

234. **Lundroff P, Hahlini P, Kallfelt B, et al.** Adhesion formation after laparoscopic surgery in tubal pregnancy: a randomized trial after laparotomy. *Fertil Steril* 1991;55:911–915.

235. **Diamond E.** A comparison of gross and microsurgical techniques for the repair of cornual occlusion in infertility: a retrospective study, 1968–1978. *Fertil Steril* 1979;32:370–376.

236. **Lavy G, Diamond MP, DeCherney AH.** Pregnancy following tubo-cornual anastomosis. *Fertil Steril* 1986;46:21–25.

237. **Donnez J, Casanas-Roux F, Nisolle-Pochet M, et al.** Surgical management of tubal obstruction at the uterotubal junction. *Acta Eur Fertil* 1987;18:5–9.

238. **Gomel V.** An odyssey through the oviduct. *Fertil Steril* 1983;39:144–156.

239. **Deaton JL, Gibson M, Riddick DH, et al.** Diagnosis and treatment of cornual obstruction using a flexible tip guidewire. *Fertil Steril* 1990;53:232–236.

240. **Ransom M, Garcia A.** Surgical management of cornual-isthmic tubal obstruction. *Fertil Steril* 1997;68:887–891.

241. **Das K, Nagel T, Malo J.** Hysteroscopic cannulation for proximal tubal obstruction: a change for the better? *Fertil Steril* 1995;63:1009–1015.

242. **Sakumoto T, Shinkawa T, Izena H, et al.** Treatment of infertility associated with endometriosis by selective tubal catheterization under hysteroscopy and laparoscopy. *Am J Obstet Gynecol* 1993;169:744–747.

243. **Confino E, Tur-Kaspa I, DeCherney A, et al.** Transcervical balloon tuboplasty: a multicenter study. *JAMA* 1990;264:2079–2082.

244. **Thurmond AS.** Selective salpingography and fallopian tube recanalization. *AJR Am J Roentgenol* 1991;156:33–38.

245. **Woolcott R, Petchpud A, O'Donnell P, et al.** Differential impact on pregnancy rate of selective salpingography, tubal catheterization and wire-guide recanalization in the treatment of proximal fallopian tube obstruction. *Hum Reprod* 1995;10:1423–1426.

246. **Capitanio GL, Ferraiolo A, Croce S, et al.** Transcervical selective salpingography: a diagnostic and therapeutic approach to cases of proximal tubal injection failure. *Fertil Steril* 1991;55:1045–1050.

247. **Ferraiolo A, Ferraro F, Remorgida V, et al.** Unexpected pregnancies after tubal recanalization failure with selective catheterization. *Fertil Steril* 1995;63:299–302.

248. **Rock JA.** Infertility: surgical aspects. In: **Yen SSC, Jaffe RB,** eds. *Reproductive endocrinology: physiology and clinical management.* 3rd ed. Philadelphia: WB Saunders, 1991.

249. **Schlaff WD, Hassiakos DK, Damewood MD, et al.** Neosalpingostomy for distal tubal obstruction: prognostic factors and impact of surgical technique. *Fertil Steril* 1990;54:984–990.

250. **Dobuisson JB, Chapron C, Morice P, et al.** Laparoscopic salpingostomy: fertility results according to the tubal mucosal appearance. *Hum Reprod* 1994;9:334–339.

251. **Eyraud B, Erny R, Vergnet F.** Chirugie tubaire distale par coelioscopie. *J Gynecol Obstet Biol Reprod (Paris)* 1993;22:9–14.

252. **Kasia JM, Raiga J, Doh AS, et al.** Laparoscopic fimbrioplasty and neosalpingostomy: experience of the Yaounde General Hospital, Cameroon (report of 194 cases). *Eur J Obstet Gynecol Reprod Biol* 1997;73: 71–77.

253. **Singhal V, Li TC, Cooke ID.** An analysis of factors influencing the outcome of 232 consecutive tubal microsurgery cases. *Br J Obstet Gynaecol* 1991;98:628–636.

254. **Wilcox LS, Chu SY, Peterson HB.** Characteristics of women who considered or obtained tubal reanastomosis: results from a prospective study of tubal sterilization. *Obstet Gynecol* 1990;75:661–665.

255. **TeVelde ER, Boer ME, Looman CWN, et al.** Factors influencing success or failure after reversal of sterilization. *Fertil Steril* 1990;54:270–277.

256. **Silber SJ, Cohen R.** Microsurgical reversal of female sterilization, the role of tubal length. *Fertil Steril* 1980;33:598–601.

257. **Novy MJ.** Reversal of Kroener fimbriectomy sterilization. *Am J Obstet Gynecol* 1980;137:198–206.

258. **Yoon TK, Sung HR, Kang HG, et al.** Laparoscopic tubal anastomosis: fertility outcome in 202 cases. *Fertil Steril* 1999;72:1121–1126.

259. **Bissonnette F, Lapensee L, Bouzayen R.** Outpatient laparoscopic tubal anastomosis and subsequent fertility. *Fertil Steril* 1999;72:549–552.

260. **Falcone T, Goldberg JM, Margossian H, et al.** Robotic-assisted laparoscopic microsurgical tubal anastomosis: a human pilot study. *Fertil Steril* 2000;73:1040–1042.

261. **Kovacs GT, Newman GB, Henson GL.** The postcoital test: what is normal? *BMJ* 1978;1:818.

262. **Jette NT, Glass RH.** Prognostic value of the postcoital test. *Fertil Steril* 1972;23:29–32.

263. **Collins JA, So Y, Wilson EH, et al.** The postcoital test as a predictor of pregnancy among 355 infertile couples. *Fertil Steril* 1984;41:703–708.

264. **Griffith CS, Grimes DA.** The validity of the postcoital test. *Am J Obstet Gynecol* 1990;162:615–620.

265. **Glatstein IZ, Best CL, Palumbo A, et al.** The reproducibility of the postcoital test: a prospective study. *Obstet Gynecol* 1995;85:396–400.

266. **Oei SG, Helmerhorst FM, Bloemenkamp KWM, et al.** Effectiveness of the postcoital test: randomised controlled trial. *BMJ* 1998;317:502–505.

267. **Bronson R, Cooper G, Rosenfeld D.** Sperm antibodies: their role in infertility. *Fertil Steril* 1984;42:171–183.

268. **Mazumdar S, Levine AS.** Antisperm antibodies: etiology, pathogenesis, diagnosis, and treatment. *Fertil Steril.* 1998;70(5):799–810.

269. **Wolfe JP, DeAlmeida M, Ducot B, et al.** High levels of sperm-associated antibodies impair human sperm oolemma interaction after aubzonal insemination. *Fertil Steril* 1995;63:584–590.

270. **Naz RK.** Effects of antisperm antibodies on early cleavage of fertilized ova. *Biol Reprod* 1992;46:130–139.

271. **Ford WCL, Williams KM, McLaughlin EA, et al.** The indirect immunobead test for seminal antisperm antibodies and fertilization rates at in-vitro fertilization. *Hum Reprod* 1996;11:1418–1422.

272. **Lahteenmaki A, Reima I, Hovatta O.** Treatment of severe male immunological infertility by intracytoplasmic sperm injection. *Hum Reprod* 1995;10:2824–2828.

273. **Pagidas K, Hemmings R, Falcone R, et al.** The effect of antisperm autoantibodies in male or female partners undergoing in vitro fertilization-embryo transfer. *Fertil Steril* 1994;62:363–369.

274. **Jager S, Kermer J, van Slochteren-Draeisma T.** A simple method of screening for antisperm antibodies in the human male: detection of spermatozoan surface IgG with the direct mixed agglutination reaction carried out on untreated fresh human semen. *Int J Fertil* 1978;23:12–21.

275. **Kremer J, Jager S.** The significance of antisperm antibodies for sperm-cervical mucus interaction. *Hum Reprod* 1992;7:781–784.

276. **Collin JA, Burrows EA, Yeo J, et al.** Frequency and predictive value of antisperm antibodies among infertile couples. *Hum Reprod* 1993;8:592–598.

277. **Haas GG Jr, Manganiello P.** A double-blind, placebo-controlled study of these of methylprednisolone in infertile men with sperm-associated immunoglobulins. *Fertil Steril* 1997;47:295–301.

278. **Nagy ZP, Verheyen G, Liu J, et al.** Results of 55 intracytoplasmic sperm injection cycles in the treatment of male-immunological infertility. *Hum Reprod* 1995;10:1775–1780.

279. **Soares SR, dos Reis MMBB, Camargos AF.** Diagnostic accuracy of sonohysterography, transvaginal sonography, and hysterosalpingography in patients with uterine cavity diseases. *Fertil Steril* 2000;73:406–411.

280. **Alatas C, Aksoy E, Akarsu C, et al.** Evaluation of intrauterine abnormalities in infertile patients by sonohysterography. *Hum Reprod* 1997;12:487–490.

281. **Schwarzler P, Concin H, Bosch H, et al.** An evaluation of sonohysterography and diagnostic hysteroscopy for the assessment of intrauterine pathology. *Ultrasound Obstet Gynecol* 1998;11:337–342.

282. **Kamel HS, Darwish AM, Mohamed SA.** Comparison of transvaginal ultrasonography and vaginal sonohysterography in the detection of endometrial polyps. *Acta Obstet Gynecol Scand* 2000;79:60–64.

283. **Raga F, Bauset C, Remohi J, et al.** Reproductive impact of congenital mullerian anomalies. *Hum Reprod* 1997;12(10):2277–2281.

284. **Heinonen PK, Pystnen PP.** Primary infertility and uterine anomalies. *Fertil Steril* 1983;40:311–316.

285. **Georgakopoulos PA, Gogas CG.** Zur Fertilitat bei Uterusmissbildungen. *Geburtshilfe Frauenheilkd* 1982;42:533–536.

286. **Homer HA, Li TC, Cooke ID.** The septate uterus: a review of management and reproductive outcome. *Fertil Steril* 2000;73:1–14.

287. **Goldberg JM, Falcone T.** Effect of diethylstilbestrol on reproductive function. *Fertil Steril* 1999;72:1–7.

288. **Kaufman RH, Adam E, Binder GL, et al.** Upper genital tract changes and pregnancy outcome in offspring exposed in utero to diethylstilbestrol. *Am J Obstet Gynecol* 1980;137:299–308.

289. **Dieckmann WJ, Davis ME, Rynkiewicz LM, et al.** Does the administration of diethylstilbestrol during pregnancy have therapeutic value? *Am J Obstet Gynecol* 1953;66:1062–1081.

290. **Berger MJ, Goldstein DP.** Impaired reproductive performance in DES-exposed women. *Obstet Gynecol* 1980;55:25–27.

291. **Senekjian EK, Potkul RK, Frey K, et al.** Infertility among daughters either exposed or not exposed to diethylstilbestrol. *Am J Obstet Gynecol* 1988;158:493–498.

292. **Berger MJ, Alper MM.** Intractable primary infertility in women exposed to diethylstilbestrol in utero. *J Reprod Med* 1986;31:231–235.

293. **Pal L, Shifren JL, Isaacson KB, et al.** Outcome of IVF in DES–exposed daughters: experience in the 90's. *J Assist Reprod Genet* 1997;14:513–517.

294. **Richards PA, Richards PD, Tiltman AJ.** The ultrastructure of fibromyomatous myometrium and its relationship to infertility. *Hum Reprod Update* 1998;4:520–525.

295. **Bulletti C, De Zieglre D, Polli V, et al.** The role of leiomyomas in infertility. *J Am Assoc Gynecol Laparosc* 1999;6:441–445.

296. **Vercellini P, Maddalena S, De Giorgi O, et al.** Abdominal myomectomy for infertility: a comprehensive review. *Hum Reprod* 1998;13:873–879.

297. **Vercellini P, Maddalena S, De Giorgi O, et al.** Determinants of reproductive outcome after abdominal myomectomy for infertility. *Fertil Steril* 1999;72:109–114.

298. **Ribeiro SC, Reich H, Rosenberg J, et al.** Laparoscopic myomectomy and pregnancy outcome in infertile patients. *Fertil Steril* 1999;71:571–574.

299. **Darai E, Deval B, Darles C, et al.** Myomectomie: coelioscopie ou laparotomie? *Contracept Fertil Sex* 1996;24:751–756.

300. **Dubuisson JB, Chapron C, Chavat X, et al.** Fertility after laparoscopic myomectomy of large intramural myomas: preliminary results. *Hum Reprod* 1996;11:518–522.

301. **Shalev J, Meizner I, Bar–Hava I, et al.** Predictive value of transvaginal sonography performed before routine diagnostic hysteroscopy for evaluation of infertility. *Fertil Steril* 2000;73:412–417.

302. **Lass A, Williams G, Abusheikha N, et al.** The effect of endometrial polyps on outcomes of in vitro fertilization (IVF) cycles. *J Assist Reprod Genet* 1999;16:410–415.

303. **Oosthuizen AP, Wessels PH, Hefer JN.** Tuberculosis of the female genital tract in patients attending an infertility clinic. *S Afr Med J* 1990;77:562–564.

304. **Varma TR.** Genital tuberculosis and subsequent fertility. *Int J Gynecol Obstet* 1991;35:1–11.

305. **Isamjovich B, Lindor A, Confino E, et al.** Treatment of minimal and moderate intrauterine adhesions (Asherman's syndrome). *J Reprod Med* 1985;30:769–772.

306. **Rousseau S, Lord J, Lepage Y, et al.** The expectancy of pregnancy for "normal" infertile couples. *Fertil Steril* 1983;40:768–772.

307. **Soules MR, McLachlan RI, Ek M, et al.** Luteal phase deficiency: characterization of reproductive hormones over the menstrual cycle. *J Clin Endocrinol Metab* 1989;69:804–812.

308. **Ma L, Yao M, Maas RL.** Genetic control of uterine receptivity during implantation. *Semin Reprod Endocrinol* 1999;17:205–216.

309. **Dey SK.** Implantation. In: **Adashi EY, Rock JA, Rosenwaks Z,** eds. *Reproductive endocrinology, surgery, and technology.* Philadelphia: Lippincott–Raven, 1996:421–434.

310. **Benson GV, Lim H, Paria BC, et al.** Mechanisms of female infertility in Hoxa-10 mutant mice: uterine homeosis versus loss of maternal Hoxa-10 expression. *Development* 1996;122:2687–2696.

311. **Gendron RL, Paradis H, Hsieh-Li HM, et al.** Abnormal uterine stromal and glandular function associated with maternal reproductive defects in Hoxa-11 null mice. *Biol Reprod* 1997;56:1097–1105.

312. **Lim H, Ma L, Ma W, et al.** Hoxa-10 regulates uterine stromal cell responsiveness to progesterone during implantation and decidualization in the mouse. *Mol Endocrinol* 1999;13:1005–1017.

313. **Lim H, Paria BC, Das SK, et al.** Multiple female reproductive failures in cyclooxygenase-2 deficient mice. *Cell* 1997;91:197–208.

314. **Stewart CL, Kaspar P, Brunet LJ, et al.** Blastocyst implantation depends on maternal expression of leukemia inhibitory factor. *Nature* 1992;359:76–79.

315. **Taylor HS, Arici A, Olive DL, et al.** *HOXA-10* is expressed in response to sex steroids at the time of implantation in the human endometrium. *J Clin Invest* 1998;101:1379–1384.

316. **Wilcox AJ, Baird DD, Weinberg CR.** Time of implantation of the conceptus and loss of pregnancy. *N Engl J Med* 1999;340:1796–1799.

317. **Lessey BA, Castelbaum AJ, Buck CA, et al.** Further characterization of endometrial integrins during the menstrual cycle and in pregnancy. *Fertil Steril* 1994;62:497–506.

318. **Acosta AA, Elberger L, Borghi M, et al.** Endometrial dating and determination of the window of implantation in healthy fertile women. *Fertil Steril* 2000;73:788–798.

319. **Lessey BA, Castelbaum A, Wolf L, et al.** Use of integrins to date the endometrium. *Fertil Steril* 2000;73:779–787.

320. **Davis OK, Berkeley AS, Naus GJ, et al.** The incidence of luteal phase defect in normal fertile women determined by serial endometrial biopsies. *Fertil Steril* 1989;51:582–586.

321. **Wentz AC, Kossoy LR, Parker RA.** The impact of luteal phase inadequacy in an infertile population. *Am J Obstet Gynecol* 1990;162:937–945.

322. **Balasch J, Fabregues F, Creus M, et al.** The usefulness of endometrial biopsy for luteal phase evaluation in infertility. *Hum Reprod* 1992;7:973–977.

323. **Soules MR, Clifton DK, Steiner RA, et al.** The corpus luteum: determinants of progesterone secretion in the normal menstrual cycle. *Obstet Gynecol* 1988;71:659 656.

324. **Wentz AC, Herbert CM, Maxson WS, et al.** Outcome of progesterone treatment of luteal phase insufficiency. *Fertil Steril* 1984;41:856–862.

325. **Toth A, Lesser ML, Brooks C, et al.** Subsequent pregnancies among 161 couples treated for T–mycoplasma genital tract infection. *N Engl J Med* 1983;308:505–507.

326. **Gaudoin M, Rekha P, Morris A, et al.** Bacterial vaginosis and past chlamydial infection are strongly and independently associated with tubal infertility but do not affect in vitro fertilization success rates. *Fertil Steril* 1999;72:730–732.

327. **Ralph SG, Rutherford AJ, Wilson JD.** Influence of bacterial vaginosis on conception and miscarriage in the first trimester: cohort study. *BMJ* 1999;319:220–223.

328. **Gump DW, Gibson M, Ashikaga T.** Lack of association between genital mycoplasmas and infertility. *N Engl J Med* 1984;310:937–941.

329. **Harrison RF, de Louvois J, Blades M, et al.** Doxycycline treatment and human infertility. *Lancet* 1975;1:605–607.

330. **Chilcott IT, Margara R, Cohen H, et al.** Pregnancy outcome is not affected by antiphospholipid antibody status in women referred for in vitro fertilization. *Fertil Steril* 2000;73:526–530.

331. **Hornstein MD, Davis OK, Massey JB, et al.** Antiphospholipid antibodies and in vitro fertilization success: a meta–analysis. *Fertil Steril* 2000;73:330–333.

332. **Corson SL, Cheng A, Gutmann JN.** Laparoscopy in the "normal" infertile patient: a question revisited. *J Am Assoc Gynecol Laparosc* 2000;7:317–324.

333. **Strathy JH, Molgaard CA, Coulam CB, et al.** Endometriosis and infertility: a laparoscopic study of endometriosis among fertile and infertile women. *Fertil Steril* 1982;38:667–672.

334. **Halme J.** Role of peritoneal inflammation in endometriosis–associated infertility. *Ann N Y Acad Sci* 1991;622:266–274.

335. **Selam B, Arici A.** Implantation defect in endometriosis: endometrium or peritoneal fluid. *J Reprod Fertil Suppl* 2000;55:121–128.

336. **Pellicer A, Albert C, Garrido N, et al.** The pathophysiology of endometriosis–associated infertility: follicular environment and embryo quality. *J Reprod Fertil Suppl* 2000;55:109–119.

337. **Guzick DS, Yao YAS, Berga SL, et al.** Endometriosis impairs the efficacy of gamete intrafallopian transfer: results of a case–control study. *Fertil Steril* 1994;62:1186–1191.

338. **Arici A, Oral E, Bukulmez O, et al.** The effect of endometriosis on implantation: results from the Yale University in vitro fertilization and embryo transfer program. *Fertil Steril* 1996;65:603–607.

339. **Jansen RP.** Minimal endometriosis and reduced fecundability: prospective evidence from an artificial insemination by donor program. *Fertil Steril* 1986;46:141–143.

340. **Guzick DS, Silliman NP, Adamson GD, et al.** *Fertil Steril* 1997;67:822–829.

341. **Berube S, Marcoux S, Langevin M, et al.** Fecundity of infertile women with minimal or mild endometriosis and women with unexplained infertility. The Canadian Collaborative Group on Endometriosis. *Fertil Steril* 1998;69:1034–1041.

342. **Marcoux S, Maheux R, Berube S.** Laparoscopic surgery in infertile women with minimal or mild endometriosis. Canadian Collaborative Group on Endometriosis. *N Engl J Med* 1997;337:217–222.

343. **Parazzini F.** Ablation of lesions or no treatment in minimal–mild endometriosis in infertile women: a randomized trial. Gruppo Italiano per lo Studio dell'Endometriosi. *Hum Reprod* 1999;14:1332–1334.

344. **Taylor HS, Olive DL.** Unexplained infertility: the role of laparoscopy. *Infertil Reprod Med Clin North Am* 1997;8:603–609.

345. **Tulandi T, al-Took S.** Reproductive outcome after treatment of mild endometriosis with laparoscopic excision and electrocoagulation. *Fertil Steril* 1998;69:229–231.

346. **Donderwinkel PF, van der Vaart H, Wolters VM, et al.** Treatment of patients with long-standing unexplained subfertility with in vitro fertilization. *Fertil Steril* 2000;73:334–337.

347. **Hughes E, Collins J, Vandkerckhove P.** Clomiphene citrate for unexplained subfertility in women. *Cochrane Database Syst Rev* 2000;3:CD000057.

348. **Gerli S, Gholami H, Manna A, et al.** Use of ethinyl estradiol to reverse the antiestrogenic effects of clomiphene citrate in patients undergoing intrauterine insemination: a comparative, randomized study. *Fertil Steril* 2000;73:85–89.

349. **Zeyneloglu HB, Arici A, Olive DL, et al.** Comparison of intrauterine insemination with timed intercourse in superovulated cycles with gonadotropins: a meta-analysis. *Fertil Steril* 1998;69:486–491.

350. **Ragni G, Maggioni P, Guermandi E, et al.** Efficacy of double intrauterine insemination in controlled ovarian hyperstimulation cycles. *Fertil Steril* 1999;72:619–622.

351. **Guzick DS, Sullivan MW, Adamson GD, et al.** Efficacy of treatment for unexplained infertility. *Fertil Steril* 1998;70:207–213.

352. **Aboulghar MA, Mansour RT, Serour GI, et al.** Management of long-standing unexplained infertility: a prospective study. *Am J Obstet Gynecol* 1999;181:371–375.

353. **Chafkin LM, Nulsen JC, Luciano AA, et al.** A comparative analysis of the cycle fecundity rates associated with combined human menopausal gonadotropin (hMG) and intrauterine insemination (IUI) versus either hMG or IUI alone. *Fertil Steril* 1991;55:252–257.

354. **Campana A, Sakkas D, Stalberg A, et al.** Intrauterine insemination: evaluation of the results according to the woman's age, sperm quality, total sperm count per insemination and life table analysis. *Hum Reprod* 1996;11:732–736.

355. **Sahakyan M, Harlow BL, Hornstein MD.** Influence of age, diagnosis and cycle number on pregnancy rates with gonadotropin-induced controlled ovarian hyperstimulation and intrauterine insemination. *Fertil Steril* 1999;72:500–504.

356. **Aboulghar M, Mansour R, Serour G, et al.** Controlled ovarian hyperstimulation and intrauterine insemination for treatment of unexplained infertility should be limited to a maximum of three trials. *Fertil Steril* 2000;75:88–91.

357. **Ruiz A, Remohi J, Minguez Y, et al.** The role of in vitro fertilization and intracytoplasmic sperm injection in couples with unexplained infertility after failed intrauterine insemination. *Fertil Steril* 1997;68:171–173.

358. **Donini P, et al.** Purification of gonadotropin from human menopausal urine. *Acta Endocrinol* 1964;45:321–328.

359. **Hughes E, Collins J, Vandekerckhove P.** Ovulation induction with urinary follicle stimulating hormone

versus human menopausal gonadotropin for clomiphene-resistant polycystic ovary syndrome. *Cochrane Database Syst Rev* 2000;(2):CD000087.

360. **Agrawal R, Holmes J, Jacobs HS.** Follicle-stimulating hormone or human menopausal gonadotropin for ovarian stimulation in in vitro fertilization cycles: a meta-analysis. *Fertil Steril* 2000;73:338–343.

361. **Daya S, Gunby J.** Recombinant versus urinary follicle stimulating hormone for ovarian stimulation in assisted reproduction. *Hum Reprod* 1999;14:2207–2215.

362. ***Physicians desk reference.*** Micromedex (R) Healthcare Series Vol. 107. Micromedex Inc, 1974–2001.

363. **Gargiulo AR. Ovulation induction.** In: **Goldstein SR** and **Benson CB,** eds. *Imaging of the infertile couple.* London, United Kingdom: Martin Dunitz, 2001:143–160.

364. **Akin JW, Shepard MK.** The effects of baseline ovarian cysts on cycle fecundity in controlled ovarian hyperstimulation. *Fertil Steril* 1993;59:453–455.

365. **Hornstein MD, Barbieri RL, Ravnikar VA, et al.** The effects of baseline ovarian cysts on the clinical response to controlled ovarian hyperstimulation in an vitro fertilization program. *Fertil Steril* 1989;52:437–440.

366. **Penzias AS, Jones EE, Seifer DB, et al.** Baseline ovarian cysts do not affect clinical response to controlled ovarian hyperstimulation for in vitro fertilization. *Fertil Steril* 1992;57:1017–1021.

367. **Thatcher SS, Jones E, DeCherney AH.** Ovarian cysts decrease the success of controlled ovarian stimulation and in vitro fertilization. *Fertil Steril* 1989;52:812–816.

368. **Segal S, Shifren JL, Isaacson KB, et al.** Effect of a baseline ovarian cyst on the outcome of in vitro fertilization-embryo transfer. *Fertil Steril* 1999;71:274–277.

369. **Lanes SF, Birmann B, Walker AM, et al.** Oral contraceptive type and functional ovarian cysts. *Am J Obstet Gynecol* 1992;166:956.

370. **Holt VL, Daling JR, McKnight B, et al.** Functional ovarian cysts in relation to the use of monophasic and triphasic oral contraceptives. *Obstet Gynecol* 1992;79:529.

371. **Land JA, Yarmolinskaya MI, Dumoulin JC, et al.** High-dose human menopausal gonadotropin stimulation in poor responders does not improve in vitro fertilization outcome. *Fertil Steril* 1996;65:961–965.

372. **Benadiva CA, Davis O, Kligman I, et al.** Withholding gonadotropin administration is an effective alternative for the prevention of ovarian hyperstimulation syndrome. *Fertil Steril* 1997;67:724–727.

373. **Al-Shawaf T, Zosmer A, Hussain S, et al.** Prevention of severe ovarian hyperstimulation syndrome in IVF with or without ICSI and embryo transfer: a modified 'coasting' strategy based on ultrasound for identification of high-risk patients. *Hum Reprod* 2001;16:24–30.

374. **Fluker MR, Hooper WM, Yuzpe AA.** Withholding gonadotropins ("coasting") to minimize the risk of ovarian hyperstimulation during superovulation and in vitro fertilization – embryo transfer cycles. *Fertil Steril* 1999;71:294–301.

375. **MacDougall MJ, Tan SH, Balen A, et al.** A controlled study comparing patients with and without polycystic ovaries undergoing in vitro fertilization. *Hum Reprod* 1993;8:233–237.

376. **MacLeod AF, Wheeler MH, Gordon P, et al.** Effect of long-term inhibition of gonadotropin secretion by the gonadotropin-releasing hormone agonist, buserelin, on sex steroid secretion and ovarian morphology in polycystic ovary syndrome. *J Endocrinol* 1990;125:317–325.

377. **Dodson WC, Hughes CL Jr, Yancy SE, et al.** Clinical characteristics of ovulation induction with human menopausal gonadotropins with and without leuprolide acetate in polycystic ovary syndrome. *Fertil Steril* 1989;52:915–918.

378. **Damario MA, Barmat L, Liu HC, et al.** Dual suppression with oral contraceptives and gonadotrophin releasing-hormone agonists improves in-vitro fertilization outcome in high responder patients. *Hum Reprod* 1997;12:2359–2365.

379. **De Leo V, la Marca A, Ditto A, et al.** Effects of metformin on gonadotropin-induced ovulation in women with polycystic ovary syndrome. *Fertil Steril* 1999;72:282–285.

380. **Dor J, Itzkowic DH, Mashiach S, et al.** Cumulative conception rates following gonadotropin therapy. *Am J Obstet Gynecol* 1980;136:102–105.

381. **Shoham Z, Balen A, Patel A, et al.** Results of ovulation induction using human menopausal gonadotropin or purified follicle-stimulating hormone in hypogonadotropic hypogonadism patients. *Fertil Steril* 1991;56:1048–1053.

382. **Shoham Z, Conway GS, Patel A, et al.** Polycystic ovaries in patients with hypogonadotropic hypogonadism: similarity of ovarian response to gonadotropin stimulation in patients with polycystic ovarian syndrome. *Fertil Steril* 1992;58:37–45.

383. **Hall JE, Martin KA, Whitney HA, et al.** Potential for fertility with replacement of hypothalamic gonadotropin-releasing hormone in long term female survivors of cranial tumors. *J Clin Endocrinol Metab* 1994;79:1166–1172.

384. **Jansen RP.** Pulsatile intravenous gonadotropin releasing hormone for ovulation induction: determinants of follicular and luteal phase response. *Hum Reprod* 1993;8:193–196.

385. **Martin KA, Hall JE, Adams JM, et al.** Comparison of exogenous gonadotropins and pulsatile gonadotropin-releasing hormone for the induction of ovulation in hypogonadotropic amenorrhea. *J Clin Endocrinol Metab* 1993;77:125–129.

386. **Braat DD, Schoemaker R, Schoemaker J.** Life table analysis of fecundity of intravenously gonadotropin-releasing hormone-treated patients with normogonadotropic and hypogonadotropic amenorrhea. *Fertil Steril* 1991;55:266–271.

387. **Skarin G, Ahlgren M.** Pulsatile gonadotropin releasing hormone (GnRH)-treatment for hypothalamic amenorrhea causing infertility. *Acta Obstet Gynecol Scand* 1994;73:482–485.

388. **Seminara SB, Beranova M, Oliveira LM, et al.** Successful use of pulsatile gonadotropin-releasing hormone (GnRH) for ovulation induction and pregnancy in a patient with GnRH receptor mutations. *J Clin Endocrinol Metab* 2000;85:556–562.

389. **Ron-El R, Herman A, Golan A, et al.** Gonadotropins and combined gonadotropin-releasing hormone agonist: gonadotropin protocols in a randomized prospective study. *Fertil Steril* 1991;55:574–578.

390. **Maroulis GB, Emery M, Verkauf BS, et al.** Prospective randomized study of human menotropin versus a follicular and a luteal phase gonadotropin-releasing hormone analog-human menotropin stimulation protocols for in vitro fertilization. *Fertil Steril* 1991;55:1157–1164.

391. **Tan SL, Kingsland C, Campbell S, et al.** The long protocol of administration of gonadotropin-releasing hormone agonist is superior to the short protocol for ovarian stimulation for in vitro fertilization. *Fertil Steril* 1992;57:810–814.

392. **Hazout A, Fernandez H, Ziegler DD, et al.** Comparison of short 7-day and prolonged treatment with gonadotropin-releasing hormone agonist desensitization for controlled ovarian hyperstimulation. *Fertil Steril* 1993;59:596–600.

393. **Kingsland C, Tan SL, Bickerton N, et al.** The routine use of gonadotropin releasing hormone agonists for all patients undergoing in vitro fertilization. Is there any medical advantage? A prospective randomized study. *Fertil Steril* 1992;57:804–809.

394. **San Roman GA, Surrey ES, Judd HL, et al.** A prospective randomized comparison of luteal phase versus concurrent follicular phase initiation of gonadotropin-releasing hormone agonist for in vitro fertilization and gamete intrafallopian transfer cycles. *Fertil Steril* 1992;58:744–749.

395. **Hughes EG, Fedorkow DM, Daya S, et al.** The routine use of gonadotropin-releasing hormone agonists prior to in vitro fertilization and gamete intrafallopian transfer: a meta-analysis of randomized, controlled trials. *Fertil Steril* 1992;58:888–896.

396. **Cramer DW, Powers DR, Oskowitz SP, et al.** Gonadotropin-releasing hormone agonist use in assisted reproduction cycles: the influence of long and short regimens on pregnancy rates. *Fertil Steril* 1999;72:83–89.

397. **Devroey P.** GnRH antagonists. *Fertil Steril* 2000;73:15–17.

398. **Tan SL, Balen A, El Hussein E, et al.** A prospective randomized study of the optimum timing of human chorionic gonadotropin administration after pituitary desensitization in in vitro fertilization. *Fertil Steril* 1992;57:1259–1264.

399. **Gonen Y, Powell WA, Casper RF.** Effect of follicular aspiration on hormonal parameters in patients undergoing ovarian stimulation. *Hum Reprod* 1991;6:356–358.

400. **Forman RG, Frydman R, Egan D, et al.** Severe ovarian hyperstimulation using agonists of gonadotropin-releasing hormone for in vitro fertilization: European series and a proposal for prevention. *Fertil Steril* 1990;53:502–509.

401. **Franco JG, Baruffi RL, Coelho J, et al.** A prospective and randomized study of ovarian stimulation for ICSI with recombinant FSH versus highly purified urinary FSH. *Gynecol Endocrinol* 2000;14:5–10.

402. **Lenton E, Soltan A, Hewitt J, et al.** Induction of ovulation in women undergoing assisted reproductive techniques: recombinant human FSH (follitropin alpha) versus highly purified urinary FSH (urofollitropin HP). *Hum Reprod* 2000;15:1021–1027.

403. **Schats R, Sutter PD, Bassil S, et al.** Ovarian stimulation during assisted reproduction treatment: a comparison of recombinant and highly purified urinary human FSH. On behalf of The Feronia and Apis Study Group. *Hum Reprod* 2000;15:1691–1697.

404. **Frydman R, Howles CM, Truong F.** A double-blind, randomized study to compare recombinant human follicle stimulating hormone (FSH; Gonal-F) with highly purified urinary FSH (Metrodin HP) in women undergoing assisted reproductive techniques including intracytoplasmic sperm injection. The French Multicentre Trialists. *Hum Reprod* 2000;15:520–525.

405. **Bergh C, Howles CM, Borg K, et al.** Recombinant human follicle stimulating hormone (r-hFSH; Gonal-F) versus highly purified urinary FSH (Metrodin HP): results of a randomized comparative study in women undergoing assisted reproductive techniques. *Hum Reprod* 1997;12:2133–2139.

406. **Hoomans EH, Andersen AN, Loft A, et al.** A prospective, randomized clinical trial comparing 150IU recombinant follicle stimulating hormone (Puregon (R)) and 225 IU highly purified urinary follicle stimulating hormone (Metrodin-HP(R)) in a fixed-dose regimen in women undergoing ovarian stimulation. *Hum Reprod* 1999;14:2442–2447.

407. **Hedon B, Out HJ, Hugues JN, et al.** Efficacy and safety of recombinant FSH (Puregon) in infertile women pituitary-suppressed with triptorelin undergoing in-vitro fertilisation: a prospective, randomised, assessor-blind, multicentre trial. *Hum Reprod* 1995;10:3102–3106.

408. **Out HJ, Mannaerts BMJL, Driessen SGAJ, et al.** A prospective, randomized, assessor-blind, multicenter study comparing recombinant and urinary follicle-stimulating hormone (Puregon vs Metrodin) in in-vitro fertilization. *Hum Reprod* 1995;10:2534–2540.

409. **Rubinstein M, Marazzi A, Polak de Fried E.** Low-dose aspirin treatment improves ovarian responsiveness, uterine and ovarian blood flow velocity, implantation, and pregnancy rates in patients undergoing in vitro fertilization: a prospective, randomized, double-blind placebo-controlled assay.

410. **Sills ES, Levy DP, Moomjy M, et al.** A prospective, randomized comparison of ovulation induction using highly purified follicle-stimulating hormone alone and with recombinant human luteinizing hormone in in-vitro fertilization. *Hum Reprod* 1999;14:2230–2235.

411. **Hammadeh ME, Wilhelm W, Huppert A, et al.** Effects of general anaesthesia versus sedation on fertilization, cleavage and pregnancy rates in an IVF program. *Arch Gynecol Obstet* 1999;263:56–59.

412. **Casati A, Valentini G, Zangrillo A, et al.** Anaesthesia for ultrasound guided oocyte retrieval: midazolam/remifentanil versus propofol/fentanyl regimens. *Eur J Anaesthesiol* 1999;16:773–778.

413. **Martin R, Tsen LC, Tzeng G, et al.** Anesthesia for in vitro fertilization: the addition of fentanyl to lidocaine. *Anesth Analg* 1999;88:523–526.

414. **van Os HC, Roozenburg BJ, Janssen-Caspers HA, et al.** Vaginal disinfection with povidone iodine and the outcome of in-vitro fertilization. *Hum Reprod* 1992;7:349–350.

415. **Egbase PE, Udo EE, Al-Sharhan M, et al.** Prophylactic antibiotics and endocervical microbial inoculation of the endometrium at embryo transfer. *Lancet* 1999;354:651–652.

416. **Eisenbach M, Ralt D.** Pre-contact mammalian sperm-egg communication and role in fertilization. *Am J Physiol* 1992;262:C1095–1101.

417. **Licciardi FL, Kwiatkowski A, Noyes NL, et al.** Oral versus intramuscular progesterone for in vitro fertilization: a prospective randomized study. *Fertil Steril* 1999;71:614–618.

418. **Croxatto HB, Ortiz MS.** Egg transport in the fallopian tube. *Gynecol Invest* 1975;6:215–225.

419. **Plachot M, Mandelbaum J, Junca AM, et al.** Cytogenic analysis and developmental capacity of normal and abnormal embryos after IVF. *Hum Reprod* 1989;4:99–103.

420. **Del Marek MA, Langley M, Gardner DK, et al.** Introduction of blastocyst culture and transfer for all patients in an in vitro fertilization program. *Fertil Steril* 1999;72:1035–1040.

421. **Gardner KD, Lane M, Stevens J, et al.** Blastocyst score affects implantation and pregnancy outcome: towards a single blastocyst transfer. *Fertil Steril* 2000;73:1155–1158.

422. **Racowsky C, Jackson KV, Cekleniak NA, et al.** The number of eight-cell embryos is a key determinant for selecting day 3 or day 5 transfer. *Fertil Steril* 2000;73:558–564.

423. **Coskun S, Hollanders J, Al-Hassan S, et al.** Day 5 versus day 3 embryo transfers: a controlled randomized trial. *Hum Reprod* 2000;15:1947–1952.

424. **Mansour RT, Aboulghar MA, Serour GI, et al.** Dummy embryo transfer using methylene blue dye. *Hum Reprod* 1994;9:1257–1259.

425. **Wood EG, Batzer FR, Go KJ, et al.** Ultrasound-guided soft catheter embryo transfers will improve pregnancy rates in in-vitro fertilization. *Hum Reprod* 2000;15:107–112.

426. **Wisanto A, Janssens R, Deschacht J, et al.** Performance of different embryo transfer catheters in a human in vitro fertilization program. *Fertil Steril* 1989;52:79–84.

427. **Moore DE, Soules MR, Klein NA, et al.** Bacteria in the transfer catheter tip influence the live-birth rate after in vitro fertilization. *Fertil Steril* 2000;74:1118–1124.

428. **Egbase PE, al-Sharhan M, al-Othman S, et al.** Incidence of microbial growth from the tip of the embryo transfer catheter after embryo transfer in relation to clinical pregnancies following in-vitro fertilization and embryo transfer. *Hum Reprod* 1996;11:1687–1689.

429. **Ghazzawi IM, Al-Hasani S, Karaki R, et al.** Transfer technique and catheter choice influence the incidence of transcervical embryo expulsion and the outcome of IVF. *Hum Reprod* 1999;14:677–682.

430. **Egbase PE, Al-Sharhan M, Grudzinskas JG.** Influence of position and length of uterus on implantation and clinical pregnancy rates in IVF and embryo transfer treatment cycles. *Hum Reprod* 2000;15:1943–1946.

431. **Lesny P, Killick SR, Robinson J, et al.** Transcervical embryo transfer as a risk factor for ectopic pregnancy. *Fertil Steril* 1999;72:305–309.

432. **Goudas VT, Hammitt DG, Damario MA, et al.** Blood on the embryo transfer catheter is associated with decreased rates of embryo implantation and clinical pregnancy with the in vitro fertilization-embryo transfer. *Fertil Steril* 1998;70:878–882.

433. **Tur-Kaspa I, Yuval Y, Bider D, et al.** Difficult or repeated sequential embryo transfers do not adversely affect in-vitro fertilization pregnancy rates or outcome. *Hum Reprod* 1998;13:2452–2455.

434. **Groutz A, Lessing JB, Wolf Yoram Yovel I, et al.** A. Cervical dilatation during ovum pick-up in patients with cervical stenosis: effect on pregnancy outcome in an in vitro fertilization-embryo transfer program. *Fertil Steril* 1997;67:909–911.

435. **Noyes N, Licciardi F, Grifo J, et al.** In vitro fertilization outcome relative to embryo transfer difficulty: a novel approach to the forbidding cervix. *Fertil Steril* 1999;72:261–265.

436. **Yanushpolsky EH, Ginsburg ES, Fox JH, et al.** Transcervical placement of a Malecot catheter after hysteroscopic evaluation provides for easier entry into the endometrial cavity for women with histories of difficult intrauterine inseminations and/or embryo transfers: a prospective case series. *Fertil Steril* 2000;73:402–405.

437. **Society for Assisted Reproductive Technology and American Society for Reproductive Medicine.** Assisted reproductive technology in the United States: 1997 results generated from the American Society for Reproductive Medicine/Society for Assisted Reproductive Technology Registry. *Fertil Steril* 2000;74:641–653.

438. **Visser A, Hann G, Zalmstra H, et al.** Psychosocial aspects of in vitro fertilization. *Psychosom Obstet Gynecol* 1994;15:35–43.

439. **Damewood MD, Shen W, Zacur HA, et al.** *Fertil Steril* 1989;52:398–400.

440. **Homan G, Brown S, Moran J, et al.** Human chorionic gonadotropin as a predictor of outcome in assisted reproductive technology pregnancies. *Fertil Steril* 2000;73:270–274.

441. **Paulson RJ, Hatch IE, Lobo RA, et al.** Cumulative conception and live birth rates after oocyte donation: implications regarding endometrial receptivity. *Hum Reprod* 1997;12:835–839.

442. **Quigley MM, Collins RL, Schover LR.** Establishment of an oocyte donor program: donor screening and selection. *Ann N Y Acad Sci* 1991;626:445–451.

443. **Toth TI, Baka SG, Veeck LL, et al.** Fertilization and in vitro development of cryopreserved human prophase I oocytes. Fertil Steril 1994;61:891–894.

444. **Sauer MV, Paulson RJ, Moyer DL.** Assessing the importance of endometrial biopsy prior to oocyte donation. *J Assist Reprod Genet* 1997;14:125–127.

445. **Kalfoglou AL, Gittelsohn J.** A qualitative follow-up study of women's experiences with oocyte donation. *Hum Reprod* 2000;15:798–805.

446. **The Ethics Committee of the American Society for Reproductive Medicine.** Financial incentives in recruitment of oocyte donors. *Fertil Steril* 2000;74:216–220.

447. **Ahuja KK, Simons EG, Edwards RG.** Money, morals and medical risks: conflicting notions underlying the recruitment of egg donors. *Hum Reprod* 1999;14:279–284.

448. **Martin JA, Park MM.** Trends in twin and triplet births: 1980–97. *National Vital Statistics Report.* Vol. 47, no.24. Hyattsville, MD: US Department of Health and Human Services, CDC, National Center for Health Statistics, 1999.

449. **Martin JA, MacDorman MF, Mathews TJ.** Triplet births: trends and outcomes, 1971–94. *Vital Health Stat* 1997;21:55.

450. **Guttmacher AF.** The incidence of multiple births in man and some other unipara. *Obstet Gynecol* 1953;2:22–35.

451. **Contribution of assisted reproductive technology and ovulation-inducing drugs to triplet and higher-order multiple births—United States, 1980–1997.** *MMWR Morb Mortal Wkly Rep* 2000;49:535–538.

452. **Davidson KM, Simpson LL, Knox TA, et al.** Acute fatty liver of pregnancy in triplet gestation. *Obstet Gynecol* 1998;91:806–808.

453. **Hardardottir H, Kelly K, Bork MD, et al.** Atypical presentation of preeclampsia in high-order multifetal gestations. *Obstet Gynecol* 1996;87:370–374.

454. **Borlum KG.** Third-trimester fetal death in triplet pregnancies. *Obstet Gynecol* 1991;77:6–9.

455. **Sassoon DA, Castro LC, Davis JL, et al.** Perinatal outcome in triplet versus twin gestations. *Obstet Gynecol* 1990;75:817–820.

456. **Elliott J, Bergauer N, Coleman S, et al.** Impact of gestational age at delivery on perinatal outcomes in triplets. *Obstet Gynecol* 2000;95:S66.

457. **Kaufman GE, Malone FD, Harvey-Wilkes KB, et al.** Neonatal morbidity and mortality associated with triplet pregnancies. *Obstet Gynecol* 1998;91:342–348.

458. **Callahan TL, Hall JE, Ettner SL, et al.** The economic impact of multiple-gestation pregnancies and the contribution of assisted-reproduction techniques to their incidence. *N Engl J Med* 1994;331:244–249.

459. **Guzick DS, Carson SA, Coutifaris C, et al.** Efficacy of superovulation and intrauterine insemination in the treatment of infertility. *N Engl J Med* 1999;340:177–183.

460. **Gleicher N, Oleske DM, Tur-Kaspa I, et al.** Reducing the risk of high-order multiple pregnancy after ovarian stimulation with gonadotropins. *N Engl J Med* 2000;343:2–7.

461. **American Society for Reproductive Medicine.** *A practice committee report: guidelines on number of embryos transferred.* 1999.

462. **Templeton A, Morris JK.** Reducing the risk of multiple births by transfer of two embryos after in vitro fertilization. *N Engl J Med* 1998;339:573–577.

463. **Bhattacharya S, Templeton A.** In treating infertility, are multiple pregnancies unavoidable? *N Engl J Med* 2000;343:58–59.

464. **Engmann L, Maconoshi N, Bekir JS, et al.** Cumulative probability of clinical pregnancy and live birth after a multiple cycle IVF package: a more realistic assessment of overall and age-specific success rates? *Br J Obstet Gynaecol* 1999;106:165–170.

465. **Jones HW, Schnorr JA.** Multiple pregnancies: a call for action. *Fertil Steril* 2001;75:11–13.

466. **Grifo J, Hoffman D, NcNamee PI.** We are due for a correction . . . and we are working to achieve one. *Fertil Steril* 2001:75:14.

467. **Paulson RJ, Ory SJ, Giudice LC, et al.** Multiple pregnancies: what action should we take? *Fertil Steril* 2000;14–15.

468. **Soules MR, Chang RJ, Lipshultz LI, et al.** Multiple pregnancies: action is taking place. *Fertil Steril* 2001.75.15–16.

469. **Delhanty JD, Handyside AH.** The origin of genetic defects in the human and their detection in the preimplantation embryo. *Hum Reprod Update* 1995;201–215.

470. **Munne S, Sandalinas M, Esudera T, et al.** Outcome of preimplantation genetic diagnosis of translocations. 2000;73:1209–1218.

471. **Griffin DK, Wilton LJ, Handyside AH, et al.** Dual fluorescent in situ hybridization for the simultaneous detection of X and Y chromosome specific probes for the sexing of human preimplantation embryonic nuclei. *Hum Genetic* 1992;89:18–22.

472. **Gianaroli L, Magli C, Ferraretti AP, et al.** Preimplantation diagnosis for aneuploidies in patients undergoing in vitro fertilization with a poor prognosis: identification of the categories for which for which it should be proposed? *Fertil Steril* 1999;72:837–844.

473. **Haning RV, Seifer DB, Wheeler CA, et al.** Effects of fetal number and multifetal reduction on length of in vitro fertilization pregnancies. *Obstet Gynecol* 1996;87:964–968.

474. **Leondires MP, Ernst SD, Miller BT, et al.** Triplets: outcomes of expectant management versus multifetal reduction for 127 pregnancies. *Am J Obstet Gynecol* 2000;183:454–459.

475. **Depp R, Macones GA, et al.** Multifetal pregnancy reduction: evaluation of fetal growth in the remaining twins. *Am J Obstet Gynecol* 1996;174:1238.

476. **Lipitz S, Uval J, Achiron R, et al.** Outcome of twin pregnancies reduced from triplets compared to nonreduced twin gestations. *Obstet Gynecol* 1996;87:511–514.

477. **Smith-Levitin M, A Kowalik, Birnholz J, et al.** Selective reduction of multifetal pregnancies to twins improves outcome over non-reduced triplet gestations. *Am J Obstet Gynecol* 1996;175: 878.

478. **Yaron Y, Bryant-Greenwood PK, Dave N, et al.** Multifetal pregnancy reductions of triplets to twins: comparison with nonreduced triplets and twins. *Am J Obstet Gynecol* 1999;180:1268–1271.

479. **Boulot P, Vignal J, Vergnes C, et al.** Multifetal reduction of triplets to twins: a prospective comparison of pregnancy outcome. *Hum Reprod* 2000;15:1619–1623.

480. **Lipitz S, Shalev, et al.** Late selective termination of fetal abnormalities in twin pregnancies: a multicentre report. *Br J Obstet Gynecol* 1996;103:1212.

481. **Evans MI, Goldberg JD, Horenstein J, et al.** Selective termination for structural, chromosomal, and mendelian anomalies: international experience. *Am J Obstet Gynecol* 1999;181:893–897.

482. **Garel M, Starck C, et al.** Psychological effects of embryonal reduction: from the decision making to 4 months after delivery. *J Gynecol Obstet Biol Reprod* 1995;24:119.

483. **Enskog A, Henriksson M, Unander M, et al.** Prospective study of the clinical and laboratory parameters of patients in whom ovarian hyperstimulation syndrome developed during controlled ovarian hyperstimulation for in vitro fertilization. *Fertil Steril* 1999;71:808–814.

484. **Blankstein J, Shalev J, Saadon T, et al.** Ovarian hyperstimulation syndrome: prediction by number and size of preovulatory ovarian follicles. *Fertil Steril* 1987;47:597–602.

485. **Navot D, Relou A, Birkenfeld A, et al.** Risk factors and prognostic variables in the ovarian hyperstimulation syndrome. *Am J Obstet Gynecol* 1988;159:210–215.

486. **MacDougall MJ, Tan SL, Jacobs HS.** In-vitro fertilization and the ovarian hyperstimulation syndrome. *Hum Reprod* 1992;7:597–600.

487. **Buyalos RP, Lee CT.** Polycystic ovary syndrome: pathophysiology and outcome with in vitro fertilization. *Fertil Steril* 1996;65:1–10.

488. **Delvigne A, Demoulin A, Smitz J, et al.** The ovarian hyperstimulation syndrome in in-vitro fertilization: a Belgian multicentric study. I. Clinical and biological features. *Hum Reprod* 1993;8:1353–1360.

489. **Haning RV Jr, Austin CW, Carlson IH, et al.** Plasma estradiol is superior to ultrasound and urinary estriol glucuronide as a predictor of ovarian hyperstimulation during induction of ovulation with menotropins. *Fertil Steril* 1983;40:31–36.

490. **Gustafson O, Carlstrom K, Nylund L.** Androstenedione as a predictor of ovarian hyperstimulation syndrome. *Hum Reprod* 1992;7:918–921.

491. **Chenette PE, Sauer MV, Paulson RJ.** Very high serum estradiol levels are not detrimental to clinical outcome of in vitro fertilization. *Fertil Steril* 1990;54:858–863.

492. **Asch RH, Li HP, Balmaceda JP, et al.** Severe ovarian hyperstimulation syndrome in assisted reproductive technology: definition of high risk groups. *Hum Reprod* 1991;6:1395–1399.

493. **Wheelan JG, Vlahos NF.** The ovarian hyperstimulation syndrome. *Fertil Steril* 2000;73:883–896.

494. **Paulson RJ, Do YS, Hsueh WA, et al.** Ovarian renin production in vitro and in vivo: characterization and clinical correlation. *Fertil Steril* 1989;51:634–638.

495. **Lightman A, Tarlatzis BC, Rzasa PJ, et al.** The ovarian renin-angiotensin system: renin-like activity and angiotensin II/III immunoreactivity in gonadotropin-stimulated and unstimulated human follicular fluid. *Am J Obstet Gynecol* 1987;156:808–816.

496. **Sealey JE, Glorioso N, Itskovitz J, et al.** Prorenin as a reproductive hormone: new form of the renin system. *Am J Med* 1986;81:1041–1046.

497. **Glorioso N, Atlas SA, Laragh JH, et al.** Prorenin in high concentrations in human ovarian follicular fluid. *Science* 1986;233:1422–1424.

498. **Derkx FH, Alberda AT, Zeilmaker GH, et al.** High concentrations of immunoreactive renin, prorenin and enzymatically-active renin in human ovarian follicular fluid. *Br J Obstet Gynaecol* 1987;92:4–9.

499. **Robertson AL, Khairallah PA.** Effects of angiotensin II and some analogues on vascular permeability in the rabbit. *Circ Res* 1972;31:923–931.

500. **Ong AC, Eisen V, Rennie DP, et al.** The pathogenesis of the ovarian hyperstimulation syndrome (OHS): a possible role for ovarian renin. *Clin Endocrinol* 1991:34:43–49.

501. **Navot D, Margalioth EJ, Laufer N, et al.** Direct correlation between plasma renin activity and severity of the ovarian hyperstimulation syndrome. *Fertil Steril* 1987;48:57–61.

502. **Morris RS, Wong IL, Kirkman E, et al.** Inhibition of ovarian-derived prorenin to angiotensin cascade in the treatment of ovarian hyperstimulation syndrome. *Hum Reprod* 1995;10:1355–1358.

503. **Loret de Mola JR, Baumgardner GP, Goldfarb JM, et al.** Ovarian hyperstimulation syndrome: pre-ovulatory serum concentrations of interleukin-6, interleukin-1 receptor antagonist and tumour necrosis factor-alpha cannot predict its occurrence. *Hum Reprod* 1996;11:1377–1380.

504. **Abramov Y, Schenker JG, Lewin A, et al.** Plasma inflammatory cytokines correlate to the ovarian hyperstimulation syndrome. *Hum Reprod* 1996;11:1381–1386.

505. **Knox GE.** Antihistamine blockade of the ovarian hyperstimulation syndrome. *Am J Obstet Gynecol* 1974;118:992–994.

506. **Knox GE, Dowd AJ, Spiesel SA, et al.** Antihistamine blockade of the ovarian hyperstimulation syndrome. II. Possible role of antigen-antibody complexes in the pathogenesis of the syndrome. *Fertil Steril* 1975;26:418–421.

507. **Gergely RZ, Paldi E, Erlik Y, et al.** Treatment of ovarian hyperstimulation syndrome by antihistamine. *Obstet Gynecol* 1976;47:83–85.

508. **Schenker JG, Polishuk WZ.** The role of prostaglandins in ovarian hyperstimulation syndrome. *Eur J Obstet Gynecol Reprod Biol* 1976;6:47–52.

509. **Pride SM, Yuen BH, Moon YS, et al.** Relationship of gonadotropin-releasing hormone, danazol, and prostaglandin blockade to ovarian enlargement and ascites formation of the ovarian hyperstimulation syndrome in the rabbit. *Am J Obstet Gynecol* 1986;154:1155–1160.

510. **Neulen J, Yan Z, Raczek S, et al.** Human chorionic gonadotropin-dependent expression of vascular endothelial growth factor/vascular permeability factor in human granulosa cells: importance in ovarian hyperstimulation syndrome. *J Clin Endocrinol Metab* 1995;80:1967–1971.

511. **Levin ER, Rosen GF, Cassidenti DL, et al.** Role of vascular endothelial cell growth factor in ovarian hyperstimulation syndrome. *J Clin Invest* 1998;102:1978–1985.

512. **Agrawal R, Tan SL, Wild S, et al.** Serum vascular endothelial growth factor concentrations in in vitro fertilization cycles predict the risk of ovarian hyperstimulation syndrome. *Fertil Steril* 1999;71: 287–293.

513. **Nakamura Y, Smith M, Krishna A, et al.** Increased number of mast cells in the dominant follicle of the cow: relationships among luteal, stromal, and hilar regions. *Biol Reprod* 1987;37:546–549.

514. Zaidise I, Friedman M, Lindenbaum ES, et al. Serotonin and the ovarian hyperstimulation syndrome. *Eur J Obstet Gynecol Reprod Biol* 1983;15:55–60.

515. Mathur RS, Akande AV, Keay SD, et al. Distinction between early and late ovarian hyperstimulation syndrome. *Fertil Steril* 2000;73:901–907.

516. Golan A, Ron-El R, Herman A, et al. Ovarian hyperstimulation syndrome: an update review. *Obstet Gynecol* Surv 1989;44:430–440.

517. Aboulghar MA, Mansour RT, Serour GI, et al. Ultrasonically guided vaginal aspiration of ascites in the treatment of severe ovarian hyperstimulation syndrome [published erratum appears in *Fertil Steril* 1990;54:957]. *Fertil Steril* 1990;53:933–935.

518. Rizk B, Aboulghar M. Modern management of ovarian hyperstimulation syndrome. *Hum Reprod* 1991;6:1082–1087.

519. Ferraretti AP, Gianaroli L, Magli C, et al. Elective cryopreservation of all pronucleate embryos in women at risk of ovarian hyperstimulation syndrome: efficiency and safety.

520. Queenan JT, Veeck LL, Toner JP, et al. Cryopreservation of all prezygotes in patients at risk of severe hyperstimulation does not eliminate the syndrome, but the chances of pregnancy are excellent with subsequent frozen-thaw transfers.

521. Queenan JT. Embryo freezing to prevent ovarian hyperstimulation syndrome. *Mol Cell Endocrinol* 2000;169:79–83.

522. Cha KY, Han SY, Chung HM, et al. Pregnancies and deliveries after in vitro maturation culture followed by in vitro fertilization and embryo transfer without stimulation in women with polycystic ovary syndrome. *Fertil Steril* 2000;73:978–983.

523. Chian RC, Buckett WM, Tulandi T, et al. Prospective randomized study of human chorionic gonadotrophin priming before immature oocyte retrieval from unstimulated women with polycystic ovarian syndrome. *Hum Reprod* 2000;15:165–170.

524. Chian RC, Gulekli B, Buckett WM, et al. Priming with human chorionic gonadotropin before retrieval of immature oocytes in women with infertility due to the polycystic ovary syndrome. *N Engl J Med* 1999;341:1624, 1626.

525. Ectopic pregnancy—United States, 1990–1992. *MMWR Morb Mortal Wkly Rep* 1995;44:46–48.

526. Strandell A, Thorburn J, Hamberger L. Risk factors for ectopic pregnancy in assisted reproduction. *Fertil Steril* 1999;71:282–286.

527. Tal J, Haddad S, Gordon N, et al. Heterotopic pregnancy after ovulation induction and assisted reproductive technologies: a literature review from 1971 to 1993. *Fertil Steril* 1996;66:1–12.

528. Louis-Sylvestre C, Morice P, Chapron C, et al. The role of laparoscopy in the diagnosis and management of heterotopic pregnancies. *Hum Reprod* 1997;12:1100–1102.

529. Whittemore AS, Harris R, Itnyre J. Characteristics relating to ovarian cancer risk: collaborative analysis of 12 US case-control studies. II. Invasive epithelial ovarian cancers in white women. Collaborative Ovarian Cancer Group. *Am J Epidemiol* 1992;136(10):1184–2203.

530. Wakeley KE, Grendys EC. Reproductive technologies and risk of ovarian cancer. *Curr Opin Obstet Gynecol.* 2000;12(1):43–47.

531. Potashnik G, Lerner-Geva L, Genkin L, et al. Fertility drugs and the risk of breast and ovarian cancers: results of a long-term follow-up study. *Fertil Steril* 1999;71(5):853–859.

532. Venn A, Watson L, Bruinsma F, et al. Risk of cancer after use of fertility drugs with in-vitro fertilisation. *Lancet* 1999;354(9190):1586–1590.

533. Domar AD, Broome A, Zuttermeister PC, et al. The prevalence and predictability of depression in infertile women. *Fertil Steril* 1992;58:1158–1163.

534. Demyttenaere K, Nijs P, Steeno O, et al. Anxiety and conception rates in donor insemination. *J Psychosom Obstet Gynaecol* 1998;8:175–181.

535. Lapane LK, Zierler S, Lasatar TM, et al. Is a history of depressive symptoms associated with an increased risk of infertility in women? *Psychosom Med* 1995;57:509–513.

536. Domar AD, Clapp D, Slawsby EA, et al. Impact of group psychological interventions on pregnancy rates in infertile women. *Fertil Steril* 2000;73:805–812.

537. Barbieri RL, Domar Ad, Loughlin KR. *6 Steps to increased fertility: an integrated medical and mind/body program to promote conception.* New York, NY: Simon & Schuster, 1992.

538. Lass A, Akagbosu F, Abusheikha N, et al. A programme of semen cryopreservation for patients with malignant disease in a tertiary infertility centre: lessons from 8 years' experience. *Hum Reprod* 1998;13:3256–3261.

539. Hallak J, Kolettis PN, Sekhon VS, et al. Sperm cryopreservation in patients with testicular cancer. *Urology* 1999;54:894–899.

540. **Anderson RA, Kinniburgh D, Baird DT.** Preliminary experience of the use of a gonadotropin-releasing hormone antagonist in ovulation induction/in-vitro fertilization prior to cancer treatment. *Hum Reprod* 1999;14:2665–2668.

541. **Meirow D, Fasouliotis SJ, Nugent D, et al.** A laparoscopic technique for obtaining ovarian cortical biopsy specimens for fertility conservation in patients with cancer. *Fertil Steril* 1999;71:948–951.

542. **Donnez J, Godin PA, Qu J, et al.** Gonadal cryopreservation in the young patient with gynaecological malignancy. *Curr Opin Obstet Gynecol* 2000;12:1–9.

543. **Oktay K, Newton H, Aubard Y, et al.** Cryopreservation of immature human oocytes and ovarian tissue: an emerging technology? *Fertil Steril* 1998;69:1–7.

544. **Pantos K, Meimeth-Damianaki T, Vaxevanogou T, et al.** Prospective study of a modified gonadotropin-releasing hormone agonist long protocol in an in vitro fertilization program. *Fertil Steril* 1994;61:709–713.

545. **Scott RT, Navot D.** Enhancement of ovarian responsiveness with microdoses of gonadotropin-releasing hormone agonist during ovulation induction for in vitro fertilization. *Fertil Steril* 1994;61:880–885.

546. **Surrey ES, Bower J, Hill DM, et al.** Clinical and endocrine effects of a microdose GnRH agonist flare regimen administered to poor responders who are undergoing in vitro fertilization. *Fertil Steril* 1998;69:419–424.

28 Recurrent Pregnancy Loss

Daniel J. Schust
Joseph A. Hill

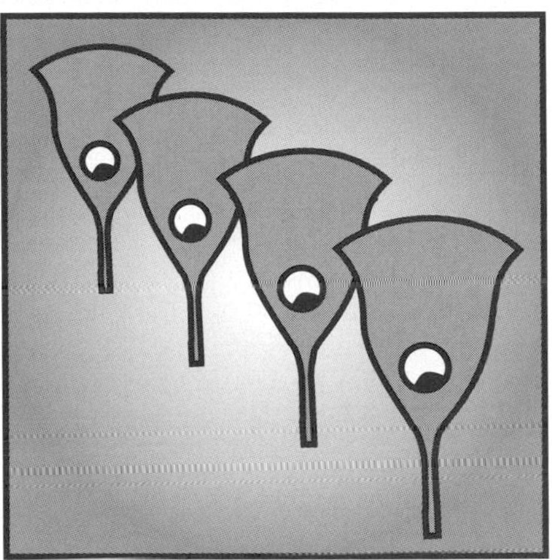

Advances in the ability to document and diagnose early pregnancy have revealed that spontaneous pregnancy loss is a common event. Spontaneous pregnancy loss is, in fact, the most common complication of pregnancy. About 70% of human conceptions fail to achieve viability, and an estimated 50% are lost before the first missed menstrual period (1). Most of these pregnancy losses are unrecognized. Studies using sensitive assays for human chorionic gonadotropin (hCG) indicate that the actual rate of pregnancy loss after implantation is 31% (2). Of pregnancies that are clinically recognized, loss occurs in 15% before 20 weeks of gestation (from last menstrual period) (3,4).

Traditionally, recurrent abortion has been defined as the occurrence of three or more clinically recognized pregnancy losses before 20 weeks from the last menstrual period. Using this definition, recurrent pregnancy loss occurs in about 1 in 300 pregnancies (2). **Clinical investigation of pregnancy loss, however, should be initiated after two consecutive spontaneous abortions, especially when fetal heart activity is identified before any of the pregnancy losses, when the woman is older than 35 years of age, or when the couple has had difficulty conceiving.** If clinical intervention is undertaken in the form of investigation after two spontaneous abortions, about 1% of pregnant women require evaluation (3). Even with a history of recurrent pregnancy loss, a patient is more likely to carry her next pregnancy to term than to miscarry. For patients with a history of recurrent pregnancy loss, the risk for subsequent pregnancy loss is estimated to be 24% after two clinically recognized losses, 30% after three losses, and 40% to 50% after four losses (5). These data make clinical study of recurrent pregnancy loss and its treatment difficult because very large groups of patients must be studied to demonstrate the effects of any proposed therapeutic intervention.

Etiology

Parental chromosomal abnormalities and thrombotic complications of the antiphospholipid antibody syndrome (APAS) are the only undisputed causes of recurrent abortion. However, collectively these abnormalities account for less than 10% to 15% of recurrent pregnancy losses. Although the exact proportion of patients diagnosed with a particular abnormality may vary among the populations studied, other associations have been made with anatomic abnormalities (12% to 16%), endocrine problems (17% to 20%), infections (0.5% to 5%), and immunologic factors, including those associated with APAS (20% to 50%). Other miscellaneous factors have been implicated and account for about 10% of cases. Even after a thorough evaluation, however, the potential cause remains unexplained in about half of cases (6) (Table 28.1).

Genetic Factors

The most common inborn parental chromosomal abnormalities contributing to recurrent abortion are balanced translocations (7–9), in which one parent carries an overall normal gene content but has a piece of one chromosome inappropriately attached to another. Depending on the nature of the translocation (reciprocal or robertsonian), the gametes produced by the translocation carrier are either normal (reciprocal only), balanced, or unbalanced for the translocated DNA. Once fertilized by a chromosomally normal gamete, the resulting embryos may be either chromosomally normal (reciprocal only) or balanced or unbalanced carriers of the translocation. Most gametes and their resulting embryos with abnormal chromosomal status do not survive. Of those that do, live offspring are either carriers of a balanced translocation or, for robertsonian translocations, monosomic or trisomic for the translocated chromosomal DNA.

Among the possible chromosomal monosomies, only that of the X chromosome typically permits viable offspring. On careful examination, however, many of these offspring may, in fact, exhibit mosaicism. Recent evidence also suggests that embryonic chromosomal monosomy may be particularly prevalent among patients with a history of recurrent pregnancy loss who are undergoing *in vitro* fertilization (10). Compared with monosomies, chromosomal trisomies (e.g., trisomies 13, 18, and 21) appear to be tolerated a bit more readily, although mosaicism may be implicated with these abnormalities as well.

Neither family history alone nor a history of prior term births is sufficient to rule out a potential parental chromosomal abnormality. Whereas the frequency of detecting a parental chromosomal abnormality is inversely related to the number of previous spontaneous losses (9), the chance of detecting a parental chromosomal abnormality also is increased among couples who have never experienced a live birth. Of course, abnormalities may be detected upon parental karyotype analysis of some couples with a history of spontaneous abortions interspersed with stillbirths and live births (with or without congenital anomalies) as well. Unfortunately, the use of parental karyotyping in evaluating structural chromosomal etiologies of recurrent pregnancy loss may soon become an insufficient screening modality. Evidence now suggests that, in some cases, paternal chromosomal abnormalities may be isolated within a particular fertilizing spermatozoa (11). Further, aneuploid spermatozoa may be particularly motile (12).

Other structural chromosome anomalies, such as inversions and insertions, also may contribute to recurrent abortion, as can chromosomal mosaicism and single gene defects. X-linked disorders uncommonly may result in recurrent abortion of male but not female offspring (13). Single gene defects and their resulting disorders (e.g., the delta f 508 mutation and cystic fibrosis) typically are recognized through either analysis of detailed family histories or the identification of some pattern of anomalies characteristic of a known heritable syndrome.

Recently, there has been a great deal of interest in the role of inherited thrombophilias in recurrent pregnancy loss (14,15). This heterogeneous group of disorders results in increased venous or arterial thrombosis. Their associations with pregnancy loss rest on both proven (16) and hypothetical alterations in placental growth and development, particularly placental vascular development. Abnormal placental vascularization and inappropriate placental thrombosis would link these thrombophilic states to pregnancy loss. Although some thrombophilic states may be acquired, most are heritable. Those heritable thrombophilias most often linked with reference to recurrent pregnancy loss include hyperhomocysteinemia,

Table 28.1. Proposed Etiologies for Recurrent Spontaneous Abortion

Etiology	*Proposed Incidence (%)*
Genetic Factors	3.5–5
1. Chromosomal	
2. Single gene defects	
3. Multifactorial	
Anatomic Factors	12–16
1. Congenital	
a. Incomplete müllerian fusion or septum resorption	
b. *DES* exposure	
c. Uterine artery anomalies	
d. Cervical incompetence	
2. Acquired	
a. Cervical incompetence	
b. Synechiae	
c. Leiomyomas	
d. Adenomyosis	
Endocrine Factors	17–20
1. Luteal-phase insufficiency	
2. Polycystic ovarian syndrome, including insulin resistance and hyperandrogenism	
3. Other androgen disorders	
4. Diabetes mellitus	
5. Thyroid disorders	
6. Prolactin disorders	
Infectious Factors	0.5–5
1. Bacteria	
2. Viruses	
3. Parasites	
4. Zoonotic	
5. Fungal	
Immunologic Factors	20–50
1. Cellular mechanisms	
a. Suppressor cell or factor deficiency	
b. Alterations in major histocompatibility antigen expression	
c. Alterations in cellular immune regulation	
i. T_H1 immune responses to reproductive antigens (embryo or trophoblast)	
ii. T_H2 cytokine or growth factor deficiency	
iii. Hormonal—progesterone and estrogen	
iv. Tryptophan metabolism	
2. Humoral Mechanisms	
a. Antiphospholipid antibodies	
b. Antithyroid antibodies	
c. Antisperm antibodies	
d. Antitrophoblast antibodies	
e. Blocking antibody deficiency	
Thrombotic Factors	Most are included among other categories (e.g., immune, genetic)
1. Heritable thrombophilias	
a. Single gene defects (*fVL, MTHFR,* factor deficiencies)	
b. Antibody-mediated thromboses (APAS, anti-β_2G1)	
Other Factors	10
1. Altered uterine receptivity (integrins, adhesion molecules)	
2. Environmental	
a. Toxins	
b. Illicit drugs	
c. Alcohol, cigarettes and caffeine	

Table 28.1.—*continued*

3. Placental abnormalities (circumvallate, marginate)
4. Medical illnesses (cardiac, renal hematologic)
5. Male factors
6. Coitus
7. Exercise
8. Dyssynchronous fertilization

activated protein C resistance associated with mutations in factor V Leiden deficiencies in proteins C and S, mutations in prothrombin, and mutations in antithrombin III.

Circulating homocysteine is derived from dietary methionine. Homocysteine, in turn, is metabolized either into cystathione or back into methionine (Fig. 28.1). The latter process involves the enzyme *methylene tetrahydrofolate reductase* (MTHFR) (15). The nutritional supplements folic acid, vitamin B_6, and vitamin B_{12} are all required for proper metabolism of homocysteine; therefore, their deficiency is associated with acquired elevations in circulating homocysteine levels (17,18). Although heritable deficiencies in the enzymes

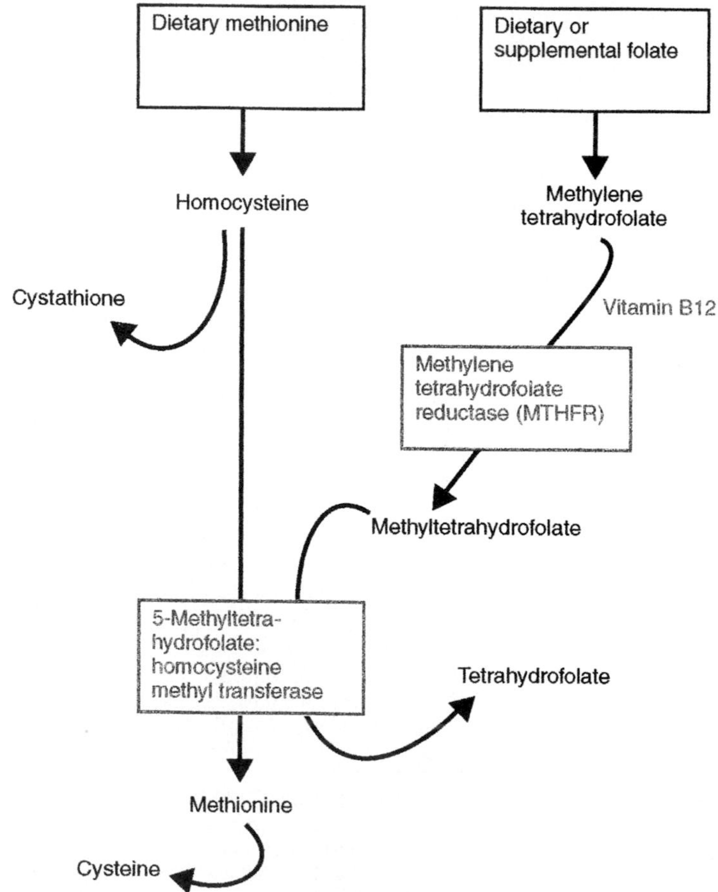

Figure 28.1 Homocysteine metabolism. Dietary methionine is metabolized either to cystathione or back into methionine. Conversion of homocysteine to methionine requires transfer of a methyl group from methyltetrahydrofolate. The conversion of folate to methyltetrahydrofolate is a multistep process requiring vitamin B_{12} and a functional enzyme, methylene tetrahydrofolate reductase (MTHFR). Vitamin B_6 is also required for metabolism of sulfur-containing amino acids such as methionine.

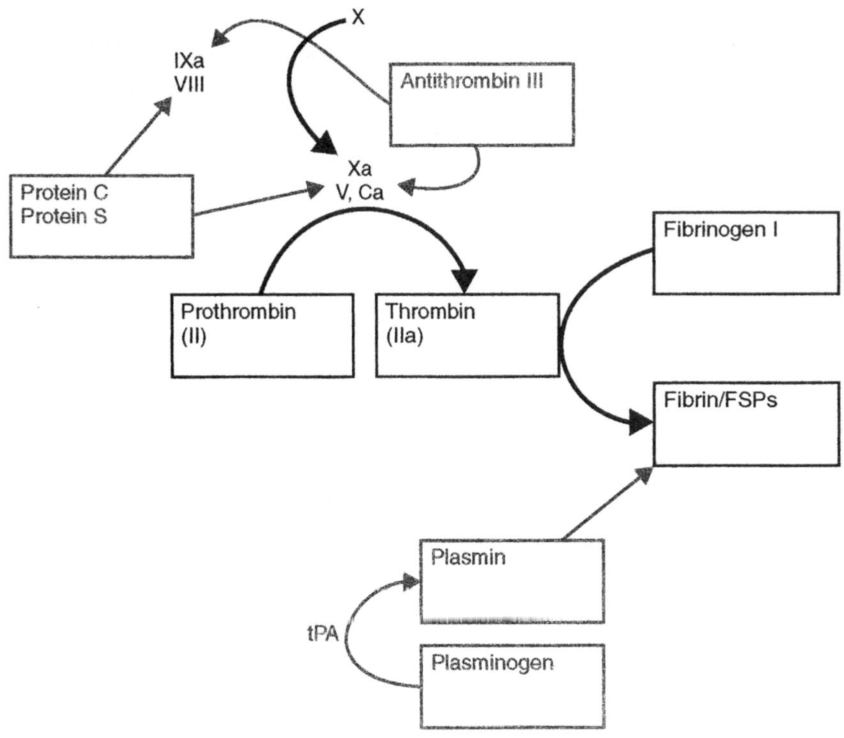

Figure 28.2 Final pathways involved in clot formation and dissolution. Pathways in *black* are part of the clotting cascade and are prothrombotic. Pathways in *red* limit or inhibit clot formation and aid in clot dissolution. FSP, fibrin split products; TPA, tissue plasminogen activator.

required for metabolism of homocysteine have been described for the pathways leading to cystathione formation and to reconversion to methionine (14,15), the latter has received considerable attention. Point mutations in MTHFR are surprisingly common (19,20), are associated with hyperhomocysteinemia, and are linked to thrombosis (15). Data directly linking hyperhomocysteinemia, folic acid, vitamin B_{12}, and MTHFR mutations to recurrent pregnancy loss have been contradictory (21–25). However, two recent studies have evaluated pooled data from previous investigations (one using metaanalysis), and both studies show these disorders to be linked to risk for recurrent pregnancy loss (15,26).

The final steps in the clotting cascade involve the conversion of factor X to factor Xa, a process catalyzed by activated factor IX (in the presence of factor VIII) (Fig. 28.2). Activated factor X (Xa), in turn, catalyzes the conversion of prothrombin (factor II) to thrombin (factor IIa). This conversion involves factor V. Thrombin, in turn, converts fibrinogen to fibrin, an essential building block for stable clot formation. A number of thrombotic control mechanisms have evolved to limit inappropriate clotting. These involve antithrombin III, protein C, and protein S. Fibrinolytic mechanisms, including plasmin-mediated clot dissolution, help limit downstream thrombotic effects.

Antithrombin III is a serine protease that inhibits the activity of thrombin as well as factors Xa, Xa, XIa, and XIIa. Although antithrombin III mutations are fairly uncommon, their association with thrombotic complications during pregnancy is quite dramatic (15). Some have demonstrated antithrombin III deficiency to represent the worst prognostic factor of all heritable thrombophilias in terms of pregnancy outcome (27). Protein C and protein S both exert their antithrombotic effects at those steps in the clotting cascade that involve conversion of factor X to Xa and conversion of prothrombin to thrombin. Heritable deficiencies in factors C and S have been demonstrated, and each is associated with thrombophilia and pregnancy complications (27). Most recently, genetic mutations in factor V have been described that disallow appropriate interactions with protein C. All mutations may be linked to recurrent fetal loss (27–29). One of the multiple mutations causing this resistance to activated protein C has been called factor V Leiden. Factor V Leiden results from a heritable point mutation at the cleavage site for factor V (30), and among white populations, it represents the most common of the genetic causes of thrombophilia (31). Although the available data are limited by studies with small patient numbers, most large studies have noted association between factor V Leiden and recurrent pregnancy loss (19,22,24,27–29,32–35).

Heritable point mutations in prothrombin (factor II) have been linked to thrombosis and, more specifically, to pregnancy loss (35,36). Factor XII deficiencies have also been reported and appear to be particularly prevalent among Japanese women with recurrent pregnancy loss (37). Associations between fibrinogen and factor XIII defects and fetal loss suggest that interactions between the clotting cascade and pregnancy maintenance involve mechanisms more complex than simple placental thrombosis and infarction (38,39).

In light of the recent completion of the human genome project and the rapid development of novel and improved molecular cytogenetic techniques (40), many advances and additional insight into the contribution of parental genetic abnormalities to recurrent pregnancy loss can be anticipated in the coming years.

Anatomic Abnormalities

Anatomic abnormalities of both the uterine cervix and the uterine body have been associated with recurrent pregnancy loss. These anatomic causes may be either congenital or acquired. During development, the uterus forms by the apposition of a portion of bilateral hollow tubes called the *müllerian ducts.* The dissolution of the walls of these ducts along their site of apposition allows formation of the intrauterine cavity, the intracervical canal, and the upper vagina. Congenital uterine anomalies may, therefore, include incomplete müllerian duct fusion, incomplete septum resorption, and uterine cervical anomalies. Although the causes underlying many of the congenital anomalies of the female reproductive tract are unclear, it has been well documented that prenatal exposure to maternally ingested *diethylstilbestrol* (*DES*) results in complex congenital uterine, cervical, and vaginal changes.

Historically, all congenital reproductive tract abnormalities have been linked to both isolated spontaneous pregnancy loss and recurrent pregnancy loss (41,42), although the presence of an intrauterine septum and prenatal exposure to *DES* demonstrate the strongest associations. In fact, women with an intrauterine septum may have as high as a 60% risk for spontaneous abortion (43). Uterine septum-related losses most frequently occur during the second trimester. However, if an embryo implants into the poorly developed endometrium overlying the uterine septum, abnormal placentation and resultant first-trimester losses may occur as well (44). The most common uterine congenital anomaly associated with *in utero DES* exposure is hypoplasia, which may contribute to first- or second-trimester spontaneous abortions, incompetent cervix, and premature labor (45,46). Congenital anomalies of the uterine arteries also may contribute to pregnancy loss through adverse alterations in blood flow to the implanted blastocyst and developing placenta (47).

Acquired anatomic anomalies have likewise been linked to both isolated and recurrent pregnancy losses. These abnormalities include such disparate conditions as intrauterine adhesions, uterine fibroids, and endometriosis. Endometrium that develops over an intrauterine synechiae or over a fibroid that impinges in the intrauterine cavity (submucous) may be inadequately vascularized (48). This may promote abnormal placentation for any embryo attempting to implant over such lesions. Although data supporting these concepts are a bit tenuous, this abnormal placentation may lead to spontaneous pregnancy loss.

Endocrine Abnormalities

The endocrinology of normal pregnancy is complex. Because spontaneous pregnancy is critically dependent on appropriately timed endocrinologic changes of the menstrual cycle, it is not surprising that those endocrine abnormalities that ultimately alter pregnancy maintenance may mediate their effects during the follicular phase of the cycle in which conception occurs, or even earlier. Modifications in follicular development and ovulation, in turn, may be reflected in abnormalities of blastocyst transport and development, alterations in uterine receptivity to the implanting blastocyst, and improper functioning of the corpus luteum. Beginning with ovulation and lasting until about 7 to 9 weeks of gestation, maintenance of early pregnancy depends on the production of progesterone by the corpus luteum. Normal pregnancies are characterized by a luteal–placental shift at about 7 to 9 weeks of gestation, during which the developing placental trophoblast cells take over progesterone production and pregnancy maintenance (49). Spontaneous pregnancy losses occurring before 10 weeks of gestation may result from a number of alterations in normal progesterone production or use. These include failure of the corpus luteum to produce sufficient quantities of progesterone, impaired delivery of progesterone to the uterus, or inappropriate use of progesterone by the uterine decidua. Pregnancy failures may also occur near the time of the expected luteal–placental shift if the trophoblast is unable to produce biologically active progesterone after demise of the corpus luteum.

Endocrinologic factors associated with recurrent abortion include luteal-phase insufficiency, diabetes mellitus thyroid disease, and potentially, hyperprolactinemia and decreased ovarian reserve. Luteal-phase insufficiency or luteal-phase defects (LPDs) are characterized by inadequate luteal milestones and most likely relate to adverse pregnancy outcome through inadequate or improperly timed endometrial development at potential implantation sites. LPD has many causes, some of which are associated with hypersecretion of luteinizing hormone. Although the mechanism underlying the association of elevated luteinizing hormone (LH) levels with recurrent pregnancy loss remains incompletely understood, abnormal LH secretion may have direct effects on the developing oocyte (premature aging), on the endometrium (dyssynchronous maturation), or both. Many patients with elevated LH levels also display physical, endocrinologic, and metabolic characteristics of polycystic ovarian syndrome (PCOS). In fact, some studies report ovarian radiologic evidence of PCOS in as many as 80% of recurrent pregnancy loss patients (50). In addition to inappropriately elevated LH levels, PCOS patients are frequently obese and often have elevated circulating androgen levels. Although not undisputed (51), both changes have been linked to recurrent pregnancy loss (50,52), and elevated androgen levels have been shown to effect markers of uterine receptivity adversely in women with a history of recurrent pregnancy loss (53).

Many women with PCOS have metabolic alterations in glycemic control characterized by insulin resistance. This too may be directly or indirectly related to adverse pregnancy outcome, and it may be related to the mechanisms for spontaneous pregnancy loss among women with type II diabetes mellitus (54). Women with overt insulin-dependent diabetes mellitus (IDDM) appear to exhibit a threshold of pregestational glycemic control above which spontaneous pregnancy loss is increased (55,56). In fact, hyperglycemia has now been directly linked to embryonic damage (57). In cases of advanced IDDM with accompanying vascular complications, compromised blood flow to the uterus may be mechanistically involved in subsequent pregnancy loss.

Patients with thyroid disease often have concomitant reproductive abnormalities, including ovulatory dysfunction and LPDs. In addition, the metabolic demands of early pregnancy mandate an increased requirement for thyroid hormones. It is therefore not surprising that hypothyroidism has been associated with spontaneous pregnancy loss and with recurrent pregnancy loss (58). Although it continues to be debated, evidence suggests that, even in clinically euthyroid patients, the presence of antithyroid antibodies might be associated with recurrent pregnancy loss (59–62). The mechanism for this association remains unclear; however, these antibodies could be markers of more generalized autoimmunity or may predict an impaired ability of the thyroid gland to respond to the demands of pregnancy.

Two additional endocrinologic abnormalities have been linked to recurrent pregnancy loss, although support for these associations and their mechanistic pathways remains shrouded in controversy. The relationship of hyperprolactinemia with recurrent pregnancy loss continues to be debated. Animal models suggest that elevated prolactin levels may adversely affect corpus luteal function; however, this concept is not well supported in humans (63,64). Some have suggested that elevated prolactin levels may promote pregnancy wastage by direct effects on the endometrium or indirect immunomodulatory mechanisms (65). Most recently, attempts have been made to correlate markers of ovarian reserve (day 3 follicle-stimulating hormone, day 3 estradiol, response to the clomiphene challenge test) with recurrent pregnancy loss (51,66,67). At present, no consensus exists concerning this potential association.

Maternal Infection

The association of infection with recurrent abortion is among the most controversial and poorly explored of the potential causes of pregnancy loss. Reproductive tract infections with bacterial, viral, parasitic, zoonotic, and fungal organisms have all been linked theoretically to pregnancy loss; however, mycoplasma, ureaplasma, chlamydia, and β-streptococcus are the most commonly studied pathogens (68,69). More recent data have directly addressed the roles of some of these proposed organisms in recurrent pregnancy loss. One prospective comparison trial involving 70 recurrent pregnancy loss patients reported no elevations in any markers for present or past infection with *Chlamydia trachomatis* when compared with controls (70). In contrast, a very large, prospective trial demonstrated a link between the detection of bacterial vaginosis and history of second-trimester pregnancy loss among 500 recurrent pregnancy loss patients (71). The risk for bacterial vaginosis detection was also positively correlated with cigarette smoking in this study.

The etiologic mechanism linking specific organisms to either isolated or recurrent pregnancy loss remains unclear and must certainly differ among infectious organisms. Certain viral organisms, such as herpes simplex virus (72) and human cytomegalovirus (73), can directly infect the placenta and fetus (72,73). The resulting villitis and related tissue destruction may lead to pregnancy disruption. Another theoretical possibility warranting study is that infection-associated early pregnancy loss may result from immunologic activation in response to pathologic organisms. A large body of evidence supports the role of this mechanism in adverse events later in gestation, such as intrauterine growth restriction (74), premature rupture of membranes, and preterm birth (75). Alternatively, mechanisms that protect the fetus from autoimmune rejection also may protect virally infected placental cells from recognition and clearance. This could potentially promote periods of unfettered infectious growth for some of the pathogenic organisms gaining entry to the reproductive tract (76).

Immunologic Phenomena

In recent years, there has been extensive information published concerning the possible immunologic causes and treatments of recurrent pregnancy loss. However, there is a lack of consensus regarding the mechanisms and the impact of therapeutic intervention because the detection of a therapeutic effect is difficult in the absence of very large studies. This situation reflects the fact that many recurrent pregnancy loss patients present after their index pregnancy has expired but before being expelled. In these cases, the physiologic immune reaction to the presence of nonviable tissue may mask any alternative, underlying immune causes of the demise itself. Finally, it is very likely that there are a wide variety of immune alterations that may result in the same end point–isolated or recurrent pregnancy loss. This latter theory is certainly supported by a recent review article that lists 10 well-supported immune mechanisms that are each potentially important in pregnancy maintenance (77).

Before launching into the most commonly accepted causes of immune-mediated pregnancy loss, a brief review of some of the important concepts in basic immunology is warranted (Table 28.2). Although these descriptions are presented in general terms and are further defined in Chapter 6, they should serve as useful reference for the ensuing information.

Immune responses classically are divided into innate and acquired responses. *Innate responses* represent the body's first line of defense against pathogenic invasion. They are

Table 28.2. Concepts in Reproductive Immunology

Cellular Immunity

1. Resident endometrial and decidual cells
   a. Few B cells
   b. TCR-$\alpha\beta^+$ and TCR-$\gamma\delta^+$ cells are present, TCR-$\gamma\delta^+$ cells increase in early pregnancy
   c. NK-like, large granular lymphocytes (decidual NK cells) accumulate at sites of implantation
   d. NKT cells and suppressor macrophage
2. Immune cell education and homing
   a. Thymic versus extrathymic education
   b. Possible *in situ* education and maintenance
   c. Integrins and vascular ligand pairs and mucosal homing
3. Antigen presentation
   a. Class II MHC molecules are not expressed in the placenta
   b. Classic class I MHC molecules HLA-A and HLA-B are not expressed in the placenta
   c. Extravillous cytotrophoblast cells express HLA-C, HLA-E, and HLA-G
4. *In situ* immunoregulation
   a. T_H1 and T_H2 cytokine microenvironments and dysregulation
   b. Hormonal immunomodulation
      i. Progesterone
      ii. Estrogen
      iii. Human chorionic gonadotropin (hCG)
      iv. Others
   c. Tryptophan metabolism and indolamine 2,3-dioxygenase (IDO)
   d. Leukemia-inhibiting factor (LIF)

Humoral Immunity

1. Fetal antigens are recognized by the maternal immune system, and humoral responses are mounted
2. Organ nonspecific autoantibodies
   a. Anticardiolipin antibodies
   b. Lupus anticoagulant
   c. Anti-β_2 glycoprotein 1 and (anti-β_2G) antibodies
   d. Antiphosphatidlyserine antibodies
3. Organ-specific autoantibodies
   a. Antithyroid antibodies
   b. Antisperm antibodies
   c. Antitrophoblast antibodies
      i. Blocking antibodies
      ii. HLA sharing
      iii. Trophoblast and lymphocyte cross-reactive antibodies (TLX)

TCR, T-cell receptor; NK, natural killer; MHC, major histocompatibility complex; HLA, human leukocyte antigen

rapid and are not antigen specific. Cell types and mechanisms typically considered vital to innate immunity include complement activation, phagocytosis by macrophage, and lysis by natural killer (NK) cells and possibly by T-cell receptor-$\gamma\delta$–positive (TCR-$\gamma\delta^+$) T cells (see later). *Acquired immune responses,* in contrast, are antigen specific and are largely mediated by T cells and B cells. Acquired responses can be further divided into *primary* (response associated with initial antigen contact) and *secondary* (rapid and powerful amnestic response associated with subsequent contact to the same antigen).

Antigen specificity is generally regulated by two sets of genes in the major histocompatibility complex (MHC), located on chromosome 6 in humans. Class I MHC molecules [human leukocyte antigens (HLA) A, B, and C] are present on the surface of nearly every cell in the human body and are important in defense against intracellular pathogens, such as viral infection and oncogenic transformation. Class I MHC molecules act as important ligands for both the TCR on CD8$^+$ cytotoxic and suppressor T cells and for a variety of receptors on NK cells (78). Class II MHC molecules (HLA-DR, HLA-DP, and HLA-DQ), in contrast, are present on the surface of a limited number of antigen-presenting cells, including dendritic cells, macrophage-monocytes, B cells, and tissue-specific cells, such as the Langerhans cells in the skin. These molecules are important in defense against extracellular pathogens, such as bacterial invaders. The major ligand for class II MHC is the TCR on $CD4^+$ T-helper cells.

One very important concept in immunology that has particular application to pregnancy is that of immune tolerance. It has been well described that bone marrow–derived T cells pass through the fetal thymus during early development. During this developmental interval, the T cells encounter a process termed *thymic education.* During thymic education, T cells are chosen that express either the CD4 or the CD8 co-receptor, and autoreactive cells are effectively eliminated. In short, this education promotes T-cell tolerance, allowing selection and survival only of those T cells that can recognize nonself but will not react against self.

These immunologic characteristics have all been thoroughly described and investigated for the immune effector cells populating the peripheral immune system. The peripheral immune system consists of the spleen and peripheral blood, and it is generally responsible for protection against blood-borne pathogens. Pathogens that enter through the extensive surface areas of the lacrimal ducts, respiratory system, gastrointestinal tract, mammary ducts, and genitourinary tract encounter a very distinct and important immune environment—that of the mucosal immune system. Although the mucosal immune system may be primarily responsible for the initial protection against most exogenous pathogens, an understanding of its immune characteristics has lagged far behind that of the peripheral immune system. Insight into the specific characteristics of immunity within the reproductive tract is even further limited.

Cellular Immune Mechanisms

Many of the immune theories surrounding the causes of isolated and recurrent spontaneous pregnancy losses have stemmed from attempts to define immunologic rules as they apply specifically to the mucosal reproductive tract. Four main questions summarize much of the theoretical thinking surrounding pregnancy maintenance and reproductive immunology:

1. Which immune cells populate the reproductive tract, particularly at implantation sites?
2. How do these cells arrive at this mucosal immune site, and are they educated in the same way as those populating the periphery?
3. How do the characteristics of antigen presentation differ at the maternal–fetal interface?
4. What regulatory mechanisms specifically affect reproductive tract immune cells?

Resident Cells Immune cells populating the reproductive tract exhibit many characteristics that distinguish them from their peripheral counterparts. In particular, the human endometrium is populated by T cells, macrophage, and NK-like cells, but very few B cells are present (79,80). The relative proportions of these resident cells vary with the menstrual cycle and change dramatically during early pregnancy. In fact, surrounding the time of implantation, one particular cell type composes between 70% to 80% of the total endometrial lymphocyte populations (79,80). This cell type is called a variety of names, including *decidual granular lymphocytes, large granular lymphocytes,* and *decidual NK cells.* This heterogeneity of names reflects the fact that this particular cell type differs from similar cells isolated from the periphery, although most believe it to be an NK cell variant. If we do consider them to be NK cells, the implantation site represents the largest accumulation of NK cells in any state of human health or disease. The true function of these cells remains unclear, but their remarkable abundance at the maternal–fetal interface makes their further study compelling (81,82). Other immune cells have been described in the periphery that have characteristics of both NK cells and T cells. These NKT cells have recently been demonstrated to play a role in pregnancy loss in animal models (83), and their presence in the decidua in humans is now being investigated.

In the peripheral immune compartment, most T cells express a TCR composed of an $\alpha\beta$ heterodimer (TCR-$\alpha\beta^+$). In addition to TCR-$\alpha\beta^+$ T cells, the human reproductive tract also is populated by a subset of T cells with a distinctive TCR composed of the $\gamma\delta$ heterodimer (TCR-$\gamma\delta^+$), and the numbers of these cells increases in early pregnancy (84–86). TCR-$\gamma\delta^+$ T cells appear to fulfill functions quite distinct from their TCR-$\alpha\beta^+$ counterparts; functions that may include direct, non–MHC-restricted recognition of antigens within tissues (87). In fact, TCR-$\gamma\delta^+$ T cells may fill a protective niche missed or poorly covered by B cells and TCR-$\alpha\beta^+$ T cells. The role and importance of TCR-$\gamma\delta^+$ cells in the reproductive tract and, more particularly, in pregnancy maintenance deserves further attention.

Finally, it has been suggested that a subset of macrophage, termed *suppressor macrophage,* may be implicated in pregnancy maintenance. These specific cells differ from typical macrophage in their promotion of antiinflammatory effects, and they have been detected in normal murine placenta (88). Their presence in human decidual specimens requires further investigation.

The human decidua is populated by characteristic immune effector cells. To date, investigations into whether alterations in these cells (including T cells, decidual NK cells, and NKT cells) determine pregnancy outcome have been hampered by insufficient patient numbers to allow meaningful conclusions. Still, these immune cell populations have been repeatedly reported to be altered in recurrent pregnancy loss patients (89–93) but not in patients experiencing isolated spontaneous pregnancy losses (86).

Immune Cell Education and Homing to the Reproductive Tract The implanting fetus represents the most common model of allograft acceptance. How the maternal immune system avoids rejection of the implanting fetus in an uncomplicated pregnancy invokes the presence of some manifestation of immune tolerance. This, in turn, begs the questions of how the resident decidual immune effector cells are selected and educated, how they home to reproductive sites, and how they are maintained once they reach this destination. Animal studies have suggested that the rules for selection and maintenance of these cells, in terms of their requirement for MHC and their education within the thymus, may be distinct from those governing either peripheral immune cells or cells within other mucosal sites, including the intestine (94). Although the results of most studies are preliminary, it appears that the human reproductive tract displays similar characteristics—the immunophenotypes of immune cells populating the human reproductive tract are distinct from both the periphery and from other mucosal sites (95). The education of TCR-$\gamma\delta^+$ cells populating epithelial sites may occur outside the thymus and might involve mechanisms that substitute for or modify interaction with MHC (86,96). The development of MHC specificity among NK cells is presently being carefully dissected in animal models (97,98) with the hope that these investigations will shed light on similar processes in humans and, more specifically, on the selection and maintenance characteristics of decidual NK cells.

It is now becoming increasingly evident that the cells populating mucosal immune tissues select these sites through interactions between cell surface molecules on the immune cell (integrins) and cell surface molecules on the endothelial cells of blood vessels within the mucosal tissues (e.g., selectins, vascular all adhesion molecule VCAM). This cellular recruitment process, called homing, has been most thoroughly described for the intestine (99,100). However, both murine (99,101) and human (102) reproductive tract tissues do express these integrin–vascular ligand pairs. The extension of these findings to pregnancy maintenance will surely prove fruitful. Solving the mechanisms of selection, education, and maintenance of reproductive tract immune effector cells is of paramount importance. Until we understand these vital processes in the normal state, we cannot define the effects that alterations will have on human disease, nor can we develop therapeutic interventions.

Antigen Presentation at the Maternal–Fetal Interface Historically, it was proposed that one method by which the implanting trophoblastic allograft could potentially avoid immune detection by the maternal host would be by making itself antigenically invisible. It could downregulate its expression of the MHC-encoded transplantation antigens (some of which would be of paternal origin) and thereby avoid recognition as nonself. Although current knowledge of immunology now makes this theory somewhat obsolete (103), the implanting fetus does, in fact, use this strategy to some extent. It is certainly true that placental trophoblast cells do not express class II MHC molecules (104,105).

Unlike nearly every other cell in the human body, trophoblast cells do not express the classic class I MHC transplantation antigens HLA-A and -B. Rather, a subpopulation of placental cells, specifically the extravillous cytotrophoblast cells, express the classic class MHC I HLA-C products and the nonclassic HLA-E and -G products (76,106–111). These extravillous cytotrophoblast cells are of particular interest because they are characterized by remarkable invasive potential (112). In fact, these cells move from the tips of the anchoring villi of the human placenta and invade deeply into the maternal decidua. Further, they can replace cells within the walls of decidual arterial vessels (112,113). Although the invasive characteristics of extravillous cytotrophoblast may reflect non–MHC-related mechanisms, including well-described integrin switching (114), the intimate contact of these fetal-derived cells with maternal immune effector cells certainly exposes the fetus to recognition as nonself.

It is not known why all placental cells downregulate expression of HLA-A and -B, whereas invasive extravillous cytotrophoblast cells express HLA-C, -E, and -G. However, this area of investigation is ripe with hypotheses and study. Because NK cells of the innate immune system recognize and kill cells that express no MHC (103), the complete downregulation of MHC would cause trophoblast cells to act as targets for those NK cells that are pervasive at sites of implantation. In addition to possible protection from direct NK cell–mediated killing, the expression of HLA-C, -E, and -G by trophoblast cells may serve a variety of alternative roles. NK cell receptor–mediated interactions with extravillous cytotrophoblast MHC could modulate cytokine expression profiles at the maternal–fetal interface (81,82). MHC expression may aid in decidual and vascular invasion by the trophoblast, an activity essential for proper placental development (115). Whereas definitive correlations between placental class I MHC expression patterns and recurrent pregnancy loss have yet to be reported, trophoblast expression of HLA-G has been linked to other disorders of placental invasion, such as preeclampsia (115,116). Finally, soluble or secreted trophoblast MHC products may aid in the development of maternal immune tolerance toward the placenta (117).

To date, the study of newly described trophoblast class I MHC products in recurrent pregnancy loss remains limited. However, the results of two small studies investigating the possible association between polymorphisms in these MHC products and recurrent pregnancy loss have been negative (118,119). Aberrant expression of class II MHC determinants, or enhanced expression of class I MHC on syncytiotrophoblasts occurring in response to interferon-γ (IFN-γ), could mediate abortion by enhancing cytotoxic T-cell attack (120,121). This theory appears unlikely, however, because the expression of classic MHC antigens does not appear to be induced on aborted tissues from women experiencing one or more pregnancy losses (122). Finally, class II MHC genotypes appear to affect susceptibility to a variety of diseases, including diabetes and other autoimmune diseases. A similar link between MHC class II typing and adverse pregnancy outcome has been reported for recurrent pregnancy loss (123,124).

Regulation of Decidual Immune Cells The characteristics of the interactions between decidual immune effector cells and the implanting fetus may be determined by factors other than those already mentioned. Local regulation of the cells that populate the human decidua will further modify the effects of selection, maintenance, and homing as well as the distinctive characteristics of antigen presentation at the maternal–fetal interface. As might be predicted, these regulatory effects are often targets for investigative efforts because they may offer more direct insight into potential therapies for immune-mediated disorders of pregnancy maintenance. Three such regulatory mechanisms are discussed here: (a) alterations in T-helper cell phenotypes, (b) reproductive hormones and immunosuppression, and (c) tryptophan metabolism.

As discussed in Chapter 6, antigen-stimulated immune responses involving $CD4^+$ T cells can be divided into two major classes: T-helper cell subset 1 (T_H1) responses and T-helper cell subset 2 (T_H2) responses. This subclassification is based on the characteristics of the $CD4^+$ cells present as well as on their associated cytokines. The production of these responses rests on the environment in which relatively undifferentiated $CD4^+$ T_H0 cells become differentiated. Thus, T_H0 cells exposed to IFN-γ become T_H1-type cells, and those exposed to interleukin-4 (IL-4) become T_H2-type cells (125). T_H1 responses are associated with inflammation and primarily involve IFN-γ and IL-12 but also involve IL-2 and tumor necrosis factor-β (TNF-β). T_H2 cell responses are associated with antibody production and the cytokines IL-10, IL-4, IL-5, and IL-6 (126–128). Although TNF-α can be secreted by both T_H1 and T_H2 cells, it is most often characteristic of a T_H1 response (129,130). A reciprocal regulating relationship exists between T_H1 and T_H2 cells and cytokines (131–134), with one response supporting its own persistence while averting conversion to the other.

Extending these immune regulatory phenomena to pregnancy, the type of $CD4^+$ cellular response to the implanting fetus is controlled not only by the types of cells (e.g., T-helper cells) in the decidua but also by the cytokine environment at the maternal–fetal interface. As mentioned previously, the human endometrium and decidua are replete with immune and inflammatory cells capable of cytokine secretion (135–139). Cytokines may affect reproductive events either directly or indirectly, depending on the specific cytokines secreted, their concentrations, and the differentiation stage of potential reproductive target tissues. It is now well documented that T_H1-type cytokines can be harmful to an implanting embryo (140–142). Further, most agree that some patients with recurrent pregnancy loss exhibit a dysregulation of their T-helper cellular immune response to antigens at the site of implantation, with typical shifts toward T_H1 inflammatory responses (143–146). Depending on the individual series, 60% to 80% of nonpregnant women with a history of otherwise unexplained recurrent spontaneous abortion have been found to have evidence of abnormal *in vitro* T_H1 cellular immune responses. Fewer than 3% of women with normal reproductive histories demonstrate these responses (143,145–147). Rather, most women with normal pregnancies have a T_H2 immune response to trophoblast antigens (146).

Methods for the documentation of cytokine dysregulation among recurrent pregnancy loss patients also vary among investigators, but groups have recently confirmed this abnormality within the endometrium (148–150) or among immune cells isolated from the decidua (151) of these patients. Others use peripheral lymphocytes from women with a history of recurrent pregnancy loss and stimulate them *in vitro* with trophoblast antigens (146,152,153). One study documented aberrant cytokine secretion when peripheral blood lymphocytes (PBLs) from recurrent pregnancy loss patients were stimulated *in vitro* by HLA-G bearing cells (154), whereas another study demonstrated that decidual and peripheral immune cells exhibit a shift toward the T_H2 phenotype when exposed to HLA-G (155). Whether peripheral cytokine levels reflect T-helper cell dysregulation at the maternal–fetal interface or whether this dysregulation affects peripheral as well as local immune response during pregnancy remains controversial (156–158). Finally, as with all immune theories, there appears to be significant redundancy in the necessity for particular cytokines and soluble immunoregulatory factors at the site of implantation. To date, animal models with directed gene deletions have shown only one of these factors to be absolutely essential to pregnancy maintenance—leukemia inhibitory factor (LIF) is required for blastocyst implantation (159), but not for subsequent embryogenesis (160). Interestingly, LIF induces the transcription of HLA-G *in vitro* in human placental cells (161).

Although many mechanisms are aimed at avoiding maternal immune recognition of the implanting fetus, research in both humans and animals indicates that immune responses to fetal antigens can be detected (162–164). Thus, the regulation of this response at the maternal–fetal interface may be critical. The concept that successful pregnancy requires some form of generalized suppression of maternal immune response is supported by reports that failure to downregulate maternal responses to recall antigens, such as tetanus toxoid and influenza, is associated with poor pregnancy outcome among recurrent pregnancy loss patients (165). Reproductive hormones have dramatic effects on peripheral cell-mediated immunity, as demonstrated by well-documented and notable gender differences in immune responsiveness (166). The levels of these potentially immunosuppressive hormones are quite elevated in pregnant women. The fact that the levels of these hormones at the maternal–fetal interface may be far above those in the maternal circulation during pregnancy (167) may explain an apparent inconsistency: overall immune responsiveness during pregnancy appears to change little, whereas local suppression at the maternal–fetal interface may be vital.

It has been suggested for some time that the immunosuppressive effects of progesterone within the reproductive tract are at least partially responsible for the maintenance of the semiallogeneic implanting fetus (168). *In vitro* studies have shown that the progesterone mediates its suppression of T-cell effector function by alterations in membrane-resident potassium channels and cell membrane depolarization. This action, in turn, affects intracellular calcium signaling cascades and gene expression (169) and may be non–receptor mediated (170). Progesterone-mediated changes in T-cell gene expression have been associated with the development of T_H2-type responses and with increased LIF expression (151,171). Because a shift in the intrauterine immune environment from T_H2 to T_H1 has been linked to early spontaneous pregnancy loss (146,151), the elevated intrauterine concentrations of progesterone characteristic of early pregnancy may promote an immune environment favoring pregnancy maintenance. To this point, recent *in vitro* evidence indicates that progesterone can inhibit both mitogen-induced proliferation of and cytokine secretion by $CD8^+$ T cells (172).

Levels of estrogen also rise dramatically during pregnancy, and attention has focused on the role of estrogen in immune modulation. A group of animal studies has shown that estrogens improve immune responses in males after significant trauma and hemorrhage (173), suppress cell-mediated immunity after thermal injury (174), and protect against chronic renal allograft rejection (175). *In vitro,* estrogens appear to downregulate delayed-type hypersensitivity reactions and promote the development of T_H2-type immune responses, particularly at the elevated estrogen concentrations typical of pregnancy (176,177).

One additional regulatory mechanism proposed for the induction of maternal tolerance to the fetal allograft involves the amino acid tryptophan and its catabolizing enzyme indolamine 2,3-dioxygenase (IDO). The IDO hypothesis of tolerance in pregnancy rests on data that T cells need tryptophan for activation and proliferation (178) and that local alterations in tryptophan metabolism at the maternal–fetal interface could either activate or fail to suppress maternal antifetal immunoreactivity (179). Recent studies in mice have shown that the inhibition of IDO leads to loss of allogeneic, but not syngeneic, fetuses and that this effect is mediated by lymphocytes (180). Further support lies in studies demonstrating that hamsters fed diets high in tryptophan have increased rates of fetal wastage (181). Extending this theory to humans requires further investigation. However, the demonstration of IDO expression in human uterine decidua (182) and the documentation of alterations in serum tryptophan levels with increasing gestational age during human pregnancy (183) both support further interest in this potential local immunoregulatory mechanism.

Endometriosis is the growth of both endometrial glands and stroma outside of the intrauterine cavity. Although associations between the development of endometriosis and immunologic abnormalities are now being defined (184), the link between endometriosis and recurrent pregnancy loss remains contentious. Recurrent pregnancy loss in the presence of endometriosis certainly would involve the interaction of complex mechanisms, some of which may involve cellular or humoral dysfunction (185,186).

Humoral Immune Mechanisms

Humoral responses to pregnancy-specific antigens exist, and patients with recurrent pregnancy loss can display altered humoral responses to endometrial antigens (187) (Table 28.2). Nevertheless, most of literature surrounding humoral immune responses and recurrent pregnancy loss focus on organ-nonspecific autoantibodies associated with APAS. Historically, these immunoglobulin G (IgG) and IgM antibodies were thought to be directed against negatively charged phospholipids. Those phospholipids most often implicated in recurrent pregnancy loss are cardiolipin and phosphatidylserine. Most recently, however, it has been shown that antiphospholipid antibodies often are directed against a protein cofactor, called β_2 glycoprotein 1, that assists antibody association with the phospholipid (188,189). Antiphospholipid antibodies were originally characterized by prolonged phospholipid-dependent coagulation tests *in vitro* [activated partial thromboplastin time (aPTT), Russell viper venom time] and by thrombosis *in vivo*. The association of these antiphospholipid antibodies with thrombotic complications has been termed the *antiphospholipid syndrome,* and although many of these complications are systemic, some are pregnancy specific—spontaneous abortion, preterm labor, premature rupture of membranes, stillbirth, intrauterine growth retardation, and preeclampsia (190). A recent reassessment of the criteria used to diagnose APAS was undertaken during a postconference workshop after the Eighth International Symposium on Antiphospholipid Antibodies held in 1998 in Sapporo, Japan (191). This reassessment resulted in the Sapporo criteria for diagnosis of APAS, which include adverse pregnancy outcomes. These criteria, which have been validated clinically (192), are as follows:

For a patient to be diagnosed with antiphospholipid antibody syndrome, one or more clinical and one or more laboratory criteria must be present:

Clinical

1. One or more confirmed episodes of vascular thrombosis of any type
   - Venous
   - Arterial
   - Small vessel

2. Pregnancy complications
   - Three or more consecutive spontaneous pregnancy losses at less than 10 weeks of gestation
   - One or more fetal deaths at greater than 10 weeks of gestation
   - One or more preterm births at less than 34 weeks of gestation secondary to severe preeclampsia or placental insufficiency

Laboratory (testing must be positive on two or more occasions, 6 weeks or more apart)

1. Positive plasma levels of anticardiolipin antibodies of the IgG or IgM isotype at medium to high levels

2. Positive plasma levels of lupus anticoagulant

The presence of antiphospholipid antibodies (anticardiolipin or lupus anticoagulant) during pregnancy is a major risk factor for adverse pregnancy outcome (193). In large series of couples with recurrent abortion, the incidence of the antiphospholipid syndrome was between 3% and 5% (68). The presence of anticardiolipin antibodies among patients with known systemic lupus erythematosus portends less favorable pregnancy outcome (194).

A number of mechanisms have been proposed by which antiphospholipid antibodies might mediate pregnancy loss. Antibodies against phospholipids could increase thromboxane and decrease prostacyclin synthesis within placental vessels. The resultant prothrombotic environment could promote vascular constriction, platelet adhesion, and placental infarction (195–197). Alternatively, *in vitro* evidence from trophoblast cell lines indicates that IgM action against phosphatidylserine inhibits formation of syncytial trophoblast (198). Syncytialization is, of course, required for proper placental function. One study demonstrated that both extravillous cytotrophoblast and syncytiotrophoblast cells synthesize β_2 glycoprotein 1, the essential cofactor for antiphospholipid antibody binding (199). Although it has been investigated, data surrounding the prognostic value of serum levels of specific antibodies against β_2 glycoprotein 1 with respect to pregnancy outcome among recurrent pregnancy loss patients remain inconsistent (200,201). Some have proposed that sera from antibody-positive recurrent pregnancy loss patients is particularly adept at inhibiting trophoblast adhesion to endothelial cells *in vitro* (202). Others have noted rapid development of atherosclerosis in the decidual spiral arteries of patients who test positive for antiphospholipid antibodies (203). Finally, still others have suggested that levels of the placental antithrombotic molecule—annexin V—are reduced within the placental villa from those women with recurrent pregnancy loss who are antiphospholipid antibody positive (204). It must be mentioned, however, that placental pathologic evidence supporting causal involvement of the antiphospholipid antibody syndrome in pregnancy loss is often equivocal. The characteristic lesions for this syndrome (placental infarction, abruption, and hemorrhage) are often missing in women with antiphospholipid antibodies (205), and these same pathologic lesions can be found in placentas from women with recurrent abortion who do not have biochemical evidence of antiphospholipid antibodies (206).

One additional group of autoantibodies that have been linked to recurrent pregnancy loss is the antithyroid antibodies (ATAs). Although the data remain somewhat controversial (207,208), one large retrospective study has demonstrated an increased prevalence of these antibodies among women with a history of recurrent pregnancy loss, even in the absence of thyroid endocrinologic abnormalities (62). The overall significance of ATAs, however, is unclear. In fact, one study recently reported that the presence of serum ATA had no effect on pregnancy outcome in euthyroid pregnant patients with a history of recurrent pregnancy loss (60).

Other antibody-mediated mechanisms for recurrent abortion have been proposed, including antisperm and antitrophoblast antibodies, as well as blocking antibody deficiency. Although each hypothesis has been shown to have minimal relevance to recurrent pregnancy loss (68,121), their discussion is warranted because therapies aimed at these disorders persist. Historically, the blocking antibody deficiency hypothesis has received the most attention. This hypotheses is based on a supposition that blocking factors (presumably antibodies) were required to prevent a maternal, cell-mediated, antifetal immune response that was believed to occur in all pregnancies. It was therefore proposed that, in the absence of these blocking antibodies, abortion occurred (209,210). This supposition has never been consistently substantiated (211,212). For instance, maternal hyporesponsiveness in mixed lymphocyte culture with paternal stimulator cells was originally proposed to identify women with deficient blocking activity (210). Investigations based on this type of testing were continued by others (213,214), who proposed that parental HLA sharing resulted in a predisposition to blocking antibody deficiency. These reports were of limited sample size, were retrospective in nature, and lacked population-based controls. One prospective, population-based control study conclusively demonstrated that HLA heterogeneity was not essential for successful pregnancy (215). However, follow-up studies have now shown that, in the exceedingly rare case of complete sharing of the entire HLA region, spontaneous pregnancy losses do increase (216). This particular 10-year prospective trial concluded, however, that HLA typing is of no use in outbred populations because only isolated and significantly inbred populations have such HLA homogeneity. Further evidence refuting the blocking antibody hypothesis for recurrent abortion comes from reports of successful pregnancies both among women who do not produce serum factors capable of mixed lymphocyte culture inhibition (210) and among women who do not produce antipaternal cytotoxic antibodies (211). Those mixed lymphocyte culture results that demonstrate hyporesponsiveness in some recurrent pregnancy loss patients are now believed to represent the effect of the pregnancy loss rather than the cause of recurrent abortion (164,210–212).

One last theory that arose out of the blocking antibody investigations involved a novel HLA-linked alloantigen system. The finding that polyclonal rabbit antisera could recognize both lymphocytes and trophoblast cells suggested to some the presence of trophoblast–lymphocyte cross-reactive alloantigens (called *TLXes*) (217). These TLXes were, in turn, linked to maternal blocking antibody deficiency and recurrent pregnancy loss. The TLX hypothesis is now of historical relevance only because this theory was invalidated when TLX was found to be identical to CD46, a complement receptor that is thought to protect the placenta from complement-mediated attack (218). CD46 was not a novel alloantigen. It can be found on a wide variety of cells, thus explaining the cross-reactive nature of the original rabbit antisera.

It is important to conclude this in-depth discussion of the immune-mediated mechanisms of isolated and recurrent pregnancy loss by suggesting that pregnancy may not require an intact maternal immune system. Supporting this concept are data showing that agammaglobulinemic animals and women can successfully reproduce (219). Further, viable births also occur among women with severe immune deficiencies and in murine models that lack T and B cells (SCID mice) and those that display a congenital absence of their thymus (nude mice). Still, immune factors may play important roles in a significant proportion of patients with recurrent pregnancy loss, and their presence is the subject of immense amounts of research. Until this role is better defined, an understanding of the contemporary immunologic hypotheses allows for the informed consideration of novel findings.

Other Factors

It is now becoming increasingly evident that the implantation of the blastocyst within the uterine decidua represents an exquisitely scripted cross-talk between embryo and mother. Alterations in this dialogue often result in improper implantation and placental development. For instance, recurrent pregnancy loss has been linked to a dysregulation in the expression patterns of vascular endothelial growth factors on the developing placenta and their requisite receptors within the maternal decidua (220). Cellular and extracellular matrix adhesion properties may also be involved in this dialogue. Lessey recently reviewed the concept of uterine receptivity, with particular emphasis on the importance of integrins and the timing of integrin switching in implantation (221). Others have reported decreased levels of endometrial mucin secretion (222) and reductions in the endometrial release of soluble intercellular adhesion molecule I (223) among women with a history of recurrent pregnancy loss. Programmed cell death (apoptosis) may also play an essential role in normal placental development. Alterations in two important apoptotic pathways—Fas-Fas ligand and bcl2—have both been linked to recurrent pregnancy loss and poor pregnancy outcome (77,224).

A variety of environmental factors have been linked to sporadic and recurrent early spontaneous pregnancy loss. These are difficult studies to perform because, in humans, they must all be retrospective and are all confounded by alternative or additional environmental exposures. Nevertheless, the following factors have been linked to pregnancy loss: exposure to medications (e.g., antiprogestogens, antineoplastic agents, and inhalation anesthetics), exposure to ionizing radiation, prolonged exposure to organic solvents, and exposure to environmental toxins, especially heavy metals (225–228). The latter has recently been demonstrated to have both endocrine and immune effects that could lead to poor placentation and subsequent pregnancy loss (229). Associations between spontaneous pregnancy loss and exposures to video display terminals, microwave ovens, high-energy electric power lines, and high altitudes (e.g., flight attendants) have not been substantiated (230,231). There is no compelling evidence that moderate exercise during pregnancy is associated with spontaneous abortion. In the absence of cervical anatomic abnormalities or incompetent cervix, coitus does not appear to increase the risk for spontaneous pregnancy loss (232,233).

Exposure to three particular substances—alcohol, cigarettes, and caffeine—deserves specific attention. Although some conflicting data exist (234,235), one very large epidemiologic study has shown that alcohol consumption during the first trimester of pregnancy, at levels as low as three drinks per week, is associated with an increased incidence of spontaneous pregnancy loss (236). Cigarette smoking has also been linked to early spontaneous pregnancy loss (237,238); however, this is also not without controversy (239). Interestingly, alcohol and tobacco intake in the male partner correlates with the incidence of domestic violence, which in turn is associated with early pregnancy loss (240). Finally, recent evidence adds to a growing body of literature that consumption of coffee and other caffeinated beverages during early pregnancy is linked to adverse pregnancy outcome (238,241). In fact, this most recent report casts doubt on the definition of a lower limit for safe use of caffeine in the first trimester of pregnancy (238).

Preconception Evaluation

Investigative measures that are potentially useful in the evaluation of recurrent spontaneous abortion include obtaining a thorough history from both partners and performing a physical assessment of the woman with attention to the pelvic examination and laboratory testing (Table 28.3).

History

Descriptions of all prior pregnancies and their sequence, as well as whether histologic assessment and karyotype determinations were performed on previously aborted tissues, are important aspects of the history. About 60% of abortuses lost before 8 weeks of gestation have been reported to be chromosomally abnormal (242); most of these pregnancies are affected by some type of trisomy, particularly trisomy 16 (243). The most common single chromosomal abnormality is monosomy X (45X), especially among anembryonic conceptuses (244). Although somewhat controversial, the detection of aneuploidy in miscarriage specimens may be less when the couple experiencing recurrent abortions is euploidic. Alternatively, some investigators have suggested that, because aneuploidy is common among miscarriage specimens from patients experiencing both isolated and recurrent spontaneous pregnancy losses, the documentation of aneuploidy among tissues from recurrent pregnancy loss patients does not affect their prognosis for future pregnancy maintenance (9).

Most women with recurrent pregnancy losses tend to experience spontaneous abortion at about the same gestational age in sequential pregnancies. Unfortunately, the gestational age when pregnancy loss occurred, as determined by last menstrual period, may not be informative, because there is often a 2- to 3-week delay between fetal demise and signs of pregnancy expulsion (245). The designation of couples experiencing recurrent abortion into either primary or secondary categories is also not helpful in either the diagnosis or management of women with recurrent abortion. About 10% to 15% of couples cannot even be classified into either the primary or secondary categories because, although their first pregnancy resulted in a loss, this was followed by a term delivery before subsequent losses.

It is important to evoke any history of subfertility or infertility among couples with recurrent pregnancy loss. This is defined by the inability to conceive after 12 months of unprotected intercourse. By definition, 15% of all couples meet this criteria; this number increases to 33% among couples with recurrent pregnancy losses. In fact, because many pregnancies are lost before or near the time of missed menses, subfertility among recurrent pregnancy loss patients may in some cases reflect preclinical losses. Menstrual cycle history also may provide information about the possibility of oligoovulation or other relevant endocrine abnormalities in recurrent pregnancy loss patients. An assessment of the timing of intercourse relative to ovulation should be reviewed with couples in an effort to detect dyssynchronous fertilization that could contribute to pregnancy loss (246). A personal and family history of thrombotic events or renal abnormalities may provide vital information.

Table 28.3. Investigative Measures Useful in the Evaluation of Recurrent Early Pregnancy Loss

History

1. Pattern, trimester and characteristics of prior pregnancy losses
2. History of subfertility or infertility
3. Menstrual history
4. Prior or current gynecologic or obstetric infections
5. Signs or symptoms of thyroid, prolactin, glucose tolerance, and hyperandrogenic disorders (including PCOS)
6. Personal or familial thrombotic history
7. Features associated with the antiphospholipid syndrome (thrombosis, false-positive test results for syphilis)
8. Other autoimmune disorders
9. Medications
10. Environmental exposures, illicit and common drug use (particularly caffeine, alcohol, cigarettes, and *in utero* DES exposure)
11. Genetic relationship between reproductive partners
12. Family history of recurrent spontaneous abortion, obstetric complications, or any syndrome associated with embryonic or fetal losses
13. Previous diagnostic tests and treatments

Physical Examination

1. General physical examination with particular attention to:
   a. Obesity
   b. Hirsuitism and acanthosis
   c. Thyroid examination
   d. Breast examination and galactorrhea
   e. Pelvic examination
      - Anatomy
      - Infection
      - Trauma
      - Estrogenization

Laboratory

1. Parental peripheral blood karyotype
2. Hysterosalpingography, followed by hysteroscopy or laparoscopy, if indicated
3. Luteal-phase endometrial biopsy
4. Thyroid-stimulating hormone level, serum prolactin level if indicated
5. Anticardiolipin antibody level
6. Lupus anticoagulant (activated partial thromboplastin time or Russell viper venom)
7. Complete blood count with platelets

A family history of pregnancy losses and obstetric complications should be addressed specifically. Detailed information about drug and environmental exposure should also be obtained.

Physical Examination

A general physical examination should be performed to detect signs of metabolic illness, including PCOS, diabetes, hyperandrogenism, and thyroid or prolactin disorders. During the pelvic examination, signs of infection, DES exposure, and previous trauma should be ascertained. Estrogenization of mucosal tissues, cervical and vaginal anatomy, and the size and shape of the uterus should also be determined.

Laboratory Assessment

Laboratory assessment of couples with recurrent pregnancy losses should include the following:

1. Parental peripheral blood karyotyping with banding techniques

2. Assessment of the intrauterine cavity with either office hysteroscopy or hysterosalpingography, followed by operative hysteroscopy if a potentially correctable anomaly is found

3. A well-timed luteal-phase endometrial biopsy, ideally 10 days after the LH surge or after cycle day 24 of an idealized 28-day cycle. If the cycle is abnormal by 3 or more days, the assessment should be repeated in a subsequent cycle. If endometrial histology is out of phase, the biopsy should be repeated in the subsequent cycle. Confirmed out-of-phase biopsies warrant further testing with serum prolactin and androgen profiles.

4. Thyroid function testing, including serum thyroid-stimulating hormone levels

5. Platelet assessment

6. Anticardiolipin and a lupus anticoagulant testing (aPTT or Russell viper venom testing)

A number of laboratory assessment tools are under investigation for use in patients with a history of recurrent pregnancy loss. At present, results are either too preliminary to warrant recommendation or studies of their use have been too contradictory to allow final determination of their value. Tests with unproven or unknown utility include the following:

1. Evaluation of ovarian reserve using day 3 serum follicle-stimulating hormone levels or the clomiphene challenge test. It appears that decreased ovarian reserve may portend poor outcome in all patients, including those with recurrent pregnancy loss (247,248).

2. Testing for serologic evidence of PCOS using LH or androgen values may be useful (50–53,249).

3. Testing for peripheral evidence of T_H1 and T_H2 cytokine dysregulation. Although large studies have failed to demonstrate an association between peripheral cytokine alterations and pregnancy outcome among patients with recurrent pregnancy loss (156), smaller studies have reported peripheral shifts toward T_H1 profiles only in those recurrent pregnancy loss patients who subsequently lose their pregnancy (158). One study documented a shift toward T_H1 profiles at the time of fetal demise in these patients; however, it is particularly difficult to determine cause and effect in this situation (157).

4. Testing for hypercoagulability using the aPTT (14) or for the presence of a hereditary thrombophilia (250) in patients with otherwise unexplained recurrent pregnancy loss has been suggested.

5. Preconceptional testing for the prevalence and activity of peripheral NK cells has been reported in small studies to reflect prognosis and to assist in patient counseling (251,252).

6. Testing for antithyroid antibodies, even among women with recurrent pregnancy loss who are euthyroid, remains controversial. Although some have shown no association between their presence and recurrent loss (207), others have demonstrated an increased prevalence among patients with a history of recurrent pregnancy loss (62,208). However, even if the prevalence of antithyroid antibodies is increased among these patients, the significance of their presence has been questioned (209).

7. Testing for the presence of a variety of autoantibodies (other than lupus anticoagulant and anticardiolipin antibody) has been hotly debated, but without consensus (253,254). Testing for some antiphospholipid antibodies, such as antiphosphatidylserine and anti-β_2 glycoprotein 1 (anti-β_2G1), are particularly attractive

because mechanistic connections between their presence and placental pathology have been made (198–201). One recent, large series has demonstrated anti-β_2G1 to be associated with risk for recurrent pregnancy loss (255). Among patients with known autoimmune diseases and recurrent pregnancy loss, additional antiphospholipid testing may be warranted (256).

8. Testing for congenital or acquired defects in homocysteine metabolism may play a role in the evaluation of some patients with recurrent pregnancy loss. The most common methods involve the measurement of blood levels of homocysteine, either fasting or after methionine loading (15). Methionine loading may increase the usefulness of results; however, it has been associated with acute endothelial dysfunction (257), which could pose potential problems if testing is performed during early pregnancy.

9. Cervical cultures for mycoplasma, ureaplasma, and chlamydia may be considered.

The following investigations have no place in modern clinical care of patients with recurrent spontaneous pregnancy loss:

1. Evaluations that involve extensive testing for serum or site-specific autoantibodies or alloantibodies (including antinuclear antibodies and antipaternal cytotoxic antibodies) are both expensive and unproven. Their use often serves only to verify the statistical tenet that if the number of tests performed reaches a critical limit, the results of at least one will be positive in every patient.

2. Testing for parental HLA profiles is never indicated in outbred populations. Findings that HLA sharing is associated with poor pregnancy outcomes are strictly limited to those specific populations studied, which have very high and sustained levels of marriage within a limited community (214).

3. Mixed lymphocyte cultures have not proved useful. Use of other immunologic tests also is unnecessary unless these studies are performed, with informed consent, under a specific study protocol in which the costs of these experimental tests are not borne by the couple or their third-party payers.

4. Further work is necessary before suppressor cell and factor determinations; cytokine, oncogene, and growth factor measurements; or embryotoxic factor assessment can be clinically justified.

Postconception Evaluation

After conception, close monitoring of patients with a history of recurrent pregnancy loss is advised to provide psychological support and to confirm intrauterine pregnancy and its viability. The incidence of ectopic pregnancy (258,259) and complete molar gestation (259,260) is increased in women with a history of recurrent spontaneous pregnancy loss. Although somewhat controversial (259), some data suggest that the risk for pregnancy complications other than spontaneous abortion are not significantly different between women with and without a history of recurrent losses (261,262). Two exceptions to this observation are those women who have antiphospholipid antibodies and those who have an intrauterine infection.

Determining serum levels of β-hCG may be helpful in monitoring early pregnancy until an ultrasonographic examination can be performed; however, not all investigators have found inadequate β-hCG levels in pregnancies that ultimately abort (263). Other hormonal determinations are rarely of benefit because levels are often normal until fetal death or abortion occurs (264).

The best method for monitoring in early pregnancy is ultrasonography. If used, serum β-hCG levels should be serially monitored from the time of a missed menstrual period until the level is about 1,500 mIU/mL, at which time an ultrasonographic scan is performed and blood sampling is discontinued. Ultrasonographic assessment is then performed every 2 weeks until the gestational age at which previous pregnancies were aborted. The prognostic value of serial ultrasonography and a variety of hormonal and biochemical measurements during early pregnancy in women with a history of recurrent losses has been recently investigated (265).

If a pregnancy has been confirmed, but fetal cardiac activity cannot be documented by about 6 to 7 weeks of gestation (by sure menstrual or ultrasonographic dating), intervention is recommended to expedite pregnancy termination and to obtain tissue for karyotype analysis. Maternal serum is obtained for α-fetoprotein assessment at 16 to 18 weeks of gestation. Amniocentesis is recommended to assess the fetal karyotype after the pregnancy has progressed past the time of prior losses.

The importance of obtaining karyotypic analysis from tissues obtained after pregnancy demise in a woman experiencing recurrent losses cannot be overemphasized. Results may suggest karyotypic anomalies in the parents. The documentation of aneuploidy may have important prognostic implications and may direct future interventions. A cost analysis has even demonstrated that karyotypic analysis is financially prudent among patients with histories of recurrent pregnancy loss (266). Of course, obtaining karyotypic data from aborted specimens has many hindrances, including difficulties in culturing cells from tissues that may have significant inflammation or necrosis and contamination of specimens with maternal cells. Efforts to develop methods that avoid such difficulties include the application of comparative genomic hybridization technology to recurrent pregnancy loss (267). This technology has even been used successfully on archived and paraffin-embedded pregnancy tissues (268). In the future, fetal karyotype assessment may also be performed using DNA isolated from nucleated fetal erythrocytes in maternal blood (269).

Therapy

Advances in the treatment of patients with recurrent pregnancy loss have been regrettably slow. Although we have experienced a rapid expansion in our understanding of the molecular and subcellular mechanisms involved in implantation and early pregnancy maintenance, extension of these concepts to prevention of recurrent early pregnancy loss has lagged. In addition to these limitations, progress toward treatment of most causes of recurrent pregnancy loss has been hampered by a variety of factors. The condition itself has been inconsistently defined. The results of clinical trials involving recurrent pregnancy loss patients are therefore often nearly impossible to compare and evaluate. Trial design is frequently substandard, with lack of rationale, lack of appropriate controls, and poor statistical analysis, limiting the ability to draw rational conclusions from reported results. Finally, epidemiologic data indicate that most patients with a history of recurrent pregnancy loss will, in fact, have a successful pregnancy the next time they conceive (5). For these reasons, with few exceptions, most therapies for recurrent pregnancy loss must be considered experimental. Until further study is completed, these treatment protocols should be undertaken only with informed consent and in the setting of a well-designed, double-blind, placebo-controlled clinical trial.

Common therapeutic options that currently exist for patients with recurrent pregnancy loss include the use of donor oocytes or sperm, the use of preimplantation genetic diagnosis (PGD), the use of antithrombotic interventions, the repair of anatomic anomalies, the correction of any endocrine abnormalities, the treatment of infections, and a variety of immunologic interventions and drug treatments. Psychological counseling and support should be recommended for all patients.

Genetic Abnormalities

No therapies are presently available to address directly those parental chromosomal anomalies that potentially contribute to recurrent abortion. Three alternative approaches exist when genetic factors are linked to recurrent pregnancy loss. Some, such as antithrombotic therapy for patients with inherited thrombophilias, address the effects of the genetic abnormality. Others attempt to identify those particular embryos that are affected by chromosomal disorders and select against them. This approach involves the technique of PGD. Recent evidence suggests that, in women with a history of two or more spontaneous pregnancy losses, a subsequent pregnancy loss has a 60% chance of chromosomal abnormality. This raises the genetic etiology of recurrent pregnancy loss to new prominence. If the incidence of chromosomal abnormalities among the conceptuses of recurrent pregnancy loss patients is indeed this high, it could be argued that the use of assisted reproductive technologies, including PGD, might be indicated for all patients with unexplained recurrent pregnancy loss.

PGD involves the removal of a single cell from an *in vitro*–matured embryo. Genetic testing can be performed on this cell to rule out gross chromosomal abnormalities or the presence of specific genetic diseases (e.g., cystic fibrosis). Embryos that are diagnosed with genetic abnormalities would not be chosen for replacement into the uterine cavity. Those demonstrated to be genetically normal would be considered appropriate for transfer into the uterus. Use of preimplantation genetic diagnosis, therefore, has the potential to reduce dramatically the incidence of pregnancy loss arising from a genetic etiology. Use of PGD in patients with known heritable genetic disorders (e.g., cystic fibrosis, X-linked disorders) is presently in widespread use in internationally recognized assisted reproductive technology centers. Efficacy of PGD in the treatment of patients with recurrent pregnancy loss is now under investigation (270–272). The third approach to patients with genetic factors and recurrent pregnancy loss is particularly relevant to those with robertsonian translocations involving homologous chromosomes. In these patients, their genetic anomaly always results in embryonic aneuploidy. Therefore, use of either donor oocyte or donor sperm, depending on the affected partner, is recommended. Use of donor gametes among patients with a history of recurrent pregnancy loss has been demonstrated to be as effective as its use in matched patients without such a history (273). Synchronization of intercourse with ovulation may benefit some patients with genetic factor recurrent pregnancy loss (246). In all cases, genetic counseling is warranted.

Anatomic Anomalies

Hysteroscopic resection represents state-of-the-art therapy for submucous leiomyomas, intrauterine adhesions, and intrauterine septa. This approach appears to limit postoperative sequelae while maintaining efficacy in terms of reproductive outcome (43). Use may even be safely extended to patients with *DES* exposure, hypoplastic uteri, and complicating septal anomalies (274). Attempts to improve on standard hysteroscopic metroplasty, which is typically performed in the operating room using general anesthesia, often with laparoscopic guidance, are presently under investigation. Ultrasonographically guided transcervical metroplasty has been reported to be safe and effective (275). Ambulatory, office-based procedures (276), including septum resection under fluoroscopic guidance (277), are also becoming attractive options.

For patients with a history of loss secondary to cervical incompetence, placement of a cervical cerclage is indicated. This is usually performed early in the second trimester, and certainly after documentation of fetal viability. Cervical cerclage should be considered as a primary intervention for women with *DES*-associated uterine anomalies. If endometriosis is encountered during a diagnostic evaluation, it should be resected laparoscopically.

Endocrine Abnormalities

Some investigators have proposed the use of ovulation induction for the treatment of recurrent pregnancy loss (278,279). The theory behind its use in these patients rests on hypotheses that ovulation induction is associated with healthier oocytes. Healthier oocytes, in turn, may decrease the incidence of luteal-phase insufficiency, which should result in improved pregnancy maintenance. This approach grossly oversimplifies the mechanisms involved in implantation and early pregnancy maintenance. Until appropriately studied, use of empiric ovulation induction for treatment of unexplained recurrent pregnancy loss should be viewed with caution. Recent evidence from small studies indicates that such use is not effective (279). Use of ovulation induction in some subsets of patients with recurrent pregnancy loss could be of benefit. For instance, stimulating folliculogenesis with ovulation induction or luteal-phase support with progesterone should be considered for women with luteal-phase insufficiency. The efficacy of these therapies, however, has never been substantiated (280). Ovulation induction might also be beneficial for women with hyperandrogen and LH hypersecretion disorders, especially following pituitary desensitization with gonadotropin-releasing hormone agonist therapy (68). This treatment also remains controversial because the only large, prospective, randomized controlled trial to date reports no therapeutic efficacy, either for prepregnancy pituitary suppression or for luteal-phase progesterone supplementation (281).

Recent links between PCOS, hyperandrogenism, hyperinsulinemia, and recurrent pregnancy loss (50–53) make use of insulin-sensitizing agents in the treatment of recurrent pregnancy loss associated with PCOS attractive. At present, their use for this application is limited to case reports (282). Prepregnancy glycemic control may be particularly important for women with overt diabetes mellitus (54,55). Thyroid hormone replacement with synthroid may be helpful in cases of hypothyroidism. There is no place in the medical management of recurrent abortion for either thyroid medication or bromocriptine for women who do not have a thyroid or prolactin disorder.

Infections

Empiric antibiotic treatment has been used for couples with recurrent abortion. Its efficacy is unproven. Thus, elaborate testing for infectious factors among recurrent pregnancy loss patients and use of therapeutic interventions are not justified unless a patient is immunocompromised or a specific infection has been documented (69). For cases in which an infectious organism has been identified, appropriate antibiotics should be administered to both partners, followed by posttreatment culture to verify eradication of the infectious agent before attempting conception.

Immunologic Factors

Immune-mediated recurrent pregnancy loss has received more attention than any other single etiologic classification of recurrent pregnancy loss. Nevertheless, the diagnosis and subsequent treatment of most cases remain unclear (121,283–285). Most therapies for proposed immune-related recurrent pregnancy loss must be considered experimental. As stated earlier, it is known that the developing conceptus contains paternally inherited gene products and tissue-specific differentiation antigens and that there is maternal recognition of these antigens (162–164). Historically, it has been speculated that both inappropriately weak immune responses to these antigens and unusually strong responses could result in early pregnancy loss. As a consequence, both immunostimulating and immunosuppressive therapies have been proposed.

Immunostimulating Therapies—Leukocyte Immunization

Stimulation of the maternal immune system using alloantigens on either paternal or pooled donor leukocytes has been promoted for patients with immune recurrent pregnancy loss, and a number of reports support possible mechanisms for potential therapeutic value (286–289). Both individual clinical trials and metaanalyses, however, continue to report conflicting results concerning the efficacy of leukocyte alloimmunization in patients with recurrent pregnancy loss (290–294). This most certainly reflects the remarkable heterogeneity in study design, patient selection, and therapeutic protocols, as well as the typically small numbers of enrolled subjects in these investigations. One published analysis reported that about 11 women with unexplained recurrent abortion would need to be immunized with alloantigenic lymphocytes before one additional live birth was achieved (292). About 92% of successful pregnancy outcomes in this study were not attributable to leukocyte immunization. Whether the 8% successful pregnancy rate achieved in leukocyte-immunized women is clinically relevant remains uncertain. One of the most recent and largest trials evaluating the efficacy of leukocyte immunization in patients with unexplained recurrent pregnancy loss is a part of the Recurrent Miscarriage (REMIS) study (294). This investigation was large (more 90 patients per treatment arm), prospective, placebo controlled, randomized, and double blinded. It demonstrated no efficacy for paternal leukocyte immunization in couples with unexplained recurrent pregnancy loss. Despite the unsubstantiated rationale for this therapy and the controversial reports concerning its efficacy, paternal leukocyte transfusion has been widely used, often in response to patient demand that some form of therapy be initiated. Unfortunately, entrepreneurial interests have also clouded the rational assessment of couples experiencing recurrent abortion, resulting in a growing number of financially lucrative leukocyte immunization clinics. However, there is no credible clinical or laboratory method to identify a specific individual who may benefit from such therapy. Further, leukocyte immunization also poses significant risk to both the mother and her fetus (295,296). Several cases of graft-versus-host disease, severe intrauterine growth retardation, and autoimmune and isoimmune complications have been reported (68,291,292,295–298). In addition, alloimmunization to platelets contained in the paternal leukocyte preparation has been associated with cases of potentially fatal fetal thrombocytopenia. The routine use of this therapy for recurrent abortion (that, at best, will only be efficacious in 1 of 11 women treated) cannot be clinically justified.

Other immunostimulating therapies have been proposed and abandoned. Intravenous preparations consisting of syncytiotrophoblast microvillous plasma membrane vesicles have been used to mimic the fetal cell contact with maternal blood that normally occurs in pregnancy (299). The efficacy of this therapy has not been established (299). The use of third-party seminal plasma suppositories has also been attempted (300), based on the misconception that TLX was part of an idiotype–antiidiotype control system (301). Third-party seminal plasma suppositories for recurrent abortion have no scientifically credible rationale and should not be used.

Immunosuppressive Therapies

Immunosuppressive and other immunoregulating therapies have been advocated for cases in which abortion was believed to be due to antiphospholipid antibodies or to inappropriate cellular immunity toward the implanting fetus. Again, study design problems, including small numbers of recruited patients, lack of prestratification by maternal age and number of prior losses before randomization, and other methodologic and statistical inaccuracies preclude definitive statements regarding therapeutic efficacy for most of the proposed immunosuppressive approaches.

Intravenous Immunoglobulin Intravenous immunoglobulins (IVIgs) are composed of pooled samples of immunoglobulins harvested from a large number of blood donors. Studies on the use of IVIg therapy in the treatment of recurrent pregnancy loss are based on the theory that some recurrent pregnancy loss patients have an overzealous immune reactivity to their implanting fetus. IVIgs do have immunosuppressive effects, but the mechanisms underlying this immune modulation are only partially understood. These mechanisms may include decreased autoantibody production and increased autoantibody clearance, T-cell and Fc receptor regulation (302), complement inactivation (303), enhanced T-cell suppressor function, decreased T-cell adhesion to the extracellular matrix (304), and downregulation of T_H1 cytokine synthesis (305). Based an a large number of relatively small studies using a variety of treatment protocols, there remains no conclusive evidence to suggest that use of IVIg in the treatment of patients with unexplained (and presumed immunologic) recurrent pregnancy loss has any benefit (306–313). However, improved post-treatment pregnancy rates may be seen when IVIg is used in those specific patients with autoimmune-mediated pregnancy loss associated with antiphospholipid syndrome (APS) (314,315). Therapy with IVIgs for recurrent pregnancy loss is expensive, invasive, and time-consuming, requiring multiple intravenous infusions over the course of pregnancy. Side effects of IVIg therapy include nausea, headache, myalgias, and hypotension. More serious adverse effects include anaphylaxis (particularly in patients with IgA deficiency) (316).

Progesterone As mentioned earlier, progesterone also has known immunosuppressive effects (166–168). A number of studies using *in vitro* cellular systems relevant to the maternal–fetal interface have now demonstrated that progesterone either inhibits T_H1 immunity or causes a shift from T_H1- to T_H2-type responses (151,171,172,317,318). Progesterone has been administered both intramuscularly and intravaginally for the treatment of recurrent pregnancy loss. It is thought that vaginal administration may increase local, intrauterine concentrations of progesterone better than systemic administration. Vaginal formulations may therefore provide a better method of attaining local immunosuppressive levels of progesterone while averting any adverse systemic side effects. Although both vaginal and intramuscular progesterone therapy are associated with few minor side effects, their efficacy in the treatment of either unexplained recurrent pregnancy loss or recurrent pregnancy loss associated with T-helper cell dysregulation has never been appropriately investigated.

Other immunoregulating therapies theoretically useful in treating recurrent pregnancy loss include the use of *cyclosporine, pentoxifylline,* and *nifedipine,* although maternal and fetal risks with these agents preclude their clinical use. Plasmapheresis has also been used to treat women with recurrent abortion suspected to be caused by antiphospholipid antibodies (319). Generalized immunosuppression with corticosteroids, such as *prednisone,* has been advocated during pregnancy for women with recurrent losses and APAS. Although corticosteroids have shown some treatment promise in these patients (320), maternal and fetal side effects and the availability of alternative therapies have limited their use. The efficacy and side effects of *prednisone* plus low-dose *aspirin* were examined in a recent, large, randomized, placebo-controlled trial treating patients with autoantibodies and recurrent pregnancy losses. Pregnancy outcomes for treated and control patients were similar; however, the incidence of maternal diabetes and hypertension and the risk for premature delivery were all increased among those treated with *prednisone* and *aspirin* (321).

Antithrombotic Therapy

Therapy for patients with recurrent pregnancy losses associated with either the APAS or other thrombophilic disorders has now shifted toward the use of antithrombotic medications. Unlike immunosuppressive treatments, this approach mainly addresses the effect (hypercoagulability), but not the underlying cause (e.g., genetic, APAS), of recurrent pregnancy loss. However, there are reports that *heparin,* one typical anticoagulant, may exert direct immunomodulatory effects by binding to antiphospholipid antibodies (322). The combined use of low-dose aspirin (75 to 80 mg/d) and subcutaneous unfractionated *heparin* (5,000 units twice daily) during pregnancy has been best studied among women with APAS and appears to be efficacious (323–325). A typical regimen for women with antiphospholipid antibody syndrome would include use of *aspirin* (80 mg every day) beginning with any attempts to conceive. After pregnancy has been confirmed, 5,000 IU unfractionated sodium *heparin* is administered subcutaneously twice daily, throughout gestation. An aPTT should be obtained weekly, and dosages of *heparin* should be adjusted until anticoagulation is achieved. Patients using this therapy should be treated in conjunction with a perinatologist because of their increased risk for preterm labor, premature rupture of the membranes, intrauterine growth restriction, intrauterine fetal demise, and preeclampsia. Other potential risks include gastric bleeding, osteopenia, and abruptio placenta.

Attempts have recently been made to extend the finding that antithrombotic therapy is efficacious when used to treat patients with APAS and recurrent pregnancy loss in a number of directions. These directions include the use of *low-molecular weight heparin* (*LMWH*) and the use of antithrombotic therapy in non-APAS patients with thrombophilia and recurrent pregnancy loss and even among recurrent pregnancy loss patients without thrombophilia (unexplained recurrent losses).

New formulations of *heparin* (*LMWH*) have been demonstrated to be superior to unfractionated heparin in the treatment of many clotting disorders (326,327). *LMWH* has the advantage of an increased antithrombotic ratio when compared with unfractionated heparin. This results in improved treatment of inappropriate clotting but fewer bleeding side effects. In addition, *LMWH* has been associated with a decreased incidence of thrombocytopenia and osteoporosis when compared with its unfractionated counterpart. Finally, *LMWH* has a long half-life and requires less frequent dosing and monitoring, thereby improving patient compliance. Although its safe use in pregnancy is only now being fully evaluated, *LMWH* has shown promise when combined with low-dose aspirin in the treatment of recurrent pregnancy loss associated with APAS (324). Efficacy has also been suggested for similar treatment of recurrent pregnancy loss associated with other thrombophilias, including activated protein C resistance associated with factor V Leiden (328–330).

The prophylactic use of daily low-dose *aspirin* has become common practice within the lay public based on its perceived cardiovascular effects combined with its low incidence of side effects. Its sole use in the treatment of recurrent pregnancy loss has likewise gained momentum, and many patients with a history of recurrent loss will either be self-prescribing this therapy or will inquire about its usefulness. At present, there are no good data supporting its use either in patients with thrombophilia or in the general recurrent pregnancy loss population. In fact, although studies are small, the use of low-dose *aspirin* alone has not been shown to be effective in the treatment of recurrent pregnancy loss associated with APAS (323,331). One large study recently addressed the therapeutic efficacy of empiric low-dose aspirin among 805 patients with unexplained recurrent pregnancy losses. The authors conclude that such therapy cannot be justified (332).

More directed antithrombotic therapies have also been described for the treatment of recurrent pregnancy loss among patients with thrombophilias. For instance, the use of protein C concentrates has been reported to be associated with favorable pregnancy outcome in a patient with a history of thrombosis, recurrent fetal losses, and protein C deficiency (333).

As mentioned previously, vitamins B_6, B_{12}, and folate are important in homocysteine metabolism (17,18), and hyperhomocysteinemia is linked to recurrent pregnancy loss (15,16,26). Use of folate or B vitamin supplementation in patients with heritable or acquired disorders in homocysteine metabolism has been suggested (14).

Psychological Support

Despite commonly held biases that anxiety, stress, depression, and other psychological variables might be related to the occurrence of miscarriage, a number of recent studies have reported no causal association (334,335). It is important to discuss this misconception, which may otherwise promote inappropriate feelings of guilt among patients with recurrent losses. There is no doubt, however, that experiencing both isolated and recurrent losses can be emotionally devastating. The risk for major depression is increased greater than twofold among women with spontaneous pregnancy loss; in most women, it arises in the first weeks after delivery (336).

A caring and empathetic attitude is prerequisite to all healing. The acknowledgment of the pain and suffering couples have experienced as a result of recurrent abortion can be a cathartic catalyst enabling them to incorporate their experience of loss into their lives rather than their lives into their experience of loss (68). Referrals to support groups and counselors should be offered. Self-help measures, such as meditation, yoga, exercise, and biofeedback, may also be useful.

Prognosis

The prognosis for successful pregnancy depends both on the potential underlying cause of pregnancy loss and (epidemiologically) on the number of prior losses (Table 28.4). As previously discussed, epidemiologic surveys indicate that the chance of a viable birth even after four prior losses may be as high as 60%. Depending on the study, the prognosis for successful pregnancy in couples with a cytogenetic etiology for reproductive loss varies from 20% to 80% (337–339). Women with corrected anatomic anomalies may expect a successful pregnancy in 60% to 90% of cases (337,338,340,341). A success rate higher than 90% has been reported for women with corrected endocrinologic abnormalities (337). Between 70% and 90% of pregnancies reported among women receiving therapy for antiphospholipid antibodies have been viable (342,343).

Many forms of preconceptional and postconceptional tests have been proposed to help predict pregnancy outcome (147,165,250,252,344); none has been fully substantiated in large, prospective trials. The documentation of fetal cardiac activity on ultrasound may offer prognostic value; however, it appears that its predictions may be greatly affected by any underlying diagnosis. In one study, the live birth rate following documentation of fetal cardiac activity between 5 and 6 weeks from the last menstrual period was about 77% in women with two or more unexplained spontaneous abortions (345). It may be important to note that most of the patients in this study had evidence of inappropriate antitrophoblast cellular immunity. Others have shown that 86% of patients with antiphospholipid antibodies and recurrent pregnancy loss had fetal cardiac activity detected before subsequent demise (346). Most recently, however, a prospective, longitudinal, observational study of 325 patients with unexplained recurrent pregnancy losses demonstrated that only 3% of

Table 28.4. Prognosis for a Viable Birth

Following:	
One spontaneous loss	76%
Two spontaneous losses	70%
Three spontaneous losses	65%
Four spontaneous losses	60%
With:	
Genetic factors	20%–80%
Anatomic factors	60%–90%
Endocrine factors	>90%
Infectious factors	70%–90%
Antiphospholipid antibodies	70%–90%
T_H1 cellular immunity	70%–87%
Unknown factors	40%–90%
Following Detection of Fetal Cardiac Activity:	
Unexplained RPL	77%–97%
APAS and RPL	30%–70%

RPL, recurrent pregnancy loss; APAS, antiphospholipid antibody syndrome.

55 miscarriages occurred after the detection of fetal cardiac activity using transvaginal ultrasonography (347).

References

1. **Edmonds DK, Lindsay KI, Miller JF.** Early embryonic mortality in women. *Fertil Steril* 1982;38:447–453.
2. **Wilcox AJ, Weinberg CR, O'Connor JF, et al.** Incidence of early loss of pregnancy. *N Engl J Med* 1988;319:189–194.
3. **Alberman E.** The epidemiology of repeated abortion. In: **Beard RW, Sharp F,** eds. *Early pregnancy loss: mechanisms and treatment.* New York: Springer-Verlag, 1988:9–17.
4. **Warburton D, Fraser FC.** Spontaneous abortion rate in man: data from reproductive histories collected in a medical genetics unit. *Am J Hum Genet* 1963;16:1–25.
5. **Regan L, Braude PR, Trembath PL.** Influence of post reproductive performance on risk of spontaneous abortion. *BMJ* 1989;299:541–545.
6. **Stephenson MD.** Frequency of factors associated with habitual abortion in 197 couples. *Fertil Steril* 1996;66:24–29.
7. **Daniel A, Hook EB, Wolf G.** Risks of unbalanced progeny at amniocentesis of carriers of chromosome rearrangements: data from United States and Canadian laboratories. *Am J Hum Genet* 1989;33:14–53.
8. **Fryns JP, Van Buggenhout G.** Structural chromosome rearrangements in couples with recurrent fetal wastage. *Eur J Obstet Gynecol Reprod Biol* 1998.81.171–176.
9. **Ogasawara M, Aoki K, Okada S, et al.** Embryonic karyotype of abortuses in relation to the number of previous miscarriages. *Fertil Steril* 2000;73:300–304.
10. **Simon C, Rubio C, Vidal F, et al.** Increased chromosomal abnormalities in human preimplantation embryos after in vitro fertilization in patients with recurrent miscarriage. *Reprod Fertil Dev* 1998;10:87–92.
11. **Egozcue S, Blanco J, Vendrell JM, et al.** Human male infertility: chromosomal abnormalities, meiotic disorders, abnormal spermatozoa and recurrent abortion. *Hum Reprod Update* 2000;6:93–105.
12. **Giorlandino C, Calugi G, Iaconianni L, et al.** Spermatozoa with chromosomal abnormalities may result in a higher rate of recurrent abortion. *Fertil Steril* 1998;70:576–577.
13. **Lanasa MC, Hogge WA.** X chromosome defects as an etiology of recurrent spontaneous abortion. *Semin Reprod Med* 2000;18:97–103.
14. **Blumenfeld Z, Brenner B.** Thrombophilia-associated pregnancy wastage. *Fertil Steril* 1999;72:765–774.
15. **Girling J, de Swiet M.** Inherited thrombophilia and pregnancy. *Curr Opin Obstet Gynecol* 1998;10:135–144.
16. **Nelen WL, Bulten J, Steegers EA, et al.** Hereditary thrombophilia as a cause of fetal loss. *Obstet Gynecol* 2000;95[Suppl 4]:S11–12.
17. **Bauters A, Zawadzki C, Bura A, et al.** Homozygous variant of antithrombin with lack of affinity for heparin: management of severe thrombotic complications associated with fetal demise. *Blood Coagul Fibrinolysis* 1996;7:705–710
18. **De Stefano V, Finazzi G, Manucci PM.** Inherited thrombophilia: pathogenesis, clinical syndromes and management. *Blood* 1996;87:3531–3544.
19. **Murphy RP, Donoghue C, Nallen RJ, et al.** Prospective evaluation of the risk conferred by factor V Leiden and thermolabile methelenetetrahydrofolate reductase polymorphisms in pregnancy. *Arterscler Thromb Vasc Biol* 2000;20:266–270.
20. **Molloy AM, Daly S, Millis JL, et al.** Thermolabile variant of 5,10-methylenetetrahydrofolate reductase associated with red cell folates: implications for folate intake recommendations. *Lancet* 1997;349:1591–1593.
21. **Nelen WL, Blom HJ, Steegers EA, et al.** Homocyteine and folate levels as risk factors for recurrent pregnancy loss. *Obstet Gynecol* 2000;95:519–524.
22. **Durnwald CP, Flora R, Agamanolis D, et al.** Hereditary thrombophilia as a cause of fetal loss. *Obstet Gynecol* 2000;95[Suppl 1]:S11–S12.
23. **Holmes ZR, Regan L, Chilcott I, et al.** The C677T MTHFR gene mutation is not predictive of risk for recurrent fetal loss. *Br J Haematol* 1999;105:98–101.
24. **Kutteh WH, Park VM, Deitcher SR.** Hypercoagulable state mutation analysis in white patients with early first-trimester recurrent pregnancy loss. *Fertil Steril* 1999;71:1048–1053.
25. **Ray JG, Laskin CA.** Folic acid and homocyst(e)ine metabolic defects and the risk of placental abruption, pre-eclampsia and spontaneous pregnancy loss: a systemic review. *Placenta* 1999;20:519–529.
26. **Nelen WL, Blom HJ, Steegers EA, et al.** Hyperhomocyscysteinemia and recurrent early pregnancy loss: a meta-analysis. *Fertil Steril* 2000;74:1196–1199.

27. **Preston FE, Rosendaal FR, Walker ID, et al.** Increased fetal loss in women with heritable thrombophilia. *Lancet* 1996;348:913–916.

28. **Brenner B, Mandel H, Lanir N, et al.** Activated protein C resistance can be associated with recurrent fetal loss. *Br J Haematol* 1997;97:551–554.

29. **Tal J, Schliamser LM, Leibovitz Z, et al.** A possible role for activated protein C resistance in patients with first and second trimester pregnancy failure. *Hum Reprod* 1999;14:1624–1627.

30. **Bertina RM, Koeleman BPC, Koster T, et al.** Mutation in blood coagulation factor V associated with resistance to activated protein C. *Nature* 1994;369:64–67.

31. **Zivelin A, Griffen JH, Xu X, et al.** A single genetic origin for a common Caucasion risk factor for venous thrombosis. *Blood* 1997;89:397–402.

32. **Foka ZJ, Lambropoulos AF, Saravelos H, et al.** Factor V Leiden and prothrombin G20210A mutations, but not methylenetetrahydrofolate reductase C677T, are associated with recurrent miscarriages. *Hum Reprod* 2000;15:458–462.

33. **Ridker PM, Miletich JP, Buring JE, et al.** Factor V Leiden mutation as a risk factor for recurrent pregnancy loss. *Ann Intern Med* 1998;128:1000–1003.

34. **Coumans AB, Huijgens PC, Jakobs C, et al.** Haemostatic and metabolic abnormalities in women with unexplained recurrent abortion. *Hum Reprod* 1999;14:211–214.

35. **Souza SS, Ferriani RA, Pontes AG, et al.** Factor V Leiden and factor II G20210A mutations in patients with recurrent abortion. *Hum Reprod* 1999;14:2448–2450.

36. **Poort SW, Rosendall FR, Reitsma PH, et al.** A common genetic variation in the 3′-untranslated region of the prothrombin geneis associated with elevated plasma prothrombin levels and an increase in venous thrombosis. *Blood* 1996;88:3698–3703.

37. **Yamada H, Kato EH, Ebina Y, et al.** Factor XII deficiency in women with recurrent miscarriage. *Gynecol Obstet Invest* 2000;49:80–83.

38. **Goodwin TM.** Congenital hypofibrinogenemia in pregnancy. *Obstet Gynecol Surv* 1989;44:157–161.

39. **Egbring R, Kroninger A, Seitz R.** Factor XIII deficiency: pathogenic mechanisms and clinical significance. *Semin Thromb Hemost* 1996;22:419–425.

40. **Wakui K, Tanemura M, Suzumori K, et al.** Clinical applications of two-color telomeric fluorescence in situ hybridization for prenatal diagnosis: identification of chrosomal translocation in five families with recurrent miscarriage or a child with multiple congenital anomalies. *J Hum Genet* 1999;44:85–90.

41. **Taylor HS.** The role of HOX genes in the development and function of the female reproductive tract. *Semin Reprod Med* 2000;18:81–90.

42. **Raga F, Bauset C, Remohi J, et al.** Reproductive impact of congenital Müllerian anomalies. *Hum Reprod* 1997;12:2277–2281.

43. **Homer HA, Li T-C, Cooke ID.** The septate uterus: a review of management and reproductive outcome. *Fertil Steril* 2000;73:1–14.

44. **Mizuno K, Koske K, Ando K.** Significance of Jones operation on double uterus: vascularity and dating of endometrium in uterine septum. *Jpn J Fertil Steril* 1978;29:9.

45. **Barnes AB, Colton T, Gundersen J, et al.** Fertility and outcome of pregnancy in women exposed in utero to diethylstilbestrol. *N Engl J Med* 1980;302:609–613.

46. **Kaufman RH, Adam E, Hatch EE, et al.** Continued follow-up of pregnancy outcomes in diethylstilbesterol-exposed offspring. *Obstet Gynecol* 2000;96:483–489.

47. **Burchell RC, Creed F, Rasoulpour M, et al.** Vascular anatomy of the human uterus and pregnancy wastages. *Br J Obstet Gynaecol* 1978;85:698–706.

48. **Buttram VC, Reiter RC.** Uterine leiomyomata: etiology, symptomology and management. *Fertil Steril* 1981;76:433–455.

49. **Csapo AI, Pulkkinen MO, Ruttner B, et al.** The significance of the corpus luteum in pregnancy maintenance. I. Preliminary studies. *Am J Obstet Gynecol* 1972;112:1061–1067.

50. **Watson H, Kiddy DS, Hamilton-Fairley D, et al.** Hypersecretion of luteinizing hormone and ovarian steroids in women with recurrent early miscarriages. *Hum Reprod* 1993;8:829–833.

51. **Rai R, Backos M, Rushworth F, et al.** Polycystic ovaries and recurrent miscarriage-a reappraisal. *Hum Reprod* 2000;15:612–615.

52. **Bussen S, Sutterlin M, Steck T.** Endocrine abnormalities during the follicular phase in women with recurrent spontaneous abortion. *Hum Reprod* 1999;14:18–20

53. **Okon MA, Laird SM, Tuckerman EM, et al.** Serum androgen levels in women who have recurrent miscarriages and their correlation with markers of endometrial function. *Fertil Steril* 1998;69: 682–690.

54. **Brydon P, Smith T, Proffitt M, et al.** Pregnancy outcome in women with type 2 diabetes mellitus needs to be addressed. *Int J Clin Pract* 2000;54:418–419.

55. **Langer O, Conway DL.** Level of glycemia and perinatal outcome in pregestational diabetes. *J Matern Fetal Med* 2000;9:35–41.

56. **Greene MF.** Spontaneous abortions and major malformations in women with diabetes mellitus. *Semin Reprod Endocrinol* 1999;17:127–136.

57. **Moley KH, Chi MM, Knudson CM, et al.** Hyperglycemia induces apoptosis in pre-implantation embryos through cell death effector pathways. *Nat Med* 1998;4:1421–1424.

58. **Vaquero E, Lazzarin N, DeCarolis C, et al.** Mild thyroid abnormalities and recurrent spontaneous abortion: diagnostic and therapeutical approach. *Am J Reprod Immunol* 2000;43:204–208.

59. **Stagnaro-Green A, Roman SH, Cobin RH, el-Harazy E, et al.** Detection of at risk pregnancy by means of highly sensitive assays for thyroid auto-antibodies. *JAMA* 1990;264:1422–1425.

60. **Rushworth FH, Backos M, Rai R, et al.** Prospective pregnancy outcome in untreated recurrent miscarriers with thyroid antibodies. *Hum Reprod* 2000;15:1637–1639.

61. **Esplin MS, Branch DW, Silver R, et al.** Thyroid autoantibodies are not associated with recurrent pregnancy loss. *Am J Obstet Gynecol* 1998;179:1583–1586.

62. **Kutteh WH, Yetman DL, Carr AC, et al.** Increased prevalence of antithyroid antibodies identified in women with recurrent pregnancy loss but not in women undergoing assisted reproduction. *Fertil Steril* 1999;71:843–848.

63. **Dlugi A.** Hyperprolactinemic recurrent spontaneous pregnancy loss: a true clinical entity or a spurious finding? *Fertil Steril* 1998;70:253–255.

64. **Soules MR, Bremner WJ, Steiner RA, et al.** Prolactin secretion and corpus luteum function in women with luteal phase deficiency. *J Clin Endocrinol Metab* 1991;72:986–992.

65. **Hirahara F, Andoh N, Sawai K, et al.** Hyperprolactinemic recurrent miscarriage and results of randomized bromocriptine treatment trials. *Fertil Steril* 1998;70:246–252.

66. **Trout SW, Seifer DB.** Do women with unexplained recurrent pregnancy loss have higher day 3 serum FSH and estradiol values? *Fertil Steril* 2000;74:335–337.

67. **Hofmann GE, Khoury J, Thie J.** Recurrent pregnancy loss and diminished ovarian reserve. *Fertil Steril* 2000;74:1192–1195.

68. **Hill JA.** Sporadic and recurrent spontaneous abortion. *Curr Probl Obstet Gynecol Fertil* 1994;17:114–162.

69. **Summers PR.** Microbiology relevant to recurrent miscarriage. *Clin Obstet Gynecol* 1994;37:722–729.

70. **Paukku M, Tulppala M, Puolakkainen M, et al.** Lack of association between serum antibodies to Chlamidia trachomatis and recurrent pregnancy loss. *Fertil Steril* 1999;72:427–430.

71. **Llahi-Camp JM, Rai R, Ison C, et al.** Association of bacterial vaginosis with a history of second trimester miscarriage. *Hum Reprod* 1996;11:1575–1578.

72. **Robb J, Benirshke K, Barmeyer R.** Intrauterine latent herpes simplex virus infection: spontaneous abortion. *Hum Pathol* 1986;17:1196–209.

73. **Altshuler G.** Immunologic competence of the immature human fetus: morphologic evidence from intrauterine cytomegalovirus infection. *Obstet Gynecol* 1974;43:811–816.

74. **Heyborne KD, Wilkin SS, McGregor JA.** Tumor necrosis factor-α in midtrimester amniotic fluid is associated with impaired intrauterine fetal growth. *Am J Obstet Gynecol* 1992;167:920–925.

75. **Romero R, Mazor M, Sepulueda W, et al.** Tumor necrosis factor in preterm and term labor. *Am J Obstet Gynecol* 1992;166:1576–1587.

76. **Furman MH, Ploegh HL, Schust DJ.** Can viruses help us to understand and classify the MHC class I molecules at the maternal-fetal interface? *Hum Immunol* 2000;61:1169–1176.

77. **Thellin O, Coumans B, Zorzi W, et al.** Tolerance of the feto-placental "graft": ten ways to support a child for nine months. *Curr Opin Immunol* 2000;12:731–737.

78. **Lanier LL.** Activating and inhibitory NK cell receptors. *Ann Rev Immunol* 1998;452:13–18.

79. **Johnson PM, Christmas PE, Vince GS.** Immunological aspects of implantation and implantation failure. *Hum Reprod* 1999;14[Suppl 2]:26–36.

80. **Vince GS, Johnson PM.** Leukocyte populations and cytokine regulation in human uteroplacental tissues. *Biochem Soc Trans* 2000;28:191–195.

81. **Loke YW, King A.** Decidual natural-killer-cell interaction with trophoblast: cytolysis or cytokine production? *Biochem Soc Trans* 2000;28:196–198.

82. **King A, Hiby SE, Gardner L, et al.** Recognition of trophoblast HLA class I molecules by decidual NK cell receptors–a review. *Placenta* 2000;21[Suppl A]14:S81–S85.

83. **Ito K, Karasawa M, Kawano T, et al.** Involvement of decidual Valpha14 NKT cells in abortion. *Proc Natl Acad Sci U S A* 2000;97:740–744.

84. **Mincheva-Nilsson L, Baranov V, Yeung M, et al.** Immunomorphologic studies of human decidus-associated lymphoid cells in normal early pregnancy. *J Immunol* 1994;152:2020–2032.

85. **Christmas SE, Brew R, Thornton SM, et al.** Extensive TCR junctional diversity of V gamma 9/V delta 2 clones from human reproductive tract tissues. *J Immunol* 1995;155:2453–2458.

86. **Vassiliadou N, Bulmer JN.** Characterization of endometrial T lymphocyte subpopulations in spontaneous early pregnancy loss. *Hum Reprod* 1998;13:44–47.

87. **Hayday AC.** $\gamma\delta$ Cells: a right time and a right place for a conserved third way of protection. *Ann Rev Immunol* 2000;18:975–1026.

88. **Chang MD, Pollard JW, Khalili H, et al.** Mouse placental macrophages have a decreased ability to present antigen. *Proc Natl Acad Sci U S A* 1993;90:462–466.

89. **Clifford K, Flanagan AM, Regan L.** Endometrial $CD56^+$ natural killer cells in women with recurrent miscarriage: a histomorphometric study. *Hum Reprod* 1999;14:2727–2730.

90. **Quenby S, Bates M, Doig T, et al.** Pre-implantation endometrial leukocytes in women with recurrent miscarriage. *Hum Reprod* 1999;14:2836–2891.

91. **Yamamoto T, Takahashi Y, Kase N, et al.** Proportion of $CD56^+3^+$ T cells in decidual and peripheral lymphocytes of normal pregnancy and spontaneous abortion with and without history of recurrent abortion. *Am J Reprod Immunol* 1999;42:355–360.

92. **Yamamoto T, Takahashi Y, Kase N, et al.** Decidual natural killer cells in recurrent spontaneous abortion with normal chromosomal content. *Am J Reprod Immunol* 1999;41:337–342.

93. **Lachapelle MH, Miron P, Hemmings R, et al.** Endometrial T, B, and NK cells in patients with recurrent spontaneous abortion. Altered profile and pregnancy outcome. *J Immunol* 1996;156: 4027–4034.

94. **Gould DS, Ploegh HL, Schust DJ.** Murine female reproductive tract intraepithelial lymphocytes display selection characteristics distinct from both peripheral and other mucosal T cells. *J Reprod Immunol* 2001;52:85–99.

95. **Pudney J, Quayle AJ, Anderson DJ.** Immunology of the human cervix and vagina (submitted).

96. **McVay LD, Carding SR.** Extrathymic origin of human gamma delta T cells during fetal development. *J Immunol* 1996;157:2873–2882.

97. **Dorfman JR, Raulet DH.** Major histocompatibility complex genes determine natural killer cell tolerance. *Eur J Immunol* 1996;26:151–155.

98. **Salcedo M, Diehl AD, Olsson-Alheim MY, et al.** Altered expression of Ly49 inhibitory receptors on natural killer cells from MHC class-I deficient mice. *J Immunol* 1997;158:3174–3180.

99. **Schon MP, Arya A, Murphy EA, et al.** Mucosal T lymphocyte numbers are selectively reduced in integrin α_E (CD103)-deficient mice. *J Immunol* 1999;162:6641–6649.

100. **Kruse A, Hallman R, Butcher EC.** Specialized patterns of vascular differentiation antigens in the pregnant mouse uterus and the placenta. *Biol Reprod* 1999;61:1393–1401.

101. **Perry LL, Feilzer K, Portis JL, et al.** Distinct homing pathways direct T lymphocytes to the genital and intestinal tmucosae in Chlamydia-infected mice. *J Immunol* 1998;160:2905–2914.

102. **Pudney J, Anderson DJ.** Immunobiology of the human penile urethra. *Am J Pathol* 1995;147:155–165.

103. **Ljunggren HG, Karre K.** In search of the "missing self": MHC molecules and NK cell recognition. *Immunol Today* 1990;11:237–244.

104. **Mattson R.** The non-expression of MHC class II in trophoblast cells. *Am J Reprod Immunol* 1998;40:385–394.

105. **Murphy SP, Tomasi TB.** Absence of MHC class II antigen expression in trophoblast cells results from a lack of class II transactivator (CIITA) gene expression. *Mol Reprod Dev* 1998;51:1–12.

106. **Kovats S, Main EK, Librach C, et al.** A class I antigen HLA-G expressed in human trophoblasts. *Science* 1990;248:220–223.

107. **Ellis SA, Palmer MS, McMichael AJ.** Human trophoblast and the choriocarcinoma cell line BeWo express a truncated HLA class I molecule. *J Immunol* 1990;144:731–735.

108. **Wei X, Orr HT.** Differential expression of HLA-E, -F, and-G transcripts in human tissue. *Hum Immunol* 1990;29:131–142.

109. **Sernee MF, Ploegh HL, Schust DJ.** Why certain antibodies cross-react with HLA-A and HLA-G: epitope mapping of two common MHC class I reagents. *Mol Immunol* 1998;35:177–188.

110. **King A, Burrows TD, Hiby SE, et al.** Surface expression of HLA-C antigen by human extravillous cytotrophoblast. *Placenta* 2000;21;376–387.

111. **King A, Allen DS, Bowen M, et al.** HLA-E is expressed on trophoblast and interacts with CD94/NKG2 receptors on decidual NK cells. *Eur J Immunol* 2000;30:1623–1631.

112. **Kam EPY, Gardner L, Loke YW, et al.** The role of trophoblast in the physiological changes in the decidual spiral arteries. *Hum Reprod* 1999;14:2131–2138.

113. **Damsky CH, Fisher SJ.** Trophoblast pseudo-vasculogenesis: faking it with endothelial adhesion receptors. *Curr Opin Cell Biol* 1998;10:660–666.

114. **Zhou Y, Fisher SJ, Janatpour M, et al.** Human cytotrophoblasts adopt a vascular phenotype as they differentiate. *J Clin Invest* 1997;99:2139–2151.

115. **Lim KH, Zhou Y, Janatpour M, et al.** Human cytotrophoblast differentiation/invasion is abnormal in pre-eclampsia. *J Clin Invest* 1997;99:2139–2151.

116. **Goldman-Wohl DS, Ariel I, Greenfield C, et al.** Lack of human leukocyte antigen-G expression in extravillous trophoblasts is associated with pre-eclampsia. *Mol Hum Reprod* 2000;6:88–95.

117. **Hunt JS, Jadhav L, Chu W, et al.** Soluble HLA-G circulates in maternal blood during pregnancy. *Am J Obstet Gynecol* 2000;183:682–688.

118. **Yamashita T, Fujii T, Tokunaga K, et al.** Analysis of human leukocyte antigen-G polymorphism including intron 4 in Japanese couples with habitual abortion. *Am J Reprod Immunol* 1999;41:159–163.

119. **Steffensen R, Christiansen OB, Bennett EP, et al.** HLA-E polymorphism in patients with recurrent spontaneous abortion. *Tissue Antigens* 1998;52:569–572.

120. **Feinman MA, Kliman JH, Main EK.** HLA antigen expression and induction by a-interferon in cultured human trophoblast. *Am J Obstet Gynecol* 1987;157:1429–1434.

121. **Hill JA.** Immunological mechanisms of pregnancy maintenance and failure: a critique of theories and therapy. *Am J Reprod Immunol* 1990;22:33–42.

122. **Hill JA, Melling GC, Johnson PM.** Immunohistochemical studies of human uteroplacental tissues from first trimester spontaneous abortion. *Am J Obstet Gynecol* 1995;173:90–96.

123. **Christiansen OB, Anderson HH, Hojbjerre M, et al.** Maternal HLA class II alogenotypes are markers for the predisposition to fetal losses in families of women with unexplained recurrent fetal loss. *Eur J Immunogenet* 1995;22:323–334.

124. **Christiansen OB, Rasmussen KL, Jerslid C, et al.** HLA class II alleles confer susceptibility to recurrent fetal losses in Danish women. *Tissue Antigens* 1994;44:225–233.

125. **Palmer EM, Seventer GA.** Human helper T cell differentiation is regulated by the combined action of cytokines and accessory cell-dependent co-stimulatory signals. *J Immunol* 1997;158:2654–2662.

126. **O'Garra A, Arai N.** The molecular basis of T helper 1 and T helper 2 cell differentiation. *Trends Cell Biol* 2000;10:542–550.

127. **Kurt-Jones EA, Hamberg S, Ohara J, et al.** Heterogeneity of helper/inducer T lymphocytes. I. Lymphokine production and lymphokine responsiveness. *J Exp Med* 1987;166:1774–1787.

128. **Romagnani S.** Human TH1 and TH2 subsets: doubt no more. *Immunol Today* 1991;8:256–257.

129. **Mosmann TR, Coffman RL.** Heterogeneity of cytokine secretion patterns and functions of helper T cells. *Adv Immunol* 1989;46:111–147.

130. **Ramagnani S.** Human TH1 and TH2 subsets: regulation of differentiation and role in protection and immunopathology. *Int Arch Allergy Immunol* 1992;4:279–285.

131. **Mosmann TR, Coffman RL.** TH1 and TH2 cells: different patterns of lymphokine secretion lead to different functional properties. *Annu Rev Immunol* 1989;7:145–173.

132. **Maggi E, Parronchi P, Monetti R, et al.** Reciprocal regulatory effects of IFN-α and IL-4 in in vitro development of human TH1 and TH2 clones. *J Immunol* 1992;148:2142–2147.

133. **Fiorentino DF, Bond MW, Mosmann TR.** Two types of mouse T helper cell IV. TH2 clones secrete a factor that inhibits cytokine production by TH1 clones. *J Exp Med* 1989;170:2081–2095.

134. **Mosmann TR, Moore KW.** The role of IL-10 in cross regulation of TH1 and TH2 responses. *Immunol Today* 1991;12:A49–53.

135. **Sen DR, Fox H.** The lymphoid tissue of the endometrium. *Gynecol Pathol* 1967;163:371.

136. **Kearns M, Lala PH.** Bone marrow origin of decidual cell precursors in the pseudopregnant mouse uterus. *J Exp Med* 1982;155:1537.

137. **Bulmer JN, Sunderland CA.** Immunohistological characterization of lymphoid cell populations in the early human placental bed. *Immunology* 1984;52:349–357.

138. **Tabibzadeh S.** Human endometrium: an active site of cytokine production and action. *Endocr Rev* 1991;12:272–290.

139. **Klentzeris LD, Bulmer JN, Warren A, et al.** Endometrial lymphoid tissue in the timed endometrial biopsy: morphometric and immunohistochemical aspects. *Am J Obstet Gynecol* 1992;167:667–674.

140. **Berkowitz RS, Hill JA, Kurtz CB, et al.** Effects of products of activated leukocytes (lymphokines and monokines) on the growth of malignant trophoblast cells in vitro. *Am J Obstet Gynecol* 1988;158:199–204.

141. **Hunt JS, Soales MJ, Lei MG, et al.** Products of lipopolysaccharide-activated macrophages (tumor necrosis factor-a, transforming growth factor-b) but not lipopolysaccharide modify DNA synthesis by rat trophoblast cells exhibiting the 80-KDa LPS-binding protein. *J Immunol* 1989;143:1606–1613.

142. **Hill J, Haimovici F, Anderson DJ.** Products of activated lymphocytes and macrophages inhibit mouse embryo development in vitro. *J Immunol* 1987;139:2250–2254.

143. **Hill JA, Polgar K, Harlow BL, Anderson DJ.** Evidence of embryo- and trophoblast-toxic cellular immune response(s) in women with recurrent spontaneous abortion. *Am J Obstet Gynecol* 1992;166:1044–1052.

144. **Mallmann P, Werner A, Krebs D.** Serum levels of interleukin-2 and tumor necrosis factor-α in women with recurrent abortion. *Am J Obstet Gynecol* 100;163:1367.

145. **Yamada H, Polgar K, Hill JA.** Cell-mediated immunity to trophoblast antigens in women with recurrent spontaneous abortion. *Am J Obstet Gynecol* 1994;170:1339–1344.

146. **Hill JA, Polgar K, Anderson DJ.** T Helper 1-type immunity to trophoblast antigens in women with recurrent spontaneous abortion. *JAMA* 1995;273:1933–1936.

147. **Ecker JL, Laufer MR, Hill JA.** Measurement of embryotoxic factors is predictive of pregnancy outcome in women with a history of recurrent abortion. *Obstet Gynecol* 1993;81:84–87.

148. **Lea RG, Tulppala M, Critchley HO.** Deficient syncytiotrophoblast tumor necrosis factor-alpha characterizes failing first trimester pregnancies in a subgroup of recurrent miscarriage patients. *Hum Reprod* 1997;12:1313–1320.

149. **von Wolff M, Thaler CJ, Strowitzki T, et al.** Regulated expression of cytokines in the human endometrium throughout the menstrual cycle: dysregulation in habitual abortion. *Mol Hum Reprod* 2000;6:627–634.

150. **Lim KJ, Odukoya OA, Ajjan RA, et al.** The role of T-helper cytokines in human reproduction. *Fertil Steril* 2000;73:136–142.

151. **Piccini MP, Beloni L, Livi C, et al.** Defective production of both leukemia inhibiting factor and type 2 cytokine production by decidual T cells in unexplained recurrent abortion. *Nat Med* 1998;4:1020–1024.

152. **Raghupathy R, Makhseed M, Azizieh F, et al.** Cytokine production by maternal lymphocytes during normal human pregnancy and in unexplained recurrent spontaneous abortion. *Hum Reprod* 2000;15:713–718.

153. **Raghupathy R, Makhseed M, Azizieh F, et al.** Maternal Th1- and Th2-type reactivity to placental antigens in normal human pregnancy and unexplained recurrent spontaneous abortions. *Cell Immunol* 1999; 196:122–130.

154. **Hamai Y, Fujii T, Yamashita T, et al.** Peripheral blood mononuclear cells from women with recurrent spontaneous abortion exhibit an aberrant reaction to release cytokines upon the direct contact of human leukocyte antigen-G-expressing cells. *Am J Reprod Immunol* 1998;40:408–413.

155. **Kanai T, Fujii T, Unno N, et al.** Human leukocyte antigen-G-expressing cells differently modulate the release of cytokines from mononuclear cells present in the decidua versus peripheral blood. *Am J Reprod Immunol Microbiol* 2001;45:94–99.

156. **Schust DJ, Hill JA.** Correlation of serum cytokine and adhesion molecule determinations with pregnancy outcome. *J Soc Gynecol Invest* 1996;3:259–261.

157. **Makhseed M, Raghupathy R, Azizieh F, et al.** Circulating cytokines and CD30 in normal human pregnancies and recurrent spontaneous abortions. *Hum Reprod* 2000;15:2011–2017.

158. **Jenkins C, Roberts J, Wilson R, et al.** Evidence of a T(H)1 type response associated with recurrent miscarriage. *Fertil Steril* 2000;73:1206–1208.

159. **Stewart CL, Kaspar P, Brunet LJ, et al.** Blastocyst implantation depends on maternal expression of leukemia inhibiting factor. *Nature* 1992;358:76–79.

160. **Chen JR, Cheng JG, Shatzer T, et al.** Leukemia inhibiting factor can substitute for nidatory estrogen and is essential to inducing a receptive uterus for implantation but is not essential for subsequent embryogenesis. *Endocrinology* 2000;141:4365–4372.

161. **Bamberger AM, Jenatschke S, Schulte HM, et al.** Leukemia inhibitory factor (LIF) stimulates the human HLA-G promoter in Jeg 3 choriocarcinoma cells. *J Clin Endocrinol Metab* 2000;85:3932–3936.

162. **Billington WD, Davies M, Bell SC.** Maternal antibody to foetal histocompatibility and trophoblast-specific antigens. *Ann Immunol (Paris)* 1984;135D:331–335.

163. **Tafuri A, Alferink J, Moller P, et al.** T cell awareness of paternal alloantigens during pregnancy. *Science* 1995:270630.

164. **Sargent IL, Wilkins T, Redman CWG.** Maternal immune responses to the fetus in early pregnancy and recurrent miscarriage. *Lancet* 1994;2:1099–1104.

165. **Bermas BL, Hill JA.** Proliferative responses to recall antigens are associated with pregnancy outcome in women with a history of recurrent spontaneous abortion. *J Clin Invest* 1997;100:1330–1334.

166. **Grossman CJ.** Possible underlying mechanisms of sexual dimorphism in the immune response: fact and hypothesis. *J Steroid Biochem* 1989;34:241–251.

167. **Runnebaum B, Stober I, Zander J.** Progesterone, 20 alpha-dihydroprogesterone, and 20 beta-dihydroprogesterone in mother and child at birth. *Acta Endocrinol* 1975;80:569–576.

168. **Siiteri PK, Febres F, Clemens LE, et al.** Progesterone and maintenance of pregnancy: is progesterone nature's immunosuppressant? *Ann N Y Acad Sci* 1977;286:384–397.

169. **Ehring GR, Kerschbaum HH, Eder C, et al.** A nongenomic mechanism for progesterone-mediated immunosuppression: inhibition of K+ channels, Ca2+ signalling, and gene expression in lymphocytes. *J Exp Med* 1998;188:1593–1602.

170. **Schust DJ, Anderson DJ, Hill JA.** Progesterone-induced immunosuppression is not mediated through the progesterone receptor. *Hum Reprod* 1996;11:980–985.

171. **Hunt JS, Miller L, Roby KF, et al.** Female steroid hormones regulate production of pro-inflammatory molecules in uterine leukocytes. *J Reprod Immunol* 1997;35:87–99.

172. **Vassiliadou N, Tucker L, Anderson DJ.** Progesterone-induced inhibition of chemokine receptor expression on peripheral blood mononuclear cells correlates with reduced HIV-1 infectability in vitro. *J Immunol* 1999;14:2252–2256.

173. **Knoferi MW, Diodato MD, Angele MK, et al.** Do female sex steroids adversely or beneficially effect the depressed immune responses in males after trauma-hemorrhage? *Arch Surg* 2000;135:425–433.

174. **Gregory MS, Duffner LA, Faunce DE, et al.** Estrogen mediates the sex difference in post-burn immunosuppression. *J Endocrinol* 2000;164:129–138.

175. **Muller V, Szabo A, Viklicky O, et al.** Sex hormones and gender-related differences: their influence on chronic renal allograft rejection. *Kidney Int* 1999;55:2011–2020.

176. **Salem ML, Matsuzaki G, Kishihara K, et al.** Beta-estradiol suppresses T cell-mediated delayed-type hypersensitivity through suppression of antigen-presenting cell function and Th1 induction. *Int Arch Allergy Immunol* 2000;121:161–169.

177. **Correale J, Arias M, Gilmore W.** Steroid hormone regulation of cytokine secretion by proteolipid protein-specific CD4+ T cell clones isolated from multiple sclerosis patients and normal control subjects. *J Immunol* 1998;161;3365–3374.

178. **Munn DH, Shafizadeh E, Attwood JT, et al.** Inhibition of T cell proliferation by macrophage tryptophan metabolism. *J Exp Med* 1999;189:1363–1372.

179. **Mellor AL, Munn DH.** Immunology at the maternal-fetal interface: lessons for T cell tolerance and suppression. *Ann Rev Immunol* 2000;18:367–391.

180. **Munn DH, Zhou M, Atwood JT, et al.** Prevention of allogeneic fetal rejection by tryptophan catabolism. *Science* 1998;281:1191–1193.

181. **Meier AH, Wilson JM.** Tryptophan feedind adversely influences pregnancy. *Life Sci* 1983;32:1193–1196.

182. **Kamimura S, Eguchi K, Yonezawa M, et al.** Localization and developmental change of indolamine 2,3-dioxygenase activity in the human placenta. *Acta Med Okayama* 1991;45:135–139.

183. **Schrocksnadel H, Baier-Bitterlich G, Dapunt O, et al.** Decreased plasma tryptophan in pregnancy. *Obstet Gynecol* 1996;88:47–50.

184. **Lebovic DI, Mueller MD, Taylor RN.** Immunobiology of endometriosis. *Fertil Steril* 2001;75:1–10.

185. **Hill JA.** Endometriosis: immune cells and their products. In: Hunt JS, ed. *Immunobiology of reproduction. Serono Symposium, USA*. New York: Springer-Verlag, 1994:23–33.

186. **Somigliana E, Vigano P, Vignali M.** Endometriosis and unexplained recurrent spontaneous abortion: pathologic states resulting from aberrant modulation of natural killer cell function? *Hum Reprod Update* 1999;5:40–51.

187. **Eblen AC, Gercel-Taylor C, Shields LB, et al.** Alterations in humoral immune responses associated with recurrent pregnancy loss. *Fertil Steril* 2000;73:305–313.

188. **Galli M, Comfurius P, Maassen C, et al.** Anticardiolipin antibodies (ACA) directed not to cardiolipin but to plasma protein cofactor. *Lancet* 1990;335:1544–1547.

189. **McNeil HP, Simpson RJ, Chesterman CN, et al.** Anti-phospholipid antibodies are directed against a complex antigen that includes a lipid-binding inhibitor of coagulation: beta 2-glycoprotein I (apolipoprotein H). *Proc Natl Acad Sci U S A* 1990;87:4120–4124.

190. **Harris EN.** Syndrome of the black swan. *Br J Rheumatol* 1986;26:324–326.

191. **Wilson WA, Gharavi AE, Koike T, et al.** International consensus statement on preliminary classification criteria for definite antiphospholipid syndrome: report of an international workshop. *Arthritis Rheum* 1999;42:1309–1311.

192. **Lockshin MD, Sammaritano LR, Schwartzman S.** Validation of the Sapporo criteria for antiphospholipid syndrome. *Arthritis Rheum* 2000;43:440–443.

193. **Out HJ, Bruinse HW, Christians CML, et al.** A prospective, controlled multicenter study of the obstetric risks of pregnant women with antiphosphalipid antibodies. *Br J Obstet Gynaecol* 1992;167:26–32.

194. **Kutteh WH, Lyda EC, Abraham SM, et al.** Association of anticardiolipin antibodies and pregnancy loss in women with systemic lupus erythematosus. *Fertil Steril* 1993;60:449–455.

195. **Harris EN, Asherson RA, Gharavi AE, et al.** Thrombocytopenia in SLE and related disorders: association with anticardiolipin antibodies. *Br J Haematol* 1985;59:227–230.

196. **Cariou R, Tobelem G, Soria C, et al.** Inhibition of protein C activation by endothelial cells in the presence of lupus anticoagulant. *N Engl J Med* 1986;314:1193–1194.

197. **Freyssinet JM, Wiesel ML, Gauchy J, et al.** An IgM lupus anticoagulant that neutralizes the enhancing effect of phospholipid on purified endothelial thrombomodulin activity: a mechanism for thrombosis. *Thromb Haemost* 1986;55:309–313.

198. **Lyden TW, NG AK, Rote NJ.** Modulation of phosphatidyl-serine epitope expression on BeWo cells during forskolin treatment. *Am J Reprod Immunol* 1992;27:24.

199. **Chamley LW, Allen JL, Johnson PM.** Synthesis of beta2 glycoprotein 1 by the human placenta. *Placenta* 1997;18:403–410.

200. **Lee RM, Emlen W, Scott JR, et al.** Anti-beta2-glycoprotein I antibodies in women with recurrent spontaneous abortion, unexplained fetal death, and antiphospholipid syndrome. *Am J Obstet Gynecol* 1999;181:642–648.

201. **Ogasawara M, Aoki K, Katano K, et al.** Prevalence of autoantibodies in patients with recurrent miscarriage. *Am J Reprod Immunol* 1999;41:86–90.

202. **Bulla R, de Guarrini F, Pausa M, et al.** Inhibition of trophoblast adhesion to endothelial cells by the sera of women with recurrent spontaneous abortion. *Am J Reprod Immunol* 1999;42:116–123.

203. **Rand JH, Wu X-X, Andree HAM, et al.** Pregnancy loss in the antiphospholipid-antibody syndrome—a possible thrombogenic mechanism. *N Engl J Med* 1997;337:154–160.

204. **Rand JH, Wu X-X, Guller S, et al.** Reduction of annexin-V (placental anticoagulant protein-I) on placental villi of women with antiphospholipid antibodies and recurrent spontaneous abortion. *Am J Obstet Gynecol* 1994;171:1566–1572.

205. **Hanly JG, Gladman DD, Rose TH, et al.** Lupus pregnancy: a prospective study of placental changes. *Arthritis Rheum* 1988;31:358–366.

206. **Lockshin MD, Druzin ML, Goei S, et al.** Antibody to cardiolipin as a predictor of fetal distress or death in pregnant patients with systemic lupus erythematosus. *N Engl J Med* 1985;313:152–156.

207. **Esplin MS, Branch DW, Silver R, et al.** Thyroid autoantibodies are not associated with recurrent pregnancy loss. *Am J Obstet Gynecol* 1998;179:1583–1586.

208. **Bussen SS, Steck T.** Thyroid antibodies and their relation to antithrombin antibodies, anticardiolipin antibodies and lupus anticoagulant in women with recurrent spontaneous abortion (antithyroid, anticardiolipin and antithrombin autoantibodies and lupus anticoagulant in habitual aborters). *Eur J Obstet Gynecol Reprod Biol* 1997;74:139–143.

209. **Rushworth FH, Backos M, Rai R, et al.** Prospective pregnancy outcome in untreated recurrent miscarriers with thyroid autoantibodies. *Hum Reprod* 2000;15:1637–1639.

210. **Rocklin RE, Kitzmiller JL, Garvey MR.** Maternal-fetal relation: further characterization of an immunologic blocking factor that develops during pregnancy. *Clin Immunol Immunopathol* 1982;22:305–315.

211. **Amos DB, Kostyn DD.** HLA: a central immunological agency of man. *Adv Hum Genet* 1980;10:137–141.

212. **Coulam CB.** Immunological tests in the evaluation of reproductive disorders: a critical review. *Am J Obstet Gynecol* 1992;167:1844–1851.

213. **Beer AE, Quebbeman JF, Ayers JW, et al.** Major histocompatibility complex antigens, maternal and paternal immune responses and chronic habitual abortion in humans. *Am J Obstet Gynecol* 1981;141:987–999.

214. **McIntyre JA, Faulk WP.** Recurrent spontaneous abortion in human pregnancy: results of immunogenetical, cellular and humoral tests. *Am J Reprod Immunol* 1983;4:165–170.

215. **Ober CL, Martin AO, Simpson JL, et al.** Shared HLA antigens and reproductive performance among Hutterites. *Am J Hum Genet* 1983;35:994–1004.

216. **Ober C, Hyslop T, Elias S, et al.** Human leukocyte antigen matching and fetal loss: results of a 10 year prospective study. *Hum Reprod* 1998;13:33–38.

217. **McIntyre JA, Faulk WP, Verhulst ST, et al.** Human trophoblast-lymphocyte cross-reactive (TLX) antigens define a new alloantigen system. *Science* 1983;222:1135–1137.

218. **Purcell DF, McKenzie IF, Lublin DM, et al.** The human cell surface glycoproteins Hu Ly-M5, membrane co-factor protein (MCP) of the complement system, and trophoblast leukocyte common (TLX) antigen are CD46. *Immunology* 1990;70:155–161.

219. **Rodger C.** Lack of a requirement for a maternal humoral immune response to establish and maintain successful allogenic pregnancy. *Transplantation* 1985;40:372–375.

220. **Vuorela P, Carpen O, Tulppala M, et al.** VEGF, its receptor and the tie receptors in recurrent pregnancy loss. *Mol Hum Reprod* 2000;6:276–282.

221. **Lessey, BA.** Endometrial integrins and the establishment of uterine receptivity. *Hum Reprod* 1998;13[Suppl]:247–258; discussion, 259–261.

222. **Alpin JD, Hey NA, Li TC.** MUC1 as a cell surface and secretory component of endometrial epithelia: reduced levels in recurrent miscarriage. *Am J Reprod Immunol* 1996;35:261–266.

223. **Gaffuri B, Airoldi L, DiBlasio AM, et al.** Unexplained habitual abortion is associated with a reduced endometrial release of soluble intercellular adhesion molecule-1 in the luteal phase of the cycle. *Eur J Endocrinol* 2000;142:477–480.

224. **Lea RG, al-Sharekh N, Tulppala M, et al.** The immunolocalization of bcl-2 at the maternal-fetal interface in healthy and failing pregnancies. *Hum Reprod* 1997;12;153–158.

225. **Polifka JE, Friedmann JM.** Environmental toxins and recurrent pregnancy loss. *Infert Reprod Med Clin North Am* 1991;2:195–213.

226. **Sharara FI, Seifer DB, Flaws JA.** Environmental toxicants and female reproduction. *Fertil Steril* 1998;70:613–622.

227. **Valanis B, Vollmer WM, Steele P.** Occupational exposure to antineoplastic agents: self-reported miscarriages and stillbirths among nurses and pharmacists. *J Occup Environ Med* 1999;41:632–638.

228. **Xu X, Cho SI, Sammel M, You L, et al.** Association of petrochemical exposure with spontaneous abortion. *J Occup Environ Med* 1998;33:31–36.

229. **Gerhard I, Waibel S, Daniel V, et al.** Impact of heavy metals on hormonal and immunological factors in women with repeated miscarriages. *Hum Reprod Update* 1998;4:301–309.

230. **Schnorr TM, Grajewski BA, Hornung RW, et al.** Video display terminals and the risk of spontaneous abortions. *N Engl J Med* 1991;324:727–733.

231. **Cone JE, Vaughan LM, Huete A, et al.** Reproductive health outcomes among female flight attendants: an exploratory study. *J Occup Environ Med* 1998;40:210–216.

232. **Naeye RL.** Coitus and associated amniotic-fluid infections. *N Engl J Med* 1979;301:1198–1200.

233. **Kwki T, Ylikorkala O.** Coitus during pregnancy is not related to bacterial vaginosis or preterm birth. *Am J Obstet Gynecol* 1993;169:1130–1134.

234. **Parazzini F, Tozzi L, Chatenoud L, et al.** Alcohol and risk of spontaneous abortion. *Hum Reprod* 1994;9:1950–1953.

235. **Abel EL.** Maternal alcohol consumption and spontaneous abortion. *Alcohol* 1997;32:211–219.

236. **Windham GC, Von Behren J, Fenster L, et al.** Moderate maternal alcohol consumption and risk of spontaneous abortion. *Epidemiology* 1997;8:509–514.

237. **Ness RB, Grisso JA, Hirschinger N, et al.** Cocaine and tobacco use and the risk of spontaneous abortion. *N Engl J Med* 1999;340:333–339.

238. **Cnattingius S, Signorello LB, Anneren G, et al.** Caffeine intake and the risk of first-trimester spontaneous abortion. *N Engl J Med* 2000;343:1839–1845.

239. **Kline J, Levin B, Kinney A, et al.** Cigarette smoking and spontaneous abortion of known karyotype: precise data but uncertain inferences. *Am J Epidemiol* 1995;141:417–427.

240. **Hedin LW, Janson PO.** Domestic violence during pregnancy: the prevalence of physical injuries, substance use, abortions, and miscarriage. *Acta Obstet Gynecol Scand* 2000;79:625–630.

241. **Mills JL, Holmes LB, Aarons JH, et al.** Moderate caffeine use and the risk of spontaneous abortion and intrauterine growth retardation. *JAMA* 1993;269:593–597.

242. **Boue J, Bove A, Laser P.** Retrospective and prospective epidemiologic studies of 1,500 karyotyped spontaneous abortions. *Teratology* 1975;11:11–26.

243. **Stein Z.** Early fetal loss. *Birth Defects* 1981;17:95–111.

244. **Hook EB, Warburton D.** The distribution of chromosomal genotypes associated with Turner's syndrome: live birth prevalence rates and evidence for administered fetal mortality and severity in genotypes associated with structural X abnormalities of mosaicism. *Hum Genet* 1983;64:24–27.

245. **Miller JF, Williamson E, Glue J, et al.** Fetal loss after implantation: a prospective study. *Lancet* 1980;2:554–556.

246. **Boue J, Boue A.** Increased frequency of chromosomal anomalies in abortions after induced ovulation. *Lancet* 1973;7804:679–680.

247. **Trout SW, Seifer DB.** Do women with unexplained recurrent pregnancy loss have higher day 3 serum FSH and estradiol levels? *Fertil Steril* 2000;74:335–337.

248. **Hofmann GE, Khoury J, Thie J.** Recurrent pregnancy loss and diminished ovarian reserve. *Fertil Steril* 2000;74:1192–1195.

249. **Watson H, Kiddy DS, Hamilton-Fairley D, et al.** Hypersecretion of luteinizing hormone and ovarian steroids in women with recurrent early miscarriage. *Hum Reprod* 1993;8:829–833.

250. **Ogasawara M, Aoki K, Katano K, et al.** Activated partial thromboplastin time is a predictive parameter for further miscarriages in cases of recurrent fetal loss. *Fertil Steril* 1998;70:1081–1084.

251. **Aoki K, Kajiura S, Matsumoto Y, et al.** Preconceptional natural-killer-cell activity as a predictor of miscarriage. *Lancet* 1995;345:1340–1342.

252. **Emmer PM, Nelen WL, Steegers EA, et al.** Peripheral natural killer cell cytotoxicity and CD56(pos)CD16(pos) cells increase during early pregnancy in women with a history of recurrent spontaneous abortion. *Hum Reprod* 2000;15:1163–1169.

253. **Yetman DL, Kutteh WH.** Antiphospholipid antibody panels and recurrent pregnancy loss: prevalence of anticardiolipin antibodies compared with other antiphospholipid antibodies. *Fertil Steril* 1996;66:540–546.

254. **Branch DW, Silver R, Pierangeli S, et al.** Antiphospholipid antibodies other than lupus anticoagulant and anticardiolipin antibodies in women with recurrent pregnancy loss, fertile controls, and antiphospholipid syndrome. *Obstet Gynecol* 1997;89:549–555.

255. **Gris JC, Quere I, Sanmarco M, et al.** Antiphospholipid and antiprotein syndromes in non-thrombotis, non-autoimmune women with unexplained recurrent primary early foetal loss. The Nimes Obstetricians and Haematologists Study—NOHA. *Thromb Haemost* 2000;84:228–236.

256. **Mavragani CP, Ionnidis JP, Tzioufas AG, et al.** Recurrent pregnancy loss and autoantibody profile in autoimmune diseases. *Rheumatology* 1999;38:1228–1233.

257. **Chambers JC, McGregor A, Jean-Marie J, et al.** Acute hyperhomocysteinaemia and endothelial dysfunction. *Lancet* 1998;351:36–37.

258. **Fedele L, Acaia B, Parazzini F, et al.** Ectopic pregnancy and recurrent spontaneous abortion: two associated reproductive failures. *Obstet Gynecol* 1989;73:206–208.

259. **Coulam CB, Wagenknecht D, McIntyre JA, et al.** Occurrence of other reproductive failures among women with recurrent spontaneous abortion. *Am J Reprod Immunol* 1991;25:96–98.

260. **Acaia B, Parazzini F, La Vecchia C, et al.** Increased frequency of complete hydatidiform mole in women with repeated abortion. *Gynecol Oncol* 1988;31:310–314.

261. **Hughes N, Hamilton EF, Tulandi T.** Obstetric outcome in women after multiple spontaneous abortions. *J Reprod Med* 1991;36:165–166.

262. **Martius JA, Steck T, Oehler MK, et al.** Risk factors associated with preterm (<37 weeks) and early preterm birth (<32 weeks): univariate and multivariate analysis of 106,345 singleton births from the 1994 statewide perinatal survey of Bavaria. *Eur J Obstet Gynecol Reprod Biol* 1998;80:183–189.

263. **Lird T, Whittaker PG.** The endocrinology of early pregnancy failure. In: **Huisjes HJ, Lird T,** eds. *Early pregnancy failure.* New York: Churchill Livingstone, 1990:39–54.

264. **Westergaard JG, Teisner B, Sinosich MJ, et al.** Does ultrasound examination render biochemical tests obsolete in the predicting of early pregnancy failure? *Br J Obstet Gynaecol* 1985;92:77–83.

265. **Li TC, Spring PG, Bygrave C, et al.** The value of biochemical and ultrasound measurements in predicting pregnancy outcome in women with a history of recurrent miscarriage. *Hum Reprod* 1998;13:3525–3529.

266. **Wolf GC, Horger EO 3rd.** Indications for examination of spontaneous abortion specimens. *Am J Obstet Gynecol* 1995;173:1364–1368.

267. **Tachdjian G, Aboura A, Lapierre JM, et al.** Cytogenetic analysis from DNA by comparative genomic hybridization. *Ann Genet* 2000;43:147–154.

268. **Bell KA, Van Deerlin PG, Feinberg RF, et al.** Diagnosis of aneuploidy in archival, paraffin-embedded pregnancy-loss tissues by comparative genomic hybridization. *Fertil Steril* 2001;75:374–379.

269. **Bianchi DW, Flint AF, Pizzimenti MF, et al.** Isolation of fetal DNA from nucleated erythrocytes in maternal blood. *Proc Natl Acad Sci U S A* 1990;87:3279–3283.

270. **Vidal F, Rubio C, Simon C, et al.** Is there a place for preimplantation genetic screening in recurrent miscarriage patients? *J Reprod Fertil Suppl* 2000;55:143–146.

271. **Vidal F, Gimenez C, Rubio C, et al.** FISH preimplantation diagnosis of chromosome aneuploidy in recurrent pregnancy wastage. *J Assist Reprod Genet* 1998;15:310–313.

272. **Pellicer A, Rubio C, Vidal F, et al.** In vitro fertilization plus preimplantation genetic diagnosis in patients with recurrent miscarriage: an analysis of chromosome abnormalities in human preimplantation embryos. *Fertil Steril* 1999;71:1033–1039.

273. **Remohi J, Gallardo E, Levy M, et al.** Oocyte donation in women with recurrent pregnancy loss. *Hum Reprod* 1996;11:2048–2051.

274. **Garbin O, Ohl J, Bettahar-Lebugle K, et al.** Hysteroscopic metroplasty in diethylstilboestrol-exposed and hypoplastic uterus: a report on 24 cases. *Hum Reprod* 1998;13:2751–2755.

275. **Querlen D, Brasme TL, Parmentier D.** Ultrasound-guided transcervical metroplasty. *Fertil Steril* 1990;54:995–998.

276. **Serden SP.** Diagnostic hysteroscopy to evaluate the cause of abnormal uterine bleeding. *Obstet Gynecol Clin North Am* 2000;27:277–286.

277. **Karande VC, Gleicher N.** Resection of uterine septum using gynaecoradiological techniques. *Hum Reprod* 1999;14:1226–1229.

278. **Fedele L, Bianchi S.** Habitual abortion: endocrinological aspects. *Curr Opin Obstet Gynecol* 1995;7:351–356.

279. **Raziel A, Herman A, Strassburger D, et al.** The outcome of in vitro fertilization in unexplained habitual aborters concurrent with secondary infertility. *Fertil Steril* 1997;67:88–92.

280. **Karamardin LM, Grimes DA.** Luteal phase deficiency: effect of treatment on pregnancy rates. *Am J Obstet Gynecol* 1992;167:1391–1398.

281. **Clifford K, Rai R, Watson H, et al.** Does suppressing luteinising hormone secretion reduce the miscarriage rate? Results of a randomised controlled trial. *BMJ* 1996;312:1508–1511.

282. **Glueck CJ, Awadalla SG, Phillips H, et al.** Polycystic ovary syndrome, infertility, familial thrombophilia, familial hypofibrinolysis, recurrent loss of in vitro fertilized embryos, and miscarriage. *Fertil Steril* 2000;74:394–397.

283. **Hill JA.** Immunotherapy for recurrent pregnancy loss: "standard of care or buyer beware." *J Soc Gynecol Invest* 1997;4:267–273.

284. **Stovall DW, Van Voorhis BJ.** Immunologic tests and treatments in patients with unexplained infertility, IVF-ET, and recurrent pregnancy loss. *Clin Obstet Gynecol* 1999;42:979–1000.

285. **Kutteh WH.** Recurrent pregnancy loss: an update. *Curr Opin Obstet Gynecol* 1999;11:435–439.

286. **Agrawal S, Pandey MK, Pandey A.** Prevalence of MLR blocking antibodies before and after immunotherapy. *J Hematother Stem Cell Res* 2000;9:257–262.

287. **Prigoshin N, Tambutti ML, Redal MA, et al.** Microchimerism and blocking activity in women with recurrent spontaneous abortion (RSA) after alloimmunization with the partner's lymphocytes. *J Reprod Immunol* 1999;44:41–54.

288. **Ito K, Tanaka T, Tsutsumi N, et al.** Possible mechanisms of immunotherapy for maintaining pregnancy in recurrent spontaneous aborters: analysis of anti-idiotypic antibodies directed against autologous T-cell receptors. *Hum Reprod* 1999;14:650–655.

289. **Gafter U, Sredni B, Segal J, et al.** Suppressed cell-mediated immunity and monocyte and natural killer cell activity following allogenic immunization of women with spontaneous recurrent abortion. *J Clin Immunol* 1997;17:408–419.

290. **Mowbray JF, Gibbings C, Liddell H, et al.** Controlled trial of treatment of recurrent spontaneous abortion by immunostimulation with paternal cells. *Lancet* 1985;1:941–943.

291. **Fraser EJ, Grimes DA, Schulz KF.** Immunization as therapy for recurrent spontaneous abortion: a review and meta-analysis. *Obstet Gynecol* 1993;82:854–859.

292. **The Recurrent Miscarriage Immunotherapy Trialist Group.** Worldwide collaborative observational study and meta-analysis of allogenic leukocyte immunotherapy for recurrent spontaneous abortion. *Am J Reprod Immunol* 1994;32:55–72.

293. **Daya S, Gunby J.** The effectiveness of allogeneic leukocyte immunization in unexplained primary recurrent spontaneous abortion. Recurrent Miscarriage Immunotherapy Trialists Group. *Am J Reprod Immunol* 1994;32:294–302.

294. **Ober C, Karrison T, Odem RR, et al.** Mononuclear-cell immunization in prevention of recurrent miscarriages: a randomized trial. *Lancet* 1999;354:365–369.

295. **Hill JA, Anderson DJ.** Blood transfusions for recurrent abortion? Is the treatment worse than the disease? *Fertil Steril* 1986;46:152–153.

296. **Hormeyr GJ, Jaffe MI, Bezwoda WR, et al.** Immunologic investigation of recurrent pregnancy loss and consequences of immunization with husbands leukocytes. *Fertil Steril* 1987;48:681–684.

297. **Katz I, Fisch B, Amit S, et al.** Cutaneous graft-versus host-like reaction after paternal lymphocyte immunization for prevention of recurrent abortion. *Fertil Steril* 1992;57:927–929.

298. **Christiansen OB, Mathiesen O, Husth M, et al.** Placebo controlled trial of active immunization with third party leukocytes in recurrent miscarriage. *Acta Obstet Gynecol Scand* 1994;73:261–268.

299. **Johnson PM, Ramsden GH.** Recurrent miscarriage. *Baillieres Clin Immunol Allergy* 1992;2:607–624.

300. **Coulam CB, Stern JJ.** Seminal plasma treatment of recurrent spontaneous abortion. In: Dondero F, Johnson PM, eds. *Reproductive immunology. Serono Symposia 97.* New York: Raven Press, 1993:205–216.

301. **Thaler CJ.** Immunologic role for seminal plasma in insemination and pregnancy. *Am J Reprod Immunol* 1989;21:147.

302. **Samuelsson A, Towers TL, Ravetch JV.** Anti-inflammatory activity of IVIG mediated through the inhibitory Fc receptor. *Science* 2001;291:484–486.

303. **Mollnes TE, Hogasen K, De Carolis C, et al.** High-dose intravenous immunoglobulin treatment activates complement in vivo. *Scand J Immunol* 1998;48:312–317.

304. **Jerzak M, Gorski A, Jerzak M, et al.** Intravenous immunoglobulin therapy influences T cell adhesion to extracellular matrix in women with a history of recurrent spontaneous abortion. *Am J Reprod Immunol Microbiol* 2000;44:336–441.

305. **Dwyer JM.** Manipulating the immune system with immunoglobulin. *N Engl J Med* 1992;326:107–116.

306. **Müeller-Eckhart G, Huni O, Poltrin B.** IVIG to prevent recurrent spontaneous abortion. *Lancet* 1991;1:424–425.

307. **Stricker RB, Steinleitner A, Bookoff CN, et al.** Successful treatment of immunologic abortion with low-dose intravenous immunoglobulin. *Fertil Steril* 2000;73:536–540.

308. **Jablonowska B, Selbing A, Palfi M, et al.** Prevention of recurrent spontaneous abortion by intravenous immunoglobulin: a double-blind placebo-controlled study. *Hum Reprod* 1999;14:838–841.

309. **Daya S, Gunby J, Porter F, et al.** Critical analysis of intravenous immunoglobulin therapy for recurrent miscarriage. *Hum Reprod Update* 1999;5:475–482.

310. **Stephenson MD, Dreher K, Houlihan E, et al.** Prevention of unexplained recurrent spontaneous abortion using intravenous immunoglobulin: a prospective, randomized, double-blinded, placebo-controlled trial. *Am J Reprod Immunol* 1998;39:82–88.

311. **Christiansen OB.** Intravenous immunoglobulin in the prevention of recurrent spontaneous abortion: the European experience. *Am J Reprod Immunol* 1998;39:77–81.

312. **Perino A, Vassiliadis A, Vucetich A, et al.** Short-term therapy for recurrent abortion using intravenous immunoglobulins: results of a double-blind placebo-controlled Italian study. *Hum Reprod* 1997;12:2388–2392.

313. **Coulam CB, Krysa L, Stern JJ, et al.** Intravenous immunoglobulin for treatment of recurrent pregnancy loss. *Am J Reprod Immunol* 1995;34:333–337.

314. **Vaquero E, Valensise H, Menghini S, et al.** Pregnancy outcome in recurrent spontaneous abortion associated with antiphospholipid antibodies: a comparative study of intravenous immunoglobulin versus prednisone plus low-dose aspirin. *Am J Reprod Immunol Microbiol* 2001;45:174–179.

315. **Harris EN, Pierangeli SS.** Utilization of intravenous immunoglobulin therapy to treat recurrent pregnancy loss in the antiphospholipid syndrome: a review. *Scand J Rheumatol Suppl* 1998;107:97–102.

316. **Thornton CA, Ballow M.** Safety of intravenous immunoglobulin. *Arch Neurol* 1993;50:135–136.

317. **Polgar K, Hill JA.** Progesterone inhibits in vitro embryotoxic factor production in women with recurrent spontaneous abortion. *Proc Soc Gynecol Invest* 1994;41:22–26.

318. **Choi BC, Polgar K, Xiao L, et al.** Progesterone inhibits in vitro embryotoxic Th1 cytokine production to trophoblast in women with recurrent pregnancy loss. *Hum Reprod* 2000;15[Suppl 1]:46–59.

319. **Ferro D, Quintarelli C, Russo G, et al.** Successful removal of antiphospholipid antibodies using repeated plasma exchanges and prednisone. *Clin Exp Rheumatol* 1989;7:103–104.

320. **Lubbe WF, Butler WS, Palmer SJ, et al.** Fetal survival after prednisone suppression of maternal lupus-anticoagulant. *Lancet* 1983;1:1361–1363.

321. **Laskin CA, Bombardier C, Hannah ME, et al.** Prednisone and aspirin in women with autoantibodies unexplained recurrent fetal loss. *N Engl J Med* 1997;337:148–153.

322. **Ermel LD, Marshburn PB, Kutteh WH.** Interaction of heparin with antiphospholipid antibodies (APA) from the sera of women with recurrent pregnancy loss. *Am J Reprod Immunol* 1995;33:14–20.

323. **Kutteh WH.** Antiphospholipid antibody-associated recurrent pregnancy loss: treatment with heparin and low-dose aspirin is superior to aspirin alone. *Am J Obstet Gynecol* 1996;174:1584–1589.

324. **Lima F, Khamashta MA, Buchanan NM, et al.** A study of sixty pregnancies in patients with the antiphospholipid syndrome. *Clin Exp Rheumatol* 1996;14:131–136.

325. **Rai R, Cohen H, Dave M, et al.** Randomised controlled trial of aspirin and aspirin plus heparin in pregnant women with recurrent miscarriage associated with phospholipid antibodies (or antiphospholipid antibodies). *BMJ* 1997;314:253–257.

326. **Bijsterveld NR, Hettiarachchi R, Peters R, et al.** Low-molecular weight heparins in venous and arterial thrombotic disease. *Thromb Haemost* 1999;82[Suppl 1]:139–147.

327. **Bates SM, Ginsberg JS.** Anticoagulation in pregnancy. *Pharm Pract Manag Q* 1999;19:51–60.

328. **Bar J, Cohen-Sacher B, Hod M, et al.** Low-molecular-weight heparin for thrombophilia in pregnant women. *Int J Gynaecol Obstet* 2000;69:209–213.

329. **Younis JS, Ohel G, Brenner B, et al.** The effect of thromboprophylaxis on pregnancy outcome in patients with recurrent pregnancy loss associated with factor V Leiden mutation. *Br J Obstet Gynecol* 2000;107:415–419.

330. **Brenner B, Hoffman R, Blumenfeld Z, et al.** Gestational outcome in thrombophilic women with recurrent pregnancy loss treated with enoxaparin. *Thromb Haemost* 2000;83:693–697.

331. **Pattison NS, Chamley LW, Birdsall M, et al.** Does aspirin have a role in improving pregnancy outcome for women with the antiphospholipid syndrome? A randomized controlled trial. *Am J Obstet Gynecol* 2000;183:1008–1012.

332. **Rai R, Backos M, Baxter N, et al.** Recurrent miscarriage—an aspirin a day? *Hum Reprod* 2000;15:2220–2223.

333. **Richards EM, Makris M, Preston FE.** The successful use of protein C concentrate during pregnancy in a patient with type 1 protein C deficiency, previous thrombosis, and recurrent fetal loss. *Br J Haematol* 1997;98:660–661.

334. **Milad MP, Klock SC, Moses S, et al.** Stress and anxiety do not result in pregnancy wastage. *Hum Reprod* 1998;13:2296–2300.

335. **Bergant AM, Reinstadler K, Moncayo HE, et al.** Spontaneous abortion and psychomatics: a prospective study on the impact of psychological factors as a cause for recurrent spontaneous abortion. *Hum Reprod* 1997;12:1106–1110.

336. **Neugebauer R, Kline J, Shrout P, et al.** Major depressive disorder in the 6 months after miscarriage. *JAMA* 1997;277:383–388.

337. **Tho PT, Byrd JR, McDonough PG.** Etiologic and subsequent reproductive performance of 100 couples with a prior history of habitual abortion. *Fertil Steril* 1979;32:389–395.

338. **Harger JH, Archer DF, Marchese SG, et al.** Etiology of recurrent pregnancy loss and outcome of subsequent pregnancies. *Obstet Gynecol* 1983;62:574–581.

339. **Vlaadneren W, Treffers PE.** Prognosis of subsequent pregnancies after recurrent spontaneous abortion in first trimester. *BMJ* 1987;295;92–93.

340. **March CM, Israel R.** Hysteroscopic management of recurrent abortion caused by septate uterus; with discussion. *Am J Obstet Gynecol* 1987;156:834–842.

341. **DeCherney AH, Russell JB, Graebe RA, et al.** Resectoscopic management of müllerian fusion defects. *Fertil Steril* 1986;45:726.

342. **Lubbe WF, Liggins GC.** Role of lupus anticoagulant and autoimmunity in recurrent pregnancy loss. *Semin Reprod Endocrinol* 1988;6:161–190.

343. **Branch DW, Silver RM, Blackwell JL, et al.** Outcome of treated pregnancies in women with antiphospholipid syndrome: an update of the Utah experience. *Obstet Gynecol* 1992;80:614–620.

344. **Pratt DE, Kaberlein G, Dudkiewicz A, et al.** The association of antithyroid antibodies in euthyroid nonpregnant women with recurrent first trimester abortions in the next pregnancy. *Fertil Steril* 1993;60:1001–1005.

345. **Laufer MR, Ecker JL, Hill JA.** Pregnancy outcome following ultrasound detected fetal cardiac activity in women with history of multiple spontaneous abortion. *J Soc Gynecol Invest* 1994;1:138–142.

346. **Rai RS, Clifford K, Cohen H, et al.** High prospective fetal loss rate in untreated pregnancies of women with recurrent miscarriage and antiphospholipid antibodies. *Hum Reprod* 1995;10:3301–3304.

347. **Brigham SA, Conlon C, Farquharson RG.** A longitudinal study of pregnancy outcome following idiopathic recurrent miscarriage. *Hum Reprod* 1999;14:2868–2871.

29 Menopause

William W. Hurd
Lawrence S. Amesse
John F. Randolph, Jr.

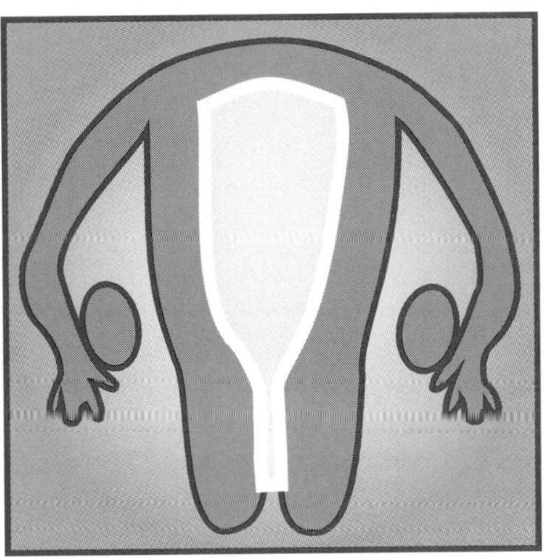

More than 30% of the female population of the United States is postmenopausal, and this percentage is increasing (1). Despite the universality of "the change of life," the importance of its medical and psychological implications has only recently been appreciated. Each woman's response to menopause may be different; as a result, management must be individualized to each woman's needs.

Menopause is defined as the permanent cessation of menses for 1 year and is physiologically correlated with the decline in estrogen secretion resulting from the loss of follicular function. It is the most identifiable event of the perimenopausal period. The years immediately preceding and the decades afterward, however, are of far greater clinical significance. The perimenopausal period encompasses the time before, during, and after menopause. This period of hormonal transition is sometimes known as the menopausal transition period. Perimenopause usually begins in the mid- to late 40s; it often is insidious and uneventful but may be abrupt and symptomatic. Symptoms that begin with the menopausal transition usually continue into the postmenopausal period.

The postmenopausal period is associated with a significant increase in the incidence of age-related medical conditions. Some of these conditions, specifically osteoporosis and cardiovascular disease, are related to estrogen deficiency as well. For this reason, hormone replacement therapy should be a part of gynecologic care of postmenopausal women.

Perimenopausal Phases

The perimenopause is the period surrounding the menopause—before, during, and after. The length of this period varies, but it is usually considered to last approximately 7 years, beginning with the decline in ovarian function in a woman's 40s, and continuing until she has not had a menstrual period for 1 year.

Menopausal Transition

The period that precedes menopause is characterized by a varying degree of somatic changes that reflect alterations in the normal functioning of the ovary. Early recognition of the symptoms and the use of appropriate screening tests can minimize the impact of this potentially disruptive period. In many cases, however, it is difficult to differentiate stress-related symptoms from those associated with decreasing levels of estrogen. For this reason, both stress and relative estrogen deficiency should be considered when managing problems associated with the menopausal transition.

In some women, menstrual irregularity is the most significant symptom of the menopausal transition (2). Because abnormal bleeding is one of the most common symptoms of uterine problems, menstrual irregularity during the perimenopause should be evaluated carefully. Often uterine bleeding associated with this transition period is secondary to normal physiologic estrogen fluctuations rather than underlying pathology and may be treated medically (3).

Menopause

The cessation of menses resulting from the loss of ovarian function is a natural event, a part of the normal process of aging. Menopause is associated with the cessation of menses resulting from the loss of ovarian follicular function, and should be characterized as an event rather than a period of time. **The time of menopause is determined genetically and occurs at a median age of 51 years** (2–4). It is related neither to race nor nutritional status. However, menopause occurs earlier in nulliparous women, in those who smoke tobacco, and in some women who have had hysterectomies (4,5).

With the depletion of ovarian follicles that are able to respond to gonadotropins, follicular development and cyclic estrogen production cease. The ovaries, however, continue indefinitely to produce small amounts of androgens postmenopausally. Traditionally, menopause has been diagnosed retrospectively based on the lack of menstrual periods. With the advent of modern laboratory testing, menopause may now be more precisely defined as amenorrhea, with signs of hypoestrogenemia, and an elevated serum follicle-stimulating hormone (FSH) level of greater than 40 IU/L. Menopause can also be diagnosed on the basis of subjective symptoms, such as hot flashes, or on the basis of provocative studies such as the progesterone withdrawal test. Hot flashes and other acute symptoms associated with the perimenopausal period often become more intense near menopause when the levels of circulating estrogen suddenly drop. These symptoms are especially intense in patients who experience premature ovarian failure or surgical menopause, which are accompanied by gradual drops in circulating estrogens.

Postmenopausal Period

The postmenopausal period is one of relative ovarian quiescence following menopause. Given the current lifespan of women in the United States, this period can comprise more than one-third of the average woman's life. During this prolonged period, women are vulnerable to conditions caused by estrogen deficiency. Even though the long-term health impact of estrogen deficiency may be similar to that of thyroid or adrenal disorders, relatively little attention has been paid to this problem until recently. For this reason hormone replacement therapy is one of the primary concerns of many postmenopausal women's health care.

Reasons for this lack of attention are many. Health problems associated with estrogen deficiency tend to be chronic rather than acute. For example, osteoporosis is not clinically apparent until decades after menopause, when unfortunately it becomes harder to treat. Second, the impact of estrogen deficiency on cardiovascular disease is often confused with age-related changes. Third, because of the peripheral conversion of both ovarian and adrenal androgens to estrogen, the loss of ovarian function does not result in an absolute estrogen deficiency. As a result, some women are less affected by estrogen deficiency than others.

Premature Ovarian Failure

As previously stated, loss of ovarian function is usually a gradual process that occurs over a number of years and culminates in menopause. Ovarian function is lost earlier and more suddenly than expected in some women as a result of natural causes, chemotherapy, or surgery.

Premature ovarian failure is defined as menopause occurring spontaneously before 40 years of age (6). Because of the relatively young age and the unexpected nature of the event, both psychological and hormonal support may be necessary. Although most practitioners are not adequately prepared to offer comprehensive psychological support, asking appropriate questions and making support services available can be helpful. The possibility of associated endocrine abnormalities should also be considered in women who develop premature ovarian failure. This is further addressed in Chapter 25.

In more than 40% of women who have hysterectomies, both ovaries are removed (3). As a result, many of these women undergo surgical menopause at a significantly younger age than do their counterparts who undergo natural menopause. The relatively young age of these women and the abrupt onset of associated symptoms create special problems (7).

The most obvious problem with surgical menopause is the acute onset of hot flashes (8). After several months, these hot flashes may be followed by signs of vaginal atrophy. In addition, long-term surgical menopause has been associated with significantly higher risk for both osteoporosis and cardiovascular disease than has natural menopause (9,10). The risk of osteoporosis can be decreased with estrogen replacement therapy. Because long-term hormone replacement may expose women to other types of risks, the relative risks and benefits of oophorectomy in conjunction with estrogen replacement therapy should be thoroughly discussed with any woman considering bilateral oophorectomy at the time of hysterectomy.

Hormonal Changes

Changes in hormone production and metabolism occur gradually during the menopausal transition. After almost 4 decades of cyclic production of estrogen and progesterone, the ovaries decrease their production of estrogen and will eventually cease any cyclic activity.

Menopausal Transition

During the menopausal transition, ovarian follicles become increasingly resistant to FSH stimulation even though levels of estradiol remain relatively constant. This process is most clearly demonstrated even before the onset of clinically apparent perimenopause by the relative resistance to gonadotropins in women undergoing ovulation stimulation for *in vitro* fertilization. In the average woman younger than 30 years, levels of estradiol higher than 1,000 pg/ml are easily attainable using stimulation of approximately 225 IU of FSH per day. In contrast, most women older than 40 years rarely attain estradiol levels this high, despite stimulation with up to 3 times as much gonadotropin per day. This degree of ovarian resistance to stimulation may explain the hot flashes experienced by some women, despite what appear to be normal levels of estradiol. It suggests that hot flashes may be the result of gonadotropin surges related to fluctuating estradiol levels or low levels of other ovarian hormones such as inhibin.

Progesterone is produced almost exclusively by granulosa cells and is highest in the mid-luteal phase. During the menopausal transition, ovulation becomes less frequent, with a decrease in overall progesterone production (11). In some women ovulation continues to occur, but the luteal levels of progesterone are lower than those observed in younger women (12).

Menopause

Near the time of the menopause, the levels of hormones, the way they are produced, and their roles change. Hormones most affected are those produced by the ovaries and include estrogen, progesterone, and androgens.

Estrogen

Even though the amount of estrogen secreted by the postmenopausal ovary is negligible, postmenopausal women continue to have measurable amounts of both estrone and estradiol (13). Prior to menopause, estradiol levels range from 50 to 300 pg/ml. However, even with cessation of ovarian function levels of estradiol may remain as high as 100 pg/ml (14). The answer to this apparent paradox lies in the ability of peripheral tissue to aromatize adrenal and ovarian androgens.

Androstenedione is produced by the adrenal and ovary and is aromatized to estrogen primarily by muscle and adipose tissue (15,16). Obese women have an increased level of circulating estrogens, and the unopposed estrogen places them at an increased risk for endometrial cancer (17). In contrast, thin women have a decreased level of circulating estrogens and are at an increased risk for developing osteoporosis (18). Surprisingly, the increased levels of estrogen often seen in obese women do not appear to protect them from acute menopausal symptoms; however, the higher levels do provide some skeletal protection (19).

Progesterone

After menopause, progesterone production ceases (20). The absence of cyclic changes in progesterone is usually associated with the absence of premenstrual symptoms (21). Decreased progesterone levels affect organs that are responsive to gonadal hormones, such as endometrium and breasts. During the reproductive years, progesterone protects the endometrium from excess estrogen stimulation by directly regulating estrogen receptors. It also exerts a direct intranuclear effect by inhibiting the trophic effects of estrogen on the endometrium (22).

Because circulating levels of estrogen can remain high enough to stimulate the endometrium both pre- and postmenopausally, unopposed stimulation of the endometrium may be a relatively common problem just prior to and after menopause (12). This probably explains the higher risk of endometrial hyperplasia and cancer found during this time (23).

Breast tissue also is known to be extremely sensitive to gonadal hormones. Although the relationship is less clear with breast than with endometrial tissue, unopposed stimulation of the breast ductal epithelium by estrogen in the absence of progesterone may play a role in the development of breast cancer (24). There are data that suggest that the use of combined estrogen and progestin replacement therapy may decrease the risk of breast cancer; however, a more recent large study does not support this conclusion (25).

Androgens

The third class of steroids produced by the ovaries is androgens, most notably testosterone and androstenedione. The role of ovaries in androgen production, especially postmenopausally, has only recently been appreciated (11).

Prior to menopause, the ovaries produce approximately 50% of the circulating androstenedione and 25% of the testosterone produced by a woman's body. Circulating concentration of testosterone in women is less than one-tenth that in men (0.50 ng/ml versus 6 ng/ml) and the amount of biologically active testosterone in women is only one-third that in men. In part, this is accounted for by the amount of sex hormone–binding globulin, which is relatively higher in women (30 to 90 nmol/L) than men (10 to 50 nmol/L) (26).

After menopause, total androgen production decreases, mainly because ovarian production decreases but also because adrenal production decreases (11). The circulating levels of androstenedione and testosterone after menopause are approximately 0.53 and 0.23 ng/ml, respectively (27). After ovulation has ceased, the ovaries are responsible for 20% of the androstenedione and 40% of the testosterone as a result of continued gonadotropin stimulation of ovarian stromal cells (28). Although oophorectomy also results in a marked reduction in androgen production, the significance of these decreases will remain uncertain until the physiologic role of these hormones becomes more fully elucidated (12).

Patient Concerns about Menopause

A broad spectrum of emotions often is associated with hormonal and bodily changes characteristic of this period (29,30). A patient's response to menopause may be affected by factors such as lifestyle and regulation of the aging process. The loss of fertility and menstrual function that accompany natural or surgical menopause may have an impact on a woman's sense of well-being. The physician should be sensitive to the potentially significant emotional distress faced by women entering menopause and be prepared to offer psychological support. Subtle signs of the menopausal transition may be overlooked, because a woman may be hesitant to report unusual and potential hormonally related symptoms. Unless asked about directly, these symptoms often go undetected and result in a delay in diagnosis and treatment.

Loss of Childbearing Capacity

The effect of the loss of the ability to have children may depend on many factors, including the role childbearing has played in a woman's life. For some women in whom childbearing and childrearing have been a major source of status and self-esteem, the loss of fertility may cause great distress (30). For other women who have delayed childbearing for various reasons and are now unable to become pregnant, menopausal symptoms may represent tangible evidence of their inability to have children. One study suggests, however, that single and childless women are less likely to be depressed than their parous counterparts (31).

Loss of Youth

Regardless of the effect of the loss of childbearing capacity, the distress produced by the loss of youth symbolized by menopause may be subtle yet disturbing (29). In our society, youth is highly prized whereas maturity often is not; thus, tangible evidence of aging may be traumatic. The degree to which this may affect a woman may be related to the value she places on personal appearance. Aging may not be important to many women, but the possibility that this may cause anxiety or depression should be considered.

Skin Changes

The apparent acceleration of the skin changes associated with aging, especially after menopause, is a concern for many women. Evidence suggests that estrogen deficiency may play a role in these changes and that estrogen therapy may help to maintain skin thickness (32). Mechanisms underlying this effect are not completely understood but appear related to the ability of estrogen to both prevent and restore age-related skin collagen (33,34). Certainly, estrogen therapy cannot completely prevent the effects of aging on skin, nor can it counteract the effects of environmental stresses on skin, such as sun exposure and cigarette smoking.

Changes in Mood and Behavior

Depression

Depression is a particularly common problem for women and older patients. It accounts for more than 20% of visits of those who seek medical care (35). Although it is a widely held belief that depression is increased during the perimenopausal period, studies have failed to show a relationship between clinical depression and hormonal status (36). This finding would suggest that many psychiatric symptoms occurring during this period may be more related to psychosocial events such as changes in relationships with children, marital status, and other life events than to changes in hormonal status (37).

Anxiety and Irritability

Many women report an increased level of anxiety and irritability during the perimenopausal period; thus, these symptoms have become a prominent part of what is sometimes termed the *climacteric syndrome* (38). These feelings can be exacerbated by sleep deprivation as a result of vasomotor symptoms. Although the incidence of overt psychiatric disorders may not be increased, these complaints become more frequent following menopause. A popular notion is that anxiety and irritability associated with menopause are the result of estrogen deficiency (30). Multiple studies, however, have found no evidence to suggest that psychological symptoms experienced during the menopausal transition are related to estrogen changes (39,40). Increased anxiety and irritability associated with the perimenopausal period are more clearly associated with psychosocial factors than with estrogen status (41). It is important not only to investigate and treat the constellation of symptoms associated with the menopausal transition, but also to realize that psychological intervention may be helpful for some women.

Decreased Libido

A major concern for some women is a decrease in libido or sexual satisfaction that may occur with natural or surgical menopause. Sexual activity, however, remains relatively stable in menopausal women (42). However, only one-half of menopausal women report being sexually active (43). This may be related to a decrease in the number of available male partners in an aging population (1).

Vaginal changes associated with menopause may also contribute to decreased sexual satisfaction. Approximately one-third of postmenopausal woman not taking estrogen supplements will experience vaginal atrophy (44). Discomforts resulting from a lack of vaginal lubrication can also lead to dyspareunia. Atrophy can be treated easily with oral or vaginal estrogen therapy. Vaginal lubricants, especially those that are water soluble, are specifically useful for vaginal dryness.

The role androgens play in libido before and after menopause is uncertain. Although testosterone levels have been reported to be lower in postmenopausal than in premenopausal women, circulating concentrations do not change at menopause, and free testosterone levels might actually increase for several months before they decrease to levels lower than those of premenopausal women (45). In contrast, there is a marked drop in androgen levels following oophorectomy (11). In men, the relationship of androgens to libido is well established. For this reason, some clinicians have advocated androgen therapy in women experiencing decreased libido (46). In women, however, the decrease in circulating androgens following menopause has not been shown to consistently alter libido. Available evidence suggests that sexual satisfaction among postmenopausal women is not decreased over time, making treatment with androgens controversial (47).

Menopausal Transition

Beginning at the age of 40 years, routine health maintenance should include screening for problems related to hormonal changes. Questions concerning changes in menstrual function, abnormal bleeding, hot flashes, sleep disturbances, and sexual function should be asked routinely.

Abnormal Bleeding

Menstrual irregularity occurs in more than one-half of all women during the menopausal transition (48). **Uterine bleeding can be irregular, heavy, or prolonged. In most cases, this bleeding is related to anovulatory cycles. This disruption of normal**

menstrual flow has been attributed to a gradual decrease in the number of normally functioning follicles and is reflected by a gradual increase in early follicular-phase FSH levels (49).

Although anovulation is one of the more common causes of abnormal uterine bleeding, pregnancy must always be considered. There are numerous reports of pregnancies in women in their late 40s who did not consider themselves fertile. In these women, abnormal bleeding may be the first indicator of an unexpected pregnancy.

Endometrial cancer should be suspected in any perimenopausal women with abnormal uterine bleeding. After menopause, the overall incidence of endometrial cancer is approximately 0.1% of women per year, but in women with abnormal uterine bleeding, it is about 10% (50–53). This risk is increased at least fivefold in women with a history of unopposed estrogen use (52,53) and decreased by more than two-thirds in women taking a combination of estrogen and a progestin (50).

Malignant precursors such as complex endometrial hyperplasia become more common during the menopausal transition. Because early diagnosis is the most effective way to improve a woman's prognosis, perimenopausal women with abnormal uterine bleeding should undergo an endometrial biopsy to exclude a malignant condition. Other causes that should be considered when a woman experiences abnormal uterine bleeding include cervical cancer, polyps, or leiomyomata.

Evaluation

The goal of evaluation of abnormal uterine bleeding is to achieve the greatest accuracy with the least risk and expense for the patient. In the past, when few diagnostic options were available, this condition was routinely managed with inpatient uterine curettage (54). However, with the development of less invasive office procedures and more accurate outpatient surgical approaches, uterine curettage without hysteroscopy is seldom done (Fig. 29.1).

Vaginal Ultrasonography

With the advent of newer diagnostic modalities, vaginal ultrasonography has become an established first step in the evaluation of perimenopausal bleeding. In premenopausal women, vaginal ultrasonography is extremely useful for identifying leiomyomata and endometrial asymmetry suggestive of endometrial polyps. When combined with saline injection, sonohysterography can accurately visualize polyps and other focal intrauterine lesions (55).

In postmenopausal women, vaginal ultrasonography, with or without saline injection, is even more helpful than in premenopausal women. An endometrial stripe <5 mm thick has been shown to be associated with an extremely low risk of endometrial hyperplasia or cancer (55–57). A thickened or asymmetric endometrial lining or an obvious intrauterine lesion is an indication for more thorough evaluation (Fig. 29.1) (55). Likewise, refractory abnormal uterine bleeding in a high-risk patient is an indication for endometrial biopsy even in the presence of reassuring ultrasonographic findings.

Endometrial Sampling

The importance of the endometrial biopsy cannot be overemphasized for the pre- or postmenopausal woman with abnormal uterine bleeding. It is well accepted that endometrial biopsy performed in the office is just as accurate as dilation and curettage and certainly more economical (54). Although vaginal ultrasonography has changed the way patients with abnormal uterine bleeding are evaluated, endometrial biopsy continues to be the most accurate screening method available for these patients. **Dilation and curettage in the operating room with adequate anesthesia should be reserved for patients with abnormal endometrial biopsies or for conditions that preclude performing an office biopsy, such as cervical stenosis.**

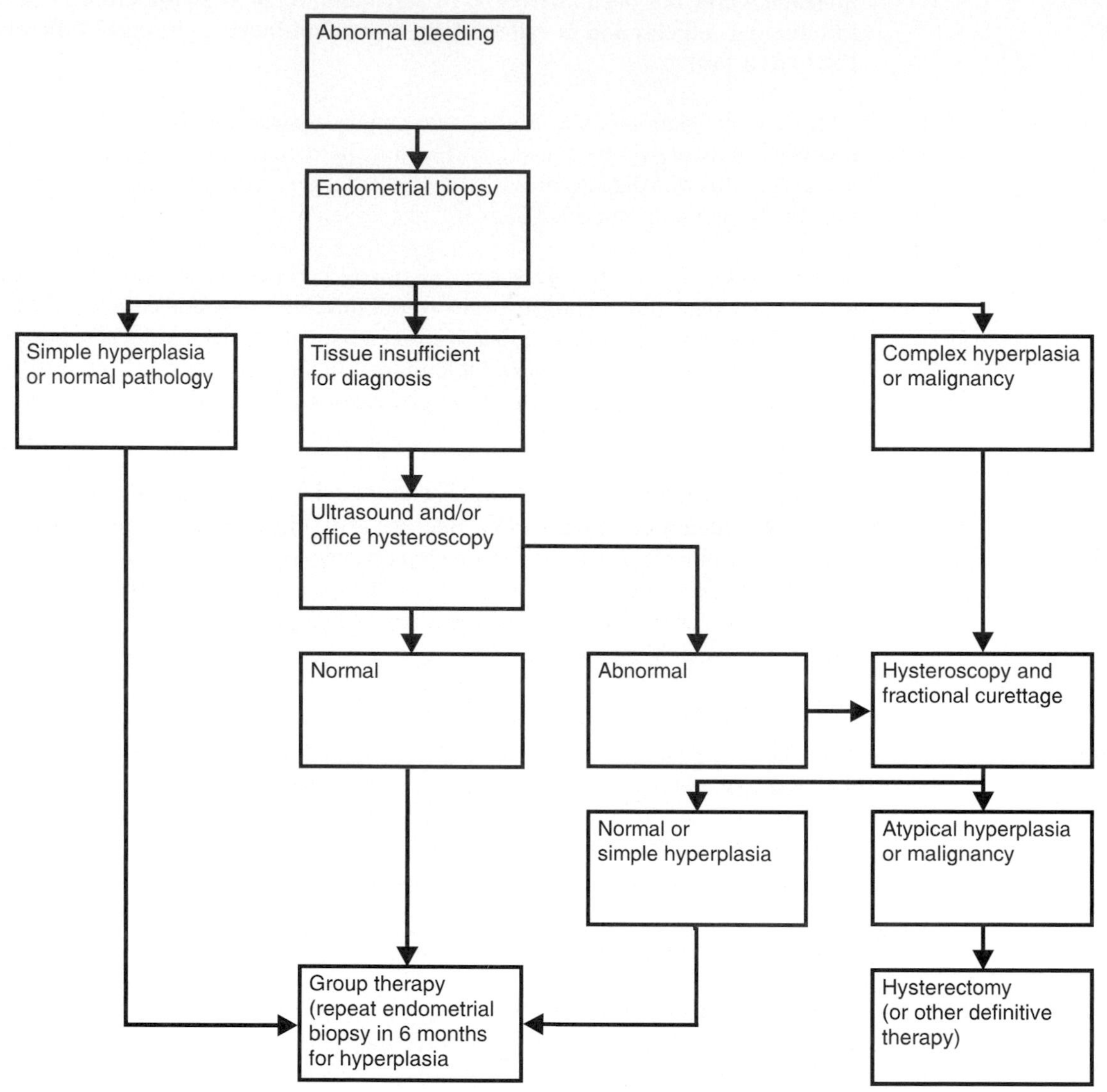

Figure 29.1 Management of postmenopausal abnormal uterine bleeding.

Hysteroscopy with Uterine Curettage

The addition of hysteroscopy to uterine curettage has greatly improved diagnostic accuracy in the evaluation of focal intrauterine lesions (58,59). It allows for visual inspection of the endometrial cavity and gives the physician the opportunity to perform directed biopsies (59). Endometrial polyps or submucosal leiomyomas can easily be identified by hysteroscopy. As with many high-technology approaches, however, hysteroscopy requires appropriate training and equipment to ensure patient safety. If hysteroscopy is unavailable, dilation and curettage remains an accepted method for evaluation of the endometrium (54) (see Chapter 13).

Treatment

Treatment of perimenopausal abnormal uterine bleeding may be either hormonal or surgical, depending on the patient's symptoms and diagnosis. Because anovulation is one of the most common causes of abnormal uterine bleeding during menopause, hormonal therapy is the first approach after the presence of intrauterine pathology has been excluded.

Hormonal Therapy

Oral Contraceptives In low-risk premenopausal women with hormone-related symptoms, modern low-dose (0.35 mg *ethinyl estradiol*) oral contraceptives offer many advantages with minimal risk (60). New formulations contain as little as 20 mg of *ethinyl estradiol* and 1 mg of *desogestrel*. In addition to preventing undesired pregnancies, these formulations are associated with a high degree of menstrual regularity and can be used to treat symptoms associated with relative estrogen deficiency. The use of oral contraceptives until menopause has been found to be safe in women with no risk factors for cardiovascular disease (61).

Before starting the administration of oral contraceptives in this age group, patients should be free of the following risk factors: hypertension, hypercholesterolemia, cigarette smoking, previous thromboembolic disorders, cerebral vascular disease, or coronary artery disease. Because the estrogen dose in these pills is approximately 4 times the dose used after the menopause, women taking this therapy should be switched to traditional estrogen therapy by 50 years of age or sooner if symptoms occur. If the estradiol level is <20 pg/ml on day 7 of the pill-free interval, it may be appropriate to switch from oral contraceptives to estrogen replacement therapy (62).

Cyclic Progestins Some women may not be candidates for oral contraceptives, because their use is contraindicated or unacceptable based on the presence of other symptoms or because of fear of complications. In these patients, alternative methods of hormonal therapy can be used. A standard approach is cyclic progestin therapy (*medroxyprogesterone* 10 mg daily for 10 days each month) to induce withdrawal bleeding and to decrease the risk of endometrial hyperplasia. It may be difficult to control abnormal uterine bleeding with cyclic progestin during the menopausal transition, because the ovaries continue to cycle intermittently. Progestin administration may be difficult to synchronize with spontaneous ovulation.

Surgical Therapy

During the menopausal transition, surgery may be required for treatment of conditions causing abnormal uterine bleeding.

Dilation and Curettage When endometrial polyps are determined to be the cause of abnormal uterine bleeding, curettage can be both therapeutic and diagnostic. Because polyps can be missed by curettage alone, it has been recommended that diagnostic hysteroscopy be performed prior to uterine curettage for abnormal uterine bleeding (58). With the exception of endometrial polyps, uterine curettage has not been shown to have any long-term benefit in the treatment of abnormal uterine bleeding.

Hysterectomy Although removal of the uterus is the most common and effective surgical treatment for abnormal uterine bleeding (63), hysterectomy is associated with a certain degree of morbidity and cost. Prior to recommending hysterectomy, an adequate preoperative evaluation must include endometrial sampling and an adequate trial of hormonal therapy to control the bleeding.

A special consideration is whether normal ovaries should be removed (see Chapter 22). It is now standard practice for postmenopausal women undergoing hysterectomy to have their ovaries removed to avoid the subsequent risk of ovarian cancer (64). Oophorectomy has been recommended in women older than 40 to 45 years for the same reason. In premenopausal women, however, there are some disadvantages to oophorectomy. First, immediate hormone replacement is necessary and may be somewhat more difficult to manage because of the sudden and precipitous drop in estrogen levels. In addition, oophorectomy results in a decrease in androgen production, which may have as yet unknown long-term effects (11). After 40 years of age, the decision to remove normal ovaries during hysterectomy should be discussed carefully and the patient should be made aware of the potential known advantages and disadvantages.

Endometrial Ablation A relatively new and potentially advantageous approach to dysfunctional uterine bleeding during the menopausal transition is endometrial ablation. This relatively minor surgical procedure involves destroying the functioning endometrium with electrical energy using a hysteroresectoscope, as discussed in Chapter 21. The risks of uterine perforation, bowel injury, and fluid overload related to the nonconducting distention media are low if the technique is used correctly (65).

In response to these problems, a nonsurgical thermal balloon endometrial ablation technique has been developed that requires a substantially lower level of technical skill (65). First reported in 1994, this method is performed by blind placement in the uterus of a single-use saline-filled balloon catheter that is warmed rapidly to cause thermal damage to the endometrium. Most patients report either decreased bleeding or amenorrhea, and both intraoperative and postoperative complications are uncommon.

The risk of uterine malignancy after any type of endometrial ablation procedure remains uncertain. The concern is that as the injured endometrial lining remodels, glandular tissue may be buried under scar tissue. Theoretically, this situation could delay uterine bleeding, which is the earliest sign of endometrial cancer. However, subsequent endometrial cancer after endometrial ablation has been reported only in women who had preexisting endometrial hyperplasia (66). For this reason, a thorough fractional curettage should be performed prior to the procedure. Monthly progestin therapy could be used thereafter in an attempt to decrease the risk in these potentially anovulatory women. Until long-term data become available, women considering this therapy should be informed about the potential risk of endometrial ablation.

Menopause

Most women experience some effects of estrogen deficiency during menopause. Other symptoms often associated with menopause may not be directly related to estrogen deficiency but rather are multifactorial or the results of aging. Effects can range from short-term discomfort to long-term changes that can have a profound effect on a woman's health. Both short-term and chronic effects respond to hormone replacement therapy.

Diagnosis of Estrogen Deficiency

The determination of ovarian function is based primarily on clinical criteria. If a woman's body is producing enough hormones to sustain regular menstruation, her estrogen level is presumed to be sufficient to protect against osteoporosis and heart disease. In the years prior to menopause, many women experience symptoms of estrogen deficiency due to declining ovarian function even while they are having relatively regular menses. These symptoms typically begin with a break in the regular pattern of ovulatory cycles and often include irregular vaginal bleeding, hot flashes, night sweats, mood swings, vaginal dryness, insomnia, heart palpitations, headache, and fatigue. Even though measurable levels of circulating hormones are still present, hormone replacement therapy in these women can be extremely helpful in controlling symptoms (67).

If a woman who is almost 50 years old stops menstruating completely, a presumptive diagnosis of estrogen insufficiency can be made. However, because chronic anovulation is common during this time and can also cause amenorrhea, a progestin challenge test is frequently used as a bioassay of estrogen status (68). If a nonpregnant woman has amenorrhea but no other symptom of estrogen deficiency, administration of *medroxyprogesterone* (10 mg orally for 10 days) will produce withdrawal bleeding in women who have levels of circulating estrogen adequate to produce endometrial proliferation.

Estradiol

In women who have amenorrhea along with other symptoms of estrogen deficiency or in whom progestin withdrawal bleeding does not occur, measurement of serum estradiol levels can be helpful. In a menstruating woman, normal estradiol levels range from 40 to 300 pg/ml. In an oligoovulatory woman, an estradiol level of 30 pg/ml usually indicates some degree of residual ovarian function. Women over 70 years of age occasionally have levels this high, presumably as a result of peripheral conversion (30). For this reason, **the absolute estradiol level should not be the deciding factor when considering hormone replacement therapy.**

During the menopausal transition, relative ovarian resistance with fluctuating estrogen secretion may result in hot flashes and related symptoms despite relatively normal serum estradiol levels. Because many of the symptoms of the menopausal transition are central nervous system in origin, treatment is sometimes indicated for symptoms alone and should not be withheld simply because the serum estradiol levels are in the normal range.

Follicle-stimulating Hormone

The most consistent finding in the menopausal transition is an elevation of serum FSH levels. In fertile menstruating women, FSH on cycle day 3 should be 5 to 10 IU/L, with normally functioning ovaries (69). Elevated FSH levels (10 to 25 IU/L) suggest relative ovarian resistance consistent with the menopausal transition, even if estradiol levels are in the normal range. Physiologically, this is believed to be the result of decreased inhibin production by the ovarian follicles during the last decade of menstrual function. FSH levels >40 IU/L are consistent with complete cessation of ovarian function. However, ovarian function can wax and wane over several years, and levels can fluctuate accordingly. Therefore, women with amenorrhea and FSH >40 IU/L may resume menstruating for a short time in the future and occasionally may achieve pregnancy (70).

Luteinizing Hormone

Evaluation of luteinizing hormone (LH) levels appears to be of somewhat less value than other hormone assessments during the menopausal transition. Prior to menopause, LH levels are usually in the range of 5 to 20 IU/L. Although LH levels increase during the menopausal transition in a manner similar to those of FSH, LH is also significantly elevated during the midcycle surge and in cases of chronic anovulation. Because individuals rarely may have amenorrhea as a result of gonadotropin-secreting pituitary adenomas, it is reasonable to check both LH and FSH in women, especially young patients, with apparent loss of ovarian function (71).

Symptoms

Amenorrhea

The most obvious symptom of cessation of cyclic ovarian function is prolonged amenorrhea. The cessation of menstruation indicates that the amount of estrogen produced by the ovaries is no longer enough to promote endometrial proliferation, and the absence of cyclic progesterone production is accompanied by the absence of withdrawal bleeding.

This is an advantageous situation for several reasons. First, the sometimes-disabling discomfort and anemia suffered by many women as a result of cyclic bleeding is no longer a problem. Second, any abnormal bleeding that may occur later serves as a warning for potential malignancy and is obvious to both the patient and her physician.

Unfortunately, hormone replacement therapy results in vaginal bleeding in most women (72). Not only is this effect a common reason for discontinuing hormone replacement therapy, but bleeding that would normally be interpreted as a warning sign is attributed to the hormone therapy, potentially delaying diagnosis of a malignancy.

Hot Flashes

The classic symptom associated with estrogen deficiency is the hot flash, also known as a *hot flush*. This symptom is described as "recurrent, transient periods of flushing, sweating, and a sensation of heat, often accompanied by palpitations, feelings of anxiety, and sometimes followed by chills" (73). The entire episode usually lasts no more than 1 to 3 minutes and may recur as many as 30 times per day, although 5 to 10 times per day is probably more common (8). Hot flashes are experienced by at least one-half of all women during natural menopause and by even more women after surgical menopause (73,74).

Although most women do not report these events as particularly disturbing, as many as 25% complain of severe or frequent hot flashes, especially after surgical menopause. In these cases, hot flashes may be accompanied by fatigue, nervousness, anxiety, irritability, depression, and memory loss (75). These sensations may result in part from hot flashes that occur at night, referred to as *night sweats,* which are believed to exert their effect by the interruption of sleep patterns. Early in the menopausal transition, vasomotor instability may manifest as an intermittent sleep disturbance in the absence of obvious hot flashes.

Physiologically, hot flashes correspond to marked, episodic increases in the frequency and intensity of gonadotropin-releasing hormone (GnRH) pulses from the hypothalamus. Although it has not been firmly established, it is believed that these symptoms are not the result of increased GnRH secretion. Instead, the increased pulsatile activity is a marker for the same central disturbance of the body temperature regulation center that is responsible for the hot flashes (76).

Estrogen replacement therapy results in the resolution of hot flashes in most women in a matter of days. In some women, especially after oophorectomy, a higher dose of estrogen is commonly needed. In the case of women without risk factors for cardiovascular disease, low-dose oral contraceptives can be used with excellent results. Alternatively, the daily estrogen dose can be increased stepwise to as high as the equivalent of 2.5 mg of *conjugated estrogens* to resolve persistent hot flashes. The estrogen dose should be tapered slowly over a period of months to no more than 1.25 mg of *conjugated estrogen* per day, because the risk of cardiovascular disease actually may be increased in women taking larger doses (77).

In women for whom hormone replacement is contraindicated, multiple alternative treatments for hot flashes have been developed. Somewhat effective alternatives may be progestins such as *medroxyprogesterone* (10 to 30 mg daily orally) (78) or *megestrol acetate* (20 to 40 mg daily orally) (79). If either of these progestins results in intolerable side effects, the use of alternative progestins may be considered, although few data exist regarding their efficacy.

In addition to the progestins, other nonsteroidal treatments for hot flashes have been developed. One of the best studied is the α_2-adrenergic agonist, *clonidine.* This drug probably works through both central and peripheral mechanisms and can be given either orally (0.05 mg twice daily) or by transdermal patch (0.1 mg weekly) (80).

In the past, night sweats were treated with a formulation that contained a combination of *phenobarbital, ergotamine,* and *belladonna.* However, this combination has a marked sedative effect and potentially can be habit forming. In addition, controlled studies show little long-term effectiveness of this treatment (81). For these reasons, this formulation is not currently recommended as a treatment for hot flashes.

Many women have mild hot flashes that they do not feel require therapy. The patients can be advised that, without treatment, the symptoms usually subside slowly over 3 to 5 years (73).

Sleep Disturbances

Changes in sleep patterns occur in both sexes with age. However, during the menopausal transition, many women experience increasing sleep difficulties and insomnia that appear to be related to estrogen deficiency (38). Hot flashes may disrupt sleep and sleep patterns, a problem that may be markedly improved by hormone therapy (82).

Long-term Health Problems Associated with the Menopause

Low estrogen levels have a cumulative effect on many tissues. Prolonged estrogen deficiency may contribute to the development of potentially reversible conditions, such as genitourinary atrophy, or more life-threatening and irreversible conditions, such as cardiovascular disease and osteoporosis. Prevention and early detection remain the cornerstones of health maintenance in this age group.

Vaginal and Urinary Tract Changes

Vaginal tissue and the tissues of the urethra and bladder base are known to be estrogen sensitive. Within 4 to 5 years of menopause, approximately one-third of women who are not taking hormone therapy develop symptomatic atrophy (83). Vaginal symptoms include dryness, dyspareunia, and recurrent vaginal infections. Fortunately, these symptoms are reversible with estrogen therapy (84).

Urinary symptoms may include dysuria, urgency, and recurrent urinary tract infections (44). In addition, genuine stress urinary incontinence may be related to estrogen deficiency. Urethral shortening associated with postmenopausal atrophic changes may result in urinary incontinence. Estrogen therapy may improve or cure stress urinary incontinence in more than 50% of treated women, presumably by exerting a direct effect on urethral mucosa (85). A trial of hormone therapy should be undertaken prior to a surgical approach in any woman with vaginal atrophy.

Central Nervous System

Estrogen deficiency appears to have effects on the central nervous system that have only recently been appreciated. Perimenopausal women often experience difficulty concentrating and loss of short-term memory. These symptoms have been attributed to either the effects of aging alone or subtle sleep deprivation associated with hot flashes (86). Estrogen appears to have direct effects on mental function, and replacement therapy has been shown to improve both short-term and long-term memory in postmenopausal women (87,88).

One of the most intriguing areas of research is the potential role of estrogen therapy in the prevention or treatment of Alzheimer's disease. Evidence suggests that the risk of developing Alzheimer's disease can be decreased by estrogen therapy (89,90), but prospective trials to verify this are lacking. Although the precise role of estrogen deficiency in Alzheimer's disease has yet to be defined, the implications of this finding for the aging population are readily apparent.

Cardiovascular Disease

Cardiovascular disease, including coronary artery disease and cerebrovascular disease, continues to be the leading public health problem in this country. Combined, these diseases account for more than 50% of all deaths in women over 50 years of age (91).

Cardiovascular disease has been associated with multiple causes, the most important of which may be age. The risk of cardiovascular disease increases for men and women throughout their lifetimes (91). Although the risk of death from coronary artery disease is at least 3 times as great for men as for women before menopause, the relative risk for women increases significantly after menopause. It is essential to be aware of preventable risk factors for cardiovascular disease and to encourage women to minimize these risk factors.

One of the most pervasive and treatable risk factors after the menopause is hypoestrogenemia. In the past, it was believed that age alone explained the increased risk of cardiovascular disease observed after menopause (92). Recent data have indicated that estrogen deficiency significantly increases the risk of cardiovascular disease and that this risk may be reduced by hormone replacement therapy (93). Postmenopausal women taking estrogen replacement therapy have less than one-half the risk of either myocardial infarction or stroke as women who are not taking estrogen therapy (77,91,94). However, long-term prospective trials of the cardiovascular benefits and risks of estrogen replacement therapy are lacking. This potentially substantial but controversial benefit of estrogen therapy should be made known to patients, especially those who may be reluctant to take estrogens for other reasons. On the other hand, a short-term trial suggested no overall decrease in mortality and an increase in early venous thrombotic events in women with preexisting cardiovascular disease (95).

Although hypoestrogenemia is apparently a major contributing factor to cardiovascular disease in women, other risk factors that are amenable to change may be equally important. Probably the most significant risk factors are hypertension and cigarette smoking (55). Studies suggest that hypertension increases the risk of cardiovascular disease by 10-fold and cigarette smoking increases the risk by at least threefold (96). Other risk factors include diabetes mellitus, hypercholesterolemia, and a sedentary lifestyle. To decrease cardiovascular disease in postmenopausal women, screening for these risk factors must be performed and lifestyle changes must be recommended.

Osteoporosis

The association between both natural and surgical menopause and osteoporosis has been clearly established. By definition, osteoporosis is the reduction in the quantity of bone. Because this definition may be too broad to be clinically useful, some authors have narrowed the definition to include only bone loss that has progressed to a point that specific parts of the skeleton are so thin that they have an enhanced susceptibility to fractures or that fractures are actually present (97). The degree of cortical and trabecular bone loss necessary to meet this criterion is uncertain in those who have not yet had a bone fracture. The numbers of elderly women who have osteoporosis-related crush fractures of spinal vertebrae or fractures of either the radius or the neck of the femur have reached epidemic proportions (98). With the aging of the population, the problem is likely to increase.

Although the rate of bone loss significantly increases at the time of menopause, the maximal incidence of osteoporosis-related fractures appears to occur several decades later. It is estimated that more than 30% of all women older than 90 years will experience hip fractures (99), and approximately 20% of these women will die within 3 months, most commonly from complications related to prolonged immobilization (100). By the time signs of osteoporosis become apparent, treatment is difficult.

Pathophysiology

The cause of osteoporosis is multifactorial. The primary factors associated with osteoporosis include heredity, age, estrogen status, and dietary calcium intake.

Age is the most important factor associated with bone loss (101). All women begin losing bone mass in their early 30s, and this loss continues throughout their lives. Before menopause, the rate of loss is less than 1% of total bone tissue per year. After menopause, the rate of bone loss increases to as high as 5% per year in estrogen-deficient women. Evidence suggests that this may be related to the gradual decrease in growth hormone levels associated with age (102).

Heredity plays a role primarily by determining the peak bone mass that a woman will attain during her life and the subsequent rate of bone loss. On average, African American women have a higher bone mass than white women, and this may explain the low risk of osteoporosis-related fractures observed in African Americans (103). A family history of osteoporosis is a strong risk factor (104).

Table 29.1. Radiographic Techniques to Screen for Osteoporosis

Test	*Advantages*	*Disadvantages*
Standard radiograph	Lowest total radiation exposure	Detects only bone losses of >30–40%
Single photon absorptiometry, hand	Does not closely correlate with vertebral bone density	—
Dual-energy x-ray absorptiometry	Measures radius, hip, and spine	—
Quantitative computed tomography	—	Highest total radiation exposure

A third factor associated with bone loss is estrogen status. For women not taking hormone replacement, bone loss after menopause is accelerated to a rate of 3% to 5% per year (105). This loss is most rapid during the first 5 years after menopause, when up to 20% of the expected lifetime loss from the femoral neck may occur (106). Depending on the age at surgery, surgical menopause poses a higher risk than natural menopause because a woman experiences a longer period with low estrogen levels (107). Hypoestrogenemia has a direct effect on osteoblast function and appears to exert its adverse effects by altering calcium balance (108,109).

A fourth factor affecting bone loss is dietary calcium. Dietary intake of calcium, primarily in the form of dairy products, has been shown to be associated with decreased bone loss in premenopausal women (110). In postmenopausal women taking estrogen therapy, calcium supplementation of 1,000 mg/day appears to be sufficient to decrease bone loss (111). Combined with the average dietary intake of calcium in the United States of only 500 mg/day for adults (110), the total requirement of 1,500 mg/day is provided by diet plus supplementation. Calcium therapy can be given as calcium carbonate (oyster shell) tablets or as calcium citrate. Fortunately, this amount of calcium supplementation does not appear to increase the risk of kidney stones (112). However, it may be associated with gastrointestinal complaints such as constipation or increased flatus.

Other factors that preserve bone density and decrease the risk of osteoporosis include physical activity (113) and avoidance of cigarette smoking (114). There have been no controlled studies of these factors to determine their impact on osteoporosis-related fractures in later life.

Methods for Detection

After a prolonged period of hypoestrogenemia, bone loss is only partially reversible. For these reasons, it is more practical and effective in most women to implement therapy to prevent bone loss at the time of menopause than to screen for early signs of osteoporosis.

In some women, hormone replacement therapy may be contraindicated or not desired by the patient. In these women, an alternative approach would be to screen for bone loss at set intervals and institute therapy if a defined threshold of osteopenia is reached (Table 29.1). No standard guideline for significant osteopenia has been established, but recommendations for screening have been published (115).

Hormone Replacement Therapy

Estrogen deficiency has been considered by many to be a physiologic rather than a pathologic condition, probably because ovarian failure is genetically programmed. With the increased life expectancy of women, however, the negative impact of prolonged estrogen deficiency

Table 29.2. Indications and Contraindications for Estrogen Replacement Therapy

Indications	*Contraindications*
Menopause	**Absolute**
Hot flashes	Pregnancy
Vaginal atrophy	Undiagnosed uterine bleeding
Urinary tract symptoms	Active thrombophlebitis
High risk for osteoporosis	Current gallbladder disease
Family history	Liver disease
Cigarette smoker	**Relative**
Low body weight	History of breast cancer
Radiographic evidence	History of recurrent thrombophlebitis or thromboembolic disease
High risk for cardiovascular disease	
Previous myocardial infarction or angina	
Hypertension	
Family history	
Cigarette smoker	

becomes more significant. Although estrogen deficiency is treatable, fewer than 20% of postmenopausal women take estrogen (116). Although hormone replacement therapy is not completely risk free, the health benefits appear to outweigh the risks for most women.

Benefits

Hormone replacement therapy is indicated for any woman with signs or symptoms of hypoestrogenemia (Table 29.2). Because of the health risks associated with estrogen deficiency, replacement therapy should be offered to all postmenopausal women who have no contraindications. Women with known risk factors for osteoporosis should be encouraged to consider taking estrogen to minimize their risks. Some of the benefits of estrogen are felt immediately, but the long-term benefits may not be apparent for several decades.

Hot Flashes

Relief of hot flashes is the most common reason motivating women to start and continue hormone replacement. Hot flashes may interfere with the normal sleep cycle resulting in insomnia (86) and, in severe cases, they may also interfere with concentration (73). Although oral estrogen therapy usually is effective in reducing the severity and frequency of hot flashes within a few days, patients should be advised that it might be several weeks before maximal relief is achieved.

Osteoporosis

Hormone replacement therapy helps maintain bone mass and skeletal integrity, thereby protecting against osteoporosis (117). Estrogen conserves calcium by both enhancing the efficiency of intestinal absorption and by improving renal calcium conservation (108). In addition, estrogen appears to have a direct effect on osteoclast function (109). Estrogen can effectively slow bone loss and, to a limited degree, it can reverse the bone loss associated with osteoporosis (118). For this reason, hormone replacement therapy should be initiated at menopause and should be given for a long term, although the optimal duration is unclear.

Recent evidence has suggested that progesterone also has a role in maintaining bone density (119). Progesterone appears to promote bone formation by increasing osteoblast activity, either directly or indirectly, by inhibiting the corticosteroid effect on osteoblasts. This finding supports the use of a progestin alone in women who are unable to take estrogen therapy.

Cardiovascular Disease

Estrogen replacement therapy may protect against cardiovascular disease, including coronary artery disease and stroke, although the issue has not been settled. Multiple cohort and case-control studies have suggested that estrogen decreases the risk of both myocardial infarction and stroke by 50% (76,90,93). Even when there is angiographic evidence of coronary artery disease, estrogen enhances survival (120). However, carefully controlled prospective trials to rule out the possibility of selection bias and other confounding factors must be completed to fully understand the cardiovascular benefits and risks of hormone replacement therapy.

There are several mechanisms by which estrogen could protect the heart. The most important mechanism appears to be the effect of estrogen on serum lipids and lipoproteins. Estrogen decreases circulating levels of low-density lipoproteins (121,122) and increases levels of high-density lipoproteins. Both the absolute decrease in total cholesterol and the increase in the high-density to low-density lipoprotein ratio appear to retard progression of coronary artery disease. Although these effects are attenuated by concomitant progestin use, this effect appears to decrease over time (123). It has been estimated that estrogen accounts for 20% to 50% of the total protective effect for cardiovascular disease. The degree to which progestins may diminish this effect, if any, is unknown.

Estrogen also exerts an antiarteriosclerotic effect on blood vessels (124). This appears to result, in part, from a direct effect on blood vessels that is not reversed by progestin. Estrogen appears to be an antioxidant that decreases the formation of lipid peroxidases, which may prevent arteriosclerosis by minimizing the oxidation of low-density lipoprotein cholesterol, a potent inducer of plaque formation in vessels (125).

A third beneficial effect is that of vasodilation (126). There appears to be a direct effect on blood vessel endothelial cells that results in immediate vasodilation, perhaps mediated by estrogen receptors (127).

A final beneficial effect is on coagulation. Low-dose estrogen therapy (i.e., 0.625 mg daily of *conjugated estrogens*) results in a subclinical decrease in coagulability by decreasing platelet aggregation and fibrinogen and by inhibiting plasminogen formation (128). This effect appears to be lost with higher doses of estrogen (i.e., 1.25 mg of *conjugated estrogens*). At even higher doses, equivalent to those used in oral contraceptives, there is an increase in coagulability. Therefore, doses of estrogen equivalent to 0.625 mg of *conjugated estrogens* should be used for long-term therapy.

Potential Health Risks

The risks of estrogen therapy appear to be dose related. Many of the side effects of high-dose oral contraceptives have not occurred with the lower doses of estrogen used for hormone replacement therapy. Because of the sensitivity of some tissues to estrogen, the potential risks of estrogen for postmenopausal women must be considered.

Breast Cancer

Numerous retrospective and prospective observational studies have evaluated whether exogenous estrogens in the form of either oral contraceptives or estrogen replacement therapy have an impact on the incidence of breast cancer. Although some recent meta-analyses have concluded that there is no increased risk of this malignancy among women who receive hormone replacement (129,130), others have demonstrated a significant increase in breast cancer risk that may be related to the duration of estrogen use (24,131,132). One of these studies showed a relative risk for the development of breast cancer of 1.46 in women who took postmenopausal estrogens for 5 years or longer (24). However, large prospective clinical trials are incomplete and the benefits of hormone replacement may outweigh this potential risk in some patients.

Endometrial Cancer

A well-established risk of estrogen replacement therapy is endometrial hyperplasia and endometrial cancer. Early observational studies found that women who used estrogen alone were 4 to 7 times more likely to develop endometrial cancer than women who did not (53). The simultaneous use of progestins effectively prevents this problem in most cases (133,134). However, it should be kept in mind that even women taking progestin therapy can develop endometrial cancer, especially if they have used unopposed estrogens in the past (135). Therefore, endometrial evaluation remains an important part of management for all women with irregular vaginal bleeding.

Gallbladder Disease

The risk of symptomatic gallbladder disease is increased by the use of oral contraceptives (135). In a recent questionnaire study of postmenopausal women, hormone replacement therapy doubled the risk of gallbladder disease compared with women taking no hormones (136). However, in two case-control studies, no increased risk could be appreciated (135,137).

Thrombophlebitis

There is no increased risk of thrombophlebitis associated with hormone replacement therapy, despite the well-established association with the use of oral contraceptives. With the standard doses of conjugated estrogens normally used, there is no increased risk of either venous thrombosis or pulmonary embolism in healthy women (138), although there appears to be some increased risk in women with preexisting cardiovascular disease (95). Hormone replacement therapy does not significantly alter clotting factors (139).

No study has specifically addressed the risk of recurrent thrombophlebitis for women taking estrogen. Therefore, women who have a history of thrombophlebitis should be offered hormone replacement therapy with the understanding that it is unlikely, but uncertain, that this therapy alters the risk of recurrent thrombophlebitis (140).

Hypertension

Hypertension has been one of the relative contraindications to oral contraceptives because the higher-dose formulations were found to further increase blood pressure (141). In contrast, at the dosages used for hormone replacement therapy, conjugated estrogens appear to have little effect on blood pressure (142). Because chronic hypertension is a well-established risk factor for myocardial infarction and stroke, women with this disorder should be encouraged to maintain low blood pressure levels and to consider the potential protective effect of hormone replacement therapy for cardiovascular disease.

Side Effects

Vaginal Bleeding

Any vaginal bleeding may be distressing; therefore, hormone replacement regimens associated with amenorrhea are preferable. Daily use of estrogen and cyclic use of progestin produces cyclic bleeding in most women. In an effort to avoid cyclic bleeding, the daily use of estrogen and progestin has been advocated. After several months, daily progestin therapy will result in amenorrhea in more than one-half of women with minimal risk of hyperplasia (72).

Irregular bleeding may be an early warning sign of endometrial hyperplasia or malignancy. More commonly, it is a sign of endometrial atrophy or asynchronous shedding. Because of the known association of estrogen replacement therapy with endometrial cancer, endometrial biopsy is indicated when irregular uterine bleeding occurs postmenopausally.

Breast Tenderness

Breast tenderness can occur with hormone replacement therapy (143). This effect may be related to both estrogen and progesterone stimulation of breast tissue. The symptoms of fibrocystic breast changes may be increased (143,144). The initial approach to relieving breast symptoms is to decrease the daily estrogen dose to the equivalent of 0.625 mg of *conjugated equine estrogen,* and reduce progestin to the equivalent of 2.5 mg of *medroxyprogesterone.* If this is ineffective, the type of estrogen may be changed.

Mood Changes

Progestins are known to cause mood disturbances similar to those of premenstrual syndrome, including anxiety, irritability, or depression (145,146). Because of the significant protective effect of progestins against endometrial cancer, a dose or formulation of progestin that has the fewest side effects should be sought.

Weight Gain and Water Retention

Some women are extremely sensitive to exogenous estrogens and experience symptoms such as weight gain or water retention (147). Although few data are available regarding these problems, alternative doses and formulations of both estrogen and progestins should be used to find the combination with the fewest side effects.

Special Cases

In some women, the standard approach to hormone replacement therapy may not be appropriate or sufficient. Despite the benefits of estrogen administration after menopause, for some this therapy is contraindicated (Table 29.2).

History of Breast Cancer

One of the most controversial subjects concerning hormone replacement therapy is whether a woman with a history of successfully treated breast cancer can receive estrogen. Because it appears that estrogen replacement therapy may increase the risk of breast cancer, there has been a fear that estrogen may increase the risk of recurrent breast cancer. The limited data available suggest no increased risk of recurrent breast cancer among postmenopausal estrogen users (148,149). Until more long-term data are available, estrogen should be used with caution in women with a history of breast cancer. In a woman with nonmetastatic (node-negative) estrogen receptor–negative breast cancer, particularly one who has a strong family history of osteoporosis and heart disease, the benefits of estrogen may outweigh the low theoretic risk that the hormone will predispose her to the development of recurrent cancer.

History of Endometrial Cancer

Although, theoretically, estrogen and progestin therapy should not increase the risk of recurrent endometrial cancer, there are few data regarding estrogen or progestin therapy in women who have been treated for endometrial cancer (150). Progestins have been used to treat recurrent endometrial cancer (151). One study of women successfully treated for stage I endometrial cancer revealed that a combination of estrogen and progestin therapy does not increase the risk of recurrence (152). Because of the limited information available, any woman with a history of endometrial cancer should be informed of the unknown risk of recurrence with hormone therapy.

Endometriosis

There have been anecdotal reports of recurrent endometriosis (153,154) or malignant transformation of endometriosis in women with endometriosis who take hormone replacement therapy following bilateral oophorectomy (155). Therefore, such women should be treated with continuous estrogen and progestin. In women with severe endometriosis, especially when the bowel, bladder, or ureter is involved, a hormone-free period for up to 6 months immediately after surgery may also be advisable prior to instituting combined estrogen and progestin therapy.

Liver Disease

Hormone replacement therapy has not been associated with the development of liver disease. However, estrogens are metabolized in the liver, and women with normal ovarian function and chronic liver disease are known to have significantly elevated levels of circulating estrogens (156). Likewise, normal doses of conjugated estrogens could lead to a substantially higher level of circulating estrogens than expected in these women. Therefore, hormone replacement therapy should be avoided in women with active or chronic liver disease.

Replacement Hormones and Regimens

The mainstay of hormone replacement in the absence of ovarian function is estrogen, usually with the addition of a progestin. Standard replacement therapy has consisted of concurrent estrogen and progestin in anyone with an intact uterus. Estrogen only was given to women who had had hysterectomies. Better understanding of the effects hormones have on the body has altered these classic approaches to therapy.

Types of Estrogen and Progesterone

Estrogens are available in oral and parenteral forms (Table 29.3). The most commonly prescribed oral estrogen preparation is *conjugated equine estrogen,* a combination of estrone (50%), equilin (23%), 17α-dihydroequilin (13%), and various other estrogens extracted from the urine of pregnant mares (157). This formulation has been available in the United States for more than 50 years; thus, most of the data regarding the safety and efficacy of estrogen replacement therapy have been gathered from women taking *conjugated estrogens.* Several other estrogen preparations have been developed, and data are accumulating regarding their comparable effectiveness. There is, at present, no compelling reason to recommend one preparation over others based on risks or side effects. If side effects become a problem with one formulation, a woman should be encouraged to try a different dose or estrogen formulation rather than abandon estrogen replacement altogether.

Estrogens are used orally as the first line of therapy in most women. Transdermal estradiol patches have also been found to be an effective method for hormone administration. However, there are several potential drawbacks to this approach. On a physiologic level, it is uncertain whether the same benefit is achieved in terms of reduction of cardiovascular disease risks, because changes in lipoprotein profiles do not occur as rapidly as with oral therapy (158). Transdermal patches are more expensive than oral preparations and result in some skin irritation at the site of placement in one-third of users (159). In women in whom oral estrogen therapy does not alleviate symptoms or is poorly tolerated or in whom oral preparations create a problem with hypertriglyceridemia, estrogen patches may offer some advantage (121).

A special situation is the vaginal use of conjugated estrogens. Apparently, the rate of vaginal absorption of estrogen is similar to that of oral absorption (160). This has two important implications. First, when women who have contraindications to oral estrogen therapy use vaginal estrogen for atrophic vaginitis, the amount of systemically absorbed estrogen must be considered. In these women, it is recommended that the smallest dose needed to maintain the vaginal tissue effect be used. This is usually approximately one-third of an applicator (0.2 mg) used 2 to 3 times weekly. Second, women who desire estrogen therapy but are unable to take oral estrogen can try vaginal administration. This route of administration appears to be less effective in resolving symptoms of estrogen deficiency (161) and may not alter serum lipids to the same degree as oral estrogens (162).

Progestins are also available in several different formulations (Table 29.3). The most common progestin used is *medroxyprogesterone* given orally. In the doses prescribed to protect the endometrium (2.5 to 10 mg daily), some women experience psychological effects such as anxiety, irritability, or depression (142,143). Although these problems may be associated to some degree with all progestins, few studies have evaluated them. Many progestin formulations have been evaluated for the treatment of irregular bleeding and have been found to be effective. No single progestin is clearly superior to another. If a woman has significant side

Table 29.3. Standard Dosages Used for Hormone Replacement Therapy

Hormone	*Usual Initial Dose*
Estrogens	
Oral	
Conjugated equine estrogens	0.625–1.25 mg daily
Synthetic conjugated estrogens	0.625–1.25 mg daily
Micronized estradiol	1–2 mg daily
Esterified estrogens	0.625–1.25 mg daily
Estropipate	0.625–1.25 mg daily
Ethinyl estradiol	0.02 mg daily
Topical patch	
17β-Estradiol	0.025–0.1-mg patch once or twice weekly (depending on brand)
Vaginal	
Conjugated equine estrogens	0.2–0.625 mg, 2–7 times per week
17β-Estradiol	1.0 mg, 1–3 times per week
Injectable	
Estrone	0.1–1.0 mg weekly
Estradiol cypionate in oil	1–5 mg IM weekly for 3–4 weeks
Estradiol valerate in oil	10–20 mg IM every 4 weeks
Progestins (oral)	
Medroxyprogesterone acetate	2.5–5 mg daily or 10 mg, 12–14 days/month
Norethindrone	5 mg daily
Norethindrone acetate	2.5–5 mg daily
Norgestrel	0.15 mg daily
Micronized progesterone	100–300 mg daily
Estrogen/progesterone combinations	
Oral	
Conjugated equine estrogens/ medroxyprogesterone acetate	0.625 mg/5 mg or 0.625 mg/2.5 mg daily; or 0.625 mg estrogens followed by 0.625 mg/5 mg (14 days each)
Ethinyl estradiol/norethindrone acetate	0.05 mg/1 mg daily
Estradiol/norgestimate	1 mg estradiol followed by 1 mg estradiol/0.09 mg norgestimate (3 days each)
17β-Estradiol/norethindrone acetate	1 mg/0.5 mg daily
Topical patch	
17β-Estradiol/norethindrone acetate	0.05 mg/0.25 mg daily
Estrogen/androgen combinations (oral)	
Esterified estrogen/methyl testosterone	1.25 mg/2.5 mg or 0.625 mg/1.25 mg daily
Selective estrogen receptor modulators (oral)	
Raloxifene	60 mg daily

IM, intramuscular.

effects with one progestin dose, a lower dose or a different progestin formulation should be given.

Estrogen Alone

Whenever possible, unopposed estrogen therapy should be avoided in a woman with a uterus (163). However, some women experience intolerable side effects from progestin therapy. If no dose or formulation of progestin can be found that has acceptable side effects, estrogen alone may be given. A reasonable approach is the use of the lowest effective dose of estrogen daily coupled with yearly surveillance of the endometrium by endometrial biopsy. The use of vaginal ultrasonography for endometrial surveillance may prove ultimately to be effective for this use.

Daily estrogen alone has been recommended for women after hysterectomy. Progestins have been avoided because they may partially reverse the beneficial effects of oral estrogens on serum lipids. However, the effects of progestins on lipids appear to be short term (122), and only part of the protective effect of estrogens on the cardiovascular system are derived from lipid effects. Therefore, it is controversial whether progestins should be used in combination with estrogen for these women (24).

Estrogen plus Cyclic Progesterone

Methods have been sought to avoid the risks of estrogen therapy while retaining the benefits. The addition of a progestin to estradiol minimizes the risk of endometrial hyperplasia and cancer (164). The use of 12 to 14 days per month of *medroxyprogesterone* results in a risk of endometrial cancer less than that for the population at large.

Initially, in the United States, estrogen was given for only 21 to 25 days per month and progestins were given for the last 7 to 10 days of the estrogen therapy (164), followed by a monthly period of 6 to 8 days when no hormones were given. Although this had the theoretic advantage of giving all hormonally responsive tissue a rest, no study has ever shown a benefit to this hormone-free period. However, data from Great Britain suggest that 10 days of progestin therapy per month may not be enough to prevent endometrial hyperplasia in some women (165). Therefore, when cyclic progestins are used, they should be given for 12 to 14 days per month. With 14 days of therapy (10 mg *medroxyprogesterone* or equivalent), endometrial hyperplasia is uncommon (166).

Estrogen plus Continuous Progesterone

Although cyclic progestins given at appropriate doses can protect the endometrium from hyperplasia, this approach also results in cyclic endometrial shedding and menstruation in most women (167). Vaginal bleeding is one of the most common reasons that women discontinue hormone replacement therapy (168). In addition, the relatively high dose of progestin used may result in significant symptoms in some women (142). These may include physical symptoms such as breast tenderness, fluid retention, and edema and psychological symptoms such as anxiety, irritability, or depression. Therefore, regimens using lower daily doses of progestins have been developed (164,169). **Daily progestin therapy (2.5 to 5.0 mg medroxyprogesterone acetate or equivalent) protects against endometrial hyperplasia to a degree similar to that of cyclic administration at higher doses** (Fig. 29.2) (166).

More than 50% of women who take a daily combination of estrogen and progestin will experience irregular bleeding, even after 1 year of therapy (72). This group of women may be better served by continuous estrogen accompanied by cyclic progesterone. For many women, regular bleeding may be preferable to unpredictable bleeding.

Selective Estrogen Receptor Modulators

In 1995, an estrogen receptor, ER-β, was cloned (170). This receptor displayed similar but distinct ligand-binding specificities to that of ER-α but had a different tissue distribution. With this discovery came the search for the optimal long-term female hormone replacement for women. It resulted in the development of selective estrogen-receptor modulators known as SERMS.

Raloxifene, a benzothiopene compound is of particular interest (171). This SERM binds with higher affinity to the estrogen receptor α than β. Clinically, *raloxifene* produces a effect similar to estrogen on the skeletal and cardiovascular system while behaving as an estrogen antagonist in the uterus and the breast. *Raloxifene* maintains a favorable lipid

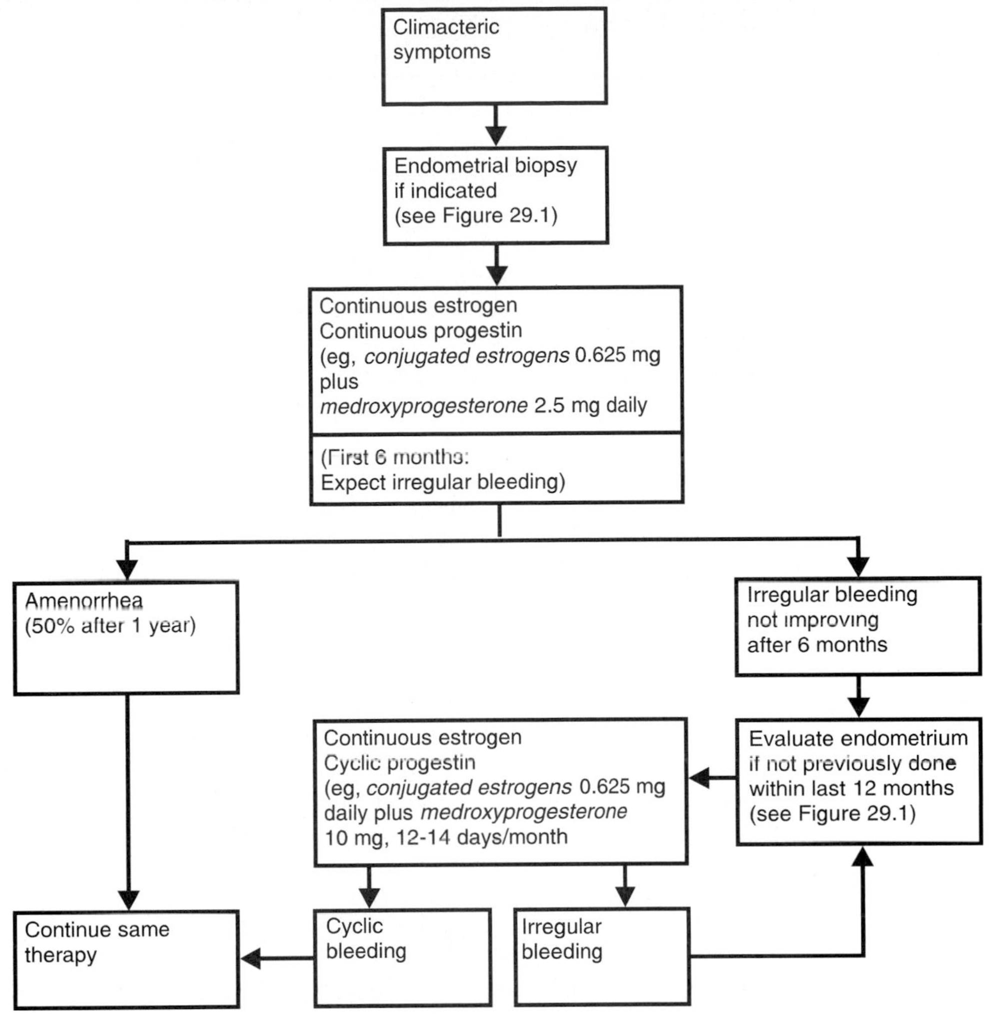

Figure 29.2 Administration of hormone replacement therapy.

profile and does not exert a proliferative effect on the endometrium. More importantly, effects on bone remodeling are similar to those of estrogen. Unfortunately, *raloxifene* does not relieve hot flushes. *Raloxifene* may be particularly useful for decreasing the risk of osteoporosis in women who are unwilling or unable to take hormone replacement therapy because of persistent benign bleeding, a history of severe endometriosis, or a high risk for primary or recurrent breast cancer (172).

Testosterone

Testosterone has been used in women, especially after surgical menopause, to alleviate specific symptoms (173). In the United States, testosterone is available in an injectable form (*testosterone enanthate* 75 to 150 mg intramuscular every month), and as a combined oral formulation (*methyltestosterone* 2.5 to 5 mg, plus conjugated or esterified estrogens 0.625 to 1.25 mg). In Great Britain, a subcutaneous *testosterone* implant is also available.

The most common indication for androgens is loss of libido (174). Studies of testosterone administration have shown mixed results in terms of libido improvement (173–178). One 6-month study of the oral preparation showed an adverse effect on the estrogen-induced changes in lipoproteins (176). Because of a lack of long-term studies of any of these agents, the effects on heart disease and other organ systems are unknown. Until studies establish a benefit for this type of therapy, androgens should be prescribed with caution. For women who experience decreased sexual responsiveness, appropriate counseling appears to be the most effective therapy (177,180).

Patient Monitoring

Continued monitoring of patients taking hormone replacement therapy relies heavily on self-reporting of symptoms and bleeding patterns. Postmenopausal women also should undergo routine assessments that should include evaluation and counseling regarding risk factors.

Symptoms

In women for whom the standard doses of estrogen do not seem to be sufficient to control hot flashes, doses as high as 2.5 mg of *conjugated estrogens* per day can be used. In premenopausal women who have undergone oophorectomy, oral contraceptives may offer relief in difficult cases (65), but they have more side effects than hormone replacement therapy (61).

Vaginal dryness responds somewhat slower than hot flashes to hormone replacement therapy. Even at the lowest therapeutic doses, however, complete resolution of vaginal dryness is usually seen after 3 to 6 weeks (181). Any symptoms of atrophic vaginitis will decrease over the same period.

Vaginal Bleeding

The bleeding patterns associated with estrogen therapy depend on the type of hormone protocol used. The most common pattern with unopposed estrogen is amenorrhea (72). If breakthrough bleeding occurs, endometrial biopsy should be performed. Even with no vaginal bleeding, yearly endometrial evaluation is recommended for women taking unopposed estrogen because of the risk of endometrial cancer.

With continuous estrogen and cyclic *medroxyprogesterone,* cyclic estrogen withdrawal bleeding almost always occurs monthly (167). If irregular or intermenstrual bleeding occurs, endometrial biopsy should be performed (Fig. 29.2). Although endometrial hyperplasia or cancer occurs only rarely, risk is not completely eliminated with progestin therapy.

When continuous estrogen and continuous progestins are used, the bleeding pattern is more variable. Many women taking this therapy will develop amenorrhea (72). One-half of women will have some degree of irregular bleeding even after 1 year. The best method for evaluation of the endometrium has not been determined. Although the bleeding is almost always light, the significance of it cannot be determined without endometrial evaluation. It is reasonable to consider a baseline endometrial biopsy for anyone taking this agent who has irregular bleeding. If irregular bleeding persists for 6 months, further evaluation with ultrasonography and possibly hysteroscopy may be of benefit.

Nonhormonal Drugs

In addition to estrogen, calcium, vitamin D, *calcitonin,* and bisphosphonates (especially *etidronate* and *alendronate*) have been used for the treatment of postmenopausal osteoporosis. Calcium can slow bone loss but does not increase bone mass (182), and calcium intake of 1,500 mg daily is considered a mainstay of both prevention and treatment of osteoporosis in postmenopausal women. Fluoride is the only known agent that can stimulate bone formation and substantially increase bone density (183), but the bone formed is actually more fracture prone, and fluoride is not recommended therapy. *Calcitonin* is probably as effective as estrogen in reducing fracture risk and is a consideration for women who cannot take oral medication (184). *Calcitriol,* a vitamin D analog, can increase lumbar bone mass and decrease the rate of vertebral fractures (185) in women with low vitamin D levels despite adequate daily intake of 400 IU vitamin D. Although *raloxifene* does not appear to slow bone loss as effectively as conventional hormone replacement therapy, it does appear to be effective in reducing fracture risk (186).

Of the bisphosphonates, *alendronate* is approximately 1,000 times more potent than *etidronate* in terms of the inhibition of bone resorption. Newer bisphosphonates, *pamidronate* and *risedronate,* are being evaluated and appear to be equally effective in increasing bone mineral density and reducing fracture risk with fewer side effects. In a randomized study, *alendronate* was given orally 5 to 20 mg/day for 3 years, or 20 mg/day for 2 years followed by 5 mg/day for the third year, along with 500 mg/day of calcium (187). Compared with placebo, the rate of vertebral fracture was approximately one-half: 3.2% for those receiving *alendronate* versus 6.2% for the placebo group.

In general, all women with documented osteoporosis, either by densitometry or previous fracture, are candidates for aggressive antiresorptive therapy in addition to calcium and vitamin D replacement.

References

1. **Kingkade WW, Torrey BB.** The evolving demography of aging in the United States of America and the former USSR. *World Health Stat Q* 1992;45:15–28.
2. **McKinlay SM, Brambilla DJ, Posner JG.** The normal menopause transition. *Maturitas* 1992;14:103–115.
3. **Whelan EA, Sandler DP, McConnaughey DR, et al.** Menstrual and reproductive characteristics and age at natural menopause. *Am J Epidemiol* 1990;131:625–628.
4. **Brambrilla DJ, McKinlay SM.** A prospective study of factors affecting age at menopause. *J Clin Epidemiol* 1989;42:1031–1039.
5. **Siddle N, Sarrel P, Whitehead M.** The effect of hysterectomy on the age at ovarian failure: identification of a subgroup of women with premature loss of ovarian function and literature review. *Fertil Steril* 1987;47:94–100.
6. **Coulam CB, Anderson SC, Annegan JF.** Incidence of premature ovarian failure. *Obstet Gynecol* 1986;67:604–606.
7. **Wilcox LS, Koonin LM, Pokras R, et al.** Hysterectomy in the United States, 1988–1990. *Obstet Gynecol* 1994;83:549–555.
8. **Feldman BM, Voda A, Gronseth E.** The prevalence of hot flash and associated variables among perimenopausal women. *Res Nurs Health* 1985;8:261–268.
9. **Hreshchyshyn MM, Hopkins A, Zylstra S, et al.** Effects of natural menopause, hysterectomy, and oophorectomy on lumbar spine and femoral neck bone densities. *Obstet Gynecol* 1988;72: 631–638.
10. **Centerwall BS.** Premenopausal hysterectomy and cardiovascular disease. *Am J Obstet Gynecol* 1981; 139:58–61.
11. **Hee J, MacNaughton J, Bangah M, et al.** Perimenopausal patterns of gonadotrophins, immunoreactive inhibin, oestradiol and progesterone. *Maturitas* 1993;18:9–20.
12. **Reyes FI, Winter JS, Faiman C.** Pituitary-ovarian relationships preceding the menopause. I. A cross-sectional study of serum follicle-stimulating hormone, luteinizing hormone, prolactin, estradiol, and progesterone levels. *Am J Obstet Gynecol* 1977;129:557–564.
13. **Adashi EY.** The climacteric ovary as a functional gonadotropin-driven androgen-producing gland. *Fertil Steril* 1994;62:20–27.
14. **Judd HL.** Hormonal dynamics associated with the menopause. *Clin Obstet Gynecol* 1976;19:775–788.
15. **Grodin JM, Siiteri PK, MacDonald PC.** Source of estrogen production in postmenopausal women. *J Clin Endocrinol Metab* 1973;36:207–214.
16. **MacDonald PC, Edman CD, Hemsell DL, et al.** Effect of obesity on conversion of plasma androstenedione to estrone in postmenopausal women with and without endometrial cancer. *Am J Obstet Gynecol* 1978;130:448–455.
17. **Harlap S.** The benefits and risks of hormone replacement therapy: an epidemiologic overview. *Am J Obstet Gynecol* 1992;166:1986–1992.
18. **Daniell HW.** Osteoporosis of the slender smoker. Vertebral compression fractures and loss of metacarpal cortex in relation to postmenopausal cigarette smoking and lack of obesity. *Arch Intern Med* 1976;136:298–304.
19. **Sherman BM, Wallace RB, Bean JA, et al** The relationship of menopausal hot flushes to medical and reproductive experience. *J Gerontol* 1981;36:306–309.

20. **Dennefors BL, Janson PO, Knutson F, et al.** Steroid production and responsiveness to gonadotropin in isolated stromal tissue of human postmenopausal ovaries. *Am J Obstet Gynecol* 1980;136:997–1002.

21. **Gath D, Osborn M, Bungay G, et al.** Psychiatric disorder and gynaecological symptoms in middle aged women: a community survey. *BMJ* 1987;294:213–218.

22. **Gambrell R Jr, Bagnell CA, Greenblatt RB.** Role of estrogens and progesterone in the etiology and prevention of endometrial cancer: review. *Am J Obstet Gynecol* 1983;146:696–707.

23. **de Aloysio D, Rocca G, Miliffi L.** Cyto-histologic evaluation of the endometrium in climacteric women at risk for endometrial carcinoma. *Tumori* 1986;72:431–437.

24. **Colditz GA, Hankinson SE, Hunter AJ, et al.** The use of estrogens and progestins and the risk of breast cancer in postmenopausal women. *N Engl J Med* 1995;332:1589–1593.

25. **Nachtigall MJ, Smilen SW, Nachtigall RD, et al.** Incidence of breast cancer in a 22-year study of women receiving estrogen-progestin replacement therapy. *Obstet Gynecol* 1992;80:827–830.

26. **Lecomte P, Lecureuil N, Lecureuil M, et al.** Sex differences in the control of sex-hormone-binding globulin in the elderly: role of insulin-like growth factor-I and insulin. *Eur J Endocrinol* 1998;139:178–183.

27. **Meldrum DR, Davidson BJ, Tataryn IV, et al.** Changes in circulating steroids with aging in postmenopausal women. *Obstet Gynecol* 1981;57:624–628.

28. **Deutsch S, Benjamin F, Seltzer V, et al.** The correlation of serum estrogens and androgens with bone density in the late postmenopause. *Int J Gynaecol Obstet* 1987;25:217–222.

29. **Sheehy G.** *The silent passage: menopause.* New York: Simon & Schuster, 1991.

30. **Nadelson CC.** Psychosomatic aspects of obstetrics and gynecology. *Psychosomatics* 1983;24:878–880.

31. **Hunter MS.** Psychological and somatic experience of the menopause: a prospective study. *Psychosom Med* 1990;52:357–367.

32. **Maheux R, Naud F, Rioux M, et al.** A randomized, double-blind, placebo-controlled study on the effect of conjugated estrogens on skin thickness. *Am J Obstet Gynecol* 1994;170:642–649.

33. **Brincat M, Versi E, Moniz CF, et al.** Skin collagen changes in postmenopausal women receiving different regimens of estrogen therapy. *Obstet Gynecol* 1987;70:123–127.

34. **Imayama S, Braverman IM.** A hypothetical explanation for the aging of skin. Chronologic alteration of the three-dimensional arrangement of collagen and elastic fibers in connective tissue. *Am J Pathol* 1989;134:1019–1025.

35. **Zung WW, Broadhead WE, Roth ME.** Prevalence of depressive symptoms in primary care. *J Fam Pract* 1993;37:337–344 (erratum, 1989;11:169).

36. **Dennerstein L, Lehert P, Burger H, et al.** Mood and the menopausal transition. *J Nerv Ment Dis* 1999;187:685–691.

37. **Ballinger SE.** Psychosocial stress and symptoms of menopause: a comparative study of menopause clinic patients and nonpatients. *Maturitas* 1985;7:315–327.

38. **de Aloysio D, Fabiani AG, Mauloni M, et al.** Analysis of the climacteric syndrome. *Maturitas* 1989;11:43–53 (erratum, 1989;11:169).

39. **Holte A, Mikkelsen A.** The menopausal syndrome: a factor analytic replication. *Maturitas* 1991;13:193–203.

40. **Strickler RC, Borth R, Cecutti A, et al.** The role of oestrogen replacement in the climacteric syndrome. *Psychol Med* 1977;7:631–639.

41. **Hunter M, Battersby R, Whitehead M.** Relationships between psychological symptoms, somatic complaints and menopausal status. *Maturitas* 1986;8:217–228.

42. **Traupmann J.** Does sexuality fade over time? A look at the question and the answer. *J Geriatr Psychiatry* 1984;17:149–159.

43. **Traupmann J, Eckels E, Hatfield E.** Intimacy in older women's lives. *Gerontologist* 1982;22:493–498.

44. **Notelovitz M.** Estrogen replacement therapy: indications, contraindications, and agent selection. *Am J Obstet Gynecol* 1989;161:1832–1841.

45. **Burger HG, Dudley EC, Cui J, et al.** A prospective longitudinal study of serum testosterone, dehydroepiandrosterone sulfate, and sex hormone-binding globulin levels through the menopause transition. *J Clin Endocrinol Metab* 2000;85:2832–2838.

46. **Greenblatt RB, Karpas A.** Hormone therapy for sexual dysfunction. The only "true aphrodisiac." *Postgrad Med* 1983;74:78–80.

47. **Bachmann GA.** Correlates of sexual desire in postmenopausal women. *Maturitas* 1985;7: 211–216.

48. **Treloar AE.** Menstrual cyclicity and the pre-menopause. *Maturitas* 1981;3:249–264.

49. **Buckler HM, Evans CA, Mamtora H, et al.** Gonadotropin, steroid, and inhibin levels in women with incipient ovarian failure during anovulatory and ovulatory rebound cycles. *J Clin Endocrinol Metab* 1991;72:116–124.

50. **Gambrell R Jr.** Clinical use of progestins in the menopausal patient: dosage and duration. *J Reprod Med* 1982;27:531–538.

51. **Lidor A, Ismajovich B, Confino E, et al.** Histopathological findings in 226 women with post-menopausal uterine bleeding. *Acta Obstet Gynecol Scand* 1986;65:41–43.

52. **Jick H, Watkins RN, Hunter JR, et al.** Replacement estrogens and endometrial cancer. *N Engl J Med* 1979;300:218–222.

53. **Ernster VL, Bush TL, Huggins GR, et al.** Benefits and risks of menopausal estrogen and or progestin hormone use. *Prev Med* 1988;17:301–323.

54. **Feldman S, Berkowitz RS, Tosteson AN.** Cost-effectiveness of strategies to evaluate postmenopausal bleeding. *Obstet Gynecol* 1993;81:968–975.

55. **Goldstein SR, Zeltser I, Horan CK, et al.** Ultrasonography-based triage for perimenopausal patients with abnormal uterine bleeding. *Am J Obstet Gynecol* 1997;177:102–108.

56. **Castelo-Branco C, Puerto B, Duran M, et al.** Transvaginal sonography of the endometrium in postmenopausal women: monitoring the effect of hormone replacement therapy. *Maturitas* 1994;19:59–65.

57. **Cacciatore B, Ramsay T, Lehtovirta P, et al.** Transvaginal sonography and hysteroscopy in postmenopausal bleeding. *Acta Obstet Gynecol Scand* 1994;73:413–416.

58. **Loffer FD.** Hysteroscopy with selective endometrial sampling compared with D&C for abnormal uterine bleeding: the value of a negative hysteroscopic view. *Obstet Gynecol* 1989;73:16–20.

59. **Goldrath MH, Sherman AI.** Office hysteroscopy and suction curettage: can we eliminate the hospital diagnostic dilatation and curettage? *Am J Obstet Gynecol* 1985;152:220–229.

60. **Mishell D Jr.** Use of oral contraceptives in women of older reproductive age. *Am J Obstet Gynecol* 1988;158:1652–1657.

61. **Trussell J, Vaughan B.** Contraceptive use projections: 1990 to 2010. *Am J Obstet Gynecol* 1992;167:1160–1164.

62. **Creinin MD.** Laboratory criteria for menopause in women using oral contraceptives. *Fertil Steril* 1996;66:101–104.

63. **Lalonde A.** Evaluation of surgical options in menorrhagia. *Br J Obstet Gynaecol* 1994;11:8–14.

64. **Hartge P, Whittemore AS, Itnyre J, et al.** Rates and risks of ovarian cancer in subgroups of white women in the United States. The Collaborative Ovarian Cancer Group. *Obstet Gynecol* 1994;84:760–764.

65. **Meyer WR, Walsh BW, Grainger DA, et al.** Thermal balloon and rollerball ablation to treat menorrhagia: a multicenter comparison. *Obstet Gynecol* 1998;92:98–103.

66. **Ramey JW, Koonings PP, Given FT Jr, et al.** The process of carcinogenesis for endometrial adenocarcinoma could be short: development of a malignancy after endometrial ablation. *Am J Obstet Gynecol* 1994;170:1370–1371.

67. **Warren MP, Kulak J Jr.** Is estrogen replacement indicated in perimenopausal women? *Clin Obstet Gynecol* 1998;41:976–987.

68. **Nakano R, Hashiba N, Washio M, et al.** Diagnostic evaluation of progesterone. Challenge test in amenorrheic patients. *Acta Obstet Gynecol Scand* 1979;58:59–64.

69. **MacNaughton J, Banah M, McCloud P, et al.** Age related changes in follicle stimulating hormone, luteinizing hormone, oestradiol and immunoreactive inhibin in women of reproductive age. *Clin Endocrinol* 1992;36:339–345.

70. **Tang L, Sawers RS.** Twin pregnancy in premature ovarian failure after estrogen treatment: a case report. *Am J Obstet Gynecol* 1989;161:172–173.

71. **Okuda K, Yoshikawa M, Ushiroyama T, et al.** Two patients with hypergonadotropic ovarian failure due to pituitary hyperplasia. *Obstet Gynecol* 1989;74:498–501.

72. **Archer DF, Pickar JH, Bottiglioni F.** Bleeding patterns in postmenopausal women taking continuous combined or sequential regimens of conjugated estrogens with medroxyprogesterone acetate. Menopause Study Group. *Obstet Gynecol* 1994;83:686–692.

73. **Kronenberg F.** Hot flashes: epidemiology and physiology. *Ann N Y Acad Sci* 1990;592:52–86.

74. **Weinstein L.** Hormonal therapy in the patient with surgical menopause. *Obstet Gynecol* 1990;75:47S—50S.

75. **Utian WH.** Biosynthesis and physiologic effects of estrogen and pathophysiologic effects of estrogen deficiency: review. *Am J Obstet Gynecol* 1989;161:1828–1831.

76. **Ravnikar V.** Physiology and treatment of hot flushes. *Obstet Gynecol* 1990;75:3S—8S.

77. **Stampfer MJ, Colditz GA, Willett WC, et al.** Postmenopausal estrogen therapy and cardiovascular disease: ten-year follow-up from the Nurses' Health Study. *N Engl J Med* 1991;325:756–762.

78. **Cedars MI, Lu JK, Meldrum DR, et al.** Treatment of endometriosis with a long-acting gonadotropin-releasing hormone agonist plus medroxyprogesterone acetate. *Obstet Gynecol* 1990;75:641–645.

79. **Erlik Y, Meldrum DR, Lagasse LD, et al.** Effect of megestrol acetate on flushing and bone metabolism in post-menopausal women. *Maturitas* 1981;3:167–172.

80. **Edington RF, Chagnon JP, Steinberg WM.** Clonidine (Dixarit) for menopausal flushing. *CMAJ* 1980;123:23–26.

81. **Bergmans MG, Merkus JM, Corbey RS, et al.** Effect of Bellergal Retard on climacteric complaints: a double-blind, placebo-controlled study. *Maturitas* 1987;9:227–234.

82. **Erlik Y, Tataryn IV, Meldrum DR, et al.** Association of waking episodes with menopausal hot flushes. *JAMA* 1981;245:1741–1744.

83. **Notelovitz M.** Gynecologic problems of menopausal women: part 1. Changes in genital tissue. *Geriatrics* 1978;33:24–30.

84. **Raz R, Stamm WE.** A controlled trial of intravaginal estriol in postmenopausal women with recurrent urinary tract infections. *N Engl J Med* 1993;329:753–756.

85. **Bhatia NN, Bergman A, Karram MM.** Effects of estrogen on urethral function in women with urinary incontinence. *Am J Obstet Gynecol* 1989;160:176–181.

86. **Dennerstein L, Burrows GD, Hyman GJ, et al.** Hormone therapy and affect. *Maturitas* 1979;1:247–259.

87. **Ditkoff EC, Crary WG, Cristo M, et al.** Estrogen improves psychological function in asymptomatic postmenopausal women. *Obstet Gynecol* 1991;78:991–995.

88. **Kampen DL, Sherwin BB.** Estrogen use and verbal memory in healthy postmenopausal women. *Obstet Gynecol* 1994;83:979–983.

89. **Henderson VW, Paganini-Hill A, Emanuel CK, et al.** Estrogen replacement therapy in older women. Comparisons between Alzheimer's disease cases and nondemented control subjects. *Arch Neurol* 1994;51:896–900.

90. **Paganini-Hill A, Henderson VW.** Estrogen deficiency and risk of Alzheimer's disease in women. *Am J Epidemiol* 1994;140:256–261.

91. **Bush TL.** The epidemiology of cardiovascular disease in postmenopausal women. *Ann N Y Acad Sci* 1990;592:263–271.

92. **Colditz GA, Willett WC, Stampfer MJ, et al.** Menopause and the risk of coronary heart disease in women. *N Engl J Med* 1987;316:1105–1110.

93. **Lobo RA.** Cardiovascular implications of estrogen replacement therapy. *Obstet Gynecol* 1990;75:18S–25S.

94. **Henderson BE, Paganini-Hill A, Ross RK.** Decreased mortality in users of estrogen replacement therapy. *Arch Intern Med* 1991;151:75–78.

95. **Hulley, S Grady D, Bush T, et al.** Randomized trial of estrogen plus progestin for secondary prevention of coronary heart disease in postmenopausal women. *JAMA* 1998;280:605–613.

96. **Perlman JA, Wolf PH, Ray R, et al.** Cardiovascular risk factors, premature heart disease, and all-cause mortality in a cohort of northern California women. *Am J Obstet Gynecol* 1988;158:1568–1574.

97. **Kanis JA.** Editorial: osteoporosis and osteopenia. *J Bone Miner Res* 1990;5:209–211.

98. **Phillips S, Fox N, Jacobs J, et al.** The direct medical costs of osteoporosis for American women aged 45 and older, 1986. *Bone* 1988;9:271–279.

99. **Resnick NM, Greenspan SL.** Senile osteoporosis reconsidered. *JAMA* 1989;261:1025–1029.

100. **Riggs BL, Melton LJ III.** Involutional osteoporosis. *N Engl J Med* 1986;314:1676–1686.

101. **Riggs BL.** Pathogenesis of osteoporosis. *Am J Obstet Gynecol* 1987;156:1342–1346.

102. **Rubin CD.** Southwestern internal medicine conference: growth hormone-aging and osteoporosis. *Am J Med Sci* 1993;305:120–129.

103. **Kellie SE, Brody JA.** Sex-specific and race-specific hip fracture rates. *Am J Public Health* 1990;80:326–328.

104. **Seeman E, Hopper JL, Bach LA, et al.** Reduced bone mass in daughters of women with osteoporosis. *N Engl J Med* 1989;320:554–558.

105. **Peck WA.** Estrogen therapy (ET) after menopause. *J Am Med Wom Assoc* 1990;45:87–90.

106. **Hedlund LR, Gallagher JC.** The effect of age and menopause on bone mineral density of the proximal femur. *J Bone Miner Res* 1989;4:639–642.

107. **Richelson LS, Wahner HW, Melton LJ, et al.** Relative contributions of aging and estrogen deficiency to postmenopausal bone loss. *N Engl J Med* 1984;311:1273–1275.

108. **Heaney RP, Recker RR, Saville PD.** Menopausal changes in calcium balance performance. *J Lab Clin Med* 1978;92:953–963.

109. **Emans SJ, Grace E, Hoffer FA, et al.** Estrogen deficiency in adolescents and young adults: impact on bone mineral content and effects of estrogen replacement therapy. *Obstet Gynecol* 1990;76:585–592.

110. **Baran D, Sorensen A, Grimes J, et al.** Dietary modification with dairy products for preventing vertebral bone loss in premenopausal women: a three-year prospective study. *J Clin Endocrinol Metab* 1990;70:264–270.

111. **Reid IR, Ames RW, Evans MC, et al.** Effect of calcium supplementation on bone loss in postmenopausal women. *N Engl J Med* 1993;328:460–464.

112. **Levine BS, Rodman JS, Wienerman S, et al.** Effect of calcium citrate supplementation on urinary calcium oxalate saturation in female stone formers: implications for prevention of osteoporosis. *Am J Clin Nutr* 1994;60:592–596.

113. **Chow RK, Harrison JE, Brown CF, et al.** Physical fitness effect on bone mass in postmenopausal women. *Arch Phys Med Rehabil* 1986;67:231–234.

114. **Jensen J, Christiansen C, Rodbro P.** Cigarette smoking, serum estrogens, and bone loss during hormone-replacement therapy early after menopause. *N Engl J Med* 1985;313:973–975.

115. **Goldberg TH.** Preventive medicine and screening in the elderly: working guidelines. *Cleve Clin J Med* 2000;67:521–530.

116. **Cauley JA, Cummings SR, Black DM, et al.** Prevalence and determinants of estrogen replacement therapy in elderly women. *Am J Obstet Gynecol* 1990;165:1438–1444.

117. **Genant HK, Baylink DJ, Gallagher JC.** Estrogens in the prevention of osteoporosis in postmenopausal women. *Am J Obstet Gynecol* 1989;161:1842–1846.

118. **Lindsay R, Tohme JF.** Estrogen treatment of patients with established postmenopausal osteoporosis. *Obstet Gynecol* 1990;76:290–295.

119. **Prior JC, Vigna YM, Barr SI, et al.** Cyclic medroxyprogesterone treatment increases bone density: a controlled trial in active women with menstrual cycle disturbances. *Am J Med* 1994;96:521–530.

120. **Sullivan JM, Vander Zwaag R, Hughes JP, et al.** Estrogen replacement and coronary artery disease. Effect on survival in postmenopausal women. *Arch Intern Med* 1990;150:2557–2562.

121. **Walsh BW, Schiff I, Rosner B, et al.** Effects of postmenopausal estrogen replacement on the concentrations and metabolism of plasma lipoproteins. *N Engl J Med* 1991;325:1196–1204.

122. **Egeland GM, Kuller LH, Matthews KA, et al.** Hormone replacement therapy and lipoprotein changes during early menopause. *Obstet Gynecol* 1990;76:776–782.

123. **Fletcher CD, Farish E, Dagen MM, et al.** A comparison of the effects of lipoproteins of two progestogens used during cyclical hormone replacement therapy. *Maturitas* 1987;9:253–258.

124. **Wagner JD, Clarkson TB, St Clair RW, et al.** Estrogen and progesterone replacement therapy reduces low density lipoprotein accumulation in the coronary arteries of surgically postmenopausal cynomolgus monkeys. *J Clin Invest* 1991;88:1995–2002.

125. **Sack MN, Rader DJ, Cannon R.** Oestrogen and inhibition of oxidation of low-density lipoproteins in postmenopausal women. *Lancet* 1994;343:269–270.

126. **Williams JK, Adams MR, Herrington DM, et al.** Short-term administration of estrogen and vascular responses of atherosclerotic coronary arteries. *J Am Coll Cardiol* 1992;20:452–457.

127. **Karas RH, Patterson BL, Mendelsohn ME.** Human vascular smooth muscle cells contain functional estrogen receptor. *Circulation* 1994;89:1943–1950.

128. **Bar J, Tepper R, Fuchs J, et al.** The effect of estrogen replacement therapy on platelet aggregation and adenosine triphosphate release in postmenopausal women. *Obstet Gynecol* 1993;81:261–264.

129. **Armstrong BK.** Oestrogen therapy after the menopause—boon or bane? *Med J Aust* 1988;148:213–214.

130. **Dupont WD, Page DL.** Menopausal estrogen replacement therapy and breast cancer. *Arch Intern Med* 1991;151:67–72.

131. **Sillero-Arenas M, Delgado-Rodriguez M, Rodigues-Canteras R, et al.** Menopausal hormone replacement therapy and breast cancer: a meta-analysis. *Obstet Gynecol* 1992;79:286–294.

132. **Steinberg KK, Thacker SB, Smith SJ, et al.** A meta-analysis of the effect of estrogen replacement therapy on the risk of breast cancer. *JAMA* 1991;265:1985–1990.

133. **Persson I, Adami HO, Bergkvist L, et al.** Risk of endometrial cancer after treatment with oestrogens alone or in conjunction with progestogens: results of a prospective study. *BMJ* 1989;298:147–151.

134. **Leather AT, Savvas M, Studd JW.** Endometrial histology and bleeding patterns after 8 years of continuous combined estrogen and progestogen therapy in postmenopausal women. *Obstet Gynecol* 1991;78:1008–1110.

135. **Scragg RK, McMichael AJ, Seamark RF.** Oral contraceptives, pregnancy, and endogenous oestrogen in gall stone disease—a case-control study. *BMJ* 1984;288:1795–1799.

136. **Grodstein F, Colditz GA, Stampfer MJ.** Postmenopausal hormone use and cholecystectomy in a large prospective study. *Obstet Gynecol* 1994;83:5–11.

137. **Kakar F, Weiss NS, Strite SA.** Non-contraceptive estrogen use and the risk of gallstone disease in women. *Am J Public Health* 1988;78:564–566.

138. **Devor M, Barrett-Connor E, Renvall M, et al.** Estrogen replacement therapy and the risk of venous thrombosis. *Am J Med* 1992;92:275–282.

139. **de Aloysio D, Mauloni M, Roncuzzi A, et al.** Effects of an oral contraceptive combination containing 0.150 mg desogestrel plus 0.020 mg ethinyl estradiol on healthy premenopausal women. *Arch Gynecol Obstet* 1993;253:15–19.

140. **Young RL, Goepfert AR, Goldzieher HW.** Estrogen replacement therapy is not conducive of venous thromboembolism. *Maturitas* 1991;13:189–192.

141. **Spellacy WN, Birk SA.** The development of elevated blood pressure while using oral contraceptives: a preliminary report of a prospective study. *Fertil Steril* 1970;21:301–306.

142. **Pfeffer RI, Kurosaki TT, Charlton SK.** Estrogen use and blood pressure in later life. *Am J Epidemiol* 1979;110:469–478.

143. **McNicholas MM, Heneghan JP, Milner MH, et al.** Pain and increased mammographic density in women receiving hormone replacement therapy: a prospective study. *AJR Am J Roentgenol* 1994;163: 311–315.

144. **Pastides H, Najjar MA, Kelsey JL.** Estrogen replacement therapy and fibrocystic breast disease. *Am J Prev Med* 1987;3:282–286.

145. **Dennerstein L, Burrows G.** Psychological effects of progestogens in the postmenopausal years. *Maturitas* 1986;8:101–106.

146. **Sherwin BB.** The impact of different doses of estrogen and progestin on mood and sexual behavior in postmenopausal women. *J Clin Endocrinol Metab* 1991;72:336–343.

147. **Studd J.** Complications of hormone replacement therapy in post-menopausal women [editorial]. *J R Soc Med* 1992;85:376–378.

148. **Cobleigh MA, Berris RF, Bush T, et al.** Estrogen replacement therapy in breast cancer survivors. A time for change. Breast Cancer Committees of the Eastern Cooperative Oncology Group. *JAMA* 1994;272:540–545.

149. **Wile AG, Opfell RW, Margileth DA.** Hormone replacement therapy in previously treated breast cancer patients. *Am J Surg* 1993;165:372–375.

150. **Baker DP.** Estrogen-replacement therapy in patients with previous endometrial carcinoma. *Compr Ther* 1990;16:28–35.

151. **Lentz SS.** Advanced and recurrent endometrial carcinoma: hormonal therapy. *Semin Oncol* 1994;21:100–106.

152. **Creasman WT, Henderson D, Hinshaw W, et al.** Estrogen replacement therapy in the patient treated for endometrial cancer. *Obstet Gynecol* 1986;67:326–330.

153. **Kapadia SB, Russak RR, O'Donnell WF, et al.** Postmenopausal ureteral endometriosis with atypical adenomatous hyperplasia following hysterectomy, bilateral oophorectomy, and long-term estrogen therapy. *Obstet Gynecol* 1984;64:60S–63S.

154. **Lam AM, French M, Charnock FM.** Bilateral ureteric obstruction due to recurrent endometriosis associated with hormone replacement therapy. *Aust N Z J Obstet Gynaecol* 1992;32:83–84.

155. **Reimnitz C, Brand E, Nieberg RK, et al.** Malignancy arising in endometriosis associated with unopposed estrogen replacement. *Obstet Gynecol* 1988;71:444–447.

156. **Pentikainen PJ, Pentikainen LA, Azarnoff DL, et al.** Plasma levels and excretion of estrogens in urine in chronic lever disease. *Gastroenterology* 1975;69:20–27.

157. **Lyman GW, Johnson RN.** Assay for conjugated estrogens in tablets using fused-silica capillary gas chromatography. *J Chromatogr* 1982;234:234–239.

158. **Stanczyk FZ, Shoupe D, Nunez V, et al.** A randomized comparison of nonoral estradiol delivery in postmenopausal women. *Am J Obstet Gynecol* 1988;159:1540–1546.

159. **Fraser DI, Parsons A, Whitehead MI, et al.** The optimal dose of oral norethindrone acetate for addition to transdermal estradiol: a multicenter study. *Fertil Steril* 1990;53:460–468.

160. **Englund DE, Johansson ED.** Plasma levels of oestrone, oestradiol and gonadotrophins in postmenopausal women after oral and vaginal administration of conjugated equine oestrogens (Premarin). *Br J Obstet Gynaecol* 1978;85:957–964.

161. **Dickerson J, Bressler R, Christian CD, et al.** Efficacy of estradiol vaginal cream in postmenopausal women. *Clin Pharmacol Ther* 1979;26:502–507.

162. **Mandel FP, Geola FL, Meldrum DR, et al.** Biological effects of various doses of vaginally administered conjugated equine estrogens in postmenopausal women. *J Clin Endocrinol Metab* 1983;57:133–139.

163. **Ettinger B, Golditch IM, Friedman G.** Gynecologic consequences of long-term, unopposed estrogen replacement therapy. *Maturitas* 1988;10:271–282.

164. **Whitehead MI, Hillard TC, Crook D.** The role and use of progestogens. *Obstet Gynecol* 1990;75:59S–76S.

165. **Whitehead MI, King RJ, McQueen J, et al.** Endometrial histology and biochemistry in climacteric women during oestrogen and oestrogen/progestogen therapy. *J R Soc Med* 1979;72:322–327.

166. **Woodruff JD, Pickar JH.** Incidence of endometrial hyperplasia in postmenopausal women taking conjugated estrogens (Premarin) with medroxyprogesterone acetate or conjugated estrogens alone. The Menopause Study Group. *Am J Obstet Gynecol* 1994;170:1213–1223.

167. **MacLennan AH, MacLennan A, O'Neill S, et al.** Oestrogen and cyclical progestogen in postmenopausal hormone replacement therapy. *Med J Aust* 1992;157:167–170.

168. **Ravnikar VA.** Compliance with hormone therapy. *Am J Obstet Gynecol* 1987;156:1332–1334.

169. **Marslew U, Riis BJ, Christiansen C.** Bleeding patterns during continuous combined estrogen-progestogen therapy. *Am J Obstet Gynecol* 1991;164:1163–1168.

170. **Kuiper GG, Enmark E, Pelto-Huikko M, et al.** Cloning of a novel receptor expressed in rat prostate and ovary. *Proc Natl Acad Sci U S A* 1996;93:5925–5930.

171. **Plouffe L Jr.** Selective estrogen receptor modulators (SERMs) in clinical practice. *J Soc Gynecol Invest* 2000;7[Suppl 1]:S38–46.

172. **Mincey BA, Moraghan TJ, Perez EA.** Prevention and treatment of osteoporosis in women with breast cancer. *Mayo Clin Proc* 2000;75:821–829.

173. **Sherwin BB, Gelfand MM.** The role of androgen in the maintenance of sexual functioning in oophorectomized women. *Psychosom Med* 1987;49:397–409.

174. **Sherwin BB, Gelfand MM.** Sex steroids and affect in the surgical menopause: a double-blind, cross-over study. *Psychoneuroendocrinology* 1985;10:325–335.

175. **Sherwin BB, Gelfand MM.** Differential symptom response to parenteral estrogen and/or androgen administration in the surgical menopause. *Am J Obstet Gynecol* 1985;151:153–160.

176. **Dow MG, Gallagher J.** A controlled study of combined hormonal and psychological treatment for sexual unresponsiveness in women. *Br J Clin Psychol* 1989;28:201–212.

177. **Dow MG, Hart DM, Forrest CA.** Hormonal treatments of sexual unresponsiveness in postmenopausal women: a comparative study. *Br J Obstet Gynaecol* 1983;90:361–366.

178. **Myers LS, Dixen J, Morrissette D, et al.** Effects of estrogen, androgen, and progestin on sexual psychophysiology and behavior in postmenopausal women. *J Clin Endocrinol Metab* 1990;70:1124–1131.

179. **Hickok LR, Toomey C, Speroff L.** A comparison of esterified estrogens with and without methyltestosterone: effects on endometrial histology and serum lipoproteins in postmenopausal women. *Obstet Gynecol* 1993;82:919–924.

180. **Whitehead A, Mathews A.** Factors related to successful outcome in the treatment of sexually unresponsive women. *Psychol Med* 1986;16:373–378.

181. **Semmens JP, Tsai CC, Semmens EC, et al.** Effects of estrogen therapy on vaginal physiology during menopause. *Obstet Gynecol* 1985;66:15–18.

182. **Reid IR, Ames RW, Evans MC, et al.** Long-term effects of calcium supplementation on bone loss and fractures in postmenopausal women: a randomized controlled trial. *Am J Med* 1995;98:331–335.

183. **Riggs BL, O'Fallon WM, Lane A, et al.** Clinical trial of fluoride therapy in postmenopausal osteoporotic women: extended observations and additional analysis. *J Bone Miner Res* 1994;9:265–275.

184. **Overgaard K, Hansen MA, Jensen SB, et al.** Effect of calcitonin given intranasally on bone mass and fracture rates in established osteoporosis: a dose-response study. *BMJ* 1992;305:556–561.

185. **Tilyard MW, Spears GFS, Thomson J, et al.** Treatment of postmenopausal osteoporosis with calcitrol or calcium. *N Engl J Med* 1992;326:357–362.

186. **Ettinger B, Black DM, Mitlak BH, et al.** Multiple Outcomes of Raloxifene Evaluation (MORE) Investigators. Reduction of vertebral fracture risk in postmenopausal women with osteoporosis treated with raloxifene: results from a 3-year randomized clinical trial. *JAMA* 1999;282:637–645.

187. **Liberman UA, Weiss ST, Broll J, et al.** Effect of oral alendronate on bone mineral density and the incidence of fractures in postmenopausal osteoporosis. *N Engl J Med* 1995;333:1437–1443.

SECTION

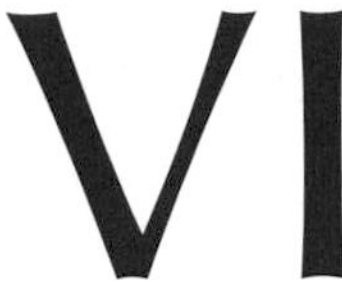

GYNECOLOGIC ONCOLOGY

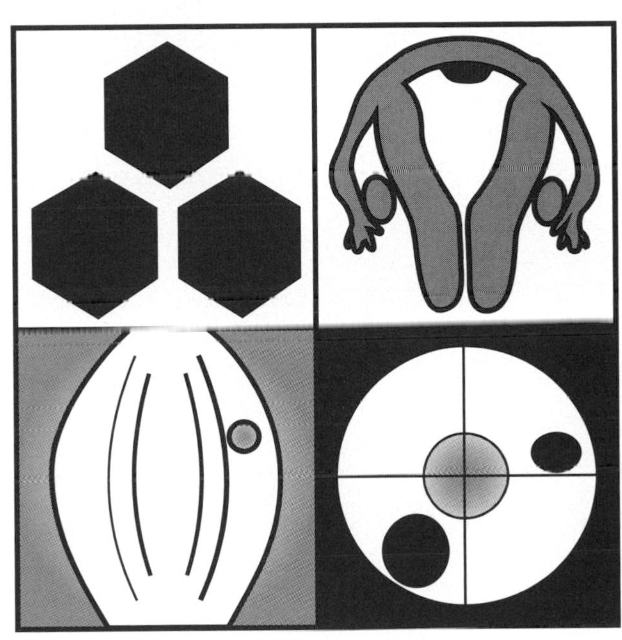

30 Uterine Cancer

John R. Lurain

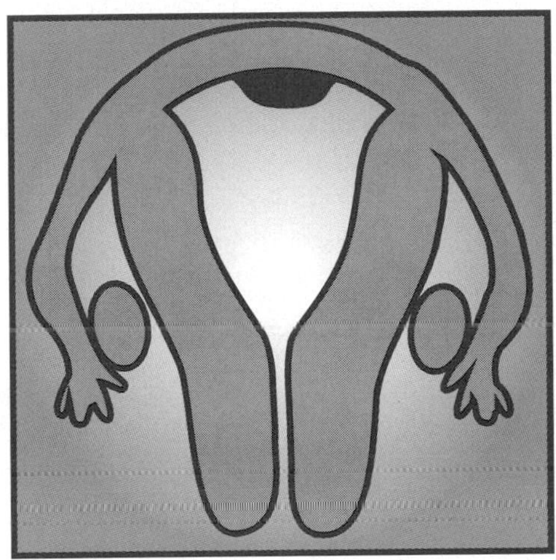

Endometrial carcinoma is the most common malignancy of the female genital tract, accounting for almost half of all gynecologic cancers in the United States. About 39,300 new cases are diagnosed annually, resulting in more than 6,600 deaths. Endometrial carcinoma is the fourth most common cancer, ranking behind breast, lung, and bowel cancers, and the seventh leading cause of death from malignancy in women. Overall, about 2% to 3% of women develop endometrial cancer during their lifetime (1).

In recent years, certain factors have led to an increasing awareness of and emphasis on diagnosis and treatment of endometrial cancer. These factors include the declining incidence of cervical cancer and related deaths in the United States, prolonged life expectancy, postmenopausal use of hormone replacement therapy, and earlier diagnosis. The availability of easily applied diagnostic tools and a clearer understanding of premalignant lesions of the endometrium have led to an increase in the number of women diagnosed with endometrial cancer. Although endometrial carcinoma usually presents as early-stage disease and can generally be managed without radical surgery or radiotherapy, deaths from endometrial carcinoma now exceed those from cervical carcinoma in the United States. **Endometrial cancer is a disease that occurs primarily in postmenopausal women and is increasingly virulent with advancing age. The role of estrogen in the development of most endometrial cancers has clearly been established; any factor that increases exposure to unopposed estrogen increases the risk for endometrial cancer.**

During the past several decades, the histopathology, spread patterns, and prognostic factors that affect the prognosis of endometrial cancers have been better defined. Management of endometrial cancer has evolved from a program of preoperative intrauterine radium packing or external pelvic irradiation followed in 6 weeks by hysterectomy, to a single brachytherapy session using an intrauterine tandem and colpostats followed immediately by hysterectomy, to an individualized approach using hysterectomy as primary therapy and employing additional postoperative treatment depending on surgical and pathologic findings. Further analysis and investigation are needed to determine whether this initial operative approach to treatment and staging, followed by targeted postoperative therapy, will translate into improved survival rates and lower morbidity.

Epidemiology and Risk Factors

There appear to be two different pathogenetic types of endometrial cancer (2). **The most common type occurs in younger, perimenopausal women with a history of exposure to unopposed estrogen, either endogenous or exogenous.** In these women, tumors begin as hyperplastic endometrium and progress to carcinoma. These "estrogen-dependent" tumors tend to be better differentiated and have a more favorable prognosis than tumors that are not associated with hyperestrogenism. **The other type of endometrial carcinoma occurs in women with no source of estrogen stimulation of the endometrium.** These spontaneously occurring cancers are not associated pathologically with endometrial hyperplasia, but may arise in a background of atrophic endometrium. They are less differentiated and associated with a poorer prognosis than estrogen-dependent tumors. These "estrogen-independent" tumors tend to occur in older, postmenopausal, thin women and are present disproportionately in African American and Asian women.

Several risk factors for the development of endometrial cancer have been identified (3–8) (Table 30.1). Most of these risk factors are related to prolonged, unopposed estrogen stimulation of the endometrium. Nulliparous women have 2 to 3 times the risk of parous women. Infertility and a history of irregular menses as a result of anovulatory cycles (prolonged exposure to estrogen without sufficient progesterone) increase the risk. Natural menopause occurring after 52 increases the risk for endometrial cancer 2.4 times compared with that in women whose menopause occurred before 49 years of age, probably as a result of prolonged exposure of the uterus to progesterone-deficient menstrual cycles. The risk for endometrial cancer is increased 3 times in women who are 21 to 50 pounds overweight and 10 times in those more than 50 pounds overweight (excess estrone as a result of peripheral conversion of adrenally derived androstenedione by aromatization in fat).

Other factors leading to long-term estrogen exposure, such as polycystic ovary syndrome and functioning ovarian tumors, also are associated with an increased risk for endometrial cancer. Menopausal estrogen replacement therapy without progestins increases the risk for endometrial cancer 4 to 8 times. This risk is greater with higher doses and with more prolonged use and can be reduced to essentially baseline levels by the addition of progestin (7). It has been noted that the use of the antiestrogen *tamoxifen* for treatment of breast cancer is associated with a twofold to threefold increased risk for the development of endometrial caner (8,9). Diabetes mellitus increases a women's risk for endometrial cancer by 1.3 to 2.8 times. Other medical conditions, such as hypertension and hypothyroidism, have been associated with endometrial cancer, but a causal relationship has not been confirmed.

Endometrial Hyperplasia

Endometrial hyperplasia represents a spectrum of morphologic and biologic alterations of the endometrial glands and stroma, ranging from an exaggerated physiologic state to

Table 30.1. Risk Factors for Endometrial Cancer

Characteristic	Relative Risk
Nulliparity	2–3
Late menopause	2.4
Obesity	
21–50 lb overweight	3
>50 lb overweight	10
Diabetes mellitus	2.8
Unopposed estrogen therapy	4–8
Tamoxifen therapy	2–3
Atypical endometrial hyperplasia	8–29

Table 30.2. Classification of Endometrial Hyperplasias

Type of Hyperplasia	*Progression to Cancer (%)*
Simple (cystic without atypia)	1
Complex (adenomatous without atypia)	3
Atypical	
Simple (cystic with atypia)	8
Complex (adenomatous with atypia)	29

From **Kurman RJ, Kaminski PF, Norris HJ.** The behavior of endometrial hyperplasia: a long term study of "untreated" hyperplasia in 170 patients. *Cancer* 1985;56:403–412, with permission.

carcinoma *in situ.* Clinically significant hyperplasias usually evolve within a background of proliferative endometrium as a result of protracted estrogen stimulation in the absence of progestin influence. Endometrial hyperplasias are important clinically because they may cause abnormal bleeding, be associated with estrogen-producing ovarian tumors, result from hormonal therapy, and precede or occur simultaneously with endometrial cancer.

The most recent classification scheme endorsed by the International Society of Gynecological Pathologists is based on architectural and cytologic features as well as long-term studies that reflect the natural history of the lesions (10) (Table 30.2). Architecturally, hyperplasias are either simple or complex; the major differing features are complexity and crowding of the glandular elements. Simple hyperplasia is characterized by dilated or cystic glands with round to slightly irregular shapes, an increased glandular-to-stromal ratio without glandular crowding, and no cytologic atypia. Complex hyperplasia has architecturally complex (budding and infolding), crowded glands with less intervening stroma without atypia. Atypical hyperplasia refers to cytologic atypia and can be categorized as simple or complex, depending on the corresponding glandular architecture. Criteria for cytologic atypia include large nuclei of variable size and shape that have lost polarity, increased nuclear-to-cytoplasmic ratios, prominent nucleoli, and irregularly clumped chromatin with parachromatin clearing (Fig. 30.1).

The risk of endometrial hyperplasia progressing to carcinoma is related to the presence and severity of cytologic atypia. Kurman and colleagues retrospectively studied endometrial curettings from 170 patients with untreated endometrial hyperplasia followed a mean of 13.4 years (11). They found that **progression to carcinoma occurred in 1% of patients with simple hyperplasia, 3% of patients with complex hyperplasia, 8% of patients with atypical simple hyperplasia, and 29% of patients with atypical complex hyperplasia.** Most of the hyperplasias seemed to remain stable (18%) or regress (74%). The premalignant potential of hyperplasia is influenced by age, underlying ovarian disease, endocrinopathy, obesity, and exogenous hormone exposure (12,13).

Of patients with atypical hyperplasia detected in an endometrial biopsy or curettage specimen, about 25% have an associated, usually well-differentiated, endometrial carcinoma seen at hysterectomy. Marked cytologic atypia, a high mitotic rate, and marked cellular stratification are features of atypical endometrial hyperplasia most often associated with the finding of an undiagnosed carcinoma at hysterectomy.

In a report of 85 menopausal women with endometrial hyperplasia treated with *medroxyprogesterone acetate* (10 to 20 mg per day), 84% of 65 who did not have cytologic atypia had complete reversal of the lesions, 6% developed recurrent hyperplasia, but none developed cancer, at a mean follow-up of 7 years (14). By contrast, of 20 patients with cytologic atypia, only 50% responded to progestin, 25% developed recurrent hyperplasia, and 25% developed adenocarcinoma. In another study, hyperplasia resolved in 94% of 32 patients with atypical endometrial hyperplasia who were treated with *megestrol acetate* (20 to 40 mg/d); however, relapse occurred in all 7 patients who discontinued progestin therapy (15).

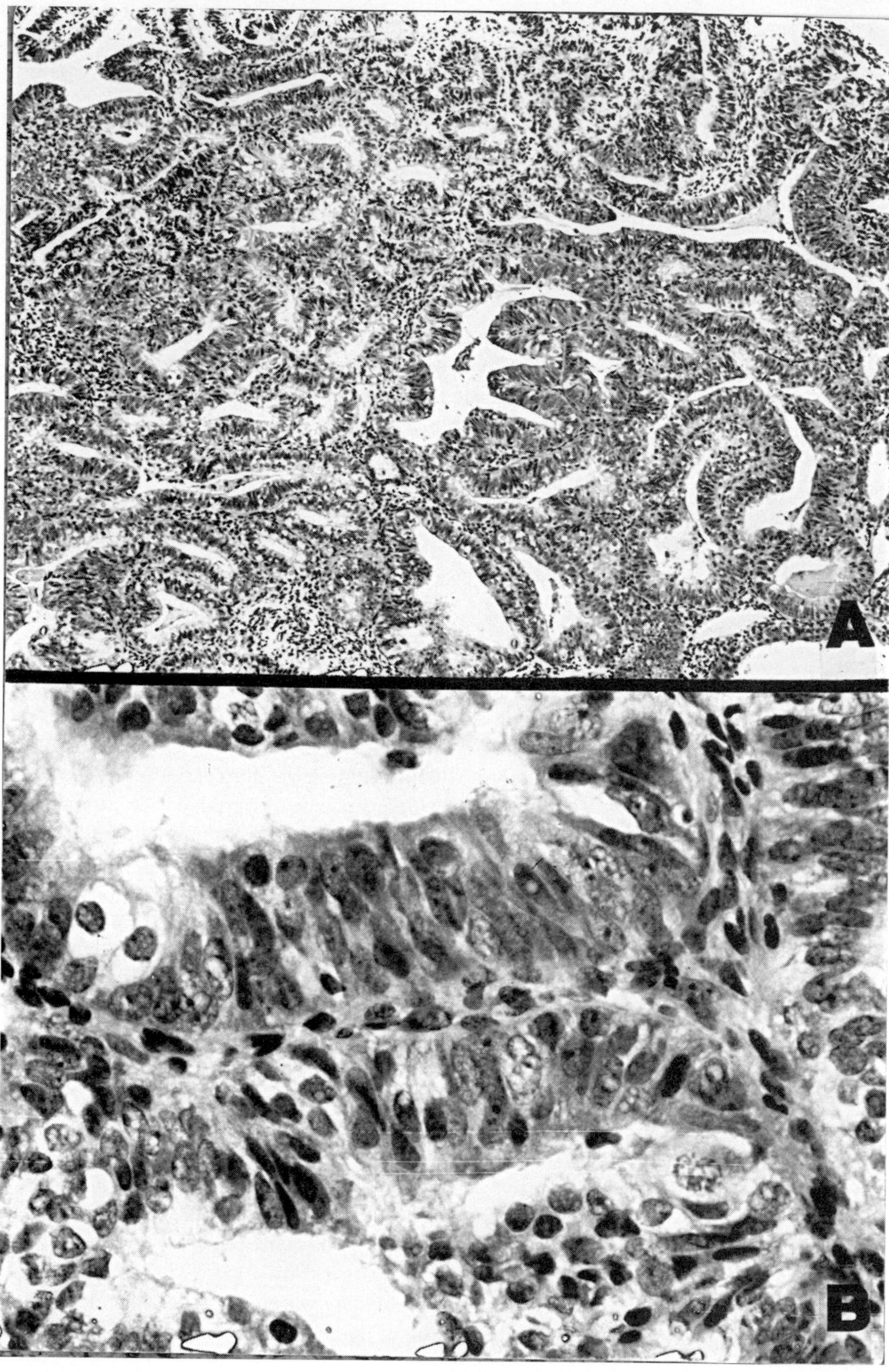

Figure 30.1 Atypical hyperplasia (complex hyperplasia with severe nuclear atypia) of endometrium. A: The proliferative endometrial glands reveal considerable crowding and papillary infoldings. The endometrial stroma, although markedly diminished, can still be recognized between the glands. **B:** Higher magnification demonstrates disorderly nuclear arrangement and nuclear enlargement and irregularity. Some contain small nucleoli. (Reproduced or modified from **Berek JS, Hacker NF.** *Practical gynecologic oncology*. 2nd ed. Baltimore: Williams & Wilkins, 1994, with permission.)

Progestin therapy is very effective in reversing endometrial hyperplasia without atypia but is less effective for endometrial hyperplasia with atypia. For women with endometrial hyperplasia without atypia, ovulation induction, cyclical progestin therapy (e.g., *medroxyprogesterone acetate,* 10 to 20 mg/d for 14 days per month), or continuous progestin therapy (e.g., *megestrol acetate,* 20 to 40 mg/d) all appear to be effective. Continuous progestin therapy with *megestrol acetate* (40 mg/d) is probably the most reliable treatment for reversing complex or atypical hyperplasia. Therapy should be continued for 2 to 3 months, and endometrial biopsy should be performed 3 to 4 weeks after completion of therapy to assess response.

Periodic endometrial biopsy or transvaginal ultrasound is advisable in patients being followed after progestin therapy for atypical hyperplasia, because of the presence of undiagnosed cancer in 25% of cases, the 29% progression rate to cancer, and the high recurrence rate after treatment with progestins.

Endometrial Cancer Screening

Screening for endometrial cancer should currently not be undertaken because of the lack of an appropriate, cost-effective, and acceptable test that reduces mortality (16–18). **Routine Papanicolaou's (Pap) test is inadequate and endometrial cytology is too insensitive and nonspecific to be useful in screening for endometrial cancer even in a high-risk population.** A progesterone challenge test reveals whether the endometrium has been primed by estrogen, but it does not identify abnormal endometrial pathology. Transvaginal ultrasound examination of the uterus and endometrial biopsy are too expensive to be employed as screening tests.

Although many risk factors for endometrial cancer have been identified, screening of high-risk individuals could at best detect only half of all cases of endometrial cancer. Furthermore, no controlled trials have been carried out to evaluate the effectiveness of screening for endometrial cancer. Screening for endometrial cancer or its precursors may be justified for certain high-risk women, such as those receiving postmenopausal estrogen replacement therapy without progestins and members of families with hereditary nonpolyposis colorectal cancer. Conversely, women taking *tamoxifen* receive no benefit from routine screening with transvaginal ultrasound or endometrial biopsy (19,20).

Fortunately, most patients who have endometrial cancer present with abnormal perimenopausal or postmenopausal uterine bleeding early in the development of the disease, when the tumor is still confined to the uterus. Application of an appropriate and accurate diagnostic test in this situation usually results in early diagnosis, timely treatment, and a high cure rate.

Endometrial Cancer

Clinical Features

Symptoms

Endometrial carcinoma most often occurs in women in the sixth and seventh decades of life, at an average age of 60 years; 75% of cases occur in women older than 50 years of age. **About 90% of women with endometrial carcinoma have vaginal bleeding or discharge as their only presenting complaint.** Most women recognize the importance of this symptom and seek medical consultation within 3 months. Some women experience pelvic pressure or discomfort indicative of uterine enlargement or extrauterine disease spread. Bleeding may not have occurred because of cervical stenosis, especially in older patients, and may be associated with hematometra or pyometra, causing a purulent vaginal discharge. This finding is often associated with a poor prognosis (21). **Less than 5% of women diagnosed with endometrial cancer are asymptomatic.** In the absence of symptoms, endometrial cancer is usually detected as the result of investigation of abnormal Pap test

Table 30.3. Causes of Postmenopausal Uterine Bleeding

Cause of Bleeding Frequency	*Percentage*
Endometrial atrophy	60–80
Estrogen replacement therapy	15–25
Endometrial polyps	2–12
Endometrial hyperplasia	5–10
Endometrial cancer	10

results, discovery of cancer in a uterus removed for some other reason, or evaluation of an abnormal finding on a pelvic ultrasound or computed tomography (CT) scan obtained for an unrelated reason. Women who are found to have malignant cells on Pap test are more likely to have a more advanced stage of disease (22).

Abnormal perimenopausal and postmenopausal bleeding should always be taken seriously and be properly investigated, no matter how minimal or nonpersistent. Causes may be nongenital, genital extrauterine, or uterine (23). Nongenital tract sites should be considered based on the history or examination, including testing for blood in the urine and stool.

Invasive tumors of the cervix, vagina, and vulva are usually evident on examination, and any tumors discovered should be biopsied. Traumatic bleeding from an atrophic vagina may account for up to 15% of all causes of postmenopausal vaginal bleeding. This diagnosis can be considered if inspection reveals a thin, friable vaginal wall, but the possibility of a uterine source of bleeding must first be eliminated.

Possible uterine causes of perimenopausal or postmenopausal bleeding include endometrial atrophy, endometrial polyps, estrogen replacement therapy, hyperplasia, and cancer or sarcoma (24–27) (Table 30.3). Uterine leiomyomas should never be accepted as a cause of postomenopausal bleeding. **Endometrial atrophy is the most common endometrial finding in women with postmenopausal bleeding, accounting for 60% to 80% of such bleeding.** Women with endometrial atrophy have usually been menopausal for about 10 years, endometrial biopsy often yields insufficient tissue or only blood and mucus, and there is usually no additional bleeding after biopsy. Endometrial polyps account for 2% to 12% of postmenopausal bleeding. Polyps are often difficult to identify with office endometrial biopsy or curettage. Hysteroscopy, transvaginal ultrasonography, or both may be useful adjuncts in identifying endometrial polyps. Unrecognized and untreated polyps may be a source of continued or recurrent bleeding, leading eventually to unnecessary hysterectomy.

Estrogen therapy is an established risk factor for endometrial hyperplasia and cancer. The risk for endometrial cancer is 4 to 8 times greater in postmenopausal women receiving unopposed estrogen replacement, and the risk increases with time and higher estrogen doses. This risk can be decreased by the addition of a progestin to the estrogen, either cyclically or continuously. Endometrial biopsy should be performed as indicated to assess unscheduled bleeding or annually in women not taking a progestin. **Endometrial hyperplasia occurs in 5% to 10% of patients with postmenopausal uterine bleeding.**

The source of excess estrogen should be considered, including obesity, exogenous estrogen, or an estrogen-secreting ovarian tumor. **Only about 10% of patients with postmenopausal bleeding have endometrial cancer.**

Premenopausal women with endometrial cancer invariably have abnormal uterine bleeding, which is often characterized as menometrorrhagia or oligomenorrhea, or cyclical bleeding that continues past the usual age of menopause. The diagnosis of endometrial cancer must be considered in premenopausal women when abnormal bleeding is persistent or recurrent or if obesity or chronic anovulation is present.

Signs

Physical examination seldom reveals any evidence of endometrial carcinoma, although obesity and hypertension are commonly associated constitutional factors. Special attention should be given to the more common sites of metastasis. Peripheral lymph nodes and breasts should be assessed carefully. Abdominal examination is usually unremarkable except in advanced cases in which ascites or hepatic or omental metastases may be palpable. On gynecologic examination, the vaginal introitus and suburethral area, as well as the entire vagina and cervix, should be carefully inspected and palpated. Bimanual rectovaginal examination should be performed specifically to evaluate the uterus for size and mobility, the adnexa for masses, the parametria for induration, and the cul-de-sac for nodularity.

Diagnosis

Office endometrial aspiration biopsy is the accepted first step in evaluating a patient with abnormal uterine bleeding or suspected endometrial pathology (28). **The diagnostic accuracy of office-based endometrial biopsy is 90% to 98% when compared with subsequent findings at dilation and curettage (D & C) or hysterectomy** (29–31).

The narrow plastic cannulas are relatively inexpensive, can often be used without a tenaculum, cause less uterine cramping, resulting in increased patient acceptance, and are successful in obtaining adequate tissue samples in more than 95% of cases. If cervical stenosis is encountered, a paracervical block can be performed, and the cervix can be dilated. Premedication with an antiprostaglandin agent can reduce uterine cramping. Complications following endometrial biopsy are exceedingly rare; uterine perforation occurs in only 1 to 2 cases per 1,000. Endocervical curettage may also be performed at the time of endometrial biopsy if cervical pathology is suspected. **A Pap test is an unreliable diagnostic test because only 30% to 50% of patients with endometrial cancer have abnormal Pap test results** (32).

Hysteroscopy and D & C should be reserved for situations in which cervical stenosis or patient tolerance does not permit adequate evaluation by aspiration biopsy, bleeding recurs after a negative endometrial biopsy, or the specimen obtained is inadequate to explain the abnormal bleeding. Hysteroscopy is more accurate in identifying polyps and submucous myomas than endometrial biopsy or D & C alone (33,34).

Transvaginal ultrasound may be a useful adjunct to endometrial biopsy for evaluating abnormal uterine bleeding and selecting patients for additional testing (35–37). Transvaginal ultrasound, with or without endometrial fluid instillation (ultrasonohysterography), may be helpful in distinguishing between patients with minimal endometrial tissue whose bleeding is due to perimenopausal anovulation or postmenopausal atrophy and patients with significant amounts of endometrial tissue or polyps who are in need of further evaluation. The finding of an endometrial thickness greater than 4 mm, a polypoid endometrial mass, or a collection of fluid within the uterus requires further evaluation. Although most studies agree that an endometrial thickness of 5 mm or less in a postmenopausal woman is consistent with atrophy, more data are needed before ultrasound findings can be considered to eliminate the need for endometrial biopsy in a patient who has symptoms.

Pathology

The histologic classification of carcinoma arising in the endometrium is shown in Table 30.4 (10,38).

Endometrioid Adenocarcinoma

The endometrioid type accounts for about 80% of endometrial carcinomas. These tumors are composed of glands that resemble normal endometrial glands; they have columnar cells with basally oriented nuclei, little or no intracytoplasmic mucin, and smooth intraluminal surfaces (Fig. 30.2). As tumors become less differentiated, they contain more solid

Table 30.4. Classification of Endometrial Carcinomas

Endometrioid adenocarcinoma
  Usual type
  Variants
    Villoglandular or papillary
    Secretory
    With squamous differentiation

Mucinous carcinoma
Papillary serous carcinoma
Clear cell carcinoma
Squamous carcinoma
Undifferentiated carcinoma
Mixed carcinoma

areas, less glandular formation, and more cytologic atypia. The well-differentiated lesions may be difficult to separate from atypical hyperplasia.

Criteria that indicate the presence of invasion and are used to diagnose carcinoma are desmoplastic stroma, glands back-to-back without intervening stoma, extensive papillary pattern, and squamous epithelial differentiation. These changes, with the exception of the infiltrating

Figure 30.2 Well-differentiated adenocarcinoma of endometrium. The glands and complex papillae are in direct contact with no intervening endometrial stroma, the so-called back-to-back pattern. (Reproduced or modified from **Berek JS, Hacker NF.** *Practical gynecologic oncology.* 2nd ed. Baltimore: Williams & Wilkins, 1994, with permission.)

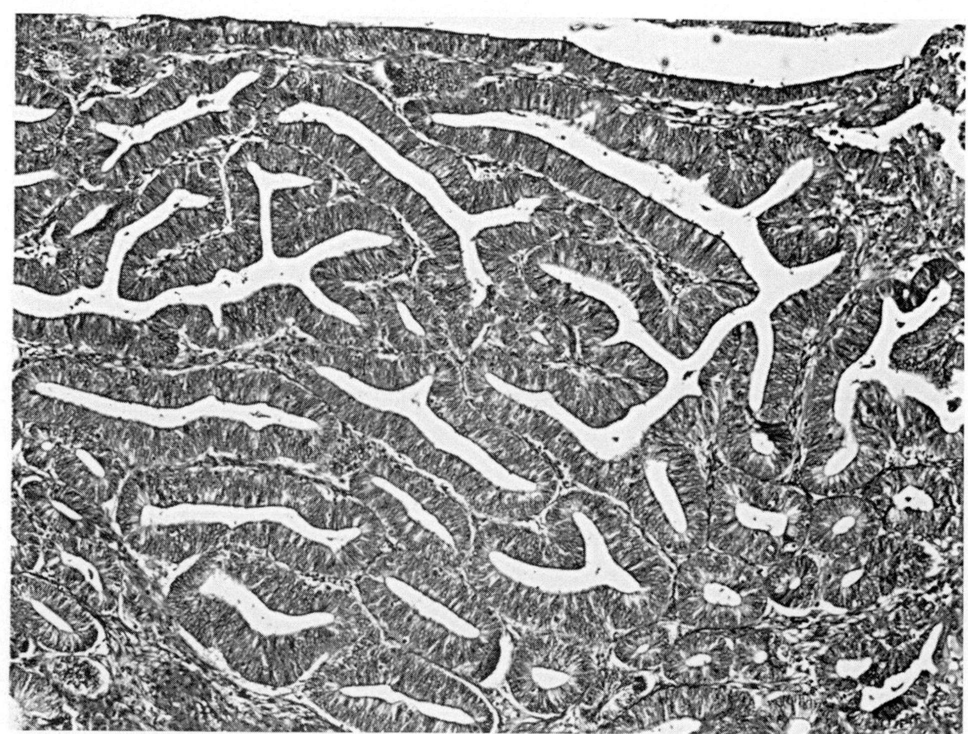

Table 30.5. FIGO Definition for Grading of Endometrial Carcinoma

Histopathologic degree of differentiation:
G1: >5% nonsquamous or nonmorular growth pattern
G2: 6%–50% nonsquamous or nonmorular growth pattern
G3: >50% nonsquamous or nonmorular growth pattern
Notes on pathologic grading:
Notable nuclear atypia, inappropriate for the architectural grade, raises a grade 1 (G1) or grade 2 (G2) tumor by one grade.
In serous adenocarcinoma, clear cell adenocarcinoma, and squamous cell carcinoma, nuclear grading takes precedence.
Adenocarcinomas with squamous differentiation are graded according to the nuclear grade of the glandular component.

FIGO, International Federation of Gynecology and Obstetrics.

pattern with desmoplastic reaction, require an area of involvement equal to or exceeding half of a low-power microscopic field (LPF) (>1 LPF; 4.2 mm in diameter) (39,40).

The differentiation of a carcinoma, expressed as its grade, is determined by architectural growth pattern and nuclear features (Table 30.5). **In the International Federation of Gynecology and Obstetrics (FIGO) grading system proposed in 1989, tumors are grouped into three grades: *grade 1,* 5% or less of the tumor shows a solid growth pattern; *grade 2,* 6% to 50% of the tumor shows a solid growth pattern; and *grade 3,* more than 50% of the tumor shows a solid growth pattern. In addition, notable nuclear atypia that is inappropriate for the architectural grade increases the tumor grade by one.**

Adenocarcinomas with squamous differentiation are graded according to the nuclear grade of the glandular component. This FIGO system is applicable to all endometrioid carcinomas, including its variants, and to mucinous carcinomas. In serous and clear cell carcinomas, nuclear grading takes precedence; however, most investigators believe that these two carcinomas should always be considered high-grade lesions, making grading unnecessary.

About 15% to 25% of endometrioid carcinomas have areas of squamous differentiation (Fig. 30.3). In the past, tumors with benign-appearing squamous areas were called *adenoacanthomas,* and tumors with malignant-looking squamous elements were called *adenosquamous carcinomas*. It is now recommended that the term *endometrial carcinoma with squamous differentiation* be used to replace these two designations because the degree of differentiation of the squamous component parallels that of the glandular component and the behavior of the tumor is largely dependent on the grade of the glandular component (41,42).

A villoglandular configuration is present in about 2% of endometrioid carcinomas (43,44). In these tumors, the cells are arranged along fibrovascular stalks, giving a papillary appearance but maintaining the characteristics of endometrioid cells. The villoglandular variants of endometrioid carcinomas are always well-differentiated lesions that behave like the regular endometrioid carcinomas, and they should be distinguished from papillary serous carcinomas.

Secretory carcinoma is a rare variant of endometrioid carcinoma that accounts for about 1% of cases (45,46). It occurs mostly in women in their early postmenopausal years. The tumors are composed of well-differentiated glands with intracytoplasmic vacuoles similar to early secretory endometrium. These tumors behave as regular well-differentiated endometrioid carcinomas and generally have an excellent prognosis. Secretory carcinoma may be an endometrioid carcinoma that exhibits progestational changes, but a history of progestational therapy is rarely elicited. Secretory carcinoma must be differentiated from clear cell

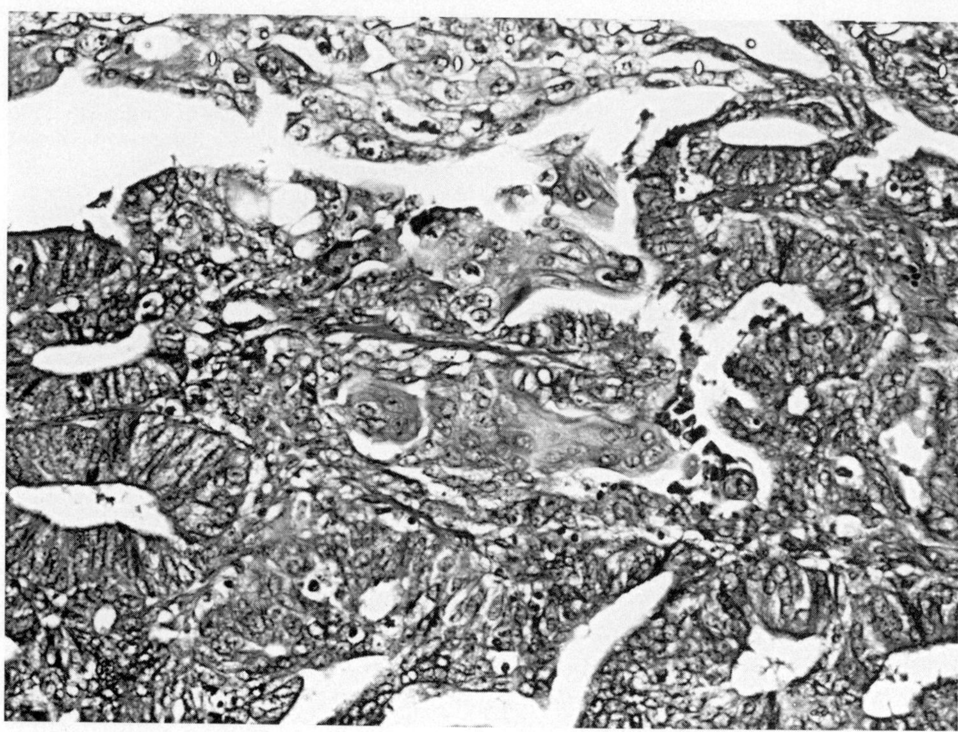

Figure 30.3 Adenocarcinoma with squamous differentiation of endometrium. This lesion is also classified as adenoacanthoma. Squamous cells with eosinophilic cytoplasm and distinct cell borders form solid clusters in the lumina of neoplastic glands. (Reproduced or modified from **Berek JS, Hacker NF.** *Practical gynecologic oncology.* 2nd ed. Baltimore: Williams & Wilkins, 1994, with permission.)

carcinoma because both tumors have predominately clear cells. These two tumors can be distinguished by their structure: secretory carcinomas have uniform glandular architecture, uniform cytology, and low nuclear grade, whereas clear cell carcinomas have more than one architectural pattern and a high nuclear grade.

Mucinous Carcinoma

About 5% of endometrial carcinomas have a predominant mucinous pattern in which more than half of the tumor is composed of cells with intracytoplasmic mucin (47,48). Most of these tumors have a well-differentiated glandular architecture; their behavior is similar to that of common endometrioid carcinomas, and the prognosis is good. It is important to recognize mucinous carcinoma of the endometrium as an entity and to differentiate it from endocervical adenocarcinoma. Features that favor a primary endometrial carcinoma are the merging of the tumor with areas of normal endometrial tissue, presence of foamy endometrial stromal cells, presence of squamous metaplasia, or presence of areas of typical endometrioid carcinoma. Positive perinuclear immunohistochemical staining with vimentin suggests an endometrial origin (49).

Papillary Serous Carcinoma

About 3% to 4% of endometrial carcinomas resemble serous carcinoma of the ovary and fallopian tube (50–53). Most often, these tumors are composed of fibrovascular stalks lined by highly atypical cells with tufted stratification (Fig. 30.4). Psammoma bodies are frequently observed.

Uterine papillary serous carcinomas (UPSCs) are all considered high-grade lesions. They are commonly admixed with other histologic patterns, but mixed tumors behave as aggressively

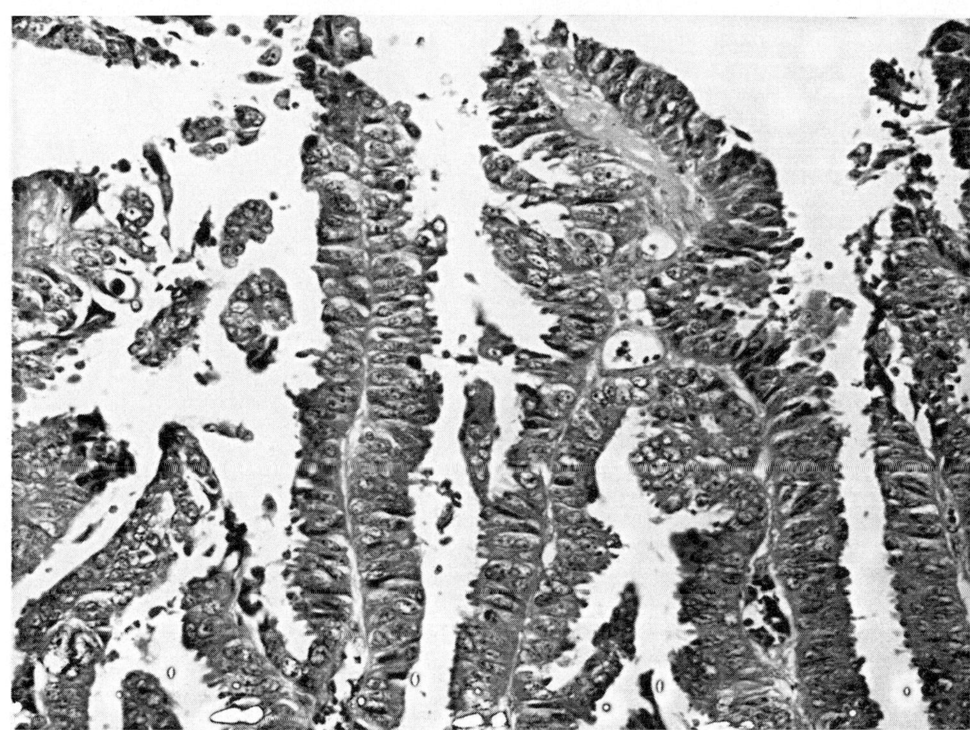

Figure 30.4 Papillary serous carcinoma of endometrium. Branching papillae are supported by delicate fibrovascular cores and lined with columnar cells with moderate nuclear atypism, multiple nucleoli, and mitotic figures. (Reproduced or modified from **Berek JS, Hacker NF.** *Practical gynecologic oncology.* 2nd ed. Baltimore: Williams & Wilkins, 1994, with permission.)

as pure serous carcinomas. Serous carcinomas are often associated with lymph–vascular space and deep myometrial invasion. Even when these tumors appear to be confined to the endometrium or endometrial polyps without myometrial or vascular invasion, they behave more aggressively than endometrioid carcinomas and have a propensity for intraabdominal spread, simulating the behavior of ovarian carcinoma. Of patients with clinical stage I disease, more than half are found to have deep myometrial invasion, three fourths manifest lymph–vascular space invasion (LVSI), and about half have extrauterine disease detected at surgery.

The first description of UPSC, in 1982, noted that this entity usually occurred in elderly, hypoestrogenic women who presented with advanced-stage disease and accounted for up to half of deaths from endometrial carcinoma (50). Since then, several reports have documented the aggressive nature and poor prognosis of UPSC. Even when the disease was confined to an endometrioid polyp without other evidence of spread, recurrence developed in more than half of patients (51,52). More recently, in a report on 50 surgically staged patients with UPSC, extrauterine disease was found in 72% (53). Presence of lymph node metastases, positive peritoneal cytology, and intraperitoneal tumor did not correlate with increasing myometrial invasion (53).

Clear Cell Carcinoma

Clear cell carcinoma accounts for less than 5% of all endometrial carcinomas (45,54). Clear cell carcinoma usually has a mixed histologic pattern, including papillary, tubulocystic, glandular, and solid types.

The cells have highly atypical nuclei and abundant clear or eosinophilic cytoplasm. Often, the cells have a hobnail configuration arranged in papillae with hyalinized stalks (Fig. 30.5).

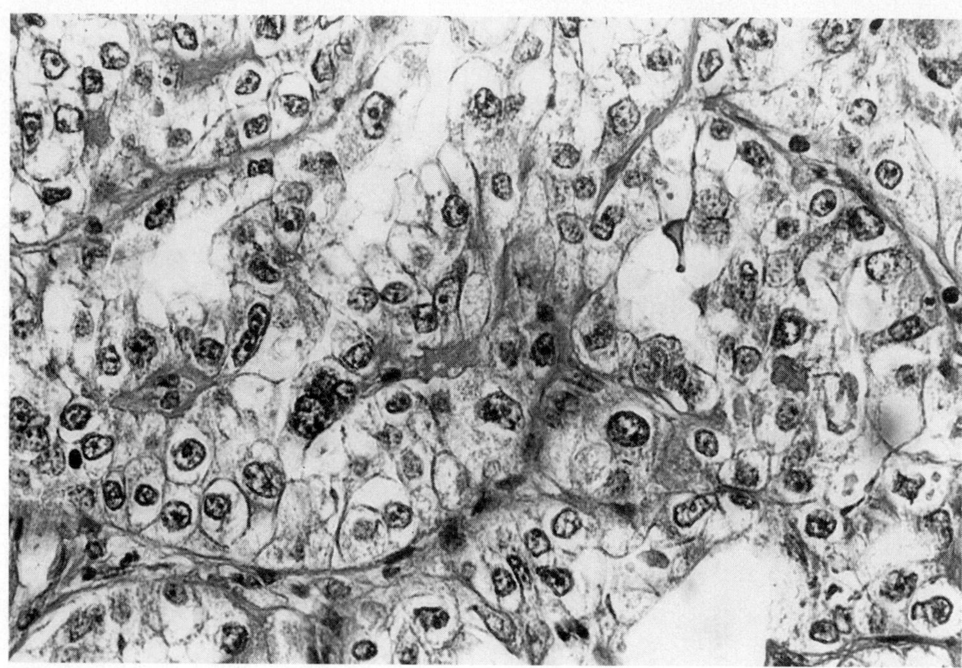

Figure 30.5 Clear cell adenocarcinoma of the endometrium. Back-to-back glands lined by polygonal to columnar cells with distinct cell membrane, abundant granular to clear cytoplasm, and variably sized nuclei (including binucleated and multinucleated forms) with prominent nucleoli (magnification × 400).

Clear cell carcinoma characteristically occurs in older women and is a very aggressive type of endometrial cancer; the prognosis is similar to or worse than that of papillary serous carcinoma. Overall survival rates of 33% to 64% have been reported. Myometrial invasion and LVSI are important prognostic indicators.

Squamous Carcinoma

Squamous carcinoma of the endometrium is rare. Some tumors are pure, but most have a few glands. To establish primary origin within the endometrium, there must be no connection with or spread from cervical squamous epithelium. Squamous carcinoma often is associated with cervical stenosis, chronic inflammation, and pyometra at the time of diagnosis. This tumor has a poor prognosis, with an estimated 36% survival rate in patients with clinical stage I disease (55).

Simultaneous Tumors of the Endometrium and Ovary

Synchronous endometrial and ovarian cancers are the most frequent simultaneously occurring genital malignancies, with a reported incidence of 1.4% to 3.8% (56–60). **Most commonly, both the ovarian and endometrial tumor are well-differentiated endometrioid adenocarcinomas of low stage, resulting in an excellent prognosis.** Patients often are premenopausal and present with abnormal uterine bleeding. The ovarian cancer usually is discovered as an incidental finding and is diagnosed at an earlier stage because of the symptomatic endometrial tumor, leading to a more favorable outcome. As many as 29% of patients with endometrioid ovarian adenocarcinomas have associated endometrial cancer. If more poorly differentiated, nonendometrioid histologic subtypes are present or if the uterine and ovarian tumors are histologically dissimilar, the prognosis is less favorable. Immunohistochemical studies, flow cytometry, and assessment of molecular DNA patterns to detect loss of heterozygosity may be helpful in distinguishing between metastatic and independent tumors, but the differential diagnosis can usually be determined by conventional clinical and pathologic criteria.

Pretreatment Evaluation

After establishing the diagnosis of endometrial carcinoma, the next step is to evaluate the patient thoroughly in order to determine the best and safest approach to management of the disease. A complete history and physical examination is of utmost importance. Patients with endometrial carcinoma are often elderly and obese and have a variety of medical problems, such as diabetes mellitus and hypertension, that affect surgical management. Any abnormal symptoms, such as bladder or intestinal complaints, should be evaluated.

On physical examination, attention should be directed to enlarged or suspicious-feeling lymph nodes, abdominal masses, and possible areas of cancer spread within the pelvis. Evidence of distant metastasis or locally advanced disease in the pelvis, such as gross cervical involvement or parametrial spread, may alter the treatment approach. Stool should be tested for occult blood.

A chest x-ray should be performed to exclude pulmonary metastasis and to evaluate the cardiorespiratory status of the patient. Other routine preoperative studies should include electrocardiography, complete blood and platelet counts, serum chemistries (including renal and liver function tests), blood type and screen, and urinalysis. Other preoperative or staging studies are neither required nor necessary for most patients with endometrial cancer. **Studies such as cystoscopy, colonoscopy, intravenous pyelography, barium enema, and CT scanning of the abdomen and pelvis are not indicated unless dictated by patient symptoms, physical findings, or other laboratory tests** (61). Ultrasonography and magnetic resonance imaging (MRI) can be used to assess myometrial invasion preoperatively with a fairly high degree of accuracy (62). This information may be of use in planning the surgical procedure with regard to whether lymph node sampling should be undertaken.

Serum CA125, an antigenic determinant that is elevated in 80% of patients with advanced epithelial ovarian cancers, also is elevated in most patients with advanced or metastatic endometrial cancer (63). In one study, 23 of 81 patients with apparently localized disease preoperatively had elevated CA125 levels (64). At surgery, 20 (87%) of these 23 patients with an elevated CA125 were found to have extrauterine disease, whereas only 1 of 58 patients with a normal CA125 had disease spread outside the uterus (64). Preoperative measurement of serum CA125 may, therefore, help determine the extent of surgical staging and, if elevated, may be useful as a tumor marker in assessing response to subsequent therapy (65).

Clinical Staging

Clinical staging, according to the 1971 FIGO system (Table 30.6), **should be performed in patients who are deemed not to be surgical candidates, because of their poor medical condition or the spread of their disease** (66). With improvements in preoperative and postoperative care, anesthesia administration, and surgical techniques, almost all patients are medically suitable for operative therapy. One study reported an operability rate of 87% in a series of 595 consecutive patients with clinical early-stage endometrial cancer (67). A small percentage of patients will not be candidates for surgical staging because of gross cervical involvement, parametrial spread, invasion of the bladder or rectum, or distant metastasis.

Surgical Staging

Most patients with endometrial cancer should undergo surgical staging based on the 1988 FIGO system (68–70) (Table 30.7). **At a minimum, the surgical procedure should include sampling of peritoneal fluid for cytologic evaluation, exploration of the abdomen and pelvis with biopsy or excision of any extrauterine lesions suggestive of metastatic cancer, extrafascial hysterectomy, and bilateral salpingo-oophorectomy. The uterine specimen should be opened and tumor size** (71), **depth of myometrial involvement** (72–74), **and cervical extension assessed. Any suspicious pelvic and paraaortic lymph nodes should be removed for pathologic examination.**

Table 30.6. FIGO Clinical Staging of Endometrial Carcinoma (1971)

Stage	Characteristic
I	Confined to the corpus
Ia G123	Uterine cavity <8 cm
Ib G123	Uterine cavity >8 cm
II	Involves the corpus and cervix but has not extended outside the uterus
III	Extends outside the uterus but not outside the true pelvis
IV	Extends outside the true pelvis or obviously involves the mucosa of the bladder or rectum
IVa	Spread to adjacent organs
IVb	Spread to distant organs

FIGO, International Federation of Gynecology and Obstetrics.

Additionally, clinically negative retroperitoneal lymph nodes should be sampled in all patients with one or more of the risk factors noted in Table 30.8. Tumor histology and depth of myometrial invasion appear to be the two most important factors in determining the risk for lymph node metastasis (69,70). The overall incidence of lymph node metastasis in clinical stage I endometrial cancer is about 3% in grade 1, 9% in grade 2, and 18% in grade 3 tumors (Table 30.9). Less than 5% of patients with no

Table 30.7. FIGO Surgical Staging for Endometrial Carcinoma (1988)

Stage	Finding
Ia G123	No myometrial invasion
Ib G123	< $^1/_2$ Myometrial invasion
Ic G123	> $^1/_2$ Myometrial invasion
IIa G123	Extension to endocervical glands
IIb G123	Cervical stromal invasion
IIIa G123	Positive uterine serosa, adnexa, and/or peritoneal cytology
IIIb G123	Vaginal metastasis
IIIc G123	Metastasis to pelvic and/or paraaortic lymph nodes
IVa G123	Tumor invasion of bladder and/or bowel mucosa
IVb	Distant metastasis including intraabdominal and/or inguinal lymph nodes

FIGO, International Federation of Gynecology and Obstetrics.

Table 30.8. Indications for Selective Pelvic and Paraaortic Lymph Node Dissection in Endometrial Cancer

Tumor histology clear cell, serous, squamous, or grade 2–3 endometrioid
Myometrial invasion >$^1/_2$
Isthmus–cervix extension
Tumor size >2 cm
Extrauterine disease

Table 30.9. Relationship of Grade to Lymph Node Mestastasis in Clinical Stage I Endometrial Carcinoma

		Pelvic Nodes		*Aortic Nodes*	
Grade	*No.*	*No.*	*%*	*No.*	*%*
1	180	5	3	3	2
2	288	25	9	14	5
3	153	28	18	17	11

From **Creasman WT, Morrow CP, Bundy BN, et al.** Surgical pathologic spread patterns of endometrial cancer. *Cancer* 1987;60:2035–2041, with permission.

myometrial invasion or with superficial (<50%) myometrial invasion have lymph node metastasis, compared with about 20% of patients with deep (>50%) myometrial invasion (Table 30.10). Pelvic lymph node metastases are present in less than 5% of grade 1 and 2 tumors with superficial myometrial invasion, in about 15% of grade 1 and 2 tumors with deep myometrial invasion or grade 3 tumors with superficial invasion, and in more than 40% of grade 3 tumors with deep myometrial invasion (Fig. 30.6). About one half to two thirds of patients with positive pelvic lymph nodes also have paraaortic lymph node metastases, but the aortic nodes are seldom involved in the absence of pelvic nodal disease. Cervical involvement is associated with about a 15% risk for pelvic or paraaortic node metastasis (70). The incidence of lymph node metastasis also correlates with tumor size (<2 cm, 4%; >2 cm, 15%; entire cavity, 35%) (71). Extrauterine spread of disease increases the risk for pelvic and paraaortic nodal metastasis. Adnexal metastasis increases the risk for pelvic and paraaortic nodal metastasis to 32% and 20%, respectively. Of patients with positive peritoneal cytology, 25% have positive pelvic nodes, and 19% have positive paraaortic nodes (70).

At a minimum, high common iliac and paraaortic lymph node dissections should be performed in the presence of adnexal or cervical involvement, a large tumor (>2 cm), deep (>50%) myometrial invasion, or a moderate to poorly differentiated endometrioid, papillary serous, or clear cell tumor. Pelvic lymph node biopsy may not be as important in patients with these risk factors because most of these patients are treated postoperatively with whole pelvis irradiation. Because fewer than 10% of patients with lymphatic metastasis have grossly enlarged nodes, palpation is not an acceptable alternative to biopsy. Conversely, because almost all patients with lymph node metastases have one or more of the aforementioned risk factors, lymph node biopsies are not required in patients at very low risk for lymphatic metastasis [i.e., patients with small (<2 cm) grade 1 and grade 2 endometrial cancers with only superficial myometrial invasion]. In addition, partial omentectomy should be considered in some high-risk patients, especially those with papillary serous and mixed müllerian tumors, which have a propensity for intraabdominal spread and upper abdominal recurrence.

Table 30.10. Relationship of Myometrial Invasion to Lymph Node Metastasis in Clinical Stage I Endometrial Carcinoma

		Pelvic Nodes		*Aortic Nodes*	
Myometrial Invasion	*No.*	*No.*	*%*	*No.*	*%*
None	87	1	1	1	1
Inner third	279	15	5	8	3
Middle third	116	7	6	1	1
Outer third	139	35	25	24	17

From **Creasman WT, Morrow CP, Bundy BN, et al.** Surgical pathologic spread patterns of endometrial cancer. *Cancer* 1987;60:2035–2041, with permission.

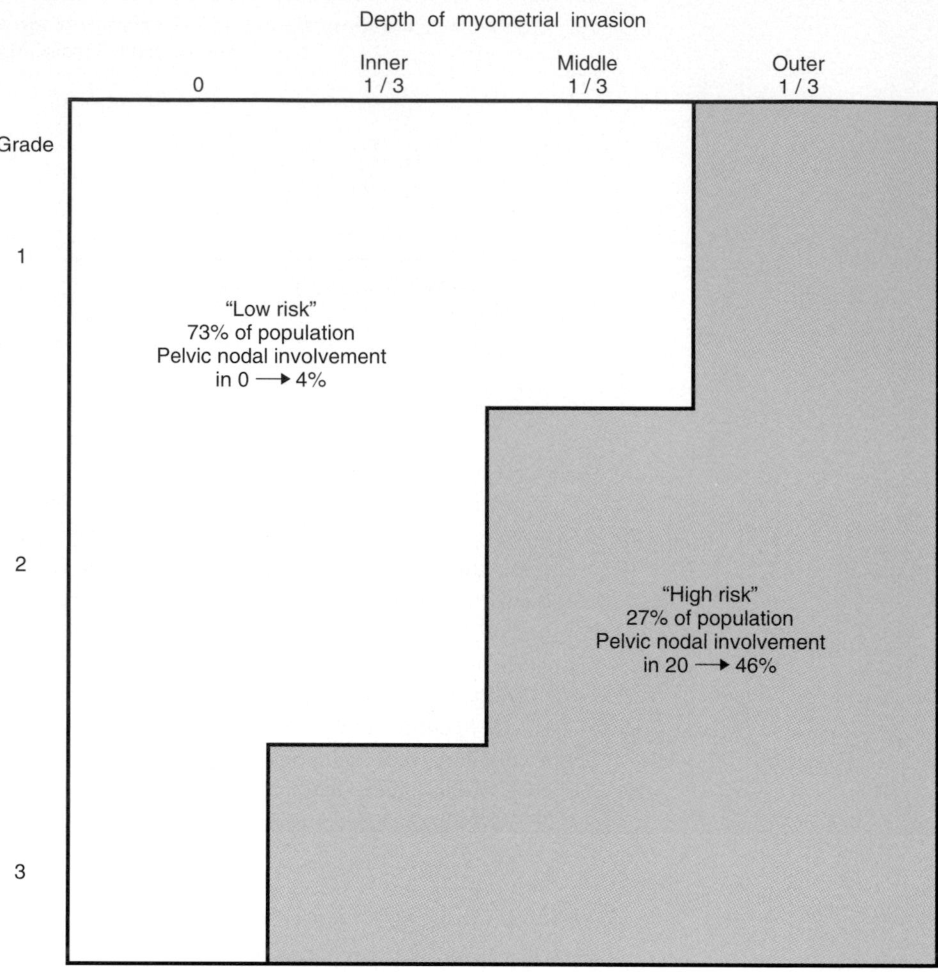

Figure 30.6 The risk for pelvic lymph node metastasis with grade and depth of myometrial penetration in clinical stage I endometrial cancer. Adjuvant pelvic irradiation is recommended for the high-risk group but not for the low-risk group. (From DiSaia PJ, Creasman WT. Management of endometrial adenocarcinoma, stage I with surgical staging followed by tailored adjuvant radiation therapy. *Clin Obstet Gynecol* 1986;13:751, with permission.)

Extended surgical staging, including selective pelvic and paraaortic lymphadenectomy, in patients with endometrial cancer does not significantly add to the morbidity from hysterectomy, which is primarily related to other factors, such as patient weight, age and race, operating time, and surgical technique. The complication rate with this type of surgery is about 20%; about 6% of these complications are serious. The most common complications are wound infection, embolic phenomena, excess blood loss, gastrointestinal injury or obstruction, and lymphocyst formation (75–79).

In addition, selective pelvic and paraaortic lymphadenectomy may have a therapeutic effect (80,81). One study noted that patients who underwent pelvic lymph node sampling had a significant survival advantage overall, as well as in both low-risk and high-risk groups (80). Likewise, paraaortic lymphadenectomy has been found to be a significant positive predictor for recurrence-free survival in patients with high-risk endometrial cancer. Among 137 high-risk patients, the 5-year progression-free survival rate was 77% for patients undergoing paraaortic lymph node dissection, compared with 62% for patients not having paraaortic lymphadenectomy (81).

Table 30.11. Surgical-Pathologic Findings in Clinical Stage I Endometrial Cancer

Surgical-Pathologic Finding	*Percentage of Patients*
Histology	
Adenocarcinoma	80
Adenosquamous	16
Other (papillary serous, clear cell)	4
Grade	
1	29
2	46
3	25
Myometrial invasion	
None	14
Inner third	45
Middle third	19
Outer third	22
Lymph–vascular space invasion	15
Isthmic tumor	16
Adnexal involvement	5
Positive peritoneal cytology	12
Pelvic lymph node metastasis	9
Aortic lymph node metastasis	6
Other extrauterine metastasis	6

Modified from **Creasman WT, Morrow CP, Bundy BN, et al.** Surgical pathologic spread patterns of endometrial cancer. *Cancer* 1987;60:2035–2041, with permission.

Surgical staging is extremely important when one considers the poor correlation of preoperative evaluation and clinical staging with surgical and pathologic findings. In a comparison of preoperative findings with surgical pathology, tumor histology was changed in 27% of patients, tumor grade was changed in 34% of patients, and stage was changed in 51% of patients (82). In the Gynecologic Oncology Group (GOG) series, 22% of 621 patients with clinical stage I endometrial cancer had evidence of extrauterine spread, including lymph node metastasis, adnexal spread, peritoneal implants, and positive peritoneal cytology, discovered at staging laparotomy (70) (Table 30.11). In two other studies, extrauterine spread was found in clinical stages I (19%) and II (40%), with an overall incidence of 23.4% (83), and in 19 (12.3%) of 154 clinical stage I and II patients (84). In a retrospective comparison of clinical and surgical stage with respect to survival in 156 patients with endometrial cancer, surgery resulted in an increase in the stage in 12.4% and 27.3% of clinical stage I and II patients, respectively (85). Surgical stage was found to be the most important factor affecting prognosis.

All patients with endometrial cancer who are taken to the operating room for primary therapy should, therefore, be prepared to undergo surgical staging. Such staging may include selective pelvic and paraaortic lymph node dissection in addition to hysterectomy and salpingo-oophorectomy, based on the intraoperative assessment of risk for lymph node metastasis or other extrauterine spread.

Surgical staging identifies most patients with extrauterine disease and has a significant impact on treatment decisions. Surgical staging also identifies patients with uterine risk factors, including deep myometrial invasion, cervical extension, and LVSI. The identification of these factors allows for a more informed approach to the use of postoperative adjuvant radiotherapy, and it is hoped that this approach will improve survival and spare many patients unnecessary exposure to radiation (86–93).

Table 30.12. Prognostic Variables in Endometrial Carcinoma
Age
Histologic type
Histologic grade
Myometrial invasion
Lymph–vascular space invasion
Isthmus–cervix extension
Adnexal involvement
Lymph node metastasis
Intraperitoneal tumor
Tumor size
Peritoneal cytology
Hormone receptor status
DNA ploidy/proliferative index
Genetic/molecular tumor markers

Prognostic Variables

Although stage of disease is the most significant variable affecting survival, a number of other individual prognostic factors for disease recurrence or survival have been identified, including tumor grade, histopathology, depth of myometrial invasion, patient age, and surgical-pathologic evidence of extrauterine disease spread (Table 30.12). Other factors, such as tumor size, peritoneal cytology, hormone receptor status, flow cytometric analysis, and oncogene perturbations, have also been implicated as having prognostic importance.

Age

In general, younger women with endometrial cancer have a better prognosis than older women. Two authors observed no deaths related to disease in patients with endometrial cancer diagnosed before 50 years of age (86,94). Others have demonstrated a 60.9% 5-year survival rate for patients older than 70 years of age, compared with 92.1% survival rate for patients younger than 50 years of age (95). Decreased survival was associated with an increased risk for extrauterine spread (38% versus 21%) and deep myometrial invasion (57% versus 24%) for these two groups. The GOG reported 5-year survival rates of 96.3% for patients 50 years of age or younger, 87.3% for patients 51 to 60 years, 78% for patients 61 to 70 years, 70.7% for patients 71 to 80 years, and 53.6% for patients older than 80 years of age (96).

Increased risk for recurrence in older patients has also been related to a higher incidence of grade 3 tumors or unfavorable histologic subtypes; however, age appears to be an independent prognostic variable. Increasing patient age is independently associated with disease recurrence in endometrial cancer (91). The mean age at diagnosis of patients who had recurrence or died of disease was 68.6 years, compared with 60.3 years for patients without recurrence. For every 1-year increase in age, the estimated rate of recurrence increased 7%. None of the patients younger than 50 years of age developed recurrent cancer, compared with 12% of patients aged 50 to 75 years and 33% of patients older than 75 years of age.

Histologic Type

Nonendometrioid histologic subtypes account for about 10% of endometrial cancers and carry an increased risk for recurrence and distant spread (97,98). In a retrospective review of 388 patients treated at the Mayo Clinic for endometrial cancer, 52 (13%) had an uncommon histologic subtype, including 20 adenosquamous, 14 papillary serous, 11 clear cell, and 7 undifferentiated carcinomas. In contrast to the 92% survival rate among patients with endometrioid tumors, the overall survival for patients with one of these more aggressive subtypes was only 33%. At the time of surgical staging, 62% of the patients with an unfavorable histologic subtype had extrauterine spread of disease (97).

Histologic Grade

Histologic grade of the endometrial tumor is strongly associated with prognosis (70,76,88–93). In one study, recurrences developed in 7.7% of grade 1 tumors, 10.5% of grade 2 tumors, and 36.1% of grade 3 tumors. Patients with grade 3 tumors were more than 5 times more likely to have a recurrence than were patients with grade 1 and 2 tumors. The 5-year disease-free survival rates for patients with grades 1 and 2 tumors were 92% and 86%, respectively, compared with 64% for patients with grade 3 tumors (91). Another study reported similar results, noting recurrences in 9% of patients with grade 1 and 2 tumors compared with 39% of patients with grade 3 lesions (89). Increasing tumor anaplasia is associated with deep myometrial invasion, cervical extension, lymph node metastasis, and both local recurrence and distant metastasis.

Myometrial Invasion

Because access to the lymphatic system increases as cancer invades into the outer one half of the myometrium, increasing depth of invasion has been associated with increasing likelihood of extrauterine spread and recurrence (69,90,93). The association of depth of myometrial invasion with extrauterine disease and lymph node metastases has been confirmed (69). Of patients without demonstrable myometrial invasion, only 1% had pelvic lymph node metastasis, compared with patients with outer one-third myometrial invasion who had 25% pelvic and 17% aortic lymph node metastases. Survival also decreases with increasing depth of myometrial invasion. In general, patients with noninvasive or superficially invasive tumors have an 80% to 90% 5-year survival rate, whereas those with deeply invasive tumors have a 60% survival rate. The most sensitive indicator of the effect of myometrial invasion on survival is distance from the tumor–myometrial junction to the uterine serosa. Patients with tumors that are less than 5 mm from the serosal surface are at much higher risk for recurrence and death than those with tumors greater than 5 mm from the serosal surface (99,100).

Lymph–Vascular Space Invasion

LVSI appears to be an independent risk factor for recurrence and death from all types of endometrial cancer (93,101–103). The overall incidence of LVSI in early endometrial cancer is about 15%, although it increases with increasing tumor grade and depth of myometrial invasion. One author reported LVSI in 2% of grade 1 tumors and 5% of superficially invasive tumors, compared with 42% of grade 3 tumors and 70% of deeply invasive tumors (101). Another reported deaths in 26.7% of patients with clinical stage I disease who had LVSI, compared with 9.1% of those without LVSI (93). Likewise, an 83% 5-year survival rate has been reported for patients without demonstrable LVSI, compared with a 64.5% survival rate for those in whom LVSI was present (102). Using multivariate analysis, only depth of myometrial invasion, DNA ploidy, and vascular invasion–associated changes correlated significantly with survival of patients with stage I endometrial adenocarcinomas (103).

Isthmus and Cervix Extension

The location of the tumor within the uterus is important. Involvement of the uterine isthmus, cervix, or both is associated with an increased risk for extrauterine disease and lymph node metastasis as well as recurrence. One study reported that if the fundus of the uterus alone was involved with tumor, there was a 13% recurrence rate, whereas if the lower uterine segment or cervix was involved with occult tumor, there was a 44% recurrence rate (88). A subsequent GOG study found that tumor involvement of the isthmus or cervix without evidence of extrauterine disease was associated with a 16% recurrence rate and a relative risk of 1.6 (76). Patients with cervical involvement also tended to have higher-grade, larger, and more deeply invasive tumors, undoubtedly contributing to the increased risk for recurrence.

Adnexal Involvement

Most patients with adnexal spread have other poor prognostic factors that place them at high risk for recurrence. For the 20% of patients with adnexal spread as their only high-risk factor, however, the survival rate has been reported to be as high as 85% (76).

Peritoneal Cytology

The significance of malignant peritoneal cytology in endometrial cancer is a controversial issue (104). Several reports in the literature have noted increased recurrence rates and decreased survival rates and, on this basis, have recommended treatment for positive cytology. In an early report, positive peritoneal cytology was noted in 26 (16%) of 167 patients with clinical stage I adenocarcinoma of the endometrium (105). Recurrent cancer developed in 10 (38%) of these 26 patients, compared with 14 (10%) of 141 patients with negative cytology. Positive peritoneal cytology was found to be associated with deep myometrial invasion, cervical involvement, adnexal spread, and lymph node metastasis as well as a propensity for intraabdominal disease recurrence. Several subsequent reports supported the observation that positive peritoneal cytology was associated with an increased risk for cancer recurrence. Most of the studies included patients with other evidence of extrauterine disease spread and were performed without appropriate multivariate analysis and with patients who were incompletely staged. The GOG study, however, critically analyzed 1,180 clinical stage I and II endometrial cancer patients in whom appropriate surgical and pathologic staging was performed (76). Considering only the 697 patients for whom peritoneal cytology status and adequate follow-up were available, 25 (29%) of 86 patients with positive cytology developed recurrence, compared with 64 (10.5%) of 611 patients with negative cytology. They noted, however, that 17 of the 25 recurrences in the positive cytology group were outside the peritoneal cavity.

In contrast to these reports, an equal number of studies have found no significant relationship between malignant peritoneal cytology and an increased incidence of disease recurrence in early endometrial cancer. In a prospective evaluation of peritoneal cytology in 157 patients with clinical stage I endometrial cancer who underwent primary surgical therapy (106), no treatment was directed specifically to positive cytology. Positive cytology was not significantly associated with disease recurrence. Recurrence developed in 5 (17%) of 30 patients with positive cytology and in 11 (9%) of 127 patients with negative cytology. Of the 5 patients with positive peritoneal cytology who had disease recurrence, only one recurrence arose within the peritoneal cavity. Patients with malignant washings often had other poor prognostic factors: 37%, deep myometrial invasion; 37%, grade 3 tumors; 17%, positive lymph nodes. Disease recurred in none of the patients with positive cytology but no other poor prognostic factors. A subsequent study confirmed by multivariate analysis that positive peritoneal cytology was not an independent prognostic factor for endometrial cancer recurrence. Only 6 (22%) of the 27 patients with positive cytology as their only evidence of extrauterine disease spread suffered a recurrence despite no therapy directed toward this finding (91). Positive peritoneal cytology seems to have an adverse effect on survival only if the endometrial cancer has spread to the adnexa, peritoneum, or lymph nodes—not if the disease is otherwise confined to the uterus (107). More grade 3 tumors (41% versus 19%), vascular invasion (18% versus 6%), adnexal spread (18% versus 4%), lymph node metastasis (29% versus 8%), and intraperitoneal spread (18% versus 2%) occurred in patients with positive peritoneal cytology, which contributed to the overall recurrence rate of 47% in these patients (107). The 5-year survival rate for patients with positive peritoneal cytology with disease otherwise confined to the uterus exceeded 90%.

The following conclusions may be reached regarding the prognostic implications of positive peritoneal cytology:

1. Positive peritoneal cytology is associated with other known poor prognostic factors.

2. Positive peritoneal cytology in the absence of other evidence of extrauterine disease or poor prognostic factors probably has no significant effect on recurrence and survival.

3. Positive peritoneal cytology, when associated with other poor prognostic factors or extrauterine disease, increases the likelihood for distant as well as intraabdominal disease recurrence and has a significant adverse effect on survival.

4. Use of several different therapeutic modalities has not resulted in any proven benefit to patients with endometrial cancer and positive peritoneal cytology.

Lymph Node Metastasis

Lymph node metastasis is the most important prognostic factor in clinical early-stage endometrial cancer. Of patients with clinical stage I disease, about 10% will have pelvic and 6% paraaortic lymph node metastases. Patients with lymph node metastases have almost a sixfold higher likelihood of developing recurrent cancer than patients without lymph node metastases. One study reported a recurrence rate of 48% with positive lymph nodes, including 45% with positive pelvic nodes and 64% with positive aortic nodes, compared with 8% with negative nodes. The 5-year disease-free survival rate for patients with lymph node metastases was 54%, compared with 90% for patients without lymph node metastases (91). The GOG found that the presence or absence of paraaortic lymph node metastases was of paramount importance in determining prognosis. Of 48 paraaortic node–positive patients, 28 (58%) developed progressive or recurrent cancer, and only 36% of these patients were alive at 5 years, compared with 85% of patients without paraaortic node involvement (76).

Intraperitoneal Tumor

Extrauterine metastasis, excluding peritoneal cytology and lymph node metastasis, occurs in about 4% to 6% of patients with clinical stage I endometrial cancer. Gross intraperitoneal spread has been highly correlated with lymph node metastases; one study noted that 51% of patients with intraperitoneal tumor had positive lymph nodes, whereas only 7% of patients without gross peritoneal spread had positive nodes (70). Extrauterine spread other than lymph node metastasis is also significantly associated with tumor recurrence. Another study found that 50% of patients with extrauterine disease developed recurrence, compared with 11% of patients without extrauterine disease, making recurrence almost 5 times more likely in patients with extrauterine disease spread. The 5-year disease-free survival rate for patients with nonlymphatic extrauterine disease was 50%, compared with 88% in the other patients (91).

Tumor Size

Tumor size is a significant prognostic factor for lymph node metastasis and survival in patients with endometrial cancer (71,108). One report determined tumor size in 142 patients with clinical stage I endometrial cancer and found lymph node metastasis in 4% of patients with tumors 2 cm or smaller, in 15% of patients with tumors larger than 2 cm, and in 35% of patients with tumors involving the entire uterine cavity (71). Tumor size better defined an intermediate-risk group for lymph nodes metastasis (i.e., patients with grade 2 tumors with less than 50% myometrial invasion). Overall, these patients had a 10% risk for lymph node metastasis, but there was no nodal metastasis associated with tumors 2 cm or smaller, compared with 18% when tumors were larger than 2 cm. Five-year survival rates were 98% for patients with tumors 2 cm or smaller, 84% for patients with tumors larger than 2 cm, and 64% for patients with tumors involving the whole uterine cavity (108).

Hormone Receptor Status

Estrogen receptor and progesterone receptor levels have been shown to be prognostic indicators for endometrial cancer independent of grade in several studies (109–115). Patients whose tumors are positive for one or both receptors have longer survival times than patients whose carcinomas lack the corresponding receptors. Even patients with metastasis have an improved prognosis with receptor-positive tumors (112). Progesterone receptor levels appear to be stronger predictors of survival than estrogen receptor levels, and the higher the absolute level of the receptors, the better the prognosis.

DNA Ploidy and Proliferative Index

About two thirds of endometrial adenocarcinomas have a diploid DNA content as determined by flow cytometric analysis (103,113,116–124). The proportion of nondiploid tumors increases with stage, lack of tumor differentiation, and depth of myometrial invasion. In several studies, DNA content has been related to clinical course of the disease, with death rates generally reported to be higher in women whose tumors contained aneuploid populations of cells. The proliferative index also is related to prognosis.

Genetic and Molecular Markers

Mutations in codons 12 or 13 of the K-*ras* oncogene have been reported in 10% to 20% of endometrial adenocarcinomas (125). In one study, the presence of mutations of K-*ras* appeared to be an independent unfavorable prognostic factor (126). Overexpression of the HER-2/*neu* oncogene, which encodes for a cell surface glycoprotein that is similar to the human epidermal growth factor receptor, has been identified in 10% to 15% of endometrial adenocarcinomas. It is more frequently found in women with metastatic disease, and overexpression has been related to diminished progression-free survival (127,128). Alteration of the tumor suppressor gene *p53* has been demonstrated in about 20% of endometrial carcinomas and has been associated with papillary serous cell type, advanced stage, and poor prognosis (123,129,130). Expression of *MIB-1 (Ki-67),* a proliferation marker, has been associated with extrauterine disease spread and decreased survival (131). Analysis of homozygous deletions on chromosome 10q23 in human cancer has led to the discovery of the *PTEN* tumor-suppressor gene. Mutations and deletions of the *PTEN* gene occur in 30% to 50% of endometrial cancers, which tend to be endometrioid, well differentiated, and minimally invasive (132). Microsatellite instability, present in about 20% of endometrial cancers, appears to be restricted to endometrioid adenocarcinomas and is associated with other molecular features that predict a favorable outcome, including *PTEN* mutation and absence of *p53* overexpression (133,134).

Treatment

An algorithm for the management of patients with clinical stage I and II endometrial cancer is presented in Fig. 30.7.

Surgery

Abdominal Hysterectomy

Total abdominal hysterectomy and bilateral salpingo-oophorectomy are the primary operative procedures for carcinoma of endometrium. The adnexa should be removed because they may be the site of microscopic metastasis, and patients with endometrial carcinoma are at increased risk for ovarian cancer occurring either simultaneously or developing later. Removal a segment of vagina below the cervix is not necessary.

Laparotomy is performed through an abdominal incision that is adequate to allow thorough intraabdominal exploration and retroperitoneal lymph node dissection, if necessary. A lower abdominal midline vertical incision is most commonly employed, although a lower abdominal transverse, muscle-dividing incision (e.g., Maylard incision) or muscle-detaching incision (e.g., Cherney incision) usually provides adequate exposure. After opening the abdomen, peritoneal washings are taken from the subdiaphragmatic area, paracolic gutters,

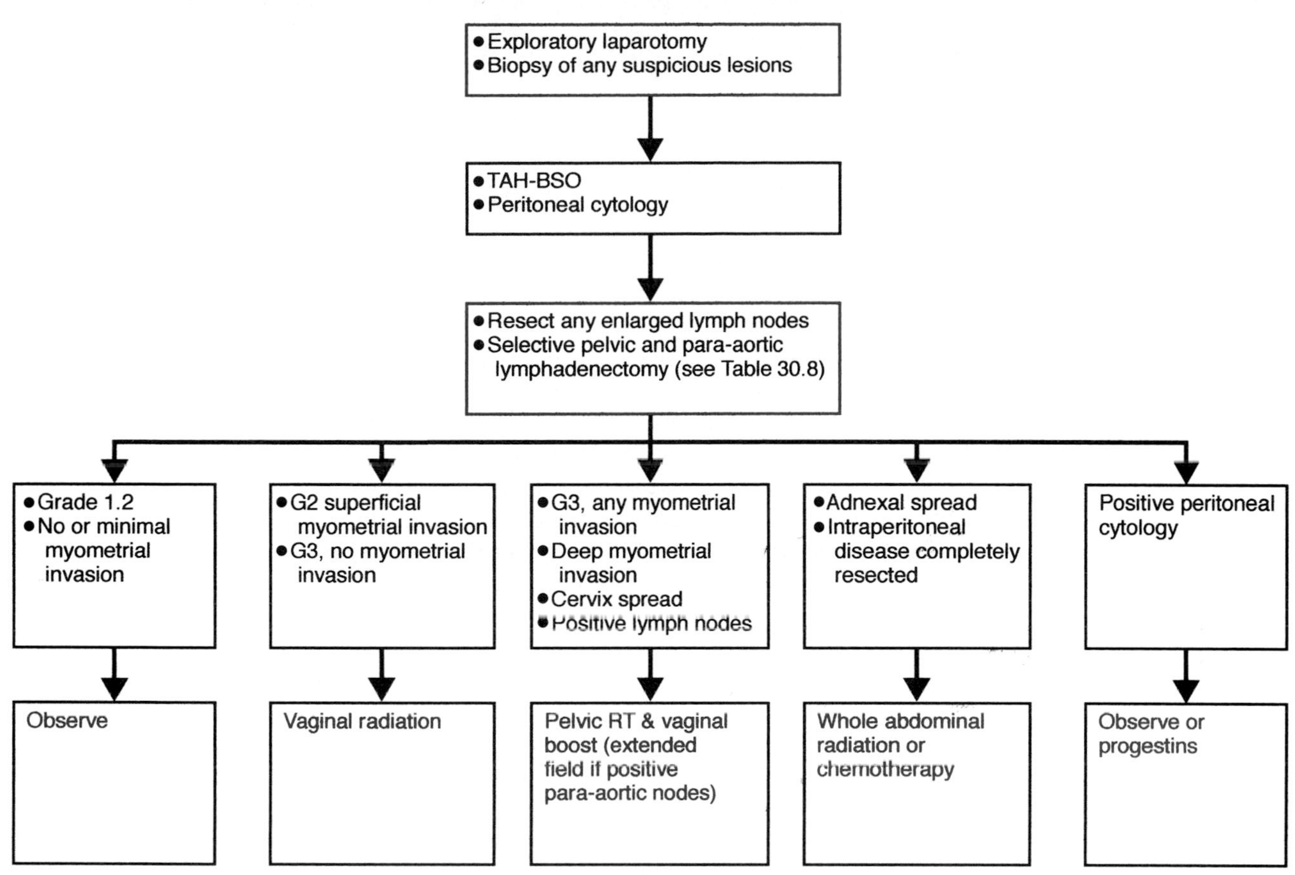

Figure 30.7 Management of patients with clinical Stage I and II endometrial carcinoma.

and pelvis using 50 mL of saline for each. These washings are sent to the cytology laboratory for examination. Exploration of the abdomen and pelvis is then performed, noting particularly the diaphragm, liver, omentum, and pelvic and aortic lymph nodes. The uterus should be observed for tumor on the serosal surface. Any suspicious-looking lesions or lymph nodes should be excised for biopsy or removed for histologic examination. The uterus is opened in the operating room, and tumor size, depth of myometrial invasion, and cervical extension are assessed. This information, along with the surgical findings and knowledge of the preoperative histology, influences whether pelvic and aortic lymph node dissection is indicated. The uterus is sent to the pathology laboratory, where tissue can be obtained for measurement of steroid hormone receptors and flow cytometry.

For patients in whom lymph node sampling is indicated, lower paraaortic lymph node resection can be accomplished by extending the pelvic peritoneal incisions over the common iliac arteries and lower aorta. A sample of lymph nodes along the upper common iliac vessels from either side and the fat pad overlying the vena cava are removed. Pelvic lymph node samples are obtained by removing nodes overlying the midportion of the external iliac artery and vein and within the obturator fossa above and along the obturator nerve. An omental biopsy or partial omentectomy may also be performed.

Vaginal Hysterectomy

Vaginal hysterectomy may be considered for selected patients who are extremely obese and have a poor medical status, or for patients with extensive uterovaginal prolapse. The disadvantages to this approach are that bilateral salpingo-oophorectomy often is technically difficult and abdominal exploration and lymph node sampling cannot be performed. Vaginal hysterectomy is, therefore, particularly suitable for patients who are at low risk for extrauterine spread of disease (i.e., those with clinical stage I, well-differentiated tumors). A 94% survival rate has been found in 56 patients with clinical stage I endometrial carcinoma treated vaginal hysterectomy, with or without postoperative radiotherapy (mostly brachytherapy). Three fourths of these patients had grade 1 lesions (135). Others have reported similar good results (136–138). Vaginal hysterectomy clearly is preferable to radiation therapy alone, but generally should be reserved for specific patients.

Laparoscopic Management

Recent advances in endoscopic surgery have allowed application of a laparoscopic approach to the management of endometrial cancer. Since 1992, there have been several reports that have documented the feasibility of laparoscopically-assisted vaginal hysterectomy with bilateral salpingo-oophorectomy and laparoscopic retroperitoneal lymph node sampling for staging and treatment of patients with endometrial cancer (139–141). In an early study of 59 patients with endometrial cancer managed laparoscopically, 29 had retroperitoneal lymph node sampling (139). In a comparison study of the results of laparoscopic versus traditional laparotomy management of 44 patients with endometrial cancer, 20 patients underwent successful laparoscopic management; 15 had both pelvic and paraaortic lymph node sampling, and 4 had pelvic node sampling only (140). There was no difference in the number of lymph nodes (19 versus 17) removed in the laparoscopy and laparotomy groups, respectively. Patients undergoing laparoscopic management had shorter hospital stays (2.5 versus 5.0 days) and a lower overall complication rate, although all three patients who had serious complications (one ureteral injury and two small bowel herniations through 12-mm trocar sites) were in the laparoscopy group. A subsequent retrospective analysis compared the clinical outcomes and hospital charges for 69 women with early-stage endometrial cancer who underwent laparoscopically-assisted vaginal hysterectomy, compared with 251 women who had traditional laparotomy. The patients managed laparoscopically had fewer complications, shorter hospital stays, and lower overall hospital charges than those who underwent laparotomy. Furthermore, there was no difference in recurrence rates between the two groups (141). Although it seems reasonable that many patients with endometrial cancer can undergo successful laparoscopic management, more experience with the technique and prospective studies are necessary to determine the specific indications for and complications of this approach.

Radical Hysterectomy

Radical hysterectomy, with removal of the parametria and upper vagina, as well as bilateral pelvic lymphadenectomy, does not improve survival of patients with clinical stage I disease compared with extrafascial hysterectomy and bilateral salpingo-oophorectomy alone (142–145). Radical hysterectomy also increases both intraoperative and postoperative morbidity and should not, therefore, be performed for treatment of apparent early endometrial cancer.

Radiation Therapy

Primary surgery followed by individualized radiation therapy has become the most widely accepted treatment for early-stage endometrial cancers. However, about 5% to 15% of endometrial cancer patients have severe medical conditions that render them unsuitable for surgery (61). These patients tend to be elderly and obese with multiple chronic or acute medical illnesses, such as hypertension, cardiac disease, diabetes mellitus, and pulmonary, renal, and neurologic diseases.

Several series have demonstrated that radiotherapy is effective treatment for patients with inoperable endometrial cancer (146–155) (Table 30.13). One reported on the treatment of 120 patients with clinical stage I and 17 patients with clinical stage II endometrial cancer with radiation alone, 85% of whom received only intracavitary irradiation. Because of the high incidence of death caused by intercurrent illness in this group of patients, the 5- and 10-year overall survival rates were only 55% and 28%, respectively, compared with disease-specific

Table 30.13. Review of Recent Series of Endometrial Carcinoma Treated with Radiation Alone

Authors	*Year*	*Stage*	*No. of Patients*	*Local Recurrence Rate (%)*	*Disease-specific Survival Rate (%)*	*Major Complication Rate (%)*
Landgren et al. (146)	1976	I–II	124	22	68	7
		III–IV	26	42	22	
Abayomi et al. (147)	1982	I–II	50	26	78	15
		III–IV	16	—	10	
Patanaphan et al. (148)	1985	I–II	42	14	64	2
		III–IV	10	60	20	
Jones & Stout (149)	1986	I–II	146	22	61	4
		III–IV	14	79	14	
Varia et al. (150)	1987	I–II	73	21	43	10
Wang et al. (151)	1987	I–II	41	22	76	5
Grigsby et al. (152)	1987	I	69	9	88	16
Taghian et al. (153)	1988	I–II	94	6	70	17
		III–IV	10	10	27	
Lehoczky et al. (154)	1991	I	171	20	75	0
Kupelian et al. (155)	1993	I–II	137	14	85	3
		III–IV	15	32	49	

From **Kupelian PA, Eifel PJ, Tornos C, et al.** Treatment of endometrial carcinoma with radiation therapy alone. *Int J Radiat Oncol Biol Phys* 1993;27:817–824, with permission.

survival rates of 87% and 85%, respectively. There was no difference in disease-specific survival rates between patients with stage I and II disease. Intrauterine cancer recurred in 14% of patients, and extrauterine pelvic disease recurred in 3%. The authors also treated 15 patients with stage III and IV disease, usually with a combination of external-beam and intracavitary radiation therapy, yielding a 5-year disease-specific survival rate of 49%. Five patients (3%) had serious late complications of radiation therapy (155).

Although it is generally agreed that intracavitary irradiation is necessary to achieve adequate local control, the indications for external-beam radiation therapy in the primary treatment of endometrial cancer are less well defined. Patients with cervical involvement and known or suspected extrauterine pelvic spread undoubtedly would benefit from external-beam radiation therapy. Theoretically, external-beam irradiation could also sterilize microscopic nodal disease and possibly increase the radiation dose to deep myometrial or subserosal uterine disease that may receive an insufficient dose from intracavitary irradiation alone. A correlation between tumor grade and recurrence has been noted by several authors. One found that the 5-year progression-free survival rate for medically inoperable patients with clinical stage I disease treated with radiotherapy alone was 94% for grade 1, 92% for grade 2, and 78% for grade 3 tumors (152). Therefore, patients with grade 3 tumors and a known propensity for deep myometrial invasion and lymph node metastasis also may benefit from external-beam therapy.

The decision to treat a patient who has endometrial cancer with radiation alone must involve a careful analysis of the relative risks and benefits of surgery. Although radiation alone can produce excellent survival and local control, it should be considered for definitive treatment only if the operative risk is estimated to exceed the 10% to 15% risk for uterine recurrence expected with radiation treatment alone.

Postoperative Adjuvant Therapy

Postoperative therapy should be based on prognostic factors determined by surgical and pathologic staging. Patients can generally be classified into three treatment categories:

Table 30.14. Postoperative Management of Endometrial Carcinoma Based on Surgical-Pathologic Findings and Stage

Surgical-Pathologic Findings	*Stage*	*Postoperative Treatment*
Low risk		
G1, G2, no myoinvasion	Ia G1, 2	None
No cervix/isthmus invasion		
Negative peritoneal cytology		
No LVSI		
No evidence of metastasis		
Intermediate risk		
G1, G2, <50% myoinvasion	Ib G1, 2	Vaginal cuff irradiation
G3, no myoinvasion	Ia G3	
G3, <50% myoinvasion	Ib G3	Pelvic versus vaginal cuff irradiation
G1, G2 isthmus/cervix extension	IIa G1, G2	
G1, G2, G3 >50% myoinvasion	Ic G1, G2, G3	Pelvic irradiation plus vaginal cuff boast
G3, isthmus/cervix extension	IIa G3	
G1, G2, G3 cervix invasion	IIb G1, G2, G3	
LVSI		
Positive peritoneal cytology	IIIa (+ cytology)	Progestin/^{32}P
High risk		
Adnexal/serosal/parametrial spread	IIIa G1, G2, G3	Pelvic and vaginal irridiation
Vaginal metastasis	IIIb G1, G2, G3	(Extended-field radiation therapy if positive aortic/common iliac lymph nodes)
Lymph node metastasis	IIIc G1, G2, G3	
Bladder/rectal invasion	IVa	Pelvic and vaginal irradiation
Intraperitoneal spread	IVb	Whole-abdomen irradiation; systemic chemotherapy

LVSI, lymph–vascular space invasion.

(1) those who show a low incidence of recurrence and a high rate of cure without any postoperative therapy (low risk), (2) those who have a reduced rate of surgical cure but may or may not benefit from additional therapy (intermediate risk), and (3) those who have a high rate of recurrence and a low survival rate without postoperative therapy (high risk) (Table 30.14). Options for postoperative management in these patients include observation, vaginal vault irradiation, external pelvic irradiation, extended-field (pelvic and paraaortic) irradiation, whole-abdomen irradiation, intraperitoneal phosphorus-32 (^{32}P), progestins, or systemic chemotherapy (Fig. 30.7).

Observation

Patients with grade 1 and 2 lesions without myometrial invasion (stage Ia, grades 1 and 2) have an excellent prognosis and require no postoperative therapy. In a GOG study, there were no recurrences and a 100% disease-free 5-year survival rate in the 91 patients in this category, 72 of whom had received no additional treatment after hysterectomy (76). Other investigators have reported equally favorable results with only surgical therapy in similar patients.

Vaginal Vault Irradiation

Numerous studies have shown that the incidence of vaginal recurrence in patients with tumors apparently confined to the uterus can be reduced from as high as 15% to 1% or 2% by the administration of vaginal irradiation. This is important because vaginal vault recurrence carries a poor prognosis. Preoperative or postoperative vaginal vault radium use has been found to decrease the incidence of vaginal recurrence from 14% to 1.7% and to improve 5-year survival rates from 75% to 90% (87). In a 10-year follow-up of a randomized trial comparing surgery alone (total abdominal hysterectomy and bilateral salpingo-oophorectomy) with preoperative and postoperative radium treatment in patients with clinical stage I endometrial adenocarcinoma, the incidence of vaginal recurrence was 7.5% with hysterectomy alone, 4.5% with preoperative intracavitary radium followed by hysterectomy, and 0% with hysterectomy followed by postoperative vaginal radium (156). In a subsequent study of 92 patients with surgical stage I disease who had grade 1 or 2 tumors with less than 50% myometrial invasion treated with total abdominal hysterectomy and bilateral salpingo-oophorectomy and postoperative vaginal cesium or radium, there were no recurrences, and the 5-year estimated disease-free survival rate was 99% (157). There was only one minor complication, proctitis, which responded to conservative treatment.

In a GOG study of surgical and pathologic risk factors and outcomes, none of the three recurrences in the vaginal radiation implant group was vaginal or pelvic, whereas 7.4% of recurrences in the pelvic radiation therapy group were vaginal, and 18.2% of recurrences were vaginal in the group that did not receive adjuvant radiation. The investigators concluded that postoperative vaginal cuff irradiation reduced local recurrence and had a therapeutic ratio superior to whole pelvis irradiation in patients at risk for isolated vaginal cuff recurrence (76).

Postoperative vaginal irradiation is most commonly administered using colpostats to deliver a surface dose of 6,000 to 7,000 cGy to the upper vagina. More recently, afterloading outpatient techniques using high-dose rate have been employed at some centers (158). Morbidity is low, although vaginal stenosis and dyspareunia may be a problem for postmenopausal patients in the absence of regular vaginal dilation. Patients most likely to benefit from vaginal irradiation are those who have surgical stage I grade 1 and 2 tumors with superficial (<50%) myometrial invasion or grade 3 tumors with no invasion and some patients with stage IIa disease who otherwise meet the aforementioned criteria.

External Pelvic Irradiation

External pelvic irradiation decreases the risk for pelvic recurrence after hysterectomy in certain high-risk groups. Patients found to benefit most from adjuvant postoperative whole pelvis irradiation are those with cervical involvement, pelvic lymph node metastases, or pelvic disease outside the uterus (adnexa, parametria), and patients with clinical stage I disease who are at significant risk for nodal metastasis [grade 3 tumors with any degree of myometrial invasion, grade 1 and 2 tumors with more than 50% myometrial invasion, large (>2 cm) grade tumors with superficial myometrial invasion, and any grade tumor with lymph-vascular space invasion] (159).

Of 41 endometrial cancer patients treated with postoperative pelvic irradiation (5,000 to 5,040 cGy) who had grade 3 tumors or deep myometrial invasion and histologically negative paraaortic lymph nodes (pelvic lymph nodes not sampled), 4 patients (9.7%) developed recurrences, but only one of the recurrences (2.4%) was within the treatment field, and the 5-year estimated disease-free survival rate was 88% (157). In the GOG study, the pelvic recurrence rate was higher in the surgery-only group of patients (31.8%) than in the patients who received postoperative external beam radiation therapy (16.8%) (76).

In 1980, the first randomized study was performed to evaluate the possible benefit of postoperative pelvic irradiation in clinical stage I endometrial cancer (93). After total abdominal hysterectomy and bilateral salpingo-oophorectomy, all 540 patients received vaginal vault radium and were then randomized to receive either 4,000 cGy of whole-pelvis irradiation or no further therapy. The addition of pelvic irradiation did not affect the overall 5-year survival rate. Patients receiving pelvic irradiation had a lower pelvic failure rate but a higher distant failure rate. Of note, patients with grade 3 tumors and more than 50% myometrial invasion had a lower rate of death from cancer if they received postoperative pelvic irradiation (18.2% versus 27.5%). This study has been criticized for a lack of complete surgical staging (no lymph node biopsies were done) and the relatively low dose of external-beam irradiation (4,000 cGy) used.

The GOG recently completed a prospective, randomized study of surgery alone versus surgery plus adjuvant pelvic irradiation in intermediate-risk endometrial cancer (stages Ib to IIb occult). Of patients accrued to the study, more than 80% were actually low-risk patients (90.6% stage I, 81.6% grade 1 to 2, 82% <50% myometrial invasion). The pelvic failure rate was 13% (22 of 171 patients) in the surgery-alone group, compared with 0.6% (1 of 179 patients) in the postoperative pelvic irradiation group. Disease-free survival was also better in the patients receiving postoperative pelvic irradiation than in those treated only with surgery (93.7% versus 84.7%, respectively) (160).

Another randomized trial of surgery and postoperative pelvic radiotherapy versus surgery alone for 714 patients with stage I endometrial carcinoma was carried out by the Netherlands PORTEC Study Group. Eligibility criteria were stage IC, grade 1 to 2 and stage IB, grade 2 to 3; patients with stage IB, grade 3 made up only 10% of the study population, and lymph node biopsies and peritoneal cytology were not required. Locoregional recurrences developed in 13.7% of the surgery group, compared with 4.2% of the postoperative pelvic irradiation group. Overall, the 5-year survival rate was no different between the two groups (85% versus 81%, respectively) (161).

Postoperative whole-pelvis external-beam radiation usually involves the delivery of 4,500 to 5,040 cGy in 180 cGy daily fractions over 5 to 6 weeks to a field encompassing the upper half of the vagina inferiorly, the lower border of the L4 vertebral body superiorly, and 1 cm lateral to the margins of the bony pelvis. The dose of radiation at the surface of the vaginal apex is usually boosted to 6,000 to 7,000 cGy by a variety of techniques. The most frequently reported side effects are gastrointestinal, usually abdominal cramps and diarrhea, although more serious complications such as bleeding, proctitis, bowel obstruction, and fistula can occur and may require surgical correction. The urinary system may also be affected in the form of hematuria, cystitis, or fistula. The overall complication rate ranges from 25% to 40%; however, the rate of serious complications requiring surgical intervention is about 1.5% to 3%.

Patients at high risk for recurrence may benefit from pelvic irradiation. The pelvic failure rate is reduced and, at least in patients with grade 3 tumors and deep myometrial invasion, survival rates also appear to be improved. Patients with cervical extension and extrauterine pelvic disease, including adnexal spread, parametrial involvement, and pelvic lymph node metastases, in the absence of extrapelvic disease, also should benefit from postoperative pelvic irradiation.

Extended-field Irradiation

Patients with histologically proven paraaortic node metastases who have no other evidence of disease spread outside the pelvis should be treated with extended-field irradiation. The entire pelvis, common iliac lymph nodes, and paraaortic lymph nodes are included within the radiation field. The paraaortic radiation dose is limited to 4,500 to 5,000 cGy. **Extended-field radiotherapy appears to improve survival in patients with endometrial cancer who have positive paraaortic lymph nodes** (76,162–165).

Five-year survival rates of 47% and 43% have been reported for patients with surgically confirmed paraaortic lymph node metastases only and for those with paraaortic as well as pelvic lymph node metastases, respectively, using postoperative extended-field irradiation. Only one case of severe enteric morbidity occurred in 48 patients, a complication rate of 2% (162). In a GOG study, 37 of 48 patients with positive paraaortic nodes received postoperative paraaortic irradiation, 36% of whom remained tumor free at 5 years (76). A comparison of patients with positive paraaortic nodes treated with megestrol acetate alone versus megestrol acetate and extended-field irradiation showed that the survival rate in the patients receiving extended-field irradiation was significantly better: 53% versus 12.5%, respectively (163). In another study of 18 patients with positive paraaortic nodes, 5-year survival rates were 67% for microscopic nodal disease and 17% for gross nodal disease (164).

Whole-abdomen Irradiation

Whole-abdomen radiation therapy usually is reserved for patients with stage III and IV endometrial cancer. It may also be considered for patients who have papillary serous or mixed müllerian tumors, which have a propensity for upper abdominal recurrence (166–171). The recommended dose to the whole abdomen is 3,000 cGy in 20 daily fractions of 150 cGy with kidney shielding at 1,500 to 2,000 cGy, along with an additional 1,500 cGy to the paraaortic lymph nodes and 2,000 cGy to the pelvis. Gastrointestinal side effects, including nausea, vomiting and diarrhea, sometimes make it necessary to interrupt therapy, but it is rare for patients not to finish treatment because of these symptoms. Hematologic toxicity can be expected to occur during whole-abdomen irradiation, but it is usually mild. The incidence of late complications, mainly chronic diarrhea and small bowel obstruction, is generally low (5% to 10%).

In a series of 27 patients treated with surgical stage III endometrial cancer with whole-abdomen irradiation, patients with spread to the adnexa, positive peritoneal cytology, or both had a 5-year, relapse-free survival of 90%, whereas all patients with macroscopic disease beyond the adnexa had recurrence (166). Similar results were reported by others (167). Some have advocated the use of adjuvant whole-abdomen radiotherapy for patients with high-risk stage I and II endometrial carcinoma, including those with deep myometrial invasion, high-grade tumors, and papillary serous histology, because of the high proportion of recurrences in the upper abdomen. A 5-year recurrence-free survival rate of 85% has been reported (169,170). With whole-abdomen irradiation in patients at increased risk for intraabdominal metastatic disease, such as those with nonnodal extrauterine disease and papillary serous histology, an actuarial 5-year relapse-free survival rate of 70% has been reported, with no significant toxicity (171). Similarly, others have noted a 3-year disease-free survival rate of 79% in patients with stage III and IV endometrial adenocarcinoma treated with whole-abdomen irradiation (172). Still other reports of using adjuvant postoperative whole-abdomen irradiation in early-stage uterine papillary serous carcinoma suggest a reduction in recurrence rates (173–175). Unfortunately, most recurrences are in the upper abdomen in all of these patients, despite this type of radiotherapy. In summary, it is reasonable to use whole-abdomen irradiation postoperatively to treat patients with adnexal or upper abdominal disease, such as in the omentum, that has been completely excised and in patients who are at very high risk for intraabdominal recurrence, such as those with papillary serous tumors, but it should not be used in patients with gross residual intraperitoneal disease.

Intraperitoneal Phosphorus-32

Apparently favorable results for the treatment of positive peritoneal cytology with intraperitoneal ^{32}P have been reported (105). In 23 patients who had positive washings, treatment with ^{32}P resulted in a lower recurrence rate than in historical controls, but the groups differed in risk factors, making conclusions regarding the efficacy of the treatment questionable. Subsequently, it was reported that when ^{32}P was combined with external pelvic irradiation, 20% of patients suffered serious bowel complications requiring surgical intervention, and two patients died of operative complications (176). At present, the role of ^{32}P in the postoperative management of endometrial cancer patients with positive cytology is limited because of the lack of evidence of a therapeutic benefit and the complications when combined with external pelvic irradiation, which these patients often receive for prevention of local pelvic recurrence.

Progestins

Because most endometrial cancers have both estrogen and progesterone receptors and progestins have been used successfully to treat metastatic endometrial cancer, postoperative adjuvant progestin therapy has been attempted to reduce the risk for recurrence. This therapy is attractive because it provides systemic treatment and has few side effects. Unfortunately, several large randomized, placebo-controlled studies have failed to identify a benefit for adjuvant progestin therapy (177–181).

Conversely, in a series of 25 patients with positive peritoneal cytology as their only evidence of disease spread outside the uterus who were treated with adjuvant progestin for 1 year postoperatively (182), 22 patients had a second-look laparoscopy, and only one patient was found to have persistent intraperitoneal malignant cells. No patient had evidence of recurrent cancer. Therefore, progestins may have a role in treating positive peritoneal cytology in this setting.

Chemotherapy

Adjuvant cytotoxic chemotherapy has been studied in a few trials. The GOG treated 181 patients who had poor prognostic factors with postoperative irradiation and then randomly assigned patients to receive no further therapy or *doxorubicin* (*Adriamycin*) chemotherapy. After 5 years of observation, there was no difference in recurrence rates between the two groups (183).

Researchers at the M. D. Anderson Cancer Center treated 62 high-risk patients with postoperative adjuvant *cisplatin, doxorubicin* and *cyclophosphamide* (PAC) chemotherapy. The presence of extrauterine disease was the only significant risk factor for recurrence, and no benefit to adjuvant chemotherapy could be demonstrated (184,185).

Clinical Stage II

Endometrial cancer involving the cervix either contiguously or by lymphatic spread has a poorer prognosis than disease confined to the corpus (186, 201). Preoperative assessment of cervical involvement is difficult. **Endocervical curettage has relatively high false-positive (50% to 80%) and false-negative rates.** Histologic proof of cancer infiltration of the cervix or presence of obvious tumor on the cervix is the only reliable means of diagnosing cervical involvement, although ultrasound, hysteroscopy, or MRI may demonstrate cervical invasion.

The relatively small number of true stage II cases in reported series and the lack of randomized, prospective studies preclude formulation of a definitive treatment plan. Three areas must be addressed in any treatment plan:

1. For optimal results, the uterus should be removed in all patients.
2. Because the incidence of pelvic lymph node metastases is about 36% in stage II endometrial cancer, any treatment protocol should include treatment of these lymph nodes.
3. Because the incidence of disease spread outside the pelvis to the paraaortic lymph nodes, adnexal structures, and upper abdomen is higher than in stage I disease, attention should be directed to evaluating and treating extrapelvic disease.

Two approaches have usually been taken to the treatment of clinical stage II disease:

1. Radical hysterectomy, bilateral salpingo-oophorectomy, and pelvic and paraaortic lymphadenectomy.
2. Combined radiation and surgery (external pelvic irradiation and intracavitary radium or cesium followed in 6 weeks by total abdominal hysterectomy and bilateral salpingo-oophorectomy).

An initial radical surgical approach to treatment of clinical stage II endometrial cancer has the advantage of allowing accurate surgical-pathologic information to be obtained. Conversely, many patients with endometrial cancer are elderly and obese and have medical problems that make this approach unsuitable. In addition, reported results are no better than with combined radiation and less radical surgical therapy. The use of radical hysterectomy may be limited to patients with anatomic problems that prevent optimum dosimetry or other conditions that conflict with the use of radiation therapy.

The most common, traditional approach to the management of clinical stage II endometrial cancer has been to use external and intracavitary irradiation followed by extrafascial hysterectomy. This combined approach has resulted in 5-year survival rates of 60% to 80%, with severe gastrointestinal or urologic complications occurring in about 10% of patients. Patients who have medically inoperable disease are usually treated with external-beam irradiation and one or two intracavitary insertions. Compared with combined radiation and surgery, the results with radiation alone are diminished, but about 50% of patients are long-term survivors (155) (Table 30.13).

Another method for management of clinical stage II endometrial cancer that is gaining favor is an initial surgical approach followed by irradiation. This method is based on the difficulty in establishing the preoperative diagnosis of cervical involvement in the absence of a gross cervical tumor, the evidence that radiation is equally effective when given after hysterectomy, and the high incidence of extrapelvic disease when the cervix is involved. Exploratory laparotomy with an extrafascial or modified radical hysterectomy, bilateral salpingo-oophorectomy, peritoneal washings for cytology, resection of grossly enlarged pelvic nodes, and selective high common iliac and lower paraaortic lymphadenectomy are performed. These procedures are followed by appropriate pelvic or extended-field external and intravaginal irradiation, depending on the results of surgical staging. Excellent results have been reported using this treatment scheme (197–199).

Clinical Stages III and IV

Clinical stage III disease accounts for about 7% to 10% of all endometrial carcinomas (202–209). Patients usually have clinical evidence of disease spread to the parametria, pelvic sidewall, or adnexal structures; less frequently, there is spread to the vagina or pelvic peritoneum. Treatment for stage III endometrial carcinoma must be individualized, but initial operative evaluation and treatment should be considered because of the high risk for occult lymph node metastases and intraperitoneal spread when disease is known to extend outside of the uterus into the pelvis. In the presence of an adnexal mass, surgery should be performed initially to determine the nature of the mass. Surgery should also be performed to determine the extent of disease and to remove the bulk of the disease if possible. This should include peritoneal washings for cytologic examination, selective paraaortic and pelvic lymphadenectomy, as well as removal of any enlarged lymph nodes, biopsy or excision of any suspicious areas within the peritoneal cavity, and partial omentectomy and peritoneal biopsies. Except in patients with bulky parametrial disease, total abdominal hysterectomy and bilateral salpingo-oophorectomy should be performed. Surgical eradication of all macroscopic disease should be the goal because this finding is of major prognostic importance in the management of patients with clinical stage III disease. Postoperative radiotherapy can then be tailored to the extent of disease.

Results of therapy depend on the extent and nature of disease. A 5-year survival rate of 54% has been reported for all patients with stage III disease; however, the survival was 80% when only adnexal metastases were present, compared with 15% when other extrauterine pelvic structures were involved (202). Patients with surgical-pathologic stage III disease have a much better survival rate (40%) than those with clinical stage III disease (16%) (194). Patients who are treated with combined surgery and irradiation fare better than patients who receive radiation therapy alone (209).

Stage IV endometrial adenocarcinoma, in which tumor invades the bladder or rectum or extends outside the pelvis, makes up about 3% of cases (209–213). Treatment of stage IV disease is patient dependent but usually involves a combination of surgery, radiation therapy, and systemic hormonal or chemotherapy. One objective of surgery and radiation therapy is to achieve local disease control in the pelvis to provide palliative relief of bleeding, discharge, and complications involving the bladder and rectum. Control of pelvic disease has been achieved in 28% of 72 patients with stage IV disease treated with radiation alone or in combination with surgery, progestins, or both (210). Several reports have noted a positive impact of cytoreductive surgery on survival, the median survival being about 3 times greater with optimal cytoreduction (18 to 34 months versus 8 to 11 months, respectively) (211–213). Pelvic exenteration may be considered in the very rare patient in whom disease is limited to the bladder, rectum, or both (214,215).

Recurrent Disease

About one fourth of patients treated for early endometrial cancer develop recurrent disease. More than half of the recurrences develop within 2 years, and about three fourths occur within 3 years of initial treatment. The distribution of recurrences is dependent in large part on the type of primary therapy: surgery alone versus surgery plus local or regional radiotherapy. In a GOG study of 390 patients with surgical stage I disease, vaginal and pelvic recurrences were noted to make up 53% of all recurrences in the group treated with surgery alone, whereas only 30% of recurrences were vaginal or pelvic in the group treated with combined surgery and radiotherapy (76). Therefore, after combined surgery and radiotherapy (vaginal or external beam), 70% or more of patients who fail treatment have distant metastases, and most of these patients do not have evidence of local or pelvic recurrence. The most common sites of extrapelvic metastases are the lung, abdomen, lymph nodes (aortic, supraclavicular, inguinal), liver, brain, and bone. In general, patients with isolated vaginal recurrences fare better than those with pelvic recurrences, who in turn have a better chance of cure than those with distant metastases. Patients who initially have well-differentiated tumors or who develop recurrent cancer more than 3 years after the primary therapy also tend to have an improved prognosis.

In a 1984 report on 379 patients with recurrent endometrial cancer seen at the Norwegian Radium Hospital from 1960 to 1976 (216), site of recurrence was local or regional in 190 patients (50%), distant in 108 patients (28%), and local and distant in 81 patients (21%). The median time to reoccur was 14 months for patients with local recurrences and 19 months for patients with distant metastases. Of all recurrences, 34% were detected within 1 year, and 76% were detected within 3 years of primary treatment. At the time of diagnosis of recurrence, 32% of patients had no symptoms. Vaginal bleeding was the most common symptom associated with local recurrence, and pelvic pain was most often present with pelvic recurrence. Hemoptysis was the initial symptom in 32% of patients with lung metastases, but 45% of cases of lung metastases were asymptomatic and picked up on routine chest x-ray. Only 9% of patients with metastases at other sites did not have symptoms; most had pain (37%) or other symptoms such as anorexia, nausea and vomiting, or ascites related to intraabdominal carcinomatosis, neurologic symptoms such as seizures from brain metastases, or jaundice caused by liver metastases.

Overall, only 29 (7.7%) of the 379 patients were alive without evidence of disease from 3 to 19 years. This included 22 patients (12%) with local or pelvic recurrence, 5 patients (5%) with distant metastases, and 2 patients (2%) with both local and distant recurrences. The best results were obtained in the 42 patients with vaginal vault recurrences who were treated with radiotherapy, resulting in a 24% survival rate. None of the 78 patients with pelvic soft tissue recurrence survived. Three patients (7%) with only lung metastases treated with progestins, two patients with lymph node metastases treated with combined radiotherapy and progestins, and two patients with local recurrence and lung metastases treated with radiotherapy, surgery, and progestins survived.

Surgery

A small subset of patients who develop recurrent endometrial cancer may benefit from surgical intervention. Pelvic or vaginal recurrence in patients who have not received prior pelvic irradiation is best treated with external irradiation plus some type of brachytherapy. Surgical resection of a metastatic nodule greater than 2 cm in diameter before irradiation, however, may improve local control. Pretherapy investigation for extrapelvic metastasis in these patients may include surgical evaluation of the peritoneal cavity and retroperitoneal lymph nodes for evidence of subclinical metastases. Upper abdominal disease has been found at laparotomy in 3 (37.5%) of 8 patients with presumed localized pelvic recurrence (217). Presence of subclinical extrapelvic metastases was associated with larger pelvic tumor size (>2 cm) and elevated serum CA125 levels. A few patients with intraperitoneal recurrence may benefit from laparotomy to relieve intestinal obstruction, or tumor-reductive surgery may be performed before whole-abdomen radiation therapy or systemic hormonal or chemotherapy.

Isolated central pelvic recurrence after irradiation is exceedingly rare. In patients with this type of recurrence, exploratory laparotomy may be performed with the plan to proceed with pelvic exenteration if there is no evidence of disease outside the pelvis and no lymph node metastases. Exenterative surgery for recurrent endometrial cancer in the pelvis has rarely been of value because of the high incidence of associated occult extrapelvic metastases. Of 36 patients who underwent pelvic exenteration for recurrent endometrial carcinoma, 75% died of their cancer within 1 year of operation, and only 14% were alive after 5 years (215).

Radiation Therapy

Patients with isolated local or regional recurrences after initial surgical treatment of endometrial cancer should be treated with radiotherapy (218–225). The best local control and subsequent cure are usually achieved by a combination of external-beam radiation therapy followed by a brachytherapy boost to deliver a total tumor dose of at least 6,000 cGy. Women with low-volume disease limited to the pelvis have the best outcome. For patients with isolated vaginal recurrence treated with irradiation, reported survival rates range from 24% to 45%. Conversely, for those patients who have pelvic extension of their disease treated with irradiation, lower survival rates from 0% to 24% have been reported. Initial endometrial cancer grade 1, younger patient age at recurrence, recurrent tumor size 2 cm or less, time to recurrence more than 1 year, vaginal versus pelvic disease, and radiation therapy that included brachytherapy vaginal boost are significant factors in determining control of pelvic disease and survival in patients with locally recurrent endometrial cancer.

Hormone Therapy

Progestational agents for treatment of metastatic endometrial cancer were first described in 1961 (226). The researchers observed an objective response rate of 29% in 21 patients. A beneficial response has been observed in 35% of 308 patients (227). Subsequent reports have noted somewhat less optimistic response rates, probably as a result of more strictly applied criteria for objective responses (228–231) (Table 30.15). Objective response rates of 16% and 11%, respectively, have been noted, with an additional 15% to 40% of patients exhibiting stable disease for at least 3 months (228,229).

Table 30.15. Response to Progestin Therapy in Advanced or Recurrent Endometrial Cancer

Study		*Progestin*	*No. of Patients*	*Response Rate (%)*
Piver et al. (228)	*HPC*	1,000 mg/wk IM	51	14
	MPA	1,000 mg/wk IM	37	19
Podratz et al. (229)	*HPC*	1–3 g/wk IM	33	9
	MA	320 mg/d PO	81	11
Thigpen et al. (230,231)	*MPA*	150 mg/d PO	219	14
		200 mg/d PO	138	26
		1,000 mg/d PO	140	18

HPC, *hydroxyprogesterone caproate* (Delalutin); *MPA, medroxyprogesterone acetate* (Provera, Depo-Provera); *MA, megestrol acetate* (Megace); IM, intramuscular; PO, oral.

In 1986, the GOG initially reported on the use of oral *medroxyprogesterone acetate* for treatment of patients with advanced or recurrent endometrial cancer (230). Of 219 patients with measurable disease, 8% had a complete response, 6% had a partial response, 52% had stable disease, and 34% developed progressive disease within 1 month. The mean survival time for the entire group was 10.4 months. In a follow-up study comparing two different doses of oral *medroxyprogesterone acetate,* similar response rates were achieved (26% for 200 mg/d and 18% for 1,000 mg/d) (231). Neither the type, dose, nor route of administration of the progestin seemed to have an effect on response in these studies.

Response of metastatic endometrial carcinoma to progestin therapy is related to several clinical and pathologic factors. Higher response rates are observed in well-differentiated tumors. A 20.5% response in low-grade tumors and only 1.4% response in high-grade tumors have been noted (229). Likewise, the probability of an objective response to progestin therapy is about 70% for tumors that are estrogen and progesterone receptor positive, compared with about 5% to 15% for tumors that are negative for both receptors. A longer disease-free interval is associated with higher response rates to progestins. The response rate to progestins has been found to range from 6% in patients with an interval from primary treatment to recurrence of less than 6 months to 65% in patients in whom disease recurred more than 5 years after initial treatment (227). Other observed, but less well documented, factors that may have an adverse effect on response to progestins are disease recurrence within a prior radiation field, large tumor burden, and advanced primary versus recurrent disease (227,229).

Tamoxifen, a nonsteroidal antiestrogen with some estrogenic properties, has been evaluated for treatment of metastatic endometrial carcinoma, based on experience in using this agent in breast cancer treatment. Its use as either a single agent or in combination with a progestin is related to its ability to inhibit the binding of estradiol to the estrogen receptor and to increase progesterone receptors. In a review of eight studies using *tamoxifen,* 20 to 40 mg/d, in patients with metastatic endometrial carcinoma, the overall response rate was 22%, with a range of 0% to 53% (232). Responses to *tamoxifen* were more likely to be observed in patients with low-grade, hormone receptor–positive tumors who had demonstrated a prior response to progestin therapy. In an attempt to reverse the hormone receptor downregulation seen with progestin therapy, *tamoxifen* has been given along with progestins, but the overall responses to combined *tamoxifen* and progestin therapy have been similar to those noted for single-agent progestin therapy.

Progestins are currently recommended as initial treatment for all patients with recurrent endometrial cancer. Radiation therapy, surgery, or both should be used whenever feasible for treatment of localized recurrent cancer such as vaginal, pelvic, bone, and peripheral lymph node disease; however, these patients should also be given long-term progestin therapy unless they are known to have a progesterone receptor–negative tumor. Patients with nonlocalized recurrent tumors, especially if progesterone receptors are known to be positive, are candidates for progestin therapy, either *megestrol acetate,* 80 mg twice daily, or *medroxyprogesterone acetate,* 50 to 100 mg three times daily. Progestin therapy should be continued for at least 2 to 3 months before assessing response. If a response is obtained, the progestin should be continued for as long as the disease is static or in remission. In the presence of a relative contraindication to high-dose progestin therapy (e.g., prior or current thromboembolic disease, severe heart disease, or inability of the patient to tolerate progestin therapy), *tamoxifen,* 20 mg twice daily, is recommended. Failure to respond to hormonal therapy is an indication for initiating chemotherapy.

Chemotherapy

Although several chemotherapeutic agents or combinations of agents are capable of inducing objective responses and even remissions in patients with metastatic endometrial carcinoma, response and survival times are short, and all cytotoxic therapy should be considered palliative (232–234). The most active chemotherapeutic agents are *doxorubicin,* the *platinum* compounds *cisplatin* and *carboplatin,* and *paclitaxel* (*Taxol*). *Doxorubicin,* in dosages of 50 to 60 mg/m^2 every 3 weeks, and *carboplatin,* 350 to 400 mg/m^2 every 4 weeks, have been associated with response rates of 21% to 29%. *Paclitaxel,* 250 mg/m^2 as a 24-hour infusion with granulocyte colony-stimulating factor support (235), or 175 mg/m^2 as a 3-hour infusion every 3 weeks (236,237), has produced response rates of about 36%. Alkylating agents such as *cyclophosphamide* and *melphalan, 5-fluoruracil,* and *altretamine* (*hexamethylmelamine*) have shown activity against endometrial cancer. Most responses obtained with use of these agents have been partial, generally averaging only 3 to 6 months, with the median survival time ranging from 4 to 8 months.

Combination chemotherapy regimens employing *doxorubicin* and *cisplatin* (AP), *cyclophosphamide, doxorubicin,* and *cisplatin* (CAP), and *paclitaxel* and *cisplatin* with or without *doxorubicin* (238,239) have resulted in response rates ranging from 38% to 76%. Most responses have been partial, with durations of 4 to 8 months. Despite these fairly impressive response rates, the median survival time has generally been less than 12 months.

Response to chemotherapy in patients with metastatic endometrial cancer does not appear to be affected by prior or concurrent progestin therapy. Metastatic site, age, disease-free interval, histology, and tumor grade also appear to have no effect on chemotherapy response. However, patients with long disease-free intervals and better performance status may live longer. Initial progestin therapy is advised before chemotherapy is undertaken, reserving the use of more toxic chemotherapy agents for situations in which endocrine therapy has failed. Alternatively, eligible patients should be entered into clinical trials.

Treatment Results

Comprehensive survival data for endometrial cancer are provided by FIGO (240). Survival in relation to clinical and surgical stage is shown in Table 30.16 and in relation to surgical stage and grade in Table 30.17. The overall 5-year survival rate was 76%. Surgically staged patients had much better 5-year survival rates than clinically staged patients across all stages (respectively): stage I, 87% versus 54%; stage II, 76% versus 41%; stage III, 57% versus 23%; stage IV, 18% versus 12%. Survival in surgical stage I disease ranged from 90% to 93% for stage Ia grades 1 and 2 and stage Ib grades 1 and 2 to 63% for stage Ic grade 3.

Follow-up after Treatment

History and physical examination remain the most effective methods of follow-up in patients treated for endometrial cancer (241–244). Patients should be examined every 3 to 4 months during the first 2 years and every 6 months thereafter. About half of patients discovered to

Table 30.16. Carcinoma of The Endometrium: Stage Distribution and Actuarial Survival by Stage (Surgical and Clinical)

	Patients Treated		*Survival (%)*	
Stage	*No.*	*%*	*3-Year*	*5-Year*
Surgical				
I	3,996	70	92	87
II	709	12	82	76
III	758	13	66	59
IV	231	4	23	18
Clinical				
I	232	61	63	54
II	64	16	53	41
III	54	14	30	23
IV	33	8	12	12
TOTAL	6,260	100	82	76

Adapted from **Creasman WT, Odicino F, Maisonneuve P, et al.** Carcinoma of the corpus uteri. FIGO Annual Report on the Results of Treatment in Gynecological Cancer. *J Epidemiol Biostat* 2001;6:45–86, with permission.

Table 30.17. Surgically Staged Endometrial Cancer: Acturial 5-Year Survival Rate (%) by Histologic Grade and Stage

	Grade		
Stage	***1***	***2***	***3***
Ia	93	90	69
Ib	90	93	84
Ic	89	81	63
IIa	91	78	57
IIb	78	75	58
IIIa	79	69	44
IIIb	77	40	21
IIIc	61	61	44
IVa	—	—	19
IVb	35	27	7

Adapted from **Creasman WT, Odicino F, Maisonneuve P, et al.** Carcinoma of the corpus uteri. FIGO Annual Report on the Results of Treatment in Gynecological Cancer. *J Epidemiol Biostat* 2001;6:45–86, with permission.

have recurrent cancer have symptoms, and 75% to 80% of recurrences are detected initially on physical examination. Particular attention should be given to peripheral lymph nodes, the abdomen, and the pelvis. Vaginal cytology should be performed at each visit. Although very few asymptomatic recurrences are detected by vaginal cytology, these early recurrences are often amendable to successful therapy.

Chest x-ray every 12 months is an important method of posttreatment surveillance. Almost half of all asymptomatic recurrences are detected by chest x-ray. Other radiologic studies, such as intravenous pyelography and CT scans, are not indicated for routine follow-up of patients who do not have symptoms.

Serum CA125 measurement has been suggested for posttreatment surveillance of endometrial cancer (245,246). Elevated CA125 levels have been documented in patients with recurrent tumor, and these levels have correlated with the clinical course of disease. However, CA125 levels may be normal in the presence of small recurrences, making the utility of CA125 measurements for follow-up of patients after treatment of early-stage disease suspect. CA125 determinations should be obtained in patients with elevated levels at the time of diagnosis or with known extrauterine disease.

Estrogen Replacement Therapy after Treatment of Endometrial Cancer

A history of endometrial cancer has long been considered a contraindication to estrogen replacement therapy because of the concern that occult metastatic disease might be activated by estrogen. Although this is a reasonable concern, the magnitude of this risk has never been quantified and, in fact, **there is no evidence that estrogen therapy after apparently successful treatment of endometrial cancer increases the risk for cancer recurrence.**

In a nonrandomized, retrospective follow-up study of 221 patients with clinical stage I endometrial cancer, 47 patients who had received estrogen after treatment were compared with 174 who had not been treated with estrogen. There were no significant differences between the two groups with respect to know risk factors for cancer recurrence. There were 26 (14.9%) recurrences in the patients not treated with estrogen, compared with only 1 (2.1%) recurrence in the patients treated with estrogen. Moreover, in the group not receiving estrogen, there were 26 deaths (16 from cancer and 10 from intercurrent disease), compared with only 1 death among those taking estrogen (247). Similarly in another report, no recurrent cancers and no intercurrent deaths were found in 44 women who took estrogen after treatment for endometrial cancer, compared with eight recurrences and eight intercurrent deaths (five from myocardial infarction) in 99 women who did not take estrogen (248). In a subsequent study of 123 surgical stage I and II endometrial cancer patients 62 (50.5%) who received estrogen replacement therapy postoperatively were identified. After controlling for risk factors for recurrence, there was no detectable difference in recurrence rate or time to recurrence between those patients who had received estrogen replacement therapy and those who had not (249). More recently, a retrospective cohort study of matched treatment-control pairs found two recurrences (1%) among the 75 women using estrogen, compared with 11 recurrences (14%) in the 75 women not using estrogen after primary therapy for endometrial cancer (250). In all of these studies, however, estrogen replacement therapy did not commence immediately after surgery in most patients.

Because many women who have been successfully treated for endometrial cancer suffer side effects of estrogen deficiency, such as vasomotor instability, vaginal dryness and dyspareunia, as well as the long-term risks of osteoporosis and atherosclerotic heart disease, treatment with estrogen is desirable. The American College of Obstetricians and Gynecologists has stated that for women with a history of endometrial cancer, hormone replacement therapy could be used for the same indications as for any other woman, except that "the selection of appropriate candidates for estrogen treatment should be based on prognostic indicators . . . and the risk she is willing to assume." A compromise between immediate postoperative estrogen replacement therapy and no hormone therapy might be to withhold estrogen for 1 to 3 years after treatment, during which time most recurrences develop, thereby minimizing the chances of administering estrogen to patients with residual cancer. In the interim, symptomatic relief of hot flashes can be achieved by prescribing progestins such a *medroxyprogesterone acetate,* 10 mg orally daily or 150 mg intramuscularly every 3 months, or nonhormonal agents such as *Bellergal, clonidine,* and *venlafaxine.*

Uterine Sarcoma

Uterine sarcomas are relatively rare tumors of mesodermal origin. They constitute 2% to 6% of uterine malignancies (251). There is an increased incidence of uterine sarcomas, usually malignant mixed müllerian tumors (MMMTs), after radiation therapy to the pelvis for either carcinoma of the cervix or a benign condition. The relative risk for uterine sarcoma after pelvic radiotherapy has been estimated to be 5.38, with an interval of usually 10 to 20 years (252). Uterine sarcomas are, in general, the most malignant group of uterine tumors and differ from endometrial cancers with regard to diagnosis, clinical behavior, pattern of spread and management.

Classification

The three most common histologic variants of uterine sarcoma are endometrial stromal sarcoma (ESS), leiomyosarcoma (LMS), and MMMTs of both homologous and heterologous type (252) (Table 30.18). Variations in the relative incidences of uterine sarcomas occur in different published series, probably related to the strictness of criteria used to classify smooth muscle and endometrial stromal tumors as sarcomas. In general, LMS and MMMT each make up about 40% of tumors, followed by ESS (15%) and other sarcomas (5%), although MMMTs predominate in more recent reports. Staging of uterine sarcomas is based on the FIGO system for endometrial carcinoma (Table 30.6 and 30.7).

Endometrial Stromal Tumors

Stromal tumors occur primarily in perimenopausal women between 45 and 50 years of age; about one third occur in postmenopausal women. There is no relationship to parity, associated diseases, or prior pelvic radiotherapy. These tumors are rare in African American

Table 30.18. Classifications of Uterine Sarcomas

I. Pure nonepithelial tumors
   A. Homologous
      1. Endometrial stromal tumors
         a. Low-grade stromal sarcoma
         b. High-grade or undifferentiated stromal sarcoma
      2. Smooth muscle tumors
         a. Leiomyosarcoma
         b. Leiomyoma variants
            (1) Cellular leiomyoma
            (2) Leiomyoblastoma (epithelioid leiomyoma)
         c. Benign metastasizing tumors
            (1) Intravenous leiomyomatosis
            (2) Benign metastasizing leiomyoma
            (3) Disseminated peritoneal leiomyomatosis
   B. Heterologous
      1. Rhabdomyosarcoma
      2. Chondrosarcoma
      3. Osteosarcoma
      4. Liposarcoma
II. Mixed epithelial–nonepithelial tumors
   A. Malignant mixed müllerian tumor
      1. Homologous (carcinosarcoma)
      2. Heterologous
   B. Adenosarcoma

Modified from **Clement P, Scully RE.** Pathology of uterine sarcomas. In: **Coppleson M, ed.** *Gynecologic oncology: principles and practice.* New York: Churchill-Livingston, 1981, with permission.

women. The most frequent symptom is abnormal uterine bleeding; abdominal pain and pressure due to an enlarging pelvic mass occur less often, and some patients do not have symptoms. Pelvic examination usually reveals regular or irregular uterine enlargement, sometimes associated with rubbery parametrial induration. The diagnosis may be determined by endometrial biopsy, but the usual preoperative diagnosis is uterine leiomyoma. At surgery, the diagnosis is suggested by the presence of an enlarged uterus filled with soft, gray-white to yellow necrotic and hemorrhagic tumors with bulging surfaces associated with wormlike elastic extensions into the pelvic veins.

Endometrial stromal tumors are composed purely of cells resembling normal endometrial stroma. They are divided into three types on the basis of mitotic activity, vascular invasion, and observed differences in prognosis: (a) endometrial stromal nodule, (b) low-grade stromal sarcoma, and (c) high-grade or undifferentiated ESS.

Endometrial stromal nodule **is an expansive, noninfiltrating, solitary lesion confined to the uterus with pushing margins, no lymphatic or vascular invasion, and usually less than 3 mitotic figures per 10 high-power microscopic fields (3 MF/10 HPF).** These tumors should be considered benign because there have been no recurrences or tumor-associated deaths reported after surgery (254).

Low-grade ESS or endolymphatic stromal myosis **is distinguished from high-grade or undifferentiated ESS microscopically by a mitotic rate of less than 10 MF/10 HPF as well as clinically by a more protracted course.** Recurrences typically occur late, and local recurrence is more common than distant metastases (255–259). Although low-grade stromal sarcoma often behaves in a histologically aggressive fashion, it lacks the aneuploid DNA content and high proliferative index associated with high-grade stromal sarcoma, and flow cytometric analysis can be used to differentiate the two conditions and predict response to therapy.

Low-grade stromal sarcoma has extended beyond the uterus in 40% of cases at the time of diagnosis, but the extrauterine spread is confined to the pelvis in two thirds of the cases. Upper abdominal, pulmonary, and lymph node metastases are uncommon. Recurrence occurs in almost half of cases at an average interval of about 5 years after initial therapy. Prolonged survival and even cure are not uncommon even after the development of recurrent or metastatic disease.

Optimum initial therapy for patients with low-grade stromal sarcoma consists of surgical excision of all grossly detectable tumor. Total abdominal hysterectomy and bilateral salpingo-oophorectomy should be performed. The adnexa should always be removed because of the propensity for tumor extension into the parametria, broad ligaments, and adnexal structures as well as the possible stimulating effect of estrogen from retained ovaries on the tumor cells. A beneficial effect of radiation therapy has been reported, and pelvic irradiation is recommended for inadequately excised or locally recurrent pelvic disease (255). There is also evidence that low-grade stromal sarcoma is hormone dependent or responsive. Objective responses to progestin therapy have been noted in 6 of 13 patients (48%) (259). Recurrent or metastatic lesions may also be amenable to surgical excision.

***High-grade or undifferentiated ESS* is a highly malignant neoplasm. Histologically, it exhibits greater than 10 MF/10 HPF and often completely lacks recognizable stromal differentiation.** This tumor has a much more aggressive clinical course and poorer prognosis than low-grade stromal sarcoma (253,255,260–262). The 5-year disease-free survival is about 25%. Treatment of high-grade stromal sarcoma should consist of total abdominal hysterectomy and bilateral salpingo-oophorectomy. The dismal therapeutic results obtained to date suggest that radiation therapy, chemotherapy, or both should be used in combination with surgery. These tumors, unlike low-grade stromal sarcoma, are not responsive to progestin therapy.

Leiomyosarcoma

The median age for women with leiomyosarcoma (43 to 53 years) is somewhat lower than that for other uterine sarcomas, and premenopausal patients have a better chance of survival. This malignancy has no relationship with parity, and the incidence of associated diseases is not as high as in MMMT or endometrial adenocarcinoma. There is a higher incidence and a poorer prognosis in African American women. A history of prior pelvic radiation therapy can be elicited in about 4% of patients with leiomyosarcoma. The incidence of sarcomatous change in benign uterine leiomyomas is reported to be between 0.13% and 0.81% (263–270).

Presenting symptoms that are usually of short duration (mean, 6 months) and that are not specific to the disease include vaginal bleeding, pelvic pain or pressure, and awareness of an abdominopelvic mass. The principal physical finding is the presence of a pelvic mass. The diagnosis should be suspected if rapid uterine enlargement occurs, especially in a postmenopausal woman. Endometrial biopsy, although not as useful as in other sarcomas, may establish the diagnosis in up to one third of cases when the lesion is submucosal.

Survival rates for patients with uterine leiomyosarcoma range from 20% to 63% (mean, 47%). The pattern of tumor spread is to the myometrium, pelvic blood vessels and lymphatics, contiguous pelvic structures, abdomen, and then distantly, most often to the lungs. The number of mitoses in the tumor has traditionally been the most reliable microscopic indicator of malignant behavior (Fig. 30.8).

Generally, tumors with less than 5 MF/10 HPF behave in a benign fashion and tumors with more than 10 MF/10 HPF are frankly malignant with a poor prognosis. Tumors with 5 to 10 MF/10 HPF, termed *cellular leiomyomas* or *smooth muscle tumors of uncertain malignant potential,* are less predictable. Therefore, in addition to mitotic index greater than 10, other histologic indicators used to classify uterine smooth muscle tumors as malignant are severe cytologic atypia and coagulative tumor cell necrosis (271). Uterine smooth muscle tumors with any two of these three features are associated with a poor prognosis. Gross presentation

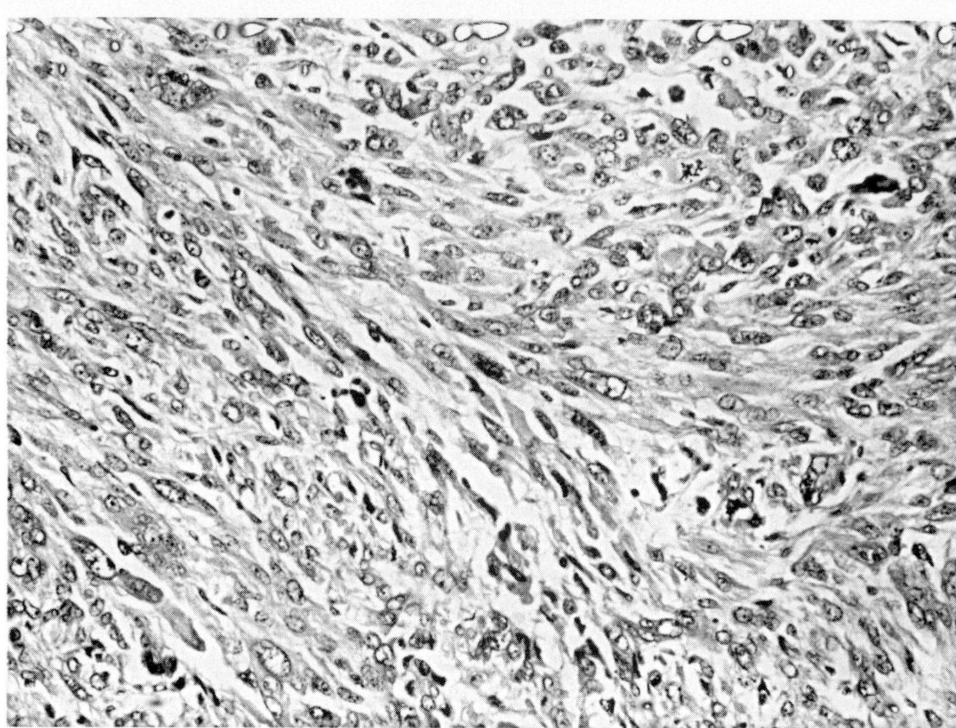

Figure 30.8 Leiomyosarcoma of the uterus. Interlacing bundles of spindle cells have fibrillar cytoplasm, irregular and hyperchromatic nuclei, and multiple mitotic figures. (Reproduced or modified from **Berek JS, Hacker NF.** *Practical gynecologic oncology.* 2nd ed. Baltimore: Williams & Wilkins, 1994, with permission.)

of the tumor at the time of surgery is also an important prognostic indicator. Tumors with infiltrating tumor margins or extension beyond the uterus are associated with poor prognosis, whereas tumors less than 5 cm in size, originating within myomas, or with pushing margins are associated with prolonged survival.

Five other clinical pathologic variants of uterine smooth muscle tumors deserve special comment: (a) myxoid leiomyosarcoma, (b) leiomyoblastoma, (c) intravenous leiomyomatosis, (d) benign metastasizing uterine leiomyoma, and (e) disseminated peritoneal leiomyomatosis.

Myxoid leiomyosarcoma is characterized grossly by a gelatinous appearance and apparent circumscribed border, but microscopically the tumors have a myxomatous stroma and extensively invade adjacent tissue and blood vessels (272). The mitotic rate is low (0 to 2 MF/10 HPF), which belies their aggressive behavior and poor prognosis. Surgical excision by hysterectomy is the mainstay of treatment. The low mitotic rate and abundance of intracellular myxomatous tissue suggest that these tumors would not be responsive to radiation therapy or chemotherapy.

Leiomyoblastoma includes smooth muscle tumors designated as epithelioid leiomyomas, clear cell leiomyomas, and plexiform tumorlets (273). This group of atypical smooth muscle tumors is distinguished by the predominance of rounded rather than spindle-shaped cells and by a clustered or cordlike pattern. These lesions should be regarding as specialized low-grade leiomyosarcomas with fewer than 5 MF/10 HPF and an excellent prognosis. Standard treatment should be hysterectomy.

Intravenous leiomyomatosis is characterized by the growth of histologically benign smooth muscle into venous channels within the broad ligament and then into uterine and iliac veins

(274–277). The intravascular growth takes the form of visible, wormlike projections that extend out from a myomatous uterus into the parametria toward the pelvic sidewalls and may be confused with low-grade stromal sarcoma. Symptoms are related to the associated uterine myomas. Most patients are in the late fifth and early sixth decades of life. The prognosis is excellent, even when tumor is left in pelvic vessels. Late local recurrences can occur, and deaths from extension into the inferior vena cava or metastases to the heart have been reported. Estrogen may stimulate the proliferation of these intravascular tumors. Treatment should be total abdominal hysterectomy and bilateral salpingo-oophorectomy with removal of as much of the tumor as possible.

Benign metastasizing uterine leiomyoma is a rare condition in which a histologically benign uterine smooth muscle tumor acts in a somewhat malignant fashion and produces benign metastases, usually to the lungs or lymph nodes (278). In most instances, intravenous leiomyomatosis is not demonstrable. The metastasizing myomas are capable of growth at distant sites, whereas the intravenous tumors spread only by direct extension within blood vessels. Both experimental and clinical evidence suggests that these tumors are stimulated by estrogen. Therefore, removing the source of estrogen, by castration or withdrawal of exogenous estrogen, or treatment with progestins, tamoxifen, or a gonadotropin agonist has an ameliorating effect (279). Surgical treatment should consist of total abdominal hysterectomy and bilateral salpingo-oophorectomy as well as resection of pulmonary metastases if possible.

Disseminated peritoneal leiomyomatosis is a rare clinical entity characterized by benign smooth muscle nodules scattered throughout the peritoneal cavity (280). This condition probably arises as a result of metaplasia of subperitoneal mesenchymal stem cells to smooth muscle, fibroblasts, myofibroblasts, and decidual cells under the influence of estrogen and progesterone. Most reported cases have occurred in 30- to 40-year-old women who are or who have recently been pregnant or who have a long history of oral contraceptive use. Intriguing features of this disease are its grossly malignant appearance, benign histology, and favorable clinical outcome. Intraoperative diagnosis requires frozen-section examination. Extirpative surgery, including total abdominal hysterectomy, bilateral salpingo-oophorectomy, omentectomy, and excision of as much gross disease as possible may be indicated after the reproductive years. Removal of the source of excess estrogen, treatment with progestins, or both treatments have resulted in regression of unresected tumor masses. Almost all patients have done well.

Malignant Mixed Müllerian Tumors

MMMTs are composed histologically of a mixture of sarcoma and carcinoma. The carcinomatous element is usually glandular, whereas the sarcomatous element may resemble the normal endometrial stroma (homologous or the so-called carcinosarcoma), or it may be composed of tissues foreign to the uterus, such as cartilage, bone, or striated muscle (heterologous). These tumors are most likely derived from totipotential endometrial stromal cells (281–283).

Almost all of these tumors occur after menopause, at a median age of 62 years. There is a higher incidence in African American women. These tumors are often found in association with other medical conditions, such as obesity, diabetes mellitus, and hypertension. A history of previous pelvic irradiation can be obtained in 7% to 37% of patients.

The most frequent presenting symptom is postmenopausal bleeding, which occurs in 80% to 90% of cases. Other less common symptoms are vaginal discharge, abdominopelvic pain, weight loss, and passage of tissue from the vagina. The duration of symptoms is usually only a few months. On physical examination, uterine enlargement is present in 50% to 95% of patients, and a polypoid mass may be seen within or protruding from the endocervical canal in up to 50% of patients. Diagnosis can usually be determined by biopsy of an endocervical mass or endometrial curettage.

The tumor grows as a large, soft, polypoid mass filling and distending the uterine cavity; necrosis and hemorrhage are prominent features. The myometrium is invaded to various degrees in almost all cases. The most frequent areas of spread are the pelvis, lymph nodes, peritoneal cavity, lungs, and liver. This metastatic pattern suggests that these neoplasms spread by local extension and regional lymph node metastasis in a manner similar to that of endometrial adenocarcinoma but behave more aggressively.

The most important single factor affecting prognosis in patients with MMMT is the extent of tumor at the time of treatment. In patients with tumor apparently confined to the uterine corpus (stage I), a 53% 2-year survival rate has been noted, whereas the survival rate dropped to 8.5% when disease had extended to the cervix, vagina, or parametria (stage II and III); no patients with disease outside the pelvis (stage IV) survived (284).

Unfortunately, disease has clinically already extended outside the uterus in 40% to 60% of cases at the time of diagnosis, indicating the highly malignant nature of this lesion. Even when disease is believed to be confined to the uterus preoperatively and potentially is still curable, surgical and pathologic staging identifies extrauterine spread of disease in a significant number of cases. In one study, 55% of women with clinical stage I MMMT had a higher surgical-pathologic stage. Only 28% of tumors were actually confined to the uterine corpus, 16% had extension to the cervix, and 56% showed extrauterine spread (285). A significant occurrence of lymph node metastases and positive peritoneal cytology, respectively, has been found in early-stage MMMT (286,287). Deep myometrial invasion, which is present in about half of stage I cases, is associated with poor prognosis. Almost all patients in whom tumor involves the outer half of the myometrium die from the disease. Patients who die from MMMT also tend to have larger tumors and a higher incidence of LVSI. Patients with a history of prior pelvic irradiation generally have a poorer prognosis. Overall, the 5-year survival rate for patients with MMMT is about 20% to 30%.

Adenosarcoma is an uncommon variant of MMMT (288,289). It consists of an admixture of benign-appearing neoplastic glands and a sarcomatous stroma. Most patients present with postmenopausal vaginal bleeding, and the disease is diagnosed or suspected based on endometrial curettage. Most adenosarcomas are well circumscribed and limited to the endometrium or superficial myometrium. The treatment is hysterectomy and bilateral salpingo-oophorectomy with or without adjuvant radiotherapy. Recurrences, mostly local pelvic or vaginal, have been reported in 40% to 50% of cases, leading some authors to recommend adjuvant postoperative intravaginal or pelvic irradiation.

Treatment of Uterine Sarcomas

Recurrences develop in more than half of cases of uterine sarcoma, even when disease is apparently localized at the time of treatment (290–292). At least half of recurrences occur outside the pelvis, with isolated pelvic failures accounting for less than 10% of recurrences. The most common sites of recurrence are the abdomen and lungs. These data emphasize that the major limitation to cure of uterine sarcomas is distant spread.

Based on this type of evidence, treatment of most stage I and II uterine sarcomas should include hysterectomy, bilateral salpingo-oophorectomy, and treatment of the pelvic lymphatics by irradiation or surgery. Strong consideration should also be given to the use of adjuvant chemotherapy to decrease the incidence of distant metastases. Stage III uterine sarcomas are probably best treated by an aggressive approach of combined surgery, radiation therapy, and chemotherapy. Stage IV disease must be treated with combination chemotherapy.

Surgery

The first step in the treatment of early uterine sarcoma should be exploratory laparotomy. Because extirpative survey is the most important aspect of treatment, and knowledge of the extent and spread of the disease is important for further management, one should not forego or delay surgery by using radiation therapy or chemotherapy first. At the time of surgery, the peritoneal cavity should be carefully explored, and special attention should be given to the pelvic and paraaortic lymph nodes. Total abdominal hysterectomy is the standard procedure, and bilateral salpingo-oophorectomy should also be performed in all patients except premenopausal women with leiomyosarcoma. Based on the surgical and pathologic findings, additional therapy with radiation therapy or chemotherapy can then be planned. Rarely, a patient may be cured by excision of an isolated pulmonary metastasis (293).

Radiation Therapy

Most studies have found adjuvant preoperative or postoperative radiation therapy to be of value in decreasing pelvic recurrences and thereby increasing quality of life in patients with localized ESS and MMMT, but not leiomyosarcoma (294–299). Radiation therapy thus appears to have a role with surgery in the combined treatment of MMMT and ESS confined to the pelvis by increasing the disease-free progression interval and by increasing pelvic control, thereby probably increasing the overall survival to some degree.

Chemotherapy

Several chemotherapeutic agents have been found to have activity in sarcomas, including *vincristine, actinomycin D, cyclophosphamide, doxorubicin,* dimethyl triazeno imidazole carboxamide (*dacarbazine, DTIC*), *cisplatin,* and *ifosfamide* (300,301). *Doxorubicin* appears to be the most active single agent in the treatment of leiomyosarcoma, producing a 25% response rate (302). *Ifosfamide* also has some lesser activity (303). On the other hand, *cisplatin* and *ifosfamide* have demonstrated clear activity in MMMTs, with responses rates of 18% to 42% and 32%, respectively (304–306). *Doxorubicin* has demonstrated less than a 10% response rate in MMMTs (302).

Combination chemotherapy with *doxorubicin* and *DTIC* or these two drugs plus *vincristine* (VAD) and *cyclophosphamide* (CYVADIC) has been reported to yield somewhat higher response rates (300,301,307). More recently, *ifosfamide* with *mesna* uroprotection, *Doxorubicin* and *DTIC* (MAID) have been combined to treat metastatic sarcomas. Combined *ifosfamide* and *cisplatin* chemotherapy has resulted in a higher response rate (54% versus 36%) and a longer progression-free survival than *ifosfamide* chemotherapy alone for treatment of advanced MMMTs (308).

Because of the relatively low survival rate in localized uterine sarcomas and the high incidence of failure due to subsequent distant metastasis, adjuvant treatment programs employing chemotherapy have been tested. Unfortunately, most reports have been unable to demonstrate a clear improvement in survival by the addition of postoperative adjuvant chemotherapy in early uterine sarcoma. The GOG conducted a trial of postoperative adjuvant *doxorubicin* in stage I and II uterine sarcoma patients. Of the 75 patients randomized to receive *doxorubicin,* 41% developed a recurrence, compared with 53% of 81 patients receiving no adjuvant chemotherapy, but these differences were not significant (309). Other smaller, nonrandomized adjuvant chemotherapy studies (310) employing CYVADIC and *cisplatin* plus *doxorubicin* reported recurrence rates of 35% and 24%, respectively (310,311).

References

1. **Jemal A, Thomas A, Murray T, et al.** Cancer statistics, 2002. *CA Cancer J Clin* 2002;52: 23–47.
2. **Bokhman JV.** Two pathogenetic types of endometrial carcinoma. *Gynecol Oncol* 1983;15:10–17.
3. **MacMahon B.** Risk factors for endometrial cancer. *Gynecol Oncol* 1974;2:122–129.
4. **Parazzini F, LaVecchia C, Bocciolone L, et al.** The epidemiology of endometrial cancer. *Gynecol Oncol* 1991;41:1–16.
5. **Parazzini F, LaVecchia C, Negri E, et al.** Reproductive factors and risk of endometrial cancer. *Am J Obstet Gynecol* 1991;64:522–527.

6. **Brinton LA, Berman ML, Mortel R, et al.** Reproductive, menstrual and medical risk factors for endometrial cancer: results from a case control study. *Am J Obstet Gynecol* 1993;81:265–271.

7. **Grady D, Gebretsadik T, Kerlikowske K, et al.** Hormone replacement therapy and cancer risk: a meta analysis. *Obstet Gynecol* 1995;85:304–313.

8. **Fisher B, Constantino JP, Redmond CK, et al.** Endometrial cancer in tamoxifen-treated breast cancer patients: findings from the National Surgical Adjuvant Breast and Bowel Project B-14. *J Natl Cancer Inst* 1994;86:527–537.

9. **Assikis VJ, Jordan VC.** Gynecologic effects of tamoxifen and the association with endometrial carcinoma. *Int J Gynecol Obstet* 1995;49:241–257.

10. **Gordon MD, Ireland K.** Pathology of hyperplasia and carcinoma of the endometrium. *Semin Oncol* 1994;21:64–70.

11. **Kurman RJ, Kaminski PF, Norris HJ.** The behavior of endometrial hyperplasia: a long term study of "untreated" hyperplasia in 170 patients. *Cancer* 1985;56:403–412.

12. **Tavassoli F, Kraus FT.** Endometrial lesions in uteri resected for atypical endometrial hyperplasia. *Am J Clin Pathol* 1978;70:770–779.

13. **Hunter JE, Tritz DE, Howell MG, et al.** The prognostic and therapeutic implications of cytologic atypia in patients with endometrial hyperplasia. *Gynecol Oncol* 1994;55:66–71.

14. **Ferenczy A, Gelfand M.** The biologic significance of cytologic atypia in progestin-treated endometrial hyperplasia. *Am J Obstet Gynecol* 1989;160:126–131.

15. **Gal D.** Hormone therapy for lesions of the endometrium. *Semin Oncol* 1986;13:33–36.

16. **Koss LG, Schreiber K, Oberlander SG, et al.** Detection of endometrial carcinoma and hyperplasia in asymptomatic women. *Obstet Gynecol* 1984;64:1–11.

17. **Abayomi O, Dritschilo A, Emami B, et al.** The value of "routine tests" in the staging evaluation of gynecologic malignancies: a cost effective analysis. *Int J Radiat Oncol Biol Phys* 1982;8:241–244.

18. **Mettlin C, Jones G, Averette H, et al.** Defining and updating the American Cancer Society guidelines for the cancer-related checkup: prostate and endometrial cancers. *CA Cancer J Clin* 1993;43:42–46.

19. **Gerber B, Krause A, Heiner M, et al.** Effects of adjuvant tamoxifen in postmenopausal women with breast cancer: a prospective long-term study using transvaginal ultrasound. *J Clin Oncol* 2000;18:3464–3470.

20. **Barakat RR, Gilewski TA, Almadrones L, et al.** Effect of adjuvant tamoxifen on the endometrium in women with breast cancer: a prospective study using office endometrial biopsy. *J Clin Oncol* 2000;18:3459–3463.

21. **Smith M, McCartney AJ.** Occult, high-risk endometrial carcinoma. *Gynecol Oncol* 1985;22:154–161.

22. **Dubeshter B, Warshal DP, Angel C, et al.** Endometrial carcinoma: the relevance of cervical cytology. *Obstet Gynecol* 1991;77:458–462.

23. **Choo YC, Mak KC, Hsu C, et al.** Postomenopausal uterine bleeding of nonorganic cause. *Obstet Gynecol* 1985;66:225–228.

24. **Pacheco JC, Kempers RD.** Etiology of postmenopausal bleeding. *Obstet Gynecol* 1968;32:40–46.

25. **Hawwa ZM, Nahhas WA, Copenhaver EH.** Postmenopausal bleeding. *Lahey Clin Found Bull* 1970;19: 61–70.

26. **Lidor A, Ismajovich B, Confino E, et al.** Histopathological findings in 226 women with postmenopausal uterine bleeding. *Acta Obstet Gynecol Scand* 1986;65:41–43.

27. **Fortier KJ.** Postmenopausal bleeding and the endometrium. *Clin Obstet Gynecol* 1986;29:440–445.

28. **Chambers JT, Chambers SK.** Endometrial sampling: When? Where? Why? With what? *Clin Obstet Gynecol* 1992;35:28–39.

29. **Grimes DA.** Diagnostic dilation and curettage: a reappraisal. *Am J Obstet Gynecol* 1982;142:1–6.

30. **Kaunitz AM, Masciello A, Ostrowski M, et al.** Comparison of endometrial biopsy with the endometrial Pipelle and Vabra aspirator. *J Reprod Med* 1988;33:427–431.

31. **Dijkuizen FPHLJ, Mol BWJ, Brolmann HAM, et al.** The accuracy of endometrial sampling in the diagnosis of patients with endometrial carcinoma and hyperplasia: a metaanalysis. *Cancer* 2000;89:1765–1772.

32. **Zucker PK, Kasdon EJ, Feldstein ML.** The validity of Pap smear parameters as predictors of endometrial pathology in menopausal women. *Cancer* 1985;56:2256–2263.

33. **Stelmachow J.** The role of hysteroscopy in gynecologic oncology. *Gynecol Oncol* 1982;14:392–395.

34. **Gimpleson RJ, Rappold HO.** A comparative study between panoramic hysteroscopy with directed biopsies and dilation and curettage: a review of 276 cases. *Am J Obstet Gynecol* 1988;158: 489–492.

35. **Bourne TH, Campbell S, Steer CV, et al.** Detection of endometrial cancer by transvaginal sonography with color flow imaging and blood flow analysis: a preliminary report. *Gynecol Oncol* 1991;40:253–259.

36. **Granberg S, Wikland M, Karlsson B, et al.** Endometrial thickness as measured by endovaginal ultrasonography for identifying endometrial abnormality. *Am J Obstet Gynecol* 1991;164:47–52.

37. **Varner RE, Sparks JM, Cameron CD, et al.** Transvaginal sonography of the endometrium in postmenopausal women. *Obstet Gynecol* 1991;78:195–199.

38. **Silverberg SG, Kurman RJ.** *Tumors of the uterine corpus and gestational trophoblastic disease* (3rd series). Washington, DC: Armed Forces Institute of Pathology, 1992.

39. **Hendrickson MR, Ross JC, Kempson RL.** Toward the development of morphologic criteria for well differentiated adenocarcinoma of the endometrium. *Am J Surg Pathol* 1983;7:819–838.

40. **Norris HJ, Tavassoli FA, Kurman RJ.** Endometrial hyperplasia and carcinoma. Diagnostic considerations. *Am J Surg Pathol* 1983;7:839–847.

41. **Zaino RJ, Kurman RJ.** Squamous differentiation in carcinoma of the endometrium: a critical appraisal of adenoacanthoma and adenosquamous carcinoma. *Semin Diagn Pathol* 1988:5:154–171.

42. **Zaino RJ, Kurman R, Herbold D, et al.** The significance of squamous differentiation in endometrial carcinoma. *Cancer* 1991;68:2293–2302.

43. **Chen JL, Trost DC, Wilkinson EJ.** Endometrial papillary adenocarcinomas: two clinicopathologic types. *Int J Gynecol Pathol* 1985;4:279–288.

44. **Sutton GP, Brill L, Michael H, et al.** Malignant papillary lesions of the endometrium *Gynecol Oncol* 1987;27:294–304.

45. **Christophenson WM, Alberhasky RC, Connelly PJ.** Carcinoma of the endometrium: a clinicopathologic study of clear cell carcinoma and secretory carcinoma. *Cancer* 1982;49:1511–1523.

46. **Tobon H, Watkins GJ.** Secretory adenocarcinoma of the endometrium. *Int J Gynecol Pathol* 1985;4:328–335.

47. **Ross JC, Eifel PJ, Cox RS, et al.** Primary mucinous adenocarcinoma of the endometrium: a clinicopathologic and histochemical study. *Am J Surg Pathol* 1983;7:715–729.

48. **Melhern MF, Tobon H.** Mucinous adenocarcinoma of the endometrium: a clinico-pathologic review of 18 cases. *Int J Gynecol Pathol* 1987;6:347–355.

49. **Dabbs DJ, Geisinger KR, Norris HT.** Intermediate filaments in endometrial and endocervical carcinomas. *Am J Surg Pathol* 1986;10:568–576.

50. **Hendrickson M, Ross J, Eifel P, et al.** Uterine papillary serous carcinoma: a highly malignant form of endometrial adenocarcinoma. *Am J Surg Pathol* 1982;6:93–108.

51. **Silva EG, Jenkins R.** Serous carcinoma in endometrial polyps. *Mod Pathol* 1990;3:120–128.

52. **Sherman ME, Bitterman P, Rosenshein NB, et al.** Uterine serous carcinoma. *Am J Surg Pathol* 1992;16:600–610.

53. **Goff BA, Kato D, Schmidt RA, et al.** Uterine papillary serous carcinoma: patterns of metastatic spread. *Gynecol Oncol* 1994;54:264–268.

54. **Abeler VM, Kjorstad KE.** Clear cell carcinoma of the endometrium: a histopathologic and clinical study of 97 cases. *Gynecol Oncol* 1991;40:207–217.

55. **Abeler VM, Kjorstad KE.** Endometrial squamous cell carcinoma: report of three cases and review of the literature. *Gynecol Oncol* 1990;36:321–326.

56. **Eifel P, Hendrickson M, Ross J, et al.** Simultaneous presentation of carcinoma involving the ovary and the uterine corpus. *Cancer* 1982;50:163–170.

57. **Zaino RJ, Unger ER, Whitney C.** Synchronous carcinomas of the uterine corpus and ovary. *Gynecol Oncol* 1984;19:329–335.

58. **Eisner RF, Nieberg RK, Berek JS.** Synchronous primary neoplasms of the female reproductive tract. *Gynecol Oncol* 1989;33:335–339.

59. **Kline RC, Wharton JT, Atkinson EN, et al.** Endometrioid carcinoma of the ovary: retrospective review of 145 cases. *Gynecol Oncol* 1990;39:337–346.

60. **Prat J, Matias-Guiu X, Barreto J.** Simultaneous carcinoma involving the endometrium and the ovary. *Cancer* 1991;68:2455–2459.

61. **Zerbe MJ, Bristow R, Crumbine FC, et al.** Inability of preoperative computed tomography scans to accurately predict the extent of myometrial invasion and extracorporeal spread in endometrial cancer. *Gynecol Oncol* 2000;78:67–70.

62. **Gordon AN, Fleischer AC, Dudley BS, et al.** Preoperative assessment of myometrial invasion of endometrial adenocarcinoma by sonography (US) and magnetic resonance imaging (MRI). *Gynecol Oncol* 1989;34:175–179.

63. **Niloff JM, Klug TL, Schaetzl E, et al.** Elevation of serum CA125 in carcinoma of the fallopian tube, endometrium, and endocervix. *Am J Obstet Gynecol* 1984;148:1057–1058.

64. **Patsner B, Mann WJ, Cohen H, et al.** Predictive value of preoperative serum CA 125 levels in clinically localized and advanced endometrial carcinoma. *Am J Obstet Gynecol* 1988;158:399–402.

65. **Dotters DJ.** Preoperative CA125 in endometrial cancer: Is it useful? *Am J Obstet Gynecol* 2000;182:1328–1334.

66. **FIGO.** Classification and staging of malignant tumors in the female pelvis. *Int J Gynecol Obstet* 1971;9:172–180.

67. **Marziale P, Atlante G, Pozzi M, et al.** 426 Cases of stage I endometrial carcinoma: a clinicopathologic analysis. *Gynecol Oncol* 189;32:278–281.

68. **FIGO.** Annual report on the results of treatment in gynecologic cancer. *Int J Gynecol Obstet* 1989;28:189–193.

69. **Boronow RC, Morrow CP, Creasman WT, et al.** Surgical staging in endometrial cancer: clinical-pathologic findings of a prospective study. *Obstet Gynecol* 1984;63:825–883.

70. **Creasman WT, Morrow CP, Bundy BN, et al.** Surgical pathologic spread patterns of endometrial cancer. *Cancer* 1987;60:2035–2041.

71. **Schink JC, Lurain JR, Wallemark CB, et al.** Tumor size in endometrial cancer: a prognostic factor for lymph node metastasis. *Obstet Gynecol* 1987;70:216–219.

72. **Doering DL, Barnhill DR, Weiser EB, et al.** Intraoperative evaluation of depth of myometrial invasion in stage I endometrial adenocarcinoma. *Obstet Gynecol* 1989;74:930–933.

73. **Goff BA, Rice LW.** Assessment of depth of myometrial invasion in endometrial adenocarcinoma. *Gynecol Oncol* 1990;38:46–48.

74. **Franchi M, Chezzi F, Melpignono M, et al.** Clinical value of intraoperative gross examination in endometrial cancer. *Gynecol Oncol* 2000;76:357–361.

75. **Moore DH, Fowler WC, Walton LA, et al.** Morbidity of lymph node sampling in cancers of the uterine corpus and cervix. *Obstet Gynecol* 1989;74:180–184.

76. **Morrow CP, Bundy BN, Kurman RJ, et al.** Relationship between surgical-pathological risk factors and outcome in clinical stage I and II carcinoma of the endometrium: a Gynecologic Oncology Group study. *Gynecol Oncol* 1991;40:55–65.

77. **Orr JW Jr, Holloway RW, Orr PF, et al.** Surgical staging of uterine cancer: an analysis of perioperative morbidity. *Gynecol Oncol* 1991;42:209–216.

78. **Larson DM, Johnson K, Olson KA.** Pelvic and para-aortic lymphadenectomy for surgical staging of endometrial cancer: morbidity and mortality. *Obstet Gynecol* 1992;79:998–1001.

79. **Homesley HD, Kadar N, Barrett RJ, et al.** Selective pelvic and peri-aortic lymph-adenectomy does not increase morbidity in surgical staging of endometrial carcinoma. *Am J Obstet Gynecol* 1992;167:1225–1230.

80. **Kilgore LC, Partridge EE, Alvarez RD, et al.** Adenocarcinoma of the endometrium: survival comparisons of patients with and without pelvic node sampling. *Gynecol Oncol* 1995;56:29–33.

81. **Mariani A, Webb MJ, Galli L, et al.** Potential therapeutic role of para-aortic lymphadenectomy in node-positive endometrial cancer. *Gynecol Oncol* 2000;76:348–356.

82. **Cowles TA, Magrina JF, Materson BJ, et al.** Comparison of clinical and surgical staging in patients with endometrial carcinoma. *Obstet Gynecol* 1985;66:413–416.

83. **Chen SS.** Extrauterine spread in endometrial carcinoma clinically confined to the uterus. *Gynecol Oncol* 1985;21:23–31.

84. **Vardi JR, Tadros GH, Anselmo MT, et al.** The value of exploratory laparotomy in patients with endometrial carcinoma according to the new International Federation of Gynecology and Obstetrics stagings. *Obstet Gynecol* 1992;80:204–208.

85. **Wolfson AH, Sightler SE, Markoe AM, et al.** The prognostic significance of surgical staging for carcinoma of the endometrium. *Gynecol Oncol* 1992;45:142–146.

86. **Christopherson WM, Connelly PJ, Aberhasky RC.** Carcinoma of the endometrium: an analysis of prognosticators in patients with favorable subtypes and stage II disease. *Cancer* 1983;51:1705–1709.

87. **Lotocki J, Copeland LJ, DePetrillo AD, et al.** Stage I endometrial adenocarcinoma: treatment results in 835 patients. *Am J Obstet Gynecol* 1983;146:141–145.

88. **DiSaia PJ, Creasman WT, Boronow RC, et al.** Risk factors and recurrent patterns in stage I endometrial cancer. *Am J Obstet Gynecol* 1985;151:1009–1015.

89. **Sutton GP, Geisler HE, Stehman FB, et al.** Features associated with survival and disease-free survival in early endometrial cancer. *Am J Obstet Gynecol* 1989;160:1385–1393.

90. **Bucy GS, Mendenhall WM, Morgan LS, et al.** Clinical stage I and II endometrial carcinoma treated with surgery and/or radiation therapy: analysis of prognostic and treatment related factors. *Gynecol Oncol* 1989;33:290–295.

91. **Lurain JR, Rice BL, Rademaker AW, et al.** Prognostic factors associated with recurrence in clinical stage I adenocarcinoma of the endometrium. *Obstet Gynecol* 1991;78:63–69.

92. **Kadar N, Malfetano JH, Homesley HD.** Determinants of survival of surgically staged patients with endometrial carcinoma histologically confined to the uterus: implications for therapy. *Obstet Gynecol* 1992;80:655–659.

93. **Aalders J, Abeler V, Kolstad P, et al.** Postoperative external irradiation and prognostic parameters in stage I endometrial carcinoma. *Obstet Gynecol* 1980;56:419–426.

94. **Crissman JD, Azoury RS, Banner AE, et al.** Endometrial carcinoma in women 40 years of age or younger. *Obstet Gynecol* 1981;57:699–704.

95. **Nilson PA, Koller O.** Carcinoma of the endometrium in Norway 1957–1960 with special reference to treatment results. *Am J Obstet Gynecol* 1969;105:1099–1109.

96. **Zaino RJ, Kurman RJ, Diana KL, et al.** Pathologic models to predict outcome for women with endometrial adenocarcinoma. *Cancer* 1996;77:1115–1121.

97. **Wilson TO, Podratz KC, Gaffey TA, et al.** Evaluation of unfavorable histologic subtypes in endometrial adenocarcinoma. *Am J Obstet Gynecol* 1990;162:418–426.

98. **Fanning J, Evans MC, Peters AJ, et al.** Endometrial adenocarcinoma histologic subtypes: clinical and pathologic profile. *Gynecol Oncol* 1989;32:288–291.

99. **Lutz MH, Underwood PB, Kreutner A Jr, et al.** Endometrial carcinoma: a new method of classification of therapeutic and prognostic significance. *Gynecol Oncol* 1978;6:83–94.

100. **Kaku T, Tsuruchi N, Tsukamoto N, et al.** Reassessment of myometrial invasion in endometrial carcinoma. *Obstet Gynecol* 1994;84:979–982.

101. **Hanson MB, Van Nagell JR, Powell DE, et al.** The prognostic significance of lymph vascular space invasion in stage I endometrial cancer. *Cancer* 1985;55:1753–1757.

102. **Abeler VM, Kjorstad KE, Berle E.** Carcinoma of the endometrium in Norway: a histopathological and prognostic survey of a total population. *Int J Gynecol Cancer* 1992;2:9–32.

103. **Ambros RA, Kurman RJ.** Identification of patients with stage I uterine endometrioid adenocarcinoma at high risk of recurrence by DNA ploidy, myometrial invasion, and vascular invasion. *Gynecol Oncol* 1992;45:235–239.

104. **Lurain JR.** The significance of positive peritoneal cytology in endometrial cancer. *Gynecol Oncol* 1992;46:143–144.

105. **Creasman WT, DiSaia PJ, Blessing J, et al.** Prognostic significance of peritoneal cytology in patients with endometrial cancer and preliminary data concerning therapy with intraperitoneal radiopharmaceuticals. *Am J Obstet Gynecol* 1981;141:921–929.

106. **Lurain JR, Rumsey NK, Schink JC, et al.** Prognostic significance of positive peritoneal cytology in clinical stage I adenocarcinoma of the endometrium. *Obstet Gynecol* 1989;74:175–179.

107. **Kadar N, Homesley HD, Malfetano JH.** Positive peritoneal cytology is an adverse factor in endometrial carcinoma only if there is other evidence of extrauterine disease. *Gynecol Oncol* 1992;46:145–149.

108. **Schink JC, Rademaker AW, Miller DS, et al.** Tumor size in endometrial cancer. *Cancer* 1991;67:2791–2794.

109. **Martin JD, Hahnel R, McCartney AJ, et al.** The effect of estrogen receptor status on survival in patients with endometrial cancer. *Am J Obstet Gynecol* 1983:147:322–324.

110. **Zaino RJ, Satyaswaroop PG, Mortel R.** The relationship of histologic and histochemical parameters to progesterone receptor status in endometrial adenocarcinomas. *Gynecol Oncol* 1983;16:196–208.

111. **Creasman WT, Soper JT, McCarty KS, et al.** Influence of cytoplasmic steroid receptor content on prognosis of early stage endometrial carcinoma. *Am J Obstet Gynecol* 1985;151:922–932.

112. **Liao BS, Twiggs LB, Leung BS, et al.** Cytoplasmic estrogen and progesterone receptors as prognostic parameters in primary endometrial carcinoma. *Obstet Gynecol* 1986;67:463–467.

113. **Geisinger KR, Homesley HD, Morgan TM, et al.** Endometrial adenocarcinoma: a multiparameter clinicopathologic analysis including the DNA profile and sex hormone receptors. *Cancer* 1986;58:1518–1525.

114. **Palmer DC, Muir IM, Alexander AI, et al.** The prognostic importance of steroid receptors in endometrial carcinoma. *Obstet Gynecol* 1988;72:388–393.

115. **Chambers JT, MacLusky N, Eisenfeld A, et al.** Estrogen and progestin receptor levels as prognosticators for survival in endometrial cancer. *Gynecol Oncol* 1988;31:65.

116. **Iverson OE.** Flow cytometric deoxyribonucleic acid index: a prognostic factor in endometrial carcinoma. *Am J Obstet Gynecol* 1986;155:770–776.

117. **Newburg J, Schuerch C, Goodspeed N, et al.** DNA content as a prognostic factor in endometrial carcinoma. *Obstet Gynecol* 1990;76:251.

118. **Stendahl U, Strang P, Wegenius G, et al.** Prognostic significance of proliferation in endometrial adenocarcinomas: a multivariate analysis of clinical and flow cytometric variables. *Int J Gynecol Pathol* 1991;10:271–284.

119. **Ikeda M, Watanabe Y, Nanjoh T, et al.** Evaluation of DNA ploidy in endometrial cancer. *Gynecol Oncol* 1993;50:25.

120. **Podratz KC, Wilson TO, Gaffey TA, et al.** Deoxyribonucleic acid analysis facilitates the pretreatment identification of high-risk endometrial cancer patients. *Am J Obstet Gynecol* 1993;168:1206.

121. **Friberg LG, Noren H, Delle U.** Prognostic value of DNA ploidy and S-phase fraction in endometrial cancer stage I and II: a prospective 5-year survival study. *Gynecol Oncol* 1994;53:64.

122. **Susini T, Rapi S, Savino L, et al.** Prognostic value of flow cytometric deoxyribonucleic acid index in endometrial carcinoma: comparison with other clinical-pathologic parameters. *Am J Obstet Gynecol* 1994;170:527.

123. **Pisani AL, Barbuto DA, Chen D, et al.** HER-2/neu, p53, and DNA analysis as prognosticators for survival in endometrial carcinoma. *Obstet Gynecol* 1995;85:729–734.

124. **Zaino RJ, Davis ATL, Ohlsson-Wilhelm BM, et al.** DNA content is an independent prognostic indicator in endometrial adenocarcinoma. *Int J Gynecol Pathol* 1998;17:312–319.

125. **Mizuuchi H, Nasim S, Kudo R, et al.** Clinical implications of K-ras mutations in malignant epithelial tumors of the endometrium. *Cancer Res* 1992;2777–2781.

126. **Fujimoto I, Shimizu Y, Hirai Y, et al.** Studies on ras oncogene activation in endometrial carcinoma. *Gynecol Oncol* 1993;48:196–202.

127. **Berchuck A, Rodriguez G, Kinney RB, et al.** Overexpression of HER-2/neu in endometrial cancer is associated with advanced stage disease. *Am J Obstet Gynecol* 1991;164:15–21.

128. **Hetzel DJ, Wilson TO, Keeney GL, et al.** HER-2/neu expression: a major prognostic factor in endometrial cancer. *Gynecol Oncol* 1992;47:179–185.

129. **Kohler MF, Berchuck A, Davidoff AM, et al.** Overexpression and mutation of p53 in endometrial carcinoma. *Cancer Res* 1992;52:1622–1627.

130. **Bur ME, Perlman C, Edelmann L, et al.** p53 Expression in neoplasms of the uterine corpus. *Am J Clin Pathol* 1992;98:81–87.

131. **Mariani A, Sebo TJ, Katzmann JA, et al.** Pretreatment assessment of prognostic indicators in endometrial cancer. *Am J Obstet Gynecol* 2000;182:1535–1544.

132. **Risinger JI, Hayes AK, Berchuck A, et al.** PTEN/MMAC1 mutations in endometrial cancers. *Cancer Res* 1997;57:250.

133. **Fiumicino S, Ercoli A, Ferrandina G, et al.** Microsatellite instability is an independent indicator of recurrence in sporadic stage I-II endometrial adeno-carcinoma. *J Clin Oncol* 2001;19:1008–1014.

134. **Maxwell GL, Risinger JI, Alvarez AA, et al.** Favorable survival associated with microsatellite instability in endometrioid endometrial cancers. *Obstet Gynecol* 2001;97:417–422.

135. **Peters WA III, Anderson WA, Thornton N Jr, et al.** The selective use of vaginal hysterectomy in the management of adenocarcinoma of the endometrium. *Am J Obstet Gynecol* 1983;146:285–289.

136. **Malkasian GD, Annegers JF, Fountain KS.** Carcinoma of the endometrium: stage. *Am J Obstet Gynecol* 1980;136:872–883.

137. **Bloss JD, Berman ML, Bloss LP, et al.** Use of vaginal hysterectomy for the management of stage I endometrial cancer in the medically compromised patient. *Gynecol Oncol* 1991;40:74–77.

138. **Chan JK, Lin YG, Monk BJ, et al.** Vaginal hysterectomy as primary treatment of endometrial cancer in medically compromised women. *Obstet Gynecol* 2001;97:707–711.

139. **Childers JM, Brzechffa PR, Hatch K, et al.** Laparoscopically-assisted surgical staging (LASS) of endometrial cancer. *Gynecol Oncol* 1993;51:33–38.

140. **Boike G, Lurain J, Burke J.** A comparison of laparoscopic management of endometrial cancer with traditional laparotomy. *Gynecol Oncol* 1994;52:105(abst).

141. **Gemignani M, Curtin JP, Zelmanovich J, et al.** Laparoscopic-assisted vaginal hysterectomy for endometrial cancer: clinical outcomes and hospital charges. *Gynecol Oncol* 1999;73:5–11.

142. **Lewis BV, Stallworthy JA, Cowdell R.** Adenocarcinoma of the body of the uterus. *J Obstet Gynecol Br Commonw* 1970;77:343–348.

143. **DeMuelenaere GFGO.** The case against Wertheim's hysterectomy in endometrial carcinoma. *J Obstet Gynecol Br Commonw* 1973;80:728–734.

144. **Rutledge F.** The role of radical hysterectomy in adenocarcinoma of the endometrium. *Gynecol Oncol* 1974;2:331–347.

145. **Jones HWIII.** Treatment of adenocarcinoma of the endometrium. *Obstet Gynecol Surv* 1975;30:147–169.

146. **Landgren R, Fletcher G, Delclos L, et al.** Irradiation of endometrial cancer in patients with medical contraindication to surgery or with unresectable lesions. *AJR Am J Roentgenol* 1976;126:148–154.

147. **Abayomi O, Tak W, Emami B, et al.** Treatment of endometrial carcinoma with radiation therapy alone. *Cancer* 1982;49:2466–2469.

148. **Patanaphan V, Salazar O, Chougule P.** What can be expected when radiation therapy becomes the only curative alternative for endometrial cancer? *Cancer* 1985;55:1462–1467.

149. **Jones D, Stout R.** Results of intracavitary radium treatment for adenocarcinoma of the body of the uterus. *Clin Radiol* 1986;169–171.

150. **Varia M, Rosenman, Halle J, et al.** Primary radiation therapy for medically inoperable patients with endometrial carcinoma-stages I–II. *Int J Radiat Oncol Biol Phys* 1987;13:11–15.

151. **Wang M, Hussey D, Vigliotti A, et al.** Inoperable adenocarcinoma of the endometrium: radiation therapy. *Radiology* 1987;165:561–565.

152. **Grigsby P, Kuske R, Perez C, et al.** Medically inoperable stage I adenocarcinoma of the endometrium treated with radiotherapy alone. *Int J Radiat Oncol Biol Phys* 1987;13:483–488.

153. **Taghian A, Pernot M, Hoffstetter S, et al.** Radiation therapy alone for medically inoperable patients with adenocarcinoma of the endometrium. *Int J Radiat Oncol Biol Phys* 1988;15:1135–1140.

154. **Lehoczky O, Busze P, Ungar L, et al.** Stage I endometrial carcinoma: treatment of nonoperable patients with intracavitary radiation therapy alone. *Gynecol Oncol* 1991;43:211–216.

155. **Kupelian PA, Eifel PJ, Tornos C, et al.** Treatment of endometrial carcinoma with radiation therapy alone. *Int J Radiat Oncol Biol Phys* 1993;27:817–824.

156. **Piver MS, Yazigi R, Blumenson L, et al.** A prospective trial comparing hysterectomy, hysterectomy plus vaginal radium and uterine radium plus hysterectomy in stage I endometrial cancer. *Obstet Gynecol* 1979;54:85–89.

157. **Piver MS, Hempling RE.** A prospective trial of postoperative vaginal radium/cesium for grade 1–2 less than 50% myometrial invasion and pelvic irradiation therapy for grade 3 or deep myometrial invasion in surgical stage I endometrial adenocarcinoma. *Cancer* 1990;66:1133–1138.

158. **Peschel RE, Healey GA, Smith RJ, et al.** High dose rate remote afterloading for endometrial cancer. *Endocurie Hyperthem Oncol* 1989;5:209–214.

159. **Stryker JA, Podczaski E, Kaminski P, et al.** Adjuvant external beam therapy for pathologic stage I and occult stage II endometrial carcinoma. *Cancer* 1991;67:2872–2879.

160. **Roberts JA, Brunetto VL, Keys HM, et al.** A phase III randomized study of surgery versus surgery plus adjuvant radiation therapy in intermediate risk endometrial adenocarcinoma. *Gynecol Oncol* 1998;68:135.

161. **Creutzberg CL, vanPatten WLJ, Kopar PCM, et al.** Surgery and postoperative radiotherapy versus surgery alone for patients with stage I endometrial carcinoma: multicenter randomized trail. *Lancet* 2000;355:1404–1411.

162. **Potish RA, Twiggs LB, Adcock LL, et al.** Para-aortic lymph node radiotherapy in cancer of the uterine corpus. *Obstet Gynecol* 1985;65:251–256.

163. **Rose PG, Cha SD, Tak WK, et al.** Radiation therapy for surgically proven paraaortic node metastasis in endometrial carcinoma. *Int J Radiat Oncol Biol Phys* 992;24:229–233.

164. **Feuer GA, Calanog A.** Endometrial carcinoma: treatment of positive para-aortic nodes. *Gynecol Oncol* 1987;27:104–109.

165. **Corn BW, Lanciano RM, Greven KM, et al.** Endometrial cancer with para-aortic adenopathy: patterns of failure and opportunities for cure. *Int J Radiat Oncol Biol Phys* 1992;24:223–227.

166. **Potish RA, Twiggs LB, Adcock LL, et al.** Role of whole abdominal radiation therapy in the management of endometrial cancer; prognostic importance of factors indicating peritoneal metastases. *Gynecol Oncol* 1985;21:80–86.

167. **Greer BE, Hamberger AD.** Treatment of intraperitoneal metastatic adenocarcinoma of the endometrium by the whole-abdomen moving-strip technique and pelvic boost irradiation. *Gynecol Oncol* 1983;16:365–373.

168. **Loeffler JS, Rosen EM, Niloff JM, et al.** Whole abdominal irradiation for tumors of the uterine corpus. *Cancer* 1988;61:1322–1335.

169. **Martinez A, Schray M, Podratz K, et al.** Postoperative whole abdomino-pelvic irradiation for patients with high-risk endometrial cancer. *Int J Radiat Oncol Biol Phys* 1989;17:371–377.

170. **Gibbons S, Martinez A, Schray M, et al.** Adjuvant whole abdominopelvic irradiation for high-risk endometrial carcinoma. *Int J Radiat Oncol Biol Phys* 1991;21:1019–1025.

171. **Small W, Mahadevan A, Roland P, et al.** Whole abdominal radiation in endometrial carcinoma: an analysis of toxicity, patterns of recurrence, and survival. *J Cancer* 2000;6:394–400.

172. **Smith RS, Kapp DS, Chen Q, et al.** Treatment of high-risk uterine cancer with whole abdominopelvic radiation therapy. *Int J Radiat Oncol Biol Phys* 2000;48:767–778.

173. **Frank AH, Tsong PC, Haffty BG, et al.** Adjuvant whole abdominal radiation in uterine papillary serous carcinoma. *Cancer* 1991;68:1561.

174. **Mallieddi P, Kapp DS, Teng NNH.** Long-term survival and adjuvant whole abdominopelvic irradiation for uterine papillary serous carcinoma. *Cancer* 1993;71:3076.

175. **Lim P, Alkushi A, Gilks B, et al.** Early stage uterine papillary serous carcinoma of the endometrium: effect of adjuvant whole abdominal radiotherapy and pathologic parameters on outcome. *Cancer* 2001;91: 752–757.

176. **Soper JT, Creasman WT, Clarke-Pearson DL, et al.** Intraperitoneal chromic phosphate 32P suspension therapy of malignant peritoneal cytology in endometrial carcinoma. *Am J Obstet Gynecol* 1985;153:191–196.

177. **Lewis GC Jr, Slack NH, Mortel R, et al.** Adjuvant progestogen therapy in the primary definitive treatment of endometrial cancer. *Gynecol Oncol* 1974;2:368–376.

178. **DePalo G, Merson M, Del Vecchio M, et al.** A controlled clinical study of adjuvant medroxyprogesterone acetate (MPA) therapy in pathologic stage I endometrial carcinoma with myometrial invasion. *Proc Am Soc Clin Oncol* 1985;4:121(abst).

179. **Vergote I, Kjorstad J, Abeler V, et al.** A randomized trail of adjuvant progestogen in early endometrial cancer. *Cancer* 1989;64:1011–1016.

180. **MacDonald RR, Thorogood J, Mason MK.** A randomized trial of progestogens in the primary treatment of endometrial carcinoma. *Br J Obstet Gynecol* 1988;95:166–174.

181. **COSA-NZ-UK Endometrial Cancer Study Groups.** Adjuvant medroxyprogesterone acetate in high-risk endometrial cancer. *Int J Gynecol Cancer* 1998;8:387–391.

182. **Piver MS, Lele SB, Gamarra M.** Malignant peritoneal cytology in stage I endometrial adenocarcinoma: the effect of progesterone therapy (a preliminary report). *Eur J Gynecol Oncol* 1988;9:187–190.

183. **Morrow CP, Bundy B, Homesley H, et al.** Doxorubicin as an adjuvant following surgery and radiation therapy in patients with high-risk endometrial carcinoma, stage I and occult stage II. *Gynecol Oncol* 1990;36:166–171.

184. **Stringer CA, Gershenson DM, Burke TW, et al.** Adjuvant chemotherapy with cisplatin, doxorubicin, and cyclophosphamide (PAC) for early-stage high-risk endometrial cancer: a preliminary analysis. *Gynecol Oncol* 1990;38:305–308.

185. **Burke TW, Gershenson DM, Morris M, et al.** Postoperative adjuvant cisplatin, doxorubicin, and cyclophosphamide (PAC) chemotherapy in women with high-risk endometrial carcinoma *Gynecol Oncol* 1994;55:47.

186. **Homesley HD, Boronow RC, Lewis JL Jr.** Stage II endometrial adenocarcinoma. Memorial Hospital for Cancer, 1949–1965. *Obstet Gynecol* 1977;49:604–608.

187. **Surwit EA, Fowler WC Jr, Rogoff EE, et al.** Stage II carcinoma of the endometrium. *Int J Radiat Oncol Biol Phys* 1979;5:323–326.

188. **Kinsella TJ, Bloomer WD, Lavin PT, et al.** Stage II endometrial carcinoma: a 10-year follow-up of combined radiation and surgical treatment. *Gynecol Oncol* 1980;10:290–297.

189. **Nahhas WA, Whitney CW, Stryker JA, et al.** Stage II endometrial carcinoma. *Gynecol Oncol* 1980;10:303–311.

190. **Onsrud M, Aalders J, Abeler V, et al.** Endometrial carcinoma with cervical involvement (stage II): prognostic factors and value of combined radiological-surgical treatment. *Gynecol Oncol* 1982;13:76–86.

191. **Berman ML, Afridi MA, Kanbour AI, et al.** Risk factors and prognosis in stage II endometrial cancer. *Gynecol Oncol* 1982;14:49–61.

192. **Nori D, Hilaris BS, Tome M, et al.** Combined surgery and radiation in endometrial carcinoma: an analysis of prognostic factors. *Int J Radiat Oncol Biol Phys* 1987;13:489–496.

193. **Larson DM, Copeland LJ, Gallager HS, et al.** Prognostic factors in stage II endometrial carcinoma. *Cancer* 1987;60:1358–1361.

194. **Larson DM, Copeland LJ, Gallager HS, et al.** Stage II endometrial carcinoma: results and complications of a combined radiotherapeutic-surgical approach. *Cancer* 1988;61:1528–1534.

195. **Boothy RA, Carlson JA, Neiman W, et al.** Treatment of stage II endometrial carcinoma. *Gynecol Oncol* 1989;33:204–208.

196. **Podczaski ES, Kaminski P, Manetta A, et al.** Stage II endometrial carcinoma treated with external-beam radiotherapy, intracavitary application of cesium, and surgery. *Gynecol Oncol* 1989;35:251–254.

197. **Mannel RS, Berman ML, Walker JL, et al.** Management of endometrial cancer with suspected cervical involvement. *Obstet Gynecol* 1990;75:1016–1022.

198. **Andersen ES.** Stage II endometrial carcinoma: prognostic factors and the results of treatment. *Gynecol Oncol* 1990;38:220–223.

199. **Lanciano RM, Curran WJ Jr, Greven KM, et al.** Influence of grade, histologic subtype, and timing of radiotherapy on outcome among patients with stage II carcinoma of the endometrium. *Gynecol Oncol* 1990;39:368–373.

200. **Higgins RV, van Nagell JR Jr, Horn EJ, et al.** Preoperative radiation therapy followed by extrafascial hysterectomy in patients with stage II endometrial cancer. *Cancer* 1991;68:1261–1264.

201. **Rubin SC, Hoskins WJ, Saigo PE, et al.** Management of endometrial adenocarcinoma with cervical involvement. *Gynecol Oncol* 1992;45:294–298.

202. **Bruckman JE, Bloomer WD, Marck A, et al.** Stage III adenocarcinoma of the endometrium: two prognostic groups. *Gynecol Oncol* 1980;9:12–17.

203. **Danoff BF, McDay J, Louka M, et al.** Stage III endometrial carcinoma: analysis of patterns of failure and therapeutic implications. *Int J Radiat Biol Phys* 1980;6:1491–1495.

204. **Aalders JG, Abeler V, Kolstad P.** Clinical (stage III) as compared with subclinical intrapelvic extrauterine tumor spread in endometrial carcinoma: a clinical and histopathological study of 175 patients. *Gynecol Oncol* 1984;17:64–74.

205. **Mackillop WJ, Pringle JF.** Stage III endometrial carcinoma. *Cancer* 1985;56:2519–2523.

206. **Genest P, Drouin P, Girard A, et al.** Stage III carcinoma of the endometrium: a review of 41 cases. *Gynecol Oncol* 1987;26:77–86.

207. **Grigsby PW, Perez CA, Kuske RR, et al.** Results of therapy, analysis of failures and prognostic factors for clinical and pathologic stage III adenocarcinoma of the endometrium. *Gynecol Oncol* 1987;27:44–57.

208. **Greven K, Curran W, Whittington R, et al.** Analysis of failure patterns in stage III endometrial carcinoma and therapeutic implications. 1989;17:35–39.

209. **Pliskow S, Penalver M, Averette HE.** Stage III and IV endometrial carcinoma: a review of 41 cases. *Gynecol Oncol* 1990;38:210–215.

210. **Aalders JG, Abeler V, Kolstad P.** Stage IV endometrial carcinoma: a clinical and histopathological study of 83 patients. *Gynecol Oncol* 1984;17:75–84.

211. **Bristow RE, Zerbe MJ, Rosenshein NB, et al.** Stage IV endometrial carcinoma: the role of cytoreductive surgery and determinants of survival. *Gynecol Oncol* 2000;78:85–91.

212. **Goff BA, Goodman A, Muntz HG, et al.** Surgical stage IV endometrial carcinoma: a study of 47 cases. *Gynecol Oncol* 1994;52:237–240.

213. **Chi DS, Welshinger M, Venkatraman ES, et al.** The role of surgical cytoreduction in stage IV endometrial carcinoma. *Gynecol Oncol* 1997;67:56–60.

214. **Rutledge F, Smith JP, Wharton JT, et al.** Pelvic exenteration: analysis of 296 patients. *Am J Obstet Gynecol* 1977;129:881–890.

215. **Barber HRK, Brunschwig A.** Treatment and results of recurrent cancer of corpus uteri in patients receiving anterior and total exoneration 1947–1963. *Cancer* 1968; 22:949–955.

216. **Aalders JG, Abeler V, Kolstad P.** Recurrent adenocarcinoma of the endometrium: a clinical and histopathological study of 379 patients. *Gynecol Oncol* 1984;17:85–103.

217. **Angel C, DuBeshter B, Dawson AE, et al.** Recurrent stage I endometrial adenocarcinoma in the nonirradiated patient: preliminary results of surgical "staging." *Gynecol Oncol* 1993;48:221–226.

218. **Phillips GL, Prem KA, Adcock LL, et al.** Vaginal recurrence of adenocarcinoma of the endometrium. *Gynecol Oncol* 1982;13:323–328.

219. **Greven K, Olds W.** Isolated vaginal recurrences of endometrial adenocarcinoma and their management. *Cancer* 1987;60:419.

220. **Curran WJ, Whittington R, Peters AJ, et al.** Vaginal recurrences of endometrial carcinoma: the prognostic value of staging by a primary vaginal carcinoma system. *Int J Radiat Oncol Biol Phys* 1988;15:803–808.

221. **Poulsen MG, Roberts SJ.** The salvage of recurrent endometrial carcinoma in the vagina and pelvis. *Int J Radiat Oncol Biol Phys* 1988;15:809–813.

222. **Kuten A, Grigsby PW, Perez CA, et al.** Results of radiotherapy in recurrent endometrial carcinoma: a retrospective analysis. *Int J Radiat Oncol Biol Phys* 1989;17:29–34.

223. **Sears JD, Greven KM, Hoen HM, et al.** Prognostic factors and treatment outcome for patients with locally recurrent endometrial cancer. *Cancer* 1994;74:1303–1308.

224. **Wylie J, Irwin C, Pintilie M, et al.** Results of radical radiotherapy for recurrent endometrial cancer. *Gynecol Oncol* 2000;77:66–72.

225. **Jereczek-Fosa B, Badzio A, Jessem J.** Recurrent endometrial cancer after surgery alone: results of salvage radiotherapy. *Int J Radiat Oncol Biol Phys* 2000;48:405–413.

226. **Kelley RM, Baker WH.** Progestational agents in the treatment of carcinoma of the endometrium. *N Engl J Med* 1961;264:216–222.

227. **Reifenstein EC Jr.** The treatment of advanced endometrial cancer with hydroxyprogesterone caproate. *Gynecol Oncol* 1974;2:377–414.

228. **Piver MS, Barlow JJ, Lurain JR, et al.** Medroxyprogesterone acetate (Depo-Provera) versus hydroxyprogesterone caproate (Delalutin) in women with metastatic endometrial adenocarcinoma. *Cancer* 1980;45:268–272.

229. **Podratz KC, O'Brien PC, Malkasian GD Jr, et al.** Effects of progestational agents in treatment of endometrial carcinoma. *Obstet Gynecol* 1985;66:106–110.

230. **Thigpen T, Blessing J, DiSaia P, et al.** Oral medroxyprogesterone acetate in advanced or recurrent endometrial carcinoma: results of therapy and correlation with estrogen and progesterone receptor levels. The Gynecologic Oncology Group experience. In: **Baulier EE, Iacobelli S, McGuire WL,** eds. *Endocrinology of malignancy.* Park Ridge, NJ: Parthenon, 1986:446–454.

231. **Thigpen T, Blessing J, Hatch K, et al.** A randomized trial of medroxyprogesterone acetate (MPA) 200 mg versus 1000 mg daily in advanced or recurrent endometrial carcinoma: a Gynecologic Oncology Group study. *Proc ASCO* 1991;10:185.

232. **Moore TD, Phillips PH, Nerenstone SR, et al.** Systemic treatment of advanced and recurrent endometrial carcinoma: current status and future directions. *J Clin Oncol* 1991;9:1071–1088.

233. **Deppe G.** Chemotherapy for endometrial cancer. In: Deppe G, ed. *Chemotherapy of gynecologic cancer.* New York: Alan R. Liss, 1990;155–174.

234. **Muss HB.** Chemotherapy of metastatic endometrial cancer. *Semin Oncol* 1994;21:107–113.

235. **Ball HG, Blessing J, Leuntz S, et al.** A phase II trial of Taxol in advanced and recurrent adenocarcinoma of the endometrium. A Gynecologic Oncology Group study. *Gynecol Oncol* 1996;62: 278–281.

236. **Woo HL, Swenerton KD, Hoskins PJ.** Taxol is active in platinum-resistant endometrial adenocarcinoma. *Am J Clin Oncol* 1996;19:290–291.

237. **Lissoini, A, Zanetta G, Losa G, et al.** Phase II study of paclitaxel as salvage treatment in advanced endometrial cancer. *Ann Oncol* 1996;7:861–865.

238. **Dimopoulos MP, Papadimitriou CA, Georgoulias V, et al.** Pactitaxel and cisplatin in advanced or recurrent carcinoma of the endometrium: long-term results of a phase II multicenter study. *Gynecol Oncol* 2000;78: 52–57.

239. **Fleming GF, Fowler JM, Waggoner SE, et al.** Phase I trial of escalating doses of paclitaxel combined with fixed doses of cisplatin and doxorubicin in advanced endometrial cancer and other gynecologic malignancies: a Gynecologic Oncology Group study. *J Clin Oncol* 2001;19:1021–1029.

240. **Creasman WT, Odicino F, Maisonneuve P, et al.** Carcinoma of the corpus uteri. FIGO Annual Report on the Results of Treatment in Gynecological Cancer, Vol 24, Pecorelli S, ed. *J Epidemiol Biostat* 2001;6:45–86.

241. **Podczaski E, Kaminski P, Gurski K, et al.** Detection and patterns of treatment failure in 300 consecutive cases of "early" endometrial cancer after primary surgery. *Gynecol Oncol* 1992;47:323–327.

242. **Shumsky AG, Stuart GE, Brasher PM, et al.** An evaluation of routine follow up of patients treated for endometrial carcinoma. *Gynecol Oncol* 1994;55: 229.

243. **Berchuck A, Auspach C, Evans AC, et al.** Postsurgical surveillance of patients with FIGO stage I/II endometrial carcinoma. *Gynecol Oncol* 1995;59:20.

244. **Reddock JM, Burke TW, Morris M, et al.** Surveillance for recurrent endometrial carcinoma: development of a follow-up scheme. *Gynecol Oncol* 1995;59:221.

245. **Patsner B, Orr JW, Mann WJ.** Use of serum CA 125 measurement in post treatment surveillance of early-stage endometrial carcinoma. *Am J Obstet Gynecol* 1990;162:427–429.

246. **Rose PG, Summers RM, Reale FR, et al.** Serial serum CA 125 measurements for evaluation of recurrence in patients with endometrial carcinoma. *Obstet Gynecol* 1994;84:12.

247. **Creasman WT, Henderson D, Hinshaw W, et al.** Estrogen replacement therapy in the patient treated for endometrial cancer. *Obstet Gynecol* 1986;67:326–330.

248. **Lee RB, Burke TW, Park RC.** Estrogen replacement therapy following treatment for stage I endometrial carcinoma. *Gynecol Oncol* 1990;36:189–191.

249. **Chapman J, DiSaia P, Osann K, et al.** Estrogen replacement in surgical stage I and II endometrial cancer survivors. *Am J Obstet Gynecol* 1996;175:1195–1200.

250. **Suriano KA, Mettale M, McLaren CE, et al.** Estrogen replacement therapy in endometrial cancer patients. *Obstet Gynecol* 2001;97:555–560.

251. **Harlow BL, Weiss NS, Lofton S.** The epidemiology of sarcomas of the uterus. *J Natl Cancer Inst* 1986;76:399–402.

252. **Czesnin K, Wronkowski Z.** Second malignancies of the irradiated area in patients treated for uterine cervix cancer. *Gynecol Oncol* 1976;6:309–315.

253. **Kempson RL, Bari W.** Uterine sarcomas: classification, diagnosis and prognosis. *Hum Pathol* 1970;1:331–349.

254. **Tavassoli FA, Norris HJ.** Mesenchymal tumors of the uterus. VII. A clinico-pathologic study of 60 endometrial stromal nodules. *Histopathology* 1981;5:1–10.

255. **Norris HJ, Taylor HB.** Mesenchymal tumors of the uterus. I. A clinical and pathologic study of 53 endometrial stromal tumors. *Cancer* 1966;19:755–766.

256. **Hart WR, Yoonessi M.** Endometrial stromatosis of the uterus. *Obstet Gynecol* 1977;49:393.

257. **Krieger PD, Gusberg SB.** Endolymphatic stromal myosis a grade 1 endometrial sarcoma. *Gynecol Oncol* 1973;1:299.

258. **Thatcher SS, Woodruff JD.** Uterine stromatosis: a report of 33 cases. *Obstet Gynecol* 1982;59:428.

259. **Piver MS, Rutledge FN, Copeland L, et al.** Uterine endolymphatic stromal myosis: a collaborative study. *Obstet Gynecol* 1984;64:173.

260. **Yoonessi M, Hart WR.** Endometrial stromal sarcomas. *Cancer* 1977;40:898.

261. **Evans HL.** Endometrial stromal sarcoma and poorly differentiated endometrial sarcoma. *Cancer* 1982;52:2170.

262. **Chang KL, Crabtree GS, Lim Tan SK, et al.** Primary uterine endometrial stromal neoplasms: a clinicopathologic study of 117 cases. *Am J Surg Pathol* 1990;14:415.

263. **Taylor HB, Norris HJ.** Mesenchymal tumors of the uterus. IV. Diagnosis and prognosis of leiomyosarcoma. *Arch Pathol* 1966;82:40.

264. **Gudgeon DH.** Leiomyosarcoma of the uterus. *Obstet Gynecol* 1968;32:96.

265. **Silverberg SG.** Leiomyosarcoma of the uterus: a clinicopathologic study. *Obstet Gynecol* 1971;38:613.

266. **Christopherson WM, Williamson EO, Gray LA.** Leiomyosarcoma of the uterus. *Cancer* 1972;29:1512.

267. **Gallup DG, Cordray DR.** Leiomyosarcoma of the uterus: case reports and a review. *Obstet Gynecol Surv* 1979;34:300.

268. **Vardi JR, Tovell HMM.** Leiomyosarcoma of the uterus: clinicopathologic study. *Obstet Gynecol* 1980;56:428.

269. **Dinh TV, Woodruff JD.** Leiomyosarcoma of the uterus. *Am J Obstet Gynecol* 1982;144:817.

270. **Berchuck A, Rubin SC, Hoskins WJ, et al.** Treatment of uterine leiomyosarcoma. *Obstet Gynecol* 1988;71:845–850.

271. **Bell SW, Kempson RL, Hendrickson MR.** Problematic uterine smooth muscle neoplasms: a clinicopathologic study of 213 cases. *Am J Surg Pathol* 1994;18:535.

272. **King ME, Dickersin GR, Scully RE.** Myxoid leiomyosarcoma of the uterus. *Am J Surg Pathol* 1982;6:589.

273. **Kurman RJ, Norris HJ.** Mesenchymal tumors of the uterus. VI. Epithelioid smooth muscle tumors including leiomyoblastoma and clear cell leiomyoma: a clinical and pathologic analysis of 26 cases. *Cancer* 1976;37:1833.

274. **Norris HJ, Parmley T.** Mesenchymal tumors of the uterus. V. Intravenous leiomyomatosis: a clinical and pathologic study. *Cancer* 1975;36:2164–2178.

275. **Scharfenberg JC, Geary WL.** Intravenous leiomyomatosis. *Obstet Gynecol* 1974;43:909–914.

276. **Evans AT III, Symmonds RE, Gaffey TA.** Recurrent pelvic intravenous leiomyomatosis. *Obstet Gynecol* 1981;57:260.

277. **Clement PB, Young RH, Scully RE.** Intravenous leiomyomatosis of the uterus: a clinicopathologic analysis of 16 cases with unusual histologic features. *Am J Surg Pathol* 1988;12:932.

278. **Abell MR, Littler ER.** Benign metastasizing uterine leiomyoma: multiple lymph node metastases. *Cancer* 1975;36:2206.

279. **Banner AS, Carrington CB, Emory WB, et al.** Efficacy of oophorectomy in lymph-angioleiomyomatosis and benign metastasizing leiomyoma. *N Engl J Med* 1981;305:204.

280. **Tavassoli FA, Norris HJ.** Peritoneal leiomyomatosis (leiomyomatosis peritoneal disseminata): a clinicopathologic study of 20 cases with ultrastructural observations. *Int J Gynecol Pathol* 1982;1:59.

281. **Norris HJ, Roth E, Taylor HB.** Mesenchymal tumors of the uterus. II. A clinical and pathologic study of 31 mixed mesodermal tumors. *Obstet Gynecol* 1966;28:57.

282. **Norris HJ, Taylor HB.** Mesenchymal tumors of the uterus. III. A clinical pathologic study of 31 carcinosarcomas. *Cancer* 1966;19:1459.

283. **Silverberg SG, Major FJ, Blessing JA, et al.** Carcinosarcoma (malignant mixed mesodermal tumor) of the uterus: a Gynecologic Oncology Group pathologic study of 203 cases. *Int J Gynecol Pathol* 1990; 9:1.

284. **DiSaia PJ, Castro JR, Rutledge FN.** Mixed mesodermal sarcoma of the uterus. *AJR Am J Roentgenol* 1973;117:632.

285. **Macasaet MA, Waxman M. Fruchter RG, et al.** Prognostic factors in malignant mesodermal (mullerian) mixed tumors of the uterus. *Gynecol Oncol* 1985;20:32.

286. **DiSaia PJ, Morrow CP, Boronow R, et al.** Endometrial sarcoma: lymphatic spread pattern. *Am J Obstet Gynecol* 1978;130:104.

287. **Geszler G, Szpak CA, Harris RE, et al.** Prognostic value of peritoneal washings in patients with malignant mixed mullerian tumors of the uterus. *Am J Obstet Gynecol* 1986;155:83.

288. **Clement PB, Scully RE.** Mullerian adenosarcoma of the uterus; a clinico-pathologic analysis of 100 cases with a review of the literature. *Hum Pathol* 1990;21:363.

289. **Kaku T, Silverberg SG, Major FJ.** Adenosarcoma of the uterus: a Gynecologic Oncology Group study of 31 cases. *Int J Gynecol Pathol* 1992;11:75.

290. **Salazar OM, Bonfiglio TA, Patten SF, et al.** Uterine sarcomas: analysis of failures with special emphasis on the use of adjuvant radiation therapy. *Cancer* 1978;42:1161.

291. **Spanos WJ, Peters LJ, Oswald MJ.** Patterns of recurrence in malignant mixed mullerian tumors of the uterus. *Cancer* 1986;57:155.

292. **Vongtama V, Karlen JR, Piver MS, et al.** Treatment results and prognostic factors in stage I and II sarcomas of the corpus uteri. *AJR Am J Roentgenol* 1976;126:139.

293. **Levenback C, Rubin SC, McCormack PM, et al.** Resection of pulmonary metastases from uterine sarcomas. *Gynecol Oncol* 1992;45:202–205.

294. **Belgrad R, Elbadawi N, Rubin P.** Uterine sarcomas. *Radiology* 1975;114:181.

295. **Salazar OM, Bonfiglio TA, Patten SF, et al.** Uterine sarcomas: natural history, treatment, and prognosis. *Cancer* 1978;42:1152–1160.

296. **Perez CA, Askin F, Baglan RJ, et al.**Effects of irradiation on mixed mullerian tumors of the uterus. *Cancer* 1979;43:1274.

297. **Hornback NB, Omura G, Major FJ.** Observations on the use of adjuvant radiation therapy in patients with stage I and II uterine sarcoma. *Int J Radiat Oncol Biol Phys* 1986;12:2127.

298. **Knocke TH, Kucera H, Dotfler D, et al.** Results of postoperative radiotherapy in the treatment of sarcoma of the corpus uteri. *Cancer* 1998;83:1972–1979.

299. **Molpus KL, Redlin-Frazier S, Reed G, et al.** Postoperative pelvic irradiation in early stage uterine mixed mullerian tumors. *Eur J Gynecol Oncol* 1998;19:541–546.

300. **Gottlieb JA, Baker LH, O'Bryan RM, et al.** Adriamycin used alone and in combination for soft tissue and bony sarcomas. *Cancer Chemother Rep Part 3* 6:271.

301. **Blum RH, Corson JM, Wilson RE, et al.** Successful treatment of metastatic sarcomas with cyclophosphamide, Adriamycin, and DTIC (CAD). *Cancer* 1980;46:1722.

302. **Omura GA, Blessing JA, Major F, et al.** A randomized study of Adriamycin with and without triazenoimidazole carboxamide in advanced uterine sarcomas. *Cancer* 1983;52:626.

303. **Sutton G, Blessing J, Barrett R, et al.** Phase II trial of ifosfamide and mesna in leiomyosarcoma of the uterus: a Gynecology Oncology Group study. *Am J Obstet Gynecol* 1992;166:556.

304. **Thigpen JT, Blessing JA, Beecham J, et al.** Phase II trial of cisplatin as first-line chemotherapy in patients with advanced or recurrent uterine sarcomas: a Gynecologic Oncology Group study. *J Clin Oncol* 1991;9:1962.

305. **Gershenson DM, Kavanagh JJ, Copeland LJ, et al.** Cisplatin therapy for a disseminated mixed mesodermal sarcoma of the uterus. *J Clin Oncol* 1987;5:618.

306. **Sutton GP, Blessing JA, Rosenshein N, et al.** Phase II trial of ifosfamide and mesna in mixed mesodermal tumors of the uterus. *Am J Obstet Gynecol* 1989;161:309.

307. **Piver MS, DeEulis TG, Lele SB, et al.** Cyclophosphamide, vincristine, Adriamycin, and dimethyltriazenoimidazole carboxamide (CYVADIC) for sarcomas of the female genital tract. *Gynecol Oncol* 1981;14:319.

308. **Sutton G, Brunetto VL, Kilgore L, et al.** A phase III trial of ifosfamide with or without cisplatin in carcinosarcoma of the uterus: a Gynecologic Oncology Group study. *Gynecol Oncol* 2000;79: 47–53.

309. **Omura GA, Blessing JA, Major F, et al.** A randomized clinical trial of adjuvant Adriamycin in uterine sarcomas: a Gynecologic Oncology Group study. *J Clin Oncol* 1985;3:1240.

310. **Hempling RE, Piver MS, Baker TR.** Impact on progression-free survival of adjuvant cyclophosphamide, vincristine, doxorubicin (Adriamycin), and dacarbazine (CYVADIC) chemotherapy for stage I uterine sarcoma: a prospective trial. *Am J Clin Oncol* 1995;18:282–286.

311. **Peters WA, III, Rivkin SE, Smith MR, et al.** Cisplatin and Adriamycin combination chemotherapy for uterine stromal sarcomas and mixed mesodermal tumors. *Gynecol Oncol* 1989;34:323.

31 Cervical and Vaginal Cancer

Thomas C. Krivak
John W. McBroom
John C. Elkas

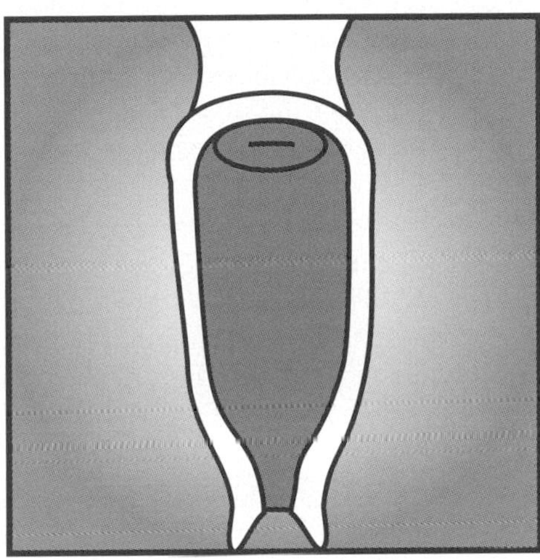

Invasive cervical cancer in the United States is relatively infrequent, and the low incidence of cervical cancer is attributable to the effectiveness of screening with Papanicolaou's (Pap) test and detecting premalignant precursors. However, cervical carcinoma remains a significant health care problem worldwide. In Third World countries where no screening programs exist, cervical carcinoma is a significant cause of mortality. Because cervical cancer is potentially preventable, it is imperative that gynecologists and other primary care providers who administer health care to women be familiar with screening techniques, diagnostic procedures, and risk factors for cervical cancer, especially its premalignant precursors. Vaginal cancer is a relatively uncommon tumor.

Cervical Cancer

Epidemiology and Risk Factors

Invasive cancer of the cervix has been considered a preventable cancer because it has a long preinvasive state, because cervical cytology screening programs are available, and because the treatment of preinvasive lesions is effective. However, 13,000 new cases of invasive cervical cancer resulting in about 4,100 deaths were anticipated in the United States in 2002 (1). Although cervical cancer has not been eliminated, the incidence of invasive disease is decreasing, and it is being diagnosed earlier, leading to better survival rates (1,2). The mean age for cervical cancer is 52.2 years, and the distribution of cases is bimodal, with peaks at 35 to 39 years and 60 to 64 years of age (1).

There are numerous risk factors for cervical cancer: young age at first intercourse (<16 years), multiple sexual partners, cigarette smoking, race, high parity, and low socioeconomic status. The relationship to oral contraceptive use has been debated in the literature. Some investigators have proposed that use of oral contraceptives may increase the incidence of cervical glandular abnormalities of the cervix (3,4); however, this hypothesis has not been consistently supported. Many of these risk factors are linked to sexual activity and exposure to sexually transmitted diseases. Infection with herpes virus was previously thought to be the initiating event in cervical cancer. However, infection with the human papillomavirus (HPV) has now been determined to be involved in the development of cervical cancer.

The initiating event in cervical dysplasia and carcinogenesis is likely to be infection with HPV. HPV infection has been detected in up to 99% of women with squamous cervical carcinoma (5). There are more than 80 different types of HPV, 25 of which affect the lower genital tract. There are 13 high-risk HPV subtypes; two of the high-risk subtypes, 16 and 18, are found in up to 62% of cervical carcinomas. The mechanism by which HPV affects cellular growth and differentiation is by interactions of viral E6 and E7 proteins with p53 and Rb, resulting in gene inactivation (6). The role of human immunodeficiency virus (HIV) in cervical cancer is thought to be mediated through immune suppression. The Centers for Disease Control and Prevention have described cervical cancer as an illness that defines acquired immune deficiency syndrome (AIDS) in patients infected with HIV (7).

Evaluation

Vaginal bleeding is the most common symptom occurring in patients with cancer of the cervix. Most often, this is postcoital bleeding, but it may occur as irregular or postmenopausal bleeding. Patients with advanced disease may have a malodorous vaginal discharge, weight loss, or obstructive uropathy.

On general physical examination, the supraclavicular and groin lymph nodes should be palpated to exclude the presence of metastatic disease. On pelvic examination, a speculum is inserted into the vagina, and the cervix is inspected for suspicious areas. The vagina is inspected for extension of disease. With invasive cancer, the cervix is usually firm and expanded, and these features should be evaluated by digital examination. Rectal examination is important to help establish cervical consistency and size, particularly in patients with endocervical carcinomas. It is the only way to determine cervical size if the vaginal fornices have been obliterated by menopausal changes or by the extension of disease. Parametrial extension of disease is best determined by the finding of nodularity beyond the cervix on rectal examination.

When obvious tumor growth is present, cervical biopsy performed on an outpatient basis is usually sufficient for diagnosis. Colposcopy may be helpful in directing the examiner toward the most invasive area for biopsy. If the diagnosis cannot be established conclusively with outpatient biopsy, diagnostic conization may be necessary.

Cervical conization is required to assess correctly the depth and the linear extent of involvement of microinvasion. The earliest invasion is characterized by a protrusion from the stromoepithelial junction. This focus consists of cells that appear better differentiated than the adjacent noninvasive cells and have abundant pink-staining cytoplasm, hyperchromatic nuclei, and small- to medium-sized nucleoli (8). **These early invasive lesions in the form of tonguelike processes without measurable volume are classified as International Federation of Gynecology and Obstetrics (FIGO) stage Ia1.** With further progression, more tonguelike processes and isolated cells occur in the stroma (Fig. 31.1). The stroma responds by a proliferation of fibroblasts (desmoplasia) and a bandlike infiltration of chronic inflammatory cells. **With increasing depth of invasion, lesions occur at multiple sites, and the growth becomes measurable by depth and linear extent. Lesions that are smaller than 3 mm are classified as FIGO stage Ia1. Lesions that are 3 to 5 mm or more in depth and up to 7 mm in linear extent are classified as FIGO stage Ia2** (9). With increasing stromal invasion, the involvement of capillary–lymphatic spaces is increased. Dilated capillaries, lymphatic spaces, and foreign-body multinucleated giant cells containing keratin debris often are seen in the stroma.

The depth of invasion should be measured with the micrometer from the base of the epithelium to the deepest point of invasion. **The depth of invasion is significant for the development of pelvic lymph node metastasis and tumor recurrence. Although lesions that have invaded 3 mm or less rarely metastasize, patients in whom lesions invade**

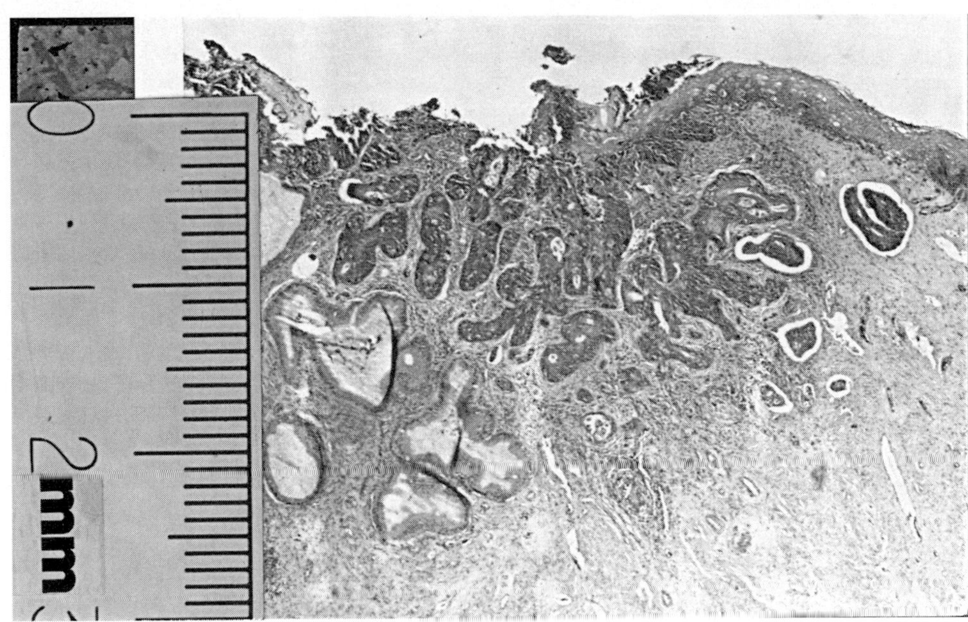

Figure 31.1 Microinvasive squamous carcinoma. Multiple irregular tonguelike processes and isolated nests of malignant cells are seen, some surrounded by clear spaces, simulating capillary lymphatic invasion. This is an artifact caused by tissue shrinkage. The depth of stromal invasion is measured from the basement membrane of the overlying cervical intraepithelial neoplasia (CIN). In this case, it is 1.5 mm. (From **Berek JS, Hacker F.** *Practical gynecologic oncology.* 2nd ed. Baltimore: Williams & Wilkins, 1994, with permission.)

more than 3 to 5 mm have positive pelvic lymph nodes in 3% to 8% of cases (10). Although the significance of the cutoff at 3 mm has not been identified completely, it may be postulated that capillary–lymphatic spaces are extremely small at this level, and it is unclear whether they can carry tumor cells beyond the specific zone. Uneven shrinkage of tissue by fixative often creates space between the tumor nests and the surrounding fibrous stroma, stimulating vascular lymphatic invasion (Fig. 31.1). A suspected vascular involvement with invasion of less than 3 mm should be interpreted with care. A lack of endothelial lining indicates that the space is an artifact of shrinkage rather than true vascular invasion.

Colposcopic Findings

For patients with suspected early invasive cancer based on Pap test results and a grossly normal-appearing cervix, colposcopic examination is mandatory. Colposcopic findings that suggest invasion are (a) abnormal blood vessels, (b) irregular surface contour with loss of surface epithelium, and (c) color tone change. Colposcopically directed biopsies may permit the diagnosis of frank invasion and thus avoid the need for diagnostic cone biopsy, allowing treatment to be administered without delay. If there is debate about the depth of invasion based on the cervical biopsies, and if the clinical stage may be upstaged to stage Ia2 or Ib1, the patient should undergo cold knife conization. A large cervical biopsy showing invasion greater than 3 mm or two biopsy specimens separated by 7 mm showing invasive cervical carcinoma would allow no delay in therapy, and the patient could undergo a radical hysterectomy or radiation therapy.

Abnormal Blood Vessels Abnormal vessels may be looped, branching, or reticular. Abnormal looped vessels are the most common finding and arise from the punctation and mosaic vessels present in cervical intraepithelial neoplasia (CIN). As the neoplastic growth process proceeds, the need for nutrition leads to proliferation of the blood vessels, and the punctate vessels at the surface produce double and triple loops. These surface tufting vessels then proliferate and push out over the surface of the epithelium in an erratic fashion.

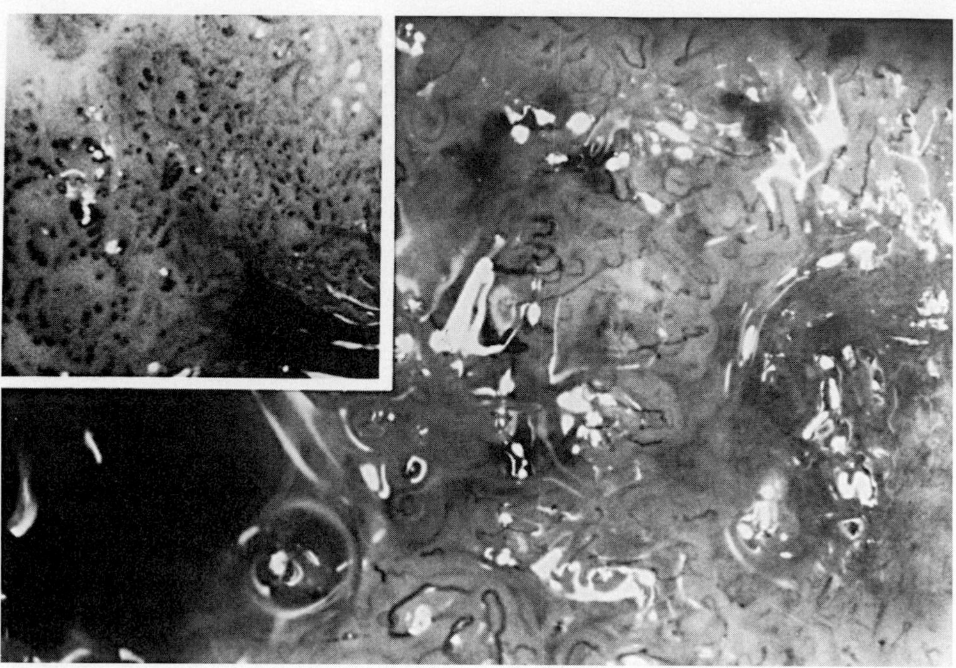

Figure 31.2 Abnormal looped vessels in invasive cervical cancer. (From **Berek JS, Hacker F.** *Practical gynecologic oncology.* 2nd ed. Baltimore: Williams & Wilkins, 1994, with permission.)

Some are straight, although most have a loop, a corkscrew, or a J-shaped pattern (Fig. 31.2). Abnormal branching vessels arise from the cervical stroma and are pushed to the surface as the underlying cancer invades and pushes upward. The normally branching cervical stromal vessels are best observed over nabothian cysts. In this area, the branches are generally at acute angles, with the caliber of vessels becoming smaller after branching, much like the arborization of a tree. The abnormal branching blood vessels seen with cancer tend to form obtuse or right angles, with the caliber sometimes enlarging after branching (Fig. 31.3). Sharp turns, dilations, and narrowings also mark the behavior of these vessels. The surface epithelium may be lost in these areas, leading to irregular surface contour and friability.

Abnormal reticular vessels represent the terminal capillaries of the cervical epithelium. Normal capillaries are best seen in a postmenopausal woman with atrophic epithelium. When cancer involves this epithelium, the surface is again eroded, and the capillary network is exposed. These vessels are very fine, short, and composed of small commas without an organized pattern (Fig. 31.4). They are not specific to invasive cancer; atrophic cervicitis may also have this appearance.

Irregular Surface Contour Abnormal surface patterns are observed as the tumor growth proceeds. The surface epithelium ulcerates as the cells lose intercellular cohesiveness secondary to the loss of desmosomes. Irregular contour also may occur because of a papillary characteristic of the lesion (Fig. 31.5). **This finding sometimes can be confused with an HPV papillary growth on the cervix; for that reason, biopsies should be performed on all papillary cervical growths.**

Color Tone Color tone may change as a result of increasing vascularity, surface epithelial necrosis, and in some cases, production of keratin. The color tone is yellow-orange rather than the expected pink of intact squamous epithelium or the red of the endocervical epithelium.

Adenocarcinoma Adenocarcinoma of the cervix does not have a specific colposcopic appearance. All of the aforementioned blood vessels may be seen in these lesions as well.

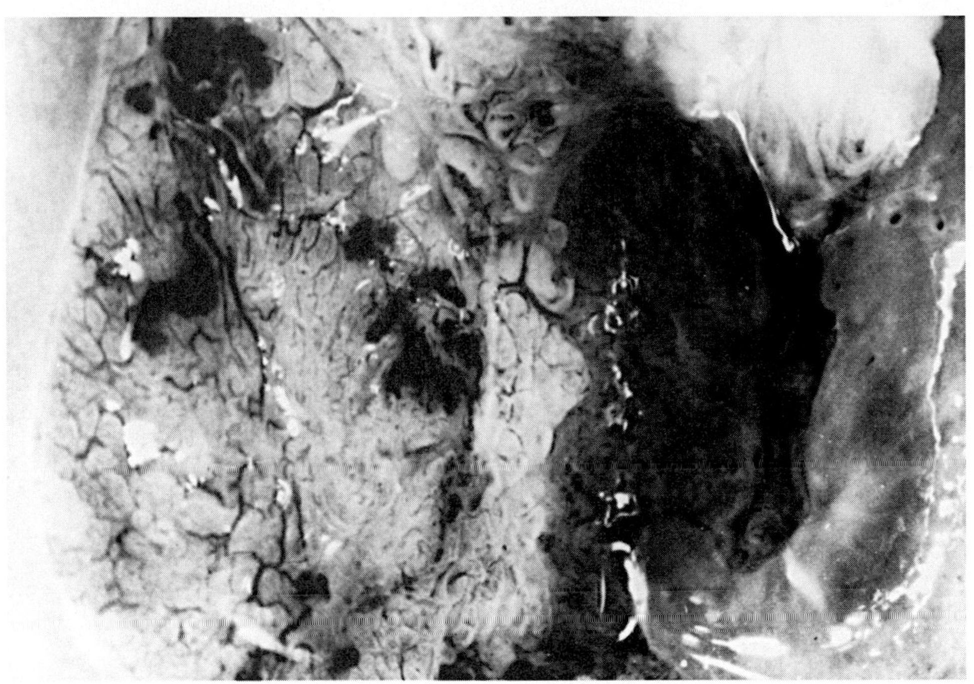

Figure 31.3 Abnormal branching vessels in invasive cervical cancer. (From **Berek JS, Hacker F.** *Practical gynecologic oncology.* 2nd ed. Baltimore: Williams & Wilkins, 1994, with permission.)

Figure 31.4 Abnormal reticular vessels in invasive cervical cancer. (From **Berek JS, Hacker F.** *Practical gynecologic oncology.* 2nd ed. Baltimore: Williams & Wilkins, 1994, with permission.)

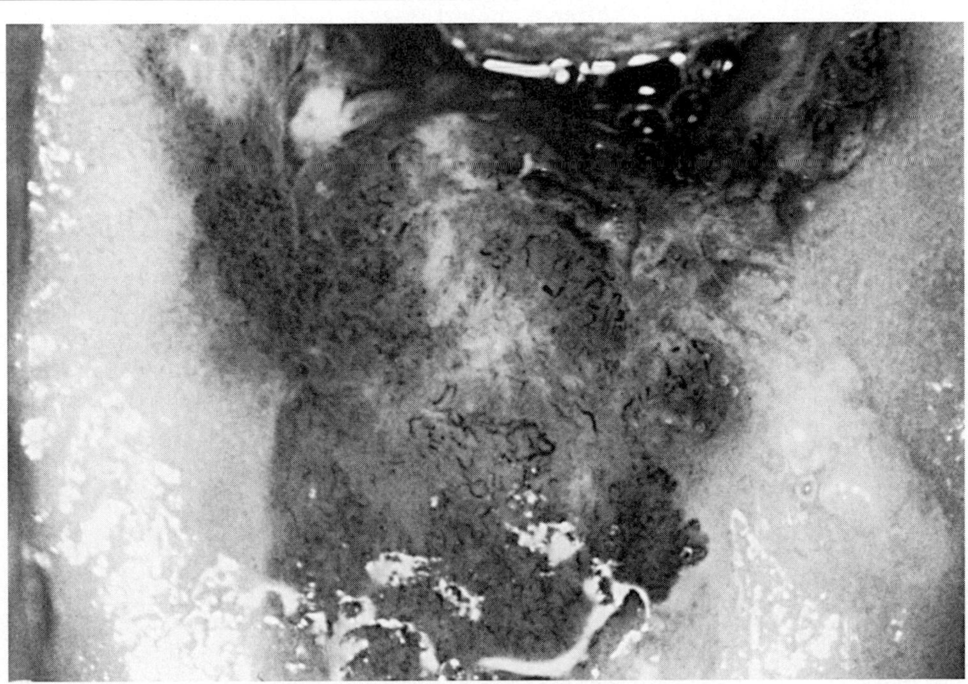

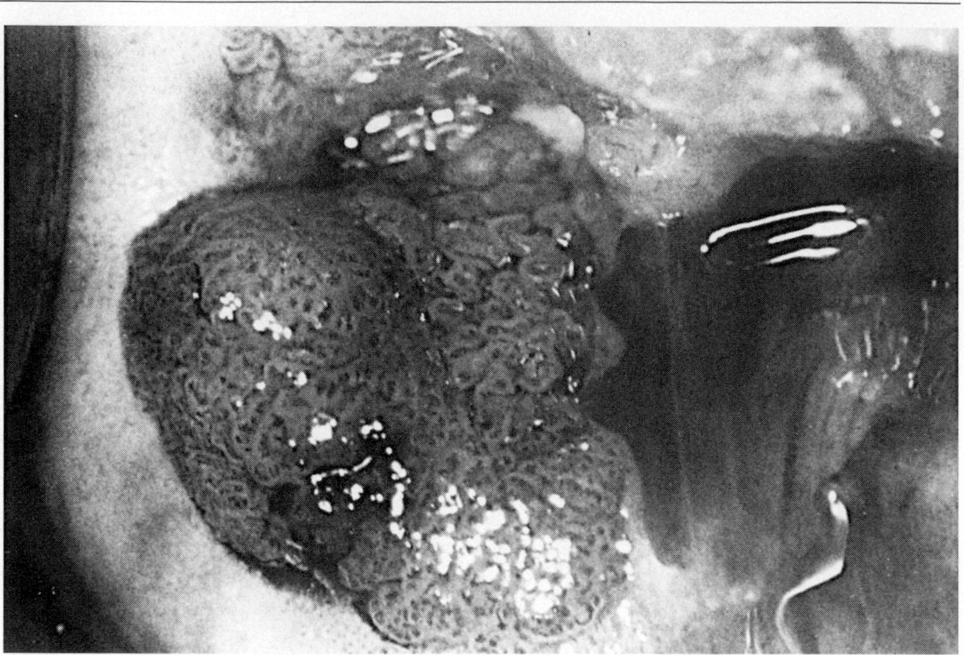

Figure 31.5 Irregular surface growth in invasive cervical cancer. (From **Berek JS, Hacker F.** *Practical gynecologic oncology.* 2nd ed. Baltimore: Williams & Wilkins, 1994, with permission.)

Because adenocarcinomas tend to develop within the endocervix, endocervical curettage is required as part of the colposcopic examination.

Clinical Staging

The current FIGO staging system is presented in Table 31.1 and Fig. 31.6. The staging procedures allowed by FIGO are listed in Table 31.2. **When there is doubt concerning the stage to which a cancer should be allocated, the earlier stage should be selected. After a clinical stage is assigned and treatment has been initiated, the stage must not be changed because of subsequent findings by either extended clinical staging or surgical staging.** The "upstaging" of patients during treatment will produce an erroneous improvement in the results of treatment of low-stage disease. Following is a breakdown of the incidence of cervical cancer by stage at diagnosis: 38%, stage I; 32%, stage II; 26%, stage III; and 4%, stage IV (2,9,12).

Extended Clinical Staging

Various investigators have used lymphangiography, computed tomography (CT), ultrasonography, and magnetic resonance imaging (MRI) in an attempt to improve clinical staging (11–16). Because these tests are not generally available throughout the world and because the interpretation of results is variable, the findings of these studies are not used for assigning the FIGO stage. However, they may be useful in planning therapy.

Evaluation of the paraaortic lymph nodes with lymphangiography is associated with a false-positive rate of 20% to 40% and a false-negative rate of 10% to 20% (11–13). The accuracy of CT scanning is 80% to 85%; the false-negative rate is 10% to 15%, and the false-positive rate is 20% to 25% (14–16). Early MRI data are comparable to CT scanning (17). When abnormalities are noted by these procedures, fine-needle aspiration (FNA) showing metastatic disease allows the radiation treatment field to be extended and obviates the need for exploratory laparotomy to determine the status of the lymph nodes.

Surgical Staging

The clinical staging system developed by FIGO is based on the belief that cervical cancer is a local disease and that, because most cases of cervical cancer occur in developing countries,

Table 31.1. FIGO Staging of Carcinoma of the Cervix Uteri

Preinvasive Carcinoma

Stage 0 Carcinoma *in situ,* intraepithelial carcinoma (cases of stage 0 should not be included in any therapeutic statistics).

Invasive Carcinoma

Stage I[a] **Carcinoma strictly confined to the cervix** (extension to the corpus should be disregarded).

- *Stage Ia* Preclinical carcinomas of the cervix, that is, those diagnosed only by microscopy.
  - *Stage Ia1* Lesion with ≤3 mm invasion.
  - *Stage Ia2* Lesions detected microscopically that can be measured. The upper limit of the measurement should show a depth of invasion of >3–5 mm taken from the base of the epithelium, either surface or glandular, from which it originates, and a second dimension, the horizontal spread, must not exceed 7 mm. Larger lesions should be staged as Ib.
- *Stage Ib* Lesions invasive >5 mm.
  - *Stage Ib1* Lesion less than or equal to 4 cm.
  - *Stage Ib2* Lesions larger than 4 cm.

Stage II[b] **The carcinoma extends beyond the cervix but has not extended onto the wall.** The carcinoma involves the vagina, but not the lower one third.

- *Stage IIa* No obvious parametrial involvement.
- *Stage IIb* Obvious parametrial involvement.

Stage III[c] **The carcinoma has extended onto the pelvic wall.** On rectal examination, there is no cancer-free space between the tumor and the pelvic wall. The tumor involves the lower one third of the vagina. All cases with hydronephrosis or nonfunctioning kidney.

- *Stage IIIa* No extension to the pelvic wall.
- *Stage IIIb* Extension onto the pelvic wall and/or hydronephrosis or nonfunctioning kidney.

Stage IV[d] **The carcinoma has extended beyond the true pelvis or has clinically involved the mucosa of the bladder or rectum.** A bullous edema, as such, does not permit a case to be allotted to stage IV.

- *Stage IVa* Spread to the growth to adjacent organs.
- *Stage IVb* Spread to distant organs.

[a]The diagnosis of both stages Ia1 and Ia2 should be based on microscopic examination of removed tissue, preferably a cone, which must include the entire lesion. The depth of invasion should not be more than 5 mm taken from the base of the epithelium, either surface or glandular, from which it originates. The second dimension, the horizontal spread, must not exceed 7 mm. Vascular space involvement, either venous or lymphatic, should not alter the staging but should be specifically recorded because it may affect treatment decisions in the future. Lesions of greater size should be staged as Ib. As a rule, it is impossible to estimate clinically whether a cancer of the cervix has extended to the corpus. Extension to the corpus should therefore be disregarded.

[b]A patient with a growth fixed to the pelvic wall by a short and indurated, but not nodular, parametrium should be allotted to stage IIb. At clinical examination, it is impossible to decide whether a smooth, indurated parametrium is truly cancerous or only inflammatory. Therefore, the case should be assigned to stage III only if the parametrium is nodular to the pelvic wall or the growth itself extends to the pelvic wall.

[c]The presence of hydronephrosis or nonfunctioning kidney due to stenosis of the ureter by cancer permits a case to be allotted to stage III even if, according to other findings, it should be allotted to stage I or II.

[d]The presence of the bullous edema, as such, should not permit a case to be allotted to stage IV. Ridges and furrows into the bladder wall should be interpreted as signs of submucous involvement of the bladder if they remain fixed to the growth at palpation (i.e., examination from the vagina or the rectum during cystoscopy). A cytologic finding of malignant cells in washings from the urinary bladder requires further examination and a biopsy specimen from the wall of the bladder.

FIGO, International Federation of Gynecology and Obstetrics.

surgical staging is not feasible with limited health care resources. The accuracy of clinical staging is somewhat limited, and surgical evaluation, which is not practical or feasible in many patients, is more accurate. Surgical staging has been advocated by providers in the United States who believe that this information details the extent of disease and affects treatment (18). Radiation oncologists may desire this information when designing treatment plans for patients. However, other providers believe that surgical staging should be limited

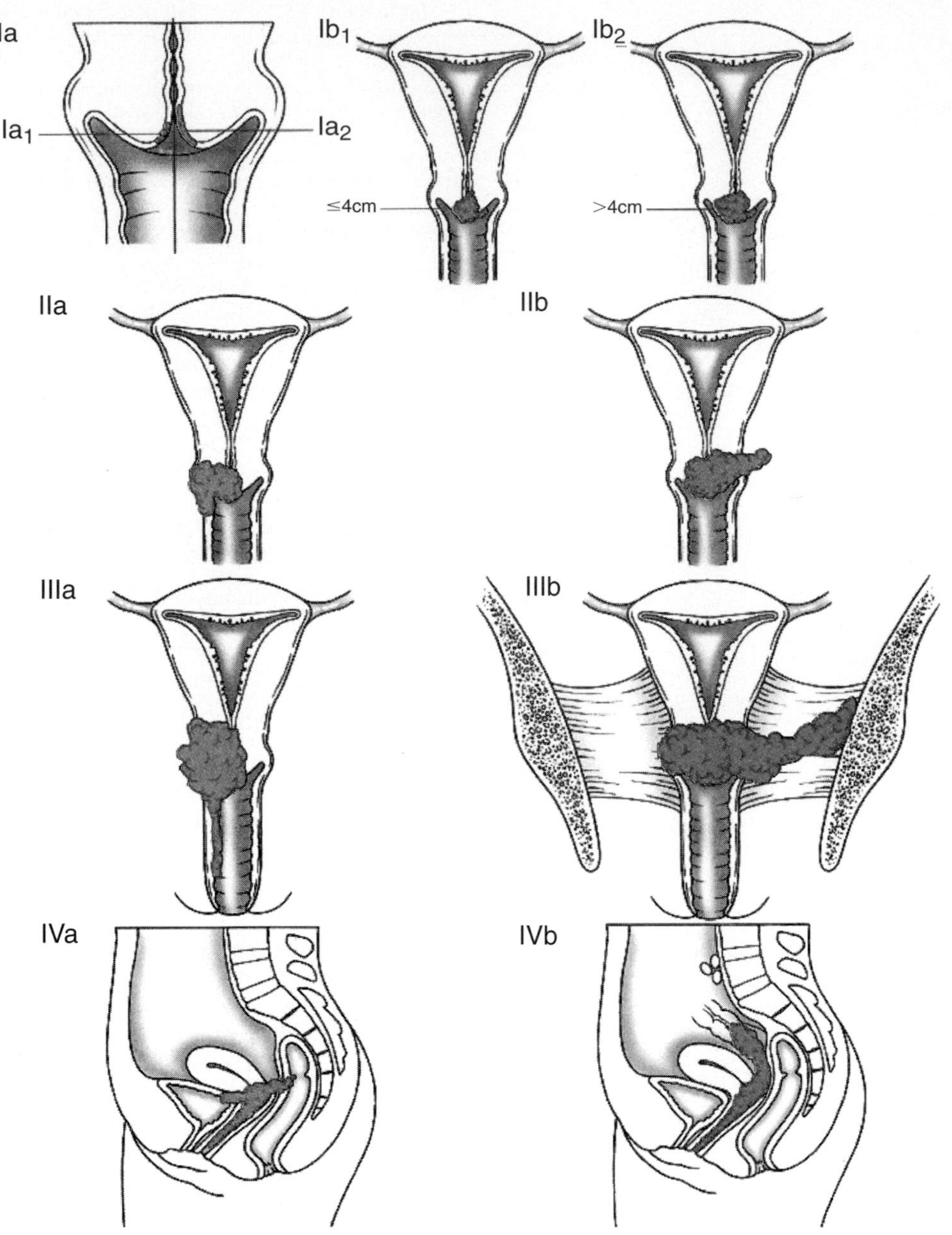

Figure 31.6 Carcinoma of the cervix uteri: staging cervical cancer (primary tumor and metastases). (From **Benedet JL, Odicino F, Maisonneuve P, et al.** Carcinoma of the cervix. *J Epidemiol Biostat* 2001;6:5–44, with permission.)

to patients who are enrolled in a clinical trial or research protocol. These beliefs are based on the fact that there is no randomized control study demonstrating a survival benefit in patients who have had surgical staging. The specifics of surgical staging are discussed later in this chapter.

Pathology

Squamous Cell Carcinoma

Invasive squamous cell carcinoma is the most common variety of invasive cancer in the cervix. Histologically, there are large cell keratinizing, large cell nonkeratinizing, and small cell types (19). Large cell keratinizing tumors are made up of tumor cells forming irregular infiltrative nests with laminated keratin pearls in the center. Large cell nonkeratinizing carcinomas reveal individual cell keratinization but do not form keratin pearls

Table 31.2. Staging Procedures

Physical examination[a]	Palpate lymph nodes Examine vagina Bimanual rectovaginal examination (under anesthesia recommended)
Radiologic studies[a]	Intravenous pyelogram Barium enema Chest x-ray Skeletal x-ray
Procedures[a]	Biopsy Conization Hysteroscopy Colposcopy Endocervical curettage Cystoscopy Proctoscopy
Optional studies[b]	Computerized axial tomography Lymphangiography Ultrasonography Magnetic resonance imaging Radionucleotide scanning Laparoscopy

[a]Allowed by the International Federation of Gynecology and Obstetrics (FIGO).
[b]Information that is not allowed by FIGO to change the clinical stage.

(Fig. 31.7). The category of small cell carcinoma includes poorly differentiated squamous cell carcinoma and small cell anaplastic carcinoma. If possible, these two tumors should be differentiated. The former contains cells that have small- to medium-sized nuclei, open chromatin, small or large nucleoli, and more abundant cytoplasm than those of the latter. The designation of small cell anaplastic carcinoma should be reserved for lesions resembling oat cell carcinoma of the lung. It infiltrates diffusely and consists of tumor cells that have scanty cytoplasm, round to oval small nuclei, coarsely granular chromatin, and high mitotic activity. The nucleoli are absent or small. Immunohistochemistry or electron microscopy differentiates the small cell neuroendocrine tumors. Patients with the large cell type of carcinoma, with or without keratinization, have a better prognosis than those with the small cell variant. Furthermore, small cell anaplastic carcinomas behave more aggressively than poorly differentiated squamous carcinomas that contain small cells. Infiltration of parametrial tissue and pelvic lymph node metastasis affect the prognosis.

Adenocarcinoma

In recent years, there has been an increasing number of cervical adenocarcinomas affecting young women in their 20s and 30s. Adenocarcinoma *in situ* is believed to be the precursor of invasive adenocarcinoma, and it is not surprising that the two often coexist (20). In addition, squamous neoplasia, intraepithelial or invasive, also occurs in 30% to 50% of cervical adenocarcinomas. It should be noted that adenocarcinoma *in situ* appears to pose a diagnostic and therapeutic dilemma when compared with squamous cell carcinoma. The incidence of residual adenocarcinoma *in situ* after conization has led some investigators to recommend hysterectomy in patients with this preneoplastic lesion. However, in two recent reports, patients with negative cone biopsy margins were followed conservatively, with few requiring repeat surgical procedures (21,22). Because cervical adenocarcinoma *in situ* tends to affect women during their reproductive years, a thorough risk and benefit discussion should take place, and treatment should be individualized.

Adenocarcinoma may be detected by cervical sampling, but less reliably so than squamous carcinomas. A definitive diagnosis may require cervical conization. Invasive adenocarcinoma may be pure (Fig. 31.8) or mixed with squamous cell carcinoma—adenosquamous carcinoma. Within the category of pure adenocarcinoma, the tumors are quite heterogeneous (19), with a wide range of cell types, growth patterns, and differentiation. About 80% of

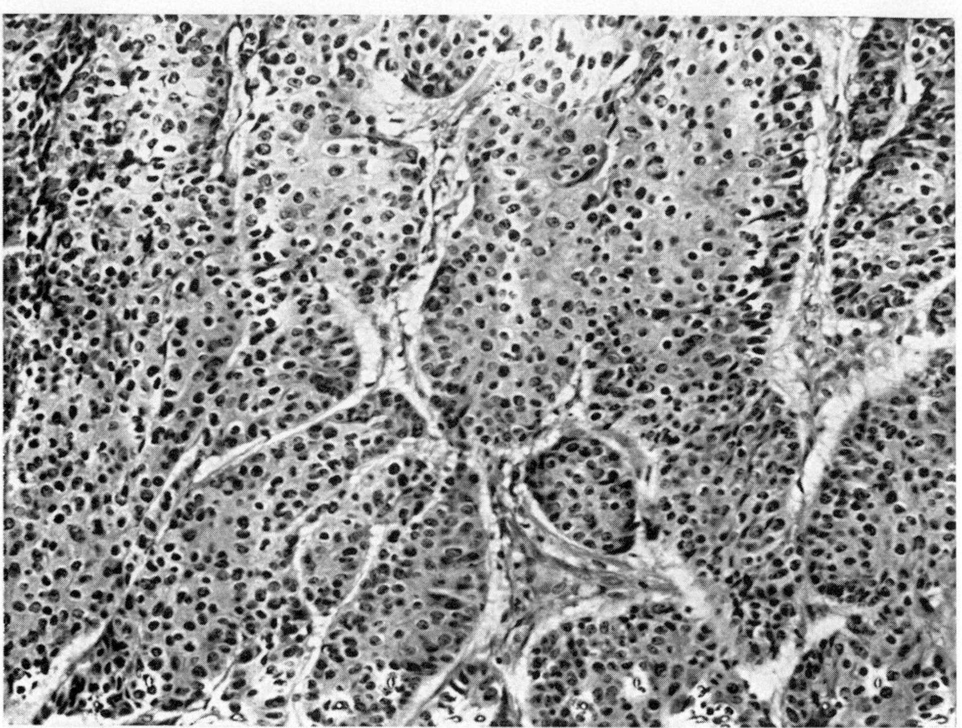

Figure 31.7 Invasive squamous cell carcinoma, large cell nonkeratinizing type. Tumor cells form irregular nests and have abundant eosinophilic cytoplasm and distinct cell borders indicative of squamous differentiation. (From **Berek JS, Hacker F.** *Practical gynecologic oncology.* 2nd ed. Baltimore: Williams & Wilkins, 1994, with permission.)

cervical adenocarcinomas are made up predominantly of cells of the endocervical type with mucin production. The remaining tumors are populated by endometrioid cells, clear cells, intestinal cells, or a mixture of more than one cell type. By histologic examination alone, some of these tumors are indistinguishable from those arising elsewhere in the endometrium or ovary.

Within each tumor type, the growth patterns and nuclear abnormalities vary according to the degree of differentiation. In well-differentiated tumors, tall columnar cells line the well-formed branching glands and papillary structures, whereas pleomorphic cells tend to form irregular nests and solid sheets in poorly differentiated neoplasms. The latter may require mucicarmine and periodic acid–Schiff (PAS) staining to confirm their glandular differentiation.

There are several special variants of adenocarcinoma. *Minimal deviation adenocarcinoma (adenoma malignum)* is an extremely well-differentiated form of adenocarcinoma in which the branching glandular pattern strongly simulates that of the normal endocervical glands. In addition, the lining cells have abundant mucinous cytoplasm and uniform nuclei (23,24). Because of this, the tumor may not be recognized as malignant in small biopsy specimens, thereby causing considerable delay in diagnosis. Earlier studies reported a dismal outcome for women with this tumor, but more recent studies have found a favorable prognosis if the disease is detected early (25). Although rare, similar tumors have also been reported in association with endometrioid, clear, and mesonephric cell types (26).

An entity described as *villoglandular papillary adenocarcinoma* also deserves special attention (27). It primarily affects young women, some of whom are pregnant or users of oral contraceptives. Histologically, the tumors have smooth, well-defined borders, are well

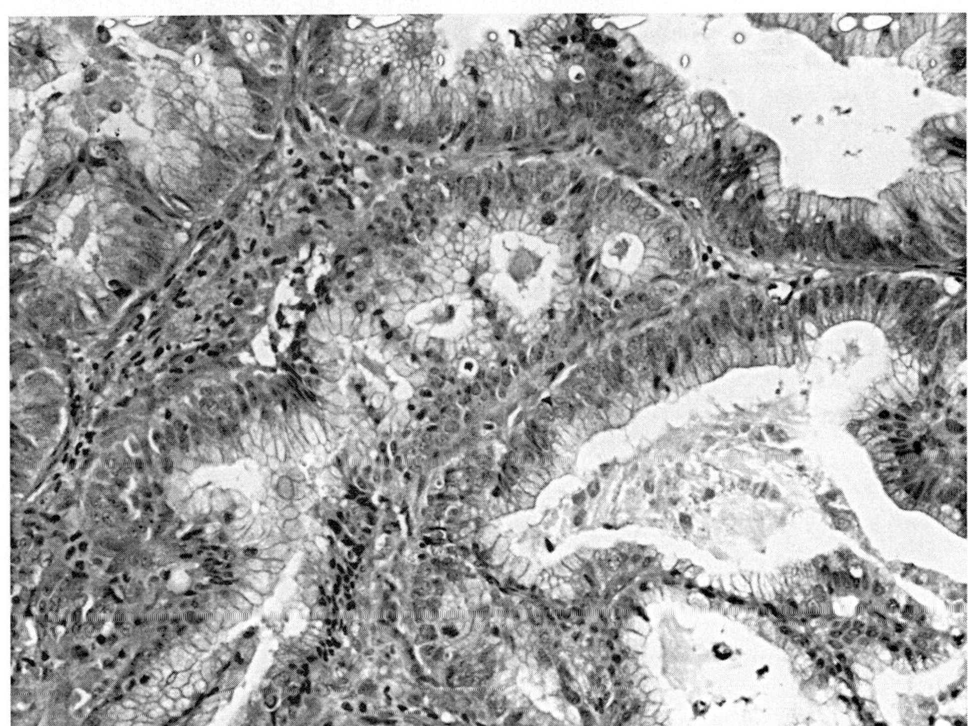

Figure 31.8 Invasive adenocarcinoma of the cervix, well-differentiated. Irregular glands are lined with tall columnar cells with vacuolated mucinous cytoplasm resembling endocervical cells. Nuclear stratification, mild nuclear atypism, and mitotic figures are evident. (From **Berek JS, Hacker F.** *Practical gynecologic oncology.* 2nd ed. Baltimore: Williams & Wilkins, 1994, with permission.)

differentiated, and are either *in situ* or superficially invasive. The follow-up information is encouraging, however; none of these tumors has recurred after cervical conization or hysterectomy. Among women undergoing pelvic nodal dissection, no metastases have been detected. This tumor appears to have limited risk for spread beyond the uterus.

In mature adenosquamous carcinomas, the glandular and squamous carcinomas are readily identified on routine histologic evaluation and do not cause diagnostic problems. In poorly differentiated or immature adenosquamous carcinomas, however, glandular differentiation can be appreciated only with special stains, such as mucicarmine and PAS. In one study (26), 30% of squamous cell carcinomas demonstrated mucin secretion when stained with mucicarmine. These squamous cell carcinomas with mucin secretion have a higher incidence of pelvic lymph node metastases than squamous cell carcinomas without mucin secretion (26) and are similar to the signet-ring variant of adenosquamous carcinoma (28).

Glassy cell carcinoma has been recognized as a poorly differentiated form of adenosquamous carcinoma (28). Individual cells have abundant eosinophilic, granular, ground-glass cytoplasm, large round to oval nuclei, and prominent nucleoli. The stroma is infiltrated by numerous lymphocytes, plasma cells, and eosinophils. About half of these tumors contain glandular structures or stain positive for mucin. The poor diagnosis of this tumor is linked to understaging and resistance to radiotherapy.

Other variants of adenosquamous carcinoma include *adenoid basal carcinoma* and *adenoid cystic carcinoma.* Adenoid basal carcinoma simulates the basal cell carcinoma of the skin (29). Nests of basaloid cells extend from the surface epithelium deep into the underlying tissue. Cells at the periphery of tumor nests form a distinct parallel nuclear arrangement, the so-called peripheral palisading. An "adenoid" pattern occasionally develops, with "hollowed-out" nests of cells. Mitoses are rare, and the tumor often extends deep into the cervical stroma.

Adenoid cystic carcinoma of the cervix behaves much like such lesions elsewhere in the body. The tumors tend to invade into the adjacent tissues and metastasize late, often 8 to 10 years after the primary tumor has been removed. Like other adenoid cystic tumors, they may metastasize directly to the lung. The pattern simulates that of the adenoid basal tumor, but there is a cystic component, and the glands of the cervix are involved (29). Mitoses may be seen but are not numerous.

Sarcoma

The most important sarcoma of the cervix is the *embryonal rhabdomyosarcoma,* which occurs in children and young adults. The tumor has grapelike polypoid nodules—the botryoid sarcoma—and the diagnosis depends on the recognition of rhabdomyoblasts (14). Leiomyosarcomas and mixed mesodermal tumors involving the cervix may be primary but are more likely to be secondary to uterine tumors. Cervical adenosarcoma has been described as a low-grade tumor with a good prognosis (30). If recurrence develops, it is generally a central recurrence that may be treated with resection and hormonal therapy.

Malignant Melanoma

On rare occasions, melanosis has been seen in the cervix. Thus, malignant melanoma may arise *de novo* in this area. Histopathologically, it simulates melanoma elsewhere, and the prognosis depends on the depth of invasion into the cervical stroma.

Metastatic Cancer

The cervix is commonly involved in cancer of the endometrium and vagina. The latter is rare, and most lesions that involve the cervix and vagina are designated *cervical primaries.* Consequently, the clinical classification is that of cervical neoplasia extending to the vagina, rather than vice versa. Endometrial cancer may extend into the cervix by three modes: direct extension from the endometrium, submucosal involvement by lymph vascular extension, and multifocal disease. The latter is most unusual, but occasionally a focus of adenocarcinoma may be seen in the cervix, separate from the endometrium. This lesion should not be diagnosed as metastasis but rather as multifocal disease. Malignancies involving the peritoneal cavity (e.g., ovarian cancer) may be found in the cul-de-sac and extend directly into the vagina and cervix. Carcinomas of the urinary bladder and colon occasionally extend into the cervix. Cervical involvement by lymphoma, leukemia, and carcinoma of the breast, stomach, and kidney is usually part of the systemic spread. However, an isolated metastasis to the cervix may be the first sign of a primary tumor elsewhere in the body.

Neuroendocrine Carcinoma

The classification of neuroendocrine cervical carcinoma includes four histologic subtypes: small cell, large cell, classical carcinoid, and atypical carcinoid (31). Neuroendocrine tumors of the cervix are rare, and treatment regimens have been based on small case series of patients. *Small cell (neuroendocrine type) carcinoma of the cervix* is aggressive in nature and is similar to cancer arising from the bronchus (32). At the time of diagnosis, it is usually disseminated, with bone, brain, liver, and bone marrow being the most common sites of metastases. In one study, 11 patients with what was apparent disease confined to the cervix and were found to have a high rate of lymph node metastasis (33). Pathologically, the diagnosis is aided by the finding of neuroendocrine granules on electron microscopy as well as by immunoperoxidase studies that are positive for a variety of neuroendocrine proteins such as calcitonin, insulin, glucagon, somatostatin, gastrin, and adrenocorticotropic hormone (ACTH). In addition to the traditional staging for cancer of the cervix, these patients should undergo bone, liver, and brain scanning as well as bone marrow aspiration and biopsy. Therapy generally consists of surgery, chemotherapy, and radiation. Patients with early-stage disease have a chance of distant metastases, and it has been recommended

Table 31.3. Incidence of Pelvic and Paraaortic Nodal Metastasis by Stage

Stage	No. of Patients	Positive Pelvic Nodes (%)	Positive Paraaortic Nodes (%)
Ia1 (≤3 mm)	179[a]	0.5	0
Ia2 (>3–5 mm)	84[a]	4.8	<1
Ib	1926[b]	15.9	2.2
IIa	110[c]	24.5	11
IIb	324[c]	31.4	19
III	125[c]	44.8	30
IVa	23[c]	55	40

[a]References 42, 47, 69, 70, 75, 79
[b]References 12, 42, 44, 49, 52, 53, 56, 57, 58, 59, 60
[c]References 11, 12, 53, 56, 57, 61, 81

that patients should have multimodal therapy. The main active chemotherapeutic agent is *etoposide.* The hallmark of neuroendocrine tumors is their aggressive malignant behavior with the propensity to metastasize.

Patterns of Spread

Cancer of the cervix spreads by (a) direct invasion into the cervical stroma, corpus, vagina, and parametrium; (b) lymphatic metastasis; (c) blood-borne metastasis; and (d) intraperitoneal implantation. The incidence of pelvic and paraaortic nodal metastasis is shown in Table 31.3.

Treatment

The treatment of cervical cancer is similar to the treatment of any other type of malignancy; that is, both the primary lesion and potential sites of spread should be treated. The therapeutic modalities for achieving this goal include primary treatment with surgery, radiotherapy, or chemoradiation. Whereas radiation therapy can be used in all stages of disease, surgery alone is limited to patients with stage I and IIa disease. The 5-year survival rate for stage I cancer of the cervix is about 85% with either radiation therapy or radical hysterectomy. A recent study using the National Cancer Institute's Surveillance Epidemiology and End Results data showed by an intent-to-treat analysis that patients who were in the surgery arm had an improved survival when compared with patients in the-intent-to treat radiation arm (34). In general, optimal therapy would consist of radiation or surgery to limit the increased morbidity when the two treatment modalities are combined. There have recently been great strides in the treatment of cervical carcinoma, including adjuvant radiation and chemoradiation in patients discovered to have high-risk cervical carcinoma after radical hysterectomy and in patients with locally advanced cervical carcinoma. The Gynecologic Oncology Group (GOG) released results from five randomized control trials evaluating radiation therapy and chemoradiation for high-risk early cervical carcinoma and advanced cervical carcinoma (discussed later).

Surgery

There are advantages to the use of surgery instead of radiotherapy, particularly in younger women for whom conservation of the ovaries is important. Chronic bladder and bowel problems that require medical or surgical intervention occur in up to 8% of patients undergoing radiation therapy (35). Such problems are difficult to treat because they result from fibrosis and decreased vascularity. This is in contrast to surgical injuries, which in general are easily repaired and without long-term complications. Sexual dysfunction after radiation therapy is more likely to occur because of vaginal shortening, fibrosis, and atrophy of the epithelium. The surgical procedure shortens the vagina, but gradual lengthening can be brought about by sexual activity. The epithelium does not become atrophic because it responds either to the patient's endogenous estrogen or to exogenous *estrogens* if the patient is postmenopausal.

Table 31.4. Surgical Management of Early Invasive Cancer of the Cervix

Stage Ia1	*≤3 mm invasion*	
	No lymph-vascular space invasion	Conization Type I hysterectomy
	With lymph-vascular space invasion	Type I or II hysterectomy with (?) pelvic lymph node dissection
Stage Ia2	*>3–5 mm invasion*	Type II hysterectomy with pelvic lymphadenectomy
Stage Ib	*>5 mm invasion*	Type III hysterectomy with pelvic lymphadenectomy

In general, radical hysterectomy is reserved for women who are in good physical condition. Chronologic age should not be a deterrent. With improvements in anesthesia, elderly patients withstand radical surgery almost as well as their younger counterparts (36). Generally, it is prudent not to operate on lesions that are larger than 4 cm in diameter because these patients will require postoperative radiation therapy. When selected in this manner, the urinary fistula rate is less than 2% (37), and the operative mortality rate is less than 1% (38). An advantage of radiotherapy is its applicability to all stages and to most patients regardless of their age, height, weight, and medical condition. A summary of the surgical management of early cervical cancer is presented in Table 31.4.

Radical Hysterectomy and Pelvic Node Dissection

The radical hysterectomy performed most often in the United States is that described by Meigs (39) in 1944. The operation includes pelvic lymph node dissection along with removal of most of the uterosacral and cardinal ligaments and the upper one third of the vagina. This operation has been referred to as the type III radical hysterectomy (40).

The hysterectomy described by Wertheim is less extensive than a radical hysterectomy and removes the medial half of the cardinal and uterosacral ligaments (40). This procedure is often referred to as the modified radical or type II hysterectomy. Wertheim's original operation did not include pelvic lymph node dissection but instead included selective removal of enlarged lymph nodes.

Radical hysterectomies can be further classified as extended radical hysterectomy (type IV). In the type IV operation, the periureteral tissue, superior vesicle artery, and up to three fourths of the vagina are removed (40). In the type V operation, portions of the distal ureter and bladder are resected. This procedure is rarely performed because radiotherapy should be used when such extensive disease is encountered (40).

The abdomen is opened through either a midline incision or a low transverse incision after the methods of Maylard or Cherney. The low transverse incision requires division of the rectus muscles and provides excellent exposure of the lateral pelvis. It allows adequate pelvic node dissection and wide resection of the primary tumor. After the abdomen is entered, the peritoneal cavity is explored to exclude metastatic disease. The stomach is palpated to ensure that it has been decompressed to facilitate packing of the intestines. The liver is palpated, and the omentum is inspected for metastases. Both kidneys are palpated to ensure their proper placement and lack of congenital and other abnormalities. The paraaortic nodes are palpated transperitoneally.

During exploration of the pelvis, the fallopian tubes and ovaries are inspected for any abnormalities. In patients younger than 40 years of age, the ovaries are generally conserved. The peritoneum of the vesicouterine fold and the rectouterine pouch should be inspected for signs of tumor extension or implantation. The cervix is then palpated between the thumb anteriorly and the fingers posteriorly to determine its extent, and the cardinal ligaments are palpated for evidence of lateral tumor extension or nodularity.

Paraaortic Lymph Node Evaluation If the patient has no evidence of disease extending beyond the cervix or vaginal fornix (i.e., surgical stage Ib or IIa), the procedure is continued. The bowel is packed to expose the peritoneum overlying the bifurcation of the aorta. The peritoneum is incised medial to the ureter and over the right common iliac artery. A retractor is placed retroperitoneally to expose the aorta and the vena cava. Any enlarged paraaortic lymph nodes are dissected, hemaclips are applied for hemostasis, and specimens are sent for analysis by frozen section. If the lymph nodes are positive for metastatic cancer, an option is to discontinue the operation and use radiation therapy (39). If the lymph nodes are negative for disease, the left side of the aorta is palpated through the peritoneal incision with a finger passed under the inferior mesenteric artery. The lymph nodes on this side of the aorta are more lateral and nearly behind the aorta and the common iliac artery. If the left paraaortic lymph nodes appear healthy and the cervical tumor is small with no suspicious pelvic lymph nodes, these additional lymph nodes are not submitted for frozen-section analysis. If they are removed, they may be dissected through the incision made for the right paraaortic nodes, or they may be dissected after reflection of the sigmoid colon medially.

Development of Pelvic Spaces The pelvic spaces are developed by sharp and blunt dissection (Fig. 31.9). The paravesical space is bordered by the following structures:

1. The obliterated umbilical artery running along the bladder medially
2. The obturator internus muscle along the pelvic sidewall laterally
3. The cardinal ligament posteriorly
4. The pubic symphysis anteriorly

The attachments of the vagina to the tendinous arch form the floor of the paravesical space.

Figure 31.9 The pelvic ligaments and spaces. (From **Berek JS, Hacker F.** *Practical gynecologic oncology.* 3rd ed. Philadelphia: Lippincott Williams & Wilkins, 2000, with permission.)

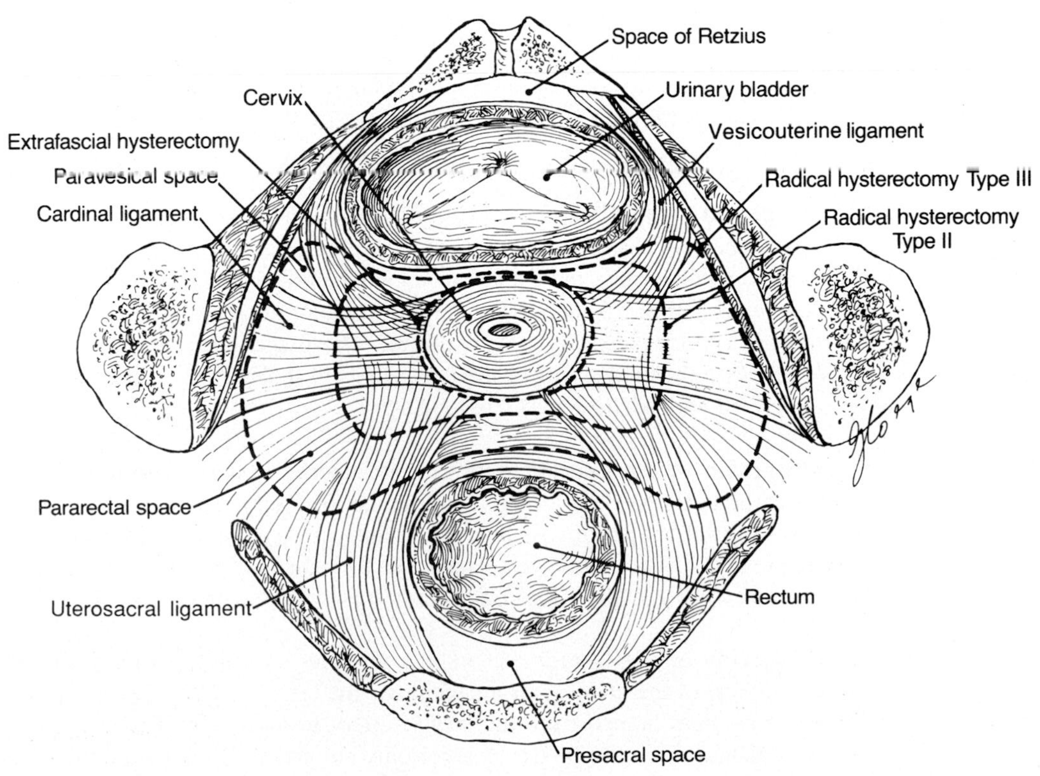

The pararectal space is bordered by the following structures:

1. The rectum medially
2. The cardinal ligament anteriorly
3. The hypogastric artery laterally
4. The sacrum posteriorly

The coccygeus (levator ani) muscle forms the floor of the pararectal space. The development of these spaces before pelvic lymphadenectomy will aid in identification and dissection of the pelvic lymph nodes as well as dissection of the ureter as it passes into the vesicouterine ligament tunnel.

Pelvic Lymphadenectomy Pelvic lymphadenectomy can proceed after lymph node evaluation or it can be deferred until the hysterectomy has been completed, depending on the preference of the surgeon. The pelvic lymph node dissection is begun by opening the round ligaments at the pelvic sidewall and developing the paravesical and pararectal spaces. The ureter is elevated on the medial flap by a Deaver retractor to expose the common iliac artery. The common iliac and external iliac nodes are dissected, with care taken to avoid injuring the genitofemoral nerve, which lies laterally on the psoas muscle. At the bifurcation of the common iliac artery, the external iliac node chain is divided into lateral and medial portions.

The lateral chain is stripped free from the artery to the circumflex iliac vein distally. A hemaclip is placed across the distal portion of the lymph node chain to reduce the incidence of lymphocyst formation. The medial chain is then dissected. The obturator lymph nodes are dissected next; for this procedure, the lymph nodes are grasped just under the external iliac vein, and traction is applied medially. Although most patients have both the obturator artery and vein dorsal to the obturator nerve, 10% have an aberrant vein arising from the external iliac vein. The node chain is separated from the nerve and vessels and clipped caudally. They are dissected cephalad to the hypogastric artery. The cephalad portion of the obturator space should be entered lateral to the external iliac artery and medial to the psoas muscle, where the remainder of the obturator node tissue can be dissected as far cephalad as the common iliac artery. In general, drainage of the pelvic and paraaortic lymph node beds is not performed because of the increase in complications in patients in whom drains have been used (41).

Dissection of the Bladder A critical step is the dissection of the bladder from the anterior part of the cervix and vagina. Occasionally, tumor extension into the base of the bladder (which cannot be detected with cystoscopy) precludes adequate mobilization of the bladder flap, leading to the abandonment of the operation. Therefore, this portion of the operation should be undertaken early in the procedure. The dissection should be performed in a manner to mobilize the bladder off of the upper third of the vagina in order to remove the tumor safely and with adequate margins.

Dissection of the Uterine Artery The superior vesicle artery is dissected away from the cardinal ligament at a point near the uterine artery. The uterine artery, which usually arises from the superior vesicle artery, is thus isolated and divided, and the vesicle arteries are preserved. The uterine vessels are then brought over the ureter by application of gentle traction. Occasionally, the uterine vein passes under the ureter.

Dissection of the Ureter The ureter is dissected free from its medial peritoneal flap at the level of the uterosacral ligament. As the ureter passes near the uterine artery, there is a consistent branch from the uterine artery to the ureter. This branch is sacrificed in the standard radical (type III) hysterectomy but preserved in the modified radical (type II)

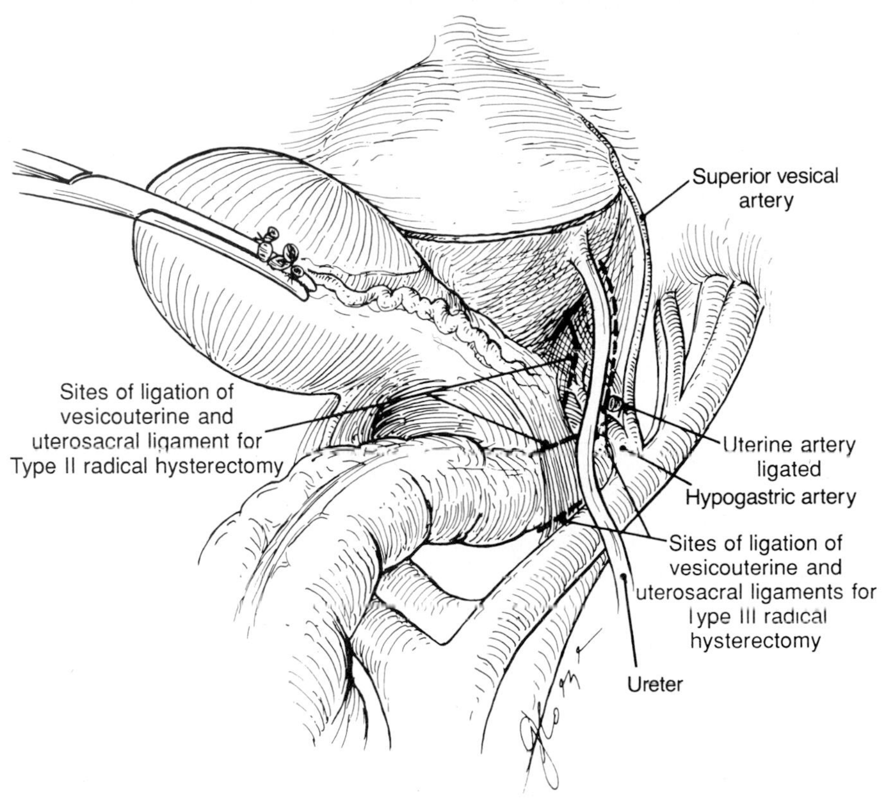

Figure 31.10 Radical hysterectomy. Uterine artery is ligated, ureter is dissected, and sites for division of the vesicouterine and uterosacral ligaments are shown. (From **Berek JS, Hacker F.** *Practical gynecologic oncology.* 3rd ed. Philadelphia: Lippincott Williams & Wilkins, 2000, with permission.)

hysterectomy. Dissection of the ureter from the vesicouterine ligament (ureteral tunnel) now may be accomplished. If the patient has a deep pelvis, ligation of the uterosacral and cardinal ligaments may be undertaken first to bring the ureteral tunnel dissection closer to the operator. The roof of the ureteral tunnel is the anterior vesicouterine ligament. It should be ligated and divided to expose the posterior ligament. This ligament is also divided in the radical (type III) hysterectomy but conserved in the modified radical (type II) hysterectomy (Fig. 31.10).

Posterior Dissection The peritoneum across the cul-de-sac is incised, exposing the uterosacral ligaments. The rectum is rolled free from the uterosacral ligaments, and these ligaments are divided midway to the sacrum in a radical (type III) hysterectomy and near the rectum in the modified radical (type II) operation. This allows the operator to develop the cardinal ligament separate from the rectum. A surgical clamp is placed on the cardinal ligament at the lateral pelvic sidewall in a radical hysterectomy and at the level of the ureteral bed in the modified radical procedure. A clamp is placed on the specimen side to maintain traction and is left on to ensure that the full cardinal ligament is excised with the specimen. A right-angled clamp then is placed caudad to this clamp across the paravaginal tissues. A second paravaginal clamp is usually needed to reach the vagina.

The vagina is entered anteriorly, and the upper one third of the vagina is removed with the specimen. More vaginal epithelium can be excised if necessary, depending on the previous colposcopic findings. The vaginal edge may be sutured in a hemostatic fashion and left open with a drain from the pelvic space or closed with a suction drain placed percutaneously. The ureteral fistula and pelvic lymphocyst rates from these two techniques are similar.

Modified Radical Hysterectomy

The modified radical hysterectomy differs from the radical hysterectomy in the following ways:

1. The uterine artery is transected at the level of the ureter, thus preserving the ureteral branch to the ureter.

2. The cardinal ligament is not divided near the sidewall but instead is divided at about its midportion near the ureteral dissection.

3. The anterior vesicouterine ligament is divided, but the posterior vesicouterine ligament is conserved.

A smaller margin of vagina is removed.

Complications of Radical Hysterectomy

Acute Complications The acute complications of radical hysterectomy include the following (42):

- Blood loss (average, 0.8 l)
- Ureterovaginal fistula (1% to 2%)
- Vesicovaginal fistula (1%)
- Pulmonary embolus (1% to 2%)
- Small bowel obstruction (1%)
- Febrile morbidity (25% to 50%)

Febrile morbidity is most often pulmonary (10%) and frequently is seen with pelvic cellulitis (7%) and urinary tract infection (6%). Wound infection, pelvic abscess, and phlebitis all occur in fewer than 5% of patients (43).

Subacute Complications The subacute effects of radical hysterectomy are postoperative bladder dysfunction and lymphocyst formation. For the first few days after radical hysterectomy, bladder volume is decreased, and filling pressure is increased. The sensitivity to filling is diminished, and the patient is unable to initiate voiding. The cause of this dysfunction is unclear. It is important to maintain adequate bladder drainage during this time to prevent overdistention. Bladder drainage is accomplished with a suprapubic catheter. It is more comfortable for the patient and allows the physician to perform cystometrography and determine residual urine volume without the need for frequent catheterization. In addition, the patient is able to accomplish trial voiding at home by clamping the catheter, voiding, and releasing to check the residual urine level. Cystometrography may be performed 3 to 4 weeks after surgery. For use of the catheter to be discontinued, the patient must be able to sense the fullness of the bladder, initiate voiding, and void with a residual urine level of less than 75 mL. Otherwise, voiding trials should continue at home until these criteria can be fulfilled.

Lymphocyst formation occurs in fewer than 5% of patients (43), and the cause is uncertain. Adequate drainage of the pelvis after radical hysterectomy may be an important step in prevention. However, routine placement of retroperitoneal drains has not been shown to reduce this morbidity (41). Ureteral obstruction and partial venous obstruction and thrombosis may occur from lymphocyst formation. Simple aspiration of the lymphocyst is generally not curative, but percutaneous catheters with chronic drainage may allow healing. If this treatment is unsuccessful, operative intervention with excision of a portion of the lymphocyst wall and placement of either large bowel or omentum into the lymphocyst should be performed.

Chronic Complications The most common chronic effect of radical hysterectomy is bladder hypotonia or, in extreme instances, atony. This condition occurs in about 3% of patients, regardless of the method of bladder drainage used (44,45). It may be a result of bladder denervation and not simply a problem associated with bladder overdistention (46). Voiding every 4 to 6 hours, increasing intraabdominal pressure with Credé's maneuver, and intermittent self-catheterization may be used to manage the hypotonic bladder.

Ureteral strictures are uncommon in the absence of postoperative radiation therapy, recurrent cancer, or lymphocyst formation (37). If the stricture is associated with lymphocyst formation, treatment of the lymphocyst usually alleviates the problem. Strictures that occur after radiation therapy should be managed with ureteral stenting. If a ureteral stricture is noted in the absence of radiotherapy or lymphocyst formation, recurrent carcinoma is the most common cause. A CT scan of the area of obstruction should be obtained and cytologic assessment by FNA cytology should be performed to exclude carcinoma if there is a target lesion. If the results of these tests are negative, a ureteral stent may be placed to relieve the stricture. Close observation for recurrent carcinoma is necessary, and the diagnosis of recurrence may ultimately require laparotomy.

Surgical Treatment of Early-stage Cervical Cancer

Stage Ia Microinvasive Carcinoma Until 1985, no FIGO recommendation existed concerning the size of lesion or the depth of invasion that should be considered microinvasive (stage Ia). This led to considerable confusion and controversy in the literature. Over the years, as many as 18 different definitions have been used to describe "microinvasion." In 1974, the Society of Gynecologic Oncologists recommended a definition that is now accepted by FIGO: **A microinvasive lesion is one in which neoplastic epithelium invades the stroma to a depth of more than 3 mm beneath the basement membrane and in which lymphatic or blood vascular involvement is not demonstrated.** The purpose of defining microinvasion is to identify a group of patients who are not at risk for lymph node metastases or recurrence and who therefore may be treated with less than radical therapy.

Diagnosis must be determined on the basis of a cone biopsy of the cervix. The treatment decision rests with the gynecologist and should be determined based on a review of the conization specimen with the pathologist. It is important that the pathologic condition be described in terms of (a) depth of invasion, (b) width and breadth of the invasive area, and (c) presence or absence of lymph–vascular space invasion. These variables are used to determine how extensive the operation should be and whether the regional lymph nodes should be treated (9).

Stage Ia1 $\leq$ 3 mm Invasion **Lesions with invasion that is less than or equal to 3 mm deep have a less than 1% incidence of pelvic node metastases.** Although this observation is controversial, it appears that the patients most at risk for nodal metastases or central pelvic recurrence are those with definitive evidence of tumor emboli in lymph vascular spaces (42,47). Therefore, patients with less than 3 mm invasion and no lymph–vascular space invasion may be treated with extrafascial hysterectomy without lymph node dissection. Therapeutic conization appears to be adequate therapy for these patients if childbearing capability is desired. Surgical margins must be free of disease. If there is lymph–vascular space invasion, an alternative is a pelvic node dissection with a type I (extrafascial) or II (modified radical) hysterectomy.

Treatment of microinvasive cervical adenocarcinoma has been complicated by a lack of agreement on approaches in the literature. Recent reports have shown that patients with stage Ia1 cervical adenocarcinoma may be treated in a fashion similar to patients with this stage and a squamous lesion. Some providers disagree with this interpretation because of the difficulty of establishing a pathologic diagnosis of microinvasion from a glandular lesion. Patients diagnosed with microinvasive cervical adenocarcinoma should have expert pathologic assessment before considering treatment with extrafascial hysterectomy.

Stage Ia2 >3–5 mm Invasion **Lesions with invasion of 3 to 5 mm have a 3.8% incidence of pelvic node metastases** (47–49); thus, pelvic node dissection is necessary for these lesions. The primary tumor may be treated with a modified radical hysterectomy (type II).

Surgical Treatment of Stage Ib to IIa

Stage Ib and IIa Invasive Cancer Stage Ib lesions are subdivided into stage Ib1, which denotes lesions that are 4 cm or smaller in maximum diameter, and stage Ib2, which denotes lesions that are larger than 4 cm. Stage IIa is direct extension to the proximal vagina. **Surgical therapy of stage Ib and IIa carcinoma of the cervix involves radical hysterectomy, pelvic lymphadenectomy, and paraaortic lymph node evaluation.**

A comparison of radical hysterectomy with radiation has resulted in similar survival rates for the two treatment modalities. A randomized study comparing patients treated by either radical hysterectomy or radiation therapy showed similar survival rates for both groups (50). Similar outcomes also were reported when patients were treated with radiation therapy or radical surgery (51). However, patients treated with type III radical hysterectomy who subsequently received postoperative radiation had a higher rate of intestinal and urinary morbidity. Therefore, many advocate using radiation and avoiding surgery in these patients because many will require adjuvant postoperative radiation. The results from the GOG showing that patients with stage Ib (>4 cm) and IIa disease treated with concurrent chemoradiation had improved survival are presented below. Thus many would advocate that the treatment of choice in patients with stage Ib and IIa disease who have a primary lesion that is larger than 5 cm should be treated with chemoradiation.

Prognostic Variables for Early-stage Cervical Cancer

The survival of patients with early-stage cervical cancer after radical hysterectomy and pelvic lymphadenectomy depends on several factors (42,51–65):

1. Status of the lymph nodes
2. Size of the tumor
3. Involvement of parametrial tissue
4. Depth of invasion
5. Presence or absence of lymph–vascular space invasion

Lymph Nodes The most dependent variable associated with survival is the status of the lymph nodes. Patients with negative nodes have an 85% to 90% 5-year survival rate (64,66), whereas the survival rate for those with positive nodes ranges from 20% to 74%, depending on the number of nodes involved and the location and size of the metastases (60–62,66–69).

Data on lymph node status can be summarized as follows:

1. When the common iliac lymph nodes are positive, the 5-year survival rate is about 25%, compared with about 65% when only the pelvic lymph nodes are involved (70–72).
2. Bilateral positive pelvic lymph nodes portend a less favorable prognosis (22% to 40% survival rate) than unilateral positive pelvic nodes (59% to 70%) (70,71).
3. The presence of more than three positive pelvic lymph nodes is accompanied by a 68% recurrence rate, compared with 30% to 50% when three or fewer lymph nodes are positive (60,67).

4. Patients in whom tumor emboli are the only findings in the positive pelvic lymph node have an 82.5% 5-year survival rate, whereas the survival rate with microscopic invasion of the lymph nodes is 62.1% and with macroscopic disease is 54% (51).

Lesion Size Lesion size is an independent predictor of survival. Patients with lesions smaller than 2 cm have a survival rate of about 90%, and patients with lesions larger than 2 cm have a 60% survival rate (54). When the primary tumor is larger than 4 cm, the survival rate drops to 40% (52,63). An analysis of a GOG prospective study of 645 patients showed a 94.6% 3-year disease-free survival rate for patients with occult lesions, 85.5% for those with tumors smaller than 3 cm, and 68.4% for patients with tumors larger than 3 cm (64).

Depth of Invasion Patients in whom depth of invasion is less than 1 cm have a 5-year survival rate of about 90%, but the survival rate falls to 63% to 78% if the depth of invasion is more than 1 cm (42,64,68). Patients with spread to the parametrium have a 5 year survival rate of 69%, compared with 95% when the parametrium is negative. When the parametrium is involved and pelvic lymph nodes are also positive, the 5-year survival rate falls to 39% to 42% (55,65).

Lymph–Vascular Space Involvement The significance of the finding of lymph vascular space involvement is somewhat controversial. Several reports have shown a 50% to 70% 5-year survival rate when lymph–vascular space invasion is present and a 90% 5-year survival rate in its absence (42,54,58,72–76). Others have found no significant difference in survival if the study is controlled for other risk factors (63,64,77–79). Lymph–vascular space involvement may be a predictor of lymph node metastasis and not an independent predictor of survival.

Postoperative Radiation

In an effort to improve survival rates, postoperative radiotherapy has been recommended for patients with high-risk factors such as metastasis to pelvic lymph nodes (42,52,66,72), invasion of paracervical tissue (55,56), deep cervical invasion (80), or positive surgical margins (67,81). Although most authors agree that postoperative radiotherapy is necessary in the presence of positive surgical margins, the use of radiation in patients with other high-risk factors is controversial. Increasing evidence supports the use of adjuvant radiation, however. Particularly controversial but best studied is the use of radiation in the presence of positive pelvic lymph nodes. The rationale for treatment is the knowledge that radiotherapy can sterilize cancer in pelvic lymph nodes and that pelvic node dissection does not remove all of the nodal and lymphatic tissue. The hesitancy to recommend postoperative radiotherapy relates to the significant rate of postradiotherapy bowel and urinary tract complications (82). Most of the data currently available are retrospective. However, the GOG has recently completed a randomized study comparing radiation with no further treatment for patients at high risk for recurrence with negative pelvic nodes (83).

Based on retrospective studies, it appears that postoperative radiation therapy for positive pelvic nodes can decrease pelvic recurrence but does not improve 5-year actuarial survival rates. One multiinstitutional study showed no difference in survival in patients with three or fewer positive pelvic nodes (59% versus 60%) (68). However, there seemed to be a benefit when radiotherapy was given to those with more than three positive nodes.

In a study of 60 pairs of irradiated and nonirradiated women matched for age, lesion size, and number and location of positive nodes after radical hysterectomy (84), no significant difference was found in projected 5-year survival rates (72% for surgery alone, 64% for surgery plus radiation). The proportion of recurrences confined to the pelvis was 67% in patients treated with surgery only and 27% in patients treated with postoperative radiation ($p = 0.03$). In a Cox regression analysis of 320 women who underwent radical hysterectomy, 72 of whom received postoperative radiation (61), there was a significant decrease in pelvic recurrence but no survival benefit. A multiinstitutional retrospective study was performed in 185 women with positive pelvic nodes after radical hysterectomy, 103 of whom received postoperative radiotherapy (63). Multivariate analysis disclosed that radiotherapy was not an independent predictor of survival, whereas age, lesion diameter, and number of positive nodes were found to influence survival. These authors concluded that additional treatment is needed to improve survival rates. Because survival is limited by distant site recurrence, the addition of chemotherapy to postoperative radiotherapy has been proposed. A 75% disease-free survival rate was reported at 3 years in 40 high-risk patients given cisplatin, vinblastine, and bleomycin after radical hysterectomy, and a 46% disease-free survival rate was found in 79 comparable patients who refused treatment (85). Only 4 (11.8%) of 34 patients with positive pelvic nodes had recurrences, whereas disease recurred in 8 (33%) of 24 untreated patients with positive nodes. An 82% rate of disease-free survival was reported at 2 years among 32 patients who were treated with postoperative radiation therapy plus cisplatin and bleomycin (86).

The location of lymph node metastases is apparently relevant to postirradiation recurrence rates. When common iliac lymph nodes are involved, the survival rate drops to 20% (73). As the number of positive pelvic nodes increases, the percentage of positive common iliac and low paraaortic nodes increases (73) (i.e., 0.6% when pelvic lymph nodes are negative, 6.3% with one positive pelvic node, 21.4% with two or three positive nodes, and 73.3% with four or more positive nodes). This information has been used to recommend extended-field radiotherapy to patients with positive pelvic lymph nodes in an attempt to treat undetected extrapelvic nodal disease (73). A 3-year disease-free survival rate of 85% occurred in patients with positive pelvic nodes and a survival rate of 51% in patients with positive common iliac nodes; these rates are better than the survival rates of 50% and 23%, respectively, for historical control groups receiving radiotherapy to the pelvis alone.

A randomized controlled trial initiated by the GOG has recently reported results of a study on patients with cervical cancer treated by radical hysterectomy and found to have at least two of the following risk factors: capillary lymphatic space invasion, more than one third stromal invasion, and larger tumor (84). A total of 277 patients were entered into the study, with 140 randomized to no further therapy and 137 patients randomized to adjuvant pelvic radiotherapy. The results showed that patients with these risk factors who were treated with postoperative radiation therapy had a statistically significant (47%) decrease in recurrent disease. The study results have not had adequate follow-up to show a statistically significant decrease in mortality. The data, however, do demonstrate improved survival rates. The morbidity with the combination of therapy was acceptable, with a low rate of enteric and urinary complications. A second GOG study reporting on patients with high-risk cervical cancer randomized patients to concurrent chemoradiation therapy or radiation therapy alone (87). The results of this study are presented in the section discussing chemoradiation.

Chemotherapy

The use of chemotherapy in the treatment of cervical carcinoma has been limited in part by the success of treating this disease with surgery or radiation therapy. However, neoadjuvant chemotherapy has been used to shrink the tumor before radical hysterectomy or radiotherapy. No randomized study on the effectiveness of this technique has been reported. However, the information available from current studies suggests that, compared with historical controls, neoadjuvant therapy can achieve a 22% to 44% complete response rate, decrease the number of positive pelvic lymph nodes, and improve the 2- and 3-year disease-free survival rates, particularly in patients with stage I or II disease. In a study in which cisplatin, vinblastine, and bleomycin were used before radical hysterectomy in 54 patients with stage I or IIa tumors larger than 4 cm, a complete response rate of 44% and a partial response rate of 50% based on evaluation of the radical hysterectomy specimen were found (88). Tumors recurred in only three patients, giving a 94% disease-free survival with a minimum of 2 years follow-up. Of the 11 patients with positive nodes, 3 had recurrences, and all had three or more positive nodes. A comparison with historical controls for a tumor of this size revealed a 40% disease-free survival rate. In treating 75 patients with stage I, II, or III disease whose tumors were larger than 4 cm, cisplatin, bleomycin, and methotrexate were administered before surgery or radiation therapy (89). Three-year disease-free survival rates of 100%, 81%, and 66% were achieved for stages I, II, and III, respectively. Initial large tumor size and parametrial infiltration significantly correlated with a lower response to neoadjuvant therapy. Recurrence was significantly correlated with FIGO stage, parametrial infiltration, and residual cervical tumor. Of the 12 recurrences, 9 involved the pelvis, indicating that additional local treatment is needed for this high-risk group.

In treating 151 patients who had stage IIb and III tumors, cisplatin, vinblastine, and bleomycin were administered before surgery plus radiation (62.5%) or radiation alone (37.7%) (90). These investigators reported a 2-year disease-free survival rate in stages II and III of 79% and 50%, respectively, compared with survival rates of 47% and 26% in historical controls treated with radiation alone. For the 25 patients (22%) who experienced a complete response to the chemotherapy, there was a 96% disease-free survival rate and a 0% incidence of lymph node metastasis. To determine the efficacy of neoadjuvant chemotherapy, randomized trials have been initiated by the GOG and other centers.

Radiation

Radiotherapy can be used to treat all stages of cervical squamous cell cancer, with cure rates of about 70% for stage I, 60% for stage II, 45% for stage III, and 18% for stage IV (2). A comparison of surgery and radiation for treatment of low-stage disease is shown in Table 31.5. The radiation treatment plan generally consists of a combination of external teletherapy to treat the regional nodes and to shrink the primary tumor and intracavitary brachytherapy to boost the central tumor. Intracavitary therapy alone may be used in patients with early disease when the incidence of lymph node metastasis is negligible.

The treatment sequence depends on tumor volume. Stage Ib lesions smaller then 2 cm may be treated first with an intracavitary source to treat the primary lesion, followed by external therapy to treat the pelvic nodes. Larger lesions require external radiotherapy first to shrink the tumor and to reduce the anatomic distortion caused by the cancer. This enables the therapist to achieve better intracavitary dosimetry. The usual doses delivered are 7,000 to 8,000 cGy to point A and 6,000 cGy to point B, limiting the bladder and rectal dosage to less than 6,000 cGy. To achieve this level, it is necessary to have adequate packing of the bladder and bowel away from the intracavitary sources. Localization films and careful calculation of dosimetry are mandatory to optimize the dose of radiation and to reduce the incidence of bowel and bladder complications. Local control depends on adequate dose to the tumor from the intracavitary source.

Clinical staging fails to predict the extension of disease to the paraaortic nodes in 7% of patients with stage Ib, 18% with stage IIb, and 28% with stage III disease (91). Such

Table 31.5. Comparison of Surgery versus Radiation for Stage Ib/IIa Cancer of the Cervix

	Surgery	*Radiation*
Survival	85%	85%
Serious complications	Urologic fistulas 1%–2%	Intestinal and urinary strictures and fistulas 1.4%–5.3%
Vagina	Initially shortened, but may lengthen with regular intercourse	Fibrosis and possible stenosis, particularly in postmenopausal patients
Ovaries	Can be conserved	Destroyed
Chronic effects	Bladder atony in 3%	Radiation fibrosis of bowel and bladder in 6%–8%
Applicability	Best candidates are younger than 65 years of age. <200 lb, and in good health	All patients are potential candidates
Surgical mortality	1%	1% (from pulmonary embolism during intracavitary therapy)

patients will have "geographic" treatment failures if standard pelvic radiotherapy ports are used. Thus, treatment plans for these patients are individualized based on CT scans and biopsy of the paraaortic lymph nodes for consideration of extended-field radiotherapy. The routine use of extended-field radiation without documentation of distant metastasis to the paraaortic nodes has been evaluated and is typically not practiced because of the increased enteric morbidity associated with this radiation.

Surgical "Staging" before Radiation

Surgical staging procedures designed to discover the presence of positive nodes have been devised. Transperitoneal exploration was first used, but it was associated with a 16% to 33% mortality rate from radiotherapy-induced bowel complications and a 5-year survival rate of only 9% to 12% (92,93). The radiotherapy dose to the paraaortic chain was 5,500 to 6,000 cGy, which is now known to be excessive. Postsurgical adhesions entrap the intestine in the radiotherapy field; therefore, the bowel receives the full dose of radiation. In the absence of postsurgical adhesions, the small bowel would move in and out of the radiotherapy field and receive a lesser dose. To avoid these postsurgical adhesions, extraperitoneal dissection of the paraaortic nodes is now recommended, and the radiation dose should be reduced to 5,000 cGy or less (94,95). When such an approach is used, postradiotherapy bowel complications occur in fewer than 5% of patients (96,97), and the 5-year survival rate is 15% to 26% in patients with positive paraaortic nodes (16,97). Survival appears to be related to the amount of disease in the paraaortic nodes and to the size of the primary tumor. In patients whose metastases to the paraaortic lymph nodes are microscopic and whose central tumor has not extended to the pelvic sidewall, the 5-year survival rate improves to 20% to 50% (98,99). Surgical staging techniques have improved to include laparascopic assessment of the paraaortic and pelvic lymph nodes. Studies have demonstrated benefit from surgical staging with improved survival and changes in treatment plans of 40% of patients (95,96).

Supraclavicular Lymph Node Biopsy

Although not standard practice, the performance of a supraclavicular lymph node biopsy has been advocated in patients with positive paraaortic lymph nodes before the initiation of extended-field irradiation as well as in patients with a central recurrence before exploration for possible exenteration. The incidence of metastatic disease in the supraclavicular lymph nodes in patients with positive paraaortic lymph nodes is 5% to 30% (100). FNA cytologic assessment can obviate the need for an excisional biopsy and thus should be performed if any enlarged nodes are present. If the scalene lymph nodes are found to be positive, the disease is incurable, and treatment is palliative.

Complications during Brachytherapy

Perforation of the uterus may occur at the time of insertion of the uterine tandem. This is a problem particularly for elderly patients and those who have had a previous diagnostic conization procedure. When perforation is recognized, the tandem should be removed, and the patient should be observed for bleeding or signs of peritonitis. Survival may be decreased in patients who have had uterine perforation (101), possibly because these patients have more extensive uterine disease, which predisposes them to perforation. Fever may occur after insertion of the uterine tandem and ovoids. Fever most often results from infection of the necrotic tumor and occurs 2 to 6 hours after insertion of the intracavitary system. If uterine perforation has been excluded by ultrasonography, intravenous broad-spectrum antibiotic coverage, usually with a cephalosporin, should be administered. If the fever does not decrease promptly or if the temperature is higher than 38.5°C, an aminoglycoside and a *Bacteroides* species–specific antibiotic should administered. If fever persists or if the patient shows signs of septic shock or peritonitis, the intracavitary system must be removed. Antibiotics are continued until the patient has recovered, and the intracavitary application is delayed for 1 to 2 weeks.

Acute Morbidity The acute effects of radiotherapy occur after 2,000 to 3,000 cGy and are caused by ionizing radiation on the epithelium of the intestine and bladder. Symptoms include diarrhea, abdominal cramps, nausea, frequent urination, and occasionally bleeding from the bladder or bowel mucosa. The bowel symptoms can be treated with a low-gluten, low-lactose, and low-protein diet. Antidiarrheal and antispasmodic agents also may help. The bladder symptoms may be treated with antispasmodic medication. Severe symptoms may require a week of rest from radiotherapy.

Chronic Morbidity The chronic effects of radiotherapy result from the induction of vasculitis and fibrosis, and they are more serious than the acute effects. These complications occur several months to several years after radiotherapy has been completed. The bowel and bladder fistula rate after pelvic radiation therapy for cervical cancer is 1.4% to 5.3% (35,37). Other serious toxicity (e.g., bowel bleeding, stricture, stenosis, or obstruction) occurs in 6.4% to 8.1% of patients (35,37).

Proctosigmoiditis Bleeding from proctosigmoiditis should be treated with a low-residue diet, antidiarrheal medications, and steroid enemas. In extreme cases, a colostomy may be required to rest the bowel completely, and occasionally resection of the rectosigmoid must be performed.

Rectovaginal Fistula Rectovaginal fistulas or rectal strictures occur in fewer than 2% of patients. The successful closure of fistulas with bulbocavernosus flaps has been reported (102), as has a technique of sigmoid colon transposition to repair rectosigmoid fistulas or rectal strictures (103). Occasionally, resection with anastomosis is feasible. Diversion resulting in colostomy may be the optimal therapy in patients who have poor vascular supply to the pelvis and a history of anastomotic leak or breakdown from prior repairs.

Small Bowel Complications Patients with previous abdominal surgery are more likely to have pelvic adhesions and thus sustain more radiotherapy complications in the small bowel. The terminal ileum may sustain chronic damage because of its relatively fixed position at the cecum. The patient typically has a long history of crampy abdominal pain, intestinal rushes, and distention characteristic of partial small bowel obstruction. Often, low-grade fever and anemia accompany the symptoms. Patients who have no evidence of disease should be treated aggressively with total parenteral nutrition, nasogastric suction, and early operation after the anemia has resolved and good nutritional status has been attained. The type of procedure performed depends on individual circumstances (104). Small bowel fistulas that occur after radiotherapy rarely close spontaneously while total parenteral nutrition is maintained. Recurrent cancer should be excluded; then aggressive fluid replacement, nasogastric suction, and wound care should be instituted. Fistulography and a barium enema should be performed to exclude a combined large and small bowel fistula. The fistula-containing loop of bowel may be either resected or isolated and left *in situ*. In the latter case, the fistula will act as its own mucous fistula.

Urinary Tract Chronic urinary tract complications occur in 1% to 5% of patients and depend on the dose of radiation to the base of the bladder. Vesicovaginal fistulas are the most common complication and usually require supravesicular urinary diversion. Occasionally, a small fistula can be repaired with either a bulbocavernosus flap or an omental pedicle. Ureteral strictures are usually a sign of recurrent cancer, and an FNA cytologic sample should be obtained at the site of the obstruction under CT scan control. If the findings are negative, the patient should undergo exploratory surgery to determine the status of the disease. If radiation fibrosis is the cause, ureterolysis may be possible, or indwelling ureteral stents may be passed through the open urinary bladder.

Treatment of Stage IIb to IVb

Traditional therapy for patients with stage IIb or greater cervical cancer was radiation therapy. In certain clinical situations, such as with patients who have stage IVa disease and present with vesicovaginal or rectovaginal fistula, urinary or rectal diversion should be performed, followed by radiation therapy. Patients with stage IVb cervical carcinoma are considered candidates for palliative radiation therapy because cure is not attainable for these patients. Control of symptoms with the least morbidity is of concern in this patient population.

Primary pelvic radiotherapy fails to control the disease in 30% to 82% of patients with cervical carcinoma (2). About two thirds of these failures occur in the pelvis (105). A variety of agents have been used in an attempt to increase the effectiveness of radiation therapy in patients with large primary tumors. *Hydroxyurea* has produced some improvement in response rate and survival rates when compared with radiation therapy alone in a controlled series of patients (106,107). The use *5-fluorouracil* (*5-FU*) and *mitomycin C* has also been reported to improve response rates for advanced cervical cancer (108). *Cisplatin* has been shown to have cytotoxic activity against cervical carcinoma (109) and recently has been demonstrated to be a radiation sensitizer (110). It has produced some improvement in response and survival rates when used with radiation therapy for cervical cancer as compared with radiation therapy alone (110,111). The results of GOG studies presented later in this chapter demonstrate that combination chemoradiation is superior to radiation therapy.

Concurrent Chemoradiation

Radiation therapy has failed to achieve control of cancer in 20% to 65% of patients with advanced cervical cancer. Chemotherapy, despite its lack of success in treating patients with cervical cancer, has been studied as neoadjuvant treatment in combination with surgery. Concomitant chemotherapy with radiation has been studied extensively by GOG, and results of five randomized studies have been reported. The concept of chemoradiation encompasses the benefits of regional therapy with radiation and the use of chemotherapy to sensitize cells to radiation therapy, thus improving locoregional control. These new results have changed the way cervical cancer is treated in many medical centers.

An intergroup trial involving the GOG, the Southwestern Oncology Group, and the Radiation Therapy Oncology Group evaluated postoperative chemoradiation therapy in patients with stage Ia2, Ib, or IIa cervical cancer who were found to have positive pelvic lymph nodes, positive parametrial extension, or positive vaginal margins at the completion of radical hysterectomy (86). A total of 243 patients were assessed in this trial, with 127 receiving chemoradiation (*cisplatin, 5-FU,* radiation therapy) and 116 receiving radiation. The results of this trial showed a statistically significant improvement in progression-free survival and overall survival at 43 months for the patients receiving concurrent chemoradiation. The 4-year survival rates for the patients receiving chemoradiation and radiation alone were 81% and 71%, respectively. The toxicity in the two groups was acceptable, with a higher rate of hematologic toxicity in the concurrent chemoradiation arm. **This study showed that in patients with these high-risk factors after radical hysterectomy for stage Ia2, Ib, and IIa disease, chemoradiation is the postoperative treatment of choice.**

Concurrent chemoradiation was evaluated in patients with advanced cervical carcinoma. The GOG protocol 85 was a prospective study that enrolled patients with stage IIb to IVa cervical cancer and compared concurrent chemoradiation (112). There were 177 patients treated with *cisplatin, 5-FU,* and radiation. These patients were compared with the 191 patients treated with *hydroxyurea* and radiation. The median follow-up of patients who were alive at the time of the analysis was 8.7 years. Patients who received concurrent chemoradiation and were treated with *cisplatin* and *5-FU* had a statistically significant improvement in progression-free interval and overall survival (112). The hematologic toxicity between the two groups was similar. This study showed that *cisplatin*-based concurrent chemoradiation was a superior treatment when compared with *hydroxyurea* and concurrent radiation.

The GOG protocol 120 was initiated to evaluate patients with negative paraaortic nodes and cervical carcinoma stage IIb to IVa and concurrent chemoradiation. The treatment arms in this study consisted of radiation plus weekly *cisplatin;* or *cisplatin, 5-FU,* and *hydroxyurea;* or *hydroxyurea.* There were 176 patients in the weekly cisplatin arm; 173 patients in the *cisplatin, 5-FU,* and *hydroxyurea* arm; and 177 patients in the *hydroxyurea* arm (113). The two treatment arms with *cisplatin*-based chemotherapy and radiation showed an improvement in progression-free interval and overall survival at a median follow-up of 35 months. The relative risks for progression of disease or death were 0.55 and 0.57, respectively, for patients treated with *cisplatin*-based chemotherapy and radiation, compared with the patients treated with *hydroxyurea* and radiation (114). **This study confirmed the findings of GOG 85 and again suggested that *cisplatin*-based concurrent chemoradiation is the treatment of choice for patients with advanced-stage cervical cancer.**

A third GOG trial evaluated patients with stage Ib to IVa cervical cancer. Of the patients enrolled in this study, 70% had stage Ib or IIa disease (115). A total of 403 patients were enrolled and evaluated. The 5-year survival rates were 73% in patients treated with chemoradiation and 58% in patients treated with radiation therapy alone. The cumulative rates of disease-free survival at 5 years were 67% in patients treated with concurrent chemoradiation and 40% in patients treated with radiation therapy alone. Survival and progression-free intervals for patients receiving concurrent chemoradiation were significantly improved (115). **The results of this study suggested that chemoradiation is the treatment for stage IIb to IVa disease and that those patients with stage Ib2 and IIa disease also may benefit from chemoradiation.** The role of extended-field radiation was evaluated in this trial, but its role in therapy for patients with no evidence of paraaortic metastasis still needs to be defined.

A GOG study of chemoradiation comparing concurrent cisplatin and radiation with radiation alone in patients with bulky Ib cervical cancer also included adjuvant hysterectomy after completion of the radiation (115). There were 183 patients assigned to the concurrent chemotherapy and radiation arm, and 186 patients treated with radiation alone. The median duration of follow-up was 36 months, with disease recurrence detected in 37% of the patients treated with radiation alone, compared with 21% who were treated with concurrent chemoradiation (114). The 3-year survival rates were 83% in the group who received concurrent chemoradiation and 74% in the group that received radiation alone (114). The study also included adjuvant hysterectomy after completion of radiation treatment. However, with the results of GOG 71 not showing an improvement in survival by using adjuvant hysterectomy, the authors concluded that adjuvant hysterectomy would not be part of their recommendations. This study supported the results of previous studies and showed that patients with bulky stage Ib and IIa cervical cancer had survival rates superior to those in patients treated with concurrent chemoradiation. **These two studies suggest that patients with bulky stage Ib and IIa disease should have primary treatment consisting of chemoradiation, with the chemotherapy agent being weekly *cisplatin.***

Patient Evaluation and Follow-up after Therapy

Patients who receive radiotherapy should be closely monitored to assess their response. Tumors may be expected to regress for up to 3 months after radiotherapy. During the pelvic examination, progressive shrinkage of the cervix and possible stenosis of the cervical os and surrounding upper vagina should be noted. During rectovaginal examination, careful palpation of the uterosacral and cardinal ligaments for nodularity is most important. FNA cytologic assessment of suspicious areas should be performed to allow early diagnosis of persistent disease. In addition to the pelvic organs, the supraclavicular and inguinal lymph nodes should be carefully examined, and cervical or vaginal cytologic assessment should be performed every 3 months for 2 years and then every 6 months for the next 3 years. Endocervical curettage may be performed in patients with large central tumors.

An x-ray film of the chest may be obtained yearly in patients who have advanced disease. Metastasis to the lung has been reported in 1.5% of cases; solitary nodules are present in 25% of cases. Resection of a solitary nodule in the absence of any other persistent disease may yield some long-term survivors (116). Although intravenous pyelography (IVP) is not a part of routine postradiotherapy surveillance, it should be performed if a pelvic mass is detected or if urinary symptoms warrant it. The finding of ureteral obstruction after radiotherapy in the absence of a palpable mass may indicate unresectable pelvic sidewall disease, but this finding should be confirmed, usually by FNA cytologic assessment (117).

Patients who have had radical hysterectomy and who are at high risk for recurrence may benefit from early recognition of recurrence because they might be saved with radiation therapy. In these patients, a routine IVP 6 to 12 months after surgery may be beneficial. After radical hysterectomy, about 80% of recurrences are detected within 2 years (118). The larger the primary lesion, the shorter the median time to recurrence (119).

Special Considerations

The incidence of adenocarcinoma of the cervix appears to be increasing relative to that of squamous cancers. Older reports indicated that 5% of all cervical cancers were adenocarcinomas (120), whereas newer reports show a proportion as high as 18.5% to 27% (121,122). The FIGO annual report indicates a poorer prognosis for adenocarcinoma than for squamous cell carcinoma in every stage. A Cox proportional hazard analysis of 203 women with adenocarcinoma and 756 women with squamous carcinoma supports these findings (122). This study showed 5-year survival rates of 90% versus 60%, 62% versus 47%, and 36% versus 8% for stages I, II, and III, respectively. Although some have attributed these rates to a relative resistance to radiation, they are more likely a reflection of the tendency of adenocarcinomas to grow endophytically and to be undetected until a large volume of tumor is present.

The clinical features of stage I adenocarcinomas have been well studied (121,123–125). These studies have identified size of tumor, depth of invasion, grade of tumor, and age of the patient as significant correlates of lymph node metastasis and survival. When matched with squamous carcinomas for lesion size, age, and depth of invasion, the incidence of lymph node metastases and the survival rate appear to be the same (123,124). Patients with stage I adenocarcinomas can be selected for treatment according to the same criteria as for those with squamous cancers (124).

The choice of treatment for bulky stage I and II tumors is controversial. Radiation alone has been advocated by some (126), but others support radiation plus extrafascial hysterectomy (127,128). In 1975, Rutledge and associates (127) reported an 85.2% 5-year survival rate for all patients with stage I disease treated with radiation alone and an 83.8% survival rate for those who had radiation plus surgery. The central persistent disease rate was 8.3%, compared with 4% for those who had radiation plus surgery. In stage II disease, the 5-year survival rate was 41.9% for radiation alone and 53.7% for radiation plus surgery. A subsequent report revealed no significant difference in survival among patients treated with radiation alone or radiation plus extrafascial hysterectomy (129).

Patients with adenosquamous carcinoma of the cervix have been reported to have a poorer prognosis than those with pure adenocarcinoma or squamous carcinoma (130). Whether this is true when corrected for size of lesion is controversial (123,124).

The association of adenocarcinoma with squamous intraepithelial neoplasia is well documented (131). A squamous intraepithelial lesion may be observed colposcopically and treated with outpatient therapy, and the coexistent adenocarcinoma in the canal may be overlooked. Performing endocervical curettage at colposcopy will help prevent such an occurrence.

Cervical Cancer during Pregnancy

A review of the literature concluded that the incidence of invasive cervical cancer associated with pregnancy was one in 2,200 (132). A Pap test should be performed on all pregnant patients at the initial prenatal visit, and any grossly suspicious lesions should be excised for biopsy. Diagnosis is often delayed during pregnancy because bleeding is attributed to pregnancy-related complications. If the results of the Pap tests are positive for malignant cells and invasive cancer cannot be diagnosed using colposcopy and biopsy, a diagnostic conization procedure may be necessary. Because conization subjects the mother and fetus to complications, it should be performed only in the second trimester and only in patients with colposcopy findings consistent with cancer and biopsy-proven microinvasive cervical cancer or strong cytologic evidence of invasive cancer. Inadequate colposcopic examination may be encountered during pregnancy in patients who have had prior ablative therapy. Close follow-up throughout pregnancy may allow the cervix to evert and develop an ectropion, allowing satisfactory colposcopy in the second or third trimester. Conization in the first trimester of pregnancy is associated with an abortion rate of up to 33% (132,133). Patients with an obvious cervical carcinoma may undergo cervical biopsy and clinical staging similar to that of nonpregnant patients.

After conization, there appears to be no harm in delaying definitive treatment until fetal maturity is achieved in patients with stage Ia cervical cancer (132,134,135). Patients with less than 3 mm of invasion and no lymphatic or vascular space involvement may be followed to term and delivered vaginally. A vaginal hysterectomy may be performed 6 weeks postpartum if further childbearing is not desired.

Patients with 3 to 5 mm of invasion and those with lymph–vascular space invasion may also be followed to term (132,135). They may be delivered by cesarean birth, followed immediately by modified radical hysterectomy and pelvic lymph node dissection. Patients with more than 5 mm invasion should be treated as having frankly invasive carcinoma of the cervix. Treatment depends on the stage of gestation and the wishes of the patient. Modern neonatal care affords a 75% survival rate for infants delivered at 28 weeks of gestation and 90% for those delivered at 32 weeks of gestation. Fetal pulmonary maturity can be determined by amniocentesis, and prompt treatment can be instituted when pulmonary maturity is documented. Although timing is controversial, it is probably unwise to delay therapy for longer than 4 weeks (134,135). The recommended treatment is classic cesarean delivery followed by radical hysterectomy with pelvic lymph node dissection. There should be a thorough discussion of the risks and options with both parents before any treatment is undertaken.

Patients with cervical cancer in stages II to IV should be treated with radiotherapy. If the fetus is viable, it is delivered by classic cesarean birth, and therapy is begun postoperatively. If the pregnancy is in the first trimester, external radiation therapy can be started with the expectation that spontaneous abortion will occur before the delivery of 4,000 cGy. In the second trimester, a delay of therapy may be entertained to improve the chances of fetal survival. If the patient wishes to delay therapy, it is important to ensure fetal pulmonary maturity before delivery is undertaken.

The clinical stage is the most important prognostic factor for cervical cancer during pregnancy. Overall survival is slightly better for patients with cervical cancer in pregnancy because an increased proportion of these patients have stage I disease. For patients with advanced disease, there is evidence that pregnancy impairs the prognosis (132,135). The diagnosis of cancer in the postpartum period is associated with a more advanced clinical stage and a corresponding decrease in survival.

Cancer of the Cervical Stump

Cancer of the cervical stump is less common today than it was several decades ago when supracervical hysterectomy was popular. Early-stage disease is treated surgically, with very little change in technique from that used when the uterus is intact (136). Advanced-stage disease may present a therapeutic problem for the radiotherapist if the length of the cervical canal is less than 2 cm. This length is necessary to allow satisfactory placement of the uterine tandem. If the uterine tandem cannot be placed, radiation therapy can be completed with vaginal ovoids or with an external treatment plan in which lateral ports are used to augment the standard anterior and posterior ports. Such a technique will reduce the dosage to the bowel and bladder and thus reduce the incidence of complications.

Pelvic Mass

The origin of a pelvic mass must be clarified before treatment is initiated. An IVP can exclude a pelvic kidney, and a barium enema helps to identify diverticular disease or carcinoma of the colon. An abdominal x-ray film may show calcifications typically associated with benign ovarian teratomas or uterine leiomyomas. Pelvic ultrasonography differentiates between solid and cystic masses and indicates uterine or adnexal origin. Solid masses of uterine origin are most often leiomyomas and generally do not need further investigation.

Pyometra and Hematometra

An enlarged fluid-filled uterine cavity may be a pyometra or a hematometra. The hematometra can be drained by dilation of the cervical canal and will not interfere with treatment. The pyometra also should be drained, and the patient should be given antibiotics to cover *Bacteroides* species, *anaerobic Staphylococcus* and *Streptococcus* species, and aerobic coliform bacterial infection. Placement of a large mushroom catheter through the cervix has been advocated, but the catheter itself may become obstructed, leading to further occlusion of the drainage. Repeated dilation of the cervix with aspiration of pus every 2 to 3 days is more effective.

If the disease is stage I, a radical hysterectomy and pelvic node dissection may be performed. However, a pyometra is usually found in patients with advanced disease, and thus radiotherapy is required. External-beam therapy can begin when the pyometra has healed. Patients often have a significant amount of pus in the uterus or a tuboovarian abscess without signs of infection; therefore, a normal temperature and a normal white blood cell count do not necessarily exclude infection. Repeat physical examination or pelvic ultrasonography is necessary to ensure adequate drainage.

Cervical Carcinoma after Extrafascial Hysterectomy

When invasive cervical cancer is found after simple hysterectomy, it may be treated with radiotherapy or reoperation involving a pelvic node dissection and radical excision of parametrial tissue, cardinal ligaments, and the vaginal stump (137).

Reoperation Reoperation is indicated particularly for a young patient who has a small lesion and in whom preservation of ovarian function is desirable. It is not indicated for patients who have positive margins or obvious residual disease (137). Survival rates after radical reoperation are similar to those after radical hysterectomy for stage I disease.

Radiation Therapy Survival after radiotherapy depends on the volume of disease, the status of the surgical margins, and the length of delay from surgery to radiotherapy. Patients with microscopic disease have a 95% to 100% 5-year survival rate; the 5-year survival rate is 82% to 84% in those with macroscopic disease and free margins, 38% to 87% in those with microscopically positive margins, and 20% to 47% in those with obvious residual cancer (138–140). A delay in treatment of more than 6 months is associated with a 20% survival rate (140).

Stage IVa

Although primary exenteration may be considered for patients with direct extension to the rectum or bladder, it is rarely performed. For patients with extension to the bladder, the survival rate with radiation therapy is as high as 30%, with a urinary fistula rate of only 3.8% (141). The presence of tumor in the bladder may prohibit cure with radiation therapy alone; thus, consideration must be given to removal of the bladder on completion of external-beam radiation treatment. This is particularly true if the disease persists at that time and the geometry is not conducive to implant therapy. Rectal extension is less commonly observed but may require diversion of the fecal stream before therapy to avoid septic episodes from fecal contamination.

Acute Hemorrhage

Occasionally, a large lesion can produce life-threatening hemorrhage. A biopsy of the lesion should be performed to verify neoplasia, and a vaginal pack soaked in Monsel's solution (*ferric subsulfate*) should be packed tightly against the cervix. After proper staging, external radiation therapy can be started with the expectation that control of bleeding may require 8 to 10 daily treatments at 180 to 200 cGy/d. Broad-spectrum antibiotics should be used to reduce the incidence of infection. If the patient becomes febrile, the pack should be removed. Rapid replacement of the pack may be necessary, and a fresh pack should be immediately available. This approach to management of hemorrhage in patients previously untreated is preferable to exploration and vascular ligation. Occasionally, vascular embolization under fluoroscopic control may be required in severe cases, and this procedure may obviate a laparotomy. However, vascular occlusion ultimately may lead to decreased blood flow and oxygenation of the tumor; because the effect of radiotherapy is dependent on tissue oxygen content, the efficacy of the radiotherapy may be compromised.

Ureteral Obstruction

Treatment of bilateral ureteral obstruction and uremia in previously untreated patients should be determined on an individual basis. Transvesical or percutaneous ureteral catheters should be placed in patients with no evidence of distant disease, and radiotherapy with curative intent should be instituted. Patients with metastatic disease beyond curative treatment fields should be presented with the options of ureteral stenting, palliative radiotherapy, and chemotherapy for the metastatic disease. A median survival rate of 17 months for these patients may be achieved with aggressive management (142).

Barrel-shaped Cervix

The expansion of the upper endocervix and lower uterine segment by tumor has been referred to as a *barrel-shaped cervix.* Patients with tumors larger than 6 cm in diameter have a 17.5% central failure rate when treated with radiotherapy alone because the tumor at the periphery of the lower uterine segment is too far from the standard intracavitary source to receive an adequate tumoricidal dose (143). Attempts have been made to overcome this problem radiotherapeutically by means of interstitial implants into the tumor with a perineal template, but high central failure rates have also been reported with this technique (144).

Most oncologists prefer a combination of radiotherapy and surgery for treatment of patients with a barrel-shaped cervix. The usual approach is to perform an extrafascial hysterectomy 6 weeks after the completion of radiation therapy in an effort to resect a small, centrally persistent tumor. The dose of external radiotherapy is reduced to 4,000 cGy, and a single intracavitary treatment is given, which is followed by an extrafascial hysterectomy (145,146). This approach appears to result in a lower rate of central failure (2%), although it is not clear that the overall survival rate is improved. There is disagreement concerning the need for extrafascial hysterectomy, and the GOG is undertaking a randomized study to compare adjuvant hysterectomy with radiotherapy alone in patients who have no evidence of occult metastases in the paraaortic nodes.

The narrow upper vagina of older patients may preclude the use of an intracavitary source of radiation. Such patients must receive their entire course of therapy from external sources, leading to a higher central failure rate and more significant bowel and bladder morbidity. If stage I disease is present in such a patient, a radical hysterectomy with pelvic node dissection is preferable if the patient's medical condition allows such an approach.

Small Cell Carcinoma

Local therapy alone gives almost no chance of cure of small cell carcinoma. Regimens of combination chemotherapy have improved the median survival rates in small cell bronchogenic carcinoma, and these regimens are now being used for treatment of small cell (neuroendocrine type) carcinoma of the cervix. Combination chemotherapy may consist of either *vincristine, doxorubicin,* and *cyclophosphamide*) (VAC) or VP-16 (*etoposide*) and *cisplatin* (EP) (147). Patients must be monitored carefully because they are at high risk for developing recurrent metastatic disease (148).

Recurrent Cervical Cancer

Treatment of recurrent cervical cancer depends on the mode of primary therapy and the site of recurrence. Patients who have been treated initially with surgery should be considered for radiation therapy, and those who have had radiation therapy should be considered for surgical treatment. Chemotherapy is palliative only and is reserved for patients who are not considered curable by the other two modalities.

Radiotherapy for recurrence after surgery consists primarily of external treatment. Vaginal ovoids also may be placed in patients with isolated vaginal cuff recurrences. Patients with a regional recurrence may require interstitial implantation with a Syed type of template in addition to external therapy. A 25% survival rate can be expected in patients treated with radiation for a postsurgical recurrence (118).

Radiation Retreatment

Retreatment of recurrent pelvic disease by means of radiotherapy with curative intent is confined to patients who had suboptimal or incomplete primary therapy. This may allow the radiotherapist to deliver curative doses to the tumor. The proximity of the bladder and rectum to the cancer and their relative sensitivity to radiation injury are the major deterrents to retreatment with radiation. The insertion of multiple interstitial radiation sources into the locally recurrent cancer through a perineal template may help overcome these dosimetric considerations (137,149). However, the fistula rates are high, and the consequences must be considered seriously before interstitial therapy is initiated. In general, for patients considered curable with interstitial implant therapy, pelvic exenteration is a better treatment choice. Radiotherapy can be palliative with localized metastatic lesions. Painful bony metastases, central nervous system lesions, and severe urologic or vena caval obstructions are specific indications.

Surgical Therapy

Surgical therapy for postirradiation recurrence is limited to patients with central pelvic disease. A few carefully selected patients with small-volume disease limited to the cervix may be treated with an extrafascial or radical hysterectomy. However, the difficulty of assessing tumor volume and the 30% to 50% rate of serious urinary complications in these previously irradiated patients have led most gynecologic oncologists to recommend pelvic exenteration as the patient's last chance for cure (150,151).

Exenteration

The operation can be an anterior exenteration (removal of the bladder, vagina, cervix, and uterus), a posterior exenteration (removal of the rectum, vagina, cervix, and uterus), or a total exenteration (removal of both bladder and rectum with the vagina, cervix, and uterus). A total exenteration that includes a large perineal phase includes the entire rectum and leaves the patient with a permanent colostomy as well as a urinary conduit. In selected patients, a total exenteration may take place above the levator muscle (supralevator), leaving a rectal stump that may be anastomosed to the sigmoid, thus avoiding a permanent colostomy.

Preoperative Evaluation and Patient Selection The search for metastatic disease is imperative. Physical examination includes careful palpation of the peripheral lymph nodes with FNA cytologic sampling of any nodes that appear suspicious. A random biopsy of nonsuspicious supraclavicular lymph nodes has been advocated but is not routinely practiced (100,152). A CT scan of the lung can detect disease missed on routine x-ray examination of the chest. Abdominal and pelvic CT scans are helpful in the detection of liver metastases and enlarged paraaortic nodes. CT-directed FNA cytologic study of any abnormality should be undertaken. If a positive cytologic diagnosis is obtained, it will obviate the need for exploratory laparotomy.

Extension of the tumor to the pelvic sidewall is a contraindication to exenteration; however, this may be difficult for even the most experienced examiner to determine because of radiation fibrosis. If any question of resectability arises, exploratory laparotomy and parametrial biopsies, the patient's last hope for cure, should be offered (153–156). **The clinical triad of unilateral leg edema, sciatic pain, and ureteral obstruction is nearly always pathognomonic of unresectable disease on the pelvic sidewall.** Preoperatively, the patient should be prepared for a major operation. Total parenteral nutrition may be necessary to place the patient in an anabolic state for optimal healing. A bowel preparation, preoperative antibiotics, and prophylaxis for deep venous thrombosis with low-dose heparin or pneumatic calf compression should be used (157). Surgical mortality increases with age, and the operation should rarely be considered in a patient who is older than 70 years of age. Other medical illnesses should be taken into account; when life expectancy is limited, exenterative surgery is unwise.

Anterior Exenteration Candidates for anterior exenteration are those in whom the disease is limited to the cervix and anterior portion of the upper vagina. Proctoscopic examination should be performed because a positive finding would mandate a total exenteration. However, a negative proctoscopic examination finding does not exclude disease in the rectal muscularis, and findings at laparotomy still must be considered. Generally, the presence of disease in the posterior vaginal mucosa directly over the rectum mandates removal of the underlying rectum.

Posterior Exenteration A posterior exenteration is rarely performed for recurrent cervical cancer. It is indicated, however, for the patient with an isolated posterior vaginal recurrence in which dissection of the ureters through the cardinal ligaments will not be necessary.

Total Exenteration Total exenteration with a large perineal phase is indicated when the disease extends down to the lower part of the vagina. Because distal vaginal lymphatics may empty into the inguinal node region, these nodes should be carefully evaluated preoperatively. A supralevator total exenteration with low rectal anastomosis is indicated in the patient whose disease is confined to the upper vagina and cervix (158,159). Frozen-section margins of the rectal edge should be obtained because occult metastases to the muscularis may occur.

The development of techniques to establish continent urinary diversion has helped improve a woman's physical appearance after exenteration (160–162). When both a rectal anastomosis and a continent diversion are performed, the patient has no permanent external appliance, and the associated psychological trauma is avoided. Every effort should be made to create a neovagina simultaneously with the exenteration (163). This procedure also helps in the reconstruction of the pelvic floor after extirpation of the pelvic viscera. Whether or not a neovagina is constructed, it is desirable to mobilize the omentum on the left gastroepiploic artery and use it to create a new pelvic floor.

Surgical mortality has steadily decreased to an acceptable level of less than 10%. The most common causes of postoperative death are sepsis, pulmonary thromboembolism, and hemorrhage. Fistulas of the gastrointestinal and genitourinary tract are serious surgical complications, with a 30% to 40% mortality rate despite attempts at surgical repair. The risk for such fistulas has been decreased by the use of nonirradiated segments of bowel for formation of the urinary conduit (157). The 5-year survival rate is 33% to 60% for patients undergoing anterior exenteration and 20% to 46% for those undergoing total exenteration (154,153–163). Survival rates are poorer for patients with recurrent disease larger than 3 cm, invasion into the bladder, positive pelvic lymph nodes, and recurrence diagnosed within 1 year after radiotherapy (156). The 5-year survival rate of patients with positive pelvic lymph nodes is less than 5%. Thus, the performance of an extensive lymphadenectomy in the irradiated field is not warranted, but discontinuation of the procedure is advisable if any nodes are positive for metastatic cancer. Patients who have any disease in the peritoneal cavity have no chance of survival.

Chemotherapy for Recurrent Cervical Cancer

Recurrent cervical cancer is not considered curable with chemotherapy. The delivery of chemotherapy to recurrent tumor in a prior radiated field may be compromised because of altered blood supply caused by radiation. *Topotecan* has been reported to have a response rate of 17%, with a median duration of 14 months (164). Many other agents have shown activity against cervical cancer and may used in attempt to help control symptoms of the cancer. A number of clinical trials with various drugs have shown response rates of up to 45% (165). Complete responses are unusual and are generally limited to patients with chest metastases, in whom the dose of drug delivered to the disease is stronger than that delivered to the fibrotic postirradiation pelvis (166).

In a review of the literature on the role of chemotherapy in cervical cancer, the author concludes that present data do not support the claim that toxic combination chemotherapy regimens are superior to cisplatin alone in terms of survival benefit, although further studies are required to determine whether combination chemotherapy may offer a benefit for certain subgroups of patients (16,17). The response rates for single-agent chemotherapy in cervical cancer are about 10% to 25%; *cisplatin* and *carboplatin* are among the most active agents. The response rate for *cisplatin* combination therapies is about 20% to 40% (167). The GOG currently has completed two trials (GOG 149 and 169) evaluating recurrent cervical carcinoma. GOG 169 is comparing *cisplatin* to *cisplatin* with *paclitaxel.* Results of these studies may alter first-line therapy for recurrent cervical carcinoma.

Vaginal Carcinoma

Primary vaginal cancer is a relatively uncommon tumor, representing only 1% to 2% of malignant neoplasms of the female genital tract (168,169). The incidence of invasive vaginal cancer is 0.42 per 100,000 women and has remained relatively unchanged since the 1980s (170). Primary vaginal cancer should be differentiated from cancers metastatic to the vagina. Metastatic cancers constitute the majority of vaginal cancers (80%% to 90%) (171).

Staging

The FIGO staging of vaginal cancer requires that a tumor that has extended to the vagina from the cervix be regarded as a cancer of the cervix, whereas a tumor that involves both the vulva and the vagina should be classified as a cancer of the vulva.

The FIGO staging for vaginal carcinoma is shown in Table 31.6. Staging is done by clinical examination and, if indicated, cystoscopy, proctoscopy, chest x-rays, and skeletal x-ray. Information derived from lymphangiography, CT, and MRI cannot be used to change the FIGO stage, but it can be used for planning treatment. Unfortunately, 75% of patients present with stage II to IV disease, indicating delay in diagnosis and complicating the treatment and subsequent cure rates (172–174).

Surgical staging and resection of enlarged lymph nodes may be indicated in selected patients. FIGO staging does not include a category for microinvasive disease. Because vaginal cancer is rare and treatment is generally by radiotherapy, there is very little information concerning the spread of disease in relation to depth of invasion, lymph–vascular space invasion, and size of the lesion.

Table 31.6. FIGO Staging of Vaginal Cancer

Stage 0	Carcinoma *in situ,* intraepithelia carcinoma.
Stage I	The carcinoma is limited to the vaginal wall.
Stage II	The carcinoma has involved the subvaginal tissue but has not extended to the pelvic wall.
Stage III	The carcinoma has extended to the pelvic wall.
Stage IV	The carcinoma has extended beyond the true pelvis or has involved the mucosa of the bladder or rectum.
Stage IVa	Spread of the growth to adjacent organs.
Stage IVb	Spread to distant organs.

FIGO, International Federation of Gynecology and Obstetrics.

Etiology

The cause of squamous cell carcinoma of the vagina is unknown. The association of cervical cancer with HPV suggests that vaginal cancer may have a similar association (175). In addition, up to 30% of women with vaginal cancer have a history of cervical cancer treated at least 5 years earlier (176–178). Similar to cervical cancer, there appears to be a premalignant phase called *vaginal intraepithelial neoplasia* (VAIN) (see Chapter 16). The exact incidence of progression to invasive vaginal cancer from VAIN is not known; however, there are documented cases of invasive disease occurring despite adequate treatment of VAIN (179,180).

By convention, any new vaginal carcinoma developing at least 5 years after the cervical cancer should be considered a new primary lesion. There are three possible mechanisms for the occurrence of vaginal cancer after cervical neoplasia:

1. Residual disease in the vaginal epithelium after treatment of the cervical neoplasia
2. New primary disease arising in a patient with increased susceptibility to lower genital tract carcinogenesis; the role of HPV in this setting is suspected.
3. Increased susceptibility of carcinogenesis caused by radiation therapy

Screening

Routine screening of all patients for vaginal cancer is inappropriate. For women who have had a cervical or vulvar neoplasm, the Pap test is an important part of routine follow-up with each physician visit. This increased risk for vaginal cancer continues for the lifetime of the patient. It is recommended that Pap test surveillance for vaginal cancer be performed yearly after the patient has completed surveillance for cancer of the cervix or vulva. For women who have had a hysterectomy for benign disease, Pap testing every 3 to 5 years has been standard practice in the United States. When adjusted for age and prior cervical disease, the incidence of vaginal cancer is not increased in women who have had hysterectomy for benign disease (181).

Symptoms

Painless vaginal bleeding and discharge are the most common symptoms of vaginal cancer. With more advanced tumors, urinary retention, bladder spasm, hematuria, and frequency of urination may occur. Tumors developing on the posterior vaginal wall may produce rectal symptoms, such as tenesmus, constipation, or blood in the stool.

Diagnosis

The diagnostic workup includes a complete history and physical examination, careful speculum examination and palpation of the vagina, and bimanual pelvic and rectal examinations.

It is important to rotate the speculum to obtain a careful view of the entire vagina because posterior wall lesions frequently occur and may be overlooked.

In early squamous cell lesions, the diagnosis is suggested by an abnormal Pap test result; however, this is not true for clear cell adenocarcinomas, which are characterized by submucosal growth. In these cases, the diagnosis is confirmed by a targeted biopsy using the same instruments as those used for cervical biopsies. The most common site of vaginal cancer is in the upper one third of the vagina on the posterior wall. The developing tumor may be missed during initial inspection because the speculum blades may have obscured it (182). Colposcopy is valuable in evaluating patients with abnormal Pap test results, unexplained vaginal bleeding, or ulcerated erythematous patches in the upper vagina. A colposcopically targeted biopsy may not allow a definitive diagnosis, and a partial vaginectomy to determine invasion may be necessary. Occult invasive carcinoma may be detected by such an excision, particularly in patients who had previous hysterectomies, in whom the vaginal vault closure may bury some of the vaginal epithelium that is at risk for cancer (183).

Pathology

Cancer of the vagina spreads most often by direct extension into the pelvic soft tissues and adjacent organs. Metastases to the pelvic and, subsequently, the paraaortic lymph nodes may occur in advanced disease. Lesions in the lower one third of the vagina may spread directly to the inguinal femoral lymph nodes as well as the pelvic nodes (184). Hematogenous dissemination to the lungs, liver, or bone may occur as a late phenomenon.

Squamous cell carcinomas are the most common form of vaginal cancer, occurring in 80% to 90% of vaginal cancers. These tumors most commonly occur in the upper, posterior wall of the vagina. The mean age of patients with squamous cell cancer is 60 years (185,186). Malignant melanoma is the second most common cancer of the vagina, accounting for 2.8% to 5% of all vaginal neoplasms (187–189). Other histologic subtypes include adenocarcinoma and sarcoma.

Primary adenocarcinoma of the vagina is rare, constituting 9% of primary tumors of the vagina. However, the most common adenocarcinoma of the vagina is metastatic. Metastatic adenocarcinoma of the vagina may originate from the colon, endometrium, ovary, or rarely, pancreas and stomach. In general, they affect a younger population of women, regardless of whether they were exposed to *diethylstilbestrol* (*DES*) *in utero* (190). Adenocarcinomas may arise in wolffian rest elements, periurethral glands, and foci of endometriosis (191). In women exposed to *DES in utero,* adenocarcinoma may develop in vaginal adenosis.

DES was used in the United States from 1940 until 1971 to maintain high-risk pregnancies in women with a history of spontaneous abortions. In 1970, Herbst and Scully reported on seven young women with clear cell adenocarcinoma of the vagina (Fig. 31.11). Later, an association between this cancer and maternal ingestion of *DES* during pregnancy was identified (192). Subsequently, more than 500 cases of clear cell cancer of the vagina and cervix have been reported to the Registry for Research on Hormonal Transplacental Carcinogenesis.

The estimated risk for developing clear cell adenocarcinoma from an exposed offspring is 1 in 1,000 or less. The mean age of diagnosis is 19 years (193). Clear cell adenocarcinoma in women with a history of *in utero* exposure to *DES* typically presents in the exocervix or upper third of the vagina. These tumors vary greatly in size, and are most frequently exophytic and superficially invasive. Stage is the most important prognostic factor. Other statistically significant factors include a tubulocystic growth pattern, size less than 3 cm^2, and less than 3 mm stromal invasion. Because the use of *DES* in pregnant women was discontinued in 1971, most of these tumors probably have been discovered. It is uncertain, however, what will happen to this cohort of women as they move into their fifth, sixth, and seventh decades of life. Continued surveillance of these women is indicated.

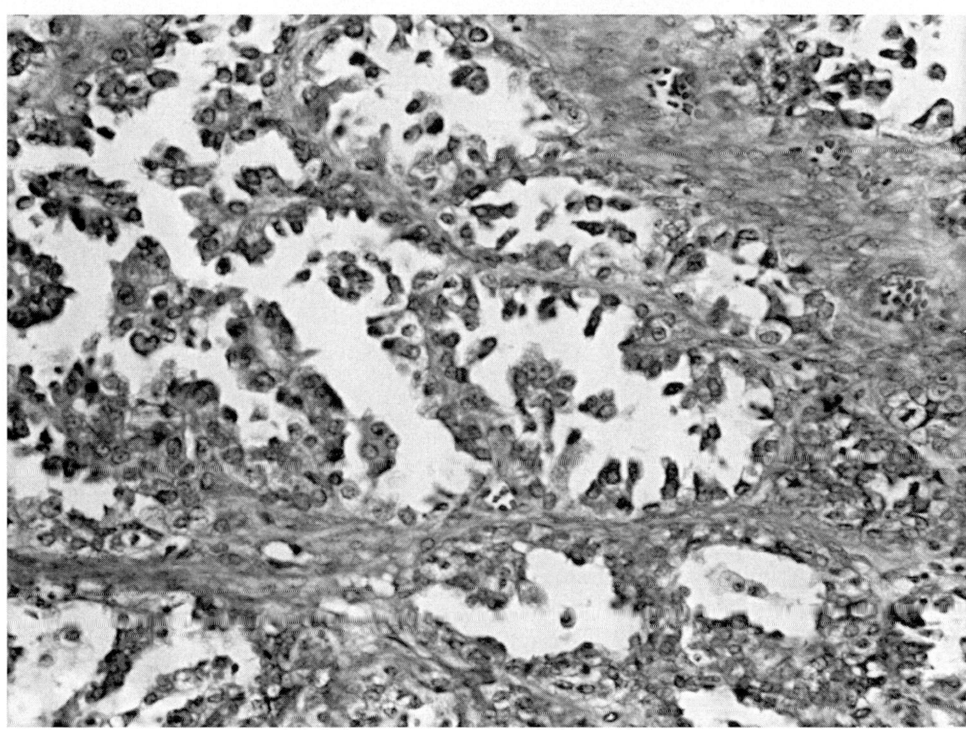

Figure 31.11 Vaginal clear cell carcinoma. Note the formation of tubules with hobnail cells lining the lumen. These cells are characterized by nuclear protrusion into the apical cytoplasm. (From **Berek JS, Hacker F.** *Practical gynecologic oncology.* 2nd ed. Baltimore: Williams & Wilkins, 1994, with permission.)

Ninety-seven percent of cases of vaginal clear cell adenocarcinoma are associated with adenosis. Adenosis is characterized by the presence of persistent müllerian-type glandular epithelium. Although adenosis is the most common histologic abnormality in women exposed to *DES in utero,* adenosis can also be found in women without a history of exposure. Adenosis typically appears as red, grapelike clusters in the vagina.

Malignant melanoma of the vagina is rare and extremely lethal. The average age of these patients is 58 years, and malignant melanoma occurs most often in white women (194). Most lesions are deeply invasive, corresponding to a level IV when compared with the staging for vulvar melanomas. The most common location of these tumors is in the lower third of the vagina (195). Melanomas have a wide variety of size, color, and growth patterns (193,196). Radical excision (vaginectomy, hysterectomy, and pelvic lymphadenectomy) has been the mainstay of treatment. The goal of treatment is to avoid local (vaginal) recurrence, which is the most common site of recurrence (194,195). The need to dissect regional lymph nodes is uncertain. Because the disease is deeply invasive, hematogenous spread is the most common lethal recurrence. This finding is consistent with more conservative local excision because there is no difference in overall survival of patients with local as opposed to radical excision (194). The survival rate is about 10% at 5 years.

The most common benign and malignant mesenchymal tumors of the vagina in adult women are smooth muscle tumors (197). Vaginal sarcomas are usually fibrosarcomas or leiomyosarcomas and are extremely rare. Radical local excision, followed by adjuvant chemotherapy or radiation therapy, is the indicated treatment.

The most common malignant mesenchymal tumor of the vagina in children and infants is botryoid rhabdomyosarcoma (Fig. 31.12). Botryoid sarcoma is usually found in the vagina during infancy and early childhood, in the cervix during the reproductive years, and in

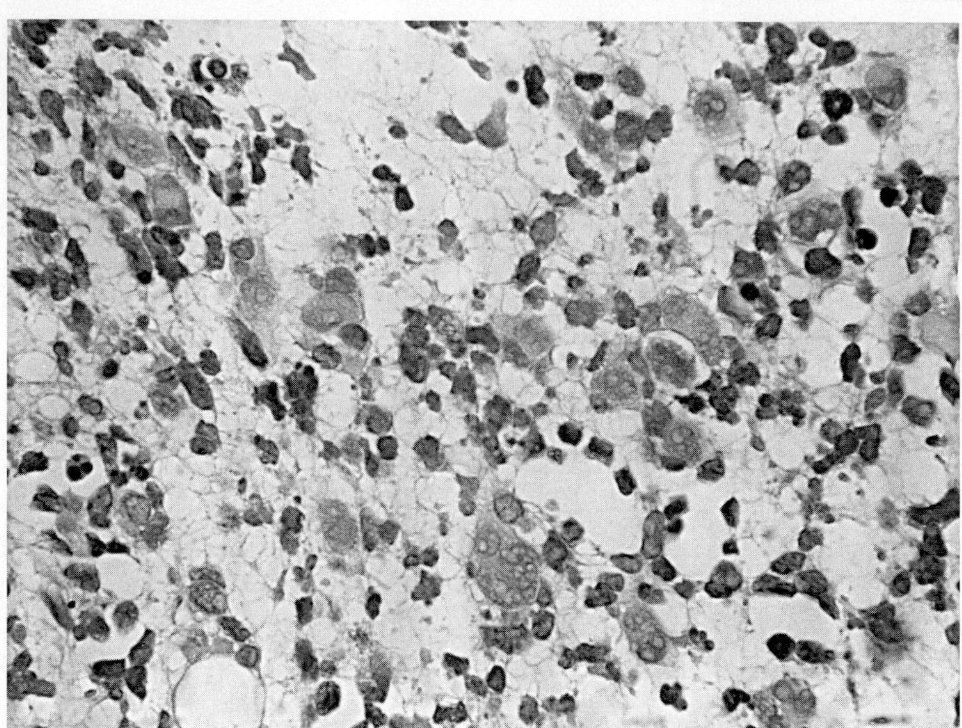

Figure 31.12 Embryonal rhabdomyosarcoma of the vagina (botryoid sarcoma). This lesion consists of primitive mesenchymal cells and rhabdomyoblasts, which have abundant eosinophilic cytoplasm. With further differentiation, cross striations may become evident. (From **Berek JS, Hacker F.** *Practical gynecologic oncology.* 2nd ed. Baltimore: Williams & Wilkins, 1994, with permission.)

the corpus uteri during postmenopausal years. Preoperative chemotherapy with *vincristine, actinomycin D,* and *cyclophosphamide,* followed by conservative surgery or radiation, has led to improved survival as well as organ preservation.

Treatment

Treatment selection is based on the clinical examination, CT scan results, chest x-ray results, age, and condition of the patient. Most tumors are treated by radiation therapy. Surgery is limited to highly selective cases.

Women with stage I disease involving the upper posterior vagina may be treated by radical vaginectomy and pelvic lymphadenectomy. If the uterus is *in situ,* it is removed as a radical hysterectomy specimen. When margins are clear and lymph nodes are negative, no additional therapy is necessary. Patients with stage IV disease with either rectovaginal or vesicovaginal fistula may be candidates for primary pelvic exenteration with pelvic and paraaortic node dissection (193). Low rectal anastomosis, continent urinary diversion, and vaginal reconstruction are indicated and are more successful in these nonirradiated patients than in patients who received prior radiation therapy (163).

Women with central pelvic recurrence after radiation therapy are candidates for pelvic exenteration similar to that for cervical cancer. Surgical staging with resection of enlarged lymph nodes may improve the control of pelvic disease by radiotherapy techniques. Surgical exploration or laparoscopy at the time of insertion of Syed interstitial implants defines more precisely the placement of the needles and ensures that needles do not pass into adherent loops of bowel.

Radiation therapy is the treatment of choice for all patients except those described previously. Small superficial lesions may be treated with intracavitary radiation alone (193). Larger,

Table 31.7. Primary Vaginal Carcinoma: 5-year Survival

Stage	No. of Patients	No. Surviving 5 Years	Percentage
I	172	118	68.6
II	236	108	45.8
III	203	62	30.5
IV	114	20	17.5
TOTAL	**725**	**308**	**42.5**

Data compiled from **Benedet et al.,** 1983 (173); **Rubin et al.,** 1985 (175); **Kucera et al.,** 1985 (196); **Houghton and Iversen,** 1982 (197); **Eddy et al,** 1991 (198); and **Pride et al.,** 1979 (199).

thicker lesions should be treated first with external teletherapy to decrease tumor volume and to treat the regional pelvic nodes, followed by intracavitary and interstitial therapy to deliver a high dose to the primary tumor (186,194). If the uterus is intact and the lesion involves the upper vagina, an intrauterine tandem and ovoids can be used. If the uterus has been previously removed, a vaginal cylinder may be used for superficial irradiation. If the lesion is more than 0.5 cm thick, interstitial radiation techniques can improve the dose distribution to the primary tumor. Extended-field radiation may be used for vaginal cancer in a manner similar to its use for cervical carcinoma. There is no experience reported with this technique in the treatment of vaginal cancer. Likewise, there is no reported experience with combination chemoradiation treatment. However, concurrent use of *5-FU* and *cisplatin* has been highly successful in anal and cervical cancer and should be considered.

Sequelae

The proximity of the rectum, bladder, and urethra leads to a major complication rate of 10% to 15% for both surgery and radiation treatment. For large tumors, the risk for bladder or bowel fistula is significant. Radiation cystitis and proctitis are common, as are rectal strictures or ulcerations. Radiation necrosis of the vagina occasionally occurs, requiring débridement and often leading to fistula formation. Vaginal fibrosis, stenosis, and stricture are common after radiation therapy. Use of vaginal dilators and resumption of regular sexual relations should be encouraged, along with the use of topical estrogen to maintain adequate vaginal function.

Survival

The overall 5-year survival rate for patients with vaginal cancer is 42% (Table 31.7). Even for patients with stage I disease, the 5-year survival rate is less than 70%, which is 15% lower than that for comparable stages of cervical or vulvar cancer (195–199). Most recurrences are in the pelvis, either from enlarged regional nodes or from large central tumors to which it is difficult to deliver an adequate dose of radiation. Radiation techniques, such as interstitial implants with Syed applicator and combination chemoradiation, may improve these results. Careful evaluation of patients who receive radiation therapy to detect central recurrence may allow some patients to be salvaged by pelvic exenteration. Because of the rarity of vaginal cancer, these patients should be treated in a center that is familiar with the complexity of treatment and modalities of therapy.

References

1. **Jemal A, Thomas A, Murray T, et al.** Cancer statistics, 2002. *CA Cancer J Clin* 2002;52:23–47.
2. **Pettersson F.** *Annual report on the results of treatment in gynecological cancer.* Radiumhemmet, Stockholm, Sweden: International Federation of Gynecology and Obstetrics (F.I.G.O.), 1994:132–168.
3. **Meland MR, Flehinger BJ.** Early incidence rates of precancerous cervical lesions in women using contraceptives. *Gynecol Oncol* 1973;1:290–294.
4. **Ursin G, Peters RK, Henderson BE, et al.** Oral contraceptive use and adenocarcinoma of the cervix. *Lancet* 1994;344:1390–1393.
5. **Walboomers JM, Jacobs MV, Manos MM, et al.** Human papillomavirus is a necessary cause of invasive cervical cancer worldwide. *J Pathol* 1999;189:12–19.

6. **Munger K, Scheffner M, Huibregtse JM, et al.** Interactions of HPV E6 and E7 oncoproteins with tumor suppressor gene products. *Cancer Surv* 1992;12:197–217.

7. **Centers for Disease Control.** Sexually transmitted disease guidelines. *MMWR Morb Mortal Wkly Rep* 1993;42:90–100.

8. **Fu YS, Berek JS.** Minimal cervical cancer: definition and histology. In: **Grundmann E, Beck L,** eds. *Minimal neoplasia—diagnosis and therapy. Recent results in cancer research.* Vol. 106. Berlin: Springer-Verlag, 1988:47–56.

9. **Creasman W.** New gynecologic cancer staging. *Gynecol Oncol* 1995;58:157–158.

10. **Fu YS, Reagan JW.** *Pathology of the uterine cervix, vagina and vulva.* Philadelphia: WB Saunders, 1989.

11. **Lagasse LD, Ballon SC, Berman ML, et al.** Pretreatment lymphangiography and operative evaluation in carcinoma of the cervix. *Am J Obstet Gynecol* 1979;134:219–224.

12. **Averette HE, Ford JH Jr, Dudan RC, et al.** Staging of cervical cancer. *Clin Obstet Gynecol* 1975;18:215–232.

13. **Koehler PR.** Current status of lymphangiography in patients with cancer. *Cancer* 1976;37:503–516.

14. **King LA, Talledo OE, Gallup DG, et al.** Computed tomography in evaluation of gynecologic malignancies: a retrospective analysis. *Am J Obstet Gynecol* 1986;155:960–964.

15. **Bandy LC, Clarke-Pearson DL, Silverman PM, et al.** Computed tomography in evaluation of extrapelvic lymphadenopathy in carcinoma of the cervix. *Obstet Gynecol* 1986;65:73–76.

16. **Hacker NF, Berek JS.** Surgical staging. In: **Surwit E, Alberts D,** eds. *Cervix cancer.* Boston: Martinus Nijhoff, 1987:43–57.

17. **Worthington JL, Balfe DM, Lee JK, et al.** Uterine neoplasms: MR imaging. *Radiology* 1986;159:725–730.

18. **Cosin JA, Fowler JM, Chen MD, et al.** Pretreatment surgical staging of patients with cervical carcinoma: the case for lymph node debulking. *Cancer* 1998;82:2241–2248.

19. **Robert ME, Fu YS.** Squamous cell carcinoma of the uterine cervix: a review with emphasis on prognostic factors and unusual variants. *Semin Diagn Pathol* 1990;7:173–189.

20. **Fu YS, Berek JS, Hilborne LH.** Diagnostic problems of cervical in situ and invasive adenocarcinoma. *Appl Pathol* 1987;5:47–56.

21. **Shin CH, Schorge JO, Lee KR, et al.** Conservative management of adenocarcinoma in situ of the cervix. *Gynecol Oncol* 2000;69:6–10.

22. **Ostor AG, Duncan A, Quinn M, et al.** Adenocarcinoma in situ of the uterine cervix: an experience with 100 cases. *Gynecol Oncol* 2000;79:207–210.

23. **Kaku T, Enjoji M.** Extremely well-differentiated adenocarcinoma ("adenoma malignum"). *Int J Gynecol Pathol* 1983;2:28–41.

24. **Gilks CB, Young R, Aguirre P, et al.** Adenoma malignum (minimal deviation adenocarcinoma) of the uterine cervix. *Am J Surg Pathol* 1989;13:717–729.

25. **Kaminski PF, Norris HJ.** Minimal deviation carcinoma (adenoma malignum) of the cervix. *Int J Gynecol Pathol* 1983;2:141–152.

26. **Benda JA, Platz CE, Buchsbaum H, et al.** Mucin production in defining mixed carcinoma of the uterine cervix: a clinicopathologic study. *Int J Gynecol Pathol* 1985;4:314–327.

27. **Young RH, Scully RE.** Villoglandular papillary adenocarcinoma of the uterine cervix: a clinicopathologic analysis of 13 cases. *Cancer* 1989;63:1773–1779.

28. **Glucksmann A, Cherry CP.** Incidence, histology and response to radiation of mixed carcinomas (adenoacanthomas) of the uterine cervix. *Cancer* 1956;9:971–979.

29. **Ferry JA, Scully RE.** "Adenoid cystic" carcinoma and adenoid basal carcinoma of the uterine cervix: a study of 28 cases. *Am J Surg Pathol* 1988;12:134–144.

30. **Rotmensch J, Rosenshein NB, Wodruff JD.** Cervical sarcoma: a review. *Obstet Gynecol Surv* 1983;38:456–461.

31. **Albores-Saavedra J, Gersell D, Gilks CB, et al.** Terminology of endocrine tumors of the uterine cervix: results of a workshop sponsored by the College of American Pathologists and National Cancer Institute. *Arch Pathol Lab Med* 1997;121:34–39.

32. **Van Nagell JR Jr, Donaldson ES, Wood EC, et al.** Small cell carcinoma of the cervix. *Cancer* 1979;40:2243–2249.

33. **Sheets EE, Berman ML, Hrountas CE, et al.** Surgically treated, early stage neuroendocrine small-cell cervical carcinoma. *Obstet Gynecol* 1988;7:10–14.

34. **Brewster WR, Monk BJ, Ziogas A, et al.** Intent-to-treat analysis of stage Ib and IIa cervical cancer in the United States: radiotherapy or surgery 1988–1995.

35. **Van Nagell JR Jr, Parker JC Jr, Maruyama Y, et al.** Bladder or rectal injury following radiation therapy for cervical cancer. *Am J Obstet Gynecol* 1974;119:727–732.

36. **Lawton FG, Hacker NF.** Surgery for invasive gynecologic cancer in the elderly female population. *Obstet Gynecol* 1990;76:287–289.

37. **Hatch KD, Parham G, Shingleton HM, et al.** Ureteral strictures and fistulae following radical hysterectomy. *Gynecol Oncol* 1984;19:17–23.

38. **Webb M, Symmonds R.** Wertheim hysterectomy: a reappraisal. *Obstet Gynecol* 1979;54:140–145.

39. **Meigs J.** Radical hysterectomy with bilateral pelvic node dissections: a report of 100 patients operated five or more years ago. *Am J Obstet Gynecol* 1951;62:854–870.

40. **Piver M, Rutledge F, Smith J.** Five classes of extended hysterectomy for women with cervical cancer. *Obstet Gynecol* 1974;44:265–272.

41. **Morice P, Lassau N, Pautier P, et al.** Retroperitoneal drainage after complete para-aortic lymphadenectomy for gynecologic cancer: a randomized trial. *Obstet Gynecol* 2001;97:243–247.

42. **Boyce J, Fruchter R, Nicastri A.** Prognostic factors in stage I carcinoma of the cervix. *Gynecol Oncol* 1981;12:154–165.

43. **Orr JW Jr, Shingleton HM, Hatch KD.** Correlation of perioperative morbidity and conization to radical hysterectomy interval. *Obstet Gynecol* 1982;59:726–731.

44. **Potter ME, Alvarez RD, Shingleton HM, et al.** Early invasive cervical cancer with pelvic lymph node involvement: to complete or not to complete radical hysterectomy? *Gynecol Oncol* 1990;37:78–81.

45. **Mann WJ Jr, Orr JW Jr, Shingleton HM, et al.** Perioperative influences on infectious morbidity in radical hysterectomy. *Gynecol Oncol* 1981;11:207–212.

46. **Green T.** Ureteral suspension for prevention of ureteral complications following radical Wertheim hysterectomy. *Obstet Gynecol* 1966;28:1–11.

47. **Simon NL, Gore H, Shingleton HM, Soong SJ, et al.** Study of superficially invasive carcinoma of the cervix. *Obstet Gynecol* 1986;68:19–24.

48. **Lowe J, Mauger G, Carmichael J.** The effect of Wertheim hysterectomy upon bladder and urethral function. *Am J Obstet Gynecol* 1981;139:826–834.

49. **Delgado G, Bundy BN, Fowler WC, et al.** A prospective surgical pathological study of stage I squamous carcinoma of the cervix: a Gynecologic Oncology Group study. *Gynecol Oncol* 1989;35:314–320.

50. **Landoni F, Maneo A, Columbo A, et al.** Randomised study of radical surgery versus radiotherapy for stage Ib–IIa cervical cancer. *Lancet* 1997;350:535–540.

51. **Morely GW, Seski JC.** Radial pelvic surgery versus radiation therapy for stage I carcinoma of the cervix (exclusive of microinvasion). *Am J Obstet Gynecol* 1976;126:785–798.

52. **Baltzer J, Lohe K, Kopke W, et al.** Histologic criteria for the prognosis of patients with operated squamous cell carcinoma of the cervix. *Gynecol Oncol* 1982;13:184–194.

53. **Chung C, Nahhas W, Stryker J, et al.** Analysis of factors contributing to treatment failures in stage Ib and IIa carcinoma of the cervix. *Am J Obstet Gynecol* 1980;138:550–556

54. **Creasman W, Soper J, Clarke-Pearson D.** Radical hysterectomy as therapy for early carcinoma of the cervix. *Am J Obstet Gynecol* 1986;155:964–969.

55. **Van Nagell J, Donaldson E, Parker J.** The prognostic significance of cell type and lesion size in patients with cervical cancer treated by radical surgery. *Gynecol Oncol* 1977;5:142–151.

56. **Inoue T, Okumura M.** Prognostic significance of parametrial extension in patients with cervical carcinoma stage Ib, IIa, and IIIb. *Cancer* 1984;54:1714–1719.

57. **Bleker O, Ketting B, Wayjean-eecen B, et al.** The significance of microscopic involvement of the parametrium and/or pelvic lymph nodes in cervical cancer stages Ib and IIa. *Gynecol Oncol* 1983;16:56–62.

58. **Gauthier P, Gore I, Shingleton HM.** Identification of histopathologic risk groups in stage Ib squamous cell carcinoma of the cervix. *Obstet Gynecol* 1985;66:569–574.

59. **Van Nagell J, Donaldson E, Wood E, et al.** The significance of vascular invasion and lymphocytic infiltration in invasive cervical cancer. *Cancer* 1978;41:228–234.

60. **Nahhas W, Sharkey F, Whitney C.** The prognostic significance of vascular channel involvement in deep stromal penetration in early cervical carcinoma. *Am J Clin Oncol* 1983;6:259–264.

61. **Soisson AP, Soper JT, Clarke-Pearson DL, et al.** Adjuvant radiotherapy following radical hysterectomy for patients with stage Ib and IIa cervical cancer. *Gynecol Oncol* 1990;37:390–395.

62. **Tinga DJ, Timmer PR, Bouma J, et al.** Prognostic significance of single versus multiple lymph node metastases in cervical carcinoma stage Ib. *Gynecol Oncol* 1990;39:175–180.

63. **Alvarez RD, Soong SJ, Kinney WK, et al.** Identification of prognostic factors and risk groups in patients found to have nodal metastasis at the time of radical hysterectomy for early stage squamous carcinoma of the cervix. *Gynecol Oncol* 1989;35:130–135.

64. **Fuller AF, Elliott N, Kosloff C, et al.** Determinants of increased risk for recurrence in patients undergoing radical hysterectomy for stage Ib and IIa carcinoma of the cervix. *Gynecol Oncol* 1989;33:34–39.

65. **Delgado G, Bundy B, Zaino R, et al.** Prospective surgical-pathological study of disease free interval in patients with stage Ib squamous cell carcinoma of the cervix: a Gynecologic Oncology Group study. *Gynecol Oncol* 1990;38:352–357.

66. **Gonzalez DG, Ketting BW, Van Bunningen B, et al.** Carcinoma of the uterine cervix stage Ib and IIa: results of postoperative irradiation in patients with microscopic infiltration in the parametrium and/or lymph node metastasis. *Int J Radiat Oncol Biol Phys* 1989;16:389–395.

67. **Martinbeau P, Kjorstad K, Iversen T.** Stage Ib carcinoma of the cervix: the Norwegian Radium Hospital. II. Results when pelvic nodes are involved. *Obstet Gynecol* 1982;60:215–218.

68. **Morrow P.** Panel report: is pelvic irradiation beneficial in the postoperative management of stage Ib squamous cell carcinoma of the cervix with pelvic node metastases treated by radical hysterectomy and pelvic lymphadenectomy? *Gynecol Oncol* 1980;10:105–110.

69. **Inoue T.** Prognostic significance of the depth of invasion relating to nodal metastases, parametrial extension, and cell types. *Cancer* 1984;54:3035–3042.

70. **Piver M, Chung W.** Prognostic significance of cervical lesion size and pelvic node metastases in cervical carcinoma. *Obstet Gynecol* 1975;46:507–510.

71. **Hsu CT, Cheng YS, Su SC.** Prognosis of uterine cervical cancer with extensive lymph node metastasis. *Am J Obstet Gynecol* 1972;114:954–962.

72. **Pilleron J, Durand J, Hamelin J.** Prognostic value of node metastasis in cancer of the uterine cervix. *Am J Obstet Gynecol* 1974;119:458–462.

73. **Inoue T, Chihara T, Morita K.** Postoperative extended field irradiation in patients with pelvic and/or common iliac node metastasis from cervical carcinoma stages Ib to IIb. *Gynecol Oncol* 1986;25:234–243.

74. **Larsson G, Alm P, Gullberg B, et al.** Prognostic factors in early invasive carcinoma of the uterine cervix. *Am J Obstet Gynecol* 1983;146:145–153.

75. **Lohe KJ, Burghardt E, Hillemanns HG, et al.** Early squamous cell carcinoma of the uterine cervix. II. Clinical results of a cooperative study in the management of 419 patients with early stromal invasion and microcarcinoma. *Gynecol Oncol* 1978;6:31–50.

76. **Burghardt E, Holzer E.** Diagnosis and treatment of microinvasive carcinoma of the cervix uteri. *Obstet Gynecol* 1977;49:641–653.

77. **Van Nagell J Jr, Greenwell N, Powell D, et al.** Microinvasive carcinoma of the cervix. *Am J Obstet Gynecol* 1983;145:981–991.

78. **Leman M, Benson W, Kurman R, et al.** Microinvasive carcinoma of the cervix. *Obstet Gynecol* 1976;48:571–578.

79. **Seski JC, Abell MR, Morley GW.** Microinvasive squamous cell carcinoma of the cervix: definition, histologic analysis, late results of treatment. *Obstet Gynecol* 1977;50:410–414.

80. **Roche WO, Norris HC.** Microinvasive carcinoma of the cervix. *Cancer* 1975;36:180–186.

81. **Nahhas WA, Sharkey FE, Whitney CW, et al.** The prognostic significance of vascular channel involvement and deep stromal invasion in early cervical cancer. *Am J Clin Oncol* 1983;6:259–264.

82. **Shingleton HM, Orr JW Jr.** Primary surgical and combined treatment. In: **Singer A, Jordan J,** eds. *Cancer of the cervix.* New York: Churchill Livingstone, 1983:76–100.

83. **Barter JF, Soong SJ, Shingleton HM, et al.** Complications of combined radical hysterectomy: postoperative radiation therapy in women with early stage cervical cancer. *Gynecol Oncol* 1989;32:292–296.

84. **Kinney WK, Alvarez RD, Reid GC, et al.** Value of adjuvant whole-pelvic irradiation after Wertheim hysterectomy for early-stage squamous carcinoma of the cervix with pelvic nodal metastasis: a matched-control study. *Gynecol Oncol* 1989;34:258–262.

85. **Lai CH, Lin TS, Soong YK, et al.** Adjuvant chemotherapy after radical hysterectomy for cervical carcinoma. *Gynecol Oncol* 1989;35:193–198.

86. **Wertheim MS, Hakes TB, Daghestani AN, et al.** A pilot study of adjuvant therapy in patients with cervical cancer at high risk of recurrence after radical hysterectomy and pelvic lymphadenectomy. *J Clin Oncol* 1985;3:912–916.

87. **Peters WA, Liu PY, Barrett RJ, et al.** Concurrent chemotherapy and pelvic radiation therapy compared with pelvic radiation therapy alone as adjuvant therapy after radical surgery in high-risk early-stage cancer of the cervix. *J Clin Oncol* 2000:18;1606–1613.

88. **Kim DS, Moon H, Kim KT, et al.** Two-year survival: preoperative adjuvant chemotherapy in the treatment of cervical cancer stages Ib and II with bulky tumor. *Gynecol Oncol* 1989;33:225–230.

89. **Panici PB, Scambia G, Baiocchi G, et al.** Neoadjuvant chemotherapy and radical surgery in locally advanced cervical cancer: prognostic factors for response and survival. *Cancer* 1991;67:372–379.

90. **Sardi J, Sananes C, Giaroli A, et al.** Neoadjuvant chemotherapy in locally advanced carcinoma of the cervix uteri. *Gynecol Oncol* 1990;38:486–493.

91. **Berman M, Keys N, Creasman W, et al.** Survival and patterns of recurrence in cervical cancer metastatic to para-aortic lymph nodes. *Gynecol Oncol* 1984;19:8–16.

92. **Piver MS, Barlow JJ, Krishnamsetty R.** Five-year survival (with no evidence of disease) in patients with biopsy-confirmed aortic node metastasis from cervical carcinoma. *Am J Obstet Gynecol* 1981;193: 575–578.

93. **Wharton JT, Jones HW III, Day TG, et al.** Preirradiation celiotomy and extended field irradiation for invasive carcinoma of the cervix. *Obstet Gynecol* 1977;49:333–338.

94. **Ballon SC, Berman ML, Lagasse LD, et al.** Survival after extraperitoneal pelvic and paraaortic lymphadenectomy and radiation therapy in cervical carcinoma. *Obstet Gynecol* 1981;57:90–95.

95. **Twiggs LB, Potish RA, George RJ, et al.** Pretreatment extraperitoneal surgical staging in primary carcinoma of the cervix uteri. *Surg Gynecol Obstet* 1984;158:243–250.

96. **Weiser EB, Bundy BN, Hoskins WJ, et al.** Extraperitoneal versus transperitoneal selective paraaortic lymphadenectomy in the pretreatment surgical staging of advanced cervical carcinoma (a Gynecologic Oncology Group study). *Gynecol Oncol* 1989;33:283–289.

97. **Stehman FB, Bundy BN, DiSaia PJ, et al.** Carcinoma of the cervix treated with radiation therapy. I. A multi-variate analysis of prognostic variables in the Gynecologic Oncology Group. *Cancer* 1991;67:2776–2785.

98. **Lovecchio JL, Averette HE, Donato D, et al.** 5-Year survival of patients with periaortic nodal metastases in clinical stage Ib and IIa cervical carcinoma. *Gynecol Oncol* 1990;38:446.

99. **Rubin SC, Brookland R, Mikuta JJ, et al.** Paraaortic nodal metastases in early cervical carcinoma: long-term survival following extended-field radiotherapy. *Gynecol Oncol* 1984;18:213–217.

100. **Stehman FB, Bundy BN, Hanjani P, et al.** Biopsy of the scalene fat pad in carcinoma of the cervix uteri metastatic to the periaortic lymph nodes. *Surg Gynecol Obstet* 1987;165:503–506.

101. **Kim RY, Levy DS, Brascho DJ, et al.** Uterine perforation during intracavitary application: prognostic significance in carcinoma of the cervix. *Radiology* 1983;147:249–251.

102. **White AJ, Buchsbaum HJ, Blythe JG, et al.** Use of the bulbocavernosus muscle (Martius procedure) for repair of radiation-induced rectovaginal fistulas. *Obstet Gynecol* 1982;60:114–118.

103. **Bricker EM, Johnston WD.** Repair of postirradiation rectovaginal fistula and stricture. *Surg Gynecol Obstet* 1979;148:499–506.

104. **Smith ST, Seski JC, Copeland LJ, et al.** Surgical management of irradiation-induced small bowel damage. *Obstet Gynecol* 1985;65:563–567.

105. **Jampolis S, Andras J, Fletcher GH.** Analysis of sites and causes of failure of irradiation in invasive squamous cell carcinoma of the intact uterine cervix. *Radiology* 1975;115:681–685.

106. **Hreshchyshyn MM, Aron BS, Boronow RC, et al.** Hydroxyurea or placebo combined with radiation to treat stage IIIb and IV cervical cancer confined to the pelvis. *Int J Radiat Oncol Biol Phys* 1979;5:317–322.

107. **Piver MS, Barlow JJ, Vongtama V, et al.** Hydroxyurea: a radiation potentiator in carcinoma of the uterine cervix. *Am J Obstet Gynecol* 1983;147:803–808.

108. **Thomas G, Dembo A, Beale F.** Concurrent radiation, mitomycin-C and 5-fluorouracil in poor prognosis carcinoma of the cervix: preliminary results of a Phase I-II study. *Int J Radiat Oncol Biol Phys* 1984;10:1785–1790.

109. **Bonomi P, Blessing JA, Stehman FB.** A randomized trial of three cisplatinum dose schedules in squamous cell carcinoma of the uterine cervix. *J Clin Oncol* 1985;3:1079–1085.

110. **Choo YC, Choy TK, Wong LC, et al.** Potentiation of radiotherapy by cisdichlorodiammine platinum (II) in advanced cervical carcinoma. *Gynecol Oncol* 1986;23:94–100.

111. **Twiggs LB, Potish RA, McIntyre S, et al.** Concurrent weekly cis-platinum and radiotherapy in advanced cervical cancer: a preliminary dose escalating toxicity study. *Gynecol Oncol* 1986;24:143–148.

112. **Whitney CW, Sause W, Bundy BN, et al.** Randomized comparison of fluorouracil plus cisplatin versus hydroxyurea as an adjunct to radiation therapy in stage IIb-IVa carcinoma of the cervix with negative para-aortic lymph nodes: a Gynecologic Oncology Group and Southwest Oncology Group study. *J Clin Oncol* 1999;17:1339–1348.

113. **Rose PG, Bundy BN, Watkins EB, et al.** Concurrent cisplatin-based radiotherapy and chemotherapy for locally advanced cervical cancer. *N Engl J Med* 1999;340:1144–1153.

114. **Morris M, Eifel PJ, Lu J, et al.** Pelvic radiation with concurrent chemotherapy compared with pelvic and para-aortic radiation for high risk cervical cancer. *N Engl J Med* 1999;340:1137–1143.

115. **Keys HM, Bundy BN, Stehman FB, et al.** Cisplatin, radiation, and adjuvant hysterectomy compared with radiation and adjuvant hysterectomy for bulky stage Ib cervical carcinoma. *N Engl J Med* 1999;340: 1154–1161.

116. **Gallousis S.** Isolated lung metastases from pelvic malignancies. *Gynecol Oncol* 1979;7:206–214.

117. **Nordqvist SR, Sevin BU, Nadji M, et al.** Fine-needle aspiration cytology in gynecologic oncology. I. Diagnostic accuracy. *Obstet Gynecol* 1979;54:719–724.

118. **Krebs HB, Helmkamp BF, Sevin B-U, et al.** Recurrent cancer of the cervix following radical hysterectomy and pelvic node dissection. *Obstet Gynecol* 1982;59:422–427.

119. **Shingleton HM, Orr JW Jr.** Posttreatment surveillance. In: **Singer A, Jordan J,** eds. *Cancer of the cervix.* New York: Churchill Livingstone, 1983:135–122.

120. **Kjorstad KE.** Adenocarcinoma of the uterine cervix. *Gynecol Oncol* 1977;5:219–223.

121. **Berek JS, Hacker NF, Fu YS, et al.** Adenocarcinoma of the uterine cervix: histologic variables associated with lymph node metastasis and survival. *Obstet Gynecol* 1985;65:46–52.

122. **Hopkins MP, Morley GW.** A comparison of adenocarcinoma and squamous cell carcinoma of the cervix. *Obstet Gynecol* 1991;77:912–917.

123. **Shingleton HM, Gore H, Bradley DH, et al.** Adenocarcinoma of the cervix. I. Clinical evaluation and pathologic features. *Am J Obstet Gynecol* 1981;139:799–814.

124. **Kilgore LC, Soong S-J, Gore H, et al.** Analysis of prognostic features in adenocarcinoma of the cervix. *Gynecol Oncol* 1988;31:137–153.

125. **Berek JS, Castaldo TW, Hacker NF, et al.** Adenocarcinoma of the uterine cervix. *Cancer* 1981;48: 2734–2741.

126. **Mayer EG, Galindo J, Davis J, et al.** Adenocarcinoma of the uterine cervix: incidence and the role of radiation therapy. *Radiology* 1976;121:725–729.

127. **Rutledge FN, Galakatos AE, Wharton JT, et al.** Adenocarcinoma of the uterine cervix. *Am J Obstet Gynecol* 1975;122:236–245.

128. **Gallup DG, Abell MR.** Invasive adenocarcinoma of the uterine cervix. *Obstet Gynecol* 1977;49:596–603.

129. **Eifel PJ, Morris M, Oswald MJ, et al.** Adenocarcinoma of the uterine cervix: prognosis and patterns of failure in 367 cases. *Cancer* 1990;65:2507–2514.

130. **Gallup DG, Harper RH, Stock RJ.** Poor prognosis in patients with adenosquamous cell carcinoma of the cervix. *Obstet Gynecol* 1985;65:416–422.

131. **Maier RC, Norris HJ.** Coexistence of cervical intraepithelial neoplasia with primary adenocarcinoma of the endocervix. *Obstet Gynecol* 1980;56:361–364.

132. **Hacker NF, Berek JS, Lagasse LD, et al.** Carcinoma of the cervix associated with pregnancy. *Obstet Gynecol* 1982;59:735–746.

133. **Averette HE, Nasser N, Yankow SL, et al.** Cervical conization in pregnancy. *Am J Obstet Gynecol* 1970;106:543–549.

134. **Lee RB, Neglia W, Park RC.** Cervical carcinoma in pregnancy. *Obstet Gynecol* 1981;58:584–589.

135. **Shingleton HM, Orr JW Jr.** Cancer complicating pregnancy. In: **Singer A, Jordan J,** eds. *Cancer of the cervix.* New York: Churchill Livingstone, 1983:193–209.

136. **Green TH, Morse WJ Jr.** Management of invasive cervical cancer following inadvertent simple hysterectomy. *Obstet Gynecol* 1969;33:763–769.

137. **Orr JW Jr, Ball GC, Soong SJ, et al.** Surgical treatment of women found to have invasive cervix cancer at the time of total hysterectomy. *Obstet Gynecol* 1986;68:353–356.

138. **Durrance FY.** Radiotherapy following simple hysterectomy in patients with stage I and II carcinoma of the cervix. *AJR Am J Roentgenol* 1968;102:165–169.

139. **Andras EJ, Fletcher GH, Rutledge F.** Radiotherapy of carcinoma of the cervix following simple hysterectomy. *Am J Obstet Gynecol* 1973;115:647–655.

140. **Heller PB, Barnhill DR, Mayer AR, et al.** Cervical carcinoma found incidentally in a uterus removed for benign indications. *Obstet Gynecol* 1986;67:187–190.

141. **Million RR, Rutledge F, Fletcher GH.** Stage IV carcinoma of the cervix with bladder invasion. *Am J Obstet Gynecol* 1972;113:239–246.

142. **Taylor PT, Andersen WA.** Untreated cervical cancer complicated by obstructive uropathy and renal failure. *Gynecol Oncol* 1981;11:162–174.

143. **Fletcher GH, Wharton JT.** Principles of irradiation therapy for gynecologic malignancy. *Curr Probl Obstet Gynecol* 1978;2:2–44.

144. **Gaddis O Jr, Morrow CP, Klement V, et al.** Treatment of cervical carcinoma employing a template for transperineal interstitial Iridium brachytherapy. *Int J Radiat Oncol Biol Phys* 1983;9:819–827.

145. **O'Quinn AG, Fletcher GH, Wharton JT.** Guidelines for conservative hysterectomy after irradiation. *Gynecol Oncol* 1980;9:68–79.

146. **Homesley HD, Raben M, Blake DD, et al.** Relationship of lesion size to survival in patients with stage Ib squamous cell carcinoma of the cervix uteri treated by radiation therapy. *Surg Gynecol Obstet* 1980;150: 529–531.

147. **Oldham RK, Greco FA.** Small cell lung cancer, a curable disease. *Cancer Chem Pharmacol* 1980;4: 173–177.

148. **Groben P, Reddick R, Askin F.** The pathologic spectrum of small cell carcinoma of the cervix. *Int J Gynecol Pathol* 1985;4:42–57.

149. **Feder BH, Syed AMN, Neblett D.** Treatment of extensive carcinoma of the cervix with the "transperineal parametrial butterfly"—a preliminary report on the revival of Waterman's approach. *Int J Radiat Oncol Biol Phys* 1978;4:735–742.

150. **Mikuta JJ, Giuntoli RL, Rubin EL, et al.** The radical hysterectomy. *Am J Obstet Gynecol* 1977;128: 119–127.

151. **Symmonds RE, Pratt JH, Welch JS.** Extended Wertheim operation for primary, recurrent, or suspected recurrent carcinoma of the cervix. *Obstet Gynecol* 1964;24:15–27.

152. **Ketcham AS, Chretien PB, Hoye RC, et al.** Occult metastases to the scalene lymph nodes in patients with clinically operable carcinoma of the cervix. *Cancer* 1973;31:180–183.

153. **Morley GW, Lindenauer SM.** Pelvic exenterative therapy for gynecologic malignancy: an analysis of 70 cases. *Cancer* 1976;38:581–586.

154. **Rutledge FN, Smith JP, Wharton JT, et al.** Pelvic exenteration: an analysis of 296 patients. *Am J Obstet Gynecol* 1977;129:881–892.

155. **Averette HE, Lichtinger M, Sevin BU, et al.** Pelvic exenteration: a 150-year experience in a general hospital. *Am J Obstet Gynecol* 1984;150:179–184.

156. **Hatch KD, Shingleton HM, Soong SJ, et al.** Anterior pelvic exenteration. *Gynecol Oncol* 1988;31: 205–216.

157. **Orr JW Jr, Shingleton HM, Hatch KD, et al.** Gastrointestinal complications associated with pelvic exenteration. *Am J Obstet Gynecol* 1983;145:325–332.

158. **Berek JS, Hacker NF, Lagasse LD.** Rectosigmoid colectomy and reanastomosis to facilitate resection of primary and recurrent gynecologic cancer. *Obstet Gynecol* 1984;64:715–720.

159. **Hatch KD, Shingleton HM, Potter ME, et al.** Low rectal resection and anastomosis at the time of pelvic exenteration. *Gynecol Oncol* 1988;31:262–267.

160. **Kock NG, Nilson AE, Nilsson LO, et al.** Urinary diversion via a continent ileal reservoir: clinical results in 12 patients. J Urol 1982;128:469–475.

161. **Penalver MA, Bejany DE, Averette HE, et al.** Continent urinary diversion in gynecologic oncology. *Gynecol Oncol* 1989;34:274–288.

162. **Mannel RS, Braly PS, Buller RE.** Indiana pouch continent urinary reservoir in patients with previous pelvic irradiation. *Obstet Gynecol* 1990;75:891–893.

163. **Berek JS, Hacker NF, Lagasse LD.** Vaginal reconstruction performed simultaneously with pelvic exenteration. *Obstet Gynecol* 1984;63:318–323.

164. **Abu-Rusteem NR, Lee S, Massad LS.** Topotecan for recurrent cervical cancer after platinum based therapy. *Int J Gynecol Cancer* 2000;10:285–288.

165. **Thigpen JT.** Single agent chemotherapy in carcinoma of the cervix. In: **Surwit EA, Alberts DS,** eds. *Cervix cancer.* Boston: Martinus Nijhoff, 1987:119–136.

166. **Barter JF, Soong SJ, Hatch KD, et al.** Diagnosis and treatment of pulmonary metastases from cervical carcinoma. *Gynecol Oncol* 1990;38:347–351.

167. **Vermorken JB.** The role of chemotherapy in squamous cell carcinoma of the uterine cervix: a review. *Int J Gynecol Cancer* 1993;3:129.

168. **Daw E.** Primary carcinoma of the vagina. *J Obstet Gynaecol Br Commonw* 1971;78:853.

169. **Herbst AL, Green TH Jr, Ulfelder H.** Primary carcinoma of the vagina. *Am J Obstet Gynecol* 1970; 106:210.

170. **Ragni MV, Tobon H.** Primary malignant melanoma of the vagina and vulva. *Obstet Gynecol* 1974;43:658.

171. **Hilborne LH, Fu YS.** Intraepithelial, invasive and metastatic neoplasms of the vagina. In: **Wilkinson EJ,** ed. *Pathology of the vulva and vagina.* New York: Churchill Livingstone, 1987:184.

172. **Weed JC, Lozier C, Daniel SJ.** Human papillomavirus in multifocal, invasive female genital tract malignancy. *Obstet Gynecol* 1986;68:333.

173. **Benedet JL, Murphy KJ, Fairey RN, et al.** Primary invasive carcinoma of the vagina. *Obstet Gynecol* 1983;62:715–719.

174. **Peters WA III, Kuman NB, Morley GW.** Carcinoma of the vagina. *Cancer* 1985;55:892–897.

175. **Rubin SC, Young J, Mikuta JJ.** Squamous carcinoma of the vagina: treatment, complications, and long-term follow up. *Gynecol Oncol* 1985;20:346–353.

176. **Benedet JL, Saunders BH.** Carcinoma in situ of the vagina. *Am J Obstet Gynecol* 1984;148:695–700.

177. **Lenehan PM, Meffe F, Lickrish GM.** Vaginal intraepithelial neoplasia: biologic aspects and management. *Obstet Gynecol* 1986;68:333–337.

178. **Herman JM, Homesley HD, Dignan MB.** Is hysterectomy a risk factor for vaginal cancer? *JAMA* 1986;256:601–603.

179. **Frick HC, Jacox HW, Taylor HC.** Primary carcinoma of the vagina. *Am J Obstet Gynecol* 1986;101:695.

180. **Hoffman MS, DeCesare SL, Roberts WS, et al.** Upper vaginectomy for in situ and occult superficially invasive carcinoma of the vagina. *Am J Obstet Gynecol* 1992;166:30–33.

181. **Al-Kurdi M, Monaghan JM.** Thirty-two years experience in management of primary tumors of the vagina. *Br J Obstet Gynaecol* 1981;88:1145–1150.

182. **Rutledge F.** Cancer of the vagina. *Am J Obstet Gynecol* 1967;97:635–655.

183. **Perez CA, Arneson AN, Dehner LP, et al.** Radiation therapy in carcinoma of the vagina. *Obstet Gynecol* 1974;44:862–872.

184. **Chung AF, Casey MJ, Flannery JT, et al.** Malignant melanoma of the vagina—report of 19 cases. *Obstet Gynecol* 1980;55:720–727.

185. **Iversen K, Robins RE.** Mucosal malignant melanomas. *Am J Surg* 1980;139:660.

186. **Norris HJ, Taylor HB.** Melanomas of the vagina. *Am J Clin Pathol* 1966;46:420.

187. **Ballon SC, Lagasse LD, Chang NH, et al.** Primary adenocarcinoma of the vagina. *Surg Gynecol Obstet* 1979;149:233–237.

188. **Herbst AL, Scully RE.** Adenocarcinoma of the vagina in adolescence. *Cancer* 1970;25:745–757.

189. **Herbst AL, Ulfelder H, Poskanzer DC.** Adenocarcinoma of the vagina: association of maternal stilbestrol therapy with tumor appearance in young women. *N Engl J Med* 1971;284:878–881.

190. **Herbst AL, Cole P, Norusis MJ, et al.** Epidemiologic aspects of factors related to survival in 384 Registry cases of clear cell adenocarcinoma of the vagina and cervix. *Am J Obstet Gynecol* 1979;135:876–886.

191. **Reid GC, Schmidt RW, Roberts JA, et al.** Primary melanoma of the vagina: a clinicopathologic analysis. *Obstet Gynecol* 1989;74:190–199.

192. **Morrow CP, DiSaia PJ.** Malignant melanoma of the female genitalia: a clinical analysis. *Obstet Gynecol Surv* 1976;31:233.

193. **Cramer DW, Cutler SJ.** Incidence and histopathology of malignancies of the female genital organs in the United States. *Am J Obstet Gynecol* 1974;118:443–460.

194. **Eddy GL, Singh KP, Gansler TS.** Superficially invasive carcinoma of the vagina following treatment for cervical cancer: a report of six cases. *Gynecol Oncol* 1990;36:376–379.

195. **Reddy S, Lee MS, Graham JE, et al.** Radiation therapy in primary carcinoma of the vagina. *Gynecol Oncol* 1987;26:19–24.

196. **Kucera H, Langer M, Smekal G, et al.** Radiotherapy of primary carcinoma of the vagina: management and results of different therapy schemes. *Gynecol Oncol* 1985;21:87–93.

197. **Houghton CRS, Iversen T.** Squamous cell carcinoma of the vagina: a clinical study of the location of the tumor. *Gynecol Oncol* 1982;13:365–372.

198. **Eddy GL, Marks RD, Miller MC III, et al.** Primary invasive vaginal carcinoma. *Am J Obstet Gynecol* 1991;165:292–296.

199. **Pride GL, Schultz AE, Chuprevich TW, et al.** Primary invasive squamous carcinoma of the vagina. *Obstet Gynecol* 1979;53:218–225.

Novak's Gynecology, 13th Edition. Edited by J.S. Berek. Lippincott Williams & Wilkins, Philadelphia © 2002

32 Ovarian Cancer

Jonathan S. Berek

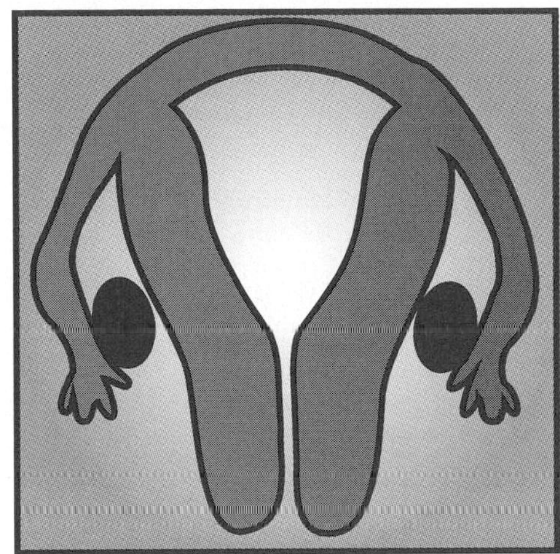

Of all the gynecologic cancers, ovarian malignancies represent the greatest clinical challenge. Epithelial cancers are the most common ovarian malignancies, and because they are usually asymptomatic until they have metastasized, patients have advanced disease at diagnosis in more than two-thirds of the cases. Ovarian cancer represents a major surgical challenge, requires intensive and often complex therapies, and is extremely demanding of the patient's psychological and physical energy. It has the highest fatality-to-case ratio of all the gynecologic malignancies. There are more than 23,300 new cases annually in the United States, and 13,900 women can be expected to succumb to their illness (1). A woman's risk at birth of having ovarian cancer sometime in her life is nearly 1.5%, and that of dying from ovarian cancer almost 1% (2).

Epithelial Ovarian Cancer

Approximately 90% of ovarian cancers are derived from tissues that come from the coelomic epithelium or mesothelium (2). The cells are a product of the primitive mesoderm, which can undergo metaplasia. A classification of the histologic types of epithelial tumors of the ovary is presented in Table 32.1. Neoplastic transformation can occur when the cells are genetically predisposed to oncogenesis or exposed to an oncogenic agent or both (3).

Pathology

Invasive Cancer

Seventy-five percent of epithelial cancers are of the serous histologic type. Less common types are mucinous (20%), endometrioid (2%), clear cell, Brenner, and undifferentiated carcinomas; each of the last three types represents less than 1% of epithelial lesions (2). Each tumor type has a histologic pattern that reproduces the mucosal features of a section of the lower genital tract (3). For example, the serous or papillary pattern has an appearance similar to that of the glandular epithelial lining and fallopian tube. Mucinous tumors contain cells that resemble the endocervical glands, and the endometrioid tumors resemble the endometrium.

Table 32.1. Epithelial Ovarian Tumors

Histologic Type	*Cellular Type*
I. Serous A. Benign B. Borderline C. Malignant	Endosalpingeal
II. Mucinous A. Benign B. Borderline C. Malignant	Endocervical
III. Endometrioid A. Benign B. Borderline C. Malignant	Endometrial
IV. Clear-cell "mesonephroid" A. Benign B. Borderline C. Malignant	Müllerian
V. Brenner A. Benign B. Borderline (proliferating) C. Malignant	Transitional
VI. Mixed epithelial A. Benign B. Borderline C. Malignant	Mixed
VII. Undifferentiated	Anaplastic
VIII. Unclassified	Mesothelioma, etc.

From **Seroy SF, Scully RE, Sobin LH.** *International histological classification of tumours no. 9. Histological typing of ovarian tumors.* Geneva: World Health Organization, 1973, with permission.

Borderline Tumors

An important group of tumors to distinguish is the *tumor of low malignant potential,* also called the *borderline tumor.* Borderline tumors are lesions that tend to remain confined to the ovary for long periods, occur predominantly in premenopausal women, and are associated with a very good prognosis (2–8). They are encountered most frequently in women between the ages of 30 and 50 years, whereas invasive carcinomas occur more often in women between the ages of 50 and 70 years (2).

Although uncommon, metastatic implants may occur with borderline tumors. Such implants have been divided into noninvasive and invasive forms. The latter group has a higher likelihood of developing into progressive, proliferative disease in the peritoneal cavity, which can lead to intestinal obstruction and death (2,6).

The criteria for the diagnosis of borderline tumors (Fig. 32.1) are as follows (7):

1. Epithelial proliferation with papillary formation and pseudostratification
2. Nuclear atypia and increased mitotic activity
3. Absence of true stromal invasion (i.e., without tissue destruction).

It should be emphasized that about 20% to 25% of borderline malignant tumors spread beyond the ovary. The diagnosis of borderline malignant versus malignant ovarian tumor must be based on the histologic features of the primary tumor (7).

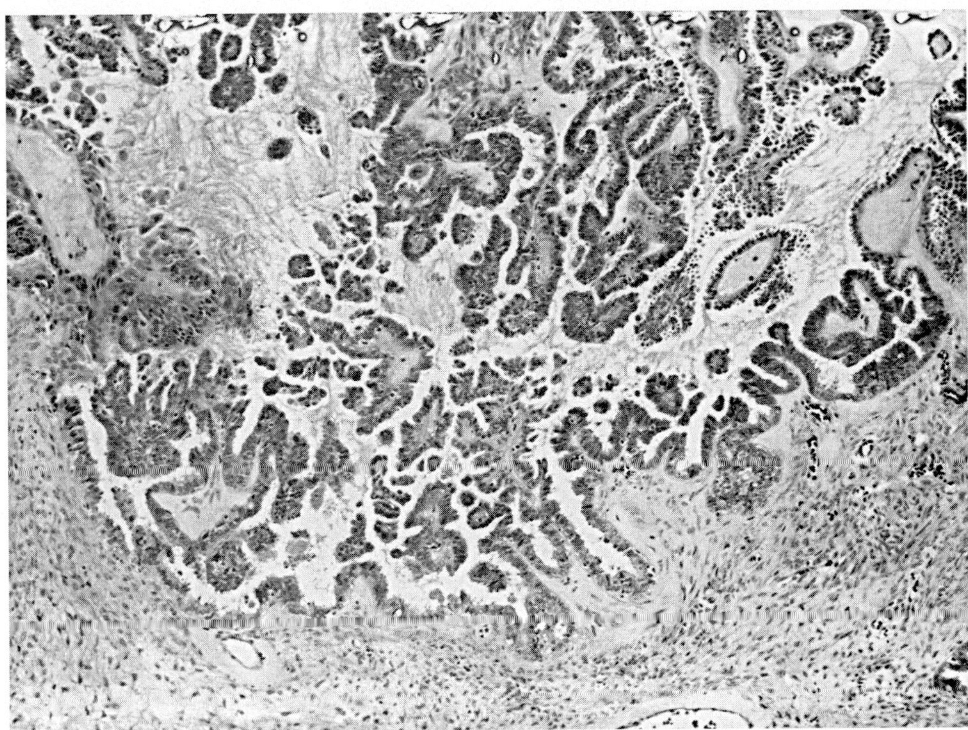

Figure 32.1 Borderline malignant serous tumor of the ovary. Complex papillary fronds are lined with pseudostratified columnar cells. The epithelium and the stroma are clearly separated by a basement membrane, indicating no stromal invasion. (From **Berek JS, Hacker NF.** *Practical gynecologic oncology,* 2nd ed. Baltimore: Williams & Wilkins, 1994:138, with permission.)

Classification of Epithelial Ovarian Tumors

Serous Tumors

Serous tumors develop by invagination of the surface ovarian epithelium and are so classified because they secrete serous fluid (as do tubal secretory cells). *Psammoma bodies,* more correctly foci of foreign material, frequently are associated with these invaginations and may be a response to irritative agents that produce adhesion formation and the entrapment of the surface epithelium. In the wall of the mesothelial invaginations, papillary ingrowths are common, representing the early stages of development of a papillary serous cystadenoma. There are many variations in the proliferation of these mesothelial inclusions. Several foci may be lined with flattened inactive epithelium; in adjacent cavities, papillary excrescences are present, often resulting from local irritants (2).

Borderline Serous Tumors Approximately 10% of all ovarian serous tumors fall into the category of a tumor of low malignant potential or borderline tumor, and 50% occur before the age of 40 years. As many as 10% of women with ovarian serous borderline tumors have extraovarian implants, and some will eventually die of the disease (9). Although multiple foci of disease have been documented in the abdominal cavity with secondary deposits in the pelvis, omentum, and adjacent tissues, including lymph nodes, metastases outside the abdominal cavity are rare. Death can occur as the result of intestinal obstruction (10–12).

The implants are divided histologically into invasive and noninvasive groups (6,10). In the noninvasive group, papillary proliferations of atypical cells involve the peritoneal surface and form smooth invaginations (6). The invasive implants resemble well-differentiated serous carcinoma and are characterized by atypical cells forming irregular glands with sharp borders. Bell and associates (6) have reported that only three of 50 women with

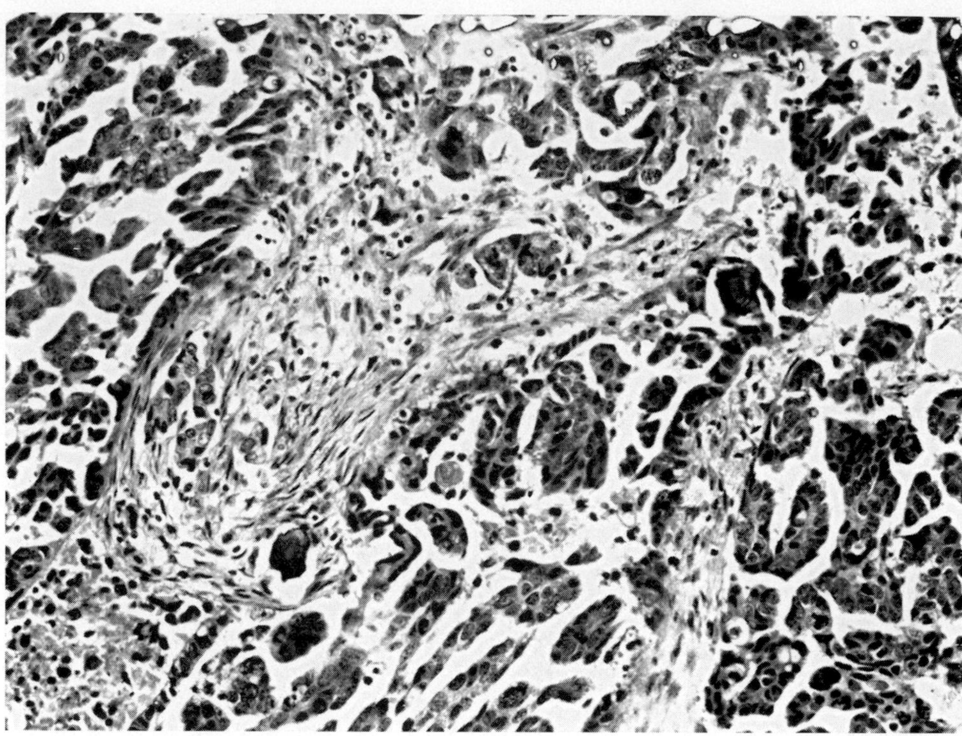

Figure 32.2 Well-differentiated serous papillary adenocarcinoma of the ovary. Clusters and papillae of malignant cells are in direct contact with fibrous stroma indicative of stromal invasion. (From **Berek JS, Hacker NF.** *Practical gynecologic oncology,* 2nd ed. Baltimore: Williams & Wilkins, 1994:140, with permission.)

noninvasive implants died, whereas four of six women with invasive implants died. In the series of McCaughey, two of 13 patients with noninvasive implants and all five patients with invasive implants died (9). Others have noted no differences in prognosis (10,11).

Rare examples of borderline malignant serous tumors with foci of microinvasion have been reported by Bell and Scully (12). Most patients are young, International Federation of Gynecology and Obstetrics (FIGO) stage I, and sometimes pregnant. Only one of 30 such patients died of disease, and she had stage III disease (12).

Malignant Serous Carcinomas In the malignant tumors, stromal invasion is present (2). The grade of tumor should be identified. In well-differentiated serous adenocarcinomas, papillary and glandular structures predominate (Fig. 32.2); poorly differentiated neoplasms are characterized by solid sheets of cells, nuclear pleomorphism, and high mitotic activity; and moderately differentiated carcinomas are intermediate between these two lesions. Laminated, calcified psammoma bodies are found in 80% of serous carcinomas.

Mucinous Tumors

These cystic tumors have loculi lined with mucin-secreting epithelium. They represent about 8% to 10% of epithelial ovarian tumors. They may reach enormous size, filling the entire abdominal cavity (2).

Borderline Mucinous Tumors The mucinous tumor of low malignant potential is often a diagnosis difficult to make. Although it is common to find a rather uniform pattern from section to section in the borderline malignant serous lesions, this is not true in the mucinous tumors. **Frequently, well-differentiated mucinous epithelium may be seen**

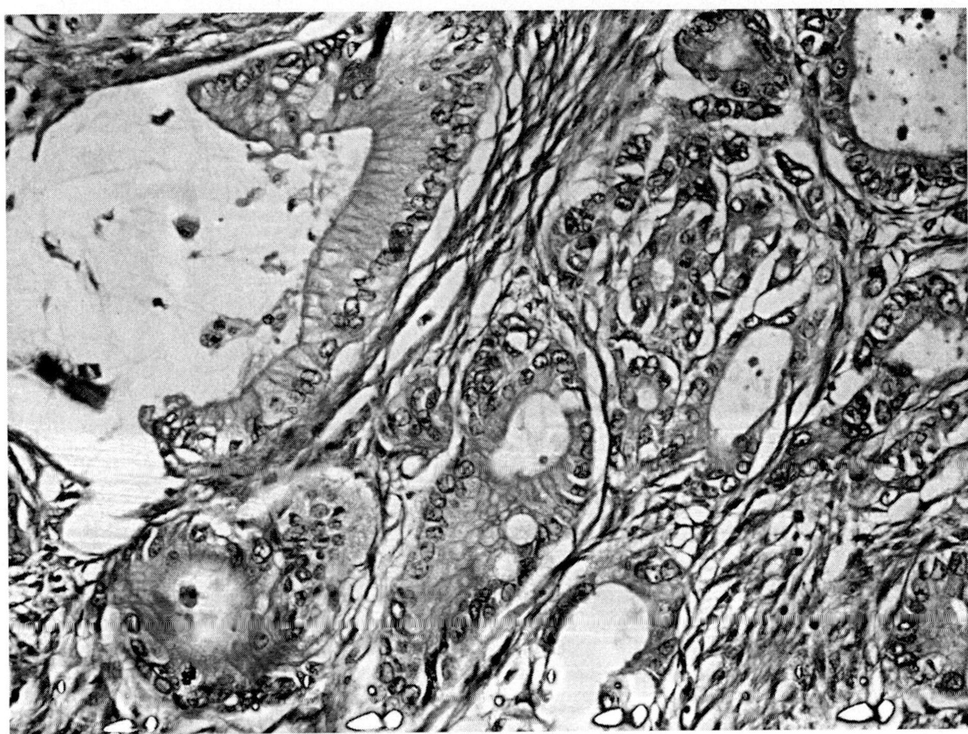

Figure 32.3 Mucinous adenocarcinoma of the ovary. Irregular glandular spaces are lined with a layer of tall columnar cells with abundant mucinous cytoplasm, resembling endocervical cells. The nuclei are mildly atypical. (From **Berek JS, Hacker NF.** *Practical gynecologic oncology,* 2nd ed. Baltimore: Williams & Wilkins, 1994:142, with permission.)

immediately adjacent to a poorly differentiated focus. Therefore, it is important to take multiple sections from many areas in the mucinous tumor to identify the most malignant alteration.

Malignant Mucinous Carcinomas **Bilateral tumors occur in 8% to 10% of cases.** The mucinous lesions are intraovarian in 95% to 98% of cases (Fig. 32.3). Because most ovarian mucinous carcinomas contain intestinal type cells, they cannot be distinguished from metastatic carcinoma of the gastrointestinal tract on the basis of histology alone. Primary ovarian neoplasms rarely metastasize to the mucosa of the bowel, although they commonly involve the serosa, whereas gastrointestinal lesions frequently involve the ovary by direct extension of vascular lymphatic spread.

Pseudomyxoma Peritonei In pseudomyxoma peritonei, the neoplastic epithelium secretes large amounts of gelatinous mucinous material. It is most commonly secondary to a well-differentiated appendiceal carcinoma, an ovarian mucinous carcinoma or, less commonly, a mucocele of the appendix.

Endometrioid Tumors

Endometrioid lesions constitute 6% to 8% of epithelial tumors. Endometrioid neoplasia includes all the benign demonstrations of endometriosis. In 1925, Sampson (13) suggested that certain cases of adenocarcinoma of the ovary probably arose in areas of endometriosis. The adenocarcinomas are similar to those seen in the uterine cavity. The malignant potential of endometriosis is very low, although a transition from benign to malignant epithelium may be demonstrated (Fig. 32.4).

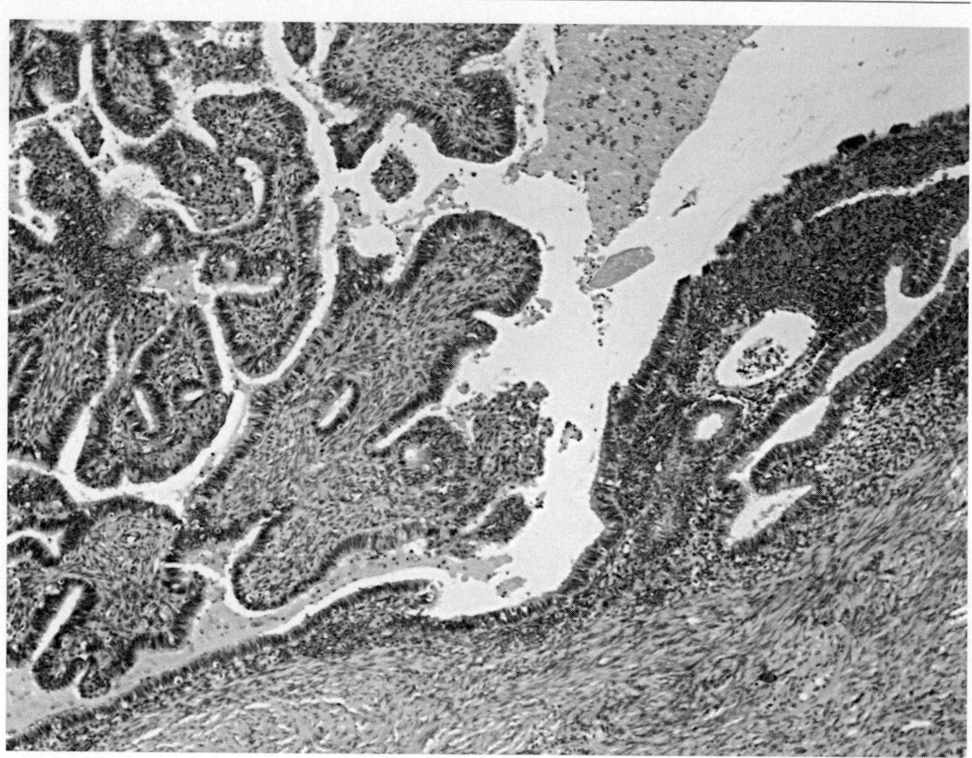

Figure 32.4 Endometrioid cancer arising in adjacent endometriosis. (From **Berek JS, Hacker NF.** *Practical gynecologic oncology,* 2nd ed. Baltimore: Williams & Wilkins, 1994:143, with permission.)

Borderline Endometrioid Tumors The endometrioid tumor of low malignant potential has a wide morphologic spectrum. Tumors may resemble an endometrial polyp or complex endometrial hyperplasia with crowding of glands. When there are back-to-back glands with no intervening stroma, the tumor is classified as a well-differentiated endometrioid carcinoma. Some borderline malignant tumors have a prominent fibromatous component. In such cases, the word *adenofibroma* is used.

Malignant Endometrioid Carcinomas Endometrioid tumors are characterized by an adenomatous pattern with all the potential variations of epithelia found in the uterus.

Multifocal Disease The *endometrial* or endometrioid tumors afford the greatest opportunity to evaluate multifocal disease. **Endometrioid tumors of the ovary are often associated with similar lesions in the endometrium.** Identification of multifocal disease is important, because patients with disease metastatic from the uterus to the ovaries have a 30% to 40% 5-year survival, whereas those with synchronous multifocal disease have a 75% to 80% 5-year survival (14). When the histologic appearance of endometrial and ovarian tumors is different, the two tumors most likely represent two separate primary lesions. When they appear similar, the endometrial tumor can be considered a separate primary tumor if it is well differentiated and only superficially invasive.

Clear Cell Carcinomas

Several basic histologic patterns are present in the clear cell adenocarcinoma (i.e., tubulocystic, papillary, and solid). The tumors are made up of clear cells and hobnail cells that project their nuclei to the apical cytoplasm. The tall clear cells have abundant clear or vacuolated cytoplasm, hyperchromatic irregular nuclei, and nucleoli of various sizes (Fig. 32.5). Focal areas of endometriosis and endometrioid carcinoma sometimes occur. The clear cell

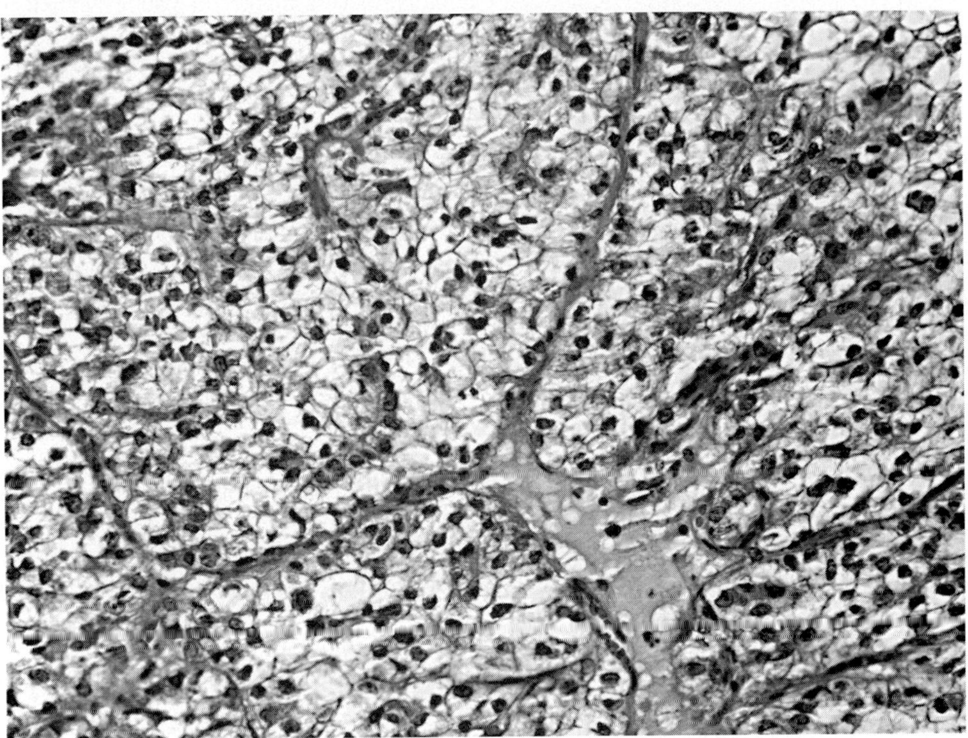

Figure 32.5 Clear cell mesonephroid carcinoma of the ovary. Note the solid variant of clear cell carcinoma with sheets of cells that have clear cytoplasm ("hobnail" cells). (From **Berek JS, Hacker NF.** *Practical gynecologic oncology,* 2nd ed. Baltimore: Williams & Wilkins, 1994:144, with permission.)

carcinoma seen in the ovary is histologically identical to that seen in the uterus or vagina of the young patient who has been exposed to diethylstilbestrol (DES) in utero.

Brenner Tumors

Borderline Brenner Tumors Borderline, or proliferating, Brenner tumors have been described. In such cases, the epithelium does not invade the stroma. Some investigators subclassify those tumors that resemble low-grade papillary transitional cell carcinoma of the urinary bladder as proliferating tumors and those with a higher grade of transitional cell carcinoma *in situ* as borderline malignant Brenner tumors (15). Complete surgical removal usually results in cure.

Malignant Brenner Tumors These are rare and are defined as benign Brenner tumors coexisting with invasive transitional cells or another type of carcinoma. The tumor infiltrates the tissue with associated destruction.

Transitional Cell Tumors

The designation *transitional cell tumor* refers to a primary ovarian carcinoma resembling transitional cell carcinoma of the urinary bladder without a recognizable Brenner tumor. An important finding is that those ovarian carcinomas that contain more than 50% of transitional cell carcinoma are more sensitive to chemotherapy and have a more favorable prognosis than other poorly differentiated ovarian carcinomas of comparable stage (16,17). Transitional cell tumors differ from malignant Brenner tumors in that they are more frequently diagnosed in an advanced stage and, therefore, are associated with a poorer survival rate (18).

Small cell carcinoma occurs mainly in young women, who may have symptoms of hypercalcemia. Immunohistochemical stains are helpful to differentiate this tumor from a lymphoma, leukemia, or sarcoma.

Peritoneal Carcinomas

Primary peritoneal tumors are histologically indistinguishable from primary ovarian serous tumors. In the case of borderline serous peritoneal tumors and serous peritoneal carcinomas, the ovaries are normal or minimally involved, and the tumors affect predominantly the uterosacral ligaments, pelvic peritoneum, or omentum. The overall prognosis for borderline serous peritoneal tumors is excellent and comparable to that of ovarian borderline serous tumors (21–23). In the review of 38 cases of peritoneal borderline serous tumors from the literature, 32 women had no persistent disease, four were well after resection of recurrence, one developed an invasive serous carcinoma, and one died from the effects of the tumor (21).

Peritoneal serous carcinomas have the appearance of a moderately to poorly differentiated serous ovarian carcinoma. Primary peritoneal endometrioid carcinoma is less common.

More than 80% of epithelial ovarian cancers are found in postmenopausal women (Fig. 32.6). These cancers are relatively uncommon in women under age 45.

Mesotheliomas

Peritoneal malignant mesotheliomas fall into the following four categories (19): (a) fibrosarcomatous, (b) tubulopapillary (papillary-alveolar), (c) carcinomatous, and (d) mixed. These lesions appear as multiple intraperitoneal masses and can develop after hysterectomy and bilateral salpingo-oophorectomy for benign disease. Malignant mesotheliomas

Figure 32.6 Ovarian cancer incidence: distribution by age. (From *J Natl Cancer Inst* 1995;87:1280, with permission.)

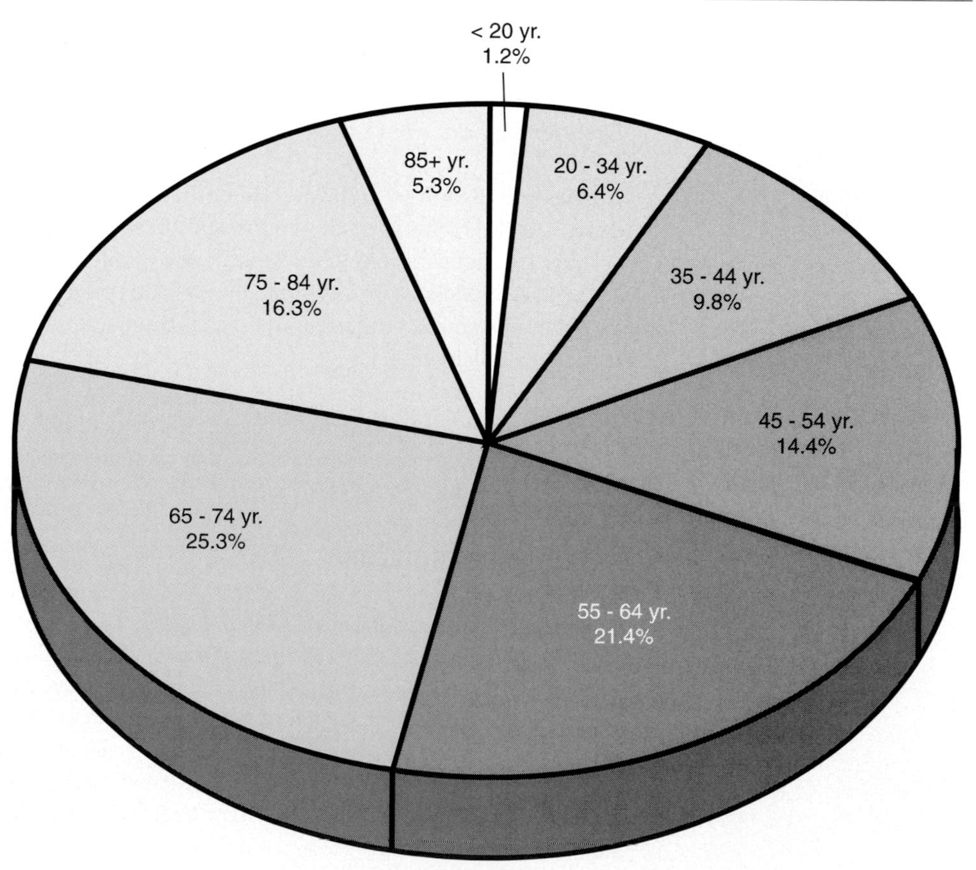

should be distinguished from ovarian tumor implants and primary peritoneal müllerian neoplasms.

The primary malignant transformation of the peritoneum has been called primary *peritoneal carcinoma* or *primary peritoneal papillary serous carcinoma.* Peritoneal carcinoma simulates ovarian cancer clinically. In patients for whom exploratory surgery is performed, there may be microscopic or small macroscopic cancer on the surface of the ovary and extensive disease in the upper abdomen, particularly in the omentum. This phenomenon can thus produce a condition in which so-called *ovarian cancer* can arise in a patient whose ovaries were surgically removed many years earlier (20).

Clinical Features

The peak incidence of invasive epithelial ovarian cancer is at 56 to 60 years of age (2,3,24). The age-specific incidence of ovarian epithelial cancer rises precipitously from 20 to 80 years of age and subsequently declines (24). Fewer than 1% of epithelial ovarian cancers occur before the age of 21 years, two-thirds of ovarian malignancies in such patients being germ cell tumors (2,24,25). About 30% of ovarian neoplasms in postmenopausal women are malignant, whereas only about 7% of ovarian epithelial tumors in premenopausal patients are frankly malignant (2,3).

The average age of patients with borderline tumors is approximately 46 years (2,3,5). Eighty to ninety percent of ovarian cancers, including borderline forms, occur after the age of 40 years, whereas 30% to 40% of malignancies occur after the age of 65 years. The chance that a primary epithelial tumor will be of borderline or invasive malignancy in a patient younger than 40 years is approximately 1 in 10, but after that age it rises to one in three (2,3). Fewer than 1% of epithelial ovarian cancers occur before the age of 20 years, with two thirds of ovarian malignancies in such patients being germ cell tumors. Approximately 30% of ovarian neoplasms in postmenopausal women are malignant, whereas only approximately 7% of ovarian epithelial tumors in premenopausal patients are frankly malignant (2).

Etiology

Ovarian cancer has been associated with low parity and infertility (26). Although there have been a variety of epidemiologic variables correlated with ovarian cancer, such as talc use, galactose consumption, and tubal ligation (see Chapter 4), none has been so strongly correlated as prior reproductive history and duration of the reproductive career (26,27). Early menarche and late menopause increase the risk of ovarian cancer (27). These factors and the relationship of parity and infertility to the risk of ovarian cancer have led to the hypothesis that suppression of ovulation may be an important factor. Theoretically, the surface epithelium undergoes repetitive disruption and repair. It is thought that this process might lead to a higher probability of spontaneous mutations that can unmask germline mutations or otherwise lead to the oncogenic phenotype (see Chapter 6).

Prevention

Because parity is inversely related to the risk of ovarian cancer, having at least one child is protective of the disease, with a risk reduction of 0.3 to 0.4. Oral contraceptive use reduces the risk of epithelial ovarian cancer (26). Women who use oral contraceptives for 5 or more years reduce their relative risk to 0.5 (i.e., there is a 50% reduction in the likelihood of development of ovarian cancer). Women who have had two children and have used oral contraceptives for 5 or more years have a relative risk of ovarian cancer as low as 0.3, or a 70% reduction (28). **Therefore, the oral contraceptive pill is the only documented method of chemoprevention for ovarian cancer, and it should be recommended to women for this purpose. When counseling patients regarding birth control options, this important benefit of oral contraceptive use should be emphasized. This is also important for women with a strong family history of ovarian cancer** (see discussion below).

Fenretinide (4-hydroxyretinoic acid), a vitamin A derivative, has been given to women with unilateral breast cancer in an effort to reduce the risk of contralateral breast cancer. In a prospective, randomized, placebo-controlled trial conducted in Italy (29), women with unilateral breast cancer were given for 6 months either fenretinide orally or a placebo. In the treatment group, no ovarian cancers developed, whereas there were six cases of ovarian cancer in the control group. A larger trial is planned in the United States in an attempt to verify these data.

The performance of a prophylactic oophorectomy reduces, but does not eliminate, the risk of ovarian cancer (20,21). Because the entire peritoneum is at risk, peritoneal carcinomas can occur even after prophylactic oophorectomy. Because the ovaries provide protection from cardiovascular and orthopedic diseases, prophylactic oophorectomy should not be routinely performed in premenopausal women at low risk for ovarian cancer.

Screening

The value of tumor markers and ultrasonography to screen for epithelial ovarian cancer has not been clearly established by prospective studies. Screening results with transabdominal ultrasonography have been encouraging (30–32), but specificity has been limited. However, advances in transvaginal ultrasonography have been shown to have a very high (>95%) sensitivity for the detection of early-stage ovarian cancer, although this test alone might require as many as 10 to 15 laparotomy procedures be performed for each case of ovarian cancer detected (30,31). Routine annual pelvic examinations have had disappointing results in the early detection of ovarian cancer (33). Transvaginal color-flow Doppler to assess the vascularity of the ovarian vessels has been shown to be a useful adjunct to ultrasonography (34,35), but it has not been shown to be useful in screening.

CA125 has been shown to contribute to the early diagnosis of epithelial ovarian cancer (36–42). Regarding the sensitivity of the test, CA125 can detect 50% of patients with stage I disease and 60% of patients if those with stage II disease are included (36). Data suggest that the specificity of CA125 is improved when the test is combined with transvaginal ultrasonography (43) or when the CA125 levels are followed over time (42,43). These data have encouraged the development of prospective screening studies in Sweden and the United Kingdom (38,39). In these studies, patients with elevated CA125 levels (>30 U/ml) have undergone abdominal ultrasonography and 14 ovarian cancers have been discovered among 27,000 women screened. About four laparotomies were performed for each case of cancer detected.

A randomized trial of nearly 22,000 women aged 45 years or older was performed in the United Kingdom (43). The patients were assigned to either a control group of routine pelvic examination (n = 10,977) or to a screening group (n = 10,958). The screening consisted of three annual screens that involved measurement of serum CA125, pelvic ultrasonography if the CA125 was 30 U/ml or higher, and referral for gynecologic examination if the ovarian volume was 8.8 ml or greater on the ultrasonography. Of the 468 women in the screened group with an elevated CA125, 29 were referred for surgery, 6 cancers were discovered, and 23 had false-positive screening results, yielding a positive predictive value of 20.7%. During a 7-year follow-up period, cancer developed in 10 additional women in the screened group, as it did in 20 women in the control group. Although the median survival of women in whom cancer developed in the screened group was 72.9 months, compared with 41.8 months in the control group ($p = 0.0112$), the number of deaths did not differ significantly between the control and screened groups [18/10,977 versus 9/10,958; relative risk 2.0 (0.78 to 5.13)]. Therefore, these data show that a multimodal approach to ovarian cancer screening is feasible, but a larger trial is necessary to determine whether this approach affects mortality. Such a three-arm randomized trial is ongoing in the United Kingdom, and the anticipated accrual is approximately 50,000 women per study arm and 100,000 women in the control arm.

Given the false-positive results for both CA125 and transvaginal ultrasonography, particularly in premenopausal women, these tests are not cost effective and should not be used routinely to screen for ovarian cancer. In the future, new markers or technologies may improve the specificity of ovarian cancer screening, but proof of this will require a large, prospective study (40,41). Screening in women who have a familial risk may have a better yield, but additional study is necessary (44,45).

Genetic Risk for Epithelial Ovarian Cancer

The lifetime risk of ovarian carcinoma for women in the United States is about 1.4% (1–3).

The risk of ovarian cancer is higher than that in the general population in women with certain family histories (46–55). **Most epithelial ovarian cancer is sporadic, with familial or hereditary patterns accounting for 5% to 10% of all malignancies** (47).

Hereditary Ovarian Cancer

BRCA1 and *BRCA2*

Most hereditary ovarian cancer is associated with mutations in the *BRCA1* gene, located on chromosome 17 (46). **A small proportion of inherited disease has been traced to another gene, *BRCA2*, located on chromosome 13** (48). Discovered through linkage analyses, these two genes are associated with the genetic predisposition to both ovarian and breast cancer. There may be other, yet undiscovered genes that predispose to ovarian and breast cancer (55).

In the past, it had been thought that there were two distinct syndromes associated with a genetic risk, *site-specific hereditary ovarian cancer and hereditary breast-ovarian cancer syndrome*. However, it is now believed that these groups essentially represent a continuum of mutations with different degrees of penetrance within a given family (50,55). In addition, there is a higher-than-expected risk of ovarian and endometrial cancer in the *Lynch II syndrome,* known also as the *hereditary nonpolyposis colorectal cancer syndrome (HNPCC syndrome)* (56).

The mutations are inherited in an autosomal dominant fashion, and therefore a full pedigree analysis (i.e., both maternal and paternal sides of the family) must be carefully evaluated (50). There are numerous distinct mutations that have been identified on each of these genes, and the mutations have different degrees of penetrance that may account for the preponderance of either breast cancer, ovarian cancer, or both, in any given family. **Based on analysis of women who have a mutation in the *BRCA1* gene and are from high-risk families, the lifetime risk of ovarian cancer may be as high as 28% to 44%, and the risk has been calculated to be as high as 27% for those women with a *BRCA2* mutation** (47,48,54). **The risk of breast cancer in women with a *BRCA1* or *BRCA2* mutation may be as high as 56% to 87%.**

Hereditary ovarian cancers in general occur in women approximately 10 years younger than those with nonhereditary tumors (47). Because the median age of epithelial ovarian cancer is in the mid- to late 50s, a woman with a first- or second-degree relative who had premenopausal ovarian cancer may have a higher probability of carrying an affected gene.

Breast and ovarian cancer may exist in a family in which there is a combination of epithelial ovarian and breast cancers, affecting a mixture of first- and second-degree relatives. Women with this syndrome tend to have these tumors at a young age, and the breast cancers may be bilateral. If two first-degree relatives are affected, this pedigree is consistent with an autosomal dominant mode of inheritance (43,46).

Founder Effect

There is a higher carrier rate of *BRCA1* and *BRCA2* mutations in women of Ashkenazi Jewish descent and in Icelandic women (52,53,55). There have been three specific mutations carried by the Ashkenazi population, 185delAG and 5382insC on *BRCA1,* and 6174delT on *BRCA2*. The total carrier rate for a patient of Ashkenazi Jewish descent to have at least one of these three mutations is 1 in 40, or 2.5%, and thus there is a substantial risk in this population. The increased risk is a result of the *founder effect,* in which a higher rate of mutations occurs in a defined geographic area.

Pedigree Analysis

The risk of ovarian cancer depends on the number of first- or second-degree relatives (or both) with a history of epithelial ovarian carcinoma or breast cancer (or both), and on the number of malignancies that occur at an earlier age. The degree of risk is difficult to determine precisely unless a full pedigree analysis is performed.

1. In families with two first-degree relatives (i.e., mother, sister, or daughter) with documented premenopausal epithelial ovarian cancer, the risk that a female first-degree relative has an affected gene could be as high as 35% to 40% (48).

2. In families with a single first-degree relative and a single second-degree relative (i.e., grandmother, aunt, first cousin, or granddaughter) with epithelial ovarian cancer, the risk that a woman has an affected gene also may be increased. The risk may be 2- to 10-fold higher than in those without a familial history of the disease (48).

3. In families with a single postmenopausal first-degree relative with epithelial ovarian carcinoma, a woman may not have an increased risk of having an affected gene because the case is most likely to be sporadic. However, if the ovarian cancer occurs in a premenopausal relative, this could be significant, and a full pedigree analysis should be undertaken.

4. Women with a primary history of breast cancer have twice the expected incidence of subsequent ovarian cancer (47).

Lynch II Syndrome

This syndrome, which includes multiple adenocarcinomas, involves a combination of familial colon cancer (known as the Lynch I syndrome), a high rate of ovarian, endometrial, and breast cancers, and other malignancies of the gastrointestinal and genitourinary systems (56). The mutations that have been associated with this syndrome are *MSH2, MLH1, PMS1,* and *PMS2.* The risk that a woman who is a member of one of these families will develop epithelial ovarian cancer depends on the frequency of this disease in first- and second-degree relatives, although these women appear to have at least 3 times the relative risk of the general population. A full pedigree analysis of such families should be performed by a geneticist to determine the risk more accurately.

Management of Women at High Risk for Ovarian Cancer

The management of a woman with a strong family history of epithelial ovarian cancer must be individualized and depends on her age, her reproductive plans, and the extent of risk. In all of these syndromes, women at risk benefit from a thorough pedigree analysis. A geneticist should evaluate the family pedigree for at least three generations. Decisions about management are best made after careful study and, whenever possible, verification of the histologic diagnosis of the family members' ovarian cancer.

The value of testing for *BRCA1* and *BRCA2* has yet to be clearly established, although some guidelines for testing now exist (50,55,57). The importance of genetic counseling cannot be overemphasized because the decision is complex. The American Society of Clinical Oncology has offered guidelines that emphasize careful evaluation by geneticists, careful maintenance of medical records, and a clear understanding in a genetic screening clinic of how to counsel and manage these patients. Concerns remain over how the information should be used, the impact on insurability, how the results will be interpreted, and how the information will be used within a specific family (e.g., to counsel children).

Although there are some conflicting data, the behavior of breast cancers arising in women with germline mutations in *BRCA1* or *BRCA2* is comparable to that of sporadic tumors (49). Women with breast cancer who carry these mutations, however, are at a greatly increased risk of ovarian cancer as well as a second breast cancer.

Although recommended by the National Institutes of Health Consensus Conference on Ovarian Cancer (58), the value of screening with transvaginal ultrasonography, CA125 levels, or other procedures has not been clearly established in women at high risk. Bourne and co-workers (45) have shown that, using this approach, tumors can be detected approximately 10 times more often than in the general population, and thus they recommend screening in high-risk women.

Data derived from a multicenter consortium of genetic screening centers indicate that the use of the oral contraceptive pill is associated with a lower risk for development of ovarian cancer in women who have a mutation in either *BRCA1* or *BRCA2* (59). The risk reduction is significant: in women who have taken oral contraceptives for 5 or more years, the relative risk of ovarian cancer is 0.4, or a 60% reduction in the incidence of the disease.

Prophylactic Oophorectomy

The value of prophylactic oophorectomy in these patients is controversial (60,61). Although the risk of ovarian cancer is significantly diminished, there remains the small risk of peritoneal carcinoma, a tumor for which women who have mutations in *BRCA1* and *BRCA2* may have a higher predisposition. Women at high risk for ovarian cancer who undergo prophylactic oophorectomy have a risk of harboring occult neoplasia. In one series of 42 such operations, four patients (9.5%) had a malignancy, one of which was noted at surgery and three that were microscopic; all were smaller than 5 mm (61).

Recommendations

Current recommendations for management of women at high risk for ovarian cancer are summarized as follows (57,58):

1. Women who appear to be at high risk for ovarian or breast cancer should undergo genetic counseling and, if the risk appears to be substantial, may be offered genetic testing for *BRCA1* and *BRCA2*.

2. Women who wish to preserve their reproductive capacity can undergo screening by transvaginal ultrasonography every 6 months, although the efficacy of this approach is not clearly established.

3. Oral contraceptives should be recommended to young women before they embark on an attempt to have a family.

4. Women who do not wish to maintain their fertility or who have completed their families may undergo prophylactic bilateral salpingo-oophorectomy. The risk should be clearly documented, preferably established by *BRCA1* and *BRCA2* testing, before oophorectomy is performed. These women should be counseled that this operation does not offer absolute protection, because peritoneal carcinomas occasionally can occur after bilateral oophorectomy (20,21).

5. In women who also have a strong family history of breast cancer, annual mammographic screening should be performed beginning at age 30 years.

6. Women with a documented HNPCC syndrome should undergo periodic screening mammography, colonoscopy, and endometrial biopsy (56).

Symptoms

Most women with epithelial ovarian cancer have no symptoms for long periods of time. When symptoms do develop, they are often vague and nonspecific (3). In early-stage disease, the patient may experience irregular menses if she is premenopausal. If a pelvic mass is compressing the bladder or rectum, she may report urinary frequency or constipation (62,63). Occasionally, she may perceive lower abdominal distention, pressure, or pain, such as dyspareunia. Acute symptoms, such as pain secondary to rupture or torsion, are unusual.

In advanced-stage disease, patients most often have symptoms related to the presence of ascites, omental metastases, or bowel metastases. The symptoms include abdominal distention, bloating, constipation, nausea, anorexia, or early satiety. Premenopausal women may complain of irregular or heavy menses, whereas vaginal bleeding may occur in postmenopausal women (64).

Signs

The most important sign of epithelial ovarian cancer is the presence of a pelvic mass on physical examination. A solid, irregular, fixed pelvic mass is highly suggestive of an ovarian malignancy. If, in addition, an upper abdominal mass or ascites is present, the diagnosis of ovarian cancer is almost certain. Because the patient usually complains of abdominal symptoms, she may not have a pelvic examination, and a tumor may be missed.

In patients who are at least 1 year past menopause, the ovaries should have become atrophic and not palpable. It has been proposed that any palpable pelvic mass in these patients should be considered potentially malignant, a situation that has been referred to as the postmenopausal palpable ovary syndrome (65). This concept has been challenged, because subsequent authors have reported that only about 3% of palpable masses measuring <5 cm in postmenopausal women are malignant (45).

Diagnosis

Ovarian epithelial cancers must be differentiated from benign neoplasms and functional cysts of the ovaries. A variety of benign conditions of the reproductive tract, such as pelvic inflammatory disease, endometriosis, and pedunculated uterine leiomyomas, can simulate ovarian cancer. Nongynecologic causes of a pelvic tumor, such as an inflammatory (e.g., diverticular) disease or neoplastic colonic mass, must be excluded (3). A pelvic kidney can simulate ovarian cancer.

Serum CA125 levels have been shown to be useful in distinguishing malignant from benign pelvic masses (66). For a postmenopausal patient with an adnexal mass and a very high serum CA125 level (>95 U/ml), there is a 96% positive predictive value for malignancy. For premenopausal patients, however, the specificity of the test is low because the CA125 level tends to be elevated in common benign conditions.

For the premenopausal patient, a period of observation is reasonable provided the adnexal mass does not have characteristics that suggest malignancy (i.e., it is mobile, mostly cystic, unilateral, and of regular contour). Generally, an interval of no more than 2 months is allowed, during which hormonal suppression with the oral contraceptive may be used. If the lesion is not neoplastic it should regress, as measured by pelvic examination and pelvic ultrasonography. If the mass does not regress or if it increases in size, it must be presumed to be neoplastic and must be removed surgically.

The size of the lesion is important. If a cystic mass is >8 cm in diameter, the probability is high that the lesion is neoplastic, unless the patient has been taking clomiphene citrate or other agents to induce ovulation (30–33). Patients whose lesions are suggestive of malignancy (i.e., predominantly solid, relatively fixed, or irregularly shaped) should undergo laparotomy, as should postmenopausal patients with adnexal masses.

The diagnosis of an ovarian cancer requires an exploratory laparotomy. Before the planned exploration, the patient should undergo routine hematologic and biochemical assessments. A preoperative evaluation in a patient undergoing laparotomy should include a radiograph of the chest and an assessment of the urinary tract with intravenous pyelography. Abdominal and pelvic computed tomography (CT) or magnetic resonance imaging (MRI) are of no value for a patient with a definite pelvic mass. A CT or MRI should be performed for patients with ascites and no pelvic mass to look for liver or pancreatic tumors. The findings only rarely preclude laparotomy (67). If the hepatic enzyme values are normal, the likelihood of liver disease is low. Liver-spleen scans, bone scans, and brain scans are unnecessary unless symptoms or signs suggest metastases to these sites.

The preoperative evaluation should exclude other primary cancers metastatic to the ovary. A barium enema or colonoscopy is indicated in some patients over 45 years of age to exclude a primary colonic lesion with ovarian metastasis. This study should be performed for any patient who has evidence of occult blood in the stool or of intestinal obstruction. An upper gastrointestinal radiographic series or gastroscopy is indicated if symptoms indicate gastric involvement (3,68). Bilateral mammography is indicated if there is any breast mass, because occasionally breast cancer metastatic to the ovaries can simulate primary ovarian cancer.

Cervical cytologic study should be performed, although its value for the detection of ovarian cancer is very limited. Patients who have irregular menses or postmenopausal vaginal bleeding should have endometrial biopsy and endocervical curettage to exclude the presence of uterine or endocervical cancer metastatic to the ovary.

Patterns of Spread

Ovarian epithelial cancers spread primarily by exfoliation of cells into the peritoneal cavity, by lymphatic dissemination, and by hematogenous spread.

Transcoelomic The most common and earliest mode of dissemination of ovarian epithelial cancer is by exfoliation of cells that implant along the surfaces of the peritoneal cavity. The cells tend to follow the circulatory path of the peritoneal fluid. The fluid tends to move with the forces of respiration from the pelvis, up the paracolic gutters, especially on the right, along the intestinal mesenteries, to the right hemidiaphragm. Therefore, metastases are typically seen on the posterior cul-de-sac, paracolic gutters, right hemidiaphragm, liver capsule, the peritoneal surfaces of the intestines and their mesenteries, and the omentum. The disease seldom invades the intestinal lumen but progressively agglutinates loops of bowel, leading to a functional intestinal obstruction. This condition is known as carcinomatous ileus (3).

Lymphatic Lymphatic dissemination to the pelvic and paraaortic lymph nodes is common, particularly in advanced-stage disease (69–71). Spread through the lymphatic channels of the diaphragm and through the retroperitoneal lymph nodes can lead to dissemination above the diaphragm, especially to the supraclavicular lymph nodes (69). Burghardt and others (71) reported that 78% of patients with stage III disease have metastases to the pelvic lymph nodes. In another series (70), the rate of paraaortic lymph nodes positive for metastasis was 18% in stage I, 20% in stage II, 42% in stage III, and 67% in stage IV.

Hematogenous Hematogenous dissemination at the time of diagnosis is uncommon. Spread to vital organ parenchyma, such as the lungs and liver, occurs in only about 2% to 3% of patients. Most patients with disease above the diaphragm when diagnosed have a right pleural effusion (3). Systemic metastases are seen more frequently in patients who have survived for some years. Dauplat and others (72) reported that distant metastasis consistent with stage IV disease ultimately occurred in 38% of the patients whose disease was originally intraperitoneal.

Prognostic Factors

The outcome of treatment can be evaluated in the context of prognostic factors, which can be grouped into pathologic, biologic, and clinical factors (73).

Pathologic Factors

The morphology and histologic pattern, including the architecture and grade of the lesion, are important prognostic variables (3). Histologic type has not generally been believed to be of prognostic significance, but several papers recently have contained suggestions that clear cell carcinomas are associated with a prognosis worse than that of other histologic types (73,74).

Histologic grade, as determined either by the pattern of differentiation or by the extent of cellular anaplasia and the proportion of undifferentiated cells, seems to be of prognostic significance (75–78). However, studies of the reproducibility of grading ovarian cancers have shown a high degree of intraobserver and interobserver variation (79,80). Because there is significant heterogeneity of tumors and observational bias, the value of histologic grade as an independent prognostic factor has not been clearly established. Baak and colleagues (81) have presented a standard grading system based on morphometric analysis, and the system seems to correlate with prognosis, especially in its ability to distinguish low-grade or borderline patterns from other tumors.

Biologic Factors

Several biologic factors have been correlated with prognosis in epithelial ovarian cancer. Using flow cytometry, Friedlander and co-workers (82) showed that ovarian cancers were commonly aneuploid. Furthermore, they and others showed that there was a high correlation between FIGO stage and ploidy; low-stage cancers tend to be diploid and high-stage tumors tend to be aneuploid (82–86). Patients with diploid tumors have a significantly longer median survival than those with aneuploid tumors: 5 years versus 1 year, respectively (82). Multivariate analyses have demonstrated that ploidy is an independent prognostic variable and one of the most significant predictors of survival (82). Flow cytometric analysis also provides data on the cell cycle, and the proliferation fraction (S phase) determined by this technique has correlated with prognosis in some studies (82–86).

More than 60 protooncogenes have been identified, and studies have focused on the amplification or expression of these genetic loci and their relationship to the development and progression of ovarian cancer (87,88). For example, Slamon and others (89) reported that 30% of epithelial ovarian tumors expressed HER-2/*neu* oncogene and that this group had a poorer prognosis, especially patients with more than five copies of the gene. Berchuck and associates (90) reported a similar incidence (32%) of HER-2/*neu* expression. In their series, patients whose tumors expressed the gene had a poorer median survival (15.7 months versus 32.8 months). Others have not substantiated this finding (92–95), and a review of the literature by Leary and others (92) revealed an overall incidence of HER-2/*neu* expression of only 11%. Thus, the prognostic value of HER-2/*neu* expression in ovarian cancer is unclear and further study is required.

The most commonly expressed tumor suppressor gene in ovarian cancer is *p53* (97–99). Indeed, as many as one-half of all epithelial ovarian cancers have evidence of mutated *p53* in the tumor.

The *in vitro* clonogenic assay has been studied in relation to ovarian cancer. A significant inverse correlation has been reported between clonogenic growth *in vitro* and survival (100–102). Multivariate analysis has found that clonogenic growth in a semisolid culture medium is a significant independent prognostic variable (102), but further study will be needed to evaluate the clinical usefulness of this essay.

Clinical Factors

In addition to stage, the extent of residual disease after primary surgery, the volume of ascites, patient age, and performance status are all independent prognostic variables

(103–111). Among patients with stage I disease, Dembo and co-workers (108) showed, in a multivariate analysis, that tumor grade and dense adherence to the pelvic peritoneum had a significant adverse impact on prognosis, whereas intraoperative tumor spillage or rupture did not. Sjövall and others (109) confirmed that **ovarian cancers that undergo intraoperative rupture or spillage do not worsen prognosis,** whereas tumors found to have already ruptured preoperatively do have a poorer prognosis. A multivariate analysis of these and several other studies was performed by Vergote (111), who found that **for early-stage disease, poor prognostic variables were tumor grade, capsular penetration, surface excrescences, and malignant ascites, but not iatrogenic rupture.**

Initial Surgery for Ovarian Cancer

Staging

Ovarian epithelial malignancies are staged according to the FIGO system listed in Table 32.2 (24). The FIGO staging is based on findings at surgical exploration. A preoperative evaluation should exclude the presence of extraperitoneal metastases.

The importance of thorough surgical staging cannot be overemphasized, because subsequent treatment will be determined by the stage of disease. For patients in whom exploratory laparotomy does not reveal any macroscopic evidence of disease on inspection and palpation of the entire intraabdominal space, a careful search for microscopic spread must be undertaken. In earlier series in which patients did not undergo careful surgical staging, the overall 5-year survival for patients with apparent stage I epithelial ovarian cancer was only about 60% (112). Since then, survival rates of 90% to 100% have been reported for patients who were properly staged and were found to have stage Ia or Ib disease (113,114).

Technique for Surgical Staging

For patients whose preoperative evaluation suggests a probable malignancy, a midline or paramedian abdominal incision is recommended to allow adequate access to the upper abdomen (3). When a malignancy is unexpectedly discovered in a patient who has a lower transverse incision, the rectus muscles can be either divided or detached from the symphysis pubis to allow better access to the upper abdomen. If this is not sufficient, the incision can be extended on one side to create a "J" incision (3).

The ovarian tumor should be removed intact, if possible, and a frozen histologic section should be obtained. If ovarian malignancy is present and the tumor is apparently confined to the ovaries or the pelvis, thorough surgical staging should be performed. Staging involves the following steps (3):

1. **Any free fluid, especially in the pelvic cul-de-sac, should be submitted for cytologic evaluation.**

2. **If no free fluid is present, peritoneal washings should be performed by instilling and recovering 50 to 100 ml of saline from the pelvic cul-de-sac, each paracolic gutter, and beneath each hemidiaphragm.** Obtaining the specimens from under the diaphragms can be facilitated with the use of a rubber catheter attached to the end of a bulb syringe.

3. **A systematic exploration of all the intraabdominal surfaces and viscera is performed,** proceeding in a clockwise fashion from the cecum cephalad along the paracolic gutter and the ascending colon to the right kidney, the liver and gallbladder, the right hemidiaphragm, the entrance to the lesser sac at the paraaortic area, across the transverse colon to the left hemidiaphragm, down the left gutter and the descending colon to the rectosigmoid colon. The small intestine and its mesentery from the Treitz ligament to the cecum should be inspected.

Table 32.2. FIGO Staging for Primary Carcinoma of the Ovary

Stage I	Growth limited to the ovaries.	
	Stage Ia	Growth limited to one ovary; no ascites containing malignant cells. No tumor on the external surface; capsule intact.
	Stage Ib	Growth limited to both ovaries; no ascites containing malignant cells. No tumor on the external surfaces; capsules intact.
	Stage Ic[a]	Tumor either stage Ia or Ib but with tumor on the surface of one or both ovaries; or with capsule ruptured; or with ascites present containing malignant cells or with positive peritoneal washings.
Stage II	Growth involving one or both ovaries with pelvic extension.	
	Stage IIa	Extension and/or metastases to the uterus and/or fallopian tubes.
	Stage IIb	Extension to other pelvic tissues.
	Stage IIc[a]	Tumor either stage IIa or IIb but with tumor on the surface of one or both ovaries; or with capsule(s) ruptured; or with ascites present containing malignant cells or with positive peritoneal washings.
Stage III	Tumor involving one or both ovaries with peritoneal implants outside the pelvis and/or positive retroperitoneal or inguinal nodes. Superficial liver metastasis equals stage III. Tumor is limited to the true pelvis, but with histologically proven malignant extension to small bowel or omentum.	
	Stage IIIa	Tumor grossly limited to the true pelvis with negative nodes but with histologically confirmed microscopic seeding of abdominal peritoneal surfaces.
	Stage IIIb	Tumor of one or both ovaries with histologically confirmed implants of abdominal peritoneal surfaces, none exceeding 2 cm in diameter. Nodes negative.
	Stage IIIc	Abdominal implants >2 cm in diameter or positive retroperitoneal or inguinal nodes or both.
Stage IV	Growth involving one or both ovaries with distant metastasis. If pleural effusion is present, there must be positive cytologic test results to allot a case to stage IV. Parenchymal liver metastasis equals stage IV.	

These categories are based on findings at clinical examination or surgical exploration or both. The histologic characteristics are to be considered in the staging, as are results of cytologic testing as far as effusions are concerned. It is desirable that a biopsy be performed on suspicious areas outside the pelvis.
[a] In order to evaluate the impact on prognosis of the different criteria for allotting cases to stage Ic or IIc, it would be of value to know if rupture of the capsule was (a) spontaneous or (b) caused by the surgeon and if the source of malignant cells detected was (a) peritoneal washings or (b) ascites.

4. **Any suspicious areas or adhesions on the peritoneal surfaces should be sampled for biopsy.** If there is no evidence of disease, multiple intraperitoneal biopsies should be performed. Tissue from the peritoneum of the pelvic cul-de-sac, both paracolic gutters, the peritoneum over the bladder, and the intestinal mesenteries should be taken for biopsy.

5. **The diaphragm should be sampled either by biopsy or by scraping with a tongue depressor and obtaining a sample for cytologic assessment.** Biopsies of any irregularities on the surface of the diaphragm can be facilitated by use of the laparoscope and the associated biopsy instrument.

6. **The omentum should be resected from the transverse colon, a procedure called an *infracolic omentectomy*.** The procedure is initiated on the underside of the greater omentum, where the peritoneum is incised just a few millimeters

away from the transverse colon. The branches of the gastroepiploic vessels are clamped, ligated, and divided, along with all the small branching vessels that feed the infracolic omentum. If the gastrocolic ligament is palpably normal, it does not need to be resected.

7. **The retroperitoneal spaces should be explored to evaluate the pelvic and paraaortic lymph nodes.** The retroperitoneal dissection is performed by incision of the peritoneum over the psoas muscles. This may be performed on the ipsilateral side only for unilateral tumors. Any enlarged lymph nodes should be resected and submitted for frozen section. If no metastases are present, a formal pelvic lymphadenectomy should be performed.

Results

Metastases in apparent stage I and II epithelial ovarian cancer occur in as many as 3 in 10 patients whose tumors appear to be confined to the pelvis but who have occult metastatic disease in the upper abdomen or the retroperitoneal lymph nodes (70,113–123). In a review of the literature (112), occult metastases were found in biopsies of the diaphragm in 7.3% of such patients, biopsies of the omentum in 8.6%, the pelvic lymph nodes in 5.9%, the aortic lymph nodes in 18.1%, and in 26.4% of peritoneal washings.

The importance of careful initial surgical staging is emphasized by the findings of a cooperative national study (113) in which 100 patients with apparent stage I and II disease who were referred for subsequent therapy underwent additional surgical staging. In this series, 28% of the patients initially believed to have stage I disease were "upstaged" and 43% of those believed to have stage II disease had more advanced lesions. A total of 31% of the patients were upstaged as a result of additional surgery, and 77% were reclassified as having stage III disease. Histologic grade was a significant predictor of occult metastasis. Sixteen percent of the patients with grade 1 lesions were upstaged, compared with 34% with grade 2 disease and 46% with grade 3 disease.

Stage I

The primary surgical treatment for stage I epithelial ovarian cancer is surgical, and patients should undergo total abdominal hysterectomy, bilateral salpingo-oophorectomy, and surgical staging (112,113). In certain circumstances, a unilateral oophorectomy may be performed. Based on the findings at surgery and the pathologic evaluation, patients with stage I ovarian cancer can be grouped into low-risk and high-risk categories (Table 32.3).

Table 32.3. Prognostic Variables in Early-stage Epithelial Ovarian Cancer

Low Risk	*High Risk*
Low grade	High grade
Non–clear cell histologic type	Clear cell histologic type
Intact capsule	Tumor growth through capsule
No surface excrecenses	Surface excrescences
No ascites	Ascites
Negative peritoneal cytologic findings	Malignant cells in fluid
Unruptured or intraoperative rupture	Preoperative rupture
No dense adherence	Dense adherence
Diploid tumor	Aneuploid tumor

From **Berek JS, Hacker NF,** eds. *Practical gynecologic oncology,* 3rd ed. Philadelphia: Lippincott Williams & Wilkins, 2000:472, with permission.

Borderline Tumors

The principal treatment of borderline ovarian tumors is surgical resection of the primary tumor. There is no evidence that either subsequent chemotherapy or radiation therapy improves survival. After a frozen section has determined that the histology is borderline, premenopausal patients who desire preservation of ovarian function may undergo a conservative operation, a unilateral oophorectomy (3,123,124). In a study of patients who underwent unilateral ovarian cystectomy only for apparent stage I borderline serous tumors, Lim-Tan and associates (124) found that this conservative operation was also safe; only 8% of the patients had recurrences 2 to 18 years later, all with curable disease confined to the ovaries. Recurrence was associated with positive margins of the removed ovarian cyst (124). Thus, hormonal function and fertility can be maintained (3,123,124). For patients in whom an oophorectomy or cystectomy has been performed and a borderline tumor is later documented in the permanent pathology, no additional immediate surgery is necessary.

Stage I Low-grade, Low-risk

For patients who have undergone a thorough staging laparotomy and for whom there is no evidence of spread beyond the ovary, abdominal hysterectomy and bilateral salpingo-oophorectomy are appropriate therapy. The uterus and the contralateral ovary can be preserved in women with stage Ia, grade 1 to 2 disease who desire to preserve fertility. The conditions of the women should be monitored carefully with routine periodic pelvic examinations and determinations of serum CA125 levels. Generally, the other ovary and the uterus are removed at the completion of childbearing.

Guthrie and others (122) studied the outcome of 656 patients with early-stage epithelial ovarian cancer. No untreated patients who had stage Ia, grade 1 cancer died of their disease; thus, adjuvant radiation and chemotherapy are unnecessary. Furthermore, the Gynecologic Oncology Group (GOG) carried out a prospective, randomized trial of observation versus melphalan for patients with stage Ia and Ib, grade 1 disease (74). Five-year survival for each group was 94% and 96%, respectively, confirming that no further treatment is needed for such patients.

Stage I High-grade, High-risk

For patients whose disease is more poorly differentiated or in whom there are malignant cells either in ascitic fluid or in peritoneal washings, complete surgical staging must be performed (3). The surgery should include the performance of a hysterectomy and bilateral salpingo-oophorectomy in addition to the staging laparotomy (3). Additional therapy is indicated, and although the optimal therapy for these patients is not known, most patients are treated with chemotherapy, as outlined below.

Cytoreductive Surgery for Advanced-stage Disease

Patients with advanced-stage epithelial ovarian cancer documented at initial exploratory laparotomy should undergo cytoreductive surgery to remove as much of the tumor and its metastases as possible (125–145) (Fig 32.7). The operation to remove the primary tumor as well as the associated metastatic disease is referred to as *debulking* surgery. The operation typically includes the performance of a total abdominal hysterectomy and bilateral salpingo-oophorectomy, along with a complete omentectomy and resection of any metastatic lesions from the peritoneal surfaces or from the intestines. The pelvic tumor often directly involves the rectosigmoid colon, the terminal ileum, and the cecum (Fig. 32.8). In a minority of

Figure 32.7 Treatment scheme for patients with advanced-stage ovarian cancer. (*under selected circumstances or clinical trials). (From **Berek JS, Hacker NF.** *Practical gynecologic oncology,* 3rd ed. Philadelphia: Lippincott Williams & Wilkins, 2000:474, with permission.)

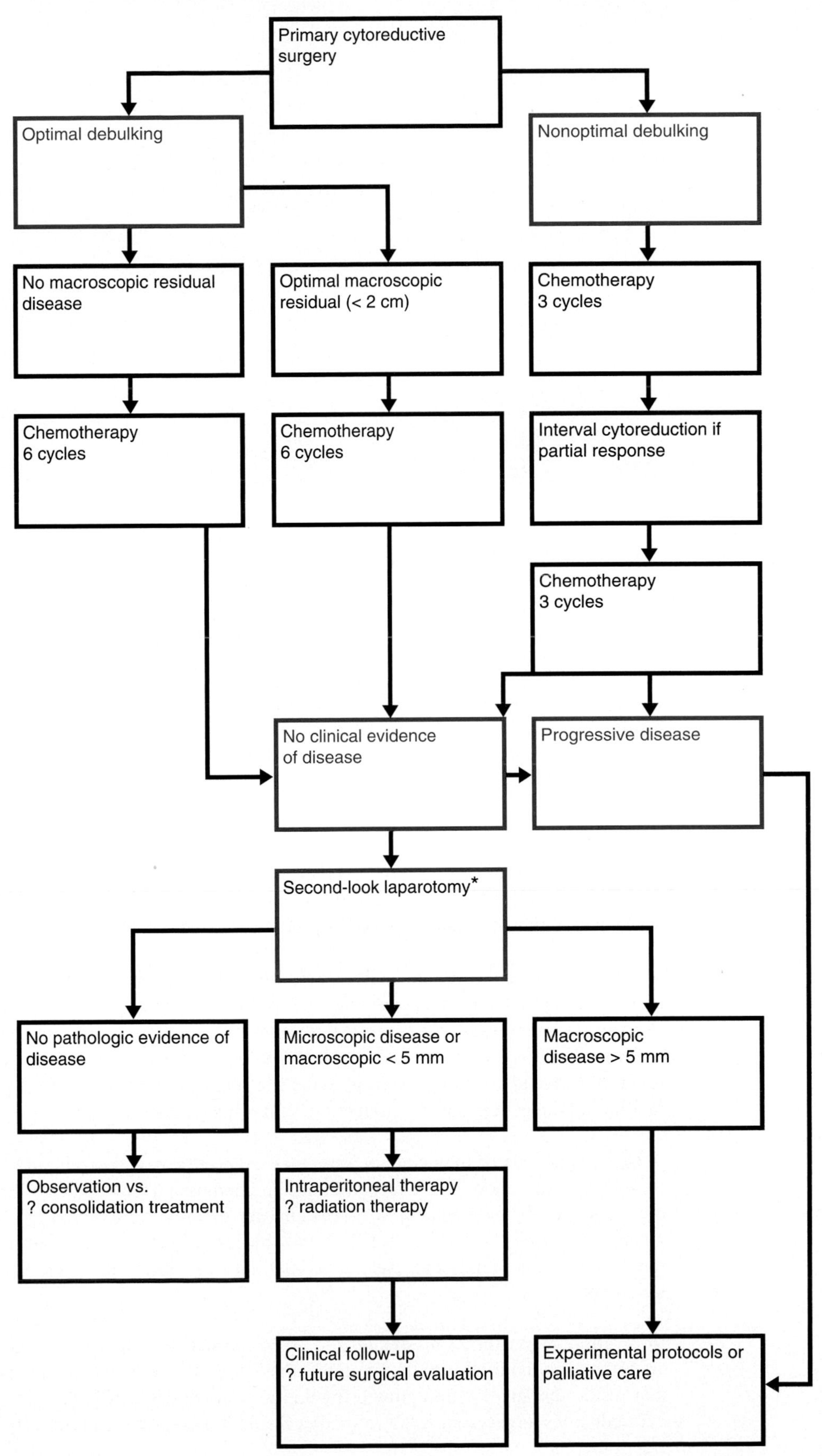
Primary cytoreductive surgery
Optimal debulking
Nonoptimal debulking
No macroscopic residual disease
Optimal macroscopic residual (< 2 cm)
Chemotherapy 3 cycles
Chemotherapy 6 cycles
Chemotherapy 6 cycles
Interval cytoreduction if partial response
Chemotherapy 3 cycles
No clinical evidence of disease
Progressive disease
Second-look laparotomy*
No pathologic evidence of disease
Microscopic disease or macroscopic < 5 mm
Macroscopic disease > 5 mm
Observation vs. ? consolidation treatment
Intraperitoneal therapy ? radiation therapy
Clinical follow-up ? future surgical evaluation
Experimental protocols or palliative care

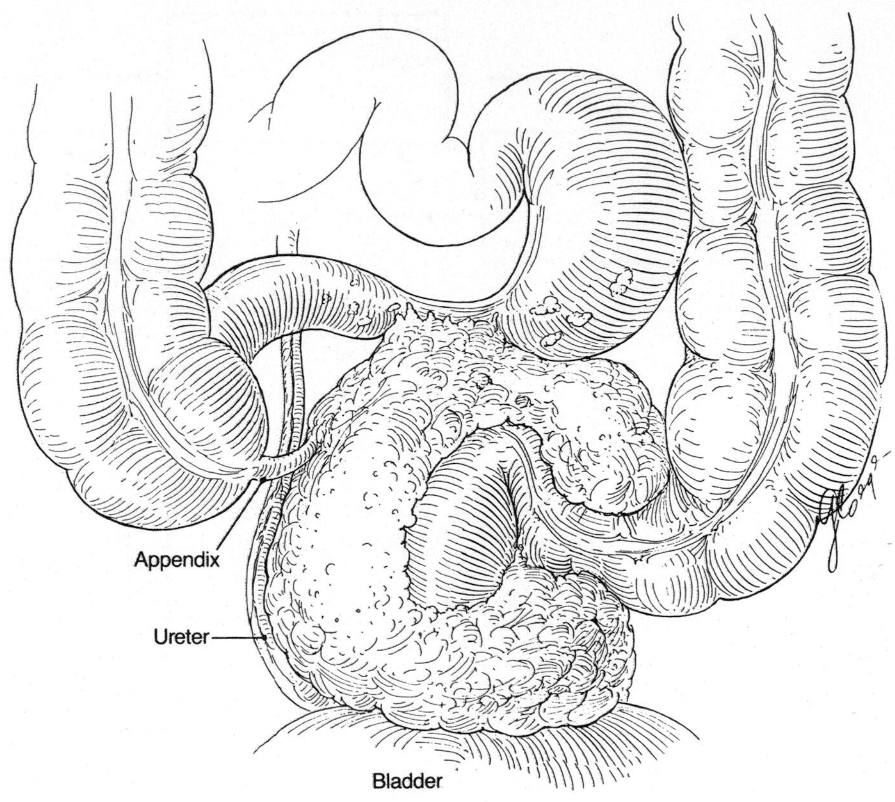

Figure 32.8 Extensive ovarian carcinoma involving the bladder, rectosigmoid, and ileocecal area. (From **Heintz APM, Berek JS.** Cytoreductive surgery for ovarian carcinoma. In: **Piver MS,** ed. *Ovarian malignancies.* Edinburgh: Churchill Livingstone, 1987:134, with permission.)

patients, most or all of the disease is confined to the pelvic viscera and the omentum, so that removal of these organs will result in extirpation of all gross tumor, a situation that is associated with a reasonable chance of prolonged progression-free survival.

The removal of bulky tumor masses may reduce the volume of ascites present. Often, ascites will completely disappear after removal of the primary tumor and a large omental "cake." Also, removal of the omental cake often alleviates the nausea and early satiety that many patients experience. Removal of intestinal metastases may restore adequate intestinal function and lead to an improvement in the overall nutritional status of the patient, thereby facilitating the patient's ability to tolerate subsequent chemotherapy.

A large, bulky tumor may contain areas that are poorly vascularized, and such areas will be exposed to suboptimal concentrations of chemotherapeutic agents. Similarly, these areas are poorly oxygenated, so that radiation therapy, which requires adequate oxygenation to achieve maximal cell kill, will be less effective. Thus, surgical removal of these bulky tumors may eliminate areas that are most likely to be relatively resistant to treatment.

In addition, larger tumor masses tend to be composed of a higher proportion of cells that are either nondividing or in the "resting" phase (i.e., G_0 cells, which are essentially resistant to the therapy). A low growth fraction is characteristic of bulky tumor masses, and cytoreductive surgery can result in smaller residual masses with a relatively higher growth fraction.

Goals of Cytoreductive Surgery

The principal goal of cytoreductive surgery is removal of all of the primary cancer and, if possible, all metastatic disease. If resection of all metastases is not feasible, the goal is to reduce the tumor burden by resection of all individual tumors to an optimal status. Griffiths (125) initially proposed that all metastatic nodules should be reduced to <1.5 cm in maximal diameter and showed that survival was significantly longer in patients for whom this was achieved.

Subsequently, Hacker and Berek (126–128) showed that patients whose largest residual lesions were <5 mm had a superior survival rate, which was substantiated by Van Lindert and co-workers (129). The median survival of patients in this category was 40 months, compared with 18 months for patients whose lesions were <1.5 cm and 6 months for patients with nodules >1.5 cm. Patients whose disease has been completely resected to no macroscopic residual disease have the best overall survival (Fig. 32.9).

The resectability of the metastatic tumor is usually determined by the location of the disease. Optimal cytoreduction is difficult to achieve in the presence of extensive disease on the diaphragm, in the parenchyma of the liver, along the base of the small-bowel mesentery, in the lesser omentum, or in the porta hepatis.

The ability of cytoreductive surgery to influence survival is limited by the extent of metastases before cytoreduction, presumably because of the presence of phenotypically resistant clones of cells in large metastatic masses. A patient whose metastatic tumor is very large (i.e., >10 cm before cytoreductive surgery) has a shorter survival than those with smaller areas of disease (128). Extensive carcinomatosis, the presence of ascites, poor tumor grade, even with lesions that measure <5 mm, may also shorten the survival (131).

Figure 32.9 Survival of patients with stage IIIc epithelial ovarian cancer based on the maximal size of residual tumor after exploratory laparotomy and tumor resection. (From **Pecoreeli S, Odicino F, Maisonneuve P, et al.** Carcinoma of the ovary. Annual Report of the Results of Treatment of Gynaecological Cancer. *J Epidemiol Biostat* 1998;3:75–102, with permission.)

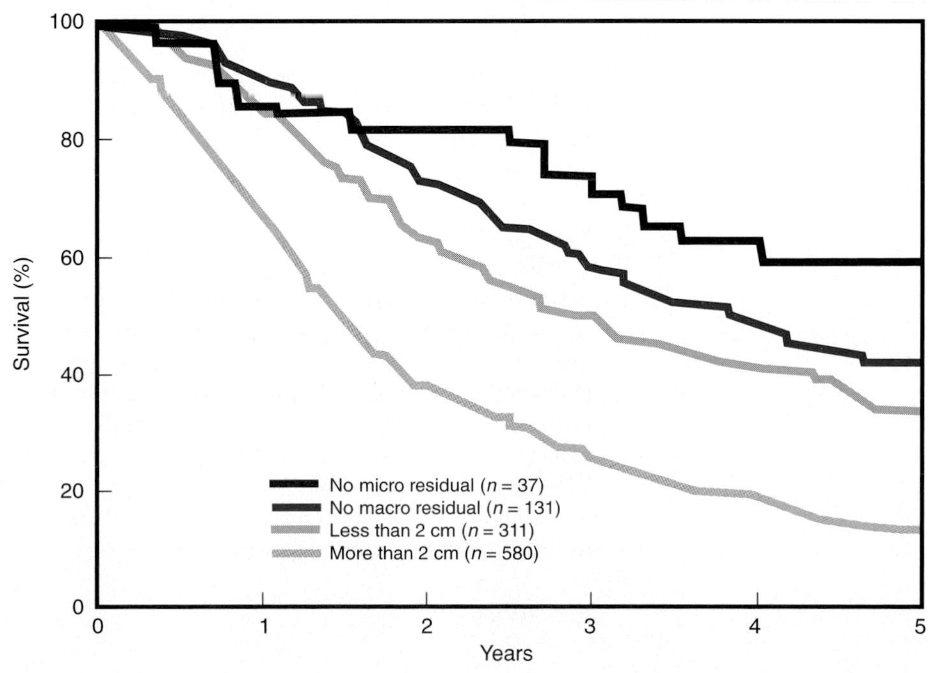

Exploration

The supine position on the operating table may be sufficient for surgical exploration of most patients. However, for those with extensive pelvic disease for whom a low resection of the colon may be necessary, the low lithotomy position should be used. Debulking operations should be performed through a vertical incision to gain adequate access to the upper abdomen as well as to the pelvis.

After the peritoneal cavity is opened, ascitic fluid, if present, should be evacuated. In some centers, fluid is submitted routinely for appropriate *in vitro* research studies, such as molecular analyses. In cases of massive ascites, careful attention must be given to hemodynamic monitoring, especially for patients with borderline cardiovascular function.

The peritoneal cavity and retroperitoneum are thoroughly inspected and palpated to assess the extent of the primary tumor and the metastatic disease. All abdominal viscera must be palpated to exclude the possibility that the ovarian disease is metastatic, particularly from the stomach, colon, or pancreas. If optimal status is not considered achievable, extensive bowel and urologic resections are not indicated, except to overcome a bowel obstruction. However, removal of the primary tumor and omental cake is usually both feasible and desirable.

Pelvic Tumor Resection

The essential principle of removal of the pelvic tumor is to use the retroperitoneal approach. To accomplish this, the retroperitoneum is entered laterally, along the surface of the psoas muscles, which avoids the iliac vessels and the ureters. The procedure is initiated by division of the round ligaments bilaterally if the uterus is present. The peritoneal incision is extended cephalad, lateral to the ovarian vessels within the infundibulopelvic ligament, and caudally toward the bladder. With careful dissection, the retroperitoneal space is explored, and the ureter and pelvic vessels are identified. The pararectal and paravesicular spaces are identified and developed as described in Chapter 31.

The peritoneum overlying the bladder is dissected to connect the peritoneal incisions anteriorly. The vesicouterine plane is identified, and with careful sharp dissection the bladder is mobilized from the anterior surface of the cervix. The ovarian vessels are isolated, doubly ligated, and divided.

Hysterectomy, which is often not a simple operation, is then performed. The ureters must be carefully displayed to avoid injury. During this procedure, the uterine vessels can be identified. The hysterectomy and resection of the contiguous tumor are completed by ligation of the uterine vessels and the remainder of the tissues within the cardinal ligaments.

Because epithelial ovarian cancers tend not to invade the lumina of the colon or bladder, it is usually feasible to resect pelvic tumors without having to resect portions of the lower colon or the urinary tract (137,138). However, if the disease surrounds the rectosigmoid colon and its mesentery, it may be necessary to remove that portion of the colon to clear the pelvic disease (Fig. 32.10) (137). This is justified if the patient will be left with optimal disease at the end of the cytoreduction. After the pararectal space is identified in such patients, the proximal site of colonic involvement is identified, the colon and its mesentery are divided, and the rectosigmoid is removed along with the uterus *en bloc*. A reanastomosis of the colon is performed. It is rarely necessary to resect portions of the lower urinary tract. Resection of a small portion of the bladder may be required and, if so, a cystotomy should be performed to assist in resection of the disease (138).

Omentectomy

Advanced epithelial ovarian cancer often completely replaces the omentum, forming an omental cake. This disease may be adherent to the parietal peritoneum of the anterior

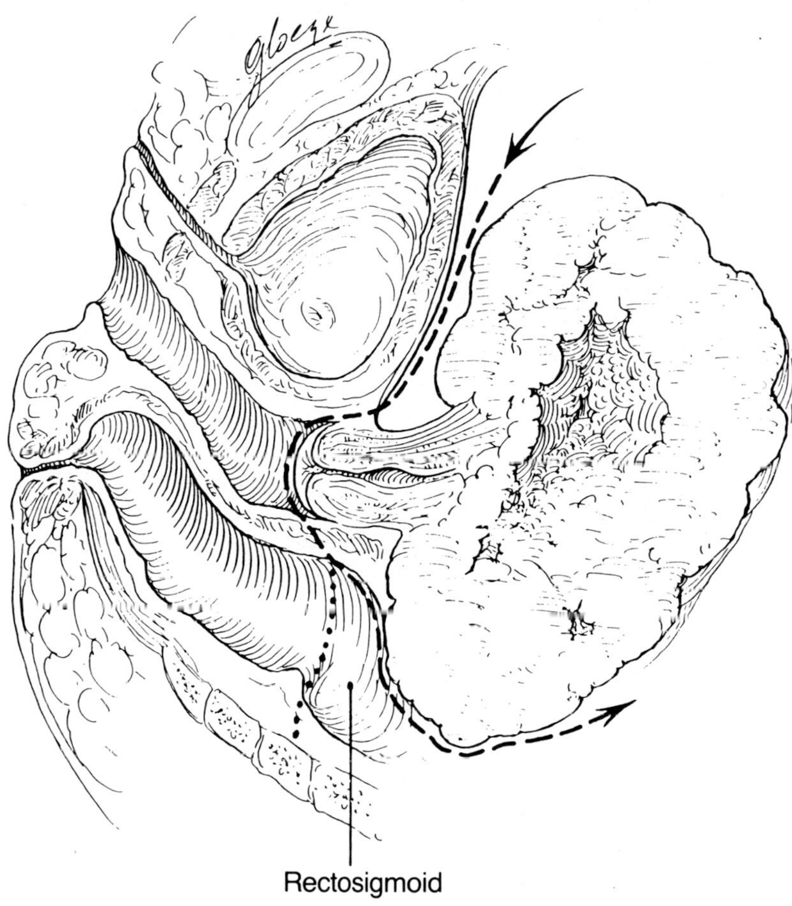

Figure 32.10 The resection of the pelvic tumor may include removal of the uterus, tubes, and ovaries, as well as portions of the lower intestinal tract. The *arrows* represent the plane of resection. (From **Berek JS, Hacker NF.** *Practical gynecologic oncology,* 3rd ed. Philadelphia: Lippincott Williams & Wilkins, 2000:480, with permission.)

abdominal wall, making entry into the abdominal cavity difficult. After freeing the omentum from any adhesions to parietal peritoneum, adherent loops of small intestine are freed by sharp dissection. The omentum is then lifted and pulled gently in the cranial direction, exposing the attachment of the infracolic omentum to the transverse colon. The peritoneum is incised to open the appropriate plane, which is developed by sharp dissection along the serosa of the transverse colon. Small vessels are ligated with hemoclips. The omentum is then separated from the greater curvature of the stomach by ligation of the right and left gastroepiploic arteries and ligation of the short gastric arteries (Fig. 32.11).

The disease in the gastrocolic ligament can extend to the hilus of the spleen and splenic flexure of the colon on the left and to the capsule of the liver and the hepatic flexure of the colon on the right. Usually, the disease does not invade the parenchyma of the liver or spleen, and a plane can be found between the tumor and these organs. However, it will occasionally be necessary to perform splenectomy to remove all the omental disease (139).

Intestinal Resection

The disease may involve focal areas of the small or large intestine, and resection should be performed if it would permit the removal of all or most of the abdominal metastases. Apart

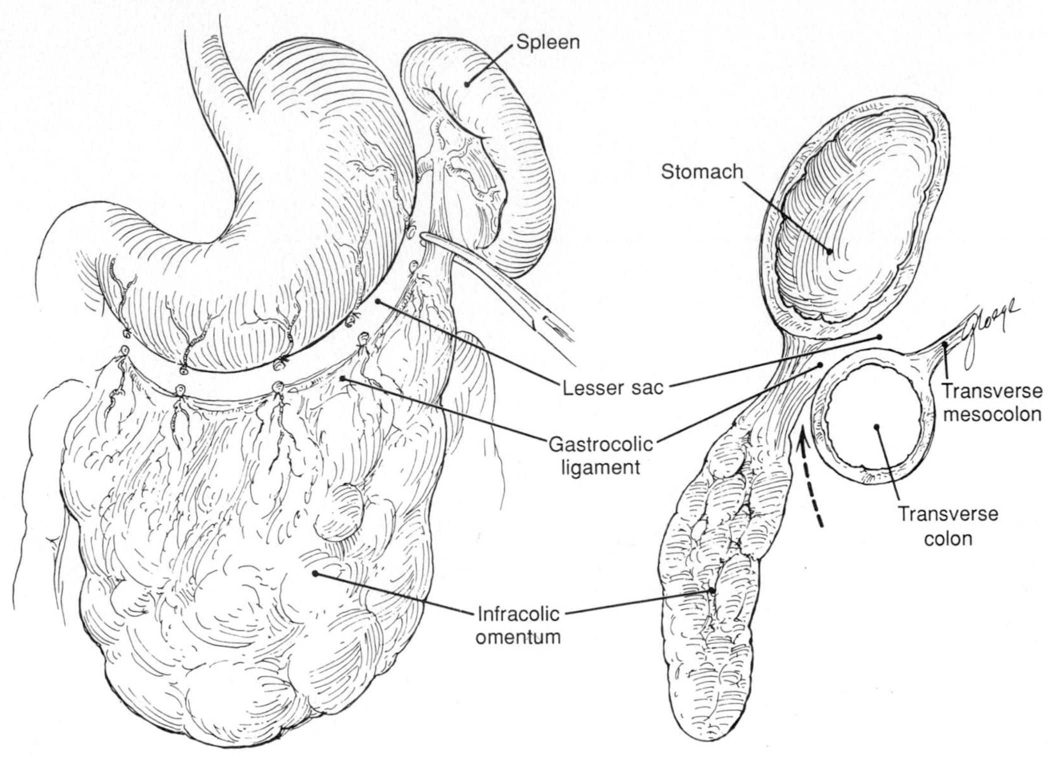

Figure 32.11 Separation of the omentum from stomach and transverse colon. (From **Heintz APM, Berek JS.** Cytoreductive surgery for ovarian carcinoma. In: **Piver MS,** ed. *Ovarian malignancies.* Edinburgh: Churchill Livingstone, 1987:134, with permission.)

from the rectosigmoid colon, the most frequent sites of intestinal metastasis are the terminal ileum, the cecum, and the transverse colon. Resection of one or more of these segments of bowel may be necessary (137,139).

Resection of Other Metastases

Other large masses of tumor that are located on the parietal peritoneum should be removed, particularly if they are isolated masses and their removal will permit optimal cytoreduction. Resection of extensive disease from the surfaces of the diaphragm is generally neither practical nor feasible, although solitary metastases may be resected, the diaphragm sutured, and a chest tube placed for a few days (140,141). The use of the Cavitron Ultrasonic Surgical Aspirator (CUSA) and the argon beam coagulator may help facilitate resection of small tumor nodules, especially those on flat surfaces (142,143).

Feasibility and Outcome

Although no randomized prospective study has ever been performed to define the value of primary cytoreductive surgery, a prospective trial of *interval* cytoreductive surgery (performed after three cycles of platinum combination chemotherapy) demonstrated a survival benefit for patients who had optimal resection of their disease at that time compared with those who did not (135). All retrospective studies indicate that the diameter of the largest residual tumor nodule before the initiation of chemotherapy is significantly related to progression-free survival in patients with advanced ovarian cancer. In addition, quality of life is likely to be significantly enhanced by removal of bulky tumor masses from the pelvis and upper abdomen (136).

An analysis of the retrospective data available suggests that these operations are feasible for 70% to 90% of patients when performed by gynecologic oncologists (133,139,144). Major morbidity is in the range of 5% and operative mortality is in the range of 1% (139,145). Intestinal resection in these patients does not appear to increase the overall morbidity caused by the operation (137,139). The performance of a pelvic lymphadenectomy in patients with stage III disease has been reported to prolong survival (71), although verification of this awaits a prospective, randomized study.

Treatment with Chemotherapy

Stage I Epithelial Ovarian Cancer

Stage I Low-grade, Low-risk

Guthrie and others (122) studied the outcome of 656 patients with early-stage epithelial ovarian cancer. No patients who had stage Ia, grade 1 cancer who did not receive radiation or chemotherapy died of their disease; thus adjuvant therapy is unnecessary. Furthermore, the GOG carried out a prospective, randomized trial of observation versus *melphalan* for patients with stage Ia and Ib, grade 1 disease (74). **Five-year survival for each group was 94% and 96%, respectively, confirming that adjuvant treatment did not improve survival. Therefore, no adjuvant chemotherapy is recommended for these patients.**

Stage I High-grade, High-risk

In patients whose disease is high-risk (e.g., more poorly differentiated or in whom there are malignant cells either in ascitic fluid or in peritoneal washings), additional therapy is indicated. Most investigators recommend chemotherapy for these patients (146–161). Chemotherapy for patients with early stage high-risk epithelial ovarian cancer can be either single agent or multiagent. Some researchers have questioned the wisdom of overly aggressive chemotherapy in women with early stage disease, suggesting that the evidence for a durable impact on survival is marginal (148,149,155). Furthermore, the risk of leukemia with alkylating agents and *platinum* make the administration of adjuvant therapy risky unless there is a significant benefit (160,161).

Because *cisplatin, carboplatin, cyclophosphamide,* and *paclitaxel* (*Taxol*) are active single agents against epithelial ovarian cancer, these drugs have been administered in various combinations. There are some series in which *cisplatin* or *cyclophosphamide* (PC) or both have been used to treat patients with stage I disease (150–152). In a GOG trial of three cycles of *cisplatin* and *cyclophosphamide* versus intraperitoneal chromic phosphate (^{32}P) in patients with stage Ib and Ic disease, the progression-free survival of women receiving the *platinum*-based chemotherapy was 31% higher than those receiving the radiocolloid (152). Similar results were also reported by a multicenter trial performed in Italy by the Gruppo Italiano Collaborativo Oncologica Ginecologica (GICOG) for progression-free survival, although there was no overall survival advantage. *Carboplatin* can be substituted for *cisplatin* in the therapy of these patients (158), although it is unclear if there is a survival benefit. The current GOG trial consists of three cycles of *carboplatin* and *paclitaxel* followed by a randomization to either observation versus 26 weeks of weekly low-dose (40 mg/m^2) *paclitaxel.*

The recommendations for therapy follow:

- **Patients with high-grade, high-risk stage I epithelial ovarian cancer be given adjuvant chemotherapy. The type depends on the patient's overall health and status.**
- **Treatment with *carboplatin* and *paclitaxel* chemotherapy for three to six cycles seems desirable in most patients, whereas a short course of a single agent, either *carboplatin* or *paclitaxel,* may be preferable for older women.**

Advanced-stage Epithelial Ovarian Cancer

Systemic multiagent chemotherapy is the standard treatment for metastatic epithelial ovarian cancer (162–180). After the introduction of cisplatin in the latter half of the 1970s, *platinum*-based combination chemotherapy became the most frequently used treatment regimen in the United States. *Paclitaxel* became available in the 1980s, and this drug was incorporated into the combination chemotherapy in the 1990s (162–167). Comparative trials of *paclitaxel, cisplatin,* and *carboplatin* are summarized below.

In a meta-analysis performed on studies of patients with advanced-stage disease, those patients given *cisplatin*-containing combination chemotherapy were compared with those treated with regimens that did not include *cisplatin* (171). Survival differences between the groups were seen from 2 to 5 years, with the *cisplatin* group having a slight survival advantage, but this difference disappeared by 8 years.

The major advance in the treatment of advanced-stage disease was the incorporation of *paclitaxel* into the chemotherapeutic regimens. A series of randomized, prospective clinical trials with *paclitaxel*-containing arms have defined the current recommended treatment protocol in advanced epithelial ovarian cancer (165,166,175,176).

Reporting the GOG data (Protocol 111), McGuire and others showed that the combination of *cisplatin* (75 mg/m^2) and *paclitaxel* (135 mg/m^2) was superior to *cisplatin* (75 mg/m^2) and *cyclophosphamide* (600 mg/m^2), each given for six cycles (165). In suboptimally resected patients, the *paclitaxel*-containing arm produced a 36% reduction in mortality. These data were verified in a trial conducted jointly by the European Organization for the Research and Treatment of Cancer (EORTC), the Nordic Ovarian Cancer Study Group (NOCOVA), and the National Cancer Institute of Canada (NCIC) in which patients with both optimal and suboptimal disease were treated (166). In this study the *paclitaxel*-containing arm produced a significant improvement in both progression-free interval and overall survival in both optimal and suboptimal groups (Fig 32.12). **Based on these two studies, *paclitaxel* should be included in the primary treatment of all women with advanced-stage epithelial ovarian cancer, unless precluded by toxicity.**

A three-arm comparison of *paclitaxel* (T) versus *cisplatin* (P) versus PT in suboptimal stage III and IV patients (protocol 132) showed equivalency in the three groups, but crossover from one drug to the other was permitted (167). The study essentially showed that the combination regimen was better tolerated than the sequential administration of the agents in suboptimally resected patients.

The second-generation *platinum* analogue, *carboplatin,* was introduced and developed to have less toxicity than its parent compound, *cisplatin.* In early trials, *carboplatin* was shown to have lower overall toxicity (169). Fewer gastrointestinal side effects, especially nausea and vomiting, were observed than with *cisplatin,* and there was less nephrotoxicity, neurotoxicity, and ototoxicity. *Carboplatin* is, however, associated with a higher degree of myelosuppression.

The initial studies showed that *carboplatin* and *cisplatin* had approximately a 4:1 equivalency ratio. Thus a standard single-agent dose of about 400 mg/m^2 has been used in most phase II trials. **The dose is calculated by using the area under the curve (AUC) and the glomerular filtration rate (GFR) according to the *Calvert formula*** (181). The target AUC is 5–6 for untreated patients with ovarian cancer. Alternatively, a dose of approximately 350 to 450 mg/m^2 *carboplatin* can be used initially in patients with a normal serum creatinine and adjusted to toxicity. A platelet nadir of approximately 50,000/ml is a suitable target (169).

Carboplatin and Paclitaxel

Two randomized, prospective clinical studies have compared the combination of *paclitaxel* and *carboplatin* to *paclitaxel* and *cisplatin* (175,176). In both studies, the efficacy and

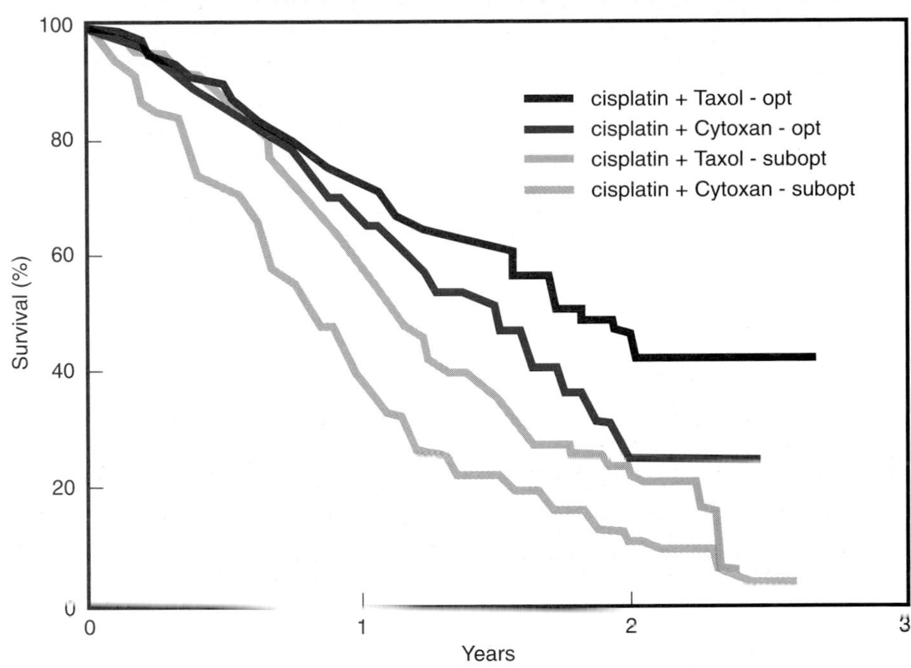

Figure 32.12 Survival of patients with stage III and IV epithelial ovarian cancer treated with *paclitaxel* and *cisplatin* or *cyclophosphamide* and *cisplatin:* results of a European cooperative group trials study. (From **Stuart G, Bertelsen K, Mangioni C, et al.** Updated analysis shows a highly significant survival for *cisplatin-paclitaxel* as first line treatment of advanced-stage epithelial ovarian cancer: mature results of the EORTC-GCCG, NOCOVA, NCIC-CTC and Scottish Intergroup Trial. *J Clin Oncol* 2000, with permission.)

survivals were similar, but the toxicity was more acceptable with the *carboplatin*-containing regimen. In the first trial, GOG Protocol 158, the randomization was *carboplatin* AUC = 7.5 and *paclitaxel* 175 mg/m^2 over 3 hours versus *cisplatin* 75 mg/m^2 and *paclitaxel* 135 mg/m^2 over 24 hours. The disease progression–free survival of the *carboplatin*-containing arm was 22 months versus 21.7 months for the control arm (175). The gastrointestinal and neurotoxicity of the *carboplatin* arm were appreciably lower than that of the *cisplatin* arm. A similar result was obtained in a large randomized trial in Germany (176), in which the dose of *carboplatin* was AUC = 6 and *paclitaxel* was 185 mg/m^2 over 3 hours compared with the same dose of *paclitaxel* and *cisplatin* 75 mg/m^2. Ongoing trials are comparing the combination of *carboplatin* and *paclitaxel* with single-agent *carboplatin* or combination *cisplatin* chemotherapy (177). **The preferred regimen in patients with advanced-stage disease is the *paclitaxel* plus *carboplatin* combination.**

Intraperitoneal Chemotherapy

A randomized, prospective trial of intraperitoneal *cisplatin* versus intravenous *cisplatin* (100 mg/m^2), each given with 750 mg/m^2 *cyclophosphamide,* has been performed jointly by the Southwest Oncology Group (SWOG) and the GOG in patients with minimal residual disease (182). The intraperitoneal *cisplatin* arm had a somewhat longer overall median survival than the intravenous arm, 49 versus 41 months ($p = 0.03$). In the patients with minimal residual disease (<0.5 cm maximal residual), however, there was no difference between the two treatments, 51 versus 46 months ($p = 0.08$).

In a follow-up trial (GOG Protocol 114), the dose-intense arm was initiated by giving a moderately high dose of *carboplatin* (dose AUC = 9) for two induction cycles, followed by intraperitoneal *cisplatin* 100 mg/m^2 and intravenous *paclitaxel* 135 mg/m^2 over 24 hours, versus intravenous *cisplatin* 75 mg/m^2 and intravenous *paclitaxel* 135 mg/m^2 (183). The dose-intense arm results were slightly better—the disease progression–free median survival was 27.6 months compared with 22.5 months for the control arm ($p = 0.02$). However, there was no difference in overall survival (52.9 months versus 47.6 months, $p = 0.056$). Thus, it is unclear if dose intensification with intraperitoneal *cisplatin* will have a sustained long-term impact on the survival of these patients. A randomized prospective GOG study is comparing intraperitoneal *cisplatin* and *paclitaxel* versus intravenous *cisplatin* and *paclitaxel.*

Based on these two studies, the value of intraperitoneal chemotherapy in the primary treatment of optimally resected stage III ovarian cancer remains unclear.

Neoadjuvant Chemotherapy

Some authors have suggested that, for patients with suboptimal stage III and stage IV disease, chemotherapy may be given in lieu of debulking surgery. A series performed by Schwartz and co-workers (184) suggested that the survival of these patients treated with neoadjuvant or cytoreductive chemotherapy was comparable to those patients historically treated in the same institution with debulking surgery followed by conventional chemotherapy. As other authors have shown a benefit to debulking patients prior to chemotherapy (135), the issue would need to be resolved by a prospective clinical trial.

However, two or three cycles of chemotherapy prior to cytoreductive surgery may be helpful in patients with massive ascites and large pleural effusions. The chemotherapy may dry up the effusions, improve the patient's performance status, and decrease postoperative morbidity, particularly chest morbidity.

Chemotherapeutic Recommendation in Advanced Epithelial Ovarian Cancer

For the treatment of advanced-stage epithelial ovarian cancer, the following is recommended (Table 32.4):

- **Combination chemotherapy with *carboplatin* and *paclitaxel* as the treatment of choice for patients with advanced disease. The recommended doses and schedule are *carboplatin* (starting dose AUC = 5 to 6) and *paclitaxel* (175 mg/m^2) given over 3 hours every 3 weeks for six cycles.**
- **In patients who cannot tolerate the combination, single-agent *carboplatin* (AUC = 5 to 6) can be given.**

Table 32.4. Combination Chemotherapy for Advanced Epithelial Ovarian Cancer: Recommended Regimens

Drugs	*Dose*	*Administration (hr)*	*Interval*	*No. of Treatments*
Standard regimens				
Paclitaxel	175 mg/m^2	24	Every 3 weeks	Six cycles
Carboplatin	AUC = 5–6			
Paclitaxel	135 mg/m^2	3	Every 3 weeks	Six cycles
Cisplatin	75 mg/m^2			
Alternative drugs[a]				
(Can be given with *platinum*)				
Cyclophosphamide	600–750 mg/m^2	—	Every 3 weeks	—
Topotecan	1.0–1.25 mg/m^2	—	Daily × 5 days every 3 weeks	—
Gemcitabine	800–1000 mg/m^2	—	Every 3 weeks	—

AUC, area under the curve dose by Calvert formula (181).
[a]Drugs that can be substituted for *paclitaxel* if hypersensitivity to that drug occurs.
From **Berek JS, Hacker NF,** eds. *Practical gynecologic oncology,* 3rd ed. Philadelphia: Lippincott Williams & Wilkins, 2000:493, with permission.

- **In those who have a hypersensitivity to *paclitaxel,* an alternative active drug can be substituted (e.g., *cyclophosphamide* or *topotecan*).**
- **In patients who cannot tolerate intravenous chemotherapy, an oral alkylating agent can be substituted.**

The treatment of all patients with advanced-stage disease is approached in a similar manner, with modifications based on the overall status and general health of the patient, as well as the extent of residual disease present at the time treatment is initiated.

Immunotherapy

There is currently a great deal of interest in the use of immunotherapies in ovarian cancer. Cytokines have been used extensively in second-line therapy, and the activity of *interferon-α, interferon-γ,* and *interleukin-2* has been demonstrated, as discussed below (3). In a recent trial of *interferon-γ* plus *cisplatin* combination chemotherapy versus chemotherapy alone, patients who received the *interferon* had a longer disease progression–free survival (185).

Trials of monoclonal antibodies directed toward ovarian cancer–associated antigens are being conducted. Antibodies directed toward CA125 and toward the HMFG (human milk fat globulin) tumor–associated antigens are underway. *Herceptin,* an antibody directed toward the extracellular protein produced when the HER-2/*neu* oncogene is overexpressed, has been used extensively in breast cancer where it has been shown to improve the response rate to chemotherapy in selected patients. Trials of this antibody in patients whose ovarian cancers overexpress HER-2/*neu* are ongoing. Antibodies against mutated *p53* tumor suppressor gene are also undergoing clinical testing (3).

Hormonal Therapy

There is no evidence that hormonal therapy alone is appropriate primary therapy for advanced ovarian cancer. The use of progestational agents in the treatment of recurrent well-differentiated endometrioid carcinomas is supported by the current data. In a study by Rendina and co-workers (186), 30 evaluable patients with recurrent epithelial cancers were treated; 17 (57%) had an objective response, and three (10%) of these patients achieved a complete response. All responding patients had well-differentiated, estrogen receptor–positive tumors. A trial of *tamoxifen* in combination with multiagent chemotherapy is being conducted.

Treatment Assessment

Many patients who undergo optimal cytoreductive surgery and subsequent chemotherapy for epithelial ovarian cancer will have no evidence of disease at the completion of treatment. Tumor markers and radiologic assessments have proven to be too insensitive to exclude the presence of subclinical disease. Therefore, a second-look surgery is often performed to evaluate these patients (112,187–196). Most often, patients have undergone formal reassessment laparotomy, although the laparoscope has also been used in this circumstance (194–196). However, there is a 35% false-negative rate if laparoscopy is used for a second-look procedure (112,195).

Tumor Markers

Tumor markers are not reliable enough to predict accurately which patients with epithelial tumors will experience complete eradication of disease with a particular therapy. Carcinoembryonic antigen (CEA) levels are often elevated in patients with ovarian cancer, but the test is too nonspecific and insensitive to have much use in the management of these patients (3).

The level of CA125, a surface glycoprotein associated with müllerian epithelial tissues, is elevated in about 80% of patients with epithelial ovarian cancers, particularly those with nonmucinous tumors. The levels frequently become undetectable after the initial surgical resection and one or two cycles of chemotherapy.

Levels of CA125 have been correlated with findings at second-look operations. Positive levels are useful in predicting the presence of disease, but negative levels are an insensitive determinant of the absence of disease. In a prospective study (197), the predictive value of a positive test was shown to be 100%; if the level of CA125 was positive (>35 U/ml), disease was always detectable in patients at the second-look procedure. The predictive value of a negative test was only 56%; if the level was <35 U/ml, disease was present in 44% of the patients at the time of the second-look surgery. A review of the literature suggests that an elevated CA125 level predicts persistent disease at second-look surgery in 97% of the cases (198), but the CA125 level is not sensitive enough to exclude subclinical disease in many patients.

Serum CA125 levels can be used during chemotherapy to follow those patients whose levels were positive at the initiation of therapy (3,198). **The change in level generally correlates with response.** Those patients with persistently elevated levels after three cycles of treatment most likely have resistant clones. When levels rise after treatment, almost invariably treatment has failed and continuation of the current regimen is futile.

Radiologic Assessment

For patients with stage I to III epithelial ovarian cancer, radiologic tests generally have been of limited value in assessing the response to therapy for subclinical disease. Ascites can be readily detected, but even quite large omental metastases can be missed on CT scan (199). If liver enzyme levels are abnormal, the liver can be evaluated with a CT scan or ultrasonography. A positive CT scan and fine-needle aspiration (FNA) cytology indicating tumor persistence could obviate the need for second-look surgery, but the false-negative rate of a CT scan is about 45% (200).

Second-look Operations

A second-look operation is one performed on a patient who has no clinical evidence of disease after a prescribed course of chemotherapy to determine the response to therapy.

Second-look Laparotomy

The technique of the second-look laparotomy is essentially identical to that for the staging laparotomy (112). The operation should be performed through a vertical abdominal incision. The incision should be initiated below the level of the umbilicus, so that if pelvic disease is detected in the absence of any palpable upper abdominal disease, a smaller incision might suffice. The incision can be extended cranially as needed.

After multiple cytologic specimens have been obtained, samples of the peritoneal surfaces should be collected for biopsy, particularly in any areas of previously documented tumor. These are the most important areas to sample for biopsy because they are most likely to give a positive result. Any adhesions or surface irregularities should be sampled. In addition, biopsy specimens should be taken from the pelvic side walls, the pelvic cul-de-sac, the bladder, the paracolic gutters, the residual omentum, and the diaphragm. A pelvic and paraaortic lymph node dissection should be performed for those patients whose nodal tissues have not been previously removed.

About 30% of patients with no evidence of macroscopic disease will have microscopic metastases (186). Also, for many patients with microscopic disease, it will be detected in only the occasional biopsy or cytologic specimen. Therefore, a large number of specimens (at least 20 to 30) should be obtained to minimize possibility of false-negative results of the operation. For selected patients in whom gross residual tumor is discovered at second-look surgery, resection of isolated masses may be performed. The removal of all macroscopic areas of disease might facilitate response to salvage therapies (201–207).

Second-look laparotomies have not been shown to influence patient survival (191,192). **Therefore, they should be performed only in a research setting, in which second-line or salvage therapies are undergoing clinical trials.**

The findings at second look correlate with subsequent outcome and survival (112,186–193). Patients who have no histologic evidence of disease have a significantly longer survival than those in whom microscopic or macroscopic disease is documented at laparotomy (192,193).

The attainment of negative findings with second-look surgery is not tantamount to a cure (184,186). Indeed, the reported probability that a patient will have a recurrence after a negative second-look laparotomy ranges from 30% to 50% at 5 years (112,186–193). Clearly, it is not possible to sample every potential site of disease. In addition, disease can become clinically apparent in sites that are occult, such as the liver parenchyma (72). Most recurrences after a negative second-look laparotomy occur in patients with poorly differentiated cancers (193).

Variables associated with the outcome of the second-look laparotomy are (a) initial stage, (b) tumor grade, (c) the size of the residual tumor and the size of the largest metastatic tumor before treatment, and (d) the type of chemotherapy. No single variable or combination of variables is sufficiently predictive to obviate a planned second-look laparotomy (3,112).

Second-look Laparoscopy

The advantage of laparoscopy is that it is less invasive than laparotomy; the disadvantage is that visibility may be limited by the frequent presence of intraperitoneal adhesions (194–196). The development of newer techniques for retroperitoneal lymph node dissection has potentially increased the utility of the endoscopic approach to a second look. The morbidity and role of this technique are currently being studied by the GOG.

One technique that has been used for second look is called *open laparoscopy.* This procedure allows placement of the scope after a cutdown to the fascia of the rectus abdominous has been performed. The peritoneum is entered under direct vision, thus avoiding the blind insertion that can be associated with intestinal injury (3,196).

The sensitivity of the laparoscopic technique has been determined by an exploratory laparotomy performed immediately after a negative laparoscopy. Thirty-five percent of those who had negative findings on laparoscopy had evidence of disease at laparotomy (196), but these patients did not undergo a lymphadenectomy at laparoscopy.

Laparoscopy has been used immediately before a planned laparotomy. If gross disease is detected and secondary resection of the tumor is not possible, a laparotomy may be omitted (196).

Thus, the role of the laparoscope for patients with epithelial ovarian cancer is still being defined. It may be used to stage disease in patients who have undergone a prior laparotomy for a tumor that was incompletely staged. Second-look laparoscopy may also be useful for patients on experimental treatment protocols, especially second-line treatments that require some evaluation of response.

Second-line Therapy

Secondary Cytoreduction

Patients with persistent or recurrent pelvic and abdominal tumors after primary therapy for ovarian cancer may be candidates for surgical excision of their disease. This operation has been referred to as *secondary cytoreductive surgery* (201–207). Tumor resection, under these circumstances, should be restricted to carefully selected patients for whom resection has a reasonable chance of either prolonging life or resulting in significant palliation of symptoms, because there is no benefit for most patients with persistent or progressive disease after primary therapy. The patient for whom secondary cytoreduction might be appropriate should be in good general medical condition. A suitable patient would be one who has no evidence of ascites, has not yet received *cisplatin* combination chemotherapy, has had at least a partial response to prior alkylating agent therapy, and has had a reasonably long interval since primary diagnosis. If the patient has previously received *cisplatin,* secondary cytoreduction is justified if there has been a long disease-free survival (longer than 12–24 months), because such patients are likely to respond again to the primary chemotherapy (185–190).

The goal of secondary debulking is to remove all residual gross tumor, if possible, or to reduce the metastatic tumor burden to <5 mm maximal dimension. Some patients with minimal residual disease will respond to second-line treatment. Those patients in whom the residual disease is completely resected have a significantly longer survival than those who do not (185).

Second-line Chemotherapy

If disease persists at the time of second-look laparotomy, or if clinically progressive disease develops during primary therapy, patients usually have been switched to an alternative treatment, often a second-line chemotherapy. The response rates for second-line chemotherapies have been 15% to 35% for most drugs tested by the oral or intravenous route (208–230). Active drugs that have been used as single agents include *cisplatin, carboplatin, paclitaxel, docetaxel* (*Taxotere*), *topotecan, gemcitabine, etoposide* (*VP-16*), *doxorubicin* (*Doxil*), *vinorelbine* (*Navelbine*), *ifosfamide, 5-fluorouracil* with *leucovorin,* and *hexamethylmelamine.* Single-agent drugs are sometimes used for second-line chemotherapy because of their relative ease of administration and low toxicity.

Platinum-sensitive Versus Platinum-resistant

Second-line therapies have been categorized by whether or not the patients responded to their initial *platinum*-based chemotherapy. Although this concept has been variously defined, *platinum* sensitivity has been related to a disease progression–free interval of 12 to 24 months. Response rates after retreatment with *cisplatin* have been shown to be higher in patients whose time to clinical relapse after prior response to *cisplatin* is at least 12 to 24 months (210–212). *Carboplatin* is active as a second-line agent in patients who have responded to prior *cisplatin* treatment, and response rates in these patients have been 20% to 30% (210). The concept of *platinum* sensitivity and *paclitaxel* sensitivity should influence the choice of second-line chemotherapy.

In patients who have *platinum-* or *paclitaxel*-sensitive tumors, retreatment with a *platinum* drug or *paclitaxel* is appropriate. Second-line responses to *paclitaxel, carboplatin,* and *cisplatin* in those patients who have responded previously to *cisplatin* have been observed in 20% to 25% of patients.

In *cisplatin*-refractory patients, response rates to second-line *carboplatin* are less than 10% (209,211). In *platinum*-resistant disease, persistent disease is best treated with non–cross-resistant agents that have different anticancer mechanisms such as the topoisomerase inhibitors (e.g., *etoposide* and *topotecan*), an anthracycline [e.g., *doxorubicin* (*Doxil*)], an alkylating agent (e.g., *ifosfamide*), or other agents, (e.g., *hexamethylmelamine*). These agents have resulted in second-line response rates of about 8% to 28% in patients with *platinum*-resistant disease (213–230).

Several new combinations of chemotherapy are now being tested in advanced epithelial ovarian cancer. The rationale for this approach is that the two agents have complementary toxicities and mechanisms of action. Combinations such as *gemcitabine* and *platinum,* and *topotecan* and *platinum* may have greater activity than either agent alone. Various neuroprotective and myelosuppressive protectors, such as *amifostine,* are being tested in *cisplatin* combination regimens.

Intraperitoneal Therapy

For patients with minimal residual (<5 mm) or microscopic disease confined to the peritoneal cavity, consideration can be given to intraperitoneal chemotherapy or immunotherapy.

The failure of second-line intravenous chemotherapy to control residual disease has led to the use of intraperitoneal therapies for small, persistent disease. Cytotoxic chemotherapeutic agents, such as *cisplatin, 5-fluorouracil, cytosine arabinoside* (*Ara-C*), *etoposide* (*VP-16*), and *mitoxantrone,* have been used for patients with persistent epithelial ovarian cancer (231–240), and complete responses have been seen in patients who begin treatment with minimal residual disease. The surgically documented response rates reported with this approach are about 20% to 40% for carefully selected patients, and the complete response rate is about 10% to 20%. *Cisplatin* seems to be the best drug, although various combinations of agents (e.g., *cisplatin* plus *etoposide*) have been shown to have significant activity (233,234). Although it has been suggested that this approach produces a significant subsequent improvement in survival (236), there are no prospective phase III data, and the patients so treated tend to be those with a more favorable prognosis regardless of subsequent therapy.

Another approach is the use of intraperitoneal immunotherapy such as *interferon* (241–247). *Interferon* has been found to have some activity for patients with minimal residual disease (241,242). Intraperitoneal administration *interferon-α, interferon-γ, tumor necrosis factor,* and *interleukin-2* has been performed. The response rate for the intraperitoneal cytokines, *interferon-α* and *interferon-γ,* is the same as that for the cytotoxic agents (i.e., about 30% to 50%) (241–247). The intraperitoneal administration of *interferon-α* has produced a 32% (9 of 28) surgically documented complete response rate, and a 50% (14 of 28) total response rate for patients with minimal residual disease after primary combination chemotherapy with *cisplatin* (241,242,246).

The interferons have been combined with cytotoxic agents in an effort to increase the overall response rates. In several trials, the combination of *cisplatin* and *interferon-α* seemed to produce a 50% complete response rate, which was greater than that produced by either single agent (244–246). However, in a prospective, single-arm, phase II trial conducted by the GOG, the intraperitoneal administration of *cisplatin* and *interferon-α* produced only a 7% response rate (247). In this GOG trial, most patients had *cisplatin*-refractory tumors with >5 mm residual disease, generalized carcinomatosis, and ascites. Surgically documented responses to intraperitoneal therapy have been generally limited to patients with minimal residual disease (i.e., <5 mm maximal tumor dimension) and patients whose tumors have been responsive to *cisplatin* chemotherapy.

Candidates for Intraperitoneal Therapy Intraperitoneal treatment is not suitable for all patients because it can be cumbersome, requiring catheters that remain functional. Neither patients with extensive intraperitoneal adhesions nor patients with extraperitoneal disease are appropriate candidates. On the basis of these issues and the failure to achieve responses in most patients with bulky, *platinum*-refractory disease, second-line intraperitoneal chemotherapy and immunotherapy should still be considered experimental.

Hormonal Therapy

Tamoxifen has been associated with response rates of 15% to 20% in well-differentiated carcinomas of the ovary (250,251). The gonadotropin agonist *leuprolide acetate* (*Lupron*) has been shown to produce a response rate of 10% in one series (252). Trials combining *tamoxifen* and *leuprolide acetate,* and *tamoxifen* and combination chemotherapy are being conducted (253). Aromatase inhibitors (e.g., *Arimidex*), which have been shown to have activity in metastatic breast cancer, are being studied in relapsed ovarian cancer (254).

Radiation Therapy

Whole-abdominal radiation therapy given as a salvage treatment has been shown to be associated with a relatively high morbidity. The principal problem associated with this approach is the development of acute and chronic intestinal morbidity. As many as 30% of patients treated with this approach develop intestinal obstruction, which will necessitate exploratory surgery with potentially morbid effects (255).

Intestinal Obstruction

Patients with epithelial ovarian cancer often develop intestinal obstruction, either at the time of initial diagnosis or, more frequently, in association with recurrent disease (112,256–264). Obstruction may be related to a mechanical blockage or to carcinomatous ileus.

The intestinal blockage can be corrected in most patients whose obstruction appears at the time of initial diagnosis. However, the decision to perform an exploratory procedure to ease intestinal obstruction in patients with recurrent disease is more difficult. For patients whose life expectancy is very short (e.g., <2 months), surgical relief of the obstruction is not indicated (256). For those whose projected lifespan is longer, features that predict a reasonable likelihood of correcting the obstruction include young age, good nutritional status, and the absence of rapidly accumulating ascites (257).

For most patients with recurrent ovarian cancer who have intestinal obstruction, initial management should include proper radiographic documentation of the obstruction, hydration, correction of any electrolyte disturbances, parenteral alimentation, and intestinal intubation. For some patients, the obstruction may be alleviated by this conservative approach. A preoperative upper gastrointestinal radiographic series and a barium enema will define possible sites of obstruction.

If exploratory surgery is deemed appropriate, the type of operation to be performed will depend on the site and the number of obstructions. Multiple sites of obstruction are not uncommon in patients with recurrent epithelial ovarian cancer. More than one-half of the patients have small-bowel obstruction, one-third have colonic obstruction, and one-sixth have both (258–262). If the obstruction is principally contained in one area of the bowel (e.g., the terminal ileum), this area can either be resected or bypassed, depending on whether a concomitant effort at secondary cytoreduction is indicated. If multiple obstructions are present, resection of several segments of intestine in patients with recurrent disease is usually not indicated, and intestinal bypass surgery or colostomy, or both, should be performed.

Intestinal bypass is generally associated with less morbidity than resection (112,258,259), and in patients with recurrent, progressive cancer, the survival time after these two operations is the same (258). Most frequently, an enteroenterostomy or an enterocolostomy is performed (260–262). Colostomy may be necessary when there is a distal large-bowel obstruction. Occasionally, the performance of an ileostomy or a jejunostomy is warranted when the large bowel is completely encased in tumor (112). In very advanced cases, a gastrostomy may be used for palliative purposes, and the gastrostomy can be placed percutaneously if there is no carcinomatosis around the stomach (263,264).

Among 268 patients reported to have undergone operations for intestinal obstruction resulting from ovarian cancer, the operative mortality was 14% and major complications were seen in 34% of the patients (256–262). The need for multiple reanastomoses and prior radiation therapy increased the morbidity, which consisted primarily of sepsis and enterocutaneous fistulas.

The median survival time for patients who have undergone intestinal surgery for obstruction secondary to ovarian cancer ranges from 2.5 to 7 months, although Castaldo and co-workers (256) reported that 17% of such patients survived longer than 12 months.

Survival

The prognosis for patients with epithelial ovarian cancer is related to several clinical variables. Survival analyses based on the most commonly used prognostic variables are presented (1,3,24,103–107). Including patients at all stages, patients less than 50 years of age have a 5-year survival rate of about 40%, compared with about 15% for patients older than 50 years. The 5-year survival rate for carefully and properly staged patients with stage I disease is 76% to 93%, depending on the tumor grade. The 5-year survival for stage II is

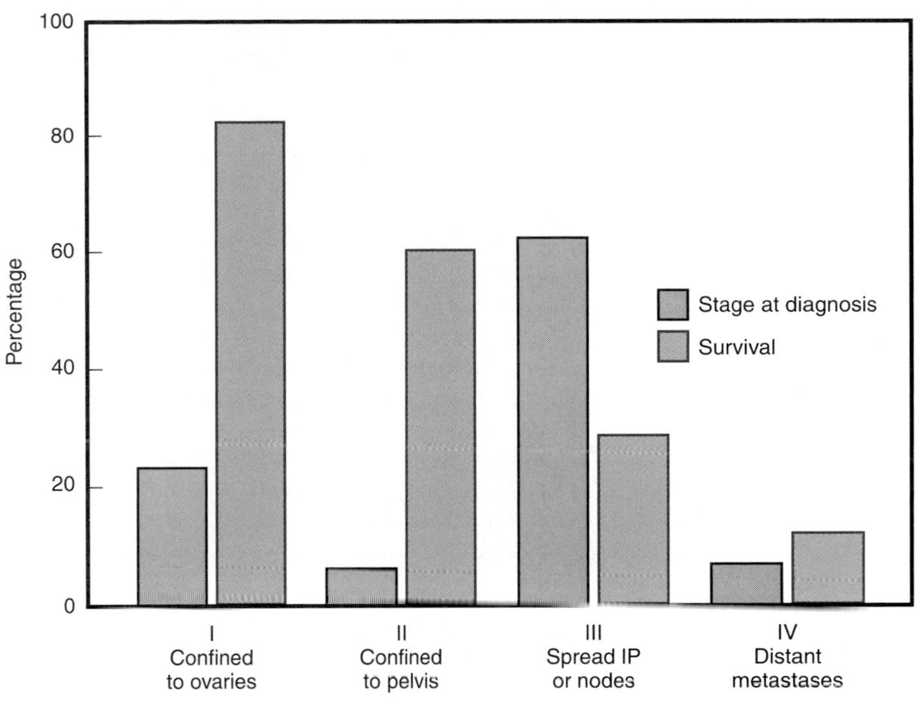

Figure 32.13 Survival of patients with epithelial ovarian cancer. The percentage of patients diagnosed at a particular stage is shown next to the 5-year survival by stage. *IP,* intraperitoneal. (From **Berek JS, Hacker NF,** eds. *Practical gynecologic oncology,* 3rd ed. Philadelphia: Lippincott Williams & Wilkins, 2000:504, with permission.)

60% to 74%. The 5-year survival rate for stage IIIa is 41%, for stage IIIb about 25%, for stage IIIc 23%, and for stage IV disease 11% (Fig 32.13).

An analysis of the National Cancer Institute's Surveillance, Epidemiology, and End Results (SEER) database reveals a trend toward improved survival for ovarian cancer in the United States during the last period of analysis (1988 to 1994). In this cohort, the survival for stage I was 93%, for stage II 70%, for stage III 37%, and for stage IV 25% (265). Compared with the interval 1983 to 1987, there was a statistically significant improvement in survival for stages I, III, and IV disease. Survival of patients with borderline tumors is excellent, with stage I lesions having a 98% 15-year survival (24). When all stages of borderline tumors are included, the 5-year survival rate is about 86% to 90%. Regarding patients with invasive cancer, the 5-year survival rate for grade 1 epithelial ovarian cancers is about 91%, compared with about 74% for grade 2 and 75% for grade 3 (24,265). For stage II disease, the survivals are 69%, 60%, and 51%, respectively, for grades 1, 2, and 3. Examining stage III to IV patients, the 5-year survivals for grades 1,2, and 3, respectively, are 38%, 25%, and 19%. Patients with stage III disease with microscopic residual disease at the start of treatment have a 5-year survival rate of about 40% to 75%, compared with about 30% to 40% for those with optimal disease and only 5% for those with nonoptimal disease (106,107,130). Patients whose Karnofsky's index (KI) is low (<70) have a significantly shorter survival than those with a KI >70 (24).

Nonepithelial Ovarian Cancers

Compared with epithelial ovarian cancers, other malignant tumors of the ovary are uncommon. Nonepithelial malignancies of the ovary account for about 10% of all ovarian cancers (2,3,266). Nonepithelial ovarian cancers include malignancies of germ cell origin, sex cord–stromal cell origin, metastatic carcinomas to the ovary, and a variety of extremely rare ovarian cancers (e.g., sarcomas, lipoid cell tumors). Although there are many similarities in the presentation, evaluation, and management of these patients, these tumors also have many unique qualities that require a special approach (2,266–269).

Germ Cell Malignancies

Germ cell tumors are derived from the primordial germ cells of the ovary. Their incidence is only about one-tenth the incidence of malignant germ cell tumors of the testis, so most of the advances in the management of these tumors have been extrapolations from experience with the corresponding testicular tumors. Although malignant germ cell tumors can arise in extragonadal sites such as the mediastinum and the retroperitoneum, most germ cell tumors arise in the gonad from undifferentiated germ cells. The variation in the site of these cancers is explained by the embryonic migration of the germ cells from the caudal part of the yolk sac to the dorsal mesentery before their incorporation into the sex cords of the developing gonads (2,3,266).

Classification

A histologic classification of ovarian germ cell tumors is presented in Table 32.5 (3,266). Both α-fetoprotein (AFP) and human chorionic gonadotropin (hCG) are secreted by some germ cell malignancies; therefore, the presence of circulating hormones can be clinically useful in the diagnosis of a pelvic mass and in monitoring the course of a patient after surgery. Placental alkaline phosphatase (PLAP) and lactate dehydrogenase (LDH) are commonly produced by dysgerminomas and may be useful for monitoring the disease. α_1-Antitrypsin (AAT) can rarely be detected in association with germ cell tumors. When the histologic and immunohistologic identification of these substances in tumors is correlated, a classification of germ cell tumors emerges (Fig. 32.14) (270).

In this scheme, embryonal carcinoma (a cancer composed of undifferentiated cells) synthesizes both hCG and AFP, and this lesion is the progenitor of several other germ cell tumors (270). More differentiated germ cell tumors, such as the endodermal sinus tumor, which secretes AFP, and the choriocarcinoma, which secretes hCG, are derived from the

Table 32.5. Histologic Typing of Ovarian Germ Cell Tumors

1. Dysgerminoma
2. Teratoma
   - A. Immature
   - B. Mature
     - 1) Solid
     - 2) Cystic
       - a. Dermoid cyst (mature cystic teratoma)
       - b. Dermoid cyst with malignant transformation
   - C. Monodermal and highly specialized
     - 1) Struma ovarii
     - 2) Carcinoid
     - 3) Struma ovarii and carcinoid
     - 4) Others
3. Endodermal sinus tumor
4. Embryonal carcinoma
5. Polyembryoma
6. Choriocarcinoma
7. Mixed forms

From **Seroy SF, Scully RE, Robin IH.** *Histological typing of ovarian tumors: international histological classification of tumors,* no. 9. Geneva: World Health Organization, 1973, with permission.

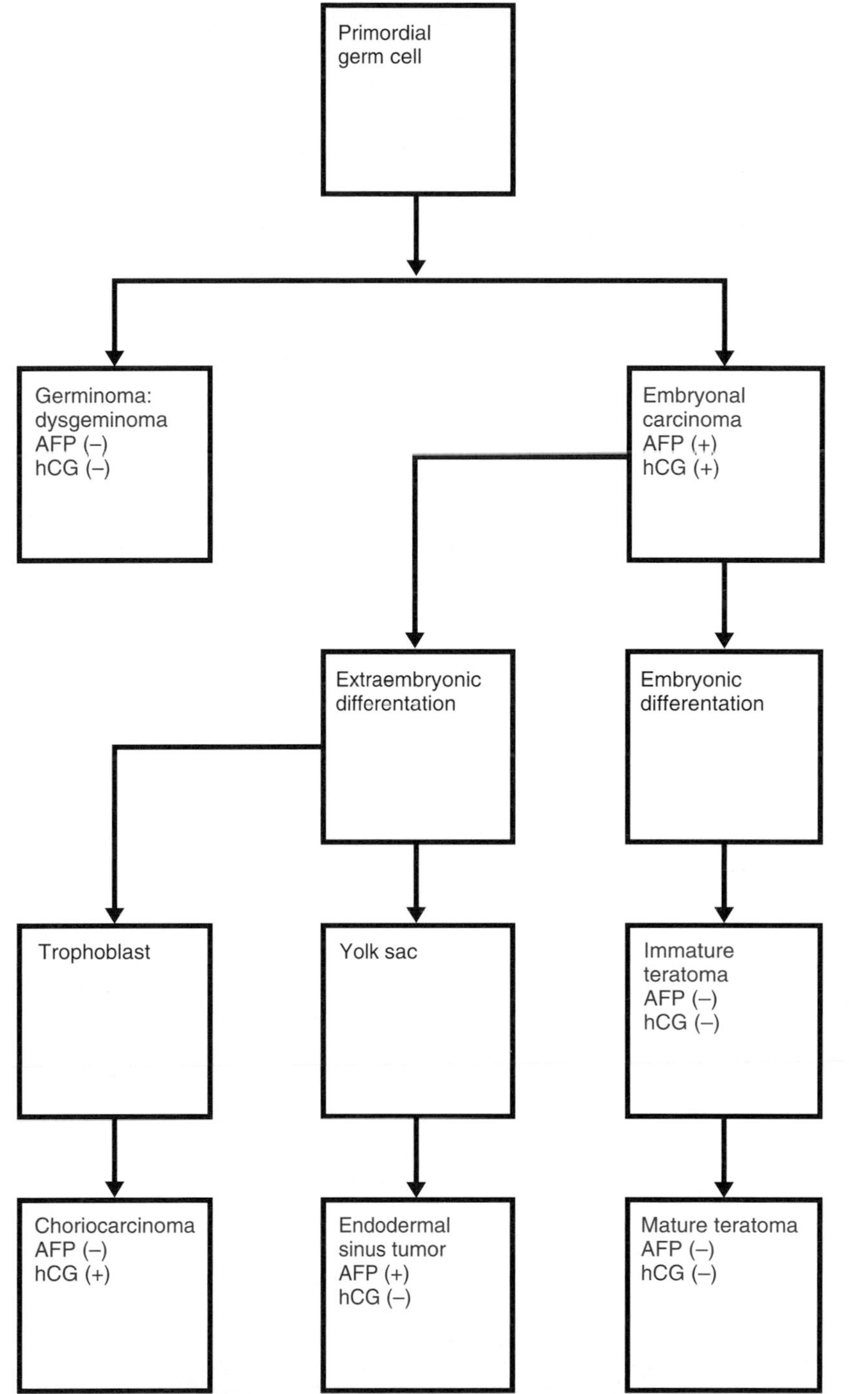

Figure 32.14 Relationship between types of pure malignant tumors. Germ cell tumors and their secreted marker substances. (From **Berek JS, Hacker NF.** *Practical gynecologic oncology,* 3rd ed. Philadelphia: Lippincott Williams & Wilkins, 2000:525, with permission.)

extraembryonic tissues; the immature teratomas derived from the embryonic cells have lost the ability to secrete these substances. Pure germinomas do not secrete these markers.

Epidemiology

Although 20% to 25% of all benign and malignant ovarian neoplasms are of germ cell origin, only about 3% of these tumors are malignant (2,3). Germ cell malignancies account for fewer than 5% of all ovarian cancers in Western countries. Germ cell malignancies represent up to 15% of ovarian cancers in Asian and African American societies, where epithelial ovarian cancers are much less common.

In the first 2 decades of life, almost 70% of ovarian tumors are of germ cell origin, and one-third of these are malignant (2,3,266). Germ cell tumors account for two-thirds of the ovarian malignancies in this age group. Germ cell cancers also are seen in the third decade, but thereafter they become quite rare.

Clinical Features

Symptoms

In contrast to the relatively slow-growing epithelial ovarian tumors, germ cell malignancies grow rapidly and often are characterized by subacute pelvic pain related to capsular distention, hemorrhage, or necrosis. The rapidly enlarging pelvic mass may produce pressure symptoms on the bladder or rectum, and menstrual irregularities also may occur in menarcheal patients. Some young patients may misinterpret the early symptoms of a neoplasm as those of pregnancy, and this can lead to a delay in the diagnosis. Acute symptoms associated with torsion or rupture of the adnexa can develop. These symptoms may be confused with acute appendicitis. In more advanced cases, ascites may develop, and the patient can have abdominal distention (268).

Signs

For a patient with a palpable adnexal mass, the evaluation can proceed as outlined. Some patients with germ cell tumors will be premenarcheal and may require examination under anesthesia. If the lesions are principally solid or a combination of solid and cystic, as might be noted on an ultrasonographic evaluation, a neoplasm is probable and a malignancy is possible (see Fig. 13.11 and Chapter 13). During the remainder of the physical examination, effort should be directed to searching for signs of ascites, pleural effusion, and organomegaly.

Diagnosis

Adnexal masses measuring 2 cm or larger in premenarcheal girls or 8 cm or larger in other premenopausal patients will usually require surgical exploration. For young patients, blood tests should include serum hCG and AFP titers, a complete blood count, and liver function tests. A radiograph of the chest is important because germ cell tumors can metastasize to the lungs or mediastinum. A karyotype should be obtained preoperatively for all premenarcheal girls because of the propensity of these tumors to arise in dysgenetic gonads (267,271). A preoperative CT scan or MRI may document the presence and extent of retroperitoneal lymphadenopathy or liver metastases; however, because these patients require surgical exploration, such extensive and time-consuming evaluation is unnecessary. If postmenarcheal patients have predominantly cystic lesions up to 8 cm in diameter, they may be observed or given oral contraceptives for two menstrual cycles (271,272).

Dysgerminoma

Dysgerminoma is the most common malignant germ cell tumor, accounting for about 30% to 40% of all ovarian cancers of germ cell origin (2,3,270). The tumors represent only 1% to 3% of all ovarian cancers, but they represent as many as 5% to 10% of ovarian cancers in patients younger than 20 years. Seventy-five percent of dysgerminomas occur between the ages of 10 and 30 years, 5% occur before the age of 10 years, and they rarely occur after 50 years of age (2,3,268). Because these malignancies occur in young women, 20% to 30% of ovarian malignancies associated with pregnancy are dysgerminomas.

Dysgerminomas are found in both sexes and may arise in gonadal or extragonadal sites. The latter include the midline structures from the pineal gland to the mediastinum and the retroperitoneum. Histologically, they represent abnormal proliferations of the basic germ cell. In the ovary, the germ cells are encapsulated at birth (the primordial follicle), and the

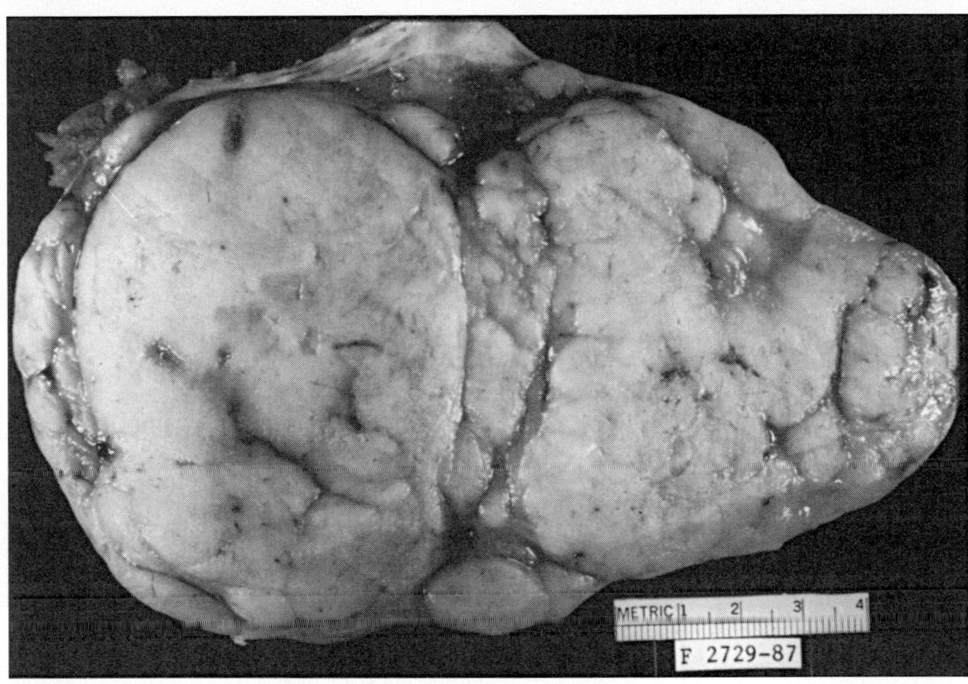

Figure 32.15 Dysgerminoma of the ovary. Note that the lesion is principally solid with some cystic areas. (From **Berek JS, Hacker NF.** *Practical gynecologic oncology,* 3rd ed. Philadelphia: Lippincott Williams & Wilkins, 2000:526, with permission.)

unencapsulated or free cells die. If either of the latter processes fails, it is conceivable that the germ cell could free itself of its normal control and multiply indiscriminately.

The size of dysgerminomas varies widely, but they are usually 5 to 15 cm in diameter (2,3). The capsule is slightly bosselated, and the consistency of the cut surface is spongy and gray-brown in color (Fig. 32.15).

The histologic characteristics of the dysgerminoma are very distinctive. The large round, ovoid, or polygonal cells have abundant, clear, very-pale–staining cytoplasm, large and irregular nuclei, and prominent nucleoli (Fig. 32.16). Mitotic figures are seen in varying numbers, although they are usually numerous. Another characteristic feature is the arrangement of the elements in lobules and nests separated by fibrous septa, which are often extensively infiltrated with lymphocytes, plasma cells, and granulomas with epitheloid cells and multinucleated giant cells. When necrosis is extensive, the lesion may be confused with tuberculosis. Occasional dysgerminomas may contain syncytiotrophoblastic giant cells and may be associated with precocious puberty or virilization. The presence of these cells does not seem to alter the behavior of the tumor (2,3).

Because the dysgerminoma is a germ cell tumor and parthenogenesis (stimulation of the basic germ cell to atypical division) is the most commonly accepted genesis for the more immature teratomas, it is logical that these two tumors may coexist. Choriocarcinoma, endodermal sinus tumor, and other extraembryonal lesions are also commonly associated with the dysgerminoma.

Approximately 5% of dysgerminomas are discovered in phenotypic females with abnormal gonads (2,271). This malignancy can be associated with patients who have pure gonadal dysgenesis (46,XY, bilateral streak gonads), mixed gonadal dysgenesis (45,X/46,XY, unilateral streak gonad, contralateral testis), and the androgen insensitivity syndrome (46,XY, testicular feminization). Therefore, for premenarcheal patients with a pelvic mass, the karyotype should be determined (see Chapter 23.)

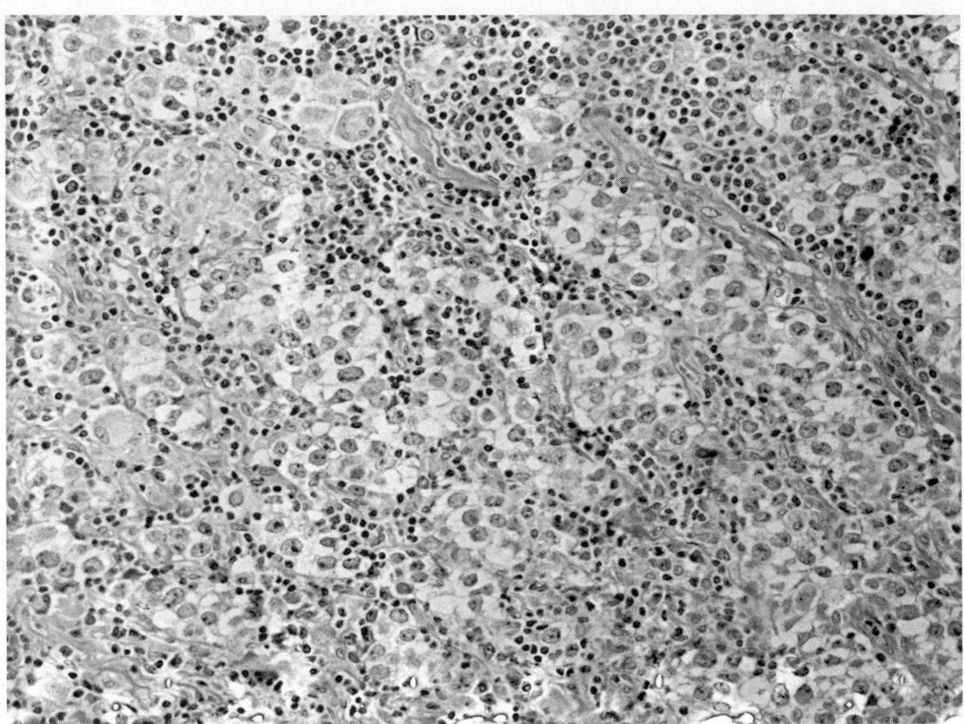

Figure 32.16 Dysgerminoma of ovary. Primitive germ cells are divided into clusters and lobules by fibrous septa rich in lymphocytes. Rare multinucleated giant cells are present in the left upper corner. (From **Berek JS, Hacker NF.** *Practical gynecologic oncology,* 3rd ed. Philadelphia: Lippincott Williams & Wilkins, 2000:147, with permission.)

For most patients with gonadal dysgenesis, dysgerminomas arise in gonadoblastomas, which are benign ovarian tumors that are composed of germ cells and sex cord stroma. If gonadoblastomas are left *in situ* in patients with gonadal dysgenesis, more than 50% will develop into ovarian malignancies (273).

About 75% of dysgerminomas are stage I (i.e., confined to one or both ovaries) at diagnosis (2,3,274–278). About 85% to 90% of stage I tumors are confined to one ovary; 10% to 15% are bilateral. In fact, dysgerminoma is the only germ cell malignancy that has this significant rate of bilaterality. Other germ cell tumors are rarely bilateral.

For patients whose contralateral ovary has been preserved, disease can develop in 5% to 10% of the retained gonads over the next 2 years (2). This figure includes those not given additional therapy, as well as patients with gonadal dysgenesis.

In the 25% of patients who are diagnosed initially with metastatic disease, the tumor most commonly spreads via the lymphatic system. It can also spread hematogenously or by direct extension through the capsule of the ovary with exfoliation and dissemination of cells throughout the peritoneal surfaces. Metastases to the contralateral ovary may be present when there is no other evidence of spread. An uncommon site of metastatic disease is bone; when metastasis to this site occurs, the lesions are seen principally in the lower vertebrae. Metastases to the lungs, liver, and brain are seen most often in patients with long-standing or recurrent disease. Metastasis to the mediastinum and supraclavicular lymph nodes is usually a late manifestation of disease (274,275).

Treatment

The treatment of patients with early dysgerminoma is primarily surgical, including resection of the primary lesion and proper surgical staging. Chemotherapy or radiation

is administered to patients with metastatic disease. Because the disease principally affects girls and young women, special consideration must be given to the preservation of fertility and use of chemotherapy as needed whenever possible. An algorithm for the management of ovarian dysgerminoma is presented in Fig. 32.17.

Surgery

The minimal surgical operation for ovarian dysgerminoma is a unilateral oophorectomy (276). If there is a desire to preserve fertility, the contralateral ovary, fallopian tube, and uterus should be left in situ, even in the presence of metastatic disease, because of the sensitivity of the tumor to chemotherapy. If fertility need not be preserved, it may be appropriate to perform a total abdominal hysterectomy and bilateral salpingo-oophorectomy for patients with advanced disease (278). For patients whose karyotype analysis reveals a Y chromosome, both ovaries should be removed, although the uterus may be left *in situ* for possible future embryo transfer. Whereas cytoreductive surgery is of unproved value, bulky disease that can be readily resected (e.g., an omental cake) should be removed during the initial operation.

For patients in whom the neoplasm appears on inspection to be confined to the ovary, a careful staging operation should be undertaken to determine the presence of any occult metastatic disease. All peritoneal surfaces should be inspected and palpated, and any suspicious lesions should be sampled for biopsy. Unilateral pelvic lymphadenectomy and at least careful palpation and biopsy of enlarged paraaortic nodes are particularly important parts of the staging. These tumors often metastasize to the paraaortic nodes around the renal vessels. Dysgerminoma is the only germ cell tumor that tends to be bilateral, and not all of the bilateral lesions are associated with obvious ovarian enlargement. Therefore, bisection of the contralateral ovary and excisional biopsy of any suspicious lesion are desirable (276–278). If a small contralateral tumor is found, it may be possible to resect it and preserve some normal ovary.

Radiation Therapy

Dysgerminomas are very sensitive to radiation therapy, and doses of 2,500 to 3,500 cGy may be curative, even for gross metastatic disease. Loss of fertility is a problem with radiation therapy, however, so radiation should rarely be used as first-line treatment (278).

Chemotherapy

Many patients with a dysgerminoma will have a tumor that is apparently confined to one ovary and will be referred for further treatment after unilateral salpingo-oophorectomy without surgical staging. The options for such patients are repeat laparotomy for surgical staging, regular pelvic and abdominal surveillance with CT scans, and adjuvant chemotherapy. Because dysgerminomas are rapidly growing tumors, regular CT surveillance is preferable. Tumor markers (AFP and hCG) should also be monitored in case occult mixed germ cell elements are present.

There have been numerous reports of successful control of metastatic dysgerminomas with systemic chemotherapy, and this technique should now be regarded as the treatment of choice (278–286). **The obvious advantage is the preservation of fertility** (287).

The most frequently used chemotherapeutic regimens for germ cell tumors are BEP (*bleomycin, etoposide,* and *cisplatin*), VBP (*vinblastine, bleomycin,* and *cisplatin*), and VAC (*vincristine, actinomycin,* and *cyclophosphamide*) (278–289) (Table 32.6).

The GOG studied three cycles of the EC regimen, consisting of *etoposide* (120 mg/m^2 intravenously on days 1, 2, and 3 every 4 weeks) and *carboplatin* (400 mg/m^2 intravenously

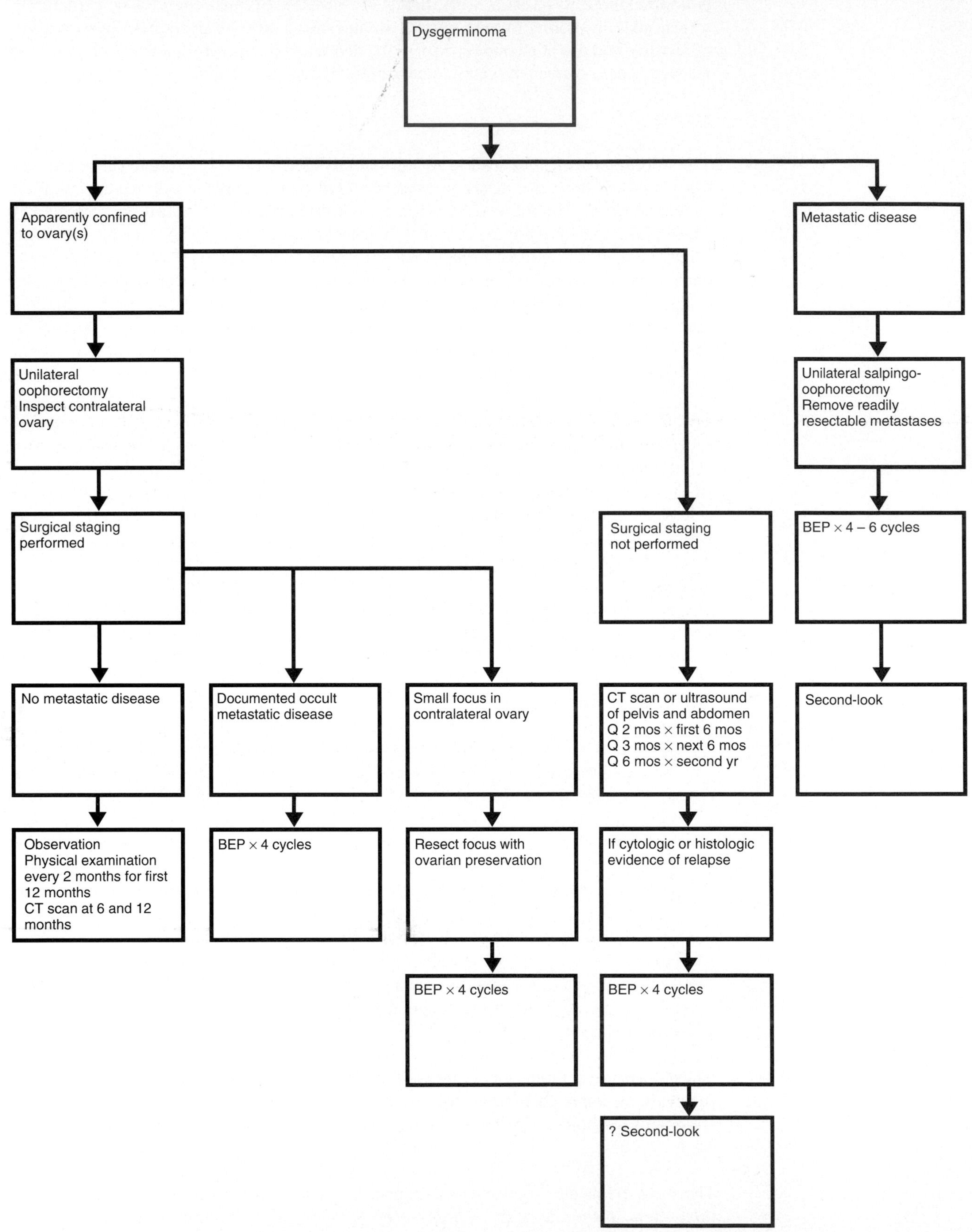

Figure 32.17 Management of dysgerminoma of the ovary. (From **Berek JS, Hacker NF.** *Practical gynecologic oncology,* 3rd ed. Philadelphia: Lippincott Williams & Wilkins, 2000:530, with permission.)

Table 32.6. Combination Chemotherapy for Germ Cell Tumors of the Ovary

Regimen and Drugs	*Dose and Schedule*[a]
BEP	
Bleomycin	15 units/m^2/week × 5; then on day 1 of course 4
Etoposide	100 mg/m^2/day × 5 days every 3 weeks
Cisplatin	20 mg/m^2/day × 5 days, or 100 mg/m^2/day × 1 day every 3 weeks
VBP	
Vinblastine	0.15 mg/kg days 1 and 2 every 3 weeks
Bleomycin	15 units/m^2/week × 5; then on day 1 of course 4
Cisplatin	100 mg/m^2 on day 1 every 3 weeks
VAC	
Vincristine	1–1.5 mg/m^2 on day 1 every 4 weeks
Actinomycin D	0.5 mg/day × 5 days every 4 weeks
Cyclophosphamide	150 mg/m^2/day × 5 days every 4 weeks

[a]All doses given intravenously.

on day 1 every 4 weeks) for patients with completely resected ovarian dysgerminoma, stages Ib, Ic, II, or III (286). The results showed a sustained disease-free remission rate of 100%.

For patients with advanced, incompletely resected germ cell tumors, the GOG studied *cisplatin*-based chemotherapy in two consecutive protocols (279,280). In the first study, patients received four cycles of *vinblastine* (12 mg/m^2 every 3 weeks), *bleomycin* (20 units/m^2 intravenously every week for 12 weeks), and *cisplatin* (20 mg/m^2 per day intravenously for 5 days every 3 weeks). Patients with persistent or progressive disease at second-look laparotomy were treated with six cycles of VAC. In the second trial, patients received three cycles of BEP initially, followed by consolidation with VAC, which was later discontinued in patients with dysgerminomas (280). The VAC consolidation after BEP in patients with tumors other than dysgerminoma is still being investigated, but VAC does not appear to improve the outcome of the BEP regimen. A total of 20 evaluable patients with stage III and IV dysgerminoma were treated in these two protocols, and 19 are alive and free of disease after 6 to 68 months (median = 26 months). Fourteen of these patients had a second-look laparotomy, and all findings were negative. Another study at M.D. Anderson Hospital (281) used BEP in 14 patients with residual disease, and all patients were free of disease during long-term follow-up. **These results suggest that patients with advanced-stage, incompletely resected dysgerminoma have an excellent prognosis when treated with *cisplatin*-based combination chemotherapy. The best regimen is four cycles of BEP based on the data from testicular cancers** (288,289).

There appears to be no need to perform a second-look laparotomy in patients with dysgerminoma whose macroscopic disease was all resected during the primary operation (290–292). In patients with macroscopic residual disease at the start of chemotherapy, we prefer to perform a second-look operation, because second-line therapy is available and the earlier persistent disease is identified, the better the prognosis should be.

Recurrent Disease

About 75% of recurrences occur within the first year after initial treatment (2,266–268), the most common sites being the peritoneal cavity and the retroperitoneal lymph nodes. These patients should be treated with either radiation or chemotherapy, depending on their primary treatment. Patients with recurrent disease who have had no therapy other than surgery should be treated with chemotherapy. If prior chemotherapy with BEP has been given, POMB-ACE (*vincristine, bleomycin, cisplatin, etoposide, actinomycin D,* and *cyclophosphamide*) may be used (Table 32.7), and consideration should be given to the use of high-dose chemotherapy (e.g., with *carboplatin* and *etoposide*). Alternatively, radiation therapy is effective for this disease, with the major disadvantage being loss of fertility if pelvic and abdominal irradiation is required.

Table 32.7. POMB-ACE Chemotherapy For Germ Cell Tumors of the Ovary

POMB	
Day 1	*Vincristine* 1 mg/m^2 IV; *methotrexate* 300 mg/m^2 as a 12-hr infusion
Day 2	*Bleomycin* 15 mg as a 24-hr infusion: *folinic acid* rescue started at 24 hrs after the start of *methotrexate* in a dose of 15 mg every 12 hrs for 4 doses
Day 3	*Bleomycin* infusion 15 mg by 24-hr infusion
Day 4	*Cisplatin* 120 mg/m^2 as a 12-hr infusion, given with hydration and 3 g magnesium sulfate supplementation
ACE	
Days 1–5	*Etoposide* (VP16-213) 100 mg/m^2, days 1–5
Days 3, 4, 5	*Actinomycin D* 0.5 mg IV, days 3, 4, and 5
Day 5	*Cyclophosphamide* 500 mg/m^2 IV, day 5
OMB	
Day 1	*Vincristine* 1 mg/m^2 IV; *methotrexate* 300 mg/m^2 as a 12-hr infusion
Day 2	*Bleomycin* 15 mg by 24-hr infusion; *folinic acid* rescue started at 24 hrs after start of *methotrexate* in a dose of 15 mg every 12 hrs for 4 doses
Day 3	*Bleomycin* 15 mg by 24-hr infusion

IV, intravenous; hCG, human chorionic gonadotropin; AFP, α-fetoprotein; PLAP, placental alkaline phosphatase; LDH, lactate dehydrogenase.
The sequence of treatment schedules is two courses of POMB followed by ACE. POMB is then alternated with ACE until patients are in biochemical remission as measured by hCG and AFP, PLAP, and LDH. The usual number of courses of POMB is three to five. Following biochemical remission, patients alternate ACE with OMB until remission has been maintained for approximately 12 weeks. The interval between courses of treatment is kept to the minimum (usually 9 to 11 days). If delays are caused by myelosuppression after courses of ACE, the first 2 days of etoposide are omitted from subsequent courses of ACE.
From **Newlands ES, Southall PJ, Paradinas FJ, et al.** Management of ovarian germ cell tumours. In: **Williams CJ, Kaikorian JG, Green MR, et al.,** eds. *Textbook of uncommon cancer.* New York: John Wiley and Sons, 1988:47, with permission.

Pregnancy

Because dysgerminomas tend to occur in young patients, they may coexist with pregnancy. When a stage Ia cancer is found, the tumor can be removed intact and the pregnancy continued. For patients with more advanced disease, continuation of the pregnancy depends on the gestational age of the fetus. Chemotherapy can be given in the second and third trimesters in the same dosages as given for the nonpregnant patient without apparent detriment to the fetus (287).

Prognosis

For patients whose initial disease is stage Ia (i.e., a unilateral encapsulated dysgerminoma), unilateral oophorectomy alone results in a 5-year disease-free survival rate of greater than 95% (277,278). The features that have been associated with a higher tendency to recur include lesions larger than 10 to 15 cm in diameter, age younger than 20 years, and a microscopic pattern that includes numerous mitoses, anaplasia, and a medullary pattern (2,270).

Although in the past, surgery for advanced disease followed by pelvic and abdominal irradiation resulted in a 5-year survival rate of 63% to83%, cure rates of 85% to 90% for this same group of patients are now being reported with the use of VBP, BEP, or EC combination chemotherapy (278–288).

Immature Teratomas

Immature teratomas contain elements that resemble tissues derived from the embryo. Immature teratomatous elements may occur in combination with other germ cell tumors as mixed germ cell tumors. The pure immature teratoma accounts for fewer than 1% of all ovarian cancers, but it is the second most common germ cell malignancy. This lesion represents 10% to 20% of all ovarian malignancies seen in women younger than 20 years and 30% of the deaths from ovarian cancer in this age group (2). About 50% of pure immature teratomas of the ovary occur in women between the ages of 10 and 20 years, and they rarely occur in postmenopausal women.

Pathology

Of fundamental importance in the understanding of the teratoma is a recognition of the maturation of the various elements. If maturation continues along normal lines, the mature or adult teratoma results, and the prognosis is excellent. Conversely, abnormal maturation of these elements produces undisciplined growth that can be fatal. Teratomas containing immature elements, although relative rate, have been recognized more commonly during the past two decades (Fig. 32.18). Among the tumors with embryonal elements, those containing neural tissues demonstrate most clearly the importance of the ability to mature. Gliomatosis peritonei is the most dramatic demonstration of the significance of maturation, because most patients with these tumors have survived, even with this disseminated disease (3).

Immature teratomas are classified according to a grading system (grades 1 to 3) that is based on the degree of differentiation and the quantity of immature tissue (241). A determination of the amount of undifferentiated neural tissue is of prognostic importance. A grade 1 tumor is one in which less than one low-power microscopic field (LPF) contains immature neural elements, a grade 2 tumor has one to three LPFs with immature elements, and a grade 3 tumor has more than three LPFs with these elements. **The prognosis can be correlated with the grade determined by the quantity of these immature neural elements; with a higher grade there is a poorer prognosis** (2,3).

Previously, most malignant teratomas were classified as secondary neoplasms developing in a primarily benign teratoma. During the last decade, lesions composed primarily of immature embryonal or extraembryonal elements have become more prevalent, and the basic demonstration of malignancy is the inability of the tissue to mature rather than the presence of individual cell anaplasia (i.e., the mitotic activity may be low). This unique aspect is demonstrated by an absence of aneuploidy in the few cases that have been studied (3).

Figure 32.18 Ovarian teratoma. This tumor contains both mature and immature neural elements with a neural tube–like structure near its center. (From **Berek JS, Hacker NF.** *Practical gynecologic oncology,* 3rd ed. Philadelphia: Lippincott Williams & Wilkins, 2000:150, with permission.)

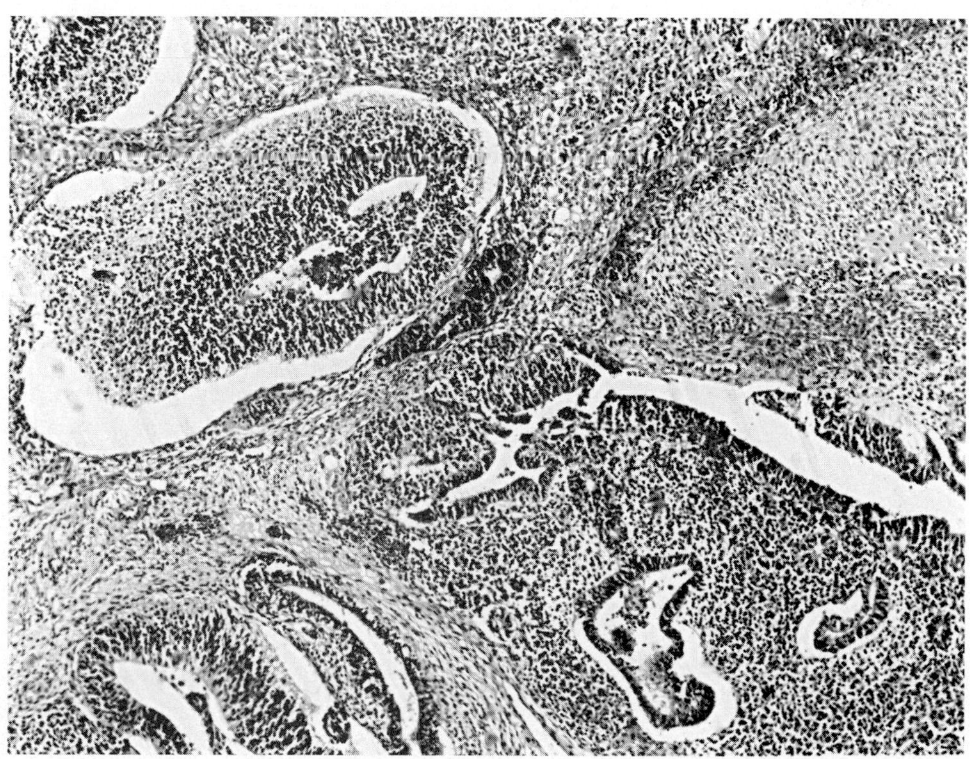

Malignant change in benign cystic teratomas has been recorded as occurring in 0.5% to 2% of cases, usually in patients over 40 years of age (293). The most common malignancy developing in the initially benign teratoma is squamous cell carcinoma. Other neoplasms have been reported (e.g., melanomas, which may arise from the skin or retinal anlage, and sarcomas, including leiomyosarcomas and mixed mesodermal tumors) (285). Carcinomas may arise from any of the epithelial elements.

Diagnosis

The preoperative evaluation and differential diagnosis of immature teratomas are the same as for other germ cell tumors. Some of these lesions will contain calcifications similar to those of mature teratomas, which can be detected by a radiograph of the abdomen or by ultrasonography. Rarely, they are associated with the production of steroid hormones and can be accompanied by sexual pseudoprecocity (268). Tumor markers are negative unless a mixed germ cell tumor is present.

Treatment

Surgery

For a premenopausal patient whose lesion appears to be confined to a single ovary, unilateral oophorectomy and surgical staging should be performed. For a postmenopausal patient, a total abdominal hysterectomy and bilateral salpingo-oophorectomy may be performed. Contralateral involvement is rare, and routine resection or wedge biopsy of the contralateral ovary is unnecessary (3,293). Any lesions on the peritoneal surfaces should be sampled and submitted for histologic evaluation. The most frequent site of dissemination is the peritoneum and, much less commonly, the retroperitoneal lymph nodes. Bloodborne metastases to organ parenchyma, such as the lungs, liver, or brain, are uncommon. When present, they are usually seen in patients with late or recurrent disease and most often in tumors that are poorly differentiated (i.e., grade 3).

Chemotherapy

Patients with stage Ia, grade 1 tumors have an excellent prognosis, and no adjuvant therapy is required. For patients whose tumors are stage Ia, grades 2 or 3, adjuvant chemotherapy should be used (281–283,290,302). Chemotherapy is also indicated for patients who have ascites, regardless of tumor grade. The most frequently used combination chemotherapeutic regimen in the past has been VAC (296–298). However, in a GOG study, the relapse-free survival rate in patients with incompletely resected disease was only 75% (298). The newer approach has been to incorporate *cisplatin* into the primary treatment of these tumors, and most of the experience has been with the VBP and BEP regimens (302). No direct comparison of these regimens with VAC has been reported, but the BEP combination can save some patients who have persistent or recurrent disease after VAC (302).

The GOG has been prospectively studying three courses of BEP therapy for patients with completely resected stage I, II, and III ovarian germ cell tumors (302). Overall, the toxicity has been acceptable, and 91 of 93 patients whose nondysgerminomatous tumors were treated are clinically free of disease. **Thus, the BEP regimen, which is used more extensively for testicular cancer, seems to be superior to the VAC regimen in the treatment of completely resected nondysgerminomatous germ cells tumors of the ovary.** Because some tumors can progress rapidly, treatment should be initiated as soon as possible after surgery, preferably within 7 to 10 days.

The switch from VBP to BEP has been prompted by the experience in patients with testicular cancer, in which the replacement of *vinblastine* with *etoposide* has been associated with a better therapeutic index (i.e., equivalent efficacy and lower morbidity), especially less neurologic and gastrointestinal toxicity. Furthermore, the use of

***bleomycin* seems to be important for this group of patients.** In a randomized study of three cycles of *etoposide* plus *cisplatin* with or without *bleomycin* (EP versus BEP) in 166 patients with germ cell tumors of the testes, the BEP regimen had a relapse-free survival rate of 84% compared with 69% for the EP regimen ($p = 0.03$) (288). In addition, *cisplatin* may be slightly better than *carboplatin* in the setting of metastatic germ cell tumors. One hundred ninety-two patients with germ cell tumors of the testes were entered into a study of four cycles of *etoposide* plus *cisplatin* (EP) versus four cycles of etoposide plus *carboplatin* (EC). There have been three relapses with the EP regimen versus seven with the EC regimen, although the overall survival of the two groups is identical thus far (289). In view of these results, **BEP is the preferred treatment regimen for patients with gross residual disease and has replaced the VAC regimen for patients with completely resected disease.**

Patients who have immature teratomas with malignant squamous elements seem to have a poorer prognosis than those whose tumors are without these elements (285). The treatment in these patients is also the BEP regimen.

Radiation Therapy

Radiation therapy is generally not used in the primary treatment of patients with immature teratomas. Furthermore, there is no evidence that the combination of chemotherapy and radiation has a higher rate of disease control than chemotherapy alone. Radiation therapy should be reserved for patients with localized persistent disease after chemotherapy (278,290).

Second-look Laparotomy

The need for a second-look operation has been questioned (291,292). It seems not to be justified in patients who have received chemotherapy in an adjuvant setting (i.e., stage Ia, grades 2 and 3), because chemotherapy in these patients is so effective. Second-look laparotomy in patients with macroscopic residual disease is of value at the start of chemotherapy, because there are no reliable tumor markers for this disease and such patients are at higher risk of failure.

If a second-look operation is performed, sampling of any peritoneal lesions should be performed and the retroperitoneal lymph nodes should be evaluated carefully. If only mature elements are found during the second-look procedure, chemotherapy should be discontinued. If the presence of persistent immature elements is documented, alternative chemotherapy should be employed. An enlarged contralateral ovary may contain a benign cyst or a mature cystic teratoma, which may be managed with an ovarian cystectomy (266,268).

Prognosis

The most important prognostic feature of the immature teratoma is the grade of the lesion (2,293). In addition, the stage of disease and the extent of tumor at the initiation of treatment have an impact on the curability of the lesion. Patients whose tumors have been incompletely resected before treatment have a significantly lower probability of 5-year survival than those whose lesions have been completely resected (i.e., 94% versus 50%) (268). Overall, the 5-year survival rate for patients with all stages of pure immature teratomas is 70% to 80%, and it is 90% to 95% for patients with surgically determined stage I lesions (290,293,294).

The degree or grade of immaturity generally correlates with the metastatic potential and curability. The 5-year survival rates for all stages combined have been reported to be 82%, 62%, and 30% for patients with grades 1, 2, and 3, respectively (293). Occasionally, these tumors are associated with mature or low-grade glial elements that have implanted throughout the peritoneum, and such patients usually have a favorable long-term survival (2,3).

Endodermal Sinus Tumors

Endodermal sinus tumors (EST) have also been referred to as *yolk sac carcinomas,* because they are derived from the primitive yolk sac (2,3). These lesions are the third most frequent malignant germ cell tumors of the ovary. ESTs occur in patients with a median age of 16 to 18 years (2,3,303,304). About one-third of the patients are premenarcheal at the time of diagnosis. Abdominal or pelvic pain is the most frequent initial symptom, occurring in about 75% of patients, whereas an asymptomatic pelvic mass is documented in 10% of patients (267).

Pathology

The gross appearance of an EST is soft grayish-brown. Cystic areas caused by degeneration are present in these rapidly growing lesions. The capsule is intact in most cases.

The EST is unilateral in 100% of cases; thus, biopsy of the opposite ovary in such young patients is contraindicated. The association of such lesions with gonadal dysgenesis must be appreciated, and chromosomal analysis should be performed preoperatively in premenarcheal patients (3).

Microscopically, the characteristic feature is the endodermal sinus, or *Schiller-Duval body* (Fig. 32.19). The cystic space is lined with a layer of flattened or irregular endothelium into which projects a glomerulus-like tuft with a central vascular core. These structures vary throughout the tumor, and the reticular, myxoid elements represent undifferentiated mesoblast. The lining of the papillary infolding and the cavity is irregular, with an occasional cell containing clear, glassy cytoplasm, simulating the hobnail appearance of the epithelium in clear cell tumors. The association of EST with dysgerminoma must be emphasized if diagnosis and therapy are to be optimal (2,3).

Figure 32.19 Endodermal sinus tumor of the ovary. Note the classic Schiller-Duval body with its central vessel and mantle of endoderm *(arrow).* (From **Berek JS, Hacker NF.** *Practical gynecologic oncology,* 2nd ed. Baltimore: Williams & Wilkins, 1994:151, with permission.)

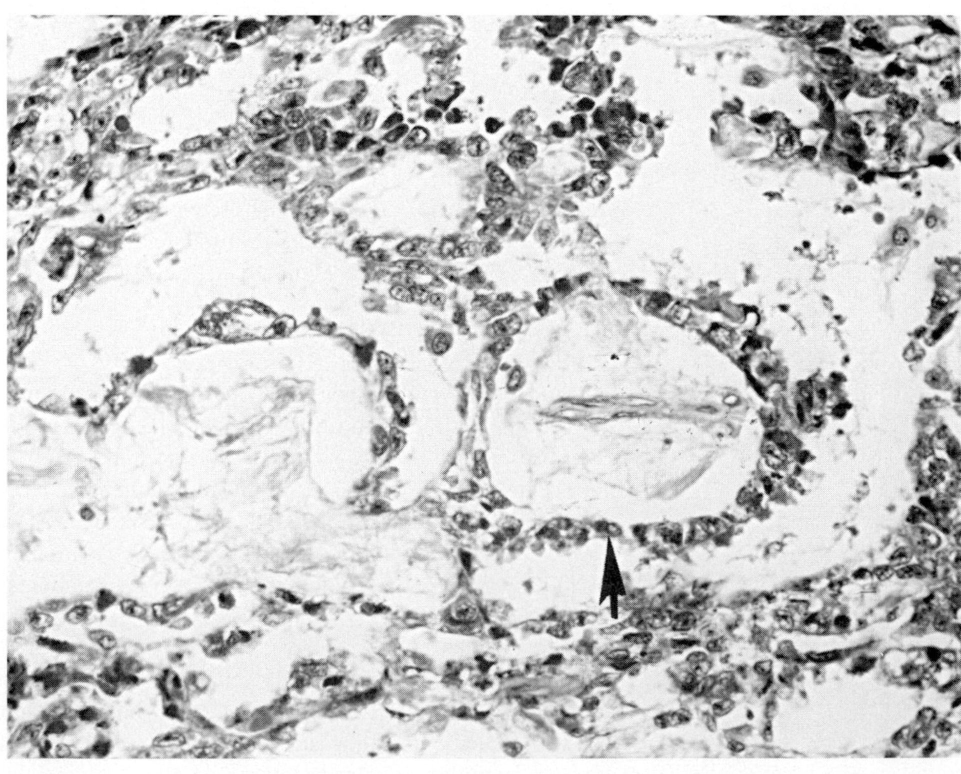

Most EST lesions secrete AFP and, rarely, they may elaborate detectable AAT. AFP can be demonstrated in the tumor by means of the immunoperoxidase technique. There is a good correlation between the extent of disease and the level of AFP, although discordance also has been observed. The serum level of these markers, particularly AFP, is useful in monitoring the patient's response to treatment (303–309).

Treatment

Surgery

The treatment of the EST consists of surgical exploration, unilateral salpingo-oophorectomy, and a frozen section for diagnosis. The addition of a hysterectomy and contralateral salpingo-oophorectomy does not alter outcome (268,307). Any gross metastases should be removed, if possible, but thorough surgical staging is not indicated because all patients need chemotherapy. At surgery, the tumors tend to be solid and large, ranging in size from 7 to 28 cm (median, 15 cm) in the GOG series (268,302). Bilaterality is not seen in these lesions, and the other ovary is involved with metastatic disease only when there are other metastases in the peritoneal cavity. Most patients have early-stage disease: 71%, stage I; 6%, stage II; and 23%, stage III (309).

Chemotherapy

All patients with ESTs are treated with either adjuvant or therapeutic chemotherapy. Before the routine use of combination chemotherapy for this disease, the 2-year survival rate was only about 25%. After the introduction of the VAC regimen, this rate improved to 60% to 70%, indicating the chemosensitivity of most of these tumors (297,298). Furthermore, with conservative surgery and adjuvant chemotherapy, fertility can be preserved as with other germ cell tumors.

VPB is a more effective regimen in the treatment of EST, particularly in the treatment of measurable or incompletely resected tumors (302). In the GOG series, only about 20% of patients with residual metastatic disease responded completely to the VAC regimen, whereas about 60% of those treated with VBP had a complete response (282). In addition, this regimen may save some patients in whom VAC therapy has failed.

Workers at the Charing Cross Hospital in London have developed the POMB-ACE regimen for high-risk germ cell tumors of any histologic type (310) (Table 32.7). This protocol introduces seven drugs into the initial management, which is intended to minimize the chances of developing drug resistance. Drug resistance is particularly relevant for patients with massive metastatic disease, and the POMB-ACE regimen may be used as primary therapy for such patients as well as for those with liver or brain metastases. The POMB schedule is only moderately myelosuppressive, so the intervals between each course can be kept to a maximum of 14 days (usually 9 to 11 days), thereby minimizing the time for tumor regrowth between courses. When *bleomycin* is given by a 48-hour infusion, pulmonary toxicity is reduced. With a maximum of 9 years of follow-up, the Charing Cross group has seen no long-term side effects for patients treated with POMB-ACE. Children have developed normally, menstruation has been physiologic, and several have completed normal pregnancies.

***Cisplatin*-containing combination chemotherapy, preferably BEP or POMB-ACE, should be used as primary chemotherapy for ESTs.** The optimal number of treatment cycles has not been established. The GOG protocols have used three to four treatment cycles given every 4 weeks (302,310). Alternatively, three cycles can be given to patients with stage I and completely resected disease, and two further cycles can be given after negative tumor marker status is achieved by patients with macroscopic residual disease before chemotherapy.

Second-look Laparotomy

The value of a second-look operation has yet to be established in patients with an EST. It seems reasonable to omit the operation for patients with pure low-stage lesions and for patients whose AFP values return to normal and remain normal for the balance of their treatment (308,309). There have been reported cases in which the AFP has returned to normal despite persistent measurable disease; some of these cases have been mixed germ cell tumors (309). For patients whose AFP levels do not return to normal, persistent disease can be assumed and alternative chemotherapy (e.g., POMB-ACE) can be offered.

Embryonal Carcinoma

Embryonal carcinoma of the ovary is an extremely rare tumor that is distinguished from a choriocarcinoma of the ovary by the absence of syncytiotrophoblastic and cytotrophoblastic cells. The patients are very young; ages ranged between 4 and 28 years (median, 14 years) in two series (311). Older patients have been reported (312). Embryonal carcinomas may secrete estrogens, with the patient exhibiting symptoms and signs of precocious pseudopuberty or irregular bleeding (2). The clinical picture is otherwise similar to that of the EST. The primary lesions tend to be large, and about two-thirds are confined to one ovary at the time of diagnosis. These lesions frequently secrete AFP and hCG, which are useful for following the response to subsequent therapy (308). **The treatment of embryonal carcinomas is the same as for the EST (i.e., a unilateral oophorectomy followed by combination chemotherapy with BEP)** (282,302). Radiation does not seem to be useful for primary treatment.

Choriocarcinoma of the Ovary

Pure nongestational choriocarcinoma of the ovary is an extremely rare tumor. Histologically, it has the same appearance as gestational choriocarcinoma metastatic to the ovaries (313). Most patients with this cancer are younger than 20 years. The presence of hCG can be useful in monitoring the patient's response to treatment. **In the presence of high hCG levels, isosexual precocity has been seen to occur in about 50% of patients whose lesions appear before menarche** (314).

There are only a few limited reports on the use of chemotherapy for nongestational choriocarcinomas, but complete responses have been reported with the MAC (*methotrexate, actinomycin D,* and *cyclophosphamide*) regimen used in a manner described for gestational trophoblastic disease (313) (see Chapter 34). Alternatively, the BEP regimen can be used. The prognosis of ovarian choriocarcinomas has been poor, with most patients having metastases to organ parenchyma at the time of diagnosis.

Polyembryoma

Polyembryoma of the ovary is another extremely rare tumor, which is composed of "embryoid bodies." This tumor replicates the structures of early embryonic differentiation (i.e., the three somatic layers: endoderm, mesoderm, and ectoderm) (2,270). The lesion tends to occur in very young, premenarcheal girls with signs of pseudopuberty and elevated AFP and hCG titers. Anecdotally, the VAC chemotherapeutic regimen has been reported to be effective (297).

Mixed Germ Cell Tumors

Mixed germ cell malignancies of the ovary contain two or more elements of the lesions described above. In one series (315), the most common component of a mixed malignancy was dysgerminoma, which occurred in 80%, followed by EST in 70%, immature teratoma in 53%, choriocarcinoma in 20%, and embryonal carcinoma in 16%. **The most frequent combination was a dysgerminoma and an EST. The mixed lesions may secrete either AFP, hCG, or both or neither of these markers, depending on the components.**

These lesions should be managed with combination chemotherapy, preferably BEP. The serum marker, if positive initially, may become negative during chemotherapy, but this finding may reflect regression of only a particular component of the mixed lesion. Therefore, for these patients, a second-look laparotomy may be indicated to determine the precise response to therapy if macroscopic disease was present at initiation of chemotherapy.

The most important prognostic features are the size of the primary tumor and the relative size of its most malignant component (315). For stage IA lesions smaller than 10 cm, survival is 100%. Tumors composed of less than one-third EST, choriocarcinoma, or grade 3 immature teratoma also have an excellent prognosis, but it is less favorable when these components constitute most of the mixed lesions.

Sex Cord–stromal Tumors

Sex cord–stromal tumors of the ovary account for about 5% to 8% of all ovarian malignancies (2,3,266,267,316–319). This group of ovarian neoplasms is derived from the sex cords and the ovarian stroma or mesenchyme. The tumors usually are composed of various combinations of elements, including the "female" cells (i.e., granulosa and theca cells), and "male" cells (i.e., Sertoli and Leydig cells), as well as morphologically indifferent cells. A classification of this group of tumors is presented in Table 32.8.

Granulosa-stromal Cell Tumors

Granulosa-stromal cell tumors include granulosa cell tumors, thecomas, and fibromas. The granulosa cell tumor is a low-grade malignancy; rarely, thecomas and fibromas have morphologic features of malignancy and then may be referred to as fibrosarcomas.

Granulosa cell tumors, which secrete estrogen, are seen in women of all ages. They are found in prepubertal girls in 5% of cases; the remainder are found in women throughout their reproductive and postmenopausal years (319). Granulosa cell tumors are bilateral in only 2% of patients.

Pathology

Granulosa cell tumors range from a few millimeters to 20 centimeters or more in diameter. The tumors are rarely bilateral, and they have a smooth, lobulated surface. The solid portions of the tumor are granular, frequently trabeculated, and are commonly yellow or gray-yellow in color. The granulosa-theca cell tumor is probably the most inaccurately diagnosed lesion of the female gonad. Of 477 ovarian tumors from the Emil

Table 32.8. Sex Cord–stromal Tumors

1. Granulosa-stromal cell tumors
- A. Granulosa cell tumor
- B. Tumors in thecoma-fibroma group
  - 1) Thecoma
  - 2) Fibroma
  - 3) Unclassified

2. Androblastomas; Sertoli-Leydig cell tumors
- A. Well-differentiated
  - 1) Sertoli cell tumor
  - 2) Sertoli-Leydig cell tumor
  - 3) Leydig cell tumor; hilus cell tumor
- B. Moderately differentiated
- C. Poorly differentiated (sarcomatoid)
- D. With heterologous elements

3. Gynandroblastoma

4. Unclassified

From **Young RE, Scully RE.** Ovarian sex cord–stromal tumors: recent progress. *Int J Gynecol Pathol* 1980;1:153, with permission.

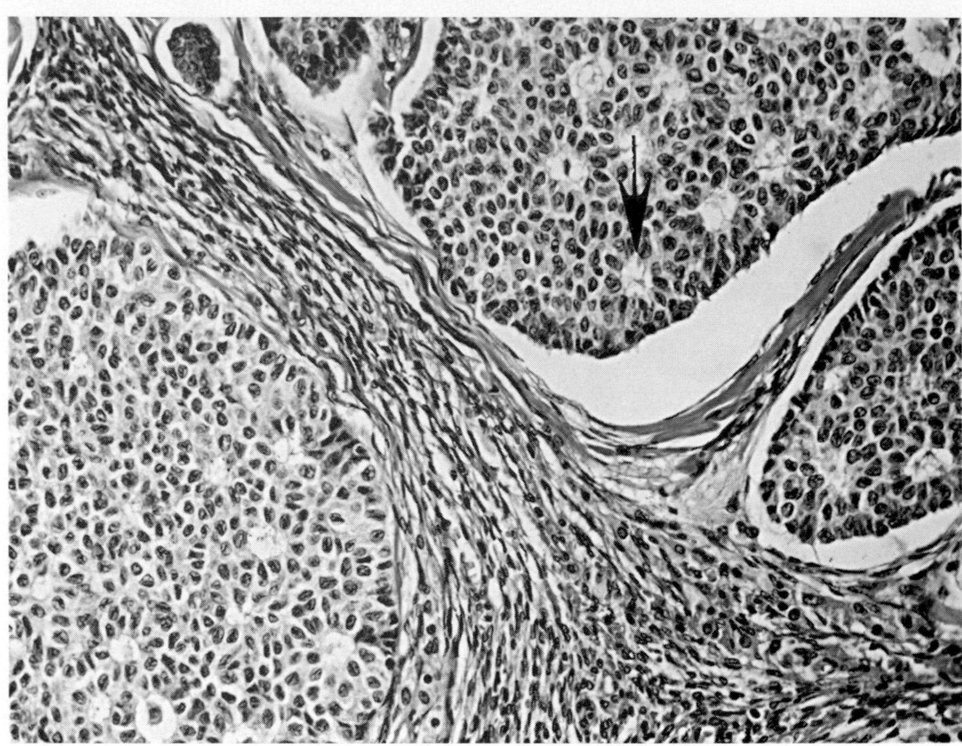

Figure 32.20 Granulosa cell tumor of the ovary. Note the classic Call-Exner bodies *(arrow)* with a minimal stromal component in this tumor of folliculoid pattern. (From **Berek JS, Hacker NF.** *Practical gynecologic oncology,* 2nd ed. Baltimore: Williams & Wilkins, 1994:153, with permission.)

Novak Ovarian Tumor Registry diagnosed initially as granulosa-theca cell tumors, almost 15% were reclassified after histologic review. Lesions misdiagnosed as granulosa cell tumors included metastatic carcinomas, teratoid tumors, and poorly differentiated mesothelial tumors (316).

The classic granulosa cell is round or ovoid with scant cytoplasm. The nucleus contains compact, finely granular cytoplasm suggesting hyperchromatism (3). "Coffee bean" grooved nuclei are common, as are mitoses, thus simulating the corresponding elements in the normal, mature follicle. Conversely, if the epithelial elements are bizarre with atypical mitoses, the lesion should not be categorized as a poorly differentiated granulosa cell tumor but instead as an undifferentiated mesothelial neoplasm. In the most common variety, the granulosa cells show a tendency to arrange themselves in small clusters or rosettes around a central cavity, so there is a resemblance to primordial follicles (i.e., *Call-Exner bodies*) (Fig. 32.20). The stroma is similar to the theca and may be luteinized. In children and adolescents, the granular cell tumors are often cystic, contain luteinized cells, and can be associated with precocious puberty.

Diagnosis

Of the rare prepubertal lesions, 75% are associated with sexual pseudoprecocity because of the estrogen secretion (319). For women of reproductive age, most patients have menstrual irregularities or secondary amenorrhea, and cystic hyperplasia of the endometrium is frequently present. For postmenopausal women, abnormal uterine bleeding is frequently the initial symptom. Indeed, the estrogen secretion in these patients can be sufficient to stimulate the development of endometrial cancer. **Endometrial cancer occurs in association with granulosa cell tumors in at least 5% of cases, and 25% to 50% are associated with endometrial hyperplasia** (2,314,316–319).

The other symptoms and signs of granulosa cell tumors are nonspecific and the same as most ovarian malignancies. Ascites is present in about 10% of cases, and rarely a pleural effusion is present (316–319). Granulosa tumors tend to be hemorrhagic; occasionally, they rupture and produce a hemoperitoneum.

Granulosa cell tumors are usually stage I at diagnosis but may recur 5 to 30 years after initial diagnosis (318). The tumors may also spread hematogenously, and metastases can develop in the lungs, liver, and brain years after initial diagnosis. When granulosa cell tumors do recur, they can progress quite rapidly. Malignant thecomas are extremely rare, and their signs and symptoms, management, and outcome are similar to those of the granulosa cell tumors (316). **Inhibin is secreted by some granulosa cell tumors and is a useful marker for the disease** (320–322).

Treatment

The treatment of granulosa cell tumors depends on the age of the patient and the extent of disease. For most patients, surgery alone is sufficient primary therapy; radiation and chemotherapy are reserved for the treatment of recurrent or metastatic disease (319–322).

Surgery

Because granulosa cell tumors are bilateral in only about 2% of patients, a unilateral salpingo-oophorectomy is appropriate therapy for stage Ia tumors in children or in women of reproductive age (317). At the time of laparotomy, if a granulosa cell tumor is identified by frozen section, a staging operation is performed, including an assessment of the contralateral ovary. If the opposite ovary appears enlarged, it should be sampled for biopsy. For perimenopausal and postmenopausal women for whom ovarian preservation is not important, a hysterectomy and bilateral salpingo-oophorectomy should be performed. For premenopausal patients in whom the uterus is left *in situ,* an endometrial biopsy should be performed, because of the possibility of a coexistent adenocarcinoma of the endometrium (319).

Radiation Therapy

There is no evidence to support the use of adjuvant radiation therapy for granulosa cell tumors, although pelvic irradiation may help to palliate isolated pelvic recurrences (319).

Chemotherapy

There is no evidence that adjuvant chemotherapy will prevent recurrence of disease. Metastatic lesions and recurrences have been treated with a variety of antineoplastic drugs. The most effective chemotherapeutic regimen appears to be BEP. In a GOG study (323), 37% (14 of 30) patients treated with BEP had a negative second-look laparotomy, and completely responding patients had a median time to progression of 24.4 months. The use of hormonal agents such as progestins or antiestrogens has been suggested, but there are no data available to suggest effectiveness (317).

Prognosis

Granulosa cell tumors have a prolonged natural history and a tendency toward late relapse, reflecting their low-grade biology. As such, 10-year survival rates of about 90% have been reported, with 20-year survival rates dropping to 75% (317–319). Most histologic types have the same prognosis, but patients with the more poorly differentiated diffuse or sarcomatoid type tend to do worse (316).

The DNA ploidy of the tumors has recently been correlated with survival. Holland and colleagues (324) reported DNA aneuploidy in 13 of 37 patients (35%) with primary granulosa cell tumors. The presence of residual disease was found to be the most important predictor of progression-free survival, but DNA ploidy was an independent prognostic factor. **Patients with residual-negative DNA diploid tumors had a 10-year progression-free survival of 96%.**

Sertoli-Leydig Tumors

Sertoli-Leydig tumors occur most frequently in the third and fourth decades of life; 75% of the lesions are seen in women younger than 40 years. These lesions are extremely rare and account for less than 0.2% of ovarian cancers (2). Sertoli-Leydig cell tumors are most frequently low-grade malignancies, although occasionally a poorly differentiated variety may behave more aggressively.

The tumors typically produce androgens, and clinical virilization is noted in 70% to 85% of patients (325). Signs of virilization include oligomenorrhea followed by amenorrhea, breast atrophy, acne, hirsutism, clitoromegaly, deepening of the voice, and a receding hairline. Measurement of plasma androgens may reveal elevated testosterone and androstenedione, with normal or slightly elevated dehydroepiandrosterone sulphate (2,325). Rarely, the Sertoli-Leydig tumor can be associated with manifestations of estrogenization (i.e., isosexual precocity, irregular or postmenopausal bleeding).

Treatment

Because these low-grade lesions are only rarely bilateral (<1%), the usual treatment is unilateral salpingo-oophorectomy and evaluation of the contralateral ovary for patients who are in their reproductive years (3,319). For older patients, hysterectomy and bilateral salpingo-oophorectomy are appropriate.

There are insufficient data to document the utility of radiation or chemotherapy for patients with persistent disease, but some responses in patients with measurable disease have been reported with pelvic irradiation and the VAC chemotherapy regimen (3,268).

Prognosis

The 5-year survival rate is 70% to 90%, and recurrences thereafter are uncommon (3,325). Most fatalities occur in the presence of poorly differentiated lesions.

Uncommon Ovarian Cancers

There are several varieties of malignant ovarian tumors that together constitute only 0.1% of ovarian malignancies (2). Two of these lesions are the lipoid (or lipid) cell tumors and the primary ovarian sarcomas.

Lipoid Cell Tumors

Lipoid cell tumors are believed to arise in adrenal cortical rests that reside in the vicinity of the ovary. More than 100 cases have been reported, and bilateral disease has been noted in only a few (2). Most are associated with virilization and, occasionally, with obesity, hypertension, and glucose intolerance reflecting corticosteroid secretion. Rare cases of estrogen secretion and isosexual precocity have been reported.

Most of these tumors have benign or low-grade behavior, but about 20%, most of which are initially larger than 8 cm in diameter, are associated with metastatic lesions. Metastases are usually in the peritoneal cavity but rarely occur at distant sites. The primary treatment is surgical extirpation of the primary lesion. There are no data regarding the effectiveness of radiation or chemotherapy for this disease.

Sarcomas

Malignant mixed mesodermal sarcomas of the ovary are extremely rare; only about 100 cases have been reported. Most lesions are heterologous, and 80% occur in postmenopausal women. The signs and symptoms are similar to those of most ovarian malignancies. These lesions are biologically aggressive, and most patients have evidence of metastases.

There is no effective treatment for ovarian sarcomas, and most patients die within 2 years. *Doxorubicin,* with or without *cyclophosphamide,* has produced an occasional partial response, and *cisplatin* is currently undergoing clinical trials (326–328). For patients in whom all macroscopic disease can be resected, we have observed disease-free survival of more than 3 years in two patients treated with six cycles of *cisplatin* and *epirubicin.*

Small Cell Carcinomas

This rare tumor occurs at an average age of 24 years (range 2 to 46 years) (389). The tumors are all bilateral. Approximately two-thirds of the tumors are accompanied by paraendocrine hypercalcemia. This tumor accounts for one-half of all of the cases of hypercalcemia associated with ovarian tumors. About 50% of the tumors have spread beyond the ovaries when they are diagnosed (329).

The management of these malignancies consists of surgery followed by platinum-based chemotherapy or radiation therapy or both. In addition to the primary treatment of the disease, control of the hypercalcemia may require aggressive hydration, loop diuretics, and the use of bisphosphonates or *calcitonin.* The prognosis tends to be poor, with most patients dying within 2 years of diagnosis in spite of treatment.

Metastatic Tumors

About 5% to 6% of ovarian tumors are metastatic from other organs, most frequently from the female genital tract, the breast, or the gastrointestinal tract (330–335). The metastases may occur from direct extension of another pelvic neoplasm, by hematogenous spread, lymphatic spread, or transcoelomic dissemination, with surface implantation of tumors that spread in the peritoneal cavity.

Gynecologic

Nonovarian cancers of the genital tract can spread by direct extension or they may metastasize to the ovaries. Tubal carcinoma involves the ovaries secondarily in 13% of cases (2,3), usually by direct extension. Under some circumstances, it is difficult to know whether the tumor originated in the tube or in the ovary when both are involved. Cervical cancer spreads to the ovary only in rare cases (<1%), and most of these are of an advanced clinical stage or are adenocarcinomas. Although adenocarcinoma of the endometrium can spread and implant directly onto the surface of the ovaries in as many as 5% of cases, two synchronous primary tumors probably occur with greater frequency. In these cases, an endometrioid carcinoma of the ovary is usually associated with the adenocarcinoma of the endometrium.

Nongynecologic

The frequency of metastatic breast carcinoma to the ovaries varies according to the method of determination, but the phenomenon is common (Fig. 32.21). **In autopsy data of women who died of metastatic breast cancer, the ovaries were involved in 24% of cases, and 80% of the involvement was bilateral** (330–333). Similarly, when ovaries are removed to palliate advanced breast cancer, about 20% to 30% of the cases reveal ovarian involvement, 60% of those bilaterally. The involvement of ovaries in early-stage breast cancer seems to be considerably lower, but precise figures are not available. In almost all cases, either ovarian involvement is occult or a pelvic mass is discovered after other metastatic disease becomes apparent.

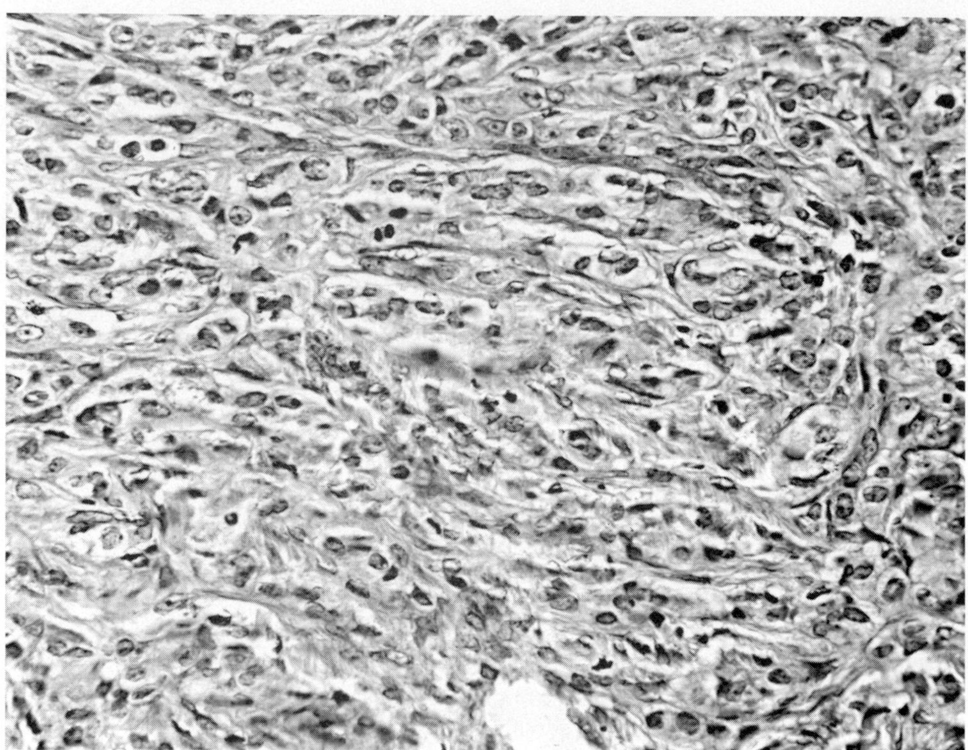

Figure 32.21 Metastatic carcinoma in the ovary. Note the "Indian file" pattern found in this metastatic breast carcinoma. (From **Berek JS, Hacker NF.** *Practical gynecologic oncology,* 2nd ed. Baltimore: Williams & Wilkins, 1994:157, with permission.)

Krukenberg Tumor

The Krukenberg tumor, which can account for 30% to 40% of metastatic cancers to the ovaries, arises in the ovarian stroma and has characteristic mucin-filled, signet-ring cells (334) (Fig. 32.22). The primary tumor is most frequently located in the stomach and less commonly in the colon, breast, or biliary tract. Rarely, the cervix or the bladder may be the primary site. Krukenberg tumors can account for about 2% of ovarian cancers at some institutions, and they are usually bilateral. The lesions are usually not discovered until the primary disease is advanced and, therefore, most patients die of their disease within 1 year. In some cases, a primary tumor is never found.

Other Gastrointestinal Tumors

In other cases of metastasis from the gastrointestinal tract to the ovary, the tumor does not have the classic histologic appearance of a Krukenberg tumor; most of these are from the colon and, less commonly, the small intestine. As many as 1% to 2% of women with intestinal carcinomas will develop metastases to the ovaries during the course of their disease (332). Before exploration for an adnexal tumor in a woman older than 40 years, a barium enema is indicated to exclude a primary gastrointestinal carcinoma with metastases to the ovaries, particularly if there are any gastrointestinal symptoms. Metastatic colon cancer can mimic a mucinous cystadenocarcinoma of the ovary histologically (331,332).

Melanoma

Rare cases of malignant melanoma metastatic to the ovaries have been reported (335). In these circumstances, the melanomas are usually widely disseminated. Removal would be warranted for palliation of abdominal or pelvic pain, bleeding, or torsion.

Carcinoid Tumors

Metastatic carcinoid tumors represent fewer than 2% of metastatic lesions to the ovaries (336). Conversely, only about 2% of patients with primary carcinoids have evidence of ovarian metastasis, and only 40% of them have the carcinoid syndrome at the time of

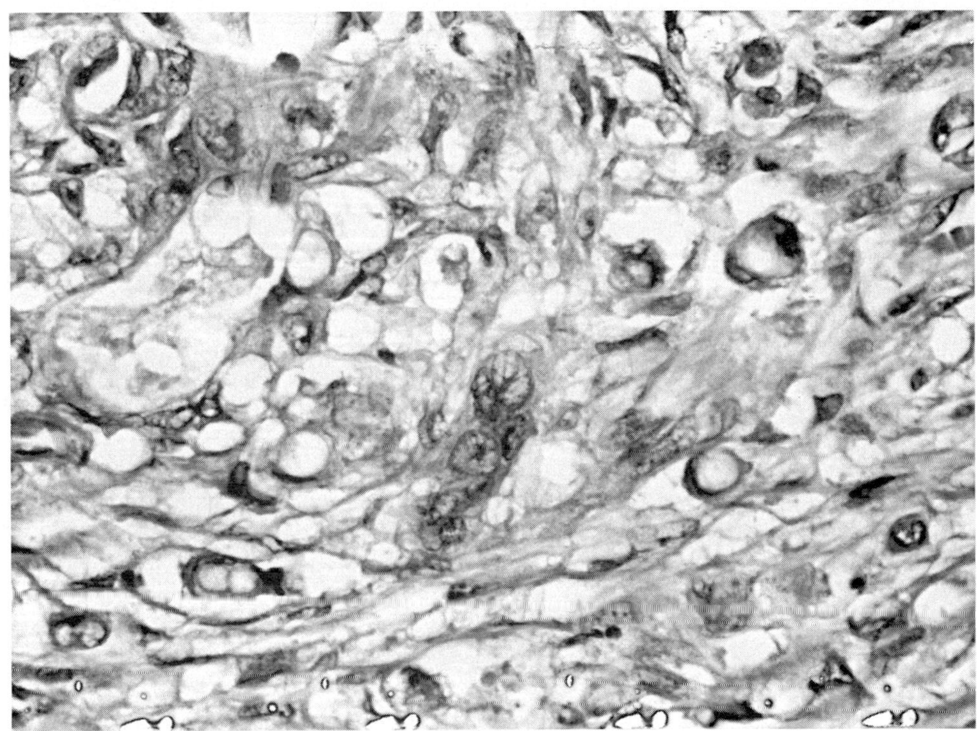

Figure 32.22 Krukenberg tumor of the ovary metastatic from a gastric carcinoma. Malignant cells have discrete vacuoles that push nuclei eccentrically, giving a signet-ring appearance. Mucicarmine stain demonstrates the cytoplasmic vacuoles to be mucin. (From **Berek JS, Hacker NF.** *Practical gynecologic oncology,* 2nd ed. Baltimore: Williams & Wilkins, 1994:158, with permission.)

discovery of the metastatic carcinoid. However, in perimenopausal and postmenopausal women explored for an intestinal carcinoid, it is reasonable to remove the ovaries to prevent subsequent ovarian metastasis. Furthermore, the discovery of an ovarian carcinoid should prompt a careful search for a primary intestinal lesion.

Lymphoma and Leukemia

Lymphomas and leukemia can involve the ovary. When they do, the involvement is usually bilateral (337,338). About 5% of patients with Hodgkin's disease will have lymphomatous involvement of the ovaries, but this involvement occurs typically with advanced-stage disease. **With Burkitt's lymphoma, ovarian involvement is very common. Other types of lymphoma involve the ovaries much less frequently, and leukemic infiltration of the ovaries is uncommon.** Sometimes the ovaries can be the only apparent site of involvement of the abdominal or pelvic viscera with a lymphoma; if this circumstance is found, a careful surgical exploration may be necessary. Intraoperatively, a hematologist-oncologist should be consulted to determine the need for these procedures if frozen section of a solid ovarian mass reveals a lymphoma. In general, most lymphomas no longer require extensive surgical staging, although biopsy of enlarged lymph nodes should generally be performed. In some cases of Hodgkin's disease, a more extensive evaluation may be necessary. Treatment involves that of the lymphoma or leukemia in general. Removal of a large ovarian mass may improve patient comfort and facilitate a response to subsequent radiation or chemotherapy.

Fallopian Tube Cancer

Carcinoma of the fallopian tube accounts for 0.3% of all cancers of the female genital tract (2,3,339–343). In histologic features and behavior, fallopian tube carcinoma is

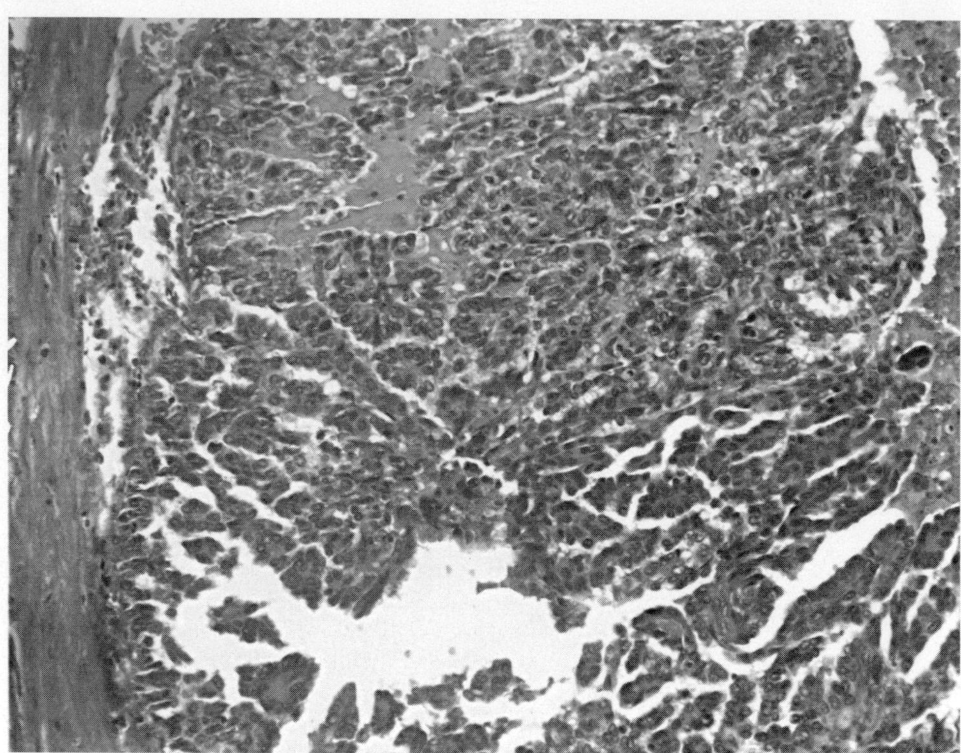

Figure 32.23 Carcinoma of the fallopian tube. This is the mixed papillary and the papillary-alveolar pattern. (From **Berek JS, Hacker NF.** *Practical gynecologic oncology,* 2nd ed. Baltimore: Williams & Wilkins, 1994:159, with permission.)

similar to ovarian cancer; thus, the evaluation and treatment are also essentially the same (Fig. 32.23). The fallopian tubes are frequently involved secondarily from other primary sites, most often the ovaries, endometrium, gastrointestinal tract, or breast. They may also be involved in primary peritoneal carcinomatosis. Almost all cancers are of epithelial origin, most frequently of serous histology. Rarely, sarcomas have also been reported.

Clinical Features

Tubal cancers are seen most frequently in the fifth and sixth decades, with a mean age of 55 to 60 years (339). There are no known predisposing factors.

Symptoms and Signs

The classic triad of symptoms and signs associated with fallopian tube cancer is (a) a prominent watery vaginal discharge (i.e., hydrops tubae profluens), (b) pelvic pain, and (c) a pelvic mass. However, this triad is noted in fewer than 15% of patients (3).

Vaginal discharge or bleeding is the most common symptom reported by patients with tubal carcinoma and is documented in more than 50% of patients (3,340). Lower abdominal or pelvic pressure and pain also are noted in many patients. However, the symptoms may be rather vague and nonspecific. For perimenopausal and postmenopausal women with unusual, unexplained, or persistent vaginal discharge, even in the absence of bleeding, the clinician should be concerned about the possibility of occult tubal cancer. Fallopian tube cancer is often found incidentally in asymptomatic women at the time of abdominal hysterectomy and bilateral salpingo-oophorectomy.

On examination, a pelvic mass is present in about 60% of patients, and ascites may be present if advanced disease exists. For patients with tubal carcinoma, the results of dilation and curettage will be negative (342), although abnormal or adenocarcinomatous cells may be seen in cytologic specimens obtained from the cervix in 10% of patients.

Spread Pattern

Tubal cancers spread in much the same manner as epithelial ovarian malignancies, principally by the transcoelomic exfoliation of cells that implant throughout the peritoneal cavity. In about 80% of the patients with advanced disease, metastases are confined to the peritoneal cavity at the time of diagnosis (341).

The fallopian tube is richly permeated with lymphatic channels, and spread to the paraaortic and pelvic lymph nodes is common. Metastases to the paraaortic lymph nodes have been documented in at least 33% of the patients with all stages of disease (343).

Staging

Fallopian tube cancer is staged according to FIGO (339). **The staging is based on the surgical findings at laparotomy** (Table 32.9). According to this system, about 20% to 25% of patients have stage I disease, 20% to 25% have stage II disease, 40% to 50% have stage III disease, and 5% to 10% have stage IV disease (339). A somewhat lower incidence of advanced disease is seen in these patients than in patients with epithelial ovarian carcinomas, presumably because of the earlier occurrence of symptoms, particularly vaginal bleeding or unusual vaginal discharge.

Treatment

The treatment of this disease is the same as that of epithelial ovarian cancer (339, 342,344). Exploratory laparotomy is necessary to remove the primary tumor, to stage the disease, and to resect metastases. After surgery, the most frequently employed treatment is combination chemotherapy, although radiation therapy is also used in selected cases.

Surgery

Patients with tubal carcinoma should undergo total abdominal hysterectomy and bilateral salpingo-oophorectomy (3). If there is no evidence of gross tumor spread, a staging operation is performed. The retroperitoneal lymph nodes should be adequately evaluated, and peritoneal cytologic studies and biopsies should be performed, along with an infracolic omentectomy.

In patients with metastatic disease, an effort should be made to remove as much tumor bulk as possible. The role of cytoreductive surgery in this disease is unclear, but extrapolation from the experience with epithelial ovarian cancer indicates that significant benefit might be expected, particularly if all macroscopic disease can be resected.

Chemotherapy

The most active combination chemotherapy for epithelial ovarian cancer is *carboplatin* and *paclitaxel,* and it is appropriate, therefore, to use the same chemotherapy for patients with epithelial tubal malignancies (3).

Data on well-staged lesions are scarce. Therefore, it is unclear whether patients with disease confined to the fallopian tube (i.e., a stage Ia, grade 1 or 2 carcinoma), benefit from additional therapy.

Radiation Therapy

Although most patients with tubal cancers have been treated with radiation therapy in the past, its role in the management of the disease remains unclear, because patients have not been treated in any consistent manner and the small numbers treated preclude any meaningful conclusions (342). Pelvic irradiation alone was once popular, but this approach seems inappropriate when the pattern of spread of this disease to the upper abdomen is

Table 32.9. Modified FIGO Staging of Fallopian Tube Cancer (Based on Operative Findings Before Debulking and Pathologic Findings)

Stage 0	Carcinoma *in situ*[a] (limited to tubal mucosa).[b]
Stage I	Growth is limited to the fallopian tubes.
Stage Ia	Growth is limited to one tube with extension into the submucosa[c] and/or muscularis but not penetrating the serosal surface; no ascites.
Stage Ib	Growth is limited to both tubes with extension into the submucosa[c] and/or muscularis but not penetrating the serosal surface: no ascites.
Stage Ic	Tumor either stage Ia or Ib but with tumor extension through or onto the tubal serosa; or with ascites present containing malignant cells or with positive peritoneal washings.
Stage II	Growth involving one or both fallopian tubes with pelvic extension.
Stage IIa	Extension and/or metastasis to the uterus and/or ovaries.
Stage IIb	Extension to other pelvic tissues.
Stage IIc	Tumor either stage IIa or IIb but with tumor extension through or onto the tubal serosa; or with ascites present containing malignant cells or with positive peritoneal washings.
Stage III	Tumor involves one or both fallopian tubes with peritoneal implants outside of the pelvis and/or positive retroperitoneal or inguinal nodes. Superficial liver metastases equals stage III. Tumor appears limited to the true pelvis but with histologically proven malignant extension to the small bowel or omentum.
Stage IIIa	Tumor is grossly limited to the true pelvis with negative nodes but with histologically confirmed microscopic seeding of abdominal peritoneal surfaces.
Stage IIIb	Tumor involving one or both tubes with histologically confirmed implants of abdominal peritoneal surfaces, none exceeding 2 cm in diameter. Lymph nodes are negative.
Stage IIIc	Abdominal implants greater than 2 cm in diameter and/or positive retroperitoneal or inguinal nodes.
Stage IV	Growth involving one or both fallopian tubes with distant metastases. If pleural effusion is present, there must be positive cytology to be stage IV. Parenchymal liver metastases equals stage IV.

FIGO, International Federation of Gynecology and Obstetrics.
[a]The staging system does not distinguish between microscopic foci or replacement of tubal epithelium by malignant epithelium and grossly evident masses in the tubal lumen that do not penetrate the wall beyond the epithelium. The former have not been reported to spread beyond the tube, whereas the latter can extend beyond the tube, recur, and be fatal.
[b]The *mucosa* presumably refers to the epithelium because involvement of the lamina propria component of the mucosa requires staging of the tumor as Ia.
[c]Because the fallopian tube has no *submucosa,* this designation presumably refers to the lamina propria.
From **Berek JS, Hacker NF,** eds. *Practical gynecologic oncology,* 3rd ed. Philadelphia: Lippincott Williams & Wilkins, 2000:546, with permission.

considered (340). Whole-abdominal irradiation with a pelvic boost has been used in patients with no evidence of gross disease in the abdomen (i.e., completely resected disease or microscopic metastases only) (3,339).

Prognosis

The overall 5-year survival for patients with epithelial tubal carcinomas is about 40%. This number is higher than for patients with ovarian cancer and reflects the somewhat higher proportion of patients diagnosed with early-stage disease. The outlook is clearly related to the stage of disease, but the available data relate to patients who have not been surgically staged. Thus, the reported 5-year survival rate for patients with stage I disease is only about 65%. The 5-year survival rate for patients with stage II disease is 50% to 60%, but it is only 10% to 20% for patients with stages III and IV disease (339).

Tubal Sarcomas

Tubal sarcomas, particularly malignant mixed mesodermal tumors, have been described but are rare. They occur mainly in the sixth decade and are typically advanced at the time of diagnosis. If all gross disease can be resected, platinum-based combination chemotherapy should be tried. However, survival is generally poor, and most patients die of their disease within 2 years (2,326).

References

1. **Jemal A, Thomas A, Murray T, et al.** Cancer statistics, 2002. *CA Cancer J Clin* 2002;52:23–47.

2. **Scully RE, Young RH, Clement PB.** Tumors of the ovary, maldeveloped gonads, fallopian tube, and broad ligament. In: Atlas of tumor pathology. Washington: Armed Forces Institute of Pathology; 1998; Fascicle 23, 3rd series.

3. **Berek JS, Hacker NF.** *Practical gynecologic oncology,* 3rd ed. Philadelphia: Lippincott Williams & Wilkins, 2000:3–38.

4. **Barnhill DR, Kurman RJ, Brady MF, et al.** Preliminary analysis of the behavior of stage I ovarian serous tumors of low malignant potential: a Gynecologic Oncology Group study. *J Clin Oncol* 1995;13:2752–2756.

5. **Seidman JD, Kurman RJ.** Subclassification of serous borderline tumors of the ovary into benign and malignant types. A clinicopathologic study of 65 advanced stage cases. *Am J Surg Pathol* 1996;20:1331–1345.

6. **Bell DA, Weinstock MA, Scully RE.** Peritoneal implants of ovarian serous borderline tumors: histologic features and prognosis. *Cancer* 1988;62:2212–2222.

7. **Bell DA.** Ovarian surface epithelial-stromal tumors. *Hum Pathol* 1991;22:750–762.

8. **Bell DA, Scully RE.** Clinical perspectives on borderline tumors of the ovary. In: **Greer BE, Berek JS,** eds. *Gynecologic oncology: treatment rationale and techniques.* New York: Elsevier Science, 1991: 119–134.

9. **McCaughey WT, Kirk ME, Lester W, et al.** Peritoneal epithelial lesions associated with proliferative serous tumours of the ovary. *Histopathology* 1984;8:195–208.

10. **Michael H, Roth LM.** Invasive and noninvasive implants in ovarian serous tumors of low malignant potential. *Cancer* 1986;57:1240–1247.

11. **Gershenson DM, Silva EG.** Serous ovarian tumors of low malignant potential with peritoneal implants. *Cancer* 1990;65:578–585.

12. **Bell DA, Scully RE.** Ovarian serous borderline tumors with stromal microinvasion: a report of 21 cases. *Hum Pathol* 1990;21:397–403.

13. **Sampson JA.** Endometrial carcinoma of the ovary. *Arch Surg* 1925;10:1.

14. **Kurman RJ, Craig JM.** Endometrioid and clear cell carcinomas of the ovary. *Cancer* 1972;29:1653–1664.

15. **Roth LM, Dallenbach-Hellweg G, Czernobilsky B.** Ovarian Brenner tumors. I. Metaplastic proliferating and of low grade potential. *Cancer* 1985;56:582–591.

16. **Robey SS, Silva EG, Gershenson DM, et al.** Transitional cell carcinoma in high-grade stage ovarian carcinoma: an indicator of favorable response to chemotherapy. *Cancer* 1989;63:839–847.

17. **Silva EG, Robey-Cafferty SS, Smith TL, et al.** Ovarian carcinomas with transitional cell carcinoma pattern. *Am J Clin Pathol* 1990;93:457–462.

18. **Austin RM, Norris HJ.** Malignant Brenner tumor and transitional cell carcinoma of the ovary: a comparison. *Int J Gynecol Pathol* 1987;6:29–34.

19. **Thor AD, Young RH, Clement PB.** Pathology of the fallopian tube, broad ligament, peritoneum, and pelvic soft tissue. *Hum Pathol* 1991;22:856–867.

20. **Tobachman JK, Greene MH, Tucker MA, et al.** Intraabdominal carcinomatosis after prophylactic oophorectomy in ovarian cancer–prone families. *Lancet* 1982;2:795–797.

21. **Piver MS, Jishi MF, Tsukada Y, et al.** Primary peritoneal carcinoma after prophylactic oophorectomy in women with a family history of ovarian cancer: a report of the Gilda Radner Familial Ovarian Cancer Registry. *Cancer* 1993;71:2751–2755.

22. **Fowler JM, Nieberg RK, Schooler TA, et al.** Peritoneal adenocarcinoma (serous) of müllerian type: a subgroup of women presenting with peritoneal carcinomatosis. *Int J Gynecol Cancer* 1994;4:43–51.

23. **Truong LD, Maccato ML, Awalt H, et al.** Serous surface carcinoma of the peritoneum: a clinicopathology study of 22 cases. *Hum Pathol* 1990;21:99–110.

24. **Pecorelli S, Odicino F, Maisonneuve P, et al.** Carcinoma of the ovary. Annual report on the results of treatment of gynaecological cancer, vol 23. International Federation of Gynecology and Obstetrics. *J Epidemiol Biostat* 1998;3:75–102.

25. **Norris HJ, Jensen RD.** Relative frequency of ovarian neoplasms in children and adolescents. *Cancer* 1972;30:713–719.

26. **Negri E, Franceschi S, Tzonou A, et al.** Pooled analysis of three European case-control studies of epithelial ovarian cancer: I. Reproductive factors and risk of epithelial ovarian cancer. *Int J Cancer* 1991;49: 50–56.

27. **Franceschi S, La Vecchia C, Booth M, et al.** Pooled analysis of three European case-control studies of epithelial ovarian cancer: II. Age at menarche and menopause. *Int J Cancer* 1991;49:57–60.

28. **Franceschi, S, Parazzini F, Negri E, et al.** Pooled analysis of three European case-control studies of epithelial ovarian cancer: III. Oral contraceptive use. *Int J Cancer* 1991;49:61–65.

29. **De Palo G, Vceronesi U, Camerini T, et al.** Can fenretinide protect women against ovarian cancer. *J Natl Cancer Inst* 1995;87:146–147.

30. **Campbell S, Bhan V, Royston P, et al.** Transabdominal ultrasound screening for early ovarian cancer. *BMJ* 1989;299:1363–1367.

31. **Higgins RV, van Nagell JR Jr, Donaldson ES, et al.** Transvaginal sonography as a screening method for ovarian cancer. *Gynecol Oncol* 1989;34:402–406.

32. **van Nagell JR Jr, DePriest PD, Puls LE, et al.** Ovarian cancer screening in asymptomatic postmenopausal women by transvaginal sonography. *Cancer* 1991;68:458–462.

33. **Rulin MC, Preston AL.** Adnexal masses in postmenopausal women. *Obstet Gynecol* 1987;70:578–581.

34. **Kurjak A, Zalud I, Jurkovic D, et al.** Transvaginal color flow Doppler for the assessment of pelvic circulation. *Acta Obstet Gynecol Scand* 1989;68:131–135.

35. **Kurjak A, Zalud I, Alfirevic Z.** Evaluation of adnexal masses with transvaginal color ultrasound. *J Ultrasound Med* 1991;10:295–297.

36. **Rustin GJS, van der Burg MEL, Berek JS.** Tumor markers. *Ann Oncol* 1993;4:S71–77.

37. **Jacobs I, Davies AP, Bridges J, et al.** Prevalence screening for ovarian cancer in postmenopausal women by CA 125 measurements and ultrasonography. *BMJ* 1993;306:1030–1034.

38. **Jacobs IJ, Skates S, Davies AP, et al.** Risk of diagnosis of ovarian cancer after raised serum CA 125 concentration: a prospective cohort study. *BMJ* 1996;313:1355–1358.

39. **Einhorn N, Sjovall K, Knapp RC, et al.** A prospective evaluation of serum CA 125 levels for early detection of ovarian cancer. *Obstet Gynecol* 1992;80:14–18.

40. **Jacobs IJ, Oram DH, Bast RC Jr.** Strategies for improving the specificity of screening for ovarian cancer with tumor-associated antigens CA125, CA15-3, and TAG 72.3. *Obstet Gynecol* 1992;80:396–399.

41. **Berek JS, Bast RC Jr.** Ovarian cancer screening: the use of serial complementary tumor markers to improve sensitivity and specificity for early detection. *Cancer* 1995;76:2092–2096.

42. **Skates SJ, Xu FJ, Yu YH, et al.** Towards an optimal algorithm for ovarian cancer screening with longitudinal tumour markers. *Cancer* 1995;76:2004–2010.

43. **Jacobs IJ, Skates SJ, MacDonald N, et al.** Screening for ovarian cancer: a pilot randomised controlled trial. *Lancet* 1999;353:1207–1210.

44. **Genetic risk and screening techniques for epithelial ovarian cancer.** ACOG Committee Opinion 1992;117.

45. **Bourne TH, Campbell S, Reynolds KM, et al.** Screening for early familial ovarian cancer with transvaginal ultrasonography and colour blood flow imaging. *BMJ* 1993;306:1025–1029.

46. **Easton DF, Ford D, Bishop DT.** Breast Cancer Linkage Consortium: breast and ovarian cancer incidence in *BRCA1*-mutation carriers. *Am J Hum Genet* 1995;56:265–271.

47. **Whittemore AS, Gong G, Itnyre J.** Prevalence and contribution of *BRCA1* mutations in breast cancer and ovarian cancer: results from three U.S. population-based case-control studies of ovarian cancer. *Am J Hum Genet* 1997;60:496–504.

48. **Frank TS, Manley SA, Olopade OI, et al.** Sequence analysis of *BRCA1* and *BRCA2:* Correlation of mutations with family history and ovarian cancer risk. *J Clin Oncol* 1998;16:2417–2425.

49. **Johannsson OT, Ranstam J, Borg A, et al.** Survival of *BRCA1* breast and ovarian cancer patients: a population-based study from southern Sweden. *J Clin Oncol* 1998;16:397–404.

50. **Burke W, Daly M, Garber J, et al.** Recommendations for follow-up care of individuals with an inherited predisposition to cancer. II. *BRCA1* and *BRCA2.* Cancer Genetics Studies Consortium. *JAMA* 1997;277: 997–1003.

51. **Berchuck A, Cirisano F, Lancaster JM, et al.** Role of *BRCA1* mutation screening in the management of familial ovarian cancer. *Am J Obstet Gynecol* 1996;175:738–746.

52. **Struewing JP, Hartge P, Wacholder S, et al.** The risk of cancer associated with specific mutations of *BRCA1* and *BRCA2* among Ashkenazi Jews. *N Engl J Med* 1997;336:1401–1408.

53. **Beller U, Halle D, Catane R, et al.** High frequency of *BRCA1* and *BRCA2* germline mutations in Ashkenazi Jewish ovarian cancer patients, regardless of family history. *Gynecol Oncol* 1997;67:123–126.

54. **Lerman C, Narod S, Schulman K, et al.** *BRCA1* testing in families with hereditary breast-ovarian cancer: a prospective study of patient decision making and outcomes. *JAMA* 1996;275:1885–1892.

55. **Ponder B.** Genetic testing for cancer risk. *Science* 1997;278:1050–1058.

56. **Lynch HT, Cavalieri RJ, Lynch JF, et al.** Gynecologic cancer clues to Lynch Syndrome II diagnosis: a family report. *Gynecol Oncol* 1992;44:198–203.

57. **Statement of the American Society of Clinical Oncology: genetic testing for cancer susceptibility.** *J Clin Oncol* 1996;14:1730–1736.

58. **NIH Consensus Development Panel on Ovarian Cancer: Ovarian Cancer.** Screening, treatment and follow-up. *JAMA* 1995;273:491–497.

59. **Narod SA, Risch H, Moslehi R, et al.** Oral contraceptives and the risk of hereditary ovarian cancer. *N Engl J Med* 1998;339:424–428.

60. **Averette HE, Nguyen HN.** The role of prophylactic oophorectomy in cancer prevention. *Gynecol Oncol* 1994;55:S38–41.

61. **Lu KH, Garber JE, Cramer DW, et al.** Prophylactic oophorectomies in women at high risk for ovarian cancer. *Proc Soc Gynecol Oncol* 1999;30(abst).

62. **Goff BA, Mandel LS, Muntz HG, et al.** Ovarian cancer diagnosis: results of a national ovarian cancer survey. *Cancer* 2000;89:2068–2075.

63. **Olson SSH, Mignone L, Nakraseive C, et al.** Symptoms of ovarian cancer. *Obstet Gynecol* 2001;98: 212–217.

64. **Smith EM, Anderson B.** The effects of symptoms and delay in seeking diagnosis on stage of disease at diagnosis among women with cancers of the ovary. *Cancer* 1985;56:2727–2732.

65. **Barber HK, Grober EA.** The PMPO syndrome (postmenopausal palpable ovary syndrome). *Obstet Gynecol* 1971;138:921–923.

66. **Malkasian GD, Knapp RC, Lavin PT, et al.** Preoperative evaluation of serum CA 125 levels in premenopausal and postmenopausal patients with pelvic masses: discrimination of benign from malignant disease. *Am J Obstet Gynecol* 1988;159:341–346.

67. **Lewis E, Wallace S.** Radiologic diagnosis of ovarian cancer. In: **Piver MS,** ed. *Ovarian malignancies.* Edinburgh: Churchill Livingstone, 1987:59–80.

68. **Hacker NF, Berek JS, Lagasse LD.** Gastrointestinal operations in gynecologic oncology. In: **Knapp RE, Berkowitz RS,** eds. *Gynecologic oncology,* 2nd ed. New York, McGraw-Hill, 1993:361–375.

69. **Plentl AM, Friedman EA.** *Lymphatic system of the female genitalia.* Philadelphia: WB Saunders, 1971.

70. **Chen SS, Lee L.** Incidence of paraaortic and pelvic lymph node metastasis in epithelial ovarian cancer. *Gynecol Oncol* 1983;16:95–100.

71. **Burghardt E, Pickel H, Lahousen M, et al.** Pelvic lymphadenectomy in operative treatment of ovarian cancer. *Am J Obstet Gynecol* 1986;155:315–319.

72. **Dauplat J, Hacker NF, Neiberg RK, et al.** Distant metastasis in epithelial ovarian carcinoma. *Cancer* 1987;60:1561–1566.

73. **Krag KJ, Canellos GP, Griffiths CT, et al.** Predictive factors for long term survival in patients with advanced ovarian cancer. *Gynecol Oncol* 1989;34:88–93.

74. **Young RC, Walton LA, Ellenberg SS, et al.** Adjuvant therapy in stage I and stage II epithelial ovarian cancer: results of two prospective randomized trials. *N Engl J Med* 1990;322:1021–1027.

75. **Bjorkholm E, Pettersson F, Einhorn N, et al.** Long term follow-up and prognostic factors in ovarian carcinoma. The Radiumhemmet series 1958 to 1973. *Acta Radiol Oncol* 1982;21:413–419.

76. **Malkasian GD, Decker DG, Webb MJ.** Histology of epithelial tumours of the ovary: clinical usefulness and prognostic significance of histologic classification and grading. *Semin Oncol* 1975;2:191–201.

77. **Silverberg SG.** Prognostic significance of pathologic features of ovarian carcinoma. *Curr Top Pathol* 1989;78:85–109.

78. **Jacobs AJ, Deligdisch L, Deppe G, et al.** Histologic correlations of virulence in ovarian adenocarcinoma. 1. Effects of differentiation. *Am J Obstet Gynecol* 1982;143:574–580.

79. **Baak JP, Langley FA, Talerman A, et al.** Interpathologist and intrapathologist disagreement in ovarian tumor grading and typing. *Anal Quant Cytol Histol* 1986;8:354–357.

80. **Hernandez E, Bhagavan BS, Parmley TH, et al.** Interobserver variability in the interpretation of epithelial ovarian cancer. *Gynecol Oncol* 1984;17:117–123.

81. **Baak JP, Chan KK, Stolk JG, et al.** Prognostic factors in borderline and invasive ovarian tumours of the common epithelial type. *Pathol Res Pract* 1987;182:755–774.

82. **Friedlander ML, Heldey DW, Swanson C, et al.** Prediction of long term survivals by flow cytometric analysis of cellular DNA content in patients with advanced ovarian cancer. *J Clin Oncol* 1988;6: 282–290.

83. **Reles AE, Conway G, Schellerschmidt I, et al.** Prognostic significance of DNA content and S-phase fraction in epithelial ovarian carcinomas analyzed by image cytometry. *Gynecol Oncol* 1998;71:3–13.

84. **Kaern J, Tropé CG, Kristensen GB, et al.** Flow cytometric DNA ploidy and S-phase heterogeneity in advanced ovarian carcinoma. *Cancer* 1994;73:1870–1877.

85. **Conte PF, Alama A, Rubagotti A, et al.** Cell kinetics in ovarian cancer: relationship to clinicopathologic features, responsiveness to chemotherapy and survival. *Cancer* 1989;64:1188–1191.

86. **Kuhn W, Kaufmann M, Feichter GE, et al.** DNA flow cytometry, clinical and morphological parameters as prognostic factors for advanced malignant and borderline tumors. *Gynecol Oncol* 1989;33:360–367.

87. **Berek JS, Martínez-Maza O.** Molecular and biological factors in the pathogenesis of ovarian cancer. *J Reprod Med* 1994;39:241–248.

88. **Berek JS, Martínez-Maza O, Hamilton T, et al.** Molecular and biological factors in the pathogenesis of ovarian cancer. *Ann Oncol* 1993;4:S3–16.

89. **Slamon DJ, Godolphin W, Jones LA, et al.** Studies of the *HER-2/neu* protooncogene in human breast and ovarian cancer. *Science* 1989;244:707–712.

90. **Berchuck A, Kamel A, Whitaker R, et al.** Overexpression of *HER-2/neu* is associated with poor survival in advanced epithelial ovarian cancer. *Cancer Res* 1990;50:4087–4091.

91. **Rubin SC, Finstad CL, Wong GY, et al.** Prognostic significance of HER-2/*neu* expression in advanced epithelial ovarian cancer: a multivariate analysis. *Am J Obstet Gynecol* 1993;168:162–169.

92. **Leary JA, Edwards BG, Houghton CRS.** Amplification of HER-2/*neu* oncogene in human ovarian cancer. *Int J Gynecol Oncol* 1993;2:291.

93. **Meden H, Marx D, Rath W, et al.** Overexpression of the oncogene *c-erb B2* in primary ovarian cancer: evaluation of the prognostic value in a Cox proportional hazards multiple regression. *Int J Gynecol Pathol* 1994;13:45–53.

94. **Makar AP, Holm R, Kristensen GB, et al.** The expression of *c-erbB-2 (her-2/neu)* oncogene in invasive ovarian malignancies. *Int J Gynecol Cancer* 1994;4:194–199.

95. **Rubin SC, Finstad CL, Federici MG, et al.** Prevalence and significance of *HER-2/neu* expression in early epithelial ovarian cancer. *Cancer* 1994;73:1456–1459.

96. **Singleton TP, Perrone T, Oakley G, et al.** Activation of *c-erb-B-2* and prognosis in ovarian carcinoma. Comparison with histologic type, grade, and stage. *Cancer* 1994;73:1460–1466.

97. **Hutson R, Ramsdale J, Wells M.** *p53* Protein expression in putative precursor lesions of epithelial ovarian cancer. *Histopathology* 1995;27:367–371.

98. **Gotlieb WH, Watson JM, Rezai BA, et al.** Cytokine-induced modulation of tumor suppressor gene expression in ovarian cancer cells: upregulation of *p53* gene expression and induction of apoptosis by tumor necrosis factor-α. *Am J Obstet Gynecol* 1994;170:1121–1128.

99. **Kohler MF, Kerns BJ, Humphrey PA, et al.** Mutation and overexpression of *p53* in early-stage ovarian cancer. *Obstet Gynecol* 1993;81:643–650.

100. **Dittrich C, Dittrich E, Sevelda P, et al.** Clonogenic growth *in vitro:* an independent biologic prognostic factor in ovarian carcinoma. *J Clin Oncol* 1991;9:381–388.

101. **Sevin BU, Perras JP, Averette HE, et al.** Chemosensitivity testing in ovarian cancer. *Cancer* 1993;71: 1613–1620.

102. **Federico M, Alberts DS, Garcia DJ, et al.** *In vitro* drug testing of ovarian cancer using the human tumor colony-forming assay: comparison of in vitro response and clinical outcome. *Gynecol Oncol* 1994;55: S156–63.

103. **Omura GA, Brady MF, Homesley HD, et al.** Long-term follow-up and prognostic factor analysis in advanced ovarian carcinoma: the Gynecologic Oncology Group experience. *J Clin Oncol* 1991;9: 1138–1150.

104. **Voest EE, van Houwelingen JC, Neijt JP.** A meta-analysis of prognostic factors in advanced ovarian cancer with median survival and overall survival measured with log (relative risk) as main objectives. *Eur J Cancer Clin Oncol* 1989;25:711–720.

105. **van Houwelingen JC, ten Bokkel Huinink WW, van der Burg ATM, et al.** Predictability of the survival of patients with ovarian cancer. *J Clin Oncol* 1989;7:769–773.

106. **Berek JS, Bertlesen K, du Bois A, et al.** Advanced epithelial ovarian cancer: 1998 consensus statement. *Ann Oncol* 1999;10:S1:87–92.

107. **Sharp F, Blackett AD, Berek JS, et al.** Conclusions and recommendations from the Helene Harris Memorial Trust sixth biennial international forum on ovarian cancer. *Int J Gynecol Cancer* 1997;7:416–424.

108. **Dembo AJ, Davy M, Stenwig AE, et al.** Prognostic factors in patients with stage I epithelial ovarian cancer. *Obstet Gynecol* 1990;75:263–273.

109. **Sjövall K, Nilsson B, Einhorn N.** Different types of rupture of the tumor capsule and the impact on survival in early ovarian cancer. *Int J Gynecol Cancer* 1994;4:333–336.

110. **Sevelda P, Dittich C, Salzer H.** Prognostic value of the rupture of the capsule in stage I epithelial ovarian carcinoma. *Gynecol Oncol* 1989;35:321–322.

111. **Vergote I, Fyles A, Bertelsen K, et al.** Analysis of prognostic factors in 1287 patients with FIGO stage I invasive ovarian cancer. *Proc Am Soc Clin Oncol* 1998;1839(abst).

112. **Berek JS, Hacker NF.** Staging and second-look operations in ovarian cancer. In: **Alberts DS, Surwit EA,** eds. *Ovarian cancer.* Boston: Martinus Nijhoff, 1985:109–127.

113. **Young RC, Decker DG, Wharton JT, et al.** Staging laparotomy in early ovarian cancer. *JAMA* 1983;250:3072–3076.

114. **Buchsbaum HJ, Lifshitz S.** Staging and surgical evaluation of ovarian cancer. *Semin Oncol* 1984;11: 227–237.

115. **Yoshimuna S, Scully RE, Bell DA, et al.** Correlation of ascitic fluid cytology with histologic findings before and after treatment of ovarian cancer. *Am J Obstet Gynecol* 1984;148:716–721.

116. **Piver MS, Barlow JJ, Lele SB.** Incidence of subclinical metastasis in stage I and II ovarian carcinoma. *Obstet Gynecol* 1978;52:100–104.

117. **Delgado G, Chun B, Caglar H.** Paraaortic lymphadenectomy in gynecologic malignancies confined to the pelvis. *Obstet Gynecol* 1977;50:418–423.

118. **Rosenoff SH, Young RC, Anderson T, et al.** Peritoneoscopy: a valuable staging tool in ovarian carcinoma. *Ann Intern Med* 1975;83:37–41.

119. **Knapp RC, Friedman EA.** Aortic lymph node metastases in early ovarian cancer. *Am J Obstet Gynecol* 1974;119:1013–1017.

120. **Keettel WC, Pixley EL, Buchsbaum HJ.** Experience with peritoneal cytology in the management of gynecologic malignancies. *Am J Obstet Gynecol* 1974;120:174–182.

121. **Creasman WT, Rutledge F.** The prognostic value of peritoneal cytology in gynecologic malignant disease. *Am J Obstet Gynecol* 1971;110:773–781.

122. **Guthrie D, Davy MLJ, Phillips PR.** Study of 656 patients with "early" ovarian cancer. *Gynecol Oncol* 1984;17:363–369.

123. **Bostwick DG, Tazelaar HD, Ballon SC, et al.** Ovarian epithelial tumors of borderline malignancy: a clinical and pathologic study of 109 cases. *Cancer* 1986;58:2052–2065.

124. **Lim-Tan SK, Cajigas HE, Scully RE.** Ovarian cystectomy for serous borderline tumors: a follow-up study of 35 cases. *Obstet Gynecol* 1988;72:775–781.

125. **Griffiths CT.** Surgical resection of tumor bulk in the primary treatment of ovarian carcinoma. *Natl Cancer Inst Monogr* 1975;42:101–104.

126. **Hacker NF, Berek JS.** Cytoreductive surgery in ovarian cancer. In: **Albert PS, Surwit EA,** eds. *Ovarian cancer.* Boston: Martinus Nijhoff, 1986:53–67.

127. **Heintz APM, Berek JS.** Cytoreductive surgery in ovarian cancer. In: **Piver MS,** eds. *Ovarian cancer.* Edinburgh: Churchill Livingstone, 1987:129–143.

128. **Hacker NF, Berek JS, Lagasse LD, et al.** Primary cytoreductive surgery for epithelial ovarian cancer. *Obstet Gynecol* 1983;61:413–420.

129. **Van Lindert AM, Alsbach GJ, Barents JW, et al.** The role of the abdominal radical tumor reduction procedure (ARTR) in the treatment of ovarian cancer. In: **Heintz APM, Griffiths CT, Trimbos JB,** eds. *Surgery in gynecologic oncology.* The Hague, Netherlands: Martinus Nijhoff, 1984: 275–287.

130. **Hoskins WJ, Bundy BN, Thigpen TJ, et al.** The influence of cytoreductive surgery on recurrence-free interval and survival in small volume stage III epithelial ovarian cancer: a Gynecologic Oncology Group study. *Gynecol Oncol* 1992;47:159–166.

131. **Farias-Eisner R, Teng F, Oliveira M, et al.** The influence of tumor grade, distribution and extent of carcinomatosis in minimal residual stage III epithelial ovarian cancer after optimal primary cytoreductive surgery. *Gynecol Oncol* 1995;5:108–110.

132. **Hunter RW, Alexander NDE, Soutter WP.** Meta-analysis of surgery in advanced ovarian carcinoma: is maximum cytoreductive surgery an independent determinant of prognosis. *Am J Obstet Gynecol* 1992;166:504–511.

133. **Eisenkop SM, Friedman RL, Waqng HJ.** Complete cytoreductive surgery is feasible and maximizes survival in patients with advanced epithelial ovarian cancer: a prospective study. *Gynecol Oncol* 1998;69:103–108.

134. **Bristow RE, Tomacruz RS, Armstrong DK, et al.** Survival impact of maximum cytoreductive surgery for advanced ovarian carcinoma during the platinum era: a meta-analysis of 6,885 patients. Proceedings of the American Society of Clinician Oncologists 2001; Abstract .

135. **van der Burg MEL, van Lent M, Buyse M, et al.** The effect of debulking surgery after induction chemotherapy on the prognosis in advanced epithelial ovarian cancer: an EROTC Gynecologic Cancer Cooperative Group study. *N Engl J Med* 1995;332:629–634.

136. **Berek JS.** Interval debulking of epithelial ovarian cancer: an interim measure. *N Engl J Med* 1995;332:675–677.

137. **Berek JS, Hacker NF, Lagasse LD.** Rectosigmoid colectomy and reanastamosis to facilitate resection of primary and recurrent gynecologic cancer. *Obstet Gynecol* 1984;64:715–720.

138. **Berek JS, Hacker NF, Lagasse LD, et al.** Lower urinary tract resection as part of cytoreductive surgery for ovarian cancer. *Gynecol Oncol* 1982;13:87–92.

139. **Heintz AM, Hacker NF, Berek JS, et al.** Cytoreductive surgery in ovarian carcinoma: feasibility and morbidity. *Obstet Gynecol* 1986;67:783–788.

140. **Deppe G, Malviya VK, Boike G, et al.** Surgical approach to diaphragmatic metastases from ovarian cancer. *Gynecol Oncol* 1986;24:258–260.

141. **Montz FJ, Schlaerth J, Berek JS.** Resection of diaphragmatic peritoneum and muscle: role in cytoreductive surgery for ovarian carcinoma. *Gynecol Oncol* 1989;35:338–340.

142. **Brand E, Pearlman N.** Electrosurgical debulking of ovarian cancer: a new technique using the argon beam coagulator. *Gynecol Oncol* 1990;39:115–118.

143. **Deppe G, Malviya VK, Boike G, et al.** Use of Cavitron surgical aspirator for debulking of diaphragmatic metastases in patients with advanced carcinoma of the ovaries. *Surg Gynecol Obstet* 1989;168:455–456.

144. **Chen SS, Bochner R.** Assessment of morbidity and mortality in primary cytoreductive surgery for advanced ovarian cancer. *Gynecol Oncol* 1985;20:190–195.

145. **Venesmaa P, Ylikorkala O.** Morbidity and mortality associated with primary and repeat operations for ovarian cancer. *Obstet Gynecol* 1992;79:168–172.

146. **Hreshchyshyn MM, Park RC, Blessing JA, et al.** The role of adjuvant therapy in stage I ovarian cancer. *Am J Obstet Gynecol* 1980;138:139–145.

147. **Berek JS.** Adjuvant therapy for early-stage ovarian cancer. *N Engl J Med* 1990;322:1076–1078.

148. **Ahmed FY, Wiltshaw E, Hern RP, et al.** Natural history and prognosis of untreated stage I epithelial ovarian carcinoma. *J Clin Oncol* 1996;14:2968–2975.

149. **Finn CB, Luesley DM, Buxton EJ, et al.** Is stage I epithelial ovarian cancer overtreated both surgically and systemically? Results of a five-year cancer registry review. *Br J Obstet Gynaecol* 1992;99:54–58.

150. **Vergote I, Vergote S, De Vos LN, et al.** Randomized trial comparing cisplatin with radioactive phosphorus or whole abdominal irradiation as adjuvant treatment of ovarian cancer. *Cancer* 1992;69:741–749.

151. **Rubin SC, Wong GY, Curtin JP, et al.** Platinum based chemotherapy of high risk stage I epithelial ovarian cancer following comprehensive surgical staging. *Obstet Gynecol* 1993;82:143–147.

152. **Young RC, Brady MF, Nieberg RM, et al.** Randomized clinical trial of adjuvant treatment of women with early (FIGO I-IIA high risk) ovarian cancer: a Gynecologic Oncology Group study (GOG 95). *Proc Am Soc Clin Oncol* 1999;1376(abst).

153. **Bolis G, Colombo N, Pecorelli S, et al.** Adjuvant treatment for early epithelial ovarian cancer. Results of two randomized clinical trials comparing cisplatin to no further treatment or chromic phosphate (^{32}P). *Ann Oncol* 1995;6:887–893.

154. **Young RC, Pecorelli S.** Management of early ovarian cancer. *Semin Oncol* 1998;25:335–339.

155. **Colombo N, Chiari S, Maggioni A, et al.** Controversial issues in the management of early epithelial ovarian cancer: conservative surgery and the role of adjuvant therapy. *Gynecol Oncol* 1994;55:S47–51.

156. **Colombo N, Maggioni A, Bocciolone L, et al.** Multimodality therapy of early-stage (FIGO I-II) ovarian cancer: review of surgical management and postoperative adjuvant treatment. *Int J Gynecol Cancer* 1996;6:13–17.

157. **Vermorken JB, Pecorelli S.** Clinical trials in patients with epithelial ovarian cancer: past, present and future. *Eur J Surg Oncol* 1996;22:455–466.

158. **Tropé C, Kaern J, Vergote I, et al.** Randomized trials of adjuvant carboplatin versus no treatment in stage I high-risk ovarian cancer patients by the Nordic ovarian cancer study group (NOCOVA). *Proc Am Soc Clin Oncol* 1997;16:1260(abst).

159. **Gadducci A, Sartori E, Maggino T, et al.** Analysis of failure in patients with stage I ovarian cancer: an Italian multicenter study. *Int J Gynecol Cancer* 1997;7:445–450.

160. **Greene MH, Boice JD, Greer BE, et al.** Acute nonlymphocytic leukemia after therapy with alkylating agents for ovarian cancer. *N Engl J Med* 1982;307:1416–1421.

161. **Travis LB, Holowaty EJ, Bergfeldt K, et al.** Risk of leukemia after platinum-based chemotherapy for ovarian cancer. *N Engl J Med* 1999;340:351–357.

162. **Eisenhauer EA, ten Bokkel Huinink WW, Swenerton KD, et al.** European-Canadian randomized trial of paclitaxel in relapsed ovarian cancer: high-dose versus low-dose and long versus short infusion. *J Clin Oncol* 1994;12:2654–2666.

163. **McGuire WP, Rowinski EK, Rosensheim NE, et al.** Taxol: a unique antineoplastic agent with significant activity in advanced ovarian epithelial neoplasms. *Ann Intern Med* 1989;111:273–279.

164. **Bookman MA, McGuire WP, Kilpatrick D, et al.** Carboplatin and paclitaxel in ovarian carcinoma: a phase I study of the Gynecologic Oncology Group. *J Clin Oncol* 1996;14:1895–1902.

165. **McGuire WP, Hoskins WJ, Brady MF, et al.** Cyclophosphamide and cisplatin compared with paclitaxel and cisplatin in patients with stage III and stage IV ovarian cancer. *N Engl J Med* 1996;334:1–6.

166. **Stuart G, Bertelsen K, Mangioni C, et al.** Updated analysis shows a highly significant improved survival for cisplatin–paclitaxel as first-line treatment of advanced stage epithelial ovarian cancer: mature results of the EORTC-GCCG, NOCOVA, NCIC CTG and Scottish Intergroup Trial. *Proc Am Soc Clin Oncol* 1998:1394(abst).

167. **Muggia FM, Braly PS, Brady MF, et al.** Phase III randomized study of cisplatin versus paclitaxel versus cisplatin and paclitaxel in patients with suboptimal stage III or IV ovarian cancer: a Gynecologic Oncology Group study. *J Clin Oncol* 2000;18:106–115.

168. **Manetta A, MacNeill C, Lyter JA, et al.** Hexamethylmelamine as a second-line agent in ovarian cancer. *Gynecol Oncol* 1990;36:93–96.

169. **Ozols RF, Ostchega Y, Curt G, et al.** High-dose carboplatin in refractory ovarian cancer patients. *J Clin Oncol* 1987;5:197–201.

170. **Markman M, Rothman R, Hakes J, et al.** Second-line platinum therapy in patients with ovarian cancer previously treated with cisplatin. *J Clin Oncol* 1991;9:389–393.

171. **Advanced Ovarian Cancer Trialists Group.** Chemotherapy in advanced ovarian cancer: an overview of randomized clinical trials. *BMJ* 1991;303:884–891.

172. **Omura G, Bundy B, Berek JS, et al.** Randomized trial of cyclophosphamide plus cisplatin with or without doxorubicin in ovarian carcinoma: a Gynecologic Oncology Group study. *J Clin Oncol* 1989;7:457–465.

173. **Ovarian Cancer Meta-analysis Project.** Cyclophosphamide plus cisplatin versus cyclophosphamide, doxorubicin, and cisplatin chemotherapy of ovarian carcinoma: a meta-analysis. *J Clin Oncol* 1991;9:1668–1674.

174. **Swenerton K, Jeffrey J, Stuart G, et al.** Cisplatin-cyclophosphamide versus carboplatin-cyclophosphamide in advanced ovarian cancer: a randomized phase III study of the National Cancer Institute of Canada Clinical Trials Group. *J Clin Oncol* 1992;10:718–726.

175. **Ozols RF, Bundy BN, Fowler J, et al.** Randomized phase III study of cisplatin/paclitaxel versus carboplatin/paclitaxel in optimal stage III epithelial ovarian cancer: a Gynecologic Oncology Group trial (GOG 158). *J Clin Oncol* 2000.

176. **Du Bois A, Lueck HJ, Meier W, et al.** Cisplatin/paclitaxel versus carboplatin/paclitaxel in ovarian cancer: update of an Arbeitsgemeinschaft Gynaekologische Onkologie (AGO) Study Group trial. *Proc Am Soc Clin Oncol* 1999;1374(abst).

177. **Harper P and ICON Collaborators.** A randomized comparison of paclitaxel and carboplatin versus a control arm of single agent carboplatin or cyclophosphamide, doxorubicin and cisplatin: 2075 patients randomized into the 3rd International Collaborative Ovarian Neoplasm Study (ICON 3). *Proc Am Soc Clin Oncol* 1999;1375(abst).

178. **McGuire WP, Hoskins WJ, Brady MS, et al.** An assessment of dose-intensive therapy in suboptimally debulked ovarian cancer: a Gynecologic Oncology Group study. *J Clin Oncol* 1995;13:1589–1599.

179. **Alberts DS, Green S, Hannigan EV, et al.** Improved therapeutic index of carboplatin plus cyclophosphamide versus cisplatin plus cyclophosphamide: final report by the Southwest Oncology Group of a phase III randomized trial in stages III (suboptimal) and IV ovarian cancer. *J Clin Oncol* 1992;10:706–717.

180. **Kaye SB, Paul J, Cassidy J, et al.** Mature results of a randomized trial of two doses of cisplatin for the treatment of ovarian cancer. *J Clin Oncol* 1996;14:2113–2119.

181. **Calvert AH, Newell DR, Gumbrell LA, et al.** Carboplatin dosage: prospective evaluation of a simple formula based on renal function. *J Clin Oncol* 1989;7:1748–1756.

182. **Alberts DS, Liu PY, Hannigan EV, et al.** Intraperitoneal cisplatin plus intravenous cyclophosphamide versus intravenous cisplatin plus intravenous cyclophosphamide for stage III ovarian cancer. *N Engl J Med* 1996;335:1950–1955.

183. **Markman M, Bundy B, Benda J, et al.** Randomized phase III study of intravenous cisplatin/paclitaxel versus moderately high dose intravenous carboplatin followed by intraperitoneal paclitaxel and intraperitoneal cisplatin in optimal residual ovarian cancer: an intergroup trial (GOG, SWOG, ECOG). *J Clin Oncol* 2000.

184. **Schwartz PE, Rutherford TJ, Chambers JT, et al.** Neoadjuvant chemotherapy for advanced ovarian cancer: long-term survival. *Gynecol Oncol* 1999;72:93–99.

185. **Windbichler GH, Hausmaninger H, Stummvoll W, et al.** Interferon-γ in the first-line therapy of ovarian cancer: a randomized phase III trial. *Br J Cancer* 2000;82:1138–1144.

186. **Rendina GM, Donadio C, Giovanni M.** Steroid receptors and progestinic therapy in ovarian endometrioid carcinoma. *Eur J Gynaecol Oncol* 1982;3:241–246.

187. **Berek JS, Hacker NF, Lagasse LD, et al.** Second-look laparotomy in stage III epithelial ovarian cancer: clinical variables associated with disease status. *Obstet Gynecol* 1984;64:207–212.

188. **Copeland LJ, Gershenson DM, Wharton JT, et al.** Microscopic disease at second-look laparotomy in advanced ovarian cancer. *Cancer* 1985;55:472–478.

189. **Gershenson DM, Copeland LJ, Wharton JT, et al.** Prognosis of surgically determined complete responders in advanced ovarian cancer. *Cancer* 1985;55:1129–1135.

190. **Smira LR, Stehman FB, Ulbright TM, et al.** Second-look laparotomy after chemotherapy in the management of ovarian malignancy. *Am J Obstet Gynecol* 1985;152:661–668.

191. **Freidman JB, Weiss NS.** Second thoughts about second-look laparotomy in advanced ovarian cancer. *N Engl J Med* 1990;322:1079–1082.

192. **Berek JS.** Second-look versus second-nature. *Gynecol Oncol* 1992;44:1–2.

193. **Rubin SC, Hoskins WJ, Hakes TB, et al.** Recurrence after negative second-look laparotomy for ovarian cancer: analysis of risk factors. *Am J Obstet Gynecol* 1988;159:1094–1098.

194. **Berek JS, Griffith CT, Leventhal JM.** Laparoscopy for second-look evaluation in ovarian cancer. *Obstet Gynecol* 1981;58:192–198.

195. **Berek JS, Hacker NF.** Laparoscopy in the management of patients with ovarian carcinoma. In: **DiSaia P,** ed. *The treatment of ovarian cancer.* Philadelphia: WB Saunders, 1983:213–222.

196. **Lele S, Piver MS.** Interval laparoscopy prior to second-look laparotomy in ovarian cancer. *Obstet Gynecol* 1986;68:345–347.

197. **Berek JS, Knapp RC, Malkasian GD, et al.** CA125 serum levels correlated with second-look operations among ovarian cancer patients. *Obstet Gynecol* 1986;67:685–689.

198. **Lavin PT, Knapp RC, Malkasian GD, et al.** CA125 for the monitoring of ovarian carcinoma during primary therapy. *Obstet Gynecol* 1987;69:223–227.

199. **De Rosa V, Mangioni di Stefano ML, et al.** Computed tomography and second-look surgery in ovarian cancer patients: correlation, actual role and limitations of CT scan. *Eur J Gynaecol Oncol* 1995;16:123–129.

200. **Lund B, Jacobson K, Rasch L, et al.** Correlation of abdominal ultrasound and computed tomography scans with second- or third-look laparotomy in patients with ovarian carcinoma. *Gynecol Oncol* 1990;37:279–283.

201. **Berek JS, Hacker NF, Lagasse LD, et al.** Survival of patients following secondary cytoreductive surgery in ovarian cancer. *Obstet Gynecol* 1983;61:189–193.

202. **Hoskins WJ, Rubin SC, Dulaney E, et al.** Influence of secondary cytoreduction at the time of second-look laparotomy on the survival of patients with epithelial ovarian carcinoma. *Gynecol Oncol* 1989;34:365–371.

203. **Bristow RE, Lagasse LD, Karlan BY.** Secondary surgical cytoreduction in advanced epithelial ovarian cancer. Patient selection and review of the literature. *Cancer* 1996;78:2049–2062.

204. **Berek JS, Tropé C, Vergote I.** Surgery during chemotherapy and at relapse of ovarian cancer. *Ann Oncol* 1999;10:S3–7.

205. **Eisenkop SM, Friedman RL, Spirtos NM.** The role of secondary cytoreductive surgery in the treatment of patients with recurrent epithelial ovarian carcinoma. *Cancer* 2000;88:144–153.

206. **Gadducci A, Iacconi P, Cosio S, et al.** Complete salvage surgical cytoreduction improves further survival of patients with late recurrent ovarian cancer. *Gynecol Oncol* 2000;79:344–349.

207. **Munkarah A, Levenback C, Wolf JK, et al.** Secondary cytoreductive surgery for localized intra-abdominal recurrences in epithelial ovarian cancer. *Gynecol Oncol* 2001;81:237–241.

208. **Ozols RF, Ostchega Y, Myers CE, et al.** High dose cisplatin in hypertonic saline in refractory ovarian cancer. *J Clin Oncol* 1985;3:1246–1250.

209. **Gershenson DM, Kavanagh JJ, Copeland LJ, et al.** Retreatment of patients with recurrent epithelial ovarian cancer with cisplatin-based chemotherapy. *Obstet Gynecol* 1989;73:798–802.

210. **Ozols RF, Ostchega Y, Curt G, et al.** High dose carboplatin in refractory ovarian cancer patients. *J Clin Oncol* 1987;5:197–201.

211. **Markman M, Rothman R, Hakes T, et al.** Second-line platinum therapy in patients with ovarian cancer previously treated with cisplatin. *J Clin Oncol* 1991;9:389–393.

212. **Gore ME, Fryatt I, Wiltshaw E, et al.** Treatment of relapsed carcinoma of the ovary with cisplatin or carboplatin following initial treatment with these compounds. *Gynecol Oncol* 1990;36:207–211.

213. **Shapiro JD, Millward MJ, Rischin D, et al.** Activity of gemcitabine in patients with advanced ovarian cancer: responses seen following platinum and paclitaxel. *Gynecol Oncol* 1996;63:89–93.

214. **Eisenhauer EA, Vermorken JB, van Glabbeke M.** Predictors of response to subsequent chemotherapy in platinum pretreated ovarian cancer: a multivariate analysis of 704 patients. *Ann Oncol* 1997;8:963–968.

215. **Muggia F, Hainsworth J, Jeffers S, et al.** Phase II study of liposomal doxorubicin in refractory ovarian cancer: antitumor activity and toxicity modification by liposomal encapsulation. *J Clin Oncol* 1997;15:987–993.

216. **Thigpen JT, Blessing JA, Ball H, et al.** Phase II trial of paclitaxel in patients with progressive ovarian carcinoma after platinum-based chemotherapy: a Gynecologic Oncology Group study. *J Clin Oncol* 1994;12:1748–1753.

217. **Trimble EL, Adams JD, Vena D, et al.** Paclitaxel for platinum-refractory ovarian cancer: results from the first 1000 patients registered to National Cancer Institute Treatment Referral Center 9103. *J Clin Oncol* 1993;11:2405–2410.

218. **Kohn EC, Sarosy G, Bicher A, et al.** Dose-intense Taxol: high response rate in patients with platinum-resistant recurrent ovarian cancer. *J Natl Cancer Inst* 1994;86:18–24.

219. **Greco FA, Hainsworth JD.** One-hour paclitaxel infusion schedules: a phase I/II comparative trial. *Semin Oncol* 1995;22:118–123.

220. **Chang AY, Boros L, Garrow G, et al.** Paclitaxel by 3-hour infusion followed by 96-hour infusion on failure in patients with refractory malignant disease. *Semin Oncol* 1995;22:124–127.

221. **Piccart MJ, Gore M, ten Bokkel Huinink W, et al.** Docetaxel: an active new drug for treatment of advanced epithelial ovarian cancer. *J Natl Cancer Inst* 1995;87:676–681.

222. **Francis P, Schneider J, Hann L, et al.** Phase II trial of docetaxel in patients with platinum-refractory advanced ovarian cancer. *J Clin Oncol* 1994;12:2301–2308.

223. **Bookman MA, Malstrom H, Bolis G, et al.** Topotecan for the treatment of advanced epithelial ovarian cancer: an open-label phase II study in patients treated after prior chemotherapy that contained cisplatin or carboplatin and paclitaxel. *J Clin Oncol* 1998;16:3345–3352.

224. **ten Bokkel Huineink W, Gore M, Carmichael J, et al.** Topotecan versus paclitaxel for the treatment of recurrent epithelial ovarian cancer. *J Clin Oncol* 1997;15:2183–2193.

225. **Hoskins P, Eisenhauer E, Beare S, et al.** Randomized phase II study of two schedules of topotecan in previously treated patients with ovarian cancer: a National Cancer Institute of Canada Clinical Trials Group study. *J Clin Oncol* 1998;16:2233–2237.

226. **Moore DH, Valea F, Crumpler LS, et al.** Hexamethylmelamine (altretamine) as second-line therapy for epithelial ovarian carcinoma. *Gynecol Oncol* 1993;51:109–112.

227. **Look KY, Muss HB, Blessing JA, et al.** A phase II trial of 5-fluorouracil and high-dose leucovorin in recurrent epithelial ovarian carcinoma: a Gynecologic Oncology group study. *Am J Clin Oncol* 1995;18:19–22.

228. **Hoskins PJ, Swenerton KD.** Oral etoposide is active against platinum-resistant epithelial ovarian cancer. *J Clin Oncol* 1994;12:60–63.

229. **Rose PG, Blessing JA, Mayer AR, et al.** Prolonged oral etoposide as second-line therapy for platinum-resistant and platinum-sensitive ovarian carcinoma: a Gynecologic Oncology Group study. *J Clin Oncol* 1998;16:405–410.

230. **Sorensen P, Pfeiffer P, Bertelsen K.** A phase II trial of ifosfamide/mesna as salvage therapy in patients with ovarian cancer refractory to or relapsing after prior platinum-containing chemotherapy. *Gynecol Oncol* 1995;56:75–78.

231. **Hacker NF, Berek JS, Pretorius G, et al.** Intraperitoneal cisplatin as salvage therapy in persistent epithelial ovarian cancer. *Obstet Gynecol* 1987;70:759–764.

232. **Markman M, Howell SB, Lucas WE, et al.** Combination intraperitoneal chemotherapy with cisplatin, cytarabine, and doxorubicin for refractory ovarian carcinoma and other malignancies principally confined to the peritoneal cavity. *J Clin Oncol* 1984;2:13–16.

233. **Howell SB, Kirmani S, Lucas WE, et al.** A phase II trial of intraperitoneal cisplatin and etoposide for primary treatment of ovarian epithelial cancer. *J Clin Oncol* 1990;8:137–145.

234. **Kirmani S, Lucas WE, Kim S, et al.** A phase II trial of intraperitoneal cisplatin and etoposide as salvage treatment for minimal residual ovarian carcinoma. *J Clin Oncol* 1991;9:649–657.

235. **Markman M, Hakes T, Reichman B, et al.** Phase II trial of weekly or biweekly intraperitoneal mitoxantrone in epithelial ovarian cancer. *J Clin Oncol* 1991;9:978–982.

236. **Howell SB, Zimm S, Markman M, et al.** Long-term survival of advanced refractory ovarian carcinoma patients with small-volume disease treated with intraperitoneal chemotherapy. *J Clin Oncol* 1987;5:1607–1612.

237. **Braly PS, Berek JS, Blessing JA, et al.** Intraperitoneal administration of cisplatin and 5-fluorouracil in residual ovarian cancer: a phase II Gynecologic Oncology Group trial. *Gynecol Oncol* 1995;34:143–147.

238. **Francis P, Rowinsky E, Schneider J, et al.** Phase I feasibility study and pharmacologic study of weekly intraperitoneal Taxol: a Gynecologic Oncology Group study. *J Clin Oncol* 1995;13:2961–2967.

239. **Feun LG, Blessing JA, Major FJ, et al.** A phase II study of intraperitoneal cisplatin and thiotepa in residual ovarian carcinoma: a Gynecologic Oncology Group study. *Gynecol Oncol* 1998;71:410–415.

240. **Markman M, Hakes T, Reichman B, et al.** Phase II trial of weekly or biweekly intraperitoneal mitoxantrone in epithelial ovarian cancer. *J Clin Oncol* 1991;9:978–982.

241. **Berek JS, Hacker NF, Lichtenstein A, et al.** Intraperitoneal recombinant α_2 interferon for "salvage" immunotherapy in stage III epithelial ovarian cancer immunotherapy in stage III: a Gynecologic Oncology Group study. *Cancer Res* 1985;45:4447–4453.

242. **Willemse PHB, De Vries EGE, Mulder NH, et al.** Intraperitoneal human recombinant interferon α-2b in minimal residual ovarian cancer. *Eur J Cancer* 1990;26:353–358.

243. **Nardi M, Lognetti F, Pallera F, et al.** Intraperitoneal α-2-interferon alternating with cisplatin as salvage therapy for minimal residual disease ovarian cancer: a phase II study. *J Clin Oncol* 1990;6:1036–1041.

244. **Bezwoda WR, Golombick T, Dansey R, et al.** Treatment of malignant ascites due to recurrent/refractory ovarian cancer: the use of interferon-α or interferon-α plus chemotherapy. In vivo and in vitro observations. *Eur J Cancer* 1991;27:1423–1429.

245. **Berek JS, Markman M, Blessing JA, et al.** Intraperitoneal α-interferon alternating with cisplatin in residual ovarian cancer: a phase II Gynecologic Oncology Group study. *Gynecol Oncol* 1999;74:48–52.

246. **Berek JS, Markman M, Stonebraker B, et al.** Intraperitoneal interferon-α in residual ovarian carcinoma: a phase II Gynecologic Oncology Group study. *Gynecol Oncol* 1999;75:10–14.

247. **Pujade-Lauraine E, Guastella JP, Colombo N, et al.** Intraperitoneal recombinant human interferon γ (IFNγ) in residual ovarian cancer: efficacy is independent of previous response to chemotherapy. *Proc Am Soc Clin Oncol* 1991;713:225.

248. **Steis RG, Urba WJ, Vandermolen LA, et al.** Intraperitoneal lymphokine-activated killer cell and interleukin 2 therapy for malignancies limited to the peritoneal cavity. *J Clin Oncol* 1990;10: 1618–1629.

249. **Markman M, Berek JS, Blessing JA, et al.** Characteristics of patients with small-volume residual ovarian cancer unresponsive to cisplatin-based ip chemotherapy: lessons learned from a Gynecologic Oncology Group phase II trial of ip cisplatin and recombinant α-interferon. *Gynecol Oncol* 1992;45:3–8.

250. **Hatch KD, Beecham JB, Blessing JA, et al.** Responsiveness of patients with advanced ovarian carcinoma to tamoxifen: a Gynecologic Oncology Group study of second-line therapy in 105 patients. *Cancer* 1991;68:269–271.

251. **Van der Velden J, Gitsch G, Wain GV, et al.** Tamoxifen in patients with advanced epithelial ovarian cancer. *Int J Gynecol Cancer* 1995;5:301–305.

252. **Miller DS, Brady MF, Barrett RJ.** A phase II trial of leuprolide acetate in patients with advanced epithelial ovarian cancer. *J Clin Oncol* 1992;15:125–128.

253. **Lopez A, Tessadrelli A, Kudelka AP, et al.** Combination therapy with leuprolide acetate and tamoxifen in refractory ovarian cancer. *Int J Gynecol Cancer* 1996;6:15–19.

254. **Vanden Bossche HV, Moereels H, Koymans LM.** Aromatase inhibitors- mechanisms for nonsteroidal inhibitors. *Breast Cancer Res Treat* 1994;30:43–55.

255. **Hacker NF, Berek JS, Burnison CM, et al.** Whole abdominal radiation as salvage therapy for epithelial ovarian cancer. *Obstet Gynecol* 1985;65:60–66.

256. **Castaldo TW, Petrilli ES, Ballon SC, et al.** Intestinal operations in patients with ovarian carcinoma. *Am J Obstet Gynecol* 1981;139:80–84.

257. **Krebs HB, Goplerud DR.** Surgical management of bowel obstruction in advanced ovarian cancer. *Obstet Gynecol* 1983;61:327–330.

258. **Tunca JC, Buchler DA, Mack EA, et al.** The management of ovarian cancer caused bowel obstruction. *Gynecol Oncol* 1981;12:186–192.

259. **Piver MS, Barlow JJ, Lele SB, et al.** Survival after ovarian cancer induced intestinal obstruction. *Gynecol Oncol* 1982;13:44–49.

260. **Clarke-Pearson DL, DeLong ER, Chin N, et al.** Intestinal obstruction in patients with ovarian cancer: variables associated with surgical complications and survival. *Arch Surg* 1988;123:42–45.

261. **Fernandes JR, Seymour RJ, Suissa S.** Bowel obstruction in patients with ovarian cancer: a search for prognostic factors. *Am J Obstet Gynecol* 1988;158:244–249.

262. **Rubin SC, Hoskins WJ, Benjamin I, et al.** Palliative surgery for intestinal obstruction in advanced ovarian cancer. *Gynecol Oncol* 1989;34:16–19.

263. **Malone JM Jr, Koonce T, Larson DM, et al.** Palliation of small bowel obstruction by percutaneous gastrostomy in patients with progressive ovarian carcinoma. *Obstet Gynecol* 1986;68:431–433.

264. **Campagnutta E, Cannizzaro R, Gallo A, et al.** Palliative treatment of upper intestinal obstruction by gynecologic malignancy: the usefulness of percutaneous endoscopic gastrostomy. *Gynecol Oncol* 1996;62:103–105.

265. **Trimble EL, Kosary CA, Cornelison TL, et al.** Improved survival for women with ovarian cancer. *Proc Soc Gynecol Oncol* 1999:136(abst).

266. **Chen LM, Berek JS.** Ovarian and fallopian tubes. In: **Haskell CM,** ed. *Cancer treatment,* 5th ed. Philadelphia: WB Saunders, 2000.

267. **Imai A, Furui T, Tamaya T.** Gynecologic tumors and symptoms in childhood and adolescence: 10-years' experience. *Int J Gynaecol Obstet* 1994;45:227–234.

268. **Gershenson DM.** Management of early ovarian cancer: germ cell and sex-cord stromal tumors. *Gynecol Oncol* 1994;55:S62–72.

269. **Gershenson DM.** Update on malignant ovarian germ cell tumors. *Cancer* 1993;71:1581–1590.

270. **Kurman RJ, Scardino PT, Waldmann TA, et al.** Malignant germ cell tumors of the ovary and testis: an immunohistologic study of 69 cases. *Ann Clin Lab Sci* 1979;9:462–466.

271. **Obata NH, Nakashima N, Kawai M, et al.** Gonadoblastoma with dysgerminoma in one ovary and gonadoblastoma with dysgerminoma and yolk sac tumor in the contralateral ovary in a girl with 46XX karyotype. *Gynecol Oncol* 1995;58:124–128.

272. **Spanos WJ.** Preoperative hormonal therapy of cystic adnexal masses. *Am J Obstet Gynecol* 1973;116: 551–556.

273. **Bremer GL, Land JA, Tiebosch A, et al.** Five different histologic subtypes of germ cell malignancies in an XY female. *Gynecol Oncol* 1993;50:247–248.

274. **Mayordomo JI, Paz-Ares L, Rivera F, et al.** Ovarian and extragonadal malignant germ-cell tumors in females: a single-institution experience with 43 patients. *Ann Oncol* 1994;5:225–231.

275. **Piura B, Dgani R, Zalel Y, et al.** Malignant germ cell tumors of the ovary: a study of 20 cases. *J Surg Oncol* 1995;59:155–161.

276. **Gordon A, Lipton D, Woodruff JD.** Dysgerminoma: a review of 158 cases from the Emil Novak Ovarian Tumor Registry. *Obstet Gynecol* 1981;58:497–504.

277. **Thomas GM, Dembo AJ, Hacker NF, et al.** Current therapy for dysgerminoma of the ovary. *Obstet Gynecol* 1987;70:268–275.

278. **Gershenson DM.** Update on malignant ovarian germ cell tumors. *Cancer* 1993;71:1581–1590.

279. **Williams SD, Birch R, Einhorn LH, et al.** Treatment of disseminated germ cell tumors with cisplatin, bleomycin and either vinblastine or etoposide. *N Engl J Med* 1987;316:1435–1440.

280. **Williams SD, Blessing JA, Hatch K, et al.** Chemotherapy of advanced ovarian dysgerminoma: trials of the Gynecologic Oncology Group. *J Clin Oncol* 1991;9:1950–1955.

281. **Williams SD, Blessing JA, Moore DH, et al.** Cisplatin, vinblastine, and bleomycin in advanced and recurrent ovarian germ-cell tumors. *Ann Intern Med* 1989;111:22–27.

282. **Williams, Blessing JA, Liao S, et al.** Adjuvant therapy of ovarian germ cell tumors with cisplatin, etoposide, and bleomycin: a trial of the Gynecologic Oncology Group. *J Clin Oncol* 1994;12: 701–706.

283. **Gershenson DM, Morris M, Cangir A, et al.** Treatment of malignant germ cell tumors of the ovary with bleomycin, etoposide, and cisplatin. *J Clin Oncol* 1990;8:715–720.

284. **Bekaii-Saab T, Einhorn LH, Williams SD.** Late relapse of ovarian dysgerminoma: case report and literature review. *Gynecol Oncol* 1999;72:111–112.

285. **Kurtz JE, Jaeck D, Maloisel F, et al.** Combined modality treatment for malignant transformation of a benign ovarian teratoma. *Gynecol Oncol* 1999;73:319–321.

286. **Williams SD, Brady M, Burnett A, et al.** Adjuvant therapy of resected dysgerminoma with carboplatin and etoposide. *Proc Soc Gynecol Oncol* 1999;114(abst).

287. **Gershenson DM.** Menstrual and reproductive function after treatment with combination chemotherapy for malignant ovarian germ cell tumors. *J Clin Oncol* 1988;6:270–275.

288. **Loehrer PJ, Johnson D, Elson P, et al.** Importance of bleomycin in favorable-prognosis disseminated germ cell tumors: an Eastern Cooperative Oncology Group trial. *J Clin Oncol* 1995;13:470–476.

289. **Bajorin DF, Sarosdy MF, Pfister GD, et al.** Randomized trial of etoposide and cisplatin versus etoposide and carboplatin in patients with good-risk germ cell tumors: a multi-institutional study. *J Clin Oncol* 1993;11:598–606.

290. **Schwartz PE, Chambers SK, Chambers JT, et al.** Ovarian germ cell malignancies: the Yale University experience. *Gynecol Oncol* 1992;45:26–31.

291. **Williams SD, Blessing JA, DiSaia PJ, et al.** Second-look laparotomy in ovarian germ cell tumors. *Gynecol Oncol* 1994;52:287–291.

292. **Culine S, Lhomme C, Michel G, et al.** Is there a role for second-look laparotomy in the management of malignant germ cell tumors of the ovary? Experience at Institute Gustave Roussy. *J Surg Oncol* 1996;62: 40–45.

293. **O'Conner DM, Norris HJ.** The influence of grade on the outcome of stage I ovarian immature (malignant) teratomas and the reproducibility of grading. *Int J Gynecol Pathol* 1994;13:283–289.

294. **De Palo G, Zambetti M, Pilotti S, et al.** Non-dysgerminomatous tumors of the ovary treated with cisplatin, vinblastine, and bleomycin: long-term results. *Gynecol Oncol* 1992;47:239–246.

295. **Culine S, Kattan J, Lhomme C, et al.** A phase II study of high-dose cisplatin, vinblastine, bleomycin, and etoposide (PVeBV regimen) in malignant non-dysgerminomatous germ-cell tumors of the ovary. *Gynecol Oncol* 1994;54:47–53.

296. **Cangir A, Smith J, van Eys J.** Improved prognosis in children with ovarian cancers following modified VAC (vincristine sulfate, dactinomycin, and cyclophosphamide) chemotherapy. *Cancer* 1978;42: 1234–1238.

297. **Wong LC, Ngan HYS, Ma HK.** Primary treatment with vincristine, dactinomycin, and cyclophosphamide in non-dysgerminomatous germ cell tumour of the ovary. *Gynecol Oncol* 1989;34:155–158.

298. **Slayton RE, Park RC, Silverberg SC, et al.** Vincristine, dactinomycin, and cyclophosphamide in the treatment of malignant germ cell tumors of the ovary: a Gynecologic Oncology Group study (a final report). *Cancer* 1985;56:243–248.

299. **Creasman WJ, Soper JT.** Assessment of the contemporary management of germ cell malignancies of the ovary. *Am J Obstet Gynecol* 1985;153:828–834.

300. **Taylor MH, DePetrillo AD, Turner AR.** Vinblastine, bleomycin and cisplatin in malignant germ cell tumors of the ovary. *Cancer* 1985;56:1341–1349.

301. **Culine S, Lhomme C, Kattan J, et al.** Cisplatin-based chemotherapy in the management of germ cell tumors of the ovary: the Institute Gustave Roussy experience. *Gynecol Oncol* 1997;64:160–165.

302. **Williams SD, Wong LC, Ngan HYS.** Management of ovarian germ cell tumors. In: **Gershenson DM, McGuire WP,** eds. *Ovarian cancer.* New York: Churchill Livingston, 1998:399–415.

303. **Talerman A.** Germ cell tumors of the ovary. *Curr Opin Obstet Gynecol* 1997;9:44–47.

304. **Kleiman GM, Young RH, Scully RE.** Primary neuroectodermal tumors of the ovary. A report of 25 cases. *Am J Surg Pathol* 1993;17:764–778.

305. **Geisler JP, Goulet R, Foster RS, et al.** Growing teratoma syndrome after chemotherapy for germ cell tumors of the ovary. *Obstet Gynecol* 1994;84:719–721.

306. **Sasaki H, Furusata M, Teshima S, et al.** Prognostic significance of histopathological subtypes in stage I pure yolk sac tumour of the ovary. *Br J Cancer* 1994;69:529–536.

307. **Fujita M, Inoue M, Tanizawa O, et al.** Retrospective review of 41 patients with endodermal sinus tumor of the ovary. *Int J Gynecol Cancer* 1993;3:329–335.

308. **Kawai M, Kano T, Kikkawa F, et al.** Seven tumor markers in benign and malignant germ cell tumors of the ovary. *Gynecol Oncol* 1992;45:248–253.

309. **Abu-Rustum NR, Aghajanian C.** Management of malignant germ cell tumors of the ovary. *Semin Oncol* 1998;25:235–242.

310. **Newlands ES, Southall PJ, Paradinas FJ, et al.** Management of ovarian germ cell tumours. In: **Williams CJ, Krikorian JG, Green MR, et al.,** eds. *Textbook of uncommon cancer.* New York: John Wiley and Sons, 1988:37–53.

311. **Ueda G, Abe Y, Yoshida M, et al.** Embryonal carcinoma of the ovary: a six-year survival. *Gynecol Oncol* 1990;31:287–292.

312. **Kammerer-Doak D, Baurick K, Black W, et al.** Endodermal sinus tumor and embryonal carcinoma of the ovary in a 53-year-old woman. *Gynecol Oncol* 1996;63:133–137.

313. **Gershenson DM, Del Junco G, Copeland LJ, et al.** Mixed germ cell tumors of the ovary. *Obstet Gynecol* 1984;64:200–206.

314. **Simosek T, Trak B, Tunoc M, et al.** Primary pure choriocarcinoma of the ovary in reproductive ages: a case report. *Eur J Gynaecol Oncol* 1998;19:284–286.

315. **Oliva E, Andrada E, Pezzica E, et al.** Ovarian carcinomas with choriocarcinomatous differentiation. *Cancer* 1993;72:2441–2446.

316. **Young RE, Scully RE.** Ovarian sex cord-stromal tumors: problems in differential diagnosis. *Pathol Annu* 1988;23:237–296.

317. **Miller BE, Barron BA, Wan JY, et al.** Prognostic factors in adult granulosa cell tumor of the ovary. *Cancer* 1997;79:1951–1955.

318. **Malmstrom H, Hogberg T, Bjorn R, et al.** Granulosa cell tumors of the ovary: prognostic factors and outcome. *Gynecol Oncol* 1994;52:50–55.

319. **Segal R, DePetrillo AD, Thomas G.** Clinical review of adult granulosa cell tumors of the ovary. *Gynecol Oncol* 1995;56:338–344.

320. **Lappohn RE, Burger HG, Bouma J, et al.** Inhibin as a marker for granulosa-cell tumors. *N Engl J Med* 1989;321:790–793.

321. **Hildebrandt RH, Rouse RV, Longacre TA.** Value of inhibin in the identification of granulosa cell tumors of the ovary. *Hum Pathol* 1997;28:1387–1395.

322. **Richi M, Howard LN, Bratthauae GL, et al.** Use of monoclonal antibody against human inhibin as a marker for sex-cord-stromal tumors of the ovary. *Am J Surg Pathol* 1997:21:583–589.

323. **Gershenson DM, Copeland LJ, Kavanauh JJ, et al.** Treatment of metastatic stromal tumors of the ovary with cisplatin, doxorubicin, and cyclophosphamide. *Obstet Gynecol* 1987;5:765–769.

324. **Holland DR, Le Riche J, Swenerton KD, et al.** Flow cytometric assessment of DNA ploidy is a useful prognostic factor for patients with granulosa cell ovarian tumors. *Int J Gynecol Cancer* 1991;1:227–232.

325. **Roth LM, Anderson MC, Govan AD, et al.** Sertoli-Leydig cell tumors: a clinicopathologic study of 34 cases. *Cancer* 1981;48:187–197.

326. **Berek JS, Hacker NF.** Sarcomas of the female genital tract. In: **Eilber FR, Morton DL, Sondak VK, et al.,** eds. *The soft tissue sarcomas.* Orlando: Grune & Stratton, 1987:229–238.

327. **Barakat RR, Rubin SC, Wong G, et al.** Mixed mesodermal tumor of the ovary: analysis of prognostic factors in 31 cases. *Obstet Gynecol* 1992;80:660–664.

328. **Fowler JM, Nathan L, Nieberg RK, et al.** Mixed mesodermal sarcoma of the ovary in a young patient. *Eur J Obstet Gynecol Reprod Bio* 1996;65:249–253.

329. **Young RH, Oliva E, Scully RE.** Small cell sarcoma of the ovary, hypercalcemic type: a clinicopathological analysis of 150 cases. *Am J Surg Pathol* 1994;18:1102–1116.

330. **Petru E, Pickel H, Heydarfadai M, et al.** Non-genital cancers metastatic to the ovary. *Gynecol Oncol* 1992;44:83–86.

331. **Demopoulos RI, Touger L, Dubin N.** Secondary ovarian carcinoma: a clinical and pathological evaluation. *Int J Gynecol Pathol* 1987;6:166–175.

332. **Young RH, Scully RE.** Metastatic tumors in the ovary: a problem-oriented approach and review of the recent literature. *Semin Diagn Pathol* 1991;8:250–276.

333. **Curtin JP, Barakat RR, Hoskins WJ.** Ovarian disease in women with breast cancer. *Obstet Gynecol* 1994;84:449–452.

334. **Yakushiji M, Tazaki T, Nishimura H, et al.** Krukenberg tumors of the ovary: a clinicopathologic analysis of 112 cases. *Acta Obstet Gynaecol Jpn* 1987;39:479–485.

335. **Young RH, Scully RE.** Malignant melanoma metastatic to the ovary: a clinicopathologic analysis of 20 cases. *Am J Surg Pathol* 1991;15:849–860.

336. **Motoyama T, Katayama Y, Watanabe H, et al.** Functioning ovarian carcinoids induce severe constipation. *Cancer* 1991;70:513–518.

337. **Fox H, Langley FA, Govan AD, et al.** Malignant lymphoma presenting as an ovarian tumour: a clinicopathological analysis of 34 cases. *Br J Obstet Gynaecol* 1988;95:386–390.

338. **Monterroso V, Jaffe ES, Merino MJ, et al.** Malignant lymphomas involving the ovary: a clinicopathologic analysis of 39 cases. *Am J Surg Pathol* 1993;17:154–170.

339. **Pecorelli S, Odicino F, Maisonneuve P, et al.** Carcinoma of the fallopian tube. FIGO annual report on the results of treatment in gynaecological cancer. *J Epidemiol Biostat* 1998;3:363–374.

340. **Cormio G, Maneo A, Gabriele A, et al.** Primary carcinoma of the fallopian tube: a retrospective analysis of 47 patients. *Ann Oncol* 1996;7:271–275.

341. **Alvarado-Cabrero I, Young RH, Vamvakas EC, et al.** Carcinoma of the fallopian tube: a clinicopathological study of 105 cases with observations on staging and prognostic factors. *Gynecol Oncol* 1999;72:367–379.

342. **Podratz KC, Podczaski ES, Gaffey TA, et al.** Primary carcinoma of the fallopian tube. *Am J Obstet Gynecol* 1986;154:1319–1326.

343. **Hellstrom AC, Silfversward C, Nilsson B, et al.** Carcinoma of the fallopian tube. A clinical and histopathologic review. The Radiumhemmet series. *Int J Gynecol Cancer* 1994;4:395–407.

344. **Barakat RR, Rubin SC, Saigo PE, et al.** Cisplatin-based combination chemotherapy in carcinoma of the fallopian tube. *Gynecol Oncol* 1991;42:156–160.

Novak's Gynecology, 13th Edition. Edited by J.S. Berek. Lippincott Williams & Wilkins, Philadelphia © 2002

33 Vulvar Cancer

Christine H. Holschneider
Jonathan S. Berek

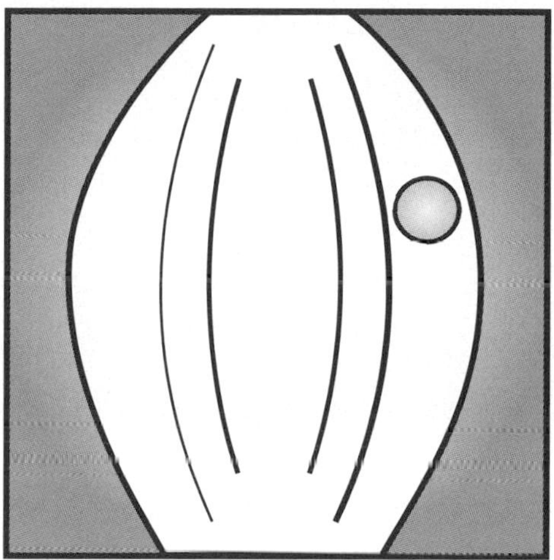

With 3,800 new cases and 800 deaths annually in the United States (1), vulvar cancer is uncommon, representing 3% to 5% of malignancies of the female genital tract. Squamous cell carcinomas account for about 90% of all primary vulvar malignancies, whereas melanomas, adenocarcinomas, basal cell carcinomas, and sarcomas are much less common. **The incidence of *in situ* vulvar cancer nearly doubled between the mid-1970s and the mid-1980s, whereas the overall rate of invasive squamous cell carcinoma has remained relatively stable** (2). However, in women younger than 50 years there has been a striking increase in the incidence of not only *in situ* but also invasive squamous cell carcinoma of the vulva (3).

Following the reports of Taussig (4) in the United States and Way (5) in Great Britain, radical vulvectomy and *en bloc* groin dissection, with or without pelvic lymphadenectomy, has been considered standard treatment for all patients who have operable disease. Postoperative morbidity was high and prolonged hospitalization common. During the past 20 years, a number of significant advances have been made in the management of vulvar cancer. The following changes have markedly decreased the physical and psychological morbidity associated with the treatment:

1. Individualization of treatment for all patients with invasive disease (6,7)
2. Vulvar conservation for patients with unifocal tumors and an otherwise normal vulva (6–10)
3. Omission of the groin dissection for patients with T_1 tumors and <1mm of stromal invasion (6,7)
4. Elimination of routine pelvic lymphadenectomy (11–15)
5. The use of separate incisions for the groin dissection to improve wound healing (16,17)
6. Omission of the contralateral groin dissection in patients with lateral T_1 lesions and negative ipsilateral nodes (7,18)

7. The use of preoperative radiation therapy to obviate the need for exenteration in patients with advanced disease (19,20)

8. The use of postoperative radiation therapy to decrease the incidence of groin recurrence in patients with multiple positive groin nodes (15).

Etiology

The etiology of vulvar cancer has been only partially elucidated and is likely to be multifactorial. Based on histopathologic and environmental factors, there appear to be at least two distinct etiologic entities of squamous cell carcinoma of the vulva.

1. *Basaloid or warty types,* which tend to be multifocal, occur generally in younger patients and are related to human papillomavirus (HPV) infection, vulvar intraepithelial neoplasia (VIN), and cigarette smoking.

2. *Keratinizing types,* which tend to be unifocal, occur predominantly in older patients, are not related to HPV, and often are found in areas adjacent to lichen sclerosus and squamous hyperplasia.

High-grade vulvar intraepithelial neoplasia (VIN 3) has been most closely studied as a potential precancerous lesion. The direct progression of VIN to cancer is difficult to document, but 10% to 20% of vulvar carcinoma *in situ* lesions harbor an occult invasive component (21,22), and VIN is found adjacent to basaloid or warty vulvar squamous cell carcinomas in more than 80% of cases. DNA of HPV has been documented in 89% of patients with VIN 3 and in up to 86% of warty or basaloid type carcinomas of the vulva, but it occurs in less than 10% of the keratinizing type of carcinomas of the vulva (23). Epidemiologic risk factors for the basaloid or warty type squamous cell carcinoma of the vulva are similar to those for cervical cancer and include a history of multiple lower genital tract neoplasias, immunosuppression, and smoking (23,24). Frequently implied as an etiologic variable for the keratinizing carcinoma is the itch–scratch cycle associated with lichen sclerosus and squamous hyperplasia, with atypical changes occurring in the repaired epithelium. In keratinizing carcinoma, associated lichen sclerosus or squamous hyperplasia is found in more than 80% of patients (25,26), yet their causative role remains controversial. Supportive evidence that some of these lesions could be precancerous comes from molecular studies that demonstrate aneuploid DNA content, *p53* overexpression, and monoclonal expansion of keratinocytes in lichen sclerosus and associated squamous hyperplasia (27,28). In the past, some studies have reported vulvar cancer to be more common in patients who are obese, have hypertension and diabetes mellitus, or are nulliparous (29,30), but a recent case-control study of vulvar cancer was unable to confirm any of these as risk factors (24).

Types of Invasive Vulvar Cancer

The varieties of invasive vulvar cancer are shown in Table 33.1.

Squamous Cell Carcinoma

Approximately 90% to 92% of all invasive vulvar cancers are of the squamous cell type. As discussed previously, squamous carcinomas of the vulva can be divided into distinct histologic subtypes designated as *basaloid carcinoma, warty carcinoma,* and *keratinizing squamous carcinoma* (25). Mitoses are noted in these malignancies, but atypical keratinization is the histologic hallmark of invasive vulvar cancer (31). Most vulvar squamous carcinomas reveal keratinization (Fig. 33.1). Histologic features that correlate with

Table 33.1. Types of Vulvar Cancer

Type	*Percent*
Squamous	92
Melanoma	2–4
Basal cell	2–3
Bartholin gland (adenocarcinoma, squamous cell, transitional cell, adenoid cystic)	1
Metastatic	1
Verrucous	<1
Sarcoma	<1
Appendage (e.g., hidradenocarcinoma)	Rare

the occurrence of inguinal lymph node metastasis are lymph–vascular space invasion, tumor thickness, depth of stromal invasion, histologic pattern of invasion (spray and stellate versus broad and pushing), and increased amount of keratin (32–35).

Microinvasive Squamous Carcinoma

Microinvasive carcinoma of the vulva has been defined as a lesion <2 cm in diameter with <1 mm stromal invasion (36). Depth of stromal invasion is measured vertically from the epithelial–stromal junction (basement membrane) of the most superficial dermal papilla to the deepest point of tumor invasion (Fig. 33.2). **When the tumor invades <1 mm, metastasis to the inguinal lymph nodes is extremely rare among reported series. However, when invasion is >1 mm, there is a significant risk of inguinal lymph node metastasis.**

Figure 33.1 Squamous cell carcinoma of the vulva, keratinizing type. The multiple pearl formations consist of laminated keratin. (From **Berek JS, Hacker NF.** *Practical gynecologic oncology,* 2nd ed. Baltimore: Williams & Wilkins, 1994, with permission.)

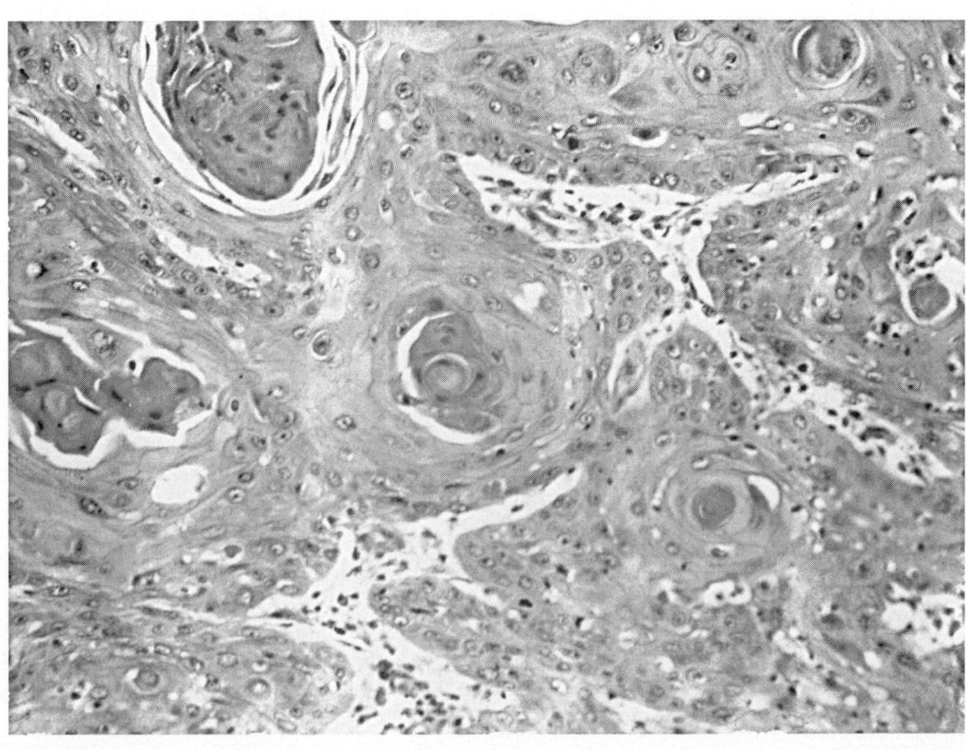

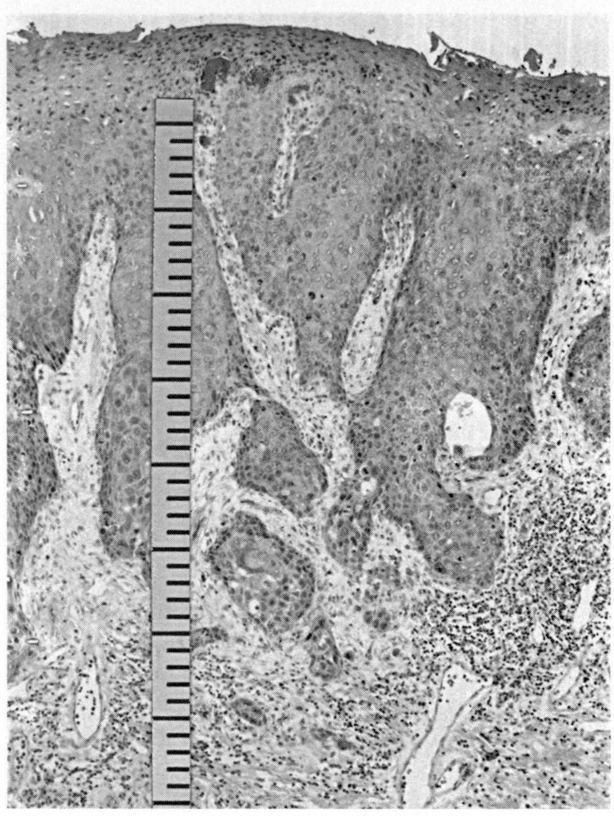

Figure 33.2 Early invasive carcinoma of vulva originating from vulvar intraepithelial neoplasia. Multiple irregular nests of malignant cells extend from the base of rete pegs. Desmoplastic stromal reaction and chronic inflammation are useful diagnostic signs of stromal invasion. The depth of stromal invasion is measured from the base of the most superficial dermal papilla vertically to the deepest tumor cells. In this tumor, it is 3.6 mm in depth. (From **Berek JS, Hacker NF.** *Practical gynecologic oncology,* 2nd ed. Baltimore: Williams & Wilkins, 1994, with permission.)

Clinical Features

Squamous cell carcinoma of the vulva is predominantly a disease of postmenopausal women; the mean age at diagnosis is about 65 years. However, 15% of patients who develop vulvar cancer do so before age 40. There may be a long-standing history of an associated vulvar intraepithelial disorder, such as lichen sclerosus, squamous hyperplasia, or VIN. Up to 27% of patients with vulvar cancer are reported to have a second primary malignancy, most commonly cervical cancer, followed by cancer of the breast, extragenital skin, and gastrointestinal tract (37–39).

Most patients are asymptomatic at the time of diagnosis. If symptoms exist, vulvar pruritus, a lump, or a mass are the most common findings. Less frequent symptoms include a bleeding or ulcerative lesion, discharge, pain, or dysuria. Occasionally, a large metastatic mass in the groin may be the initial complaint.

A careful inspection of the vulva should be part of every gynecologic examination. On physical examination, vulvar carcinoma is usually raised and may be fleshy, ulcerated, leukoplakic, or warty in appearance. It may be pigmented, red or white, tender or painless. The lesion may be clinically indistinct, especially in the presence of VIN or vulvar dystrophies (22,40). Thus, any lesion of the vulva warrants a biopsy.

Most squamous carcinomas of the vulva occur on the labia majora and minora (60%), but the clitoris (15%) and perineum (10%) also may be primary sites. Approximately 10% of the cases are too extensive to determine a site of origin, and about 5% of the cases are multifocal.

As part of the clinical evaluation, a careful assessment of the extent of the lesion, including whether it's unifocal or multifocal, should be performed. The groin lymph nodes should be evaluated carefully, and a complete pelvic examination should be performed. A cytologic sample should be taken from the cervix for Papanicolaou testing, and colposcopy of the cervix and vagina should be performed because of the common association with other squamous intraepithelial or invasive neoplasms of the lower genital tract.

Diagnosis

Diagnosis requires a wedge biopsy specimen, which usually can be obtained in the office using local anesthesia. If the lesion is only about 1 cm in diameter, excisional biopsy is preferable.

Physician delay is a common problem in the diagnosis of vulvar cancer, particularly if the lesion has a warty appearance. Any confluent warty lesion requires biopsy before medical or ablative therapy is initiated.

Routes of Spread

Vulvar cancer spreads by the following routes:

1. Direct extension, to involve adjacent structures such as the vagina, urethra, and anus
2. Lymphatic embolization to the regional inguinal and femoral lymph nodes
3. Hematogenous spread to distant sites, including the lungs, liver, and bone.

Lymphatic metastases may occur early in the disease. Twelve percent of T_1 tumors have regional metastases (37,41). Initially, spread is usually to the inguinal lymph nodes, which are located between Camper's fascia and the fascia lata (8). From these superficial groin nodes, the disease will spread to the deep femoral nodes, which are located medially along the femoral vessels (Fig. 33.3). *Cloquet's* or *Rosenmüller's node,* situated beneath the inguinal ligament, is the most cephalad of the femoral node group. **Metastases to the femoral nodes without involvement of the inguinal nodes have been reported** (42–45), and intraoperative lymphatic mapping studies find the sentinel node to be deep to the cribriform fascia in 5% of cases (46).

From the inguinal-femoral nodes, the cancer spreads to the pelvic nodes, particularly the external iliac group. Although direct lymphatic pathways from the clitoris and Bartholin gland to the pelvic nodes have been described, these channels seem to be of minimal clinical significance (11,47,48). The lymphatics of the vulva from either side form a rich network of anastomoses along the midline. Lymphatic drainage from the clitoris, anterior labia minora, and perineum is bilateral. For lateral vulvar tumors, metastases to contralateral lymph nodes in the absence of ipsilateral nodal involvement is rare (0.4% for T_1 tumors) (41).

The overall incidence of inguinal-femoral lymph node metastases is reported to be about 30% (9,10,45–51) (Table 33.2). Metastases to pelvic nodes occur in about 12% of cases. Pelvic nodal metastases are rare (0.6 %) in the absence of groin node involvement, but they occur on average in about 16% of cases with positive groin nodes (Table 33.2). The risk increases to 33% in the presence of clinically suspicious groin nodes (12), and to about 50% if there are three or more pathologically positive inguinal-femoral nodes (12,15,38). The incidence of lymph node metastases in relation to depth of invasion is shown in Table 33.3. Hematogenous spread usually occurs late in the course of vulvar cancer and is rare in the absence of lymph node metastases.

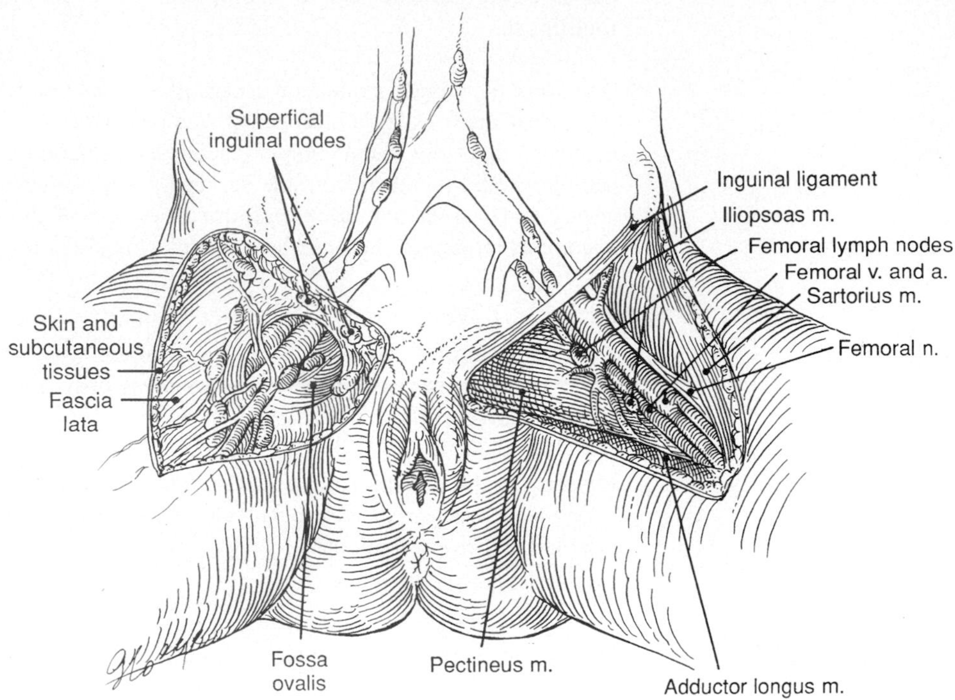

Figure 33.3 Inguinal-femoral lymph nodes. (From **Berek JS, Hacker NF.** *Practical gynecologic oncology,* 3rd ed. Philadelphia: Lippincott Williams & Wilkins, 2000, pg 558, with permission.)

Staging

Previously, vulvar carcinoma was staged clinically based on tumor size and location, palpable regional lymph node status, and a limited search for distant metastases. The prognostic importance of the lymph node status is significant, yet the accuracy of the clinical assessment of the lymph nodes is limited. Microscopic metastases may be present in nodes that are not clinically suspicious, and suspicious nodes may be enlarged because of inflammation only. **When compared with surgical staging, the percentage of error in clinical staging increases from 18% for stage I disease to 44% for stage IV disease** (38).

These factors led the Cancer Committee of the International Federation of Gynecology and Obstetrics (FIGO) in 1988 to introduce a surgical staging system for vulvar cancer, which was revised in 1995 to separate T_1 lesions invasive to 1 mm or less as stage Ia (Table 33.4). This surgical staging system offers much improvement over the previous clinical staging system, but there remains need for further refinements. One major problem is that stage III represents a very heterogeneous group of patients. It includes patients ranging from those with a small tumor involving the distal urethra or vagina and negative nodes and those with one microscopically involved groin node, who should have a good prognosis, to those with multiple positive groin nodes, who have a very poor prognosis.

Prognosis and Survival

Survival of patients with vulvar cancer correlates with FIGO stage. The prognosis for patients with early-stage disease is generally very good (Table 33.5). **The single most important prognostic factor is lymph node status, followed by lesion size** (57). Histologic grade, tumor thickness, depth of stromal invasion, and lymph–vascular space involvement contribute to the risk of lymph node involvement but are not independent predictors of survival (58). Patients with negative lymph nodes have a 5-year survival rate greater than 90%, compared with about 50% for patients with positive lymph nodes (57). The number of positive inguinal-femoral lymph nodes is an important prognostic factor. Patients with only one microscopically involved node have a prognosis comparable to those with negative

Table 33.2. Incidence of Lymph Node Metastases in Squamous Cell Carcinoma of the Vulva

Author	*Positive Inguinal femoral LN*	*Positive Pelvic LN/Patients with Pelvic LND*	*Positive Pelvic LN/ Patients with Negative Inguinal-femoral LN*	*Positive Pelvic LN/ Patients with Positive Inguinal-femoral LN*
Rutledge, 1970 (37)	33/86 (38%)	12/72 (17%)	0/53 (0%)	12/33 (36%)
Collins, 1971 (49)	27/98 (28%)	11/98 (11%)	4/71 (6%)	7/27 (26%)
Morley, 1976 (50)	67/180 (37%)	6/23 (26%)	0/113 (0%)	6/67 (9%)
Krupp, 1978 (51)	40/195 (21%)	10/195 (5%)	1/155 (0.6%)	9/40 (23%)
Benedet, 1979 (52)	34/120 (28%)	4/51 (8%)	N/A	N/A
Curry, 1980 (11)	57/191 (30%)	9/52 (17%)	0/134 (0%)	9/57 (16%)
Iversen, 1980 (53)	90/262 (34%)	7/100 (7%)	1/172 (0.6%)	6/90 (7%)
Hacker, 1983 (12)	31/113 (27%)	6/18 (33%)	0/82 (0%)	6/31 (19%)
Podratz, 1983 (38)	59/175 (34%)	7/114 (6%)	0/116 (0%)	7/59 (12%)
Monaghan, 1984 (13)	37/134 (28%)	3/80 (4%)	N/A	N/A
Hopkins, 1991 (54)	61/145 (42%)	13/38 (34%)	0/84 (0%)	13/61 (21%)
Keys, 1993 (55)	203/588 (35%)	15/53 (28%)	N/A	N/A
Total	739/2,287 (32%)	103/894 (12%)	6/980 (0.6%)	75/465 (16%)

LN, lymph node; LND, lymph node dissection; N/A, data not available.

lymph nodes (10,12), whereas the 2-year survival rate is 20% for patients with three or more metastatic lymph nodes (12). In a Gynecologic Oncology Group (GOG) study, patients with N_0 or N_1 nodes had a 2-year survival rate of 78%, compared with 52% for patients with N_2 nodes and 33% for patients with N_3 nodes (15). The survival rate for patients with positive pelvic nodes is about 11% (59). Tumor ploidy is another important prognostic factor. Data from the Norwegian Radium Hospital (60) demonstrate a 5-year crude survival rate of 62% for diploid and 23% for the aneuploid tumors ($p < 0.001$). In a multivariate Cox regression analysis, tumor ploidy was the second most important prognostic factor after lymph node status.

Table 33.3. Nodal Status in T_1 Squamous Cell Carcinoma of the Vulva Versus Depth of Stromal Invasion

Depth of Invasion	*No.*	*Positive Nodes*	*Nodes*
<1 mm	163	0	0
1.1–2 mm	145	11	7.7
2.1–3 mm	131	11	8.3
3.1–5 mm	101	27	26.7
>5 mm	38	13	34.2
Total	578	62	10.7

From **Berek JS, Hacker NF.** Practical gynecologic oncology. 3rd ed. Philadelphia: Lippincott Williams & Wilkins 2000, pg. 560, with permission.

Table 33.4. Revised FIGO Surgical Staging for Vulvar Cancer (36)

FIGO Stage	*TNM Classification*	*Clinical/Pathologic Findings*
0	Tis[a]	Carcinoma *in situ,* intraepithelial carcinoma
I	$T_1N_0M_0$	Tumor confined to vulva and/or perineum, ≤2 cm in greatest dimension, nodes are negative
Ia[b]		Stromal invasion ≤1 mm
Ib		Stromal invasion >1 mm
II	$T_2N_0M_0$	Tumor confined to vulva and/or perineum, >2 cm in greatest dimension, nodes are negative
III	$T_3N_0M_0$ $T_{1-3}N_1M_0$	Tumor of any size with 1. Adjacent spread to lower urethra, vagina, or anus or 2. Unilateral regional lymph node metastases
IVa	$T_4N_{any}M_0$ $T_{any}N_2M_0$	Tumor of any size with 1. Adjacent spread to upper urethra, bladder mucosa, rectal mucosa, pelvic bone or 2. Bilateral regional lymph node metastases
IVb	$T_{any}N_{any}M_1$	Any distant metastases, including pelvic lymph nodes

[a]TNM Classification:

T: Primary tumor
Tx: Primary tumor cannot be assessed
T_0: No evidence of primary tumor
Tis: Carcinoma *in situ* (preinvasive carcinoma)
T_1: Tumor confined to the vulva and/or perineum, ≤2 cm in greatest dimension
T_2: Tumor confined to the vulva and/or perineum, >2 cm in greatest dimension
T_3: Tumor invades any of the following: lower urethra, vagina, anus
T_4: Tumor invades any of the following: bladder mucosa, rectal mucosa, upper urethra, pelvic bone

N: Regional lymph nodes
Regional lymph nodes are the femoral and inguinal nodes
Nx Regional lymph nodes cannot be assessed
N_0 No lymph node metastases
N_1 Unilateral regional lymph node metastases
N_2 Bilateral regional lymph node metastases

M Distant metastases
Mx Presence of distant metastases cannot be assessed
M_0 No distant metastases
M_1 Distant metastases (including pelvic lymph node metastases)

[b]The depth of stromal invasion is measured from the epithelial–stromal junction of the adjacent most superficial dermal papilla to the deepest point of invasion.

Treatment

After the pioneering work of Taussig (4) in the United States and Way (5) in Great Britain, *en bloc* radical vulvectomy and bilateral dissection of the groin and pelvic nodes became the standard treatment for most patients with operable vulvar cancer. If the disease involved the anus, rectovaginal septum, or proximal urethra, some type of pelvic exenteration was combined with the dissection.

Although the survival rate improved markedly with this aggressive surgical approach, several factors have led to modifications of this treatment plan during the past 20 years. These

Table 33.5. Five-year Survival for Patients with Vulvar Carcinoma (57)

FIGO Stage	*No. of Patients*	*Corrected 5-Year Survival (%)*
I	148 (26%)	98%
II	191 (33%)	85%
III	176 (31%)	74%
IV	62 (11%)	31%
All stages	577	79%

factors are summarized as follows:

1. An increasing proportion of patients with early-stage disease—up to 50% of patients in many centers—have T_1 tumors.
2. There were concerns about the postoperative morbidity and associated long-term hospitalization common with the *en bloc* radical dissection.
3. Increasing awareness has emerged of the psychosexual consequences of radical vulvectomy.

In order to individualize the patient's care and determine the appropriate therapy, it is necessary to determine independently the primary lesion as well as groin lymph nodes.

Before initiation of therapy, all patients should undergo colposcopy of the cervix, vagina, and vulva. Preinvasive (and rarely invasive) lesions may be present at other sites along the lower genital tract.

Management of the Primary Lesion

Early Vulvar Cancer (T_1) **The modern approach to the management of patients with T_1 carcinoma of the vulva should be individualized** (6,7). There is no standard approach applicable to every patient, and emphasis is on performing the most conservative operation that is consistent with cure of the disease.

Radical vulvectomy has been considered the standard treatment for primary vulvar lesions, but this operation is associated with significant surgical morbidity and disturbances of sexual function and body image. Psychosexual sequelae are a major long-term morbidity associated with the treatment of vulvar cancer (8). One study reported that sexual arousal was reduced to the eighth percentile and body image was reduced to the fourth percentile for women who had undergone vulvectomy when compared with healthy adult women (61).

Traditionally, there has been concern that, without an *en bloc* resection, intervening tissue left between the primary tumor and the regional lymph nodes may contain microscopic tumor foci in draining lymphatics. However, experience with a separate incision technique for node dissection has confirmed that metastases rarely occur in the skin bridge in patients without clinically suspicious nodes in the groin (17).

During the past 20 years, several investigators have advocated a radical local excision rather than a radical vulvectomy for the primary lesion for patients with T_1 tumors (6–9). Regardless of whether a radical vulvectomy or a radical local excision is performed, the surgical margins adjacent to the tumor will be the same. An analysis of the available literature indicates that the incidence of local invasive recurrence after radical local excision is not higher than that after radical vulvectomy (9,41,59,62). This finding suggests that in the presence of an otherwise normal-appearing vulva, radical local excision is a safe surgical option, regardless of the depth of invasion. A recent review of 135 patients with all stages of disease assessed the surgical margin that must be obtained to prevent local disease recurrence. In this study, a 1-cm tumor-free surgical margin on the vulvar specimen (0.8-cm on pathologic specimen) resulted in a very high rate of local control (63). Neither clinical tumor size nor the presence of coexisting benign vulvar pathology correlated with local recurrence. It is important to bear in mind that paraffin-embedded tissue shrinks by about 25%. Thus, at the time of radical local excision, at least a 1- to 1.5-cm grossly negative margin, which should extend down to the level of the inferior fascia of the urogenital diaphragm, should be obtained.

When vulvar cancer arises in the presence of VIN or some nonneoplastic epithelial disorder, treatment will be influenced by the patient's age. Elderly patients who often have had many

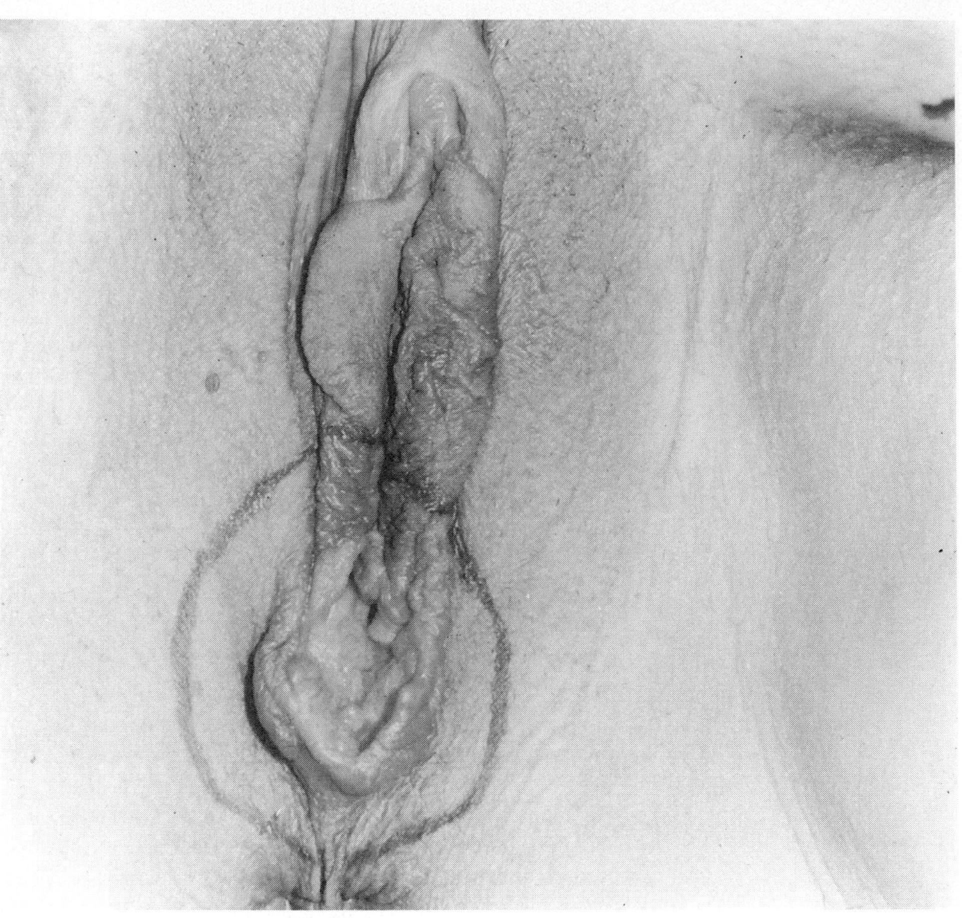

Figure 33.4 Small (T_1) vulvar carcinoma at the posterior fourchette. (From **Berek JS, Hacker NF.** *Practical gynecologic oncology,* 3rd ed. Philadelphia: Lippincott Williams & Wilkins 2000, pg. 565, with permission.)

years of chronic itching may not be disturbed by the prospect of a vulvectomy. In younger women, it will be desirable to conserve as much of the vulva as possible. Thus, radical local excision should be performed for the invasive disease, and the associated intraepithelial disease should be treated in the manner most appropriate to the patient. For example, topical steroids may be required for lichen sclerosus or squamous hyperplasia, whereas VIN may require superficial local excision and primary closure.

Radical local excision is most appropriate for lesions on the lateral or posterior aspects of the vulva (Fig. 33.4). Midline lesions pose special challenges due to their proximity to clitoris, urethra, or anus. For anterior lesions that involve the clitoris or that are in proximity to it, any type of surgical excision will have psychosexual consequences. In addition, marked edema of the posterior vulva may occur. For young patients with periclitoral lesions, the primary lesion can be treated with a small field of radiation therapy, possibly with concomitant sensitizing chemotherapy. Small vulvar lesions should respond very well to about 5,000 cGy external radiation, and biopsy can be performed after therapy to confirm the absence of any residual disease (64).

T_2 and T_3 Vulvar Cancer

In recent years, the indications for vulvar conservation have been extended by some surgeons to selected patients with T_2 and early T_3 tumors. Although the reported experience is limited (9,10,65), a recent study suggests that the local recurrence rate for patients with conservatively treated T_2 tumors is identical to that for patients with T_1 tumors (66) as long as surgical margins of at least 1 cm are obtained. The tumor-free margin should be the same, whether or not a radical vulvectomy or a radical local excision is performed, so it would seem to be both feasible and desirable to extend the indications for vulvar conservation, particularly for younger patients. **Tumors that are most suitable to a more conservative resection are those involving the posterior half of the vulva, where preservation of the clitoris and mons pubis is feasible.**

For patients with more advanced T_2 and T_3 lesions, management consists of radical vulvectomy and bilateral inguinal-femoral lymphadenectomy. If the disease involves the distal urethra, vagina, or anus, partial resection of these organs will be required. Alternatively, it may be preferable to give preoperative radiation therapy to allow for a less radical resection (see below).

Closure of Large Defects

After radical local excision, primary closure without tension often can be accomplished for smaller defects. However, if a more extensive dissection has been required to treat a large primary lesion, a number of options are available to repair the defect.

1. An area may be left open to granulate, which it will usually do over a period of 6 to 8 weeks (67).

2. Full-thickness skin flaps may be devised (68–71). The rhomboid flap is best suited to covering large defects of the posterior vulva (71), whereas for lateral defects, a mons pubis pedicle flap has been advocated (68).

3. Myocutaneous flaps may be developed to cover the defect. Unilateral or bilateral gracilis myocutaneous grafts are most useful when an extensive area from the mons pubis to the perianal area has been resected. Because the graft brings a new blood supply to the area, it is particularly applicable if the vulva is poorly vascularized from prior surgical resection or radiation (72).

4. If extensive defects exist in the groin and vulva, the tensor fascia lata myocutaneous graft may be the most applicable (73).

Advanced Disease—Large T_3 and T_4 Primary Tumors

To achieve primary surgical clearance for tumors involving the upper urethra, anus, rectum, or rectovaginal septum, pelvic exenteration is needed in addition to radical vulvectomy and inguinal-femoral lymphadenectomy, which carries an extremely high physical and psychological morbidity (61,74). Reported 5-year survival rates are about 50% (75–78). For many of these patients, a combined approach of surgery and radiation therapy offers improved survival and reduced morbidity. Numerous small prospective and retrospective series report on the use of external beam radiation, often with concomitant chemotherapy to shrink the primary tumor. Reported initial response rates to chemoradiation approximate 90% (79–81). It is important that this chemoradiation is followed by a more limited resection of the tumor bed and lymphadenectomy on an individualized basis. About one-half of the specimens will contain residual tumor (20,82), and local relapse rates are as high as 50% to 79% with external radiation alone (with or without concomitant chemotherapy) (83,84), emphasizing the need for a combined approach that involves radiation and surgery.

As experience with this combination therapy has evolved, it appears that external beam therapy is generally appropriate for most cases, with more selective use of brachytherapy. The extensiveness of the surgery has also been significantly modified. A more limited vulvar resection is now advocated, and bulky N_2 and N_3 nodes are resected without full groin dissection to avoid the leg edema associated with groin dissection and radiation. With this combined radiation-surgical approach, 5-year survival rates as high as 76% have been reported (82). With the experience now accrued, preoperative radiation, with or without concurrent chemotherapy, should be regarded as the treatment of first choice for patients with advanced vulvar cancer who would otherwise require some type of pelvic exenteration.

Management of the Lymph Nodes

Groin dissection is associated with postoperative wound infection and breakdown, as well as chronic leg edema. Although the incidence of wound breakdown is reduced significantly when separate incisions are used for the groin dissection (Fig. 33.5) (17), chronic leg edema remains a major problem. When assessing a patient for groin dissection, the following three facts should to be kept in mind:

1. The only patients with virtually no risk of lymph node metastases are those whose tumor invades the stroma to <1 mm.
2. Patients who develop recurrent disease in an undissected groin have a >90% mortality (88).
3. Based on the laterality of the vulvar lesions, an ipsilateral or bilateral lymphadenectomy becomes necessary.

Appropriate groin dissection is the single most important factor in decreasing the mortality for early vulvar cancer.

Figure 33.5 Skin incision for groin dissection through a separate incision. A line is drawn 1 cm below and parallel to the groin crease, and a narrow ellipse of skin is removed. (From **Berek JS, Hacker NF.** *Practical gynecologic oncology,* 2nd ed. Baltimore: Williams & Wilkins, 1994, with permission.)

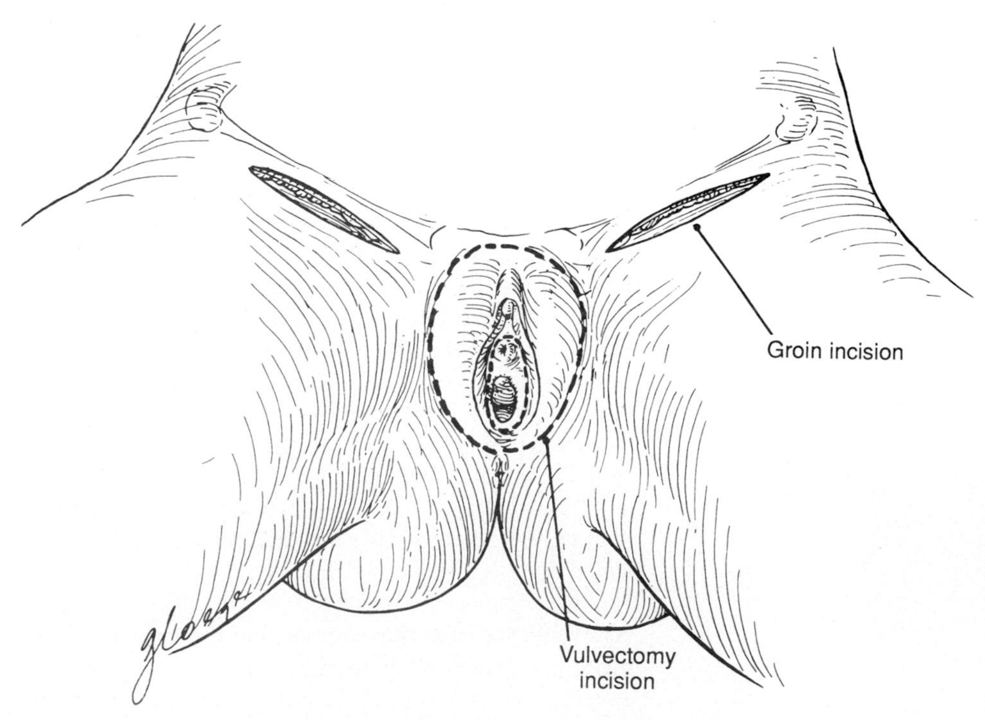

Microinvasive Carcinoma **All patients whose tumors demonstrate more than 1 mm of stromal invasion require inguinal-femoral lymphadenectomy.** A wedge biopsy specimen of the primary tumor should be obtained, and the depth of invasion should be determined. If it is smaller than 1 mm on the wedge biopsy specimen, the entire lesion should be locally excised and analyzed histologically to determine the depth of invasion. If there is still no invasive focus larger than 1 mm, groin dissection may be omitted provided there is no lymph–vascular space invasion and there are no clinically suspicious groin lymph nodes. Although an occasional patient with less than 1 mm of stromal invasion has had documented groin node metastases (89), the incidence is so low that it is of no practical significance.

Inguinal-femoral Lymphadenectomy **If groin dissection is indicated in patients with early vulvar cancer, it should be a thorough inguinal-femoral lymphadenectomy.** The GOG recently reported six groin recurrences among 121 patients with T_1 N_0 tumors after a superficial (inguinal) dissection, even though the removed inguinal nodes were negative (45). Whether all of these recurrences were in the femoral nodes is unclear, but this large multicenter study does indicate that an incomplete groin dissection will increase the number of groin recurrences and, therefore, mortality. Comparable failure rates have been reported by Burke and colleagues (9). Furthermore, GOG data indicate that radiation therapy cannot substitute for groin dissection followed by selective radiation as indicated, even in patients with clinically nonsuspicious lymph nodes (90). This GOG study was closed early because a significantly higher incidence of recurrences occurred in women who were receiving groin radiation therapy only (19% versus 0%). The dose of radiation was 5,000 cGy given in daily 200-cGy fractions to a depth of 3 cm below the anterior skin surface. Although the radiation regimen prescribed has been criticized extensively, the therapeutic effects of an alternative radiation regimen remain to be determined.

Unilateral Versus Bilateral Groin Dissection **It is clear that it is not necessary to perform a bilateral groin dissection if the primary lesion is unilateral and the ipsilateral lymph nodes are negative.** In a patient with unilateral T_1 lesion and negative ipsilateral groin nodes, the risk of contralateral lymph node metastasis is 0.4% (41). However, there is an increase in the risk of contralateral nodal involvement proportional to the number of positive ipsilateral inguinal nodes (15). Thus, it is recommended that patients with any bulky or multiple microscopically positive ipsilateral groin lymph nodes undergo contralateral inguinal-femoral lymphadenectomy as well. Bilateral inguinal-femoral lymphadenectomy should be performed for midline lesions (clitoris, anterior labia minora, posterior fourchette) or those within 2 cm of the midline, because of the more frequent contralateral lymph flow from these regions (91).

Management of Pelvic Lymph Nodes In the past, pelvic lymphadenectomy has been considered part of the routine surgery for invasive vulvar cancer. However, the incidence of pelvic lymph node metastasis is rare in the absence of groin node involvement (Table 33.2), thus a more selective approach is preferred. Patients most prone to pelvic lymph node metastasis are those with clinically suspicious or three or more pathologically positive groin nodes (11,12,14,38). In these patients, the pelvis requires treatment by pelvic lymphadenectomy or radiation. If a preoperative pelvic imaging study reveals enlarged pelvic lymph nodes, resection of these nodes should be performed via an extraperitoneal approach because of the inability of external beam radiation therapy to sterilize bulky positive pelvic nodes.

Sentinel Lymph Node Studies A number of investigators have explored the use of intraoperative lymphatic mapping using lymphoscintigraphy or blue dye to identify a sentinel node that would predict the presence or absence of regional nodal metastases (46,92–94). Small preliminary studies suggest that a sentinel node can be identified in most patients. Reliable identification of the sentinel node and foregoing a full node dissection in patients with clinically nonsuspicious groin lymph nodes and a negative sentinel node may significantly reduce the number of patients who undergo unnecessary, extensive lymphadenectomy in the absence of disease. However, until the accuracy of the negative predictive value of an uninvolved sentinel node is documented in well-designed and sufficiently powered clinical trials, complete inguinal-femoral lymphadenectomy remains indicated in all but stage Ia disease, given the high mortality of recurrence in an undissected groin.

Postoperative Management

Despite the age and general medical condition of many elderly patients with vulvar cancer, surgery is usually remarkably well tolerated. Patients should be able to commence eating a low-residue diet on the first postoperative day. In the past, bedrest had been advised for 3 to 5 days postoperatively to allow for immobilization of the wounds and foster healing. Because radical local excisions are being performed with increasing frequency and groin dissections are done through separate incisions, patients generally begin ambulation on postoperative day 1 or 2. Pneumatic calf compression or subcutaneous heparin should be given to help prevent deep venous thrombosis, and active leg movements are to be encouraged. Frequent dressing changes are performed to keep the vulvar wound dry. Meticulous perineal hygiene is maintained. Suction drainage of each side of the groin is continued until output is minimal to help decrease the incidence of groin seromas. It is not uncommon for suction drainage to continue for 10 or more days. The Foley catheter is removed once the patient is ambulatory. If there is significant periurethral swelling, prolonged bladder drainage may be advisable. If there is breakdown of the vulvar wound, sitz baths or whirlpool therapy is helpful, followed by drying of the perineum with a hair dryer.

Early Postoperative Complications

The major immediate morbidity is related to groin wound infection, necrosis, and breakdown. This complication has been reported in as many as 53% to 85% of patients having an *en bloc* operation (37,38). With the separate-incision approach, the incidence of wound breakdown can be reduced to about 44%; major breakdown occurs in about 14% of patients (17,39,95). With appropriate antibiotics, debridement, and wound dressings, the area will granulate and reepithelialize over the next several weeks and may be managed with home nursing. Whirlpool therapy is effective for areas of extensive breakdown.

Other early postoperative complications include urinary tract infection, seromas in the femoral triangle, deep venous thrombosis, pulmonary embolism, myocardial infarction, hemorrhage and, rarely, osteitis pubis. Lymphocysts or groin seromas occur in about 10% to 15% of cases and should be managed by periodic sterile aspiration. Anesthesia of the anterior thigh resulting from femoral nerve injury is common and usually resolves slowly.

Late Complications

One major late complication is chronic lymphedema, which occurs on average in about 30% of patients (37–39,95,96). Recurrent lymphangitis or cellulitis of the leg develops in about 10% of patients and usually responds to oral antibiotics. Urinary stress incontinence, with or without genital prolapse, occurs in about 10% of patients after radical vulvectomy and may require corrective surgery. Introital stenosis can lead to dyspareunia and may require a vertical relaxing incision, which is sutured transversely. An uncommon late complication is femoral hernia, which usually can be prevented intraoperatively by closure of the femoral canal with a suture from the inguinal ligament to Cooper's ligament. Pubic osteomyelitis and rectovaginal or rectoperineal fistulas are rare late complications.

Other major long-term treatment complications associated with the extent of vulvar surgery include depression, altered body image, and sexual dysfunction (61,74). Modifications in the radical extent of the surgical approach and appropriate preoperative and postoperative counseling may help lessen some of the psychological trauma.

Role of Radiation Therapy

Radiation therapy traditionally has been considered to have a limited role in the management of patients with vulvar cancer. In the orthovoltage era, local tissue tolerance was poor and vulvar necrosis was common, but with megavoltage therapy, tolerance has improved significantly. Thus, radiation therapy, with or without concurrent chemotherapy, is likely to have an increasingly important role in the management of patients with vulvar cancer. It is important to remember, though, that with a rare exception, radiation therapy alone has little place in the primary management of vulvar cancer. It is generally indicated in conjunction with surgery.

The indications for radiation therapy for patients with primary vulvar cancer are still evolving. At present, radiation seems to be clearly indicated in the following situations:

1. Preoperatively, in patients with advanced disease who would otherwise require pelvic exenteration (19,20)
2. Postoperatively, to treat the pelvic lymph nodes and groin of patients with two or more microscopically positive or one grossly positive groin node (15).

Possible roles for radiation therapy include the following:

1. Postoperatively, to help prevent local recurrences in patients with involved or close surgical margins (97,98,103)
2. As primary therapy for patients with small primary tumors, particularly clitoral or periclitoral lesions in young and middle-aged women, for whom surgical resection would have significant psychological consequences (64).

No additional treatment is recommended if one microscopically positive groin node is found. The prognosis for this group of patients is excellent (12), and only careful observation is required. Even if a unilateral groin dissection has been performed for a lateral lesion, there seems to be no indication for dissection of the other side, because contralateral lymph node involvement is likely only if there are multiple microscopic or any gross ipsilateral inguinal node metastases (12,15).

If clinically evident groin metastases or two or more microscopically positive groin nodes are found, which is unusual in patients with T_1 vulvar cancer, the patient is at increased risk of groin and pelvic recurrence and should receive postoperative groin and pelvic irradiation. In 1977, the GOG initiated a prospective trial in which patients with positive groin nodes were randomized to either ipsilateral pelvic node dissection or bilateral pelvic node dissection plus groin irradiation (15). Radiation therapy consisted of 4,500 to 5,000 cGy to the midplane of the pelvis at a rate of 180 to 200 cGy per day. The survival rate for the radiation group (68% at 2 years) was significantly better than the survival rate for the pelvic lymphadenectomy group (54% at 2 years) ($p = 0.03$). The survival advantage was limited to patients with clinically evident groin nodes or more than one positive groin node. Groin recurrence occurred in 3 of 59 patients (5%) treated with radiation, compared with 13 of 55 (23.6%) patients treated with lymphadenectomy ($p = 0.02$). Four patients who received radiation had a pelvic recurrence, compared with one who had lymphadenectomy. These data indicate no benefit from pelvic irradiation compared with pelvic lymphadenectomy for the prevention of pelvic recurrence, but they do highlight the value of prophylactic groin irradiation in preventing groin recurrence in patients with multiple positive groin nodes.

Recurrent Vulvar Cancer

Approximately two-thirds of recurrences of vulvar cancer occur within the first 2 years from initial therapy (99), with groin recurrences occurring sooner (median time to recurrence 6 months) than vulvar recurrences (median time to recurrence 3 years) (100).

Recurrence of vulvar cancer correlates most closely with the number of positive groin nodes (12). Patients with fewer than three positive nodes, particularly if the nodes are only microscopically involved, have a low incidence of recurrence at any site, whereas patients with three or more positive nodes have a high incidence of local, regional, and systemic recurrences (12,15).

Local Recurrence Margin status at the time of radical resection of the vulvar cancer is the most powerful predictor of local vulvar recurrence, with an almost 50% recurrence risk with margins closer than 0.8 cm (63). Margin status does not, however, predict survival (57). Local vulvar recurrences are likely in patients with primary lesions larger than 4 cm in diameter, especially if lymph–vascular space invasion is present (97,101). When detected early, isolated local failure is usually salvageable by additional surgical therapy (9,17,39,45,102), often with a gracilis myocutaneous graft to cover the defect. Radiation therapy, particularly a combination of external beam therapy plus interstitial needles, at times combined with chemotherapy, has also been used to treat vulvar recurrences (104). One study reported on 10 patients treated in this manner, nine of whom were still alive with a mean follow-up of 28 months (105). However, 6 of the 10 patients developed severe radionecrosis at a median of 8.5 months after radiation, and the authors concluded that, although this treatment was highly effective, it also had a high degree of morbidity.

Regional and Distant Recurrence Regional and distant recurrences are difficult to manage and are associated with a poor prognosis (97,99,100). Radiation therapy may be used in conjunction with surgery for groin recurrence, whereas chemotherapeutic agents that have activity against squamous carcinomas may be offered for distant metastases. The literature on the use of chemotherapy for recurrent vulvar cancer consists of mainly small series. The most extensively studied regimens contain *bleomycin* and *methotrexate,* with or without *cisplatin* or *CCNU* (a nitrosourea) and *bleomycin* and *mitomycin C* (106,107), but response rates are low and the duration of response is usually disappointing. Long-term survival is very uncommon with regional or distant recurrence.

Melanoma

Vulvar melanomas are rare, with an incidence of 0.1 to 0.19 per 100,000 women (108,109). They account for 4% to 10% of all cases and are the second most common form of vulvar malignancy (36). Most melanomas arise *de novo* (110), but they may arise from a preexisting junctional nevus. Vulvar melanomas occur predominantly in postmenopausal white women. The incidence of cutaneous melanomas worldwide is increasing significantly. Vulvar melanomas appear to behave in a manner similar to that of other cutaneous melanomas (111–113).

Most patients with vulvar melanoma have no symptoms except for a pigmented lesion that may be enlarging. Some patients have itching or bleeding, and a few have a groin mass. Vulvar melanomas occur most frequently on the labia minora or the clitoris (Fig. 33.6), and extension into the urethra or vagina at discovery is not uncommon. Any pigmented lesion on the vulva should be excised or, if the lesion is large, sampled for biopsy unless it is known to have been present and unchanged for some years. Most vulvar nevi are junctional and may be precursor lesions to melanoma; thus, any nevus of the vulva should be removed.

Histopathology

There are three basic histologic types of vulvar melanoma (Fig. 33.7).

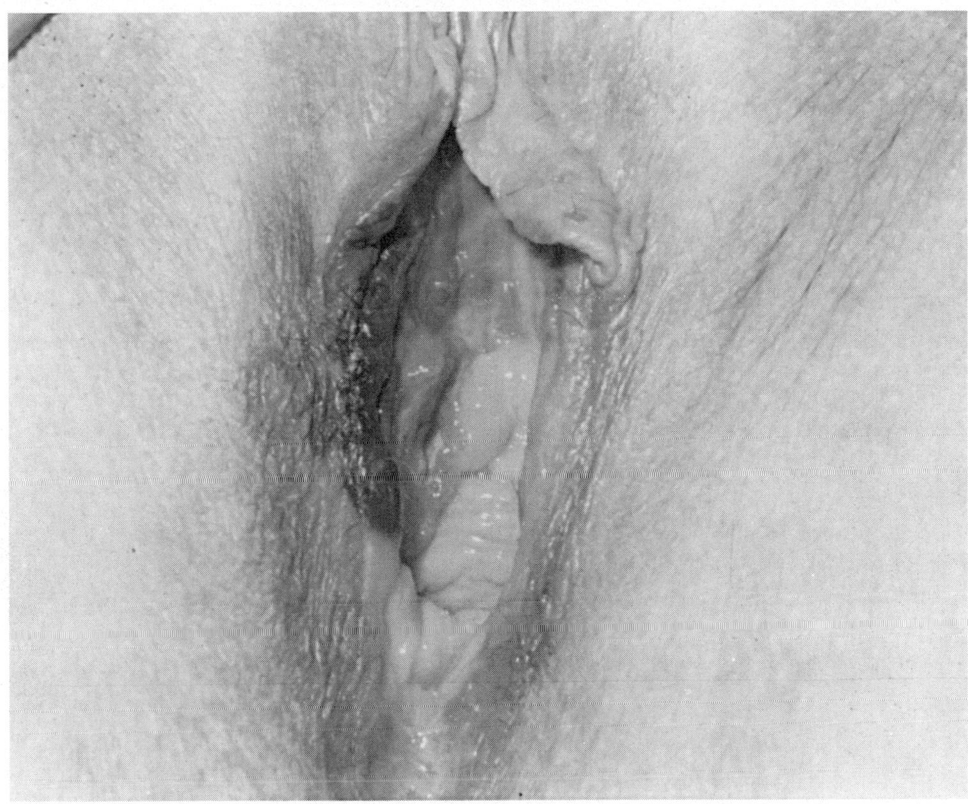

Figure 33.6 Melanoma of the vulva involving the right labium minus. (From **Berek JS, Hacker NF.** *Practical gynecologic oncology,* 3rd ed. Philadelphia: Lippincott Williams & Wilkins, 2000, pg. 582, with permission.)

1. The *mucosal lentiginous melanoma* is a flat freckle that may become quite extensive but tends to remain superficial.

2. The most common type is the *superficial spreading melanoma,* which tends to remain relatively superficial early in its development.

3. The *nodular melanoma,* which is the most aggressive, is characterized by a raised lesion that penetrates deeply and may metastasize widely.

In the largest series reported to date, more than one-fourth of the cases of melanomas were macroscopically amelanotic (108). Vulvar melanoma tends to spread early, not only lymphatically but also hematogenously.

Staging

The FIGO staging used for squamous lesions is not applicable to melanomas, because the lesions are usually much smaller and the prognosis is related to the depth of tumor invasion rather than to the diameter of the lesion (111,115,117). The leveling system established by Clark and others (117) for cutaneous melanomas is less readily applicable to vulvar lesions because of the different skin morphology. The vulvar skin lacks a well-defined papillary dermis. Breslow (118) measured the thickest portion of the melanoma from the surface of intact epithelium to the deepest point of invasion. This system is more adequate for the vulva. Chung and colleagues (115) proposed a modified system that retained Clark's definitions for levels I and V but arbitrarily defined levels II, III, and IV, using measurements in millimeters. The 1992 American Joint Committee on Cancer (AJCC)

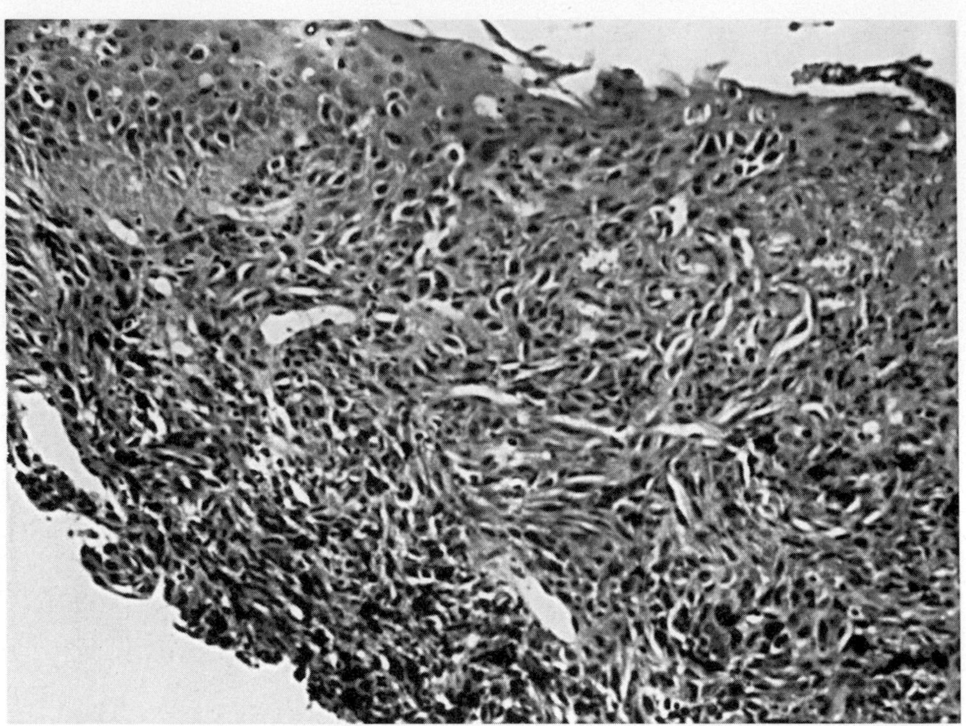

Figure 33.7 Vulvar melanoma. Spindle-shaped melanoma cells form interlacing bundles, and some contain melanin pigment (left lower corner). Epidermal invasion is evident in the form of Pagetoid migration (left upper corner). (From **Berek JS, Hacker NF.** *Practical gynecologic oncology,* 2nd ed. Baltimore: Williams & Wilkins, 1994, with permission.)

staging for melanoma combined the Clark and Breslow systems with clinical staging (119). A comparison of these systems is shown in Table 33.6.

Treatment

With better understanding of the prognostic significance of the microstage, some individualization of treatment has developed. However, treatment of vulvar melanoma continues to be controversial, in part because of the lack of large retrospective studies, which makes it difficult to draw conclusions regarding the behavior and best treatment of vulvar melanoma. Currently used treatments are guided by experience from cutaneous melanoma in general and squamous cell carcinomas of the vulva. Paralleling the trend toward more conservative

Table 33.6. Microstaging of Vulvar Melanoma

	Clark Level (117)	*Chung Depth of Invasion (115)*	*Breslow Tumor Thickness (118)*
I	Intraepithelial	Intraepithelial	<0.76 mm
II	Into papillary dermis	<1 mm from granular layer	0.76–1.5 mm Superficial invasion
III	Filling dermal papillae	1.1–2.0 mm from granular layer	1.51–2.25 mm Intermediate invasion
IV	Into reticular dermis	>2 mm from granular layer	2.26–3.0 mm Intermediate invasion
V	Into subcutaneous fat	Into subcutaneous fat	>3 mm Deep invasion

surgical management of cutaneous melanoma, there is a shift toward more conservative management of vulvar melanoma (112,113,120,121).

It is generally accepted that lesions with less than 1 mm of invasion may be treated with radical local excision alone (115,116). With more invasive lesions, *en bloc* resection of the primary tumor and regional groin nodes has traditionally been recommended. In the last 15 years, however, radical vulvectomy has been performed less frequently and survival does not seem to be compromised (122). One study reported on 32 patients with vulvar melanoma who underwent local excision (n = 14), simple vulvectomy (n = 7), or radical resection (n = 11) (123). No group had a superior survival rate, although the overall survival rate at 5 years was only 25%. More recently, another study reported on 59 patients who underwent radical vulvectomy and 19 who underwent more conservative resections (112). Survival was not improved by the more radical approach, and they recommended radical local excision for the primary tumor, with groin dissection for tumors with a thickness of more than 1 mm. Current literature on cutaneous melanoma suggests that a 1-cm margin of skin and subcutaneous tissue is sufficient for the treatment of superficial localized melanoma (Breslow tumor thickness <0.76 mm), whereas a 2-cm margin suffices for intermediate-thickness lesions (1 to 4 mm) (124,125).

Because melanomas commonly involve the clitoris and labia minora, the vaginourethral margin of resection is a common site of failure, and care should be taken to obtain an adequate "inner" resection margin (126). A 10-year survival rate of 61% has been shown for lateral lesions, compared with 37% for medial lesions ($p = 0.027$) (111).

Controversy exists as to which patients may benefit from inguinal-femoral lymphadenectomy. A prospective study by the GOG demonstrated that the risk of inguinal-femoral lymph node metastasis correlated with the Breslow microstage (113). As with cutaneous melanoma, it appears that for superficial lesions (Breslow tumor thickness <0.76 mm) the risk for nodal spread is so low that routine lymphadenectomy is not indicated as long as the nodes appear clinically to be free of disease. For intermediate-thickness (1 to 4 mm) cutaneous melanoma, a randomized controlled trial of elective lymph node dissection versus observation showed a 5-year survival advantage for patients who underwent elective lymph node dissection, who were younger than 60 years, and whose tumors were characterized by 1- to 2-mm thickness and no ulcerations (127). Patients with deeply invasive cutaneous melanomas (>4-mm tumor thickness) have a high risk of regional and systemic metastases and are unlikely to benefit from regional lymphadenectomy (128). Given some of the epidemiologic, histologic, and prognostic differences between vulvar and cutaneous melanoma (114), extrapolation of these data to the vulva should be done with caution. Specific to patients with vulvar melanoma, there is a small body of literature to suggest that there may be a clinical benefit in elective groin lymphadenectomy and the resection of clinically positive nodes (111,112).

Pelvic node metastases do not occur in the absence of groin node metastases (126,129,130). In addition, the prognosis for patients with positive pelvic nodes is so poor that there seems to be no value in performing pelvic lymphadenectomy for this disease.

Chemotherapy and immunotherapy for vulvar melanoma have disappointing results. *Interferon-α* has been used with some improvement in survival rates for patients with deep invasive (>4 mm) cutaneous melanoma and those with lymph node metastases, but morbidity is significant (131,132). Estrogen receptors have been demonstrated in human melanomas (133), and an occasional response to *tamoxifen* has been reported (134,135). Cancer vaccines are currently under investigation (136).

Prognosis

The behavior of melanomas can be quite unpredictable, but the overall prognosis is poor. The reported 5-year survival rate for vulvar melanoma ranges from 25% (123) to 50% (108,109). Because vulvar melanoma has a propensity for late recurrences, 5-year survival may not

Table 33.7. Prognosis for Patients with Vulvar Melanoma Stratified by Breslow Microstaging

Breslow Tumor Thickness	*No. of Patients*	*% DOD*
<0.76 mm	31 [19]	7 (23%) [1 (5%)][a]
0.76–1.5 mm	35	6 (17%)
1.51–3.0 mm	42	23 (55%)
>3.0 mm	195	131 (67%)

DOD, died of disease.
[a]All but one of these seven deaths were reported in one study with an unusually low 5-year survival of 48% for 12 patients with superficial melanomas of Breslow thickness <0.76 mm. If these 12 cases were excluded, 5% of patients with superficial melanoma of the vulva died of disease.
From references 108, 112, 116, 129, 130, 137–140, with permission.

reflect cure. Prognosis is best predicted by microstaging. Patients with lesions invading to 1 mm or less have a good prognosis, but as depth of invasion increases, the prognosis worsens (Table 33.7). Tumor volume has been reported to correlate with prognosis; patients whose lesions have a volume under 100 mm^3 have an excellent prognosis (130). Additional prognostic factors are the patient's age, AJCC stage, presence of multifocal or satellite lesions, tumor ulceration, central tumor location, histologic growth pattern, lymph–vascular space involvement, and aneuploidy (108,111–113,138).

Bartholin Gland Carcinoma

Epidemiology

Primary carcinoma of the Bartholin gland is a rare form of vulvar cancer, which accounts for about 2% to 7% of vulvar malignancies (141). Because of its rarity, individual experience with the tumor is limited, and recommendations for management must be based on the review of small published series. To date, only about 300 cases have been reported (47,141,142). Bartholin gland carcinoma is 5 times more common in postmenopausal than in premenopausal women (143).

Histopathology

The bilateral Bartholin glands are greater vestibular glands situated posterolaterally in the vulva. Their main duct is lined with stratified squamous epithelium, which changes to transitional epithelium as the terminal ducts are reached. Because tumors may arise from the gland or the duct, a variety of histologic types occur, including adenocarcinomas, squamous carcinomas and, rarely, transitional cell, adenosquamous, and adenoid cystic carcinomas.

Classification of a vulvar tumor as a Bartholin gland carcinoma has typically required that it fulfill Honan's criteria, which are as follows:

1. The tumor is in the correct anatomic position.
2. The tumor is located deep in the labium majus.
3. The overlying skin is intact.
4. There is some recognizable normal gland present.

Strict adherence to these criteria will result in underdiagnosis of some cases. Large tumors may ulcerate through the overlying skin and obliterate the residual normal gland. Although transition between normal and malignant tissue is the best criterion, some cases will be diagnosed on the basis of their histologic characteristics and anatomic location.

Table 33.8. Survival of Patients with Bartholin Gland Carcinoma

FIGO Stage	*No. of Patients*	*No. of Patients with Recurrent Disease*	*No. of Patients NED at last F/U*[a]
I	15 (21%)	3 (20%)	14 (93%)
II	16 (23%)	2 (13%)	15 (94%)
III	30 (42%)	11 (37%)	22 (73%)
IV	10 (14%)	5 (50%)	5 (50%)
Total	71	21	56 (79%)

FIGO, International Federation of Gynecology and Obstetrics; NED, no evidence of disease; F/U, follow-up.
[a]Median follow-up in each study was at least 5 years.
From references 47, 141, 142, 145, with permission.

Signs and Symptoms

The most common initial symptom of Bartholin gland carcinoma is a vulvar mass or perineal pain. About 10% of patients have a history of inflammation of the Bartholin gland and malignancies may be mistaken for benign cysts or abscesses. Therefore, delay of diagnosis is common, particularly for premenopausal patients. The differential diagnosis of any pararectovaginal neoplasm should include cloacogenic carcinoma and secondary neoplasm (142).

Treatment

Traditionally, treatment has been radical vulvectomy with bilateral groin and pelvic node dissection (144). However, there seems to be no indication for dissection of the pelvic nodes in the absence of positive groin nodes, and good results have been reported with hemivulvectomy or radical local excision for the primary tumor (142). Because these lesions are deep in the vulva, extensive dissection is required in the ischiorectal fossa; even then, surgical margins are often close. Postoperative radiation to the vulva decreased the likelihood of local recurrence from 27% (6 of 22 patients) to 7% (1 of 14 patients) (142). If the ipsilateral groin nodes are positive, bilateral groin and pelvic irradiation may decrease regional recurrence. If the tumor is fixed to the inferior pubic ramus or involves adjacent structures, such as the anal sphincter or rectum, preoperative radiation and chemotherapy is preferable to avoid ultraradical surgery.

Prognosis

Because of the deep location of the gland, disease tends to be more advanced than squamous carcinomas at the time of diagnosis but, stage for stage, the prognosis is similar. Five-year disease-free survival rates by stage are summarized in Table 33.8.

Adenoid Cystic Carcinoma of the Bartholin Gland

The adenoid cystic variety accounts for 15% of Bartholin gland carcinomas. It is less likely to metastasize to lymph nodes and carries a somewhat better prognosis (47,146) (Fig. 33.8). Local recurrences are common, however, and metastases may occur, particularly to the lungs. The slowly progressive nature of these tumors and the tendency for late recurrences is reflected in the disparity between progression-free interval and survival curves (146).

Other Adenocarcinomas

Adenocarcinomas of the vulva usually arise in a Bartholin gland or occur in association with Paget's disease. They may rarely arise from the skin appendages, paraurethral glands, minor vestibular glands, aberrant breast tissue, endometriosis, or a misplaced cloacal remnant (147).

Adenosquamous Carcinoma

A particularly aggressive type of carcinoma is the adenosquamous carcinoma. This tumor has a number of synonyms, including cylindroma, pseudoglandular squamous cell

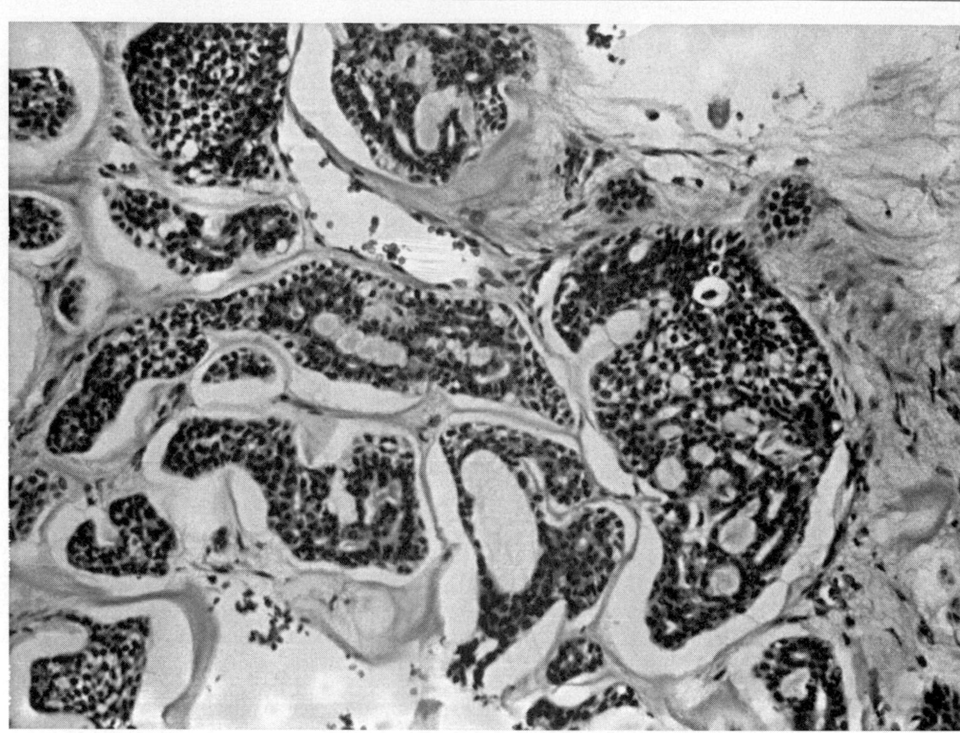

Figure 33.8 Adenoid cystic tumor of the Bartholin gland. Basaloid cells form cribriform, sieve-like spaces containing mucinous material. The hyaline stroma is another distinct feature of this tumor. (From **Berek JS, Hacker NF.** *Practical gynecologic oncology,* 2nd ed. Baltimore: Williams & Wilkins, 1994, with permission.)

carcinoma, adenoid squamous cell carcinoma, and adenoacanthoma of the sweat gland of Lever. The tumor has a propensity for perineural invasion, early lymph node metastasis, and local recurrence. One study noted a crude 5-year survival rate of 5.5% (1 of 18) for adenosquamous carcinoma of the vulva, compared with 62.3% (48 of 77) for patients with squamous cell carcinoma (148). Treatment should be radical vulvectomy and bilateral groin dissection. Postoperative radiation therapy may be appropriate.

Basal Cell Carcinoma

Basal cell carcinomas represent about 2% of vulvar cancers. As with other basal cell carcinomas, vulvar lesions commonly appear as a "rodent ulcer" with rolled edges, although nodules and macules are other morphologic varieties that occur. Most lesions are smaller than 2 cm in diameter and are usually situated on the anterior labia majora. Giant lesions occasionally occur (149). Basal cell carcinoma usually affects postmenopausal white women and is locally aggressive. Symptoms are frequently present for a prolonged period and most frequently include pruritus, soreness, and irritation (150). It is diagnosed by biopsy, and radical local excision is generally adequate treatment. Metastasis to regional lymph nodes has been reported but is rare (151–153). The local recurrence rate is about 10% to 20% (150,154). Basal cell carcinoma of the vulva is associated with a high incidence of antecedent or concomitant malignancies elsewhere (150). In a series of 28 women with vulvar basal cell carcinoma, 10 patients had other basal cell carcinomas, and 10 patients suffered from other primary malignancies (150).

About 3% to 5% of basal cell carcinomas contain a malignant squamous component, the so-called *basosquamous carcinoma.* These lesions are more aggressive and should be treated as squamous carcinomas (153). Another subtype of basal cell carcinoma is the adenoid basal cell carcinoma, which must be differentiated from the more aggressive adenoid cystic carcinoma arising in a Bartholin gland or the skin (153).

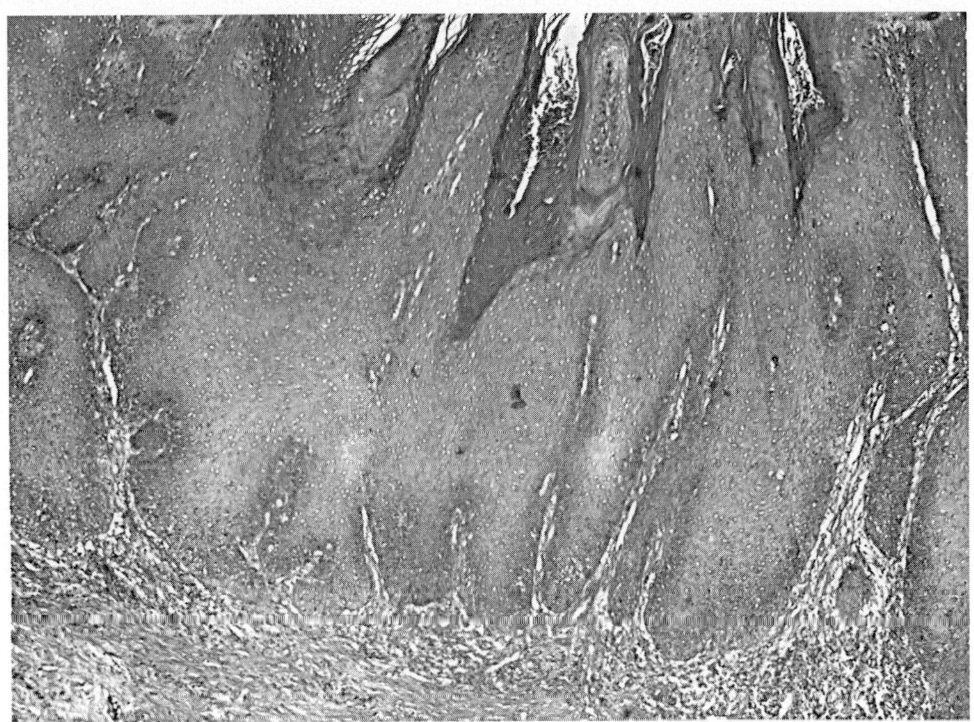

Figure 33.9 Verrucous carcinoma of the vulva. Note the exophytic hyperkeratotic papillary fronds and endophytic bulky rete pegs with smooth borders. (From **Berek JS, Hacker NF.** *Practical gynecologic oncology,* 2nd ed. Baltimore: Williams & Wilkins, 1994, with permission.)

Verrucous Carcinoma

Verrucous carcinoma is a variant of squamous cell carcinoma and has distinctive clinical and pathologic characteristics (155). Although most commonly found in the oral cavity, verrucous lesions may be found on any moist membrane composed of squamous epithelium (156). In the female genital tract, these lesions may develop on the cervix, vulva, and vagina. The cause of the lesion in the female genital tract is not fully understood, but associated HPV-6 and HPV-11 have been found (157).

Grossly, the tumors have a cauliflower-like appearance; microscopically, they contain multiple papillary fronds that lack the central connective tissue core that characterizes condylomata acuminata (Fig. 33.9). The gross and microscopic features of a verrucous carcinoma are very similar to those of the giant condyloma of Buschke-Loewenstein, and they probably represent the same disease entity (147). Adequate biopsy from the base of the lesion is required to differentiate a verrucous carcinoma from a benign condyloma acuminatum or a squamous cell carcinoma with a verrucous growth pattern.

Verrucous carcinomas usually occur in postmenopausal women, and they are slow-growing but locally destructive lesions. Even bone may be invaded. Metastasis to regional lymph nodes is rare but has been reported (158). Radical local excision is the basic treatment, although any palpably suspicious groin nodes should be evaluated with fine-needle aspiration cytology or excisional biopsy. Usually, enlarged nodes will be caused by inflammatory hypertrophy (159). If the nodes contain metastases, radical vulvectomy and bilateral inguinal-femoral lymphadenectomy are indicated.

Several small studies failed to document any therapeutic advantage with radiation therapy (159,160). In addition, there is concern that radiation may induce anaplastic transformation with subsequent regional and distant metastasis (161). One study reported a corrected 5-year survival rate of 94% for 17 patients treated with surgery alone, compared with 42% for 7 patients treated with surgery and radiation (159). The latter patients had, however, more advanced disease. If there is a recurrence, further surgical excision is the treatment of choice, which occasionally may necessitate some type of exenteration.

Vulvar Sarcoma

Sarcomas represent 1% to 2% of vulvar malignancies and constitute a heterogenous group of tumors. Leiomyosarcomas are the most common, and other histologic types include fibrosarcomas, neurofibrosarcomas, liposarcomas, rhabdomyosarcomas, angiosarcomas, epithelioid sarcomas, and malignant schwannomas (147).

Leiomyosarcomas usually appear as enlarging, often painful masses, usually in the labium majus. Smooth muscle tumors of the vulva that show at least three of the following four criteria should be regarded as sarcomas: (a) diameter >5 cm, (b) infiltrating margins, (c) 5 or more mitotic figures per 10 high-power fields, (d) moderate-to-severe cytological atypia (162). The absence of one, or even all, of these features does not guarantee against recurrence (163). Lymphatic metastases are uncommon, and radical local excision is the usual treatment.

Epithelioid sarcomas characteristically develop in the soft tissues of the extremities of young adults but rarely may occur on the vulva. In a description of two cases and review of three other reports, the authors concluded that these tumors may mimic a Bartholin cyst, thus leading to inadequate initial treatment (164). They also believed that vulvar epithelioid sarcomas behave more aggressively than their extragenital counterparts, with four of the five patients dying of metastatic disease. They suggested that early recognition and wide excision should improve the prognosis.

Rhabdomyosarcomas are the most common soft tissue sarcomas in childhood, and 20% involve the pelvis or genitourinary tract (165). Dramatic gains have been made in the treatment of these tumors during the past 20 years. Previously, radical pelvic surgery was the standard approach, but results were poor. More recently, a multimodal approach has evolved, and survival rates have improved significantly, with a corresponding decrease in morbidity. In a report of the experience of the Intergroup Rhabdomyosarcoma Study I and II (1972 to 1984) with primary tumors of the female genital tract, nine patients aged 1 to 19 years had primary vulvar tumors, and these tumors were often regarded as a form of Bartholin gland infection before biopsy (166). They were all managed with chemotherapy (*vincristine,* or *actinomycin D* and *cyclophosphamide* and *doxorubicin*), with or without radiotherapy. Wide local excision of the tumor, with or without inguinal-femoral lymphadenectomy, was carried out before or after the chemotherapy. Seven of the nine patients were free of disease 4 or more years from diagnosis, one patient was free of disease when lost to follow-up at 5 years, and one patient was alive with disease.

Rare Vulvar Malignancies

In addition to the previously mentioned tumors, a number of malignancies more commonly seen in other areas of the body may rarely occur as isolated vulvar tumors.

Lymphomas

The genital tract may be involved primarily by malignant lymphomas but, more commonly, involvement is a manifestation of systemic disease. In the lower genital tract, the cervix is most often involved, followed by the vulva and the vagina (147). Most patients are in their third to sixth decade of life, and about three-fourths of the cases involve diffuse large cell or histiocytic non-Hodgkin's lymphomas. The remainder are nodular or Burkitt's lymphomas (134). Treatment is by surgical excision followed by chemotherapy and radiation or both, and the overall 5-year survival rate is about 70% (167).

Endodermal Sinus Tumor

There have been four case reports of endodermal sinus tumor of the vulva, and three of the four patients died of distant metastases (147,168). All patients were in their third decade of life, but none was treated with modern chemotherapy.

Merkel Cell Carcinoma

Merkel cell carcinomas are primary small cell carcinomas of the skin, which resemble oat cell carcinomas of the lung. They metastasize widely and have a very poor prognosis (169,170). They should be locally excised and treated with cisplatin-based chemotherapy.

Dermatofibrosarcoma Protuberans

This rare, low-grade cutaneous malignancy occasionally involves the vulva. It has a marked tendency for local recurrence but a low risk of systemic spread (171). Radical local excision should be sufficient treatment.

Metastatic Tumors of the Vulva

Eight percent of vulvar tumors are metastatic (147). The most common primary site is the cervix, followed by the endometrium, kidney, and urethra. Most patients in whom vulvar metastases develop have advanced primary tumors when diagnosed, and in about one-fourth of the patients the primary lesion and the vulvar metastasis are diagnosed simultaneously (172).

References

1. **Jemal A, Thomas A, Murray T, et al.** Cancer statistics, 2002. *CA Cancer J Clin* 2002;52:23–47.
2. **Sturgeon SR, Brinton LA, Devesa SS, et al.** In situ and invasive vulvar cancer incidence trends (1973 to 1987). *Am J Obstet Gynecol* 1992;166:1482–1485.
3. **Jones RW, Baranyai J, Stables S.** Trends in squamous cell carcinoma of the vulva: the influence of vulvar intraepithelial neoplasia. *Obstet Gynecol* 1997;90:448–452.
4. **Taussig FJ.** Cancer of the vulva: an analysis of 155 cases. *Am J Obstet Gynecol* 1940;40:764–778.
5. **Way S.** Carcinoma of the vulva. *Am J Obstet Gynecol* 1960;79:692–697.
6. **Iversen T, Abeler V, Aalders J.** Individualized treatment of stage I carcinoma of the vulva. *Obstet Gynecol* 1981;57:85–89.
7. **Hacker NF, Berek JS, Lagasse LD, et al.** Individualization of treatment for stage I squamous cell vulvar carcinoma. *Obstet Gynecol* 1984;63:155–162.
8. **DiSaia PJ, Creasman WT, Rich WM.** An alternative approach to early cancer of the vulva. *Am J Obstet Gynecol* 1979;133:825–832.
9. **Burke TW, Levenback C, Coleman RL, et al.** Surgical therapy of T1 and T2 vulvar carcinoma: further experience with radical wide excision and selective inguinal lymphadenectomy. *Gynecol Oncol* 1995;57:215–220.
10. **Burrell MO, Franklin EW III, Campion MJ, et al.** The modified radical vulvectomy with groin dissection. An eight-year experience. *Am J Obstet Gynecol* 1988;159:715–722.
11. **Curry SL, Wharton JT, Rutledge F.** Positive lymph nodes in vulvar squamous carcinoma. *Gynecol Oncol* 1980;9:63–67.
12. **Hacker NF, Berek JS, Lagasse LD, et al.** Management of regional lymph nodes and their prognostic influence in vulvar cancer. *Obstet Gynecol* 1983;61:408–412.
13. **Monaghan JM, Hammond IG.** Pelvic node dissection in the treatment of vulval carcinoma—is it necessary? *Br J Obstet Gynaecol* 1984;91:270–274.
14. **Hoffman JS, Kumar NB, Morley GW.** Prognostic significance of groin lymph node metastases in squamous carcinoma of the vulva. *Obstet Gynecol* 1985;66:402–405.
15. **Homesley HD, Bundy BN, Sedlis A, et al.** Radiation therapy versus pelvic node resection for carcinoma of the vulva with positive groin nodes. *Obstet Gynecol* 1986;68:733–740.
16. **Byron RL, Mishell DR, Yonemoto RH.** The surgical treatment of invasive carcinoma of the vulva. *Surg Gynecol Obstet* 1965;121:1243–1251.
17. **Hacker NF, Leuchter RS, Berek JS, et al.** Radical vulvectomy and bilateral inguinal lymphadenectomy through separate groin incisions. *Obstet Gynecol* 1981;58:574–579.
18. **Figge DC, Gaudenz R.** Invasive carcinoma of the vulva. *Am J Obstet Gynecol* 1974;119:382–395.

19. **Boronow RC.** Therapeutic alternative to primary exenteration for advanced vulvo-vaginal cancer. *Gynecol Oncol* 1973;1:223–230.

20. **Hacker NF, Berek JS, Juillard GJF, et al.** Preoperative radiation therapy for locally advanced vulvar cancer. *Cancer* 1984;54:2056–2061.

21. **Hording U, Junge J, Poulsen H, et al.** Vulvar intraepithelial neoplasia III: a viral disease of undetermined progressive potential. *Gynecol Oncol* 1995;56:276–279.

22. **Modesitt SC, Waters AB, Walton L, et al.** Vulvar intraepithelial neoplasia III: occult cancer and the impact of margin status on recurrence. *Obstet Gynecol* 1998;92:962–966.

23. **Trimble CL, Hildesheim A, Brinton LA, et al.** Heterogeneous etiology of squamous carcinoma of the vulva. *Obstet Gynecol* 1996;87:59–64.

24. **Brinton LA, Nasco PC, Mallin K, et al.** Case-control study of cancer of the vulva. *Obstet Gynecol* 1990;75:859–866.

25. **Kurman RJ, Toki T, Schiffman MH.** Basaloid and warty carcinomas of the vulva: Distinctive types of squamous cell carcinoma frequently associated with human papillomaviruses. *Am J Surg Pathol* 1993;17:133–145.

26. **Vilmer C, Cavelier-Balloy B, Nogues C, et al.** Analysis of alterations adjacent to invasive vulvar carcinoma and their relationship with the associated carcinoma: a study of 67 cases. *Eur J Gynaecol Oncol* 1998;19: 25–31.

27. **Carlson JA, Ambros R, Malfetano J, et al.** Vulvar lichen sclerosus and squamous cell carcinoma: a cohort, case control, and investigational study with historical perspective; implications for chronic inflammation and sclerosis in the development of neoplasia. *Hum Pathol* 1998;29: 932–948.

28. **Tate JE, Mutter GL, Boynton KA, et al.** Monoclonal origin of vulvar intraepithelial neoplasia and some vulvar hyperplasias. *Am J Pathol* 1997;150:315–322.

29. **Franklin EW, Rutledge FD.** Epidemiology of epidermoid carcinoma of the vulva. *Obstet Gynecol* 1972;39:165–172.

30. **Green TH Jr, Ulfelder H, Meigs JV.** Epidermoid carcinoma of the vulva: an analysis of 238 cases. Parts I and II. *Am J Obstet Gynecol* 1958;73:834–864.

31. **Woodruff JD.** Early invasive carcinoma of the vulva. *Clin Oncol* 1982;1:349.

32. **Binder SW, Huang I, Fu YS, et al.** Risk factors for the development of lymph node metastasis in vulvar squamous cell carcinoma. *Gynecol Oncol* 1990;37:9–16.

33. **Boyce J, Fruchter RG, Kasambilides E, et al.** Prognostic factors in carcinoma of the vulva. *Gynecol Oncol* 1985;20:364–377.

34. **Donaldson ES, Powell DE, Hanson MB, et al.** Prognostic parameters in invasive vulvar cancer. *Gynecol Oncol* 1981;11:184–190.

35. **Buscema J, Woodruff JD.** Progressive histobiologic alterations in the development of vulvar cancer. *Am J Obstet Gynecol* 1980;138:146–150.

36. **Shepherd J, Sideri M, Benedet J, et al.** FIGO annual report on the results of treatment in gynecological cancer: carcinoma of the vulva. *J Epidemiol Biostat* 1998;3:111–127.

37. **Rutledge F, Smith JP, Franklin EW.** Carcinoma of the vulva. *Am J Obstet Gynecol* 1970;106:1117–1130.

38. **Podratz KC, Symmonds RE, Taylor WF, et al.** Carcinoma of the vulva: analysis of treatment and survival. *Obstet Gynecol* 1983;61:63–74.

39. **Cavanagh D, Fiorica JV, Hoffman MS, et al.** Invasive carcinoma of the vulva: changing trends in surgical management. *Am J Obstet Gynecol* 1990;163:1007–1115.

40. **Chafe W, Richards A, Morgan L, et al.** Unrecognized invasive carcinoma in vulvar intraepithelial neoplasia (VIN). *Gynecol Oncol* 1988;31:154–162.

41. **Hacker NF, Van der Velden J.** Conservative management of early vulvar cancer. *Cancer* 1993;71:1673–1677.

42. **Hacker NF, Nieberg RK, Berek JS, et al.** Superficially invasive vulvar cancer with nodal metastases. *Gynecol Oncol* 1983;15:65–77.

43. **Chu J, Tamimi HK, Figge DC.** Femoral node metastases with negative superficial inguinal nodes in early vulvar cancer. *Am J Obstet Gynecol* 1981;140:337–339.

44. **Podczaski E, Sexton M, Kaminski P, et al.** Recurrent carcinoma of the vulva after conservative treatment for "microinvasive" disease. *Gynecol Oncol* 1990;39:65–68.

45. **Stehman FB, Bundy BN, Dvoretsky PM, et al.** Early stage I carcinoma of the vulva treated with ipsilateral superficial inguinal lymphadenectomy and modified radical hemivulvectomy: a prospective study of the Gynecologic Oncology Group. *Obstet Gynecol* 1992;79:490–497.

46. **Levenback C, Burke TW, Morris M, et al.** Potential applications of intraoperative lymphatic mapping in vulvar cancer. *Gynecol Oncol* 1995;59:216–220.

47. **Leuchter RS, Hacker NF, Voet RL, et al.** Primary carcinoma of the Bartholin gland: a report of 14 cases and a review of the literature. *Obstet Gynecol* 1982;60:361–368.

48. **Piver MS, Xynos FP.** Pelvic lymphadenectomy in women with carcinoma of the clitoris. *Obstet Gynecol* 1977;49:592–595.

49. **Collins CG, Lee FY, Roman-Lopez JJ.** Invasive carcinoma of the vulva with lymph node metastases. *Am J Obstet Gynecol* 1971;109:446–452.

50. **Morley GW.** Infiltrative carcinoma of the vulva: results of surgical treatment. *Am J Obstet Gynecol* 1976;124:874–888.

51. **Krupp PJ, Bohm JW.** Lymph gland metastases in invasive squamous cell cancer of the vulva. *Am J Obstet Gynecol* 1978;130:943–952.

52. **Benedet JL, Turko M, Fairey RN, et al.** Squamous carcinoma of the vulva: results of treatment, 1938 to 1976. *Am J Obstet Gynecol* 1979;134:201–207.

53. **Iversen T, Aalders JG, Christensen A, et al.** Squamous cell carcinoma of the vulva: a review of 424 patients, 1956–1974. *Gynecol Oncol* 1980;9:271–279.

54. **Hopkins MP, Reid CG, Vettrano I, et al.** Squamous cell carcinoma of the vulva: prognostic factors influencing survival. *Gynecol Oncol* 1991;43:113–117.

55. **Keys H.** Gynecologic Oncology Group randomized trials of combined technique therapy of vulvar cancer. *Cancer* 1993;71:1691–1696.

56. **Paladini D, Cross P, Lopes A, et al.** Prognostic significance of lymph node variables in squamous cell carcinoma of the vulva. *Cancer* 1994;74:2491–2496.

57. **Homesley HD, Bundy BN, Sedlis A, et al.** Assessment of current International Federation of Gynecology and Obstetrics staging of vulvar carcinoma relative to prognostic factors for survival (a Gynecologic Oncology Group study). *Am J Obstet Gynecol* 1991;164:997–1003.

58. **Homesley HD, Bundy BN, Sedlis A, et al.** Prognostic factors for groin node metastasis in squamous cell carcinoma of the vulva (a Gynecologic Oncology Group Study). *Gynecol Oncol* 1993;49:279–283.

59. **van der Velden J, Hacker NF.** Update on vulvar carcinoma. In: **Rothenberg ML,** ed. *Gynecologic oncology. Controversies and new developments.* Boston: Kluwer Academic Publishers, 1994:101–119.

60. **Kaern J, Iversen T, Tropé C, et al.** Flow cytometric DNA measurements in squamous cell carcinoma of the vulva: an important prognostic method. *Int J Gynecol Cancer* 1992;2:169–174.

61. **Andersen BL, Hacker NF.** Psychological adjustment after vulvar surgery. *Obstet Gynecol* 1983;62:457–462.

62. **Stehman FB, Bundy BN, Droretsky PM, et al.** Early stage I carcinoma of the vulva treated with ipsilateral superficial inguinal lymphadenectomy and modified radical hemivulvectomy: a prospective study of the Gynecologic Oncology Group. *Obstet Gynecol* 1992;79:490–497.

63. **Heaps JM, Fu YS, Montz FJ, et al.** Surgical-pathologic variables predictive of local recurrence in squamous cell carcinoma of the vulva. *Gynecol Oncol* 1990;38:309–314.

64. **Hacker NF.** Vulvar cancer. In: **Berek JS, Hacker NF,** eds. *Practical gynecologic oncology,* 3rd ed. Philadelphia: Lippincott Williams & Wilkins, 2000:553–596.

65. **Andrews SJ, Williams BT, De Priest PD, et al.** Therapeutic implications of lymph node spread in lateral T1 and T2 squamous cell carcinoma of the vulva. *Gynecol Oncol* 1994;55:41–46.

66. **Farias-Eisner R, Cirisano FD, Grouse D, et al.** Conservative and individualized surgery for early squamous carcinoma of the vulva: the treatment of choice for stages I and II (T1–2, N0–1, M0) disease. *Gynecol Oncol* 1994;53:33–38.

67. **Simonsen E, Johnsson JE, Tropé C.** Radical vulvectomy with warm-knife and open-wound techniques in vulvar malignancies. *Gynecol Oncol* 1984;17:22–31.

68. **Potkul RK, Barnes WA, Barter JF, et al.** Vulvar reconstruction using a mons pubis pedicle flap. *Gynecol Oncol* 1994;55:21–24.

69. **Trelford JD, Deer DA, Ordorica E, et al.** Ten-year prospective study in a management change of vulvar carcinoma. *Am J Obstet Gynecol* 1984;150:288–296.

70. **Julian CG, Callison J, Woodruff JD.** Plastic management of extensive vulvar defects. *Obstet Gynecol* 1971;38:193–198.

71. **Barnhill DR, Hoskins WJ, Metz P.** Use of the rhomboid flap after partial vulvectomy. *Obstet Gynecol* 1983;62:444–447.

72. **Ballon SC, Donaldson RC, Roberts JA.** Reconstruction of the vulva using a myocutaneous graft. *Gynecol Oncol* 1979;7:123–127.

73. **Chafe W, Fowler WC, Walton LA, et al.** Radical vulvectomy with use of tensor fascia lata myocutaneous flap. *Am J Obstet Gynecol* 1983;145:207–213.

74. **Andersen BL, Hacker NF.** Psychosexual adjustment following pelvic exenteration. *Obstet Gynecol* 1983;61:457–462.

75. **Kaplan AL, Kaufman RH.** Management of advanced carcinoma of the vulva. *Gynecol Oncol* 1975;3:220–232.

76. **Phillips B, Buchsbaum HJ, Lifshitz S.** Pelvic exenteration for vulvovaginal carcinoma. *Am J Obstet Gynecol* 1981;141:1038–1044.

77. **Cavanagh D, Shepherd JH.** The place of pelvic exenteration in the primary management of advanced carcinoma of the vulva. *Gynecol Oncol* 1982;13:318–322.

78. **Grimshaw RN, Aswad SG, Monaghan JM.** The role of anovulvectomy in locally advanced carcinoma of the vulva. *Int J Gynecol Cancer* 1991;1:15.

79. **Moore DH, Thomas GM, Montana GS, et al.** Preoperative chemoradiation for advanced vulvar cancer: a phase II study of the GOG. *Int J Radiat Oncol Biol Phys* 1998;42:79–85.

80. **Cunningham MJ, Goyer RP, Gibbons SK, et al.** Primary radiation, cisplatin, and 5-fluorouracil for advanced squamous carcinoma of the vulva. *Gynecol Oncol* 1997;66:258–261.

81. **Eifel PJ, Morris M, Burke TW, et al.** Prolonged continuous infusion cisplatin and 5-fluorouracil for advanced squamous carcinoma of the vulva. *Gynecol Oncol* 1995;59:51–56.

82. **Boronow RC, Hickman BT, Reagan MT, et al.** Combined therapy as an alternative to exenteration for locally advanced vulvovaginal cancer. II. Results, complications and dosimetric and surgical considerations. *Am J Clin Oncol* 1987;10:171–181.

83. **Backstrom A, Edsmyr F, Wicklund H.** Radiotherapy of carcinoma of the vulva. *Acta Obstet Gynecol* 1972;51:109–115.

84. **Thomas G, Dembo A, DePetrillo A, et al.** Concurrent radiation and chemotherapy in vulvar carcinoma. *Gynecol Oncol* 1989;34:263–267.

85. **Hoffman JS, Kumar NB, Morley GW.** Microinvasive squamous carcinoma of the vulva: search for a definition. *Obstet Gynecol* 1983;61:615–618.

86. **Magrina JF, Webb MJ, Gaffey TA, et al.** Stage I squamous cell cancer of the vulva. *Am J Obstet Gynecol* 1979;134:453–459.

87. **Lingard D, Free K, Wright RG, et al.** Invasive squamous cell carcinoma of the vulva: behaviour and results in the light of changing management regimes. *Aust N Z J Obstet Gynaecol* 1992;32:137–145.

88. **Marsden DE, Hacker NF.** Contemporary management of primary carcinoma of the vulva. *Surg Clin North Am* 2001;81:799–813.

89. **Atamdede F, Hoogerland D.** Regional lymph node recurrence following local excision for microinvasive vulvar carcinoma. *Gynecol Oncol* 1989;34:125–128.

90. **Stehman FB, Bundy BN, Thomas G, et al.** Groin dissection versus groin radiation in carcinoma of the vulva: a Gynecologic Oncology Group study. *Int J Radiat Oncol Biol Phys* 1992;24:389–396.

91. **Iversen T, Aas M.** Lymph drainage from the vulva. *Gynecol Oncol* 1983;16:179–189.

92. **Terada K, Shimizu D, Wong J.** Sentinel node dissection and ultrastaging in squamous cell carcinoma of the vulva. *Gynecol Oncol* 2000;76:40–44.

93. **Ansink AC, Sie-Go DM, van der Velden J, et al.** Identification of sentinel lymph nodes in vulvar carcinoma patients with the aid of a patent blue V injection: a multicenter study. *Cancer* 1999;86:652–656.

94. **De Cicco C, Sideri M, Bartolomei M, et al.** Sentinel node biopsy in early vulvar cancer. *Br J Cancer* 2000;82:295–299.

95. **Hopkins MP, Reid GC, Morley GW.** Radical vulvectomy: the decision for the incision. *Cancer* 1993;72:799–803.

96. **Gould N, Kamelle S, Tillmanns T, et al.** Predictors of complications after inguinal lymphadenectomy. *Gynecol Oncol* 2001;82:329–332.

97. **Podratz KC, Symmonds RE, Taylor WF.** Carcinoma of the vulva: analysis of treatment failures. *Am J Obstet Gynecol* 1982;143:340–351.

98. **Malfetano J, Piver MS, Tsukada Y.** Stage III and IV squamous cell carcinoma of the vulva. *Gynecol Oncol* 1986;23:192–198.

99. **Puira B, Masotina A, Murdoch J, et al.** Recurrent squamous cell carcinoma of the vulva: a study of 73 cases. *Gynecol Oncol* 1993;48:189–195.

100. **Stehman FB, Bundy BN, Ball H, et al.** Sites of failure and time to failure in carcinoma of the vulva treated conservatively: a GOG study. *Am J Obstet Gynecol* 1996;174:1128–1133.

101. **Homesley HD.** Management of vulvar cancer. *Cancer* 1995;76[Suppl 1]:2159–2170.

102. **Hopkins MP, Reid GC, Morley GW.** The surgical management of recurrent squamous cell carcinoma of the vulva. *Obstet Gynecol* 1990;75:1001–1005.

103. **Faul CM, Mirmow D, Huang Q, et al.** Adjuvant radiation for vulvar carcinoma: improved local control. *Int J Radiat Oncol Biol Phys* 1997;38:381–389.

104. **Hruby G, MacLeod C, Firth I.** Radiation treatment in recurrent squamous cell cancer of the vulva. *Int J Radiat Oncol Biol Phys* 2000;46:1193–1197.

105. **Hoffman M, Greenberg S, Greenberg H, et al.** Interstitial radiotherapy for the treatment of advanced or recurrent vulvar and distal vaginal malignancy. *Am J Obstet Gynecol* 1990;162:1278–1282.

106. **Wagenaar HC, Colombo N, Vergote I, et al.** Bleomycin, methotrexate, and CCNU in locally advanced or recurrent, inoperable, squamous-cell carcinoma of the vulva: an EORTC Gynaecological Cancer Cooperative Group Study. *Gynecol Oncol* 2001;81:348–354.

107. **Tropé C, Johnsson JE, Larsson G, et al.** Bleomycin alone or combined with mitomycin C in treatment of advanced or recurrent squamous cell carcinoma of the vulva. *Cancer Treat Rev* 1980;64: 639–642.

108. **Ragnarsson-Olding BK, Nilsson BR, Kanter-Lewensohn LR, et al.** Malignant melanoma of the vulva in a nationwide, 25-year study of 219 Swedish females: clinical observations and histopathologic features. Predictors of survival. *Cancer* 1999;86:1273–1293.

109. **Weinstock MA.** Malignant melanoma of the vulva and vagina in the United States: patterns of incidence and population-based estimates of survival. *Am J Obstet Gynecol* 1994;171:1225–1230.

110. **Dunton CJ, Kautzky M, Hanau C.** Malignant melanoma of the vulva: a review. *Obstet Gynecol Surv* 1995;50:739–746.

111. **Podratz KC, Gaffey TA, Symmonds RE, et al.** Melanoma of the vulva: an update. *Gynecol Oncol* 1983;16:153–168.

112. **Trimble EL, Lewis JL Jr, Williams LL, et al.** Management of vulvar melanoma. *Gynecol Oncol* 1992;45:254–258.

113. **Phillips GL, Bundy BN, Okagaki T, et al.** Malignant melanoma of the vulva treated by radical hemivulvectomy: a prospective study by the Gynecologic Oncology Group. *Cancer* 1994;73:2626–2632.

114. **Dunton JD, Berd D.** Vulvar melanoma, biologically different from other cutaneous melanomas. *Lancet* 1999;354:2013–2014.

115. **Chung AF, Woodruff JM, Lewis JL Jr.** Malignant melanoma of the vulva: a report of 44 cases. *Obstet Gynecol* 1975;45:638–646.

116. **Phillips GL, Twiggs LB, Okagaki T.** Vulvar melanoma: a microstaging study. *Gynecol Oncol* 1982;14:80–88.

117. **Clark WH, From L, Bernardino EA, et al.** The histogenesis and biologic behavior of primary human malignant melanomas of the skin. *Cancer Res* 1969;29:705–727.

118. **Breslow A.** Thickness, cross-sectional area and depth of invasion in the prognosis of cutaneous melanoma. *Ann Surg* 1970;172:902–908.

119. **Baehrs OH, Henson DE, Hutter RVP, et al.**, eds. *American Joint Committee on Cancer: manual for the staging of cancer,* 4th ed. Philadelphia: JB Lippincott, 1992:143–145.

120. **Aitken DR, Clausen K, Klein JP, et al.** The extent of primary melanoma excision—a re-evaluation. How wide is wide? *Ann Surg* 1983;198:634–641.

121. **Day CL, Mihm MC Jr, Sober AJ, et al.** Narrower margins for clinical stage I malignant melanoma. *N Engl J Med* 1982;306:479–482.

122. **Rose PG, Piver MS, Tsukada Y, et al.** Conservative therapy for melanoma of the vulva. *Am J Obstet Gynecol* 1988;159:52–55.

123. **Davidson T, Kissin M, Wesbury G.** Vulvovaginal melanoma—should radical surgery be abandoned? *Br J Obstet Gynaecol* 1987;94:473–476.

124. **Veronesi U, Cascinelli N.** Narrow excision (1-cm margin): a safe procedure for thin cutaneous melanoma. *Arch Surg* 1991;126:438–441.

125. **Balch CM, Urist MM, Karakousis CP, et al.** Efficacy of 2-cm surgical margins for intermediate-thickness melanoma (1–4 mm): results of a multi-institutional randomized surgical trial. *Ann Surg* 1993;218: 262–269.

126. **Morrow CP, Rutledge FN.** Melanoma of the vulva. *Obstet Gynecol* 1972;39:745–752.

127. **Balch CM, Soong SJ, Bartolucci AA, et al.** Efficacy of an elective regional lymph node dissection of 1–4 mm thick melanomas for patients 60 years of age or younger. *Ann Surg* 1996;224:255–263.

128. **Balch CM, Soong SJ, Milton GW, et al.** A comparison of prognostic factors and surgical results in 1,786 patients with localized (stage I) melanoma treated in Alabama, USA, and New South Wales, Australia. *Ann Surg* 1982;196:677–684.

129. **Jaramillo BA, Ganjei P, Averette HE, et al.** Malignant melanoma of the vulva. *Obstet Gynecol* 1985;66:398–401.

130. **Beller U, Demopoulos RI, Beckman EM.** Vulvovaginal melanoma: a clinicopathologic study. *J Reprod Med* 1986;31:315–319.

131. **Agarwala SS, Kirkwood JM.** Adjuvant interferon treatment for melanoma. *Hematol Oncol Clin North Am* 1998;12:823–833.

132. **Kirkwood JM, Strawderman MH, Ernstoff MS, et al.** Interferon alfa-2b adjuvant therapy of high-risk resected cutaneous melanoma: the Eastern Cooperative Oncology Group Trial EST 1684. *J Clin Oncol* 1996;14:7–17.

133. **Fisher RI, Neifeld JP, Lippman ME.** Oestrogen receptors in human malignant melanoma. *Lancet* 1976;2:337–339.

134. **Masiel A, Buttrick P, Bitran J.** Tamoxifen in the treatment of malignant melanoma. *Cancer Treat Rep* 1981;65:531–532.

135. **Nesbit RA, Woods RL, Tattersall MH, et al.** Tamoxifen in malignant melanoma. *N Engl J Med* 1979;301:1241–1242.

136. **Thompson LW, Brinckerhoff L, Slingluff CL Jr.** Vaccination for melanoma. *Curr Oncol Rep* 2000;2:292–299.

137. **Woolcott RJ, Henry RJW, Houghton CRS.** Malignant melanoma of the vulva. Australian experience. *J Reprod Med* 1988;33:699–702.

138. **Scheistroen M, Tropé C, Kaern J, et al.** Malignant melanoma of the vulva: evaluation of prognostic factors with emphasis on DNA ploidy in 75 patients. *Cancer* 1995;75:72–80.

139. **Piura B, Egan M, Lopes A, et al.** Malignant melanoma of the vulva: a clinicopathologic study of 18 cases. *J Surg Oncol* 1992;50:234–240.

140. **Look KY, Roth LM, Sutton GP.** Vulvar melanoma reconsidered. *Cancer* 1993;72:143–146.

141. **Cardosi RJ, Speights A, Fiorica JV, et al.** Bartholin's gland carcinoma: a 15-year experience. *Gynecol Oncol* 2001;82:247–251.

142. **Copeland LJ, Sneige N, Gershenson DM, et al.** Bartholin gland carcinoma. *Obstet Gynecol* 1986;67:794–801.

143. **Visco AG, Del Priore G.** Postmenopausal Bartholin gland enlargement: a hospital-based cancer risk assessment. *Obstet Gynecol* 1996;87:286–290.

144. **Barclay DL, Collins CG, Macey HB.** Cancer of the Bartholin gland: a review and report of 8 cases. *Obstet Gynecol* 1964;24:329–336.

145. **Wheelock JB, Goplerud DR, Dunn LJ, et al.** Primary carcinoma of the Bartholin gland: a report of 10 cases. *Obstet Gynecol* 1984;63:820–824.

146. **Copeland LJ, Sneige N, Gershenson DM, et al.** Adenoid cystic carcinoma of Bartholin gland. *Obstet Gynecol* 1986;67:115–120.

147. **Fu YS, Reagan JW.** Benign and malignant epithelial tumors of the vulva. In: **Fu YS, Reagan JW,** eds. *Pathology of the uterine cervix, vagina, and vulva.* Philadelphia: WB Saunders, 1989:138–192.

148. **Underwood JW, Adcock LL, Okagaki T.** Adenosquamous carcinoma of skin appendages (adenoid squamous cell carcinoma, pseudoglandular squamous cell carcinoma, adenoacanthoma of sweat gland of Lever) of the vulva: a clinical and ultrastructural study. *Cancer* 1978;42:1851–1858.

149. **Dudzinski MR, Askin FB, Fowler WC.** Giant basal cell carcinoma of the vulva. *Obstet Gynecol* 1984;63:57S–60S.

150. **Benedet JL, Miller DM, Ehlen TG, et al.** Basal cell carcinoma of the vulva: clinical features and treatment results in 28 patients. *Obstet Gynecol* 1997;90:765–768.

151. **Jimenez HT, Fenoglio CM, Richart RM.** Vulvar basal cell carcinoma with metastasis: a case report. *Am J Obstet Gynecol* 1975;121:285–286.

152. **Sworn MJ, Hammond GT, Buchanan R.** Metastatic basal cell carcinoma of the vulva: a case report. *Br J Obstet Gynaecol* 1979;86:332–334.

153. **Hoffman MS, Roberts WS, Ruffolo EH.** Basal cell carcinoma of the vulva with inguinal lymph node metastases. *Gynecol Oncol* 1988;29:113–119.

154. **Palladino VS, Duffy JL, Bures GJ.** Basal cell carcinoma of the vulva. *Cancer* 1969;24:460–470.

155. **Isaacs JH.** Verrucous carcinoma of the female genital tract. *Gynecol Oncol* 1976;4:259–269.

156. **Partridge EE, Murad R, Shingleton HM, et al.** Verrucous lesions of the female genitalia. II. Verrucous carcinoma *Am J Obstet Gynecol* 1980;137:419–424.

157. **Kondi-Paphitis A, Deligeorgi-Politi H, Liapis A, et al.** Human papillomavirus in verrucous carcinoma of the vulva: an immunopathological study of three cases. *Eur J Gynecol Obstet* 1998;19:319–320.

158. **Gallousis S.** Verrucous carcinoma: report of three vulvar cases and a review of the literature. *Obstet Gynecol* 1972;40:502–507.

159. **Japaze H, Van Dinh TV, Woodruff JD.** Verrucous carcinoma of the vulva: study of 24 cases. *Obstet Gynecol* 1982;60:462–466.

160. **Gallouis S.** Verrucous carcinoma. Report of 3 vulvar cases and review of the literature. *Obstet Gynecol* 1972;40:502–507.

161. **Demian SDE, Bushkin FL, Echevarria RA.** Perineural invasion and anaplastic transformation of verrucous carcinoma. *Cancer* 1973;32:395–401.

162. **Nielsen GP, Rosenberg AE, Koerner FC, et al.** Smooth-muscle tumors of the vulva: a clinicopathological study of 25 cases and review of the literature. *Am J Surg Pathol* 1996;20:779–793.

163. **Tavassoli FA, Norris HJ.** Smooth muscle tumors of the vulva. *Obstet Gynecol* 1979;53:213–217.

164. **Ulbright TM, Brokaw SA, Stehman FB, et al.** Epithelioid sarcoma of the vulva. *Cancer* 1983;52:1462–1469.

165. **Bell J, Averette H, Davis J, et al.** Genital rhabdomyosarcoma: current management and review of the literature. *Obstet Gynecol Surv* 1986;41:257–263.

166. **Hays DM, Shimada H, Raney RB Jr, et al.** Clinical staging and treatment results in rhabdomyosarcoma of the female genital tract among children and adolescents. *Cancer* 1988;61:1893–1903.

167. **Harris NL, Scully RE.** Malignant lymphoma and granulocytic sarcoma of the uterus and vagina. *Cancer* 1984,53:2530–2545.

168. **Dudley AG, Young RH, Lawrence WD, et al.** Endodermal sinus tumor of the vulva in an infant. *Obstet Gynecol* 1983;61:76S–79S.

169. **Bottles K, Lacy CG, Goldberg J, et al.** Merkel cell carcinoma of the vulva. *Obstet Gynecol* 1984;63:61S–65S.

170. **Husseinzadeh N, Wesseler T, Newman N, et al.** Neuroendocrine (Merkel cell) carcinoma of the vulva. *Gynecol Oncol* 1988;29:105–112.

171. **Bock JE, Andreasson B, Thorn A, et al.** Dermatofibromasarcoma protuberans of the vulva. *Gynecol Oncol* 1985;20:129–135.

172. **Dehner LP.** Metastatic and secondary tumors of the vulva. *Obstet Gynecol* 1973;42:47–57.

34 Gestational Trophoblastic Disease

Ross S. Berkowitz
Donald P. Goldstein

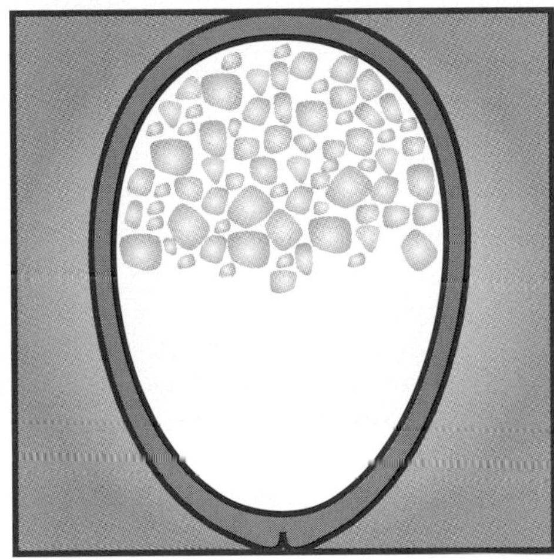

Gestational trophoblastic disease (GTD) is among the rare human tumors that can be cured even in the presence of widespread dissemination (1,2). This classification includes a spectrum of interrelated tumors, including complete and partial hydatidiform mole, placental-site trophoblastic tumor, and choriocarcinoma, which have varying propensities for local invasion and metastasis. Although persistent gestational trophoblastic tumors (GTTs) most commonly follow a molar pregnancy, they may ensue after any gestational event, including therapeutic or spontaneous abortion, ectopic pregnancy, or term pregnancy. Advances in the understanding of the pathogenesis, natural history, and treatment of GTD and the current approach to management are reviewed.

Hydatidiform Mole

Epidemiology

Estimates of the incidence of GTD vary dramatically in different regions of the world. For example, the incidence of molar pregnancy in Japan (2 per 1,000 pregnancies) has been reported to be about threefold higher than the incidence in Europe or North America (about 0.6 to 1.1 per 1,000 pregnancies) (3). The variation in the incidence rates of molar pregnancy may in part result from differences between reporting population-based versus hospital-based data. The incidences of both complete and partial mole have been investigated in Ireland by reviewing all products of conception from first- and second-trimester abortions (4). Based on a complete pathologic review, the incidence of complete and partial mole was found to be 1 per 1,945 and 1 per 695 pregnancies, respectively.

Case-control studies have been undertaken to identify risk factors for both complete and partial molar pregnancy. The high incidence of molar pregnancy in some populations has been attributed to nutritional and socioeconomic factors. **Case-control studies from Italy and the United States have shown that low dietary intake of carotene may be associated with an increased risk of complete molar pregnancy** (5,6). **Areas with a high incidence of molar pregnancy also have a high frequency of vitamin A deficiency. Dietary factors, therefore, may partly explain regional variations in the incidence of complete mole.**

Table 34.1. Features of Complete and Partial Hydatidiform Moles

Features	*Complete Mole*	*Partial Mole*
Fetal or embryonic tissue	Absent	Present
Hydatidiform swelling of chorionic villi	Diffuse	Focal
Trophoblastic hyperplasia	Diffuse	Focal
Scalloping of chorionic villi	Absent	Present
Trophoblastic stromal inclusions	Absent	Present
Karyotype	46,XX (90%); 46,XY	Triploid (90%)

Maternal age older than 35 years has consistently been shown to be a risk factor for complete mole. Ova from older women may be more susceptible to abnormal fertilization. In one study, the risk for complete mole was increased 2.0-fold for women older than 35 years and 7.5-fold for women older than 40 years (7).

Limited information is available concerning risk factors for partial molar pregnancy. However, the epidemiologic characteristics of complete and partial mole may differ. There is no association between maternal age and the risk for partial mole (7). The risk for partial mole has been reported to be associated with the use of oral contraceptives and a history of irregular menstruation, but not with dietary factors (8).

Complete Versus Partial Hydatidiform Mole

Hydatidiform moles may be categorized as either complete or partial moles on the basis of gross morphology, histopathology, and karyotype (Table 34.1).

Complete Hydatidiform Mole

Pathology **Complete moles lack identifiable embryonic or fetal tissues, and the chorionic villi exhibit generalized hydatidiform swelling and diffuse trophoblastic hyperplasia** (Fig. 34.1).

Figure 34.1 Photomicrograph of complete mole demonstrating diffusely hydropic chorionic villi and diffuse trophoblastic hyperplasia.

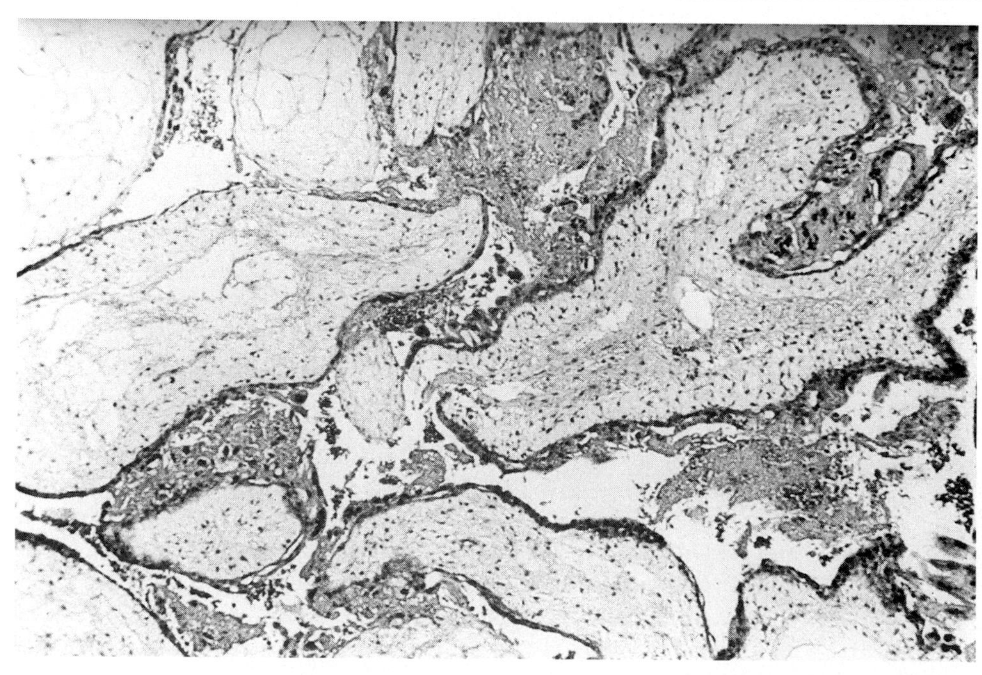

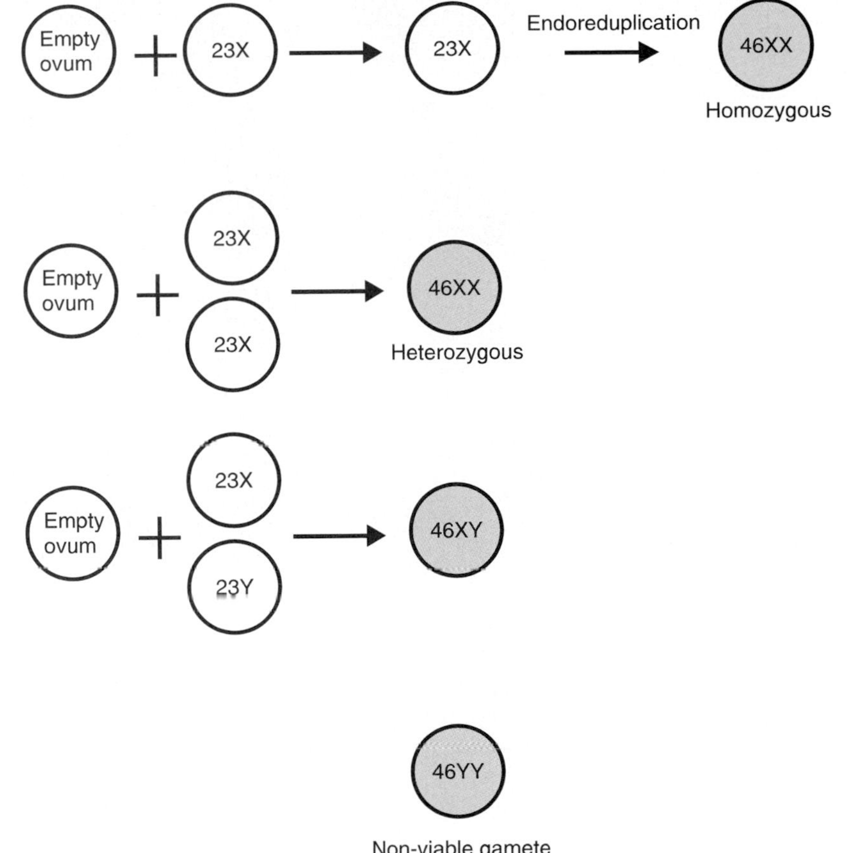

Figure 34.2 The karyotype of complete hydatidiform mole.

Chromosomes **Cytogenetic studies have demonstrated that complete hydatidiform moles usually have a 46,XX karyotype, and the molar chromosomes are entirely of paternal origin** (Fig. 34.2) (9). **It appears that complete moles usually arise from an ovum that has been fertilized by a haploid sperm, which then duplicates its own chromosomes. The ovum nucleus may be either absent or inactivated** (10). **Although most complete moles have a 46,XX chromosomal pattern, about 10% have a 46,XY karyotype** (11). Chromosomes in a 46,XY complete mole also appear to be entirely of paternal origin, although mitochondrial DNA is of maternal origin (12).

Partial Hydatidiform Mole

Pathology Partial hydatidiform moles are characterized by the following pathologic features (13) (Fig. 34.3):

1. Chorionic villi of varying size with focal hydatidiform swelling, cavitation, and trophoblastic hyperplasia
2. Marked villous scalloping
3. Prominent stromal trophoblastic inclusions
4. Identifiable embryonic or fetal tissues.

Chromosomes **Partial moles generally have a triploid karyotype (69 chromosomes); the extra haploid set of chromosomes usually is derived from the father** (Fig. 34.4) (14). One study reported that 93% of partial moles were triploid (14), whereas another

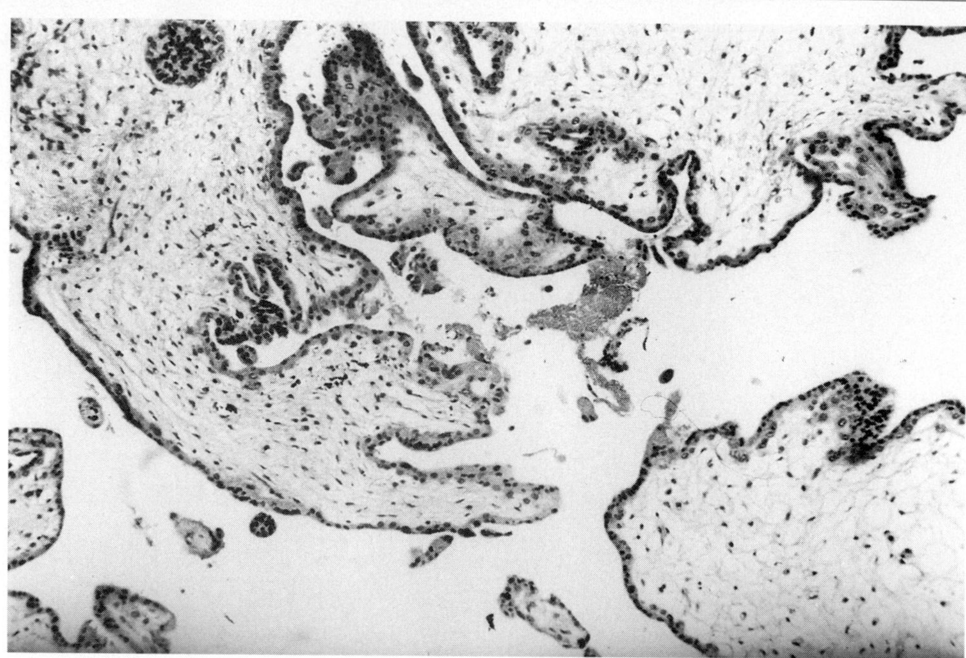

Figure 34.3 Photomicrograph of partial mole showing varying-sized chorionic villi with focal trophoblastic hyperplasia, stromal trophoblastic inclusions, and villous scalloping. (From **Berkowitz RS, Goldstein OP.** Gestational trophoblastic diseases. In: **Ryan KJ, Berkowitz R, Barbieri R,** eds. *Kistner's gynecology principles and practice,* 5th ed. Chicago: Year Book Medical Publishers, 1990:433, with permission.)

found 90% to be triploid (15). When a fetus is present in conjunction with a partial mole, it generally exhibits the stigmata of triploidy, including growth restriction and multiple congenital malformations such as syndactyly and hydrocephaly (Fig. 34.5).

Clinical Features

Increasingly, patients with complete molar pregnancy are being diagnosed earlier in pregnancy and are being treated before they develop the classic clinical signs and symptoms. This may be due to changes in clinical practice, such as the frequent use of vaginal probe ultrasonography in early pregnancy in women with vaginal staining and even asymptomatic women. Following is a description of the classic and current clinical features of complete molar pregnancy based on the authors' experience (16).

Complete Hydatidiform Mole

Vaginal Bleeding **Vaginal bleeding is the most common symptom causing patients to seek treatment for complete molar pregnancy.** Previously, it was reported to occur in 97% of cases, whereas currently it is reported to occur in 84% of patients (17). Molar tissues may separate from the decidua and disrupt maternal vessels, and large volumes of retained blood may distend the endometrial cavity. Because vaginal bleeding may be considerable and prolonged, one-half of these patients had anemia (hemoglobin <10 g/100 ml). Currently anemia is present in only 5% of patients.

Excessive Uterine Size **Excessive uterine enlargement relative to gestational age is one of the classic signs of a complete mole, although it was present in only about one-half of patients.** The endometrial cavity may be expanded by both chorionic tissue and retained blood. Excessive uterine size is generally associated with markedly elevated levels of human chorionic gonadotropin (hCG), because uterine enlargement results in part from trophoblastic overgrowth. Currently, excessive uterine size is present at diagnosis in only 28% of patients.

Figure 34.4 The karyotype of partial hydatidiform mole.

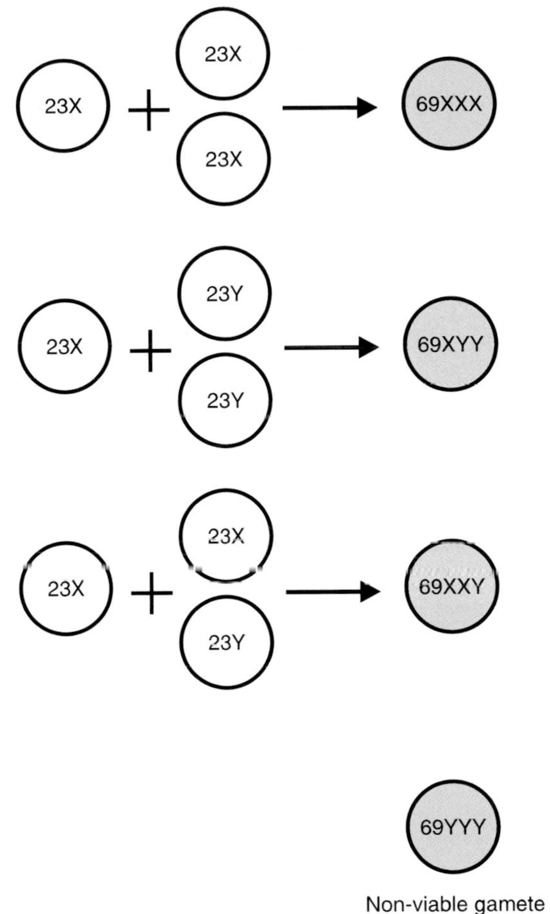

Figure 34.5 Photomicrograph of a fetal hand demonstrating syndactyly. The fetus had a triploid karyotype and the chorionic tissues were a partial mole.

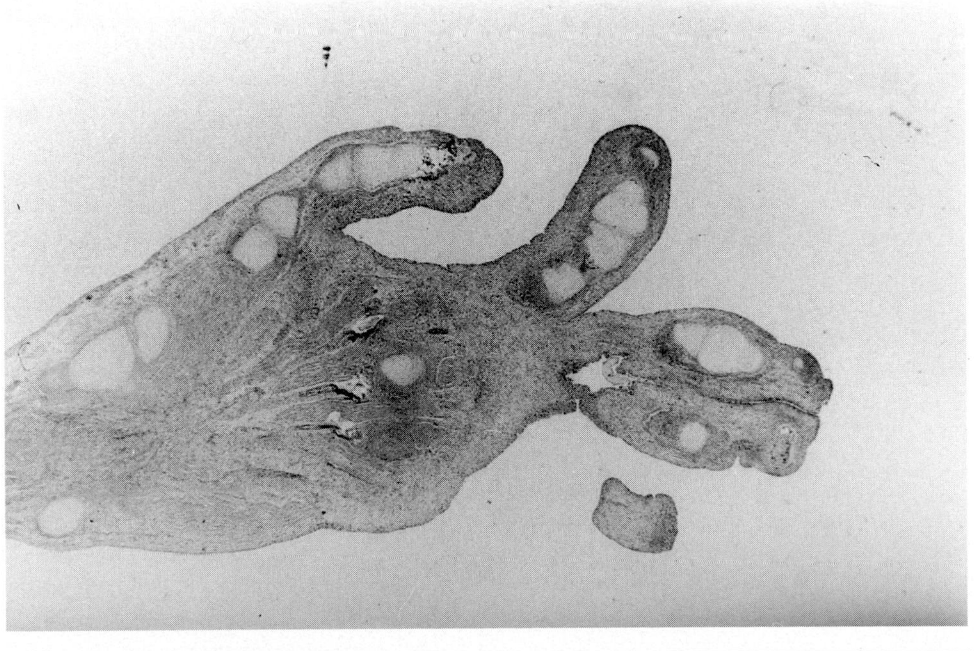

Preeclampsia **Preeclampsia was once observed in 27% of patients with a complete hydatidiform mole.** However, at one center between 1988 and 1993, only 1 of 74 patients with complete mole had preeclampsia at the initial visit (17). Although preeclampsia is associated with hypertension, proteinuria, and hyperreflexia, eclamptic convulsions rarely occur. Preeclampsia develops almost exclusively in patients with excessive uterine size and markedly elevated hCG levels. Hydatidiform mole should be considered whenever preeclampsia develops early in pregnancy.

Hyperemesis Gravidarum Hyperemesis requiring antiemetic or intravenous replacement therapy once occurred in one-fourth of women with a complete mole, particularly those with excessive uterine size and markedly elevated hCG levels. Severe electrolyte disturbances may develop and require treatment with parenteral fluids. Currently, only 8% of patients have hyperemesis.

Hyperthyroidism Clinically evident hyperthyroidism was once observed in 7% of patients with a complete molar gestation. These women may have tachycardia, warm skin, and tremor, and the diagnosis can be confirmed by detection of elevated serum levels of free thyroxine (T_4) and triiodothyronine (T_3). Between 1988 and 1993, none of the author's 74 patients with complete mole had clinical evidence of hyperthyroidism.

If hyperthyroidism is suspected before the induction of anesthesia for molar evacuation, β-adrenergic blocking agents should be administered because anesthesia or surgery may precipitate thyroid storm. Thyroid storms may be manifest by hyperthermia, delirium, convulsions, tachyrhythmia, high-output heart failure, or cardiovascular collapse. Administration of β-adrenergic blocking agents prevents or rapidly reverses many of the metabolic and cardiovascular complications of thyroid storm. After molar evacuation, thyroid function test results return rapidly to normal.

Hyperthyroidism develops almost exclusively in patients with very high hCG levels. Some investigators have suggested that hCG is the thyroid stimulator in women with GTD, because positive correlations between serum hCG and total T_4 or T_3 concentrations have been observed. However, one study in which thyroid function was measured in 47 patients with a complete mole reported no significant correlation between serum hCG levels and serum values of free T_4 index or free T_3 index (18). Although some investigators have speculated about a separate chorionic thyrotropin, this substance has not yet been isolated.

Trophoblastic Embolization Respiratory distress developed in 2% of patients with a complete mole in the past, but it has occurred in none of the authors' patients. Respiratory distress is usually diagnosed in patients with excessive uterine size and markedly elevated hCG levels. These patients may have chest pain, dyspnea, tachypnea, and tachycardia and may experience severe respiratory distress during and after molar evacuation. Auscultation of the chest usually reveals diffuse rales, and chest radiographic evaluation may demonstrate bilateral pulmonary infiltrates. Respiratory distress usually resolves within 72 hours with cardiopulmonary support. In some circumstances, patients may require mechanical ventilation. Respiratory insufficiency may result from trophoblastic embolization or from the cardiopulmonary complications of thyroid storm, preeclampsia, and massive fluid replacement.

Theca Lutein Ovarian Cysts Prominent theca lutein ovarian cysts (6 cm in diameter) develop in about one-half of patients with a complete mole (19). Theca lutein ovarian cysts result from high serum hCG levels, which cause ovarian hyperstimulation (20). Because the uterus also may be excessively enlarged, theca lutein cysts may be difficult to palpate during physical examination; however, ultrasonography can accurately document their presence and size. After molar evacuation, theca lutein cysts normally regress spontaneously within 2 to 4 months.

Prominent theca lutein cysts may cause symptoms of marked pelvic pressure, and they may be decompressed by laparoscopic or ultrasonographically directed aspiration. If acute pelvic pain develops, laparoscopy should be performed to assess possible cystic torsion or rupture.

Partial Hydatidiform Mole

Patients with partial hydatidiform mole usually do not have the dramatic clinical features characteristic of complete molar pregnancy. **In general, these patients have the signs and symptoms of incomplete or missed abortion, and partial mole can be diagnosed after histologic review of the tissue obtained by curettage** (21).

In a survey of 81 patients with a partial mole, the main initial sign was vaginal bleeding, which occurred in 59 patients (72.8%) (22). Excessive uterine enlargement and preeclampsia were present in only three patients (3.7%) and two (2.5%) patients, respectively. No patients had theca lutein ovarian cysts, hyperemesis, or hyperthyroidism. The initial clinical diagnosis was an incomplete or missed abortion in 74 patients (91.3%) and hydatidiform mole in only five patients (6.2%). Preevacuation hCG levels were measured in 30 patients and were higher than 100,000 mIU/ml in only two patients (6.6%).

Natural History

Complete Hydatidiform Mole

Complete moles have a potential for local invasion and dissemination. **After molar evacuation, local uterine invasion occurs in 15% of patients and metastasis occurs in 4%** (19).

A review of 858 patients with complete hydatidiform mole revealed that two-fifths of the patients had the following signs of marked trophoblastic proliferation at the time they sought treatment (19):

1. hCG level >100,000 mIU/ml
2. Excessive uterine enlargement
3. Theca lutein cysts 6 cm in diameter.

Patients with any one of these signs were considered at high risk. After molar evacuation, local uterine invasion occurred in 31% and metastases developed in 8.8% of the 352 high-risk patients. For the 506 low-risk patients, local invasion was found in only 3.4%, and metastases developed in 0.6%.

Older patients are also at increased risk of developing postmolar GTT. One study reported that persistent tumor developed after a complete molar pregnancy in 37% of women older than 40 years (23), whereas in another study this finding occurred in 56% of women older than 50 years (23,24).

Partial Hydatidiform Mole

Persistent tumor, usually nonmetastatic, develops in approximately 4% of patients with a partial mole, and chemotherapy is required to achieve remission (25). **Patients who develop persistent disease have no distinguishing clinical or pathologic characteristics** (26). Additionally, it has been reported that 11 (85%) of 13 patients with partial moles who developed persistent tumor had a triploid karyotype (27).

Diagnosis

Ultrasonography is a reliable and sensitive technique for the diagnosis of complete molar pregnancy. Because the chorionic villi exhibit diffuse hydropic swelling, complete moles produce a characteristic vesicular ultrasonographic pattern.

Ultrasonography also may contribute to the diagnosis of partial molar pregnancy by demonstrating focal cystic spaces in the placental tissues and an increase in the transverse diameter of the gestational sac (28). **When both of these criteria are present, the positive predictive value for partial mole is 90%.**

Treatment

After molar pregnancy is diagnosed, the patient should be evaluated carefully for the presence of associated medical complications, including preeclampsia, hyperthyroidism, electrolyte imbalance, and anemia. After the patient's condition has been stabilized, a decision must be made concerning the most appropriate method of evacuation.

Hysterectomy

If the patient desires surgical sterilization, a hysterectomy may be performed with the mole *in situ*. The ovaries may be preserved at the time of surgery, even though prominent theca lutein cysts are present. Large ovarian cysts may be decompressed by aspiration. Hysterectomy does not prevent metastasis; therefore, patients still require follow-up with assessment of hCG levels.

Suction Curettage

Suction curettage is the preferred method of evacuation, regardless of uterine size, for patients who desire to preserve fertility. It involves the following steps:

1. *Oxytocin infusion*—This procedure is begun in the operating room before the induction of anesthesia.

2. *Cervical dilation*—As the cervix is being dilated, the surgeon frequently encounters increased uterine bleeding. Retained blood in the endometrial cavity may be expelled during cervical dilation. However, active uterine bleeding should not deter the prompt completion of cervical dilation.

3. *Suction curettage*—Within a few minutes of commencing suction curettage, the uterus may decrease dramatically in size, and the bleeding is generally well controlled. The use of a 12-mm cannula is strongly advised to facilitate evacuation. If the uterus is larger than 14 weeks of gestation, one hand should be placed on top of the fundus, and the uterus should be massaged to stimulate uterine contraction and reduce the risk of perforation.

4. *Sharp curettage*—When suction evacuation is believed to be complete, gentle sharp curettage is performed to remove any residual molar tissue.

Because trophoblast cells express RhD factor, patients who are Rh negative should receive Rh immune globulin at the time of evacuation.

Prophylactic Chemotherapy

The use of prophylactic chemotherapy at the time of molar evacuation is controversial (29). The debate concerns the wisdom of exposing all patients to potentially toxic treatment when only about 20% are at risk of developing persistent tumor.

In a study of 247 patients with complete molar pregnancy who received prophylactically a single course of *actinomycin D* at the time of evacuation, local uterine invasion subsequently developed in only 10 patients (4%), and no patients experienced metastasis (29). Furthermore, all 10 patients with local invasion achieved remission after only one additional course of chemotherapy. **Prophylactic chemotherapy, therefore, not only prevented metastasis but also reduced the incidence and morbidity of local uterine invasion.**

In a prospective randomized study of prophylactic chemotherapy in patients with a complete mole, a significant decrease in persistent tumor was detected in patients with high-risk mole who received prophylactic chemotherapy (47% versus 14%) (30). **Prophylaxis may be particularly useful in the management of high-risk complete molar pregnancy, especially when hormonal follow-up is unavailable or unreliable.**

Follow-up

Human Chorionic Gonadotropin

After molar evacuation, patients should be monitored with weekly determinations of β-subunit hCG levels until these levels are normal for 3 consecutive weeks, followed by monthly determinations until the levels are normal for 6 consecutive months. The average time to achieve the first normal hCG level after evacuation is about 9 weeks (31). At the completion of follow-up, pregnancy may be undertaken.

Contraception

Patients are encouraged to use effective contraception during the entire interval of hCG follow-up. Because of the potential risk of uterine perforation, intrauterine devices should not be inserted until the patient achieves a normal hCG level. If the patient does not desire surgical sterilization, the choice is to use either oral contraceptives or barrier methods.

The incidence of postmolar persistent tumor has been reported to be increased among patients who used oral contraceptives before gonadotropin remission (32). However, more recent data indicate that oral contraceptives do not increase the risk of postmolar trophoblastic disease (33,34). **It appears that oral contraceptives may be used safely after molar evacuation during the entire interval of hormonal follow-up.**

Persistent Gestational Trophoblastic Tumor

Nonmetastatic Disease

Locally invasive GTT develops in about 15% of patients after molar evacuation and infrequently after other gestations (1). These patients usually are seen clinically with the following symptoms:

1. Irregular vaginal bleeding
2. Theca lutein cysts
3. Uterine subinvolution or asymmetric enlargement
4. Persistently elevated serum hCG levels.

The trophoblastic tumor may perforate through the myometrium, causing intraperitoneal bleeding, or erode into uterine vessels, causing vaginal hemorrhage. Bulky, necrotic tumor may involve the uterine wall and serve as a nidus for infection. Patients with uterine sepsis may have a purulent vaginal discharge and acute pelvic pain.

After molar evacuation, persistent GTT may exhibit the histologic features of either hydatidiform mole or choriocarcinoma. After a nonmolar pregnancy, however, persistent GTT always has the histologic pattern of choriocarcinoma. Histologically, choriocarcinoma is characterized by sheets of anaplastic syncytiotrophoblast and cytotrophoblast without chorionic villi.

Placental-site Trophoblastic Tumor

Placental-site trophoblastic tumor is an uncommon but important variant of choriocarcinoma that consists predominantly of intermediate trophoblast (35). Relative to their mass, these tumors produce small amounts of hCG and human placental lactogen (hPL), and they tend to remain confined to the uterus, metastasizing late in their course. **In contrast to other trophoblastic tumors, placental-site tumors are relatively insensitive to chemotherapy.**

Metastatic Disease

Metastatic GTT occurs in about 4% of patients after evacuation of a complete mole, but it is seen more often when GTT develops after nonmolar pregnancies (1). Metastasis is usually associated with choriocarcinoma, which has a tendency toward early vascular invasion with widespread dissemination. Because trophoblastic tumors often are perfused by fragile vessels, they are frequently hemorrhagic. Symptoms of metastases may result from spontaneous bleeding at metastatic foci. The most common sites of metastases are lung (80%), vagina (30%), pelvis (20%), liver (10%), and brain (10%).

Pulmonary

At the time of diagnosis, lung involvement is visible on chest radiographs of 80% of patients with metastatic GTT. Patients with pulmonary metastasis may have chest pain, cough, hemoptysis, dyspnea, or an asymptomatic lesion on chest radiograph. Respiratory symptoms may be acute or chronic, persisting over many months.

GTT may produce four principal pulmonary radiographic patterns:

1. An alveolar or "snowstorm" pattern
2. Discrete rounded densities
3. Pleural effusion
4. An embolic pattern caused by pulmonary arterial occlusion.

Because respiratory symptoms and radiographic findings may be dramatic, the patient may be thought to have a primary pulmonary disease. Some patients with extensive pulmonary involvement have minimal, if any, gynecologic symptoms because the reproductive organs may be free of trophoblastic tumor. Unfortunately, the diagnosis of GTT may be confirmed only after thoracotomy has been performed, particularly in patients with a nonmolar antecedent pregnancy.

Pulmonary hypertension may develop in patients with GTT secondary to pulmonary arterial occlusion by trophoblastic emboli. The development of early respiratory failure requiring intubation is associated with a dismal clinical outcome (36,37).

Vaginal

Vaginal metastases occurs in 30% of the patients with metastatic tumor. These lesions are usually highly vascular and may bleed vigorously if a sample is taken for biopsy. Metastases to the vagina may occur in the fornices or suburethrally and may produce irregular bleeding or a purulent discharge.

Hepatic

Liver metastases occur in 10% of patients with disseminated trophoblastic tumor. Hepatic involvement is encountered almost exclusively in patients with protracted delays in diagnosis and extensive tumor burdens. Epigastric or right upper quadrant pain may develop if metastases stretch the hepatic capsule. Hepatic lesions may be hemorrhagic, causing hepatic rupture and exsanguinating intraperitoneal bleeding.

Table 34.2. Staging of Gestational Trophoblastic Tumors

Stage I	**Disease confined to uterus**
Stage IA	Disease confined to uterus with no risk factors
Stage IB	Disease confined to uterus with one risk factor
Stage IC	Disease confined to uterus with two risk factors
Stage II	**Gestational trophoblastic tumor extending outside uterus but limited to genital structures (adnexa, vagina, broad ligament)**
Stage IIA	Gestational trophoblastic tumor involving genital structures without risk factors
Stage IIB	Gestational trophoblastic tumor extending outside uterus but limited to genital structures with one risk factor
Stage IIC	Gestational trophoblastic tumor extending outside uterus but limited to genital structures with two risk factors
Stage III	**Gestational trophoblastic disease extending to lungs with or without known genital tract involvement**
Stage IIIA	Gestational trophoblastic tumor extending to lungs with or without genital tract involvement and with no risk factors
Stage IIIB	Gestational trophoblastic tumor extending to lungs with or without genital tract involvement and with one risk factor
Stage IIIC	Gestational trophoblastic tumor extending to lungs with or without genital tract involvement and with two risk factors
Stage IV	**All other metastatic sites**
Stage IVA	All other metastatic sites without risk factors
Stage IVB	All other metastatic sites with one risk factor
Stage IVC	All other metastatic sites with two risk factors

Risk factors affecting staging include the following: (a) human chorionic gonadotropin > 100,000 mIU/ml and (b) duration of disease longer than 6 months from termination of antecedent pregnancy.
The following factors should be considered and noted in reporting: (a) prior chemotherapy has been given for known gestational trophoblastic tumor, (b) placental site tumors should be reported separately and (c) histologic verification of disease is not required.

Central Nervous System

Metastatic trophoblastic disease involves the brain in 10% of patients. Cerebral involvement is generally seen in patients with advanced disease; virtually all patients with brain metastasis have concurrent pulmonary or vaginal involvement or both. Because cerebral lesions may hemorrhage spontaneously, patients may develop acute focal neurologic deficits.

Staging

An anatomic staging system for GTT has been adopted by the International Federation of Gynecology and Obstetrics (FIGO) (Table 34.2). It is hoped that this staging system will encourage the objective comparison of data among various centers.

Stage I: Patients have persistently elevated hCG levels and tumor confined to the uterine corpus.

Stage II: Patients have metastases to the vagina and pelvis or both.

Stage III: Patients have pulmonary metastases with or without uterine, vaginal, or pelvic involvement. The diagnosis is based on a rising hCG level in the presence of pulmonary lesions on chest radiograph.

Stage IV: Patients have advanced disease and involvement of the brain, liver, kidneys, or gastrointestinal tract. These patients are in the highest risk category, because they are most likely to be resistant to chemotherapy. The histologic pattern of choriocarcinoma is usually present, and disease commonly follows a nonmolar pregnancy.

Prognostic Scoring System

In addition to anatomic staging, it is important to consider other variables to predict the likelihood of drug resistance and to assist in selecting appropriate chemotherapy (38).

Table 34.3. Scoring System Based on Prognostic Factors

	Score			
	0	*1*	*2*	*4*
Age (years)	≤39	>39	—	—
Antecedent pregnancy	Hydatidiform mole	Abortion	Term	—
Interval between end of antecedent pregnancy and start of chemotherapy (months)	<4	4–6	7–12	>12
Human chorionic gonadotropin (IU/liter)	$<10^3$	10^3–10^4	10^4–10^5	$>10^5$
ABO groups	—	O or A	B or AB	—
Largest tumor, including uterine (cm)	<3	3–5	>5	—
Site of metastases	—	Spleen, kidney	Gastrointestinal tract, liver	Brain
Number of metastases	—	1–3	4–8	>8
Prior chemotherapy	—	—	1 drug	≥2 drugs

The total score for a patient is obtained by adding the individual scores for each prognostic factor. Total score: <4, low risk; 5–7, middle risk; ≥8, high risk.

A prognostic scoring system proposed by the World Health Organization reliably predicts the potential for resistance to chemotherapy (Table 34.3).

When the prognostic score is higher than 7, the patient is categorized as high risk and requires intensive combination chemotherapy to achieve remission. Patients with stage I disease usually have a low-risk score, and those with stage IV disease have a high-risk score. The distinction between low and high risk applies mainly to patients with Stage II or III disease.

Diagnostic Evaluation

Optimal management of persistent GTT requires a thorough assessment of the extent of the disease prior to the initiation of treatment. **All patients with persistent GTT should undergo a careful pretreatment evaluation, including the following:**

1. Complete history and physical examination
2. Measurement of the serum hCG value
3. Hepatic, thyroid, and renal function tests
4. Determination of baseline peripheral white blood cell and platelet counts.

The metastatic workup should include the following:

1. Chest radiograph or computed tomography (CT) scan
2. Ultrasonography or CT scan of the abdomen and pelvis
3. CT or magnetic resonance imaging (MRI) scan of the head.

When the pelvic examination and chest radiographic findings are negative, metastatic involvement of other sites is uncommon.

Liver ultrasonography and CT scanning will document most hepatic metastases in patients with abnormal liver function tests. CT or MRI scan of the head has facilitated the early diagnosis of asymptomatic cerebral lesions (39). Chest CT scans may demonstrate micrometastases not visible on a chest radiograph.

Table 34.4. Protocol for Treatment of GTT

Stage I	
Initial	Single-agent chemotherapy or hysterectomy with adjunctive chemotherapy
Resistant	Combination chemotherapy Hysterectomy with adjunctive chemotherapy Local resection Pelvic infusion
Stages II and III	
Low risk [a]	
Initial	Single-agent chemotherapy
Resistant	Combination chemotherapy
High risk [a]	
Initial	Combination chemotherapy
Resistant	Second-line combination chemotherapy
Stage IV	
Initial	Combination chemotherapy
Brain	Whole-heat irradiation (3,000 cGy) Craniotomy to manage complications
Liver	Resection to manage complications
Resistant[a]	Second-line combination chemotherapy Hepatic arterial infusion

[a] Local resection optional.
GTT, gestational trophoblastic tumor.

In patients with choriocarcinoma or metastatic disease, hCG levels may be measured in the cerebrospinal fluid (CSF) to exclude cerebral involvement if the results of CT scanning of the brain are normal. The ratio of plasma-to-CSF hCG tends to be lower than 60 in the presence of cerebral metastases (40). However, a single plasma-to-CSF hCG ratio may be misleading, because rapid changes in plasma hCG levels may not be reflected promptly in the CSF (41).

Pelvic ultrasonography appears to be useful in detecting extensive trophoblastic uterine involvement and may also aid in identifying sites of resistant uterine tumor (42). Because ultrasonography can accurately and noninvasively detect extensive uterine tumor, it may help identify patients who would benefit from hysterectomy.

Management of Persistent GTT

A protocol for the management of GTT is presented in Table 34.4.

Stage I

In patients with stage I disease, the selection of treatment is based primarily on whether the patient desires to retain fertility.

Hysterectomy plus Chemotherapy

If the patient does not wish to preserve fertility, hysterectomy with adjuvant single-agent chemotherapy may be performed as primary treatment. Adjuvant chemotherapy is administered for three reasons:

1. To reduce the likelihood of disseminating viable tumor cells at surgery
2. To maintain a cytotoxic level of chemotherapy in the bloodstream and tissues in case viable tumor cells are disseminated at surgery
3. To treat any occult metastases that may already be present at the time of surgery.

Chemotherapy can be administered safely at the time of hysterectomy without increasing the risk of bleeding or sepsis. In a series of 30 patients treated with primary hysterectomy and a single course of adjuvant chemotherapy, all have achieved complete remission with no additional therapy.

Hysterectomy is also performed in all patients with stage I placental-site trophoblastic tumor. Because placental-site tumors are resistant to chemotherapy, hysterectomy for presumed nonmetastatic disease is the only curative treatment. To date, only a small number of patients with metastatic placental-site tumor have been reported to be in sustained remission as a result of chemotherapy (43).

Chemotherapy Alone

Single-agent chemotherapy is the preferred treatment in patients with stage I disease who desire to retain fertility. When primary single-agent chemotherapy was administered to 468 patients with stage I GTT, 431 patients (92.1%) attained complete remission. The remaining 37 resistant patients subsequently achieved remission after combination chemotherapy or surgical intervention.

When patients are resistant to single-agent chemotherapy and desire to preserve fertility, combination chemotherapy should be administered. If the patient is resistant to both single-agent and combination chemotherapy and wants to retain fertility, local uterine resection may be considered. When local resection is planned, a preoperative ultrasonography, MRI, or arteriography may help to define the site of the resistant tumor.

Stages II and III

Low-risk patients are treated with primary single-agent chemotherapy, and high-risk patients are treated with primary intensive combination chemotherapy.

Vaginal and Pelvic Metastasis

In one series, 27 treated patients with stage II disease achieved remission. Single-agent chemotherapy induced complete remission in 16 (84.2%) of 19 low-risk patients. In contrast, only two of eight high-risk patients achieved remission with single-agent treatment; the others required combination chemotherapy.

Vaginal metastases may bleed profusely because they are highly vascular and friable. When bleeding is substantial, it may be controlled by packing the vagina or by wide local excision. Infrequently, arteriographic embolization of the hypogastric arteries may be required to control hemorrhage from vaginal metastases.

Pulmonary Metastasis

Of 143 patients treated with stage III disease, 142 (99%) attained complete remission. Gonadotropin remission was induced with single-agent chemotherapy in 80 of 97 (82.5%) patients with low-risk disease. All patients who were resistant to single-agent treatment subsequently achieved remission with combination chemotherapy.

Thoracotomy Thoracotomy has a limited role in the management of stage III disease. **If a patient has a persistent viable pulmonary metastasis despite intensive chemotherapy, however, thoracotomy may be attempted to excise the resistant focus.** A thorough metastatic workup should be performed before surgery to exclude other sites of persistent disease. Evidence of fibrotic pulmonary nodules may persist indefinitely on chest radiographs, even after complete gonadotropin remission has been attained. In patients undergoing thoracotomy for resistant disease, chemotherapy should be administered postoperatively to treat potential occult sites of micrometastasis.

Hysterectomy

Hysterectomy may be required in patients with metastatic disease to control uterine hemorrhage or sepsis. Furthermore, in patients with extensive uterine tumor, hysterectomy may substantially reduce the trophoblastic tumor burden and thereby limit the need for multiple courses of chemotherapy.

Follow-up

All patients with stage I through stage III disease should receive follow-up with:

1. Weekly measurement of hCG levels until they are normal for 3 consecutive weeks
2. Monthly measurement of hCG values until levels are normal for 12 consecutive months
3. Effective contraception during the entire interval of hormonal follow-up.

Patients with stage IV disease are at greatest risk of developing rapidly progressive and unresponsive tumors despite intensive multimodal therapy. They should preferably be referred to centers with special expertise in the management of trophoblastic disease.

Stage IV

All patients with stage IV disease should be treated with primary intensive combination chemotherapy and the selective use of radiation therapy and surgery. Before 1975, only 6 of 20 patients (30%) treated with stage IV disease attained complete remission, whereas after that time, 14 of 18 patients (77.8%) achieved remission. This improvement in survival has resulted from the use of primary combination chemotherapy in conjunction with radiation and surgical treatment.

Hepatic Metastasis

The management of hepatic metastasis is particularly difficult. If a patient is resistant to systemic chemotherapy, hepatic arterial infusion of chemotherapy may induce complete remission in selected cases. Hepatic resection may also be required to control acute bleeding or to excise a focus of resistant tumor. New techniques of arterial embolization may reduce the need for surgical intervention.

Cerebral Metastasis

If cerebral metastases are diagnosed, whole-brain irradiation (3,000 cGy in 10 fractions) can be instituted promptly. The risk of spontaneous cerebral hemorrhage may be lessened by the concurrent use of combination chemotherapy and brain irradiation, because irradiation may be both hemostatic and tumoricidal. However, excellent remission rates (86%) have been reported in patients with cranial metastases treated with intensive intravenous combination chemotherapy and intrathecal *methotrexate* (*MTX*) (44).

Craniotomy Craniotomy may be required to provide acute decompression or to control bleeding. It should be performed to manage life-threatening complications in the hope that the patient ultimately will be cured with chemotherapy. In one study (45), the use of craniotomy to control bleeding in six patients resulted in complete remission in three patients. Infrequently, cerebral metastases that are resistant to chemotherapy may be amenable to local resection. Fortunately, patients with cerebral metastases who achieve sustained remission generally have no residual neurologic deficits.

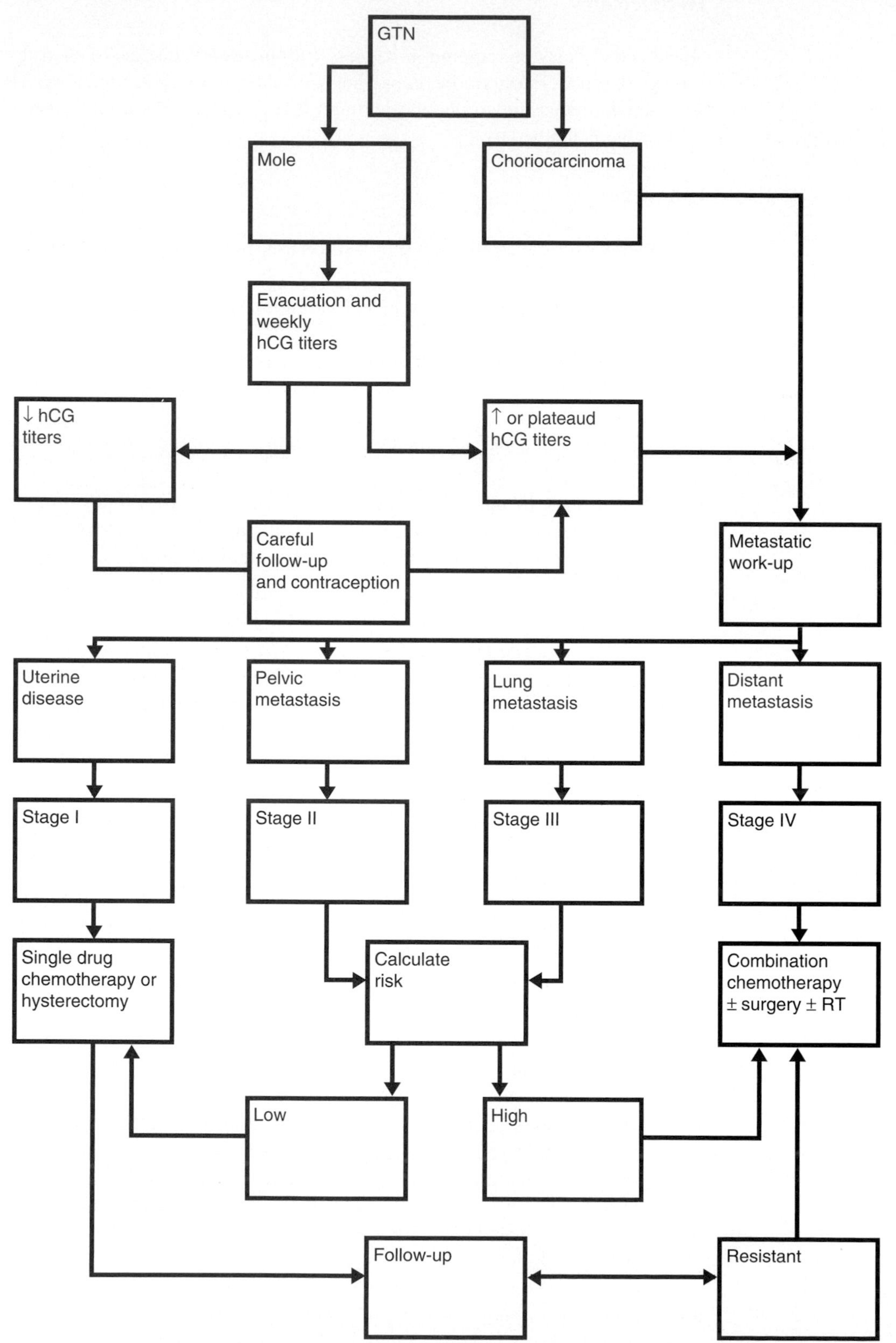

Figure 34.6 Algorithm for the management of persistent gestational trophoblastic tumor. (From **Berkowitz RS, Goldstein DP.** Gestational trophoblastic neoplasia. In: **Berek JS, Hacker NF,** eds. *Practical gynecologic oncology,* 3rd ed. Philadelphia: Lippincot Williams & Wilkins, 2000;632, with permission.)

Follow-up

Patients with stage IV disease should receive follow-up with:

1. Weekly determination of hCG levels until they are normal for 3 consecutive weeks
2. Monthly determination of hCG levels until they are normal for 24 consecutive months.

These patients require prolonged gonadotropin follow-up because they are at increased risk of late recurrence.

An algorithm for the management of persistent GTT is presented in Fig. 34.6.

Chemotherapy

Single-agent Treatment

Single-agent chemotherapy with either *actinomycin D* (*Act-D*) or *MTX* has achieved comparable and excellent remission rates in both nonmetastatic and low-risk metastatic GTT (46). Several protocols using these agents are available. *Act-D* can be given every other week as a 5-day regimen or in a pulsatile fashion; similarly, *MTX* can be given either in a 5-day regimen or pulsatile weekly. No study has compared all of these protocols with regard to success. An optimal regimen should maximize the response rate while minimizing morbidity and cost.

The administration of *methotrexate* with *folinic acid* (*MTX-FA*) in GTT to limit systemic toxicity was first reported in 1964 (47). Subsequently, it has been confirmed that *MTX-FA* is both effective and safe in the management of GTT (48).

MTX-FA has been the preferred single agent in the treatment of GTT. An evaluation of 185 patients treated in this manner revealed that complete remission was achieved in 162 patients (87.6%); of these patients, 132 (81.5%) required only one course of *MTX-FA* to attain remission (48). *MTX-FA* induced remission in 147 of 163 patients (90.2%) with stage I GTT and in 15 of 22 patients (68.2%) with low-risk stages II and III GTT. Resistance to therapy was more common in patients with choriocarcinoma, metastasis, and pretreatment serum hCG levels higher than 50,000 mIU/ml. After treatment with *MTX-FA*, thrombocytopenia, granulocytopenia, and hepatotoxicity developed in only 3 (1.6%), 11 (5.9%), and 26 (14.1%) patients, respectively. Thus, *MTX-FA* achieved an excellent therapeutic outcome with minimal toxicity and attained this goal with limited exposure to chemotherapy.

Technique of Single-agent Treatment

The serum hCG level is measured weekly after each course of chemotherapy, and the hCG regression curve serves as the primary basis for determining the need for additional treatment.

After the first treatment:

1. Further chemotherapy is withheld as long as the hCG level is falling progressively.
2. Additional single-agent chemotherapy is not administered at any predetermined or fixed interval.

A second course of chemotherapy is administered under the following conditions:

1. If the hCG level plateaus for more than 3 consecutive weeks or begins to rise again

2. If the hCG level does not decline by 1 log within 18 days after completion of the first treatment.

If the patient's response to the first treatment was adequate and a second course of *MTX-FA* is required the dosage of *MTX* is unaltered. An adequate response is defined as a fall in the hCG level by 1 log after a course of chemotherapy.

If the response to the first treatment is inadequate, the dosage of *MTX* is increased from 1.0 mg/kg per day to 1.5 mg/kg per day for each of the 4 treatment days. If the response to two consecutive courses of *MTX-FA* is inadequate, the patient is considered to be resistant to *MTX*, and *Act-D* is promptly substituted. If the hCG levels do not decline by 1 log after treatment with *Act-D*, the patient also is considered resistant to *Act-D* as a single agent. She must then be treated intensively with combination chemotherapy to achieve remission.

Combination Chemotherapy

Triple Therapy

Triple therapy with *MTX, Act-D,* and *cyclophosphamide* is inadequate as an initial treatment in patients with metastasis and a high-risk prognostic score. Collectively, data from various centers indicate that triple therapy induced remission in only 21 (49%) of 43 patients with metastasis and a high-risk score (score >7) (49–51).

Etoposide has been reported to induce complete remission in 56 (95%) of 60 patients with nonmetastatic and low-risk metastatic GTT (52). A new combination regimen described in 1984 included *etoposide, MTX, Act-D, cyclophosphamide,* and *vincristine* (*EMA-CO*) and had an 83% remission in patients with metastasis and a high-risk score (53). Another study (54) confirmed that primary *EMA-CO* induced complete remission in 76% of the patients with metastatic GTT and a high-risk score (54). Still another study reported that *EMA-CO* induced complete sustained remission in 61 (94%) of 65 patients with high-risk (score >5) GTT (55). Furthermore, remission occurred with *EMA-CO* in 13 (86%) of 15 patients with brain metastasis (44).

The *EMA-CO* regimen is generally well tolerated, and treatment seldom has to be suspended because of toxicity. The *EMA-CO* regimen is the preferred primary treatment in patients with metastasis and a high-risk prognostic score. However, the optimal combination drug protocol for management of GTT has not yet been clearly defined. If patients experience resistance to *EMA-CO,* they may then be treated successfully by substituting *etoposide* and *cisplatin* on day 8 (*EMA-EP*). *EMA-EP* has induced remission alone or with surgery in 16 (76%) of 21 patients who were resistant to *EMA-CO* (56). The optimal combination drug protocol will most likely include *etoposide, MTX,* and *Act-D* and perhaps other agents administered in the most dose-intensive manner.

Duration of Therapy

Patients who require combination chemotherapy must be treated intensively to attain remission. Combination chemotherapy should be given as often as toxicity permits until the patient achieves three consecutive normal hCG levels. After normal hCG levels are attained, at least two additional courses of chemotherapy are administered to reduce the risk of relapse.

Subsequent Pregnancies

Pregnancies After Hydatidiform Mole **Patients with hydatidiform moles can anticipate normal reproduction in the future** (57). From 1965 until 1999, patients who were treated for complete mole had 1,239 subsequent pregnancies that resulted in 850 term live births (68.6%), 93 premature deliveries (7.5%), 11 ectopic pregnancies (0.9%),

7 stillbirths (0.5%), and 17 repeat molar pregnancies (1.4%). First- and second-trimester spontaneous abortions occurred in 205 (16.5%) and 18 (1.5%) pregnancies, respectively. Major and minor congenital malformations were detected in 38 infants (4.0%), and primary cesarean delivery was performed in 56 of 345 (16.2%) term or preterm births from 1979 to 1999.

Although data regarding pregnancies after partial mole are limited (205 subsequent pregnancies), the information is reassuring (57). **Patients with both complete and partial mole should be reassured that they are at no increased risk of complications in later gestations.**

When a patient has had a molar pregnancy, she is at an increased risk of having a molar gestation in subsequent conceptions (58). **After one molar pregnancy, the risk of having molar disease in a future gestation is about 1%.** Of 29 patients with at least two documented molar pregnancies, every possible combination of repeat molar pregnancy was observed. After two molar gestations, these 29 patients had 34 later conceptions resulting in 19 (55.9%) term deliveries, 7 (20.6%) moles (6 complete, 1 partial), 3 spontaneous abortions, 3 therapeutic abortions, 1 intrauterine fetal death, and 1 ectopic pregnancy. In six patients, the medical records indicated that the patient had a different partner at the time of different molar pregnancies (59).

Therefore, for any subsequent pregnancy, it seems prudent to undertake the following approach:

1. Perform pelvic ultrasonographic examination during the first trimester to confirm normal gestational development.

2. Obtain a thorough histologic review of the placenta or products of conception.

3. Obtain an hCG measurement 6 weeks after completion of the pregnancy to exclude occult trophoblastic neoplasia.

Pregnancies After Persistent GTT **Patients with GTT who are treated successfully with chemotherapy can expect normal reproduction in the future.** Patients who were treated with chemotherapy at the authors' institution from 1965 to 1999 had 522 subsequent pregnancies that resulted in 358 term live births (68.6%), 30 preterm deliveries (5.8%), 6 ectopic pregnancies (1.1%), 8 stillbirths (1.5%), and 6 repeat molar pregnancies (1.1%) (57). First- and second-trimester spontaneous abortions occurred in 81 (15.5%) and 7 (1.4%) pregnancies, respectively. Major and minor congenital malformations were detected in 10 infants (2.5%). Primary cesarean delivery was performed in 57 (19.4%) of 294 subsequent term and preterm births from 1979 to 1999. It is particularly reassuring that the frequency of congenital anomalies is not increased, although chemotherapeutic agents are known to have teratogenic and mutagenic potential.

References

1. **Berkowitz RS, Goldstein DP.** The management of molar pregnancy and gestational trophoblastic tumors. In: **Knapp RC, Berkowitz RS,** eds. *Gynecologic oncology,* 2nd ed. New York: McGraw-Hill, 1993:328–338.
2. **Bagshawe KD.** Risks and prognostic factors in trophoblastic neoplasia. *Cancer* 1976;38:1373–1385.
3. **Palmer JR.** Advances in the epidemiology of gestational trophoblastic disease. *J Reprod Med* 1994;39:155–162.
4. **Jeffers MD, O'Dwyer P, Curran B, et al.** Partial hydatidiform mole: a common but underdiagnosed condition. *Int J Gynecol Pathol* 1993;12:315–323.
5. **Parazzini F, La Vecchia C, Mangili G, et al.** Dietary factors and risk of trophoblastic disease. *Am J Obstet Gynecol* 1988;158:93–99.
6. **Berkowitz RS, Cramer DW, Bernstein MR, et al.** Risk factors for complete molar pregnancy from a case-control study. *Am J Obstet Gynecol* 1985;52:1016–1020.

7. **Parazzini F, La Vecchia C, Pampallona S.** Parental age and risk of complete and partial hydatidiform mole. *Br J Obstet Gynaecol* 1986;93:582–585.

8. **Berkowitz RS, Bernstein MR, Harlow BL, et al.** Case-control study of risk factors for partial molar pregnancy. *Am J Obstet Gynecol* 1995;173:788–794.

9. **Kajii T, Ohama K.** Androgenetic origin of hydatidiform mole. *Nature* 1977;268:633–634.

10. **Yamashita K, Wake N, Araki T, et al.** Human lymphocyte antigen expression in hydatidiform mole: androgenesis following fertilization by a haploid sperm. *Am J Obstet Gynecol* 1979;135:597–600.

11. **Pattillo RA, Sasaki S, Katayama KP, et al.** Genesis of 46XY hydatidiform mole. *Am J Obstet Gynecol* 1981;141:104–105.

12. **Azuma C, Saji F, Tokugawa Y, et al.** Application of gene amplification by polymerase chain reaction to genetic analysis of molar mitochondrial DNA: the detection of anuclear empty ovum as the cause of complete mole. *Gynecol Oncol* 1991;40:29–33.

13. **Szulman AE, Surti U.** The syndromes of hydatidiform mole. I. Cytogenetic and morphologic correlations. *Am J Obstet Gynecol* 1978;131:665–671.

14. **Lawler SD, Fisher RA, Dent J.** A prospective genetic study of complete and partial hydatidiform moles. *Am J Obstet Gynecol* 1991;164:1270–1277.

15. **Lage JM, Mark SD, Roberts DJ, et al.** A flow cytometric study of 137 fresh hydropic placentas: correlation between types of hydatidiform moles and nuclear DNA ploidy. *Obstet Gynecol* 1992;79: 403–410.

16. **Soto-Wright V, Bernstein MR, Goldstein DP, et al.** The changing clinical presentation of complete molar pregnancy. *Obstet Gynecol* 1995;86:775–779.

17. **Goldstein DP, Berkowitz RS.** Current management of complete and partial molar pregnancy. *J Reprod Med* 1994;39:139–146.

18. **Amir SM, Osathanondh R, Berkowitz RS, et al.** Human chorionic gonadotropin and thyroid function in patients with hydatidiform mole. *Am J Obstet Gynecol* 1984;150:723–728.

19. **Berkowitz RS, Goldstein DP.** Presentation and management of molar pregnancy. In: **Hancock BW, Newlands ES, Berkowitz RS,** eds. *Gestational trophoblastic disease.* London: Chapman and Hall, 1997: 127–142.

20. **Osathanondh R, Berkowitz RS, de Cholnoky C, et al.** Hormonal measurements in patients with theca lutein cysts and gestational trophoblastic disease. *J Reprod Med* 1986;31:179–183.

21. **Szulman AE, Surti U.** The clinicopathologic profile of the partial hydatidiform mole. *Obstet Gynecol* 1982;59:597–602.

22. **Berkowitz RS, Goldstein DP, Bernstein MR.** Natural history of partial molar pregnancy. *Obstet Gynecol* 1985;66:677–681.

23. **Tow WSH.** The influence of the primary treatment of the hydatidiform mole on its subsequent course. *J Obstet Gynaecol Br Commonw* 1966;73:545–552.

24. **Tsukamoto N, Iwasaka T, Kashimura Y, et al.** Gestational trophoblastic disease in women aged 50 or more. *Gynecol Oncol* 1985;20:53–61.

25. **Berkowitz RS, Goldstein DP.** Chorionic tumors. *N Engl J Med* 1996;335:1740–1748.

26. **Rice LW, Berkowitz RS, Lage JM, et al.** Persistent gestational trophoblastic tumor after partial hydatidiform mole. *Gynecol Oncol* 1990;36:358–362.

27. **Lage JM, Berkowitz RS, Rice LW, et al.** Flow cytometric analysis of DNA content in partial hydatidiform moles with persistent gestational trophoblastic tumor. *Obstet Gynecol* 1991;77:111–115.

28. **Fine C, Bundy AL, Berkowitz RS, et al.** Sonographic diagnosis of partial hydatidiform mole. *Obstet Gynecol* 1989;73:414–418.

29. **Goldstein DP, Berkowitz RS.** Prophylactic chemotherapy of complete molar pregnancy. *Semin Oncol* 1995;22:157–160.

30. **Kim DS, Moon H, Kim KT, et al.** Effects of prophylactic chemotherapy for persistent trophoblastic disease in patients with complete hydatidiform mole. *Obstet Gynecol* 1986;67:690–694.

31. **Genest DR, LaBorde O, Berkowitz RS, et al.** A clinicopathologic study of 153 cases of complete hydatidiform mole (1980–1990): histologic grade lacks prognostic significance. *Obstet Gynecol* 1991;78: 402–409.

32. **Stone M, Dent J, Kardana A, et al.** Relationship of oral contraception to development of trophoblastic tumour after evacuation of a hydatidiform mole. *Br J Obstet Gynaecol* 1976;83:913–916.

33. **Berkowitz RS, Goldstein DP, Marean AR, et al.** Oral contraceptives and postmolar trophoblastic disease. *Obstet Gynecol* 1981;58:474–477.

34. **Curry SL, Schlaerth JB, Kohorn EI, et al.** Hormonal contraception and trophoblastic sequelae after hydatidiform mole (a Gynecologic Oncology Group study). *Am J Obstet Gynecol* 1989;160:805–809.

35. **Finkler NJ, Berkowitz RS, Driscoll SG, et al.** Clinical experience with placental site trophoblastic tumors at the New England Trophoblastic Disease Center. *Obstet Gynecol* 1988;71:854–857.

36. **Kelly MP, Rustin GJ, Ivory C, et al.** Respiratory failure due to choriocarcinoma: a study of 103 dyspneic patients. *Gynecol Oncol* 1990;38:149–154.

37. **Bakri YN, Berkowitz RS, Khan J, et al.** Pulmonary metastases of gestational trophoblastic tumor—risk factors for early respiratory failure. *J Reprod Med* 1994;39:175–178.

38. **Goldstein DP, Vzanten-Przybysz I, Bernstein MR, et al.** Revised FIGO staging system for gestational trophoblastic tumors: recommendations regarding therapy. *J Reprod Med* 1998;43:37–43.

39. **Athanassiou A, Begent RHJ, Newlands ES, et al.** Central nervous system metastases of choriocarcinoma: 23 years' experience at Charing Cross Hospital. *Cancer* 1983;52:1728–1735.

40. **Bagshawe KD, Harland S.** Immunodiagnosis and monitoring of gonadotropin-producing metastases in the central nervous system. *Cancer* 1976;38:112–118.

41. **Bakri Y, Al-Hawashim N, Berkowitz RS.** Cerebrospinal fluid/serum β-subunit human gonadotropin ratio in patients with brain metastases of gestational trophoblastic tumor. *J Reprod Med* 2000;45:94–96.

42. **Berkowitz RS, Birnholz J, Goldstein DP, et al.** Pelvic ultrasonography and the management of gestational trophoblastic disease. *Gynecol Oncol* 1983;15:403–412.

43. **Newland ES, Bower M, Fisher RA, et al.** Management of placental site trophoblastic tumors. *J Reprod Med* 1998;43:53–59.

44. **Rustin GJ, Newlands ES, Begent RHJ, et al.** Weekly alternating etoposide, methotrexate, actinomycin D/ vincristine and cyclophosphamide chemotherapy for the treatment of CNS metastases of choriocarcinoma. *J Clin Oncol* 1989;7:900–903.

45. **Weed JC Jr, Hammond CB.** Cerebral metastatic choriocarcinoma: intensive therapy and prognosis. *Obstet Gynecol* 1980;55:89–94.

46. **Homesley HD.** Single-agent therapy for nonmetastatic and low-risk gestational trophoblastic disease. *J Reprod Med* 1998;43:69–74.

47. **Bagshawe KD, Wilde CE.** Infusion therapy for pelvic trophoblastic tumors. *J Obstet Gynaecol Br Commonw* 1964;71:565–570.

48. **Berkowitz RS, Goldstein DP, Bernstein MR.** Ten years' experience with methotrexate and folinic acid as primary therapy for gestational trophoblastic disease. *Gynecol Oncol* 1986;23:111–118.

49. **Curry SL, Blessing JA, DiSaia PJ, et al.** A prospective randomized comparison of methotrexate, dactinomycin and chlorambucil versus methotrexate, dactinomycin, cyclophosphamide, doxorubicin, melphalan, hydroxyurea and vincristine in "poor prognosis" metastatic gestational trophoblastic disease: a Gynecologic Oncology Group study. *Obstet Gynecol* 1989;73:357–362.

50. **Gordon AN, Gershenson DM, Copeland LJ, et al.** High-risk metastatic gestational trophoblastic disease: further stratification into clinical entities. *Gynecol Oncol* 1989;34:54–56.

51. **DuBeshter B, Berkowitz RS, Goldstein DP, et al.** Metastatic gestational trophoblastic disease: experience at the New England Trophoblastic Disease Center, 1965–1985. *Obstet Gynecol* 1987;69:390–395.

52. **Wong LC, Choo YC, Ma HK.** Primary oral etoposide therapy in gestational trophoblastic disease: an update. *Cancer* 1986;58:14–17.

53. **Bagshawe KD.** Treatment of high-risk choriocarcinoma. *J Reprod Med* 1984;29:813–820.

54. **Bolis G, Bonazzi C, Landoni F, et al.** EMA-CO regimen in high-risk gestational trophoblastic tumor (GTT). *Gynecol Oncol* 1988;31:439–444.

55. **Quinn M, Murray J, Friedlander M, et al.** EMACO in high risk gestational trophoblastic disease—the Australian experience. *Aust N Z J Obstet Gynaecol* 1994;34:90–92.

56. **Bower M, Newlands ES, Holden L, et al.** EMA-CO for high-risk gestational trophoblastic tumors: results from a cohort of 272 patients. *J Clin Oncol* 1997;15:2636–2643.

57. **Berkowitz RS, Tuncer ZS, Bernstein MR, et al.** Management of gestational trophoblastic diseases: subsequent pregnancy experience. *Semin Oncol* 2000;27:678–685.

58. **Schorge JO, Goldstein DP, Bernstein MR, et al.** Recent advances in gestational trophoblastic disease. *J Reprod Med* 2000;45:692–700.

59. **Tuncer ZS, Bernstein MR, Wang J, et al.** Repetitive hydatidiform mole with different male partners. *Gynecol Oncol* 1999;75:224–226.

35 Breast Cancer

Dean T. Nora
Armando E. Giuliano

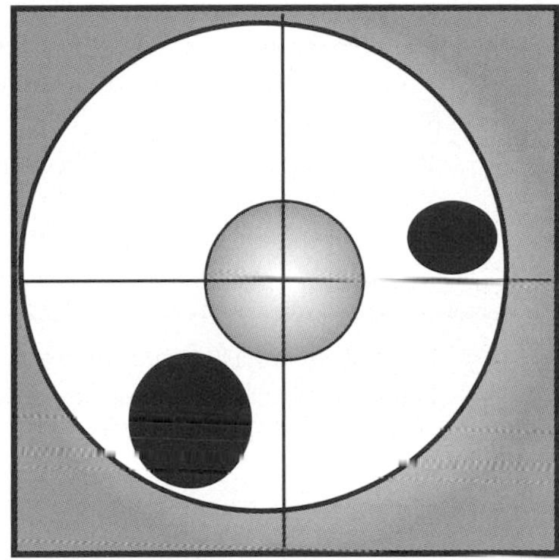

Breast cancer accounts for approximately one-third of all cancers in women and is second only to lung cancer as the leading cause of cancer deaths in women. Breast cancer, however, has the highest incidence rate of all cancers. According to estimates from the American Cancer Society, in the United States during 2002 there will be 203,500 new cases of breast cancer and 39,600 deaths from this disease in women (1). During the past 50 years, the incidence of breast cancer in this country has increased significantly; nearly one in every eight women in the United States will develop breast cancer. Fortunately, the mortality rate actually declined between 1993 and 1997, implying an increased success in earlier diagnosis and treatment.

Predisposing Factors

Less than 1% of all breast cancers occur in women less than 25 years of age. After 30 years of age, however, there is a sharp increase in the incidence of breast cancer. Except for a short plateau between the ages of 45 and 50 years, the incidence increases steadily with age (2).

Family History

Only 20% of women who develop breast cancer have a family history of the disease. **Any family history of breast cancer increases the overall relative risk** (3). However, the risk is not increased significantly in women whose mothers or sisters had breast cancer after menopause, whereas women whose mothers or sisters had bilateral breast cancer premenopausally have at least a 40% to 50% lifetime risk. If the patient's mother or sister had unilateral breast cancer premenopausally, her lifetime risk of developing breast cancer is approximately 30%. The increased incidence in this group is probably due to inherited oncogenes.

Approximately 5% to 10% of all breast cancers have an inherited basis. All inherited genes are autosomal dominant but have variable penetrance. Males can carry the gene 50% of the time. Carriers of these germline mutations have up to a 4%-per-year risk of developing breast cancer and a lifetime risk of up to 85% (4). The most common gene mutations are the *BRCA1* (chromosome 17q21) and *BRCA2* (chromosome 13q12–13) gene deletions. These mutations are rare in the general public (0.1%) but are more commonly identified in Jews of Ashkenazi descent (1% to 2%) (5). Testing should be performed only if there is a high likelihood that results will be positive, can be interpreted accurately, and will be used to influence decisions regarding medical management of the patient and family.

Diet, Obesity, and Alcohol

Marked geographic differences in the incidence of breast cancer may be related to diet, in particular with regard to variations in fat intake (6). It is not clear, however, that a high-fat diet is a specific risk factor, because most studies have not clearly separated obesity from other known risk factors (7). Alcohol consumption may increase the risk of breast cancer, but again this relationship is not clear (8).

Reproductive and Hormonal Factors

The risk of breast cancer increases with the length of a woman's reproductive phase (9). Thus, the median age at menarche is lower for women who develop breast cancer, and either natural or artificial early menopause protects against the development of breast cancer (10). Artificial menopause as a result of oophorectomy lowers the risk of breast cancer farther than does early natural menopause. There is no clear association between the risk of breast cancer and menstrual irregularity and duration of menses. There is some evidence that these reproductive factors, although decreasing the risk of developing breast cancer, may adversely affect a patient's prognosis (11).

Lactation does not affect the incidence of breast cancer, but women who have never been pregnant have a higher risk of breast cancer than those who are multiparous. Also, women who bear their first child later in life have a higher incidence of breast cancer than do younger primigravida females (12).

A well-controlled study from the Centers for Disease Control and Prevention showed that oral contraceptive use does not increase the risk of breast cancer, regardless of duration of use, family history, or coexistence of benign breast disease (13). However, a recent pooled analysis from 54 epidemiologic studies showed current users of oral contraceptives had a small, but real, increased risk when compared with nonusers. Ten years after discontinuation, the risk of past users declined to that of the normal population (14).

Although short-term estrogen treatment for menopausal symptoms probably does not increase the risk of breast cancer, prolonged use (longer than 10 years) or higher dosages of estrogen may increase the risk. Current data suggest that postmenopausal estrogen administration is a risk factor (15). The current consensus is that, postmenopausally, estrogen should be given in a relatively low dose either cyclically or in combination with progestins when the uterus is present. Although estrogens may slightly increase the incidence of breast cancer, this risk should be weighed against the possible benefits in preventing osteoporosis and heart disease.

History of Cancer

Women with a history of breast cancer have an approximately 50% risk of developing microscopic breast cancer and about a 20% risk of developing clinically apparent cancer in the contralateral breast, which occurs at a rate of 1% to 2% per year (16). Lobular carcinoma has a higher incidence of bilaterality than does ductal carcinoma. A history of endometrial carcinoma, ovarian carcinoma, or colon cancer has also been associated with an increased risk of breast cancer.

Diagnosis

Breast cancer most commonly arises in the upper outer quadrant, where there is more breast tissue. Breast masses are most often discovered by the patient and less frequently by the physician during routine breast examination. The increasing use of screening mammography has expanded the ability to detect nonpalpable abnormalities. Rarely metastatic breast cancer may be found as an axillary mass without obvious malignancy.

Mammography and physical examination, the standard screening modalities, are complementary. In the past, most cases of breast cancer were discovered as a palpable mass. However, **10% to 50% of cancers detected mammographically are not palpable. Conversely, physical examination detects 10% to 20% of cancers not seen on mammography** (17). The purpose of screening is to detect cancers when they are small (<1 cm) and have the highest potential for surgical cure. Most trials have shown a 20% to 30% reduction in breast cancer mortality for women age 50 and older who undergo annual screening mammography. Data for screening of women under 40 have been more controversial. However, recent data from the Gothenburg screening trial showed a 45% reduction in mortality for women screened between the ages 40 and 49 (18). Because of these findings, it is recommended that all women undergo screening mammography starting at age 40, along with clinical breast examination and breast self-examination. No other tests, such as ultrasonography, magnetic resonance imaging (MRI), computed tomography (CT) scans, sestamibi scans, positron emission tomography (PET) scans, or serum blood markers, are effective screening modalities, and these tests should be used only when indicated. Screening guidelines recommended by the American College of Radiology and the American Cancer Society are presented in Table 35.1.

Masses are easier to palpate in older women with fatty breasts than in younger women with dense, often nodular breasts. An area of thickening amid normal nodularity may be the only clue to an underlying malignancy. Skin dimpling, nipple retraction, or skin erosion is usually obvious, but these are later-stage disease signs. Algorithms for the evaluation of breast masses in premenopausal and postmenopausal women are presented in Chapter 18.

A dominant breast mass must be considered a possible carcinoma, and biopsy is essential for diagnosis. **About 30% to 40% of lesions believed clinically to be malignant will be benign on histologic examination** (19). Conversely, 20% to 25% of clinically benign-appearing lesions will be proven malignant by biopsy (20).

Table 35.1. Official Screening Recommendations

Bilateral mammograms:
- By age 40: baseline mammogram
- Age 40–49: every 1–2 years
- Age >50: every year
- If family history of breast cancer, may consider baseline mammogram age 35, or 10 years younger than earliest family member was diagnosed, whichever is younger.

Self-examination:
- Premenopausal: 5–7 days after menstrual period monthly
- Postmenopausal: same day every month

Clinical breast examination:
- Age 20–40: exam by physician every 3 years
- Age ≥ 40: exam by physician every 2–3 years
- (May do annually if there is a positive family history)

Tumor markers (CA27–29, CA15–3): not recommended as screening tests

From American Cancer Society, Workshop on Guidelines for Breast Cancer Detection; March 7–9, 1997; Chicago, 11. National Cancer Institute Advisory Board issues on mammography screening recommendations; Bethesda, MD NIH; March 27, 1997; **Dodd GD.** Screening for breast cancer: practical considerations. *J Surg Oncol* 1995;60:1–3, with permission.

Biopsy Techniques

For patients with obvious malignancy, it may be reasonable to obtain a biopsy specimen and a frozen section immediately before mastectomy or other definitive treatment. It is preferable for the patient to be involved in the planning of her therapy. Initial biopsy is better followed by subsequent definitive treatment in the two-step approach. This approach allows the physician to discuss alternative forms of therapy with the patient who has a malignancy, and it gives the patient an opportunity to obtain a second opinion before undergoing definitive treatment.

Fine-needle Aspiration Cytology

Fine-needle aspiration (FNA) cytology is performed with a 20- or 22-gauge needle. The technique has a high level of diagnostic accuracy, with a 10% to 15% false-negative rate and rare, but persistent, false-positive results (21). If a mass appears to be malignant on physical examination or mammography or both, FNA cytology results can be useful in discussing alternatives with the patient. Negative FNA cytologic results do not exclude malignancy and usually are followed by excisional biopsy or careful observation. In young women, it is prudent to follow a benign-appearing mass for one or two menstrual cycles. Furthermore, confirmation of a clinically apparent fibroadenoma with FNA can serve as the basis for observational follow-up without excision.

Open Biopsy

Open biopsy may be performed if FNA cytology has not been performed or if the results are negative or equivocal. **An unequivocal histologic diagnosis of cancer should be obtained before treatment of breast cancer is undertaken.** Cytologic diagnosis may be relied on if the mass clinically or mammographically appears to be malignant. In equivocal cases, a partial mastectomy can be performed, and a frozen section can be obtained to confirm the diagnosis of cancer before the axillary dissection is started. An alternative to open biopsy is removal of a core of tissue through a Vim-Silverman–type cutting needle. If a definitive diagnosis is not obtained, these procedures must also be followed by open biopsy.

Open biopsy can usually be performed in an outpatient setting with the patient under light sedation, in conjunction with the use of local anesthesia, in the following manner:

1. The patient is positioned and the location of the mass confirmed.
2. Local anesthesia is used to infiltrate the skin and subcutaneous tissue surrounding the palpable mass.
3. An incision is made directly over the mass. Planning should include an ellipse of skin to be either excised with the mastectomy or placed cosmetically so that partial mastectomy can be performed through the same incision. Paraareolar incisions are appropriate only for lesions in proximity to the nipple–areolar complex.
4. After the skin and underlying tissue are incised, the mass is gently grasped with Allis forceps or with a stay suture and moved into the operative field.
5. The mass should be excised completely whenever possible. Large masses that are difficult to excise totally with local anesthesia can be incised. When an incisional biopsy is used, a frozen section should be obtained to confirm that tissue is malignant. Such masses, however, are preferably sampled with FNA or core biopsy.
6. Once the mass is removed, adequate hemostasis is achieved and the incision is closed. A cosmetically superior result will be achieved if the breast parenchyma is not reapproximated deeply. The most superficial subcutaneous fat can be

reapproximated with fine absorbable sutures. The skin should be closed with a subcuticular suture and adhesive strips to achieve the most cosmetically pleasing result. Usually a drain is not necessary.

Mammographic Localization Biopsy

Biopsy of nonpalpable lesions is a potentially difficult procedure that requires close cooperation between the surgeon and the mammographer. The mammographer places a needle or specialized wire into the breast parenchyma at or near the site of the suspected abnormality. Many mammographers will also inject a biologic dye to assist localization further. The surgeon then reviews the films with the mammographer and localizes the abnormality with respect to the tip of the wire or needle. An incision is made directly over this area, and a small portion of the breast that is suspected of containing the abnormality is excised. A mammogram of the surgical specimen is obtained to ensure that the abnormality has been excised. Often, the mammographer can place a needle in the specimen at the site of the abnormality to facilitate histologic evaluation and ensure that the pathologist examines the site of the abnormality.

Stereotactic Core Biopsy

Mammographic units with computerized stereotactic modifications can be used to localize abnormalities and perform needle biopsy without surgery. Under mammographic guidance, a biopsy needle is inserted into the lesion and a core of tissue is removed for histologic examination. Ultrasonography may also be used to obtain a core biopsy of a nonpalpable lesion. Because it is less invasive and less expensive than mammographic localization biopsy, core biopsy is preferred for accessible lesions.

Pathology and Natural History

Breast cancer may arise in the intermediate-sized ducts or terminal ducts and lobules. In most cases, the diagnosis of lobular and intraductal carcinoma is based more on histologic appearance than site of origin. The cancer may be either invasive (infiltrating ductal carcinoma, infiltrating lobular carcinoma) or *in situ* (ductal carcinoma *in situ* or lobular carcinoma *in situ*). Morphologic subtypes of infiltrating ductal carcinoma can be described as scirrhous, tubular, medullary, and mucinous.

Infiltrating ductal carcinoma of unspecified type accounts for 60% to 70% of the breast cancers in the United States (22). Mammographically, it is characterized by a stellate density or by microcalcifications. Macroscopically, there are gritty, chalky streaks within the tumor that most likely represent a desmoplastic response; microscopically, there is invasion of the surrounding stroma and fat. There is often a fibrotic response surrounding the invasive carcinoma.

Other types of infiltrating ductal carcinoma are far less common. Medullary carcinoma, which accounts for approximately 5% to 8% of breast carcinomas, arises from larger ducts within the breast and has a dense lymphocytic infiltrate. The tumor appears to be a slow-growing, less aggressive malignancy than the infiltrating ductal carcinoma.

Mucinous (colloid) carcinoma accounts for 5% of all breast cancers. Grossly, the tumor may have areas that appear mucinous or gelatinous. Infiltrating comedo carcinoma accounts for 1% of breast malignancies. It is an invasive cancer characterized by foci of necrosis that exude a comedonecrosis-like substance when biopsied. Usually, comedocarcinomas are *in situ* malignancies. Papillary carcinoma is predominantly a noninvasive ductal carcinoma; when invasive components are present, it should be specified as invasive papillary carcinoma. Tubular carcinoma is a well-differentiated breast cancer that accounts for 1% of all breast malignancies. Tubular carcinomas tend to have a better prognosis than infiltrating ductal carcinomas and rarely metastasize to axillary lymph nodes. Adenoid cystic carcinomas are extremely rare and are similar histologically to those seen in the salivary glands. They tend to be well differentiated and slow to metastasize.

Growth Patterns

The growth potential of breast cancer and the patient's resistance to malignancy vary widely with the individual and the stage of disease. The doubling time of breast cancer can range from several weeks for rapidly growing tumors to months or years for slowly growing ones. If the doubling time of a breast tumor was constant and a tumor originated from one cell, a doubling time of 100 days would result in a 1-cm tumor in about 8 years (Fig. 35.1) (23). During the preclinical phase, tumor cells may be circulating throughout the body.

Because of the long preclinical tumor growth phase and the tendency of infiltrating lesions to metastasize early, many clinicians view breast cancer as a systemic disease at the time of diagnosis. Although cancer cells may be released from the tumor prior to diagnosis,

Figure 35.1 Growth rate of breast cancer indicating long preclinical phase. (From **Gullino PM.** Natural history of breast cancer: progression from hyperplasia to neoplasia as predicted by angiogenesis. *Cancer* 1977;39:2697–2703, with permission.)

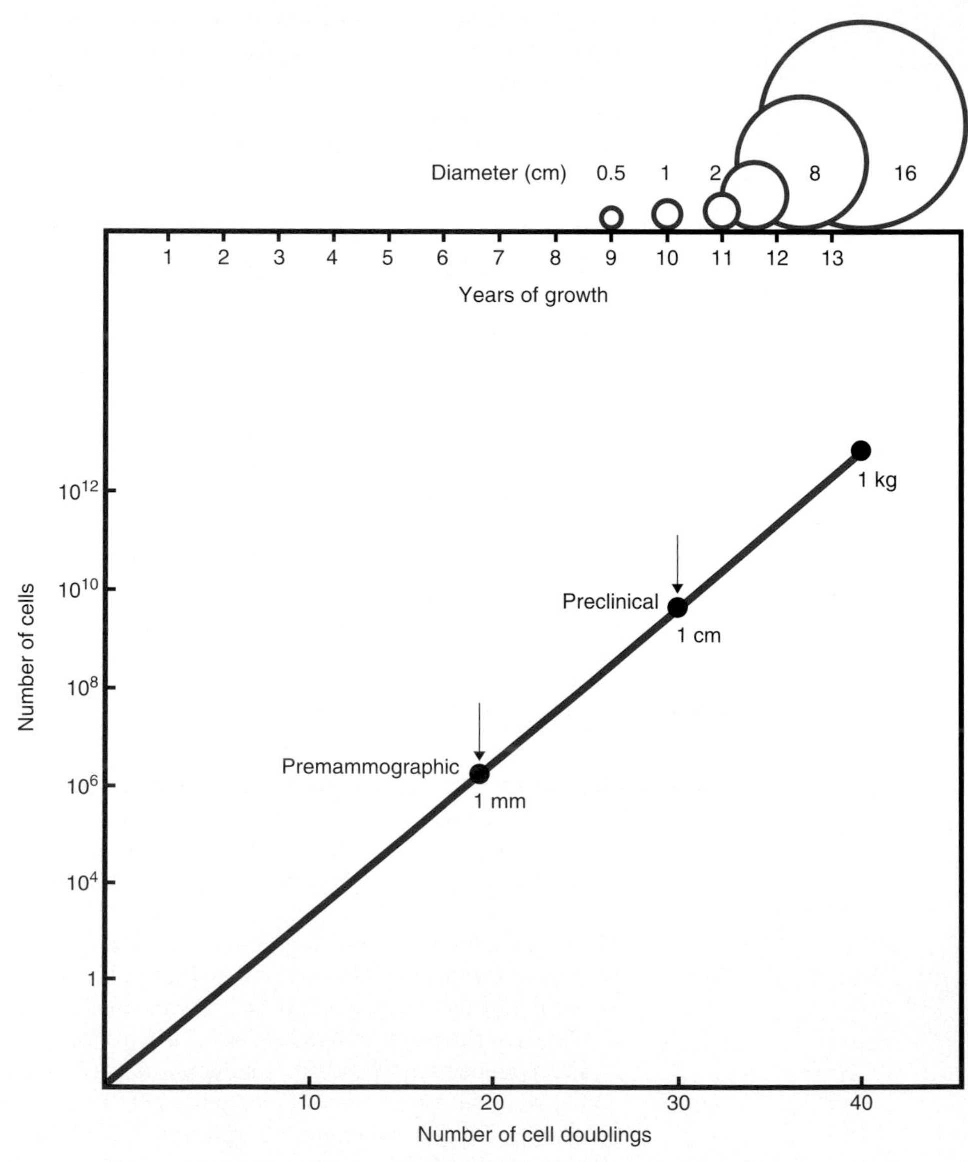

variations in the tumor's ability to grow in other organs and the host's response to the tumor may inhibit dissemination of the disease. Many women with breast cancer can be treated successfully with surgery alone, and some women have been cured even in the presence of palpable axillary disease. Thus, a pessimistic attitude that breast cancer is systemic and incurable at the time of diagnosis is unwarranted. A more realistic approach may be to view breast cancer as a two-component disease: one is the primary tumor in the breast, with all the inherent problems of local and regional extension and primary tumor control, and the other consists of the systemic metastases with their life-threatening consequences.

Although the natural history of breast cancer can involve metastases to any organ, involvement of bone, lungs, or liver occurs in 85% of women with metastatic breast cancer (24–26). If any of these sites is involved, metastases to other organs are highly likely. The use of systemic chemotherapy affects the sites of metastases, and currently metastases are occurring in more unusual sites with greater frequency.

Staging

After the diagnosis of breast cancer has been established, either cytologically or histologically, the clinical stage of disease should be determined. The Columbia Clinical Staging System was widely used for many years (27) but has been replaced by the tumor–nodes–metastases (TNM) system recommended by the International Union Against Cancer (UICC) and the American Joint Committee on Cancer (28). This system allows both preoperative clinical staging and postoperative pathologic staging (Tables 35.2 and 35.3).

Preoperative Evaluation

The extent of preoperative workup varies with the initial stage of the disease (29). For most patients with small tumors, no palpable lymph nodes (TNM stage I), and no symptoms of metastasis, the preoperative evaluation should consist of bilateral mammography, chest radiograph, complete blood count, and screening blood chemistry tests. Bone, CT, and MRI scanning are not necessary unless symptoms or abnormal blood chemistry suggest bone or liver metastasis. For patients with clinical stage II disease, a bone scan should be obtained, but a CT scan of the liver is not necessary unless symptoms or liver function tests suggest liver metastasis. Patients with clinical stage III or IV disease should undergo both bone and liver scanning. A bone marrow biopsy should be performed if there is obvious bone marrow dysfunction but metastases are not evident on a bone scan.

Treatment

Mastectomy

Traditionally, treatment of breast cancer has been surgical, but the type of operation employed has remained a controversial and highly emotional issue. During the nineteenth century, surgical treatment of breast cancer was haphazard, varying from local excision alone to total mastectomy. Halsted devised the radical mastectomy in an attempt to treat carcinoma of the breast as a local infiltrative process (30). Thus, radical mastectomy removes the entire breast, the underlying pectoral muscles, and the contiguous axillary lymph nodes in continuity (31) (Fig. 35.2A). Haagensen and Bodian reported a 51-year experience with radical mastectomy. Their data, which included 1,036 patients with a follow-up of 47 years, remain unequalled in evaluating any single method of treating breast cancer (32).

During the twentieth century, extensions and modifications of the radical mastectomy procedure were devised that involved removal of more local and regional tissue. Supraclavicular

Table 35.2. Tumor–Nodes–Metastasis (TNM) System for Staging of Breast Cancer

Primary tumor (T)	
TX	Primary tumor cannot be assessed
T_0	No evidence of primary tumor
Tis	Carcinoma *in situ:* intraductal carcinoma, lobular carcinoma *in situ,* or Paget's disease of the nipple with no tumor
T_1	Tumor 2 cm or less in greatest dimension
T_{1A}	0.5 cm or less in greatest dimension
T_{1B}	More than 0.5 cm but not more than 1 cm in greatest dimension
T_{1C}	More than 1 cm but not more than 2 cm in greatest dimension
T_2	Tumor more than 2 cm but not more than 5 cm in greatest dimension
T_3	Tumor more than 5 cm in greatest dimension
T_4	Tumor of any size with direct extension to chest wall or skin
T_{4A}	Extension to chest wall
T_{4B}	Edema (including *peau d'orange*) or ulceration of the skin of breast or satellite skin nodules confined to same breast
T_{4C}	Both T_{4A} and T_{4B}
T_{4D}	Inflammatory carcinoma
Lymph node (N)	
NX	Regional lymph nodes cannot be assessed (e.g., previously removed)
N_0	No regional lymph node metastasis
N_1	Metastasis to movable ipsilateral axillary lymph node(s)
N_2	Metastasis to ipsilateral axillary lymph node(s) fixed to one another or to other structures
N_3	Metastasis to ipsilateral internal mammary lymph node(s)
Pathologic classification (pN)	
pNX	Regional lymph nodes cannot be assessed (e.g., previously removed or removed but not for pathologic study)
pN_0	No regional lymph node metastasis
pN_1	Metastasis to movable ipsilateral axillary lymph node(s)
pN_{1A}	Only micrometastasis (none larger than 0.2 cm)
pN_{1B}	Metastasis to lymph nodes, any larger than 0.2 cm
pN_{1bi}	Metastasis in one to three lymph nodes, any more than 0.2 cm and all less than 2 cm in greatest dimension
pN_{1bii}	Metastasis to four or more lymph nodes, any more than 0.2 cm and all less than 2 cm in greatest dimension
pN_{1biii}	Extension of tumor beyond the capsule of a lymph node metastasis less than 2 cm in greatest dimension
pN_{1biv}	Metastasis to a lymph node 2 cm or more in greatest dimension
pN_2	Metastasis to ipsilateral axillary lymph nodes that are fixed to one another or to other structures
pN_3	Metastasis to ipsilateral internal mammary lymph node(s)
Distant metastasis (M)	
MX	Presence of distant metastasis cannot be assessed
M_0	No distant metastasis
M_1	Distant metastasis (includes metastasis to ipsilateral supraclavicular lymph node[s]).

From **Fleming ID, Cooper JS, Henson DE, et al.,** eds. *AJCC cancer staging manual,* 5th ed. Philadelphia: JB Lippincott, 1997:171–180, with permission.

node dissections were added to the radical mastectomy (33). In addition, supraclavicular, mediastinal, and internal mammary lymph node dissections were performed (34).

Urban added *en bloc* internal mammary lymph node dissection to the standard radical mastectomy (35). This technique became popular and is the operation commonly referred to as the *extended radical mastectomy.* The extended radical mastectomy did not enhance overall survival rates (36). About 5% to 10% of patients in whom axillary lymph nodes are not involved will have involvement of internal mammary nodes. Locally destructive surgery is not justified, however, based on current understanding of the biologic behavior of breast cancer.

Table 35.3. Staging of Breast Carcinoma

	TNM Classification[a]		
	Tumor	*Node*	*Metastasis*
Stage 0	Tis	N_0	M_0
Stage I	T_1	N_0	M_0
Stage IIa	T_0	$N_1{}^b$	M_0
	T_1	$N_1{}^a$	M_0
	T_2	N_0	M_0
Stage IIb	T_2	N_1	M_0
	T_3	N_0	M_0
Stage IIIa	T_0	N_2	M_0
	T_1	N_2	M_0
	T_2	N_2	M_0
	T_3	N_1	M_0
	T_3	N_2	M_0
Stage IIIb	T_4	Any N	M_0
	Any T	N_3	M_0
Stage IV	AnyT	Any N	M_1

[a]See Table 35.2.
[b]Note: The prognosis of patients with N1A is similar to that of patients with pN_0.
From **Fleming ID, Cooper JS, Henson DE, et al.**, eds. *American Joint Committee on Cancer: manual for staging of cancer*, 5th ed. Philadelphia: JB Lippincott, 1997;171–180, with permission.

Modified Radical Mastectomy

Modified radical mastectomy preserves the pectoralis major muscle (37,38) (Fig. 35.2B). The breast is removed in a manner similar to that of the radical mastectomy; however, removal of the skin and the axillary lymph node dissection are not as extensive, and there is no need for skin grafting. There is no difference in survival rates between radical mastectomy and modified radical mastectomy, but the latter procedure has a better functional and cosmetic result (39). Modified radical mastectomy has replaced radical mastectomy and remains the procedure most often performed for breast cancer despite the proven equivalence of breast conservation therapy.

Total Mastectomy

Total mastectomy is the removal of the entire breast, nipple, and areolar complex without the underlying muscles or axillary lymph nodes. Axillary nodes are not removed intentionally. However, low-lying lymph nodes in the upper outer portion of the breast and low axilla usually are included in the specimen. Total mastectomy has local control rates comparable with those of radical or modified radical mastectomy but has a higher risk of axillary recurrence. Because the axillary lymph nodes are not examined microscopically, this operation generally is less desirable than modified radical mastectomy. Regional recurrence will occur in at least 15% to 20% of patients treated with total mastectomy alone.

Adjuvant Radiation Therapy

McWhirther developed the combination of total mastectomy with radiation therapy (40). Many have advocated adjuvant radiation therapy in combination with various operative procedures. Studies claiming improvements in overall survival usually are flawed by the use of historical controls and inaccurate preoperative staging. Earlier trials, both prospective randomized studies and historical control studies, show that adjuvant radiation therapy improves local control but not survival rates (41–44). In contrast, a recent randomized control study demonstrated a 9% absolute increase in 10-year overall survival (45). The researchers concluded that the addition of postoperative radiation to mastectomy and chemotherapy prolongs survival in high-risk premenopausal women with breast cancer.

In a prospective randomized trial performed by the National Surgical Adjuvant Breast Project (NSABP), the roles of postoperative radiation therapy and axillary treatment were examined (46). Patients were randomly assigned to therapy consisting of total mastectomy, radical mastectomy, or total mastectomy with radiation therapy. This trial showed no

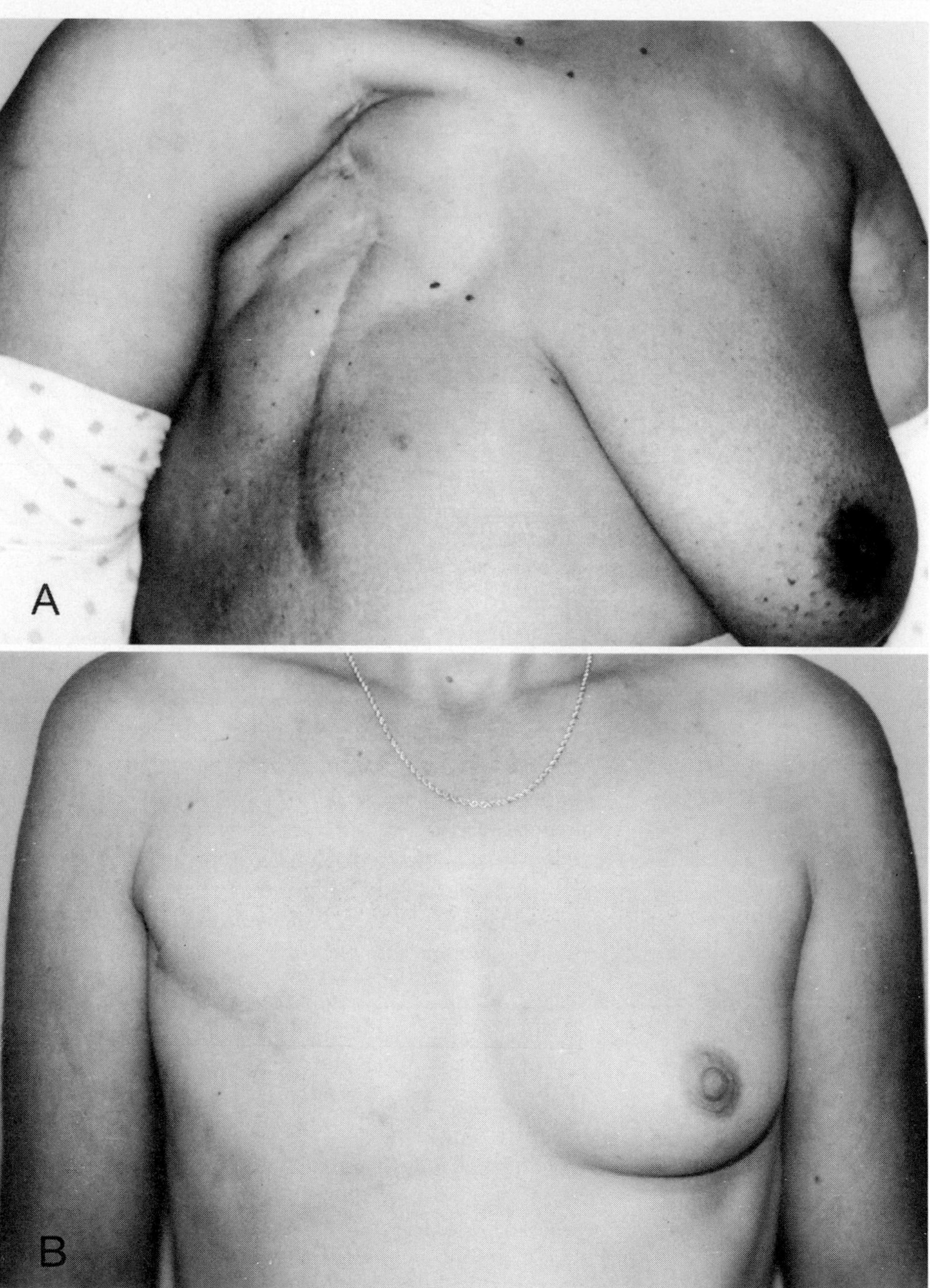

Figure 35.2 Appearance of breast after radical mastectomy (A) versus modified mastectomy (B). (From **Haigh PI, Giuliano AE.** Breast disease. In: **Berek JS, Hacker NF,** eds. *Practical gynecologic oncology,* 3rd ed. Philadelphia: Lippincott Williams & Wilkins, 2000:660, with permission.)

difference in survival rates among the three groups of patients, whereas radiation therapy and axillary treatment improved local and regional control.

Conservative Therapy with or without Radiation Therapy

Radiation therapy alone, without excision of the tumor, is associated with a high local failure rate (47–50). Similarly, local excision without radiation has a high local failure rate. A major prospective randomized trial compared radical surgery with a combination of conservative surgery and modern radiotherapeutic techniques (51,52). Patients were randomly assigned to treatment with either standard Halsted radical mastectomy or a combination of quadrantectomy, axillary lymph node dissection, and postoperative radiation therapy. Only patients in whom tumors were smaller than 2 cm and not centrally located and who had no clinical evidence of axillary lymph node disease (T_1 N_0 M_0) were considered for this trial. All 701 women in the study were comparable in age, tumor size, menopausal status, and histologic involvement of the axillary lymph nodes (52). After more than 15 years of follow-up, there has been no statistically significant difference between the two groups in either local control or overall survival rates.

The NSABP conducted a trial that extended these observations and provided further information (53). Eligible patients could have a primary tumor $\leq$4 cm, with or without palpable axillary lymph nodes, provided that the lymph nodes were not fixed (i.e., stage I or stage II, T_1 or T_2, and N_0 or N_1). Patients were assigned randomly to one of three groups: (a) modified radical mastectomy; (b) segmental mastectomy (lumpectomy) and axillary lymph node dissection; or (c) segmental mastectomy, axillary lymph node dissection, and postoperative radiation therapy. Unlike the quadrantectomy, segmental mastectomy or "lumpectomy" consists of removing only the tumor and a small rim of normal surrounding tissue and is cosmetically superior (Fig. 35.3). Patients were considered ineligible if they were found to have microscopic involvement of the margins. A total of 1,843 women were randomized among the three treatment arms, and the groups were comparable. The lowest local recurrence rate was seen among patients treated with segmental mastectomy and postoperative radiation therapy. Of these patients, 90% were free of local recurrence after 8 years of observation, whereas 39% of the patients undergoing segmental mastectomy without radiation therapy had a local recurrence. Although the addition of radiation therapy clearly improved the local control rate, no significant difference in overall survival rates or disease-free survival could be seen among the three treatment arms; there was a trend, however, in favor of patients who received radiation. **This NSABP study clearly shows that the combination of segmental mastectomy, axillary lymph node dissection, and postoperative radiation therapy was**

Figure 35.3 Appearance of breast after lumpectomy, axillary dissection, and radiation therapy. (From **Haigh PI, Giuliano AE.** Breast disease. In: **Berek JS, Hacker NF,** eds. *Practical gynecologic oncology,* 3rd ed. Philadelphia: Williams & Wilkins, 2000:662, with permission.)

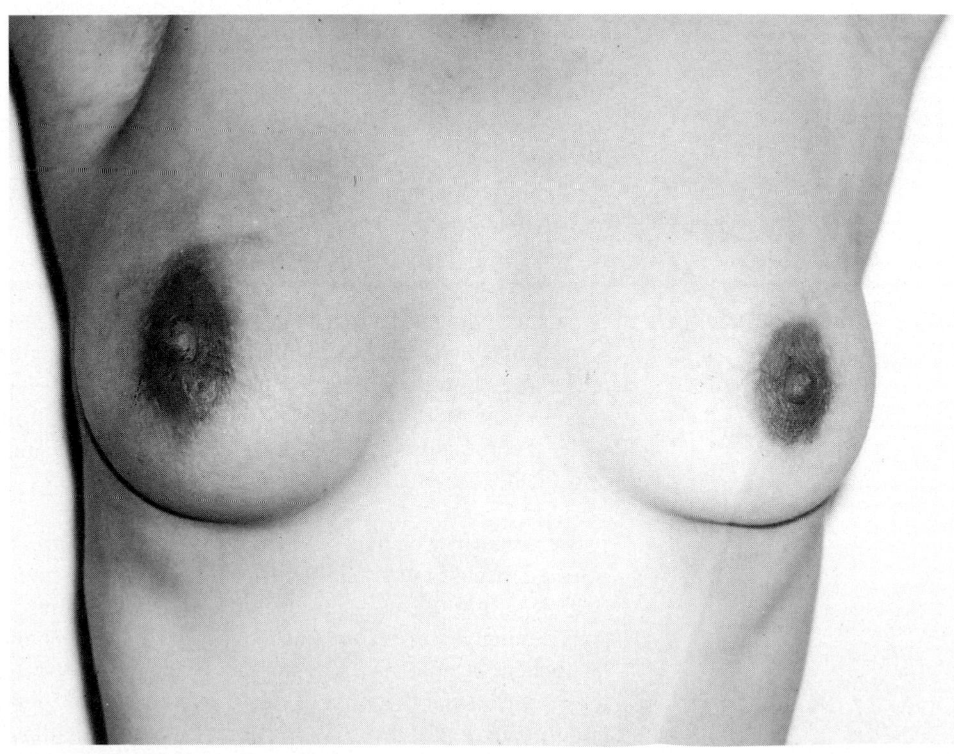

as effective as modified radical mastectomy for the management of patients with stage I and II breast cancer. These findings have since been updated; after 12 years of follow-up, no difference was seen in survival among the three groups (54). The high local recurrence rate without radiation therapy makes limited surgery alone generally unacceptable except in unusual circumstances.

Axillary lymph node status and the number of involved nodes is the most important prognostic indicator for patients with primary breast cancer (55–57). For these reasons, axillary lymphadenectomy is used to detect and quantify the extent of nodal metastasis (58). Axillary lymph node dissection (ALND) is performed routinely on all patients with breast cancer for the purposes of staging and the planning of adjuvant chemotherapy. Axillary dissection is associated with a very low risk of regional recurrence (1% to 3%) but at the cost of significant morbidity (59). The rate of acute complication is 20% to 30%. Similarly, the risk of chronic lymphedema is reportedly as high as 20% to 30% (60). Limiting the dissection to level I nodes or random sampling is associated with unacceptably high false-negative rates (61).

Only one-third of patients with a clinically negative axilla will be found to have nodal metastasis after histopathologic examination of all lymph nodes (62). This means that two-thirds of patients will undergo the morbidity of ALND without proven benefit.

In 1991, intraoperative lymphatic mapping and selective lymph node sampling was introduced in an effort to address these problems (63). The concept behind sentinel lymph node dissection (SLND) is best described by the definition of a sentinel node (SN). The SN is the lymph node that has the greatest potential to harbor metastasis if present. The SLND accurately predicts the status of the entire nodal basin by removing only one or two lymph nodes with minimal morbidity. If the SN is found to be negative, this directed approach can be used to distinguish patients who would not benefit from ALND and its morbidity. **In a study of 107 patients with T1 and T2 breast cancer who underwent SLND followed by ALND, the SLN was successfully identified in 100 patients (93.5%). There were no false-negative results and the sentinel node accurately predicted axillary status in all 100 patients.**

The technique of SLND has been validated by a number of authors using a variety of techniques (64,65). The information obtained from SLND appears to be equivalent to that of ALND in the few small trials conducted to date. Furthermore, a recent prospective study demonstrated that in node-negative patients undergoing SLND only, the recurrence rate in the axilla was zero at a median follow up of 39 months (66). The degree of accuracy in predicting axillary metastasis, combined with a very low morbidity rate, makes SLND an attractive alternative to ALND.

Adjuvant Systemic Therapy

For many patients, local and regional control of breast cancer is achieved readily with surgery and radiation therapy alone. About 90% of patients will never experience a local recurrence; however, patients may still develop metastatic disease. The goal of adjuvant systemic therapy is to eliminate occult metastases during the early postoperative period while theoretically they are most vulnerable to anticancer agents (67). This approach, in turn, reduces the risk of local and distant recurrence.

It is currently well accepted that adjuvant systemic therapy will prolong survival in selected breast cancer patients. However, in patients with favorable tumors and a low risk of recurrence and subsequent death, such as those who have node-negative cancers smaller than 1 cm or node-negative cancers smaller than 2 cm with grade 1 histology, this benefit is small and may not justify the risks of systemic therapy. **Adjuvant systemic therapy reduces the odds of death by about 25% per year in both node-negative and node-positive patients** (68). Because this risk reduction is relatively constant, patients with favorable, node-negative disease have a much smaller absolute benefit as compared with patients who have node-positive disease and a high risk of recurrence. For patients with node-negative disease, the absolute benefit may only be a few percent versus 10% to 20% for those with node-positive disease.

Cytotoxic chemotherapy and hormonal therapy have inherent risks that must be considered when choosing which patients should receive them. Not only are there known acute side effects with current standard regimens, but also there is growing evidence that patients who undergo chemotherapy more frequently report chronic neurocognitive deficits (69). The impact of these deficits remains undefined. Similarly, systemic therapy with tamoxifen has an appreciable long-term morbidity. Adverse effects include an increased incidence of uterine cancer, vaginal dryness, and hot flashes. Choosing the patients who should receive adjuvant therapy can be a difficult decision. This decision entails analyzing a variety of prognostic and predictive factors, identifying patients at risk for recurrence, and quantifying that risk. **In general, adjuvant chemotherapy is currently recommended for women with a greater than 10% chance of relapse within 10 years.** In practice, systemic adjuvant therapy is offered to many patients with early-stage breast cancer. The choice of therapy generally depends on an evaluation of specific risk factors.

Factors that determine the patient's risk of recurrence are nodal involvement, tumor size, estrogen and progesterone receptor status, nuclear grade, histologic type, proliferative rate, and a variety of biologic markers. These prognostic factors and their effects on recurrence are summarized in Table 35.4. The assumption is made that patients with high-risk prognostic factors are more likely to benefit from adjuvant cytotoxic or hormonal therapy; thus, these patients are generally offered such treatment.

It is generally accepted that patients with lymph node metastasis have a higher risk of recurrence than patients with node-negative disease. The 10-year survival rate for women with palpable metastatic axillary lymph nodes who receive no systemic therapy is only about 50% to 60%. Even when they are not clinically palpable, lymph node metastases portend an unfavorable course. The number of lymph nodes involved and the presence of extracapsular invasion are important indicators of poor prognosis.

Another important prognostic indicator of relapse is tumor size. In an evaluation of 767 patients with node-negative disease who underwent radical or modified radical mastectomy without adjuvant chemotherapy, the relapse rate in patients with tumors larger than 1 cm or special tumor types larger than 3 cm (tubular, mucinous or papillary) was 27% at 10 years (70). For tumors smaller than 1 cm, the relapse rate was only 9% at 10 years.

Hormone receptor status is an important predictor not only of prognosis but also of response to hormonal therapy. Several studies demonstrated that patients who are estrogen and progesterone positive have overall improved survival (71,72). The status of these receptors should be known when determining the need for and choice of adjuvant therapy.

Table 35.4. Prognostic Factors in Node-negative Breast Carcinoma

Factor	*Increased Risk of Recurrence*
Size	Larger tumors
Histologic grade	High-grade tumors
DNA ploidy	Aneuploid tumors
Labeling index	High index (>3%)
S phase fraction	High fraction (>5%)
Lymphatic-vascular invasion	Present
Cathepsin D	High levels
HER-2/*neu* oncogene expression	High expression
Epidermal growth factor	High levels

From **Tierney LM, McPhee SJ, Papadakis MA.** *Current medical diagnosis and treatment.* Lange, 1995, with permission.

Table 35.5. Year Survival According to Stage of Breast Cancer

AJCC Stage	*Breast Cancer Cases (%)*	*5-Year Survival (%)*
0	9.4	99
I	40.9	82
II	36.6	73
III	8.9	55
IV	4.2	23

AJCC, American Joint Committee on Cancer.
From **Osteen RT, Karnell LH.** Breast cancer. In: **Steele GD Jr, Winchester DP, Menck HR, et al.,** eds. *National cancer database annual review of patient care, 1993.* Atlanta: American Cancer Society, 1993:10–9, with permission.

Histologic grade appears to predict overall survival as well. Those patients with favorable, well-differentiated tumors tend to fare better than those with poorly differentiated ones (Table 35.5). In a British study of 1,168 women, histologic grade was an independent predictor of overall survival at 10 years. Among multiple factors analyzed, only tumor size, lymph node status, and histologic grade had independent significance (73).

Specific tumor biologic markers are now gaining research interest because of their possible role in predicting which patients will respond to chemotherapy regimens. The most research has been performed with HER-2/*neu*. In an NSABP study, patients with HER-2/*neu* overexpression fared worse if they were not treated with anthracycline-based regimens (74). Another study showed that the addition of *trastuzumab* (*Herceptin*), an antibody directed against the HER-2/*neu* receptor, significantly increased the response rate to therapy over standard chemotherapy alone in the presence of metastases (75). Current research is focusing on the role of *trastuzumab* as adjuvant therapy. Other prognostic indicators such as *p53,* Ki-67, and S-phase fraction are also being investigated.

Over the course of several decades, more than 100 prospective, randomized trials have been conducted examining the role of adjuvant chemotherapy in breast cancer (76). From this work, a variety of systemic regimens have emerged. Systemic therapy includes cytotoxic agents and hormonal agents, used alone or in combination. Following is a brief description of the more commonly used regimens. A comprehensive review of all available modalities is beyond the scope of this chapter but is readily available in standard medical oncology texts.

Initially, trials involved a single perioperative course of chemotherapy in an attempt to eradicate circulating tumor cells. The Nissen-Meyer study from Norway showed that a single course of *cyclophosphamide* improved overall survival rates (77). Subsequently, numerous trials have shown the benefit of adjuvant chemotherapy for certain subgroups of patients (78). In the initial NSABP adjuvant trial, a 2-year course of *melphalan* was shown to be superior to no treatment (79). Subsequent trials have shown the enhanced beneficial effect of multiple drugs and a combination of hormonal manipulation with chemotherapy (80).

Historically, the most frequently used adjuvant combination chemotherapy has been CMF: *cyclophosphamide, methotrexate,* and *5-fluorouracil* (*5-FU*). In the original study by Bonadonna and associates, patients with positive axillary lymph nodes were randomized to receive either 12 monthly cycles of CMF or no therapy after radical mastectomy (81). A statistically significant benefit was found with CMF for premenopausal patients, especially those with one to three positive nodes. A subsequent study showed six cycles of CMF to be as effective as 12 cycles (82). However, no significant effect was seen for postmenopausal women. This was thought to be because postmenopausal women were less likely to tolerate the full course of CMF (83). **After 20 years of follow-up, this trial demonstrated a persistent survival advantage for premenopausal women receiving CMF adjuvant therapy** (84). **In a later study of node-negative, estrogen receptor–negative breast cancer patients, adjuvant CMF also had a beneficial effect. After 12 years of follow-up, 71% of**

treated patients remained disease free in comparison with 48% in the control group. Both premenopausal and postmenopausal women benefited from adjuvant CMF (85).

Today, anthracylines (A) are commonly used more often than in the adjuvant and metastatic treatment of breast cancer. They are among the most active drugs and have been used in the adjuvant setting since 1973 (86). A large randomized NSABP study compared CMF versus AC regimens in node-positive patients. This study demonstrated similar treatment outcomes in the AC and CMF treatment groups. However, the AC regimen was preferred because of the shorter duration (four cycles for 3 months versus six cycles for 6 months) and better reported tolerance (87).

Taxanes are also being used frequently in a variety of multiple-agent chemotherapy regimens because of their demonstrated activity in metastatic breast cancer patients (88). In a randomized trial of 3,170 node-positive patients who received AC 4 times followed by *paclitaxel* 4 times for 4 weeks or no additional therapy, there was an absolute improvement in survival from 84% to 87% at 36 months of follow-up. Benefits were similar in both premenopausal and postmenopausal women (89). In contrast, no benefits were seen in large studies conducted elsewhere (90,91). Currently, there are no definitive data that demonstrate any benefit to the addition of taxanes over CMF or AC in node-negative patients. Ongoing clinical studies are under way in an attempt to define the role of taxanes in the adjuvant setting.

Hormonal Therapies

Hormonal manipulation used alone and in combination with cytotoxic regimens is beneficial in select groups of women. *Tamoxifen,* an estrogen analogue, offers substantial benefits in both premenopausal and postmenopausal women. **Taken at a dose of 20 mg per day for 5 years, *tamoxifen* reduces the annual odds of recurrence by about 50% and the annual odds of death by about 25%. These benefits were seen in women with estrogen receptor–positive disease despite the presence or absence of chemotherapy** (92). The possibility of substituting *tamoxifen* for radiotherapy in patients with small (<1 cm) tumors is also being evaluated prospectively.

There are data to suggest that *tamoxifen,* when used in combination with cytotoxic chemotherapy, improves survival in women with positive axillary lymph nodes and positive estrogen receptor expression (93). In patients with node-negative, estrogen receptor–positive disease, the addition of *tamoxifen* to chemotherapy improved disease-free survival after 5 years of follow-up (94). In NSABP study B-14, 2,644 patients with estrogen receptor–positive tumors and no axillary metastases were randomized, double blinded to either *tamoxifen* (10 mg orally twice daily for 5 years) or a placebo control. After a 4-year median follow-up, the disease-free survival rate for the 1,318 patients treated with *tamoxifen* was 82% compared with 77% for the 1,326 patients treated with placebo ($p = 0.00001$). An advantage existed for both premenopausal and postmenopausal women.

The Early Breast Cancer Trialists' Collaborative Group performed a metaanalysis of adjuvant systemic therapy for breast cancer. They analyzed randomized trials involving adjuvant systemic hormonal, cytotoxic, or immune therapy administered to more than 75,000 women with stage I or II carcinoma. The investigators concluded that, for postmenopausal women with estrogen receptor–positive tumors, *tamoxifen* in a dose of 20 mg daily for at least 2 years had a significant beneficial effect on disease-free survival rates. This beneficial effect lasted up to 10 years. Data demonstrated a decreased incidence of carcinoma in the contralateral breast and a decreased death rate from heart disease.

General Recommendations

Adjuvant systemic therapy, either with *tamoxifen* or multiple-chemotherapy agents, lowers the incidence of recurrence by about 30%. It is important to understand that the

Table 35.6. Effect of Systemic Therapy on Recurrence and Survival from Breast Cancer

Age	*Therapy*	*Reduction in Annual Odds of Recurrence %*	*Reduction in Annual Odds of Death %*
<50	*Tamoxifen* × 5yrs	45 ± 8	32 ± 10
50–59	*Tamoxifen* × 5yrs	37 ± 6	11 ± 8
60–69	*Tamoxifen* × 5yrs	54 ± 5	33 ± 6
<40	Polychemotherapy	37 ± 7	27 ± 8
40–49	Polychemotherapy	35 ± 5	27 ± 5
50–59	Polychemotherapy	22 ± 4	14 ± 4
60–69	Polychemotherapy	18 ± 4	8 ± 4

From **Early Breast Cancer Trialists' Collaborative Group.** Polychemotherapy for early breast cancer: an overview of the randomised trials. *Lancet* 1998;352:930; **Early Breast Cancer Trialists' Collaborative Group.** Tamoxifen for early breast cancer: an overview of the randomised trials. *Lancet* 1998;352:930, with permission.

proportional reduction in risk of relapse is relatively constant regardless of absolute risk (95) (Table 35.6). As mentioned earlier, adjuvant cytotoxic chemotherapy appears to affect the natural history of patients with axillary node–negative breast cancer. A 2000 consensus statement from the National Institutes of Health on early-stage breast cancer advised that all patients be considered for clinical trials and offered the opportunity to participate (96). Furthermore, node-negative patients who are not candidates for clinical trials should be made aware of the benefits and potential risks of adjuvant systemic therapy. Most high-risk patients with node-negative disease are now being treated with adjuvant cytotoxic therapy.

In postmenopausal women, chemotherapy is about one-half as effective as *tamoxifen* in the adjuvant setting (97). For most postmenopausal women with hormone-responsive disease (estrogen- and progesterone-responsive positivity), including node-positive patients, *tamoxifen* alone may be adequate therapy. High-risk patients with hormone-resistant disease may benefit from cytotoxic systemic therapy. In patients over age 70 years, there are little data available regarding the benefits of adjuvant cytotoxic therapy because of the eligibility criteria of many large trials. Because of the inherent toxicity of chemotherapeutic regimens, patients in this age group must be carefully selected with regard to treatment.

Caution should be exercised when using chemotherapeutic agents. Patients in whom the risk of recurrence is low are likely to derive little overall benefit from the use of adjuvant systemic therapy, whereas those with an overall high risk of recurrence are likely to receive the greatest benefit. When the risk of recurrence is extremely low, as would be expected for tumors smaller than 1 cm with no lymph node metastasis, the reduction in the risk of recurrence may not justify the side effects of the drugs. Current studies are under way to investigate whether this assumption is true.

The current recommendations for adjuvant systemic therapy in breast cancer are summarized as follows:

1. **Premenopausal women with lymph node involvement should be treated with adjuvant combination chemotherapy. *Tamoxifen* may be added to the regimen for patients with estrogen receptor–positive tumors following cytotoxic therapy.**

2. **Premenopausal women without evidence of axillary lymph node involvement but with risk factors such as large (>1 cm), aneuploid, or estrogen receptor–negative tumors should be treated with combination chemotherapy. *Tamoxifen* should be added for patients with estrogen receptor–positive tumors.**

3. **Postmenopausal patients who have negative lymph nodes and positive hormone receptor levels should receive adjuvant *tamoxifen* therapy. Those**

with positive lymph nodes may receive *tamoxifen* alone, multidrug cytotoxic therapy, or a combination thereof.

4. **Postmenopausal women who have lymph node metastasis and negative hormone receptor levels may be treated with adjuvant chemotherapy.**

5. **Adjuvant systemic therapy is not recommended for patients with favorable, small nonpalpable tumors or palpable tumors smaller than 1 cm. The toxicity of chemotherapy and its effect on quality of life must be carefully evaluated, especially in older postmenopausal women.**

Prognosis

The treatment of advanced, metastatic breast cancer is largely palliative. For most physicians who treat this disease, quality of life issues are paramount when choosing which type of therapy is offered. In patients with locally advanced disease in conjunction with distant metastasis, palliative radiotherapy may be advised. Palliative radiotherapy is most widely used in the treatment of certain soft tissue or bony metastases to control pain or avoid fracture. This approach is best exemplified in the treatment of isolated bone metastases, chest wall recurrences, brain metastases, and spinal cord compression.

Systemic disease may be controlled by hormonal or cytotoxic therapy. Because the quality of life during a remission induced by endocrine manipulation usually is superior to a remission following cytotoxic chemotherapy, it usually is preferable to try endocrine manipulation first. Disseminated disease may respond favorably after endocrine therapy such as functional organ ablation (ovary, pituitary, adrenal glands) or administration of drugs that block hormonal function. A favorable response occurs in about one-third of patients with metastatic disease. For those patients whose tumors express estrogen receptors, this response rate may be as high as 60%. Because only 5% to 10% of women whose tumors do not contain estrogen receptors respond to treatment, they should not receive hormonal therapy except in unusual cases such as elderly patients who are unable to tolerate cytotoxic therapy (98).

Cytotoxic chemotherapy should be considered for the treatment of metastatic breast cancer in the following instances: (a) if organ involvement is potentially life-threatening (brain, lung, or liver) (b) if hormonal treatment is unsuccessful or the disease has progressed after an initial response to hormonal manipulation, or (c) if the tumor is estrogen receptor–negative. The most useful single chemotherapeutic agent is an anthracycline such as *doxorubicin,* which has an estimated response rate of 40% to 50%. Combination therapy using multiple agents has proved to be more effective, with response rates as high as 60% to 80% (99). Clinical trials are under way to examine a variety of combinations for stage IV disease. The side effects of nausea and vomiting, which can be devastating, are now well controlled with central-acting antiemetics. The importance of controlling these side effects cannot be overemphasized.

Special Breast Cancers

Paget's Disease

Sir James Paget described a nipple lesion similar to eczema and recognized that this nipple change was associated with an underlying breast malignancy (100). The erosion results from invasion of the nipple and surrounding areola by characteristic large cells with irregular nuclei, now called Paget cells. The origin of these cells has been much debated by pathologists. However, they are probably extensions of an underlying carcinoma into the major ducts of the nipple–areolar complex. There may be no visible changes associated with the initial invasion of the nipple. Often, the patient will notice a nipple discharge, which is actually a combination of serum and blood from the involved ducts.

The overall prognosis for patients with Paget's disease depends on the underlying malignancy. In patients who have an intraductal carcinoma alone, the prognosis is favorable, whereas in those with infiltrating ductal carcinoma metastatic to the regional lymph nodes, the prognosis is poor. Traditionally, treatment has almost always been total mastectomy and lymph node dissection, although radiotherapy with resection of the tumor and nipple–areolar complex is being performed (101).

Inflammatory Carcinoma

Inflammatory carcinoma of the breast initially appears to be an acute inflammation with redness and edema. Inflammatory cancer, rather than infiltrating ductal carcinoma, should be diagnosed when more than one-third of the breast is involved with erythema and edema and when biopsy of this area shows metastatic cancer in the subdermal lymphatics. There may be no distinct palpable mass, because the tumor infiltrates through the breast with ill-defined margins, or there may be a dominant mass. There may even be satellite nodules within the parenchyma. Most of the tumors are poorly differentiated, and mammographically the breast shows skin thickening with an infiltrative process.

Except for biopsy of the lesion, surgery usually should not be used in the initial management of inflammatory carcinoma. Mastectomy in the face of inflammatory carcinoma usually fails locally and does not improve survival rates. The best results are achieved with a combination of chemotherapy and radiation therapy. Mastectomy may be indicated for patients who remain free of distant metastatic disease after initial chemotherapy and radiation (102,103).

In Situ Carcinomas

Both lobular carcinoma and ductal carcinoma may be confined by the basement membrane of the ducts. These carcinomas do not invade the surrounding tissue and, theoretically, lack the ability to spread. Indeed, lobular carcinoma *in situ* is not a malignancy. Untreated it may not become a new cancer, whereas ductal carcinoma *in situ* will. A more appropriate nomenclature for lobular carcinoma *in situ* is lobular neoplasia, and it should be considered a risk factor for the development of cancer in either breast (104). Because of their unusual natural history, they represent a special form of breast cancer. If treated by biopsy alone, 25% to 30% of patients with lobular carcinoma *in situ* will subsequently develop invasive cancer.

Lobular Carcinoma *In Situ*

Most women with lobular carcinoma *in situ* are premenopausal. The tumor typically is not a discrete mass, but rather it is a multifocal lesion within one or both breasts found incidentally at biopsy of a mass or mammographic assessment of an abnormality not related to the lobular carcinoma *in situ.* Lobular carcinoma *in situ* usually is managed with excisional biopsy followed by careful observation and mammography. It should not be considered a malignancy but rather a risk factor for malignancy. Patients should be informed that they have a higher risk of developing invasive breast cancer. Occasionally, a patient may request bilateral prophylactic mastectomy.

Ductal Carcinoma *In Situ*

Ductal carcinoma *in situ* is more common in postmenopausal women. It may manifest as a palpable mass with features typical of an invasive ductal carcinoma but usually is detected mammographically as a cluster of branched or Y-shaped microcalcifications. By definition, the intraductal disease does not invade beyond the basement membrane. Unlike patients with lobular carcinoma *in situ,* however, at least 30% to 50% of patients with ductal carcinoma *in situ* will develop invasive cancer within the same breast when treated by excisional biopsy alone (105).

Although modified radical mastectomy has been standard treatment for intraductal carcinoma, more conservative surgery, with or without radiation therapy, can yield good results (106). In NSABP trial B17, 818 patients were randomly assigned to treatment with excision alone or excision followed by radiation therapy (107). The mean extent of ductal carcinoma *in situ* lesions was 13 mm, and 88% were larger than 20 mm. All lesions were completely resected with negative margins. After a median follow-up of 43 months, the actuarial 5-year local recurrence rate was 10.4% without radiation versus 7.5% with radiation ($p = 0.055$) for noninvasive cancers, and 10.5% without radiation versus 2.9% with radiation ($p > 0.001$) for invasive cancers. Of 83 recurrences, only 9 (11%) were not in the index quadrant. A recent reanalysis with a mean follow up of 90 months confirmed these results (108). These data suggest that segmental mastectomy offers excellent local control.

Axillary metastases occur in fewer than 5% of patients, indicating that an invasive component has been missed during biopsy. For small, true ductal carcinoma *in situ,* axillary dissection is not indicated. About 5% of patients whose initial biopsy results show intraductal carcinoma will be found to have infiltrating ductal carcinoma when treated with mastectomy. The incidence of contralateral breast cancer in women with intraductal carcinoma is the same as in those with invasive ductal carcinoma (5% to 8%) (109).

Breast Cancer in Pregnancy

Breast cancer complicates approximately one in 3,000 pregnancies (110–112). It is the second most common malignancy seen in association with pregnancy, surpassed only by cervical cancer (113). Initial studies suggested a significantly worse prognosis for patients with breast cancer diagnosed during pregnancy, but more recent data indicate that the hormonal changes associated with pregnancy seem to have little, if any, influence on prognosis. **When pregnant patients are matched stage for stage with nonpregnant patients, survival rates seem equivalent** (114).

The treatment of breast cancer in pregnant women must be highly individualized. Considerations include the patient's age and desire to have the child. The overall prognosis should be considered, especially when axillary lymph nodes are involved, because adjuvant chemotherapy can be teratogenic or lethal, particularly during the first trimester, but may be given later in the pregnancy. It is not known whether interruption of pregnancy alters the prognosis for patients with potentially curable breast cancer.

Following are recommendations for treatment of pregnant women with breast cancer:

1. Localized disease found during the first or second trimester of pregnancy is probably best treated with definitive surgery and radiation therapy similar to that done for nonpregnant patients. Radiation therapy is relatively safe to give provided the abdomen is shielded. Adjuvant chemotherapy can be given after the first trimester. However, most oncologists prefer not to give it to pregnant women.

2. Localized tumors found during the third trimester of pregnancy must be managed on an individual basis. Initially, tumors should be excised early in the third trimester using local anesthesia. If delivery is imminent, standard therapy can be performed immediately postpartum.

3. If the breast cancer is diagnosed during lactation, lactation should be suppressed and the cancer should be treated definitively.

4. Advanced, incurable cancer should be treated with palliative therapy, and the pregnancy may be continued or interrupted depending on the therapy necessary and the desires of the mother.

Counseling regarding future childbearing is important for women who have had carcinoma of the breast. Although it generally has been assumed that subsequent pregnancies are detrimental because of the high levels of circulating estrogens, **there is no clear difference in survival for women who become pregnant after the diagnosis of breast cancer.** A recent study evaluated the effect of subsequent pregnancy on overall survival after the diagnosis of early-stage breast cancer. Although approximately 40% of the women in the study had node-positive disease, 5- and 10-year survival rates were better in women who became pregnant than in matched pair controls who did not. This study suggests that subsequent pregnancy does not adversely affect the prognosis of early-stage breast cancer (115). Theoretically, it may be that only women with estrogen receptor–positive or progesterone-positive tumors would be affected deleteriously by subsequent pregnancy, but this possibility has not been studied. Because recurrences are most frequent within the first 2 to 3 years after diagnosis, patients with receptor-positive tumors and advanced-stage disease probably should wait before becoming pregnant again (if ever).

References

1. **Jemal A, Thomas A, Murray T, et al.** Cancer Statistics, 2002. *CA Cancer J Clin* 2002;52:23–47.
2. **Brian DD, Melton LJ, Goellner JR, et al.** Breast cancer incidence, prevalence, mortality, and survivorship in Rochester, Minnesota. *Mayo Clin Proc* 1980;55:355–359.
3. **Mesko TW, Dunlap JN, Sutherland CM, et al.** Risk factors for breast cancer. *Compr Ther* 1990;16:3–9.
4. **Greene MH.** Genetics of breast cancer. *Mayo Clin Proc* 1997;72:54–65.
5. **FitzGerald MG, MacDonald DJ, Krainer M, et al.** Germ-line *BRCA1* mutations in Jewish and non-Jewish women with early-onset breast cancer. *N Engl J Med* 1996;334:143–149.
6. **Van't Veer P, Van Leer EM, Rietdijk A, et al.** Combination of dietary factors in relation to breast cancer occurrence. *Int J Cancer* 1991;47:649–653.
7. **Hsieh CC, Trichopoulos D, Katsouyanni K, et al.** Age at menarche, age at menopause, height and obesity as risk factors for breast cancer: associations and interactions in an international case-control study. *Int J Cancer* 1990;46:796–780.
8. **Schatzkin A, Jones Y, Hoover RN, et al.** Alcohol consumption and breast cancer in the epidemiologic follow up: study of the first national health and nutrition examination survey. *N Engl J Med* 1987;316:1169–1173.
9. **Pike MC, Krailo MD, Henderson BE, et al.** "Hormonal" risk factors, "breast tissue age" and the age-incidence of breast cancer. *Nature* 1983;303:767–770.
10. **Brinton LA, Hoover R, Fraumeni JF Jr.** Reproductive factors in the etiology of breast cancer. *Br J Cancer* 1983;47:757–762.
11. **Korzeniowski S, Dyba T.** Reproductive history and prognosis in patients with operable breast cancer. *Cancer* 1994;14:1591–1594.
12. **Trapido EJ.** Age at first birth, parity, and breast cancer risks. *Cancer* 1983;51:946–948.
13. **The Cancer and Steroid Hormone Study of the Centers for Disease Control and the National Institute of Child Health and Human Development.** Oral-contraceptive use and the risk of breast cancer. *N Engl J Med* 1986;315:405–411.
14. **Collaborative Group on Hormonal Factors in Breast Cancer.** Breast cancer and hormonal contraceptives: collaborative reanalysis of individual data on 53 297 women with breast cancer and 100 239 women without breast cancer from 54 epidemiological studies. *Lancet* 1996;347:1713–1727.
15. **Schairer C, Lubin J, Troisi R, et al.** Estrogen-progestin replacement and risk of breast cancer. *JAMA* 2000;284:691–694.
16. **Nielsen M, Christensen L, Andersen J.** Contralateral cancerous breast lesions in women with clinical invasive breast carcinoma. *Cancer* 1986;57:897–903.
17. **Baker LH.** The Breast Cancer Detection Demonstration Project: 5 year summary report. *Cancer* 1982;32:194.
18. **Bjurstam N, Bjorneld L, Duffy SW, et al.** The Gothenburg Breast Cancer Screening Trial: preliminary results on breast cancer mortality for women aged 39–49. *J Natl Cancer Inst Monogr* 1997;22:53–55.
19. **Bassett LW, Liu TH, Giuliano AE, et al.** The prevalence of carcinoma in palpable vs nonpalpable mammographically detected lesions. *Am J Roentgenol* 1991;157:21–24.
20. **Miller AB, Bulbrook RD.** Screening, detection and diagnosis of breast cancer. *Lancet* 1982;1:1109–1111.
21. **Frable WJ.** Fine-needle aspiration biopsy: a review. *Hum Pathol* 1983;14:9–28.
22. **McDivitt RW, Stewart FW, Bert JW.** *Atlas of tumor pathology tumors of the breast. Second series, fascicle 2.* Washington DC: Armed Forces Institute of Pathology, 1968.

23. **Tubiana M, Pejovic JM, Renaud A, et al.** Kinetic parameters and the course of the disease in breast cancer. *Cancer* 1981;47:937–943.

24. **Lee YT.** Breast carcinoma: pattern of metastasis at autopsy. *J Surg Oncol* 1983;23:175–180.

25. **Giuliano A.** The pattern of recurrence of early stage breast cancer. *J Surg Oncol* 1989;31:152–158.

26. **Bloom HJG, Richardson MB, Harris EJ.** Natural history of untreated breast cancer (1805–1933). *BMJ* 1962;47:937.

27. **Haagensen CD.** *Diseases of the breast,* 3rd ed. Philadelphia: WB Saunders, 1986.

28. **American Joint Committee on Cancer.** In: **Fleming ID, Cooper JS, Henson DE, et al.,** eds. *AJCC cancer staging manual,* 5th ed. Philadelphia: JB Lippincott, 1997:171–180.

29. **Bassett LW, Giuliano AE, Gold RH.** Staging for breast carcinoma. *Am J Surg* 1989;157:250–255.

30. **Halsted WS.** The results of radical operation for cure of carcinoma of the breast. *Ann Surg* 1907;46:1–19.

31. **Meyer W.** Carcinoma of the breast; ten years experience with my method of radical operation. *JAMA* 1905;45:297–313.

32. **Haagensen CD, Bodian C.** A personal experience with Halsted's radical mastectomy. *Ann Surg* 1984;199:143–150.

33. **Dahl-Iversen E, Tobiassen T.** Radical mastectomy with parasternal and supraclavicular dissection for mammary carcinoma. *Ann Surg* 1963;157:170–173.

34. **Lewis FJ.** Extended or super radical mastectomy for cancer of the breast. *Minn Med* 1953;36:763–766.

35. **Urban JA.** Extended radical mastectomy for breast cancer. *Ann Surg* 1963;106:399.

36. **Veronesi U, Valagussa P.** Inefficacy of internal mammary node dissection in breast cancer surgery. *Cancer* 1981;47:170–173.

37. **Handley RS.** The conservative radical mastectomy of Patey: 10-year results in 425 patients. *Breast* 1976;2:16–19.

38. **Maier WP, Leber D, Rosemond GP, et al.** The technique of modified radical mastectomy. *Surg Gynecol Obstet* 1977;145:68–74.

39. **Robinson GN, Van Heerden JA, Payne SW, et al.** The primary surgical treatment of carcinoma of the breast: a changing trend toward modified radical mastectomy. *Mayo Clin Proc* 1976;51:433–442.

40. **McWhirter R.** Should more radical treatment be attempted in breast cancer? *AJR* 1964;92:3–13.

41. **Montague ED.** Radiation therapy and breast cancer. Past, present and future. *Am J Clin Oncol* 1985;8: 455–462.

42. **Montague ED, Fletcher GH.** The curative value of irradiation in the treatment of nondisseminated breast cancer. *Cancer* 1980;46:995–998.

43. **Wallgren A, Arner O, Bergstrom J, et al.** The value of preoperative radiotherapy in operable mammary carcinoma. *Int J Radiat Oncol Biol Phys* 1980;6:287–290.

44. **Nevin JE, Baggerly JT, Laird TK.** Radiotherapy as an adjuvant in the treatment of cancer of the breast. *Cancer* 1982;49:1194–1200.

45. **Overgaard M, Hansen P, Overgaard J, et al.** Postoperative radiotherapy in high-risk premenopausal women with breast cancer who receive adjuvant chemotherapy. *N Engl J Med* 1997;337: 949–955.

46. **Fisher B, Redmond C, Fisher ER, et al.** Ten-year results of a randomized clinical trial comparing radical mastectomy and total mastectomy with or without radiation. *N Engl J Med* 1985;312:674–681.

47. **Keynes G.** Conservative treatment of cancer of the breast. *BMJ* 1937;2:643–647.

48. **Calle R, Pilleron JP, Schlienger P, et al.** Conservative management of operable breast cancer: ten years' experience at the Foundation Curie. *Cancer* 1978;42:2045–2053.

49. **Prosnitz LR, Goldenberg IS, Packard RA, et al.** Radiation therapy as initial treatment for early stage cancer of the breast without mastectomy. *Cancer* 1977;39:917–923.

50. **Harris JR, Hellman S, Silen W.** *Conservative management of breast cancer.* Philadelphia: JB Lippincott, 1983.

51. **Veronesi U, Saccozzi R, Del Veccio M, et al.** Comparing radical mastectomy with quadrantectomy, axillary dissection and radiotherapy in patients with small cancers of the breast. *N Engl J Med* 1981;305: 6–11.

52. **Veronesi U, Zucali R, Luini A.** Local control and survival in early breast cancer: the Milan trial. *Int J Radiat Oncol Biol Phys* 1986;12:717–720.

53. **Fisher B, Bauer M, Margolese R, et al.** Five-year results of a randomized clinical trial comparing total mastectomy and segmental mastectomy with or without radiation in the treatment of cancer. *N Engl J Med* 1989;320:822–828.

54. **Fisher B, Anderson S, Redmond CK, et al.** Reanalysis and results after 12 years of follow-up in a randomized clinical trial comparing total mastectomy with lumpectomy with or without irradiation in the treatment of breast cancer. *N Engl J Med* 1995;333:1456–1461.

55. **Carter CL, Allen C, Henson DE.** Relation of tumor size, lymph node status, and survival in 24,740 breast cancer cases. *Cancer* 1989;63:181–187.

56. **Fisher ER, Sass R, Fisher B.** Pathologic findings from the National Surgical Adjuvant Project for Breast Cancers (protocol no. 4). X. Discriminants for tenth year treatment failure. *Cancer* 1984;53:712–723.

57. **Rosen PP, Groshen S, Saigo PE, et al.** Pathological prognostic factors in stage I (T1N0M0) and stage II (T1N1M0) breast carcinoma; a study of 644 patients with median follow-up of 18 years. *J Clin Oncol* 1989;7:1239–1251.

58. **National Institutes of Health.** NIH consensus conference on the treatment of early-stage breast cancer. *JAMA* 1991;265:391–395.

59. **Ivens D, Hoe AL, Podd TJ, et al.** Assessment of morbidity from complete axillary dissection. *Br J Cancer* 1992;66:136–138.

60. **Kissin MW, Querci della Rovere G, Easton D, et al.** Risk of lymphoedema following the treatment of breast cancer. *Br J Surg* 1986;73:580–584.

61. **Davies GC, Millis RR, Hayward JL.** Assessment of axillary lymph node status. *Ann Surg* 1980;192: 148–151.

62. **Sacre RA.** Clinical evaluation of axillary lymph nodes compared to surgical and pathological findings. *Eur J Surg Oncol* 1986;12:169–173.

63. **Giuliano AE, Kirgan DM, Guenther JM, et al.** Lymphatic mapping and sentinel lymphadenectomy for breast cancer. *Ann Surg* 1994;220:391–401.

64. **Krag DN, Weaver DL, Alex JC, et al.** Surgical resection and radiolocalization of the sentinel lymph node in breast cancer using a gamma probe. *Surg Oncol* 1993;2:335–339.

65. **Veronesi U, Paganelli G, Galimberti V, et al.** Sentinel-node biopsy to avoid axillary dissection in breast cancer with clinically negative lymph-nodes. *Lancet* 1997;349:1864–1867.

66. **Giuliano AE, Haigh PI, Brennan MB, et al.** Prospective observational study of sentinel lymphadenectomy without further axillary dissection in patients with sentinel node-negative breast cancer. *J Clin Oncol* 2000;13:2553–2559.

67. **Schabel FM Jr.** Rationale for adjuvant chemotherapy. *Cancer* 1977;39:2875–2882.

68. **Murphy GP, Lawrence W, Lenhard RE, eds.** *American Cancer Society textbook of clinical oncology.* Atlanta, GA: American Cancer Society, 1995:213.

69. **Brezden C, Phillips KA, Abdolell M, et al.** Cognitive function in breast cancer patients receiving adjuvant chemotherapy. *J Clin Oncol* 2000;18:2695–2701.

70. **Rosen PP, Groshen S, Kinne DW, et al.** Factors influencing prognosis in node-negative breast carcinoma: analysis of 767 T1N0M0/T2N0M0 patients with long-term follow-up. *J Clin Oncol* 1993;11: 2090–2100.

71. **Adami H-O, Graffman S, Lindgren A, et al.** Prognostic implication of estrogen receptor content in breast cancer. *Breast Cancer Res Treat* 1985;5:293–300.

72. **Mason BH, Holdaway IM, Mullins PR, et al.** Progesterone and estrogen receptors as prognostic variables in breast cancer. *Cancer Res* 1983;43:2985–2990.

73. **Kollias J, Elston CW, Ellis IO, et al.** Early-onset breast cancer—histopathological and prognostic considerations. *Br J Cancer* 1997;75:1318–1323.

74. **Paik S, Bryant J, Park C, et al.** ErbB-2 and response to doxorubicin in patients with node-positive breast cancer. *J Natl Cancer Inst* 1998;90:1346.

75. **Slamon DJ, Leyland-Jones B, Shak S, et al.** Use of chemotherapy plus a monoclonal antibody against HER2 for metastatic breast cancer that overexpresses HER2. *N Engl J Med* 2001;344:783–792.

76. **Winer EP, Morrow M, Osborne CK, et al.** Malignant tumors of the breast. In: **Devita VT, Hellman S, Rosenberg S,** eds. *Cancer principles and practice of oncology,* 6th ed. Philadelphia: Lippincott Williams & Wilkins, 2001:1688–1689.

77. **Nissen-Meyer R.** The Scandinavian clinical trials. *Experientia Suppl* 1982;41:571–579.

78. **Bonadonna G, Valagussa P.** Adjuvant systemic therapy for resectable breast cancer. *J Clin Oncol* 1985;3:259–275.

79. **Fisher B, Carbone P, Economou SG, et al.** L-phenylalanine mustard in the management of primary breast cancer. A report of early findings. *N Engl J Med* 1975;292:117–122.

80. **Mueller CB, Lesperance ML.** NSABP trials of adjuvant chemotherapy for breast cancer. A further look at the evidence. *Ann Surg* 1991;214:206–211.

81. **Bonadonna G, Rossi A, Valagussa P.** Adjuvant CMF chemotherapy in operable breast cancer: ten years later. *World J Surg* 1985;9:707–713.

82. **Tancine G, Bonadonna G, Valagussa P, et al.** Adjuvant CMF in breast cancer: comparative 5-year results of 12 versus 6 cycles. *J Clin Oncol* 1983;1:2–10.

83. **Bonadonna G, Valagussa P.** Dose-response effect of adjuvant chemotherapy in breast cancer. *N Engl J Med* 1981;304:10–15.

84. **Bonadonna G, Valagussa P, Moliterni A, et al.** Adjuvant cyclophosphamide, methotrexate, and fluorouracil in node-positive breast cancer: the results of 20 years of follow-up. *N Engl J Med* 1995;332:901–906.

85. **Zambetti M, Valagussa P, Bonadonna G.** Adjuvant CMF in node-negative and estrogen receptor negative breast cancer: updated results. *Ann Oncol* 1996;7:481–485.

86. **Buzdar AU, Gutterman JU, Blumenschein GR, et al.** Intensive postoperative chemoimmunotherapy for patients with stage II and stage III breast cancer. *Cancer* 1978;41:1064–1075.

87. **Fisher B, Brown AM, Dimitrov NV, et al.** Two months of doxorubicin-cyclophosphamide with and without interval reinduction therapy compared with 6 months of cyclophosphamide, methotrexate, and fluorouracil in positive-node breast cancer patients with tamoxifen-nonresponsive tumors: results from the National Surgical Adjuvant Breast and Bowel Project B-15. *J Clin Oncol* 1990;8:1483–1496.

88. **Nabholtz JM, Senn HJ, Bezwoda WR, et al.** Prospective randomized trial of docetaxel versus mitomycin plus vinblastine in patients with metastatic breast cancer progressing despite previous anthracycline-containing chemotherapy. 304 Study Group. *J Clin Oncol* 1999;17:1413–1424.

89. **Henderson IC, Berry D, Demetri G, et al.** Improved disease free survival and overall survival from the addition of sequential paclitaxel but not from the escalation of doxorubicin dose level in the adjuvant chemotherapy of patients with node-positive breast cancer. *Proc Am Soc Clin Oncol* 1998; 17:101(abst).

90. **Thomas E, Buzdar A, Theriault R, et al.** Role of paclitaxel in adjuvant therapy of operable breast cancer: preliminary results of a prospective randomized clinical trial. *Proc Am Soc Clin Oncol* 2000;19:74(abstr).

91. **Mamounas EP.** Evaluating the use of paclitaxel following doxorubicin/cyclophosphamide in patients with breast cancer and positive axillary nodes. Paper presented at: NIH Consensus Development Conference on Adjuvant Therapy for Breast Cancer; November 1–3, 2000; Washington, DC.

92. **Early Breast Cancer Trialists' Collaborative Group.** Polychemotherapy for early breast cancer: an overview of the randomised trials. *Lancet* 1998;352:930–942.

93. **Albain K, Green S, Ravdin P, et al.** Overall survival after cyclophosphamide, adriamycin, 5-FU, and tamoxifen is superior to tamoxifen alone in post-menopausal, receptor(+), node(+) breast cancer: new findings from phase III Southwest Oncology Group Intergroup Trial S8814 (INT-0100). *Proc Am Soc Clin Oncol* 2001;20(abstr).

94. **Fisher B, Digman J, Wolmark N, et al.** Tamoxifen and chemotherapy for lymph node-negative, estrogen receptor-positive breast cancer. *J Natl Cancer Inst* 1997;89:1673–1682.

95. **Winer EP, Morrow M, Osborne CK, et al.** Malignant tumors of the breast. In: **Devita VT, Hellman S, Rosenberg S,** eds. *Cancer principles and practice of oncology,* 6th ed. Philadelphia: Lippincott Williams & Wilkins, 2001:1651–1717.

96. **National Institutes of Health Consensus Development Conference Statement: Adjuvant chemotherapy for breast cancer; November 1–3, 2000; Washington, DC.** Available at: http://odp.od.nih.gov/consensus/cons/114/114_statement.htm. Accessed .

97. **Early Breast Cancer Trialists' Collaborative Group.** Systemic treatment of early breast cancer by hormonal, cytotoxic or immune therapy: 133 randomised trials involving 31,000 recurrences and 24,000 deaths among 75,000 women. *Lancet* 1992;339:1–15, 71–85.

98. **Dhodapkar MV, Ingle JN, Cha SS, et al.** Prognostic factors in elderly women with metastatic breast cancer treated with tamoxifen: an analysis of patients entered on four prospective clinical trials. *Cancer* 1996;77:683–690.

99. **Valero V.** Combination docetaxel/cyclophosphamide in patients with advanced solid tumors. *Oncology* 1997;11:34–36.

100. **Paget J.** Disease of the mammary areola preceding cancer of the mammary gland. *St Bart Host Rep* 1874;10:89.

101. **Bulens P, Vanuytsel L, Rijnders A, et al.** Breast conserving treatment of Paget's disease. *Radiother Oncol* 1990;17:305–309.

102. **Droulias CA, Sewell CW, McSweeney MB, et al.** Inflammatory carcinoma of the breast: a correlation of clinical, radiologic and pathologic findings. *Ann Surg* 1976;184:217–222.

103. **Donegan WL, Padrta B.** Combined therapy for inflammatory breast cancer. *Arch Surg* 1990;125:578–582.

104. **Sunshine JA, Moseley HS, Fletcher WS, et al.** Breast carcinoma *in situ:* a retrospective review of 112 cases with a minimum 10-year follow up. *Am J Surg* 1985;150:44–51.

105. **Barth A, Brenner RJ, Giuliano AE.** Current management of ductal carcinoma *in situ. West J Med* 1995;163:360–366.

106. **Stotter AT, McNeese M, Oswald MJ, et al.** The role of limited surgery with irradiation in primary treatment of ductal *in situ* breast cancer. *Int J Radiat Oncol Biol Phys* 1990;18:283–287.

107. **Fisher B, Constantino J, Redmond C, et al.** Lumpectomy compared with lumpectomy and radiation therapy for the treatment of intraductal breast cancer. *N Engl J Med* 1993;328:1581–1586.

108. **Fisher B, Dignam J, Wolmark N, et al.** Lumpectomy and radiation therapy for the treatment of intraductal breast cancer: findings from the National Surgical Adjuvant Breast and Bowel Project B-17. *J Clin Oncol* 1998;16:441–452.

109. **Kinne DW, Petrek JA, Osborne MP, et al.** Breast carcinoma *in situ. Arch Surg* 1989;124:33–36.

110. **Donegan WL.** Cancer and pregnancy. *CA Cancer J Clin* 1983;33:194–214.

111. **Hornstein E, Skornick Y, Rozin R.** The management of breast carcinoma in pregnancy and lactation. *J Surg Oncol* 1982;21:179–182.

112. **Hoover HC Jr.** Breast cancer during pregnancy and lactation. *Surg Clin North Am* 1990;70:1151–1163.

113. **Antonelli NM, Dotters DJ, Katz VL, et al.** Cancer in pregnancy: a review of the literature. Part I. *Obstet Gynecol Surv* 1996;51:125–134.

114. **Petrek JA.** Breast cancer and pregnancy. *J Natl Cancer Inst Monogr* 1994;16:113–121.

115. **Gelber S, Coates A, Goldhirsch A, et al.** Effect of pregnancy on overall survival after the diagnosis of early stage breast cancer. *J Clin Oncol* 2001;19:1671–1675.

Appendix: Reference Values

Measure	SI	Conventional (C)	Conversion Factor (CF) C × CF = SI
Acetoacetate, plasma	<100 μmol/l	<1.0 mg/dl	97.95
Adrenal steroids, plasma			
Aldosterone, supine, saline suppression	<220 pmol/l	<8 ng/dl	27.74
Cortisol			
8:00 AM	220–660 nmol/l	8–24 μg/dl	27.59
4:00 PM	50–410 nmol/l	2–15 μg/dl	27.59
Overnight dexamethasone suppression	<140 nmol/l	<5 μg/dl	27.59
Dehydroepiandrosterone (DHEA)	0.6–70 nmol/l	0.2–20 μg/l	3.467
Dehydroepiandrosterone sulfate (DHEAS)	5.4–9.2 μmol/l	820–3380 ng/ml	0.002714
11-Deoxycortisol (compound S)	<60 nmol/l	<2 μg/dl	28.86
17α-Hydroxyprogesterone, women	1–13 nmol/l	0.3–4.2 μg/l	3.026
Adrenal steroids, urinary excretion			
Aldosterone	15–70 nmol/d	5–26 μg/d	2.774
Cortisol, free	30–300 nmol/d	10–100 μg/d	2.759
17-Hydroxycorticosteroids	5.5–28 μmol/d	2–10 mg/d	2.759
17-Ketosteroids, women	14–52 μmol/d	4–15 mg/d	3.467
Ammonia (as NH_3), venous whole blood	6–45 μmol/l	10–80 μg/dl	0.5872
Angiotensin II, plasma, 8 AM	10–30 ng/l	10–30 pg/ml	1.0
Arginine vasopressin (AVP), plasma, random fluid intake	2.3–7.4 pmol/l	2.5–8 ng/l	0.92
Bicarbonate, serum	18–23 mmol/l	18–23 meq/l	1.0
Calciferols (see vitamin D)			
Calcitonin, serum	<50 ng/l	<50 pg/ml	1.0
Calcium			
Ionized serum	1–1.5 mmol/l	4–4.6 mg/dl	0.2495
Total serum	2.2–2.6 mmol/l	9–10.5 mg/dl	0.2495
β-Carotene, serum	0.9–4.6 μmol/l	50–250 μg/dl	0.01863
Catecholamines, plasma			
Epinephrine, basal supine	170–520 pmol/l	30–95 pg/ml	5.458
Norepinephrine, basal supine	0.3–2.8 nmol/l	15–475 pg/ml	0.005911
Catecholamines, urinary			
Epinephrine	<275 nmol/d	<50 μg/d	5.458
Normetanephrine	0–11 μmol/d	0–2.0 mg/d	5.458
Total catecholamines (as norepinephrine)	<675 nmol/d	<120 μg/d	5.911
Vanillylmandelic acid (VMA)	<35 μmol/d	<68 mg/d	5.046
Chloride, serum	98–106 mmol/l	98–106 meq/l	1.0
Cholesterol, plasma			
Total cholesterol			
Desirable	<5.20 mmol/l	<200 mg/dl	0.02586
Borderline high	5.2–6.18 mmol/l	200–239 mg/dl	0.02586
High	≥6.21 mmol/l	≥240 mg/dl	0.02586
High–density lipoprotein (HDL) cholesterol			
Desirable	≥1.29 mmol/l	≥50 mg/dl	0.02586
Borderline high	0.9–1.27 mmol/l	36–49 mg/dl	0.02586
High	≤0.91 mmol/l	≤35 mg/dl	0.02586
Low-density lipoprotein (LDL) cholesterol			
Desirable	<3.36 mmol/l	<130 mg/dl	0.02586
Borderline high	3.39–4.11 mmol/l	131–159 mg/dl	0.02586
High	≥4.14 mmol/l	≥160 mg/dl	0.02586
Corticotropin (ACTH), plasma	4–22 pmol/l	20–100 pg/ml	0.2202
C peptide, plasma	0.5–2 μg/l	0.5–2 ng/ml	1.0
Creatinine, serum	<133 μmol/l	<1.5 mg/dl	88.40
Fatty acids, nonesterified or free (FFA), plasma	<0.7 mmol/l	<18 mg/dl	0.03906
Gastrin, serum	<120 ng/l	<120 pg/ml	1.0
Glucagon, plasma	50–100 ng/l	50–100 pg/ml	1.0
Glucose, plasma			
Overnight fast, normal	4.2–6.4 mmol/l	75–115 mg/dl	0.05551
Overnight fast, diabetes mellitus	7.8 mmol/l	>140 mg/dl	0.05551
72-hour fast, normal women	>2.2 mmol/l	>40 mg/dl	0.05551
Glucose tolerance test, 2–hour postprandial plasma glucose			
Normal	<7.8 mmol/l	<140 mg/dl	0.05551
Imparied glucose tolerance	7.8–11.1 mmol/l	140–200 mg/dl	0.05551
Diabetes mellitus	>11.1 mmol/l	>200 mg/dl	0.05551

Measure	*SI*	*Conventional (C)*	*Conversion Factor (CF) C × CF = SI*
Gonadal steroids, plasma			
Androstenedione, women	3.5–7.0 nmol/l	1–2 ng/ml	3.492
Estradiol, women			
Basal	70–220 pmol/l	20–60 pg/ml	3.671
Ovulatory surge	>740 pmol/l	>200 pg/ml	3.671
Dihydrotestosterone, women	0.17–1.0 nmol/l	0.05–3 ng/ml	3.467
Progesterone, women			
Luteal phase	6–64 nmol/l	2–20 ng/ml	3.180
Follicular phase	<6 nmol/l	<2 ng/ml	3.180
Testosterone			
Women	<3.5 nmol/l	<1 ng/ml	3.467
Prepubertal boys and girls	0.2–0.7 nmol/l	0.05–0.2 ng/ml	3.467
Gonadotropins, plasma			
Women, basal			
Follicle-stimulating hormone	5–20 IU/l	5–20 mIU/ml	1.0
Luteinizing hormone	5–25 IU/l	5–25 mIU/ml	1.0
Women, ovulatory peak			
Follicle-stimulating hormone	12–30 IU/l	12–30 mIU/ml	1.0
Luteinizing hormone	25–100 IU/l	25–100 mIU/ml	1.0
Prepubertal boys and girls			
Follicle-stimulating hormone	<5 IU/l	<5 mIU/ml	1.0
Luteinizing hormone	<5 IU/l	<5 mIU/ml	1.0
Growth hormone, plasma			
After 100 g glucose orally	<5 μg/l	<5 ng/ml	1.0
After insulin-induced hypoglycemia	>9 μg/l	>9 ng/ml	1.0
Human chorionic gonadotropin, beta subunit, plasma; nonpregnant women	<3 IU/l	<3 mIU/ml	1.0
β-Hydroxybutyrate, plasma	<300 nmol/l	<3.0 mg/dl	96.05
Insulin, plasma			
Fasting	35–145 pmol/l	5–20 μU/ml	7.175
During hypoglycemia (plasma glucose <2.8 nmol/l [<50 mg/dl])	<35 pmol/l	<5 μU/ml	7.175
Insulin-like growth factor I (IGF I, somatomedin-C), women	0.45–2.2 kU/l	0.45–2.2 U/ml	1.0
Lactate, plasma	0.56–2.2 mmol/l	5–20 mg/dl	0.111
Magnesium, serum	0.8–1.20 mmol/l	1.8–3.0 mg/dl	0.4114
Osmolality, plasma	285–295 mmol/kg	285–295 mosm/kg	1.0
Oxytocin, plasma			
Random	1–4 pmol/l	1.25–5 ng/l	0.80
Ovulatory peak in women	408 pmol/l	5–10 ng/l	0.80
Parathyroid hormone, serum (intact PTH using immunoradiometric assay [IRMA])	10–65 ng/l	10–65 pg/ml	1.0
Phosphorus, inorganic, serum	1–1.5 mmol/l	3.0–4.5 mg/dl	0.3229
Potassium, serum	3.5–5.0 mmol/l	3.5–5.0 meq/l	1.0
Prolactin, serum	2–15 μg/l	2–15 ng/ml	1.0
Pyruvate, blood	39–102 μmol/l	0.3–0.9 mg/dl	0.01129
Renin activity, plasma, normal-sodium diet			
Supine	3.2 ± 1 μg/l/h	3.2 ± 1.1 ng/ml/h	1.0
Standing	9.3 ± 4.3 μg/l/h	9.3 ± 4.3 ng/ml/h	1.0
Sodium, serum	136–145 mmol/l	136–145 meq/l	1.0
Thyroid function tests			
Radioactive iodine uptake, 24 hours	0.05–0.30	5–30%	—
Reverse triiodothyronine (rT_3), serum	0.15–0.61 nmol/l	10–4 ng/dl	0.01536
Thyrotropin (TSH), highly sensitive assay, serum	0.6–4.6 mU/l	0.6–4.6 μU/ml	1.0
Thyroxine (T_4), serum	51–42 nmol/l	4–11 μg/dl	12.87
Thyroxine-binding globulin, serum (as thyroxine)	150–360 nmol/l	12–28 μg/ml	12.87
Triiodothyronine (T_3), serum	1.2–3.4 nmol/l	75–220 ng/dl	0.01536
Triiodothyronine resin uptake, serum	0.25–0.35	25–35%	—
Triglycerides, plasma (as Triolein)	<1.80 mmol/l	<160 mg/dl	0.01129
Uric acid, serum	120–420 μmol/l	2–7 mg/dl	59.48
Vitamin D (as vitamin D_3, cholecalciferol), plasma			
1,25-Dihydroxycholecalciferol (1,25$(OH)_2$D)	36–144 pmol/l	15–60 pg/ml	2.400
25-Hydroxycholecalciferol (25-OHD)	20–100 nmol/l	8–40 ng/ml	2.496

Modified with permission from **Wilson JD, Foster DW.** *Williams textbook of endocrinology,* 8th ed. Philadelphia: WB Saunders, 1991.

Index

Page numbers followed by "f" denote figures; those followed by "t" denote tables.